Jason Heckman, M.D.

SURGERY REVIEW ILLUSTRATED

SURGERY REVIEW ILLUSTRATED

Amit D. Tevar, MD

Transplant Surgery Fellow
Division of Transplantation
Department of Surgery
University of Cincinnati
Cincinnati, Ohio

Rafael E. Azuaje, MD

Minimally Invasive and Endoscopic Surgery Fellow
Department of Surgery
University of Miami
Jackson Memorial Hospital
Miami, Florida

Larry T. Micon, MD, FACS

Clinical Assistant Professor of Surgery
Indiana University School of Medicine
Assistant Director, Surgery Education
Methodist Hospital of Indiana
Indianapolis, Indiana

McGraw-Hill

Medical Publishing Division

New York   Chicago   San Francisco   Lisbon   London   Madrid
Mexico City   Milan   New Delhi   San Juan   Seoul
Singapore   Sydney   Toronto

Surgery Review Illustrated

Notice

Medicine is an ever-changing science. As new research and clinical experience broaden our knowledge, changes in treatment and drug therapy are required. The authors and the publisher of this work have checked with sources believed to be reliable in their efforts to provide information that is complete and generally in accord with the standards accepted at the time of publication. However, in view of the possibility of human error or changes in medical sciences, neither the authors nor the publisher nor any other party who has been involved in the preparation or publication of this work warrants that the information contained herein is in every respect accurate or complete, and they disclaim all responsibility for any errors or omissions or for the results obtained from use of the information contained in this work. Readers are encouraged to confirm the information contained herein with other sources. For example and in particular, readers are advised to check the product information sheet included in the package of each drug they plan to administer to be certain that the information contained in this work is accurate and that changes have not been made in the recommended dose or in the contraindications for administration. This recommendation is of particular importance in connection with new or infrequently used drugs.

This book was set in Palatino by International Typesetting and Composition.
The editors were Marc Strauss and Marsha Loeb.
The production supervisor was Sherri Souffrance.
Project management was provided by International Typesetting and Composition.
Quebecor Dubuque was printer and binder.

This book is printed on acid-free paper.

Library of Congress Cataloging-in-Publication Data

Tevar, Amit D.
   Surgery review illustrated / Amit D. Tevar, Rafael Azuaje, Larry Micon.
      p. ; cm.
   Includes bibliographical references and index.
   ISBN 0-07-141654-4
      1. Surgery—Examinations, questions, etc. I. Azuaje, Rafael. II. Micon, Larry. III. Title.
   [DNLM: 1. Surgery—Examination Questions. 2. Surgical Procedures,
   Operative—Examination Questions. WO 18.2 T353s 2004]
   RD37.T39 2004
   617′.0076—dc22
                                                                                    2004049909

ISBN: 0-07-111473-4 (International Edition)
Copyright © 2005. Exclusive rights by The McGraw-Hill Companies, Inc., for manufacture and export. This book cannot be re-exported from the country to which it is consigned by McGraw-Hill. The International Editoin is not available in North America.

Contents

Contributors

John D. Abad, MD (*Chapter 10*)
General Surgery Resident
Department of Surgery
Indiana University School of Medicine
Indianapolis, Indiana

Rafael E. Azuaje, MD
Fellow, Minimally Invasive and Endoscopic Surgery
Department of Surgery
University of Miami
Jackson Memorial Hospital
Miami, Florida

Christa Balanoff, MD (*Chapter 15*)
Staff Breast Surgeon
Department of Surgery
St. Vincent Hospital
Indianapolis, Indiana
Department of Surgery
Women's Hospital
Indianapolis, Indiana

Christopher M. Bearden, MD (*Chapter 5*)
General Surgery Resident
Department of Surgery
Indiana University School of Medicine
Indianapolis, Indiana

Matthew W. Blanton, MD (*Chapter 10*)
General Surgery Resident
Department of Surgery
Indiana University School of Medicine
Indianapolis, Indiana

Edward J. Brizendine, MS (*Chapter 7*)
Biostatistician
Division of Biostatistics
Department of Medicine
Indiana University School of Medicine
Indianapolis, Indiana

Thomas A. Broadie, MD, PhD, FACS (*Chapter 19*)
Frederick W. Taylor Professor of Surgery
Department of Surgery
Indiana University School of Medicine
Indianapolis, Indiana

Michael T. Broman, MD (*Chapter 1*)
MD/PhD Student
Department of Surgery
University of Illinois at Chicago
Chicago, Illinois

David Camp, MD (*Chapter 36*)
Anesthesia Resident
Department of Anesthesia
Indiana University School of Medicine
Indianapolis, Indiana

Rabih A. Chaer, MD (*Chapter 28*)
General Surgery Chief Resident
Department of Surgery
University of Illinois at Chicago
Chicago, Illinois

Joseph Chao, MD (*Chapter 1*)
Medical Student
Department of Surgery
University of Illinois at Chicago
Chicago, Illinois

Jennifer Choi, MD (*Chapter 23*)
General Surgery Resident
Department of Surgery
Indiana University School of Medicine
Indianapolis, Indiana

John P. Clark, MD (*Chapter 42*)
Department of Family Medicine
Methodist Hospital
St. Louis Park, Minnesota
William Mitchell College of Law
St. Paul, Minnesota

John J. Coleman III, MD (*Chapter 11*)
James E. Bennett Professor of Plastic Surgery
Director, Division of Plastic Surgery
Indiana University School of Medicine
Indianapolis, Indiana
Department of Surgery
Indiana University Medical Center
Indianapolis, Indiana

Michael Dalsing, MD, FACS (*Chapter 32*)
Professor of Surgery
Director, Section of Vascular Surgery
Indiana University School of Medicine
Indianapolis, Indiana

Akinsansoye K. Dosekun, MD (*Chapter 8*)
Associate Professor of Medicine
Division of Renal Diseases and Hypertension
Department of Internal Medicine
University of Texas Health Science Center at
    Houston Medical School
Houston, Texas

Tyler Emley, MD (*Chapter 39*)
Urology Resident
Department of Urology
Indiana University School of Medicine
Indianapolis, Indiana

Terrence J. Endres, MD (*Chapter 37*)
Staff Orthopedic Surgeon
Orthopaedic Associates of Grand Rapids
Spectrum Health—Butterworth
Grand Rapids, Michigan

Andrew C. Eppstein, MD (*Chapter 41*)
General Surgery Resident
Department of Surgery
Indiana University School of Medicine
Indianapolis, Indiana

Mauricio Antonio Escobar, MD (*Chapter 4*)
Staff General Surgeon
Frio Regional Hospital
Pearsall, Texas

Mauricio Antonio Escobar Jr., MD
General Surgery Resident
Department of Surgery
Indiana University School of Medicine
Indianapolis, Indiana

N. Joseph Espat, MD, MS, FACS (*Chapters 1, 28, 30*)
Associate Professor
Hepatobiliary and Oncologic Surgery
University of Illinois at Chicago
University Hospitals and Clinics
Chicago, Illinois

Kevin W. Finkel, MD, FACP (*Chapter 8*)
Associate Professor of Medicine
Division of Renal Disease and Hypertension and
    Section of Nephrology
The University of Texas-Houston Medical School
Houston, Texas
The University of Texas-MD Anderson Cancer Center
Houston, Texas

Earl A. Gage, MD (*Chapter 19*)
General Surgery Resident
Department of Surgery
Indiana University School of Medicine
Indianapolis, Indiana

Satinderjit Singh Gill, MD (*Chapter 12*)
General Surgery Chief Resident
Department of Surgery
Spartanburg Regional Medical Center
Spartanburg, South Carolina

Sunil Gollapudi, MD (*Chapter 8*)
Staff Physician
Department of Nephrology
Methodist Hospital
Indianapolis, Indiana

Julius M. Goodman, MD (*Chapters 18, 35*)
Clinical Professor of Neurological Surgery
Indiana University School of Medicine
Indianapolis, Indiana
Clarian Health-Methodist-Indiana University—Riley
Indianapolis Neurosurgical Group
Indianapolis, Indiana

Christian S. Hinrichs, MD (*Chapter 33*)
Surgical Oncology Fellow
State University of New York at Buffalo
Buffalo, New York
Roswell Park Cancer Institute
Buffalo, New York

Thomas J. Howard, MD (*Chapter 29*)
Associate Professor of Surgery
Department of Surgery
Indiana University School of Medicine
Indianapolis, Indiana

David H. Jho, MD (*Chapter 1*)
MD/PhD Student
Department of Surgery
University of Illinois at Chicago
Chicago, Illinois

Olaf B. Johansen, MD, FACS, FASCRS (*Chapter 25*)
Clinical Assistant Professor
Department of Surgery
Indiana University School of Medicine
Indianapolis, Indiana
Department of Colorectal Surgery
St. Francis Hospital
Mooreseville, Indiana

Anthony Keever, MD (*Chapter 36*)
Anesthesia Resident
Department of Anesthesia
Indiana University School of Medicine
Indianapolis, Indiana

Kenneth A. Kesler, MD (*Chapter 21*)
Professor of Surgery
Thoracic Surgery Division
Indiana University School of Medicine
Indianapolis, Indiana

Myung Kim, MD (*Chapter 31*)
General Surgery Resident
Department of Surgery
Indiana University School of Medicine
Indianapolis, Indiana

Mike Koch, MD (*Chapter 39*)
Professor of Surgery
Chairman, Department of Urology
Indiana University School of Medicine
Indianapolis, Indiana

Maria Korchagin
Medical Illustrator
University of Chicago
Chicago, Illinois

Priya D. Krishna, MD (*Chapter 14*)
Laryngology Fellow
Division of Laryngology and Voice Disorders
Department of Otolaryngology
University of Pittsburgh
Eye and Ear Institute
Pittsburgh, Pennsylvania

Alan P. Ladd, MD (*Chapter 34*)
Assistant Professor of Surgery
Section of Pediatric Surgery
Indiana University School of Medicine
Indianapolis, Indiana
Riley Children's Hospital
Division of Pediatric Surgery
Indiana University School of Medicine
Indianapolis, Indiana

Peter Lawrence, MD (*Chapter 39*)
Urology Chief Resident
Department of Urology
Indiana University School of Medicine
Indianapolis, Indiana

Eugene K. Lee, MD (*Chapter 1*)
Visiting Research Specialist
Department of Surgery
University of Illinois at Chicago
Chicago, Illinois

Kristine A.K. Lombardozzi, MD (*Chapters 6, 13*)
Staff Trauma Surgeon
Department of Surgery
Methodist Hospital of Indiana
Indianapolis, Indiana

Joao A. Lopes, MD (*Chapter 26*)
General Surgery Chief Resident
Department of Surgery
Indiana University School of Medicine
Indianapolis, Indiana

Derek C. Lou, MD (*Chapter 27*)
General Surgery Chief Resident
Department of Surgery
Indiana University School of Medicine
Indianapolis, Indiana

Jason Lowrey, MD (*Chapter 36*)
Anesthesia Resident
Department of Anesthesia
Indiana University School of Medicine
Indianapolis, Indiana

Richard S. Mangus, MD, MS (*Chapter 24*)
General Surgery Chief Resident
Department of Surgery
Indiana University School of Medicine
Indianapolis, Indiana

Marisa A. Mastropietro, MD, FACOG (*Chapter 40*)
Chief, Section of Urogynecology and Reconstructive
    Pelvic Surgery
Department of Obstetrics and Gynecology
New York Methodist Hospital
Brooklyn, New York

John McGregor, MD (*Chapter 9*)
Assistant Professor of Clinical Neurosurgery
Department of Neurological Surgery
The Ohio State University Medical Center
Columbus, Ohio

R. Barry Melbert, MD, FACS, FASCRS (*Chapter 25*)
Clinical Instructor
Department of Surgery
Indiana University School of Medicine
Indianapolis, Indiana
Department of Colorectal Surgery
St. Francis Hospital
Mooresville, Indiana

Larry T. Micon, MD, FACS (*Chapters 15, 23*)
Clinical Assistant Professor of Surgery
Indiana University School of Medicine
Assistant Director, Surgery Education
Methodist Hospital of Indiana
Indianapolis, Indiana

Joshua Miller, MD (*Chapter 9*)
Neurosurgery Resident
Department of Neurological Surgery
The Ohio State University Medical Center
Columbus, Ohio

Michael D. Miller, MD (*Chapter 36*)
Anesthesia Resident
Department of Anesthesia
Indiana University School of Medicine
Indianapolis, Indiana

Charles Morrison, MD (*Chapter 24*)
General Surgery Resident
Department of Surgery
Indiana University School of Medicine
Indianapolis, Indiana

Charles E. Morrow, Jr., MD (*Chapter 12*)
Director of Trauma/Critical Care
Department of Surgery
Spartanburg Regional Medical Center
Spartanburg, South Carolina

Carol Palachko, MD (*Chapter 23*)
General Surgery Resident
Department of Surgery
Indiana University School of Medicine
Indianapolis, Indiana

Lucio Giovanni M. Palanca, MD (*Chapter 26*)
General Surgery Resident
Department of Surgery
Indiana University School of Medicine
Indianapolis, Indiana

Frederick J. Rescorla, MD (*Chapter 34*)
Professor of Surgery
Section of Pediatric Surgery
Indiana University School of Medicine
Indianapolis, Indiana
Riley Children's Hospital
Division of Pediatric Surgery
Indiana University School of Medicine
Indianapolis, Indiana

Richard B. Rodgers, MD (*Chapters 18, 35*)
Neurosurgery Resident
Department of Neurosurgery
Indiana University School of Medicine
Indianapolis, Indiana

Lori Rolando, MD (*Chapter 32*)
Vascular Surgery Fellow
Section of Vascular Surgery
Indiana University School of Medicine
Indianapolis, Indiana

Michael Rowe, MS, MD (*Chapter 4*)
Faculty
Department of General Surgery
Indiana University School of Medicine
Indianapolis, Indiana
Surgical Attending
Department of Surgery
Methodist Hospital
Indianapolis, Indiana

Bridget M. Sanders, MD (*Chapter 25*)
General Surgery Chief Resident
Department of Surgery
Indiana University School of Medicine
Indianapolis, Indiana

John A. Sandoval, MD (*Chapter 34*)
General Surgery Resident
Department of Surgery
Indiana University School of Medicine
Indianapolis, Indiana

Chansamone Saysana, MD (*Chapter 36*)
Anesthesia Resident
Department of Anesthesia
Indiana University School of Medicine
Indianapolis, Indiana

L.R. Scherer III, MD (*Chapter 13*)
Director
Kiwanis-Riley Regional Pediatric Trauma Center
Associate Professor
Section of Pediatric Surgery
Indiana University School of Medicine
Indianapolis, Indiana

Valerie Schissler, MSN, CRNP (*Chapter 40*)
Institute for Female Pelvic Medicine and
   Reconstructive Surgery
Allentown, Pennsylvania

C. Max Schmidt, MD (*Chapters 17, 22*)
Assistant Professor
Department of Surgery
Indiana University School of Medicine
Indianapolis, Indiana

Jeffrey E. Schreiber, MD (*Chapter 38*)
Plastic Surgery Fellow
Division of Plastic Surgery
Johns Hopkins University School of Medicine
University of Maryland School of Medicine
Baltimore, Maryland

Don Seltzer, MD (*Chapter 41*)
Assistant Professor
Department of Surgery
Indiana University School of Medicine
Indianapolis, Indiana

Kevin Sheridan, MD (*Chapter 4*)
General Surgery Resident
Department of Surgery
Indiana University
Indianapolis, Indiana

Clark J. Simons, MD (*Chapters 3, 26*)
Assistant Professor of Surgery
Indiana University School of Medicine
Indianapolis, Indiana
Faculty
Indiana University Hospital
Wishard Memorial Hospital
Richard L. Roudebush Veterans
   Administration Medical Center
Indianapolis, Indiana

Navin K. Singh, MD, FACS (*Chapter 38*)
Assistant Professor of Plastic Surgery
Johns Hopkins University School of Medicine
University of Maryland School of Medicine
Baltimore, Maryland

Cord Sturgeon, MD (*Chapter 30*)
Clinical Instructor
Endocrine Surgical Oncology
University of California
San Francisco, California
Department of Surgery
UCSF Comprehensive Cancer Center at Mt. Zion
San Francisco, California

Ursula M. Szmulowicz, MD (*Chapter 6*)
General Surgery Resident
Department of Surgery
Indiana University School of Medicine
Indianapolis, Indiana

Rahul D. Tevar, MD (*Chapter 2*)
General Surgery Resident
Department of Surgery
George Washington University
Washington, DC

Amit D. Tevar, MD (*Chapters 2, 16*)
Transplant Surgery Fellow
Division of Transplantation
Department of Surgery
University of Cincinnati
Cincinnati, Ohio

Dinesh P. Tevar, MD (*Chapter 16*)
Staff General Surgeon
McDonough District Hospital
Macomb, Illinois

Ben M. Tsai, MD (*Chapter 21*)
General Surgery Resident
Department of Surgery
Indiana University School of Medicine
Indianapolis, Indiana

Carlos A. Vieira, MD (*Chapter 3*)
General Surgery Chief Resident
Department of Surgery
Indiana University School of Medicine
Indianapolis, Indiana

Maria A.S. Vieira, MD (*Chapter 3*)
Pathology Resident
Department of Pathology
Indiana University School of Medicine
Indianapolis, Indiana

Nicolas Villanustre, MD (*Chapter 29*)
General Surgery Resident
Indiana University School of Medicine
Department of Surgery
Indianapolis, Indiana

Robert Vire, MD (*Chapter 20*)
Attending Physician
Department of Surgery
Porter Memorial Hospital
Valparaiso, Indiana

Patrice M. Weiss, MD, FACOG (*Chapter 40*)
Residency Program Director
Director of Medical Education
Medical Co-Director of Risk Management
Department of Obstetrics and Gynecology
Lehigh Valley Physician Group
Lehigh Valley Hospital
Allentown, Pennsylvania

Chad Wiesenauer, MD (*Chapters 17, 22*)
General Surgery Resident
Department of Surgery
Indiana University School of Medicine
Indianapolis, Indiana

Nathalie C. Zeitouni, MDCM, FRCPC (*Chapter 33*)
Associate Professor of Clinical Dermatology
State University of New York at Buffalo
Buffalo, New York
Roswell Park Cancer Institute
Department of Dermatology
Buffalo, New York

Madeline J. Zieger, PA-C (*Chapter 11*)
Physician Assistant
Plastic Surgery Division
Indiana University School of Medicine
Indianapolis, Indiana

Foreword

There is likely no other period of education in any profession that can match a surgical residency with respect to the total amount of knowledge that must be acquired. Not only must a surgical trainee achieve the technical skills necessary to become a surgeon, but also acquire the judgment and knowledge of the principals and pathophysiology, management, and outcomes of surgical disease. The evaluation of these skills and knowledge has become a key element of the education and certification process of a surgeon. The process begins with the American Board of Surgery in-training/surgical basic science exams and culminates with the board's qualifying and certifying examinations. Appropriately, the process now continues on well into a surgeon's career with the ABS recertification process and exam.

No surgical text or journal can replace the hands-on experience of surgical training and practice and the acquisition of surgical knowledge. But, to quote Sir William Osler, "It is astonishing with how little reading a doctor can practice medicine, but it is not astonishing how badly he can do it." A surgeon who does not read or fails to prepare for the examination process, no matter how well trained, may encounter significant risk of failure. It is for these reasons that this text, *Surgical Review Illustrated*, is such an important contribution. The editors, Drs. Tevar, Azuaje, and Micon have covered the entire breadth of surgical basic science and clinical practice in the preparation of this text, which I believe will become an essential tool for surgeons for the accumulation of factual knowledge both for practice and examination preparation.

As Chairman of the Department of Surgery at Indiana University I am extremely proud of the contributions of so many of our residents, faculty, and staff in this project. As a surgical educator and program director I know that it will become an important part of our educational mission at IU. Finally as the Director of the American Board of Surgery, I feel confident that it will serve to raise the level of surgical knowledge for future generations.

Keith D. Lillemoe, MD
Jay L. Grosfeld Professor and Chairman
Department of Surgery
Indiana University School of Medicine
Indianapolis, Indiana

Preface

One of the requirements of becoming a successful surgeon is the development and maintenance of a broad and encyclopedic fund of knowledge. This is first accomplished during general surgery residency with a systematic and thorough study of the classic textbooks and a complete review of the current literature. This process does not end with the completion of residency and fellowship, as the more important step is to maintain this knowledge base with disciplined and systematic self-education throughout the entirety of a surgeon's career.

The American Board of Surgery's written and oral board examinations serve as a test of the newly trained surgeon's knowledge base. The recertification examination functions as a test of the level and quality of self-education that the seasoned surgeon has pursued throughout his career.

The concept for this manuscript began several years ago and was spurred by the lack of any review text that was comprehensive in nature. Our goal, from the onset, was to provide an all-inclusive source for review of the broad expanse of general surgery. This meant that every topic that could be tested during the ABS certification examinations would be reviewed during the course of the book. We chose the format of the text to be a palatable "question and answer" layout with information taken from gold standard surgery textbooks, complemented with recent literature from the leading journals in the field.

We are quite pleased with the final product. Each chapter has been carefully designed to cover all of the topics encountered in each given field. The comments following each answer provide a succinct appraisal of each topic. The information emphasizes the clinical science most commonly seen on licensure examinations, but also contains basic science, including physiology, anatomy, and pathology. The authors for each chapter were carefully chosen and include surgeons with extensive expertise and academic interests in their fields. The publishing team at McGraw-Hill was gracious enough to allow us the abundant use of illustrations. As such, each chapter is filled with radiographs, gross pathology pictures, histology slides, anatomy and physiology diagrams, algorithms, and countless tables and charts.

In all, we were impressed with the caliber of work each author contributed to this first edition. It cannot be emphasized enough that this *review* is not a replacement for the study of fundamental general surgery textbooks and journals in building a fund of knowledge. Instead, we present this text as a valuable resource for senior surgical residents and young surgeons preparing for their licensure examinations as well as for the seasoned practitioner wishing to periodically review the field of general surgery.

Good luck.

Amit D. Tevar, MD

SURGERY REVIEW ILLUSTRATED

CHAPTER 1

Cell Physiology and Structure

*David H. Jho, Michael T. Broman, Eugene K. Lee,
Joseph Chao, and N. Joseph Espat*

Questions

1. What is/are the function(s) of the various phospho-lipids that compose the lipid bilayer of cell membranes?

   (A) separates the intracellular space from the extracellular space

   (B) serve as substrates for the formation of signal transduction molecules

   (C) serve as signals to induce the phagocytosis of apoptotic cells

   (D) A and B only

   (E) all of the above

2. Which of the following plasma membrane molecules are exclusively located on the extracellular side of the lipid bilayer?

   (A) glycolipids

   (B) glycoproteins

   (C) glycosylphosphatidylinositol (GPI)-anchored proteins

   (D) prenylated membrane proteins

   (E) A, B, and C

3. Which of these is *not* a function that is carried out by an integral membrane protein in a plasma membrane?

   (A) receptor for growth factors

   (B) pump for K^+

   (C) channel for macromolecules

   (D) structural protein

   (E) determinant of membrane fluidity

4. Using freeze-fracture electron microscopy, RBCs are frozen in liquid nitrogen and fractured with a blade. The fracture plane passes between the lipid bilayers, dividing the membrane into two monolayers. The fracture faces are then shadowed with platinum and examined under an electron microscope (EM). The cytosolic or plasma face (P face) is the outer surface of the inner membrane leaflet, and the extracellular face (E face) is the inner surface of the outer leaflet. Which of the following statements is true?

   (A) The P face contains more integral proteins than the E face.

   (B) The E face contains more integral proteins than the P face.

   (C) Only the P face contains integral proteins.

   (D) Only the E face contains integral proteins.

   (E) No integral proteins can be seen on either the P face or the E face.

5. Which of the following statements about osmolarity, electrochemical gradient, and membrane transport is *incorrect*?

   (A) Large intracellular macromolecules such as proteins do not make any direct or indirect contributions to osmolarity.

   (B) Treating a human cell with ouabain would cause the cell to swell and burst.

   (C) Ionophores can cause collapse of the electrochemical gradient in cells and can ultimately result in cell death.

   (D) Multidrug resistance (MDR) proteins can pump hydrophobic drugs out of the cell and are responsible for the resistance of cancer cells to certain chemotherapeutics.

   (E) None of the statements is incorrect.

6. Cystic fibrosis (CF) is an autosomal recessive disorder in which three nucleotides are deleted, resulting in the absence of a key amino acid in a channel protein. What amino acid is deleted and which channel is affected in most cases of CF?

   (A) phenylalanine, CFTR chloride channel
   (B) glutamine, CFTR chloride channel
   (C) lysine, CFTR sodium channel
   (D) valine, CFTR sodium channel
   (E) alanine, CFTR sodium-chloride channel

7. Relative to a normal nerve cell, in which one of these conditions would depolarization be facilitated or prolonged?

   (A) doubling the number of Na^+-K^+ ATPase pumps
   (B) increasing Na^+ permeability across leak channels
   (C) increasing K^+ permeability across leak channels
   (D) changing the resting membrane potential to -100 mV
   (E) none of the above

8. Which of these scenarios is an example of secondary active transport?

   (A) Na^+-K^+ ATPase pump
   (B) linked movement of glucose and Na^+ down their electrochemical gradients
   (C) movement of ethanol across the cell membrane
   (D) amino acid crossing the cell membrane utilizing a carrier protein
   (E) Ca^+ ATPase and H^+ ATPase working together on the same membrane

9. What are the calcium-dependent proteins responsible for intercellular adhesion, and in which segment of the junctional complex are they located?

   (A) calcineurin at the zonula adherens
   (B) calmodulin at the macula adherens
   (C) ZO-1 at the zonula occludens
   (D) desmosomes at the macula adherens
   (E) cadherins at the zonula adherens

10. A tissue sample was obtained from a patient and was determined to be of neural origin using a stain for a glial-specific protein. To what group of cytoskeletal elements does this protein belong, and what is its main function in the cell?

   (A) neurofilaments involved in axonal transport
   (B) microtubules involved in cell motility and intracellular transport
   (C) actin filaments involved in cell motility and intracellular transport
   (D) intermediate filaments for providing structure and mechanical support
   (E) vimentins for providing structure and mechanical support

11. In a culture of electrically coupled cells, a water-soluble dye is injected into one cell, and the dye spreads laterally from cell to cell at a constant rate. How could one increase the rate of the spread of the dye from one cell to another?

   (A) lowering the pH of the intracellular compartments
   (B) lowering the pH of the extracellular compartment
   (C) increasing intracellular $[Ca^{2+}]$
   (D) decreasing intracellular $[Ca^{2+}]$
   (E) increasing the size of the dye

12. Which of the following are classified as apical cytoskeletal specializations?

   (A) cilia composed of microtubules
   (B) stereocilia composed of actin microfilaments
   (C) microvilli composed of actin microfilaments
   (D) all of the above
   (E) only A and C

13. Which of these drugs are *not* microtubule-specific?

   (A) paclitaxel
   (B) colchicine and colcemid
   (C) vinblastine and vincristine
   (D) nocodazole
   (E) latrunculin and phalloidin

14. Which of the following is *not* a molecular motor protein?

   (A) myosin
   (B) kinesin
   (C) dynein
   (D) actin
   (E) all of the above are molecular motor proteins

15. In the skeletal muscle sarcomere, which of the following bands or lines shorten in length during contraction of the myofibrils?

    (A) H band and I band
    (B) H band and A band
    (C) M line and A band
    (D) Z line and I band
    (E) none of the above

16. Which of the following statements about receptors is *not* true?

    (A) Ion channel-linked receptors activate the opening of an ion channel with the binding of ligand, which is the method of signaling used by most neurotransmitters.
    (B) G protein-linked receptors activate heterotrimeric GTPases in response to ligand-binding, such as in the action of neuropeptide Y.
    (C) Enzyme-linked receptors include receptor tyrosine kinases (RTKs) and receptor serine/threonine kinases, which are the receptors used by endothelial growth factor (EGF) and transforming growth factor beta (TGF-β).
    (D) Steroid hormone receptors are usually found in the cytosol, and the functions of vitamins A and D are dependent on this class of receptors.
    (E) All of the above statements are true.

17. When RTKs are activated by ligands (e.g., insulin, epidermal growth factor, fibroblast growth factor, and other growth factors), they are autophosphorylated at intracellular tyrosine receptors by oligomerization. Which of the following intracellular signaling molecules or pathways are activated as a result?

    (A) Src family of protein kinases which contain SH_2 domains
    (B) PLC and PKC pathway
    (C) Ras, Raf, and MAPK pathway
    (D) PI3K, PDK1, and PKB/Akt pathway
    (E) all of the above

18. Which of the following signaling pathways is most directly activated in response to γ-interferon?

    (A) phosphatidylinositol 3'-kinase/Akt pathway
    (B) MAPK pathway
    (C) Jak-STAT pathway
    (D) PLC pathway
    (E) none of the above

19. Which of the following statements about low density lipoprotein (LDL) and transferrin receptors is *not* true?

    (A) Both types of receptors are recycled.
    (B) Both promote recycling of their ligands.
    (C) Both are transmembrane receptors.
    (D) Both are endocytosed via clathrin-coated pits.
    (E) Both associate with endosomes.

20. Which of the following motifs is important in steroid receptor structure?

    (A) transmembrane domain
    (B) zinc finger
    (C) catalytic domain
    (D) multiple C-terminal tyrosine residues
    (E) SH_2 domain

21. A eukaryotic cell is lysed and fractionated into plasma membrane, cytosolic, and nuclear fractions. Which of the following hormones would most likely be found in the nuclear fraction of the cell?

    (A) human chorionic gonadotrophin
    (B) glucagon
    (C) aldosterone
    (D) gastrin
    (E) histamine

22. Which of the following statements about organelle function is *incorrect*?

    (A) The rough endoplasmic reticulum (rER) is the site of protein synthesis and the cotranslational modification of proteins.
    (B) The smooth endoplasmic reticulum (sER) is the site of phospholipid synthesis, steroid hormone synthesis, drug detoxification, and calcium store release.
    (C) The Golgi complex is the site of vesicular packaging of proteins, membrane component recycling, and posttranslational modification of proteins.
    (D) The mitochondrion functions in acetyl-CoA production, tricarboxylic acid (TCA) cycle, oxidative phosphorylation, and fatty acid oxidation.
    (E) The lysosome contains amino acid oxidase, urate oxidase, catalase, and other oxidative enzymes relating to the production and degradation of hydrogen peroxide and oxidation of fatty acids.

23. Which one of the following lysosomal storage diseases is X-linked recessive in inheritance?

    (A) Fabry's disease
    (B) Krabbe's disease
    (C) Gaucher's disease
    (D) Niemann-Pick disease
    (E) Tay-Sachs disease

24. Which one of the following lysosomal storage diseases is X-linked recessive in inheritance?

    (A) Hurler's syndrome
    (B) Hunter's syndrome
    (C) Sanfilippo's syndrome
    (D) Scheie's syndrome
    (E) Sly's syndrome

25. A polypeptide newly synthesized in the rER has the C-terminal sequence of Lys-Asp-Glu-Leu or KDEL. What is the final fate of this polypeptide?

    (A) secretion outside of the cell
    (B) translocation into the nucleus
    (C) transport into the Golgi apparatus
    (D) bound to the cell membrane
    (E) localization to the ER

26. Cellular proteins processed mainly in the Golgi apparatus include all of the following *except*

    (A) lysosomal enzymes
    (B) peroxisomal enzymes
    (C) membrane receptors
    (D) secreted proteins
    (E) all of the above are mainly processed in the Golgi

27. Which of these cell types might be expected to have an extensive sER?

    (A) adrenal zona glomerulosa cell
    (B) adrenal chromaffin cell
    (C) pancreatic acinar cell
    (D) keratinocyte
    (E) hepatic Küpffer cell

28. Which of the following examples describe the correct direction of movement through a nuclear pore?

    (A) Messenger RNA is recycled from the cytoplasm to the nucleus.
    (B) Free ribosomes are transported from the cytoplasm to the nucleus.

    (C) New histone proteins are pumped from the nucleus to the cytoplasm.
    (D) New lamins are transported from the cytoplasm to the nucleus.
    (E) None of the above statements are true.

29. Which of the following statements about the regulation of gene expression is *incorrect*?

    (A) Promoter and enhancer sequences govern the binding of specific TFs and GRPs.
    (B) Common DNA-binding motifs on TFs and GRPs include helix-turn-helix, helix-loop-helix, leucine zippers, and zinc fingers.
    (C) NF-κB activation involves the phosphorylation of IκB and its subsequent degradation by the ubiquitin-proteasome proteolytic (UPP) pathway.
    (D) The NF-κB pathway is activated by specific proinflammatory cytokines such as tumor necrosis factor-alpha (TNF-α) and interleukin-1 (IL-1) but not by bacterial products such as LPS.
    (E) All of the statements are correct.

30. DNA fluorescent *in situ* hybridization of a cell isolated from human tissue displays an extremely long series of short tandem repeats (TTAGGG) at the end of the chromosomes. What type of cell would this most likely be?

    (A) neuron
    (B) kidney cell
    (C) lymphocyte
    (D) spermatozoa
    (E) hepatocyte

31. Which of the following is *not* a mechanism of DNA mismatch repair or DNA excision repair?

    (A) When DNA is damaged by ultraviolet (UV) light, DNA mismatch repair proteins recognize and remove the altered nucleotides, followed by repair of the sequence with DNA polymerase and ligase.
    (B) Errors made by the DNA polymerase, which are missed by its proofreading exonuclease, are corrected by DNA mismatch repair proteins that recognize and degrade the mismatched base pair on the newly synthesized strand.
    (C) A single damaged purine base can be excised via nicks produced by AP endonuclease and a phosphodiesterase for removal of the damaged base, followed by repair with DNA polymerase and ligase.

(D) When cytosines are spontaneously deaminated unto uracils, they are recognized by uracil-DNA glycosidase then repair proceeds with AP endonuclease, a phosphodiesterase, DNA polymerase, and DNA ligase.

(E) Pyrimidine dimers are repaired by uvrABC enzymes, which excise a 12-residue sequence around the dimer, followed by repair with DNA polymerase and ligase.

32. Which of these is a characteristic common to *both* meiosis and mitosis?

(A) final daughter cells produced have half the number of chromosomes

(B) homolog synapse and crossover recombination create genetic variability

(C) original parent cells undergo a single round of cytokinesis

(D) synthesis of new DNA only occurs once during the entire process

(E) none of the above

33. Which is the shortest phase of the normal cell cycle?

(A) G_1 phase

(B) S phase

(C) G_2 phase

(D) M phase

(E) all of the above are approximately equal in length

34. Which of the following are *not* either proto-oncogene or oncogene products?

(A) Vhl and Apc

(B) Ras and Sis

(C) Erb and Neu

(D) Myc and Abl

(E) Jun and Fos

35. A biopsy was performed on an aggressive tumor, and assays of various protein levels and enzyme activities were performed on the tumor cells. Which of the following proteins would likely *not* show either increased expression or activity?

(A) telomerase

(B) Fas receptor

(C) Myc

(D) Ras

(E) Bcl-2

36. Which protein is not involved in the stimulation and/or prolongation of the apoptosis pathway?

(A) cytochrome c

(B) Bcl-X_L

(C) Apaf-1

(D) Bad

(E) Bax

37. Damaged or misfolded proteins in the cytosol will most likely be _____ and degraded in a _____.

(A) glycosylated, lysosome

(B) farnesylated, peroxisome

(C) ubiquitylated, proteasome

(D) solubilized, lysosome

(E) none of the above

38. Which of these is *not* a function of heat shock proteins (HSP)?

(A) aiding protein folding in intracellular compartments

(B) preventing protein aggregation

(C) facilitating the translocation of proteins across membranes

(D) facilitating the degradation of unstable proteins

(E) increasing the rate of protein synthesis

39. Which of the following are necessary to import a mitochondrial precursor protein into the mitochondrial matrix?

(A) TOM complex

(B) TIM complex

(C) mitochondrial signal sequence

(D) chaperone proteins

(E) all of the above

40. Which of the following statements about cellular metabolic pathways is *not* true?

 (A) Glycogenolysis in liver and muscle is responsible for supplying glucose to tissues in the first 8 h after a meal.
 (B) Gluconeogenesis in the liver supplies glucose from amino acid and fatty acid substrates 8–30 h after a meal.
 (C) Defects in protein metabolism can be because of organ dysfunction or inherited enzyme deficiencies.
 (D) Glucokinase is found throughout the body, whereas hexokinase is a high capacity enzyme only found in the liver.
 (E) Even if the urine ketone test is negative, there can be a significant level of ketogenesis occurring in the liver.

41. Which glycogen storage disease (GSD) is a process that primarily affects glycogen storage in the muscles?

 (A) type I GSD (Von Gierke's disease)
 (B) type II GSD (Pompe's disease)
 (C) type III GSD (Cori's disease)
 (D) type IV GSD (Andersen's disease)
 (E) type V GSD (McArdle's disease)

42. Which of the following reactions is unique to gluconeogenesis in the liver and is not a directly reversed step of glycolysis?

 (A) conversion of pyruvate to oxaloacetate by pyruvate carboxylase
 (B) conversion of oxaloacetate to phosphoenolpyruvate (PEP) by PEP-carboxykinase (PEPCK)
 (C) conversion of fructose-1,6-bisphosphate (F-1,6-BP) to fructose-6-phosphate (F6P) by fructose-1,6-bisphosphatase (F-1,6-BPase)
 (D) conversion of glucose-6-phosphate to glucose by glucose-6-phosphatase
 (E) all of the above

43. Which intermediate is common to both cholesterol synthesis and ketogenesis?

 (A) acetoacetate
 (B) β-hydroxybutyrate
 (C) β-hydroxy-β-methylglutaryl-CoA (HMG-CoA)
 (D) mevalonate
 (E) none of the above

44. Which of the following statements about the urea cycle is *not* true?

 (A) The urea cycle is main pathway responsible for the excretion of nitrogenous wastes derived from protein metabolism.
 (B) The nitrogens in urea are directly derived from ammonia, alanine, and glutamate by reactions of the urea cycle.
 (C) Urea cycle reactions occur in both the mitochondria and cytosol of hepatocytes.
 (D) The urea cycle uses ATP as energy in the formation of urea and is also known as the Krebs-Henseleit cycle or the Krebs ornithine cycle.
 (E) The fumarate by-product of the urea cycle is converted into energy by the TCA cycle.

45. Which of the following statements is *not* true?

 (A) Selectins are Ca^{2+}-dependent cell-cell adhesion molecules in the bloodstream that mediate transient binding.
 (B) Collagen fiber formation begins at approximately three days after a wound occurs and is responsible for providing tensile strength and pliability to the healing wound.
 (C) Mutations in the fibrillin component of elastic fibers is responsible for Marfan's syndrome.
 (D) TIMPs are proteases that breakdown the extracellular matrix for cell migration.
 (E) All of the above are true.

46. Which of the following statements about integrins is *not* true?

 (A) Integrins are structural proteins that function to anchor cells to the extracellular matrix and do not play a major role in signal transduction.
 (B) Integrins are the major receptors for binding extracellular matrix proteins such as collagens, laminins, and fibronectins, and they are dependent on extracellular divalent cations such as Ca^{2+} or Mg^{2+} for binding.
 (C) Integrins exist as transmembrane heterodimers with alpha and beta subunits that are noncovalently associated.
 (D) Integrins serve as transmembrane linkers between the extracellular matrix and actin cytoskeleton but cannot directly activate cell shape changes.
 (E) All of the above statements are true.

47. Which of the following correctly depicts a complement activation pathway?

    (A) The alternate pathway is activated by IgG or IgM bound to the surface of a microbe and involves the sequential activation of C1, C2, and C4.

    (B) The classical pathway involves the spontaneous activation of C3 by factors B and D.

    (C) The lectin pathway involves the activation of early complement components by mannan-binding lectin (MBL).

    (D) The final common pathway is the assembly of late complement components to form a membrane attack complex (MAC).

    (E) Both C and D are correct.

48. What is the role of the TLR pathway?

    (A) The TLR pathway mediates the inflammatory response to pathogenic substances such as LPS by activating the transcription of proinflammatory genes.

    (B) The TLR pathway is responsible for deactivating phagocytic cells after they have engulfed target pathogens.

    (C) The TLR pathway activates apoptosis in virus-infected cells as part of the innate and adaptive immune responses.

    (D) The TLR pathway is involved in signal transduction for activating inflammatory genes in response to hypoxia-inducible factors.

    (E) None of the above are correct.

49. Which of the following statements is *incorrect*?

    (A) There are two major isoforms of the cyclooxygenase (COX) enzyme, with COX-1 being consitutively expressed and COX-2 being inducible in inflammation.

    (B) Eicosapentaenoic acid (EPA) and aspirin inhibit the AA pathway in the same manner.

    (C) EPA is considered to be anti-inflammatory in its actions while AA generally produces proinflammatory effects.

    (D) When EPA and AA are used as substrates for COX through the AA pathway, they result in different sets of prostenoid products.

    (E) All of the above are correct.

50. Which of the following are considered proangiogenic factors?

    (A) vascular endothelial growth factor and angiopoietin-1 (Ang1)

    (B) vascular endothelial growth factor and angiopoietin-2 (Ang2)

    (C) Ang1 and Ang2

    (D) vascular endothelial growth factor and angiostatin

    (E) all are proangiogenic factors

Answers and Explanations

1. **(E)** Although phospholipids are commonly thought of only as the structural components of the cell membrane, they serve many signaling functions as well. Phospholipids are involved in the PLA-arachidonic acid pathway, the phospholipase C (PLC) pathway, the marking of apoptotic cells for phagocytosis, and as self-antigens in autoimmune disorders. There are several phospholipids in the cell membrane that include phosphatidylcholine, phosphatidylethanolamine, phosphatidylinositol (PI), phosphatidylserine, and sphingomyelin. These are all amphipathic molecules without a net charge except for phosphatidylserine, which has a net negative charge. The hydrophilic heads and hydrophobic tails impart a property to phospholipids that cause them to spontaneously form lipid bilayers or spherical micelles to shield their hydrophobic tails from the aqueous environment in an energetically favorable conformation. The formation of the phospholipid bilayer plasma membrane results in the separation of the intracellular space from the extracellular space and controls the permeability of the cell to ions and molecules. The inclusion of cholesterol and glycolipids in the phospholipid bilayer additionally enhance the barrier properties and modify the fluidity of the membrane. Thus, one of the main functions of phospholipids is to provide a fluid barrier between the cytosol and the extracellular environment.

However, many phospholipids in the plasma membrane also serve as substrates for cell signaling, primarily in the conversion of extracellular signals to intracellular signals. Phosphatidylinositol 3'-kinase (PI3K) is a lipid kinase that phosphorylates inositol phospholipids, derivatives of phosphotidylinositol, to transmit intracellular signals in response to growth factors and cytokines. Phospholipases are another example of enzymes in the plasma membrane that are activated in response to a variety of extracellular ligands. Phospholipase A cleaves arachidonic acid (AA) or its relatives from the two-position on membrane phospholipids to result in the eventual formation of inflammatory leukotrienes and prostaglandins. PLC cleaves an inositol phospholipid (i.e., PIP_2) on the cytosolic side of the plasma membrane to form two fragments (i.e., DAG and IP_3). 1,2-Diacylglycerol (DAG) remains in the membrane to activate protein kinase C (PKC), and cytosolic IP_3 stimulates the release of Ca^{2+} from the endoplasmic reticulum (ER). PKC remains bound to the cytosolic side of the plasma membrane where there is a concentration of negatively charged phosphatidylserines, which are necessary for its activity. PKC and cytosolic Ca^{2+} are involved in many signaling functions of the cell.

The asymmetrical distribution of the charged phosphatidylserine molecules are also used to distinguish cells that have undergone apoptosis. Phosphatidylserines are normally maintained on the cytosolic side of the plasma membrane in living cells. The altered activities of phospholipid translocators in apoptotic cells results in the translocation of phosphotidylserines to the outer face of the cell membrane. The exposed phosphotidylserines serve as signals to induce the phagocytosis of apoptotic cells by macrophages.

Bibliography

Alberts B, Johnson A, Lewis K, et al. Membrane structure. In: Alberts B, Johnson A, Lewis K, et al. (eds.), *Molecular Biology of the Cell*, 4th ed. New York, NY: Garland Science, 2002, 583–592.

Aoki J, Nagai Y, Hosono H, et al. Structure and function of phosphatidylserine-specific phospholipase A1. *Biochim Biophys Acta* 2002;1582:26–32.

Bell RM, Hannun YA, Loomis CR. Mechanism of regulation of protein kinase C by lipid second messengers. *Symp Fundam Cancer Res* 1986;39:145–156.

Bevers EM, Comfurius P, Dekkers DW, et al. Lipid translocation across the plasma membrane of mammalian cells. *Biochim Biophys Acta* 1999;1439:317–330.

Devaux PF, Zachowski A, Morrot G, et al. Control of the transmembrane phospholipid distribution in eukaryotic cells by aminophospholipid translocase. *Biotechnol Appl Biochem* 1990;12:517–522.

Dygas A, Baranska J. Lipids and signal transduction in the nucleus. *Acta Biochim Pol* 2001;48:541–549.

McCarty-Farid GA. Antiphospholipid antibodies in systemic lupus erythematosus and Sjogren's syndrome. *Curr Opin Rheumatol* 1993;5:596–603.

Schlegel RA, Callahan M, Krahling S, et al. Mechanisms for recognition and phagocytosis of apoptotic lymphocytes by macrophages. *Adv Exp Med Biol* 1996;406:21–28.

Schlegel RA, Williamson P. Phosphatidylserine, a death knell. *Cell Death Differ* 2001;8:551–563.

Yedgar S, Lichtenberg D, Schnitzer E. Inhibition of phospholipase A(2) as a therapeutic target. *Biochim Biophys Acta* 2000;1488:182–187.

2. **(E)** Glycosylated proteins are located exclusively on the extracellular side of the cell membrane, whereas membrane proteins with covalently attached lipid chains such as prenyl groups are located only on the cytosolic or intracellular side. Lipid-linked proteins are synthesized first as proteins on free cytosolic ribosomes and are directed to the intracellular side of the plasma membrane by the attachment of the lipid group. Sugar residues are added to proteins or lipids in the lumen of the ER or Golgi apparatus, which are topologically analogous to the exterior of the cell. Vesicles that carry proteins or lipids from the ER or Golgi to the plasma membrane fuse with the lipid bilayer in a manner that result in the lumen of the vesicle becoming the extracellular face of the cell membrane. The sugar residues on glycolipids are important for modulating interactions with each other in lipid rafts and in altering the electrical effects in the membrane transport of ions.

Most transmembrane proteins are actually glycoproteins; the glycosylation of these proteins is a post-transcriptional modification that adds an essential structural component for their various functions. Both glycolipids and glycoproteins are also important in cell-cell adhesion, as they bind to membrane-bound lectin or selectin molecules especially in the rolling interaction of neutrophils with the endothelium. Glycosylphosphatidylinositol anchors are added to designated proteins in the ER, which are then associated with the extracellular side of the plasma membrane by a covalent linkage to PI. GPI-anchored proteins are important in immune function, and mutations in the GPI anchor are associated with immune dysfunctions such as paroxysmal nocturnal hemoglobinuria (PNH). PNH is the result of an acquired mutation in the phosphatidylinositol glycan A (PIGA) gene that is necessary for the synthesis of the GPI anchor. Since GPI-anchored proteins are necessary for the inactivation of complement, the mutation renders affected red blood cells (RBCs), granulocytes, and platelets hypersensitive to lysis by complement.

Therefore, the significance of glycolipids, glycoproteins, and GPI-anchored proteins being located exclusively on the extracellular face of the cell membrane is a result of the topographic location of the glycosylation process and is related to their function.

Bibliography

Alberts B, Johnson A, Lewis K, et al. Membrane structure. In: Alberts B, Johnson A, Lewis K, et al. (eds.), *Molecular Biology of the Cell*, 4th ed. New York, NY: Garland Science, 2002, 592–589.

Bessler M, Schaefer A, Keller P. Paroxysmal nocturnal hemoglobinuria: insights from recent advances in molecular biology. *Transfus Med Rev* 2001;15:255–267.

Butikofer P, Malherbe T, Boschung M, et al. GPI-anchored proteins: now you see 'em, now you don't. *FASEB J* 2001;15:545–548.

Cotran R, Kumar V, Collins T. Red cells and bleeding disorders. In: Cotran R, Kumar V, Collins T (eds.), *Robbins Pathologic Basis of Disease*, 6th ed. Philadelphia, PA: W.B. Saunders, 1999, 619–620.

Emmelot P, Van Hoeven RP. Phospholipid unsaturation and plasma membrane organization. *Chem Phys Lipids* 1975;14:236–246.

Hooper NM. Determination of glycosyl-phosphatidylinositol membrane protein anchorage. *Proteomics* 2001;1:748–755.

Rothman JE, Lenard J. Membrane asymmetry. *Science* 1977;195:743–753.

Rosse WF. New insights into paroxysmal nocturnal hemoglobinuria. *Curr Opin Hematol* 2001;8:61–67.

Sinensky M. Recent advances in the study of prenylated proteins. *Biochim Biophys Acta* 2000;1484:93–106.

3. **(E)** Plasma membrane fluidity is determined by lipid composition involving phospholipid chain lengths, fatty acid chain saturation, and cholesterol content; it is not a function of integral proteins. Integral proteins are structures firmly embedded in the cell membrane and are difficult to dissociate without the use of detergents. Transmembrane proteins are subtypes of integral proteins that physically span the entire lipid bilayer and often serve as receptor proteins to transduce outside-in or inside-out signaling pathways. Ion channels, transport proteins, and many receptors are integral proteins. In contrast to integral proteins, peripheral proteins are weakly associated with the membrane by covalent bonds or adaptor proteins and can be removed by altering the pH. Peripheral proteins can be found on either the intracellular or extracellular side of the cell membrane; hormone receptors are usually peripheral proteins.

Integral proteins have three general categories of function: (1) receptors, (2) channels or pumps, and (3) structural proteins. Receptor proteins can be subdivided by their methods of signal transduction into

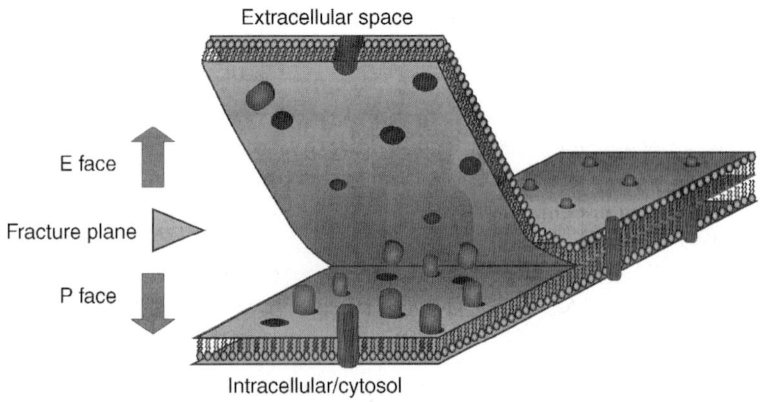

Cell membrane

Extracellular space

E face

Fracture plane

P face

Intracellular/cytosol

FIG. 1-1   Diagram illustrating the concept of P face and E face.

those linked to ion channels (i.e., neurotransmitter-gated, mechanical-gated, voltage-gated ion channels), G proteins (i.e., heterotrimeric GTP-binding proteins), or enzymes (i.e., tyrosine kinases, serine-threonine kinases). Integral proteins are also involved as receptors in immune function and in receptor-mediated endocytosis. Passive ion channels or active transport pumps are often integral proteins themselves. An example of structural function is the involvement of integral proteins with polysaccharide attachments in forming the glycocalyx layer on cell surfaces, which is involved in cell protection and lectin-mediated cell-cell adhesion.

Bibliography

Alberts B, Bray D, Johnson A, et al. Programmed cell death is mediated by an intracellular proteolytic cascade. In: Alberts B, Bray D, Johnson A, et al. (eds.), *Essential Cell Biology*. New York, NY: Garland Publishing, 1998, 347–367.

Boon JM, Smith BD. Chemical control of phospholipid distribution across bilayer membranes. *Med Res Rev* 2002;22(3):251–281.

Cheng KH, Somerharju P, Virtanen A, Cheng KH. Lateral organization of membrane lipids. The superlattice view. *Biochim Biophys Acta* 1999;1440(1):32–48.

Cribier S, Morrot G, Zachowski A. Dynamics of the membrane lipid phase. *Prostaglandins Leukot Essent Fatty Acids* 1993;48(1):27–32.

Ross MH, Romrell LJ, Kaye GI. Plasma membrane. In: Ross MH, Romrell LJ, Kaye GI (eds.), *Histology: A Text and Atlas*, 3rd ed. Baltimore, MD: Williams & Wilkins, 1995, 20–22.

Subczynski WK, Wisniewska A. Physical properties of lipid bilayer membranes: relevance to membrane biological functions. *Acta Biochim Pol* 2000;47(3):613–625.

4. **(A)** The integral proteins tend to remain in the monolayer or leaflet that contains the greater bulk of the protein. There is a greater density of integral proteins on the P face (protoplasmic or cytoplasmic leaflet) than the E face (external or extracellular leaflet) after freeze-fracture in most human cells, including RBCs. The large number of integral proteins on the P face can be visualized as bumps under EM, whereas the E face contains many more pits than bumps. But although the P face contains many more integral proteins after freeze-fracture than the E face, the E face still contains a small number of integral proteins. In fact, a few integral proteins (e.g., glycophorin in RBCs) can be found exclusively in the E face (see Fig. 1-1).

Bibliography

Alberts B, Johnson A, Lewis K, et al. Membrane structure. In: Alberts B, Johnson A, Lewis K, et al. (eds.), *Molecular Biology of the Cell*, 4th ed. New York, NY: Garland Science, 2002, 605–606.

Morrison M, Mueller TJ, Edwards HH. Protein architecture of the erythrocyte membrane. *Prog Clin Biol Res* 1981;51: 17–34.

Severs NJ. Freeze-fracture cytochemistry: a simplified guide and update on developments. *J Microsc* 1991;161: 109–134.

5. **(A)** Intracellular macromolecules contribute little to osmolarity directly because of their relatively low numbers and large sizes, but their indirect contribution is significant. The charges on intracellular macromolecules attract many small counterions, which then contribute to osmolarity and the Donnan effect. The tenets of the Donnan equilibrium are that nondiffusible and diffusible substances are distributed on the two sides of the membrane so that the products of their concentrations are equal and ionic charges are

balanced on both sides. However, only the distribution of diffusible ions creates a potential difference across the membrane. The Donnan effect results in a higher concentration of diffusible ions intracellularly, and the membrane potential is maintained by the Na^+-K^+ ATPase pump. Treating human cells with ouabain or digitalis glycosides inhibits the Na^+-K^+ ATPase pump. At the cellular level, the prolonged inhibition of the pump results in the accumulation of intracellular Na^+, which causes the cell to swell and burst.

Polar or charged molecules have difficulty traversing cell membranes and must be transported by carrier or channel proteins. Channel proteins and some carrier proteins allow passive transport or facilitated transport down an electrochemical gradient. Some carrier proteins act in active transport to pump molecules against the electrochemical gradient. Ionophores are hydrophobic molecules released by microorganisms to form carriers or channels in host cell membranes to cause the rapid flow of ions down the electrochemical gradient. For example, gramicidin A is an antibiotic produced by certain bacteria that functions as a channel-forming ionophore to collapse the H^+, Na^+, and K^+ gradient of other bacteria sensitive to its effects. FCCP is a mobile carrier ionophore that dissipates the H^+ gradient across the mitochondrial inner membrane. Valinomycin dissipates K^+ gradients, and A23187 or ionomycin causes a massive influx of Ca^{2+} and can activate the apoptotic signaling pathway.

The automated blood counts (ABC) transporter superfamily consists of membrane channel proteins with two adenosine triphosphate (ATP)-binding cassettes or domains. The cystic fibrosis transmembrane conductance regulator (CFTR) is a member of the ABC transporter superfamily, whose members are also known as traffic ATPases. The binding of ATP to the domains leads to conformational changes that help transport molecules across the membrane, and ATP hydrolysis leads to dissociation of the domains to repeat the cycle. MDR proteins are ABC transporters that pump hydrophobic drugs out of the cytosol. MDR proteins are overexpressed in certain human cancer cells, making the cells resistant to many chemotherapeutic agents. An ABC transporter is also involved in many cases of *Plasmodium falciparum* infections, which are resistant to conventional malaria drugs such as chloroquine.

Bibliography

Alberts B, Johnson A, Lewis K, et al. Carrier proteins and active membrane transport. In: Alberts B, Johnson A, Lewis K, et al. (eds.), *Molecular Biology of the Cell*, 4th ed. New York, NY: Garland Science, 2002, 615–657.

Borst P, Elferink RO. Mammalian ABC transporters in health and disease. *Annu Rev Biochem* 2002;71:537–592.

Cantiello HF. Electrodiffusional ATP movement through CFTR and other ABC transporters. *Pflugers Arch* 2001;443(Suppl 1):S22–S27.

Doris PA. Regulation of Na,K-ATPase by endogenous ouabain-like materials. *Proc Soc Exp Biol Med* 1994;205:202–212.

Efferth T. The human ATP-binding cassette transporter genes: from the bench to the bedside. *Curr Mol Med* 2001;1:45–65.

Kipp H, Arias IM. Trafficking of canalicular ABC transporters in hepatocytes. *Annu Rev Physiol* 2002;64:595–608.

Poelarends GJ, Mazurkiewicz P, Konings WN. Multidrug transporters and antibiotic resistance in *Lactococcus lactis*. *Biochim Biophys Acta* 2002;1555:1–7.

Skatrud PL. The impact of multiple drug resistance (MDR) proteins on chemotherapy and drug discovery. *Prog Drug Res* 2002;58:99–131.

Yaroshchuk AE. Dielectric exclusion of ions from membranes. *Adv Colloid Interface Sci* 2000;85:193–230.

6. (A) The CF gene is 230 kb in length and codes for 1480 amino acids, yet a single phenylalanine deletion is usually the cause of dysfunction in the CFTR chloride channel. CFTR is an ATP-dependent transport protein that includes two membrane-spanning domains, two nucleotide-binding domains that interact with ATP, and one regulatory domain with several phosphorylation sites. This channel is located on the luminal plasma membrane of epithelial cells in many different tissues. In the regulation of Cl^- transport, CFTR is normally closed and only opens when it is phosphorylated by protein kinase A. There have been about 400 different mutations found in the CFTR gene since 1989; however, about 70% of individuals who have CF are linked to the deletion of three nucleotides encoding phenylalanine-508. The mutant CFTR is not glycosylated or transported to the cell surface, and the mutant CFTR eventually becomes degraded within the ER.

CF afflicts 1 in 2000 live births making it the most fatal inherited disease of Whites. The disease affects exocrine glands in multiple organs, but its most devastating effects occur in the respiratory system. The thick, chloride-deficient mucous clogs airways and produce chronic infections. CFTR dysfunction also results in malabsorption and infertility. The lungs, pancreas, and bile ducts in CF demonstrate dysfunction in secreting Cl^-, resulting in a hyperviscous secretion product. In contrast, sweat glands are unable to reabsorb Cl^- properly before final secretion. The resulting increase in sweat NaCl content allows for diagnosis using the sweat chloride test with Cl^-

concentration above 50 meq/L (children) or 60 meq/L (adults) being positive.

Bibliography

Abély M, Bajolet O, Puchelle E. Airway mucus in cystic fibrosis *Paediatr Respir Rev* 2002;3(2):115–119.

Aps JK, Delanghe J, Martens LC. Salivary electrolyte concentrations are associated with cystic fibrosis transmembrane regulator genotypes. *Clin Chem Lab Med* 2002;40(4):345–350.

Devlin TM. Cystic fibrosis. In: Devlin TM (ed.), *Textbook of Biochemistry with Clinical Correlations*, 4th ed. New York, NY: Wiley-Liss, 1997, 1066–1067.

Fujiki K, Naruse S, Kitagawa M, Ishiguro H, Hayakawa T. Cystic fibrosis and related diseases of the pancreas. *Best Pract Res Clin Gastroenterol* 2002;16(3):511–526.

Puchelle E. Early bronchial inflammation in cystic fibrosis. *J Soc Biol* 2002;196(1):29–35.

7. **(B)** The Na^+-K^+ ATPase pump transfers three intracellular Na^+ ions out of the cell and two extracellular K^+ ions into the cell per ATP molecule. This process serves three main purposes. First, an electrochemical gradient is created to energetically link the transport of other ions and molecules into and out of the cell against their concentration gradients. Second, the active transport of Na^+ out of the cell prevents the cell from swelling and bursting from osmosis. Third, the movement and diffusion of the ions involved are critical to regulating the electrical activity in nerves and in muscles by rapidly restoring the resting potential. Therefore, digitalis toxicity causing excessive blockage of the pump results in symptoms and signs occurring in the nervous, cardiovascular, and musculoskeletal systems as cells have difficulty repolarizing. Doubling the number of pumps would theoretically result in the facilitation of repolarization rather than depolarization.

The Na^+-K^+ pump creates a gradient of ions across the nerve membrane, with a general distribution of 142 meq/L extracellular Na^+, 14 meq/L intracellular Na^+, 4 meq/L extracellular K^+, and 140 meq/L intracellular K^+. Ions diffuse through leak channels based on these gradients. Therefore, increasing the Na^+ leak current would theoretically facilitate depolarization whereas increasing the K^+ leak current would facilitate repolarization. Since the ratio between extracellular and intracellular K^+ is about 1:35, there is an electrical potential of –94 mV according to the Nernst equation. The ratio between extracellular and intracellular Na^+ is 10:1, giving a calculated potential of +61 mV. According to the Goldman equation, which takes into account that K^+ is 100x more permeable than Na^+, the calculated resting membrane potential equals –86 mV. Active ion transport by Na^+-K^+ pumps contributes –4 mV to the resting membrane potential, bringing the final resting membrane potential to –90 mV in large nerve cells. Large skeletal muscle fibers have a similar resting potential, but small nerve and muscle fibers have resting potentials ranging from –40 to –60 mV, making them easier to depolarize. Conversely, changing the resting membrane potential to –100 mV would make depolarization more difficult.

Bibliography

Alberts B, Bray D, Johnson A, et al. Membrane transport. In: Alberts B, Bray D, Johnson A, et al. (eds.), *Essential Cell Biology*. New York, NY: Garland Publishing, 1998, 371–404.

Bamberg E, Clarke RJ, Fendler K. Electrogenic properties of the Na^+,K^+-ATPase probed by presteady state and relaxation studies. *J Bioenerg Biomembr* 2001;33(5):401–405.

Devlin TM. Active mediated transport systems. In: Devlin TM (ed.), *Textbook of Biochemistry with Clinical Correlations*, 4th ed. New York, NY: Wiley-Liss, 1997, 206–211.

Grossmann M, Joubert PH. Local and systemic effects of Na^+/K ATPase inhibition. *Eur J Clin Invest* 2001;31:1–4.

Guyton AC, Hall JE. Membrane potentials and action potentials. In: Guyton AC, Hall JE (eds.), *Textbook of Medical Physiology*, 10th ed. Philadelphia, PA: W.B. Saunders, 2000, 52–65.

Kashiwaya Y, King MT, Veech RL. The resting membrane potential of cells are measures of electrical work, not of ionic currents. *Integr Physiol Behav Sci* 1995;30(4):283–307.

Offner FF. Ion flow through membranes and the resting potential of cells. *J Membr Biol* 1991;123(2):171–182.

Pastor J. Biophysical foundations of the neuronal activity. *Rev Neurol* 2000;30(8):741–755.

Scheiner-Bobis G. The sodium pump. Its molecular properties and mechanics of ion transport. *Eur J Biochem* 2002;269(10):2424–2433.

8. **(B)** Solutes cross cell membranes by passive diffusion, facilitated diffusion, primary active transport, or secondary active transport. The major difference between diffusion (or passive transport) and active transport is that the latter requires the use of energy. Passive transport is the movement of molecules down its electrochemical gradient without the active mobilization of a metabolic energy source. Passive transport can be subdivided into simple diffusion and facilitated diffusion. In simple or free diffusion, permeable molecules are able to move down their electrochemical gradients and freely across cell membranes. Some examples of free diffusers are ethanol, nitric oxide, carbon dioxide, oxygen, and steroid hormones. In facilitated diffusion, slowly permeable molecules undergo rapid transport down their electrochemical gradient with the aid of channels or carrier proteins. Facilitated diffusion is more rapid than simple diffusion but demonstrates saturation. Carrier proteins are

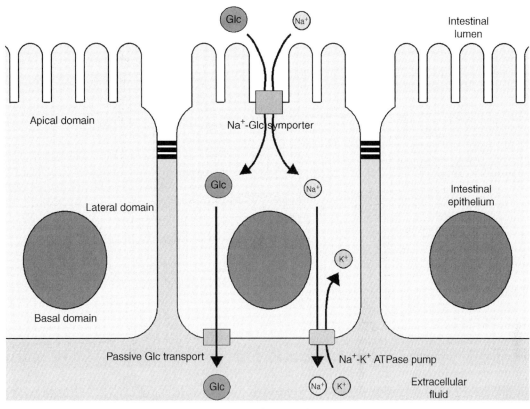

FIG. 1-2   Active and passive transport of Na$^+$ and glucose in intestinal epithelial cells.

often highly selective and stereospecific but can demonstrate competition with similar ligands. Some examples of molecules that undergo facilitated diffusion include sugars, amino acids, and nucleotides.

Sometimes solutes must go up their electrochemical gradients with the use of energy in an active transport process. Active transport is subdivided into primary and secondary active transport. Primary transporters use a direct metabolic energy source, usually ATP hydrolysis, to move solutes against an electrochemical gradient. A well-known example is the Na$^+$-K$^+$ pump, which uses the hydrolysis of ATP to transport Na$^+$ and K$^+$ against their gradients. Other examples of primary active transport include the Ca^{2+} ATPase pump, the H$^+$ ATPase proton pump, and the H$^+$-K$^+$ ATPase proton pump. Secondary active transport can be further subdivided into synport (also called cotransport) and antiport (also called countertransport). Secondary transporters indirectly use metabolic energy for transport by utilizing the gradients of molecules created by the ATP hydrolysis of primary active transport, usually the Na$^+$ gradient formed by the Na$^+$-K$^+$ pump. Synport involves the transport of a molecule in the same direction as the linked downhill Na$^+$ gradient, whereas antiport involves the transport of a molecule in the opposite direction. Examples of synport include the Na$^+$-glucose cotransporter in the small intestine and Na$^+$-K$^+$-2Cl$^-$ cotransporter in the thick ascending limb of the nephron. An example of antiport is the Na$^+$-Ca^{2+} exchanger, which is ubiquitous in cell membranes.

Transcellular transport of glucose across an intestinal epithelial cell is accomplished by Na$^+$-glucose symporters on the apical cell membrane. These symporters pump glucose from its relatively low concentration in the intestinal lumen into the high glucose concentration of the epithelial cytosol through secondary active transport. Passive glucose carrier proteins in the basal membrane then transport glucose down its concentration gradient from the cytosol to the extracellular fluid, where it can eventually pass into the circulation (see Fig. 1-2).

Bibliography

Alberts B, Bray D, Johnson A, et al. Carrier proteins and their functions. In: Alberts B, Bray D, Johnson A, et al. (eds.), *Essential Cell Biology*. New York, NY: Garland Publishing, 1998, 373–385.

Avila J, Brownleader MD, Cozar-Castellano I, et al. Na$^+$, K$^+$-ATPase isozyme diversity; comparative biochemistry and physiological implications of novel functional interactions. *Biosci Rep* 2000;20(2):51–91.

Brown GK. Glucose transporters: structure, function, and consequences of deficiency. *J Inherit Metab Dis* 2000;23(3): 237–246.

Devlin TM. Active mediated transport systems. In: Devlin TM (ed.), *Textbook of Biochemistry with Clinical Correlations*, 4th ed. New York, NY: Wiley-Liss, 1997, 206–207.

Gerencser GA, Zhang J. Cl(-)-ATPases: novel primary active transporters in biology. *J Exp Zool* 2001;289(4):215–223.

Loo DD, Wright EM. Coupling between Na$^+$, sugar, and water transport across the intestine. *Ann N Y Acad Sci* 2000;915:54–66.

Zeuthen T. General models for water transport across leaky epithelia. *Int Rev Cytol* 2002;215:285–317.

9. **(E)** Cadherins are calcium-binding integral membrane glycoproteins crucial for cell-cell adhesion and are located at the zonula adherens. The cadherin family is divided into two major types: the classic cadherins associated with catenins intracellularly and the non-classic cadherins unassociated with catenins. Classic cadherins are anchored to the actin cytoskeleton of the cell by intracellular intermediates called catenins. The major classic cadherins include E-cadherins (aka uvomorulin) on epithelial cells, N-cadherins on neural cells, VE-cadherins on vascular endothelial cells, and P-cadherins on several cell types. Cadherins undergo *cis*-dimerization with other cadherins on the same plasma membrane to form strand dimers and undergo calcium-dependent *trans*-dimerization with cadherins on adjacent plasma membranes to form adhesion dimers.

The junctional complex consists of three major regions: zonula occludens, zonula adherens, and macula adherens. The zonula occludens is also called the tight junction because it is highly resistant to the passage of molecules and is composed of occludins, ZO-1, ZO-2, and claudins. The zonula adherens or belt desmosome is primarily composed of cadherins, and along with the zonula occludens, is highly tissue specific. The macula adherens is composed of desmosome proteins forming spot desmosomes and are distinct from the gap junctions, which are composed of connexons functioning in cell-cell communication. They are also distinct from hemidesmosomes, which anchor the cell to the basal lamina or basement membrane.

The other answers are incorrect because ZO-1 and desmosomes are not calcium dependent, and neither calcineurin nor calmodulin is directly involved in cell-cell adhesion. Calcineurin is a calmodulin-binding protein found in the mammalian brain, which acts as a phosphatase in the regulation of calcium channels. Calmodulin is an intracellular protein that binds calcium and regulates various cell signaling functions, including phospholipase A$_2$ (PLA$_2$), actin cytoskeleton formation, various kinases, and adenylate and guanylate cyclases.

Of clinical interest, the disassembly of VE-cadherins results in increased vascular permeability and may be involved in various vascular pathologies. The loss of function of E-cadherin is associated with increased invasiveness and metastases of epithelial tumors. Cadherins and catenins are also associated with heritable cancer predispositions. Familial adenomatous polyposis (FAP) is caused primarily by inactivation of the adenomatous polyposis coli (APC) tumor suppressor gene or mutations in β-catenins. β-Catenins, which associate with the intracellular region of classic cadherins, also function to sequester APC in the cytosol. In FAP, β-catenin degradation by the ubiquitin-proteasome pathway is prevented by mutations in β-catenin or APC that increase the strength of their interaction. As a consequence, the degradation of β-catenin is dramatically reduced, resulting in the increased sequestration of APC. Increased levels of β-catenin also result in interaction with lymphoid enhancer-binding factor (LEF-1) and other transcription factors (TFs) to increase gene proliferation or block apoptosis in various forms of cancer (see Fig. 1-3).

Bibliography

Gumbiner BM, McCrea PD. Catenins as mediators of the cytoplasmic functions of cadherins. *J Cell Sci Suppl* 1993;17:155–158.

Hajra KM, Fearon ER. Cadherin and catenin alterations in human cancer. *Genes Chromosomes Cancer* 2002;34:255–268.

Hinck L, Nathke IS, Papkoff J, et al. Beta-catenin: a common target for the regulation of cell adhesion by Wnt-1 and Src signaling pathways. *Trends Biochem Sci* 1994; 19:538–542.

Hirohashi S. Inactivation of the E-cadherin-mediated cell adhesion system in human cancers. *Am J Pathol* 1998;153:333–339.

Jankowski JA, Bruton R, Shepherd N, et al. Cadherin and catenin biology represent a global mechanism for epithelial cancer progression. *Mol Pathol* 1997;50:289–290.

Miyaguchi K. Ultrastructure of the zonula adherens revealed by rapid-freeze deep-etching. *J Struct Biol* 2000;132:169–178.

Ozawa M, Baribault H, Kemler R. The cytoplasmic domain of the cell adhesion molecule uvomorulin associates with three independent proteins structurally related in difference species. *EMBO J* 1989;8:1711–1717.

Shapiro L, Fannon AM, Kwong PD, et al. Structural basis of cell-cell adhesion by cadherins. *Nature* 1995;374:327–337.

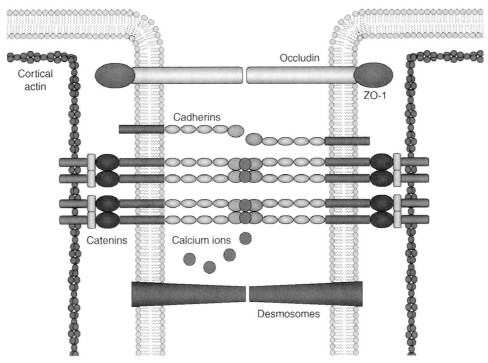

FIG.1-3 Diagram demonstrating cadherins at the zonula adherens and its relationship to other components of the junctional complex.

Su LK, Vogelstein B, Kinzler KW. Association of the APC tumor suppressor proteins with catenins. *Science* 1993;262:1734–1737.

10. **(D)** The glial-specific stain used was a stain for glial fibrillary acidic protein (GFAP), a type of intermediate filament, which plays a role in imparting mechanical strength to the cell. Intermediate filaments are long, tough fibers 10 nm in diameter that play a structural role in the cell and are composed of a heterogenous group of proteins, which tend to be tissue-specific. The peptide monomer for intermediate filaments is elongated in shape with a long α-helical coil region that winds together with another identical monomer to form a coiled-coil dimer. The dimer associates with another dimer, which is oriented with its N- and C-terminus in the opposite direction, to create a staggered tetramer conformation. The staggered tetramer can then bind other tetramers and twist into a final rope-like filament composed of eight tetramers. Nuclear lamins are intermediate filaments that provide mechanical support to the nuclear lamina lining the inside of the nuclear envelope. There are also many other tissue-specific types of intermediate filament proteins including keratins in skin, desmin in muscle, and neurofilament proteins in neurons. Many different types of keratins are responsible for the tensile strength of skin. Keratin filaments form structural networks in epithelium within each cell, which are then linked to networks of neighboring cells by desmosomes. Abnormalities of intermediate filaments are associated with several human diseases, including epidermolysis bullosa simplex and amyotrophic lateral sclerosis (ALS). Keratin mutations are responsible for genetic forms of epidermolysis bullosa, in which blisters form in response to mild mechanical stress. Abnormal assembly and accumulation of neurofilaments have been associated with motoneuron dysfunction in some forms of ALS.

Microtubules are hollow tubes, 25 nm in diameter, composed of many individual α- and β-tubulin monomers. The α-tubulin monomers bind β-tubulin monomers to form tubulin heterodimers, which are also known as microtubule subunits. Each α- or β-tubulin monomer can bind one GTP molecule, but only the GTP associated with β-tubulin is exchangeable. Microtubule subunits bind to form long, threadlike protofilaments with alternating α- and β-tubulins. Protofilaments demonstrate structural polarity with α-tubulin exposed on one end and β-tubulin on the other. The β-tubulin end is called the plus end and the α-tubulin end is called the minus end; the plus end is the more dynamic of the two, undergoing rapid growth and shrinkage. The hollow

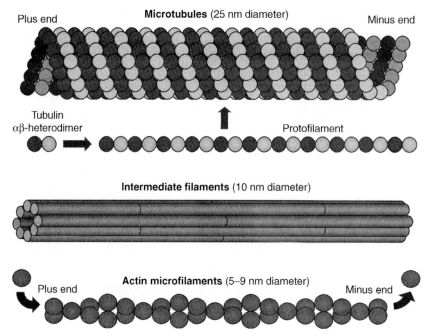

FIG. 1-4   Diagram demonstrating the structures of microtubules, intermediate filaments, and actin microfilaments.

microtubules are then assembled from 13 protofilaments attached in parallel strands. Microtubules play an important role in structure and transport, especially during cell division.

Actin filaments are double-stranded helical polymers, 5–9 nm in diameter, composed of actin protein subunits. They are also known as microfilaments and are abundantly dispersed throughout the cell, although they are most abundant just beneath the cell membrane. Actin monomers (also known as globular- or G-actin) bind ATP molecules at their minus ends or "pointed" ends and form double-helix filamentous- or F-actin strands toward their plus ends or "barbed" ends (see Fig. 1-4).

Bibliography

Alberts B, Johnson A, Lewis K, et al. The cytoskeleton. In: Alberts B, Johnson A, Lewis K, et al. (eds.), *Molecular Biology of the Cell*, 4th ed. New York, NY: Garland Science, 2002, 907–982.

Eng L. Glial fibrillary acidic protein (GFAP): the major protein of glial intermediate filaments in differentiated astrocytes. *J Neuroimmunol* 1985;8:203–214.

Osborn M, Weber K. Tumor diagnosis by intermediate filament typing: a novel tool for surgical pathology. *Lab Invest* 1983;48:372–394.

Tilney L. The role of actin in nonmuscle cell motility. *Soc Gen Physiol Ser* 1975;30:339–388.

Wittmann T, Hyman A, Desai A. The spindle: a dynamic assembly of microtubules and motors. *Nat Cell Biol* 2001;3:E28–E34.

11. **(D)** Cell junctions in general can be classified into three main functional divisions: (1) occluding junctions, (2) anchoring junctions, and (3) communicating junctions. Anchoring junctions can be subdivided into those with actin filament attachment sites (e.g., adherens junction in cell-cell interactions or focal adhesions in cell-matrix interactions) and those with intermediate filament attachment sites (e.g., desmosomes in cell-cell junctions and hemidesmosomes in cell-matrix junctions). The main form of communicating junction is the gap junction.

Gap junctions are specialized channels found between many different types of cells that permit the transfer of small molecules and ions from one cell to another. These protein complexes are especially prevalent in populations of cells that are electrically coupled, such as cardiac myocytes and smooth muscle. The flow of intracellular ions from cell to cell allows for coordinated contraction of the heart or visceral smooth muscles. Gap junctions also function in the transfer of second messengers from cell to cell, even in cells that are not electrically excitable. This communication prevents random fluctuations in response to extracellular signaling in a population of cells. Therefore, gap junctions allow a population of cells to maintain a coherent intracellular environment during signaling events.

Gap junctions are composed of integral membrane structures arranged in two halves, each found

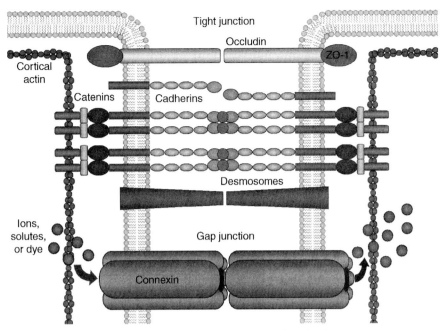

FIG. 1-5 Diagram illustrating the concept of gap junctions.

on two neighboring cells. These halves are called connexons, and each connexon is made up of six subunits of the protein connexin. Connexins are a diverse group of proteins with cell type-specific isoforms that, when mutated or missing, can cause specific disease entities. The mutation of connexin 32 in Schwann cells is the cause of the X-linked form of Charcot-Marie-Tooth disease, which is a peripheral neuromuscular disorder associated with severe wasting of distal extremities, especially peroneal muscle groups. Mutations of various connexins are also associated with cardiac abnormalities, heritable deafness, and dermatologic disorders.

One of the inherent dangers in the coupling of cells is the possibility that one cell could become damaged; allowing the neighboring cell's contents to spill into the extracellular space through the gap junction. To prevent this catastrophe, the gap junction changes its conformation and decreases the intracellular pore size in response to high levels of Ca^{2+}, which occurs during apoptotic signaling or cell death and normally remains at low levels intracellularly. Thus, flow of solutes through the gap junction decreases in response to high levels of Ca^{2+} ion (see Fig. 1-5).

Bibliography

Abrams CK, Oh S, Ri Y, et al. Mutations in connexin 32: the molecular and biophysical bases for the X-linked form of Charcot-Marie-Tooth disease. *Brain Res Brain Res Rev* 2000;32:203–214.

Carystinos GD, Bier A, Batist G. The role of connexin-mediated cell-cell communication in breast cancer metastasis. *J Mammary Gland Biol Neoplasia* 2001;6:431–440.

Garcia-Dorado D, Ruiz-Meana M, Padilla F, et al. Gap function-mediated intercellular communication in ischemic preconditioning. *Cardiovasc Res* 2002;55:456–465.

Kamholz J, Menichella D, Jani A, et al. Charcot-Marie-Tooth disease type 1: molecular pathogenesis to gene therapy. *Brain* 2000;123:222–233.

Lefebvre PP, Van De Water TR. Connexins, hearing, and deafness: clinical aspects of mutations in the connexin 25 gene. *Brain Res Brain Res Rev* 2000;32:159–162.

Nicholson SM, Ressot C, Gomes D, et al. Connexin 32 in the peripheral nervous system. Functional analysis of mutations associated with X-linked Charcot-Marie-Tooth syndrome and implications for the pathophysiology of the disease. *Ann N Y Acad Sci* 1999;883:168–185.

Omori Y, Zaidan-Dagli ML, Yamakage K, et al. Involvement of gap junctions in tumor suppression: analysis of genetically-manipulated mice. *Mutat Res* 2001;477:191–196.

Rabionet R, Lopez-Bigas N, Arbones ML, et al. Connexin mutations in hearing loss, dematological and neurological disorders. *Trends Mol Med* 2002;8:205–212.

Severs NJ. Gap junction remodeling and cardiac arrhythmogenesis: cause or coincidence? *J Cell Mol Med* 2001;5:355–366.

Shibata Y, Kumai M, Nishii K, et al. Diversity and molecular anatomy of gap junctions. *Med Electron Microsc* 2001;34:153–159.

12. **(D)** Epithelial cells can have apical cytoskeletal specializations such as cilia, stereocilia, or microvilli. Cilia are microtubule structures that function in motility using dynein ATPase to provide energy and are composed of the axoneme (i.e., a microtubule core of nine doublets circumferentially and two singlets centrally) attached at its base to a basal body (i.e., nine triplet microtubules circumferentially and none centrally). Cilia beat in waves to transport external materials in tissues such as the respiratory epithelium and oviducts.

Stereocilia are long, irregular microvilli composed of actin microfilaments, functioning in signal transduction in hair cells of the inner ear or absorptive function in epididymal cells. Microvilli are composed of actin microfilaments anchored to the terminal web (i.e., apical actin network that connects to the zonula adherens) and greatly increase the surface area of cells important for absorption. Microvilli form the brush border of renal proximal tubular cells and the striated border of intestinal epithelial cells. In the intestinal epithelium, the microvilli are also coated with a glycocalyx layer that aids in carbohydrate digestion and physical protection.

Bibliography

Bretscher A. Microfilament organization in the cytoskeleton of the intestinal brush border. *Cell Muscle Motil* 1983;4:239–268.

DeRosier DJ, Tilney LG. F-actin bundles are derivatives of microvilli: what does this tell us about how bundles might form? *J Cell Biol* 2000;148:1–6.

Hackney CM, Furness DN. Mechanotransduction in vertebrate hair cells: structure and function of the stereociliary bundle. *Am J Physiol* 1995;268:C1–C13.

Heintzelman MB, Mooseker MS. Assembly of the intestinal brush border cytoskeleton. *Curr Top Dev Biol* 1992; 26:93–122.

Lange K. Regulation of cell volume via microvillar ion channels. *J Cell Physiol* 2000;185:21–35.

Lange K, Gartzke J. Microvillar cell surface as a natural defense system against xenobiotics: a new interpretation of multidrug resistance. *Am J Physiol Cell Physiol* 2001;281:C369–C385.

Tilney LG, Tilney MS, DeRosier DJ. Actin filaments, stereocilia, and hair cells: how cells count and measure. *Annu Rev Cell Biol* 1992;8:257–274.

13. **(E)** Latrunculin and phalloidin do not act at the microtubules. Latrunculin, derived from a sea sponge, binds and stabilizes globular actin monomers to prevent actin polymerization. Phalloidin, derived from a poisonous mushroom, binds and stabilizes microfilaments of actin to result in excessive actin polymerization. Both latrunculin and phalloidin are highly poisonous to humans. The other drugs listed are microtubule-specific drugs. Paclitaxel (trade name, Taxol) is an alkaloid derived from the bark of the Pacific yew tree, and it binds and stabilizes microtubules to result in

excessive tubulin polymerization. Paclitaxel is sometimes used in the treatment of ovarian or breast cancer. Colchicine and colcemid are alkaloids derived from the autumn crocus, which bind and stabilize free tubulin subunits to prevent microtubule polymerization. Colchicine is used in the treatment of acute gout and pseudogout. Vinblastine and vincristine are vinka alkaloids extracted from the periwinkle plant, which also function to bind tubulin subunits and prevent their polymerization into microtubules, arresting mitotic cells in metaphase. Vinblastine is used in the treatment of various neoplastic diseases including Hodgkin's disease, choriocarcinoma, and various forms of leukemia. Vincristine does not demonstrate any cross-resistance with vinblastine and is able to penetrate the blood-brain barrier, making it a useful form of chemotherapy in neoplasms of the central nervous system as well as various forms of leukemia. Nocodazole also binds tubulin subunits and prevent microtubule polymerization. As a balance of microtubule assembly and disassembly are necessary for mitosis, drugs that cause the net polymerization of microtubules or the net depolymerization of microtubules both preferentially kill actively dividing cells.

Bibliography

Alberts B, Johnson A, Lewis K, et al. The cytoskeleton. In: Alberts B, Johnson A, Lewis K, et al. (eds.), *Molecular Biology of the Cell*, 4th ed. New York, NY: Garland Science, 2002, 952–960.

Hastie SB. Interactions of colchicine with tubulin. *Pharmacol Ther* 1991;51:377–401.

Jordan A, Hadfield JA, Lawrence NJ, et al. Tubulin as a target for anticancer drugs: agents which interact with the mitotic spindle. *Med Res Rev* 1998;18:259–296.

Kumar N. Taxol-induced polymerization of purified tubulin. Mechanism of action. *J Biol Chem* 1981;256;10435–10441.

Levy M, Spino M, Read SE. Colchicine: a state-of-the-art review. *Pharmacotherapy* 1991;11:196–211.

Luduena RF, Roach MC. Tubulin sulfhydryl groups as probes and targets for antimitotic and antimicrotubule agents. *Pharmacol Ther* 1991;49:133–152.

Rieder CL, Palazzo RE. Colcemid and the mitotic cycle. *J Cell Sci* 1992;102:387–392.

14. **(D)** Actin is a cytoskeletal filament and not a molecular motor protein; the rest are motor proteins. Molecular motor proteins are defined as proteins that bind to polarized cytoskeletal filaments (e.g., microtubules or actin) and use energy from ATP hydrolysis to move along the filament to generate molecular level movements such as those involved in muscle contraction, the transport of intracellular cargo, cell division, and ciliary motion. Most motor proteins are

associated with cytoskeletal filaments via a motor head domain, which binds and hydrolyzes ATP to undergo cycles of "walking" movements. For example, the myosin contraction cycle begins with the myosin head bound tightly to an actin filament in a *rigor* configuration (named for *rigor mortis*). The binding of an ATP molecule to the myosin head results in a conformational change that releases myosin from the actin filament. The hydrolysis of ATP occurs with an additional conformational change that cocks the myosin head to displace the head about 5 nm further toward the plus end of the actin filament. The force-generating power stroke is created by the weak binding of the myosin head to the new site on the actin filament associated with the release of inorganic phosphate from ATP hydrolysis then the strong binding of the myosin head to actin associated with the release of ADP. The motor head domain resumes its prior conformation rebound at a portion of the cytoskeletal filament a few nanometers away to repeat the cycle. Other motor proteins such as kinesin and dynein undergo similar walking cycles coupling nucleotide hydrolysis with conformational changes, utilizing two motor head domains that dimerize before alternately binding and unbinding cytoskeletal filaments.

Myosin was the first motor protein identified and was determined to be the skeletal muscle protein responsible for contraction. Myosin was later discovered to be present in nonmuscle cells and was found to function in different types of cell contraction in nonmuscle cells as well as in cytokinesis or cell division. This type of myosin consists of two heavy chains, each consisting of an N-terminal motor head domain and elongated C-terminal coiled-coil α-helical domain for dimerization; each heavy chain is associated with two different forms of light chains at its motor head region. This dimeric form of myosin was later renamed myosin II after the discovery of a monomeric form of myosin named myosin I in protozoa. Several additional monomeric and dimeric forms of myosin were later discovered and named myosin III through XVIII in order of discovery. There are about 40 myosin genes in humans with several structural classes being represented. Myosin is a conventional motor protein, using ATP hydrolysis to walk toward the plus ends of actin filaments; myosin VI is the only exception in that it moves toward the minus end.

Kinesin is a microtubule motor protein that belongs to the kinesin superfamily of kinesin-related proteins (KRPs). Kinesin contains an N-terminal motor domain, responsible for ATP-dependent transport toward the plus end of the microtubule, and a C-terminal coiled-coil domain responsible for dimerization and binding to cargo. The dimerization of kinesin allows the connection of two N-terminal "feet" that alternately bind and unbind to "walk" along the microtubule in an anterograde fashion.

The dyneins belong to a separate family of microtubule motors that mediate transport in the retrograde direction, toward the minus end of the microtubule. The *cytoplasmic dyneins* form homodimers with two motor domain heads and are responsible for vesicle trafficking and localization of the Golgi within the cell. The *axonemal dyneins* form heterodimers and heterotrimers responsible for the fast sliding movement of microtubules in the beating of cilia and flagella (see Fig. 1-6).

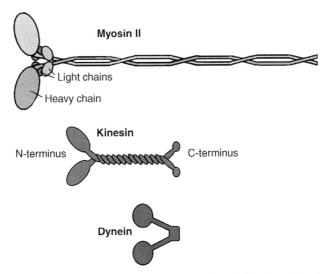

FIG. 1-6 Diagram demonstrating the structures of myosin, kinesin, and dynein.

Bibliography

Alberts B, Johnson A, Lewis K, et al. The cytoskeleton. In: Alberts B, Johnson A, Lewis K, et al. (eds.), *Molecular Biology of the Cell*, 4th ed. New York, NY: Garland Science, 2002, 952–960.

Hackney DD. The kinetic cycles of myosin, kinesin, and dynein. *Annu Rev Physiol* 1996;58:731–750.

Huitorel P. From cilia and flagella to intracellular motility and back again: a review of a few aspects of microtubule-based motility. *Biol Cell* 1988;63:249–258.

Schnapp BJ, Reese TS. Dynein is the motor for retrograde axonal transport of organelles. *Proc Natl Acad Sci USA* 1989;86:1548–1552.

Vale RD, Reese TS, Sheetz MP. Identification of a novel force-generating protein, kinesin, involved in micro-tubule-based motility. *Cell* 1985;42:39–50.

15. **(A)** Only the H band and I band shorten during contraction while the A band, Z line, and M line remain the same. In skeletal muscle, the myofibrils are organized into bundles that contain thick and thin filaments, which interdigitate to form sarcomeres. The striated pattern in skeletal muscle is the result of the regular repeating pattern of the longitudinal sarcomeres. Each sarcomere unit runs from one Z line (also called Z disk) to the next Z line, which is composed of connective tissue molecules such as α-actinin and serve to anchor the thin filaments. The thin filaments are composed of actin microfilaments (or F-actin) with tropomyosin and troponin, which run parallel to and interdigitate with the myosin thick filaments anchored at the Z lines by titin molecules. The M line is an imaginary line that hemisects each sarcomere. The H band is defined as the length of thick filaments that do not overlap with the thin filaments and is hemisected by the M line. The A band is the length of thick filament including the portions that overlap with thin filaments and is also hemisected by the M line. The I band is the length of thin filaments that do not overlap with thick filaments, is hemisected by the Z line, and traverses two sarcomere units.

During contraction of the myofibrils in response to action potentials, the depolarization of the muscle end plate at the neuromuscular junction causes an electrical potential to spread through the T tubules, transmitting the signal from the sarcomlemmal membrane to the sarcoplasmic reticulum (SR) in the cell's interior. The T tubules are invaginations of the cell membrane overlying the junctions of the A and I bands where terminal cisternae of the SR border on opposite sides of the T tubule invaginations to form a triad arrangement. The contact between the T tubules and SR allow for direct coupling of the voltage-sensitive dihydropyridine receptors on the T tubules with ryanodine receptor channels on the SR in a 4:1 ratio. Ca^{2+} is then released to the sarcomere through ryanodine receptor channels to result in excitation-contraction coupling. The released Ca^{2+} binds troponin C on the troponin complex and releases the inhibition on actomyosin interactions imposed by troponin I and tropomyosin. Troponin T, which binds the troponin complex to tropomyosin, changes conformation to allow the tropomyosin chains to shift away from the myosin binding sites on the actin microfilaments. The exposed myosin binding sites allow for the cross-bridge formation between the myosin heavy chains heads and actin filaments. The myosin heads use ATP hydrolysis to break and reform cross-bridges resulting in the sliding of the thick filament over the thin filament. The sliding movement continues until Ca^{2+} sequestration by the sarcoplasmic reticulum Ca^{2+}-ATPase (SERCA) pump back into the SR lowers cytosolic Ca^{2+} levels back to resting levels. The M and Z lines serve as anchors that attach the sarcomeres to fixed points on the cytoskeleton of the muscle cell. Since the overall length of the thick filament itself does not change during contraction, the length of the A band remains the same. The increasing overlap of the thick and thin filaments during contraction results in the shortening of the H and I bands.

Hypertrophic cardiomyopathy, central core disease, nemaline myopathy, and limb-girdle muscular dystrophy are examples of heritable disorders involving mutations in sarcomere proteins and disarrays in sarcomere structure (see Fig. 1-7).

Bibliography

Constanzo LS. Cell physiology. In: Constanzo LS (ed.), *Board Review Series: Physiology*, 2nd ed. Baltimore, MD: Williams & Wilkins, 1998, 18–23.

Cooke P. A periodic cytoskeletal lattice in striated muscle. *Cell Muscle Motil* 1985;6:287–313.

Goldstein MA, Schroeter JP, Michael LH. Role of the Z band in the mechanical properties of the heart. *FASEB J* 1991;5:2167–2174.

Labeit S, Kolmere B, Linke WA. The giant protein titin. Emerging roles in physiology and pathophysiology. *Circ Res* 1997;80:290–294.

Laing NG. Inherited disorders of contractile proteins in skeletal and cardiac muscle. *Curr Opin Neurol* 1995;8:391–396.

Schroder RR, Hofmann W, Menetret JF, et al. Cyro-electron microscopy of vitrified muscle samples. *Electron Microsc Rev* 1992;5:171–192.

16. **(E)** Signaling molecules bind to specific receptors to activate signal transduction pathways inside target cells, which are then modified and terminated by complex feedback and regulatory mechanisms. The signal can also be terminated by ligand degradation,

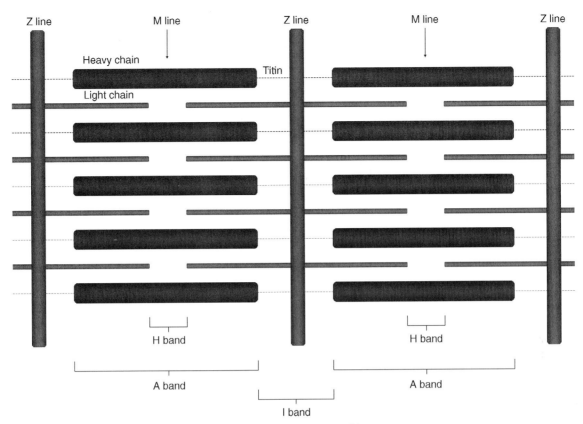

Z line   M line   Z line   M line   Z line

Heavy chain   Titin

Light chain

H band   H band

A band   A band

I band

FIG. 1-7   Diagram showing the structure of the sarcomere.

inactivation, or reuptake. Signal transduction is achieved by five general types of ligand-binding receptors: (1) ion channel-linked receptors, (2) G protein-linked receptors, (3) enzyme-linked receptors, (4) intracellular steroid hormone receptors, and (5) intracellular receptor guanylate cyclases. Signaling can also be accomplished without ligands in certain cases through direct voltage-gated or mechanical-gated ion channels.

Ion channel-linked receptors are multisubunit, single-pass transmembrane proteins that function by opening selective ion channels in response to ligand-binding and include most of the major neurotransmitter receptors (NTRs). These include both excitatory NTRs (i.e., glutamate receptor, nicotinic acetylcholine receptor (nAChR), and serotonin receptor) and inhibitory NTRs (i.e., $GABA_A$ receptor and glycine receptor). As an example, the nAChR contains two ACh binding sites and is composed of five subunits that form an ion channel permeable to many cations (e.g., Na^+, K^+, Ca^{2+}). On binding of two ACh molecules, nAChR undergoes a conformational change to open the channel gate, primarily allowing the rapid influx of Na^+ ions to depolarize the postsynaptic membrane. At the neuromuscular junction,

nAChR transmits the signal to contract from nerve cells to muscle cells. The glutamate NMDA receptor also forms an ion channel permeable to cations, but the NMDA receptor is blocked at resting membrane potential by extracellular Mg^{2+} ions. Both voltage-dependent membrane depolarization and glutamate binding are necessary to remove the Mg^{2+} plug and to open the channel gate, allowing the influx of Ca^{2+} ions important in long-term potentiation in the hippocampus. $GABA_A$ receptors are permeable to Cl^- ions, resulting in membrane hyperpolarization, and act as the major inhibitory NTR in the brain. Glycine receptors are also permeable to Cl^- ions and serve as the major inhibitory NTR in the spinal cord.

G protein-coupled receptors (GPCRs) traverse the cell membrane seven times and are linked to heterotrimeric GTP-binding proteins with α-, β-, and γ-subunits. There are several known G proteins, which include G_s, G_i, G_o, G_q, and $G_{12/13}$. Ligand-binding results in dissociation of heterotrimeric G protein subunits and activation of downstream signaling, usually through the adenylate cyclase (AC) or PLC pathway. On binding of ligand, the associated G protein exchanges its GDP for GTP to become activated and is inactivated when its GTPase activity hydrolyzes the bound GTP to GDP. Activation of G_s protein results in the dissociation of the α_s-subunit, which stimulates AC and increases cAMP levels. Cholera toxin ADP-ribosylates the α_s-subunit to block its GTPase activity and overactivates AC activity to cause high cAMP levels and oversecretion in intestinal epithelium. In contrast, activation of G_i protein results in the dissociation of the α_i-subunit, which inhibits AC and decreases cAMP levels. Pertussis toxin ADP-ribosylates the α_i-subunit to block its dissociation from the other subunits and prevents AC inhibition to cause high cAMP levels and oversecretion in respiratory epithelium. Activation of G_q protein results in stimulation of PLC, which cleaves PIP_2 into DAG and IP_3 to activate PKC and elevation of cytosolic Ca^{2+}. Multiple G protein subtypes can be activated by a single GPCR, causing the activation of multiple signal transduction pathways. A number of ligands activate GPCRs including the adrenergic receptors, dopamine receptors, $GABA_B$ receptor, PAR-1 thrombin receptor, purinergic receptors (e.g., A-type adenosine receptor, P-type ATP receptor), glucagon receptor, neuropeptide receptors (e.g., NPY, VIP, opiate, bradykinin, ADH, oxytocin), and pituitary hormone receptors (e.g., TSH, ACTH, LH).

Enzyme-linked receptors have extracellular domains that bind ligand and intracellular domains that serve as enzymes to activate intracellular signaling. Enzyme-linked receptors are subdivided into RTKs (e.g., insulin receptor and various growth factor receptors), tyrosine kinase-associated receptors (e.g., GH receptor, prolactin receptor, and many cytokine receptors), receptor serine-threonine kinases (e.g., TGF-β), receptor tyrosine phosphatases (e.g., CD45), and receptor guanylate cyclases (e.g., ANP receptor). RTKs oligomerize and autophosphorylate each other in response to binding oligomerized ligands. The phosphotyrosine residues interact with SH_2 domain-containing proteins, which activate son-of-sevenless (Sos) proteins, then Ras proteins, then Raf protein kinases, and finally the mitogen-activated protein kinase (MAPK) pathway to phosphorylate gene regulatory proteins (GRPs) in the nucleus. RTKs also activate the PLC-γ and PI3K pathways. Tyrosine kinase-associated receptors can phosphorylate other intracellular proteins such as Src to transduce its signal. Receptor serine-threonine kinases transmit their intracellular signal through the Smad pathway. Receptor tyrosine phosphatases dephosphorylate tyrosine residues in certain intracellular proteins to regulate their activities. Activation of receptor guanylate cyclases results in increased cGMP levels and activation of protein kinase G (PKG) to phosphorylate serine and threonine residues on certain intracellular proteins.

Intracellular steroid hormone receptors are distinctive in that their hydrophobic ligands can pass through the cell membrane to bind receptors in the cytosol and to induce nuclear translocation, activating the transcription of specific genes. Steroid hormone receptors are themselves GRPs that contain zinc finger motifs as their DNA-binding domains, which are composed of four cysteine residues bound to a zinc atom. Inactive steroid hormone receptors are complexed to the heat shock proteins Hsp90 and Hsp56 in the cytosol, which are released on binding of ligand to expose the DNA-binding region. The ligand-and-receptor complex translocates to the nucleus to activate the transcription of specific genes within 30 min, termed the primary response. The products of the primary response can then activate the transcription of other genes, termed the secondary response. Ligands for steroid hormone receptors include glucocorticoids, estrogen, progesterone, thyroid hormone, retinoic acid (vitamin A_1), and vitamin D_3.

Special intracellular receptor guanylate cyclases (aka soluble guanylyl cyclase or sGC) bind the unique gaseous ligand nitric oxide (NO) to activate cGMP production, PKG activation, and the phosphorylation of serine or threonine on intracellular proteins to activate signaling. NO is formed from arginine precursors by nitric oxide synthases (i.e., iNOS, eNOS, nNOS) with the half-life of NO being approximately 5 s. The gaseous nature of NO and its brief half-life mean that it only acts in a local fashion and is primarily regulated at the level of NOS activity. NO is an important neurotransmitter in the central and peripheral nervous systems, participates in the immune function of leukocytes, and causes blood vessel dilatation by smooth muscle relaxation. Many cardiovascular drugs for reducing blood pressure depend on the NO-cGMP pathway, including nitroglycerin and nitroprusside. Although originally studied as a drug for hypertension, sildenafil exploits the downstream portions of the NO-cGMP pathway in achieving penile erection by inhibiting PDE_5 (which normally breaks down cGMP in the corpus cavernosum) (see Fig. 1-8).

Bibliography

Anderson NG, Ahmad T. ErbB receptor tyrosine kinase inhibitors as therapeutic agents. *Front Biosci* 2002;7:1926–1940.

Bellamy TC, Garthwaite J. The receptor-like properties of nitric oxide-activated soluble guanylyl cyclase in intact cells. *Mol Cell Biochem* 2002;230:165–176.

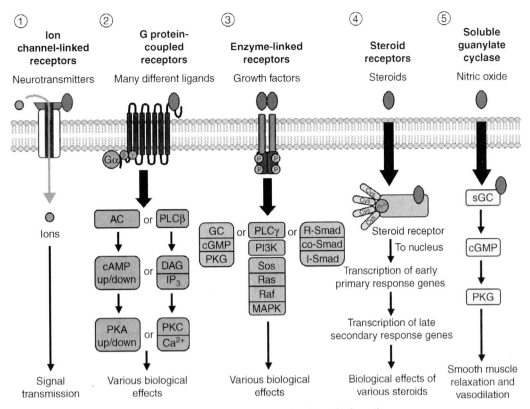

FIG. 1-8   Diagram illustrating general signal transduction pathways.

Brioni JD, Nakane M, Hsieh GC, et al. Activators of soluble guanylate cyclase for the treatment of male erectile dysfunction. *Int J Impot Res* 2002;14:8–14.

Chawla A, Repa JJ, Evans RM, et al. Nuclear receptors and lipid physiology: opening the X-files. *Science* 2001;294: 1866–1870.

Corbin JD, Francis SH, Webb DJ. Phosphodiesterase type 5 as a pharmacologic target in erectile dysfunction. *Urology* 2002;60:4–11.

Franklin WA, Veve R, Hirsch FR, et al. Epidermal growth factor receptor family in lung cancer and premalignancy. *Semin Oncol* 2002;29:3–14.

Gewaltig MT, Kojda G. Vasoprotection by nitric oxide: mechanisms and therapeutic potential. *Cardiovasc Res* 2002;55:250–260.

Hall RA, Lefkowitz RJ. Regulation of G-protein-coupled receptor signaling by scaffold proteins. *Circ Res* 2002;91:672–680.

Hanafy KA, Krumenacker JS, Murad F. NO, nitrotyrosine, and cycle GMP in signal transduction. *Med Sci Monit* 2001;7:801–819.

Hao D, Rowinsky EK. Inhibiting signal transduction: recent advances in the development of receptor tyrosine kinase and Ras inhibitors. *Cancer Invest* 2002;20:387–404.

Klabunde T, Hessler G. Drug design strategies for targeting G-protein-coupled receptors. *Chembiochem* 2002;3:928–944.

Steeg PS. Metastasis suppressors alter the signal transduction of cancer cells. *Nat Rev Cancer* 2003;3(1):55–63.

17. **(E)** RTKs activate several signaling molecules and three major signaling pathways. The primary ligands of RTKs are growth factors that stimulate cell division and proliferation. Therefore, it is no surprise that the signaling pathways listed are involved in cell proliferation and oncogenesis. The most proximal molecules phosphorylated by RTKs are the Src protein kinases, which contain *src* (Rous sarcoma virus) homology domains SH_2 or SH_3. Cytosolic signaling proteins that contain phosphotyrosine-binding (PTB) domains are also directly activated. The activation of the proximal signaling molecules secondary to RTK autophosphorylation then activates three major downstream signaling pathways: PLC, MAPK, and PI3K.

The PLC pathway involves the phosphorylation of PLC-γ, which hydrolyzes phosphatidylinositol-(4,5)-bisphosphate $[PI(4,5)P_2]$ into membrane-bound DAG and cytosolic inositol-(1,4,5)-trisphosphate $[Ins(1,4,5)P_3]$. DAG then activates various PKC isoforms, and $[Ins(1,4,5)P_3]$ stimulates the release of Ca^{2+} from intracellular stores, which is involved in various signaling functions including cell contraction and proliferation. Some PKC isoforms are activated by Ca^{2+}, thus resulting in downstream crosstalk between the two branches of the PLC pathway.

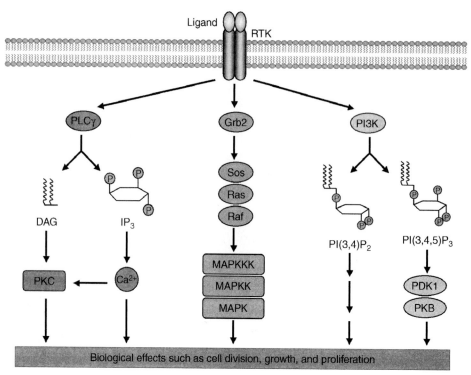

FIG. 1-9   Diagram illustrating the three main RTK pathways.

In the MAPK pathway, Grb2 serves as an adaptor protein containing SH_2 and SH_3 domains to interact directly with the RTK and with son-of-sevenless, which is a guanine nucleotide exchange factor (GEF) that goes on to activate Ras kinase. Ras activates Raf kinase, which then activates the downstream MAPK pathway. This involves the activation of MAP-kinase-kinase-kinase to phosphorylate MAP-kinase-kinase, which then phosphorylates MAP-kinase, which activates activated protein 1 (AP-1) (i.e., a heterodimer of Jun/Fos TFs) to translocate to the nucleus and enhance the transcription of growth-related genes.

Whereas the MAPK pathway is primarily mitogenic since its main function is to activate cell division, the PI3K pathway participates primarily in cell growth during active division to aid in cell survival and proliferation. PI3K phosphorylates phosphatidylinositol at the 3-position of the inositol ring to generate $PI(3,4)P_2$ and $PI(3,4,5)P_3$ products. Although the PI substrate is similar for PI3K and PLC, note that the products are different in that PLC cleaves $PI(4,5)P_2$ to form DAG and $[Ins(1,4,5)P_3]$. Intracellular proteins that have Pleckstrin homology (PH) domains interact with the $PI(3,4)P_2$ and $PI(3,4,5)P_3$ products of PI3K. Such proteins include PDK1 and protein kinase B (PKB, also known as

Akt), which are recruited to the plasma membrane to interact resulting in the phosphorylation of PKB by PDK1. Active PKB then dissociates to phosphorylate and inactivate BAD, resulting in the inhibition of apoptotic signaling. The PI3K downstream pathway for cell growth is complex and still poorly understood (see Figs. 1-9 and 1-10).

Bibliography

Alberts B, Johnson A, Lewis K, et al. Cell communication. In: Alberts B, Johnson A, Lewis K, et al. (eds.), *Molecular Biology of the Cell*, 4th ed. New York, NY: Garland Science, 2002, 882–884.

Andrechek ER, Muller WJ. Tyrosine kinase signalling in breast cancer: tyrosine kinase-mediated signal transduction in transgenic mouse models of human breast cancer. *Breast Cancer Res* 2000;2:211–216.

Avruch K, Khokhlatchev A, Kyriakis JM, et al. Ras activation of the Raf kinase: tyrosine kinase recruitment of the MAP kinase cascade. *Recent Prog Horm Res* 2001;56: 127–155.

Cantrell DA. Phosphoinositide 3-kinase signalling pathways. *J Cell Sci* 2001;114:1439–1445.

Dudek R. Cell biology. In: Dudek R (ed.), *High-yield Histology*, 2nd ed. Baltimore, MD: Lippincott, Williams & Wilkins, 2000, 8–9.

Hao D, Rowinsky EK. Inhibiting signal transduction: recent advances in the development of receptor tyrosine kinase and Ras inhibitors. *Cancer Invest* 2002;20:387–404.

centromeres as in mitosis, but homologous pairs can synapse. Crossover recombination occurs during prophase I making it possible for genetic variations. Metaphase I is characterized by each homologous pair of sister chromatids lining up in the middle of the cell. During anaphase I, each sister chromatid pair is pulled to opposite ends of the cell. Cytokinesis occurs during telophase I before the cell proceeds directly into meiosis II. The daughter cells at this stage are still diploid but become haploid by the end of meiosis II because no new DNA synthesis occurs. Meiosis II proceeds with prophase II then metaphase II, during which sister chromatid pairs align themselves along the equator of the cell. It is during anaphase II that centromeres are pulled apart and the sister chromatids separate to opposite poles of the cell. Telophase II is marked by nuclear reformation and results in four daughter cells containing half the number of original chromosomes.

Bibliography

Alberts B, Bray D, Johnson A, et al. Cell division. In: Alberts B, Bray D, Johnson A, et al. (eds.), *Essential Cell Biology*. New York, NY: Garland Publishing, 1998, 547–567.

Andersen SS, Wittmann T. Toward reconstitution of in vivo microtubule dynamics in vitro. *Bioessays* 2002;24(4):305–307.

Compton DA, Kapoor TM. Searching for the middle ground: mechanisms of chromosome alignment during mitosis. *J Cell Biol* 2002;157(4):551–556.

Griffiths AJF, Gelbart WM, Miller JH, et al. The inheritance of genes. In: Griffiths AJF, Gelbart WM, Miller JH, et al. (eds.), *Modern Genetic Analysis*. New York, NY: WH Freeman, 1999, 85–125.

Nasmyth K. Segregating sister genomes: the molecular biology of chromosome separation. *Science* 2002;297 (5581):559–565.

Stack SM, Anderson LK. A model for chromosome structure during the mitotic and meiotic cell cycles. *Chromosome Res* 2001;9(3):175–198.

Uhlmann F. Chromosome cohesion and segregation in mitosis and meiosis. *Curr Opin Cell Biol* 2001;13(6):754–761.

33.   (D) The cell cycle is subdivided into interphase and mitosis (M phase). Interphase consists of the G_0, G_1, and G_2 (gap) phases and the S phase between the G_1 and G_2 phases. The G_0 phase is a resting phase in which the cell cycle is suspended; many mature adult cells are in this phase, and this phase can last indefinitely. Organelle, RNA, and protein synthesis occurs during the G_1 phase (lasting for 5/16th of the cell cycle length) to prepare for cell division. This is followed by the G_1 checkpoint, at which progression of the cell cycle is regulated by cyclin-dependent kinase 2 (Cdk2). Cdk2-cyclin D and Cdk2-cyclin E are produced during G_1 to mediate the transition to the S phase. DNA replication occurs during the S phase (lasting for 7/16th of the cell cycle length) and doubles the number of chromosomes in the parent cell preparing the cell for division; centrosomes of the MTOC and histones also duplicate. ATP synthesis and Cdk1 production occur during the G_2 phase (lasting for 3/16th of the cell cycle length). Cdk1-cyclin A and Cdk1-cyclin B regulate the G_2 to M phase transition at the G_2 checkpoint.

The M phase is the shortest phase (lasting 1/16th of the cell cycle length) and is subdivided into prophase, metaphase, anaphase, and telophase. The MTOC consists of a centrosome complex that splits and moves to opposite poles of the cell during prophase. The mitotic spindle forms a network of microtubules between the centrosomes and connects to kinetochores on the centromeres of chromosome pairs. Chromosomes align at the central metaphase plate during metaphase, and the kinetochores separate to allow the split chromosome pairs to move to opposite poles during anaphase. The chromosomes decondense into chromatin as the nuclear envelopes and nucleoli reform at each pole during telophase. Cytokinesis occurs to divide the cytoplasmic contents at the cleavage furrow by the action of the contractile ring, composed of actin and myosin.

The M phase is very rapid in normal cells, and few cells can be caught in mitosis at any specific timepoint; however, cancer cells with altered cell cycles show increased frequency of mitosis and can often be seen in the M phase. Tumor suppressors such as p53 can arrest the cell cycle at the G_1 or G_2 checkpoints in cells with DNA damage by modulation of Cdk and cyclin production. The cells are suspended at the G_1 phase by p53 until DNA excision repair pathways can fix the damage. Apoptotic signaling can be activated in cells with irreparable DNA or organelle damage to prevent the uncontrolled proliferation of mutated or dysfunctional cells.

Bibliography

Danova M, Riccardi A, Mazzini G. Cell cycle-related proteins and flow cytometry. *Haematologica* 1990;75:252–264.

Dudek RW. The cell cycle. In: Dudek RW (ed.), *Hi-yield Cell and Molecular Biology*. Baltimore, MD: Lippincott, Williams & Wilkins, 1999, 80–84.

Funk JO. Cancer cell cycle control. *Anticancer Res* 1999;19:4772–4780.

Lacombe F, Belloc F. Flow cytometry study of cell cycle, apoptosis and drug resistance in acute leukemia. *Hematol Cell Ther* 1996;38:495–504.

Smith ML, Seo YR. p53 regulation of DNA excision repair pathways. *Mutagenesis* 2002;17:149–156.

The DNA excision repair process is used to correct DNA damage, which can be because of induced or spontaneous mutations unrelated to replication. DNA excision repair involves excision of the damaged sequence, synthesis of the proper sequence, and ligation. There are two major DNA excision repair pathways, base excision repair (BER) and nucleotide excision repair (NER). BER involves the removal of a single base and filling of the resulting nucleotide gap, whereas NER involves the removal of large portion of the nucleotide sequence followed by repair. The most common forms of DNA damage that occur are depurination of a single base, deamination of cytosine to uracil, or pyrimidine dimerization. Depurination involves the breaking of the *N*-glycosyl bond between the purine base and the deoxyribose sugar phosphate. The damaged purine is repaired by the BER pathway with excision by the AP endonuclease and a phosphodiesterase; DNA polymerase and ligase then restore the correct sequence. Deamination of cytosine occurs spontaneously about 100 times per day, and the conversion of C-G to U-A pairs would occur at replication in the absence of repair. Uracil-DNA glycosidase recognizes and removes the abnormal uracil in the DNA sequence, followed by repair through the BER pathway with AP endonuclease and a phosphodiesterase excising the remaining deoxyribose sugar phosphate. DNA polymerase and ligase restore the original sequence. Pyrimidine dimerization is caused by UV radiation, causing covalent linkage of neighboring pyrimidine bases, especially thymines. The uvrABC enzyme excises a 12-residue sequence that includes the pyrimidine dimer before DNA polymerase and ligase restore the correct sequence.

Genetic defects in DNA excision repair enzymes result in severe disorders that include xeroderma pigmentosum (XP), ataxia-telangiectasia (AT), Fanconi's anemia, and Bloom's syndrome. All are autosomal recessive in inheritance and result in high susceptibilities to cancers. XP results in UV radiation hypersensitivity with skin lesions, severe neurologic abnormalities, and high risk of skin malignancies causing early death. AT causes hypersensitivity to ionizing radiation with neurologic abnormalities, cerebellar ataxia, oculocutaneous telangiectasias, immunodeficiency, and susceptibility to lymphoid malignancies. Fanconi's anemia is characterized by hypersensitivity to DNA cross-linking agents with pancytopenia, bone marrow hypoplasia, and congenital anomalies. Bloom's syndrome causes hypersensitivity to many DNA-damaging agents and manifests in telangiectasia, immunodeficiency, growth retardation, and cancer predisposition.

Bibliography

Alberts B, Johnson A, Lewis K, et al. DNA replication, repair, and recombination. In: Alberts B, Johnson A, Lewis K, et al. (eds.), *Molecular Biology of the Cell*, 4th ed. New York, NY: Garland Science, 2002, 235–250.

Cotran RS, Kumar V, Collins T. Neoplasia. In: Cotran RS, Kumar V, Collins T (eds.), *Robbins Pathologic Basis of Disease*. Philadelphia, PA: W.B. Saunders, 1999, 295–296.

Dudek RW. Chromosome replication and DNA synthesis. In: Dudek RW (ed.), *Hi-yield Cell and Molecular Biology*. Baltimore, MD: Lippincott, Williams & Wilkins, 1999, 6–11.

Jacob S, Praz F. DNA mismatch repair defects: role in colorectal carcinogenesis. *Biochimie* 2002;84:27–47.

Marti TM, Kunz C, Fleck O. DNA mismatch repair and mutation avoidance pathways. *J Cell Physiol* 2002; 191:28–41.

32. (E) Some major differences between mitosis and meiosis are as follows: meiosis results in final daughter cells with half the number of chromosomes as the parent cell while mitosis results in cells with the same number of chromosomes, crossover recombination with synapsis of homologous alleles happen in meiosis but not in mitosis, and original parent cells undergo two rounds of cytokinesis in meiosis but only one round in mitosis. Although sister chromatid exchange may occur during mitosis, this only happens in chromosomes with abnormal fragility. Synthesis of new DNA technically does not occur during meiosis or mitosis (M phase of the cell cycle); DNA synthesis only occurs once during the S (synthesis) phase per each round of the cell cycle whether the cell undergoes meiosis or mitosis.

In brief, mitosis is generally subdivided into prophase, metaphase, anaphase, and telophase. Prophase is the first step, during which chromosomes become visible and the nucleoli disappear. Metaphase is characterized by nuclear spindle formation, which are protein fibers made of tubulin that run from the centrosomes of microtubule organizing centers (MTOC) at each pole of the cell. The chromosomes line up in the middle of the cell and two spindle fibers, each originating from opposite sides of the cell, attach to each chromosome pair. The chromatid pairs separate during anaphase, and the nuclear membrane reforms around each new daughter nucleus during telophase. Cytokinesis occurs to divide the cytoplasm into two separate compartments, forming two new daughter cells each having the same number of chromosomes as the original cell.

Meiosis is basically the same process as mitosis but has two rounds of divisions, meiosis I and meiosis II. In meiosis, sister chromatids are attached at the

Vermeulen L, De Wilde G, Notebaert S, et al. Regulation of the transcriptional activity of the nuclear factor-kappaB p65 subunit. *Biochem Pharmacol* 2002;64:963–970.

Zhang G, Ghosh S. Molecular mechanisms of NF-kappaB activation induced by bacterial lipopolysaccharide through Toll-like receptors. *J Endotoxin Res* 2000;6:453–457.

30. **(D)** The series of short tandem repeats at the end of the chromosomes described is a telomere sequence. Telomeres are repeating DNA sequences (TTAGGG in humans) that are bound by specialized protein complexes, which confer stability and provide a protective role to the ends of chromosomes. Without these sequences, human chromosomes undergo progressive degradation of their ends because of the nature of DNA replication (i.e., the *End Replication Problem* described in 1972 by James Watson). Protection is also provided from nuclease attack, end to end joining of the chromosomes, and recombination. Eventually because of chromosomal instability, the replicative potential of these cells become limited, and the cells undergo apoptosis or enter a state of cellular senescence in which cells are neither dividing nor dying.

Telomerase is a ribonucleoprotein enzyme that functions in elongating telomere sequences at the ends of chromosomes through DNA reverse transcriptase activity. Telomerase expression is absent in most normal somatic cells but is present in germ cells and most cancers. Telomerase activity is high in germ cells such as a spermatozoa that are consistently being renewed and nearly absent in somatic cells. High telomerase activity results in long TTAGGG repeats on the chromosome ends of spermatozoa and allows indefinite replication without chromosome shortening. Low telomerase activity in somatic cells is believed to contribute to the aging process as the chromosomes progressively shorten with each round of replication. High telomerase expression and activity is also associated with cancer cells as they are able to replicate continuously at abnormally high frequencies. It is believed that inhibiting telomerase in cancer cells could be a prospective form of antineoplastic therapy.

Bibliography

Bree RT, Stenson-Cox C, Grealy M, et al. Cellular longevity: role of apoptosis and replicative senescence. *Biogerontology* 2002;3:195–206.

Cong YS, Wright WE, Shay JW. Human telomerase and its regulation. *Microbiol Mol Biol Rev* 2002;66:407–425.

De Lange T. Activation of telomerase in a human tumor. *Proc Natl Acad Sci U S A* 1994;91:2882–2885.

Doyle LA, Highsmith WE. Telomerase as a diagnostic and therapeutic target for cancer. *Expert Rev Anticancer Ther* 2002;2:217–225.

Falchetti ML, Larocca LM, Pallini R. Telomerase in brain tumors. *Child Nerv Syst* 2002;18:112–117.

Li H, Liu JP. Signaling on telomerase: a master switch in cell aging and immortalization. *Biogerontology* 2002;3:107–116.

McCaul JA, Gordon KE, Clark LJ, et al. Telomerase inhibition and the future management of head-and-neck cancer. *Lancet Oncol* 2002;3:280–288.

Stewart SA, Hahn WC. Prospects for anti-neoplastic therapies based on telomere biology. *Curr Cancer Drug Targets* 2002;2:1–17.

Watson JD. Origin of concatemeric T7 DNA. *Nat New Biol* 1972;239(94):197–201.

31. **(A)** There are two major points at which DNA errors are repaired using two different repair processes: (1) DNA mismatch repair and (2) DNA excision repair. The DNA mismatch repair process corrects errors in DNA sequences that are produced during the replication process whereas DNA excision repair is used to correct errors because of direct DNA damage. Therefore, in DNA damage induced by UV light, the DNA excision repair proteins are activated rather than DNA mismatch repair proteins.

In DNA mismatch repair, DNA replication errors that occur during the action of DNA polymerase are initially corrected by the 3′-to-5′ proofreading exonucleolytic domain of the polymerase as it synthesizes new strands in the 5′-to-3′ direction. However, some mistakes escape this initial proofreading mechanism and are corrected by strand-directed DNA mismatch repair. New strands are initially marked with nicks that allow DNA mismatch repair proteins to recognize and correct any remaining errors. DNA mismatch repair proteins recognize and bind a mismatched base pair before activating degradation of the newly synthesized strand from the nearest nick back to the mismatch, and then the removed sequence is repolymerized.

Hereditary nonpolyposis colorectal cancer (HNPCC) is due to one inherited defective copy of any of four DNA mismatch repair genes (i.e., *hMSH2*, *hMLH1*, *hPMS1*, and *hPMS2*). Mutations can be detected by microsatellite instability, which is the term for widespread alterations in the thousands of dinucleotide repeat sequences normally present in the human genome. Although one normal copy of mismatch repair genes can provide sufficient repair activity, the normal copy is susceptible to inactivating somatic mutations. Defects in mismatch repair result in a 1000-fold increase of the frequency of replication errors, which results in increased risk of colon cancer (especially cecum and proximal colon) even without extensive polyp formation.

Bibliography

Adam SA. Transport pathways of macromolecules between the nucleus and the cytoplasm. *Curr Opin Cell Biol* 1999;11(3):402–406.

Alberts B, Bray D, Johnson A, et al. Proteins enter the nucleus through nuclear pores. In: Alberts B, Bray D, Johnson A, et al. (eds.), *Essential Cell Biology*. New York, NY: Garland Publishing, 1998, 455–457.

Corbett AH, Quimby BB. Nuclear transport mechanisms. *Cell Mol Life Sci* 2001;58(12–13):1766–1773.

Corbett AH, Silver PA. Nucleocytoplasmic transport of macromolecules. *Microbiol Mol Biol Rev* 1997;61(2):193–211.

Devlin TM. Channels and pores. In: Devlin TM (ed.), *Textbook of Biochemistry with Clinical Correlations*, 4th ed. New York, NY: Wiley-Liss, 1997, 201–204.

Macara IG. Transport into and out of the nucleus. *Microbiol Mol Biol Rev* 2001;65(4):570–594.

Ross MH, Romrell LJ, Kaye GI. Nuclear envelope. In: Ross MH, Romrell LJ, Kaye GI (eds.), *Histology: A Text and Atlas*, 3rd ed. Baltimore, MD: Williams & Wilkins, 1995, 48–49.

29. (D) Gene expression or regulation is determined at the transcriptional level by promoter and enhancer sequences. There are two main types of genes, which are regulated differently. Housekeeping genes are constitutively transcribed at a constant rate into housekeeping proteins necessary for common cellular function, such as metabolic enzymes and cytoskeletal components. Specialized genes are cell type-specific and are usually tightly regulated at the transcriptional level, such as inflammatory cytokines and glucocorticoids. Promoters commonly containing TATA box, CAAT box, or GC box sequences are usually located upstream of the regulated gene near the transcription initiation site. Promoters bind RNA polymerase II and TFs to form the transcription-initiation complex. Enhancer sequences or response elements are usually located far upstream or downstream from the gene of interest and bind GRPs to repress or activate the transcription-initiation complex.

The term *gene regulatory protein* generally applies to any protein that binds DNA regulatory enhancer sequences, activating or inhibiting transcription of selected sets of genes. The term *transcription factor* applies to any protein required to initiate or regulate transcription, including the TFs that bind to the initiation complex at the promoter site or GRPs that bind to distant enhancer sites. Often the two terms are used interchangeably. There are thousands of GRPs, many of which combine to form homodimers or heterodimers. Most TFs or GRPs contain common DNA-binding structural motifs such as the helix-turn-helix (e.g., Pit-1 homeodomain protein), helix-loop-helix (e.g., HLH homodimer), leucine zippers (e.g., Jun-Jun homodimer, Jun-Fos heterodimer or AP-1), and zinc fingers (e.g., glucocorticoid receptor, other steroid receptors). TFs or GRPs such as nuclear factor kappa-B (NF-κB) usually remain inactive in the cytosol complexed to inhibitor proteins. On stimulation, inhibitory proteins unbind to expose NLS and DNA-binding domains on GRPs to stimulate their translocation into the nucleus and modification of gene expression.

Proinflammatory cytokines, such as TNF-α and IL-1, bind their cell-surface receptors and activate normally latent NF-κB in the cytosol to stimulate the transcription of over 60 genes involved in the inflammatory response. Activation of TNF-α receptor involves trimerization and recruitment of adaptor proteins that activate IKK kinase (IKKK), which activates IκB kinase (IKK) to remove the inhibitory IκB from NF-κB. There are five major varieties of NF-κB proteins that form a variety of homodimers and heterodimers to activate specific sets of genes. NF-κB dimers remain complexed to the inhibitory protein IκB until a proinflammatory signal activates the phosphorylation of IκB by a serine/threonine kinase called IKK, which is followed by ubiquitylation and targeted degradation of IκB by the UPP pathway. A nuclear localization signal on NF-κB then becomes exposed, which allows NF-κB to translocate into the nucleus and stimulate the transcription of selected genes. Toll-like receptors (TLRs) mediate the innate immunity response to lipopolysaccharide (LPS) and also activate the NF-κB pathway through a number of intermediate signaling molecules.

Bibliography

Alberts B, Johnson A, Lewis K, et al. The cytoskeleton. In: Alberts B, Johnson A, Lewis K, et al. (eds.), *Molecular Biology of the Cell*, 4th ed. New York, NY: Garland Science, 2002, 952–960.

Bharti AC, Aggarwal BB. Nuclear factor-kappaB and cancer: its role in prevention and therapy. *Biochem Pharmacol* 2002;64:883–888.

Bowie A, O'Neill LA. The interleukin-1 receptor/Toll-like receptor superfamily: signal generators for pro-inflammatory interleukins and microbial products. *J Leukoc Biol* 2000;67:508–514.

Caamano J, Hunter CA. NF-kappaB family of transcription factors: central regulators of innate and adaptive immune function. *Clin Microbiol Rev* 2002;15:414–429.

Dudek RW. Control of gene expression. In: Dudek RW (ed.), *Hi-yield Cell and Molecular Biology*. Baltimore, MD: Lippincott, Williams & Wilkins, 1999, 36–41.

Klug A. Gene regulatory proteins and their interaction with DNA. *Ann N Y Acad Sci* 1995;758:143–160.

Richmond A. Nf-kappa B, chemokine gene transcription and tumour growth. *Nat Rev Immunol* 2002;2:664–674.

sequences will simply enter the ER lumen. Some proteins that contain multiple transmembrane sequences include ion channels and G protein-coupled receptors. Lipid vesicles, containing proteins from the rER, are shuttled to the *cis*-Golgi network, where they enter the Golgi apparatus. The Golgi modifies proteins it receives from the rER through addition and removal of sugar groups as well as phosphorylation and sulfation. The amino acid code of the protein will dictate its specific Golgi modifications. For example, lysosomal hydrolases are given a M6P group, which serves as a ligand for a Golgi receptor for M6P. This receptor binds these enzymes and carries them to lysosomes, where they are activated. In I-cell disease, this phosphorylation of mannose in the Golgi is defective, and these hydrolase enzymes cannot localize to lysosomes, so the lysosomal enzymes are mistakenly secreted by the cell.

Bibliography

Issa LL, Leong GM, Eisman JA. Molecular mechanism of vitamin D receptor action. *Inflamm Res* 1998;47:451–475.

Voeltz, GK, Rolls MM, Rapoport TA. Structural organization of the endoplasmic reticulum. *EMBO Rep* 2002;3:944–950.

Yang L, Guan T, Gerace L. Integral membrane proteins of the nuclear envelope are dispersed throughout the endoplasmic reticulum during mitosis. *J Cell Biol* 1997;137: 1199–1210.

27. **(A)** Regions of a cell's ER that lack ribosomes and have a less coarse appearance on electron microscopy are called sER. sER is not a major organelle in most cells, but is pronounced in other types of cells that carry out specific processes. Some of these processes include steroid hormone synthesis (in adrenal cortex cells and Leydig cells of the testes), detoxification (in hepatocytes), and calcium sequestration (in muscle). The sER (called sarcoplasmic reticulum in muscle cells) contains integral membrane proteins called sER Ca^{2+}-ATPase pumps that shuttle Ca^{2+} ions into the ER lumen from the cytosol. Thus, the sER also serves as a Ca^{2+} storage compartment that can be released during certain signaling cascades.

Bibliography

Issa LL, Leong GM, Eisman JA. Molecular mechanism of vitamin D receptor action. *Inflamm Res* 1998;47:451–475.

Voeltz, GK, Rolls MM, Rapoport TA. Structural organization of the endoplasmic reticulum. *EMBO Rep* 2002;3:944–950.

Yang L, Guan T, Gerace L. Integral membrane proteins of the nuclear envelope are dispersed throughout the endoplasmic reticulum during mitosis. *J Cell Biol* 1997;137: 1199–1210.

28. **(D)** Nuclear pore complexes are octagonal structures located throughout the nuclear envelope and are composed of over 50 different proteins called nucleoporins. The nuclear envelope has an outer membrane that is continuous with the ER membrane and the intermembranous space is continuous with the ER lumen. The outer and inner membranes of the nuclear envelope converge together to form the edges of the nuclear pore. Nuclear pores traverse the perinuclear cisterna, which is the space between the inner and outer nuclear membranes. The nuclear lamina is a network of intermediate filaments composed of lamin A, B, and C, which line the inner nuclear membrane and provide structure to the nuclear envelope.

The job of a nuclear pore is to regulate the bidirectional passage of particles between the cytoplasm and nucleus. Essential nuclear proteins (e.g., lamins and histones) are made in the ER or cytoplasm and need to be imported into the nucleus. RNA (e.g., mRNA, rRNA, tRNA) and ribosomal subunits assembled in the nucleus need to be exported to the ER or cytoplasm. Import and export of these macromolecules through the nuclear pores are regulated by GTP hydrolysis and nuclear receptors. The nuclear pore also acts as the last monitoring step in RNA control in the nucleus; incomplete or damaged RNA will have difficulties passing through a nuclear pore.

Some tiny particles such as ions and proteins less than ~60 kDa can pass through the nuclear pores by simple diffusion. The limiting factor for diffusion is the 9–10 nm functional diameter of the pore (although the actual physical pore diameter is about 70–80 nm). Larger particles depend on a receptor-mediated process driven by a GTP hydrolysis cycle involving Ran GTPases, which provides energy and directionality to nuclear transport. Large proteins destined for the nucleus must possess a NLS for import, and RNA molecules and assembled ribosomal subunits must possess a nuclear export signal in order to pass through the pores. The 4–8 amino acid sequence usually contains many positively charged lysine or arginine residues in nuclear import and many leucine and isoleucine residues in nuclear export. Also necessary are nuclear import and export receptors that assist in molecular movement through pores by continually shuttling between the nucleus and cytoplasm. Surprisingly, some tiny nuclear proteins (<10 nm diameter) have also been found to use receptor-mediated passage. It is believed that this method of movement is faster and more efficient than simple diffusion in many cases.

Hopwood JJ, Morris CP. The mucopolysaccharidoses. Diagnosis, molecular genetics and treatment. *Mol Biol Med* 1990;7:381–404.

Kachur E, Del Maestro R. Mucopolysaccharidoses and spinal cord compression: case report and review of the literature with implications of bone marrow transplantation. *Neurosurgery* 2000;47:223–228.

Kakkis ED. Enzyme replacement therapy for the mucopolysaccharide storage disorders. *Expert Opin Investig Drugs* 2002;11:675–685.

Kelly TE. The mucopolysaccharidoses and mucolipidoses. *Clin Orthop* 1976;114:116–133.

Schiffmann R, Brady RO. New prospects for the treatment of lysosomal storage diseases. *Drugs* 2002;62:733–742.

Sly WS, Vogler C. Brain-directed gene therpay for lysosomal storage disease: going well beyond the blood-brain barrier. *Proc Natl Acad Sci USA* 2002;99:5760–5762.

Wraith JE. The mucopolysaccharidoses: a clinical review and guide to management. *Arch Dis Child* 1995;72:263–267.

Wraith JE. Enzyme replacement therapy in mucopolysaccharidosis type I: progress and emerging difficulties. *J Inherit Metab Dis* 2001;24:245–250.

25. (E) The polypeptide described has the sequence KDEL at the end of its C-terminus when the amino acids are expressed in single letter code. The KDEL sequence acts as a signal that leads ultimately to the localization of a protein to the ER. There exists a KDEL receptor in the Golgi apparatus, which binds KDEL-tagged proteins. On binding of its ligand, the KDEL receptor complex undergoes a conformational change that leads to retrograde transport of the protein back to the ER. If the sequence was to be deleted or more amino acids were to be added to the C-terminus to extend the sequence, the protein would be secreted from the cell. Even though the protein does traverse the Golgi apparatus as part of its trafficking, localization in the Golgi is not its final fate. Polypeptides that are destined to become transmembrane proteins contain the sequence KKXX (di-lysine signal motif) at the C-terminus. Proteins destined for transport into the nucleus are involved in a different system from the ER-Golgi system of vesicular transport. These proteins contain nuclear localization signals (NLS) that are short basic amino acid sequences that do not show much conservation. The NLS is recognized by importin-α which is associated with importin-β and nuclear pores. Nuclear transport is an energy requiring process that is carried out by a monomeric GTPase called Ran.

Bibliography

Komeili A, O'Shea EK. New perspectives on nuclear transport. *Annu Rev Genet* 2001;35:341–364.

Pelham HR. Recycling of proteins between the endoplasmic reticulum and Golgi complex. *Curr Opin Cell Biol* 1991;3:585–591.

Pelham HR. The dynamic organisation of the secretory pathway. *Cell Struct Funct* 1996;21:413–419.

Teasdale RD, Jackson MR. Signal-mediated sorting of membrane proteins between the endoplasmic reticulum and the Golgi apparatus. *Annu Rev Cell Dev Biol* 1996;12:27–54.

26. (B) The Golgi works in conjunction with the ER for the production and processing of many proteins. The ER is a multifunctional contiguous intracellular membrane structure that encompasses many vital roles of the cell. The luminal compartment of the ER is a distinct cellular compartment that houses specific proteins and often a different chemo-osmotic milieu. One fluid membrane bilayer makes up at least three specific domains in the cell: the rER, the sER, and the outer nuclear envelope. Each domain has unique characteristics that are mainly determined by the proteins contained in each domain. During mitosis, these domains are lost and both daughter cells receive an equal portion of the ER. During interphase, the ER again subspecializes into its three domains as proteins become compartmentalized.

The rER has a granular appearance on electron micrographs because of the many ribosomes that are attached to the external portion of the membrane. These ribosomes contain a messenger RNA that is being actively transcribed into specific types of proteins found throughout the cell. Proteins translated in the rER include all transmembrane proteins, secreted proteins, and lysosomal enzymes; however, peroxisomal enzymes are imported from the cytosol directly into peroxisomes and are not synthesized in the rER. Only proteins translated in the rER can be shuttled to the Golgi for processing. Proteins to be translated in the rER contain a signal-recognition sequence of amino acids that is recognized during translation on a free ribosome by a protein called signal-recognition peptide (SRP). SRP halts cytosolic translation and brings the ribosome-mRNA complex to the rER, where there is a receptor for the SRP. The ribosome binds to a protein translocator pore on the external leaflet of the rER membrane, and translation is allowed to continue as the protein is fed through the pore into the ER lumen.

As proteins are fed into the ER, hydrophobic amino acid regions of the protein may remain embedded in the ER membrane. These will become membrane proteins and may localize to either the external plasma membrane or an intracellular organelle. Proteins that do not contain these membrane-spanning causes an accumulation of GM$_2$ ganglioside with death occurring before age 3, is associated with cherry-red spots on the maculae, and is especially prevalent in Ashkenazi Jews. Niemann-Pick disease is due to a deficiency in sphingomyelinase with accumulation of sphingomyelin in the RES, resulting in death before age 3. Cherry-red spots can also occur in Niemann-Pick although less frequently than in Tay-Sachs, which are because of lipid infiltration leading to the visualization of the red vascular choroids surrounded by white retinal edema. Metachromatic leukodystrophy is the deficiency of arylsulfatase A with accumulation of sulfatide in the brain, peripheral nerves, liver, and kidneys, resulting in spasticity and death before puberty. The minor sphingolipidoses include GM$_1$ gangliosidosis (resembling Tay-Sachs), Sandhoff's disease (resembling a rapid form of Tay-Sachs), and Farber's disease (a fatal accumulation of ceramide in joints and subcutaneous tissues).

Bibliography

Abe A, Wild SR, Lee WL, et al. Agents for the treatment of glycosphingolipid storage disorders. *Curr Drug Metab* 2001;2:331–338.

Barranger JA, O'Rourke E. Lessons learned from the development of enzyme therapy for Gaucher disease. *J Inherit Metab Dis* 2001;24(Suppl 2):89–96.

Champe PC, Harvey RA. Sphingolipidoses: an alternate fuel for cells. In: Champe PC, Harvey RA (eds.), *Lippincott's Illustrated Reviews: Biochemistry*, 2nd ed. Philadelphia, PA: JB Lippincott, 1994, 202–203.

Cox TM. Gaucher disease: understanding the molecular pathogenesis of sphingolipidoses. *J Inherit Metab Dis* 2001;24(Suppl 2):106–121.

Desnick RJ, Banikazemi M, Wasserstein M. Enzyme replacement therapy for Fabry disease in inherited nephropathy. *Clin Nephrol* 2002;57:1–8.

Desnick RJ, Kaback MM. Future perspectives for Tay-Sachs disease. *Adv Genet* 2001;44:349–356.

Devlin TM. Sphingolipids. In: Devlin TM (ed.), *Textbook of Biochemistry with Clinical Correlations*, 4th ed. New York, NY: Wiley-Liss, 1997, 420–431.

Siatskas C, Medin JA. Gene therapy for Fabry disease. *J Inherit Metab Dis* 2001;24(Suppl 2):25–41.

Wenstrup RJ, Roca-Espiau M, Weinreb NJ, et al. Skeletal aspects of Gaucher disease: a review. *Br J Radiol* 2002;75:A2–A12.

Zhao H, Grabowski GA. Gaucher disease: perspectives on a prototype lysosomal disease. *Cell Mol Life Sci* 2002;59:694–707.

24. **(B)** Lysosomal storage diseases are the result of a deficiency in one of many lysosomal enzymes and can be subdivided into five glycosaminoglycan (GAG) degradation disorders (aka MPSs), nine forms of sphingolipidoses, and I-cell disease. I-cell disease is the deficiency of phosphotransferase, resulting in the accumulation of mucopolysaccharide with aberrant secretion of all newly synthesized lysosomal proteins in the absence of mannose-6-phosphate (M6P) localizing signals.

MPSs occur because of enzyme deficiencies that affect mucopolysaccharide metabolism and usually involve neurons and the RES. The five major MPSs include Hurler's (type I MPS), Hunter's (type II MPS), Sanfilippo's (type III MPS), Scheie's (type V MPS), and Sly's syndrome (type VII MPS). All are autosomal recessive in inheritance except for Hunter's syndrome, which is X-linked recessive. Hurler's is a deficiency in α-L-iduronidase, resulting in the accumulation of heparan sulfate and dermatan sulfate. Corneal clouding and severe mental retardation are usually present along with skeletal abnormalities, cardiomegaly, and hepatosplenomegaly. Hunter's is iduronate sulfatase deficiency and is not as severe as Hurler's, demonstrating milder skeletal abnormalities and milder mental retardation. There is no corneal clouding in Hunter's, although deafness may be present. Sanfilippo's syndrome is a deficiency of heparan sulfamidase with an accumulation of heparan sulfate and results in severe mental retardation with mild hepatomegaly and skeletal abnormalities. Scheie's syndrome is also a form of α-L-iduronidase deficiency (like Hurler's) with corneal clouding, hand deformities, and aortic valve abnormalities, but mental retardation is absent. Sly's syndrome is the deficiency of β-glucuronidase, with accumulation of heparan sulfate and dermatan sulfate, resulting in physical deformity and hepatosplenomegaly.

The three minor MPSs include Morquio's syndrome (type IV MPS), Maroteaux-Lemy's syndrome (type VI MPS), and Di Ferrante's syndrome (type VIII MPS), which all present with the secretion of heparin, keratan, or dermatan sulfate in the urine and severe skeletal abnormalities similar to Sly's syndrome. A specific diagnosis and clinical assessment should be performed in MPSs to ensure an accurate prognosis because some of these disorders are compatible with near-normal life expectancy and intelligence. The number of various heritable disorders associated with deficiencies of various lysosomal enzymes demonstrates the abundance, diversity, and importance of lysosomal function.

Bibliography

Caillaud C, Poenaru L. Gene therapy in lysosomal diseases. *Biomed Pharmacother* 2000;54:505–512.

Diaz JH, Belani KG. Perioperative management of children with mucopolysaccharidoses. *Anesth Analg* 1993;77: 1261–1270.

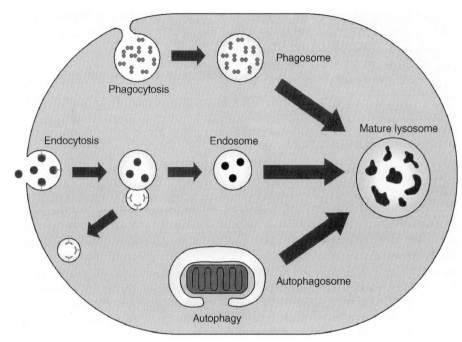

FIG. 1-13   Diagram illustrating lysosome formation.

Bibliography

Alberts B, Johnson A, Lewis K, et al. Intracellular compartments and protein sorting. In: Alberts B, Johnson A, Lewis K, et al. (eds.), *Molecular Biology of the Cell*, 4th ed. New York, NY: Garland Science, 2002, 658–746.

Brosius U, Gartner J. Cellular and molecular aspects of Zellweger syndrome and other peroxisome biogenesis disorders. *Cell Mol Life Sci* 2002;59:1058–1069.

Brunk UT, Terman A. The mitochondrial-lysosomal axis theory of aging: accumulation of damaged mitochondria as a result of imperfect autophagocytosis. *Eur J Biochem* 2002;269:1996–2002.

Dudek R. Cell biology. In: Dudek R (ed.), *High-yield Histology*, 2nd ed. Baltimore, MD: Lippincott, Williams & Wilkins, 2000, 2–6.

Hasilik A. The early and late processing of lysosomal enzymes: proteolysis and compartmentation. *Experientia* 1992;48:130–151.

Lazarow PB. The role of peroxisomes in mammalian cellular metabolism. *J Inherit Metab Dis* 1987;10(Suppl 1):11–22.

Moser HW. New approaches in peroxisomal disorders. *Dev Neurosci* 1987;9:1–18.

Pillay CS, Elliott E, Dennison C. Endolysosomal proteolysis and its regulation. *Biochem J* 2002;363:417–429.

23. (A) Lysosomal storage diseases are the result of a deficiency in one of many lysosomal enzymes and can be subdivided into nine forms of sphingolipidoses, five mucopolysaccharidoses (MPSs), and I-cell disease. It is also possible to include Pompe's disease (type II glycogen storage disease) as a lysosomal disorder.

Of the nine forms of sphingolipidoses, the six major forms are Fabry's, Krabbe's, Gaucher's, Tay-Sachs, Niemann-Pick, and metachromatic leukodystrophy. All are autosomal recessive in inheritance except for Fabry's disease, which is X-linked recessive. Fabry's disease occurs in 3 of 100,000 births, is because of a deficiency in α-galactosidase A, and causes an accumulation of ceramide trihexoside. Fabry's is characterized by renal and cardiac failure, cerebrovascular complications, severe pain in the lower extremities, and angiokeratomas.

Krabbe's is also known as globoid leukodystrophy, results in the deficiency of galactosylceramide β-galactosidase with galactocerebroside (aka galactosylceramide) accumulation in the brain, and leads to neurologic problems with early death. Gaucher's disease is the most common sphingolipidosis occurring in 166 of 100,000 births, is caused by the deficiency of β-glucocerebrosidase, and results in the accumulation of glucocerebroside in the brain and reticuloendothelial system (RES). Enlarged Gaucher's cells with a characteristic "crinkled tissue paper" appearance is pathognomonic, and the most common type I form does not affect lifespans. To give a relative idea of the frequency of occurrence, Down's syndrome has a prevalence of 125 in 100,000 births.

The next most common sphingolipidosis is Tay-Sachs, which occurs in 33 of 100,000 births. Tay-Sachs occurs because of a deficiency in hexosaminidase A,

34. (A) Proto-oncogenes encode proteins that normally stimulate the cell cycle, and tumor suppressor genes encode proteins that suppress the cell cycle. Oncogenes are mutated proto-oncogenes that are transcribed into oncoproteins, which alter the normal cell cycle, often causing cancer. Proto-oncogenes (e.g., *c-ras*) can become tumorigenic in four major ways: insertional mutagenesis by promoter or enhancer insertion, point mutation, chromosomal translocation, or gene amplification. By convention, proto-oncogenes and oncogenes are designated by three-letter abbreviations in italics with a prefix denoting its cellular or viral origin (e.g., *c-ras* and v-*ras*); the name of the protein product is not italicized and the first letter is capitalized (e.g., Ras). Tumor suppressor genes (e.g., *p53*, *Rb*, *BRCA-1*, *VHL*, *APC*, *DCC*, *NF-1*, *WT-1*) do not follow the same convention except that the gene is italicized and the protein is not, and their mutations result in a variety of familial cancer syndromes.

Oncogenes encode four different types of signaling products to accelerate the cell cycle: (1) growth factor mimics, (2) mutant growth factor receptors, (3) altered signal transducers, and (4) altered nuclear TFs. For instance, the *sis* oncogene is a mutated form of PDGF that acts as a growth factor mimic to stimulate the formation of astrocytomas and osteosarcomas. The *erb* and *neu* oncogenes are mutated EGF receptors with increased activity compared to the wild-type, resulting in various cancers, especially breast cancer. At the intracellular signal transduction level, the *ras* oncogene encodes a p21 protein, which functions like a G protein except that the mutated form binds GTP irreversibly because of loss of GTPase activity, resulting in continuous stimulation of the cell cycle. The *abl* proto-oncogene, named after a pediatrician named Abelson, also acts as an altered signal transducer when *abl* from chromosome 9 translocates to the major breakpoint cluster region *bcr* on chromosome 22. The t(9:22) translocation results in a fusion gene that encodes a constitutively-active Bcr-Abl hybrid called P210, which is an abnormal intracellular tyrosine kinase found in chronic myelocytic leukemia (CML). Again at the signal transduction level, some forms of follicular lymphoma have a translocation of the immunoglobulin (Ig) heavy chain locus on chromosome 14 to the *bcl-2* locus on chromosome 18, resulting in increased expression of Bcl-2 and inhibition of apoptosis. At the TF level in the nucleus, the *c-myc* proto-oncogene encodes a helix-loop-helixTF, which can be mutated into an overactive form. The *c-myc* proto-oncogene on chromosome 8 can also be translocated to the Ig heavy chain locus on chromosome 14 in some forms of Burkitt's lymphoma, resulting in Myc overexpression.

Also at the transcriptional level, mutations of *jun* or *fos* proto-oncogenes can result in overactive leucine zipper TFs in their homodimeric forms or their heterodimeric form, the latter of which is also called activated protein-1.

Tumor suppressor genes usually encode GRPs or regulators of GRPs, which either inhibit the gene expression of products that stimulate the cell cycle or activate the expression of products that suppress the cell cycle. Therefore, tumor suppressors generally act at the transcriptional level. For instance, *p53* encodes a zinc finger GRP that increases the production of inhibitors of Cdk2-cyclin D and Cdk2-cyclin E, arresting cells with damaged DNA at the G_1 phase of the cell cycle. The *p53* gene is named for the molecular weight of its protein product and is mutated in the majority of known cancers. In retinoblastoma, the Rb protein product binds and inhibits a GRP, preventing the expression of certain gene products that stimulate the cell cycle. Rb is the prototype for the Knudson two-hit hypothesis, which states that two separate mutagenic events are necessary to induce alterations on both *rb* chromosomes. In familial forms of retinoblastoma, one defective *rb* chromosome is inherited and only one somatic mutation is needed. In sporadic cases of retinoblastoma, two somatic mutations are required to produce loss-of-function in both gene copies.

Bibliography

Dudek RW. Proto-oncogenes, oncogenes, and anti-oncogenes. In: Dudek RW (ed.), *Hi-yield Cell and Molecular Biology*. Baltimore, MD: Lippincott, Williams & Wilkins, 1999, 73–79.

Holmila R, Fouquet C, Cadranel J, et al. Splice mutations in the p53 gene: case report and review of the literature. *Hum Mutat* 2003;21(1):101–102.

Jass JR. Pathogenesis of colorectal cancer. *Surg Clin North Am* 2002;82(5):891–904.

Masood S, Bui MM. Prognostic and predictive value of HER2/neu oncogene in breast cancer. *Microsc Res Tech* 2002;59(2):102–108.

Moynahan ME. The cancer connection: BRCA1 and BRCA2 tumor suppression in mice and humans. *Oncogene* 2002;21(58):8994–9007.

Robbins DH, Itzkowitz SH. The molecular and genetic basis of colon cancer. *Med Clin North Am* 2002;86(6): 1467–1495.

Schneider AS, Szanto PA. Neoplasia. In: Schneider AS, Szanto PA (eds.), *Board Review Series: Pathology*, 2nd ed. Baltimore, MD: Lippincott, Williams & Wilkins, 1993, 92–95.

35. (B) All of the above except for Fas receptor, which is involved in proapoptotic signaling, may have increased expression or activity in transformed cells.

Telomerase activity allows for stabilization and prevention of degradation of chromosomal ends through continual cycles of replication of a cell, and high levels of telomerase expression have been shown in a wide variety of human tumors. The c-*myc* gene is termed an immediate-early gene encoding for a TF that can rapidly cause continual growth and replication of the cell on its overexpression. Such an example can be seen with Burkitt's lymphoma, where a translocation between the Ig heavy chain locus on chromosome 14 and the c-*myc* gene on chromosome 8 leads to high levels of Myc protein expression. Ras, a monomeric G protein, commonly acts as an oncogene when point mutations occur which lower its GTPase activity. Thus, Ras being left in a constant "on" state leads to upregulation of signal transduction pathways causing increased expression of growth factors and tumor induction. Ras mutations can be seen in such cancers as pancreatic adenocarcinoma and cholangiocarcinoma. The gene for *bcl-2* encodes an antiapoptotic factor, in which increased levels of Bcl-2 dimers in a cell favors cellular survival. B-cell lymphomas are examples of malignancies in which translocation of the *bcl-2* gene on chromosome 18 with the Ig heavy chain locus on chromosome 14 causes overexpression of the Bcl-2 protein, promoting cellular survival and growth of indolent tumors.

Bibliography

Cotran RS, Kumar V, Collins T. Cellular pathology I: cell injury and cell death. In: Cotran RS, Kumar V, Collins T (eds.), *Robbins Pathologic Basis of Disease*, 6th ed. Philadelphia, PA: W.B. Saunders, 1999, 19–25.

Hamad NM, Elconin JH, Karnoub AE, et al. Distinct requirements for Ras oncogenesis in human versus mouse cells. *Genes Dev* 2002;16(16):2045–2057.

Hoffman B, Amanullah A, Shafarenko M, et al. The proto-oncogene c-myc in hematopoietic development and leukemogenesis. *Oncogene* 2002;21(21):3414–3421.

Maser RS, DePinho RA. Connecting chromosomes, crisis, and cancer. *Science* 2002;297(5581):565–569.

Selim AG, El-Ayat G, Wells CA. Expression of c-erbB2, p53, Bcl-2, Bax, c-myc and Ki-67 in apocrine metaplasia and apocrine change within sclerosing adenosis of the breast. *Virchows Arch* 2002;441:449–455.

Vousden KH. Switching from life to death: the Miz-ing link between Myc and p53. *Cancer Cell* 2002;2:351–352.

Wajant H. The Fas signaling pathway: more than a paradigm. *Science* 2002;296(5573):1635–1636.

36. (B) Apoptosis, also known as programmed cell death, is the regulated suicide of a cell in response to damage or stress in the absence of inflammation or involvement of neighboring cells. The function of apoptosis is to efficiently remove one's own cells that are unnecessary or may be a threat to overall health. The two main apoptotic pathways are the extrinsic pathway initiated by an extracellular ligand and the intrinsic pathway initiated by intracellular events. In both pathways, there are four main phases of apoptic progression: (1) the initial signal, (2) the control phase, (3) the execution phase, and (4) the removal of dead cell debris.

The initial signal can be triggered by various mechanisms such as decreased survival stimuli (e.g., decreased hormones, growth factors, or cytokines), receptor-ligand interactions (e.g., tumor necrosis factor receptor, Fas death receptor), or specific injurious agents (e.g., heat, radiation, or hypoxia). The control phase can involve the regulation of Fas receptor-Fas ligand signaling for targeted cell death by killer lymphocytes in the extrinsic pathway or can involve regulation of cytochrome *c* release by the Bcl-2 family in the intrinsic pathway.

The extrinsic pathway of apoptosis involves the production of Fas ligand by killer lymphocytes and the activation of Fas receptor. The activated Fas death receptor clusters and recruits adaptor proteins to activate procaspase-8 to initiate the caspase cascade and targeted cell death by cytotoxic T-lymphocytes. The intrinsic pathway of apoptosis involves the release of cytochrome *c* from mitochondria to bind to the adaptor protein Apaf-1, which activates procaspase-9 to trigger the caspase cascade and cell death.

In the intrinsic pathway, apoptotic signals increase the permeability of mitochondria by forming pores and stimulate the release of cytochrome *c* from the mitochondria. Especially at this step, the Bcl-2 family of intracellular proteins can promote or hinder the apoptotic process. Bcl-2 itself and Bcl-X_L are members of the Bcl-2 family that inhibit the apoptotic pathway partly by preventing the release of cytochrome *c*, while Bax and Bak are members that promote apoptosis by stimulating the release of cytochrome *c*. Bad is a member that also functions in promoting apoptosis by binding and inactivating inhibitory members of the Bcl-2 family.

The execution phase of apoptosis is regulated by caspases, which are involved in an amplifying intracellular proteolytic cascade to transmit the death signal throughout the cell. Caspases normally exist as inactive procaspases in the cytosol, which may be activated by adaptor proteins recruited by the initiating signal. The activation of a small number of initiator caspases leads to an amplifying cascade as each initiator caspase cleaves more procaspases, which in turn cleave other procaspases. Some activated caspases can eventually cleave downstream signaling proteins and are known as effector caspases.

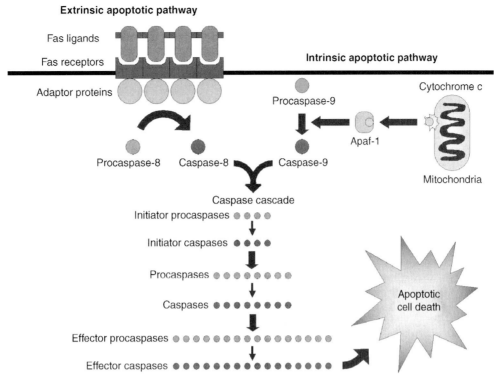

Extrinsic apoptotic pathway

Fas ligands

Fas receptors

Intrinsic apoptotic pathway

Adaptor proteins

Cytochrome c

Procaspase-9

Apaf-1

Procaspase-8   Caspase-8   Caspase-9

Mitochondria

Caspase cascade

Initiator procaspases

Initiator caspases

Procaspases

Caspases

Apoptotic
cell death

Effector procaspases

Effector caspases

FIG. 1-14   Diagram depicting the extrinsic and intrinsic apoptotic signaling pathways.

Members of the inhibitor of apoptosis (IAP) family can regulate the caspase cascade by binding to specific procaspases to prevent their activation and to caspases to inhibit their activity.

The final step in apoptosis is the removal of dead cellular debris by phagocytes. This process is fast, complete, and does not leave any signs of inflammation (see Fig. 1-14).

Bibliography

Adams JM, Cory S. The Bcl 2 family: regulators of the cellular life-or-death switch. *Nat Rev Cancer* 2002;2(9): 647–656.

Aigner T. Apoptosis, necrosis, or whatever: how to find out what really happens? *J Pathol* 2002;198(1):1–4.

Alberts B, Bray D, Johnson A, et al. Programmed cell death is mediated by an intracellular proteolytic cascade. In: Alberts B, Bray D, Johnson A, et al. (eds.), *Essential Cell Biology*. New York, NY: Garland Publishing, 1998, 585–587.

Belka C, Budach W. Anti-apoptotic Bcl-2 proteins; structure function and relevance for radiation biology. *Int J Radiat Biol* 2002;78(8):643–658.

Bree RT, Stenson-Cox C, Grealy M, et al. Cellular longevity: role of apoptosis and replicative senescence. *Biogerontology* 2002;3(4):195–206.

Cotran RS, Kumar V, Collins, T. Apoptosis. In: Cotran RS, Kumar V, Collins T (eds.), *Pathologic Basis of Disease*, 6th ed. Philadelphia, PA: W.B. Saunders, 1999, 18–25.

Fadok VA, Geske FJ, Monks J, et al. The role of the macrophage in apoptosis: hunter, gatherer, and regulator. *Int J Hematol* 2002;76(1):16–26.

Griffiths AJF, Gelbart WM, Miller JH, et al. Controlling the cell proliferation and death machinery. In: Griffiths AJF, Gelbart WM, Miller JH, et al. (eds.), *Modern Genetic Analysis*. New York, NY: WH Freeman, 1999, 472–478.

Schneider AS, Szanto PA. Apoptosis. In: Schneider AS, Szanto PA (eds.), *Board Review Series: Pathology*, 2nd ed. Baltimore, MD: Lippincott, Williams & Wilkins, 2002, 7–9.

37. **(C)** A cell produces many types of proteins that are constantly being turned over in the microenvironment of the cell. Proteins can become damaged, may disassemble from multipeptide complexes, or be misfolded because of inherent errors in ribosomal translation. Quality control of protein components is important to all cells, and there are many mechanisms by which a cell may dispose of proteins that are no longer functional.

The major way by which a cell is able to dispose of damaged proteins is through the UPP pathway, which is the major nonlysosomal pathway for the breakdown of proteins. The pathway is initiated by the ATP-dependent activation of ubiquitin by the ubiquitin-activating enzyme (E1). Ubiquitin is a

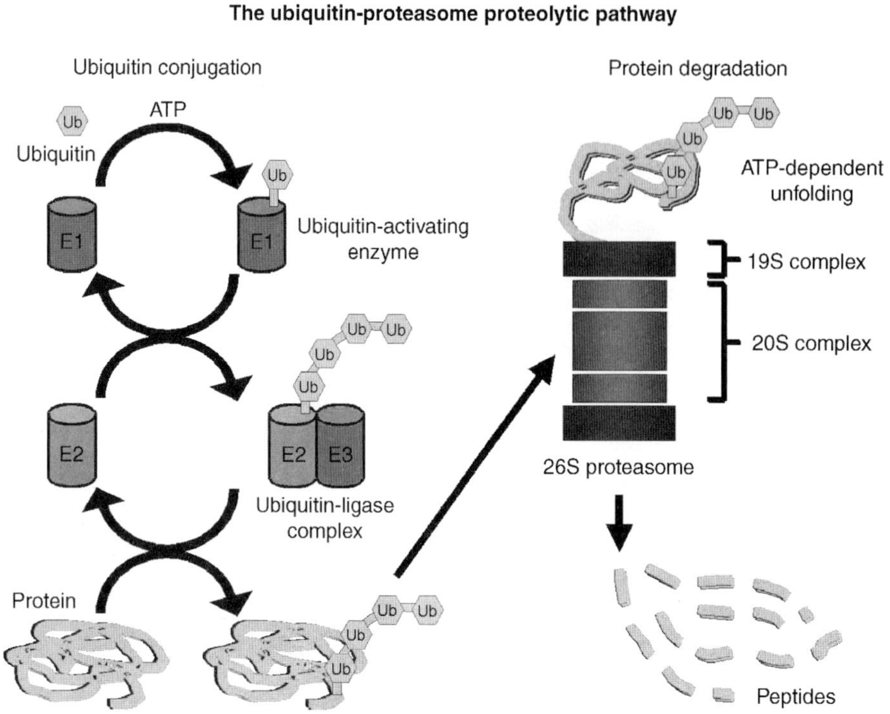

The ubiquitin-proteasome proteolytic pathway

FIG. 1-15   Diagram illustrating the ubiquitin-proteasome proteolytic pathway.

small polypeptide that can be covalently bonded to targeted proteins through special conjugating enzymes. E1 links to ubiquitin and transfers activated ubiquitin to the ubiquitin-conjugating enzyme (E2). Through the repeated action of E1, multiple ubiquitins become linked to the E2 enzyme to form a multiubiquitin chain. E2 can then transfer the multiubiquitin chain to targeted proteins at lysine residues, a process termed polyubiquitination or polyubiquitylation. This process requires the formation of ubiquitin-ligase complex (E2-E3), with accessory proteins (E3) that bind specific degradation signals in protein substrates. There are at least 30 different E2 enzymes and at least 100 different E3 enzymes, which target proteins through the nature of their N-terminal amino acids (N-end rule). The multiubiquitylated protein is specifically targeted for degradation by the 26S proteasome. The 26S proteasome is composed of 19S regulatory caps on both ends that selectively bind ubiquitylated proteins, unfolding and feeding them in an ATP-dependent manner into the barrel-shaped 20S catalytic core for cleavage into short peptides. Upregulation of gene expression or activity of the UPP pathway has been associated with muscle cachexia and trauma. The UPP system may also play a role in MHC class I antigen processing and in apoptosis.

Other important protein degradation pathways exist in the cell, notably in the rER and in lysosomal compartments. The rER is responsible for degrading misfolded or misassembled proteins that originate in the ER, not the cytoplasm. Lysosomal protein degradation occurs mainly through autophagy of senescent organelles, and does not involve farnesylation. Proteins with a KFERQ(lys-phe-glu-arg-gln) signal peptide may become attached to senescent organelles destined for degradation through lysosomes. The inability to eliminate misfolded proteins results in intracellular aggregates that interfere with the normal functioning of the cell, resulting in various pathologies (see Fig. 1-15).

Bibliography

Blaise R, Masdehors P, Lauge A, et al. Chromosomal DNA and p53 stability, ubiquitin system and apoptosis in B-CLL lymphocytes. *Leuk Lymphoma* 2001;42:1173–1180.

Bucciantini M, Giannoni E, Chiti F, et al. Inherent toxicity of aggregates implies a common mechanism for protein misfolding diseases. *Nature* 2002;416:507–511.

Garcia-Echeverria C. Recent advances in the identification and development of 20S proteasome inhibitors. *Mini Rev Med Chem* 2002;2:247–259.

Glickman MK, Ciechanover A. The ubiquitin-proteasome proteolytic pathway: destruction for the sake of construction. *Physiol Rev* 2002;82:373–428.

Goldberg AL, Cascio P, Saric T, et al. The importance of the proteasome and subsequent proteolytic steps in the generation of antigenic peptides. *Mol Immunol* 2002;39:147–164.

Jesenberger V, Jentsch S. Deadly encounter: ubiquitin meets apoptosis. *Nat Rev Mol Cell Biol* 2002;3:112–121.

Naujokat C, Hoffmann S. Role and function of the 26S proteasome in proliferation and apoptosis. *Lab Invest* 2002;82:965–980.

Sijts A, Zaiss D, Kloetzel PM. The role of the ubiquitin-proteasome pathway in MHC class I antigen processing: implications for vaccine design. *Curr Mol Med* 2001;1:665–676.

Wickner S, Maurizi MR, Gottesman S. Posttranslational quality control: folding, refolding, and degrading proteins. *Science* 1999;286:1888–1893.

38. **(E)** HSP, which tend to be activated by high temperatures or other stresses, are chaperone proteins that mainly function to aid the proper folding and unfolding of proteins inside the cell. HSP do not affect the rate of protein synthesis, but aid proteins in reaching their complex conformations during and after synthesis. HSP are also involved in refolding proteins after they cross the membranes of certain organelles such as the ER or mitochondria. HSP perform other cytoprotective functions such as correcting misfolded proteins, preventing protein aggregation, facilitating the degradation of unstable proteins, and aiding the translocation of proteins across membranes. The protective nature of HSP is especially necessary in stressful situations such as recovery from light-induced damage to the retina and ischemia-reperfusion injury to various organs. HSP synthesis is increased dramatically in the liver after resuscitation involving cardiac shock.

The HSP chaperones include the Hsp70 and chaperonin families. Both are significant contributors to protein folding during normal and adverse conditions. One of the important functions of the Hsp70 family in adverse conditions is thermotolerance. This is an organism's ability to become resistant to heat stress after a sublethal heat exposure. The cell can also develop tolerance for other stresses such as hypoxia, ischemia, acidosis, energy depletion, cytokines, and UV radiation. This heat tolerance will usually develop after a few hours and last approximately 3–5 days. Hsp70 chaperones promote the proper folding of proteins by blocking hydrophobic peptide segments around non-native polypeptides. In contrast, chaperonins enclose proteins within a central cavity to enhance efficient folding of certain proteins by shielding them from their local environments.

Bibliography

Benjamin IJ, Christians ES, Yan LJ. Heat shock factor 1 and heat shock proteins: critical partners in protection against acute cell injury. *Crit Care Med* 2002;30:43–50.

Devlin TM. Steroid hormone receptors. In: Devlin TM (ed.), *Textbook of Biochemistry with Clinical Correlations*, 4th ed. New York, NY: Wiley-Liss, 1997, 909–914.

Edwards M, Grantham J, Oosterum MV, et al. The role of heat shock proteins in mammalian differentiation and development. *Environ Med* 1999;43(2):79–87.

Hartl FU, Hayer-Hartl M. Molecular chaperones in the cytosol: from nascent chain to folded protein. *Science* 2002;295(5561):1852–1858.

Hartl FU, Naylor DJ. Contribution of molecular chaperones to protein folding in the cytoplasm of prokaryotic and eukaryotic cells. *Biochem Soc Symp* 2001;68:45–68.

Kregel KC. Heat shock proteins: modifying factors in physiological stress responses and acquired thermotolerance. *J Appl Physiol* 2002;92(5):2177–2186.

Srivastava P. Interaction of heat shock proteins with peptides and antigen presenting cells: chaperoning of the innate and adaptive immune responses. *Annu Rev Immunol* 2002;20:395–425.

39. **(E)** Although mitochondria are capable of synthesizing some of their own proteins since they contain their own DNA (of maternal inheritance) and ribosomes, they import most of their proteins, which are encoded by nuclear DNA. Mitochondrial precursor proteins (MCPPs) do not fold into their native conformation until after they are imported into the mitochondria. Immediately after synthesis, MCPPs remain unfolded by interacting with cytosolic chaperone proteins such as members of the cytosolic Hsp70 family. The MCPPs bind to import receptor proteins of the TOM complex by virtue of their mitochondrial signal sequences, which are fed first into the translocation channel with dissociation of cytosolic chaperone proteins by ATP hydrolysis. The 18-amino acid signal sequence on the N-terminus of a MCPP is recognized by the receptor portion of the TOM complex for import and are cleaved by signal peptidases in the mitochondrial matrix following translocation.

Translocation across the mitochondrial membranes is accomplished by the concerted action of the translocases of the outer and inner mitochondrial membranes (TOM and TIM, respectively). The TOM complex can import all nucleus-encoded mitochondrial proteins from the cytosol into the intermembrane space and can also insert transmembrane proteins into the outer mitochondrial proteins. The coupled action of the TIM23 complex completes the transport of proteins from the intermembrane space into the mitochondrial matrix and can insert transmembrane proteins into the inner mitochondrial proteins. Unlike the

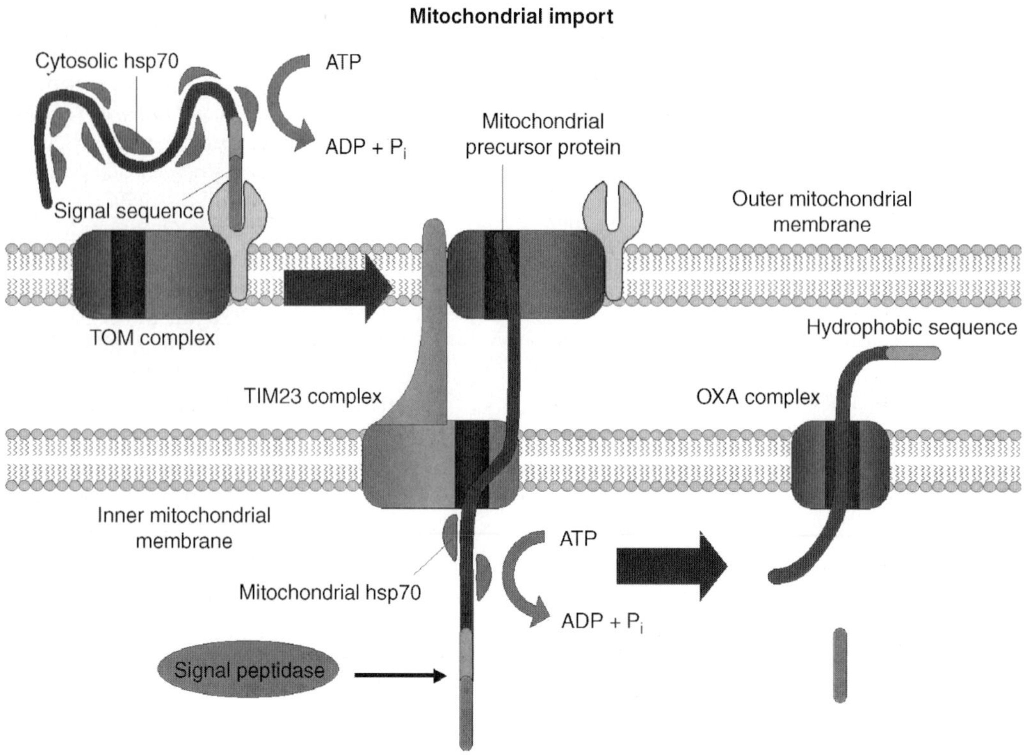

Mitochondrial import

FIG. 1-16   Diagram illustrating import of mitochondrial precursor proteins.

TIM23 complex, which spans both mitochondrial membranes and can physically couple to the TOM complex, the TIM22 complex only spans the inner mitochondrial membrane and is necessary for inserting a subset of inner mitochondrial membranes into the membrane.

Mitochondrial Hsp70 binds to polypeptide sequences of MCPPs as they emerge from the TIM23 complex to help pull MCPPs into the matrix. The mitochondrial Hsp70 chaperone proteins are released by ATP hydrolysis to allow the mitochondrial proteins to fold into their proper three-dimensional conformations. Other chaperone proteins such as mitochondrial Hsp60 may help some MCPPs fold by binding and unbinding different conformations through repeated cycles of ATP hydrolysis.

MCPPs that are designated for the intermembrane space have a second hydrophobic signal sequence following the N-terminal signal sequence. This can act as a stop-transfer sequence, preventing translocation into the matrix by the TIM23 complex. An alternate pathway taken by some MCPPs is initially the same as matrix proteins by translocation through TOM and TIM23. But after the cleavage of the N-terminal signal sequence by matrix signal peptidase, the hydrophobic sequence acts as the new signal sequence to translocate back across the inner mitochondrial membrane through OXA complexes. The OXA complex can also insert mitochondrion-encoded mitochondrial proteins into the inner membrane. MCPPs designated for the intermembrane space rather than the inner membrane have their hydrophobic sequences cleaved by proteases in the intermembrane space.

Mitochondrial diseases show maternal inheritance patterns and tend to affect tissues that constantly require high levels of ATP such as nervous tissue, eyes, heart muscle, and skeletal muscle (see Fig. 1-16).

Bibliography

Alberts B, Johnson A, Lewis K, et al. Intracellular compartments and protein sorting. In: Alberts B, Johnson A, Lewis K, et al. (eds.), *Molecular Biology of the Cell*, 4th ed. New York, NY: Garland Science, 2002, 678–684.

Bauer MF, Neupert W. Import of proteins into mitochondria: a novel pathomechanism for progressive neurodegeneration. *J Inherit Metab Dis* 2001;24(2):166–180.

Koehler CM. Protein translocation pathways of the mitochondrion. *FEBS Lett* 2000;476(1–2):27–31.

Lithgow T. Targeting of proteins to mitochondria. *FEBS Lett* 2000;476(1–2):22–26.

Rehling P, Wiedemann N, Pfanner N, et al. The mitochondrial import machinery for preproteins. *Crit Rev Biochem Mol Biol* 2001;36(3):291–336.

40. (D) Hexokinase is found in all cells and performs the first step of glycolysis. Glucokinase can also perform the first step of glycolysis but has a low affinity for glucose substrate and is predominantly found in the liver. Only hexokinase is inhibited by its glucose-6-phosphate product because the role of glucokinase is to provide a high capacity system to rapidly breakdown glucose when excess exists.

Problems with cellular metabolic pathways such as glycolysis, glycogenolysis, gluconeogenesis, glycogen storage, protein metabolism, and fatty acid oxidation can be the result of organ dysfunction or rare inherited metabolic disorders. Defects in protein metabolism can specifically be the result of liver or kidney failure as well as inherited enzyme deficiencies such as in phenylketonuria. When there are nutritional problems in specific pathways, the timing of the signs and symptoms may hint at the biochemical pathways affected. For instance, if a catabolic process such as glycolysis or β-oxidation were deficient, the patient would have neuromuscular symptoms unrelated to meals. If the defect was in glycogen storage, the patient could present with hepatomegaly and problems maintaining blood glucose levels for the first 8 h postprandial. Gluconeogenesis abnormalities result in a drop in blood glucose between 8 and 30 h postprandial.

Highly active tissues such as the brain, eyes, liver, muscles, RBCs, and kidneys need a continuous supply of glucose in order to survive. The brain, liver, and RBCs do not need insulin for glucose transport and utilization, whereas muscles and adipocytes have insulin-dependent glucose transporters inhibited by fasting. This serves to provide glucose to the most essential cells necessary for survival during periods of prolonged fasting. The breakdown of liver and muscle glycogen via glycogenolysis can supply the entire body for an average of 8 h (sometimes up to 18 h) without any carbohydrate intake. The Cori cycle cooperates with glycogenolysis as the glucose from glycogenolysis in the muscles is converted into lactate during muscular activity. The lactate is transported through the circulation to the liver where it is converted into pyruvate and glycogen with the use of ATP. The pyruvate is converted into glucose to be transported back to the muscles through the circulation along with the glucose from glycogenolysis in the liver. After the glycogen stores are exhausted, the body relies on gluconeogenesis in the liver to provide glucose fuel from different substrates such as lactate, pyruvate, α-ketoacids, glycerol, and acetyl-CoA.

When gluconeogenesis occurs in the liver to provide glucose fuel for other organs, glycolysis is inhibited in the liver but not in other organs. Although a low level of gluconeogenesis can occur in the kidney and intestinal epithelia, the liver is the primary center for gluconeogenesis. Since the glycogen stores are exhausted, proteins and fats are primarily used as substrates to convert into glucose. One significant supply of pyruvate substrate for gluconeogenesis is the breakdown of branched chain amino acids (BCAAs) in muscles, which include leucine, isoleucine, and valine. Lactate, glutamine, and alanine can be transported to the liver from muscles to serve as substrates for gluconeogenesis. Glycerol and acetyl-CoA are derived from fatty acid breakdown to be converted into pyruvate for gluconeogenesis.

In extremely prolonged starvation, ketogenesis in the liver converts fatty acids and amino acids into acetoacetate. Acetoacetate is then reduced into β-hydroxybutyrate (β-HB) by the enzyme β-HB dehydrogenase, with the utilization of NADH. Some of the acetoacetate is spontaneously converted into acetone instead, which is responsible for the fruity breath odor in diabetic ketoacidosis (DKA). Ketone bodies can be used by the brain, heart muscle, and skeletal muscle in the absence of glucose or free fatty acids. The urine ketone test only detects acetoacetate and acetone in ketoacidosis, which can be misleading because the β-HB product is favored by high redox states that produce an excess of NADH (see Fig. 1-17).

Bibliography

Brosnan JT. Comments on metabolic needs for glucose and the role of gluconeogenesis. *Eur J Clin Nutr* 1999;53:107–111.

Champe PC, Harvey RA. Gluconeogenesis. In: Champe PC, Harvey RA (eds.), *Lippincott's Illustrated Reviews: Biochemistry*, 2nd ed. Philadelphia, PA: JB Lippincott, 1994, 99–104.

Corssmit EP, Romijn JA, Sauerwein HP. Regulation of glucose production with special attention to nonclassical regulatory mechanisms: a review. *Metabolism* 2001;50(7):742–755.

Devlin TM. Gluconeogenesis. In: Devlin TM (ed.), *Textbook of Biochemistry with Clinical Correlations*, 4th ed. New York, NY: Wiley-Liss, 1997, 200–312.

Foster JD, Nordlie RC, Lange AJ. Regulation of glucose production by the liver. *Annu Rev Nutr* 1999;19:379–406.

Pye S, Radziuk J. Hepatic glucose uptake, gluconeogenesis and the regulation of glycogen synthesis. *Diabetes Metab Res Rev* 2001;17(4):250–272.

41. (E) Glycogen storage disease or glycogenosis is the result of defects in one or more enzymes involved in the synthesis or degradation of glycogen. Most often, the tissues that are affected by these abnormalities are the liver, heart, and muscle. The types of disorders

Starvation with depleted glycogen

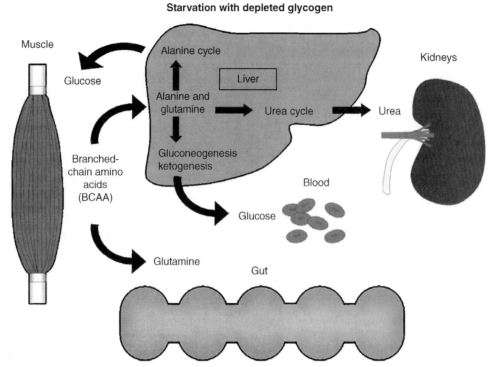

FIG. 1-17   Gluconeogenesis and ketogenesis are activated in the liver in response to glycogen depletion and prolonged starvation.

are broken down into 12 subcategories based on the enzyme deficiency, but only types I through VIII will be briefly discussed.

Type I GSD (Von Gierke's) is caused by a deficiency in the enzyme glucose-6-phosphatase. Glycogen accumulates in the liver and kidneys, enlarging these organs, and severe hypoglycemia with growth retardation is observed. No glucose can be released from the liver; instead glucose-6-phosphate becomes a substrate for hepatic glycolysis and lactic acid production as occur in the muscles. This leads to the severe lactic acidemia often seen in these patients. Glycolysis and the pentose phosphate pathway (a.k.a. hexose monophosphate pathway) also increases phosphorylated intermediate compounds and inhibits the rephosphorylation of adenine nucleotides. This activates nucleic acid degradation into uric acid, causing hyperuricemia and gout. The hypoglycemia that results from this disorder stimulates epinephrine. This in turn activates lipoprotein lipase and free fatty acid movement to the liver for triglyceride synthesis; however, malonyl-CoA inhibits the fatty acids from entering the mitochondria and the β-oxidation of fatty acids to support the hypoglycemia does not occur.

Type II GSD (Pompe's) is caused by a deficiency of α-1,4-glucosidase, which is usually found in lysosomes and can also be classified as a lysosomal enzyme disorder. Without this enzyme, there is a build up of glycogen in almost all tissues, and the heart is especially affected, resulting in early death.

Type III GSD (Cori's) is caused by a deficiency of the glycogen debranching enzyme, α-1,6-glucosidase. Only the outer branches of glycogen can be degraded by glycogen phosphorylase, resulting in the accumulation of glycogen with many short branches. Clinically, Cori's disease can resemble Von Gierke's but is usually less severe since gluconeogenesis is unaffected. The growth retardation is controllable with frequent ingestion of glucose sources to prevent hypoglycemia.

Type IV GSD (Andersen's) is due to the deficiency of glucosyl α-4,6-transferase, resulting in the accumulation of glycogen with few long branches in the liver and spleen. Although infants may appear normal at birth, Andersen's disease results in early death, usually before age two.

Type V GSD (McArdle's) is caused by a deficiency in muscle glycogen phosphorylase, which is involved in removing 1,4-glucosyl groups to release glucose-1-phosphate. Although not lethal, the inability to breakdown muscle glycogen leads to painful cramps and myoglobinuria with strenuous exercise. Muscle enzymes such as creatine kinase and aldolase may also be elevated in these patients.

Type VI GSD (Hers') is because of the deficiency of liver glycogen phosphorylase, which is the rate-limiting enzyme of glycogenolysis, resulting in glycogen accumulation in hepatocytes and leukocytes. Type VII GSD is the deficiency of phosphofructokinase in muscle and blood cells, resulting in muscle cramps and myoglobinuria on extreme exertion; the clinical picture resembles the muscle specificity of McArdle's disease. Type VIII GSD is the deficiency of phosphorylase kinase in the liver, which resembles Hers' disease.

Bibliography

Andreu AL, Bruno C, Dimaur S, et al. Myophosphorylase deficiency (glycogenosis type V; McArdle disease). *Curr Mol Med* 2002;2(2):189–196.

Burchell A. Glycogen storage diseases and the liver. *Baillieres Clin Gastroenterol* 1998;12(2):337–354.

Byrne BJ, Plotz P, Raben N. Acid alpha-glucosidase deficiency (glycogenosis type II, Pompe disease). *Curr Mol Med* 2002;2(2):145–166.

Champe PC, Harvey RA. Glycogen storage diseases. In: Champe PC, Harvey RA (eds.), *Lippincott's Illustrated Reviews: Biochemistry*, 2nd ed. Philadelphia, PA: JB Lippincott, 1994, 236–239.

Chen YT, Chou JY, Mansfield BC, et al. Type I glycogen storage diseases: disorders of the glucose-6-phosphatase complex. *Curr Mol Med* 2002;2(2):121–143.

Chou JY. The molecular basis of type 1 glycogen storage diseases. *Curr Mol Med* 2001;1(1):25–44.

Devlin TM. Degradation of glycogen. In: Devlin TM (ed.), *Textbook of Biochemistry with Clinical Correlations*, 4th ed. New York, NY: Wiley-Liss, 1997, 139–141.

Janecke AR, Mayatepek E, Utermann G. Molecular genetics of type 1 glycogen storage disease. *Mol Genet Metab* 2001;73(2):117–125.

42. **(E)** For the most part, the gluconeogenesis pathway is just the reversal of glycolysis; however, there are three key steps in glycolysis that cannot be reversed and must be bypassed by four steps that are unique to gluconeogenesis. The first step that must be circumvented in gluconeogenesis is the irreversible conversion of phosphoenolpyruvate to pyruvate in glycolysis by the pyruvate kinase enzyme. In order to prevent both the forward glycolysis reaction and reverse gluconeogenesis reaction from occurring simultaneously in a futile cycle, liver pyruvate kinase is inactivated by protein kinase A-dependent phosphorylation during prolonged fasting. The lack of upstream F-1,6-BP reactant or the presence of excess ATP or alanine products also inhibit pyruvate kinase activity. Only the liver performs gluconeogenesis with the inhibition of glycolysis, and the other tissues such as the brain or RBCs continue glycolysis utilizing the glucose supplied by the liver reactions.

The gluconeogenesis reaction at first step involves the carboxylation of pyruvate to form oxaloacetate or oxaloacetic acid (OAA) in liver mitochondria by pyruvate carboxylase with CO_2, biotin, Mg^{2+}, Mn^{2+}, and ATP. OAA is then reduced to malate because OAA is unable to cross the mitochondrial membrane to the cytosol. Once in the cytosol, malate is then converted back into OAA. OAA is then converted to PEP by PEPCK, using the energy of GTP hydrolysis. Pyruvate carboxylase is activated by the presence of acetyl-CoA from fatty acid breakdown, amino acid breakdown, or lactate metabolism.

The second step that must be bypassed in glycolysis is the irreversible rate-limiting reaction of phosphofructokinase-1 (PFK-1), which is activated by AMP or insulin-stimulated fructose-2,6-bisphosphate formation (by PFK-2) and inhibited by ATP or citrate. PFK-1 converts fructose-6-phosphate (F6P) into F-1,6-BP. The circumventing gluconeogenesis reaction at this step is performed by F-1,6-BPase in liver cytosol, which hydrolyzes F-1,6-BP into F6P. The third step that must be bypassed is the hexokinase reaction (glucokinase in liver) of glycolysis. To form free glucose molecules, glucose-6-phosphate is hydrolyzed by glucose-6-phosphatase in the liver cytosol.

Bibliography

Brosnan JT. Comments on metabolic needs for glucose and the role of gluconeogenesis. *Eur J Clin Nutr* 1999;53:107–111.

Champe PC, Harvey RA. Gluconeogenesis. In: Champe PC, Harvey RA (eds.), *Lippincott's Illustrated Reviews: Biochemistry*, 2nd ed. Philadelphia, PA: JB Lippincott, 1994, 99–104.

Corssmit EP, Romijn JA, Sauerwein HP. Review article: regulation of glucose production with special attention to nonclassical regulatory mechanisms: a review. *Metabolism* 2001;50(7):742–755.

Devlin TM. Gluconeogenesis. In: Devlin TM (ed.), *Textbook of Biochemistry with Clinical Correlations*, 4th ed. New York, NY: Wiley-Liss, 1997, 200–312.

Foster JD, Nordlie RC, Lange AJ. Regulation of glucose production by the liver. *Annu Rev Nutr* 1999;19:379–406.

Pye S, Radziuk J. Hepatic glucose uptake, gluconeogenesis and the regulation of glycogen synthesis. *Diabetes Metab Res Rev* 2001;17(4):250–272.

43. **(C)** Both cholesterol synthesis and ketogenesis occur in the liver mitochondria. Ketogenesis is the process by which the liver can take acetyl-CoA and produce ketone bodies for use by extrahepatic tissues such as brain, cardiac muscle, skeletal muscle, and renal cortex when glucose is unavailable. The compounds that are considered ketone bodies include acetoacetate, acetone, and β-hydroxybutyrate. The common steps of

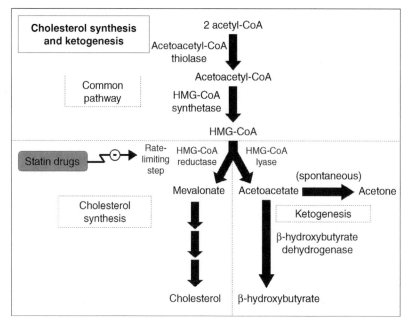

FIG. 1-18   Diagram showing cholesterol synthesis and ketogenesis.

cholesterol synthesis and ketogenesis begin with the conversion of two acetyl-CoA molecules into one ace-toacetyl-CoA molecule by the enzyme acetoacetyl-CoA thiolase. Acetoacetyl-CoA is then converted by HMG-CoA synthase into HMG-CoA, which is the branching point where cholesterol synthesis and keto-genesis diverge. In cholesterol synthesis, the rate-limiting step is the conversion of HMG-CoA to mevalonate by HMG-CoA reductase, which is inhib-ited by statin drugs. In ketogenesis, HMG-CoA is cleaved into acetoacetate by HMG-CoA lyase. Some of the acetoacetate is reduced to β-hydroxybutyrate by the enzyme β-hydroxybutyrate dehydrogenase. This reaction is dependent on the NADH/NAD⁺ ratio. Some of the acetoacetate can also undergo sponta-neous decarboxylation to acetone, but the amount of acetone produced is normally very small.

Under normal conditions, the body does not need significant ketogenesis; however, in times of severe starvation the amount of ketone body forma-tion increases drastically. This allows organs such as the heart and the skeletal muscles to conserve glu-cose in order to provide the central nervous system with enough fuel. As the process is prolonged, the higher levels of acetoacetate and β-hydroxybutyrate in the blood result in the additional utilization of ketone bodies by the brain. DKA is a condition marked by low insulin, excess glucagon, and excess ketone bodies. The overabundance of ketone bodies in this condition is the result of dysfunctional glucose transport in muscles and adipocytes, which are

insulin-dependent. The increased glucagon/insulin ratio additionally stimulates fatty acid oxidation and ketone body production. In normal starvation ketosis, insulin is present to antagonize the breakdown of fatty acids, but there is no mechanism in DKA to halt this process, leading to significant ketosis and dan-gerous acidosis (see Fig. 1-18).

Bibliography

Bruyette DS. Diabetic ketoacidosis. *Semin Vet Med Surg* 1997;12(4):239–247.

Champe PC, Harvey RA. Ketone bodies: an alternate fuel for cells. In: Champe PC, Harvey RA (eds.), *Lippincott's Illustrated Reviews: Biochemistry*, 2nd ed. Philadelphia, PA: JB Lippincott, 1994, 187–188.

Devlin TM. Methods of interorgan transport of fatty acids and their primary products. In: Devlin TM (ed.), *Textbook of Biochemistry with Clinical Correlations*, 4th ed. New York, NY: Wiley-Liss, 1997, 378–391.

Gerber PP, Keller U, Lustenberger M, et al. Human ketone body production and utilization studied using tracer techniques: regulation by free fatty acids, insulin, cate-cholamines, and thyroid hormones. *Diabetes Metab Rev* 1989;5(3):285–298.

Hanas R, Rosenbloom AL. Diabetic ketoacidosis (DKA): treatment guidelines. *Clin Pediatr (Phila)* 1996;35(5):261–266.

Scharrer E. Control of food intake by fatty acid oxidation and ketogenesis. *Nutrition* 1999;15(9):704–714.

44. (B) The urea cycle is a series of biochemical reactions performed by the liver to rid nitrogenous wastes from the body and accounts for about 90% of the nitrogen

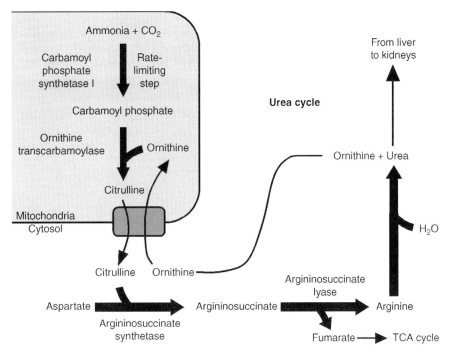

FIG. 1-19 Diagram depicting reactions of the urea cycle.

in urine. Urea is produced within the liver and is carried through the blood to the kidneys where it is excreted. Dysfunction of the liver or kidneys can result in the accumulation of ammonia or urea and its metabolites, resulting in uremia and metabolic encephalopathy. The first nitrogen of urea is derived from ammonia while the second nitrogen is from aspartate; both are products of protein metabolism. Transaminases or aminotransferases, glutamate dehydrogenase, and argininosuccinate synthetase are the enzymes responsible for supplying the nitrogen from ammonia and aspartate. Ammonia is the result of glutamate breakdown since most amino acids undergo transamination reactions linked with α-ketoglutarate. Aspartate is derived from oxaloacetate via a transamination reaction linked with glutamate.

The urea cycle begins with carbamoyl phosphate synthetase I utilizing ATP and *N*-acetylglutamate to convert ammonia and CO_2 (or bicarbonate) to carbamoyl phosphate. This reaction occurs in the mitochondrial matrix of hepatocytes and is considered to be the rate-limiting step. Carbamoyl phosphate synthetase I in the mitochondria should not be confused with carbamoyl phosphate synthetase II in the cytosol, which is responsible for catalyzing the first step in pyrimidine synthesis. The second step of the urea cycle also occurs in the mitochondrial matrix and involves the combination of carbamoyl phosphate

and ornithine into citrulline by ornithine transcarbamoylase. Citrulline is transported from the mitochondria to the cytosol (by the citrulline-ornithine exchange transporter) where it is combined with aspartate by the ATP-dependent argininosuccinate synthetase enzyme to form argininosuccinate. Argininosuccinate is then broken down into fumarate and arginine by argininosuccinate lyase. Fumarate is recycled into energy by the TCA cycle (aka citric acid or Krebs cycle), whereas arginine is hydrolyzed into urea and ornithine. The urea molecule is excreted in the urine, and the ornithine molecule is recycled to the urea cycle at the second step. Recycled ornithine is able to efficiently enter the mitochondrial matrix via the citrulline-ornithine exchange transporter, which also serves to transport citrulline out to the cytosol after the second step of the urea cycle (see Fig. 1-19).

Bibliography

Champe PC, Harvey RA. Urea cycle. In: Champe PC, Harvey RA (eds.), *Lippincott's Illustrated Reviews: Biochemistry*, 2nd ed. Philadelphia, PA: JB Lippincott, 1994, 236–239.

Devlin TM. Urea cycle. In: Devlin TM (ed.), *Textbook of Biochemistry with Clinical Correlations*, 4th ed. New York, NY: Wiley-Liss, 1997, 453–456.

Leonard JV, Morris AA. Urea cycle disorders. *Semin Neonatol* 2002;7(1):27–35.

Shambaugh GE III. Urea biosynthesis I. The urea cycle and relationships to the citric acid cycle. *Am J Clin Nutr* 1977;30(12):2083–2087.

Watford M. The urea cycle: a two-compartment system. *Essays Biochem* 1991;26:49–58.

45. (D) Selectins or lectins are carbohydrate-binding proteins located on the surface of many different types of cells. There are at least three different types of lectins, which include E-selectin (on endothelial cells), L-selectin (on leukocytes), and P-selectin (on platelets and endothelial cells). Selectins are especially important in the binding of leukocytes to endothelial walls, which enables them to migrate from blood vessels into tissues. For instance, activated endothelial cells at sites of inflammation can express E-selectins for binding and slowing down leukocytes and platelets. Lymphocytes can express L-selectin to bind oligosaccharides on endothelial cells of lymphoid organs to result in the accumulation of lymphocytes. In the migration of white blood cells (WBCs) out of blood vessels, selectins and integrins act in sequence to modulate the weak rolling adhesion and firm binding adhesion, respectively. The Ig protein superfamily modulates Ca^{2+}-independent cell-cell adhesion, in contrast to cadherins, selectins, and integrins, which are dependent on Ca^{2+} or Mg^{2+}. There are several members of the Ig superfamily, which include the intercellular adhesion molecules (ICAM) on endothelial cells and neural cell adhesion molecules (N-CAM). ICAMs bind to integrins on WBCs for firm adhesion before migration, and N-CAMs bind cells together by homophilic interactions.

The extracellular matrix is made up of two main classes of extracellular macromolecules: GAGs and fibrous proteins. GAGs are further subdivided into four main groups that include hyaluronan, heparan sulfate, keratan sulfate, and chondroitin or dermatan sulfate. GAGs are usually found covalently attached to core proteins in the form of proteoglycans, except hyaluronan. Fibrous proteins include collagen, elastin, fibronectin, and laminin. Collagen can be even further subdivided into at least 18 types with specific characteristics and tissue distributions. Collagen is the most important matrix protein for providing tensile strength and pliability to the extracellular matrix. Members of the fibroblast family of cells are mainly responsible for secreting matrix macromolecules, which are then assembled into an intricate network that interconnects cells within various tissues. The nature of the matrix molecules and the organization of the network determine the characteristics of the extracellular matrix in different tissues.

Elastin is the main component of elastic fibers and is somewhat similar to collagen except for the random coil structure and the lack of hydroxylysine or glycosylation. Elastic fibers are composed of elastin cores covered by microfibrils, which contain fibrillin. Mutations in the fibrillin gene are responsible for Marfan's syndrome.

Fibronectin is a glycoprotein dimer that is a component of the extracellular matrix and is composed of domains or modules that occur commonly in many other ligands and receptors. For instance, the type III fibronectin repeat can bind integrins and is also found in many growth factor receptors. A crucial Arg-Gly-Asp sequence (RGD) is responsible for the binding properties of fibronectin, and snakes exploit this quality in their venom, which contains RGD sequence anticoagulants called disintegrins.

Extracellular proteolytic enzymes can degrade the extracellular matrix and can be divided into two general classes: matrix metalloproteases (MMPs) and serine proteases. MMPs exist in over 19 forms and depend on Ca^{2+} or Zn^{2+} for activity. MMPs and serine proteases work together to breakdown matrix proteins such as collagen, fibronectin, and laminin. Specific MMPs such as the collagenases are selective for certain matrix proteins. This allows the structure of the matrix to be retained while allowing cell migration through a cleared portion of the matrix. To localize the action of matrix proteases, many are secreted as inactive precursors, allowing their action to be confined to a local area and activated only when needed. Cell-surface receptors can also bind and localize protease to specific sites of action, and protease inhibitors such as tissue inhibitors of metalloproteases (TIMPs) and serine protease inhibitors (serpins) can also help limit the area of protease activation.

Bibliography

Alberts B, Johnson A, Lewis K, et al. Cell junctions, cell adhesion, and the extracellular matrix. In: Alberts B, Johnson A, Lewis K, et al. (eds.), *Molecular Biology of the Cell*, 4th ed. New York, NY: Garland Science, 2002, 1065–1113.

Cawston T, Carrere S, Catterall J, et al. Matrix metalloproteinases and TIMPs: properties and implications for the treatment of chronic obstructive pulmonary disease. *Novartis Found Symp* 2001;234:205–218.

Hocking DC. Fibronectin matrix deposition and cell contractility: implications for airway remodeling in asthma. *Chest* 2002;122(Suppl 6):275S–278S.

Hornebeck W, Emonard H, Monboisse JC, et al. Matrix-directed regulation of pericellular proteolysis and tumor progression. *Semin Cancer Biol* 2002;12(3):231–241.

Ohbayashi H. Matrix metalloproteinases in lung diseases. *Curr Protein Pept Sci* 2002;3(4):409–421.

Ushiki T. Collagen fibers, reticular fibers and elastic fibers. A comprehensive understanding from a morphological viewpoint. *Arch Histol Cytol* 2002;65(2):109–126.

46. (A) Integrins are transmembrane heterodimers composed of noncovalently associated alpha and beta subunits, dependent on divalent cations for binding ligands. They serve as the major receptors for extracellular matrix proteins and link the extracellular matrix to the actin cytoskeleton of cells without directly affecting cell shape changes. Integrins provide both structural and signaling functions through their extracellular ligand-binding and intracellular domains. The structural function of integrins is because of their transmembrane linking of extracellular matrix proteins and intracellular anchor proteins that are bound to the actin cytoskeleton at focal adhesions. However, the integrins also serve as signal transducers by activating outside-in and inside-out signaling. Integrins exist in large numbers on the cell surface and bind extracellular molecules with low affinity, activating intracellular signaling pathways that communicate to the cell the nature of the extracellular matrix to which the cell is bound, termed outside-in signaling. Integrins also must be activated by the cell before mediating adhesion especially in platelets and leukocytes, termed inside-out signaling. Changes in integrin conformation can be promoted by signals coming from the cell, promoting stronger adhesion and binding.

Leukocyte adhesion deficiency is due to the absence of β_2-integrin subunits, resulting in the lack of LFA-1 (i.e., $\alpha_L \beta_2$ integrin), which mediates firm leukocyte binding to vessel walls and migration into the tissues. Patients with this deficiency suffer repeated bacterial infections and impaired healing. Glanzmann's thrombasthenia is a bleeding disorder because of the deficiency of β_3 integrin, causing problems with platelet-fibrinogen interactions.

Bibliography

Alberts B, Johnson A, Lewis K, et al. Cell junctions, cell adhesion, and the extracellular matrix. In: Alberts B, Johnson A, Lewis K, et al. (eds.), *Molecular Biology of the Cell*, 4th ed. New York, NY: Garland Science, 2002, 1113–1118.

Bokel C, Brown NH. Integrins in development: moving on, responding to, and sticking to the extracellular matrix. *Dev Cell* 2002;3(3):311–321.

Hogg N, Bates PA. Genetic analysis of integrin function in man: LAD-1 and other syndromes. *Matrix Biol* 2000; 19(3):211–222.

Hynes RO. Integrins: bidirectional, allosteric signaling machines. *Cell* 2002;110(6):673–687.

Hynes RO. A reevaluation of integrins as regulators of angiogenesis. *Nat Med* 2002;8(9):918–921.

Liddington RC, Ginsberg MH. Integrin activation takes shape. *J Cell Biol* 2002;158(5):833–839.

Tomiyama Y. Glanzmann thrombasthenia: integrin alpha IIb beta 3 deficiency. *Int J Hematol* 2000;72(4):448–454.

47. (E) The complement system involves the interaction of serum proteins produced by the liver as a component of innate immunity. The complement system can assist the action of antibodies or contribute directly to pathogen elimination. The early complement components consist of C1, C2, and C4, with the cleavage of C3 complex being the crucial and common point of the early cascade. The cascade of C3 activation through sequential proteolytic cleavage occurs through three different pathways: (1) the classical pathway, (2) the alternative pathway, and (3) the lectin pathway. The resulting fragments of complement such as C3a, C4a, and C5a act as chemoattractants that can recruit phagocytes to sites of infection or inflammation. The C3b component can bind covalently to pathogen surfaces and acts in opsonization to facilitate phagocytosis or to activate late complement activation.

The classical pathway is activated by IgG or IgM antibodies binding to microbe surfaces, resulting in the binding and cleavage of C1, C2, C4, and eventually C3. The alternative pathway involves the spontaneous activation of C3 with the assistance of complexes involving factors B and D. Human cells produce proteins that prevent this spontaneous reaction from proceeding on their surfaces, but pathogenic cells do not. MBL is also called mannose-binding protein (MBP) and recognizes carbohydrates such as mannose and N-acetylglucosamine on pathogen surfaces. MBL forms a complex with serine proteases called MBL-associated serine proteases (MASP) that proteolytically cleave C2, C4, and C3. Thus, MBL is able to activate the complement pathway through the MBL-MASP or lectin pathway independent of the classical and alternative pathways. The liver usually produces MBL, and MBL deficiency has been associated with many disease states.

The late complement components are activated by the cleavage of C5 by membrane-bound C3b. The fragment C5b remains on the cell surface and binds late complement components C6, C7, and C8 to form the C5678 complex. This complex can bind C9 to induce a conformational change in C9 to cause its insertion into the target cell membrane. The C9 molecule continues to bind other C9 molecules until a large transmembrane channel is formed, resulting in the lysis of the cell. The C5-9 complex is also called the MAC. Deficiency in MAC results in increased susceptibility to bacterial infections, especially *Neisseria meningitidis*.

There are also several inhibitors and regulators of the complement pathways, including soluble control

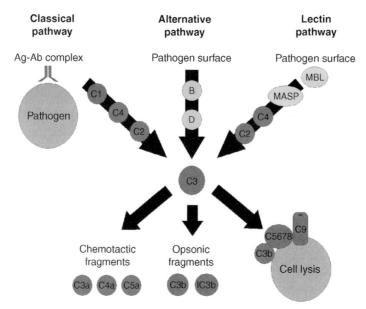

FIG. 1-20   Diagram showing the complement activation pathways.

proteins (e.g., C1 inhibitor, factor H, factor I, C4b binding proteins, and protein S) and membrane regulatory proteins (e.g., CD55 or DAF, CD59, MCP). Deficiency in C1 inhibitor results in hereditary angioedema because of complement overactivation, and deficiency in GPI anchors for CD55 and CD59 results in paroxysmal nocturnal hemoglobinuria because of complement-mediated lysis of RBCs (see Fig. 1-20).

Bibliography

Alberts B, Johnson A, Lewis K, et al. Pathogens, infection, and innate immunity. In: Alberts B, Johnson A, Lewis K, et al. (eds.), *Molecular Biology of the Cell*, 4th ed. New York, NY: Garland Science, 2002, 1456–1457.

Bessler M, Schaefer A, Keller P. Paroxysmal nocturnal hemoglobinuria: insights from recent advances in molecular biology. *Transfus Med Rev* 2001;15(4):255–267.

Laufer J, Katz Y, Passwell JH. Extrahepatic synthesis of complement proteins in inflammation. *Mol Immunol* 2001;38(2–3):221–229.

Nielsen CH, Fischer EM, Leslie RG. The role of complement in the acquired immune response. *Immunology* 2000;100(1):4–12.

Nonaka M. Evolution of the complement system. *Curr Opin Immunol* 2001;13(1):69–73.

Nzeako UC, Frigas E, Tremaine WJ. Hereditary angioedema: a broad review for clinicians. *Arch Intern Med* 2001;161 (20):2417–2429.

Sturfelt G. The complement system in systemic lupus erythematosus. *Scand J Rheumatol* 2002;31(3):129–132.

48. (A) The TLR family of receptors activates host cell gene expression in response to pathogens. There are at least 10 TLRs, many of which play important roles in the innate immune system for the recognition of pathogenic particles such as LPS. LPS is bound by circulating LPS-binding protein (LBP), and the complex is recognized by CD14 on macrophage surfaces. The resulting complex can then stimulate TLR4 for the activation of nuclear factor-kappaB (NF-κB) through the adaptor proteins and signaling mediators of the MAPK pathway called MyD88, IRAK, TRAF6, and TAK1. NF-κB normally remains bound to inhibitory kappaB (IκB) until phosphorylated by IκB kinase (IKK), which is activated by TAK1 in the TLR4 pathway. Phosphorylation of IκB induces its degradation and frees NF-κB. The activated NF-κB then translocates to the nucleus, as does the AP-1 TF (i.e., Jun and Fos heterodimer), which is activated in parallel to NF-κB by TAK1, and ERK/JNK. The final result is the activated transcription of genes involved in the inflammatory or immune response (see Fig. 1-21).

Bibliography

Alberts B, Johnson A, Lewis K, et al. Pathogens, infection, and innate immunity. In: Alberts B, Johnson A, Lewis K, et al. (eds.), *Molecular Biology of the Cell*, 4th ed. New York, NY: Garland Science, 2002, 1456–1457.

Beutler B. TLR4 as the mammalian endotoxin sensor. *Curr Top Microbiol Immunol* 2002;270:109–120.

Bowie A, O'Neill LA. Oxidative stress and nuclear factor-kappaB activation: a reassessment of the evidence in the light of recent discoveries. *Biochem Pharmacol* 2000; 59(1):13–23.

Calandra T. Pathogenesis of septic shock: implications for prevention and treatment. *J Chemother* 2001;13(1):173–180.

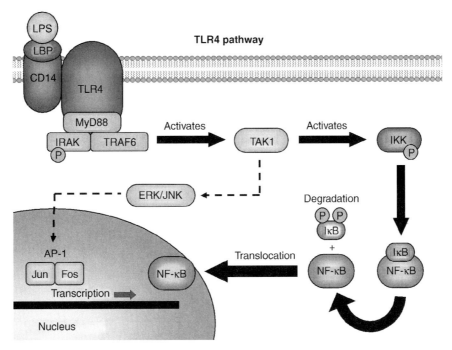

FIG. 1-21 Diagram of the TLR4 and NF-κB pathways.

Heumann D, Roger T. Initial responses to endotoxins and Gram-negative bacteria. *Clin Chim Acta* 2002;323(1–2): 59–72.

Hwang D. Modulation of the expression of cyclooxygenase-2 by fatty acids mediated through toll-like receptor 4-derived signaling pathways. *FASEB J* 2001;15(14): 2556–2564.

Kaisho T, Akira S. Toll-like receptors as adjuvant receptors. *Biochim Biophys Acta* 2002;1589(1):1–13.

Li Q, Verma IM. NF-kappaB regulation in the immune system. *Nat Rev Immunol* 2002;2(10):725–734.

Raetz CR, Whitfield C. Lipospolysaccharide endotoxins. *Annu Rev Biochem* 2002;71:635–700.

Royds JA, Dower SK, Owarnstrom EE, et al. Response of tumour cells to hypoxia: role of p53 and NFkB. *Mol Pathol* 1998;51(2):55–61.

49. (B) There are two major isoforms of the COX enzyme: COX-1 is constitutively and ubiquitously expressed in the human body, whereas the inducible COX-2 is upregulated by inflammatory stimuli. Corticosteroids and other steroidal anti-inflammatory agents block the arachidonate pathway at the level of PLA_2, aspirin irreversibly acetylates the COX enzyme, and other nonsteroidal anti-inflammatory drugs reversibly inhibit COX. While COX inhibitors and steroidal agents also block the formation of TXA_2, only EPA additionally produces PGI_3.

In 1978, a landmark epidemiologic study by Dyerberg and Bang showed that the Eskimos of Northwest Greenland had a strikingly low incidence of acute myocardial infarction and demonstrated delayed atherosclerosis associated with a high dietary intake of ω-3 polyunsaturated fatty acids (PUFAs) of marine origin. The Eskimos had a dramatic shift of plasma lipids from the ω-6 PUFAs of dietary vegetable oil origin to the ω-3 PUFAs found in a variety of fish oils. Specifically, the Eskimo people had high plasma concentrations of EPA, a biologically active ω-3 PUFA, but an extremely low concentration of AA, the primary ω-6 PUFA in most humans. This was in stark contrast to the high AA and extremely low EPA composition of the plasma lipids found in European and Western populations. Subsequent studies in Japan, Sweden, and The Netherlands found decreased incidences of atherosclerotic diseases (i.e., coronary heart disease, ischemic heart disease, and cerebrovascular accidents) among consumers of fish.

There are two essential fatty acids in the human diet, linoleic acid (C18:2; $\Delta^{9,12}$, ω-6 PUFA) and α-linolenic acid (C18:3; $\Delta^{9,12,15}$, ω-3 PUFA). In the human body, the majority of linoleic acid is converted into AA, which is also known as eicosatetraenoic acid (C20:4; $\Delta^{5,8,11,14}$, ω-6 PUFA). Briefly, the fatty acid nomenclature indicates that AA contains 20 carbons and 4 double bonds at locations that are 5, 8, 11, and 14 bonds away from the carboxy end of the fatty acid, and the omega-6 designation signifies that the final double bond is 6 bonds away from the terminal ω-carbon. EPA (C20:5; $\Delta^{5,8,11,14,17}$, ω-3 PUFA) likewise contains 20 carbons but 5 double bonds with the fifth double bond located 17 bonds away from the carboxy end and 3 bonds away from the ω-carbon. In contrast to AA, EPA is not endogenously produced in humans; ω-3 or ω-6 PUFAs cannot be synthesized *de novo* and the two families cannot be interconverted in animals. Although phytoplankton and other relatively simple life forms have the ability to convert α-linolenic acid into EPA, human and most other animals lack the enzymes necessary to elongate and desaturate α-linolenic acid into the more biologically active longer chain species, EPA and docosahexaenoic acid. Marine animals derive their EPA from ingesting phytoplankton or other fish, while humans must ingest EPA in the form of fish oils (e.g., salmon, mackerel, cod liver oil, anchovy).

EPA acts at three levels of the arachidonate pathway: (1) membrane incorporation, (2) competitive inhibition of COX, and (3) conversion to a unique set of prostanoids. First, EPA competes with linoleic acid and AA to become incorporated into the two-position of membrane phospholipids, from which they are liberated by PLA_2 to serve as a substrate for COX. Additionally, the administration of dietary fish oil led to the incorporation of EPA into the membranes of vascular endothelial cells in surgical patients. Second, EPA competes with AA for the membrane-bound COX enzymes but does not have the kinetic profile of a typical competitive inhibitor because of its slow release from the COX enzyme. The x-ray crystallographic structure of the interaction shows that EPA may bind within the COX active site and hairpin turn in a strained conformation because of the additional double bond (producing increased electron density and different structural *cis-trans* isomers), resulting in the slow release of EPA and the low observed rate of EPA oxygenation. Third, COX enzymes normally act to convert AA into prostaglandins of the two-series, but COX converts EPA into prostaglandins of the three-series. The two-series prostaglandins include thromboxane A_2 (TXA_2), a potent vasoconstrictor and platelet agonist produced by platelet COX, and prostaglandin I_2 (PGI_2 or prostacyclin), an extremely potent vasodilator and platelet antagonist produced by endothelial COX. In contrast, many of the three-series prostanoids (TXA_3, PGG_3, PGH_3) have no biological activity, with the exception of PGI_3, which is nearly as active as prostacyclin in its vasodilatory and platelet antagonistic activities. Thus, EPA products result in a shift of platelet function toward antiaggregation.

EPA has been shown to reduce the severity of tumors and other chronic inflammatory conditions. It is hypothesized that the effects of EPA on atherosclerosis, malignancies, and chronic inflammatory diseases may be linked. One argument links the three by pathogenic theory, and postulates that the EPA's main effects are as an anti-inflammatory, antiproliferative agent.

Bibliography

Babcock T, Helton WS, Espat NJ. Eicosapentaenoic acid (EPA): an antiinflammatory omega-3 fat with potential clinical applications. *Nutrition* 2000;16(11–12):1116–1118.

Demaison L, Moreau D. Dietary *n*-3 polyunsaturated fatty acids and coronary heart disease-related mortality: a possible mechanism of action. *Cell Mol Life Sci* 2002;59(3):463–477.

Dyerberg J, Bang HO, Stoffersen E, et al. Eicosapentaenoic acid and prevention of thrombosis and atherosclerosis? *Lancet* 1978;2(8081):117–119.

Kelley DS. Modulation of human immune and inflammatory responses by dietary fatty acids. *Nutrition* 2001;17(7–8):669–673.

Nordoy A, Marchioli R, Arnesen H, et al. *n*-3 polyunsaturated fatty acids and cardiovascular diseases. *Lipids* 2001;36(Suppl):S127–S129.

Senzaki H, Tsubura A, Takada H. Effect of eicosapentaenoic acid on the suppression of growth and metastasis of human breast cancer cells in vivo and in vitro. *World Rev Nutr Diet* 2001;88:117–125.

Tisdale MJ. Cancer anorexia and cachexia. *Nutrition* 2001;17(5):438–442.

50. (A) Vascular endothelial growth factor (VEGF) was originally discovered in the 1980s as vascular permeability factor (VPF) and has dual effects of increasing blood vessel permeability as well as promoting angiogenesis. Ang1 was discovered in the mid-1990s as a proangiogenic factor that also decreases vascular permeability. Embryologic studies have shown that VEGF is necessary for vasculogenesis (i.e., the *de novo* formation of vessels) and the early morphogenic phase of angiogenesis (i.e., the formation of vessels from existing vessels). The blood vessels formed by VEGF compose a leaky, primitive vascular network of tubes without fine capillary branching. Ang1 acts on these primitive vessels to promote interactions between endothelial cells, pericytes, and smooth muscle cells, inducing extensive capillary branching and forming the tight vessels characteristic of normal mature vasculature. VEGF and Ang1 are both proangiogenic growth factors that act via tyrosine kinase receptors.

There are several isoforms and splice variants of VEGF that have been discovered since the original identification of VEGF-A_{165}. The isoforms VEGF-A through VEGF-D exist, and VEGF-A can be subdivided into five splice variants with different heparin-binding properties. The biological action of VEGF-A$_{165}$ has already been described, much less is known about VEGF-B, and VEGF-C plus VEGF-D are known to be lymphangiogenic factors. References to VEGF in this discussion indicate the original VEGF-A$_{165}$. Most of the biological actions of VEGF are through the receptors VEGFR-1 and more importantly VEGFR-2. The neuropilin coreceptor can aid VEGF receptor binding, and VEGFR-3 is found on lymph vessels for the specific binding of VEGF-C and VEGF-D. VEGF gene transcription is upregulated by the activation of a gene regulatory protein called hypoxia-inducible factor 1 (HIF-1), which is activated by hypoxia in tissues.

Ang1 acts through the Tie-2 receptor (Tie-1 is an orphan receptor), which is endothelial cell-specific. Ang1 remains constitutively bound to its receptor on mature vessels and is only displaced by Ang2, its natural antagonist, in areas of vessel damage and repair such as in wound healing, the female menstruation cycle, and in inflammation (including tumors). The displacement of Ang1 by Ang2 allows regression of the blood vessels to their leaky primitive state, which primes them for repair by VEGF and Ang1. Thus, VEGF has concerted action with the antiangiogenic factor, Ang2, in tumor angiogenesis. Ang2 is necessary to destabilize the normal host vasculature back to the primitive state, and VEGF is then immediately necessary to facilitate growth of the vessels toward the tumor. Ang1 can act on the blood vessels following VEGF, similar to their synergistic actions during embryologic angiogenesis. However, VEGF often acts alone during tumor angiogenesis, and tumor vessels tend to be more leaky than normal blood vessels. Without the immediate availability of VEGF, Ang2 alone causes the regression of vessels. So although the concerted action of Ang2 and VEGF can be considered proangiogenic, Ang2 is really an antiangiogenic factor while VEGF is a proangiogenic factor. Ang1 and Ang2 do not show a similar synergistic relationship since they bind to the same receptor with comparable affinities and tend to directly antagonize each other.

Endostatin and angiostatin are endogenous antiangiogenic factors. Preclinical studies have shown that endostatin can cause the shrinkage of existing tumor vessels and inhibit tumor growth; however, angiogenic inhibitors such as angiostatin and endostatin can be activated by tumors to modulate angiogenesis both at the primary site and at downstream sites of metastasis. This gave rise to the theory that removing the primary tumor could allow the enhanced growth of satellite lesions that were held in check by antiangiogenic factors secreted by the primary tumor. Therefore, instead of the theory that a tumor can only produce proangiogenic factors, the evolving idea is that a tumor can produce both antiangiogenic and proangiogenic factors to direct the flow of blood away from other tissues and toward itself. Besides directing the supply of nutrients, the guiding of blood vessel growth by tumor is also believed to be important in metastatic processes (see Figs. 1-22 and 1-23).

Bibliography

Brock CS, Lee SM. Anti-angiogenic strategies and vascular targeting in the treatment of lung cancer. *Eur Respir J* 2002;19(3):557–570.

Cao Y. Therapeutic potentials of angiostatin in the treatment of cancer. *Haematologica* 1999;84(7):643–650.

Conti CJ. Vascular endothelial growth factor: regulation in the mouse skin carcinogenesis model and use in antiangiogenesis cancer therapy. *Oncologist* 2002;7(Suppl 3):4–11.

Ellis LM, Ahmad S, Fan F, et al. Angiopoietins and their role in colon cancer angiogenesis. *Oncology* 2002;16 (4 Suppl 3):31–35.

Ferrara N. Role of vascular endothelial growth factor in physiologic and pathologic angiogenesis: therapeutic implications. *Semin Oncol* 2002;29(6 Suppl 16):10–14.

Folkman J. Role of angiogenesis in tumor growth and metastasis. *Semin Oncol* 2002;29(6 Suppl 16):15–18.

Guppy M. The hypoxic core: a possible answer to the cancer paradox. *Biochem Biophys Res Commun* 2002;299(4):676–680.

Jain RK. Tumor angiogenesis and accessibility: role of vascular endothelial growth factor. *Semin Oncol* 2002;29(6 Suppl 16):3–9.

Lie W, Reinmuth N, Stoeltzing O, et al. Antiangiogenic therapy targeting factors that enhance endothelial cell survival. *Semin Oncol* 2002;29(3 Suppl 11):96–103.

Qin LX, Tang ZY. The prognostic molecular markers in hepatocellular carcinoma. *World J Gastroenterol* 2002;8(3):385–392.

Ribatti D, Vacca A, Presta M. The discovery of angiogenic factors: a historical review. *Gen Pharmacol* 2000;35(5):227–231.

Thurston G. Complementary actions of VEGF and angiopoietin-1 on blood vessel growth and leakage. *J Anat* 2002;200(6):575–580.

Zetter BR. Angiogenesis and tumor metastasis. *Annu Rev Med* 1998;49:407–424.

Roles of VEGF & Ang1 in angiogenesis

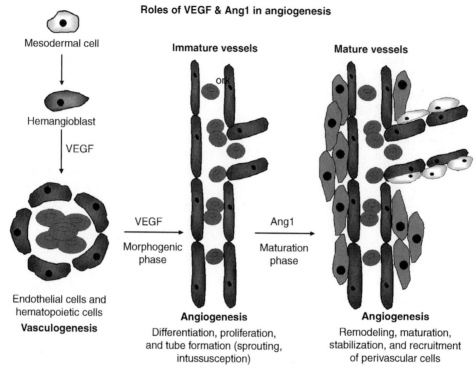

Mesodermal cell

Hemangioblast

VEGF

Endothelial cells and
hematopoietic cells
Vasculogenesis

Immature vessels

Mature vessels

VEGF
Morphogenic
phase

Ang1
Maturation
phase

Angiogenesis
Differentiation, proliferation,
and tube formation (sprouting,
intussusception)

Angiogenesis
Remodeling, maturation,
stabilization, and recruitment
of perivascular cells

FIG. 1-22   Diagram illustrating the synergistic action of VEGF and Ang1 during angiogenesis.

Role of Ang2 in angiogenesis

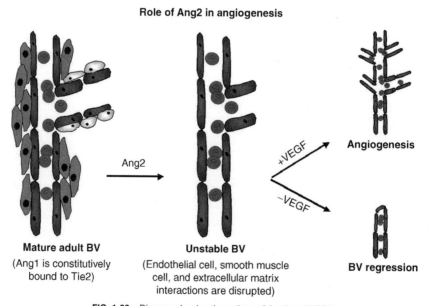

Mature adult BV
(Ang1 is constitutively
bound to Tie2)

Ang2

Unstable BV
(Endothelial cell, smooth muscle
cell, and extracellular matrix
interactions are disrupted)

+VEGF

−VEGF

Angiogenesis

BV regression

FIG. 1-23   Diagram showing the actions of Ang2 and VEGF.

SUMMARY

A human can be subdivided into organs, tissues, and eventually down to the single cell, which is the smallest living unit of the body able to survive independently. Each human being is the end result of the coordinated performance of countless trillions of cells working both individually and together. Although different cells can vary vastly in structure and function, each cell has essentially the same general internal organization and operates on similar principles of molecular communication.

The cell uses phospholipid membranes to form borders and intracellular subdivisions. The cell membrane helps establish electrochemical gradients and activates signaling pathways in addition to providing a protective barrier and delineating the borders of intracellular space. The resulting electrochemical gradients allow passive or facilitated diffusion of small molecules through the cell membrane along their gradients, and the membrane Na^+-K^+ pump allows coupled active transport of molecules against their gradients. Intracellular membranes compartmentalize the nucleus and organelles within the human cell to provide functional subdivisions, allowing the cell to operate as a miniature organism. Mitochondria and cytosolic enzymes provide oxidative pathways for the digestion of organic molecules to generate energy. The nucleus, ribosomes, RER, SER, and Golgi participate in synthetic pathways for the generation of molecules that function in cell structure and signaling. Endosomes, phagosomes, lysosomes, and peroxisomes are intracellular vesicles specialized for the breakdown of wastes and foreign particles. Substances can·be specifically transported from one organelle to another using signal sequences and molecular motors. Various signal sequences are used as tags to localize substances to the nucleus or to a specific organelle, and molecular chaperones assist proteins in assuming their proper conformations in passing from one organelle to another. As each organelle performs specific activities, organelle dysfunction results in corresponding changes as in maternally-inherited mitochondrial disorders, lysosomal storage disorders, and ALD.

Cellular metabolism is accomplished through the oxidation of sugars, proteins, and fats by mitochondria and cytosolic enzymes to chemical forms of energy, primarily ATP and NADH. For glucose, there are three stepwise reaction cycles: glycolysis in the cytosol, TCA cycle in the mitochondrial matrix, and oxidative phosphorylation on the inner mitochondrial membrane. Oxidation of fatty acids also occurs between the cytosol and mitochondria, with the resulting acetyl-CoA breakdown products entering the TCA cycle. Excess fuels are stored as glycogen and adipose, which are released by glycogenolysis and lipolysis during periods of fasting. In prolonged starvation, gluconeogenesis and ketogenesis are activated in hepatocytes to provide glucose and ketone bodies to cells most essential for survival. Carbon dioxide waste from oxidative metabolism is expelled through respiration and bicarbonate buffering. Nitrogenous waste from protein metabolism is eliminated via the urea cycle in hepatocytes and excreted through the renal system. Dysfunctions in cellular metabolism are often because of disease states causing organ failure or rarely because of heritable enzyme deficiencies.

Several specialized cellular structures function in the establishment of cell shape, cell-cell adhesion, and cell-matrix adhesion. Cell shape is established by the cytoskeleton, which is composed of microtubules, intermediate filaments, and actin microfilaments. The cytoskeleton can coordinate changes in cell shape to allow migratory movement of the entire cell. Microtubules also function in the movement of chromosomes during reproduction, motion of cilia, and movement of vesicles during endocytosis or exocytosis. Molecular motor proteins can transport intracellular cargo directionally along various cytoskeletal filaments and are especially important in vesicular movement along microtubules. Various cell type-specific intermediate filaments act as cytoplasmic links between the nucleus, cytoplasm, and extracellular matrix. Actin microfilaments function in cell locomotion, cytokinesis, and vesicular movement; actin also functions in contraction by associating with myosin molecular motors. Cell-cell adhesion is regulated by the junctional complex, which is composed of tight junctions (i.e., zonula occludens) and adherens junctions (i.e., zonula adherens and macula adherens). The junctional complex forms a paracellular barrier to the movement of molecules, helps establish apical-basal polarity, and participates in signaling pathways. Gap junctions allow the electrical and metabolic coupling of cells to coordinate contraction or rapid multicellular functional regulation. Cell-matrix adhesions are regulated by transmembrane proteins called integrins, which are components of hemidesmosomes connecting the cytoskeleton to the extracellular matrix or basal lamina. Integrins also serve important roles in signal transduction from the extracellular milieu to the intracellular milieu (i.e., outside-in signaling) and vice versa (i.e., inside-out signaling). Cell-matrix interactions can be modified by matrix metalloproteinases, collagenases, or other degradation enzymes produced and secreted by the cell.

Cells can regulate the levels of specific proteins by altering the rate of protein synthesis and breakdown. Protein synthesis and gene expression is regulated at the mRNA transcriptional level by TFs (which bind to DNA promoter sequences) and gene regulatory elements (which bind to DNA enhancer sequences or response elements). The stability of a specific mRNA sequence can also determine the amount of corresponding protein production. Protein breakdown can determine the half-life or activity of a specific protein and can occur through two major pathways, lysosomal and nonlysosomal. The UPP pathway is the major nonlysosomal pathway responsible for targeted protein degradation and can also indirectly regulate mRNA transcription by the targeted destruction of TFs or associated proteins. For instance, the inhibitory IκB protein is degraded by the UPP system to activate the NF-κBTF, resulting in increased transcription of many inflammatory proteins. Also the majority of signaling molecules are proteins or peptides, nucleotides such as adenosine, lipids such as phosphatidylserine, and gases such as nitric oxide can also serve as signaling molecules. A cell can produce signaling molecules that act on itself (autocrine action), on local cells (paracrine action), or on distant cells by traveling through the circulation (endocrine action).

Signaling molecules bind to specific receptors to activate signal transduction pathways inside target cells, which are then modified and terminated by complex feedback and regulatory mechanisms. The signal can also be terminated by ligand degradation, inactivation, or reuptake. Signal transduction is governed by five main classes of ligand-binding receptors: (1) ion channel-linked receptors, (2) GPCRs, (3) enzyme-linked receptors, (4) intracellular steroid hormone receptors, and (5) intracellular receptor guanylate cyclases. Ion channel-linked receptors function by opening selective ion channels in response to ligand-binding and include most of the major excitatory and inhibitory NTRs. GPCRs traverse the cell membrane seven times (i.e., heptaspan) and are linked to heterotrimeric GTP-binding proteins with α-, β-, and γ-subunits. Ligand-binding results in the dissociation of G protein subunits and activation of downstream signaling, usually through the AC or PLC pathway. A number of ligands activate GPCRs including the adrenergic receptors, dopamine receptors, $GABA_B$ receptor, glucagon receptor, neuropeptide receptors, and pituitary hormone receptors. Enzyme-linked receptors have extracellular domains that bind ligand and intracellular domains that serve as enzymes to activate intracellular signaling. Enzyme-linked receptors are subdivided into RTKs (e.g., insulin receptor and various growth factor receptors), tyrosine kinase-associated receptors (e.g., GH receptor, prolactin receptor, and many cytokine receptors), receptor serine-threonine kinases (e.g., TGF-β), receptor tyrosine phosphatases (e.g., CD45), and receptor guanylate cyclases (e.g., ANP receptor). Intracellular steroid hormone receptors are distinctive in that their hydrophobic ligands can pass through the cell membrane to bind receptors in the cytosol and induce nuclear translocation

to activate the transcription of specific genes. Ligands for steroid hormone receptors include glucocorticoids, estrogen, progesterone, thyroid hormone, retinoic acid, and vitamin D_3. Special intracellular receptor guanylate cyclases bind nitric oxide to activate cGMP production, PKG activation, and the phosphorylation of serine or threonine on intracellular proteins to transduce a signal. Signaling can also be accomplished without ligands in certain cases through direct voltage-gated or mechanical-gated ion channels.

Reproduction of cells is achieved through activation of mitosis and cell cycle progression. Chromosomal DNA replication is accomplished during the S phase of the cell cycle, during which DNA and histones expand into euchromatin form, with transcriptional complexes acting at numerous replication origins. Telomerases are needed to replicate DNA to its full length since removal of RNA primers, which were necessary for initiation of replication, leaves shortened lagging strands. The integrity of DNA replication is double-checked by DNA repair and proofreading enzymes. Cells then enter the G_2 phase during which ATP synthesis occurs, followed by the M phase during which mitosis or meiosis occurs. This is followed by either the G_0 resting phase of cell cycle suspension or the G_1 phase of RNA, protein, lipid, and carbohydrate synthesis. The cell cycle is regulated at the G_1 and G_2 checkpoints by cyclin-dependent kinases (Cdks), cyclins, and tumor suppressors such as p53 and Rb. Uncontrolled cell cycle activation through the activation of oncogenes or inactivation of tumor suppressor genes underlies many forms of malignancy.

Cell death occurs through various forms of cellular necrosis or by apoptotic programmed cell death. In contrast with necrosis, apoptosis results in cell death without the extensive involvement of neighboring cells or signs of inflammation. Apoptosis can be initially triggered by viral infection or irreparable cellular damage. Extrinsic Fas ligand-Fas receptor and intrinsic cytochrome c signaling pathways can activate the caspase proteolytic cascade for apoptosis.

The compartmentalization of cell structure into organelles, cellular metabolic pathways, synthetic and degradation pathways, signaling or communication, replication, and cellular death are processes that characterize the activity of a cell as the basic unit of life. There are some pathologic processes such as malignancy or diabetes that are best considered at the organism, organ, tissue, and cellular levels combined. In this genomic and proteomic era of scientific discovery, a firm grasp of basic cell physiology and structure will aid the clinician in gaining a deeper understanding of pathology and future therapeutic developments.

CHAPTER 2

Surgical Nutrition

Rahul D. Tevar and Amit D. Tevar

Questions

1. A 67-year-old woman with rectal cancer is admitted to a general surgical floor. Which of the following laboratory studies should be included in the surgeon's initial nutritional assessment?

   (A) transferrin
   (B) prealbumin
   (C) albumin
   (D) glutamine
   (E) all of the above

2. A 34-year-old male is mechanically ventilated in the intensive care unit at a community hospital after a closed head injury. He is 5 ft 11 in. tall and weighs 176 lb. He has no burns, has not had surgery, and shows no signs of sepsis. Estimate his caloric requirement per 24 h.

   (A) cannot be estimated with the given data
   (B) 1840 kcal
   (C) 2200 kcal
   (D) 2390 kcal
   (E) 2570 kcal

3. A 35-year-old trauma victim with malabsorption requires hyperalimentation. The patient's injuries include a stable nondisplaced fracture of the third thoracic vertebra, a closed head injury, multiple upper and lower extremity fractures and bilateral pulmonary contusions requiring ventilatory support. Which of the following are the most appropriate site and type of venous access in this patient?

   (A) bilateral antecubital fossae, 18G peripheral intravenous catheters
   (B) femoral vein, central venous catheter (CVC)
   (C) dorsum of one foot, single 16G peripheral intravenous catheter
   (D) subclavian vein, CVC

4. In which of the following conditions is the enteral route appropriate for nutrition?

   (A) upper gastrointestinal bleed
   (B) complete small bowel obstruction
   (C) acute flare-up of Crohn's disease
   (D) low output colonic fistula

5. A 45-year-old male has sustained a closed head injury and multiple rib fractures in a motor vehicle collision. The patient requires maximal ventilatory support because of bilateral pulmonary contusions and aspiration pneumonitis. His Glasgow Coma Scale score is 5. Which of the following would be the most appropriate method of artificial nutrition?

   (A) parenteral nutrition with a protein sparing formula through a CVC
   (B) intragastric tube feeding
   (C) parenteral nutrition through a peripheral venous catheter
   (D) postpyloric tube feeding
   (E) any of the above with appropriate calories

6. A 63-year-old male with end-stage renal disease requiring hemodialysis three times per week presents with bone pain and several pathologic fractures of the extremities. Which is the most likely electrolyte abnormality in this patient?

   (A) hypokalemia
   (B) hypernatremia
   (C) hyperphosphatemia
   (D) hypercalcemia
   (E) hypochloremia

7. A 35-year-old male trauma patient is being considered for extubation from a 10-day course of ventilatory support after a motor vehicle accident in which he suffered several hollow viscus injuries requiring an exploratory laparotomy. The patient has been receiving parenteral nutrition and currently has a tidal volume of 400 mL and a respiratory rate of 40 breaths/min. What changes in his hyperalimentation may improve this patient's minute ventilation?

    (A) adding long-acting insulin to the mixture
    (B) increasing the proportion of glucose calories
    (C) decreasing the total volume with a more concentrated solution
    (D) increasing the proportion of fat calories
    (E) adding fat soluble vitamins A, D, E, and K

8. Which of the following would most accurately reflect the metabolic stress on a 45-year-old female undergoing an elective open cholecystectomy?

    (A) albumin of 3.6 g/dL
    (B) weight loss of 400 g
    (C) urine nitrogen loss of 8 g per day
    (D) retinal-binding protein of 6 mg/dL

9. An obese patient requires nutritional support. Which objective measure should be used to determine the patient's nutritional requirement?

    (A) ideal body weight
    (B) adjusted body weight
    (C) actual body weight
    (D) actual body weight after allowing for usage of fat stores

10. Which is the most commonly cultured hospital acquired organism in critical care patients with aspiration pneumonia?

    (A) *Streptococcus pneumoniae*
    (B) *Staphylococcus aureus*
    (C) anaerobic species
    (D) *Pseudomonas aeruginosa*
    (E) *Haemophilus influenzae*

11. What is the most appropriate single agent for emperic coverage of the above patient?

    (A) metronidazole
    (B) clindamycin
    (C) piperacillin-tazobactam
    (D) vancomycin
    (E) first generation penicillin

12. A 28-year patient with a closed head injury requires ventilatory and nutritional support. The patient has no evidence of bowel obstruction, is receiving enteral feeds through a gastric tube, and is found to have aspirated gastric contents. The patient has no immediate pulmonary compromise. Which of the following therapies is appropriate to treat this condition in the first 12 h?

    (A) corticosteroids
    (B) oral and gastric suctioning
    (C) empiric antibiotics
    (D) gastric content culture
    (E) endotracheal tube replacement

13. A 45-year-old male with alcoholic liver disease and short gut syndrome was previously on chronic parenteral nutrition. He has been switched to an elemental enteral diet for the past 6 months, which has been poorly tolerated. He has complained of generalized weakness for several months and now has erythematous, scaly and symmetrical lesions on his upper extremities, stomatitis, and glossitis. What is the most appropriate treatment for these symptoms?

    (A) addition of fat soluble vitamins A, D, E, and K
    (B) thiamine replacement
    (C) niacin replacement
    (D) change to a lactose-free enteral feed
    (E) addition of tincture of opium

14. Which of the following dietary changes will improve the Child-Pugh classification in end-stage liver patients with protein-calorie malnutrition?

    (A) lactoalbumin supplementation
    (B) oral intake of fat soluble vitamin K
    (C) maltodextrin supplementation
    (D) branched chain amino acid supplementation
    (E) long-term parenteral nutrition

15. Which of the following trace element deficiencies are associated with glucose intolerance and peripheral neuropathy?

    (A) copper
    (B) iron
    (C) fluorine
    (D) chromium
    (E) selenium

16. Which of the following statements about vitamins is true?

(A) vitamins are essential and cannot be produced by the body

(B) fat soluble vitamins are stored in fat

(C) cholecalciferol is converted to calcitriol in the kidney and liver

(D) fat soluble vitamin deficiency can result in coagulopathy

(E) all of the above

17. An adult male develops acute nectrotizing pancreatitis after an endoscopic retrograde cholangiopancreaticogram. The patient requires ventilatory support and is in need of nutritional support. Which is the best route of providing nutrition?

(A) parenteral nutrition through peripheral access

(B) parenteral nutrition through central access

(C) enteral nutrition through jejunal feeding tube

(D) oral elemental supplementation

18. A 35-year female presents with a small bowel obstruction 9 months after a duodenal switch procedure. She has been unable to tolerate oral intake for 6 days.

Parenteral nutrition is started and 48 h later she is noted to have paresthesias, ocular disturbances, and seizures. Which of the following are responsible for her neurologic changes?

(A) hyperkalemia

(B) hypophosphatemia

(C) vitamin B_1 deficiency

(D) hyperkalemia

(E) hypomagnesemia

19. An 18-year-old male undergoes extensive small bowel resection after a gunshot wound to the abdomen. Despite his resultant short gut, his remaining colonic function allows him to subsist on an oral high-carbohydrate diet. What substrate is the preferred fuel for colonocytes?

(A) short chain fatty acids (SCFAs)

(B) glutamate

(C) luminal oligopeptides

(D) ketones

(E) fructose

Answers and Explanations

1. **(C)** The nutritional assessment of the surgical patient consists of a subjective assessment combined with objective measures. The *subjective* assessment may be informal, such as in the "eyeball" assessment that a patient appears well nourished or poorly nourished. It may also be more formalized, as in the subjective global assessment (SGA), which uses five guidelines (weight loss, dietary intake, gastrointestinal symptoms, functional capacity, and physical signs) to categorize the patient into one of three groups (well nourished, moderately nourished, or severely malnourished).

While many different *objective* measures of nutritional status have been shown to be accurate and reproducible in clinical studies, body mass index (BMI) and albumin concentration are the most commonly used. Their popularity lies in the fact that they are inexpensive, simple, and reasonably accurate.

BMI is defined as weight (kg) divided by the square of height (m^2). It is considered a more accurate indicator than ideal body weight (IBW) because it is less dependent on comparison to control populations. A BMI of less than 18.5 kg/m^2 is associated with increased morbidity in hospitalized patients.

The serum albumin concentration correlates with global protein synthesis, degradation, and exchange between fluid compartments. However, albumin does not reflect acute changes in nutritional status because of its long half-life (18–21 days) and as a negative acute phase reactant it is decreased in acute inflammatory states. Despite these limitations it is widely used as part of the initial nutritional assessment because of its ready availability and its accuracy as a marker of global nutritional status. A serum albumin level of less than 3.5 g/dL is associated with increased morbidity in hospitalized patients.

While other markers such as prealbumin and transferrin have greater sensitivity to acute changes in nutritional status, their expense and their unpredictable responses to stress and inflammation make them less practical for general clinical use, and they are not recommended for initial screening.

Glutamine is an important nutrient for the maintenance of gut mucosa during stress; however, it has been proposed as an additive to feeding solutions, and not as a nutritional marker.

Bibliography

Baker JP, Detsky AS, Wesson DE, et al. Nutritional assessment: a comparison of clinical judgment and objective measurements. *N Engl J Med* 1982;306:969–972.

Carney DE, Meguid MM. Current concepts in nutritional assessment. *Arch Surgery* 2002;137:42–45.

Hedlund JU, Hansson LO, Ortqvist AB. Hypoalbuminemia in hospitalized patients with community-acquired pneumonia. *Arch Intern Med* 1995;155:1438–1442.

LeLeiko NS, Walsh MJ. The role of glutamine, short-chain fatty acids, and nucleotides in intestinal adaptation to gastrointestinal disease. *Pediatr Clin North Am* 1996;43(2):451–469.

2. **(D)** Critically ill patients require accurate determination of nutritional needs to avoid the complications of both under- and overfeeding (Table 2-1).

Nutritional needs are determined by measuring energy expenditure (EE), and the most accurate

TABLE 2-1 Accurate Determination of Nutritional Needs to Avoid the Complications of Both Under- and Overfeeding

Overfeeding	Underfeeding
Physiologic stress	Increased complications
Hyperosmolar state	Immune suppression
Hyperglycemia	Prolonged hospitalization
Hepatic dysfunction	Poor wound healing
Excessive cost	Nosocomial infection
Fluid overload	Respiratory compromise
Azotemia	Prolonged mechanical ventilation
Respiratory compromise	
Prolonged mechanical ventilation	

method of determining EE is by indirect calorimetry (IC). Unfortunately, the equipment necessary for IC is expensive and requires skilled personnel. In clinical settings where IC is unavailable, a common practice is the use of standardized equations to estimate EE based on factors such as height, weight, age, and sex. Different equations have been developed for specific populations and clinical situations; in fact, over 200 have been published. The more notable of these include the Harris-Benedict, Frankenfeld, Swinamer, Penn State and Ireton-Jones equations. The Harris-Benedict equation is the most frequently applied because of its ease of use and because of its good correlation with IC in diverse patient populations.

The Harris-Benedict equation provides an estimate of resting energy expenditure (REE) as follows:

Men:

$$66.5 + [13.75 \times \text{weight (kg)}] + [5.0 \times \text{height (cm)}] - [6.78 \times \text{age (years)}]$$

Women:

$$655 + [9.56 \times \text{weight (kg)}] + [1.85 \times \text{height (cm)}] - [4.68 \times \text{age (years)}]$$

The calculated REE is adjusted to simulate the patient's actual clinical state by multiplying by an estimated stress factor; the commonly used stress factors are 1.2 for minor surgery and cancer, 1.3 for fracture and multiple trauma, and 1.4 for sepsis.

The calculation for our ventilated trauma patient is as follows:

$$\text{REE} = 66.5 + [13.75 \times 80 \text{ kg}] + [5.0 \times 180 \text{ cm}] - [6.78 \times 34 \text{ years}] = 1836 \text{ kcal per day}$$

Multiplying by the stress factor of 1.3 for fracture/trauma, we obtain the answer of 2386 kcal per day.

Bibliography

Cheng CH, Chen CH, Wong Y, Lee BJ, Kan MN, Huang YC. Measured versus estimated energy expenditure in mechanically ventilated critically ill patients. *Clin Nutr* 2002;21(2):165–172.

MacDonald A, Hildebrandt L. Comparison of formulaic equations to determine energy expenditure in the critically ill patient. *Nutrition* 2003;19(3):233–239.

McClave SA, McClain CJ, Snider HL. Should indirect calorimetry be used as part of nutritional assessment? *J Clin Gastroenterol* 2001;33(1):14–19.

3. **(D)** Obtaining central venous access in the critically ill patient remains a common dilemma for the surgeon. Unfortunately, site selection for CVC placement is often based on the comfort level of the technician, rather than on the complication rates of the different sites.

Central venous catheterization is performed using the Seldinger technique and usually employs a 15–17 cm polyurethane catheter with two to four lumens. All lines should be placed under maximal sterile precautions including hand wash, mask and cap, and sterile drapes, gowns and gloves. Thorough insertion site cleansing should be undertaken as well, preferably with 2% chlorhexidine.

Site selection is important in minimizing the most commonly seen complications: infection, venous thrombosis, and mechanical adverse events (arterial puncture, pneumothorax, hemothorax, mediastinal hematoma, malposition, and air embolism). In a large series reviewing femoral and subclavian CVC placement, thrombotic complications were the most common adverse events.

Femoral vein catheters are associated with an overall higher rate of infectious complications (19.8%) in comparison with subclavian vein catheters (4.5%). In patients with and without bacteremia, coagulase negative staphylococcus was the most common organism isolated.

Mechanical complications have been found to occur with similar frequency in both subclavian and femoral line placement. The most common mechanical injuries include arterial puncture and minor bleeding. The complication of pneumothorax occurs in only 1.5–2.3% of subclavian CVC placements. Several studies have demonstrated that the risk factors for mechanical complications include increased time for insertion, nighttime placement, more than two needle passes for insertion, BMI greater than 30 and previous catheterization or surgery near the site of placement. Ultrasound guidance was not found to significantly decrease incidence of complications in subclavian vein catheterization.

Thrombotic complications have been shown to occur more frequently in patients with femoral lines. Catheter-related thrombosis has been shown to occur in 21.5% of femoral lines versus 1.9% of subclavian lines. A large single study trial found the absolute risk reduction of subclavian catheters in comparison to femoral catheters to be 33% for all complications. This would imply that for every three subclavian CVCs placed instead of femoral CVCs, one complication is avoided.

Bibliography

Mansfield PF, Hohn DC, Fornage BD, et al. Complications and failures of subclavian vein catheterization. *N Engl J Med* 1994;331:1735–1738.

Merrer J, Jonghe BD, Golliot F, et al. Complication of femoral and subclavian venous catheterization in critically ill patients. *JAMA* 2001;286:700–707.

Sitzmann JV, Townsend TR, Siler MC, et al. Septic and technical complications of central venous catheterization: a prospective study of 200 consecutive patients. *Ann Surg* 1985;202:766–770.

4. **(D)** Patients who present with objective markers of malnutrition or will be unable to provide themselves with oral nutrition for 7–10 days benefit from synthetic feeding. Enteral feeding has been found to have several key benefits over parenteral nutrition.

First, there are the decreased costs of providing long-term feeds via the enteral route. The solution itself is less expensive than parenteral nutrition solutions, daily electrolyte adjustments are not required, and administration costs are minimized. Another benefit is the trophic effect of enteral feeds on small and large bowel mucosa. Parenteral nutrition can lead to intestinal mucosal atrophy and a resultant increase in bacterial translocation, which may contribute to the known increase in incidence of septic complications in parenterally fed patients.

Most physicians routinely prefer enteral feeding over parenteral when possible. It is important that the surgeon recognize those patients who will not be able to tolerate or maximally benefit from enteral feeding. The absolute contraindication to enteral nutrition is complete bowel obstruction. The relative contraindications include high output intestinal fistula, acute inflammatory bowel disease, severe ileus, massive gastrointestinal hemorrhage, and hemodynamic instability with resultant decrease in mesenteric blood flow.

Bibliography

Grimble GK. The adequacy of enteral nutrition. *Curr Opin Gastroenterol* 1996;12:174–182.

Keating K. Nutritional support of the critically ill patient. In: Cameron JL (ed.), *Current Surgical Therapy*, 7th ed. St. Louis, MO: Mosby, 2001.

MacFie J. Enteral versus parenteral nutrition. *Br J Surg* 2000;87:1121–1122.

5. **(D)** The enteric route should be used for nutritional supplementation whenever it is not contraindicated. The route of enteric feeds must be carefully chosen to provide adequate calories quickly while minimizing the risk for aspiration. Options include intragastric, transpyloric, gastrostomy, jejunostomy, and gastojejunostomy tube feeding.

Contraindications for tube gastric feedings include nasogastric tube output greater than 600 mL in 24 h, known history of aspiration, lack of adequate airway protection, severe pulmonary dysfunction, recent regurgitation and inability to be maintained in 30° reverse Trendelenburg position. If any of these contraindications exist the patient should receive a transpyloric feeding catheter, which can be placed under fluoroscopic guidance or using a bedside technique.

If patient is an acceptable candidate for gastric feeding, full strength feeding should be started at 30–50 mL/h. Feeding intolerance should be assessed by checking for residual feeds. Any residual volume greater than 150–200 mL should be discarded and tube feeds should be held for 4 h before they are resumed at the previous rate. While monitoring the patient closely for osmotic diarrhea and/or abdominal distention, advance the rate of tube feeds every 4–8 h by an amount calculated to reach the caloric goal in 72 h. If patient does show signs of feeding intolerance or is unable to attain goal feeds a transpyloric route of feeding should be used.

Postpyloric feeds should be advanced in a manner similar to intragastric feeds, and patients should also be assessed for signs of feeding intolerance such as abdominal distention and/or diarrhea. Parenteral feeding is an option if the patient is unable to tolerate transpyloric catheter feeding.

Patients who will require enteral feeding for an extended period of time should be considered for gastrostomy tube placement. Those who cannot tolerate gastric feeding should be considered for gastrojejunal or jejunostomy tube placement.

Bibliography

Keating K. Nutritional support of the critically ill patient. In: Cameron JL (ed.), *Current Surgical Therapy*, 7th ed. St. Louis, MO: Mosby, 2001.

6. **(C)** Hyperphosphatemia is a prevalent and often preventable disease among the chronic renal failure and dialysis patient population. The total body phosphate content of an average male is approximately 10 g/kg and 85% is found in the skeleton. The extracellular portion of total body phosphorus is less than 1% and 10% is protein bound with approximately 33% fixed to sodium, calcium, and magnesium. Daily intake of phosphate is 1000–1500 mg. Fecal and urinary output are usually regulated to maintain a total body phosphate balance of zero. The small bowel, primarily the jejunum, is responsible for absorption of 60–70% of phosphate intake.

Parathyroid hormone plays a key role in phosphate homeostasis in the renal failure patient. Hyperphosphatemia and the resultant decrease in the levels of ionized calcium act directly to increase the secretion of parathyroid hormone. Parathyroid hormone in turn stimulates osteoclast activity to promote bone resorption of calcium and phosphorus. In addition, there is greater metabolization of calcidol to calcitrol leading to improved small bowel absorption of calcium. Finally parathyroid hormone acts directly on the renal tubules to increase calcium reabsorption and phosphate excretion, resulting in phosphaturia. The kidney is able to adequately maintain normal phosphate levels until the glomerular filtration rate is less than 25 mL/min.

Although acute and chronic renal failure remain the most common causes of hyperphosphatemia, others to consider in the differential diagnosis include parathyroid dysfunction, hyperthyroidism, juvenile hypogonadism, menopause, vitamin D toxicity, enemas, laxatives, phosphorus burns, diabetic ketoacidosis, lactic acidosis, rhabdomyolysis, malignant hyperthermia, chemotherapy, and familial disease.

Hyperphosphatemia is a disease that deserves immediate attention so as to avoid its short- and long-term complications. The most commonly seen effect is secondary hyperparathyroidism. Complications from calcium deposits include: vascular wall calcification, calciphylaxis, and cardiac tissue calcification. Approximately 50% of all deaths in the dialysis patient population are from cardiovascular complications. Persistently elevated phosphate is an independent risk factor for cardiovascular complications, possible through the calcium deposits to vascular and cardiac tissue. Patients with phosphorus levels above 6.5 mg/dL have a 27% greater mortality risk than those with a level between 2.4 and 6.5 mg/dL.

The treatment of hyperphosphatemia in the dialysis patient begins with dietary control of phosphate without restriction of protein intake. This means avoiding milk, cheese, eggs, red meats, fatty fish, shellfish, peas, beans, lentils, brans, and coarse grains. Dialysis removal of phosphate is the next action taken. The difficulty with this method is the intracellular nature of phosphate and the rapidly rising level 3–4 h after dialysis.

Next in the treatment is the use of oral phosphate binding agents such as aluminum carbonate, calcium carbonate, and acetate. Aluminum salts remain the most effective phosphate binders, but there is still no satisfactory method to reliable reduce phosphate levels in the dialysis patient. The known increase in cardiovascular complications in those patients with chronically elevated phosphorus levels makes this an active avenue for continued research.

Bibliography

Albaaj D, Hutchison A. Hyperphosphataemia in renal failure: causes, consequences and current management. *Drugs* 2003;63:577–596.

Blacher J, Guerin AP, Pannier B, et al. Arterial calcifications, arterial stiffness and cardiovascular risk in end-stage renal disease. *Hypertension* 2001;38:938–942.

Block GA, Port FK. Re-evaluation of risks associated with hyperphosphatemia and hyperparathyroidism in dialysis patients: recommendations for a change in management. *Am J Kidney Dis* 2000;35:1226–1237.

7. **(D)** A commonly used tool to determine substrate oxidation and utilization is the respiratory quotient. The respiratory quotient is determined by following-formula:

$$\text{Respiratory quotient} = \frac{CO_2 \text{ produced}}{O_2 \text{ consumed}}$$

The respiratory quotient for protein oxidation is 0.85, fat oxidation is 0.7, glucose oxidation is 1.0, and lipogenesis is >1.0.

The patient above has a minute ventilation of 16 L/min which is likely because of increased CO_2 production from the caloric distribution and quantity of the parenteral nutrition. The first hyperalimentation error is in providing too many nonprotein calories distributed as glucose. Glucose has a respiratory quotient of 1.0 versus fat's respiratory quotient of 0.7 and therefore causes greater production of CO_2. Compounding the problem, the excess nonprotein calories are converted into fat. The respiratory quotient of lipogenesis is >1, contributing to elevated CO_2 and the compensatory increased minute ventilation.

The hyperalimentation mixture in this patient should be adjusted to provide fewer calories and a greater portion of those calories as lipid.

Clinicians should also perform a thorough evaluation for other potential nonmetabolic sources of failure to wean. An unfortunate complication of decreasing calories in a patient who may be undergoing continued metabolic stress from an evolving inflammatory process is inadvertent and unnecessary malnutrition.

Bibliography

Moore FA, McQuiggan M. Nutritional support of the stressed intensive care unit patient. In: Hall JB, Freid EB (eds.), *Society of Critical Care Medicine and American College of Chest Physicians 4th Combined Critical Care Course*. New York, NY, 2002.

Rombeau JL, Rolandelli RG, Wilmore DW. Nutritional support. In: Wilmore DW, Brennan MF, Harken AH (eds.), *Scientific American Surgery*. New York, NY, 1995.

Talpers S, Romberger D, Bunce S, et al. Nutritionally associated increased carbon dioxide production: excess total calories versus high proportion of carbohydrate calories. *Chest* 1992;102:551–555.

8. **(C)** Urine area nitrogen balance is an excellent measure of metabolic stress. A negative nitrogen balance denotes that inadequate protein is being supplied to offset the nitrogen excreted as the breakdown product of protein metabolism. Nitrogen balance in the clinical setting is assessed by measuring 24-h urine urea output.

$$\text{Nitrogen balance} = \text{nitrogen (g)}_{\text{Intake}}$$
$$- \text{nitrogen (g)}_{\text{Output}}$$

$$\text{Nitrogen balance} = \frac{\text{protein (gm)}_{\text{Intake}}}{6.25 - \text{nitrogen (gm)}_{\text{Output}}}$$

The goal of nutritional support should be to maintain neutral or positive nitrogen balance.

The measurement of serum albumin reflects long-term nutritional status (18–21 days) and therefore does not accurately measure the acute metabolic stress of surgery. Weight loss is also not an accurate measure of short-term stress; additionally, small fluctuations in body weight are readily attributable to changes in fluid status. While retinol binding protein (RBP) has been promoted as a measure of nutritional status, its ability to accurately reflect acute metabolic stress is limited by its variable response to other stimuli such as infection.

Bibliography

Pingleton SK. Nutrition in chronic critical illness. *Clin Chest Med* 2001;22(1):149–163.

9. **(B)** Obesity is a health problem with increasing prevalence in the United States. Obesity affects approximately one-third of all Americans and in those with heart failure it has been found to be the sole risk factor in 11% of men and 14% of women. The appropriate calculation of nutritional requirements is crucial to the obese critical care patient.

Height-to-weight tables should be used to determine the IBW. Obesity is defined as 120% above the calculated IBW. The nutritional calculations should be done using the adjusted body weight.

$$\text{Adjusted weight} = \text{ideal body weight}$$
$$+ 0.25 \text{ (actual body weight}$$
$$- \text{ideal body weight)}$$

The obese critical care patient should have caloric needs calculated and nutritional supplementation initiated using the same guidelines and timelines as nonobese patients.

Bibliography

Kenchaiah S, Evans JC, Levy D, et al. Obesity and the risk of heart failure. *N Engl J Med* 2002;347:305–313.

Moore FA, McQuiggan M. Nutritional support of the stressed intensive care unit patient. In: Hall JB, Freid EB (eds.), *Society of Critical Care Medicine and American College of Chest Physicians 4th Combined Critical Care Course*. New York, NY, 2002.

10. **(D)**

11. **(C)** Several large trials performed in the 1990s determined bacterial species of critical care patients with aspiration pneumonia using protected brush specimens. Only 19% of patients grew an identifiable organism in quantities sufficient for identification. It was determined that in contrast to previous trials, anaerobic infection was not the most common type and the identifiable organism was dependent on if the pneumonia was community acquired or hospital acquired.

The most common community acquired organisms are *Streptococcus pneumonia*, *Staphylococcus aureus*, *Haemophilus influenzae*, and enterobacter species. In the aspiration pneumonia suffered by hospitalized patients, *Pseudomonas aeruginosa* and other gram-negative species were the most common.

For patients with an aspiration pneumonia antibiotic therapy must be started at once. Empiric therapy should be started immediately and directed toward the most likely organisms and the spectrum narrowed once the pneumonia has been speciated.

In the hospitalized patient, empiric antibiotics must be directed toward gram-negative organisms. Antibiotic choices include third generation cephalosporins, fluouroquinolones, and piperacillins. Both large trials showed there to be no patients that speciated to an anaerobic organism. It is not recommended to start an anaerobic antibiotic agent unless there is evidence of pulmonary abscess or periodontal disease. Commonly chosen single coverage antibiotics such as clindamycin and penicillin have inappropriate gram-negative coverage spectrums for hospitalized patients with aspiration pneumonia.

Bibliography

Marik PE. Aspiration pneumonitis and aspiration pneumonia. *N Engl J Med* 2001;344:665–671.

Marik PE, Careau P. The role of anaerobes in patients with ventilator-associated pneumonia and aspiration pneumonia: a prospective study. *Chest* 1999;115:178–183.

Mier L, Dreyfuss D, Darchy B, et al. Is penicillin G an adequate initial treatment for aspiration pneumonia? A prospective evaluation using a protected specimen brush and quantitative cultures. *Intensive Care Med* 1993;19:279–284.

12. **(B)** Aspiration pneumonitis is defined as aspiration of gastric contents resulting in acute lung injury. The risk of this adverse event is increased as the level of consciousness decreases. Referred to as Mendelson's syndrome, the level of lung injury is proportional to the acidity of the gastric contents and the presence of particulate matter. Gastric acid prevents the growth of bacteria and therefore bacterial contamination in aspiration pneumonitis is less frequently a concern. The exception to this is when there is an elevation in the pH of gastric contents as occurs with proton pump inhibitors and H2 blockers and with increased colonization, which may be seen with small bowel obstruction.

The most appropriate initial treatment option is immediate suctioning of the oropharynx to prevent further aspiration. Enteral feeds with a nasogastric tube or gastric tube should be held and the stomach aspirated. The use of empiric antibiotics in this condition is widespread and unnecessary. Antibiotic therapy is also *not* recommended in those who develop fever or leukocytosis in the first 24 h after an aspiration event, so as to avoid selection of more resistant organisms. Antibiotic management is recommended for those who may have colonization of their gastric contents or for those who fail to improve after 48 h.

Another commonly used treatment that has no proven benefit is corticosteroids. Two randomized multicenter trials have failed to show a benefit in patients with acute respiratory distress disorder treated with corticosteroid. It has been shown that there is a higher rate of gram-negative pneumonia in aspiration pneumonitis patients treated with corticosteroids. Given the current data, corticosteroid therapy cannot be recommended.

Bibliography
Bernard GR, Luce JM, Sprung CL, et al. High-dose corticosteroids in patients with the adult respiratory distress syndrome. *N Engl J Med* 1987;317:1565–1570.

Marik PE. Aspiration pneumonitis and aspiration pneumonia. *N Engl J Med* 2001;344:665–671.

Sukumaran M, Granada MJ, Berger HW, et al. Evaluation of corticosteroid treatment in aspiration of gastric contents: a controlled clinical trial. *Mt Sinai J Med* 1980; 47:335–340.

13. **(C)** This patient is suffering from niacin deficiency. Niacin is a B vitamin that is obtained from dietary sources and is primarily absorbed in the stomach and ileum. Animal protein breakdown remains the greatest source of natural dietary niacin (1.5% of tryptophan is converted into niacin). This conversion increases in deficiency states. Nicotinamide adenine dinucleotide (NAD+) and nicotinamide adenine dinucleotide phosphate (NADPH) are both coenzymes that require niacin for production. These coenzymes are necessary for glycolysis, lipid synthesis, and oxidative phosphorylation.

The U.S. Recommended Daily Allowance of niacin is 45–80 μg for men and 45–65 μg for women. In enteral support niacin intake should be 12–20 mg per day and for parenteral nutrition 40 mg per day is recommended.

The symptoms of niacin deficiency begin with nonspecific changes such as anorexia, weight loss, and weakness. Signs of later stages include the classic erythematous, scaly lesions of the extremities. Also commonly seen are stomatitis, glossitis, enteritis, and diarrhea. Malabsorption and diarrhea can facilitate greater niacin deficiency. Central nervous system symptoms include insomnia, amnesia, anxiety, depression, seizures, and psychosis. Peripheral paresthesias may also be noted.

The treatment of acute deficiency states is niacin replacement with doses of 100 mg per day. Symptoms completely and quickly resolve with correction of niacin stores.

Bibliography
Sriram K, Jayanthi V, Suchitra D. Acute niacin deficiency. *Nutrition* 1996;12:355–357.

14. **(D)** Malnutrition in the end-stage liver failure patient plays a significant role in outcome. The nutritional deficiencies are mainly because of protein malnutrition and have been shown to be an independent risk factor for mortality and life-threatening complication. The factors causing the protein loss and failure of intake are the hypermetabolism associated with end-stage liver failure necessitating a greater protein intake. A protein load in these patients can, in turn, lead to worsening encephalopathic changes.

Branched chain amino acid supplements have been used successfully in cirrhotic patients to increase the protein intake to combat nitrogen losses, while avoiding encephalopathic changes.

Long-term studies assessing the benefits of oral branched chain amino acid supplementation in these patients have found that there is no statistically significant difference in mortality. When compared with equivalent caloric and protein oral supplementation there have been shown to be significant improvements in Child-Pugh score, number of required hospital admissions, bilirubin, anorexia, and health-related quality of life. Nutritional support with branched chain amino acids has improved anthropometric measurements in this subset of malnourished patients and this correction has been proven to prolong life.

The major downside to branched chain amino acid supplementation is that the supplements are notoriously unpalatable and this had led to noncompliance and patient withdrawal from trials.

Bibliography

Fabbri A, Magrini N, Bianchi G, et al. Overview of randomized clinical trials of oral branched-chain amino acid treatment in chronic hepatic encephalopathy. *JPEN J Parenter Enteral Nutr* 1996;20:159–164.

Italian multicentre cooperative project in nutrition in liver cirrhosis. Nutritional status in cirrhosis. *J Hepatol* 1994;21:317–325.

Marchesini G, Bianchi G, Merli M, et al. Nutritional supplementation with branched-chain amino acids in advanced cirrhosis: a double-blind, randomized trial. *Gastroenterology* 2003;124:1792–1801.

Plauth M, Merli M, Kondrup J, et al. ESPEN guidelines for nutrition in liver disease and transplantation. *Clin Nutr* 1997;16:43–55.

15. **(D)** Trace elements represent less than 0.1% of the average diet. Deficiencies are found mostly in malnourished patients and those receiving hyperalimentation without trace elements. Although not commonly seen, the clinician should be familiar with the function of each of the trace elements and the key signs of their deficiencies.

Zinc deficiencies develop in patients who have a persistently catabolic state or chronic diarrhea. Normal daily zinc requirements are 3–6 mg. Greater amounts are required in patients with excessive diarrhea or short bowel syndrome. When zinc stores are depleted patients will often present with alopecia, hypogonadism, olfactory dysfunction, darkening of the skin creases, perioral pustular rash, impaired wound healing, and growth arrest.

Selenium deficiency is a rare condition and is associated with cardiomyopathy.

Copper is a key component of intracellular and extracellular enzymes. Deficiency is seen in chronic parenteral nutrition patients without adequate replacement. Symptoms of deficiency are hypochromic microcytic anemia, neutropenia, and diarrhea.

Chromium deficiency is almost always seen in patients on parenteral nutrition without appropriate replacement. The daily amount of chromium required in parenteral nutrition to avoid insufficient states is 15–20 μg per day. The classic presentation of deficient patients is a suddenly hyperglycemic state with peripheral neuropathy and encephalopathy.

Fluorine is a known to be essential in structural support for bones and teeth. Lack of adequate fluorine results in dental caries.

Iron is known to be essential for the production of hemoglobin. Patients with inadequate iron supplies, along with microcytic anemia, will often demonstrate glossitis and stomatitis.

Molybdenum is another rare trace element; patients show neurologic abnormalities and night blindness in molybdenum-deficient states.

Bibliography

Fischer JE. Metabolism in surgical patients: protein, carbohydrate, and fat utilization by oral and parenteral routes. In: Townsend CM, Beauchamp RD, Evers BM, Mattox KL (eds.), *Sabiston Textbook of Surgery: The Biologic Basis of Modern Surgical Practice*, 16th ed. Philadelphia, PA: W.B. Saunders, 1997, 90–130.

Szeto WY, Buzby GP. Nutrition, digestion and absorption. In: Kreisel D, Krupnick AS, Kaiser LR (eds.), *The Surgical Review: An Integrated Basic and Clinical Science Study Guide*. Philadelphia, PA: Lippincott, Williams & Wilkins, 2001, 272–291.

16. **(E)** Vitamins are essential elements of nutrition and cannot be synthesized by the body. The fat soluble vitamins are vitamins A, D, E, and K and are stored in body fat. Deficiencies in vitamin A (retinol) cause xerophthalmia and keratomalacia. Vitamin D (cholecalciferol) plays a key role in calcium absorption. It is converted to calcitrol in the kidney and liver; insufficient supply of vitamin D leads to rickets in children and osteomalacia in adults. Deficiency of vitamin E (α–tocopherol), an antioxidant, results in hemolytic anemia and neurologic changes. Vitamin K (naphthoquinone) plays a role in the function of certain coagulation factors (II, VII, IX, X, protein C, and protein S).

The water soluble vitamins include those in the B complex and vitamin C. Thiamine (vitamin B_1) deficiency leads to heart failure, beriberi, neuropathy, and fatigue. Riboflavin (vitamin B_2) is involved in oxidation-reduction reactions and glossitis and dermatitis are the most common features of its deficiency. Pyridoxal phosphate (vitamin B_6) deficiency leads to neuropathy, glossitis, and anemia. Dermatitis and alopecia are the features of biotin (vitamin B_7) deficiency. Folate (vitamin B_9) plays a role in DNA synthesis and its deficiencies are associated with megaloblastic anemia and glossitis. Cyanocobalamin (vitamin B_{12}) is involved in DNA synthesis and myelination and predictably megaloblastic anemia and neuropathy are the signs associated with its deficiency.

Vitamin C (ascorbic acid) hydroxylates proline in collagen synthesis. Scurvy is seen in those lacking artificial or organic supplies of vitamin C.

Bibliography

Szeto WY, Buzby GP. Nutrition, digestion and absorption. In: Kreisel D, Krupnick AS, Kaiser LR (eds.), *The Surgical Review: An Integrated Basic and Clinical Science Study Guide*. Philadelphia, PA: Lippincott, Williams & Wilkins, 2001, 272–291.

17. (C) The controversy over the appropriate route for nutrition in the acute pancreatitis patient is still a topic of heated discussion. The physiologic insult resulting from acute and even chronic pancreatitis induces a state of stress metabolism. This is generally compounded with prehospitalization starvation because of poor oral intake secondary to gastroparesis, small bowel ileus, and/or nausea and vomiting. Also a factor is the malabsorption and often alcoholism seen frequently in the chronic pancreatitis patient. These factors all contribute to the importance of promptly starting and continuing nutritional support in these patients.

In the past, patients with episodes of acute pancreatitis requiring nutrition were given parenteral nutrition in order to avoid excess exocrine stimulation of the pancreas. The avoidance of enteral feeding has not been shown to improve patient outcomes, other than decreased pain. Clinical studies have shown that feeds into the jejunum result in clinically insignificant levels of pancreatic exocrine stimulation when compared to feeds to more proximal segments of small bowel and the stomach. There has also been evidence that elemental enteral formulas, in comparison to intact protein formulas decrease exocrine stimulation of the pancreas.

The need for nutrition in these patients is essential and a persistently negative nitrogen balance in acute pancreatitis patient has been shown to increase mortality. Several prospective randomized studies have demonstrated that in comparison with parenteral feeding, transpyloric enteral feeding has fewer total and infectious complications and was well tolerated in the study groups. The cost of parenteral nutrition is significantly more than enteral feeding as well. It is now recommended that in pancreatitis patients without an ileus, transpyloric feeding is a more efficacious and economical form of nutrition.

Bibliography

Baron TH, Morgan DE. Acute necrotizing pancreatitis. *N Engl J Med* 1999;340:1412–1417.

Kalfarentzos F, Kehagias J, Mead N, et al. Enteral nutrition is superior to parenteral nutrition in severe acute pancreatitis: results of a randomized prospective trial. *Br J Surg* 1997;84:1665–1669.

McClace SA, Snider H, Owens N, et al. Clinical nutrition in pancreatitis. *Dig Dis Sci* 1997;42:2035–2044.

Windsor AC, Kanwar S, Li AG, et al. Compared with parenteral nutrition, enteral feeding attenuates the acute phase response and improves disease severity in acute pancreatitis. *Gut* 1998;42:431–435.

18. (B, C, E) The patient is suffering from refeeding syndrome. This is a potentially morbid condition associated with electrolyte and fluid shifts in the malnourished patient resuming feeds.

This syndrome can be seen after the onset of parenteral or enteral feeding in any chronically malnourished patient, especially those in which there has been a greater than a 15% weight loss over several months. The patients studied who had conditions for which this has been described include: prisoners of war, prolonged fasting, weight loss in patients after obesity surgery, alcoholics, malnourished elderly, those undergoing chemotherapy, and patients with eating disorders.

Fluid balance abnormalities, vitamin B_1 deficiency, hypophosphatemia, hypomagnesemia, and hypokalemia are the main features seen with refeeding syndrome. The physiology centers on the conversion of starvation lipid metabolism to refeeding carbohydrate metabolism. The insulin release causes intracellular uptake of glucose, phosphate, potassium, magnesium, water, and protein.

The fluid disturbances center on dehydration and resultant prerenal azotemia. Compounding this problem is the glucose disturbance of hyperglycemia which can cause osmotic diuresis and hyperosmolar nonketotic coma.

Decrease in phosphate is the most commonly seen electrolyte abnormality in refeeding syndrome. The clinical manifestations are impaired skeletal muscle function, diaphragmatic muscle weakness, cardiomyopathy, thrombocytopenia, decreased chemotaxis, hemolysis, paresthesias, and seizures. Thiamine deficiency is also often noted and presents with Wernicke's encephalopathy, ocular disturbances, short-term memory loss, confusion ataxia, and coma. Hypomagnesemia is also seen and presents with cardiac arrhythmias (torsade de pointes) and neurologic changes. Cardiac arrhythmias including cardiac arrest are the most commonly seen manifestations of hypokalemia, another electrolyte abnormality that is seen with refeeding syndrome.

The treatment of patients with electrolyte abnormalities because of refeeding syndrome should be prompt correction of deficiencies and frequent electrolyte monitoring. Prevention should be an important aspect of avoiding severe complications of this syndrome. All patients who are malnourished should have electrolytes corrected before starting feeding and should be monitored frequently after the start of either parenteral or enteral nutrition. Patients that are at high risk for refeeding syndrome should have a gradual increase in feeds from 20 kcal/kg per day to goal over a period of 5–7 days, or until the patient is metabolically stable.

Bibliography

Blackburn GL, Jensen GL. Severe hypophosphatemia related to refeeding. *Nutrition* 1996;12:538–539.

Crook MA, Hally V, Panteli JV. The importance of the refeeding syndrome. *Nutrition* 2001;17:632–637.

Solomon SM, Kirby DF. The refeeding syndrome: a review. *JPEN J Parenter Enteral Nutr* 1990;14:90–96.

19. **(A)** Carbohydrates in the diet that reach the colon unabsorbed by the small bowel are fermented by anaerobic bacteria to form SCFAs. The most abundant SCFAs are butyrate, propionate, and acetate, with butyrate being the preferred substrate for the colonocyte. SCFAs are rapidly absorbed from the colonic lumen, and their oxidation inside the colonocyte is the major energy source of the colorectal epithelium.

In patients with normal small bowel function, colonic SCFAs provide only 5–10% of daily calories; however, some studies have shown that the colon can be an energy salvage organ in patients with decreased small bowel function. In one study, preservation of half of colon length decreased parenteral energy requirements by half in patients with short gut syndrome.

In addition to being an energy source, SCFAs have been proposed to be involved in various cell-signaling systems in the colonocyte. Impaired metabolism of SCFAs has been implicated in the pathogenesis of ulcerative colitis.

Bibliography

Clausen MR, Mortensen PB. Kinetic studies on colonocyte metabolism of short chain fatty acids and glucose in ulcerative colitis. *Gut* 1995;37:684–689.

Jeppesen PB, Mortensen PB. Significance of a preserved colon for parenteral energy requirements in patients receiving home parenteral nutrition. *Scand J Gastroenterol* 1998;33:1175–1179.

Ohkusa T, Okayasu I, Ogihara T, Morita K, Ogawa M, Sato N. Induction of experimental ulcerative colitis by *Fusobacterium varium* isolated from colonic mucosa of patients with ulcerative colitis. *Gut* 2003;52:79–83.

CHAPTER 3

Wound Healing and Care

Carlos A. Vieira, Maria A.S. Vieira, and Clark Simons

Questions

1. Regarding Fig. 3-1, which of the following statements is *correct*?

    (A) Lymphocytes play a major role in phase I.
    (B) Wound healing is definitive by 6 months.
    (C) Epithelialization occurs in phase III.
    (D) Granulation tissue formation develops in phase II.
    (E) Myofibroblasts produce contracture of the wound in phase II.

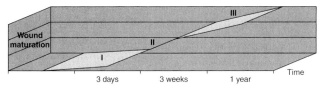

FIG. 3-1 Phases of wound maturation: I-Inflammation, II-Proliferation, and III-Maturation.

2. A 39-year-old male underwent a ventral hernia repair with prosthetic mesh. The peak of collagen production in his wound will be achieved by day

    (A) 2
    (B) 7
    (C) 14
    (D) 21
    (E) 28

3. The maximum net collagen content for the patient in Question 2 will be achieved by day

    (A) 7
    (B) 14
    (C) 21
    (D) 42
    (E) 90

4. The greatest burst strength of the wound will be achieved by

    (A) 1 week
    (B) 3 weeks
    (C) 6 weeks
    (D) 12 weeks
    (E) 6 months

5. The same patient comes back for a 3-week follow-up visit. Figure 3-2 depicts the patient's wound after removal of the staples. The next step on the management of this patient is as follows:

    (A) primary closure of the skin with stitches
    (B) mesh irrigation with antibiotic solution daily and closure of the wound by secondary intention
    (C) wound debridement and placement of a new PTFE mesh
    (D) removal of PTFE mesh and placement of polypropylene mesh
    (E) removal of PTFE mesh and closure of the wound with Vicryl mesh

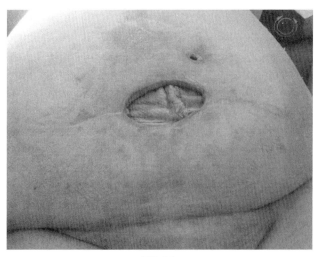

FIG. 3-2

6. The same patient comes back to your office for a follow-up visit. His skin was left open after the second repair and he is doing wet to dry dressing changes with normal saline twice a day. It seems that the wound didn't decrease in size since the last visit. An alternative to manage this patient wound is

   (A) tell the patient that there is nothing else to do and continue to do dressing changes with normal saline twice a day
   (B) increase frequency of dressing changes to three times a day
   (C) closure of the wound with stitches
   (D) closure of the wound with staples
   (E) placement of a vacuum-assisted device system (V.A.C.)

7. A 35-year-old female underwent a ventral hernia repair around 6 months ago. She comes back complaining of a nodule at the incision site. The nodule is excised and microscopically revealed macrophages, collagen, and giant cells. Also a polarized refractile material is present in the nodule. What is the most likely diagnosis (see Fig. 3-3)?

   (A) normal wound healing
   (B) abscess formation
   (C) suture granuloma
   (D) hypertrophic scar
   (E) keloid

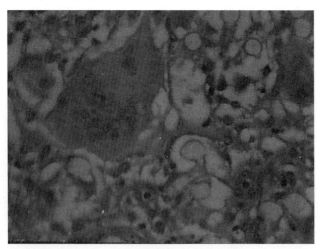

FIG. 3-3

8. A 60-year-old male underwent an elective, uncomplicated femoral hernia repair. The appearance of this wound section in Fig. 3-4 is most likely to be seen how long after the surgery?

   (A) 1 day
   (B) 2 days
   (C) 7 days
   (D) 14 days
   (E) 1 month

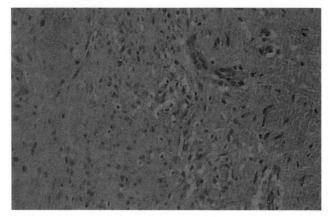

FIG. 3-4

9. A 45-year-old male undergoes an exploratory laparotomy because of a perforated duodenal ulcer. Intraoperatively 1.5 L of turbid fluid is found. After closing fascia the best management of his wound is

   (A) closure of skin with staples
   (B) interrupted skin closure
   (C) closure of skin with Dermabond
   (D) wound left open and local wound care
   (E) subcuticular skin closure

10. A 70-year-old male underwent a total gastrectomy. His chances of developing wound dehiscence are increased due to all of the following except:

   (A) decrease cellular migration and proliferation
   (B) decreased rate of wound capillary growth
   (C) decrease epithelialization
   (D) delayed wound contraction
   (E) decreased elastin degradation

11. Patients with chronic granulomatous disease (CGD) are more susceptible to infections. Which is the mechanism responsible for their immunosupression?

   (A) defective lysosome release
   (B) decreased synthesis of interleukin (IL)-1 and tumor necrosis factor-alpha (TNF-α)
   (C) lack of opsonization
   (D) lack of oxygen-dependent killing of bacteria by neutrophils
   (E) deficiency of selectins

12. A 5-year-old male present with a recurrent history of pyogenic infections. He always has a normal white blood cell count. An analysis of the patient's neutrophils is performed and revealed a defect in neutrophil rolling. Which of the following is the most likely diagnosis?

    (A) decreased neutrophil rolling is normal in children
    (B) chronic granulomatous disease
    (C) selectin deficiency
    (D) integrin deficiency
    (E) immunoglobulin deficiency

13. A 65-year-old male underwent a colectomy because of colon cancer. Just after surgery, you found out that he has been taking aspirin daily. Which one of the following features of the inflammatory response will be ablated in this patient?

    (A) chemotaxis
    (B) vasodilatation
    (C) cytokine release
    (D) collagen synthesis
    (E) fibroblastic proliferation

14. A 45-year-old female underwent a kidney transplant 6 months ago and has been taking cyclosporine and steroids. She developed cholelithiasis and requires a laparoscopic cholecystectomy. She wants to know if her chance to have a wound infection is increased. The best answer to her question is

    (A) No, steroids and cyclosporine do not increase the chance to have wound infection when used chronically
    (B) Yes, because of inhibition of collagen synthesis and fibroblast proliferation
    (C) Yes, because of persistent vasoconstriction and hypoxia
    (D) Yes, because of structural nuclear changes and decreased DNA synthesis
    (E) Yes, mainly because of cyclosporine, which blocks IL-2 and decrease migration of macrophages

15. A 65-year-old male underwent a placement of a split thickness skin graft for a chronic wound on his thigh. You are concerned with adherence of the graft to the wound bed. Which of the following factors will downregulate wound angiogenesis?

    (A) lactate
    (B) von Hippel-Lindau protein
    (C) acidic pH
    (D) cytokines
    (E) Prostaglandins

16. With regards to cytokines, which of the following alternatives is *correct*?

    (A) IL-1 is secreted mainly by lymphocytes and mediates inflammation.
    (B) IL-10 is involved in cell division and activation.
    (C) IL-8 is secreted by macrophages and promotes chemotaxis.
    (D) IL-2 is a major inhibitor of cell division.
    (E) TNF-α is produced by T cells and is associated with a rise of immature neutrophils in the blood circulation.

17. Regarding growth factors, which one of the following statements is *correct*?

    (A) Epidermal growth factor (EGF) inhibits metalloproteanases.
    (B) Platelet-derived growth factor (PDGF) is a powerful chemoattractant and influence in the deposition of extracellular matrix.
    (C) Fibroblast growth factor is secreted by lymphocytes and promotes angiogenesis.
    (D) Vascular endothelial growth factor promotes angiogenesis in healthy tissue only.
    (E) Transforming growth factor-beta (TGF-β) inhibit expression of PDGF in low doses.

18. What is the most common type of collagen in this wound (see Fig. 3-5)?

    (A) I
    (B) II
    (C) III
    (D) IV
    (E) V

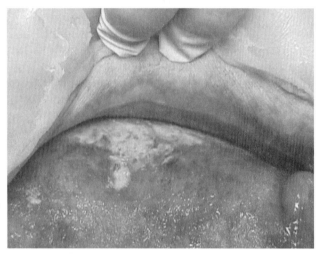

FIG. 3-5

19. In reference to Fig. 3-5, which one of the following statements is *correct*?

    (A) This tissue is rich in mature vessels.
    (B) Fibroblasts are scarce.
    (C) Exuberant granulation or proud flesh is called the excessive amount of granulation tissue deposition.
    (D) Reepithelialization occurs before granulation tissue formation.
    (E) After complete healing, skin will regain hair follicles.

20. A 35-year-old female with breast cancer underwent lumpectomy and radiation therapy. She had recurrence of the tumor and underwent a modified radical mastectomy. Regarding radiotherapy and wound healing, all of the following statements are true, *except*:

    (A) Can cause fibroblast injury.
    (B) Decrease amount of collagen deposition is seen.
    (C) Effects are reversible after 1 year of last treatment.
    (D) Radiation therapy increases the risk of wound infection.
    (E) Wound healing is impaired because of vascular damage.

21. Regarding nitric oxide (NO), which one of the following statements is *incorrect*?

    (A) Macrophages synthesized NO in the inflammatory phase of wound healing.
    (B) Arginine is substrate for NO synthesis.
    (C) Inhibition of NO decreases collagen deposition.
    (D) L-Arginine as well as NO can partially reverse the impaired healing of chronic diabetic ulcers.
    (E) NO increases cyclic adenosine monophosphate (cAMP).

22. A 32-year-old male comes back to your clinic for a 6-month follow-up after an appendectomy. He is an alcoholic, lives by himself, and states that since surgery he hasn't eaten any fruits or vegetables. On physical examination, his skin is dry with reddish spots. His appendectomy scar, which was healed 3 months after surgery, is dehisced. His gum is red, swollen, and shiny. Regarding this condition, which one of the following alternatives is *correct*?

    (A) Laboratory studies should be performed to confirm clinical diagnosis.
    (B) Leukopenia is associated in 30% of the cases.
    (C) Abnormalities are not reverse by vitamin supplementation.
    (D) Ingestion of dairy products can reverse this condition.
    (E) Dehiscence of the wound was caused most likely by infection of the wound.

23. Which of the following patients is a suitable candidate to undergo hyperbaric oxygenation (HBO) therapy because of chronic nonhealing wound at the right thorax?

    (A) 56-year-old male with untreated pneumothorax
    (B) 35-year-old male receiving cisplatinum for testicular carcinoma
    (C) 45-year-old female 35% burn patient treated with sulfamylon
    (D) 55-year-old male alcoholic treated with disulfiram
    (E) 65-year-old female s/p chest radiation, heart transplant with wound dehiscence because of infection

24. Regarding matrix metalloproteinases (MMPs), which one of the following statements is *correct*?

    (A) MMPs are always present in chronic wounds.
    (B) Disruption of basal membrane apparently is a critical determinant for collagenases activity.

(C) Cytokines down regulate the activity of MMPs.

(D) MMPs are secreted in their active form.

(E) MMPs are stored intracellularly for long periods of time.

25. The differences between a keloid and a hypertrophic scar include all of the following *except*

(A) presence of antinuclear antibodies against fibroblast

(B) levels of adenosine triphosphate

(C) collagen bundles with a glazed appearance

(D) scar limits

(E) the predominate collagen is type I

26. Regarding the condition illustrated by Fig. 3-6, which alternative is *correct*?

(A) It is limited to the area of wound healing.

(B) It is preventable.

(C) It is most common on lower extremities, lower back, and abdomen.

(D) Histologically, keloid scar and hypertrophic scar are no different.

(E) Collagen type I is the predominant type of collagen found in keloid scar.

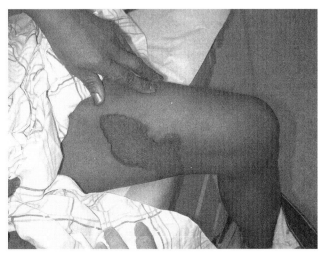

FIG. 3-6

27. Regarding Fig. 3-7, which one of the following statements is *incorrect*?

(A) It is a preventable condition.

(B) Tension during closure is a contributory factor.

(C) Scar parallel to the underlying muscle may prevent this condition.

(D) Infection is a common cause for this condition.

(E) Fibroblasts in this type of scar produce more TGF-β-1.

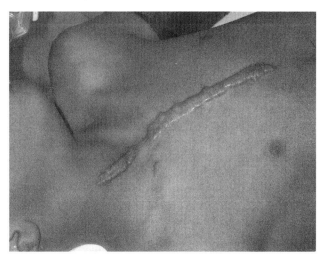

FIG. 3-7

28. A 65-year-old white male sustained a gunshot wound to his right lower extremity at the Vietnam War. He is being seen in your clinic because of intermittent drainage from his chronic leg wound (see Fig. 3-8). The most appropriate management of this patient is

(A) wet to dry dressing changes with normal saline and follow-up in 1 month.

(B) Silvadene to the wound and follow-up in 1 month

(C) x-ray of the lower extremity

(D) biopsy of the wound

(E) exploration of the wound

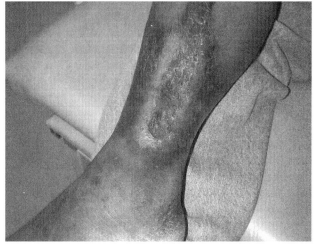

FIG. 3-8

29. Which of the statements is *incorrect* regarding the cell represented in Fig. 3-9?

    (A) This cell uses fibronectin as provisional stroma for ingrowth.

    (B) Cell proliferation is non-cytokine-dependent.

    (C) Collagen synthesis by this cell starts around 3rd day postinjury.

    (D) Matrix metalloproteases (MMPs) are secreted by this cell.

    (E) Participates actively in wound contraction.

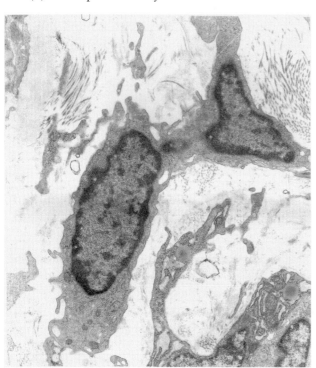

FIG. 3-9

30. Regarding vitamins and wound healing, which one of the following statements is false?

    (A) Reverse of vitamin C deficiency can be obtained with ingestion of 100 mg of ascorbic acid per day.

    (B) Vitamin A can reduce the poor impact of steroids in wound healing.

    (C) Zinc deficiency can reduce bursting strength of the wound.

    (D) Catabolic bioproducts of arginine can retard wound healing.

    (E) Vitamin E has anti-inflammatory properties.

31. Regarding the inflammatory phase of wound healing, which one of the following alternatives is *correct*?

    (A) After initial injury, the first cells to arrive to the wound are neutrophils.

    (B) Immediately vasodilatation occurs in order to increase cellular inflow to the wound.

    (C) Neutrophils are essential for wound healing.

    (D) Lymphocytes play a major role in wounds critically contaminated.

    (E) IL-2 down regulates the initial inflammatory process.

32. Regarding knot-tying techniques, which one of the following statements is true about Fig. 3-10?

    (A) This knot-tying technique is as efficient as square knots.

    (B) Crossing of the hands is necessary to tie down this knot.

    (C) Greater knot security is achieved when tension is applied during knot throws.

    (D) Equal distribution of forces is applied during this knot throw.

    (E) Multifilament sutures tend to slip more than monofilament sutures.

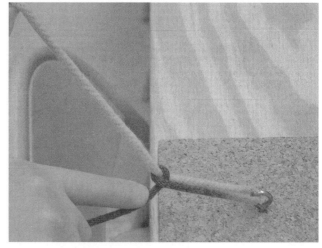

FIG. 3-10

33. Regarding biodegradation of suture material, which one of the following alternatives is *incorrect*?

    (A) Degradation of suture materials is mainly through hydrolysis.

    (B) Profile of strength loss always proceeds the profile of mass or weight loss in sutures.

(C) Variation of pH has little effect on suture biodegradation.

(D) Gamma-irradiation accelerates loss of tensile strength of different sutures.

(E) Because of the lack of hydrolysable bounds, polyethylene and polypropylene are not subjected to hydrolytic degradation.

34. What is the predominant type of collagen in this wound (see Fig. 3-11)?

(A) I

(B) II

(C) III

(D) IV

(E) V

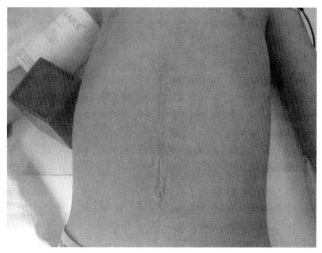

FIG. 3-11

35. What is most abundant type of collagen in the human body?

(A) I

(B) II

(C) III

(D) IV

(E) V

36. Regarding collagen, which one of the following statements is *incorrect*?

(A) Collagen is the principal component of the extracellular matrix.

(B) Collagen type I replaces collagen type III during maturation of the wound.

(C) Deposition of collagen type I starts around the 14th day postinjury.

(D) Hypoxia and accumulation of lactate stimulate increase collagen production.

(E) Exposure of fibrillar collagen to blood promotes aggregation and activation of platelets.

37. Regarding collagen structure and synthesis, which one of the following statements is *incorrect*?

(A) Prolyl hydroxylase is one of the rate-limiting enzymes for the synthesis of this molecule.

(B) Precursor forms are manufactured intracellular.

(C) Final molecule is a three alpha-peptide chain in a right-handed helix.

(D) Fibroblast actively secretes collagen, which is ready to be used.

(E) Accumulation of collagen depends on the ratio of collagen synthesis and collagen degradation.

38. Regarding the event depicted in Fig. 3-12, which of the following statements is *correct*?

(A) It is always a pathologic event.

(B) Failure to exclude vital dye is observed.

(C) There is an early disruption of membranes.

(D) Ladder pattern of DNA fragments is observed.

(E) Chromatin is loose and nucleolus is absent.

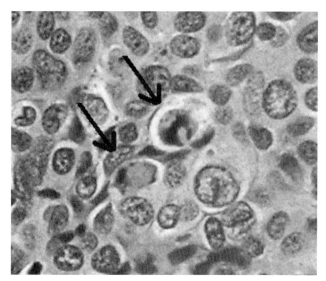

FIG. 3-12

39. Which one of the following statements is *incorrect* about fibronectin?

(A) Fibronectins are encoded by a single gene.

(B) Major functions are to mediate cellular adhesion and to promote cell migration.

(C) Tissue plasminogen activator (TPA) competes with fibronectin for fibrin-binding domains.

(D) Collagen usually serves as a template for fibronectin deposition.

(E) Fibronectin matrix is easily degraded by proteases.

40. Regarding proteoglycans, which one of the following statements is *incorrect*?

(A) Contain a core protein to which at least one glycosaminoglycan chain is covalently bound.

(B) Can be found in secretory granules, extracellular matrix, or as an intrinsic or extrinsic cell membrane protein.

(C) Functions of these molecules include extracellular organization, promotion of growth factor receptor binding, regulation of blood coagulation.

(D) Condroitin-4-sulfate occurs in high levels in mature scar.

(E) Proteoglycans levels during wound healing sustained minimal variation.

41. Regarding laminin, which one of the following statements is *incorrect*?

(A) Laminin is the most abundant glycoprotein of the basal membrane.

(B) Basal membrane is rich in collagen type IV.

(C) In endothelial cell cultures exposed to fibroblast growth factor (FGF), laminin causes alignment of endothelial cells.

(D) Laminin is not secreted by tumor cells.

(E) Fifty percent of classic type congenital muscular dystrophy (CMD) cases are associated with a deficiency of the basal lamina protein alpha$_2$-laminin.

Answers and Explanations

1. **(D)** Wound healing can be divided into three phases: inflammation, proliferation, and maturation. During the inflammatory phase, injury to the skin promotes cell migration (in order of appearance: platelets, neutrophils, lymphocytes, and fibroblasts). Macrophages play a key role during the inflammatory phase; cleaning debris, releasing cytokines, and promoting chemotaxis.

Once the provisional extracellular matrix with fibronectin has been made cells continue to migrate until they reach other migrating cells, leading to contact inhibition. By 48 h the wound is completely epithelialized (and the surgical dressing can be safely removed). Cellular proliferation continues, as epidermis is reconstructed. The inflammatory phase resolves after 72 h.

The appearance of fibroblasts marks the beginning of the proliferative phase. Collagen starts releasing and turnover of the extracellular matrix is an ongoing process until the wound is mature (1–2 years after injury). Granulation tissue formation is characteristic of the proliferative phase and serves as bridge for wound maturation, especially in open wounds.

Initially, angiogenesis parallels the deposition of collagen. New capillaries that reconstruct the vasculature are stimulated by high lactate levels, acidic pH, and low oxygen tension. The migration and revascularization of endothelial cells is facilitated by the formation of a new extracellular matrix formation of new capillary vessels.

Wound contraction begins 4–5 days after injury. Myofibroblasts are modified fibroblasts that interact with extracellular matrix, leading to wound contraction. It appears that wound contraction is more dependent of myofibroblasts than collagen synthesis.

During maturation phase (remodeling), fibroblasts and macrophages disappear and the wound collagen content stabilizes. Old collagen is broken and new collagen is synthesized in a denser, more organized fashion. The number of intermolecular cross-links between collagen molecules increased significantly. Slowly, as wound matures, collagen type III is replaced by collagen type I.

Bibliography

Cotran RS, Kumar V, Collins T. Robbins. *Pathologic Basis of Disease*, 6th ed. St. Louis, MO: W.B. Saunders, 1999.

2. **(B)**

3. **(D)**

4. **(E)**

Explanations 2 through 4

Collagen secretion by fibroblasts begins 10–72 h after injury. Production of collagen increases rapidly, achieving its peak by 7 days. After 3 weeks the rate of collagen synthesis decline and a balance between the rates of collagen deposition/degradation will be achieved. The maximum net collagen deposition normally is achieved by 6 weeks.

As collagen deposition continues with scar remodeling wounds will gradually increase their burst strength.

After 3 weeks, wound burst/tensile strength is only 15–30%. After the initial phase of the maturation process this number increases to 80%, and plateaus around 90% after 6 months.

Although collagen turnover is an ongoing process, the wound will never regain the tensile strength of normal skin (see Fig. 3-13).

Bibliography

Lawrence WT. Wound healing biology and its application to wound management. In: O'Leary JP (ed.), *The Physiologic Basis of Surgery*, 2nd ed. Baltimore, MD: Williams & Wilkins, 1996, 118–140.

5. **(E)** Many different techniques have been employed to close abdominal wall defects. Primary repairs of ventral hernia have been associated with an incidence of recurrence of as high as 50%. Significantly better results have

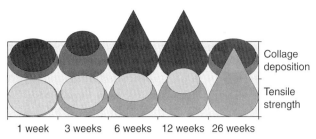

FIG. 3-13   Relation of collagen deposition and tensile strength. By 26 weeks the wound reaches 90% of its tensile strength with minimal collagen deposition.

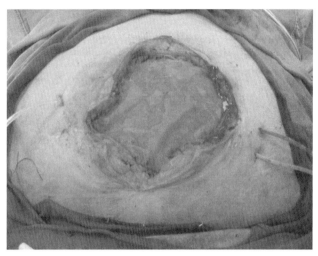

FIG. 3-15   Placement of Vicryl mesh on a large ventral hernia defect after removal of permanent mesh.

been achieved with mesh repairs with recurrence rates of around 6%. Although the use of mesh decreases the risk of recurrence, complications such as wound infection and intestinal fistula formation (see Fig. 3-14) occur more frequent when a foreign body material is used.

Polyethylene terephthalate (Mersilene), polytetrafluoroethylene (PTFE) and polypropylene (Marlex, Prolene) are some of the commercially nonabsorbable materials available for hernia repair.

In case of wound infection, mesh exposure, or enteric fistula formation, the best alternative of treatment is removal of the foreign material and primary closure of the fascia when possible, or placement of an absorbable mesh such as polyglactin 910 (see Fig. 3-15). The use of an absorbable mesh provides safe coverage of the abdominal contents, and decreases the incidence of abdominal compartment syndrome. Unlike permanent mesh, absorbable mesh does not chronically harbor infection, allowing local and systemic clearance of the infectious process. Unfortunately, the use of absorbable mesh will universally lead to ventral hernia recurrence, which will be cared for at a later date.

Bibliography

Scott DJ, Jones DB. Hernias and abdominal wall defects. In: Norton J, et al. (eds.), *Surgery, Basic Science and Clinical Evidence.* New York, NY: Springer, 2001, 814–817.

6. **(E)** A novel approach to improve healing of open abdominal wounds is the V.A.C. system (see Fig. 3-16). The V.A.C. therapy system consists of a computer-controlled therapy unit, canister, sterile plastic tubing, foam dressing, and clear V.A.C. drape dressing. The foam dressing is placed into the wound. One end of the tube is connected to the foam, the other end to a

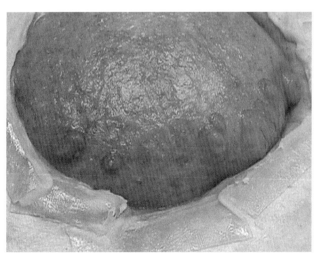

FIG. 3-14   Open wound with multiple enterocutaneous fistuale.

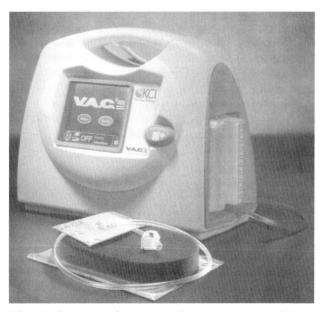

FIG. 3-16   Complete V.A.C. system, including the computer-controlled unit, canister, plastic tubing, foam dressing, and clear tape dressing.

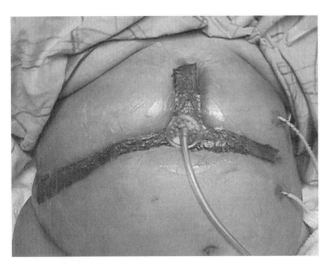

FIG. 3-17   V.A.C. dressing place on an open wound.

canister that connects to the V.A.C. control unit. The wound area is sealed with the clear V.A.C. drape, similar to a large bandage (see Fig. 3-17). The V.A.C. system pulls infectious materials and other fluids from the wound through the tube and collects them inside the canister.

The V.A.C system can be used in dehisce wounds, flaps and skin grafts, chronic wounds (diabetic or pressure ulcers), and for temporary abdominal wall closure.

V.A.C. promotes healing applying controlled negative pressure (vacuum) to the wound. It also helps to debride and to clean the contaminated wound bed. It does not replace sharp debridement of contaminated wounds and should not be used in wounds with necrotic or scar tissue.

Bibliography

Banwell PE. Topical negative therapy in wound care. J Wound Care 1999;8(2):79–84.

7. **(C)** Typically, giant cells are seen in the presence of foreign bodies. The polarize refractile material, however, is diagnostic of a suture granuloma. No inflammatory infiltrate is seen, characteristic of abscess formation. Hypertrophic and keloid scars present normally with thickening of the scar and increased collagen deposition at the wound.

Suture granuloma is a well-recognized surgical complication that can mislead clinicians. Suture granulomas can be responsible for chronic open wounds or for persistent hematuria on kidney transplant recipients, or can be the cause of infection after a ventral hernia repair with mesh. Enterocutaneus fistula formation can also be attributed to suture granuloma.

Suture granulomas can lead to false-positive results when staging tumors with positron emission tomography (PET) scan because of the uptake by histiocytes of F 2-fluoro-2-deoxy-D-glucose (FDG). The diagnosis of suture granuloma is clinical and the treatment consists of granuloma resection. Most of the symptoms associated with suture granuloma will fade away after resection of the foreign body.

Bibliography

Cotran RS, Kumar V, Collins T, Robbins S. *Pathologic Basis of Disease*, 6th ed. St. Louis, MO: W.B. Saunders, 1999, 110.
Holder WD, White RL, Zuger JH, Easton EJ, Greene FL. Effectiveness of Positron Emisson Tomography for the Detection of Melanoma Metastases. *Ann Surg* 1998;227(5):764–771.

8. **(E)** This patient underwent an elective procedure, with primary closure of the wound. After 1 month of the initial injury, dense collagen deposition can be seen as shown in Fig. 3-4.

On the first 24 h an inflammatory infiltrate would be noticed. By 72 h granulation tissue is seen followed by neovascularization. By the second to third week, collagen is prominent and inflammatory cells are seen, but scarce.

Intrinsic and extrinsic factors have a direct impact on how fast a wound will heal. Loss of tissue, bacteria contamination, and the presence of foreign body are all extrinsic factors that can limit the process of healing. Cardiovascular disease, renal failure, nutrition, age are some of the intrinsic factors that can retard significantly wound healing.

Wound closure can be divided in three categories: primary, secondary, and tertiary. Primary or first-intention closures are wounds immediately sealed by suturing, stapling, skin grafting, or by flap placement. Secondary closure involves no active sealing of the wound. The wound is left open because of gross contamination of the surgical field. Closure of the wound will be achieved by contraction and epithelialization. Wound closure by tertiary intention involves delay closure of an infected wound after debridement, and local and systemic antibiotic treatment. It is also known as delay primary closure.

Bibliography

Cotran RS, Kumar V, Collins T, Robbins S. *Pathologic Basis of Disease*, 6th ed. St. Louis, MO: W.B. Saunders, 1999, 98–99.

9. **(D)** Secondary intention healing occurs because of the interaction of multiple forces. Wound contraction is the most important factor. Decrease edema, collagen

TABLE 3-1   Traditional Classification of Operative Wounds

Clean (class I)	Nontraumatic, uninfected wounds; no inflammation; primarily closed; no break in aseptic technique
Clean-contaminated (class II)	Alimentary, respiratory or genitourinary tract entered under controlled conditions; no contamination; minor break in aseptic technique
Contaminated (class III)	Fresh traumatic wounds; gross spillage from gastrointestinal tract; acute, nonpurulent inflammation; major break in technique
Dirty/infected (class IV)	Traumatic wounds with retained devitalized tissue, foreign bodies or fecal contamination; perforated viscus; acute, purulent bacterial inflammation

synthesis, and deposition of granulation tissue are contributor factors. A wound left open will fill with granulation tissue and contraction will help to pull normal, healthy tissue to close the defect. Wounds are normally left open after gross contamination of the surgical field.

In 1964, the National Research Council (NRC) proposed the idea of using wound classification to predict risk for surgical site infection.

Wounds were divided as clean, clean/contaminated, contaminated, and dirty/infected (Table 3-1).

Wound infection rates for these four wound classes are 1.5–2.9% for clean, 2.8–7.7% for clean-contaminated, 6.4–15.2% for contaminated, and 7.1–40% for dirty wounds.

Bibliography

Altemeier WA, Burke JF, Pruitt BA, Sandusky WR (eds.). *Manual on Control of Infection in Surgical Patients.* Philadelphia, PA: Lippincott-Raven, 1984.

Cotran RS, Kumar V, Collins T. Robbins. *Pathologic Basis of Disease*, 6th ed. St. Louis, MO: W.B. Saunders, 1999, 108–110.

Dellinger EP, Ehrenkranz NJ. Surgical infections. In: Bennett JV, Brachman PS (eds.), *Hospital Infections*, 4th ed. Philadelphia, PA: Lippincott-Raven, 1998, 571–585.

Howard JM, Barker WF, Culbertson WR, et al. Postoperative wound infections: the influence of ultraviolet irradiation of the operating room and of various other factors. *Ann Surg* 1964;160(Suppl):1–192.

Mangram AJ, Horan TC, Pearson ML, et al. Hospital Infection Control Practices Advisory Committee. Guideline for the prevention of surgical site infection. *Infect Control Hosp Epidemiol* 1999;20:247–280.

10. **(E)** Several studies have shown that the rate of wound dehiscence in patients over 70 years is two to three times higher. Delayed wound contraction, decrease epithelialization, delayed cellular migration and proliferation, decreased rate of wound capillary growth, decreased solubility and increased sclerotic connective tissue are factors that lead to decreased wound breaking strength and increased dehiscence rate.

Dermal changes that occur with aging include decreased cellularity (especially macrophages) and decreased amounts of collagen and ground substance, leading to decreased dermal thickness. In addition, dermal collagenase activity increases, and the appearance of the elastin fibers suggests increased elastin degradation. These changes also contribute to impaired wound healing in the elderly.

Aging affects all stages of wound healing, but macrophages are particularly impacted.

Histologic features of skin aging include flattened dermal-epidermal junction, occasional nuclear atypia, fewer melanocytes, fewer Langerhans cells, fewer fibroblasts, fewer mast cells, fewer blood vessels, shortened capillary loops, abnormal nerve endings, depigmented hair, loss of hair, conversion of terminal to vellus hair, abnormal nail plates, and fewer glands.

Bibliography

Mulder GD, et al. Factors complicating wound repair. In: McCulloch JM, Kloth LC, Feedar JA (eds.), *Wound Healing Alternatives in Management*, 2nd ed. Philadelphia, PA: FA Davis, 1996, 51.

Yaar M, Gilchrest BA. Skin aging postulated mechanisms and consequent changes in structure and function. *Clin Geriatr Med* 2001;17(4):661–672.

11. **(D)** Patients with CGD characteristically experience recurrent and often severe pyogenic infections, a granulomatous tissue response, and impaired phagocyte microbicidal activity because of the absence of respiratory burst oxidase activity. Although initially described as an X-linked disorder, with males affected and mothers and sisters serving as heterozygous carriers, CGD can be transmitted with the inheritance pattern of either an autosomal or an X-linked disease, depending on the molecular defect.

CHD is characterized by reduced killing of ingested microbes because of a defective NADPH oxidase system. This system produces superoxide anions, essential for production of H_2O_2, OH, and HOCl.

The most characteristic pathogens are *Staphylococcus aureus*, *Serratia marcescens*, *Pseudomonas cepacia*, and *Aspergillus* spp., although a wide variety of other catalase-positive bacteria and fungi may cause disease as well.

The management of patients with CGD is based largely on the early recognition and aggressive treatment of infections.

Prophylactic use of antimicrobial agents is of well-established benefit in patients with CGD, and trimethoprim-sulfamethoxazole is generally preferred.

Bibliography

Nauseef WM, Clark RA. Granulocytic phagocytes. In: Mandell GL, Bennett JE, Dolin R (eds.), *Mandell: Principles and Practice of Infectious Diseases*, 5th ed. Philadelphia, PA: Churchill Livingstone, 2000, 102–103.

12. (C) This patient has a defective neutrophil rolling, the first step for transmigration of neutrophils from the vasculature to the tissues. Rolling depends on the interaction between selectins and their sialylated ligand molecules. Selectins (CD11) mediate neutrophil binding and beta$_2$-integrins (CD18) are required for further activation-induced firm sticking and emigration. Patients usually present as children with multiple recurrent pyogenic infections and a normal white blood cell count and a normal differential.

Some investigators suggest that resuscitation of patients with hypertonic saline decreases neutrophil rolling and adherence to the endothelium and reduces *in vivo* vascular leakage.

Also studies have shown that patients with systemic inflammatory response (SIRS), neonates with bacterial infections, children undergoing cardiopulmonary bypass have decrease expression of selectins, causing impaired neutrophil rolling.

Bibliography

Ahmed NA, Yee J, Giannias B, Kapadia B, Christou NV. Expression of human neutrophil L-selectin during the systemic inflammatory response syndrome is partly mediated by tumor factor alpha. *Arch Surg* 1996; 131(1):31–35; discussion 35–36.

Buhrer C, Graykucg J, Stibenz D, Dudenhausen JW, Obladen M. L-Selectin is down-regulated in umbilical cord blood granulocytes and monocytes of newborn infants with acute bacterial infections. *Pediatr Res* 1994;36:799–804.

Cotran RS, Kumar V, Collins T. Robbins. *Pathologic Basis of Disease*, 6th ed. St. Louis, MO: W.B. Saunders, 1999, 56–57.

Pascual JL, Ferri LE, Seely AJ, et al. Hypertonic saline resuscitation of hemorrhagic shock diminishes neutrophil rolling and adherence to endothelium and reduces in vivo vascular leakage. *Ann Surg* 2002;236(5): 634–642.

13. (B) Searching for a better anti-inflammatory medication for his father, Dr. Felix Hoffmann discovered acetylsalicylic acid (ASA) in 1897. ASA is hydrolyzed in the liver and excreted in the urine. As a result of the rapid hydrolysis, ASA levels are always low. The peak of salicylates level for uncoated ASA is 2 h. Prostaglandins are potent mediators of the inflammatory response. The first and committed step in the production of prostaglandins from arachidonic acid is the bis-oxygenation of arachindonate to prostaglandin, followed by reduction to PGH2. Both reactions are catalyzed by cyclooxygenase (COX), also know as PGH synthase. There are two isoforms of COX in animals: COX-1, which carries out normal, physiologic production of prostaglandins, and COX-2, which is induced by cytokines, mitogens, and endotoxins in inflammatory cells, and which is responsible for the production of prostaglandins in inflammation.

ASA is a nonselective inhibitor of COX, which blocks the COX pathway of arachidonic acid metabolism, which results in decrease prostaglandin output. Prostaglandins promote vasodilatation at the inflammatory site. Cytokine release is partially ablated by the use of aspirin. Release of IL-1 and TNF-α will not be blocked. Collagen synthesis can start as early as 10 h of the initial injury. Collagen synthesis or fibroblast proliferation is not directly affected by the use of aspirin.

Bibliography

Cotran RS, Kumar V, Collins T, Robbins S. *Pathologic Basis of Disease*, 6th ed. St. Louis, MO: W.B. Saunders, 1999, 71–72.

14. (B) During the past two decades the survival rate of solid organ recipients has improved dramatically. The major factor in improved clinical outcome is the decline in death secondary to infection. Currently, 1-year mortality caused by infection has decreased to less than 5% for renal transplant patients. Better immunosuppression and understanding by the clinician of drug pharmacodynamics and pharmacokinetics are responsible for decrease morbidity and mortality after solid organ transplantation.

Steroids reduce the inflammatory process blocking transcription of cytokine genes (especially IL-1) leading to nonspecific inhibition of T lymphocytes and macrophages. It is well documented that steroids decrease fibroblast migration and collagen synthesis. Topical steroids also inhibit wound healing.

Cyclosporine is a potent immunosuppressant used to suppress transplant rejection. Experimental evidence suggests that the effectiveness of cyclosporine is because of specific and reversible inhibition of immunocompetent lymphocytes in the G$_0$- or G$_1$-phase of the cell cycle. T lymphocytes are preferentially inhibited. The T-helper cell is the main target, although the T-suppressor cell may also be suppressed. Cyclosporine also inhibits lymphokine production and release of IL-2. Cyclosporine does not significantly affect hydroxyproline content and macrophages migration, although there is some evidence that cyclosporine impairs wound healing. Studies in rats have shown that activin-β expression and matrix metalloproteinases (MMPs) activity by fibroblast is reduced.

Bibliography

Mulder GD et al. Factors complicating wound repair. In: McCulloch JM, Kloth LC, Feedar JA (eds.), *Wound Healing Alternatives in Management*, 2nd ed. Philadelphia, PA: FA Davis, 1996, 51.

Petri JB, Schurk S, Gebauer S, Haustein U. Cyclosporine A delays wound healing and apoptosis and suppresses activin BA expression in rats. *Eur J Dermatol* 1998;8(2): 104–113.

15. **(B)** Angiogenesis is an important intermediate wound healing event. It occurs 2–4 days after the initial injury. It reconstructs the vasculature that was damaged locally. Small capillary sprouts initially develop on venules at the periphery of the devascularized area. Eventually these capillary sprouts will interconnect forming vascular loops.

    Angiogenesis is stimulated directly by high lactate levels, acidic pH, decrease oxygen tension, cytokines (fibroblast growth factor, FGF, is the most potent angiogenic stimulant identified), and prostaglandins.

    Heparin appears to stimulate angiogenesis. Heparin also binds to angiogenic factors such as tumor angiogenesis factor, endothelial cell growth factor, retina- and eye-derived growth factor, and cartilage-derived growth factor. Also matrix components, such as fibronectin and hyalurinic acid can stimulate angiogenesis.

    Hypoxia induces the vascular endothelial growth factor (VEGF) paracrine system by increasing the transcription of VEGF and its receptor, VEGFR-1 (Flt-1) and by stabilizing VEGF mRNA. The hypoxia-inducible transcription factor 1 (HIF-1) complex mediates these effects. An important regulator of this complex is the von Hippel-Lindau tumor suppressor protein, which serves as a cellular oxygen sensor. In the presence of oxygen, HIF-1α binds to von Hippel-Lindau protein. This leads to the rapid degradation of HIF-1α and the ensuing down regulation of VEGF transcription leading to inhibition of angiogenesis. Von Hippel-Lindau gene activity is lost in some sporadic cases of renal cell carcinoma and in tumors of patients with von Hippel-Lindau's syndrome. This leads to the deregulated expression of VEGF even under normoxic conditions, emphasizing the importance of von Hippel-Lindau protein in the oxygen-dependent regulation of VEGF expression. Angiogenesis is a key factor for tumor growth. Without blood vessel supply tumors cannot grow more than 2–3 mm.

Bibliography

Kaban K, Herbst RS. Angiogenesis as a target for cancer therapy. *Hematol Oncol Clin North Am* 2002;16(5): 1125–1171.

Lawrence WT. Wound healing biology and its application to wound management. In: O'Leary JP (ed.), *The Physiologic Basis of Surgery*, 2nd ed. Baltimore, MD: Williams & Wilkins, 1996, 118–140.

16. **(C)** IL-8 is secreted by macrophages and is a potent chemotactic agent. IL-1 and TNF-α are cytokines that mediate the acute inflammatory phase. Their secretion by macrophages results in fever and rise of immature neutrophils in the blood circulation.

    IL-2 is responsible for cell division. It is produced by T cells and has as major targets T, B, and NK cells.

    IL-10 down regulates the immune response. It is produced by and immunomodulates T cells.

Cytokine	Source	Effect
IL-1	Macrophage	Inflammation
IL-2	Helper T	Cell division
IL-6	Helper T	Activation, differentiation
IL-8	Macrophage	Chemotaxis
IL-10	Helper T	Inhibit cellular immunity
TNF-α	Macrophage	Inflammation

Bibliography

Cotran RS, Kumar V, Collins T, Robbins S. *Pathologic Basis of Disease*, 6th ed. St. Louis, MO: W.B. Saunders, 1999, 73.

17. **(B)** Growth factors have effects on cell locomotion, contractility, and differentiation.

    EGF is secreted by monocytes and macrophages, and promotes reepithelialization and angiogenesis. EGF also promotes extracellular matrix turnover stimulating collagenases.

    Platelets, monocytes, macrophages, and endothelial cells secrete PDGF. PDGF is a powerful chemoattractant that promotes deposition of intracellular matrix.

    Monocytes, macrophages, and endothelial cells produce FGF. FGF promotes reepithelialization and angiogenesis.

    VEGF also promotes angiogenesis in cancer, chronic inflammatory states, and healing wounds.

    TGF-β is secreted by platelets endothelial cells, lymphocytes, and macrophages. In low concentrations, it induces the synthesis and secretion of PDGF and is thus indirectly mitogenic. In high concentrations, it is growth inhibitory, owing to its ability to inhibit the expression of PDGF receptors.

Bibliography

Cotran RS, Kumar V, Collins T, Robbins S. *Pathologic Basis of Disease*, 6th ed. St. Louis, MO: W.B. Saunders, 1999, 104–106.

18. (C)

19. (C)

Explanations 18 and 19

Granulation tissue is a red beefy tissue deposited by fibroblasts. The histologic features of granulation tissue are the formation of new small blood vessels (angiogenesis) and the proliferation of fibroblasts. These new vessels are leaky, allowing the passage of proteins and red cells into the extravascular space. Thus, new granulation tissue is often edematous. Type III collagen is the most common type of collagen present in granulation tissue.

An excessive amount of granulation tissue deposition is called exuberant granulation or proud flesh.

Granulation tissue will allow reepithelialization of the skin. After complete scar maturation, hair follicles will not be regained.

Bibliography

Cotran RS, Kumar V, Collins T, Robbins S. *Pathologic Basis of Disease*, 6th ed. St. Louis, MO: W.B. Saunders, 1999, 108–110.

20. (C) Patients undergoing radiation therapy may present a challenge to heal. The effects of radiation therapy are variable and depend on a number of factors, including dose, frequency, and location. Cells display differential sensitivity to radiation in various phases of the cell cycle. In general, cells are more sensitive in early S and in mitosis, while they are less sensitive in late S and G_2. Rapid dividing cells are more susceptible to radiation.

Conversely, cells that do not divide rapidly, such as neurons or muscle cells tend to be resistant to radiation. The DNA of the nucleus is the main target of radiation therapy. The radiation effects on DNA can be direct or indirect. The direct effect is particularly damaging to the DNA and often results in damage to both DNA strands. Far more often, the effects on DNA are indirect. The ionization cellular fluid by radiation produces hydroxyl radicals (OH·), peroxide (H_2O_2), hydrated electrons (e_{aq}), and oxygen radicals (O·). These radicals will react with DNA to disrupt

the backbone of sugars or directly damage the pyrimidine and purine bases causing cell damage.

Injury to fibroblasts, leading to decreased amount of collagen deposition, and injury to endothelial cells are the most common effects caused by radiation resulting abnormal wound healing. Fibrosis and obliterative endarteritis are progressive and irreversible, causing lifetime wound impairment.

Bibliography

Lawrence WT. Wound healing biology and its application to wound management. In: O'Leary JP (ed.), *The Physiologic Basis of Surgery*, 2nd ed. Baltimore, MD: Williams & Wilkins, 1996, 118–140.

Mulder GD, et al. Factors complicating wound repair. In: McCulloch JM, Kloth LC, Feedar JA (eds.), *Wound Healing Alternatives in Management*, 2nd ed. Philadelphia, PA: FA Davis, 1996, 53.

21. (E) NO is a short-lived free radical that is involved in many important biological functions. NO is formed from the terminal guanidino nitrogen atom of arginine. Macrophages are responsible for the presence of most of the NO in the inflammatory phase of wound healing. Fibroblasts, keratinocytes, and endothelial cells contribute to ongoing NO synthesis but to a lesser degree. Inhibition of NO decreases collagen deposition and breaks strength of the wounds. Studies have shown that when rats are fed an arginine-free diet, wound healing is impaired. Also animal model studies have shown that NO can partially reversed the impaired healing of diabetes.

NO activates soluble guanate cyclase, which increases cellular cyclic guanosine monophosphate (cGMP) concentrations (see Fig. 3-18).

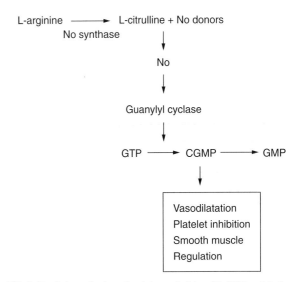

FIG. 3-18 Schematic view of arginine and nitric oxide (NO) metabolism.

Bibliography

Witte MB, Barbul A. Role of nitric oxide in wound repair. *Am J Surg* 2002;183(4):406–412.

22. **(B)** Scurvy is caused by the deficiency of vitamin C (ascorbic acid) intake. Ascorbic acid is present in vegetables and fruits, and absent in dairy products, poultry, and eggs.

Diagnosis is primarily clinical. Mucocutaneous manifestations, including change of skin color (pale), hyperkeratosis, reddish, bluish or black spots, gingival hypertrophy, and edema. Leukopenia is present in 30% of the patients. Treatment constitutes of initial replacement with 100 mg of vitamin C a day. Abnormalities are usually reversible and complete recovery is achieved in most of the cases by 3 months.

Vitamin C is one of the most important cofactors for collagen synthesis. Chronic nonhealing wounds, opening of well heal wounds, and fascial dehiscence can be caused by deficiency of vitamin C.

Bibliography

Raugi GJ. Adult scurvy. *J Am Acad Dermatol* 1999;41(6): 895–906.

23. **(E)** HBO is a therapeutic modality, which employs air or other gas mixtures at greater-than-atmospheric pressure for short intervals, over days or months, to treat various disease states. Gas gangrene, necrotizing fasciitis, osteomyelitis, decompression sickness, air or gas embolism, carbon monoxide and cyanide poisoning, radiation osteonecrosis, crush injury, selected nonhealing chronic wounds, smoke inhalation are conditions shown to improve with hyperbaric oxygen therapy.

Oxygen chambers are flooded with 100% oxygen with pressures varying from 3 to 6 ATA.

HBO effects are several, including

1. decrease of the bubble size (governed by Boyle's law, which states that the volume of gas in an enclosed space is inversely proportional to the pressure exerted on it)
2. increase leukocyte bactericidal and bacteriostatic function
3. stimulation of fibroblast growth, which results in increased collagen formation and resultant neovascularization
4. inhibition of neutrophil adherence to ischemic vessel walls
5. reduction of postischemic vasoconstriction
6. reduction of lipid peroxidation.

The most common adverse effects associated with HBO are barotrauma of the middle ear, cranial sinuses, teeth, or lungs.

Contraindications of HBO are patients receiving cisplatinum, bleomycin, sulfamylon, disulfiram, and patients with untreated pneumothorax.

Other relative contraindications include pregnancy, known malignancy, emphysema, pneumonia, bronchitis, and hyperthermia.

Bibliography

Frantz RA. Adjuvant therapy for ulcer care. *Clin Geriatr Med* 1997;13(3):553–564.

Mulinde JM, Caplan ES. Hyperbaric oxygen. In: Mandell GL, Bennett JE, Dolin R (eds.), *Mandell: Principles and Practice of Infectious Diseases*, 5th ed. Philadelphia, PA: Churchill Livingstone, 2000, 501–504.

24. **(B)** MMPs comprise a gene family of enzymes, including collagenases, gelatinases, stromelysins, matrilysin, and metalloelastase. These enzymes share important common properties. They are secreted as inactive zymogens, are rapidly secreted and not stored for long periods of time, and inhibited by tissue-derived inhibitors (TIMPs).

MMPs are upregulated by cytokines, especially TNF-α and IL-1. MMPs play a key role in degradation of collagen, but usually are not found in chronic wounds. The confinement of collagenase expression to the basal epidermal cells suggests that disruption of the basal membrane with subsequent exposure of keratinocytes is a critical determinant for epidermal collagenolytic activity.

Bibliography

Mignatti P, Rifkin DB, Welgus HG, Parks WC. Proteinases and tissue remodeling. In: Clark RAF (ed.), *The Molecular and Cell Biology of Wound Repair*, 2nd ed. New York, NY: Plenum Press, 1996, 427–461.

25. **(E)**

26. **(E)**

Explanations 25 and 26

Unfortunately, keloid scar is not preventable. A keloid scar extends beyond the limits of the original wound, differently from hypertrophic scar that usually is contained within the limits of the original wound. Histologically (see Fig. 3-19), keloid scar and hypertrophic scar are similar but minimal differences can still be found under the microscope. Collagen bundles with a glazed appearance, presence of antinuclear antibodies against fibroblast, epithelial, and endothelial cells, and higher levels of adenosine triphosphate are found in keloid scar, but not in hypertrophic scar.

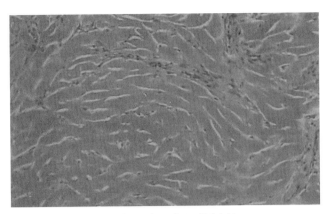

FIG. 3-19   Slide of a patient with keloid scar.

Collagen type I is the predominant type of collagen in both keloid and hypertrophic scars, differently from a normal nonmature scar where the predominant type of collagen is type III.

Bibliography

Shaffer JJ, Taylor SC, Cook-Bolden F. Keloidal scars: a review with a critical look at therapeutic options. *J Am Acad Dermatol* 2002;46(2): 563–597.

27. **(C)** Hypertrophic scar is defined as an increase ratio collagen deposition/degradation within the limits of the primary wound. It occurs anywhere and it is a preventable condition.

Infection, prolonged inflammation, insufficient resurfacing, increased wound tension, poor surgical technique, and delayed suture removal can lead to deposition of excessive collagen and formation of a hypertrophic scar. Scars that are close perpendicular to the underlying muscle fibers tend to be flatter and narrower than those where closure is done parallel to the underlying muscle fibers. As muscle fibers contract, easier reapproximation of the wound edges occurs if the scar is perpendicular to the underlying muscle. If, however, the scar is parallel to the underlying muscle, then contraction of the muscle will tend to cause gapping of the wound edges and lead to more tension and scar formation.

Bibliography

Philips LG. Wound healing. In: Townsend CM (ed.), *Sabiston: The Biological Basis of Modern Surgical Practice*, 16th ed. St. Louis, MO: W.B. Saunders, 2001, 140–141.

28. **(D)** Marjolin's ulcer is a rare neoplasm that occurs in chronic nonhealing wounds. Squamous cell carcinoma is the most common cancer associated with Marjolin's ulcer. Latency period for development of the cancer is variable ranging from 1 to 75 years.

Potential patients to developed Marjolin's ulcer are patients with burn or chronic open wounds, open orthopedic fractures, and chronic osteomyelitis.

Bibliography

Philips LG. Wound healing. In: Townsend CM (ed.), *Sabiston: The Biological Basis of Modern Surgical Practice*, 16th ed. St. Louis, MO: W.B. Saunders, 2001, 245.

29. **(B)** Fibroblasts are key cells in every step of wound healing. These cells are present by 3rd day postinjury in the wound. These cells use fibronectin as provisional stroma for ingrowth and scaffold for collagen deposition.

Fibroblasts are cytokine-dependent and once competent will produce collagen only under stimulation by growth factors such as EGF or insulin-like growth factor (IGF)-1.

MMPs are secreted by fibroblasts and monocytes. These enzymes degraded elastin. Elastin turnover in nonwounded circumstances is extremely low, lasting the life of the individual.

Fibroblasts are also essential during wound contraction. When stimulated they develop cytoplasmic actin-myosin contractile activity called myofibroblasts.

Bibliography

Cotran RS, Kumar V, Collins T, Robbins S. *Pathologic Basis of Disease*, 6th ed. St. Louis, MO: W.B. Saunders, 1999, 56–57.

30. **(D)** Vitamin C is essential for wound healing. Patients with ascorbic acid deficiency will require 100 mg orally daily for about 3 months to correct their deficiency.

Deficiency of vitamin A will impair monocyte activation, fibronectin deposition that further affects cellular adhesion, and impairment of the TGF-β receptors. Vitamin A contributes to lysosomal membrane destabilization and directly counteracts the effect of glucocorticoids. The recommended dietary allowance (RDA) of vitamin A is 900 retinol activity equivalents (RAE) for men and 700 RAE for women per day. This corresponds approximately to 3000 international units (IU) and 2300 IU, respectively. The Nutrition Advisory Group of the American Medical Association recommends 3300 IU of vitamin A for adult intravenous multivitamin formulations to prevent deficiency. Some investigators have recommended 25,000–50,000 IU per day orally and 10,000 IU intravenously for severely to moderately injured patients or for malnourished patients prior to and after elective surgery. The use of corticosteroids is associated with delayed wound healing and a higher risk of developing wound infection. Vitamin A supplementation antagonizes steroid-induced delays in wound healing. Studies with rabbits and rats have indicated that high doses of vitamin A reverse the anti-inflammatory effect of steroids and increase the tensile strength of the wound.

Zinc is an essential trace element required for protein synthesis and the function of several hundred zinc metalloenzymes and zinc finger proteins. Zinc is normally bound in the plasma; approximately 70% is bound loosely to albumin, 25% is more tightly bound to alpha$_2$-macroglobulin, and the remaining is bound to peptides and amino acids. The serum zinc concentration is the most frequently used method of assessing zinc status. Major food sources for zinc are proteins, such as red meat, and there is a direct correlation between dietary protein and dietary zinc intake. Patients with zinc deficiency will present with a wide variety of signs and symptoms, including diarrhea, impaired wound healing and impaired protein metabolism, hypogonadism, altered visual function, altered mental status, altered immune function, and impaired taste or anorexia. Zinc deficiency can be caused by chronic inflammatory states, poor zinc intake, poor absorption or increased excretion. Zinc deficiency can be associated with decreased wound burst strength.

Arginine may contribute to the wound healing process in multiple ways. When administered at pharmacologic levels it will cause secretion of anabolic hormones, insulin and growth hormone. Additionally, arginine present in the wound can be catabolized by immune cells to nitric oxide or ornithine. Nitric oxide is a powerful vasodilator, an autocrine stimulator of fibroblast-contractile and collagen-synthetic activities, and a mediator of macrophage-induced bacterial killing. Ornithine can be converted to proline and used for collagen synthesis, or converted to polyamines, which are important for cellular proliferation and differentiation.

Administration of arginine orally has been shown to enhance hydroxyproline deposition.

Vitamin E or tocopherol is an essential fat soluble vitamin. Vitamin E acts as an antioxidant in the human body and has become a popular nutrient in skin care products. It has anti-inflammatory properties, with a theoretical effect of inhibition of collagen deposition. Studies are still controversial regarding the true effect of tocopherol on wound healing.

Bibliography

Philips LG. Wound healing. In: Townsend CM (ed.), *Sabiston: The Biological Basis of Modern Surgical Practice*, 16th ed. St. Louis, MO: W.B. Saunders, 2001, 140–141.

Scholl D, Langkamp-Henken B. Nutrient recommendations for wound healing. [Review] *J Intraven Nurs* 2001;24(2):124–132.

31. (D) After initial injury, vasoconstriction occurs followed by the entrapment of platelets. Platelets will degranulate, releasing several different substances, including homeostasis factors (i.e., von Willebrand's factor, thrombospondin), growth factors (IGF-1, PDGF, TGF-β), proteases and hydrolases that will cause protein and cell degradation. Vasodilatation occurs after homeostasis followed by inflow of neutrophils, monocytes, macrophages, and lymphocytes.

Although not essential for the wound healing process, neutrophils scavenge necrotic tissue, foreign material, and bacteria.

Lymphocytes can play a major role in the resolution of the inflammatory process, especially in contaminated wounds. Lymphocytes produce interferon-λ, which decreases synthesis of prostaglandins and stimulates production of cytokines. T cells also stimulate IL-2 release, an up regulator of the immune system and inflammatory response, which directly stimulates monocytes to release free radicals against bacteria.

Bibliography

Philips LG. Wound healing. In: Townsend CM (ed.), *Sabiston: The Biological Basis of Modern Surgical Practice*, 16th ed. St. Louis, MO: W.B. Saunders, 2001, 245.

32. (C) Knowing how to tie a knot is one of the most important fundamentals of surgery. The weakest link in the surgical suture is the knot and the second weakest point is next to the knot.

Surgical knots can be divided in two groups: symmetric and asymmetric. Symmetric knots are square knots (see Fig. 3-20), granny, and surgeon's knot. Asymmetric knots are sliding knots characterized by an unequal distribution of friction during knot tying. Sliding knots are tied by holding one strand under a

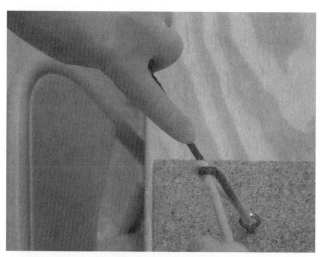

FIG. 3-20 Tie of a square knot.

constant region and tension while the other strand is wrapped around. No crossing of the hands is necessary, which turns this technique more attractive. Unfortunately sliding knots are not as effective as symmetric knots because of their tendency to unravel. Greater knot security is achieved when a tension of 1500 g or more is applied to the suture while tying.

Square knots are achieved when equal distribution of forces is applied during the throw. Symmetric knots are safer and less likely to unrevealed.

Multifilament suture material exhibited higher values of coefficient of friction, which decreases the chances of knot slippage when comparing with monofilament sutures.

Bibliography

Fraunhofer JA, Chu CC. Mechanical properties. In: Fraunhofer JA, Greisler HP (eds.), *Wound Closure Biomaterials and Device*, 2nd ed. Boca Raton, FL: CRC Press, 1996, 107–130.

33. **(C)** Degradation of suture materials is mainly through hydrolysis, although thermal, mechanical, ultraviolet radiation, and oxidation also can cause degradation of polymeric materials. Three important properties are used to describe biodegradation of suture materials: tensile strength, mass profile, and type of degradation products release into surrounding tissues. The profile of strength loss always occurs before the profile of mass or weight loss.

Variation of the pH has major impact on biodegradation of suture material. For example, in polyglactil 910 sutures (Vicryl) the curve of breaking strength has a convex shape with maximum retention strength at pH 7.0 and low retention strength at strong acidic or alkaline pH.

Gamma-irradiation causes loss of tensile strength of different sutures. Studies done by Chu (1996) have shown that tensile strength of suture materials decrease with an increase of the radiation dose.

Among nonabsorbable sutures, silk and cotton are the most susceptible to degradation. Because of the lack of hydrolysable bounds, polyethylene and polypropylene are not subjected to hydrolytic degradation and retained their tensile strength *in vivo* for long periods of time.

Bibliography

Chu CC. Biodegradation properties. In: Fraunhofer JA, Greisler HP (eds.), *Wound Closure Biomaterials and Device*, 2nd ed. Boca Raton, FL: CRC Press, 1996, 131–235.

34. **(A)**

35. **(A)**

36. **(C)**

37. **(D)**

Explanations 34 through 37

Collagen is an essential component for wound healing and the main component of the extracellular matrix. Collagens are triple-helix structural proteins divided in XII subgroups or types. The most important types with their tissue distribution are shown below. Type I collagen is the most abundant form of collagen and accounts for a total of 90% of the total body collagen. It is present in all connective tissues, but cartilage and basal membranes. Collagen type III is initially deposited after an injury and will be replaced by collagen type I during maturation of the wound. Deposition of type I collagen starts by the 7th day postinjury.

During the inflammatory phase, the exposure of fibrillar collagen to blood promotes aggregation and activation of platelets.

During collagen synthesis (see Fig. 3-21), fibroblasts produce procollagen molecules (tropocollagen) intracellular, which are packed in the complex of Golgi and subsequently excreted. Once released to the extracellular space, cleavage of the nonhelical segments will occur. Prolyl hydroxylase is a rate-limiting enzyme for the synthesis of collagen and has as cofactors vitamin C, oxygen, iron, alpha-ketoglutarate. Lactate and hypoxia also indirectly stimulate prolyl hydroxylase synthesis.

Type	Tissue distribution
I	All connective tissues, except cartilage and basement membranes
II	Cartilage, vitreous humor, intervertebral disc
III	Skin, blood vessels, granulation tissue, internal organs
IV	Basement membranes

Bibliography

Cotran RS, Kumar V, Collins T, Robbins S. *Pathologic Basis of Disease*, 6th ed. St. Louis, MO: W.B. Saunders, 1999, 56–57.

38. **(D)** Death of a cell can be categorized in two groups: necrosis (incidental cell death) or apoptosis (programmed cell death).

Necrosis is characterized by loss of membrane function and abnormal permeability (observed by the cell's inability to exclude vital dye such as trypan blue). Disruption of organelles is seen early in the process. Most of the time, the effect of necrosis is seen in a large number of cells.

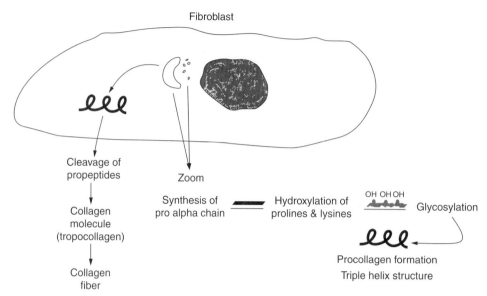

FIG. 3-21   Schematic representation of collagen synthesis and excretion.

Apoptosis is considered a programmed cell death. It is a physiologic event and has been compared to "the falling of leaves from a tree during autumn." During apoptosis, the cells decrease in size, lose microvillae, and develop deep invaginations on the surface. The cell membranes and organelles remain intact and are able to exclude vital dye until the very end of the process. The nucleus also undergoes structural modifications. Chromatin becomes dense with a prominent nucleolus.

A key biochemical feature of apoptosis is internucleosomal cleavage of chromatin in a pattern indicative of endogenous endonuclease activation. This creates low molecular-sized fragments of DNA. A characteristic "ladder" pattern of DNA fragments is seen when DNA extracted from apoptotic cells is submitted to electrophoresis.

Bibliography

Haslett C, Henson P. Resolution of inflammation. In: Clark RA (ed.), *The Molecular and Cellular Biology of Wound Repair*, 2nd ed. New York, NY: Plenum Press, 1996, 153–168.

39. (D) Fibronectin is a cell adhesion protein found in blood and in matrices. Although encoded by a single gene, fibronectins exist in a number of different forms. Major functions include mediating cellular adhesion, promoting cell migration and chemotaxis, and regulating cell growth and gene expression.

Each fibronectin molecule consists of a series of structural and functional domains. Six or more peptides are present, and are capable of mediating cell adhesion. They are located in three general regions: the central cell-binding domain, the alternatively spliced IIICS region, and the heparin-binding domain.

Fibronectin plays a major role in the capacity of cells to interact with fibrin, containing at least two fibrin-binding domains.

Fibronectin major fibrin-binding domain is homologous to the finger domain of TPA. Competition between TPA and fibronectin to bind on this homologous domain might be an important regulator of fibrinolysis.

Fibronectin is usually deposited before collagen, serving as matrix for further collagen deposition. Fibronectin matrix will be degraded by proteases as collagen is deposited and as the wound matures.

Bibliography

Yamad KM, Clark RAF. Provisional matrix. In: Clark RA (ed.), *The Molecular and Cellular Biology of Wound Repair*, 2nd ed. New York, NY: Plenum Press, 1996, 153–168.

40. (D) Proteoglycans are a heterogeneous group of protein-carbohydrate complexes containing at least one glycosaminoglycan chain covalently bound. Proteoglycans are named after the most prevalent glycosaminoglycan in the structure.

Proteoglycans are versatile molecules found in secretory granules, or as an intrinsic or extrinsic membrane protein, and in the extracellular matrix.

Many different functions are attributed to these molecules including blood coagulation regulators, promotion of extracellular organization, storage of growth factors, and promotion of growth factor receptor binding.

Chondroitin-4 sulfate occurs in high levels in granulation tissue, but it is not found in the mature scar. Levels of proteoglycans in general vary according to the degree of wound maturation.

Bibliography

Gallo RL, Bernfield M. Proteoglycans and their role in wound repair. In: Clark RA (ed.), *The Molecular and Cellular Biology of Wound Repair*, 2nd ed. New York, NY: Plenum Press, 1996, 475–488.

41. (D) Laminin is the most abundant glycoprotein in basal membrane. Laminin binds with specific receptors on the surface of cells and functions as a bridge between surface receptors and matrix components, such as collagen type IV and heparan sulfate. Laminin is also believed to mediate cell attachment to connective tissue substrates; in culture it alters the growth, survival, morphology, differentiation, and motility of various cell types. In endothelial cell cultures exposed to FGF, laminin causes alignment of endothelial cells, critical for angiogenesis. Laminin is found in and secreted by colon cancer cells. Fifty percent of classic type CMD cases are associated with a deficiency of the basal lamina protein alpha$_2$-laminin, known as merosin.

Bibliography

Fidler I. Cancer biology: invasion and metastases. In: Abeloff MD (ed.), *Clinical Oncology*, 2nd ed. New York, NY: Churchill Livingstone, 2000, 31.

CHAPTER 4

Preoperative Evaluation

*Mauricio Antonio Escobar Jr., Kevin Sheridan,
Mauricio Antonio Escobar, and Michael Rowe*

Questions

1. What is the single most important data/test to ascertain a patient's risk assessment and preparation prior to a surgical procedure?

   (A) history
   (B) physical
   (C) chest x-ray (CXR)
   (D) electrocardiogram (ECG)
   (E) stress test

2. The patient is a 2-year-old Hispanic female who presents for elective bilateral inguinal hernia repair. Which of the following would cancel the case?

   (A) history of ventricular-peritoneal shunt placement 8 weeks ago
   (B) history of a 1-month stay in the neonatal intensive care unit
   (C) history of trisomy 21
   (D) history of patent ductus arteriosus
   (E) persistent chronic otitis media with continued nasal clear discharge

3. The patient is a 48-year-old White male who presents with a history of hypertension, diabetes mellitus, and one block right lower extremity claudication. He smokes four packs of cigarettes per day. He works as a top executive in a major advertising firm. He has never had chest pain. Routine evaluation includes a resting ECG that reveals Q waves 0.04 s wide in V5 and V6 and one-half the height of the R waves. What should this be interpreted as?

   (A) normal variation of a patient with hypertension
   (B) coronary artery disease (CAD)
   (C) normal variation of a patient with diabetes mellitus
   (D) normal variation of a patient with Berger's disease
   (E) No evidence of CAD because the patient has never had chest pain

4. Which of the following will immediately delay or cancel an elective surgical case if not obtained appropriately preoperatively?

   (A) CBC
   (B) urinalysis
   (C) CXR
   (D) informed consent
   (E) ECG

5. A 48-year-old Hispanic male with a history of gastroesophageal reflux disease refractory to medical management is advised to undergo an elective Nissen fundoplication. An extensive preoperative history and physical reveals no evidence of cardiac or pulmonary disease. What would be the most appropriate preoperative laboratory studies to obtain given the fact the patient has no significant past medical history?

   (A) CBC
   (B) CBC, ECG
   (C) CBC, ECG, blood glucose
   (D) CBC, ECG, CXR, basic metabolic panel, glucose
   (E) none

6. The patient is a 67-year-old Asian-American male with history of CHF, diabetes mellitus, hypertension (HTN), CAD, chronic renal insufficiency, and peripheral vascular disease. Although not yet on dialysis, it is likely within 2 months he will start. The patient has undergone all appropriate preoperative evaluation and testing and is ready for his arteriovenous fistula creation. Which of the following medications he is taking should be stopped preoperatively?

   (A) glyburide
   (B) glucophage
   (C) atenolol
   (D) aspirin
   (E) digoxin

7. The patient is a 36-year-old White female. Which of the following preoperative conditions would *not* lead the patient to experience extracellular fluid volume depletion?

   (A) fistula loss
   (B) small bowel obstruction
   (C) peritonitis
   (D) pancreatitis
   (E) closed head injury

8. A 68-year-old Black female on dialysis presents 12 weeks after an episode of diverticulitis requiring percutaneous drainage of an abscess. The plan is to perform an elective sigmoidectomy. Which of the following medications started now would reduce her risk of perioperative MI?

   (A) metoprolol
   (B) diltiazem
   (C) hydrochlorothiazide
   (D) lisinopril
   (E) lasix

9. The patient is a 55-year-old White male without history of chronic obstructive pulmonary disease (COPD). Which of the following places the patient at highest risk for postoperative pulmonary complications?

   (A) right upper lobe resection for cancer
   (B) diaphragm repair after traumatic rupture 2 years ago
   (C) total abdominal colectomy
   (D) left radical nephrectomy
   (E) coronary artery bypass graft

10. Which of the following does not help ameliorate cardiac stress perioperatively in high-risk patients?

   (A) maintaining normal body temperature
   (B) providing epidural anesthesia
   (C) providing metoprolol perioperatively
   (D) transfusing two units of packed red blood cells
   (E) maintaining a perioperative heart rate of 50–60 bpm

11. Preoperative bowel preparation helps reduce which of the following postoperative complications by 40%?

   (A) pneumonia
   (B) urinary tract infection (UTI)
   (C) dehiscence
   (D) wound infection
   (E) intraabdominal abscess

12. When should parenteral antibiotics be given perioperatively?

   (A) the night before
   (B) 6 h prior to surgery
   (C) 30 min prior to incision
   (D) at the time of incision
   (E) 30 min after incision

13. The patient is a 50-year-old woman with history of biliary colic and gallstones noted on ultrasound. There is no evidence of biliary dilatation. A laparoscopic cholecystectomy is planned. After how much time is the patient at increased risk for deep venous thrombosis?

   (A) 30 min
   (B) 60 min
   (C) 90 min
   (D) 120 min
   (E) 150 min

14. For which of the following surgeries would you order coagulation studies?

   (A) inguinal herniorrhaphy
   (B) femoral-popliteal bypass graft
   (C) right hemicolectomy
   (D) total thyroidectomy
   (E) laparoscopic appendectomy

15. A 64-year-old Black female with history of diabetes and left great toe amputation secondary to infection presents obtunded and febrile. On examination the patient is noted to have an ulcer along the lateral aspect of her foot with cellulitis. No frank pus is expressible. Blood glucose is 843 mg/dL. Serum potassium is 4.0. Arterial blood gas (ABG) reveals pH 7.28 and PCO_2 of 38 mmHg. White blood cell (WBC) is 15.4. Urine dip is positive for ketones and glucose. What is the next step in the management of this patient?

   (A) immediate trip to the OR for debridement
   (B) immediate trip to the OR for amputation
   (C) 1 L normal saline bolus
   (D) 1 L normal saline with 1 ampule of $NaHCO_3$
   (E) 10 units of regular insulin subcutaneously

16. The patient is a 40-year-old White female diagnosed with Crohn's disease 3 weeks prior. She has been treated with Remicade and high-dose steroids. For the last 2 weeks she has experienced a lower gastrointestinal bleed for which she has required multiple blood transfusions. She finally experiences hypotension with continued bleeding and is taken urgently to the operating room and undergoes a total abdominal colectomy with ileostomy. Preoperatively, she only received antibiotics. Two hours after operation, the patient is persistently hypotensive in the 80/30s. She is not responding to fluid boluses and her postoperative hematocrit is 30%. What is the next step in this patient's management?

    (A) continue to give normal saline boluses
    (B) transfuse two units of packed red blood cells
    (C) start a dopamine drip at 5 μg/kg/min
    (D) give 100 mg IV of hydrocortisone
    (E) reexplore her immediately

17. Which of the following medications should be given first in the preoperative preparation of a patient with pheochromocytoma?

    (A) phenoxybenzamine
    (B) propranolol
    (C) nifedipine
    (D) lisinopril
    (E) hydrochlorothiazide

18. Which of the following is an independent risk factor for cardiovascular death after elective noncardiac and cardiovascular surgery?

    (A) renal insufficiency
    (B) hyperthyroidism
    (C) pheochromocytoma
    (D) adrenal insufficiency
    (E) hypertension

19. The patient is a 43-year-old White male with history of Caroli's disease and end-stage liver disease. Which of the following would optimize the patient's liver function prior to elective Nissen fundoplication?

    (A) hemodialysis
    (B) control of hypertension
    (C) right hepatic lobectomy
    (D) transjugular intrahepatic portal caval shunt (TIPS)
    (E) none of the above

20. Which of the following is *not* a manifestation of thyroid storm?

    (A) fever
    (B) tachycardia
    (C) significantly elevated levels of T_4 and T_3 compared to hyperthyroidism
    (D) atrial fibrillation
    (E) seizures

21. Which of the following heart sounds noted during physical examination would require infective endocarditis prophylaxis prior to noncardiac surgery?

    (A) fixed splitting of S2
    (B) holosystolic murmur
    (C) S3
    (D) loud A2
    (E) A2 before P2 with increased splitting on inspiration

Answers and Explanations

1. (A) A history and physical is diagnostic in 75–90% of patients. Diagnostically, the history is three times more productive than the physical examination and 11 times more effective than routine laboratory tests. Furthermore, "routine" preoperative testing results in wasted expenditure of health care funds and may result in morbidity to the patient from further work-up of false-positive results. Review of systems with identification of comorbidities (history of myocardial infarction (MI), syncope, angina, anemia, orthostatic intolerance, pulmonary edema, valvular disease, hepatic and renal failure, diabetes) reveals areas for further testing.

A recent MI is the single most important risk factor for perioperative infarction regardless if it was Q-versus non-Q-wave. The risk of having a postoperative reinfarction if the patient undergoes general anesthesia after an MI is 27% within three months of operation. A perioperative MI is associated with a 40–70% mortality rate. After an acute MI an elective operation should be postponed for six months. Emergency surgery should have invasive monitoring at the minimum.

A study involving routine coronary angiography in patients undergoing peripheral vascular surgery has revealed severe coronary artery disease in 36% of patients with aortic aneurysms, in 32% of patients with cerebrovascular disease, and in 28% of patients with lower extremity ischemia. In fact, the study demonstrated that of the population of patients scheduled to undergo peripheral vascular surgery, only 8% had normal coronary arteries.

Age, cigarette smoking, valvular heart disease, congestive heart failure (CHF), and arrhythmias all increase perioperative risk. There is a significantly increased risk of developing pulmonary edema perioperatively if the patient has a history of CHF. Patients with a history of cardiac disease and diabetes are at higher risk of developing CHF.

The increased mortality of aortic stenosis is related to the limited capacity to increase cardiac output in response to stress, vasodilatation, or hypovolemia. If the patient is symptomatic from his aortic stenosis, i.e., syncope, angina, or CHF, and is categorized as severe by echocardiogram or cardiac catheterization, elective aortic valve replacement before noncardiac surgery is indicated. Otherwise, invasive monitoring including pulmonary artery catheters and arterial lines, and caution with use of afterload-reducing agents is required. Patients with mitral stenosis and hypertrophic obstructive cardiomyopathy also require careful hemodynamic monitoring given their increased risk of perioperative pulmonary edema secondary to their disease process. Invasive monitoring should be continued postoperatively for 48 h.

The presence of an arrhythmia demands further work-up. If the patient is symptomatic or hemodynamically unstable secondary to the arrhythmia, therapy should be instituted preoperatively to address the cause and treat the arrhythmia. Of note, frequent paroxysmal ventricular contractions and/or asymptomatic nonsustained ventricular tachycardia have not been associated with increased risk of nonfatal MI or cardiac death in the perioperative period (invasive monitoring is therefore not indicated). Implantable cardiac defibrillator (ICDs) or pacemaker should be programmed off immediately before surgery and then on again postoperatively.

Bibliography

Baker RJ, Fischer JE. *Preparation of the Patient. Mastery of Surgery*, 4th ed. New York, NY: Lippincott, Williams & Wilkins, 2001, 23–54.

Christou NV, Harken AH, Wilmore DW, Arya J. Risk stratification, preoperative testing, and operative planning. *ACS Surgery: Principles & Practice*. New York, NY: WebMD, 2002.

Eagle KA, Berger PB, Calkins H, et al. ACC/AHA guideline update for preoperative cardiovascular evaluation for noncardiac surgery: executive summary. A report of the American College of Cardiology/American Heart

Association Task Force on Practice Guidelines (Committee to Update the 1996 Guidelines on Perioperative Cardiovascular Evaluation for Noncardiac Surgery). *Circulation* 2002;105:1257–1267.

Hertzer NR, Beven EG, Young JR, et al. Coronary artery disease in peripheral vascular patients: a classification of 1000 coronary angiograms and results of surgical management. *Ann Surg* 1984;199:223–233.

King MS. Preoperative evaluation. *Am Fam Physician* 2000;62(2):387–396.

Marcello PW, Roberts PL. "Routine" preoperative studies: which studies in which patients? *Surg Clin North Am* 1996;76(1):17–23.

Narr BJ, Warner ME, Schroeder DR, et al. Outcomes of patients with no laboratory assessment before anesthesia and a surgical procedure. *Mayo Clin Proc* 1997;72(6): 505–509.

Shammash JB, Ghali WA. Preoperative assessment and perioperative management of the patient with nonischemic heart disease. *Med Clin North Am* 2003;87(1): 137–152.

2. **(E)** A history in a child should include everything mentioned in an adult. Furthermore, in children, the history should also include birth history and history of recent infections. Birth history should delineate prematurity, perinatal complications, and congenital chromosomal and anatomic malformations. Recent infections include upper respiratory infections (URIs) and pneumonia. A second visit to assess the child's URI may be in order; the case may be cancelled if the patient continues to have fever, wheezing or significant nasal discharge, as URIs have been shown to complicate postoperative care.

Bibliography

Christou NV, Harken AH, Wilmore DW, et al. Risk stratification, preoperative testing, and operative planning. *ACS Surgery: Principles & Practice.* New York, NY: WebMD, 2002.

Cohen MM, Cameron CB. Should you cancel the operation when a child has an upper respiratory tract infection? *Anesth Analg* 1991;72(3):282–288.

King MS. Preoperative evaluation. *Am Fam Physician* 2000;62(2):387–396.

Maxwell LG, Yaster M. Perioperative management issues in pediatric patients. *Anesthesiol Clin North America* 2000;18(3):601–632.

McMillan JA, DeAngelis CD, Feigen RD, et al. Pediatric history and physical examination. *Oski's Pediatrics: Principles and Practice,* 3rd ed. New York, NY: Lippincott, Williams & Wilkins, 1999, 39–51.

3. **(B)** Patients with an abnormal resting ECG are three times more likely to have a fatal perioperative infarction. A Q wave 0.04 s or wider and at least one-third the height of the R wave is evidence of a prior MI.

Evidence of prior MI must be taken as evidence of CAD; however, a normal resting ECG does not rule out CAD. Further testing includes the following modalities.

Echocardiography (resting and stress) can estimate left ventricular ejection fraction (LVEF), which if reduced correlates with perioperative myocardial events. Also, wall motion abnormalities or thickening define the presence of ischemia.

Radionuclide cardiac studies assess LVEF, which correlates with the incidence of perioperative infarction and severity of CAD. Myocardial perfusion imaging analyzes and distinguishes between areas of ischemia and scars from a previous infarction as well as between ischemic and nonischemic cardiomyopathy that has excellent correlation with risk of postoperative infarctions.

However, those patients with high-risk clinical profiles with or without clinical or laboratory evidence of unstable CAD may still require preoperative coronary catheterization.

In patients with known or suspected CAD undergoing high-risk procedures, an ECG at baseline, immediately postoperatively, and on the first 2 days after surgery appears to be cost-effective. Postoperative markers should be reserved for the subset of patients with clinical, ECG, or hemodynamic evidence of cardiovascular dysfunction. Patients who sustain acute MIs in the perioperative period need to be followed closely secondary to increased risk of future cardiac events.

Bibliography

Baker RJ, Fischer JE. *Preparation of the Patient. Mastery of Surgery,* 4th ed. New York, NY: Lippincott, Williams & Wilkins, 2001, 23–54.

Charlson ME, MacKenzie CR, Ales K, et al. Surveillance for postoperative myocardial infarction after noncardiac operations. *Surg Gynecol Obstet* 1988;167:404–414.

Christou NV, Harken AH, Wilmore DW, et al. Risk stratification, preoperative testing, and operative planning. *ACS Surgery: Principles & Practice.* New York, NY: WebMD, 2002.

Cohn SL, Goldman L. Preoperative risk evaluation and perioperative management of patients with coronary artery disease. *Med Clin North Am* 2003;87(1):111–136.

Eagle KA, Berger PB, Calkins H, et al. ACC/AHA guideline update for preoperative cardiovascular evaluation for noncardiac surgery: executive summary. A report of the American College of Cardiology/American Heart Association Task Force on Practice Guidelines (Committee to Update the 1996 Guidelines on Perioperative Cardiovascular Evaluation for Noncardiac Surgery). *Circulation* 2002;105:1257–1267.

King MS. Preoperative evaluation. *Am Fam Physician* 2000;62(2):387–396.

4. (D) Informed consent is ultimately the responsibility of the operating surgeon. It is not only a legal obligation, but grounded in the ethical principle of autonomy. It provides the patient a chance to ask questions, calm fears, and strengthen trust between the surgeon and the patient. Furthermore, well-informed patients require less analgesia in the postoperative period and experience less pain. Informed consent includes explaining the risks, benefits, alternatives, and outcomes of surgery. Include as many details as possible and if possible, write them out. If the patient is not competent, then a surrogate must give informed consent in a nonemergent setting. In an emergent setting, institutions have several options for providing consent. A "three-doc consent" is a popular version of this (in which three physicians agree that a procedure is needed in an emergent situation to prevent significant morbidity or mortality and indicate so in the chart). The patient's social support and rehabilitation needs should be assessed preoperatively. Home services or rehabilitation may be needed postoperatively. Inquiry regarding health care power of attorney and do-not-resuscitate (DNR) status should life-threatening complications arise should also be discussed.

Bibliography

Baker RJ, Fischer JE. *Preparation of the Patient. Mastery of Surgery*, 4th ed. New York, NY: Lippincott, Williams & Wilkins, 2001, 23–54.

Beauchamp TL, Walters L. *Contemporary Issues in Bioethics*, 4th ed. Belmont, CA: Wadsworth, 1994, 1–38.

Christou NV, Harken AH, Wilmore DW, Arya J. Risk stratification, preoperative testing, and operative planning. *ACS Surgery: Principles & Practice*. New York, NY: WebMD, 2002.

Doukas DJ, McCullough LB. The values history. *J Fam Pract* 1991;32:145–153.

Emanuel LL, Emanuel EJ. In: Cate FH, Gill BA (eds.), *The Patient Self-Determination Act: Implementation Issues and Opportunities*. Washington, DC: The Annenberg Washington Program in Communications Policy Studies of Northwestern University, 1991, 58–64.

5. (C) In general, routine preoperative testing is not recommended, with specific testing considered useful for specific patients. Age, gender, and comorbidities are all factors to be considered when ordering tests prior to surgery. Table 4-1 summarizes recommended preoperative laboratory tests. Checking liver function tests and coagulation panels are tailored to the specific patient depending on history and physical findings.

TABLE 4-1   Recommended Preoperative Testing for Elective Surgery*

Patient status	Hemoglobin	PT/PTT	PLT	T/S	K⁺	BUN/Creat	Glucose	CXR	ECG	Additional tests
Age										
<6 months	X									
<40 years	Female only								Males > 40 years	
40–60 years	Female only								Females > 50 years	
>60 years	X					X	X	X	X	
Procedure with blood loss	X			X						
Associated conditions										
Cardiovascular disease	X					X		X	X	Stress test†
Pulmonary disease	X							X	X	PFT/ABG†
Smoker (>20 pack-years)	X							X	X	PFT/ABG†
Hepatic disease		X								AST
Renal disease	X				X	X				
Diabetes					X	X	X		X	
Bleeding disorder		X	X							
Malignancy	X							X		
Morbid obesity	X								X	Weight† PFT/ABG†
Medications										
Anticoagulant	X	X								
Digoxin					X	X	X		X	
Diuretic					X	X				
Corticosteroid					X		X			

*PT/PTT indicates prothrombin time and partial thromboplastin time; T/S, blood typing and screening; PLT, platelet count; K⁺, potassium; BUN/Creat, blood urea nitrogen and creatinine; CXR, chest x-ray; ECG, electrocardiogram; PFT, pulmonary function tests; ABG, arterial blood gas; AST, aspartate aminotransferase; and WBC, white blood cell count.

†A stress test (including exercise tolerance test, dipyridamole-thallium scintigraphy, or dobutamine echocardiography) and PFT/ABG should be individualized to the patient and procedure planned.

Source: Reprinted from Marcello PW, Roberts PL. "Routine" preoperative studies: which studies in which patients? *Surg Clin North Am* 76:11–23. Copyright 1996, with permission from Elsevier.

Bibliography

Christou NV, Harken AH, Wilmore DW, et al. Risk stratification, preoperative testing, and operative planning. *ACS Surgery: Principles & Practice*. New York, NY: WebMD Inc, 2002.

Fischer SP. Cost-effective preoperative evaluation and testing. *Chest* 1999;115(5):96S–100S

King MS. Preoperative evaluation. *Am Fam Physician* 2000;62(2):387–396.

Marcello PW, Roberts PL. "Routine" preoperative studies: which studies in which patients? *Surg Clin North Am* 1996;76(1):11–23.

Narr BJ, Hansen TR, Warner MA. Preoperative laboratory screening in healthy Mayo patients: cost-effective elimination of tests and unchanged outcomes. *Mayo Clin Proc* 1991;66(2):155–159.

Smetana GW. The case against routine preoperative laboratory testing. *Med Clin North Am* 2003; 87(1):7–40.

Velanovich V. The value of routine preoperative laboratory testing in predicting postoperative complications: a multivariate analysis. *Surgery* 1991;109(3 Pt 1):236–243.

Velanovich V. Preoperative laboratory screening based on age, gender, and comorbid diseases. *Surgery* 1994;115(1):56–61.

Wattsman TA, Davies RS. The utility of preoperative laboratory testing in general surgery patients for outpatient procedures. *Am Surg* 1997;63(1):81–90.

6. **(D)** Optimization of comorbid conditions such as CHF, diabetes, and HTN are essential. All antihypertensives should be continued through the perioperative period. Withdrawal of beta-blockade is associated with unstable angina, tachyarrhythmias, MI, or sudden death. Digoxin should be continued with careful monitoring of levels and signs of toxicity (arrhythmias, nausea, vomiting, headache, dizziness, visual disturbance). Electrolytes and volume status should also be monitored as all classes of antihypertensives and digoxin can cause disturbances in and be influenced themselves by these.

Aspirin is a nonsteroidal anti-inflammatory drug (NSAID), which irreversibly acetylates (and thus inactivates) platelet cyclooxygenase (COX). This results in inhibition of thromboxane production in platelets, with a concomitant reduction in platelet aggregation. Thus, bleeding time will be prolonged. Because this is irreversible, it lasts for the lifetime of the platelet (3–7 days). It is recommended that patients stop taking aspirin at least 7 days prior to surgery, since the circulating pool of platelets is replenished every 7–10 days.

Other NSAIDs reversibly inhibit platelet cyclooxygenase. These should be stopped 1–3 days prior to surgery based on the individual drug's half-life. Ibuprofen and indomethacin, with short half-lives between 2 and 5 h, can be stopped 1 day prior to

surgery. Naproxen and sulindac have half-lives in the 12–47 h range, and should be stopped 3 days prior to surgery. While the COX-2 inhibitors have little to no effect on platelets, they should be stopped 2–3 days prior to surgery because of their inhibition of renal prostaglandin synthesis with a potential for renal complications.

Bibliography

Christou NV, Harken AH, Wilmore DW, et al. Risk stratification, preoperative testing, and operative planning. *ACS Surgery: Principles & Practice*. New York, NY: WebMD, 2002.

Baker RJ, Fischer JE. *Preparation of the Patient. Mastery of Surgery*, 4th ed. New York, NY: Lippincott, Williams & Wilkins, 2001, 23–54.

Eagle KA, Berger PB, Calkins H, et al. ACC/AHA guideline update for preoperative cardiovascular evaluation for noncardiac surgery: executive summary. A report of the American College of Cardiology/American Heart Association Task Force on Practice Guidelines (Committee to Update the 1996 Guidelines on Perioperative Cardiovascular Evaluation for Noncardiac Surgery). *Circulation* 2002;105:1257–1267.

King MS. Preoperative evaluation. *Am Fam Physician* 2000;62(2):387–396.

Mercado DL, Petty BG. Perioperative medication management. *Med Clin North Am* 2003;87(1):41–57.

Mycek MJ, Harvey RA, Champe PC. Anti-inflammatory drugs. In: Mycek MJ, Harvey RA, Champe PC (eds.), *Lippincott's Illustrated Reviews: Pharmacology*, 2nd ed. Philadelphia, PA: Lippincott-Raven, 1997, 401–418.

Spell NO. Stopping and restarting medications in the perioperative period. *Med Clin North Am* 2001;85(5):1117–1128.

7. **(E)** Preoperative fluid assessment is critical in a surgical patient. Often times, the surgeon is required to make a rapid assessment of the patient's fluid and electrolyte imbalances and replete ongoing losses. Regardless whether the patient is managed preoperatively in the trauma bay or the clinic setting, depleted intravascular volume is best established through a thorough history and physical examination.

Multiple factors may lead a surgical patient to experience extracellular fluid volume depletion: mechanical small bowel obstruction, fistula loss, vomiting, diarrhea, peritonitis, pancreatitis, and so on. Physical examination may reveal skin tenting, dry mucous membranes, tachycardia, oliguria, or postural hypotension. Operating on a patient prior to adequate volume resuscitation may lead to cardiovascular collapse.

Monitoring renal function via urine output measured through an indwelling bladder catheter is essential to assess adequate resuscitation. Normal hourly urine output is 0.5 cc/kg in an adult, greater than or equal to 1 cc/kg in children, depending on age (in patients not receiving diuretics or experiencing glycosuria). More invasive monitoring with central venous pressure (CVP) or pulmonary artery wedge pressure may be appropriate in select cases, although their role is controversial. Other guides that may assist in difficult resuscitations include arterial pH, lactate, and base deficit.

Rate of resuscitation is guided by the urgency of need for operation (replacement of deficit and ongoing losses may be necessary in the operating room). Resolution of clinical signs of volume deficit is the best indicator of response. Correction of electrolyte imbalances follows the same principles in emergent as in nonemergent situations. Maintenance fluid requirements can be estimated as 100 cc/kg/day for the first 10 kg, 50 cc/kg/day for the second 10 kg, and 10 cc/kg/day thereafter. If bolus is required, 1000 cc of Ringer's lactate may be given in less than an hour, and safely repeated up to 3000–5000 cc with sodium replacement of 450–700 meq with careful urine output and CVP monitoring. Choosing the type of repletion solution depends on the source of existing abnormalities and ongoing losses.

Bibliography

Baker RJ, Fischer JE. *Preparation of the Patient. Mastery of Surgery*, 4th ed. New York, NY: Lippincott, Williams & Wilkins, 2001, 23–54.

Berlauk JF, Abrams JH, Gilmour IJ, et al. Preoperative optimization of cardiovascular hemodynamics improves outcome in peripheral vascular surgery. A prospective, randomized clinical trial. *Ann Surg* 1991;214(3):289–297.

DelGuercio LR, Cohn JD. Monitoring operative risk in the elderly. *JAMA* 1980;243(13):1350–1355.

Sampliner JE. Postoperative care of the pancreatic surgical patient: the role of the intensivist. *Surg Clin North Am* 2001;81(3):637–645.

8. **(A)** Current studies suggest that appropriately administered beta-blockers reduce perioperative cardiac events (ischemia) and may reduce the risk of MI and death in high-risk patients. If possible, the medication should be started sufficiently early to titrate to a dose that results in a resting heart rate between 50 and 60 bpm. Some authorities have recommended starting patients on beta-blockers 1–2 weeks prior to surgery and continuing the medication for at least 2 weeks after surgery.

Trials also suggest that alpha agonists may have similar effects, although these agents have not been evaluated as extensively as beta-blockers. Clonidine has been shown to decrease the incidence of postoperative and intraoperative myocardial ischemia in some studies. Mivazerol, an alpha agonist used outside of the United States, has been shown to reduce perioperative myocardial ischemia but had no effects on perioperative MI or death. Further trials on these agents will be necessary to validate their use perioperatively to prevent cardiac events.

Contraindications to either class of drug must be taken into account. These include severe bronchospastic disease, heart block or severe bradycardia, hypotension, and severe left ventricular dysfunction.

Bibliography

Cohn SL, Goldman L. Preoperative risk evaluation and perioperative management of patients with coronary artery disease. *Med Clin North Am* 2003;87(1):111–136.

Eagle KA, Berger PB, Calkins H, et al. ACC/AHA guideline update for preoperative cardiovascular evaluation for noncardiac surgery: executive summary. A report of the American College of Cardiology/American Heart Association Task Force on Practice Guidelines (Committee to Update the 1996 Guidelines on Perioperative Cardiovascular Evaluation for Noncardiac Surgery). *Circulation* 2002;105:1257–1267.

Nishina K, Mikawa K, Uesugi T, et al. Efficacy of clonidine for prevention of perioperative myocardial ischemia: a critical appraisal and meta-analysis of the literature. *Anesthesiology* 2002;96:323–329.

Oliver MF, Goldman L, Julian DG, et al. Effect of mivazerol on perioperative cardiac complications during noncardiac surgery in patients with coronary heart disease. *Anesthesiology* 1999;91(4):951–961.

Weitz HH. Perioperative cardiac complications. *Med Clin North Am* 2001;85(5):1151–1169.

9. **(B)** As a rule, the closer the surgery is to the diaphragm, the higher the risk of pulmonary complications.

Patients who have a history of lung disease or those in whom a pulmonary resection is contemplated, preoperative assessment of pulmonary function is of great value secondary to increased risk of mortality from pulmonary complications postoperatively. History of pulmonary disease (including smoking history and oxygen use) is key to preoperative evaluation.

Physical findings, while certainly important, are often times normal. Evidence of right heart failure should be sought.

CXR is indicated in a patient with underlying lung disease, if for nothing else to serve as a basis of comparison later.

Arterial blood gas should be checked in high-risk patients. PaO_2 less than 60 mmHg correlates with pulmonary hypertension, and a $PaCO_2$ of greater than 45 mmHg is associated with increased perioperative morbidity.

Spirometry and diffusing capacity are two techniques used to evaluate preoperative pulmonary function. In general, patients with a preoperative forced exploratory volume (FEV1) and diffusing capacity lung carbon monoxide (DLCO) greater than or equal to 80% predicted need no further pulmonary evaluation. Studies have shown that few postoperative pulmonary complications occurred in those patients with an FEV1 greater than 2 L undergoing pneumonectomy, an FEV1 greater than 1.5 L for those undergoing lobectomy, and an FEV1 greater than 0.6 L for those undergoing segmentectomy. Additionally, a DLCO less than 60% predicted has been shown to increase mortality, while a DLCO greater than 60% but less than 80% has an increased risk of postoperative pulmonary complications.

Those that do not meet initial preoperative requirements for lung resection should undergo predicted postoperative lung function testing. While studies vary as to the exact values necessary for safe pulmonary resection, current recommendations are for exercise testing to be performed in those with a percent postoperative FEV1 or DLCO less than 40%.

Cardiopulmonary exercise testing is useful in evaluating patients who are marginal candidates for pulmonary resection. Maximal oxygen consumption is a calculated value from this test that gives an indication of lung function. In general, patients with a preoperative maximal oxygen consumption of greater than 20 mL/kg/min will tolerate lung resection without an increased risk of complications. Those with a value less than 10 mL/kg/min have been shown to be at a higher risk for postoperative complications, and are deemed inoperable. Split-function studies along with a pulmonary perfusion scan can be used to evaluate patients with maximal oxygen consumption values between 10 and 20 mL/kg/min. This allows prediction of postoperative function with respect to the portion of the lung to be removed (i.e., the functional contribution of the portion of lung that is being resected).

Ideally, patients should quit smoking for 8 weeks prior to operation. This allows recovery of cilia, decreased secretions, and drop in blood carbon monoxide (CO) levels. Cessation for shorter periods may be associated with a hyperactive inflammatory response in the respiratory system. Patients who quit smoking more than 9 weeks prior to operation approach nonsmokers in terms of postoperative pulmonary complications.

Indicators of increased surgical risk for pulmonary complications include the following:

- cough
- dyspnea
- pulmonary disease

- smoking
- obesity
- abdominal or thoracic surgery
- FEV1 < 2 L
- maximum voluntary ventilation < 50% of predicted value.
- peak expiratory flow rate < 100 L or 50% of predicted value
- PCO_2 > 45 mmHg
- PO_2 < 50 mmHg

The major pulmonary complications in the perioperative period are as follows:

- atelectasis
- pneumonia
- bronchitis

Bibliography

Baker RJ, Fischer JE. *Preparation of the Patient. Mastery of Surgery*, 4th ed. New York, NY: Lippincott, Williams & Wilkins, 2001, 23–54.

Bechard DE. Pulmonary function testing. *Chest Surg Clin North Am* 1992;2(3):565–586.

Beckles MA, Spiro SG, Colice GL, et al. The physiologic evaluation of patients with lung cancer being considered for resectional surgery. *Chest* 2003;123(1):105S–114S.

King MS. Preoperative evaluation. *Am Fam Physician* 2000;62(2):387–396.

Moores L. Smoking and postoperative pulmonary complications: an evidence-based review of the recent literature. *Clin Chest Med* 2000;21(1):139–146.

Nakagawa M, Tanaka H, Tsukama H, et al. Relationship between the duration of the preoperative smoke-free period and the incidence of postoperative pulmonary complications after pulmonary surgery. *Chest* 2001; 120(3):705–710.

Powell CA, Caplan CE. Pulmonary function tests in preoperative pulmonary evaluation. *Clin Chest Med* 2001;22(4): 703–714.

Schuurmans MM, Diacon AH, Bolliger CT. Functional evaluation before lung resection. *Clin Chest Med* 2002;23(1): 159–172.

Slinger PD, Johnston MR. Preoperative assessment for pulmonary resection. *Anesthesiol Clin North America* 2001; 19(3):411–433.

Stephan F, Boucheseiche S, Hollande J, et al. Pulmonary complications following lung resection: a comprehensive analysis of incidence and possible risk factors. *Chest* 2000;118(5):1263–1270.

10. **(D)** Transfusion is not indicated unless a patient is anemic.

It is possible to ameliorate cardiac stress perioperatively. The following is an example of maneuvers available. Hypothermia causes an increase in catecholamine, cortisol, and stress hormone release. Keeping a patient normothermic helps blunt this response. Epidural anesthesia blocks afferent nervous stimulation. This results in attenuation of sympathetic nervous system stimulation. Other maneuvers that ameliorate cardiac stress include control of heart rate and blood pressure with beta-blockade.

Bibliography

Christou NV, Harken AH, Wilmore DW, et al. Risk stratification, preoperative testing, and operative planning. In: Wilmore DW, Souba WW, Fink MP, et al. (eds.), *ACS Surgery: Principles & Practice*. New York, NY: WebMD, 2002.

Frank SM, Fleisher LA, Breslow MJ, et al. Perioperative maintenance of normothermia reduces the incidence of morbid cardiac events. A randomized clinical trial. *JAMA* 1997;227:1127–1134.

Frank SM, Higgins MS, Breslow MJ, et al. The catecholamine, cortisol, and hemodynamic responses to mild perioperative hypothermia. A randomized clinical trial. *Anesthesiology* 1995;82:83–93.

Grass JA. The role of epidural anesthesia and analgesia in postoperative outcome. *Anesthesiol Clin North America* 2000;18(2):407–428.

Kehlet H, Wilmore DW. Multimodal strategies to improve surgical outcome. *Am J Surg* 2002;183(6):630–641.

Lee TW, Grocott HP, Schwinn D, et al. High spinal anesthesia for cardiac surgery: effects on beta-adrenergic receptor function, stress response, and hemodynamics. *Anesthesiology* 2003;98(2):499–510.

11. **(D)** Evidence has shown indisputably that bowel preparation significantly reduces postoperative wound complications. The goals of bowel preparation are reduction of bacterial count and activity. This is accomplished by reduction of bulk stool and bacterial counts by mechanical cleansing of the bowel and administration of antibiotics that cover aerobic gram-negative bacilli and anaerobic bacteria, respectively.

Mechanical cleansing can be accomplished by a variety of regimens to facilitate operative manipulation of the bowel. Of note, this part of the bowel preparation helps facilitate the operative procedure; there is no additional benefit if systemic antibiotic prophylaxis is used. Examples include, but are not exclusive to

clear liquid or low-residue diet the day prior to surgery
magnesium sulfate
magnesium citrate
electrolyte polyethylene glycol solution
phospho-soda
Fleet, tap water, or soapsuds enema

Antibiotics are required to lower bacterial count. The classic regimen involves use of the oral regimen of neomycin and erythromycin base (1 g PO each at 1 p.m., 2 p.m., and 11 p.m.) timed specifically so that the nadir of bacterial count coincides with the beginning of surgery. Data has emerged questioning the need for this regimen in favor of perioperative administration of parenteral antibiotics. Although the results differ in the literature, it appears there is no significant difference in surgical wound infections among many different regimens. A meta-analysis performed by the Health Technology Assessment Unit of the United Kingdom of 147 relevant trials revealed no significant difference in the rate of surgical wound infections among different regimens. Stellato et al. (1990) undertook a prospective, randomized double-blind study to compare the efficacy of three prophylactic regimens (oral neomycin and erythromycin, intravenous cefoxitin, and a combination of both oral and intravenous antibiotics) in patients undergoing elective colorectal surgery of 146 patients. No advantage was found with the use of oral antibiotics in any combination of wound infection rates. An effective intravenous regimen includes administration of second-generation cephalosporins before incision which is active against facultative gram-negative rods and obligate anaerobes and achieves high peak tissue concentrations before incision.

At this time, the preferred regimen of bowel preparation is largely the personal choice of the surgeon, although the evidence implies oral antibiotic regimens are outdated.

In an emergency situation such as obstruction or perforation, parenteral antibiotics are usually the only choice for prophylaxis.

In cases when mechanical bowel preparation is desired for noncolonic abdominal surgery (such as abdominal aortic aneurysm repair), oral antibiotics are not necessary.

Bibliography

Baker RJ, Fischer JE. *Preparation of the Patient. Mastery of Surgery*, 4th ed. New York, NY: Lippincott, Williams & Wilkins, 2001, 23–54.

Cameron JL. *Current Surgical Therapy*, 7th ed. Philadelphia, PA: Mosby, 2001, 265–266.

Lewis RT. Oral versus systemic antibiotic prophylaxis in elective colon surgery: a randomized study and meta-analysis send a message from the 1990s. *Can J Surg* 2002;45(3):173–180.

Polk HC, Jr. Prophylactic antibiotics in surgery and surgical wound infections. *Am Surg* 2000;66(2):105–111.

Stellato TA, et al. Antibiotics in elective colon surgery, a randomized trial of oral, systemic, and oral/systemic antibiotics for prophylaxis. *Am Surg* 1990;56(4):251–254.

12. **(C)** Wound infections or surgical site infections (SSI) are markedly reduced with preoperative antibiotic

administration as noted above. Wound infections are classified as superficial or deep incisional SSIs. One-third of postoperative infections are organ/space SSIs. Infection occurs within 30 days of operation (or 1 year if an implant is left) and involves either the skin and subcutaneous tissue or fascia and muscle layers, respectively. Either pus, evidence of cellulitis, fever, opening of wound, positive cultures or evidence of abscess, or diagnosis by surgeon or attending physician must be noted. Bacterial killing by neutrophils is reduced by approximately 25% and may take as long as 10 days to recover after surgery. Use of preoperative antibiotics as prophylaxis reduces the risk of wound infection, endocarditis, or prosthetic material infection. It has no role in preventing most other types of nosocomial infections.

Wounds can be classified as clean, clean-contaminated, contaminated, or dirty. The risk of infection is 1.5, 7.5, 15, and 40%, respectively. Class I or clean wounds are those that are atraumatic or operative incisions with associated blunt trauma, without associated inflammation. The respiratory, alimentary, genital, uninfected urinary tract, or biliary tracts are not entered. These are closed primarily with or without closed drainage systems. An example is a hernia operation.

Class II or clean-contaminated enter the above tracts under controlled conditions and without unusual contamination. Examples include nonruptured appendix, vaginal hysterectomy, and cholecystectomy.

Class III or contaminated cases include traumatic wounds, major breaks in sterile techniques, gross spillage from the gastrointestinal tract, and incisions where acute, nonpurulent inflammation is encountered. Open cardiac massage is an example.

Class IV or dirty wounds involve old traumatic wounds with retained devitalized tissue and those that involve existing clinical infection or perforated viscera. An example is a Hartmann's operation for perforated diverticulitis.

There are many aspects to consider for proper prophylaxis. The first is whether or not to treat. Several studies have been aimed at defining the use of preoperative antibiotics in clean cases. For the most part they have shown reduction in postoperative SSIs including percutaneous endoscopic gastrostomy tube placements, although one study did not show any difference in wound infection rates in breast surgery with or without antibiotics. The current recommendation is to reserve antibiotics for cases where infection would be catastrophic (intracranial procedures) or prosthetic material is inserted (cardiac valves, vascular cases, mesh). Breast surgery, massive obesity, and diabetes mellitus are sometimes

also considered indications for antibiotic prophylaxis regardless of wound class. The presence of an infected breast wound delays the beginning of postoperative adjuvant anticancer therapy. There is good evidence to suggest that delayed adjuvant therapy compromises the outcome for patients in terms of both local control and survival. In general, antibiotic prophylaxis should be used in all clean-contaminated cases (category IA—recommendations are strongly supported by well-designed experimental, clinical, or epidemiologic studies), although this may not be indicated in laparoscopic cholecystectomies. Class III or IV wounds require antibiotic therapy not prophylaxis.

Second, what is being treated? Different surgeries have different pathogens to consider. Wound infections after soft tissue operations primarily result from gram-positive bacteria, notably *Staphylococci*. Operation on intraabdominal viscera raises concerns for aerobic gram-negative or anaerobes. Cephalosporins are the drugs of choice. The anatomic location of operation influences the choice of a first- or second-generation cephalosporin (third generation cephalosporins provide no additional benefit and promote bacterial resistance). For clean or clean-contaminated cases, cefazolin provides cheap, safe, and appropriate coverage for the pathogens encountered. It also has a relatively long half-life. A second-generation cephalosporin such as cefoxitin or cefotetan covers colorectal surgeries quite well. A third-generation cephalosporin is almost never indicated. Vancomycin should be reserved for clinically significant penicillin-allergic patients or operations at high risk for methicillin-resistant *Staphylococcus aureus* or *epidermidis* (such as cardiac valve or total joint replacement).

Timing of the first dose is critical in relation to skin incision. Administration is ideally complete, or at least under way, when the patient enters the operating theatre to achieve appropriate tissue levels. Intravenous antibiotics should be administered 30 min before the operative incision. Antibiotics should be dosed every 4 h.

Further maneuvers such as preoperative bathing with disinfectants, proper skin preparation, careful placement of drapes, protection of the wound edges from contaminated fluids and viscera, and careful surgical technique all help reduce the risk of SSIs. Razor shaving of the skin on the evening before surgery increases wound infections. If hair must be removed, the following techniques should be used in order of preference: depilatory creams, hair clipping immediately before prepping, and finally shaving immediately before prepping. Postoperative wound management includes protecting the wound with a sterile dressing for 24–48 h postoperatively (category IB—recommendations are supported by some experimental, clinical, or epidemiologic studies and strong theoretical rationale).

Length of prophylaxis is controversial; many times no or only one postoperative dose is necessary. The goal of antibiotic prophylaxis is to maintain the operative levels of antibiotics during operative exposure of the tissue and for a short period thereafter. The indication for antibiotic prophylaxis is based on the surgeon's preoperative prediction of how the wound will be classified *at the end of* the operation. Prophylaxis beyond 24 h is not supported.

Bibliography

Baker RJ, Fischer JE. *Preparation of the Patient. Mastery of Surgery*, 4th ed. New York, NY: Lippincott, Williams & Wilkins, 2001, 23–54.

Bonow RO, Carabello B, de Leon AC Jr, et al. ACC/AHA guidelines for the management of patients with valvular heart disease: executive summary. A report of the American College of Cardiology/American Heart Association Task Force on Practice Guidelines (Committee on Management of Patients With Valvular Heart Disease). *Circulation* 1998;98:1949–1984.

Cacciola F, et al. Antibiotic prophylaxis in clean neurosurgery. *J Chemother* 2001;13 Spec No. 1(1):119–122.

Cameron JL. *Current Surgical Therapy*, 7th ed. Philadelphia, PA: Mosby, 2001, 1278–1281.

D'Amico DF. Antibiotic prophylaxis in clean surgery: breast surgery and hernia repair. *J Chemother* 2001;13 Spec No. 1(1):108–111.

Fatica CA, et al. The role of preoperative antibiotic prophylaxis in cosmetic surgery. *Plast Reconstr Surg* 2002;109(7):2570–2573; discussion 2574–2575.

Gervino L, et al. A retrospective study on the efficacy of short-term perioperative prophylaxis in abdominal surgery for hernia repair in 1,254 patients. *J Chemother* 2000;12(Suppl 3):34–37.

Gossner L, et al. Antibiotic prophylaxis in percutaneous endoscopic gastrostomy (PEG): a prospective randomized clinical trial. *Endoscopy* 1999;31(2):119–124.

Gupta R, et al. Antibiotic prophylaxis for post-operative wound infection in clean elective breast surgery. *Eur J Surg Oncol* 2000;26(4):363–366.

Ríos A, et al. Antibiotic prophylaxis in incisional hernia repair using a prosthesis. *Hernia* 2001;5(3):148–152.

Townsend CM, et al. *Sabiston Textbook of Surgery*, 16th ed. New York, NY: W.B. Saunders, 2001, 1550–1551.

13. (A) In general surgery populations, the respective incidence of pulmonary embolism/deep vein thrombosis (PE/DVT) is 1.6 and 25%. The etiology of venous thromboembolism is described by Virchow's triad: vascular wall injury, stasis, and hypercoagulation. The highest incidence of venous thromboembolism occurs within 24 h of operation. Most occur within 2 weeks of surgery. Pulmonary embolisms generally arise from lower extremity DVTs that have propagated from the calf into the popliteal vein (less than 20% of all DVTs). Two-thirds of deaths occur within 30 min of the embolic event.

Risk factors for the development of DVT include the following. Well-documented ones include antithrombin III (AT-III) deficiency, antiphospholipid antibodies, lupus anticoagulant, myeloproliferative disorders, Leiden mutation, and hyperhomocystinemia. There is increased risk of developing a DVT in any patient older than 40 undergoing general anesthesia for more than 30 min. The risk increases substantially after age 55. Patients with fracture of the pelvis or proximal femur are at the very highest risk group. Other very high-risk patients include severe trauma, spinal cord injury, paralytic stroke, elective knee or hip surgery. Other risk factors include prolonged immobilization, history of DVT or PE, malignancy, obesity, prolonged operation, varicose veins, recent MI, CHF, cigarette smoking, and pregnancy. Stratification of risk is as follows:

2 risk factors: moderate risk
3 risk factors: high risk
4+ risk factors: very high risk

Prophylaxis options include early ambulation, unfractionated heparin, low molecular weight heparin, sequential compression devices (SCDs), elastic stockings, and oral anticoagulants. Sequential compression devices work through stimulation of endothelial cell fibrinolytic activity. When continued until the patient is ambulating, they are just as effective as medications. A very rare complication is peroneal nerve injury. These should be placed prior to the beginning of a case. Heparin in its various forms is active with AT-III and against von Willebrand's factor, affecting the coagulation cascade and platelet activity, respectively. Although low-dose heparin or anticoagulation alternatives' increased risk of bleeding can make them undesirable (minor bleeding and wound hematoma occur in 6–10% of patients), they are the agents of choice in high-risk patients (reduce the risk of DVT from 25 to 8%) given their efficacy. It should be given 2 h before surgery and 8–12 h postoperatively until patients are ambulating. Class I (consistent randomized, prospective trials) evidence supports the following therapies. For low-risk patients, prophylaxis is not indicated. In moderate-risk patients, a combination of stockings, SCDs, and subcutaneous heparin q 12 h or q 8 h or low-dose low molecular weight heparin is recommended. In high-risk patients, the above with high-dose low molecular weight heparin is supported

Armas-Loughran B, et al. Evaluation and management of anemia and bleeding disorders in surgical patients. *Med Clin North Am* 2003;87(1):229–242.

Baker RJ, Fischer JE. *Preparation of the Patient. Mastery of Surgery*, 4th ed. New York, NY: Lippincott, Williams & Wilkins, 2001, 23–54.

Cameron JL. *Current Surgical Therapy*, 7th ed. Philadelphia, PA: Mosby, 2001, 1289, 1349.

Eisenberg JM, Goldfarb S. Clinical usefulness of measuring prothrombin time as a routine admission test. *Clin Chem* 1976;22:1644–1647.

Joseph AJ, Cohn SL. Perioperative care of the patient with renal failure. *Med Clin North Am* 2003;87(1):193–210.

Livio M, Gotti E, Marchesi D. Uraemic bleeding: role of anaemia and beneficial effect of red cell transfusions. *Lancet* 1982;2(8306):1013–1015.

O'Leary JP, Capote LR. *The Physiologic Basis of Surgery*, 3rd ed. Philadelphia, PA: Lippincott, Williams & Wilkins, 2002, 536.

Peterson P, et al. The preoperative bleeding time test lacks clinical benefit: College of American Pathologists' and American Society of Clinical Pathologists' position article. *Arch Surg* 1998;133:134–139.

Ramsey G, Arvan DA, Stewart S, et al. Do preoperative laboratory tests predict blood transfusion needs in cardiac operations? *J Thorac Cardiovasc Surg* 1983;85:564–569.

Rodeghiero F, et al. Epidemiological investigation of the prevalence of von Willebrand's disease. *Blood* 1987;69:454–459.

Suchman AL, Mushlin AI. How well does the activated partial thromboplastin time predict postoperative hemorrhage? *JAMA* 1986;256:750–753.

Townsend CM, et al. *Sabiston Textbook of Surgery*, 16th ed. New York, NY: W.B. Saunders, 2001, 68–78, 81.

15. (C) Optimal control of diabetes is essential in preoperative patients who are at increased risk of developing infectious, metabolic, electrolyte, renal, and cardiac complications during and after surgery. The attendant immunosuppression seen in poorly controlled diabetics increases the risk for postoperative wound infections. Neutrophil phagocytosis and chemotaxis, as well as collagen synthesis, is adversely affected when the blood glucoses are greater than 250 mg/dL. Wound infections, skin infections, pneumonia, and UTIs account for two-thirds of all postoperative complications and 20% of all postoperative deaths in diabetics. Further, many surgical emergencies can give rise to diabetic emergencies such as diabetic ketoacidosis (DKA) or hyperglycemic hyperosmolar nonketotic coma (HHNC). The best method for tightly controlling diabetes mellitus during major surgery is with a continuous IV insulin and glucose infusion.

DKA arises from a combination of effects from insulin deficiency and increase in epinephrine, norepinephrine, cortisol, glucagons, and growth hormone with resultant insulin resistance. In addition, epinephrine causes a decrease in insulin secretion. The patient's metabolism is characterized by hyperglycemia, accelerated gluconeogenesis, reduced peripheral glucose utilization, catabolism of lean tissue and lipid stores, hyperosmolar, osmotic diuresis, volume depletion, paradoxical dilutional hyponatremia, acidemia, ketonemia, and inability to metabolize long-chain fatty acids via lipogenic pathways.

Precipitants giving rise to this state include infection, pregnancy, acute MI, trauma, acute psychiatric illness, major surgery, thyrotoxicosis, and pheochromocytoma.

Signs and symptoms include dehydration, vomiting, tachypnea, severe abdominal pain, and obtundation.

Blood glucose greater than 700 mg/dL, serum osmolarity greater than 340 mOsm/L, arterial pH less than 7.3 with PCO_2 ≤40 mmHg, ketonemia, and ketonuria are diagnostic of DKA.

The differential diagnoses are lactic acidosis, uremia, intoxication (including ethanol), sepsis, cerebrovascular accident, and intraabdominal catastrophe.

Although HHNC and DKA may coexist, patients who have HHNC by definition do not have ketonemia. HHNC patients by definition do not have acidosis or ketonemia/uria. They present obtunded, dehydrated, and azotemic with extremely elevated blood glucose levels. They can be as high as 1000 mg/dL. HHNC is instigated by many of the same culprits as DKA. Pancreatitis and certain medications (beta-blockers, furosemide, parenteral nutrition, thiazides) are also implicated in HHNC. There is sufficient insulin present to suppress lipolysis, preventing ketosis. Therapy is similar to DKA. Resuscitation should be initiated immediately.

Treatment is manifold. Obtain an ECG to rule out a "silent" MI. Institute aggressive fluid resuscitation (patients may have up to a 10 L deficit); hypotonic or isotonic fluid is acceptable initially. Five percent dextrose should be added when the blood glucose drops below 250 mg/dL to prevent hypoglycemia and cerebral edema. Potassium chloride should be added with the second liter or with the first if hypokalemic while acidemic on presentation. Bicarbonate is seldom required secondary to metabolism of ketones (acetoacetate and β-hydroxybutyrate); add 100 meq of $NaHCO_3$ if pH < 7.1, HCO_3 < 10 meq/dL, or to relieve Kussmaul's respirations. Insulin therapy is as follows: 10–30 unit bolus; regular insulin drip at 5–10 units/h; discontinue drip when blood glucose ≤250 mg/dL; cover with subcutaneous regular insulin subsequently; address precipitating factor(s). In this case the patient should be resuscitated prior to being taken to the operating room, if indicated.

Bibliography

Andreoli TE, Bennet JC, Carpenter CCJ, et al. *Cecil Essentials of Medicine*, 4th ed. Philadelphia, PA: W.B. Saunders, 1997, 533–545.

Baker RJ, Fischer JE. *Preparation of the Patient. Mastery of Surgery*, 4th ed. New York, NY: Lippincott, Williams & Wilkins, 2001, 23–54.

Furnary AP, Zerr KJ, Grunkemeier GL. Continuous intravenous insulin infusion reduces the incidence of deep sternal wound infection in diabetic patients after cardiac surgical procedures. *Ann Thorac Surg* 1999;67:352–362.

Gallacher SJ, Thomson G, et al. Neutrophil bactericidal function in diabetes mellitus: evidence for association with blood glucose control. *Diabet Med* 1995;12:916–920.

Hirsch IB, McGill JB. Role of insulin in management of surgical patients with diabetes mellitus. *Diabetes Care* 1990;13:980–991.

Naito Y, Tamai S, Shingu K, et al. Responses of plasma adrenocorticotropic hormone, cortisol, and cytokines during and after upper abdominal surgery. *Anesthesiology* 1992;77:426–431.

Pomposelli JJ, Baxter JK, Babineau TJ, et al. Early postoperative glucose control predicts nosocomial infection rate in diabetic patients. *JPEN J Parenter Enteral Nutr* 1998;22:77–81.

Scherpereel PA, Tavernier B. Perioperative care of diabetic patients. *Eur J Anaesthesiol* 2001;18:277–294.

Schiff RL; Welsh GA. Perioperative evaluation and management of the patient with endocrine dysfunction. *Med Clin North Am* 2003;87(1):175–192.

16. **(D)** The production of glucocorticoids by the adrenal cortex is regulated predominantly by adrenocorticotropic hormone (ACTH) secreted by the anterior pituitary under the influence of hypothalamic corticotropin-releasing hormone (CRH). Aldosterone secretion by the adrenal gland is regulated mainly by the renin-angiotensin system. Patients with primary adrenal insufficiency (Addison's disease) have defects in cortisol and aldosterone secretion. In secondary adrenal insufficiency (e.g., from previous steroid intake), aldosterone secretion is intact. Surgery is one of the most potent activators of the hypothalamic-pituitary-adrenal (HPA) axis, resulting in increased plasma ACTH and cortisol concentrations. The patient described is in addisonian crisis, a result of adrenal insufficiency, the consequences of which if left untreated can be fatal.

Because of this risk, surgeons historically administered high-dose glucocorticoid prophylaxis preoperatively to patients currently on or having received steroids within 6 months to 1 year of surgery. Any patient who has taken more than 20 mg of prednisone or its equivalent per day for more than 3 weeks or who is clinically cushingoid has probable adrenal axis suppression. Patients taking intermediate doses (5–20 mg of prednisone) have questionable suppression. Suppression is not assumed with less frequent dosing regimens. Typically, for prophylaxis, 100 mg IV was given preoperatively and every 8 h (not to exceed 300 mg IV per day) on postoperative day 0, then tapered or weaned to off or maintenance dose over the next 72 h (day 2: 50 mg q 8 h, day 3: 25 mg q 8 h, day 4: 25 mg bid).

Several studies have shown that these doses far exceed daily endogenous cortisol production rates. A consensus paper recommended that surgeons replace glucocorticoids only in amounts equivalent to the normal physiologic response to surgical stress, which in turn depends on the type and duration of surgery. Typical cortisol levels may average 50–75 mg per day for 1–2 days in a moderate stress surgery and 100–150 mg per day for 2–3 days for major stress surgery. Up to 200–500 mg of cortisol of secretion is possible during severe stress, but rates of more than 200 mg per day in the 24 h after surgery are rare.

Based on these physiologic principles, the following are current recommendations for glucocorticoid prophylaxis. In patients with no HPA axis suppression, the usual daily dose of steroids should be given perioperatively. In patients with presumed or biochemically proven HPA axis suppression, the prophylaxis is stratified according to type of surgery: low-risk, no supplementation; moderate, 50 mg IV hydrocortisone prior to induction of anesthesia, 25 mg hydrocortisone every 8 h thereafter for 24–48 h, then resume usual dose; high-risk, 100 mg IV hydrocortisone prior to induction of anesthesia, 50 mg hydrocortisone every 8 h for 48–72 h, then resume usual dose. In patients with uncertain HPA axis suppression undergoing moderate- to high-risk procedures, if time permits check an ACTH stimulation test or to proceed as if suppressed. Although these guidelines are sound, many surgeons still use the former regimen.

It is not necessary to taper supplemental glucocorticoids. If the patient is in addisonian crisis, the taper should not begin until the patient is asymptomatic, then proceed as above.

The diagnosis of addisonian crisis is difficult, as the metabolic derangement seen can be from a variety of conditions as well as concomitant endocrinopathies including diabetes mellitus with or without DKA, hypothyroidism, thyrotoxicosis, and hypoparathyroidism.

Addisonian crisis should be suspected in a patient with sudden cardiovascular collapse.

Various abnormalities include hyperpyrexia (infection need not be present), nausea, obtundation, vomiting, abdominal pain, hypotension, decreased

vascular tone and hypovolemia, retroperitoneal (adrenal) hemorrhage (which may precipitate the crisis), hyponatremia, hyperkalemia, hypoglycemia, prerenal azotemia, metabolic acidosis, and low plasma cortisol level.

Diagnosis is made by administration of ACTH stimulation test (cosyntropin) with pre- and postcortisol levels. Baseline cortisol level in a profoundly stressed patient should be 20 μg/dL with an increase by 25–50% after ACTH stimulation. Symptomatic patients below this level should be treated with steroids; however, this should not impede prompt therapy with hydrocortisone or equivalent (dexamethasone should not interfere with the stimulation test). Approximately 300 mg of hydrocortisone per day is required to treat a patient in crisis. In addition, repletion of volume and electrolytes is mandatory.

Mineralocorticoid deficiency is rare and manifests with the above electrolyte imbalances. Glucocorticoid therapy typically exerts sufficient mineralocorticoid activity, but if the patient continues to be hypotensive, mineralocorticoid replacement may be indicated (deoxycorticosterone acetate or fluorohydrocortisone). Mineralocorticoid replacement need not be initiated until the dosage of hydrocortisone is less than 50 mg per day.

Bibliography

Andreoli TE, Bennet JC, Carpenter CCJ, et al. *Cecil Essentials of Medicine*, 4th ed. Philadelphia, PA: W.B. Saunders, 1997, 497–508.

Baker RJ, Fischer JE. *Preparation of the Patient. Mastery of Surgery*, 4th ed. New York, NY: Lippincott, Williams & Wilkins, 2001, 23–54.

Cameron JL. *Current Surgical Therapy*, 7th ed. Philadelphia, PA: Mosby, 2001, 1138–1340.

Jabbour SA. Steroids and the surgical patient. *Med Clin North Am* 2001;85(5):1311–1317.

Lamberts SW, et al. Corticosteroid treatment in severe illness. *N Engl J Med* 1997;337:1285–1292.

Salem M, Tainsh RE, et al. Perioperative glucocorticoid coverage: a reassessment 42 years after the emergence of a problem. *Ann Surg* 1994;219:416–425.

Schiff RL, Welsh GA. Perioperative evaluation and management of the patient with endocrine dysfunction. *Med Clin North Am* 2003;87(1):175–192.

SESAP 11 *Surgical Education and Self-Assessment Program 2002–2004*. American College of Surgeons, 2001, 243–274.

Zaloga GP, Marik P. Hypothalamic-pituitary-adrenal insufficiency. *Crit Care Clin* 2001;17(1):25–41.

17. (A) Pheochromocytoma is a neuroendocrine tumor of the chromaffin cell that originates from the adrenal medulla and extraadrenal paraganglia cells that most commonly produces hypertension and hypovolemia from release of catecholamines that can lead to a fatal hypertensive crisis or hypotension intraoperatively. When tumor veins are ligated during surgery, the sudden drop in circulating catecholamines can lead to vasodilatation. The catecholamine output of the contralateral adrenal may be suppressed from previous catecholamine excess. In the hypovolemic patient, this can lead to hypotension, shock, and death.

Pheochromocytoma has a varied presentation. Patients are volume-depleted. They also may complain of paroxysmal hypertension (up to 75% of patients) with or without headache, chest pain, abdominal pain, dyspnea, fever, seizures, end organ damage in a pheochromocytoma crisis, insulin resistance, normal blood pressure, and persistent hypertension (50% of patients). Left ventricular hypertrophy, dysfunction, and cardiomyopathy may result.

Treatment is aimed at controlling hypertension, expanding intravascular volume, and controlling arrhythmia. Volume expansion with oral salt and fluid intake is paramount. Normotension (140/90) is a preoperative goal. α-Adrenergic blockade with phenoxybenzamine (5–10 mg PO bid, increased by 10 mg every day to a dose of 0.5–1 mg/kg per day divided q 8 h to an average dose of 40–80 mg per day or until postural hypotension is observed) 1–3 weeks prior to surgery (phentolamine 0.5–1.0 mg bolus; then 1.0 mg/min IV drip intraoperatively) is used to treat hypertension, vasoconstriction, and hypovolemia. The patient should be hospitalized for several days before the operation when postural hypotension is present, for observation and administration of intravenous fluid. Phenoxybenzamine's side effects include somnolence, orthostatic hypotension, stuffy nose, and an inability to ejaculate. Selective alpha$_1$-receptor blockers prazosin, doxazosin, or terazosin can be used if these are not tolerated. Metyrosine competitively inhibits tyrosine hydroxylase, the rate-limiting step in catecholamine biosynthesis, and may be added when other antihypertensive agents are not effective. Second line agents include calcium channel blockers (calcium ion transport is essential for release of catecholamines from chromaffin cells) and angiotensin-converting enzyme inhibitors. β-Adrenergic blockade (propranolol, metoprolol, atenolol) should then be initiated if not contraindicated (asthma, CHF) to prevent the reflex tachycardia associated with nonselective alpha-receptor blockade, prevent perioperative arrhythmias, and cardiac complications. β-Blockade should be begun several days after alpha-blockade, and at least a few days prior to surgery, when adequate α-blockade is achieved or an unopposed α-effect of the catecholamine may occur—leading to block of beta-receptor-mediated vasodilatation in skeletal muscle with resultant vasoconstriction, hypertension crisis, CHF, or pulmonary edema. Morphine and phenothiazines may precipitate hypertensive crisis and should be avoided preoperatively.

Anesthetic drugs that precipitate catecholamine secretion should be avoided (isoflurane, enflurane, nitroprusside, nitroglycerin, phentolamine). Cardiac arrhythmias are best managed with short-acting beta-blockers (esmolol) or lidocaine perioperatively. Invasive monitoring is required, occasionally needing a Swan-Ganz catheter in patients with significant cardiac disease. Laparoscopic procedures are generally better tolerated.

Hypertension may persist for up to 2 weeks postoperatively. Urinary catecholamines should be checked to rule out residual disease. Twenty-five percent of patients have persistent hypertension from other etiologies. Hypoglycemia must be guarded against. If bilateral adrenalectomy is performed, steroid replacement will be required.

Bibliography

Baker RJ, Fischer JE. *Preparation of the Patient. Mastery of Surgery*, 4th ed. New York, NY: Lippincott, Williams & Wilkins, 2001, 23–54.

Bravo EL. Evolving concepts in the pathophysiology, diagnosis, and treatment of pheochromocytoma. *Endocrinol Rev* 1994;15:356.

Cameron JL. *Current Surgical Therapy*, 7th ed. Philadelphia, PA: Mosby, 2001, 624–630.

Plouin PF, et al. Factors associated with perioperative morbidity and mortality in patients with pheochromocytoma: analysis of 165 operations at a single center. *J Clin Endocrinol Metabol* 2001;86(4):1480–1486.

Proye C, et al. Exclusive use of calcium channel blockers in preoperative and intraoperative control of pheochromocytoma. *Surgery* 1989;106:1149.

Prys-Roberts C. Phaeochromocytoma: recent progress in management. *Br J Anaesthesia* 2000;85(1):44–57.

Schiff RL, Welsh GA. Perioperative evaluation and management of the patient with endocrine dysfunction. *Med Clin North Am* 2003;87(1):175–192.

Townsend CM, et al. *Sabiston Textbook of Surgery*, 16th ed. New York, NY: W.B. Saunders, 2001, 684–688.

Ulchaker JC, et al. Successful outcomes in pheochromocytoma surgery in the modern era. *J Urol* 1999;161:764–767.

18. (A) Renal insufficiency is an independent risk factor for cardiovascular death after elective general and cardiovascular surgery. One study found the following as predictive of perioperative MI: valvular disease, previous CHF, emergency surgery, general anesthesia, preoperative diagnosis of CAD, lower preoperative and postoperative hemoglobin concentrations, and increased intraoperative bleeding. Preexisting renal insufficiency is a risk factor for the development of acute renal failure (ARF) postoperatively. ARF is broadly defined as a sudden deterioration of renal function resulting in retention of nitrogenous wastes including urea and creatinine. Other risk factors of postoperative ARF include cardiac dysfunction, sepsis, hypovolemia, cholestatic jaundice, advanced age (suspected without definitive data), trauma surgery, procedures on the heart, aorta, and peripheral arterial system, and hepatic transplantation. Prerenal ARF results from diminished renal perfusion caused by volume depletion and/or hypotension. Renal ARF patients have diminished baseline glomerular filtration rate (GFR) because of diabetes, hypertension, or vascular disease. Acute tubular necrosis is the most common mechanism of renal failure and occurs in the setting of critical surgical illness and multiple organ failure. Postrenal ARF occurs because of tubular obstruction (sulfonamide and acyclovir crystals or bladder dysfunction). Creatinine is a simple but rough estimation of GFR, which in turn is a rough estimate of renal function. Twenty percent of patients presenting with a creatinine between 1.5 and 3.0 mg/dL have coexisting cardiovascular disease. In a patient with previously unknown renal insufficiency, it must be worked up in conjunction with an internist or nephrologist before an elective operation. Patients on dialysis should have their dialysis (within 24 h of the procedure) and fluid management carefully managed by a multidisciplinary team consisting of the surgeon, nephrologist, anesthesiologist, cardiologist, endocrinologist, primary care physician, and nutritionist. During the postoperative period, dialysis patients undergo heparin-free dialysis for at least 24 h. In patients with severe renal insufficiency (creatinine greater than 3.0 mg/dL) not on dialysis, appropriate volume resuscitation should be guided by invasive monitoring, either by CVP or pulmonary wedge pressure. Uremic patients may have platelet dysfunction resulting in an increased bleeding tendency manifested by a prolonged bleeding time. An indwelling bladder catheter is required. Nephrotoxic agents or agents that impair renal blood flow autoregulation should be avoided. Examples of these agents include contrast dye, aminoglycosides, NSAIDs, angiotensin-converting enzyme inhibitors. Low-dose dopamine has been shown to increase urine flow rate in sick postoperative patients, but a recent multicenter, randomized, double blind, placebo-controlled study found that low-dose dopamine conferred no significant protection from renal dysfunction. It is suggested that the dose of low molecular weight heparins be decreased by 50% when the GFR is lower than 10 mL/min.

Bibliography

Andreoli TE, Bennet JC, Carpenter CCJ, et al. *Cecil Essentials of Medicine*, 4th ed. Philadelphia, PA: W.B. Saunders, 1997, 235–252.

Baker RJ, Fischer JE. *Preparation of the Patient. Mastery of Surgery*, 4th ed. New York, NY: Lippincott, Williams & Wilkins, 2001, 23–54.

Bellomo R, Chapman M, et al. Low-dose dopamine in patients with early renal dysfunction: a placebo-controlled randomized trial. Australian and New Zealand Intensive Care Society (ANZICS) Clinical Trials Group. *Lancet* 2000;36(9248):2139–2143.

Flancbaum L, Choban PS, Dasta JF. Quantitative effects of low-dose dopamine on urine output in oliguric surgical intensive care unit patients. *Crit Care Med* 1994;22: 61–68.

Joseph AJ, Cohn SL. Perioperative care of the patient with renal failure. *Med Clin North Am* 2003;87(1):193–210.

Sprung J, et al. Analysis of risk factors for myocardial infarction and cardiac mortality after major vascular surgery. *Anesthesiology* 2000;93(1):129–140.

Weldon BC, Monk TG. The patient at risk for acute renal failure. Recognition, prevention, and preoperative optimization. *Anesthesiol Clin North America* 2000;18(4): 705–717.

19. **(E)** Unlike renal or pulmonary insufficiency, there is no artificial means to support hepatic function. This patient population is prone to multiple complications including gastrointestinal hemorrhage, electrolyte abnormalities (hyponatremia), renal dysfunction (hepatorenal syndromes), and encephalopathy.

In a patient with suspected liver disease secondary to history and physical, the following liver function (LFTs) and synthetic function tests should be ordered: serum bilirubin, aspartate aminotransferase (AST or SGOT), alanine aminotransferase (ALT or SGPT), alkaline phosphatase, protime (PT), and serum albumin.

The Child-Pugh classification of cirrhosis indicates surgical risk, with even low scoring individuals having an increased complication risk. Patients treated medically with improvement of their Child's classification have proportionate improvement in survival (Child's C to Child's A or B).

	Bilirubin	Albumin	Nutrition	Encephal-opathy	Ascites	Operative mortality
A	<2	>3.5	Excellent	None	None	<5%
B	2–3	3.0–3.5	Good	Minimal	Easily controlled	<15%
C	>3	<3	Poor	Severe	Poorly controlled	≈ 33%

Further evaluation of sequelae of cirrhosis may be warranted including endoscopy, pulmonary function tests, CAD, CHF, and renal function.

Variations on the criteria included different levels of albumin and inclusion of increases of PT in seconds from baseline (A: 1–3, B: 4–6, C: >6).

Care should be taken to maintain intravascular volume (Swan-Ganz catheter monitoring); control ascites; avoid hyponatremia; prevent gastrointestinal bleeding (stress ulcer prophylaxis); provide adequate nutrition (thiamine); consider reduction of intestinal flora (gut decontamination and/or lactulose).

Bibliography

Baker RJ, Fischer JE. *Preparation of the Patient. Mastery of Surgery*, 4th ed. New York, NY: Lippincott, Williams & Wilkins, 2001, 23–54.

Blackbourne LH. *Surgical Recall*, 2nd ed. New York, NY: Lippincott, Williams & Wilkins, 1998, 309.

Townsend CM, et al. *Sabiston Textbook of Surgery*, 16th ed. New York, NY: W.B. Saunders, 2001, 1062.

20. **(C)** T_3 and T_4 exert direct inotropic and chronotropic effects on cardiac muscle with increased cardiac output that may limit cardiac reserves during surgery in the hyperthyroid patient. Atrial fibrillation is present in 10–20% of patients. Thyroid storm or thyrotoxicosis may be precipitated in patients who have underlying hyperthyroidism of any cause. This entity is difficult to diagnose, and therapy most likely needs to be instituted prior to return of any lab values. Further, although thyroxine (T_4) and triiodothyronine (T_3) levels are elevated, they are not more so than in nontoxic hyperthyroidism.

Precipitants

- Burns
- Diabetic ketoacidosis
- Hyperglycemic hyperosmolar nonketotic coma
- Hypoglycemia
- Iodinated radio contrast agents
- Pulmonary embolism
- Sepsis
- Major surgery
- Trauma
- Vascular accidents

Manifestations

- Fever
- Confusion or agitation
- Tachycardia
- Seizures
- Diarrhea
- Nausea or vomiting
- Abdominal pain
- CHF
- Rapid atrial fibrillation

Differential diagnosis

- Malignant hyperthermia
- Pheochromocytoma crisis
- Sepsis
- Intoxication
  - Anticholinergic agents
  - Adrenergic agents

Treatment

- β-Blockade attenuates fever, tachycardia, dysrhythmias, anxiety, and agitation
  - Propranolol 10–40 mg qid
  - Atenolol or esmolol in patients with CHF with digitalis
- Iodine blocks release of T_4 and T_3 from the thyroid
- Iopanoic acid blocks T_4 to T_3 conversion
- Thionamides block thyroid hormone synthesis
  - Propylthiouracil (PTU) 1 h before iodine administration to prevent uptake of iodine by the thyroid as substrate for more hormone production
  - Methimazole reverses hyperthyroidism sooner than PTU
- Dexamethasone in patients with suspected adrenal insufficiency (may block peripheral conversion of T_4 to T_3 as well)
- Hydration
- Nutrition with glucose and vitamins
- Antipyretics
  - Acetaminophen
  - Aspirin may increase thyroid hormone concentrations by interfering with protein binding of T4 and T3
- Cooling blankets
- Treatment of cardiac complications such as heart failure and atrial fibrillation

Bibliography

Baker RJ, Fischer JE. *Preparation of the Patient. Mastery of Surgery*, 4th ed. New York, NY: Lippincott, Williams & Wilkins, 2001, 23–54.

Klein I, Ojamaa K. Mechanisms of disease: thyroid hormone and the cardiovascular system. *N Engl J Med* 2001;344(7):501–509.

Mazzaferri EL, Skillman TG. Thyroid storm: a review of 22 episodes with special emphasis on the use of guanethidine. *Arch Intern Med* 1969;124:684–690.

McArthur JW, Rawson RW, Means JH, et al. Thyrotoxic crisis. *JAMA* 1947;132:868.

Sawin CT, Geller A, Wolf PA. Low serum thyrotropin concentration as a risk factor for atrial fibrillation in older patients. *N Engl J Med* 1994;331:1249–1252.

Schiff RL, Welsh GA. Perioperative evaluation and management of the patient with endocrine dysfunction. *Med Clin North Am* 2003;87(1):175–192.

Woeber KA. Thyrotoxicosis and the heart. *N Engl J Med* 1992;327:94–97.

21. **(B)** The above noted cardiac sounds are associated with atrial septal defect, mitral regurgitation or ventricular septal defect, left ventricular failure or volume overload (normal in children), systemic hypertension, normal, respectively.

There is a significant prevalence of valvular heart disease amongst the population of patients undergoing elective major noncardiac procedures. The American Heart Association has published guidelines for antibiotic prophylaxis for prevention of endocarditis, the need of which is dictated by both the cardiac abnormality and type of surgical procedure. There exist no published randomized trials demonstrating that prophylaxis lowers the risk of developing endocarditis. Nevertheless, the morbidity and mortality associated with infective endocarditis are used to justify prophylaxis for patients who have high- and intermediate-risk cardiac lesions and who are to undergo bacteremia-inducing procedures.

Knowledge of the pathogens associated with types of procedures is paramount in choosing the appropriate prophylaxis agent. The target for prophylaxis in procedures involving the oral cavity, respiratory tract, or esophagus is viridans streptococci. For genitourinary and gastrointestinal cases, there is a strong association with enterococcal endocarditis. Prophylaxis against *Staphylococcus aureus* is employed when incising and draining skin or soft tissue infections.

Procedures for which prophylaxis is recommended include dental procedures which induce gingival or mucosal bleeding (especially extractions); tonsillectomy or adenoidectomy; gastrointestinal or respiratory mucosa; rigid bronchoscopy; esophageal varix sclerotherapy; esophageal dilatation; endoscopic retrograde cholangiography (ERCP) with biliary obstruction; gallbladder surgery; cystoscopy with urethral dilation; urethral catheterization if UTI present; urinary tract surgery, including prostate; incision and drainage of infected tissue.

Procedures for which prophylaxis is recommended only if patients are at highest risk include flexible bronchoscopy, gastrointestinal endoscopy, and vaginal hysterectomy. Further, in the absence of infection, the following may need prophylaxis: urethral catheterization, dilatation and curettage, uncomplicated vaginal delivery, therapeutic abortion, insertion or removal of intrauterine devices, sterilization procedures, and laparoscopy.

The following procedures are not recommended for prophylaxis: dental procedures not likely to cause bleeding, shedding of primary teeth, tympanostomy tube insertion, endotracheal tube insertion, transesophageal echocardiography, cardiac catheterization, pacemaker implantation, incision or biopsy of scrubbed skin, Cesarean section, and circumcision.

Certain preexisting cardiac disorders are associated with relatively high risk of infective endocarditis, the presence of prosthetic heart valves being the highest. Others for which prophylaxis is recommended include patent ductus arteriosus, aortic regurgitation or stenosis, mitral regurgitation with or without stenosis, ventricular septal defect, coarctation of the aorta, postoperative intracardiac lesion with residual hemodynamic abnormality or prosthetic device. Cardiac disorders with relatively high risk but not recommended for prophylaxis include previous infective endocarditis, cyanotic congenital heart disease, and surgically constructed systemic-pulmonary shunts.

Intermediate risk conditions include mitral valve prolapse with regurgitation (murmur) or thickened valve leaflets, mitral stenosis, tricuspid valve disease, pulmonary stenosis, asymmetrical septal hypertrophy, bicuspid aortic valve or calcific aortic sclerosis with minimal hemodynamic abnormality, degenerative valvular disease in elderly patients, and postoperative (less than 6 months) intracardiac lesion with minimal or no hemodynamic abnormality.

Cardiac disorders with very low or negligible risk, for which prophylaxis is not recommended include mitral valve prolapse without regurgitation (murmur) or thickened valve leaflets, trivial valvular regurgitation on echocardiogram without structural abnormality, atrial septal defect (secundum), arteriosclerotic plaques, CAD, pacemaker or implanted defibrillators, postoperative (more than 6 months) intracardiac lesion with minimal or no hemodynamic abnormality, prior coronary bypass graft surgery, and prior Kawasaki's disease or rheumatic fever without valvular dysfunction.

The following regimens are recommended for genitourinary and gastrointestinal (except esophageal) procedures. In high-risk patients give ampicillin (2 g IV/IM in adults or 50 mg/kg in children) plus gentamicin (1.5 mg/kg IV/IM not to exceed 120 mg) within 30 min of the procedure, followed by ampicillin (1 g IV/IM adult or 25 mg/kg children) or amoxicillin (1 g PO adult or 25 mg/kg children) 6 h later. For patients with a penicillin allergy, vancomycin (1 g IV adult or 20 mg/kg children over 12 h to be completed 30 min prior to operation) plus gentamicin (1.5 mg/kg IV/IM) infused or injected

30 min before the procedure without second dose is recommended.

In moderate-risk the patient amoxicillin (2 g PO adult or 50 mg/kg children) 1 h before procedure or ampicillin (2 g IM/IV adult or 50 mg/kg children) 30 min before the procedure is recommended. For those with penicillin allergies give vancomycin (1 g IV adult or 20 mg/kg children) over 1–2 h with completion 30 min before the procedure.

For dental, oral, respiratory tract, or esophageal procedures, the following regimens are recommended. Depending if the patient is able to take oral antibiotics, amoxicillin (2 g PO adult or 50 mg/kg children) 1 h before procedure or ampicillin (2 g IM/IV adult or 50 mg/kg children) 30 min before the procedure is recommended. If the patient is allergic to penicillin, then in order of preference, the following antibiotics are recommended to take orally: clindamycin 600 mg adults or 20 mg/kg children, cephalexin or cefadroxil 2 g adults or 50 mg/kg children, or azithromycin or clarithromycin 500 mg adults or 15 mg/kg children 1 h before the procedure. If this group of patients is unable to take oral antibiotics, then clindamycin 600 mg adults or 20 mg/kg children IV or cefazolin 1 g IV adult or 25 mg/kg children within 30 min before the procedure. Total children's dose should not exceed adult dose.

Penicillin-resistant flora may emerge among patients who are receiving continuous penicillin for prevention of rheumatic fever or repetitive doses for serial dental procedures. A regimen without penicillin is preferable in these patients. If prophylaxis is initiated several days before surgery, then organisms become resistant at the mucosal site.

Bibliography

Braunwald E. *Heart Disease: A Textbook of Cardiovascular Medicine*, 6th ed. Philadelphia, PA: W.B. Saunders, 2001, 1742–1745.

Dajani AS, et al. Prevention of bacterial endocarditis: recommendations by the American Heart Association. *JAMA* 1997;277:1794.

Durack DT. Prevention of endocarditis. *N Engl J Med* 1995;332:38–44.

McMillan JA, et al. *Oski's Pediatrics: Principles and Practice*, 3rd ed. Baltimore, MD: Lippincott, Williams & Wilkins, 1999, 1409–1412.

Shammash JB, Ghali WA. Preoperative assessment and perioperative management of the patient with nonischemic heart disease. *Med Clin North Am* 2003;87(1): 137–152.

CHAPTER 5

Hemostasis and Coagulation

Christopher M. Bearden

Questions

1. All of the following are true *except*

   (A) In the classic model of coagulation the intrinsic pathway initiates coagulation by interaction of circulating factors already within the blood.

   (B) In the classic model of coagulation the extrinsic pathway initiates coagulation by interaction with subendothelial tissue factor.

   (C) Defects in the intrinsic pathway lead to elevations of the activated partial thromboplastin time (aPTT).

   (D) Defects in the extrinsic pathway lead to elevations of the prothrombin time (PT).

   (E) The intrinsic pathway requires the presence of factor VII and Ca^{2+}.

2. Which one of the following substances is not known to directly activate platelets during the process of clot formation?

   (A) thrombin

   (B) adenosine triphosphate (ATP)

   (C) epinephrine

   (D) collagen

   (E) interleukin (IL)-6

3. Which of the following substances is primarily found in beta granules of platelets?

   (A) platelet factor 4

   (B) beta-thromboglobulin

   (C) thmbospondin

   (D) fibrinogen

   (E) serotonin

4. In regards to the coagulation *in vivo* which of the following statements is true (see Fig. 5-1)?

   (A) Factor XII is not included in the newer schemes.

   (B) TF does not play a role in the newer schemes.

   (C) The intrinsic pathway is the initiator of events.

   (D) The intrinsic pathway is not involved with hemostasis *in vivo*.

   (E) Thrombin acts to activate further amounts of TF-VIIa thus leading to a positive feedback mechanism.

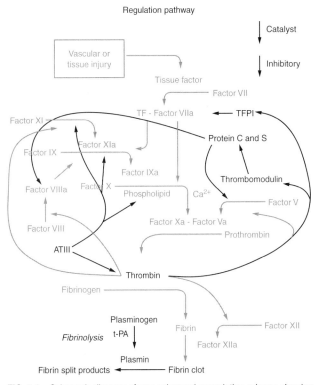

FIG. 5-1 Schematic diagram of new enhanced coagulation scheme showing major role of tissue factor in activation of coagulation.

5. In regards to the physiology of the TFPI all of the following statements are true *except*

    (A) The plasma concentration of TFPI is about 2 nM.
    (B) Platelets carry the majority of the total TFPI in blood.
    (C) Heparin infusion *in vivo* increases the circulating levels of TFPI.
    (D) Elevated levels of TFPI can be occasionally seen in septicemia and disseminated intravascular coagulation.
    (E) No individual with TFPI deficiency has been identified.

6. All of the following statements concerning the regulation of the physiologic cascade (see Fig. 5-2) are true *except*

    (A) Antithrombin III (ATIII) slowly inactivates factors IXa, Xa, and XIa.
    (B) Thrombomodulin as the name implies changes the shape of thrombin causing it to lose its ability to activate other proteins.
    (C) Protein C and S are vitamin-K-dependent factors responsible for inactivating factors Va and VIIa.

Updated coagulation pathway

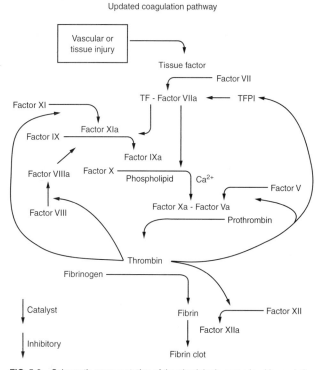

FIG. 5-2   Schematic representation of the physiologic cascade with regulation factors highlighted.

    (D) Plasmin acts to degrade the clot formation and prevent thrombosis.
    (E) Thrombin-activatable fibrinolysis inhibitor suppresses the conversion of plasminogen to plasmin.

7. Low molecular weight heparin (LMWH) produces its primary effects because of its inhibition of which factor?

    (A) IIa
    (B) IXa
    (C) Xa
    (D) XIa
    (E) XIIa

8. von Willebrand's disease (vWD)

    (A) is the second most common bleeding disorder after vitamin K deficiency
    (B) is caused by a quantitative or qualitative defect in a protein necessary for TF-VII interaction
    (C) is inherited recessively in type I
    (D) results in an elevated PT
    (E) can be treated with cryoprecipitate

9. Which of the following drugs is not known to affect platelet function?

    (A) NSAIDS
    (B) warfarin
    (C) nitroprusside
    (D) furosemide
    (E) abciximab

10. Hemophilia

    (A) type A represents a deficiency in factor VIII and comprises 20% of all coagulation factor deficiencies
    (B) type B represents a deficiency in factor IX and is the second most common inherited coagulation disorder after vWD
    (C) is transmitted as an autosomal dominant disorder
    (D) results in an elevated PT
    (E) type A can be treated with DDAVP after mild trauma or before dental procedures

11. A twenty-one-year-old Black male presents to the hospital with multiple gun shot wounds to both lower legs and right upper chest. The left lower leg was amputated below the knee and a right middle and

lower lobectomy were performed. Patient was given over 12 units of packed red blood cells (RBCs) and was sent to the ICU stable but requiring high pressure ventilation. Patient was kept sedated and paralyzed for several days during his progression to acute respiratory distress syndrome.

Within the next week the patient develops a gramnegative pneumonia and bacteremia. An underling low grade sepsis ensues require small amount of dopamine to maintain blood pressure. Patient is started on appropriate antibiotics and maintained on full ventilator management. A week after admission the patient develops a loss of palpable pulses distal to his popliteal artery on his right leg although his dorsalis pedis is dopplerable. Labs reveal the patient to be in disseminated intravascular coagulation.

Which of the following lab values correspond with acute DIC?

(A) slowly rising platelet count

(B) selective deficiency of vitamin K factors

(C) hypofibrigonemia

(D) prolonged bleeding time

(E) presence of fibrin split products

12. Which of the following platelet function test(s) most resembles *in vivo* physiologic clotting?

(A) aggregometry

(B) flow cytometry

(C) thromboelastography (TEG)

(D) bleeding time

(E) all of the above

13. A 45-year-old female presents to the emergency room (ER) after suffering a head-on collision with another vehicle at a high rate of speed. Advanced trauma life support (ATLS) is followed. Primary survey reveals an intact airway with decreased breath sound necessitating chest tube placement. Blood pressure is stable at 110/64 mmHg. Secondary survey reveals tenderness to the abdomen with some guarding but no definite peritoneal signs. Patient is transported to the CT scanner which reveals the following examination (see Fig. 5-3).

Patient is noted to have continued draining from the chest tube at 50 mL/h of dark red blood. She becomes hemodynamically unstable and undergoes exploratory laparotomy and splenectomy with the

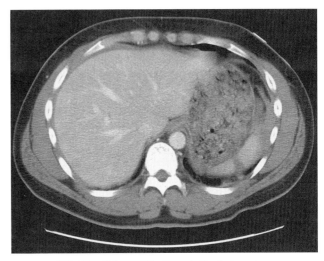

FIG. 5-3 Abdomen CT with grade III splenic rupture.

appearance of generalized oozing within the peritoneal cavity. She is taken back to the ICU where she is warmed and resuscitated.

Over the next several days she is noted to have continued oozing from her needle sticks with a slight decrease in hematocrit. Her chest tube output remains stable at approximately 50 mL/h and is still dark red in nature. She is taken back to the CT scanner where fluid accumulation is noted around the liver and spleen bed.

If coagulation studies on this patient revealed a normal PT, fibrinogen, platelet count, and an elevated aPTT all of the following statements are true *except*

(A) This could be caused by administration of heparin containing substances and can be reversed with protamine.

(B) This could be caused by administration of LMWH that is being used for deep vein thrombosis (DVT) prophylaxis.

(C) If this picture is from heparin administration then infusion of FFP could enhance her anticoagulation.

(D) vWD can be associated with an elevation in the aPTT leading to the possible use of DDAVP in this patient.

(E) Her prolonged bleeding could be caused by a factor deficiency.

14. Factor V Leiden (FVL)

    (A) is the most common inheritable disorder of
        coagulation

    (B) is associated with a defect in factor S activity

    (C) is caused by a mutation in the gene for factor C

    (D) occurs in approximately 10% of people in the
        western population

    (E) results in slightly less than two-fold increase in
        risk for thromboembolism

15. A 68-year-old female presents to the ER with com-
    plaints of right-sided abdominal pain that presented
    12 h earlier. She is diagnosed with polymyalgia
    rheumatica and takes prednisone daily. No other sig-
    nificant medical or family history was found.

    Physical examination revealed moderate right-
    sided tenderness without rebound tenderness. Mild
    hematuria was present on urinalysis, and mild ele-
    vated liver enzymes noted. Differential diagnosis
    included biliary tract disease versus appendicitis.
    Patient is sent for CT of abdomen seen in Fig. 5-4.

    This is followed by a hepatic ultrasound which
    revealed a left hepatic artery thrombosis (see Fig. 5-5).

    Further workup revealed the source of thrombo-
    sis as an antibody.

    Which of the following statements concerning
    antibodies and coagulation defects are true?

    (A) Patients must have detectable antibodies of IgE
        class against phospholipids membranes present
        in blood on several occasions to be classified as
        having antiphospholipid syndrome.

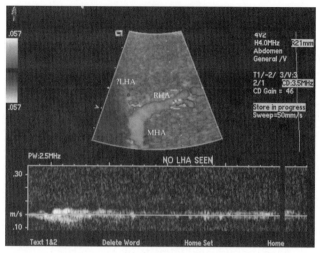

FIG. 5-5   Hepatic ultrasound revealing flow through main hepatic artery into right hepatic artery without significantly measurable blood flow into left hepatic artery.

    (B) Anticardiolipin antibodies react with a β_2-
        glycoprotein I (β_2GI) protein found in plasma.

    (C) Venereal Disease Research Laboratory (VDRL)
        test for syphilis is based on a noncomplement
        fixing antiphospholipid antibody.

    (D) Lupus anticoagulant antibodies can be ruled
        out by a single phospholipid-dependent
        coagulation assay.

    (E) Current protocols for detecting
        antiphospholipid antibodies are by using flow
        cytometric analyses.

16. Elevated levels of homocystine

    (A) lead to an increase in coronary artery disease

    (B) are caused by a deficiency in B_6 intake.

    (C) are being treated with experimental drugs
        currently in clinical trials

    (D) increase one's risk of venous disease by a factor
        of 7

    (E) are being treated with folate supplementation
        in grains by the Food and Drug Administration
        (FDA)

17. Prothrombin gene mutation

    (A) is a common genetic mutation leading to
        hemophilia (excessive bleeding)

    (B) is caused by a missense mutation

    (C) has a low relative risk <2 of causing symptoms

    (D) leads to elevated levels of prothrombin

    (E) occurs in as high as 4% of unaffected people in
        the population

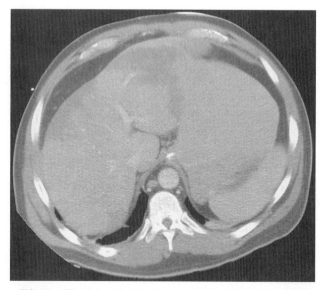

FIG. 5-4   CT showing infarction of segments of the left lobe of the liver.

18. Venous disease caused by oral contraceptives use

    (A) is caused only by the estrogen component

    (B) is not dependent on dose

    (C) is a factor of dose over time

    (D) carries a relative risk of approximately 2

    (E) is as prevalent as arterial disease in these patients

19. Which of the following diseases, if present, has the highest relative risk of developing VTE?

    (A) oral contraceptive use

    (B) heterozygous carrier of FVL

    (C) antiphospholipid syndrome

    (D) prothrombin gene mutation

    (E) heterozygous protein C deficiency

20. Oral contraceptive use in the presence of a heterozygous carrier of FVL increases the risk of developing VTE by

    (A) 2x

    (B) 4x

    (C) 10x

    (D) 20x

    (E) 30x

21. A 55-year-old previously healthy male has just received a left hemicolectomy for Dukes B colon cancer. Patient is slow to regain mobility secondary to pain issues. All of the following are accepted treatment options for DVT prophylaxis *except*

    (A) enoxoprin

    (B) sequential compression devices (SCDs)

    (C) elastic stockings (TED hose)

    (D) clopidogrel

    (E) warfarin

22. A 23-year-old female unrestrained driver was involved in a head-on collision with a pickup truck. Patient is confused (GCS 8) and hypotensive on arrival to the ER. Appropriate ATLS protocol is followed and the following x-rays (see Figs. 5-6 through 5-9) are obtained.

    Patient has appropriate operative procedure(s) and undergoes pelvic angiography with successful embolism for continued bleeding. She has external fixaters placed on femurs and pelvis. She is taken to the ICU intubated, sedated, and in critical condition. Forty-eight hours later the patient's overall condition has not changed.

    Which one of the following statements is true?

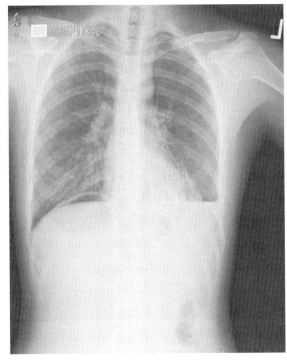

FIG. 5-6   Chest x-ray (pneumoperitoneum).

    (A) Patient should be started on warfarin for DVT prophylaxis.

    (B) Compression devices are contraindicated in this patient secondary to orthopedic fractures.

    (C) Bedside IVC filter placement requires fluoroscopic capability.

    (D) Prophylactic IVC filter is unwarranted secondary to increased morbidity.

    (E) GCS score ≤ 9 is a known risk factor for developing venous thromboembolism.

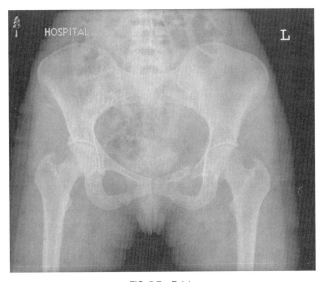

FIG. 5-7   Pelvis.

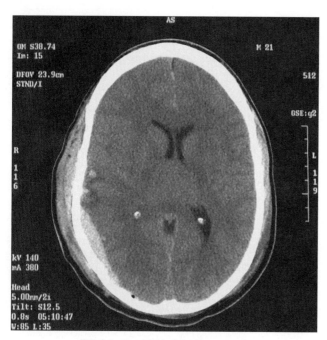

FIG. 5-8   Head CT (subdural hematoma).

23. If the previous patient had been therapeutic on warfarin prior to her injury her relative risk of mortality compared to a similarly injured person that was not anticoagulated would be

(A) 1

(B) 1.5

(C) 2

(D) 3

(E) 5

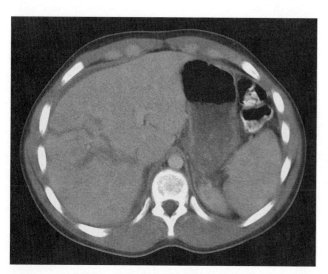

FIG. 5-9   Abdominal CT (hepatic laceration).

24. Who performed the first known successful transfusion of blood to a human?

(A) Jean-Baptiste Denis

(B) Philip Syng Physick

(C) Karl Landsteiner

(D) A. Von Decastello

(E) A. Sturli

25. A 36-year-old male involved in a motor vehicle accident is placed in the ICU for observation of a grade III liver laceration. He is infused two units of packed RBCs because of slow decline of hematocrit and blood pressure. He tolerates the first infusion without any difficulty; however, after 100 mL of the second infusion the patient becomes profoundly hypotensive, develops chest pain, shortness of breath and pain in his right arm. All of the following statements concerning this patient is correct *except*

(A) This is a complement-derived destruction of RBCs.

(B) It is often because of a clerical error.

(C) It can lead to renal failure.

(D) This would not happen if blood was from autologous source.

(E) This presentation could have been delayed for days after the infusion.

26. Donated whole blood is

(A) routinely used in trauma situations

(B) is more expensive for the hospital and the patient

(C) is usually unavailable at most hospitals and blood banks

(D) can be stored for 60 days in standard storage solutions

(E) has hematocrit > 80%

27. Which of the following statements about blood processing and storage is *incorrect*?

(A) Deglycerolized RBCs can be stored for up to 3 years.

(B) Platelets are separated from the plasma component by centrifugation.

(C) Plasma is stored at −18 to −30°C to preserve clotting factor function.

(D) Packed RBCs contain essentially no platelets and levels of factors V and VIII are stable.

(E) Leukocyte concentrate can be obtained and used in patients who are profoundly granulocytopenic.

28. Which of the following diseases is a person at the highest risk of contracting after receiving a standard unit of blood from a volunteer donor?

(A) hepatitis A

(B) hepatitis B

(C) hepatitis C

(D) human immunodeficiency virus (HIV)

(E) parvovirus B19

29. Acute lung injury following transfusion

(A) occurs in 1 in 1000 transfusions

(B) can be caused by antibody formation to the blood donor cells

(C) can be secondary to storage defects of the blood transfused

(D) leads to death in greater than 35% of affected patients

(E) usually manifests slowly and presents clinically several days after transfusion

30. The transfusion of red cells

(A) should be untaken if the hemoglobin is ≤ 7 g/dL

(B) if indicated can be performed without involving the patient decision

(C) should be transfused two units at a time if indicated

(D) can be used appropriately as a volume expander

(E) is based on clinical indications

31. A 54-year-old patient is brought to the ER for complaints of bleeding per rectum. The patient states she has lost approximately 25 lb in the last year and has had "sticky" bowel movements for months. Laboratory examination reveals hemoglobin of 6.5 g/dL after rehydration. Patient is sent for colonoscopy where a large obstructing fungating mass is noted in the sigmoid colon. Patient is approached about surgical resection and the possible need for blood transfusion. She consents for the surgery but states that she is a Jehovah's Witness and will not accept any blood products.

Which of the following statement concerning her beliefs is *incorrect*?

(A) She is likely to refuse autologous blood as well.

(B) She will refuse human albumin as a volume expander.

(C) She should be cared for by someone who is sympathetic to her beliefs.

(D) She will not accept immune globulin from animals.

(E) She is at a high risk for complications without blood transfusion.

32. Acute normovolemic hemodilution

(A) is generally safe for elective cases in young healthy individuals

(B) can be performed safely in patients with hematocrits $\leq 20\%$

(C) decreases the risk of disease transmission

(D) involves separating of blood products prior to infusion

(E) produces several physiologic changes but the end result is less oxygen delivery to the tissues

33. A 65-year-old man is seen in your clinic for possible pancreaticoduodenectomy secondary to pancreatic cancer. He is scheduled for surgery in 2 weeks. He asks you specifically about blood loss and that he wants to donate blood for himself. Which of the following statements concerning preoperative autologous blood transfusion is *correct*?

(A) Preoperative blood transfusion is safe in patients with hematocrit of 25%.

(B) Blood can be donated up to 2 months prior to surgery.

(C) Preoperative autologous blood transfusion prevents the risk of transfusion reactions.

(D) Is a cost-effective method to treat postoperative anemia.

(E) Blood can be withdrawn as quickly as every 3–4 days.

34. A 45-year-old patient contracted hepatitis C from a previous blood transfusion. The patient underwent a successful liver transplantation. The patient is given rabbit antithymocyte globulin and develops profound thrombocytopenia from the drug. Which of the following statements concerning platelet transfusion in this patient is *incorrect*?

(A) If asymptomatic a platelet count of $\leq 20,000/\text{mm}^3$ is an indication for transfusion for this patient.

(B) Apheresis units have less HLA to complicate this patient's immunosuppression.

(C) Platelets are highly immunogenic.

(D) Platelet should be withheld if the patient is symptomatic but hypothermic.

(E) It is indicated for microvascular bleeding.

35. Red blood cell substitutes

    (A) have currently been approved by the FDA

    (B) are being produced by *E. coli* through recombinant technology

    (C) all show decreased mortality in current trials

    (D) currently in use contain no human or bovine hemoglobin

    (E) include synthetic compounds based on polyethylene glycol

36. Concerning intraoperative and postoperative blood collecting, which statement is *correct*?

    (A) Cell washing machines can process up to 20 units of blood per hour for infusion.

    (B) Cell washing machines process blood intraoperatively and can be stored for up to 1 month.

    (C) Red cells obtained from cell saver machines have longer half-life once infused than do allogenic cells.

    (D) Blood from devices such as chest tubes often contain high concentrations of hemoglobin (i.e., hematocrit).

    (E) Blood from devices such as chest tubes and surgical drains can be reinfused without processing.

37. With regard to suture material which one of the following statements is *incorrect*?

    (A) Suture material is categorized as absorbable versus nonabsorbable.

    (B) Steel produces the least amount of inflammation of all the suture material.

    (C) Steel suture materials are available in braided preparations.

    (D) Braided suture passes through tissue better than monofilament ones.

    (E) Surgical hemostasis begins with good surgical technique.

38. Which one of the following devices provides the least amount of adjacent tissue damage during normal usage?

    (A) electrocautery on cutting mode

    (B) electrocautery on coagulation mode

    (C) harmonic scapel

    (D) argon beam coagulation

    (E) Nd-YAG laser

39. Topical hemostatic and tissue sealing agents

    (A) act by augmenting the coagulation cascade

    (B) can be used in the place of subcutaneous sutures

    (C) such as gelfoam do not work without the addition of thrombin

    (D) such as the cyanoacrylate derivatives are used strictly for skin closure

    (E) are not widely used

40. Fibrin preparations

    (A) are commercially available in the United States by combining human thrombin and bovine cryoprecipitate

    (B) as commercial sealants have been available in the Unites States for over 20 years

    (C) can be stabilized by the addition of aprotinin

    (D) are contraindicated in patients with vWD

    (E) require presence of thrombin from the patient for activation

Answers and Explanations

1. (E) Older textbooks divide the coagulation cascade into the intrinsic and extrinsic pathways. This traditional depiction is useful in interpreting coagulation test abnormalities, such as PT and aPTT. The intrinsic pathway can be activated without an extravascular source. The extrinsic pathway in contrast requires an extravascular component, such as tissue factor (TF) for activation. Both pathways are thought to be activated simultaneously to initiate and sustain clot formation (Fig. 5-10).

Elevations in the aPTT are thought to arise from defects in the intrinsic pathway. This pathway begins with trauma to the blood vessel, exposure of blood to collagen in a damaged vascular wall but as the name implies can also occur outside the vascular wall with most "wetable" surfaces, such as tables and glass. In response to these stimuli, factor XII (Hageman Factor) is activated to form factor XIIa. Activated factor XII then activates factor XI to factor XIa. Activated factor XI converts factor IX to factor IXa. Factor IXa then converts factor X to factor Xa. This activation of factor X is also greatly accelerated by factor VIIIa. Activated factor X converts the inactive molecule prothrombin to the active thrombin.

Elevations in the PT are thought to arise from defects in the extrinsic pathway. This pathway requires either a vascular wall to be penetrated or the presence of extravascular tissue. TF is found predominately on most nonendothelial cells. Damage to vessel walls causes the plasma to be exposed to TF. TF combines with factor VII to form the TF-VIIa complex. TF-VIIa complex in the presence of Ca^{2+} and phospholipids can activate factor X to Xa leading to thrombin formation.

Once thrombin has formed it has numerous other jobs including cleaving fibrinogen into the fibrin monomers. Fibrin monomers consist of fibrinopeptides A and B which each undergo conformation changes to expose the active components and allow for polymerization. Polymerization of fibrin occurs by cross-linking the monomers forming a mesh-like substrate where the clot will form. In addition, thrombin is able through a positive feedback mechanism to activate most of the components within the cascade thereby leading to larger amounts of thrombin and fibrin.

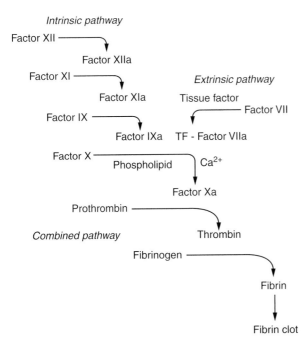

Classic coagulation pathway "waterfall hypothesis"

FIG. 5-10 Schematic representation of the traditional coagulation scheme or "Waterfall Hypothesis."

Bibliography

Davie EW, Fujikawa K, Kisiel W. The coagulation cascade: initiation, maintenance, and regulation. *Biochemistry* 1991;30(43):10363–10370.

Furie B, Furie BC. Molecular and cellular biology of blood coagulation. *N Engl J Med.* 1992;326(12):800–806.

Owings J, Gosselin R. Bleeding and transfusion. In: Wilmore D, Cheung L, Harken A, Holcroft J, Meakins J,

Soper N (eds.), *ACS Surgery: Principles and Practice*. New York, NY: WebMD, 2002, 77–90.

2. (E)

3. (E)

Explanations 2 and 3

The primary role of platelets in the process of hemostasis is providing a phospholipid layer for which the coagulation activation sequences can progress. Platelets are found in the circulation as anucleate cellular particles with both alpha granules that contain platelet factor 4, beta-thromboglobulin, thrombospondin, platelet-derived growth factor, fibrinogen and von Willebrand's factor (vWF), and beta granules that contain adenosine diphosphate (ADP), serotonin, and organelles. Their synthesis is primary controlled by IL-3, IL-6, IL-11, and thrombopoietin. The cell surface contains several glycoprotein (GP) receptors responsible for hemostasis. GPIb interacts with vWF and causes adherence of the platelet to the injured vessel wall. GPIIb-IIIa serves as a receptor for fibrinogen and helps with platelet aggregation. After activation by substances such as ATP, ADP, epinephrine, thromboxane A_2, collagen and thrombin, the platelets undergo shape changes, degranulate and provide receptors for the coagulation factors.

Once released, the granules within platelets enhance the coagulation process. They act by further activating platelets, aiding with vasoconstriction, stimulating adherence of leukocytes, and providing microparticles essential in the formation of the platelet plug. Activated platelets also act as a surface by which the coagulation cascade can occur in the presence of Ca^{2+} and the phospholipids layer needed for factor activation.

As fibrin is formed the platelets get intertwined within the cross-linking helping to form the clot. Leukocytes get trapped as well and they help initiate inflammatory responses necessary for wound healing. The final platelet plug is later replaced by endothelial cells and tissue repair occurs.

Bibliography

Fakhry S, Rutherford E, Sheldon G. Hematologic principles in surgery. In: Townsend C (ed.), *Sabiston Textbook of Surgery*, 16th ed. Philadelphia, PA: W.B. Saunders, 2001, 69–89.

Martin P, Santhouse A. von Willebrand disease: recent advances in pathophysiology and treatment. *Am J Med Sci* 1998;316(2):77–89.

Owings J, Gosselin R. Bleeding and transfusion. In: Wilmore D, Cheung L, Harken A, Holcroft J, Meakins J, Soper N (eds.), *ACS Surgery: Principles and Practice*. New York, NY: WebMD, 2002, 77–90.

4. (A) *In vivo* coagulation has been found to be a combination of the two pathways described earlier. Patients with factor XII deficiencies were not found to have inherent bleeding leading to the removal of this factor from most schemes. TF is the important initiator of coagulation. When vascular injury occurs factor VII is exposed to TF and the complex forms as described earlier. TF-VIIa complex then proceeds similarly through the extrinsic pathway leading to thrombin formation and eventually fibrin clot formation. Only limited amounts of thrombin are produced by this mechanism. Thrombin binds to and activates a protein called tissue factor pathway inhibitor (TFPI). This complex then inactivates the factor VII-TF complexes, thus inhibiting further synthesis of thrombin through this pathway, representing a negative feedback system thus controlling hemostasis.

The thrombin initially synthesized through the factor VII-TF complex pathway also has other functions that are procoagulant in nature. One of its main functions is to catalyze the activation of factors V, VIII, XI, and XIII, induce platelet aggregation, and induce expression of TF. In this manner, the intrinsic pathway is activated leading to further clot production.

In summary, the extrinsic pathway is the initiator of events through its TF-VIIa complex. This in turn produces enough thrombin to activate the intrinsic pathway leading to large amounts of clot-producing fibrin.

Bibliography

Broze GJ, Jr. Tissue factor pathway inhibitor and the revised theory of coagulation. *Ann Rev Med.* 1995;46:103–112.

Fakhry S, Rutherford E, Sheldon G. Hematologic principles in surgery. In: Townsend C (ed.), *Sabiston Textbook of Surgery*, 16th ed. Philadelphia, PA: W.B. Saunders, 2001, 69–89.

Owings J, Gosselin R. Bleeding and transfusion. In: Wilmore D, Cheung L, Harken A, Holcroft J, Meakins J, Soper N (eds.), *ACS Surgery: Principles and Practice*. New York, NY: WebMD, 2002, 77–90.

Schell S, Barbul A. Coagulopathy. In: Cameron J (ed.), *Current Surgical Therapy*, 6th ed. St. Louis, MO: Mosby, 1998, 1146–1150.

5. (B) The recent understanding of the TFPI and its effects after forming the complex with factor Xa was the basis for the new representation of the coagulation cascade. Most of the TFPI circulating in the plasma is bound to the lipoproteins to include low density lipoprotein (LDL) and high density lipoprotein (HDL). TFPI concentration in the plasma is quite low and is estimated at about 2 nM. Platelets carry only 10% of the total concentration of TFPI and their release following stimulation is important in regulating the clot formation.

Experiments conducted with *in vivo* infusion of heparin show a two- to threefold increase in the amount of circulating TFPI. This is not seen when heparin is infused *ex vivo* leading to the hypothesis that a majority of TFPI is found in an extravascular source which is likely the endothelium. This release after the infusion of heparin may augment the effects of heparin anticoagulation.

The infusion of TFPI has been studied as a possible treatment of sepsis-induced disseminated intravascular coagulopathy (DIC). It is known that levels of TFPI do not rise in the face of DIC and sepsis, although the level of TF-VIIa complex is extremely elevated. This suggests that DIC in the face of sepsis is caused by an imbalance in the ratio of TFPI and TF-VIIa. Supraphysiologic doses of TFPI have been shown to stop DIC induced by TF in rabbits and decrease mortality in baboons.

Human trials with recombinant TFPI (rTPFI-1) have shown promise in the treatment of sepsis-induced DIC. Phase I trials showed that rTFPI can be safely given to humans with no increase in bleeding. Phase II trials in patients with severe sepsis showed a reduction in the thrombin-antithrombin complexes and IL-6 levels, with no significant adverse events and a trend toward reducing mortality and length of stays. Phase III trials are currently underway.

There are no individuals who have been found to be deficient in TFPI, prompting the theory that the lack of TFPI does not cause hypercoagulability.

Bibliography

Abraham E, Reinhart K, Svoboda P, et al. Assessment of the safety of recombinant tissue factor pathway inhibitor in patients with severe sepsis: a multicenter, randomized, placebo-controlled, single-blind, dose escalation study. *Crit Care Med* 2001;29(11):2081–2089.

Broze GJ, Jr. Tissue factor pathway inhibitor and the revised theory of coagulation. *Ann Rev Med* 1995;46:103–112.

Doshi SN, Marmur JD. Evolving role of tissue factor and its pathway inhibitor. *Crit Care Med* 2002;30(Suppl 5):S241–S250.

Gando S, Kameue T, Morimoto Y, Matsuda N, Hayakawa M, Kemmotsu O. Tissue factor production not balanced by tissue factor pathway inhibitor in sepsis promotes poor prognosis. *Crit Care Med* 2002;30(8):1729–1734.

Levi M. The imbalance between tissue factor and tissue factor pathway inhibitor in sepsis. *Crit Care Med* 2002;30(8):1914–1915.

6. **(B)** Regulation of the coagulation system is a complex process involving interactions of several proteins and occurs simultaneously with the activation of the procoagulant and inhibitory factors mentioned earlier. Just as thrombin is a major factor in formation of clot it functions as the main down regulator.

Thrombomodulin is a membrane-bound molecule found on both normal and damaged endothelium. In the presence of thrombin, it binds to and changes the shape of thrombin. This conformational change causes the molecule to be a potent activator of proteins C and S thus becoming a potent anticoagulant. This also keeps clot from forming on normal endothelium.

Proteins C and S are vitamin-K-dependent molecules that once activated by the thrombin-thrombomodulin complex are potent inhibitors of factors VIIIa and Va, respectively. Formation of these two proteins highly regulate the formation of clots.

ATIII is a serine protease that requires no activation and is a slow inhibitor of thrombin and factors IXa, Xa, XIa. Undamaged endothelium cells produce a membrane-bound receptor similar to the heparin molecule that will bind ATIII. This functions to reduce clot formation in the presence of normal endothelium.

Plasminogen is converted to plasmin through plasminogen activator (t-PA and u-PA) released from the endothelium. Once activated plasmin is the primary fibrinolytic protein responsible for cleaving fibrin. Breakdown of fibrin prevents the obstruction of the blood flow within the vessel. Formation of plasmin is regulated by the protein called thrombin-activatable fibrinolysis inhibitor (TAFI). TAFI is activated by thrombin after it forms complexes with thrombomodulin thus making the thrombomodulin-thrombin complex an inhibitor fibrinolysis as well as a potent anticoagulant.

Bibliography

Davie EW, Fujikawa K, Kisiel W. The coagulation cascade: initiation, maintenance, and regulation. *Biochemistry* 1991;30(43):10363–10370.

Furie B, Furie BC. Molecular and cellular biology of blood coagulation. *N Engl J Med* 1992;326(12):800–806.

Owings J, Gosselin R. Bleeding and transfusion. In: Wilmore D, Cheung L, Harken A, Holcroft J, Meakins J, Soper N (eds.), *ACS Surgery: Principles and Practice*. New York, NY: WebMD, 2002, 77–90.

7. **(C)** Both standard heparin (SH) and LMWH exert direct effects by binding and catalyzing ATIII. This serine protease inhibitor forms a complex with heparin that is able to inhibit all of the procoagulation serine proteases listed above but primarily thrombin and Xa. SH size is approximately two to four times as big as LMWH. As the size of the molecule decreases the

TABLE 5-1   Subtypes of von Willebrand's Disease

Type	Genetic	Phenotype
I	No abnormality in vWF but relative decrease in quantity and function. Autosomal dominant trait.	70–80% of cases. Mild excessive epistaxis, mucosal bleeding. Normal PT, mildly elevated aPTT.
II	Point mutations in the coding sequence of the vWF gene. Variable inheritance and penetration.	Subdivided in four types based on gene mutation and phenotype. Severity of bleeding is relative to type and location of mutation.
III	Complete absence of gene, or catastrophic mutations lead to lack of formation of vWF. Autosomal recessive trait.	10% of cases. Present as severe bleeding. Normal PT, moderately elevated aPTT.
Platelet-type vWD	Mutation in platelet receptor for vWf.	Mild-to-moderate bleeding.

complex is less able to inhibit factor IIa (thrombin) without losing is ability to inhibit factor Xa. LMWH-ATIII has complete ability to inhibit factor Xa but has lost its ability the inhibit IIa.

Laboratory monitoring of LMWH is essentially unnecessary. LMWH has a much lower affinity for plasma proteins than does SH. This accounts for its 90% bioavailability after subcutaneous administration and less interpatient variability once dose is adjusted for weight. If monitoring is needed then anti-Xa levels can be obtained. Peak response occurs 3–4 h after injection and its plasma half-life is two to four times longer than SH.

Side effects of LMWH are small and include a 1.3% change of developing thrombocytopenia which is similar to SH. LMWH can also induce hemorrhage which is most often seen as wound hematomas. It is not recommended to be used in patients with bacterial endocarditis, congenital or acquired bleeding disorders, active ulcerative and angiodysplastic gastrointestinal disease, hemorrhagic stroke, or shortly after brain, spinal, or ophthalmologic surgery, or in patients treated concomitantly with platelet inhibitors. There is a significant increase in risk of spinal and epidural hematoma after spinal/epidural anesthesia which can lead to paralysis.

Bibliography

Horlocker TT, Heit JA. Low molecular weight heparin: biochemistry, pharmacology, perioperative prophylaxis regimens, and guidelines for regional anesthetic management. *Anesth Analg* 1997;85(4):874–885.

Lovenox Prescribing Information. Aventis Pharmaceuticals, Rev 11/01.

8. **(E)** vWD is the most common inherited bleeding disorder whose prevalence is estimated to be 1% of the population. vWF is found in specialized storage granules within endothelial cells and in alpha granules of platelets. Endothelial cells will secrete vWF and their function is to assist in platelet aggregation as well as a carrier protein for factor VIII. Patients with vWD present with symptoms of platelet dysfunction, such as mucosal bleeding, petechiae, epistaxis, and menorrhagia (see Table 5-1).

vWD can also be acquired. Most acquired forms are seen in patients with lymphoproliferative disorders, but can also be caused by drugs, malignancies, hypothyroidism, and autoimmune diseases. These patients produce antibodies directed at the vWF leading to removal of the protein by the reticuloendothelial system.

The treatment of choice in patients with mild-to-moderate type 1, acquired vWD and some patients with type II is desmopressin acetate (DDAVP). DDAVP is an analog to vasopression and it causes release of endogenous stores of vWF from the endothelial cells. Administration of DDAVP causes a shortening in the bleeding time and normalization of factor VIII-vWF complex activities. DDAVP can only be used once every 48 h to allow reformation of the used vWF and will have no effect in type III patients since they lack all forms of vWF.

Several other treatment options are available for patients who do not respond to DDAVP or have type III. Plasma purified factor VIII concentrations usually have sufficient quantity of vWF-VIII to be effective. Recombinant factor VIII does not contain any vWF and is ineffective. Cryoprecipitate also contains enough vWF to be effective. Several local preparations exist for ancillary treatment during dental procedures. These include aminocaproic acid elixir and tranexamic acid which both be administered as a

TABLE 5-2 Common Inherited Diseases of Platelet Dysfunction

Disease	Characterization
von Willebrand's disease	Caused by a defect in vWF leading to decrease in platelet aggregation.
Bernard-Soulier's syndrome	Glycoprotein IB is missing from the platelet membrane. Platelets are unable to bind to von Willebrand's factor.
Glanzmann's thrombasthenia	An abnormality of the glycoprotein IIb-IIIa complex on the cell membrane. Platelets do not bind fibrinogen properly and do not aggregate well.
Storage pool disorders	A deficiency or abnormality in the platelet granules or in their release mechanisms.
Gray platelet syndrome—alpha granules Delta storage pool deficiency—beta granules	

mouthwash. These agents work by inhibiting fibrinolysis. Topical thrombin, gelfoam, and fibrin glue have also been used.

Major surgery can be performed in these patients if appropriate precautions are taken. In one review of over 64 major surgical cases performed on patients with vWD no mortality was noted in these patients. These patients were treated with items listed above for major bleeding which occurred in only 6.7% of the population.

Bibliography

Blomback M, Johansson G, Johnsson H, Swedenborg J, Wabo E. Surgery in patients with von Willebrand's disease. *Br J Surg* 1989;76(4):398–400.

Martin P, Santhouse A. von Willebrand disease: recent advances in pathophysiology and treatment. *Am J Med Sci* 1998;316(2):77–89.

Owings J, Gosselin R. Bleeding and transfusion. In: Wilmore D, Cheung L, Harken A, Holcroft J, Meakins J, Soper N (eds.), *ACS Surgery: Principles and Practice*. New York, NY: WebMD, 2002, 77–90.

Rinder MR, Richard RE, Rinder HM. Acquired von Willebrand's disease: a concise review. *Am J Hematol* 1997;54(2):139–145.

9. **(B)** Platelet disorders are generally broken up into quantitative defects (thrombocytopenia) or qualitative defects (thrombocytopathys). Inherited disorders include vWD, and defects in the surface receptors GPIb and GPIIb-IIIa thus preventing platelet aggregation. Acquired disorders are very common occurrences and can usually be linked to food or drugs (see Tables 5-2 and 5-3).

Thrombocytopenia is a quantitative defect of platelets defined when the count is less then $100,000/mm^3$. Spontaneous bleeding may occur if platelet counts fall to less then $10,000/mm^3$. Similar to vWD this bleeding is manifested as mucosal bleeding, petechia, GI bleeding, and central nervous system (CNS) bleeding, that can sometimes be life-threatening. Thrombocytopenia can also be seen in various autoimmune disorders, acquired immunodeficiency syndrome (AIDS) patients, and after massive volume resuscitation. The goal of treatment is replacement of the platelets with transfusion. One unit of platelet should raise the platelet count by $5000/mm^3$ with a goal of maintaining the count greater than $50,000/mm^3$. Treating the underlying cause of the thrombocytopenia if known will have a greater benefit than transfusions. As more platelets are transfused the patient is more likely to produce antibodies toward the platelets and decrease the half-life of the infusion.

A common cause of thrombocytopenia in surgery patient is caused by heparin-induced autoantibodies. These patients will generally present with a precipitous drop in the platelet count that returns to normal on discontinuation. Newer drugs derived from snake venom and leaches may be used in these patients if anticoagulation is necessary.

TABLE 5-3 Substances Known to Lead to Qualitative Defects in Platelet Functions

Fish oils	Aspirin	Antihistamines
Chocolate	Ibuprofen (NSAIDs)	Phenytoin
Red wine	Ticlopidine	Dipyridamole
Garlic	Penicillins	Ethanol
Herbs	Cephalosporins	Furosemide
Abciximab	Nitrofurantoin	Thiazide diuretics
Eptifibatide	Theophyllines	Halothane
Clopidogrel	Caffeine	Nitroprusside
Chemotherapy	Estrogen	Prostaglandins

Bibliography

Fakhry S, Rutherford E, Sheldon G. Hematologic principles in surgery. In: Townsend C (ed.), *Sabiston Textbook of Surgery*, 16th ed. Philadelphia, PA: W.B. Saunders, 2001, 69–89.

Owings J, Gosselin R. Bleeding and transfusion. In: Wilmore D, Cheung L, Harken A, Holcroft J, Meakins J, Soper N (eds.), *ACS Surgery: Principles and Practice*. New York, NY: WebMD, 2002, 77–90.

Rodgers GM. Overview of platelet physiology and laboratory evaluation of platelet function. *Clin Obstet Gynecol* 1999;42(2):349–359.

Schell S, Barbul A. Coagulopathy. In: Cameron J (ed.), *Current Surgical Therapy*, 6th ed. St. Louis, MO: Mosby, 1998, 1146–1150.

10. **(E)** The two most common genetically transmitted defects in the clotting factors include the absence of factor VIII (hemophilia type A) and factor IX (hemophilia type B). Both of these diseases are inherited as X-linked recessive disorders, with males being almost exclusively affected. Hemophilias can have varying penetrance with mild cases having 5% normal factor levels to a more severe form with levels less than 1%. In contrast to patients with platelet disorders these patients will have spontaneous bleeding, deep bleeding, and hemarthroses.

Type A is the most common form and is seen in 70–80% factor-deficient patients. These patients will have a prolonged aPTT with normal PT and bleeding times. DDAVP is very effective for mild hemophilia A. As with vWD administration of DDAVP will raise the levels of factor VIII. This is sometimes the only treatment needed for minor trauma or dental procedures. For more severe cases the use of fresh frozen plasma (FFP), cryoprecipitate, or factor VIII concentrate is necessary. The use of FFP requires large amounts of volume and is therefore used as a second line treatment. Goal factor levels for minor surgery are usually 20–30% or normal whereas 50–80% of normal levels are needed for major surgery. As with vWD, DDAVP is less effective if given repeatedly.

Type B or Christmas disease is the second most common clotting factor-deficient disorder and is seen is 15% of cases. Symptoms and laboratory findings with type B are identical to type A except for a decrease in factor IX levels. DDAVP will not be effective in this disorder. Standard treatment of type B bleeding is with prothrombin complex concentrate which contains all of the vitamin K clotting factors or factor IX concentrate which is also available.

Defects in the production of other clotting factors have been noted and are generally secondary to point mutations and are extremely rare (<5%). Most cases if diagnosed can be treated effectively with

FFP. Patients in hepatic failure will also have an acquired from with deficiencies in the vitamin K clotting factors. In contrast to hemophiliacs they will have an evelated PT.

Bibliography

Bell WR, Braverman PE. Abnormal operative and postoperative bleeding. In: Cameron J (ed.), *Current Surgical Therapy*, 6th ed. St. Louis, MO: Mosby, 1998, 1086–1091.

Owings J, Gosselin R. Bleeding and transfusion. In: Wilmore D, Cheung L, Harken A, Holcroft J, Meakins J, Soper N (eds.), *ACS Surgery: Principles and Practice*. New York, NY: WebMD, 2002, 77–90.

11. **(E)** Disseminated intravascular coagulation is a systemic disease that is best illustrated as an intense activation of the coagulation cascade leading to thrombotic occlusion of macro and microvascular vessels. This intense activation of the coagulation leads to consumption of the coagulation factors, excess fibrinolysis, and depletion of platelets leading to widespread coagulapathy, bleeding, and shock (see Fig. 5-11).

DIC is caused when the formation of thrombin remains unchecked. Regulatory proteins such as ATIII, proteins C and S, thrombomodulin are also consumed quickly during DIC and are unable to keep

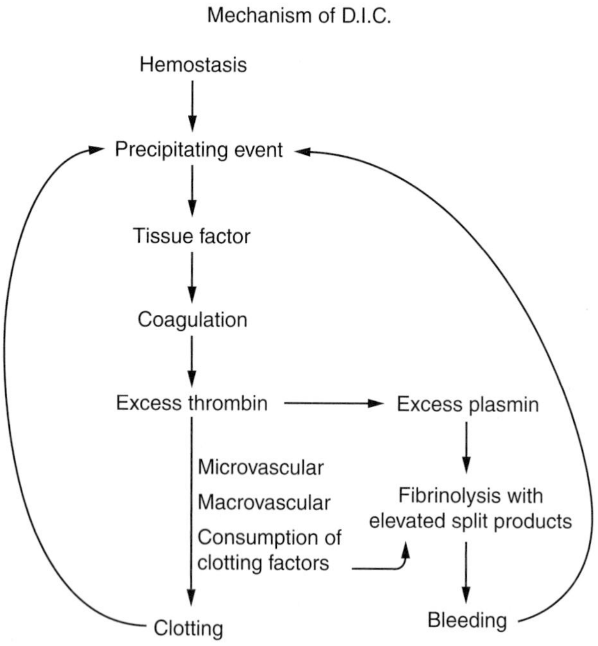

FIG. 5-11 Mechanism of disseminated intravascular coagulation depicting activation of coagulation with excess thrombin formation. Thrombin leads to excess clotting in both micro and macrovascular vessels leading to end organ damage and potentiating the effects of the cascade. Thrombin also leads to excess degradation of fibrin leading to bleeding, hypotension, shock, and vascular permeability resulting in worsening of the cascade.

TABLE 5-4 Causes of Acute DIC

Sepsis and septic shock—generally an endotoxin or exotoxin-related event
Obstetric accidents
    Amniotic fluid embolism—presence of mucus or meconium from the stressed fetus potentates the thrombotic events
    Abruptio placentae—TF-like material is released from the placenta
    Retained fetus syndrome—necrotic fetal tissue activates the procoagulant system
    Abortion induced by hypertonic saline
Hematologic and oncologic diseases
    Solid tumors—activate procoagulant systems as they become necrotic
    Acute leukemias—because of release of procoagulants from promyelocytes on administration of chemotherapy
    Intravascular hemolysis—release of ADP from red cells after transfusion reactions
    Myeloproliferative diseases—various anecdotal reports
Viremias (viral hepatitis, CMV, and varicella)
Trauma
Thermal injury
Kasabach-Merritt's syndrome (giant cavernous hemangiomata)
Metabolic abnormalities—acidosis leads to sloughing of the endothelium with activation of coagulation

up with the massive amounts of thrombin formation. Thrombin induces the formation of tumor necrosis factor (TNF), IL-1, IL-6, endothelin, and selectin inducing vascular permeability and end-organ damage. In addition to clot formation and subsequent uncheck fibrinolysis, thrombin leads to the activation of the complement cascade which produces hypotension, shock, and further exacerbation of DIC.

Several diseases are known to cause DIC (see Table 5-4). The most common surgical causes include severe trauma, burns, and infectious related entities. There is a direct relationship between injury severity and prevalence of DIC. DIC begins at the onset of injury and proceeds rapidly within the first few hours and ultimately death if not treated. Tissue damage caused by burns release TF, IL-1β, and TNF-α directly into the circulation and initiates the DIC pathway. Infections related causes are generally thought to be caused by gram-negative bacteria; however, LPS and endotoxins from gram-positive organisms are known to activate the diffuse coagulation seen in DIC.

Bibliography

Levi M, ten Cate H. Current concepts: disseminated intravascular coagulation. *N Engl J Med* 1999;341(8): 586–592.

Senno SL, Pechet L, Bick RL. Disseminated intravascular coagulopathy (DIC): pathophysiology, laboratory diagnosis, and management. *J Intensive Care Med* 2000;15: 144–158.

12. **(D)** Several commercially available tests are currently on the market for measurement of platelet function. The first and most often used test to measure platelet function is the peripheral platelet count. Modern equipment measure platelet counts through impedance measurements or through light scattering properties similar to a flow cytometer. These machines are generally easy to use, highly reproducible, and require small amount of whole blood in ethylene diamine tetra acetate (EDTA). They will often underestimate or overestimate the count in patients with certain diseases where smaller platelets are missed or larger particles are counted separately. Newer protocols utilizing flourochromes such anti-CD61 with flow cytometry have lead to more precise measurements of the platelet count. The platelet count is a poor indicator of true platelet function. A patient may have normal platelet count but a severe dysfunction of the platelets.

The most used screening of *in vivo* physiologic clotting is assessment of the bleeding time. This is performed by making a standardized incision in the skin and accessing the length of time till clot formation. This test although clinically useful is highly operator dependent, poorly reproducible, invasive, and does not correlate with certain bleeding disorders. This test is being slowly replaced by better *in vitro* measurements that simulate *in vivo* bleeding.

The "gold standard" for platelet function is based on the aggregation properties of the platelets. This is formed by obtaining platelet-rich plasma after centrifugation. Platelets are then stimulated to aggregate and as they adhere to one another the properties of the light scatter is measured and recorded. Dysfunctional platelets cause the light scatter to change slower and distinctive patterns will appear leading to a diagnosis. Several commercially available products are available that use these properties for analyses.

Hemostasis is a combination of several different factors to include platelet function, interaction of clotting factors both procoagulant and anticoagulant,

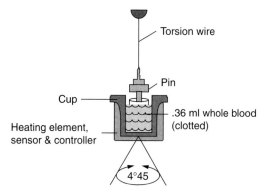

FIG. 5-12 Cross-sectional view of the current TEG system (reproduced with permission Haemoscope Corporation, Skokie, IL).

and fibrin formation to effectively seal vessel injury and develop clots. The dynamics of these interactions are complex in nature and faults in any step can lead to abnormal clot formation. TEG was developed in 1948 and is able to globally measure hemostasis by looking at the dynamics of clot formation. It is able to measure the ability of platelets to form clot and then the subsequent lysis of the clot by plasminogen.

The TEG (Haemoscope Corporation, Skokie, IL) system measures the clot's physical properties, by the use of a cylindrical cup that holds the blood as it oscillates through an angle of 4°45' (see Fig. 5-12). Each rotation cycle lasts 10 s. The pin is suspended in the blood by a torsion wire and is monitored for motion. The torque of the rotating cup is transmitted to the immersed pin only after fibrin or fibrin-platelet bonding has linked the cup and pin together. The strength and rate of these fibrin or fibrin-platelet bonds affect the magnitude of the pin motion such that strong clots move the pin directly in phase with cup motion. As the clot retracts, or lyses, these bonds are broken and transfer of cup motion is diminished. A mechanical-electrical transducer converts the rotation of the pin into an electrical signal that can be monitored by a computer.

The resulting hemostasis profile (see Figs. 5-13 and 5-14) is a measure of the time it takes for the first fibrin strand to be formed, the kinetics of clot formation, the strength of the clot (in either mm or in shear elasticity units of dyn/cm^2) and dissolution of clot. This profile is advantageous as it provides a numerical and graphic representation of coagulation and can differentiate between hyper and hypocoagulable states. One of the disadvantages to the TEG is it is not able to identify platelet dysfunction secondary to aspirin use as platelet adhesion is not tested with this system.

The TEG system has proved reliable in helping to diagnose blunt trauma patients who are more likely to need a blood transfusion within the first 24 h. Approximately 85% of patients who have a hypocoagulable tracing will need blood products compared to only 4% of patients who are hypercoagulable and almost no patients who have normal tracings. Although TEG has been used in research its usefulness in the clinical setting is underutilized by many clinicians.

Bibliography

Harrison P. Progress in the assessment of platelet function. *Br J Haematol* 2000;111(3):733–744.

Kaufmann CRMDMPH, Dwyer KMMD, Crews JDBS, Dols SJMT, Trask ALMD. Usefulness of thrombelastography in assessment of trauma patient coagulation. *J Trauma Injury Infect Crit Care* 1997;42(4):716–722.

Rodgers GM. Overview of platelet physiology and laboratory evaluation of platelet function. *Clin Obstet Gynecol* 1999;42(2):349–359.

13. **(B)** Patients who have continued bleeding after a surgical or traumatic procedure are usually evaluated with coagulation panels which consist of PT (INR, International Normalized Ratio), aPTT, platelet counts,

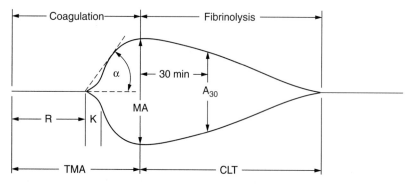

FIG. 5-13 TEG system profile (reproduced with permission Haemoscope Corporation, Skokie, IL).

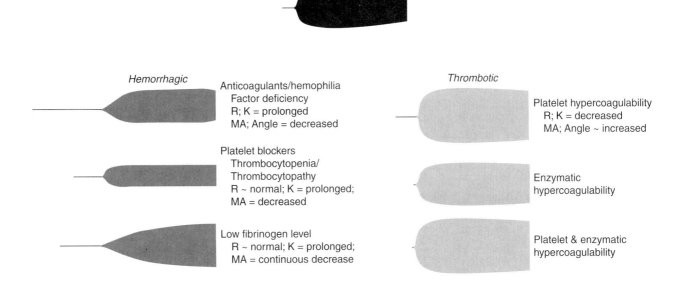

FIG. 5-14 Qualitative interpretation of results from the TEG system. DIC, disseminated intravascular coagulation; R = reaction time, R + K = time to clot formation, MA (maximum amplitude) = mm of clot or strength of clot (reproduced with permission Haemoscope Corporation, Skokie, IL).

fibrinogen, and fibrin split product levels. Based on the results of these tests a general hypothesis and treatment plan can be initiated.

An elevation of the aPTT without a concomitant rise in the PT is almost universally caused by administration of unfractionated heparin. Heparin half-life is approximately 1 h and discontinuing heparin for 4–6 h will return levels to normal. LMWH does not elevate to aPTT and its activity can be tested with anti-Xa levels. Both unfractionated and LMWH act by binding to ATIII and ultimately lowering thrombin levels. They can be reversed with the administration of protamine. Protamine is associated with anaphylactic reactions, hypotension, and pulmonary hypertension and should be used cautiously. FFP does not contain thrombin but does contain sufficient amount of ATIII which will likely potentate the effects of the heparin.

vWD will commonly cause a slight elevation in the aPTT. This can be confirmed by performing platelet function analysis. Correction can be performed with DDAVP, cryoprecipitate, or purified not recombinant factor VIII.

The most common factor deficiencies are IX and VIII. When factor levels fall below 40% then the aPTT will start to be elevated. If mixing studies are performed then the aPTT should normalize revealing this to be a factor deficiency not an inhibitor causing the problem. Specific factor deficiency tests can be performed to determine which factor is missing and appropriate therapy can be instituted. Hemophilia A and B are X-linked traits and are rare in females and would result in a passage of the allele through both X genes (see Table 5-5).

Bibliography

Horlocker TT, Heit JA. Low molecular weight heparin: biochemistry, pharmacology, perioperative prophylaxis regimens, and guidelines for regional anesthetic management. *Anesth Analg* 1997;85(4):874–885.

Martin P, Santhouse A. von Willebrand disease: recent advances in pathophysiology and treatment. *Am J Med Sci* 1998;316(2):77–89.

Owings J, Gosselin R. Bleeding and transfusion. In: Wilmore D, Cheung L, Harken A, Holcroft J, Meakins J, Soper N (eds.), *ACS Surgery: Principles and Practice*. New York, NY: WebMD, 2002, 77–90.

TABLE 5-5   Commercially Available Preparations for Treatment of Hemophilia and von Willebrand's Disease

Product name	Origin
Alphanate, Monarc-M, Hermofil M, Humate, Koate-HP, Monoclate-P	Purified factor VIII from plasma. Contains vWF for treatment of vWD
Recombinate, Kogenate, Bioclate, Helixate	Recombinant factor VIII. Does not contain any vWF
Hyate:C	Porcine plasma
Autoplex T, Feiba VH Immuno, Mononine, AlphaNine-SD, Bebulin VH Immuno, Proplex T, Konyne 80, Profilnine SD	Purified factor IX from plasma
BeneFix	Recombinant factor IX
Novo Seven	Recombinant factors IX and VIII

Schell S, Barbul A. Coagulopathy. In: Cameron J (ed.), *Current Surgical Therapy*, 6th ed. St. Louis, MO: Mosby, 1998, 1146–1150.

14. **(A)** FVL was not recognized as an entity until 1994. It is caused by a single point mutation in the gene for factor V production (FV:Q506 allele) and inherited as a autosomal dominant disorder with highly variable penetrance. Homozygous carriers are affected greater than heterozygous individuals. FVL can be found in 20–50% of patients who develop venous thrombosis with an overall prevalence in the western population of about 5%. This incidence makes it the most common inherited disorder of coagulation. The carrier frequency in Hispanic, Black, Asian, and native American populations are substantially less but are existent.

FVL mutation causes factor Va to be relatively resistant to inactivation by protein C (see Fig. 5-2). Activated protein C (APC) resistance ultimately leads to a hypercoagulable state and individuals are prone to thrombosis. This is increased in individuals who are exposed to oral contraceptives, major surgery, prolonged immobilization, and relatively sedentary individuals.

Clinically FVL presents most commonly with deep venous thrombosis, although pulmonary embolism and superficial throbophelebitis is common. Rarely does it present as arterial thromboses. Twenty percent of recurrent miscarriages in the second trimester are associated with FVL. It affects both sexes and all age groups equally. Because of its high prevalence it is often found in combination with other genetic defects, such as protein C, S, or ATIII deficiency, or antiphospholipid syndrome. These individuals are at higher risk for thrombotic disease than with a single genetic defect.

FVL can be diagnosed with a simple mixing study to determine patient's clotting time. Patient's blood either anticoagulated or not is mixed with plasma-deficient factor V to correct all other abnormalities. A standard aPTT is performed with the blood as well as with blood that has been supplemented with APC. A ratio of supplemented aPTT to unsupplemented aPTT is calculated. Patients with FVL will have a slower clotting time when APC is added compared to controls leading to a ratio that is less than 2. Normal individuals will have a ratio greater than 2. This procedure is rapid, relatively cheap, and reproducible.

Treatment of patients with venous thrombosis secondary to FVL is with anticoagulation. Long-term preventive strategies have not been determined; however, most physicians will treat patients with recurrent DVTs with warfarin anticoagulation for life. Further studies are underway to determine the duration and type of anticoagulation needed.

Bibliography

Middeldorp S, Meinardi JR, Koopman MM, et al. A prospective study of asymptomatic carriers of the factor V Leiden mutation to determine the incidence of venous thromboembolism. *Ann Intern Med* 2001;135(5):322–327.
Sheppard DR. Activated protein C resistance: the most common risk factor for venous thromboembolism. *J Am Board Fam Pract* 2000;13(2):111–115.

15. **(B)** The antiphospholipid syndrome is a collection of diseases resulting from antibodies against phospholipids membranes or associated binding cofactors in the blood. The syndrome was first noted in syphilis patients who produce a complement fixing antibody to mitochondrial phospholipids termed cardiolipin. This was later the basis for the VDRL test that is still used today.

Several types of anticardiolipin antibodies have been discovered. These antibodies are primarily of the IgG or IgM types. Some react directly with cardiolipin whereas others require the presence of the plasma phospholipid-binding protein β_2GI. This requirement for the presence of the binding protein is specific for patients with systemic lupus erythematosus (SLE) but not with syphilis patients. This has led to better tests to differentiate patients with syphilis from those with other noninfectious causes for anticardiolipin production.

Antiphospholipid antibodies are generally found among young healthy individuals with a prevalence of 1–5%. Among patients with SLE this can range as high as 12–30%. Affected patients are at a higher risk of venous thrombosis, myocardial infarction, strokes, and miscarriages, thrombocytopenia, hemolytic anemia, livedo reticularis, and rarely arterial thrombosis. Renal involvement with hypertension is almost invariably present. Virtually any organ can be involved.

The diagnosis of antiphospholipid syndrome requires the presence of one clinical and one laboratory indicator.

Clinical manifestations required for diagnosis include one of the following:

- Documented episodes of arterial, venous, or small vessel thrombosis, in any tissue.
- One or more unexplained deaths of a morphologically normal fetus beyond the 10th week of gestation.
- One or more premature births of a normal neonate before the 34th week of gestation because of preeclampsia or eclampsia, or severe placental insufficiency or three or more unexplained consecutive spontaneous abortions before the 10th week of gestation.

Laboratory diagnosis is based on enzyme-linked immunoassays that require β_2GI and IgM anticardiolipin antibodies. Several different tests and protocols exist and all must be negative in order to rule out presence of disease.

Most individuals present with isolated thrombosis. Catastrophic antiphospholipid syndrome is a rare consequence of this disease and patients will present with acute and devastating syndrome of multiple thrombosis usually leading to death. The kidney is the most common organ affected followed by lungs, CNS, heart, and skin. Thromboses of small vessels tend to predominate with a syndrome similar to DIC. The mortality rate is 50% and secondary to multiple organ system failure. Treatment is aimed at removing the antibody with plasmapheresis and steroids as well as anticoagulation and fibrinolytic therapy.

Several studies have been performed looking at the prophylactic treatment of these patients. Aspirin has generally only been shown to help female patients with recurrent miscarriages. Anticoagulation with warfarin to an INR > 2.0 has been shown to reduce both venous and arterial thrombosis; however, discontinuation can lead to recurrent thrombosis and catastrophic antiphospholipid syndrome.

Bibliography

Levine JS, Branch DW, Rauch J. The antiphospholipid syndrome. *N Engl J Med* 2002;346(10):752–763.

Rand JH. Molecular pathogenesis of the antiphospholipid syndrome. *Circ Res* 2002;90(1):29–37.

Roubey RA. Update on antiphospholipid antibodies. *Curr Opin Rheumatol* 2000;12(5):374–378.

Wilson WA, Gharavi AE, Koike T, et al. International consensus statement on preliminary classification criteria for definite antiphospholipid syndrome: report of an international workshop. *Arthritis Rheum* 1999;42(7):1309–1311.

16. **(A)** Homocystine is a sulfur-containing amino acid that occurs in the body as a result of metabolism of methionine. These reactions are used in the body to methylate amino acids, formation of adenosine and tetrahydrofolate, conversion of thymidylate from uracil, and conversion of glycine from serine. These reactions are summarized in Fig. 5-15. Any defect in these pathways can lead to an increase in homocystine leading to homocystineuria or hypercysteinemia.

Levels of homocystine can be elevated for a variety of genetic and environmental factors. Enzyme deficiencies of cysthathionine beta-synthase (CBS), methylenetetrahydrofolate reductase (MTHR), and methionine synthase (MS), chronic renal failure, hypothyroidism, neoplasms, methotrexate, phenytoin, or theophyline are known to raise levels of homocystine. Dietary or absorbptional deficiencies of B_{12} can lead to elevation of homocystine.

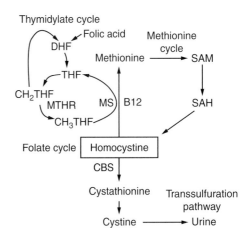

FIG. 5-15 Methionine metabolism. MS, methionine synthase; CBS, cysthathionine beta-synthase; MTHR, methylenetetrahydrofolate reductase; THR, tetrahydrofolate; DHR, dihydrofolate; SAM, S-adenosyl methionine; SAH, S-adenosyl homocysteine.

Mild hyperhomocystinemia is often seen in patients with dietary, environmental, or heterozygote deficiency of MTHR or CBS. Unlike other prothrombotic diseases, there is strong evidence that links this disease with elevated risk of both arterial and venous thrombosis. There is a two- to fourfold increase in the risk of CAD and DVTs. One meta-analyses showed that hyperhomocystinemia was found in 21.7% of CAD, 26.6% of cerebrovascular accident (CVA), 32.8% of peripheral vascular disease (PVD), and 13.8% of DVT patients.

Very high levels of homocystine are found in patients devoid of either CBS or MTHR. These patients have a high level of arterial (usually CAD) and venous thrombosis as well as increased risks of skeletal and ocular problems as well as mental retardation/developmental delay. Prevalence in United States is not fully known but thought to be quite rare.

Mechanisms by which homocystine causes thrombotic complications are not fully understood. One popular theory involves direct toxicity to the endothelium; however, homocystine is known to potentate the oxidation of low density lipoprotein cholesterol, effect arachidonic acid metabolism, cause expression of thrombomodulin, activate factor V, and inhibit protein C.

Homocystine levels are determined after fasting overnight. A postmethionine load test is often frequently performed. Homocystine levels are determined 4–6 h after oral administration of 0.1 g/kg of methionine.

Treatment of homocystine is accomplished by saturating the body of B_{12} and folate. This is designed to overcome the effects of mild enzyme deficiency and drive the pathway toward reducing homocystine levels. No trials are currently underway looking at novel enzyme replacements or other drug replacements possibilities. Folate supplementation of grains by the FDA was done to lower levels of neural tube defects and this supplementation level is too low to cause a significant decrease in homocystine levels.

Bibliography

den Heijer M, Koster T, Blom HJ, et al. Hyperhomocysteinemia as a risk factor for deep-vein thrombosis. *N Engl J Med* 1996;334(12):759–762.

Federman DG, Kirsner RS. An update on hypercoagulable disorders. *Arch Intern Med* 2001;161(8):1051–1056.

Finkelstein JD. The metabolism of homocysteine: pathways and regulation. *Eur J Pediatr* 1998;157(Suppl 2):S40–S44.

Makris M. Hyperhomocysteinemia is a risk factor for venous and arterial thrombosis. *Br J Haematol* 1998;101 (Suppl 1):18–20.

17. **(D)** Prothrombin is a vitamin-K-dependent protein that is the precursor to thrombin created during the coagulation cascade described earlier. Along with FVL, it is one of the most common genetic disorders leading to thrombophilia. It is caused by a common genetic variant of prothrombin when a transition occurs in the DNA sequence at position 20210 in the 3'-untranslated region of the gene. This leads to decreased effectiveness of the prothrombinase complex to produce thrombin. As such prothrombin levels are elevated. Heterozygous carriers were found to have approximately 30% higher levels than noncarriers. The change in ratio of prothrombin to thrombin is thought to be the cause of this disease's thrombotic effects.

The prevalence of this mutation varies greatly among the world's population. It is almost entirely a disease in Whites. The prevalence among healthy controls varies from 0.7to 4.0% whereas 4 to 8% of patients presenting with a first episode of thrombosis was found to have the mutation. This represents a relative risk of two to seven compared with the general population.

Bibliography

Brown K, Luddington R, Williamson D, Baker P, Baglin T. Risk of venous thromboembolism associated with a G to A transition at position 20210 in the 3'-untranslated region of the prothrombin gene. *Br J Haematol* 1997; 98(4):907–909.

Federman DG, Kirsner RS. An update on hypercoagulable disorders. *Arch Intern Med* 2001;161(8):1051–1056.

Poort SR, Rosendaal FR, Reitsma PH, Bertina RM. A common genetic variation in the 3'-untranslated region of the prothrombin gene is associated with elevated plasma prothrombin levels and an increase in venous thrombosis. *Blood* 1996;88(10):3698–3703.

Vicente V, Gonzalez-Conejero R, Rivera J, Corral J. The prothrombin gene variant 20210A in venous and arterial thromboembolism. *Haematologica* 1999;84(4):356–362.

18. **(C)** Oral contraceptives are the most common cause of drug-induced thrombotic disorders. Two basic types of oral contraceptive pills (OCPs) are in use today. Thrombotic events are related to the type of OCPs and whether confounding variables such as genetic defects are present.

Second generation OCPs contain primarily levonorgestrel as the progestin whereas third generation OCPs are based on either desogestrel, gestodene, or norgestimate. It is often reported in several World Health Organization (WHO) studies that normal patients on OCPs have a fourfold increase in risk of venous thrombotic events (VTE). Recently concern has been raised of an increased risk in population studies of DVTs in patients on third generation

OCPs. This raises the thought that the thrombotic events are caused by the estrogen component only and not secondary to the progestin component. More studies are being conducted to see if confounding variables may be the cause for the differences. Nonetheless, the U.K. Committee of Safety of Medicine recommended that OCPs containing third generation progestins be limited.

Age distribution curves of patients on OCPs between second and third generation are very similar with second generation patients being on average 3–4 years older. The risk of thrombotic events is a factor of how long the patient has been on a certain dose. Risk is often expressed as woman–years of exposure similar to smoking risk and cancer.

Bibliography

Farmer RD, Lawrenson RA, Thompson CR, Kennedy JG, Hambleton IR. Population-based study of risk of venous thromboembolism associated with various oral contraceptives. *Lancet* 1997;349(9045):83–88.

Federman DG, Kirsner RS. An update on hypercoagulable disorders. *Arch Intern Med* 2001;161(8):1051–1056.

Rosendaal FR. Thrombosis in the young: epidemiology and risk factors. A focus on venous thrombosis. *Thromb Haemost* 1997;78(1):1–6.

Rosing J, Tans G, Nicolaes GA, et al. Oral contraceptives and venous thrombosis: different sensitivities to activated protein C in women using second- and third-generation oral contraceptives. *Br J Haematol* 1997;97(1):233–238.

19. (C)

20. (B)

Explanations 19 and 20

The term hypercoagulable state is often used incorrectly to label a patient who has recurrent thrombotic events (usually DVTs) without an apparent source. In the last few questions the most common reasons for hypercoagulability have been discussed. They include OCP use, antiphospholipid syndrome (lupus anticoagulant), FVL (APC resistance), hyperhomocystinemia, prothrombin gene mutation, protein C, S, or ATIII deficiency. Other causes not discussed yet include pregnancy, elevated factor VIII or XI levels. All of these causes should be ruled out before labeling a patient as having an idiopathic hypercoagulable disorder.

Venous thrombosis is a common disorder. Approximately 1 in 1000 people per year in the United States will develop venous thrombosis and over 250,000 hospitalizations occur per year secondary to venous thrombosis. Of these over 50,000 people will develop fatal pulmonary embolisms. The

TABLE 5-6 Relative Risk of Venous Thrombosis with Various Prothombotic Disorders

Thrombotic disorder	Relative risk VTE*
Normal	1
Oral contraceptive (OCP) use	4
Antiphospholipid syndrome	29–55
Factor V Leiden, heterozygous	7
FVL, heterozygous + OCP	28
FVL, heterozygous + pregnancy	9
FVL, homozygous	70
FVL, homozygous + OCP	>100
Hyperhomocystinemia	2–4
Hyperhomocystinemia + FVL, heterozygous	20
Prothrombin gene mutation	2–7
Prothrombin gene mutation + OCP	16
Prothrombin gene mutation + pregnancy	15
Prothrombin gene mutation + FVL	3–5
Protein C deficiency, heterozygous	7
Protein S deficiency, heterozygous	6
ATIII deficiency, heterozygous	5
Elevated factor VIII levels >1500 IU/L	5
Elevated factor XI levels >90% percentile	2
Protein C, S, or ATIII deficiency, homozygous	Intrauterine death

*VTE, venous thrombotic events.

risk of developing venous disease depends on the disease state of the patient (see Table 5-6).

If a patient develops VTE tracking down the cause can be a daunting task. Only 5–15% of patients with VTE have deficiencies of protein C, S, or ATIII making them the least likely cause of diagnosis. FVL is one of the most common causes of VTEs occurring in approximately 20–50% of patients. Patients who also have combined OCP use with FVL are at extreme high risk for development of VTEs and should be cautioned against there use.

The risk of thromboembolism is increased during pregnancy and puberty secondary to increased estrogen production. If a concurrent inheritable disease is present the relative risk is even greater. Female patients should be counseled about their risk of thrombosis during pregnancy and the increased risk of OCPs in the presence of other disorders. Warfarin is contraindicated in these patients.

Increased levels of factor VIII and XI levels have recently been investigated as possible causes of VTEs. Elevated factor VIII levels are the most common cause of disease found in patients who were not diagnosed with one of the more common disorders; however, this factor is also elevated in other diseases and thought to be an acute phase reactant. Significance of this disease at this time is unknown. Elevated factor XI has just recently been looked at as a disease entity in humans and studies are currently under way to determine its significance and occurrence.

TABLE 5-7   Risk Factors for Developing DVT

History of DVT or PE	Prolonged immobility or paralysis	Cancer
Obesity (>20% IBW)	Varicose veins	Stroke or coma
Fractures of the pelvis, hip or leg	Inflammatory bowel disease	Nephrotic syndrome
Hormone therapy	Hypercoagulable disorders	

The question about whom to evaluate is often a question facing surgeons. Unfortunately there are no large, well-done studies that have answered this question. They fail to find a cost-effective screening method with high predictive values. Most authors recommend evaluating anybody who has a thrombotic event less than 50 years of age, has a family history of thrombosis, or recurrent thrombosis, or thrombosis at an unusual site.

ATIII, protein C and S deficiency are more likely to present before the age of 50. After age 50 these tests will be of little use in determining causes—also surgeons should wait several months after the event as these levels can be raised acutely. ATIII levels will be depressed in patients on heparin, and protein C and S can be low in vitamin-K-deficient patients. In patients with a family history of thrombosis the most likely cause will be FVL, prothrombin mutation, and hyperhomocyteinemia. Antiphospholipid syndrome can occur at any age.

Bibliography

de Bruijn SF, Stam J, Koopman MM, Vandenbroucke JP. Case-control study of risk of cerebral sinus thrombosis in oral contraceptive users and in [correction of who are] carriers of hereditary prothrombotic conditions. The Cerebral Venous Sinus Thrombosis Study Group. [Erratum appears in *BMJ* 1998 Mar 14;316(7134):822]. *BMJ* 1998;316(7131):589–592.

de Stefano V, Martinelli I, Mannucci PM, et al. The risk of recurrent deep venous thrombosis among heterozygous carriers of both factor V Leiden and the G20210A prothrombin mutation. *N Engl J Med* 1999;341(11): 801–806.

Federman DG, Kirsner RS. An update on hypercoagulable disorders. *Arch Intern Med* 2001;161(8):1051–1056.

Hansson PO, Sorbo J, Eriksson H. Recurrent venous thromboembolism after deep vein thrombosis: incidence and risk factors. *Arch Intern Med* 2000;160(6):769–774.

Martinelli I, Sacchi E, Landi G, Taioli E, Duca F, Mannucci PM. High risk of cerebral-vein thrombosis in carriers of a prothrombin-gene mutation and in users of oral contraceptives. *N Engl J Med* 1998;338(25):1793–1797.

Vandenbroucke JP, Koster T, Briet E, Reitsma PH, Bertina RM, Rosendaal FR. Increased risk of venous thrombosis in oral-contraceptive users who are carriers of factor V Leiden mutation. *Lancet* 1994;344(8935):1453–1457.

21. **(D)** General surgery patients can be classified into three groups based on their risk for DVT formation and is based on the risk factors listed in Table 5-7.

Prophylaxis of all patients includes early ambulation and the use of TED (anti-embolism stockings) hose and/or SCDs from immediately before surgery until full ambulation is achieved. Moderate-risk patients can be treated with either subcutaneous heparin or LMWH and the dose is adjusted depending on the risk factors. In both moderate- and high-risk patients the addition of dextran IV can be considered. High-risk patients should be started on warfarin the day of or day after surgery and adjusted to INR of 1.5–3 (see Table 5-8).

Major trauma patients are considered high risk from thromboembolism. All patients should be started on a heparin-based regimen unless contraindicated. The use of SCDs and/or TEDs should be used until heparin is started. If patient is at high risk for thromboembolism and patient has suboptimal prophylaxis then an inferior vena cava (IVC) filter should be considered.

Trials have been performed looking at the timing of starting LMWH. Most studies show an inherent advantage of starting LMWH 2 h before operation. This has an added benefit of preventing DVT during operation and in the immediate postoperative period. If bleeding is a concern then the dose can be given up to 12 h prior to major operations.

Clopidogrel and other antiplatelet drugs have been shown to reduce DVT in the general surgery

TABLE 5-8   DVT Risk Stratification

Low risk—uncomplicated minor surgery (general anesthesia <30 min) in patients <40 years old with no clinical risk factors
Moderate risk
    Any surgery in patients 40–60 years old with no clinical risk factors
    Major surgery in patients <40 years old with no additional risk factors
    Minor surgery in patients with risk factors
High risk
    Major surgery in patients >60 years old with no additional risk factors
    Major surgery in patients 40–60 years old with additional risk factors
    Patients with MI
Very high risk—Major surgery in patients >40 years old with prior history of DVT, PE, cancer, or hypercoagulable state

patients by as much as 37%; however, these studies appear misleading and no consensus statement on the use of these drugs have been produced at this time.

Bibliography

Bjerkeset O, Larsen S, Reiertsen O. Evaluation of enoxaparin given before and after operation to prevent venous thromboembolism during digestive surgery: play-the-winner designed study. *World J Surg* 1997;21:584–589.

Clagett GP, Anderson FA, Jr, Geerts W, et al. Prevention of venous thromboembolism. *Chest* 1998;114:531S–560S.

Cohen AT, Skinner JA, Kakkar VV. Antiplatelet treatment for thromboprophylaxis: a step forward or backward? *BMJ* 1994;309:1213–1215.

22. **(E)** Multiple-injured patients are at a significant risk for venous thrombotic disease. Major risk factors for the development of venous thromboembolism include severe head injury (GCS ≤ 9), paralysis, major pelvic fracture, major lower extremity fracture, and repair of a major lower extremity vein. These factors are in addition to the preinjury risk factors listed in Table 5-7.

Patients who are considered high risk for thromboembolic complications should undergo prophylaxis with both SCDs and LMWH. Patients who are unable to undergo full prophylaxis should be considered for prophylactic IVC filter placement within 48 h of admission. Orthopedic fractures are not a contraindication for compression devices. AVI foot pumps can be used in this situation. Intracranial bleeding is a contraindication for both LMWH and warfarin use.

IVC filter can be easily and safely placed in the ICU settings. A majority of filters are placed by experienced radiologists with the use of fluoroscopy. IVC filters have also been deployed successfully with ultrasound guidance. The morbidity and mortality with vena caval filter insertion is extremely low. Several studies have examined both short-term and long-term complication rates of prophylactic IVC filter insertions. Complications include groin hematomas, arteriovenous (AV) fistulas, incomplete opening, and misplacement and occur in approximately 1.6–2% of patients. Long-term complications include caval penetration 0–2%, migration 1–5%, filter occlusion 2–4%, and insertion site thrombosis 2–6%. Prophylactic placement can offer up to 98% protection rate from pulmonary embolism which can be fatal. The safety and added benefit of prophylactic IVC filter placement should be considered in major trauma patients who are unable to undergo full DVT prophylaxis.

Bibliography

Greenfield LJ, Proctor MC, Michaels AJ, Taheri PA. Prophylactic vena caval filters in trauma: the rest of the story. *J Vasc Surg* 2000;32(3):490–495; discussion 496–497.

Langan EM III, Miller RS, Casey WJ III, Carsten CG III, Graham RM, Taylor SM. Prophylactic inferior vena cava filters in trauma patients at high risk: follow-up examination and risk/benefit assessment. *J Vasc Surg* 1999; 30(3):484–488.

Rogers FB, Shackford SR, Wilson J, Ricci MA, Morris CS. Prophylactic vena cava filter insertion in severely injured trauma patients: indications and preliminary results. *J Trauma Injury Infect Crit Care* 1993;35(4):637–641; discussion 641–632.

Sing RF, Cicci CK, Smith CH, Messick WJ. Bedside insertion of inferior vena cava filters in the intensive care unit. *J Trauma Injury Infect Crit Care* 1999;47(6):1104–1107.

23. **(A)** Warfarin and its derivatives act by blocking the formation of the vitamin-K-dependent clotting factors (II, VII, IX, X, and proteins C and S). The proteins lack the carboxyglutamic acid residue that is necessary to bind calcium. As such, the extrinsic pathway is primarily affected with elevations seen in the PT with only slight elevations in the aPTT. Warfarin has a half-life of 40 h and its effects can be reversed quickly with the use of FFP, slightly slower with vitamin K administration, or by stopping the drug altogether.

Trauma in the face of anticoagulation with warfarin would intuitively seem to cause a greater tendency for bleeding leading to increased mortality; however, several retrospective analyses have been done to see if preinjury warfarin use correlated with increased mortality. In two case-matched series the use of warfarin did not adversely impact mortality or length of stay outcomes in both head and nonhead injured patients. It was noted that the warfarin treated cohort without a head injury was less likely to be discharged home and needing skilled nursing or rehabilitation center assistance on discharge. This was not seen in the head injured patients.

These studies, however, fail to compare mechanism of injury which could show that patients on warfarin may have lower Glasgow coma score (GCS), higher injury severity scores, and higher ASCOT (a severity characterization of trauma) scores for the same type of mechanism which would invalidate these studies.

Bibliography

Kennedy DM, Cipolle MD, Pasquale MD, Wasser T. Impact of preinjury warfarin use in elderly trauma patients. *J Trauma Injury Infect Crit Care* 2000;48(3):451–453.

Wojcik R, Cipolle MD, Seislove E, Wasser TE, Pasquale MD. Preinjury warfarin does not impact outcome in trauma patients. *J Trauma Injury Infect Crit Care* 2001;51(6):1147–1151; discussion 1151–1142.

24. **(A)** The history of blood transfusion is relatively recent. Until modern time blood letting and phlebotomy were

common practices to rid people of evil spirits. The first known successful transfusion was performed by Jean-Baptiste Denis in 1667 when he transfused three pints of sheep's blood into a patient. His latter attempts failed and blood transfusion was outlawed until the mid-1800s.

The first human-to-human blood transfusion was administered by Philip Syng Physick in 1825 and was later followed by Blundell in 1828 to a patient with postpartum hemorrhage. It wasn't until Karl Landsteiner discovered the A, B, and O blood types in 1900 and AB by A. Von Decastello and A. Sturli in 1902 that modern blood typing was performed.

Approximately 60% of all blood products used are given perioperatively and a total of 11–12 million units of packed RBCs are administered in the United States yearly.

Bibliography

Fakhry S, Rutherford E, Sheldon G. Hematologic principles in surgery. In: Townsend C (ed.), *Sabiston Textbook of Surgery*, 16th ed. Philadelphia, PA: W.B. Saunders, 2001, 69–89.

25. **(D)** Transfusion reactions occur secondary to presence of antigens on the RBCs that are infused into a patient who possesses or develops antibodies to the antigen. This activates a complement-mediated destruction of the RBCs leading to cytokine release, hypotension, decreased renal blood flow, activation of the coagulation cascade and ultimately DIC. Early signs and symptoms of a reaction is because of the histamine release and presents as pain and redness in the site of infusion, chest tightness, impeding feeling of doom and oozing from open skin sites.

Transfusion most often occur secondary to incompatibility with the major antigens A, B, O, and Rh. Clerical errors are the most common reason for mismatched blood transfusion. There are several steps along the way that errors can occur, from blood drawing and labeling specimens, laboratory processing, and matching of unit and patient prior to transfusions. Other minor antigens are also present on RBCs and can participate in reactions despite proper cross-matching and infusion of correctly assigned units.

When a reaction is suspected the infusion should be stopped immediately and the unit returned to the blood bank along with a sample of the patient's blood for detections of major and minor antigens and to see if the correct unit of blood was infused. Treatment of the patient should begin immediately with infusion of antipyretics and histamine blockers. Supportive care should be given to the patient and signs and symptoms of DIC treated aggressively.

Fluid resuscitation, oxygenation, and diuresis with manitol to prevent renal failure are mainstays of treatment. Patients who develop DIC early are at greatest risk of mortality.

Transfusion reactions are not always present immediately on infusion and can occur hours to days later with symptoms of jaundice, fever, or precipitous fall in hematocrit. One study also examined reactions given with autologous blood and noticed a reaction in 2.1% of all patients given autologous blood both in preoperative stored units and with blood salvaged during the operative procedure.

Bibliography

Bradbury M, Cruickshank JP. Blood and blood transfusion reactions: 1. *Br J Nurs* 1995;4(14):814–817.

Bradbury M, Cruickshank JP. Blood and blood transfusion reactions: 2. *Br J Nurs* 1995;4(15):861–868.

Domen RE. Adverse reactions associated with autologous blood transfusion: evaluation and incidence at a large academic hospital. *Transfusion* 1998;38(3):296–300.

Fakhry S, Rutherford E, Sheldon G. Hematologic principles in surgery. In: Townsend C (ed.), *Sabiston Textbook of Surgery*, 16th ed. Philadelphia, PA: W.B. Saunders, 2001, 69–89.

26. **(C)**

27. **(D)**

Explanations 26 and 27

Whole blood obtained from volunteers is rarely used in the United States and many blood banks do not routinely store this product. Once a unit of whole blood is donated it is quickly broken down into subcomponents for more efficient use of the blood and its products. Whole blood can be stored in citrate phosphate dextrose adenine (CPDA)-1 with a shelf life of approximately 35 days.

Packed RBCs are obtained by centrifugation of whole blood to separate the plasma and platelet components from the red cell mass. This process increases the hematocrit to approximately 80% and can be stored for 35 days in CPDA-1 or 42 days in AS-1 (Adsol) at 1–6°C. Longer storage decreases red cell viability. Packed RBCs contain essentially no platelets and levels of factors V and VIII are unstable.

The plasma component is then further centrifuged to pellet the platelets. It is then pooled with 6–10 other donors to provide one unit of pooled platelets. Alternatively a single donor unit can be obtained by apheresis. This is especially useful for patients who have developed antibodies against specific platelets types and will help prevent immune destruction of donor cells. The plasma component is

TABLE 5-9 Summary of Available Blood Components

Whole blood	Platelets—single unit from whole blood
Packed RBCs	Platelets—apheresis unit
Leukocyte-reduced RBCs	Fresh frozen plasma
Deglycerolized RBCs	Solvent/detergent-treated plasma
Leukocyte concentrate	Cryoprecipitate

immediately frozen at −18 to −30°C to preserve clotting factor function. It can be thawed to 4°C to remove the cryoprecipitate component.

Each of these components can then be specialized to meet the needs of the patients. Leukocyte-reduced RBCs can be obtained to reduce the human leukocyte antigen (HLA) components within the blood and reduce reactions and immunosuppression. Deglycerolized RBCs are available and can be stored frozen up to 3 years allowing for stockpiling of rare blood units. Leukocyte concentrate can be obtained and used in patients with profound granulocytopenic; however, some blood banks and hospitals do not carry these special units secondary to cost and lack of support for their use (see Table 5-9).

Bibliography

Fakhry S, Rutherford E, Sheldon G. Hematologic principles in surgery. In: Townsend C (ed.), *Sabiston Textbook of Surgery*, 16th ed. Philadelphia, PA: W.B. Saunders, 2001, 69–89.

28. **(E)** Transfusion of blood products are not without risk. Aside from transfusion reactions, blood products are potentially hazardous substances containing infectious agents. In the 1980s, 1 in 10 patients transfused developed a hepatitis infection. Since learning of the risks of transferring diseases in blood such as hepatitis and HIV, blood banks began to routinely screen donors and test for viral components prior to infusion of the blood. This has led to a slow steady decline in the risk of blood transfusion; however, some infected blood goes undetected and the risk is still present. Table 5-10 illustrates the current risk of receiving blood products.

Blood transfusion exposes the recipient to several immune products that can lead anywhere from graft-versus-host disease in an immunocompromised patient to increased immunosuppression in cancer patients leading to recurrence of tumors and poorer prognosis. Gamma-irradiation and leukocyte depletion of blood products can decrease the risk of graft-versus-host disease.

Bibliography

Fakhry S, Rutherford E, Sheldon G. Hematologic principles in surgery. In: Townsend C (ed.), *Sabiston Textbook of Surgery*, 16th ed. Philadelphia, PA: W.B. Saunders, 2001, 69–89.

Goodnough LT, Brecher ME, Kanter ME, AuBuchon JP. Medical progress: tranfusion medicine (first of two parts)—blood transfusion. *N Engl J Med* 1999;340(6):438–447.

29. **(C)** Acute lung injury is caused by a number of factors but usually presents within 4 h of transfusion and clinically presents as noncardiac pulmonary edema. Patients will present dyspneic and hypoxic secondary to capillary leak of fluid. There are several mechanisms that exist to increase the permeability of the

TABLE 5-10 Relative Risk of Blood Transfusion

Risk factor	Estimated frequency per million units	Per actual unit	No. of deaths per million units
Infection			
Viral			
Hepatitis A	1	1/1,000,000	0
Hepatitis B	7–32	1/30,000–1/250,000	0–0.14
Hepatitis C	4–36	1/30,000–1/150,000	0.5–17
HIV	0.4–5	1/200,000–1/2,000,000	0.5–5
HTLV types I and II	0.5–4	1/250,000–1/2,000,000	0
Parvovirus B19	100	1/10,000	0
Bacterial contamination			
Red cells	2	1/500,000	0.1–0.25
Platelets	83	1/12,000	21
Acute hemolytic reactions	1–4	1/250,000–1/1,000,000	0.67
Delayed hemolytic reactions	1000	1/1,000	0.4
Tranfusion related acute lung injury	200	1/5,000	0.2

capillary membrane within the lung. One popular mechanism involves the infusion of antibody from the donor that attacks the patient's cells, primarily the neutrophils. Another leading theory involves the formation of lipid products on the donor cells membranes during storage. Patients are at greatest risk of developing acute lung injury in the setting of sepsis as neutrophils play an important role in the pathophysiology of this disease.

The incidence of acute lung injury is quite low and estimated to be in 1 in 5000 transfusion; however, some occur subclinically or the patients die quickly and the disease is unrecognized. Despite this fact almost 90% of patients recover.

Bibliography

Goodnough LT, Brecher ME, Kanter ME, AuBuchon JP. Medical progress: tranfusion medicine (first of two parts)—blood transfusion. *N Engl J Med* 1999;340(6):438–447.

30. (E) Blood utilization is an important aspect of surgical management. With the risks of transfusion reactions, disease transmission, and immunosuppression it is imperative that blood is not infused without rational consideration of its need. Blood is primarily designed to deliver oxygen to the peripheral tissue from the lungs. Therefore, its transfusion should be aimed at raising the ability of the body to deliver oxygen to the peripheral tissue, not as a volume expander. The use of transfusion triggers based on hematocrit should be avoided. Instead, the patient should be evaluated for clinical symptoms of decreased oxygen concentration, such as tachycardia or increased cardiac output, hypoxia, decreased venous saturation (VO$_2$) (see Table 5-11).

Hospital utilization reviews and indications for transfusion vary from hospital to hospital and from surgeon to surgeon. The science of blood transfusion and indications is not an exact science but is based on clinical knowledge and experience. Table 5-12 lists some suggested guidelines for red cell transfusion.

Bibliography

Fakhry S, Rutherford E, Sheldon G. Hematologic principles in surgery. In: Townsend C (ed.), *Sabiston Textbook of Surgery*, 16th ed. Philadelphia, PA: W.B. Saunders, 2001, 69–89.

Spence RK. Surgical red blood cell transfusion practice policies. *Am J Surg* 1995;170(6S)(Suppl):3S–12S.

31. (D) Several policies were set forth during a consensus conference on blood management and Surgical Practice Guidelines in 1995 (see Table 5-13).

It is important to remember when dealing with Jehovah's Witness patients that their belief is based

TABLE 5-11   Policies Set Forth by the Consensus Conference: Blood Management and Surgical Practice Guidelines on Surgical Red Blood Cell Transfusion Policies

Policy 1	Transfusion need should be assessed on a case-by-case basis.
Policy 2	Blood should be transfused one unit at a time, followed by an assessment of benefit and further need.
Policy 3	Exposure to allogeneic blood should be limited to appropriate need.
Policy 4	Perioperative blood loss should be prevented or controlled.
Policy 5	Autologous blood should be considered for use as an alternative to allogeneic tranfusion.
Policy 6	Efforts should be made to maximize oxygen delivery in the surgical patient.
Policy 7	RBC mass should be increased or restored by means other than RBC transfusion.
Policy 8	The patient should be involved in the transfusion decision.
Policy 9	The reasons for and results of the transfusion decision should be documented contemporaneously in the patient's record.
Policy 10	Hospitals' transfusion policies and procedures should be developed as a cooperative effort that includes input from all those involved in the transfusion decision.
Policy 11	Transfusion practices, both individual and institutional, should be reassessed yearly or more often.

Source: Adapted with permission from Spence RK. Surgical red blood cell transfusion practice policies. *Am J Surg* 170(6S):3S–12S. Copyright 1995, with permission from Excerpta Medica Inc.

TABLE 5-12   Suggested Transfusion Guidelines for Red Blood Cells

Hemoglobin ≤8 g/dL or acute blood loss in an otherwise healthy patient with signs and symptoms of decreased oxygen delivery with two or more of the following:
   Estimated or anticipated acute blood loss of ≥15% of total blood volume (750 mL in 70-kg male)
   Diastolic blood pressure ≤60 mmHg
   Systolic blood pressure drop ≥30 mmHg from baseline
   Tachycardia (>100 bpm)
   Oliguria/anuria
   Mental status changes
Hemoglobin ≤10 g/dL in patients with known increased risk of coronary artery disease or pulmonary insufficiency who have sustained or are expected to sustain significant blood loss
Symptomatic anemia with any of the following:
   Tachycardia (>100 bpm)
   Mental status changes
   Evidence of myocardial ischemia including angina
   Shortness of breath or dizziness with mild exertion
   Orthostatic hypotension
Unfounded/questionable indications
   To increase wound healing
   To improve the patient's sense of well-being
   7 ≤ hemoglobin ≤ 10 in otherwise stable, asymptomatic patient
   Mere availability of predonated autologous blood without medical indication

Source: Reprinted from Fakhry S, Rutherford E, Sheldon G. Hematologic principles in surgery. In: Townsend C, (ed.), *Sabiston Textbook of Surgery*, 16th ed. Philadelphia, PA: W.B. Saunders, 69–89, with permission from Elsevier.

TABLE 5-13   Policies Set Forth by the Consensus Conference: Blood Management and Surgical Practice Guidelines on Surgical Management of Jehovah's Witnesses

Policy 1	Accept the limitation that allogeneic blood cannot be used.
Policy 2	Use alternatives to allogeneic blood whenever possible and appropriate.
Policy 3	Discuss consequences with the patient, including the potential for life-threatening hemorrhage and possible death if not transfused.
Policy 4	If unable or unwilling to treat a Jehovah's Witness patient, stabilize and transfer the patient to a sympathetic institution, such as a Center for Bloodless Surgery.
Policy 5	Contact the local Jehovah's Witness liaison committee for information and help.
Policy 6	In an emergency or if a patient is unconscious, look for an advance directive.
Policy 7	Seek legal assistance when dealing with an unconscious or incompetent adult.

Source: Adapted with permission from Spence RK. Surgical red blood cell transfusion practice policies. Appendix 2. *Am J Surg* 170(6S):14S–15S, 1995, with permission from Excerpta Medica Inc.

on their interpretation of the Bible. They believe that if blood is separated from the body it is inherently evil and that they will be eternally doomed if they receive this blood. This includes all products that are derived from human or animal blood to include FFP, cryoprecipitate, and albumin. Most patients will accept products that contain small amounts of blood products, such as immune globulin and epoetin alfa.

Patients should be counseled on their increased risk of morbidity and mortality and their consent should contain this information as well; however, one must remember that courts have held physicians liable for transfusing these patients despite life saving attempts. If this is not agreeable to the surgeon then the patient should be referred to another physician or center that is able to honor the patient's desire.

In the emergency situation the physician is often faced with difficult decisions. If a patient has an advance directive then this must be honored despite the patient condition. If no advance directive is found then life-saving blood can be given; however, one must remember that the patient may not be happy with this after the fact. Most Jehovah's Witnesses would rather die with honor than lose their right for eternal life.

Bibliography

Spence RK. Surgical red blood cell transfusion practice policies: Appendix 2. *Am J Surg* 1995;170(6S)(Suppl): 14S–15S.

32. (A) The act of acute normovolemic hemodilution was proposed by Messemer in 1975. Briefly, it involves removal of the whole blood of a patient immediately before surgery and replacement of the blood volume with a colloid or crystalloid solution to maintain normovolemia. The degree of hemodilution depends on the patient's medical status and type of operation performed. Hemodilution to a hematocrit level of 20% is generally safe in patients less than 60 years of age without contraindications. The operation is performed as usual and the whole blood is reinfused with any massive blood loss after hemostasis is achieved. Contraindications include patients with coronary heart disease, severe aortic stenosis, left ventricular impairment, significant anemia, renal disease, severe hepatic disease, pulmonary emphysema, obstructive lung disease, severe hypertension, or clotting deficiencies.

Several physiologic conditions occur as a result of hemodilution. Mechanisms include a compensatory increase in cardiac output to maintain oxygen delivery, reduction in systemic vascular resistance, increased oxygen extraction, and shift of the oxygen dissociation curve to the right. These processes work together to maintain normal oxygen delivery even at profound (HCT <20%) hemodilution.

Acute normovolemic hemodilution involves storing the whole blood in anticoagulated bags within the operating room. This reduces or nearly eliminates the worry with transfusion reactions; however, contamination of the blood can occur with poor aseptic techniques.

Bibliography

D'Ambra MN, Kaplan DK. Alternatives to allogeneic blood use in surgery: acute normovolemic hemodilution and preoperative autologous donation. *Am J Surg* 1995; 170(6S)(Suppl):49S–52S.

Fakhry S, Rutherford E, Sheldon G. Hematologic principles in surgery. In: Townsend C (ed.), *Sabiston Textbook of Surgery*, 16th ed. Philadelphia, PA: W.B. Saunders, 2001, 69–89.

Goodnough LT, Brecher ME, Kanter ME, AuBuchon JP. Medical progress: transfusion medicine (second of two parts)—blood conservation. *N Engl J Med* 1999;340(7): 525–533.

Messmer K. Hemodilution. *Surg Clin North Am* 1975;55:659.

Monk TG, Goodnough LT. Acute normovolemic hemodilution. *Clin Orthop* 1998;357:74–81.

33. (E) With the knowledge of infectious disease transmission with transfusion, preoperative autologous blood transfusion has become more popular. Patients who are scheduled for elective operations where the blood loss is expected to be greater than 1000 mL should be counseled on storing preoperative blood. Several states have made it mandatory that surgeons give patients the option of storing blood prior to surgery.

Before considering preoperative blood donations, patients should have good medical and nutritional status and a hematocrit ≥30% prior to undergoing phlebotomy. Although with monitoring this procedure is safe even in coronary artery disease patients. Predonation can occur up to one month prior to surgery with blood withdrawn every 3–4 days. Iron supplementation and erythropoietin should be given to enhance erythropoiesis and prevent preoperative anemia.

Although the risk of disease transmission is diminished, this procedure does carry risks as several studies have shown that adverse events including transfusion reactions can occur after infusion of autologous blood. Surgeons should also be cautioned against transfusion blood postoperatively just because the unit exists. Over transfusion can lead to viscosity issues, pulmonary edema, ischemic events, clerical errors, and other medical problems.

Several controversies exist as to the complete usefulness of preoperative blood donation. More blood is generally donated than used, making this procedure quite wasteful. Cost-effective models illustrate that the benefit-to-risk ratio of preoperative donation is quite low compared to volunteer donor units. Some studies have shown that preoperative autologous donation may appear to increase the risk of postoperative anemia, thus increasing the likelihood that transfusion will be necessary.

Bibliography

D'Ambra MN, Kaplan DK. Alternatives to allogeneic blood use in surgery: acute normovolemic hemodilution and preoperative autologous donation. *Am J Surg* 1995; 170(6S)(Suppl):49S–52S.

Fakhry S, Rutherford E, Sheldon G. Hematologic principles in surgery. In: Townsend C (ed.), *Sabiston Textbook of Surgery*, 16th ed. Philadelphia, PA: W.B. Saunders, 2001, 69–89.

Goodnough LT, Brecher ME, Kanter ME, AuBuchon JP. Medical progress: transfusion medicine (second of two parts)—blood conservation. *N Engl J Med* 1999;340(7): 525–533.

34. **(A)** The transfusion of platelets is indicated for symptomatic patients who are thrombocytopenic and demonstrate microvascular bleeding. Older guidelines recommend transfusion asymptomatic patients with counts ≤20,000/mm^3; however, recent studies have determined this to be excessive and patients can be watched with much lower counts. Suggested transfusion guidelines are summarized in Table 5-14.

    Platelets are available in two types of preparations. Pooled units come from separated whole blood from 6 to 10 different donors. These units are

TABLE 5-14   Suggested Transfusion Guidelines for Platelets

Recent (within 24 h) platelet count ≤10,000/mm^3 (for prophylaxis)

Recent (within 24 h) platelet count ≤50,000/mm^3 with demonstrated microvascular bleeding ("oozing") or a planned surgical/invasive procedure

Demonstrated microvascular bleeding and a precipitous fall in platelet count

Patients in the operating room who have had complicated procedures or have required more than 10 U of blood and have microvascular bleeding; giving platelets assumes adequate surgical hemostasis has been achieved

Document platelet dysfunction (e.g., prolonged bleeding time >15 min, abnormal platelet function tests) with petechiae, purpura, microvascular bleeding ("oozing"), or surgical/invasive procedure

Unwarranted indications

   Empirical use with massive transfusion when patient is not having clinically evident microvascular bleeding ("oozing")

   Prophylaxis in thrombotic thrombocytopenic purpura/hemolytic-uremic syndrome or idiopathic thrombocytopenic purpura

   Extrinsic platelet dysfunction (e.g., renal failure, von Willebrand's disease)

Source: Reprinted from Fakhry S, Rutherford E, Sheldon G. Hematologic principles in surgery. In: Townsend C, (ed.), *Sabiston Textbook of Surgery*, 16th ed. Philadelphia, PA: W.B. Saunders, 2001, 69–89, with permission from Elsevier.

highly immunogenic and contain increased risk of disease transmission and antiplatelet antibody production. Single donor units can be obtained by apheresis where the red cells mass is returned to the patient leading to higher platelet counts in the preparation. Although the unit is still immunogenic, the amount of HLA and the risk of disease transmission is less. A six-pack of pooled or one apheresis unit of platelets should raise the patient's count by 30,000/mm^3.

Bibliography

Fakhry S, Rutherford E, Sheldon G. Hematologic principles in surgery. In: Townsend C (ed.), *Sabiston Textbook of Surgery*, 16th ed. Philadelphia, PA: W.B. Saunders, 2001, 69–89.

35. **(B)** Within the last two decades several pharmaceutical companies and academic departments have been extensively researching and developing alternatives to packed red cells. This has the potential of eliminating infectious risk, decreasing transfusion reactions, providing an unlimited supply of product and possibly allowing Jehovah's Witnesses an alternative. Possible indications include trauma, hemorrhagic shock, perioperative blood loses, sepsis, stroke, myocardial infarction, cardiac arrest, and organ perfusion during transplantation all aimed at increasing the oxygen carry capacity currently available within the patient.

Products currently being tested either use animal-based hemoglobin or are purely synthetic molecules. In order to be useful, these products must have the ability to carry oxygen, have a relatively good shelf life, an acceptable half-life once infused, and at least equal mortality compared to allogenic transfusions.

Hemoglobin-based solutions are derived from either human, bovine, or through recombinant techniques. Red cells are lysed and the hemoglobin is polymerized or pyridoxylated to decrease renal excretion. These solutions have the ability to carry oxygen and stay in the circulation for 4–5 days before clearance by the kidneys. Clinical trials are currently underway for several different preparations and are being used principally in acute trauma, cardiac surgery, and septic patients. Several products have not met FDA requirements and are no longer being used for clinical purposes.

Perflurocarbons are currently the only synthetic preparations currently undergoing testing. They have the ability to carry 40 times the amount of oxygen as normal red cells. Human trials have showed limited success.

Numerous potential problems exist with red cell substitutes. Iron that is infused with these products enhances bacterial multiplication leading to increased mortality in septic animal models. It is also taken up by macrophages leading to inflammatory response similar to allogeneic transfusions. These products increase nitric oxide metabolism leading to vasoconstriction, increase pulmonary vascular resistance, oxidative damage, platelet activation, and they interfere with standard photometric blood tests. Clinical usefulness of these problems have yet to be determined (see Table 5-15).

Bibliography

Buchman TG. Augmenting the carriage of the oxygen in the emergency situation. In: Cameron JL (ed.), *Current Surgical Therapy*, 6th ed. St. Louis, MO: Mosby, 1998, 922–924.

TABLE 5-15 Synthetic Hemoglobin Preparations

Hemoglobin based currently in FDA trials
  Hemopure—bovine
  Polyethylene glycol-hemoglobin—bovine
  Polyheme—human
  Hemolink—human
  Optro—Recombinant (*E. coli*)
Hemoglobin based closed by FDA
  Diaspirin cross-linked—human (increased mortality)
Synthetic—awaiting FDA approval
  Perflubron

Creteur J, Sibbald W, Vincent JL. Hemoglobin solutions—not just red blood cell substitutes. *Crit Care Med* 2000;28(8):3025–3034.
Fakhry S, Rutherford E, Sheldon G. Hematologic principles in surgery. In: Townsend C (ed.), *Sabiston Textbook of Surgery*, 16th ed. Philadelphia, PA: W.B. Saunders, 2001, 69–89.
Goodnough LT, Brecher ME, Kanter ME, AuBuchon JP. Medical progress: transfusion medicine (second of two parts)—blood conservation. *N Engl J Med* 1999;340(7): 525–533.

36. **(E)** Intraoperative and postoperative recovery and reinfusion of patient's blood are two possible sources by which allogenic blood requirements can be diminished. Intraoperative blood recovery is performed by immediately adding heparin to the blood as it is recovered from the body. Pure erythrocytes are then washed, concentrated, and then banked in saline free of heparin and returned to the blood stream by infusion. Some devices have the ability to collect and process 10 units of blood per hour. Cells are not stored in appropriate media to allow for long-term storage and must be used within several hours of processing. Once infused the red cells have a similar half-life to that of allogenic blood transfusions.

Cell washing does not sterilize the blood. Therefore, the cell saver technique should not be used in the presence of bacterial contamination. Spreading of malignant cells is also considered a possibility and is generally contraindicated. Amniotic or ascetic fluid reintroduction can cause massive DIC and other unwarranted complications and should be avoided. Processed cells contain no plasma component and can precipitate dilutional coagulopathy.

Postoperative recovery of blood includes collections from such devices as chest tubes and surgical drains. These collections are often diluted, hemolyzed, and contain fragments of clots. Therefore, these collections must be used cautiously as the infusion of low hematocrit fluid into the system may enhance the patient's blood deficit. Contraindications are similar to intraoperative cell washing techniques.

Bibliography

Buchman TG. Augmenting the carriage of the oxygen in the emergency situation. In: Cameron JL (ed.), *Current Surgical Therapy*, 6th ed. St. Louis, MO: Mosby, 1998, 922–924.
Goodnough LT, Brecher ME, Kanter ME, AuBuchon JP. Medical progress: transfusion medicine (second of two parts)—blood conservation. *N Engl J Med* 1999;340(7): 525–533.
Polk HCJ, Cheadle W, Franklin GA. Principles of operative surgery. In: Townsend C (ed.), *Sabiston Textbook of*

TABLE 5-16   Several Commercially Available Suture Products*

	Absorbable	Nonabsorbable
Braided	Polyglactic acid (Vicryl†) Polyglycolic acid (Dexon†)	Nylon (Surgilon†, Neurolon†) Polyester (Ti-Cron†, Ethibond†, Mersiline†) Silk Steel
Monofilament	Catgut Chromic Poliglecaprone 25 (Monocryl†) Polydioxanone (PDS II†) Gylocomer 631 (Biosyn†) Polyglyconate (Maxon†)	Nylon (Ethilon†) Polyester Polypropylene (Prolene†, SurgiPro†) Steel

*Products listed in same categories do not necessary have the same tensile properties.
†Brand names are copyright of Ethicon Inc or United Surgical Steel and Davis and Geck Inc.

Surgery, 16th ed. Philadelphia, PA: W.B. Saunders, 2001, 163–170.

37. **(D)** The best method for preventing the need for blood transfusion is obviously good surgical technique and effective surgical hemostasis. Suture material should be chosen based on its properties and the result desired by the surgeon. Suture material is basically categorized as absorbable or nonabsorbable and whether it is monofilament or braided.

The choice of suture to use is based primarily on surgeon preference but also by the properties of the suture compared to the task on hand. For short-term hemostasis and approximation of soft tissue catgut, chromic and polyglactic acid sutures work the best. They have the shortest tensile strength and are usually gone within 2–4 weeks. Monofilaments tend to slide better through tissue than does the braided; however, the knots will tend to unravel if not laid down correctly. Therefore, if tissue integrity is desired then a monofilament is a better choice as it will not slice the tissue as it is passed.

All of the sutures listed in Table 5-16 have the ability to produce local and systemic irritation and inflammation. Suture made from animal products such as catgut and chromic tend to cause the highest rate of local irritation whereas steel rarely causes any local or system reaction. Steel is also available in braided and single strand preparations.

Bibliography

Polk HCJ, Cheadle W, Franklin GA. Principles of operative surgery. In: Townsend C (ed.), *Sabiston Textbook of Surgery*, 16th ed. Philadelphia, PA: W.B. Saunders, 2001, 163–170.
Product Information, Ethicon Inc.
Product Information, United Surgical Steel and Davis and Geck Suture.

38. **(C)** Electrocautery is the most used method for obtaining hemostasis in the operative field. Standard operating room electrocautery can be used either as a bipolar or unipolar instrument. Bipolar settings do not require the patient to be "grounded" and electrons pass from one side of the instrument through the tissue and back through the other side completing the circuit. Bipolar is used extensively in neurosurgical applications where passage of electrons through the brain tissue is not desired.

Unipolar settings require the patient to be "grounded" to the machine and electrons are passed from the tip of the instrument through the adjacent tissue and diffuse through the patient to the "grounding" pad completing the circuit. Typical machines can be set on "cutting" which provide a continuous current of electrons desiccating the tissue but providing little hemostasis; or set as "coagulate" where a sinusoidal pattern of electrons is passed which provide for dehydration and coagulation of vessels but the tissue is not cut itself. Some machines allow for mixing or "blending" of these two modalities.

Ligasure (Valley Lab) is a brand of bipolar electrocautery that uses heat to denature proteins within the vessel wall followed by a cool down under pressure leading to vessel occlusion. It produces a thin layer membrane that can easily be transected. Tests using this system show that bursts strength are similar if not superior to clips and sutures.

Argon Beam Coagulator produces a high flow stream of argon gas from the tip of the applicator. When placed in proximity to a organ parenchyma it spreads out over the surface blowing away debris and drying the field. Once activated the argon transmits electricity from the top along the surface of the tissue causing a superficial coagulation of tissue that the gas has spread to. This is performed without excess heat or smoke.

Ultrasonic coagulation are devices that use ultra-high frequency vibrations (>55,000) to provide cool cutting and coagulation of tissues with little damage to surrounding tissues. This device has found many uses in general surgery to include laparoscopic procedures and hemorrhoidectomy.

Also available are specialized devices that produce lasers, infrared photocoagulation, and radio frequency ablation, which have their unique properties and uses.

Bibliography

Kennedy JS, Stranahan PL, Taylor KD, Chandler JG. High-burst-strength, feedback-controlled bipolar vessel sealing. *Surg Endosc* 1998;12(6):876–878.

Polk HCJ, Cheadle W, Franklin GA. Principles of operative surgery. In: Townsend C (ed.), *Sabiston Textbook of Surgery*, 16th ed. Philadelphia, PA: W.B. Saunders, 2001, 163–170.

39. **(A)** Several devices are available to assist the surgeon in control of hemostasis intraoperatively. Gelfoam with or without thrombin is the most used device for surgical procedure. Gelfoam is water insoluble matrix derived from pork skin. It acts as a sponge and is able to absorb large quantities of blood, fluid, or thrombin. It acts as a hemostasis agent through unknown methods. It is almost completely absorbed within several weeks. It is also available as a powder which is made by milling the matrix to the desired coarseness.

Several other companies are devising similar matrix type preparations that are currently in or finishing clinical trials. They all contain proprietary matrix formulations along with thrombin. The mixture is squeezed into a wound along with thrombin to act as a hemostatic plug. It is designed to close the hole, seal the tissue, and promote clotting.

N-Butyl-2-cyanoacrylate and octyl-2-cyanoacrylate are examples of sealants that were designed strictly for skin closure. These substances are packaged sterilely and polymerized on activation and released from their containers. They are ideal for closing small wounds and can be used in conjunction with but not replacing deeper subcutaneous stitches. Prior to use the wound should be clean and dry, and not under across areas of high skin tension or unstabilized joints. The protective film will breakdown naturally over time into cyanoacrylate and formaldehyde. Several studies are looking at alternative uses of octyl-2-cyanoacrylate to include variceal injection to stop bleeding, scleral bucking in eye surgery, hand surgery, and vascular anastamosis.

Bibliography

Ang ES, Tan KC, Tan LH, Ng RT, Song IC. 2-Octylcyanoacrylate-assisted microvascular anastomosis: comparison with a conventional suture technique in rat femoral arteries. *J Reconstr Microsurg* 2001;17(3):193–201.

Hallock GG, Lutz DA. Octyl-2-cyanoacrylate adhesive for rapid nail plate restoration. *J Hand Surg [Am]* 2000;25(5): 979–981.

Mattick A, Clegg G, Beattie T, Ahmad T. A randomised, controlled trial comparing a tissue adhesive (2-octyl-cyanoacrylate) with adhesive strips (Steristrips) for paediatric laceration repair. *Emerg Med J* 2002;19(5):405–407.

Nguyen AJ, Baron TH, Burgart LJ, Leontovich O, Rajan E, Gostout CJ. 2-Octyl-cyanoacrylate (Dermabond), a new glue for variceal injection therapy: results of a preliminary animal study. *Gastrointest Endosc* 2002;55(4):572–575.

Weaver FA, Hood DB, Zatina M, Messina L, Badduke B. Gelatin-thrombin-based hemostatic sealant for intraoperative bleeding in vascular surgery. *Ann Vasc Surg* 2002;16(3):286–293.

40. **(C)** Sealants derived from fibrin preparations have been used in Europe for over 20 years. Recently the FDA has approved for use in the United States one commercially available product (Tisseel VH; Baxter/Immuno AG, Vienna Austria). Most fibrin preparations contain a combination of virally inactivated purified human fibrinogen and thrombin and can be applied in liquid or dried form to the area of injury. These two products are reconstituted in the operating room and used within seconds to minutes of mixing together and applied as a thick liquid gel or aerosolized. Several products, including the United States version, contain antifibrinolytic agents such as aprotinin or tranexamic acid to increase clot stability, and factor XIII which catalyzes cross-linking between fibrin molecules and cross-links several useful proteins. Addition of these two products to the stability of the sealant is still controversial.

Noncommercially available fibrin sealant is available and is often called "fibrin glue." It is made by mixing human cryoprecipitate with bovine thrombin and applying to the area of injury. This combination contains approximately 10% of the fibrin concentration of fibrin sealants and is not virally inactivated. Bovine thrombin has been known to cause antifactor V antibodies and severe hypotension on administration.

Usefulness of fibrin sealants are many and include most applications where bleeding or seroma formation is an issue. Fibrin sealants have been used successfully in operative and reoperative cardiac surgery, carotid endarterectomy with polytetrafluorethylene patch angioplasty, circumcisions, bowel anastomosis, tooth extractions, orthopedic surgery, dura mater closure after neurosurgical procedures to decrease cerebrospinal fluid leakage, and to decrease seroma formation after soft tissue flap formation as with mastectomies. The most useful application of fibrin sealants are in those patients with coagulopathies. Several studies have shown improved efficacy both inside and outside of the operating room with patients with factor deficiencies.

Bibliography

Carless PA, Anthony DM, Henry DA. Systematic review of the use of fibrin sealant to minimize perioperative allogeneic blood transfusion. *Br J Surg* 2002;89(6):695–703.

Jackson MR, Alving BM. Fibrin sealant in preclinical and clinical studies. *Curr Opin Hematol* 1999;6(6):415–419.

Jackson MR, Gillespie DL, Longenecker EG, et al. Hemostatic efficacy of fibrin sealant (human) on expanded poly-tetrafluoroethylene carotid patch angioplasty: a randomized clinical trial. *J Vasc Surg* 1999;30(3):461–466.

Martinowitz U, Schulman S, Horoszowski H, Heim M. Role of fibrin sealants in surgical procedures on patients with hemostatic disorders. *Clin Orthop* 1996(328):65–75.

Rousou J, Levitsky S, Gonzalez-Lavin L, et al. Randomized clinical trial of fibrin sealant in patients undergoing resternotomy or reoperation after cardiac operations. A multicenter study. *J Thorac Cardiovasc Surg* 1989;97(2):194–203.

Inflammation and Shock

Ursula M. Szmulowicz and Kristine A.K. Lombardozzi

Questions

1. A 12-year-old girl presents to her family physician, complaining of redness and swelling of an incision on her right index finger, sustained earlier in the day. On examination, the finger is seen to be erythematous and tender, with mild soft tissue swelling.

   What is the predominant cell type involved in the early stages of this acute inflammatory response?

   (A) macrophages
   (B) cells
   (C) natural killer cells
   (D) neutrophils
   (E) T cells

2. Cells of the monocyte-macrophage lineage recognize antigens by which of the following mechanisms?

   (A) lipid A
   (B) toll-like receptors (TLR)
   (C) T cell receptor
   (D) immunoglobulin G
   (E) IL-2

3. The cell type most characteristic of chronic inflammation is the

   (A) macrophage
   (B) B cell
   (C) natural killer cell
   (D) neutrophil
   (E) eosinophil

4. The resolution of an acute inflammatory process is mediated by which of the following?

   (A) apoptosis
   (B) anti-inflammatory cytokines
   (C) angiogenesis
   (D) corticosteroids
   (E) all of the above

5. The coagulation cascade is activated as part of the acute inflammatory response by means of

   (A) factor XIII
   (B) factor VII
   (C) factor VIII
   (D) prekallikrein
   (E) protein C

Questions 6 through 8
Match the lettered items with the following questions.

   (A) classic pathway of the complement cascade
   (B) alternative pathway of the complement cascade
   (C) both
   (D) neither

6. Virus-infected cells

7. Antibody-antigen reactions

8. Mannin-binding lectin

Questions 9 through 11
Match the lettered items with the following questions.

   (A) thromboxane A_2
   (B) prostacyclin
   (C) both
   (D) neither

9. Produced by mast cells

10. Results in vasodilatation

11. Promotes platelet aggregation

12. A 35-year-old male develops a fever of 38.9°C 24 hours following a motor vehicle accident in which he sustained multiple lower extremity fractures. This febrile response stems from which of the following mediators?

   (A) IL-1
   (B) IL-2
   (C) IFN-α
   (D) IL-10
   (E) IL-4

13. In combination with oxygen, which molecule is the precursor to nitric oxide?

   (A) citrulline
   (B) arginine
   (C) tryptophan
   (D) alanine
   (E) leucine

14. Anaerobic metabolism produces how many moles of ATP from 1 mol of glucose?

   (A) 1
   (B) 2
   (C) 3
   (D) 4
   (E) 5

15. The severity of hypovolemic shock has been found to correlate with the

   (A) hematocrit
   (B) pulmonary capillary wedge pressure (PCWP)
   (C) lactic acid
   (D) PaO_2
   (E) white blood cell count

Questions 16 through 18
An 80-year-old male with a history of pancreatitis undergoes pancreatic debridement. Subsequent to the procedure, his pancreatic drains are found to contain elevated levels of amylase and lipase. The output from the drains also markedly increases once the patient begins a regular diet. Two days later, the patient develops hypotension and tachycardia, accompanied by oliguria and confusion.

16. The first organ affected by the compensatory mechanisms of hypovolemic shock is the

   (A) heart
   (B) kidney
   (C) gastrointestinal tract

   (D) skin
   (E) spleen

17. An example of hypovolemia due solely to losses from the extracellular fluid compartment is

   (A) burn injury
   (B) hemorrhage
   (C) dehydration
   (D) fever
   (E) mechanical ventilation

18. The initial compensatory mechanism to hypovolemic shock is the release of

   (A) aldosterone
   (B) norepinephrine
   (C) renin
   (D) vasopressin
   (E) angiotensinogen

19. A 25-year-old white male presents to the emergency department following a motorcycle crash in which he was the unhelmeted driver. On arrival, the patient is poorly responsive. He demonstrates a systolic blood pressure of 80 mmHg with a heart rate of 125 bpm. A deep laceration, no longer bleeding, is on his left leg, with a fractured femur exposed. The patient smells strongly of alcohol. What findings are expected in an intoxicated patient with hypovolemic shock?

   (A) exaggerated hypotension
   (B) warm, flushed skin
   (C) worsened metabolic acidosis
   (D) increased IL-10
   (E) all of the above

20. A 22-year-old male presents to the emergency department after sustaining a gunshot wound to the right upper quadrant of his abdomen. On arrival, the patient is lethargic. His vital signs are significant for a systolic blood pressure of 85 mmHg with a heart rate of 130 bpm. As part of his therapy, fluid resuscitation is initiated. Which of the following is currently considered the best resuscitation fluid?

   (A) 0.9% sodium chloride
   (B) albumin
   (C) dextran
   (D) 5% dextrose in 0.45% sodium chloride
   (E) 7.5% sodium chloride

21. Hypertonic saline (7.5% sodium chloride) has been promoted as the initial fluid for acute resuscitation for which of the following reasons?

   (A) proven survival advantage over isotonic solutions
   (B) decrease in cerebral perfusion pressures in amounts smaller than that of isotonic solutions
   (C) interference with neutrophil adherence to endothelial cells
   (D) increase in pulmonary myeloperoxidase
   (E) reduced cerebral edema in the case of a compromised blood-brain barrier

22. A 33-year-old male arrives at the emergency department following a motor vehicle crash in which he was the restrained driver. The patient only noted severe left hip pain. On examination, his systolic blood pressure was 85 mmHg and his heart rate 110 bpm. The patient's pelvis was found to be unstable, with a deformity at the left hip. The next step in treatment is

   (A) norepinephrine infusion
   (B) placement of military antishock trousers (MAST)
   (C) delay of fluid resuscitation until the hemorrhage is controlled
   (D) bolus of 1–2 L of 0.9% sodium chloride
   (E) dopamine administration

23. A 41-year-old female presents to the emergency department after sustaining a gunshot wound to the abdomen, with injuries to the liver and large bowel. Despite successful resuscitation and operative intervention, the patient dies 2 weeks later of multisystem organ failure in the intensive care unit. Which organ most likely first experienced dysfunction?

   (A) liver
   (B) gastrointestinal tract
   (C) lung
   (D) kidney
   (E) heart

24. A 23-year-old male presents to the emergency department by ambulance after an altercation in which he sustained trauma to his head and neck. According to witness reports, the patient was dragged on the floor by his head. On arrival, the patient is found to have a systolic blood pressure of 65 mmHg with a heart rate of 50 bpm. His Glasgow Coma Scale level is five. A head CT reveals a large epidural hematoma while a cervical spine CT demonstrates bilateral vertebral facet dislocations at the level of C4. What is the likely cause of his hypotension?

   (A) head trauma
   (B) hypovolemia
   (C) massive vasodilatation
   (D) alcohol intoxication
   (E) blunt cardiac injury

25. The most common mechanism of spinal cord injury is

   (A) distraction
   (B) transection
   (C) impact with persisting compression
   (D) impact alone
   (E) laceration

26. In which category of shock is the Trendelenburg position considered a viable treatment option?

   (A) cardiogenic
   (B) neurogenic
   (C) hypovolemic
   (D) septic
   (E) cardiac compressive

27. A 74-year-old previously healthy woman is admitted to the hospital for intravenous antibiotics following an uneventful open appendectomy for a ruptured appendix. On postoperative day 1, the patient reports crushing substernal chest pain with radiation to the left arm. The patient appears pale, anxious, and diaphoretic. Her extremities are cold. Initial vital signs reveal a systolic blood pressure of 75 mmHg and a heart rate of 101 bpm. An electrocardiogram (ECG) is consistent with an acute anterior myocardial infarction (MI).

   What factors predict the development of cardiogenic shock in the setting of an acute MI?

   (A) ST elevations on presenting ECG
   (B) age less than 75 years old
   (C) posterior infarction
   (D) rales on physical examination
   (E) inferior infarction

28. The previous patient is transferred to the intensive care unit and judicious fluid resuscitation as well as vasopressor support is initiated. A pulmonary artery catheter is placed to guide therapy. What readings are characteristic of cardiogenic shock?

	Cardiac output	SVR	PCWP	CVP
(A)	Low	High	High	Normal to high
(B)	Low	High	Low	Low
(C)	High	Low	Low	High
(D)	Low	High	Low	High
(E)	High	Low	Low	Low

29. A transthoracic echocardiogram of this patient is obtained, demonstrating new onset mitral regurgitation. Immediately, an angiogram is performed, showing acute left main coronary artery occlusion. What is the next step in management?

    (A) thrombolytic therapy
    (B) emergent coronary artery bypass graft (CABG) with mitral valve repair
    (C) emergent percutaneous coronary intervention (PCI) (angioplasty with stenting)
    (D) medical stabilization followed by delayed PCI
    (E) placement of an intraaortic balloon pump (IABP)

30. An 89-year-old male develops cardiogenic shock following an acute MI. All of the following factors are expected to increase his myocardial oxygen requirements *except*:

    (A) elevated heart rate
    (B) aldosterone release
    (C) increased myocardial contractility
    (D) sympathetic stimulation
    (E) decreased left ventricular diastolic pressure

31. A 69-year-old woman with a history of hypertension presents to the emergency department with complaints of crushing chest pain, sudden in its onset. On physical examination, this ill-appearing woman is hypotensive and tachycardic. An ECG reveals ST elevations in the V3 and V4 leads. What is a characteristic finding on echocardiogram in this condition?

    (A) tricuspid regurgitation
    (B) left ventricular hypokinesis
    (C) mitral regurgitation
    (D) left ventricular dilatation
    (E) aortic root dilatation

32. The typical measurements demonstrated by a Swan-Ganz catheter placed in this 69-year-old woman are as follows:

	Central venous pressure	PCWP	Cardiac index
(A)	Normal	High	Low to normal
(B)	High	Low to normal	Low to normal
(C)	High	High	Low
(D)	Low	Low	High
(E)	Normal	Low	High

33. The intraaortic balloon pump

    (A) increases perfusion at the expense of elevated oxygen consumption
    (B) inflates during late diastole and deflates in late systole
    (C) is complicated by vascular damage and bleeding in 5–20% of patients
    (D) significantly improves mortality in early revascularization candidates
    (E) is contraindicated for use in patients with mitral regurgitation

34. Following an MI complicated by cardiogenic shock, thrombolytic therapy in conjunction with the IABP improves mortality. What is the mechanism of this synergism?

    (A) Reduction in the release of tissue plasminogen activator
    (B) Improvement in hemodynamic parameters
    (C) Increase in oxygen consumption
    (D) Inactivation of the coagulation cascade
    (E) Complement activation

35. Inflation of the IABP occurs at which point on an ECG?

    (A) T wave
    (B) P wave
    (C) PR interval
    (D) R wave
    (E) QRS complex

36. A 30-year-old male is involved in a motor vehicle crash in which he is the restrained driver. At the accident scene, the steering wheel is seen to be deformed. Prior to his arrival at the emergency department by ambulance, the patient is hemodynamically stable without signs of respiratory compromise; however,

on reassessment by the trauma physicians, the blood pressure is found to be 82/45 mmHg with a heart rate of 100 bpm. Fluid resuscitation is initiated with normal saline boluses, resulting in a transient increase in the blood pressure. The patient begins to complain of severe anterior chest pain. On examination, breath sounds are equal bilaterally, and a large hematoma is seen over the sternum. No abdominal tenderness is elicited. A chest x-ray is unremarkable. A focused abdominal sonogram for trauma (FAST) examination is performed, showing cardiac tamponade. Immediately following the FAST examination, the patient becomes obtunded, requiring intubation, and his blood pressure falls further. His pulse is lost and the rhythm strip reveals pulseless electrical activity. In addition to initiating advanced cardiac life support procedures, what is the next step in management while in the emergency department?

(A) continued intravenous hydration

(B) emergency department thoracotomy

(C) subxiphoid pericardial window

(D) pericardiocentesis

(E) placement of a pulmonary artery catheter

37. What readings would a pulmonary artery catheter have demonstrated in this patient prior to the advent of the pulseless electrical activity?

(A) high cardiac output

(B) equalization of the systolic pressures among the cardiac chambers

(C) equalization of the diastolic pressures among the cardiac chambers

(D) high systemic vascular resistance

(E) high PCWP

38. A 65-year-old male presents to the emergency department in obvious respiratory distress. On arrival, the patient is intubated. His vital signs are significant for marked tachycardia and hypotension. Urticarial lesions are identified. The history that is offered is that this previously healthy patient suddenly developed shortness of breath after a seafood dinner. What is the mediator of this condition?

(A) IgA

(B) IgG

(C) IgE

(D) IgM

(E) IgD

39. This patient has been taking β-blocking medications for treatment of hypertension. Epinephrine was given at the standard dosage for treatment of anaphylaxis without any improvement in his condition. What agent should be used next for treatment of his current hypotension?

(A) epinephrine in a higher dosage

(B) glucagon

(C) hydrocortisone

(D) ranitidine

(E) norepinephrine

40. An example of an anti-inflammatory cytokine is

(A) IL-2

(B) IFN-γ

(C) Lymphotoxin-α (LT-α)

(D) IL-4

(E) TNF-α

41. TNF-α features prominently in all of the following *except*:

(A) inhibition of the coagulation cascade

(B) neutrophil chemotaxis

(C) apoptosis

(D) angiogenesis

(E) protection against intracellular bacteria

42. An 80-year-old male is transferred from a nursing home to the emergency department with the complaint of altered mental status. On examination, the patient is ill-appearing, with a temperature of 35°C and a systolic blood pressure of 85 mmHg. Laboratory studies reveal a white blood cell count of 3,000 and a positive nitrite in the urinalysis. The patient is admitted to the intensive care unit for treatment of a urinary tract infection complicated by septic shock. To assist in his treatment, a right pulmonary artery catheter is placed. The findings most associated with septic shock are

	Cardiac output	Central venous pressure	PCWP
(A)	Elevated	Decreased	Normal to elevated
(B)	Elevated	Normal elevated	Normal to elevated
(C)	Decreased	Decreased	Normal to elevated
(D)	Elevated	Normal to elevated	Decreased
(E)	Decreased	Normal to elevated	Normal to elevated

43. The pathogen most commonly responsible for the onset of septic shock is

(A) Klebsiella

(B) Pseudomonas

(C) Staphylococcus

(D) Escherichia coli

(E) Bacteroides

44. Which of the following is true of oxygenation in septic shock?

(A) Oxygen delivery is elevated while oxygen extraction is decreased.

(B) Oxygen delivery is reduced while oxygen extraction is increased.

(C) Arterial-venous oxygen difference is increased.

(D) Both oxygen delivery and extraction are increased.

(E) Mixed venous oxygen is decreased.

45. Glucocorticoids influence the inflammatory response by all of the following *except*:

(A) enhanced synthesis of $I\kappa B$

(B) reduced neutrophil aggregation

(C) increased production of COX

(D) decreased IL-2 levels

(E) suppression of inducible nitric oxide synthase production

46. A 46-year-old female develops septic shock following an open cholecystectomy for a gangrenous gallbladder. She remains intubated after surgery but exhibits persistent hypoxia with maximal ventilator support. The diagnosis of acute respiratory distress syndrome (ARDS) is suggested. This condition is defined by which of the following criteria?

(A) $PaO_2/FiO_2 < 200$ and PCWP < 18 mmHg

(B) $PaO_2/FiO_2 > 200$ and PCWP < 18 mmHg

(C) $PaO_2/FiO_2 < 200$ and PCWP > 18 mmHg

(D) $PaO_2/FiO_2 > 200$ and PCWP > 18 mmHg

(E) none of the above

47. Positive end-expiratory pressure (PEEP) is added to this patient's ventilatory support with an improvement in her oxygenation. The mechanism by which PEEP functions includes

(A) reduction in the rate of pulmonary edema formation

(B) improvement in the reabsorption of edema fluid

(C) promotion of the opening of collapsed alveoli

(D) prevention of the collapse of alveoli

(E) enhancement of surfactant production

48. A 75-year-old male with a history of steroid-dependent chronic obstructive pulmonary disease undergoes a left hemicolectomy for treatment of cancer. The operation is complicated by an anastomotic dehiscence, requiring reexploration and the creation of a colostomy. Following surgery, the patient becomes febrile and exhibits a decline in his systolic blood pressure. The nitric oxide-induced vasodilatation exhibited by this patient is mediated by which intracellular messenger?

(A) cyclic adenosine monophosphate (cAMP)

(B) cyclic guanosine monophosphate (cGMP)

(C) inositol 1,4,5-trisphosphate (IP_3)

(D) diacylglycerol (DAG)

(E) inosine 5-monophosphate (IMP)

49. The effects of nitric oxide inhibition include

(A) pulmonary hypertension

(B) decreased neutrophil adhesion

(C) increased peroxynitrite production

(D) more pronounced inhibition of mitochondrial respiration

(E) elevated cardiac output

50. On postoperative day 6, following an abdominoperineal resection for rectal cancer, a 68-year-old male develops signs consistent with septic shock. His physicians consider activated protein C as a treatment modality. What is its mechanism of action?

(A) induction of apoptosis

(B) inhibition of tissue plasminogen activator

(C) promotion of the translocation of NF-κB into the nucleus

(D) inactivation of factors Va and VIIIa

(E) enhanced production of protein S

51. Among the potential complications of activated protein C administration is

(A) acute renal failure

(B) bleeding

(C) atrial fibrillation

(D) thrombosis

(E) increased susceptibility to infection

52. The pulmonary artery catheter is used to measure which variable directly?

    (A) cardiac index
    (B) systemic vascular resistance
    (C) mixed-venous oxygen saturation
    (D) left ventricular end diastolic pressure
    (E) pulmonary vascular resistance index

53. The variable directly measured by gastric tonometry is the

    (A) gastric mucosal pH
    (B) gastric mucosal PCO_2
    (C) gastric mucosal PO_2
    (D) gastric mucosal bicarbonate
    (E) splanchnic hypoperfusion

Answers and Explanations

1. **(D)** As early as 30 minutes following the initial tissue injury, neutrophils travel to the affected area to participate in the localized inflammatory response (Fig. 6-1). The number of neutrophils peaks 8–12 hours after the injury. As neutrophils are unable to replicate, their legions must be continuously replenished in the course of the inflammatory response. During periods of high demand, the overall neutrophil concentration in the blood increases. The need for these large numbers of neutrophils often requires that the bone marrow release immature cells, explaining the bandemia seen with inflammation.

Neutrophils circulate within the blood; however, the role of neutrophils in inflammation transpires within the tissues. Inflammatory mediators, such as histamine and the kinins, released from the damaged tissues and from macrophages, induce an increase in the diameter of neighboring vessels as well as in their permeability. The greater volume of blood passing through these porous vessels accounts for the characteristic features of acute inflammation: warmth (*calor*), pain (*dolor*), swelling (*tumor*), and erythema (*rubor*). More importantly, the newly penetrable vessels permit neutrophils to enter the damaged tissues. To gain admission to the injured area, the naïve neutrophil initially binds loosely and repeatedly via L-selectin adhesion molecules to the E-selectin receptors expressed by the inflamed endothelium, a process called margination. Once acted on by cytokines, the activated neutrophils generate integrin molecules which have a greater affinity for the intercellular adhesion molecule-1 (ICAM-1) receptors on endothelial cells, allowing for a stronger adherence and, ultimately, migration through the pervious endothelium (diapedesis) (Fig. 6-2). Neutrophils are guided more specifically to the injured area by a gradient of chemokines such as interleukin (IL)-8, the complement split products, and

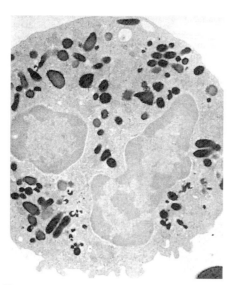

FIG. 6-1 Electron micrograph of a human neutrophil. A characteristic feature of the neutrophil is its single, elongated nucleus with multiple points of constriction. The dark cytoplasmic granules contain various preformed proteolytic enzymes, active in microbial defense. This particular neutrophil contains no rough endoplasmic reticulum: these terminally differentiated cells produce few proteins after reaching maturity.
Source: Reproduced with permission from Parslow TG, Bainton DF. Innate immunity. In: Parslow TG, Stites DP, Terr AI, Imboden JB (eds.), *Medical Immunology*, 10th ed. New York, NY: Lange, 2001, 28.

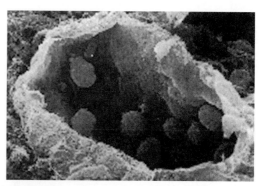

FIG. 6-2 Scanning electron micrograph (×16,000) showing acute inflammation with the adherence of leukocytes to the surface of a blood vessel.
Source: Reproduced with permission from Roitt I, Brostoff J, Male D. *Immunology*, 6th ed. Edinburgh: Mosby, 2001, 47.

prostaglandins. After reaching the inflamed tissue, neutrophils engage in engulfing a variety of target particles, including bacteria, cellular debris, and foreign material. The particles within the resulting phagosomes are then acted on by effector proteins such as lysozyme and cathepsin G, derived from intracellular granules. The breakdown of the phagosomal contents is also achieved by the superoxide anion and its free radical derivatives, produced by nicotinamide adenine dinucleotide phosphate (NADPH) oxidase, an enzyme complex assembled on the phagosome membrane itself. Unfortunately, these highly toxic metabolites do not remain confined to the phagosome, but may travel beyond the site of injury and thus extend it.

Like neutrophils, macrophages are involved in the acute inflammatory response, but appear 5–6 hours after its initiation. Natural killer cells are non-B cell, non-T cell lymphocytes that function in destroying virus-infected and tumor cells. B and T cells are active in adaptive immunity, not the innate immunity represented by the phagocytes seen early in the inflammatory process.

Bibliography

Parslow TG, Bainton DF. Innate immunity. In: Parslow TG, Stites DP, Terr AI, Imboden JB (eds.), *Medical Immunology*, 10th ed. New York, NY: McGraw-Hill, 2001, 19–39.

Roitt I, Brostoff J, Male D. *Immunology*, 6th ed. Edinburgh, UK: Mosby, 2001.

Rosenberg HF, Gallin JI. Inflammation. In: Paul WE (ed.), *Fundamental Immunology*, 4th ed. Philadelphia, PA: Lippincott-Raven, 1999, 1051–1063.

Winchester R. Principles of the immune response. In: Humes HD, DuPont HL, Gardner LB (eds.), *Kelley's Textbook of Internal Medicine*, 4th ed. Philadelphia, PA: Lippincott, Williams & Wilkins, 2000, 14–21.

2. **(B)** Phagocytic cells such as macrophages, monocytes, and neutrophils comprise the innate immune system. Unlike acquired immunity, this phytologically ancient immune process is found in most animals, both invertebrates and vertebrates. Innate immunity represents a preexisting resistance to antigens, not requiring a prior exposure. This contrasts with acquired immunity, which depends on repeated contact with the antigen to augment the immune response. Although the innate immune system commences an inflammatory reaction, its interaction with the T and B cells of acquired immunity propagate and strengthen the response.

The omnipresent cells of the monocyte-macrophage lineage are the first to encounter antigens within the blood and tissues. Until recently, the mechanism by which macrophages identify these antigens was unknown; however, studies have revealed that the specificity of the response to an antigen derives from the toll-like receptors (TLR), a family of pattern recognition molecules. This family of transmembrane protein receptors, present on the surface of macrophages and monocytes, binds various antigenic products such as bacterial flagellin and DNA. Each of the 10 known TLRs detects a particular antigen; for example, TLR-3 and TLR-4 bind viral double-stranded DNA and lipopolysaccharide (LPS), respectively. Following the attachment of LPS to the LPS binding protein, TLR-4, in conjunction with MD2 and the soluble protein CD14, activates a cascade of intracellular proteins, including the toll/IL-1 receptor-associated protein and the mitogen-activated protein (MAP) kinases, ultimately resulting in activation of nuclear factor-κB (NF-κB) (Fig. 6-3). This transcription factor promotes the expression of numerous inflammatory mediators.

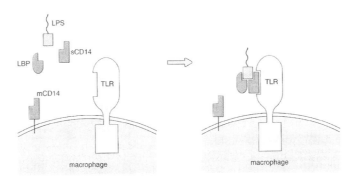

FIG. 6-3 The toll-like receptor binds lipopolysaccharide in association with lipopolysaccharide binding protein. The signal is potentiated by the protein CD14, either in its soluble or membrane-bound form. In the case of toll-like receptor 4, the protein MD2 is required for successful recognition of the antigen. TLR—toll-like receptor, LPS—lipopolysaccharide, LBP—lipopolysaccharide binding protein.
Source: Reproduced with permission from Parslow TG, Bainton DF. Innate immunity. In: Parslow TG, Sites DP, Terr AI, Imboden JB (eds.), *Medical Immunology*, 10th ed. New York, NY: Lange, 2001, 37.

Lipid A is the toxic moiety of LPS, the characteristic outer membrane component of gram-negative bacteria. Along with the inner and outer cores and the O antigen, lipid A comprises LPS. The T cell receptor detects antigens in the context of antigen-presenting cells, phagocytic cells which expose antigenic components on their surface. Immunoglobulin G is generated by B cells in response to a specific antigen; this antibody may appear on the surface membrane of B cells or free within the blood. IL-2 is a cytokine product of the inflammatory process.

Bibliography

Beutler B, Poltorak A. Sepsis and evolution of the innate immune response. *Crit Care Med* 2001;29(7):S2–S6.

Henneke P, Golenbock DT. Innate immune recognition of lipopolysaccharide by endothelial cells. *Crit Care Med* 2002;30(5):S207–S213.

Lorenz E, Mira JP, Frees KL, Schwartz DA. Relevance of mutations in the TLR4 receptor in patients with gram-negative septic shock. *Arch Intern Med* 2002;162(9):1028–1032.

Nahm MH, Apicella MA, Briles DE. Immunity to extracellular bacteria. In: Paul WE (ed.), *Fundamental Immunology*, 4th ed. Philadelphia, PA: Lippincott-Raven, 1999, 1051–1063.

Parslow TG, Bainton DF. Innate immunity. In: Parslow TG, Stites DP, Terr AI, Imboden JB (eds.), *Medical Immunology*, 10th ed. New York, NY: McGraw-Hill, 2001, 19–39.

Read RC, Wyllie DH. Toll receptors and sepsis. *Curr Opin Crit Care* 2001;7(5):371–375.

Rosenberg HF, Gallin JI. Inflammation. In: Paul WE (ed.), *Fundamental Immunology*, 4th ed. Philadelphia, PA: Lippincott-Raven, 1999, 1051–1063.

Winchester R. Principles of the immune response. In: Humes HD, DuPont HL, Gardner LB (eds.), *Kelley's Textbook of Internal Medicine*, 4th ed. Philadelphia, PA: Lippincott, Williams & Wilkins, 2000, 14–21.

Zigarelli B, Sheehan M, Wong HR. Nuclear factor-κB as a therapeutic target in critical care medicine. *Crit Care Med* 2003;31(1):S105–S111.

3. **(A)** Chronic inflammation represents the persistence of an acute inflammatory process. It may occur in the setting of multiple episodes of acute inflammation at a single site or the incomplete eradication of an initial inflammatory focus. The predominant cell type involved in chronic inflammation is the macrophage, its activity promoted by tumor necrosis factor α (TNF-α) and interferon-γ (INF-γ). Additionally, the transcription factor NF-κB is being investigated regarding its role in the induction of chronic inflammation. Mediators released from activated macrophages effect fibroblast activity and vascular formation, resulting in scarring. The prototypical lesion resulting from these factors is the granuloma—a collection of inflammatory cells encased in a fibrotic shell. Granulomata are especially associated with intracellular bacteria and inorganic pathogens, as with tuberculosis or berylliosis. These lesions confine bacteria to a single area, restrict bacterial reproduction, and limit nutrition and oxygen to the pathogens within.

While lymphocytes also take part in the chronic inflammatory process, macrophages serve as the predominant cell type. Neutrophils act in acute inflammation. The natural killer cell destroys tumor cells as well as virus-infected cells. Eosinophils are involved in allergic reactions and helminthic parasite infections.

Bibliography

Parslow TG, Bainton DF. Innate Immunity. In: Parslow TG, Stites DP, Terr AI, Imboden JB (eds.), *Medical Immunology*, 10th ed. New York, NY: McGraw-Hill, 2001, 19–39.

Roitt I, Brostoff J, Male D. *Immunology*, 6th ed. Edinburgh, NY: Mosby, 2001, 47–64.

Rosenberg HF, Gallin JI. Inflammation. In: Paul WE (ed.), *Fundamental Immunology*, 4th ed. Philadelphia, PA: Lippincott-Raven, 1999, 1051–1063.

Winchester R. Principles of the immune response. In: Humes HD, DuPont HL, Gardner LB (eds.), *Kelley's Textbook of Internal Medicine*, 4th ed. Philadelphia, PA: Lippincott, Williams & Wilkins, 2000, 14–21.

4. **(E)** Inflammation represents the complex response of vascularized tissue to damage. The initiation of the inflammatory response to injury has been well elucidated; however, the factors which result in its resolution are largely an enigma and remain an area of intense study. Pursuit of this field of inquiry may ultimately yield agents able to manage inflammation. This becomes especially important with an uncontrolled inflammatory process in which massive tissue damage occurs, as in septic shock or multiple organ failure. Until 1793, when John Hunter first described inflammation as a normal host reaction to tissue damage, inflammation was solely considered a manifestation of the disease process itself, because of its damaging effects on the subject. Now, the inflammatory process is recognized as a "double-edged sword," with beneficial as well as potentially devastating effects on the host.

A number of anti-inflammatory cytokines participate in the down-regulation of the acute inflammatory process, including IL-4, IL-10, and TGF-β. IL-4, in particular, initially acts as a proinflammatory agent, but ultimately counters production of the superoxide anion and IL-6. Programmed cell death, apoptosis, may also contribute to the resolution of inflammation. TNF-α has been shown to induce apoptosis by binding to its receptor, TNFR1, thus activating its death domain. Several other mediators demonstrate similar effects: the eicosanoids, IL-10, and the antioxidants. Attention has also focused on the hypothalamic-pituitary-adrenocortical axis, with the realization that glucocorticoids, as immunosuppressants, may moderate the inflammatory response. In studies, observations have been made of increases in adrenocorticotropic hormone (ACTH) and corticosterone in animals injected with IL-1, IL-6, and TNF-α. Finally, the mediators responsible for wound healing and angiogenesis, among them TGF-α and β, endothelial cells, epidermal growth factor, and platelet-derived growth factor, are also subjects of study for their role in the down-regulation of inflammation.

Bibliography

Roitt I, Brostoff J, Male D. *Immunology*, 6th ed. Edinburgh, NY: Mosby, 2001, 47–64.

Rosenberg HF, Gallin JI. Inflammation. In: Paul WE (ed.), *Fundamental Immunology*, 4th ed. Philadelphia, PA: Lippincott-Raven, 1999, 1051–1063.

Terr AI. Inflammation. In: Parslow TG, Stites DP, Terr AI, Imboden JB (eds.), *Medical Immunology*, 10th ed. New York, NY: Lange Medical Books, 2001, 189–203.

Winchester R. Principles of the immune response. In: Humes HD, DuPont HL, Gardner LB (eds.), *Kelley's Textbook of Internal Medicine*, 4th ed. Philadelphia, PA: Lippincott, Williams & Wilkins, 2000, 14–21.

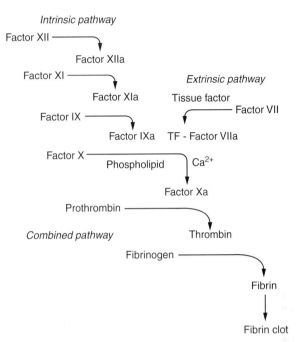

FIG. 6-4 Schematic representation of the traditional coagulation scheme or "Waterfall Hypothesis."

5. **(B)** The fundamental role of the coagulation cascade in the acute inflammatory process has been well-recognized. Tissue damage activates the extrinsic pathway of the coagulation system. In the past, it was believed that direct contact with endotoxins or microorganisms was the primary mediator of inflammation-induced thrombin generation. Recently, however, it has been discovered that this role belongs to tissue factor. This membrane-bound protein is expressed constitutively on cells normally not in direct contact with the blood. Damage to the endothelium may expose these underlying extravascular cells to the blood. Also, as part of the inflammatory process, tissue factor is induced by cytokines to appear on monocytes and endothelial cells. Following the initiation of an acute inflammatory process, tissue factor complexes with factor VII of the extrinsic coagulation pathway, resulting in factor VIIa. This complex converts factor X into its active form; in turn, prothrombin and fibrinogen are also triggered. The extrinsic pathway is augmented by the thrombin-induced activation of factor XI as well as by the induction of factor IX by the tissue factor/factor VIIa complex. Ultimately, by this pathway, fibrin is formed (Fig. 6-4). A thrombus is thus deposited in the area of tissue damage. Ostensibly, clot formation will isolate the damaged area and prevent the spread of potential pathogens; however, the same mediators that engender the coagulation cascade also initiate the fibrinolytic system in which plasmin destroys the fibrin clot. In addition, tissue factor pathway inhibitor is a potent antagonist of the tissue factor pathway inhibitor. Antithrombin III contributes to the regulation of the coagulation cascade by interfering in the action of thrombin, factor X, and factor IX. The breakdown products of the thrombus, chemotactic for inflammatory cells, act to further the inflammatory process.

Factor XIII stabilizes the fibrin strands forming a clot. Factor VIII acts as a cofactor for factor IX in the intrinsic pathway of coagulation. Prekallikrein is a precursor to bradykinin, which promotes vasodilatation, vascular permeability, and edema. Protein C serves as an inhibitor of factors Va and VIIIa.

Bibliography

Hack CE. Tissue factor pathway of coagulation in sepsis. *Crit Care Med* 2000;28(9):S25–S28.

Levi M, ten Cate H, van der Poll T. Endothelium: interface between coagulation and inflammation. *Crit Care Med* 2002;30(5):S220–S224.

Rosenberg HF, Gallin JI. Inflammation. In: Paul WE (ed.), *Fundamental Immunology*, 4th ed. Philadelphia, PA: Lippincott-Raven, 1999, 1051–1063.

Scott-Connor CEH, Rigdon EE, Rock WA, Mancino AT. Hematology. In: O'Leary JP (ed.), *The Physiologic Basis of Surgery*, 2nd ed. Philadelphia, PA: Lippincott, Williams & Wilkins, 1996, 479–506.

ten Cate H. Pathophysiology of disseminated intravascular coagulation in sepsis. *Crit Care Med* 2000;28(9):S9–S12.

6. (B)

7. (A)

8. (D)

Explanations 6 through 8

The complement system functions as an essential and early participant in the inflammatory response. There are three pathways by which complement is activated: the classical, alternative, and more recently discovered mannin-binding lectin pathways. The classical pathway is initiated by antibody-antigen complexes while the alternative pathway begins in the absence of antibody with virus-infected cells, parasites, or LPS. The mannan-binding lectin pathway commences in the presence of lectin, a protein which binds to mannan, a carbohydrate found on certain microorganisms. Despite their disparate beginnings, the three pathways converge with C3, which is cleaved into C3a and C3b by C3 convertase. The C3b fragment then acts to opsonize target particles. The C3a fragment, as well as the product of C5 convertase, C5a, serve to attract and activate leukocytes to the site of inflammation (chemotaxis) as well as to promote vasodilatation. The final product of the three pathways of the complement cascade is the membrane attack complex (MAC), comprised of C5b6789, which lyses various pathogens by incorporating itself into their cell membrane, forming a transmembrane channel by which ion displacement results in membrane disruption.

Of note, both C3a and C5a, as well as C4a, act as anaphylatoxins, promoting the release of histamine and other vasoactive substances from mast cells and basophils. Studies in which these products were injected into live subjects recreated the bronchoconstriction and circulatory collapse seen in anaphylaxis.

Bibliography

Jurusz DJ, Gilmore JY. Shock and hypoperfusion states. In: O'Leary JP (ed.), *The Physiologic Basis of Surgery*, 2nd ed. Philadelphia, PA: Lippincott, Williams & Wilkins, 1996, 84–99.

Parslow TG, Bainton DF. Innate immunity. In: Parslow TG, Stites DP, Terr AI, Imboden JB (eds.), *Medical Immunology*, 10th ed. New York, NY: McGraw-Hill, 2001, 19–39.

Roitt I, Brostoff J, Male D. *Immunology*, 6th ed. Edinburgh, NY: Mosby, 2001, 47–64.

Rosenberg HF, Gallin JI. Inflammation. In: Paul WE (ed.), *Fundamental Immunology*, 4th ed. Philadelphia, PA: Lippincott-Raven, 1999, 1051–1063.

Terr AI. Inflammation. In: Parslow TG, Stites DP, Terr AI, Imboden JB (eds.), *Medical Immunology*, 10th ed. New York, NY: Lange Medical Books, 2001, 189–203.

Walport MJ. Advances in immunology: complement (first of two parts). *N Engl J Med* 2001;344(14):1058–1066.

Walport MJ. Advances in immunology: complement (second of two parts). *N Engl J Med* 2001;344(15):1140–1144.

9. (D)

10. (B)

11. (B)

Explanations 9 through 11

The eicosanoids—the prostaglandins and leukotrienes—feature prominently in the acute inflammatory response (Fig. 6-5). In particular, thromboxane A_2 and prostacyclin—produced by platelets and endothelial cells, respectively—play central roles in inflammation. As prostaglandins, these two substances are derivatives of arachadonic acid. In response to mechanical trauma or various inflammatory stimuli, arachadonic acid is released from the cell membrane by the enzyme phospholipase A. Via the cyclooxygenase (COX) pathway, the prostaglandins are ultimately formed. Two isoforms of the COX enzyme exist: COX-1 and COX-2. COX-2 is induced in inflammation while the constitutive form, COX-1, is little affected by this process, being engaged in the basal production of prostaglandins. The two arachadonic acid derivatives, thromboxane A_2 and prostacyclin, have conflicting

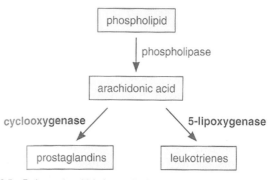

FIG. 6-5 Pathways by which the arachadonic acid derivatives are formed. *Source:* Reproduced with permission from Terr AI. Inflammation. In: Parslow TG, Stites DP, Terr AI, Imboden JB (eds.), *Medical Immunology*, 10th ed. New York, NY: Lange, 2001, 195.

actions: while the former induces platelet aggregation and vasoconstriction, the latter promotes vasodilatation, increases vascular permeability, and inhibits platelet aggregation. The ultimate effect of these two arachadonic acid metabolites depends on their relative concentrations.

Leukotrienes are also arachadonic acid derivates, produced via the lipoxygenase pathway. These are proinflammatory mediators released from neutrophils, macrophages, and mast cells. Leukotriene B$_4$, in particular, functions in promoting leukocyte adhesion to endothelial cells and neutrophil chemotaxis. Other leukotrienes foster mucus secretion and porous blood vessels. In general, the leukotrienes have been found to be important in asthma and allergy.

Bibliography

Funk CD. Prostaglandins and leukotrienes: advances in eicosanoid biology. *Science* 2001;294:1871–1875.

Jurusz DJ, Gilmore JY. Shock and hypoperfusion states. In: O'Leary JP (ed.), *The Physiologic Basis of Surgery*, 2nd ed. Philadelphia, PA: Lippincott, Williams & Wilkins, 1996, 84–99.

Rosenberg HF, Gallin JI. Inflammation. In: Paul WE (ed.), *Fundamental Immunology*, 4th ed. Philadelphia, PA: Lippincott-Raven, 1999, 1051–1063.

Terr AI. Inflammation. In: Parslow TG, Stites DP, Terr AI, Imboden JB (eds.), *Medical Immunology*, 10th ed. New York, NY: Lange Medical Books, 2001, 189–203.

12. **(A)** Localized inflammation, as with trauma, is normally accompanied by a systemic acute phase response, a common feature of which is fever. Approximately 12–24 hours following the initiation of an acute phase response, the inflammatory mediators IL-1, IL-6, and TNF-α are found in elevated levels in the blood. These three endogenous pyrogens act on the hypothalamus, raising its set point for body temperature, resulting in a fever. The effects of both IL-1 and TNF-α depend on central IL-6 activity. In IL-6 knock-out mice, Chai et al. demonstrated that the peripheral administration of exogenous pyrogens, including IL-6, does not generate a fever; however, the injection of IL-6 directly into the central nervous system results in a temperature elevation. In a study of rats, the local administration of LPS in a subcutaneous air pouch produced increased levels of TNF-α and IL-1 within the pouch and of IL-6 in the blood, indicating the pivotal role of IL-6 in fever. Banks et al. discovered an active transport mechanism by which IL-6 crosses the blood-brain barrier (BBB) in order to act on the central nervous system. Central IL-6 increases production of prostaglandin E$_2$, which directly activates the thermoregulatory center of the anterior hypothalamus; additionally, this prostaglandin induces peripheral vasoconstriction, giving an impression of "the chills," while simultaneously triggering the shiver response, again leading to the generation of body heat. Along with IL-6, neuronal afferents are believed to play a role in fever. Following a subdiaphragmatic vagotomy, animals have exhibited an attenuated fever response. Fever has been cited as directly inhibiting pathogen proliferation, with various bacteria and viruses growing more slowly at higher temperatures. In addition, fever enhances chemotaxis and leukocyte function; however, an elevated body temperature also elevates oxygen consumption, gluconeogenesis, and protein catabolism.

IFN-α, produced by leukocytes, induces the expression of class I major histocompatibility antigens on somatic cells, activates macrophages and natural killer cells, and has antiviral effects. It has no role in fever. Both IL-4 and IL-10 act as anti-inflammatory cytokines. IL-2 promotes T cell proliferation.

Bibliography

Banks WA, Kastin AJ, Gutierrez EG. Penetration of interleukin-6 across the murine blood-brain barier. *Neurosci Letters* 1994;179:53–56.

Blum FC. Fever. In: Marx JA (ed.), *Rosen's Emergency Medicine: Concepts and Clinical Practice*, 5th ed., vol. 1. St. Louis, MO: Mosby, 2002, 115–119.

Buechter KJ, Byers PM. Nutrition and metabolism. In: O'Leary JP (ed.), *The Physiologic Basis of Surgery*, 2nd ed. Philadelphia, PA: Lippincott, Williams & Wilkins, 1996, 100–117.

Chai Z, Gatti S, Toniatti C, Poli V, Bartfai T. Interleukin (IL)-6 gene expression in the central nervous system is necessary for fever response to lipopolysaccharide or IL-1α: a study on IL-6 deficient mice. *The Journal of Experimental Medicine* 1996;183:311–316.

Funk CD. Prostaglandins and leukotrienes: advances in eicosanoid biology. *Science* 2001;294(30):1871–1875.

Luheshi GN. Cytokines and fever: mechanisms and sites of action. *Ann N Y Acad Sci* 1998;856:83–89.

Oppenheim JJ, Ruscetti FW. Cytokines. In: Parslow TG, Stites DP, Terr AI, Imboden JB (eds.), *Medical Immunology*, 10th ed. New York, NY: McGraw-Hill, 2001, 148–166.

Rosenberg HF, Gallin JI. Inflammation. In: Paul WE (ed.), *Fundamental Immunology*, 4th ed. Philadelphia, PA: Lippincott-Raven, 1999, 1051–1063.

Zetterstrom M, Sundgren-Andersson AK, Ostlund P, Bartfai T. Delineation of the proinflammatory cytokine cascade in fever induction. *Ann N Y Acad Sci* 1998;856:48–52.

13. **(B)** Nitric oxide has been shown to have a potent antimicrobial effect. This reactive free radical gas is produced by activated neutrophils and macrophages via the inducible enzyme nitric oxide synthase (iNOS),

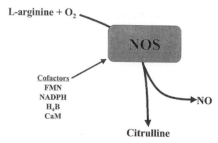

FIG. 6-6 Production of nitric oxide via the enzyme inducible nitric oxide synthase (iNOS). Unlike its constitutive isomers, neuronal, and endothelial nitric oxide synthase, iNOS is not dependent on calcium concentrations for its activity. *Source:* Reproduced with permission from Salyapongse AN, Billiar TR. Nitric oxide as a modulator of sepsis: therapeutic possibilities. In: Baue AE, Faist E, Fry DE (eds.), *Multiple Organ Failure: Pathophysiology, Prevention, and Therapy*. New York, NY: Springer, 2000, 177.

one of three NOS isoforms. Production of this inducible enzyme is stimulated by endotoxins as well as by cytokines such as IFN-γ and IL-1. The precursor molecule, L-arginine, in combination with oxygen, is converted by iNOS into nitric oxide and L-citrulline (Fig. 6-6). The cofactors participating in this reaction include flavin mononucleotide (FMN), NADPH, tetrahydrobiopterin (H_4B), and calmodulin. The production of nitric oxide is preceded by a respiratory burst from the neutrophil or macrophage, representing a transient, prominent consumption of oxygen. This metabolic burst follows phagocytosis and may last for 3 hours, highlighting the importance of nitric oxide and oxidative killing in the antimicrobial arsenal of these phagocytes. Nitric oxide diffuses into target cells infected by intracellular pathogens, where it inhibits a number of enzymes vital to cell function. For example, nitric oxide inactivates cytochrome P450 by binding to its iron complex. This free radical affects the demise of pathogens ranging from bacteria to viruses and fungi; this activity is diminished in test animals in which iNOS is inhibited. For instance, iNOS knock-out mice demonstrate a heightened susceptibility to *Mycobacterium tuberculosis* and *Leishmania major*. Additionally, in the presence of other oxidating agents, nitric oxide may be transformed into peroxynitrite, nitrogen dioxide, and the hydroxyl radical, also directly toxic to infected cells. In particular, peroxynitrite contributes to cytotoxicity by irreversibly inhibiting complexes I and III of the mitochondrial electron transport chain, responsible for adenosine triphosphate (ATP) production. Moreover, nitric oxide or its derivative, peroxynitrite, may damage single strands of DNA. Nitric oxide also serves to induce the production of proinflammatory cytokines and prostaglandins. Further studies suggest that nitric oxide plays a role in regulating apoptosis.

Bibliography

Bongard FS. Shock & resuscitation. In: Bongard FS, Sue DY (eds.), *Current Critical Care Diagnosis & Treatment*, Stamford, CT: Appleton & Lange, 1994, 14–36.

Fink MP. The role of cytokines as mediators of the inflammatory response. In: Townsend CM (ed.), *Textbook of Surgery: The Biological Basis of Modern Surgical Practice*, 16th ed. Philadelphia, PA: W.B. Saunders, 2001, 28–43.

Murray PT, Wylam ME, Umans JG. Nitric oxide and septic vascular dysfunction. *Anesth Analg* 2000;90(1):89–101.

Parslow TG, Bainton DF. Innate immunity. In: Parslow TG, Stites DP, Terr AI, Imboden JB (eds.), *Medical Immunology*, 10th ed. New York, NY: McGraw-Hill, 2001, 19–39.

Rosenberg HF, Gallin JI. Inflammation. In: Paul WE (ed.), *Fundamental Immunology*, 4th ed. Philadelphia, PA: Lippincott-Raven, 1999, 1051–1063.

Ruetten H, Thiemermann C. Shock states and nitric oxide. In: Loscalzo J, Vita JA (eds.), *Contemporary Cardiology: Nitric Oxide and the Cardiovascular System*, vol. 4. Totowa, NJ: Humana Press, 2000, 321–341.

Salyapongse AN and Billiar TR. Nitric Oxide as a Modulator of Sepsis: Therapeutic Possibilities. In: Baue AE, Faist E, and Fry DE. *Multiple Organ Failure: Pathophysiology, Prevention, and Therapy*. New York, NY: Springer; 2000: 176-187.

14. (B)

15. (C)

Explanations 14 and 15

The shock state is characterized by decreased perfusion such that the supply of oxygenated blood to the peripheral tissues is unable to maintain aerobic metabolism. Based on an expansion of the system devised by Blalock, shock is categorized into hypovolemic, cardiogenic, neurogenic, cardiac compressive, and septic. Despite its different manifestations, shock is typified by end-organ dysfunction secondary to a deficiency of oxygen and, consequentially, to a paucity of ATP in cells. On the cellular level, the hydrolysis of the high-energy phosphate bond of ATP generates the energy necessary for metabolism. Without this energy, cells become disrupted, followed by the death of the organism as a whole.

Aerobic metabolism is the basis of cellular metabolism in the presence of oxygen. With glucose as the fuel, ATP is produced via a series of metabolic pathways, including glycolysis and the tricarboxylic acid (TCA) cycle. The aerobic glycolytic pathway is comprised of 10 reactions that convert glucose to pyruvate, in the process reducing nicotinamide adenine dinucleotide (NAD^+) to NADH following the oxidation of glyceraldehyde-3-phosphate (Fig. 6-7). Two moles of ATP are produced by the glycolytic pathway. Pyruvate is then available for conversion

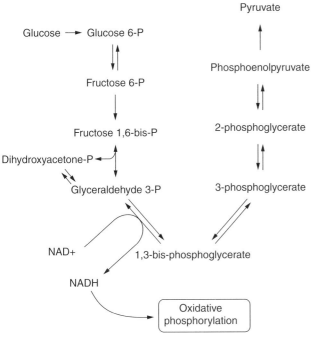

FIG. 6-7 Aerobic glycolysis.

known as oxidative phosphorylation. These electrons are then passed along the chain to complexes III and IV. As electrons are transferred between the complexes, a gradient of protons (H+) is created across the inner mitochondrial membrane, with the majority of the protons accumulating in the intermembrane space. The energy from this concentration differential powers the generation of ATP from adenosine diphosphate (ADP) and inorganic phosphate by means of the enzyme complex ATP synthase. Complete oxidation of 1 mole of glucose from glycolysis to oxidative phosphorylation results in 38 moles of ATP, making available 456,000 calories of energy.

In the absence of oxygen, cells rely solely on anaerobic metabolism to produce ATP. Cells convert to an anaerobic metabolism on reaching their anaerobic threshold, the primary determinant of which is oxygen availability. As with aerobic glycolysis, pyruvate is generated from glucose; however, in anaerobic glycolysis, pyruvate then is reduced to lactate via lactate dehydrogenase, following the donation of an electron from NADH, the species produced from the reduction of NAD by glyceraldehyde-3-phosphate dehydrogenase (Fig. 6-9). In the presence of plentiful hydrogen ion, lactic acid results from lactate. Ultimately, 2 moles of ATP are created from 1 mole of glucose. Thus, the energy available for cellular work is severely curtailed in comparison to aerobic metabolism. The energy deficit leads to cell disruption secondary to the loss of transmembrane potential and death.

The amount of lactate produced in the course of anaerobic metabolism reflects the oxygen deficit resulting from the hypoperfused state (type A lactic acidosis). Accordingly, lactic acid serves as an indicator of the severity of shock. Numerous studies have suggested that levels of lactic acid predict survival in shock patients, despite the etiology. For

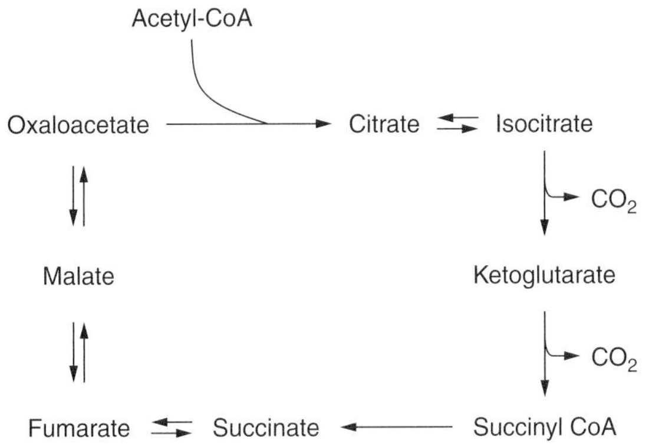

by the pyruvate dehydrogenase complex to acetyl-CoA, the initial substrate for the TCA cycle (Fig. 6-8). Acetyl-CoA also emanates from the conversion of amino acids, glycerol, and fatty acids. Within the mitochondrial matrix, the TCA cycle oxidizes acetyl-CoA to carbon dioxide and water, ultimately producing 12 moles of ATP. These diverse reactions also achieve the reduction of NAD+ and flavin adenine dinucleotide (FAD) to the energy-rich coenzymes NADH and FADH$_2$. These coenzymes become available to the electron transport chain located in the inner mitochondrial membrane. Specifically, NADH and FADH$_2$ donate their electrons to complex I and II, respectively, of the electron transport chain in a process

Oxaloacetate ——→ Citrate ⇄ Isocitrate

Malate

Fumarate ⇄ Succinate ←—— Succinyl CoA

Acetyl-CoA

→ CO$_2$

Ketoglutarate

→ CO$_2$

FIG. 6-8 Tricarboxylic acid cycle.

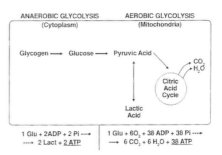

FIG. 6-9 Aerobic and anaerobic metabolism of glucose. Under anaerobic conditions, the pyruvate generated by glycolysis, instead of entering the tricarboxylic acid cycle, is converted to lactate. Fewer moles of ATP are produced by the anaerobic pathway.
Source: Reproduced with permission from Mizock BA, Falk JL. Lactic acidosis in critical illness. *Crit Care Med* 1992;20(1):80–93.

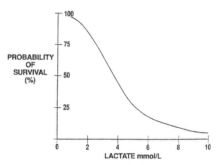

FIG. 6-10 The probability of survival decreases as the initial arterial lactate of ICU patients increases.
Source: Reproduced with permission from Mizock BA, Falk JL. Lactic acidosis in critical illness. *Crit Care Med* 1992;20(1):80–93.

example, Weil and Afifi (1970) revealed that an increase in lactate level from 2.0 to 8.0 mmol/L was associated with a decrease in survival from 90 to 10% (Fig. 6-10). Kruse et al. demonstrated a similar increase in the mortality of critically ill patients with a lactate level greater than 2.5 mmol/L. Conversely, the success of resuscitation is signaled by a decline in the lactate level.

Bibliography

Bongard FS. Shock & resuscitation. In: Bongard FS, Sue DY (eds.), *Current Critical Care Diagnosis & Treatment*, Stamford, CT: Appleton & Lange, 1994, 14–36.

Champe PC, Harvey RA. *Lippincott's Illustrated Reviews: Biochemistry*, 2nd ed. Philadelphia, PA: JB Lippincott, 1994, 61–98, 105–110.

Kruse JA, Mehta KC, Carlson RW. Definition of clinically significant lactic acidosis. *Chest.* 1987;92:100.

Maier RV. Shock. In Braunwald E, Fauci AS, Kasper DL, et al. (eds.), *Principles of Internal Medicine*, 15th ed., vol. 1. New York, NY: McGraw Hill, 2001, 222–228.

Mizock BA, Falk JL. Lactic acidosis in critical illness. *Crit Care Med* 1992;20(1):80–93.

Mullins RJ. Fluid, electrolytes, and shock. In: Townsend CM (ed.), *Textbook of Surgery: The Biological Basis of Modern Surgical Practice*, 16th ed. Philadelphia, PA: W.B. Saunders, 2001, 45–67.

Schwesinger WH, Moyer MP. Cell biology. In: O'Leary JP (ed.), *The Physiologic Basis of Surgery*, 2nd ed. Philadelphia, PA: Lippincott, Williams & Wilkins, 1996, 1–42.

Weil MH, Afifi AA. Experimental and clinical studies on lactate and pyruvate as indicators of the severity of acute circulatory failure (shock). *Circulation* 1970;41:989–1001.

16. (D)

17. (A)

18. (B)

Explanations 16 through 18

Hypovolemic shock arises from the depletion of the circulating blood volume. Trauma patients most commonly present with this category of shock. Among the many causes of hypovolemic shock are hemorrhage, emesis, diarrhea, excessive diuresis, dehydration, gastrointestinal fistula, burn injury, and anaphylaxis. The volume losses involved in hypovolemic shock emanate from any of the three fluid compartments in the body: intracellular, extracellular, and intravascular. Hemorrhage exemplifies a loss from the intravascular space while dehydration features depletion from both the intracellular and extracellular spaces. A pure extracellular fluid hypovolemia is typified by burns, diarrhea, and a gastrointestinal fistula. Despite these differences, in general, hypovolemic shock is characterized by a decrease in preload and in cardiac filling pressures, which ultimately results in a diminished cardiac output and a compromised peripheral perfusion. The severity of hypovolemic shock depends on the rate and the extent of the volume loss. The premorbid condition of the patient determines the ability of compensatory mechanisms to counteract the shock state. Hypovolemic shock is categorized into mild, moderate, and severe based on the symptoms and signs, volume of fluid losses, and the organ systems affected (Table 6-1).

With mild hypovolemia, a loss of less than 20% of the circulating blood volume, perfusion to organs such as the skin, skeletal muscle, and bone is decreased. These organs are able to sustain a relative ischemia for short periods of time, allowing blood to be shunted to organs intolerant of ischemia. The decrease in intravascular volume lessens the stimulation of baroreceptors located in the aortic arch, atria, and carotid bodies, resulting in a decreased parasympathetic but an elevated sympathetic outflow; norepinephrine is released from the postsynaptic sympathetic nerves and adrenal medulla, while epinephrine is discharged from the adrenal medulla. This adrenergic discharge achieves an increase in myocardial contractility and heart rate as well as the constriction of the vascular smooth muscle, augmenting blood pressure. Vasoconstriction of the vessels produces the pale, cold, and clammy skin characteristic of shock. Constriction of the large veins and venules—which normally contain 60% of the total blood volume—permits an increase in preload to the heart, as the blood from these capacitance vessels is redistributed to the circulation. Accordingly, the collapse of the cutaneous veins comprises another sign of hypovolemic shock. The skin manifestations of hypovolemic shock are most pronounced in the

TABLE 6-1   The Pathophysiology and Clinical Features of the Categories of Hypovolemia

	Pathophysiology	Clinical features
Mild (<20% of blood volume)	Decreased perfusion of organs that are able to tolerate ischemia (skin, fat, skeletal muscle, bone). Redistribution of blood flow to critical organs.	Subjective complaints of feeling cold. Postural changes in blood pressure and pulse. Pale, cool, clammy skin. Flat neck veins. Concentrated urine.
Moderate (deficit = 20–40% of blood volume)	Decreased perfusion of organs that withstand ischemia poorly (pancreas, spleen, kidneys).	Subjective complaint of thirst. Blood pressure is lower than normal in the supine position. Oliguria.
Severe (deficit >40% of blood volume)	Decreased perfusion of brain and heart.	Patient is restless, agitated, confused, and often obtunded. Low blood pressure with a weak and often thready pulse. Tachypnea may be present. If allowed to progress, cardiac arrest results.

Source: Reproduced with permission from Bongard FS. Shock & Resuscitation. In: Bongard FS, Sue DY (eds.), *Current Critical Care Diagnosis & Treatment. Stamford,* CT: Appleton & Lange, 1994, 15.

lower extremities, especially the plantar surfaces of the feet. More subtle signs of mild hypovolemia include minimal oliguria (urine output <0.5 cc/kg/h in adults), postural hypotension (a sustained decrease in systolic blood pressure of >10 mmHg with an alteration in position), and a subjective feeling of cold. Overall, heart rate, blood pressure, and respiratory rate are unchanged. In the absence of continued intravascular losses, the compensatory mechanisms to mild hypovolemic shock assure survival without further treatment.

Moderate hypovolemia is classified as the depletion of 20–40% of the blood volume. Perfusion of organs such as the kidney, spleen, pancreas, and gastrointestinal tract—less tolerant of ischemia—is sacrificed in order to supply the heart and brain with blood. In particular, the kidney reacts to the vasoconstriction of its afferent vessels to the cortex, induced by norepinephrine and epinephrine, by decreasing the glomerular filtration pressure below that required to maintain filtration into Bowman's capsule; as a result, oliguria ensues. The fall in renal perfusion also provokes the release of renin from the juxtaglomerular apparatus (Fig. 6-11). Renin promotes the conversion of angiotensinogen to angiotensin I in the liver, ultimately resulting in the production of angiotensin II,

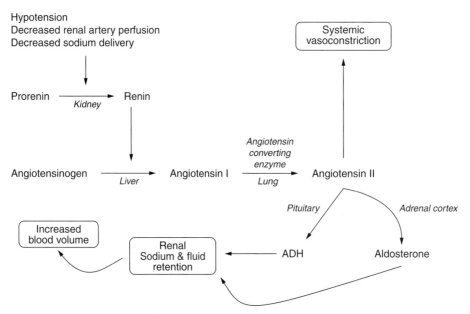

FIG. 6-11   Renin-angiotensin-aldosterone system.

a potent vasoconstrictor and catalyst for the issuance of aldosterone from the adrenal zona glomerulosa. Aldosterone participates in the compensatory mechanisms to hypovolemic shock by promoting the reabsorption of sodium in the distal convoluted tubules of the kidney and, therefore, by conserving the free water which contributes to intravascular volume. Also, in response to a decrease in intravascular volume of greater than 5% or a plasma osmolality higher than 285 mOsm, vasopressin is released from the posterior pituitary (neurohypophysis). Vasopressin, like angiotensin II, acts as a peripheral vasoconstrictor. Moreover, vasopressin promotes the reabsorption of free water in the collecting ducts of the kidney. The intravascular volume is further enhanced by fluid shifts between the extracellular and intravascular compartments, potentiated by a decrease in the hydrostatic pressure within the capillary bed. The adrenergic discharge promotes a greater degree of constriction in the precapillary than the postcapillary sphincter, resulting in a pressure differential between the extracellular and intravascular spaces: fluid and electrolytes are consequently transferred into the intravascular compartment until the oncotic pressure of the interstitum surpasses that of the intravascular space, at which point the fluid shift reverses. In sum, moderate hypovolemic shock is characterized by a normal blood pressure in conjunction with tachycardia, pronounced oliguria, incipient mental status changes, and thirst.

In severe hypovolemic shock, greater than 40% of the blood volume is depleted. Without intervention, perfusion of the heart and brain is compromised, resulting in ischemic injury and, ultimately, death, often by cardiac arrest. In particular, the blood supply to the brain remains intact until a pressure below 70 mmHg is reached. The poor perfusion exacerbates the manifestations of the shock state. The characteristic appearance of a patient in severe hypovolemic shock includes agitation, confusion, hypotension, tachycardia, tachypnea, oliguria, and a narrowed pulse pressure. Continuation of the volume depletion heightens and then eventually overwhelms the compensatory mechanisms.

Bibliography

Bongard FS. Shock & resuscitation. In: Bongard FS, Sue DY (eds.), *Current Critical Care Diagnosis & Treatment*, Stamford, CT: Appleton & Lange, 1994, 14–36.

Holcroft JW. Shock. In: Cameron JL (ed.), *Current Surgical Therapy*, 7th ed. St. Louis, MO: Mosby, 2001, 1043–1050.

Holcroft JW, Wisner DH. Shock & acute pulmonary failure in surgical patients. In: Way LW (ed.), *Current Surgical Diagnosis & Treatment*, 10th ed. Norwalk, CT: Appleton & Lange, 1994, 186–212.

Jurusz DJ, Gilmore JY. Shock and hypoperfusion states. In: O'Leary JP (ed.), *The Physiologic Basis of Surgery*, 2nd ed. Philadelphia, PA: Lippincott, Williams & Wilkins, 1996, 84–99.

Maier RV. Shock. In Braunwald E, Fauci AS, Kasper DL, et al. (eds.), *Principles of Internal Medicine*, 15th ed., vol. 1. New York, NY: McGraw Hill, 2001, 222–228.

Mullins RJ. Fluid, electrolytes, and shock. In: Townsend CM (ed.), *Textbook of Surgery: The Biological Basis of Modern Surgical Practice*, 16th ed. Philadelphia, PA: W.B. Saunders, 2001, 45–67.

Nwariaku F, Thal E. Shock. *Parkland Trauma Handbook.* London: Mosby, 1999, 37–49.

19. **(E)** The diagnosis of hypovolemic shock is often confounded by alcohol intoxication. Approximately 40–60% of trauma patients are intoxicated on admission. In addition, the presence of an elevated alcohol level is correlated with a greater severity of injury. The inebriated, hypovolemic patient displays warm, flushed skin as a result of cutaneous vasodilatation; in contrast, hypovolemic shock alone is associated with pale, cold skin. Furthermore, ethanol promotes diuresis by interfering with the action of vasopressin, whereas a hypovolemic patient is typically oliguric. Hypotension is consequently exaggerated in these intoxicated, hypovolemic patients. In a study of the impact of alcohol intoxication on hypovolemic shock, Phelan et al. (2002) used a rat model of fixed-pressure hemorrhage, treating the subjects with intragastric infusions of either ethyl alcohol or isocaloric dextrose. Among their findings, Phelan et al. (2002) revealed a significantly lower basal mean arterial blood pressure in the study group. Also, the metabolic acidosis associated with hypovolemia was greater in the alcohol group. Alcohol intoxication prevented the normal increases in the glucose and lactate levels found in hypovolemic shock. Furthermore, inebriation obviated the hemorrhage-induced elevation of TNF-α while promoting the increase of IL-10 levels. In an earlier study of alcohol administration in dogs with blunt cardiac injury, myocardial contractility was reduced while cardiac irritability was enhanced. Despite the prevalence of alcohol intoxication among trauma patients with hypovolemic shock, this phenomenon has been little studied.

Bibliography

Bongard FS. Shock & resuscitation. In: Bongard FS, Sue DY (eds.), *Current Critical Care Diagnosis & Treatment*, Stamford, CT: Appleton & Lange, 1994, 14–36.

Ivatury RR, Simon RJ, Rohman M. Cardiac complications. In: Mattox KL (ed.), *Complications of Trauma*. New York, NY: Churchill Livingstone, 1994, 409–428.

Phelan H, Stahls P, Hunt J, et al. Impact of alcohol intoxication on hemodynamic, metabolic, and cytokine responses to hemorrhagic shock. *J Trauma* 2002;52(4):675–682.

20. (A) Fluid resuscitation plays an integral role in the treatment of patients in hypovolemic shock. Crystalloid solutions are currently advocated as the best initial fluid selection. Still, this subject remains an area of great controversy, with vocal proponents of colloid fluid resuscitation. In a metaanalysis from Velanovich (1989), crystalloid therapy was associated with a 5.7% improvement in mortality as compared to colloids; with regard to the subset of trauma patients alone, this difference in mortality grew to 12.3%. Similarly, Choi et al. (1999) revealed a decrease in mortality among trauma patients treated with crystalloid solutions. A recent review of randomized and quasi-randomized trials from Alderson et al. (2002), however, did not reproduce these results, instead demonstrating no difference in mortality when comparing crystalloids and colloids. Yet, the authors promoted the use of crystalloids because of their lower cost and equal efficacy. In sum, there exists no large randomized, controlled trial to evaluate crystalloids and colloids.

Crystalloid and colloid fluids differ in the molecular weight of their component species. Crystalloid solutions contain species with a molecular weight less than 6000 while colloids are comprised of high molecular weight substances. The typical crystalloid is 0.9% sodium chloride, attractive for a sodium concentration (154 mM) similar to that of plasma. This isotonic fluid is also expected to distribute in the extravascular and intravascular compartments in proportions equivalent to that of plasma: 75 and 25%, respectively; however, only 20% of the administered fluid will remain in the intravascular space after 2 h, leading to "third spacing." In addition, the equivalent chloride concentration of 154 mM in normal saline, significantly greater than that of plasma, induces a hyperchloremic metabolic acidemia; such a mild acidemia may serve to enhance myocardial contractility. However, in the presence of a preexisting hyperchloremic metabolic acidosis, lactated or acetated Ringer's solution acts to buffer the acidemia, transforming the lactate or acetate to an organic acid which is then converted to carbon dioxide and water in the liver via the Kreb's cycle. Fluids containing dextrose, such as 5% dextrose in 0.45% sodium chloride, should be avoided because of the osmotic diuretic effect of glucose.

Colloids expand the intravascular space to an equivalent degree but in smaller volumes than crystalloids through an increase in the oncotic pressure within vessels: 1 g of albumin will draw 18 mL of fluid into the intravascular space. It is thought, however, that colloids ultimately travel to the interstitum via blood vessels made permeable by inflammation, leading to an intractable edema. Albumin, the most commonly administered colloid, has been associated with pulmonary dysfunction when given in large volumes as well as coagulopathy, hypocalcemia, and myocardial dysfunction. The colloid dextran has not been adequately studied in the setting of acute fluid resuscitation. Additionally, administration of this solution has been complicated by renal failure, anaphylaxis, and bleeding.

Bibliography

Alderson P, Schierhout G, Roberts I, Bunn F. Colloids versus crystalloids for fluid resuscitation in critically ill patients. *Cochrane Database Syst Rev* 2002;4:1–36.

Bongard FS. Shock & resuscitation. In: Bongard FS, Sue DY (eds.), *Current Critical Care Diagnosis & Treatment*, Stamford, CT: Appleton & Lange, 1994, 14–36.

Choi PT-L, Yip G, Quinonez LG, et al. Crystalloids vs. colloids in fluid resuscitation: a systematic review. *Crit Care Med* 1999;27(1):200–210.

Holcroft JW. Shock. In: Cameron JL (ed.), *Current Surgical Therapy*, 7th ed. St. Louis, MO: Mosby, 2001, 1043–1050.

Nwariaku F, Thal E. Shock. *Parkland Trauma Handbook*. London: Mosby, 1999, 37–49.

Velanovich V. Crystalloid versus colloid fluid resuscitation: a meta-analysis of mortality. *Surgery* 1989;105(1): 65–71.

21. (C) Hypertonic saline (7.5% sodium chloride) has been advocated as an alternative to isotonic solutions for acute fluid resuscitation. The practice of administering hypertonic saline to hypovolemic shock patients originated in Brazil and is widely used in South America, but is not currently approved in the United States. In a metaanalysis of 17 trials, Brown (2002) revealed no survival difference between the administration of 7.5% and 0.9% sodium chloride in acute fluid resuscitation. Yet, a multicenter trial of 7.5% sodium chloride from Vassar et al. (1993) demonstrated a notably higher mean arterial pressure (MAP) in trauma patients when using this hypertonic solution as opposed to lactated Ringer's or 7.5% sodium chloride with additives (6 or 12% dextran 70); overall survival did not vary significantly among the four trial groups but was higher than predicted by the Major Trauma Outcome Study for patients treated with hypertonic saline alone. Intense study of 7.5% normal saline continues because of its perceived benefits. This solution expands the intravascular space via an osmotic fluid shift from the extravascular compartment, to a degree greater than a similar volume of an isotonic solution, rapidly increasing blood pressure and cardiac output. A bolus of 7.5% sodium chloride produces an increase in intravascular volume equivalent to 2–3 L of an isotonic solution. This autotransfusion phenomenon is especially beneficial in patients who require acute resuscitation but

are unable to receive a large volume of fluid. For instance, with a head injury, cerebral perfusion must be maintained by means of an adequate MAP and a low ICP (CPP-MAP-ICP). Yet, the administration of a large volume of isotonic fluid serves to elevate not only the MAP but also the intracranial pressure (ICP). Hypertonic saline allows for a satisfactory cerebral perfusion pressure (CPP) in the presence of a low ICP. In one study, a single 4 mL/kg bolus of 7.5% sodium chloride was associated with an improved survival in patients with a head injury. Yet, a compromised blood-brain barrier disrupts the osmotic gradient between the intra- and extravascular compartments: the hypertonic saline instead draws fluid into the extravascular space, causing interstitial edema and thus increasing ICP. Studies suggest that hypertonic saline administration is associated with worsened bleeding, potentially because of interference with ADP-mediated platelet aggregation.

The potential role of hypertonic saline as an immunomodulatory agent has recently been subject to exploration. In 1997, Junger et al. published a study demonstrating an improvement in mortality in a mouse model following administration of 7.5% sodium chloride, attributed to the modulation of trauma-induced immunosuppression. *In vitro*, neutrophils bathed in hypertonic saline exhibit a decrease in superoxide activity, elastase production, and cytotoxicity. Rotstein et al. (2000) built on these studies, producing a mouse model of lung injury in which hemorrhagic shock in combination with LPS administration resulted in a threefold increase in lung permeability; this scenario was obviated by use of hypertonic saline, which was associated with a reduction in neutrophil infiltration of the lung via alterations in the selectin and integrin molecules on the neutrophil membrane. The specific mechanism of this change in the cellular adhesion molecules was cited to be the prevention of the up-regulation of the CD11b adhesion molecule on the neutrophil surface. In the absence of these normal adhesion molecules, neutrophils are unable to adhere to the endothelial surface and pass into the interstitial space to mediate injury. A similar study from Pascual et al. (2002, 2003) demonstrated a reduction in the adherence of neutrophils to the endothelial surface as well as in vascular permeability in a murine model of shock. Hypertonic saline thus holds promise as an agent for efficient fluid resuscitation and immunomodulation.

Bibliography

Bongard FS. Shock & resuscitation. In: Bongard FS, Sue DY (eds.), *Current Critical Care Diagnosis & Treatment*, Stamford, CT: Appleton & Lange, 1994, 14–36.

Brown MD. Hypertonic versus isotonic crystalloid for fluid resuscitation in critically ill patients. *Ann Emerg Med* 2002;40:113–114.

Bunn F, Roberts I, Tasker R, Akpa E. Hypertonic versus isotonic crystalloid for fluid resuscitation in critically ill patients. *Cochrane Database Syst Rev* 2002;4:1–20.

Holcroft JW. Shock. In: Cameron JL (ed.), *Current Surgical Therapy*, 7th ed. St. Louis, MO: Mosby, 2001, 1043–1050.

Nwariaku F, Thal E. Shock. *Parkland Trauma Handbook*. London: Mosby, 1999, 37–49.

Pascual JL, Ferri LE, Seely AJ, et al. Hypertonic saline resuscitation of hemorrhagic shock diminishes neutrophil rolling and adherence to endothelium and reduces in vivo vascular leakage. *Ann Surg* 2002;236(5):634–642.

Pascual JL, Khwaja KA, Ferri LE, et al. Hypertonic saline resuscitation attenuates neutrophil lung sequestration and transmigration by diminishing leukocyte-endothelial interactions in a two-hit model of hemorrhagic shock and infection. *J Trauma* 2003;54(1):121–132.

Rotstein OD. Novel strategies for immunomodulation after trauma: revisiting hypertonic saline as a resuscitation strategy for hemorrhagic shock. *J Trauma* 2000;49(4):580–583.

Vassar MJ, Fischer RP, O'Brien PE, et al. A multicenter trial for resuscitation of injured patients with 7.5% sodium chloride. The effect of added dextran 70. The Multicenter Group for the Study of Hypertonic Saline in Trauma Patients. *Arch Surg* 1993;128(9):1003–1011.

22. **(D)** According to the Advanced Trauma Life Support guidelines, acute hemorrhagic shock is initially treated with the rapid infusion of 1–2 L of an isotonic fluid. This approach allows for the repletion of intravascular fluid lost during hemorrhage, elevating the blood pressure and cardiac output. Tissue perfusion is regained as is vital organ function. The goal of this therapy is maintenance of a normal systolic blood pressure. Animal studies have suggested, however, that a delay in full fluid resuscitation until the hemorrhage is controlled may be associated with survival benefits; instead of the rapid bolus of 1–2 L of normal saline, fluid is administered to achieve a lower than normal systolic blood pressure. In uncontrolled hemorrhage, the rapid administration of intravenous fluids has been seen to interfere mechanically with thrombus formation, thus inducing further bleeding. Also, the dilution of the various coagulation factors and the decreased viscosity of blood following the rapid infusion of a large volume of fluid promote persistent hemorrhage. In a study of 598 trauma patients with penetrating injuries to the torso, Bickell et al. (1994) demonstrated that a delay in fluid resuscitation until the definitive management of the hemorrhage resulted in a clear survival benefit: 70% survival in the study group versus 62% in the immediate resuscitation group. Moreover, the immediate resuscitation group exhibited an increased volume of blood loss during

surgery as well as elevated coagulation factors. Furthermore, in a randomized study of 110 trauma patients, Dutton et al. (2002) performed fluid resuscitation with the goal of a systolic blood pressure greater than 100 mmHg or of 70–80 mmHg (study group), continued until hemorrhage was definitively controlled. Mortality among the two groups did not differ significantly, with survival measured at 92.7% in both; however, the authors criticized their own methodology, which featued a widely heterogeneous array of trauma patients and which produced an average systolic blood pressure of 100 mmHg in the study group. These studies do not challenge the benefit of fluid resuscitation but do debate the appropriate timing and volume of such treatment.

Vasopressor agents have no role in the initial resuscitation of patients in hemorrhagic shock. The vasoconstriction that these medications promote exacerbates the poor tissue perfusion, resulting in an increase in tissue damage. MAST, when inflated, elevate systemic vascular resistance in the periphery, thus improving the systolic blood pressure; however, this same increase in the resistance may diminish cardiac output and tissue perfusion. The trousers do not improve survival and may, in fact, delay ambulance transport because of the time involved in applying the garment. Complications of the trousers include the development of a compartment syndrome, respiratory distress, and hypotension during deflation.

Bibliography

Bickell WH, Wall MJ, Pepe PE, et al. Immediate versus delayed fluid resuscitation for hypotensive patients with penetrating torso injuries. *N Engl J Med* 1994;331(17): 1105–1109.

Bongard FS. Shock & resuscitation. In: Bongard FS, Sue DY (eds.), *Current Critical Care Diagnosis & Treatment*, Stamford, CT: Appleton & Lange, 1994, 14–36.

Dutton RP, Mackenzie CF, Scalea TM. Hypotensive resuscitation during active hemorrhage: impact on in-hospital mortality. *J Trauma* 2002;52(6):1141–1146.

Nwariaku F, Thal E. Shock. *Parkland Trauma Handbook*. London: Mosby, 1999, 37–49.

23. **(C)** Death due to trauma with hemorrhagic shock is arranged in a trimodal distribution: immediate (at the scene), within the first 24 hours, and 1 week or more following the injury. In the acute period after trauma, mortality is attributable to massive hemorrhage or neurologic injury. Direct injury to an organ contributes to a primary multiple organ dysfunction in this early period. In contrast, late deaths, occurring at least 1 week subsequent to the trauma, generally arise from secondary multiple organ dysfunction syndrome (MODS).

This condition develops in 30–60% of these trauma patients and is associated with an 80% mortality rate.

MODS is defined as the failure of multiple organs in a critically ill patient in whom the maintenance of homeostasis requires intervention. This syndrome appears as the end point in a variety of conditions, not isolated to trauma and hemorrhagic shock. In the case of trauma, the prevalence of MODS is ascribed to a two-hit phenomenon, first proposed by Partrick et al. This hypothesis suggests that trauma represents an initial insult which predisposes the immune system to react later to a lesser injury with a massive response, mediated primarily by neutrophils, resulting in great collateral damage (Fig. 6-12). The primed neutrophils mediate further tissue injury by means of proteolytic enzymes, reactive oxygen species, and vasoactive substances. A study from Fan et al. (1998) demonstrated that, in a model of murine hemorrhagic shock, intratrachial administration of LPS 1 hour after successful resuscitation provoked enhanced neutrophil sequestration and edema in the lung; this response was not generated in the absence of resuscitated hemorrhagic shock or LPS. Following traumatic hemorrhagic shock, the patient is resuscitated into not only a local but also a systemic inflammatory response syndrome (SIRS), with generalized inflammation generated within 1 hour of injury. Neutrophils and monocytes are first activated, releasing inflammatory mediators. TNF-α, IL-1, and IL-6 are particularly implicated in the evolution of MODS, found in studies to induce this syndrome and to be present in elevated levels. Additionally, the coagulation and alternative complement cascades are initiated. In the absence of further injury, SIRS is beneficial to recovery from the trauma. The second,

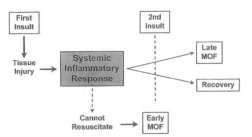

FIG. 6-12 Illustration of the two-hit model of multiple organ dysfunction in trauma. Resuscitation following the initial insult, trauma, induces a systemic inflammatory response syndrome. A second, often trivial, injury precipitates organ dysfunction due to the exuberant response of the previously primed immune system. Early, or primary, multiple organ dysfunction results from direct trauma to organs. MOF—multiple organ failure.

Source: Reproduced with permission rom Offiner PJ, Moore EE. Risk factors for MOF and pattern of organ failure following severe trauma. In: Baue AE, Faist E, Fry DE (eds.), *Multiple Organ Failure: Pathophysiology, Prevention, and Therapy*, New York, NY: Springer, 2000, 33.

often trivial, insult, however, results in an enhanced immune response from the already primed immune cells, notably neutrophils. This second hit may arise from a mild infection, pulmonary aspiration, or blood transfusion (Table 6-2). Bacterial translocation from the ischemic mucosa of the gastrointestinal tract is a focus of investigation as a potential source of contamination. Ultimately, organs not involved in the original trauma experience an alteration in function. Usually, the lung is affected prior to the kidneys, liver, and gastrointestinal tract. Offiner and Moore (2000) attribute this predilection to direct lung injury, to the lung's filtration of toxins and cytokines as well as to its sensitivity for developing vascular permeability.

Bibliography

Fan J, Marshall JC, Jimenez M, et al. Hemorrhagic shock primes for increased expression of cytokine-induced neutrophil chemoattractant in the lung: role in pulmonary inflammation following lipopolysaccharide. *J Immunol* 1998;161(1):440–447.

Lee CC, Marrill KA, Carter WA, Crupi RS. A current concept of trauma-induced multiorgan failure. *Ann Emerg Med* 2001;38(2):170–176.

Offiner PJ, Moore EE. Risk factors for MOF and pattern of organ failure following severe trauma. In: Baue AE, Faist E, Fry DE (eds.), *Multiple Organ Failure: Pathophysiology, Prevention, and Therapy*. New York, NY: Springer, 2000, 30–43.

Pascual JL, Khwaja KA, Ferri LE, et al. Hypertonic saline resuscitation attenuates neutrophil lung sequestration and transmigration by diminishing leukocyte-endothelial interactions in a two-hit model of hemorrhagic shock and infection. *J Trauma* 2003;54(1):121–132.

Partrick DA, Moore FA, Moore EE, Barnett CC, Silliman CC. Neutrophil priming and activation in the pathogenesis of postinjury multiple organ failure. *New Horiz* 1996;4:194–210.

TABLE 6-2   Risk Factors Associated with the Development of Multiple Organ Dysfunction Following Trauma

Associated with the first insult
Severity of tissue injury
Shock-ischemia/reperfusion
Severity of the systemic inflammatory response
Associated with the second insult
Infection
Transfusion
Secondary operative procedures
Host factors
Age
Preexisting conditions

Source: Reproduced with permission from Offiner PJ, Moore EE. Risk factors for MOF and pattern of organ failure following severe trauma. In: Baue AE, Faist E, Fry DE (eds.), *Multiple Organ Failure: Pathophysiology, Prevention, and Therapy*. New York, NY: Springer, 2000, 40.

24. (C)

25. (C)

Explanations 24 and 25

Neurogenic shock arises from the loss of autonomic innervation to the vasculature below the affected level. Among the causes of neurogenic shock are certain neurologic disorders, high spinal anesthesia, fainting, and medications that antagonize the adrenergic system; however, the most common cause of this phenomenon is traumatic spinal cord injury. A spinal cord injury usually results from damage to the cervical, lower thoracic, or upper lumbar regions. The most common mechanism of the injury is an impact with persistent compression, often associated with burst fractures, fracture-dislocation, missile injury, and ruptured discs (Table 6-3). The magnitude of neurogenic shock depends on the severity and level of the injury, with actual shock developing only following damage above the midthoracic level. Its manifestations emanate from the pronounced sympathetic discharge produced above the level of the denervation. Sympathetic activation results in the loss of arteriolar tone and, thus, massive vasodilatation. The venules are similarly affected: blood pools in these capacitance vessels within the denervated areas of the body. The accumulation of blood in the venous system is aggravated by the inability of the muscles of the extremities to assist in returning the blood to the heart. While the total blood volume is unchanged, the circulating blood volume— the preload—is lessened. In sum, neurogenic shock presents as central hypotension (a low systemic vascular resistance) with a decreased cardiac output, PCWP, and central venous pressure. The effect of spinal cord injury on heart rate is variable, depending on the level of denervation: bradycardia ensues from a lesion above the midthoracic sympathetic outflow tract, while

TABLE 6-3   Mechanisms of Spinal Cord Injury

Mechanical force	Mechanism of injury
Impact plus persisting compression	Burst fracture
	Fracture-dislocation
	Disc rupture
Impact alone (temporary compression)	Hyperextension
Distraction	Hyperflexion
Laceration, transection	Burst fracture
	Laminar fracture
	Fracture-dislocation
	Missile

Source: Reproduced with permission from Tator CH. Pathophysiology and pathology of spinal cord injury. In: Wilkins RH, Rengachary SS (eds.), *Neurosurgery*, 2nd ed., vol. II. New York, NY: McGraw-Hill, 1996, 2847.

lower lesions present with tachycardia. Above the midthoracic level, myocardial contractility is also depressed. The loss of autonomic reflexes to the spinal cord below the lesion is accompanied by immediate flaccid paralysis, an absence of sensation, and tendon areflexia. The condition of spinal shock has a duration of 1–6 weeks, but, in a minority of patients, is permanent. In contradistinction to hypovolemic shock, neurogenic shock features warm, pink skin in the denervated areas secondary to the cutaneous vasodilatation. Mentation is often intact. Urine output remains normal or elevated.

Treatment of neurogenic shock centers on the usual trauma protocols, with the establishment of an airway and intravenous access being of highest priority. Stabilization of the cervical spine must be ensured with a cervical collar. The diagnosis of hypovolemic shock should be entertained despite a lesion that solely suggests neurogenic shock. Resuscitation is started with intravenous fluids, which function to increase the circulating blood volume and, thus, the preload. Often, this intervention is sufficient to elevate the blood pressure. A failure of intravenous fluids to improve hypotension may point to occult bleeding. In the absence of such bleeding, vasoactive agents may be used if fluid resuscitation is insufficient to elevate the preload. Commonly, alpha-adrenergic agents such as phenylephrine or norepinephrine are relied on for this treatment, especially in the case of tachycardia; refractory hypotension with bradycardia usually requires dopamine and, often, atropine. These vasoactive medications are generally given in low doses and weaned off rapidly. An elevation in the blood pressure serves to obviate progressive spinal cord ischemia. Once the acute resuscitation phase is completed, a radiographic survey may be performed and definitive treatment of the injury pursued. For instance, an unstable spine requires surgical fixation. Past studies have suggested that corticosteroids are associated with improved motor and sensory function at 6 months if administered within 8 hours of the injury; the dosage is a 30 mg/kg bolus followed by a drip of 5.4 mg/kg/h for 24 hours. However, a more recent study of compressive spinal cord injury in dogs from Carlson et al. (2003) revealed that methylprednisolone, as compared to saline, provided no improvement in the recovery or preservation of neurologic function; following decompression of the spinal cord, three dogs in the steroid group and seven in the saline group regained somatosensory evoked potentials while four steroid-treated dogs lost their previously intact somatosensory evoked potentials. Furthermore, the authors found that the saline group evidenced a significantly higher reperfusion flow to the injured spinal cord, with a return to baseline flow 5 minutes following decompression; the methylprednisolone group, in contrast, showed no recovery of normal circulation to the spinal cord subsequent to decompression. This reduction in blood flow to the damaged spinal cord associated with steroids indicates that this treatment may worsen long-term neurologic function by enhancing ischemic injury. The spinal cord injury is dynamic, evolving over the first post-trauma days. Ultimately, these patients develop a state of heightened reflex activity weeks to months following the injury.

Head trauma itself is never a cause of hypotension. Via the Cushing reflex, the increased ICP seen with head trauma generally results in hypertension and bradycardia. Moreover, intracranial bleeding cannot alone be responsible for hypovolemic shock, as the rigid adult skull is unable to accommodate large volumes of blood; an acute increase in intracranial volume, as per the Monro-Kellie doctrine, affects a large increase in the ICP, with shifting of the brain or herniation the result.

Bibliography

Bongard FS. Shock & resuscitation. In: Bongard FS, Sue DY (eds.), *Current Critical Care Diagnosis & Treatment*, 1st ed. Stamford, CT: Appleton & Lange, 1994, 14–36.

Carlson GD, Gorden CD, Nakazawa S, et al. Sustained spinal cord compression. Part II. Effect of methylprednisolone on regional blood flow and recovery of somatosensory evoked potentials. *J Bone Joint Surg* 2003;85-A (1):95–101.

Holcroft JW. Shock. In: Cameron JL (ed.), *Current Surgical Therapy*, 7th ed. St. Louis, MO: Mosby, 2001, 1043–1050.

Holcroft JW, Wisner DH. Shock & acute pulmonary failure in surgical patients. In: Way LW (ed.), *Current Surgical Diagnosis & Treatment*, 10th ed. Norwalk, CT, 1994, 186–212.

Jurusz DJ, Gilmore JY. Shock and hypoperfusion states. In: O'Leary JP (ed.), *The Physiologic Basis of Surgery*, 2nd ed. Philadelphia, PA: Lippincott, Williams & Wilkins, 1996, 84–99.

Maier RV. Shock. In Braunwald E, Fauci AS, Kasper DL, et al. (eds.), *Principles of Internal Medicine*, 15th ed., vol. 1. New York, NY: McGraw Hill, 2001, 222–228.

Simon RP, Aminoff MJ, Greenberg DA. *Clinical Neurology*, 4th ed. Stamford, CT: Appleton & Lange, 1999.

Tator CH. Pathophysiology and pathology of spinal cord injury. In: Wilkins RH, Rengachary SS (eds.), *Neurosurgery*, 2nd ed., vol. II. New York, NY: McGraw-Hill, 1996, 2847–2859.

Victor M, Ropper AH. *Adam's and Victor's Principles of Neurology*, 7th ed. New York, NY: McGraw-Hill, 2001.

26. **(B)** The Trendelenburg position allows for the translocation of venous blood from the extremities to the heart by gravity. This method, developed in the late nineteenth century by the surgeon Friedrich Trendelenburg, became popular during World War I as an antishock position; however, this technique is of value only in neurogenic shock, where the massive dilatation of the venous system results in pooling of blood in the capacitance vessels of the extremities. The increased return of blood to the heart from these expanded vessels improves the cardiac preload and reduces the degree of hypotension. This maneuver has no application in hypovolemic shock, where the blood volume is low and the vessels are severely constricted. In this hypovolemic situation, no additional blood is transferred to the heart from the already-depleted vessels. The heart, in fact, is required to expend more energy to deliver blood to the viscera and elevated lower extremities. In a study of hypovolemic postoperative patients with pulmonary artery catheters by Sing et al. (1994), the use of the Trendelenburg position resulted in increases in the MAP, wedge pressure, and systemic vascular resistance, while the cardiac output remained unchanged. The authors attributed the increase in the PCWP to the elevated diaphragm resulting from the tilted position. The blood pressure rise was ascribed to the systemic vasoconstriction associated with hypovolemia. The failure of the Trendelenburg maneuver in hypovolemic shock rests on the high capacity of the venous system, which prevents an increase in the pressure differential between the peripheral and central veins in a low volume state while in the Trendelenburg position. Such a differential, however, is possible in the case of venous capacitance vessels that are fully distended, as with neurogenic shock.

Bibliography

Holcroft JW. Shock. In: Cameron JL (ed.), *Current Surgical Therapy*, 7th ed. St. Louis, MO: Mosby, 2001, 1043– 1050.

Marino PL. *The ICU Book*, 2nd ed. Philadelphia, PA: Lippincott, Williams & Wilkins, 1998.

Sing R, O'Hara D, Sawyer MAJ, et al. Trendelenburg position and oxygen transport in hypovolemic adults. *Ann Emerg Med* 1994;23:564–568.

27. **(D)**

28. **(A)**

29. **(B)**

Explanations 27 through 29

Cardiogenic shock represents a failure of the mechanical pump function of the heart. This condition may arise from valvular heart disease (insufficiency or stenosis), arrhythmia, obstructive myocardial hypertrophy, papillary muscle rupture, or myocardial contusion; however, the most prevalent cause of cardiogenic shock is an acute MI, especially left ventricular pump dysfunction. According to the Multicenter Investigation of Limitation of Infarct Size (MILIS) trial, cardiogenic shock occurs in 7% of subjects admitted to the hospital for MI. The Worcester Heart Attack Study revealed a rise in the incidence of MI complicated by cardiogenic shock between the years 1975 and 1988. In addition, mortality from an acute MI is most often because of cardiogenic shock; after 30 days, the death rate for a non-ST elevation MI with cardiogenic shock was found to be 66% in the platelet glycoprotein IIb/IIIa in unstable angina: receptor suppression using integrilin therapy (PURSUIT) study. Characteristics that predict cardiogenic shock following a MI are old age, an anterior infarction, diabetes mellitus, a history of infarction, and a history of angina or congestive heart failure. Approximately 40% of the left ventricle must be involved in the infarction in order for cardiogenic shock to occur; the loss of viable myocardium may be cumulative. The PURSUIT study further pointed to ST depression on the initial ECG and rales on physical examination as correlating with the development of cardiogenic shock. The should we emergently revascularize Occluded Coronaries for cardiogenic shock (SHOCK) registry measured a median time of 6 hours from the onset of the MI to the advent of cardiogenic shock; generally, these patients presented to the hospital 2 hours following the commencement of their infarction. Manifestations of cardiogenic shock emanate from hypotension and poor tissue perfusion: oliguria, altered mentation, and cool extremites, for example. This entity occurs in a setting of euvolemia, with the hypotension unresponsive to fluid resuscitation alone. The hemodynamic parameters demonstrated in cardiogenic shock include a systolic blood pressure <90 mmHg for a duration greater than 30 min, an elevated arteriovenous oxygen difference (>5.5 mL/dL), a low cardiac index (<2.2 L/min/m²), and an increased pulmonary artery wedge pressure (>15 mmHg). Diastolic function of the left ventricle is compromised prior to its systolic activity. A majority of patients in the SHOCK study—64%—demonstrated signs of pulmonary congestion. A diagnosis of cardiogenic shock is aided by an ECG, which may reveal an acute MI or other heart disease. An echocardiogram may confirm the diagnosis of MI and identify such mechanical complications as cardiac tamponade, septal rupture, aortic dissection, and severe mitral regurgitation, requiring surgical intervention. Also, left and right ventricular function is gauged by echocardiography, as is infarct size and intravascular volume. The SHOCK trial identified a

reduced left ventricular ejection fraction (<28%) and severe mitral regurgitation as echocardiographic predictors of increased mortality.

Treatment of MI associated with cardiogenic shock depends on early revascularization. In the SHOCK study, a significant improvement in the survival rate was reported with the early revascularization strategy as opposed to the initial medical stabilization with delayed revascularization group at 6 months and 1 year; however, the 13.2% reduction in mortality was not observed in subjects over the age of 75 years old. The initial goal of therapy is the avoidance of sustained end-organ damage by maintaining an adequate blood pressure, usually with vasopressor agents. An IABP provides additional hemodynamic support. Close monitoring of respiratory and cardiovascular parameters is required in an intensive care setting. Both aspirin and heparin should be administered. While angiography with PCI is advocated as the definitive strategy for revascularization, the Fibrinolytic Therapy Trialists (FTT) Collaborative Group recommended thrombolytic therapy in patients with a ST elevation MI if a delay greater than 2 hours is anticipated for PCI; this study found a 35-day mortality of 28.9% in hypotensive patients receiving thrombolytics versus a 35.1% death rate in those administered a placebo; however, patients with a non-ST elevation MI should be offered a glycoprotein IIb/IIIa inhibitor in the case of a long interval before their revascularization procedure. Ideally, PCI should be performed 48 hours following the onset of the MI or 18 hours after the development of cardiogenic shock in order to benefit. Prior to an intervention, the coronary anatomy should be delineated. Wong et al. (2000) discovered that MI complicated by cardiogenic shock is most often associated with triple vessel disease, left main disease, and left ventricular dysfunction. Once the infarct-related artery is identified, PCI is undertaken, with stenting of the vessel often performed; however, stents should be avoided in vessels demonstrating poor flow despite successful angioplasty, because of the risk of distal embolus. Instead, stenting should be pursued after improved blood flow is exhibited following administration of glycoprotein IIb/IIIa antagonists or of intracoronary nitroprusside or adenosine. Only the infarct-related stenosed vessels should be addressed in an emergent PCI; the remaining diseased vessels may be treated nonemergently with CABG. Coronary artery bypass grafting is also a viable revascularization option for a MI with cardiogenic shock, especially in the setting of left main or severe three vessel disease. Differences in mortality following CABG and PCI are insignificant; however, no randomized trials have compared the two methods of revascularization for cardiogenic shock. Yet, surgery must be performed for complications such as ventricular septal rupture and mechanical mitral regurgitation. Ventricular septal rupture occurs in 0.2% of cases according to the global utilization of streptokinase and tissue plasminogen activator for occluded coronary arteries (GUSTO-I) trial, but has a mortality of 87% in the SHOCK trial, improved to 81% with surgery. Acute mitral regurgitation is particularly associated with inferior MIs, in which compromise of the single blood supply (present in 63% of subjects) to the posterior papillary muscle interferes with the maintenance of adequate leaflet tension and opposition of the mitral valve.

The successful treatment of MI complicated by cardiogenic shock rests on identifying the condition and then intervening with a revascularization procedure. Despite the advances in therapies offered for MI and cardiogenic shock, the mortality remains high. Studies investigating novel therapies such as nitric oxide inhibitors continue.

Bibliography

Antman EM, Braunwald E. Acute myocardial infarction. In: Braunwald E, Fauci AS, Kasper DL, et al. (eds.), *Principles of Internal Medicine*, 15th ed., vol. 1. New York, NY: McGraw Hill, 2001, 1386–1398.

Appleby P, Baigent C, Collins R, et al. Fibrinolytic Therapy Trialists (FTT) Collaborative Group. Indications for fibrinolytic therapy in suspected acute myocardial infarction: collaborative overview of early mortality and major morbidity results from all randomized trials of more than 1000 patients. *Lancet* 1994;343:311–322.

Bongard FS. Shock & resuscitation. In: Bongard FS, Sue DY (eds.), *Current Critical Care Diagnosis & Treatment*, 1st ed. Stamford, CT: Appleton & Lange, 1994, 14–36.

Califf RM, Bengtson JR. Current concepts: cardiogenic shock. *N Engl J Med* 1994;330(24):1724–1730.

Holcroft JW, Wisner DH. Shock & acute pulmonary failure in surgical patients. In: Way LW (ed.), *Current Surgical Diagnosis & Treatment*, 10th ed. Norwalk, CT, 1994, 186–212.

Jurusz DJ, Gilmore JY. Shock and hypoperfusion states. In: O'Leary JP (ed.), *The Physiologic Basis of Surgery*, 2nd ed. Philadelphia, PA: Lippincott, Williams & Wilkins, 1996, 84–99.

Maier RV. Shock. In Braunwald E, Fauci AS, Kasper DL et al. (eds.), *Principles of Internal Medicine*, 15th ed., vol. 1. New York, NY: McGraw Hill, 2001, 222–228.

Menon V, Hochman J. Management of cardiogenic shock complicating acute myocardial infarction. *Heart* 2002;88(5):531–537.

Murphy JG, Reeder GS, Bresnahan JF. Mechanical complications of myocardial infarction. In: Murphy JG (ed.), *Mayo Clinic Cardiology Review*, 2nd ed. Philadelphia, PA: Lippincott, Williams & Wilkins, 2000, 231–240.

Picard MH, Davidoff R, Sleeper LA, et al. Echocardiographic predictors of survival and response to early revascularization in cardiogenic shock. *Circulation* 2003;107(2):279–284.

Wong SC, Sanborn T, Sleeper LA, et al. Angiographic findings and clinical correlates in patients with cardiogenic shock complicating acute myocardial infarction: a report from the SHOCK trial registry. *J Am Coll Cardiol* 2000;36:1077–1083.

30. **(E)** Cardiogenic shock most often arises following an acute MI. In this condition, an acute occlusion of the coronary arteries occurs because of the rupture or fissure of an atherosclerotic plaque, resulting in the formation of an occlusive thrombus. The area of myocardium at risk for infarction depends on the size of the lesion, the rate of its development, and the presence of collateral vessels. The goal of treatment in an acute MI is the limitation of the infarction size: while the central area of damage is irreversibly necrotic, the surrounding ischemic tissue may be rescued from a similar demise. However, cardiogenic shock itself promotes tissue ischemia. Oxygen demand is determined by heart rate, contractility, and systolic blood pressure whereas supply is influenced by coronary artery diameter and blood flow. The double product (heart rate × systolic blood pressure) is directly proportional to the myocardial oxygen requirement. The left ventricular dysfunction characteristic of cardiogenic shock compromises cardiac output and, thus, coronary blood flow. Similarly, coronary blood flow is lessened by the decreased left ventricular diastolic pressure: 80% of the coronary artery circulation transpires during diastole. Accompanying the reduced delivery of oxygen to the myocardium is an increased demand for oxygen due to the elevation in wall stress associated with an MI. Also, the compensatory mechanisms to shock, including the increased heart rate and contractility of sympathetic output and the activation of the renin-angiotensin-aldosterone axis with a subsequent increase in fluid preload, produces an enhanced need for oxygen by the myocardium. In sum, as cardiogenic shock progresses, the demand for oxygen grows while the supply diminishes. As a result, the ischemic zone, theoretically reversible, becomes irretrievably necrotic in the face of continued cardiogenic shock. The definitive treatment for cardiogenic shock remains a revascuarization procedure.

Bibliography

Antman EM, Braunwald E. Acute myocardial infarction. In: Braunwald E, Fauci AS, Kasper DL, et al. (eds.), *Principles of Internal Medicine*, 15th ed., vol. 1. New York, NY: McGraw Hill, 2001, 1386–1398.

Narahara K. Coronary heart diseases. In: Bongard FS, Sue DY (eds.), *Current Critical Care Diagnosis & Treatment*, Stamford, CT: Appleton & Lange, 1994, 454–467.

31. **(A)**

32. **(B)**

Explanations 31 and 32

Infarction of the right ventricle appears in one-third of acute inferior wall MIs; however, most right-sided MIs are recognized only at autopsy. This condition is suggested by the combination of an inferior wall MI and hypotension. Cardiogenic shock complicates a right ventricular MI in approximately 32% of cases. Dysfunction of the right ventricle restricts the delivery of blood to the lungs and left ventricle, causing peripheral venous congestion. In addition, the sudden dilatation of the right ventricle that accompanies a right ventricular MI produces a leftward shift in the intraventricular septum, compromising left ventricular filling. The characteristic findings on physical examination include jugular venous distension, no rales, and a positive Kussmaul sign (increased distension of the jugular veins with inspiration). A chest radiograph reveals clear lung fields. On an ECG, ST elevation of the right chest leads, V3 and V4, is found; however, this classic sign disappears several hours following the onset of the MI. Echocardiography remains the most reliable diagnostic tool for a right ventricular MI. An echocardiogram demonstrates right ventricular dilatation and hypokinesis. Tricuspid regurgitation may be evident because of the acute increase in right ventricular dimensions and, consequently, in the diameter of the tricuspid annulus. Right heart catheterization displays a high central venous pressure (>12 mmHg), low to normal PCWP, and low to normal cardiac index. The initial intervention in treating a right ventricular MI is to administer fluids, with the goal of a PCWP greater than 18 mmHg, in order to improve the preload to the left ventricle. Systemic vasodilators and diuretics are avoided to prevent further hypotension. Inotropic support with dopamine or dobutamine is initiated for hypotension resistant to fluid resuscitation. Revascularization by thrombolysis or percutaneous transluminal coronary angioplasty is the definitive therapy for right ventricular MI. The mortality of an acute MI is worsened by the involvement of the right ventricle. The right ventricle often requires 3 days to recover its function; however, intact left ventricular function in the face of a right ventricular MI improves survival.

Bibliography

Antman EM and Braunwald E. Acute myocardial infarction. In: Braunwald E, Fauci AS, Kasper DL, et al. (eds.), *Principles of Internal Medicine*, 15th ed., vol. 1. New York, NY: McGraw Hill, 2001, 1386–1398.

Murphy JG, Reeder GS, Bresnahan JF. Mechanical complications of myocardial infarction. In: Murphy JG (ed.), *Mayo Clinic Cardiology Review*, 2nd ed. Philadelphia, PA: Lippincott, Williams & Wilkins, 2000, 231–240.

Saltzberg MT, Sable JS, Parrillo JE. Acute heart failure and shock. In: Crawford MH, Dimarco JP, Asplund K, et al. (eds.), *Cardiology*. London: Mosby, 2001, 5.3.1–5.3.12.

33. (C)

34. (B)

35. (A)

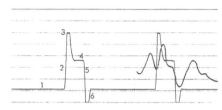

FIG. 6-13 A normal balloon pressure waveform. 1—fill pressure, 2—rapid inflation, 3—peak inflation artifact, 4—inflation plateau pressure, 5—rapid deflation, 6—peak deflation pressure.
Source: Reproduced with permission from Daily EK, Schroeder JS. *Techniques of Bedside Hemodynamic Monitoring*, 5th ed. St. Louis, MO: Mosby, 1994, 250.

Explanations 33 through 35

In the setting of cardiogenic shock, the IABP enhances hemodynamic parameters. Although surgical placement was once widely practiced, this mechanical device is now usually inserted percutaneously via the femoral artery using a modified Seldinger technique and directed into the thoracic aorta. Within the aorta, the balloon inflates in early diastole, augmenting coronary arterial perfusion, and rapidly deflates in early systole, reducing the afterload against which the left ventricle must contract (Fig. 6-13). The decrease in afterload allows the aortic valve to open at a lower systolic pressure, reducing myocardial oxygen consumption. In relation to the ECG, balloon inflation occurs on the T wave while deflation is coincident with the R wave (Fig. 6-14). The timing of counterpulsation may also be guided by the arterial waveform, with inflation commencing at the dicrotic notch and deflation at the upstroke of the waveform. Among the physiologic effects of intraaortic balloon pumping are a rise in diastolic pressure of 90% and an increase in cardiac output of 20–50%.

Counterpulsation is applied to candidates for aggressive revascularization who remain hypotensive despite maximal treatment with vasopressors. Also, IABP placement is recommended prior to transfer of a cardiogenic shock patient to a tertiary care center. This device is not a replacement for revascularization, serving only as a temporary measure to improve hemodynamic parameters. In one observational study, DeWood et al. found that counterpulsation was associated with longer survival only in patients who subsequently underwent mechanical or pharmacologic revascularization. Other studies demonstrate that, in the absence of a revascularization procedure, only 15–20% of patients treated with an IABP will be successfully weaned from the device, with 10–30% of this population

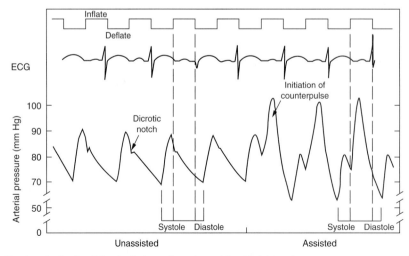

FIG. 6-14 Counterpulsation in relation to electrocardiography and the arterial waveform.
Source: Reproduced with permission from Daily EK, Schroeder JS. *Techniques of Bedside Hemodynamic Monitoring*, 5th ed. St. Louis, MO: Mosby, 1994, 253.

experiencing long-term survival; however, the second National Registry of Myocardial Infarction (NRMI-2) study revealed that the IABP does improve survival in patients treated with thrombolytic medications from 49 to 67%, a result not repeated in patients who eventually underwent PCI or coronary artery bypass grafting. Alone, thrombolytics such as streptokinase are ineffective in relieving coronary artery occlusion in acute MI complicated by cardiogenic shock. Barron et al. (2001) point to the impaired perfusion found in cardiogenic shock as preventing adequate penetration of the thrombolytic agents into the occluded coronary arteries: at systolic blood pressures below 70 mmHg, perfusion of the coronary arteries decreases, stopping completely at a mean pressure of 30 mmHg. Counterpulsation increases hemodynamic parameters such that the thrombolytic medications are able to infiltrate and dissipate the thrombus.

Despite its advantages, IABP is complicated by bleeding and vascular damage in 5–20% of cases, with injuries such as groin hematoma, aortic dissection or perforation, systemic emboli, and limb ischemia because of thromboembolism. Percutaneous insertion of the IABP is associated with a higher rate of complications than is surgical placement (20% vs. 5%). Vascular complications are more common in elderly women and diabetics. Contraindications for placement include aortic incompetence, severe peripheral vascular disease, and aortic aneurysm or dissection. In general, other indications for placement of an IABP include recurrent intractable ventricular arrhythmias complicated by hypotension; severe angina post-MI as a temporizing measure prior to revascularization; acute mitral regurgitation or ventricular septal defect coincident with a MI; and patients with large areas of myocardium at risk for ischemia secondary to pronounced coronary artery disease.

Bibliography

Antman EM, Braunwald E. Acute myocardial infarction. In: Braunwald E, Fauci AS, Kasper DL, et al. (eds.), *Principles of Internal Medicine*, 15th ed., vol. 1. New York, NY: McGraw Hill, 2001, 1386–1398.

Barron HV, Every NR, Parsons LS, et al. The use of intra-aortic balloon counterpulsation in patients with cardiogenic shock complicating acute myocardial infarction: data from the National Registry of Myocardial Infarction 2. *Am Heart J* 2001;141(6):933–939.

Califf RM, Bengtson JR. Current concepts: cardiogenic shock. *N Engl J Med* 1994;330(24):1724–1730.

Chitwood WR, Elbeery JR. Intra-aortic balloon counterpulsation: physiology, indications, and techniques. In: Sabiston DC (ed.), *Textbook of Surgery: The Modern Basis of Modern Surgical Practice*, 15th ed. Philadelphia, PA: W.B. Saunders, 1997, 2218–2228.

Daily EK, Schroeder JS. *Techniques of Bedside Hemodynamic Monitoring*, 5th ed. St. Louis, MO: Mosby, 1994.

DeWood MA, Notske KN, Hensley GR, et al. Intraaortic balloon counterpulsation with and without reperfusion of myocardial infarction shock. *Circulation* 1980;61: 1105–1112.

Kovack RJ, Rasak MA, Bates ER, et al. Thrombolysis plus aortic counterpulsation: improved survival in patients who present to community hospitals with cardiogenic shock. *J Am Coll Cardiol* 1997;29(7):1454–1458.

Murphy JG, Reeder GS, Bresnahan JF. Mechanical complications of myocardial infarction. In: Murphy JG (ed.), *Mayo Clinic Cardiology Review*, 2nd ed. Philadelphia, PA: Lippincott, Williams & Wilkins, 2000, 231–240.

36. (D)

37. (C)

Explanations 36 and 37

This patient has developed cardiac tamponade as a result of blunt trauma to his chest. Cardiac tamponade exemplifies compressive cardiogenic shock, in which the pump mechanism of the heart fails because of extrinsic factors acting on the heart or the great vessels. Impingement on these cardiovascular structures compromises diastolic filling and, consequently, cardiac output. Among the causes of compressive cardiogenic shock are air embolism, tension pneumothorax, diaphragmatic rupture, and intestinal distention.

Cardiac tamponade is a life-threatening disorder commonly resulting from penetrating chest trauma, although it is also frequently encountered with blunt injuries. Nontraumatic etiologies of cardiac tamponade include malignancy, idiopathic pericarditis, cardiac surgery, tuberculosis, and uremia. Beck's triad refers to the characteristic signs of cardiac tamponade: hypotension, muffled heart sounds, and jugular venous distension. However, these "typical" findings are discovered infrequently. Pulsus paradoxus, a reduction in the systolic blood pressure of 10 mmHg or more with inspiration, may be noted. An ECG may reveal a decrease in the amplitude of the QRS complex or electrical alternans. A globular cardiac silhouette is the distinctive radiographic finding in cardiac tamponade, rarely seen clinically. As these signs and typical study results are seldom present, a high index of suspicion must be maintained. The diagnosis may be suggested if a hypotensive patient exhibits a transient improvement in blood pressure following a fluid bolus. Confirmation of the diagnosis rests on the FAST examination, the subxiphoid pericardial window, or transesophageal and transthoracic echocardiography. Several studies have advocated the FAST examination as the preferred manner of diagnosis of cardiac tamponade, as it is

inexpensive, readily available, reliable, and quickly learned. The definitive treatment of cardiac tamponade involves the release of the pericardial fluid and repair of any cardiac or great vessel injury via an emergent thoracotomy or median sternotomy; however, in the unstable patient, pericardiocentesis may be a temporizing, albeit life-saving, maneuver, allowing for an improved cardiac output prior to surgery.

The pathophysiology of cardiac tamponade has been well-understood since the nineteenth century. At its most basic, cardiac tamponade is defined as impingement on the heart by the accumulation of pericardial effluents, including blood, pus, and air. The pericardium is an inelastic tissue which poorly tolerates increases in its volume. The intrapericardial volume is shared by the heart as well as the pericardial fluid, which normally amounts to 15–30 mL of fluid. The pericardial fluid first occupies the small pericardial reserve volume, slightly distending the pericardium (Fig. 6-15). As seen in the figure, further increases in this volume exceed the distensibility of the pericardium, manifest by the steep pressure–volume curve. The heart and the pericardial fluid are thus forced to compete for space within the unyielding pericardium. The cardiac chambers become compressed, compromising their diastolic filling and, ultimately, cardiac output. The mean diastolic pressures among the four cardiac chambers equalize, with the relatively thinner right atrium and ventricle the first to be affected. The cardiac index and pulmonary wedge pressures are reduced. Pulsus paradoxus occurs secondary to an increase in right ventricular filling during inspiration, at the expense of the left ventricle, with a shift of the intraventricular septum to the left; this pattern is reversed in expiration.

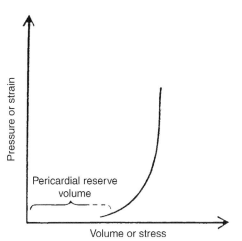

FIG. 6-15 Illustration of the relationship between pericardial volume and pressure. Prior to tamponade, the small pericardial reserve volume is occupied, distending the inelastic parietal pericardium by filling its sinuses. Tamponade occurs when the rate of volume accumulation exceeds the capacity of the parietal pericardium to accommodate it.
Source: Reproduced with permission from Spodick DH. Pathophysiology of cardiac tamponade. *Chest* 1998;113(5):1372–1378.

Bibliography

Bongard FS. Shock & resuscitation. In: Bongard FS, Sue DY (eds.), *Current Critical Care Diagnosis & Treatment.* Stamford, CT: Appleton & Lange, 1994, 14–36.

Braunwald E. Pericardial disease. In: Braunwald E, Fauci AS, Kasper DL, et al. (eds.), *Principles of Internal Medicine,* 15th ed., vol. 1. New York, NY: McGraw Hill, 2001, 1365–1372.

Carrillo EH, Schirmer TP, Sideman MJ, et al. Blunt hemopericardium detected by surgeon-performed sonography. *J Trauma* 2000;48(5):971–974.

Holcroft JW. Shock. In: Cameron JL (ed.), *Current Surgical Therapy,* 7th ed. St. Louis, MO: Mosby, 2001, 1043–1050.

Holcroft JW, Wisner DH. Shock & acute pulmonary failure in surgical patients. In: Way LW (ed.), *Current Surgical Diagnosis & Treatment.* Norwalk, CT: Appleton & Lange, 1994, 186–212.

Maier RV. Shock. In Braunwald E, Fauci AS, Kasper DL, et al. (eds.), *Principles of Internal Medicine,* 15th ed., vol. 1. New York, NY: McGraw Hill, 2001, 222–228.

Nwariaku F, Thal E. *Parkland Trauma Handbook,* 2nd ed. London: Mosby, 1999.

Oh JK. Pericardial diseases. In: Murphy JG (ed.), *Mayo Clinic Cardiology Review,* 2nd ed. Philadelphia, PA: Lippincott, Williams & Wilkins, 2000, 509–532.

Spodick DH. Pathophysiology of cardiac tamponade. *Chest* 1998;113(5):1372–1378.

38. (C)

39. (B)

Explanations 38 and 39

Anaphylactic shock represents an acute, systemic allergic reaction. This immunologically-mediated phenomenon is described as an immediate hypersensitivity reaction. This condition is an anamnestic response to an antigen through the release of pre-formed inflammatory mediators from mast cells. Agents which are responsible for anaphylactic shock include drugs (penicillins, sulfonamides), food (nuts, chocolate), and insect venom (fire ants, Hymenoptera) (Table 6-4). Anaphylactic shock because of penicillin is associated with 400–800 deaths per year in the United States. Only minute quantities of the antigen are required to instigate this potentially life-threatening reaction. IgE antibodies are formed to these various antigens. In a sensitized individual, these antibodies are bound to high affinity Fc-ε receptors (Fc-εRI) on the surface of mast cells. Although basophils possess similar receptors, their contribution to anaphylaxis is minimal. Anaphylaxis occurs when an antigen binds to the

TABLE 6-4   Etiologic Agents for Anaphylactic Shock

Haptens	Potato
Beta-lactam antibiotics	Rice
Sulfonamides	Legumes
Nitrofurantoin	Citrus fruits
Demeclocycline	Chocolate
Streptomycin	Others
Vancomycin	**Venoms**
Local anesthetics	Stinging insects,
Others	especially Hymenoptera,
Serum products	fire ants
Gamma globulin	**Hormones**
Immunotherapy for	Insulin
allergic diseases	Adrenocorticotropic
Heterologous serum	hormone
Foods	Thyroid-stimulating
Nuts	hormone
Shellfish	**Enzymes**
Buckwheat	Chymopapain
Egg white	L-Asparaginase
Cottonseed	**Miscellaneous**
Milk	Seminal fluid
Corn	Others

Source: Reproeuced with permission from Bongard FS. Shock and resuscitation. In: Bongard FS, Sue DY (eds.) *Current Critical Care Diagnosis and Treatment.* Stamford, CT: Appleton & Lange, 1994, 29.

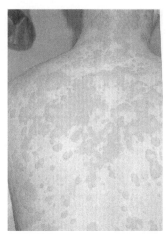

FIG. 6-16   Diffuse urticarial lesions.
Source: Reproduced with permission from Roitt I, Brostoff J, Male D. *Immunology,* 6th ed. Edinburgh: Mosby, 2001, 324.

IgE antibody-Fc-εRI complex. Following cross-linking of two or more of these complexes, a series of reactions occurs such that the mast cell releases a variety of mediators from its cytoplasmic granules. In the immediate phase of anaphylaxis, preformed mediators such as histamine as well as the arachidonic acid derivatives are liberated. The late phase features TNF-α, IL-4, and platelet-activating factor, formed following the degranulation of the mast cells. The late phase occurs approximately 6 hours after antigen contact.

This condition is characterized by vascular collapse and airway obstruction. The preformed mediators released in the immediate phase provoke a generalized vasodilatation of the arterioles, giving rise to a profound hypotension. An increase in vascular permeability further contributes to hypotension by the depletion of intravascular fluid. Accordingly, the hematocrit and blood viscosity increase. The cardiac output and, consequently, coronary artery perfusion decline secondary to the diminished preload. The coronary artery perfusion is worsened by the low systemic vascular resistance as well as by coronary artery spasm, precipitated by the stimulation of cardiac histamine H_1 receptors. The enhanced vascular permeability also promotes the development of laryngeal edema and, thus, airway obstruction. Pulmonary compromise is increased by the bronchoconstriction instigated by histamine and the leukotrienes. In the

skin, the increased vascular permeability presents as angioedema.

Following exposure to an antigen, anaphylactic shock may manifest within seconds up to 1 hour. Initially, patients note pruritis and anxiety. Palpitations and weakness precede cardiovascular signs such as tachycardia, hypotension, arrhythmias, and myocardial ischemia. The reduction in coronary artery perfusion may precipitate an MI. Respiratory symptoms commence with a feeling of a "lump in the throat," progressing to dyspnea, hoarseness, and a cough. The patient may exhibit rhinorrhea and nasal congestion. Additional complaints involve crampy abdominal pain, bloating, and nausea, with emesis and diarrhea later developing. The characteristic cutaneous manifestations are urticaria and angioedema. Urticaria is typified by swelling, erythema, and itching (Fig. 6-16). Conjunctival injection, diaphoresis, and lacrimation may also become apparent. Neurologic disturbances of syncope and seizures may occur. On laboratory evaluation, an elevated histamine and mast cell tryptase are often found. The blood eosinophil level is generally normal. Activation of the coagulation cascade may precipitate disseminated intravascular coagulation.

The treatment of anaphylactic shock relies on ventilatory and circulatory support. Intubation is performed prior to the development of laryngeal edema, ensuring a secure airway. Hypotension is counteracted with epinephrine. Epinephrine halts the production of the mediators of anaphylactic shock by increasing the intracellular concentration of cyclic adenosine monophosphate. This drug is given subcutaneously (0.3–0.5 mL) or intravenously (5–10 mL) every 5 minutes as needed. A patient who normally receives β-blocking medications may not respond to sympathomimetic drugs such as epinephrine. The alternative medication is glucagon. Bronchoconstriction is reversed with inhaled racemic epinephrine or β-adrenergic nebulizers. Antihistamine agents treat the skin and gastrointestinal manifestations of anaphylactic shock. The preferred histamine antagonists are intravenous diphenhydramine (1 mg/kg) and ranitidine (50 mg over 5 min). Vasopressor agents may be initiated for refractory hypotension. Steroids attenuate the late phase of anaphylactic shock.

Prognosis depends on the premorbid condition of the patient and the severity of the symptoms.

Bibliography

Bongard FS. Shock & resuscitation. In: Bongard FS, Sue DY (eds.), *Current Critical Care Diagnosis & Treatment*, Stamford, CT: Appleton & Lange, 1994, 14–36.

Roitt I, Brostoff J, Male D. *Immunology*, 6th ed. Edinburgh, NY: Mosby, 2001, 323–343.

Terr AI. Anaphylaxis and urticaria. In: Parslow TG, Stites DP, Terr AI, Imboden JB (eds.), *Medical Immunology*, 10th ed. New York, NY: McGraw-Hill, 2001, 370–379.

40. **(D)** Cytokines function in mediating the inflammatory response. These small proteins, produced by diverse cells, possess a myriad of important biological effects, acting locally in an autocrine or paracrine manner. A cytokine is categorized as pro- or anti-inflammatory, based on the T helper subset from which it originates. A naive CD4+ T cell (Th0) ultimately develops into a helper T cell of the Th1 or Th2 lineage following stimulation from IL-12 and IFN-γ-inducing factor or IL-4, respectively (Fig. 6-17). Additional stimuli that influence the lineage of the helper T cell include the type of

pathogen, the site of the infection, and the size of the inoculum. The Th1 cells are associated with cell-mediated immunity, protecting the host from intracellular pathogens via the cytotoxic T cell (CD8+), as well as with type IV delayed hypersensitivity. In addition, this subset of helper T cells activates macrophages and promotes antibody production. The cytokines released by the Th1 cells, including IL-2, IFN-γ, and LT-α, are regarded as proinflammatory mediators. While promoting the differentiation of Th0 cells to the Th1 lineage, IFN-γ also down-regulates Th2 production. In contrast, Th2 is responsible for humoral immunity, enhancing B cell maturation. The cytokines created by the Th2 subset include IL-4, IL-5, IL-6, IL-9, IL-10, and IL-13. In particular, IL-4, IL-10, and IL-13 play a prominent anti-inflammatory role in immune function. IL-4, generated from mast cells, eosinophils, and basophils as well as the Th2 cells, interferes with proinflammatory mediators such as IL-1 and IL-8 and inhibits the conversion of Th0 cells to the Th1 subtype. This anti-inflammatory cytokine also promotes B cell differentiation and inhibits the translocation of NF-κB to the nucleus. Cytokines such as IL-3, TNF-α, and granulocyte macrophage colony stimulating factor (GM-CSF) are generated by both cell types. The balance achieved between the poinflammatory Th1 and the anti-inflammatory Th2 cells determines the progression of the inflammatory process.

Traditionally, sepsis has been described as an uncontrolled inflammatory response. Studies have demonstrated that the proinflammatory cytokines IL-1 and TNF-α feature prominently in early sepsis; however, more recent studies suggest that the cells of the Th2 lineage as well as their anti-inflammatory cytokines become more prevalent as the septic process continues. In a study of burn and trauma patients, mononuclear cells produced significantly more of the Th2 than the Th1 cytokines; survival was improved once this preference for the Th2 cytokines was reversed. Other investigations revealed that both the Th1 and Th2 response was blunted, resulting in a state of anergy, the nonresponsiveness to antigen. The prevailing theory of sepsis as an unbridled immune response, therefore, is challenged by current research.

Bibliography

Fink MP. The role of cytokines as mediators of the inflammatory response. In: Townsend CM (ed.), *Textbook of Surgery: The Biological Basis of Modern Surgical Practice*, 16th ed. Philadelphia, PA: W.B. Saunders, 2001, 28–43.

Hotchkiss RS, Karl IE. Medical progress: the pathophysiology and treatment of sepsis. *N Engl J Med* 2003;348(2):138–150.

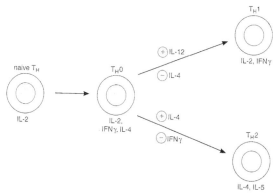

FIG. 6-17 Differentiation of Th0 cells into the Th1 or Th2 lineage.
Source: Reproduced with permission from Imboden JB, Seaman WE. T lymphocytes & natural killer cells. In: Parslow TG, Stites DP, Terr AI, Imboden JB (eds.), *Medical Immunology*, 10th ed. New York, NY: Lange, 2001, 141.

Moldawer LL, Minter RM, Rectenwald JE. Emerging evidence of a more complex role for proinflammatory and antiinflammatory cytokines in the sepsis response. In: Baue AE, Faist E, Fry DE (eds.), *Multiple Organ Failure: Pathophysiology, Prevention, and Therapy*. New York, NY: Springer, 2000, 145–154.

Parslow TG. Lymphocytes and lymphoid tissue. In: Parslow TG, Stites DP, Terr AI, Imboden JB (eds.), *Medical Immunology*, 10th ed. New York, NY: McGraw-Hill, 2001, 40–60.

Roitt I, Brostoff J, Male D. *Immunology*, 6th ed. Edinburgh, NY: Mosby, 2001.

Rosenberg HF, Gallin JI. Inflammation. In: Paul WE (ed.), *Fundamental Immunology*, 4th ed. Philadelphia, PA: Lippincott-Raven, 1999, 1051–1063.

41. (A) TNF-α is a major cytokine which, in conjunction with IL-1, has a prominent role in the acute inflammatory response. This proinflammatory cytokine is released primarily by macrophages and monocytes, but is also derived from nucleated cells such as natural killer cells and neutrophils, after proper stimulation. Mediators responsible for production of TNF-α include IL-1, IFN-γ, IFN-α, GM-CSF, IL-2, and TGF-β (Table 6-5). Other factors that induce TNF-α formation are LPS, ultraviolet light, protozoa, and viral infection. Following the initial impetus for TNF-α release, a variety of cytokines act to regulate its output.

TNF-α has a myriad of biological functions in inflammation (Table 6-6). Among these are neutrophil recruitment, augmentation of superoxide production by neutrophils, angiogenesis, and initiation of the coagulation cascade. Moreover, TNF-α is able to trigger apoptosis, cell death, via the intracellular "death domain" of its receptor, TNFR1. Studies in which knock-out mice lacking genes for TNF or

TNFR1 were inoculated with the intracellular bacteria *Listeria monocytogenes* demonstrated the rapid demise of these subjects with only small amounts of the pathogen. In contrast, the wild-type mice survived despite inoculation with the same concentration of the bacteria. This study underscores the importance of TNF-α in the host defense against intracellular bacteria; however, the beneficial effect of this proinflammatory mediator rests on its presence in moderate amounts. In higher concentrations, TNF-α becomes one of the more prominent agents in the septic response. Infusion of TNF-α in experimental animals produced alterations in perfusion, lactic acidosis, intravascular coagulation, and capillary permeability; a similar result occurred following infusions of endotoxin. Moreover, subjects with septic shock were found to have high levels of TNF-α in their blood. The link between TNF-α and the septic response is further enhanced by the protective effect of antibodies to TNF-α in septic animal subjects. In a metaanalysis of trials in which anti-TNF-α agents were used to treat sepsis, small but insignificant survival benefits were seen. The most encouraging results demonstrated a 3% improvement in survival after treatment with monoclonal antibodies against TNF-α.

TABLE 6-5   Factors Inducing TNF-α Release

Endogenous Factors
Cytokines (TNF-α, IL-1, IFN-γ, GM-CSF, IL-2)
Platelet-activating factor
Myelin P2 protein

Microbe-Derived Factors
Lipopolysaccharide
Zymosan
Peptidoglycan
Streptococcal pyrogenic exotoxin A
Streptolysin O
Lipoteichoic acid
Staphylococcal enterotoxin B
Staphylococcal toxic shock syndrome toxin-1
Lipoarabinomannan

Source: Reproduced with permission from Fink MP. The role of cytokines as mediators of the inflammatory response. In: Townsend CM, (ed.) *Textbook of Surgery: The Biological Basis of Modern Surgical Practice*, 16th ed. Philadelphia, PA: W.B. Saunders, 2001, 34.

TABLE 6-6   Physiologic Effects of the Infusion of TNF-α and IL-1 on Human Subjects

Effect	IL-1	TNF
Fever	+	+
Headache	+	+
Anorexia	+	+
Increased plasma ACTH level	+	+
Hypercortisolemia	+	+
Increased plasma nitrite/nitrate levels	+	+
Systemic arterial hypotension	+	+
Neutrophilia	+	+
Transient neutropenia	+	+
Increased plasma acute-phase protein levels	+	+
Hypoferremia	+	+
Hypozincemia		+
Increased plasma level of IL-1RA	+	+
Increased plasma level of TNF-R1 and TNF-R2	+	+
Increased plasma level of IL-6	+	+
Increased plasma level of IL-8	+	+
Activation of coagulation cascades	−	+
Increased platelet count	+	−
Pulmonary edema	−	+
Hepatocellular injury	−	+

Source: Reproduced with permission from Fink MP. The role of cytokines as mediators of the inflammatory response. In: Townsend CM (ed.) *Textbook of Surgery: The Biological Basis of Modern Surgical Practice*, 16th ed. Philadelphia, PA: W.B. Saunders, 2001, 31.

Bibliography

Bongard FS. Shock & resuscitation. In: Bongard FS, Sue DY (eds.), *Current Critical Care Diagnosis & Treatment*, Stamford, CT: Appleton & Lange, 1994, 14–36.

Fink MP. The role of cytokines as mediators of the inflammatory response. In: Townsend CM (ed.), *Textbook of Surgery: The Biological Basis of Modern Surgical Practice*, 16th ed. Philadelphia, PA: W.B. Saunders, 2001, 28–43.

Krakauer T, Vilcek J, Oppenheim JJ. Proinflammatory cytokines: TNF and IL-1 families, chemokines, TGF-β, and others. In: Paul WE (ed.), *Fundamental Immunology*, 4th ed. Philadelphia, PA: Lippincott-Raven, 1999, 775–784.

Maier RV. Shock. In Braunwald E, Fauci AS, Kasper DL, et al. (eds.), *Principles of Internal Medicine*, 15th ed., vol. 1. New York, NY: McGraw Hill, 2001, 222–228.

Oppenheim JJ, Ruscetti FW. Cytokines. In: Parslow TG, Stites DP, Terr AI, Imboden JB (eds.), *Medical Immunology*, 10th ed. New York, NY: McGraw-Hill, 2001, 148–166.

Reinhart K, Karzai W. Anti-tumor necrosis factor therapy in sepsis: update on clinical trials and lessons learned. *Crit Care Med* 2001;29(7):S121–S125.

Roitt I, Brostoff J, Male D. *Immunology*, 6th ed. Edinburgh, NY: Mosby, 2001.

42. (B)

43. (D)

Explanations 42 and 43

Sepsis and septic shock have become especially prominent in this age of high tech intervention in high-risk patients. This condition afflicts approximately 750,000 individuals and accounts for a mortality of 30–60%. Sepsis represents an unrestrained inflammatory process, arising in the setting of the SIRS. As defined by a consensus conference in 1991, SIRS is a generalized inflammatory process associated with a variety of etiologies, including pancreatitis, multiple trauma, hemorrhagic shock, and vascular occlusion (Fig. 6-18). Among the criteria for SIRS are a body temperature >38 or <36°C; a heart rate >90 bpm; a respiratory rate >20 or a $PaCO_2$ <32 mmHg; a white blood cell count >12,000 or <4000; and a bandemia >10%. Two of these criteria must be met to fulfill a diagnosis of SIRS. In the presence of a documented infection, SIRS becomes sepsis. The most common pathogen associated with the bacteremia of sepsis and septic shock is the gram-negative bacilli, most notably *E. coli*; however, other gram-negative bacterial species—*Klebsiella, Proteus,* and *Pseudomonas*—as well as the gram-positive bacteria are often isolated from the blood cultures of septic patients. A fungemia or viremia also may give rise to sepsis. Positive blood cultures are obtained in 45% of

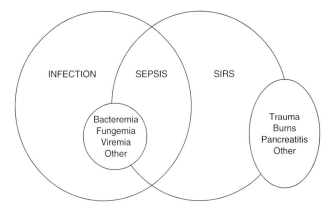

FIG. 6-18 Sepsis arises in the setting of a systemic inflammatory response syndrome (SIRS) with a documented infection. SIRS alone is induced by conditions such as trauma, burns, and pancreatitis.
Source: Reproduced with permission from Offiner PJ, Moore EE. Risk factors for MOF and pattern of organ failure following severe trauma. In: Baue AE, Faist E, Fry DE (eds.), *Multiple Organ Failure: Pathophysiology, Prevention, and Therapy.* New York, NY: Springer, 2000, 31.

septic patients. The majority of these infections emanate from the genitourinary, gastrointestinal, and biliary tracts and the tracheobronchial tree.

In the time of Hippocrates, *sepsis* signified solely death and decay. Today, sepsis exists along a continuum of disease that ranges from sepsis to MODS. The development of hypotension and organ dysfunction in a septic patient indicates severe sepsis. Once the hypotension becomes refractory to intervention with fluids and tissue perfusion is markedly reduced, septic shock ensues. In patients with a gram-negative bacteremia, 26% progressed to septic shock. Multiple organ dysfunction and, ultimately, failure follow. In the setting of sepsis, secondary, not primary, multiple organ dysfunction occurs, with the damage a consequence of the exuberant host response to the pathogen. The probability of developing MODS depends on the severity of the presentation, from sepsis to septic shock. Multiple organ dysfunction accounts for an overall mortality rate of 34% at 28 days; mortality worsens with the number of dysfunctional organ systems (Table 6-7). Death secondary to sepsis follows a bimodal distribution: early death secondary to septic shock unresponsive to pressor agents or a later demise (weeks to months) following MODS. Organ dysfunction first affects the lungs, resulting in the adult respiratory distress syndrome (ARDS).

A diagnosis of sepsis and septic shock rests on a high index of suspicion, as its manifestations are nonspecific. A patient with sepsis often presents with fever, tachypnea, and tachycardia. Septic shock develops at

TABLE 6-7   Prognosis in Multisystem Organ Dysfunction

Number of failing systems	Mortality (%)
0	3
1	30
2	50–60
3	85–100
4	72–100
5	100

Source: Reproduced with permission from Jurusz DJ, Gilmore JY. Shock and hypoperfusion states. In: O'Leary JP (ed.), *The Physiologic Basis of Surgery*, 2nd ed. Philadelphia, PA: Lippincott, Williams & Wilkins, 1996, 94.

a mean blood pressure of less than 60 mmHg or a systolic blood pressure of less than 90 mmHg. Cardiac output is supranormal while the central venous pressure and PCWP are normal to elevated. The systemic vascular resistance remains markedly diminished. Septic shock once was described as hypo- or hyperdynamic depending on the cardiac output; however, current investigations discount this division, attributing the hypodynamic scenario to inadequate fluid resuscitation. The elevated cardiac output enhances oxygen delivery to the periphery; however, the extraction of oxygen is reduced, possibly secondary to shunting of arterial blood to the venous circulation, bypassing the capillaries. A narrowing of the arterial-venous oxygen difference is the result of this shunting. Laboratory studies demonstrate either a leukopenia (<4000) or leukocytosis (>12,000). Findings consistent with disseminated intravascular coagulation may be present: increased D-dimer and fibrin split products and a decreased fibrinogen level. On an arterial blood gas, a metabolic acidosis is evident.

The treatment of septic shock focuses on eliminating the pathogen while addressing the physiologic derangements of the patient. The source of infection must be identified via cultures and, if feasible, surgically eradicated, as with drainage or debridement. Antibiotics are initiated and later tailored to the susceptibilities of the inciting agent. Resuscitation is accomplished with intravenous fluids, replacing the losses of the permeable capillaries. Refractory hypotension is countered with vasopressors such as dopamine. A right pulmonary artery catheter guides therapy, with an elevated PCWP the goal of resuscitation. As the lung is an early target of dysfunction, mechanical ventilation is commonly initiated for these patients. Dysfunction of other organ systems is similarly supported. Currently, immunotherapy is being explored as a novel method for treating septic shock.

Bibliography

Abraham E, Matthay MA, Dinarello CA, et al. Consensus conference definitions for sepsis, septic shock, acute lung injury, and acute respiratory distress syndrome: time for a reevaluation. *Crit Care Med* 2000;28(1):232–235.

Bone RC, Balk RA, Cerra FB, et al. American College of Chest Physicians/Society of Critical Care Medicine Consensus Conference: definitions for sepsis and organ failure and guidelines for the use of innovative therapies in sepsis. *Crit Care Med* 1992;20(6):864–873.

Bongard FS. Shock & resuscitation. In: Bongard FS, Sue DY (eds.), *Current Critical Care Diagnosis & Treatment*, Stamford, CT: Appleton & Lange, 1994, 14–36.

Jurusz DJ, Gilmore JY. Shock and hypoperfusion states. In: O'Leary JP (ed.), *The Physiologic Basis of Surgery*, 2nd ed. Philadelphia, PA: Lippincott, Williams & Wilkins, 1996, 84–99.

Maier RV. Shock. In Braunwald E, Fauci AS, Kasper DL et al. (eds.), *Principles of Internal Medicine*, 15th ed., vol. 1. New York, NY: McGraw Hill, 2001, 222–228.

Marshall JC. SIRS, MODS, and the Brave New World of ICU Acronyms: have they helped us? In: Baue AE, Faist E, Fry DE (eds.), *Multiple Organ Failure: Pathophysiology, Prevention, and Therapy*. New York, NY: Springer, 2000, 14–22.

Marshall JC, Papia G. The septic response. In: Cameron JL (ed.), *Current Surgical Therapy*, 7th ed. St. Louis, MO: Mosby, 2001, 1327–1332.

Mullins RJ. Fluid, electrolytes, and shock. In: Townsend CM (ed.), *Textbook of Surgery: The Biological Basis of Modern Surgical Practice*, 16th ed. Philadelphia, PA: W.B. Saunders, 2001, 45–67.

44. **(A)** Septic shock is characterized by a derangement of systemic oxygen metabolism: while oxygen delivery is elevated, its extraction at the periphery is reduced. As a result, the arterial-venous oxygen difference is reduced and mixed venous oxygenation is increased. A typical patient with septic shock demonstrates adequate oxygen delivery but exhibits signs of refractory hypoxia, notably a persistent lactic acidosis. In a study of 109 critically ill patients, Hayes et al. (1994) attempted to improve survival by increasing the cardiac index and, thus, systemic oxygen delivery to supranormal levels with dobutamine administration. Systemic oxygen delivery (DO_2) is determined by arterial oxygen content (CaO_2) and cardiac output (CO): $CaO_2 \times CO \times 10$. Despite the improved cardiac index and oxygen delivery, these patients did not experience better outcomes. Instead, the treatment group had an in-unit mortality of 50% as compared to the 30% mortality of the control group. In general, oxygen extraction was equivalent between the two groups, as the treatment group developed a decline in oxygen consumption although the supply of oxygen increased. An insufficient supply of oxygen was thus

discounted as being responsible for the persistent lactic acidosis of sepsis. In response to this scenario, an arterial to venous cutaneous shunt was proposed to be the cause of the poor peripheral oxygen extraction. Marshall and Papia (2001) attribute this shunting phenomenon to microvascular occlusion and decreased vascular tone; however, no such shunts have been demonstrated in autopsy studies. Current investigations of oxygenation in sepsis focus on cytopathic dysoxia—an altered cellular oxygen metabolism. These studies suggest that sepsis is associated with dysfunctional mitochondria that are incapable of utilizing the supplied oxygen. In a feline model of acute endotoxemia, Crouser et al. examined mitochondrial function and ultrastructure following the administration of LPS or isotonic saline. The two groups revealed similar parameters with regards to oxygen availability and hemoglobin concentration. Yet, the mitochondria of the endotoxin group were seen on electron micrographs to be injured, with swelling and disrupted membranes. Furthermore, mitochondrial respiratory activity was notably compromised in the endotoxin group, especially the adenosine-5-diphosphate-dependent (state 3) respiration at complex IV. A concurrent increase in adenosine-5-diphosphate-independent mitochondrial respiration (state 4) indicates an uncoupling of oxidative phosphorylation and impaired ATP generation in the study group. Prior studies point to TNF-α and LPS as the probable culprits in this mitochondrial damage. Further investigation of aerobic respiration on the cellular level continues based on these findings.

Bibliography

Bongard FS. Shock & resuscitation. In: Bongard FS, Sue DY (eds.), *Current Critical Care Diagnosis & Treatment*, Stamford, CT: Appleton & Lange, 1994, 14–36.

Crouser ED, Julian MW, Blaho DV, Pfeiffer DR. Endotoxin-induced mitochondrial damage correlates with impaired respiratory activity. *Crit Care Med* 2002;30(2):276–284.

Hayes MA, Timmins AC, Yau EHS, et al. Elevation of systemic oxygen delivery in the treatment of critically ill patients. *N Engl J Med* 1994;330(24):1717–1722.

Marshall JC, Papia G. The septic response. In: Cameron JL (ed.), *Current Surgical Therapy*, 7th ed. St. Louis, MO: Mosby, 2001, 1327–1332.

Ronco JJ. Tissue dysoxia in sepsis: getting to know the mitochondrion. *Crit Care Med* 2002;30(2):483–484.

45. (C) Septic shock is associated with alterations in the hypothalamic-pituitary-adrenal (HPA) axis. The mechanism by which the HPA axis is triggered has not been fully elucidated; however, both neural and inflammatory pathways are integral to its activation. The hypothalamus is directly stimulated by input from the site of inflammation, directed to the brain via central neurons. In experimental models, division of the vagus nerve diminished the response of the HPA axis to LPS, TNF-α, and IL-1. In addition, the proinflammatory cytokines TNF-α, IL-1, and IL-6 independently trigger the HPA axis but act synergistically (Table 6-8). In a study of 189 patients with severe sepsis, Annane et al. (2002) found that occult adrenal insufficiency occurred in 50%; the 28-day mortality of these patients was 75%. Further study of these septic patients with occult adrenal insufficiency revealed that the administration of corticosteroids produced an improvement in the blood pressure response to vasopressor agents. Glucocorticoids potentiate vasoconstrictor systems while counteracting the various vasodilatory mediators; also, volume expansion is achieved via the mineralocorticoid properties of glucocorticoids (Fig. 6-19). In addition to an occult adrenal insufficiency, sepsis is also accompanied by a peripheral resistance to glucocorticoids with the cytokines IL-2 and IL-4 promote alterations in the affinity of the glucocorticoid receptor via the transcription factor NF-κB.

Cortisol has many effects in modulating inflammation. This endogenous substance acts by binding to glucocorticoid receptors located in the cytoplasm or nucleus. The association of cortisol and the receptor exposes the DNA binding site, previously camouflaged by heat shock proteins, on the receptor. The cortisol-receptor complex travels to the nucleus and binds to certain DNA sequences, glucocorticoid response elements, in the promoter region of various genes. By attaching to these elements, the transcription of specific genes is either promoted or inhibited

TABLE 6-8   Cytokines that Induce Activation of the Hypothalamic-Pituitary-Adrenal Axis

Inflammatory cytokines
Tumor necrosis factor α
Interleukin-1α and interleukin-1β
Interleukin-6
Other cytokines
Interferon α
Interferon γ
Interleukin-2
Growth factors
Epidermal growth factor
Transforming growth factor β
Lipid mediators
Prostanoids
Platelet-activating factor

Source: Reproduced with permission from Chrousos GP. Seminars in Medicine of the Beth Israel Hospital, Boston: The Hypothalamic-Pituitary-Adrenal Axis and Immune-Mediated Inflammation. *N Engl J Med* 1995;332:1351–1362.

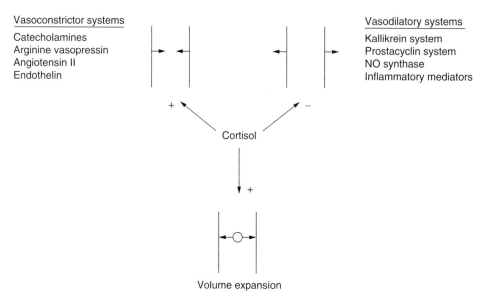

FIG. 6-19   Effect of cortisol on arterial blood pressure.
Source: Reproduced with permission from Meduri GU. Rationale for glucocorticoid treatment in septic shock and unresolving ARDS. In: Baue AE, Faist E, Fry DE (eds.), *Multiple Organ Failure: Pathophysiology, Prevention, and Therapy.* New York, NY: Springer, 2000, 516.

(Table 6-9). For instance, cortisol enhances the production of IκB, the inhibitor of the transcription factor NF-κB; the increased IκB allows NF-κB to be relocated to the cytoplasm, where it has no effect. Consequently, by restricting the synthesis of chemokines, cortisol reduces the accumulation of inflammatory cells in the tissues. In addition, cortisol reduces levels of IL-1, IL-2, IL-3, IL-6, IFN-γ, GM-CSF, and TNF-α. The inflammatory process is also

TABLE 6-9   Effect of Glucocorticoids on Gene Transcription

Increased transcription
    Lipocortin-1
    β_2-Adrenoceptor
    Endonucleases
    Secretory leukocyte protease inhibitor
    Inhibitory protein IκB
Decreased transcription
    Cytokines (TNFα, IL-1, IL-2, IL-3, IL-4, IL-5, IL-6, IL-8, IL-11, IL-12, IL-13, GM-CSF, RANTES, MIP-1α)
    Inducible nitric oxide synthase (iNOS)
    Inducible cyclooxygenase (COX-2)
    Inducible phospholipase A_2 (cPLA$_2$)
    Endothelin-1
    NK1-receptors
    Adhesion molecules (ICAM-1, E selectin)

Source: Reproduced with permission from Meduri GU. Rationale for glucocorticoid treatment in septic shock and unresolving ARDS. In: Baue AE, Faist E, Fry DE (eds.) *Multiple Organ Failure: Pathophysiology, Prevention, and Therapy.* New York, NY: Springer, 2000, 518.

interrupted by suppressing the expression of COX-2 and inducible nitric oxide synthase.

Corticosteroids were the first medications applied as immunotherapeutic agents in septic shock. These early studies of corticosteroids, given for short durations at high doses, demonstrated no survival benefit; however, interest in corticosteroids was renewed by two small randomized studies in which treatment with low doses of hydrocortisone for long durations (>5 days) was associated with a more rapid weaning of vasopressor agents. Similarly, healthy volunteers administered hydrocortisone prior to a local endotoxin challenge did not develop vasoplegia to norepinephrine. Recently, Annane et al. (2002) completed a randomized, placebo-controlled study of 300 patients with septic shock, investigating the efficacy of a 7-day course of hydrocortisone and fludrocortisone in benefiting survival. Occult adrenal insufficiency was discovered in 229 of these patients (115 placebo group, 114 corticosteroid group) based on a corticotropin test. Among the patients with occult adrenal insufficiency, mortality was 63% in the placebo group but 53% in the corticosteroid cohort. After 28 days, vasopressors were withdrawn in 40% of the placebo group and 57% of the corticosteroid group. These results were found to be statistically significant. No adverse effects were encountered.

Bibliography

Annane D. Corticosteroids for septic shock. *Crit Care Med* 2001;29(7):S117–S120.

Annane D, Sebille V, Charpentier C, et al. Effect of treatment with low doses of hydrocortisone and fludrocortisone on mortality in patients with septic shock. *JAMA* 2002;288(7):862–871.

Bongard FS. Shock & resuscitation. In: Bongard FS, Sue DY (eds.), *Current Critical Care Diagnosis & Treatment*, Stamford, CT: Appleton & Lange, 1994, 14–36.

Champe PC, Harvey RA. *Biochemistry*, 2nd ed. Philadelphia, PA: JB Lippincott, 1994.

Chrousos GP. Seminars in medicine of the Beth Israel Hospital, Boston: the hypothalamic-pituitary-adrenal axis and immune-mediated inflammation. *N Engl J Med* 1995;332(20):1351–1362.

Hotchkiss RS, Karl IE. Medical progress: the pathophysiology and treatment of sepsis. *N Engl J Med* 2003;348(2):138–150.

Marshall JC, Papia G. The septic response. In: Cameron JL (ed.), *Current Surgical Therapy*, 7th ed. St. Louis, MO: Mosby, 2001, 1327–1332.

Meduri GU. Rationale for glucocorticoid treatment in septic shock and unresolving ARDS. In: Baue AE, Faist E, Fry DE (eds.), *Multiple Organ Failure: Pathophysiology, Prevention, and Therapy.* New York, NY: Springer, 2000,514–523.

Rosenberg HF, Gallin JI. Inflammation. In: Paul WE (ed.), *Fundamental Immunology*, 4th ed. Philadelphia, PA: Lippincott-Raven, 1999, 1051–1063.

Soni A, Pepper GM, Wyrwinski PM, et al. Incidence, outcome, and relationship to peripheral cytokine levels. *Am J Med* 1995;98(3):266–271.

46. (A)

47. (D)

Explanations 46 and 47

A significant proportion of the mortality of septic shock is attributable to the subsequent MODS. The lung appears as the first target of dysfunction, followed by the kidneys, gastrointestinal tract, and liver. A series of 154 septic patients from Herbert et al. determined that ALI and ARDS were the most common manifestations of MODS. The classification of the lung damage as an acute lung injury (ALI) or ARDS depends on its severity. An ALI arises in a setting of inflammation and pronounced capillary permeability. A consensus conference defined ALI as an acute onset injury characterized by a PaO_2/FiO_2 <300 and a pulmonary artery wedge pressure of <18 mmHg with bilateral infiltrates evident on a chest radiograph. ARDS represents a more severe form of ALI, with a PaO_2/FiO_2 <200. Lung injury occurs in 30–80% of the cases of septic shock, most of which present as ARDS. In a 1996 metaanalysis, Garber et al. identified sepsis as the most common inciting factor for ARDS.

The lung dysfunction of ARDS emanates from the exaggerated immune response to the infecting pathogen. Neutrophils appear as the primary mediator of this damage, being the predominant cell type in biopsy specimens from ARDS-afflicted lungs. The presence of neutrophils is coincident with an increase in oxidant activity. Oxygen free radicals serve to inhibit surfactant activity by damage to its lipid components and to type II pneumocytes, the source of surfactant. Moreover, the cytotoxic products of neutrophils promote endothelial damage, resulting in protein-rich pulmonary edema, accumulating in both the alveoli and interstitum. Immune agents such as platelet-activating factor, prostaglandins, and the leukotrienes further contribute to this enhanced vascular permeability, which is accompanied by an increase in pulmonary vascular resistance. Activation of the coagulation cascade produces numerous microthrombi within the pulmonary circulation; hypoperfusion of the lung and right-to-left shunting thus arise. Autopsy studies of the lung reveal interstitial and alveolar edema, atelectasis, microthrombi, and hyaline membrane formation. Clinically, this is manifest as hypoxemia because of a ventilation-perfusion mismatch, decreased functional residual capacity, elevated airway resistance, and a pronounced reduction in lung compliance.

Treatment of ARDS rests on the support of pulmonary function while limiting additional lung injury. A majority of patients with ARDS require mechanical ventilation, with the goal of keeping the PaO_2 greater than 60 mmHg or the oxygen saturation higher than 90%. The ventilation-perfusion mismatch may prevent an increase in PaO_2 despite the administration of supplemental oxygen; however, a FiO_2 of less than 50% is recommended to avoid further lung injury from oxygen toxicity. The application of PEEP is essential in maximizing oxygen exchange and, thus, PaO_2. Alveoli are predisposed to collapse at end expiration because of low lung volumes, pulmonary edema, and the deficiency of surfactant. The application of PEEP prevents this collapse, making more alveoli available for gas exchange (Fig. 6-20). Additionally, studies have suggested that PEEP may redirect pulmonary artery circulation to better ventilated areas of the lung, lessening the ventilation-perfusion mismatch. Yet, PEEP may contribute to lung injury by inducing barotrauma through alveolar overdistention. Also, cardiac output may be compromised by the addition of PEEP; consequently, the systemic delivery of oxygen is reduced. Other strategies for the management of ARDS include inverse ratio ventilation, high-frequency jet ventilation, and prone positioning. In one study, corticosteroids improved survival in patients with

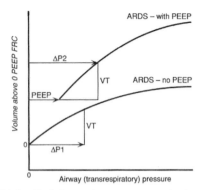

FIG. 6-20 Relationship between airway pressure and volume in a patient with adult respiratory distress syndrome (ARDS). By adding positive end expiratory pressure to the mechanical ventilation, the pressure-volume curve demonstrates greater lung compliance.
Source: Reproduced with permission from Sue DY. Respiratory failure. In: Bongard FS, Sue DY (eds.), *Current Critical Care Diagnosis & Treatment.* Stamford, CT: Appleton & Lange, 1994.

ARDS: the use of steroids was associated with a mortality of 38%, significantly less than the 67% mortality in the nonsteroid group. The utility of corticosteroids in treating ARDS, however, remains a point of contention.

Bibliography

Abraham E, Matthay MA, Dinarello CA, et al. Consensus conference definitions for sepsis, septic shock, acute lung injury, and acute respiratory distress syndrome: Time for a reevaluation. *Crit Care Med* 2000;28(1):232–235.

Bone RC, Balk RA, Cerra FB, et al. American College of Chest Physicians/Society of Critical Care Medicine Consensus Conference: definitions for sepsis and organ failure and guidelines for the use of innovative therapies in sepsis. *Crit Care Med* 1992;20(6):864–873.

Dellinger RP. Lung. In: Baue AE, Faist E, Fry DE. *Multiple Organ Failure: Pathophysiology, Prevention, and Therapy.* New York, NY: Springer, 2000, 353–363.

Forsythe RM, Sambol JT, Adams CA, Deitch EA. Multiple organ failure. In: Cameron JL (ed.), *Current Surgical Therapy,* 7th ed. St. Louis, MO: Mosby, 2001, 1354–1360.

Garber BG, Hebert PC, Yelle JD, Hodder RV, McGowan J. Adult respiratory distress syndrome: a systemic overview of incidence and risk factors. *Crit Care Med* 1996;24:687–695.

Herbert PC, Drummond AJ, Singer J, Bernard GR, Russell JA. A simple multiple system organ failure scoring system predicts mortality of patients who have sepsis syndrome. *Chest* 1993;104:230–235.

Sue DY. Respiratory failure. In: Bongard FS, Sue DY (eds.), *Current Critical Care Diagnosis & Treatment,* Stamford, CT: Appleton & Lange, 1994, 37–87.

48. (B)

49. (A)

Explanations 48 and 49

A prominent feature of septic shock is vasopressor-resistant hypotension, attributable to a pronounced systemic vasodilatation. This massive vasodilatation has been ascribed to nitric oxide, a free radical gas derived from the three isomers of the enzyme nitric oxide synthase. Under normal physiologic conditions, nitric oxide, produced from the constitutive enzyme endothelial nitric oxide synthase (eNOS), maintains a baseline of vasodilatation, regulating tissue perfusion. Inhibition of eNOS with guanidine-substituted L-arginine analogs promotes severe systemic and pulmonary hypertension. In the presence of inflammatory agents such as TNF-α, IL-1, and endotoxin, inducible nitric oxide synthase (iNOS) is generated from macrophages and vascular smooth muscle, following the tyrosine kinase-induced activation of the transcription factor NF-κB. As part of a normal inflammatory response, nitric oxide and its free radical derivatives contribute to the eradication of the invading pathogens. In addition, the nitric oxide created by iNOS promotes the dilatation of neighboring blood vessels via the intracellular messenger cGMP. Nitric oxide activates the enzyme soluble guanylate cyclase, which catalyzes the conversion of guanosine triphosphate (GTP) to cGMP by binding to its iron-heme component. This intracellular messenger induces a cGMP-dependent protein kinase within the cells of vascular smooth muscle to open calcium and potassium channels, thereby achieving vasodilatation.

With septic shock, the amount of nitric oxide generated becomes exuberant. In an *in vitro* model of sepsis, in which endothelial cells and endotoxin were placed in culture, nitrite, the stable end product of nitric oxide, was revealed in a concentration that far exceeded that associated with the baseline production of nitric oxide (millimoles vs. micromoles). Similar studies in adults with severe sepsis produced equivalent results, albeit in amounts smaller than in rodent models. However, the initial release of nitric oxide, within the first 2 hours of the onset of septic shock, is ascribed to eNOS, as iNOS is not yet present. Yet, the contribution of eNOS to the abundant output of nitric oxide is transient. Ochoa et al. measured elevated levels of nitrite in patients suffering from septic shock, correlating this finding with hypotension and an increased cardiac output. Inhibition of nitric oxide synthase in septic patients has resulted in an improved responsiveness to vasopressors. Moreover, iNOS knock-out mice afflicted with septic shock exhibit a diminished degree of hypotension, culminating in a survival advantage. Further benefits associated with the inhibition of iNOS include diminished peroxynitrite generation and attenuation of the suppression of mitochondrial respiration.

The NOS-cGMP pathway has been the subject of intense study in an effort to regulate septic shock. Intervention in the formation of nitric oxide may target the induction or activity of iNOS. In addition, the action of nitric oxide itself can be blocked. The original agent discovered to effect NOS inhibition is the N-substituted L-arginine analog L-NMMA, which was associated with improvements in blood pressure in selected animal models of septic shock. L-NMMA exerts its effects by competition with L-arginine for binding sites on NOS. A phase I trial of L-NMMA in patients with septic shock demonstrated elevations in blood pressure, an improved response to vasopressors, and a normalized cardiac index; however, a phase III trial involving L-NMMA was halted prior to completion because of a clear increase in mortality in the study group. The worsened survival associated with L-NMMA may arise from its nonselective inhibition of not only iNOS but also the isoforms eNOS and neuronal nitric oxide synthase (nNOS). Other potential agents in the blockage of the nitric oxide pathway include glucocorticoids, insulin-like growth factor 1 (IGF-1), and methylene blue. In particular, methylene blue interferes with cGMP production, resulting in vasoconstriction. A recent small uncontrolled study of intravenous methylene blue administered to patients in septic shock in a bolus of 2–4 mg/kg achieved a persistent elevation in blood pressure without influencing vascular permeability or diastolic function.

Despite its adverse effects, nitric oxide appears to play a physiologic role in maintaining tissue perfusion in the presence of septic shock. It is likely that this action is directed by the constitutive isomers of NOS, eNOS and nNOS. Septic shock is associated with a localized vasoconstriction within various organs, including the mesenteric, pulmonary, and renal circulations. This is counteracted by the vasodilatory action of nitric oxide. In a canine model of septic shock, nonselective inhibition of NOS led to a diminished splanchnic perfusion, with gastrointestinal and liver injury the result. Furthermore, patients in the phase II trial of L-NMMA were found to have an increased incidence of pulmonary hypertension. Also, iNOS knock-out mice with septic shock demonstrated liver injury despite an improvement in their hemodynamic parameters. Nitric oxide provides further benefits in septic shock, among which are a reduction in neutrophil adhesion and decreased platelet aggregation. In sum, the search for an inhibitor of nitric oxide synthesis or action must consider the detrimental as well as beneficial contributions of nitric oxide to septic shock.

Bibliography

Bongard FS. Shock & resuscitation. In: Bongard FS, Sue DY (eds.), *Current Critical Care Diagnosis & Treatment*, Stamford, CT: Appleton & Lange, 1994, 14–36.

Donati A, Conti G, Loggi S, et al. Does methylene blue administration to septic shock patients affect vascular permeability and blood volume? *Crit Care Med* 2002;30(10):2271–2277.

Fink MP. The role of cytokines as mediators of the inflammatory response. In: Townsend CM (ed.), *Textbook of Surgery: The Biological Basis of Modern Surgical Practice*, 16th ed. Philadelphia, PA: W.B. Saunders, 2001, 28–43.

Gomez-Jimenez J, Salgado A, Mourelle M, et al. L-Arginine: nitric oxide pathway in endotoxemia and human septic shock. *Crit Care Med* 1995;23(2):253–258.

Murray PT, Wylam ME, Umans JG. Nitric oxide and septic vascular dysfunction. *Anesth Analg* 2000;90(1):89–101.

Parslow TG, Bainton DF. Innate immunity. In: Parslow TG, Stites DP, Terr AI, Imboden JB (eds.), *Medical Immunology*, 10th ed. New York, NY: McGraw-Hill, 2001, 19–39.

Rosenberg HF, Gallin JI. Inflammation. In: Paul WE (ed.), *Fundamental Immunology*, 4th ed. Philadelphia, PA: Lippincott-Raven, 1999, 1051–1063.

Ruetten H, Thiemermann C. Shock states and nitric oxide. In: Loscalzo J, Vita JA (eds.), *Contemporary Cardiology: Nitric Oxide and the Cardiovascular System*, vol. 4. Totowa, NJ: Humana Press, 2000, 321–341.

Salyapongse AN, Billiar TR. Nitric oxide as a modulator of sepsis: therapeutic possibilities. In: Baue AE, Faist E, Fry DE. *Multiple Organ Failure: Pathophysiology, Prevention, and Therapy*. New York, NY: Springer, 2000, 176–187.

Sheehan M, Wong HR. Yet another potential role for nitric oxide in the pathophysiology of septic shock. *Crit Care Med* 2002;30(6):1393–1394.

50. (D)

51. (B)

Explanations 50 and 51

Sepsis has been characterized as an uncontrolled inflammatory response. In this disorder, an exuberant inflammatory process is accompanied by a pronounced coagulopathy, initiated by endotoxin and cytokines such as TNF-α, IL-1, and IL-6. These cytokines induce the expression of the transmembrane glycoprotein tissue factor on monocytes and endothelial cells. This highly thrombogenic molecule activates the extrinsic pathway of coagulation. The products of the coagulation cascade, notably the serine protease thrombin, perpetuate the inflammatory response by activating the endothelium, platelets, and smooth muscle. Microvascular thrombosis develops, manifest clinically as disseminated intravascular coagulation, compromising tissue perfusion. Ultimately, diffuse vascular injury and multiple organ dysfunction ensue. In an animal model, administration of endotoxin was followed by the formation of thrombi in the hepatic microcirculation within 5 minutes; persistent endotoxemia resulted in the deposition of multiple fibrin clots with subsequent tissue hypoperfusion and necrosis. Furthermore, biopsies of the skin lesion purpura fulminans, seen with meningococcemia, demonstrate microvascular thrombosis; these lesions are resolved following replacement therapy with the antithrombotic, anti-inflammatory-activated protein C. The intimate connection between inflammation and coagulation prompted the study of activated protein C as a therapeutic agent in sepsis.

Protein C functions as an endogenous vitamin-K-dependent plasma serine protease in the coagulation cascade, essential in regulating hemostasis. Normally, protein C exists as an inactive zymogen, circulating in the blood. Its activation is accomplished by a complex of thrombin and thrombomodulin, an endothelial surface membrane glycoprotein (Fig. 6-21). The generation of activated protein C is further promoted by the transmembrane endothelial protein C receptor (EPCR). Activated protein C, along with its cofactor protein S, inhibits both factors Va and VIIIa, thus restricting the creation of thrombin. In addition to its antithrombotic function, activated protein C enhances fibrinolysis by promoting tissue plasminogen function via tissue plasminogen activator and by impeding the activity of plasmino-

gen activator inhibitor 1 (PAI-1) and thrombin-activated fibrinolysis inhibitor.

In addition to its antithrombotic and profibrinolytic actions, activated protein C (APC) exhibits an anti-inflammatory function. In part, APC exerts its anti-inflammatory effect by inhibiting the generation of the proinflammatory agent, thrombin; however, APC itself directly interferes with inflammation. Studies have suggested that APC restricts IL-1 and TNF-α production as well as the monocyte/macrophage response to LPS and IFN-γ. In addition, translocation of the transcription factor NF-κB to the nucleus following stimulation with LPS is impeded by APC via a reduction in p50/p52 subunit expression; consequently, the production of proinflammatory agents is constrained. This protein also suppresses the adhesion of neutrophils to the endothelium via E-selectin, preventing diapedesis. Moreover, apoptosis is inhibited by APC through the increased production of the antiapoptotic factors endothelial A_1 and inhibitor of apoptosis 1.

Sepsis is associated with a disruption of the regulation of coagulation. The onset of sepsis is associated with an initial increase in the level of activated protein C; however, this protein is rapidly consumed in the early stages of the exuberant procoagulant response to sepsis, thus allowing unrestricted thrombin formation. Studies of both adult and pediatric patients with sepsis have demonstrated a marked reduction in protein C levels. The depletion of protein C likely occurs because of a decrease in its synthesis by the liver accompanied by an early increase in its expenditure. Also, the neutrophil enzyme elastase contributes to the paucity of protein C via its degradation. A deficiency of protein C often precedes clinical manifestations of sepsis, including fever, by 12 hours. Furthermore, studies have suggested that protein C levels may serve as a useful prognostic indicator of the severity of the septic process. Thrombomodulin and EPCR expression is also decreased in the course of the septic process, reducing the activation of available protein C. For this reason, activated protein C, not the inactive form, must be administered in the treatment of septic shock.

Studies have clearly demonstrated the efficacy of activated protein C replacement therapy in treating septic shock. The recombinant human activated protein C worldwide evaluation in severe sepsis (PROWESS) trial evaluated recombinant human activated protein C (drotrecogin alfa) as compared to a placebo with regards to a primary end-point of death within 28 days of the treatment. The randomized, double-blind, placebo-controlled study enrolled

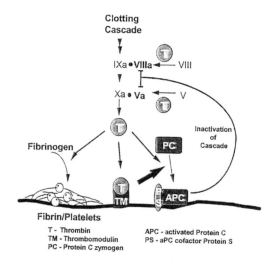

FIG. 6-21 Regulation of hemostatis by the anti-coagulant protein C. T—thrombin, TM—thrombomodulin, PC—protein C, APC—activated protein C, PS—factor S. *Source:* Reproduced with permission from Grinnell BW, Joyce D. Recombinant human activated protein C: a system modulator of vascular function for treatment of severe sepsis. *Crit Care Med* 2001;29(7):S53–S60.

1690 patients diagnosed with systemic inflammation and organ failure, 840 of whom received placebo with the remaining 850 administered drotrecogin alfa activated. A deficiency of protein C was evident in 87.6% of the 1574 patients in whom the level was obtained. Treatment consisted of an infusion of 24 mg/kg/h of drotrecogin alfa activated or a placebo for a period of 96 hours. Mortality in the study and control groups was 24.7 and 30.8%, respectively (Fig. 6-22). This absolute decrease in mortality of 6.1% was found to be statistically significant. The survival benefit was evident in the drotrecogin alfa group despite the baseline level of protein C. Moreover, the study group exhibited a significant decline in the proinflammatory cytokine IL-6 as well as in the D-dimer level as compared to the placebo group. Bleeding occurred as a complication more often in the drotrecogin alfa group than in the placebo group (3.5% vs. 2.0%), only during the administration of the drug; patients with a predisposition to bleeding, e.g., those with vascular trauma or gastrointestinal ulcerations, were more prone to develop this complication. No other side effects were discovered. The trial was suspended prior to its completion because of the evident benefits of the treatment.

Bibliography

Bernard G, Artigas A, Dellinger P, et al. Clinical expert round table discussion (session 3) at the Margaux Conference on Critical Illness: the role of activated protein C in severe sepsis. *Crit Care Med* 2001;29(7):S75–S77.

Bernard GR, Vincent J-L, Latere P-F, et al. Efficacy and safety of recombinant human activated protein C for severe sepsis. *N Engl J Med* 2001;344(10):699–709.

Dhainaut J-F, Yan SB, Cariou A, Mira J-P. Soluble thrombomodulin, plasma-derived unactivated protein C, and recombinant human activated protein C in sepsis. *Crit Care Med* 2002;30(5):S318–S324.

Finney SJ, Evans TW. Emerging therapies in severe sepsis. *Thorax* 2002;57(Suppl 2):ii8–ii14.

Fisher CJ, Yan SB. Protein C levels as a prognostic indicator of outcome in sepsis and related disease. *Crit Care Med* 2000;38(9):S49–S56.

Grinnell BW, Joyce D. Recombinant human activated protein C: a system modulator of vascular function for treatment of severe sepsis. *Crit Care Med* 2001;29(7): S53–S60.

Hack CE. Tissue factor pathway of coagulation in sepsis. *Crit Care Med* 2000;28(9):S25–S29.

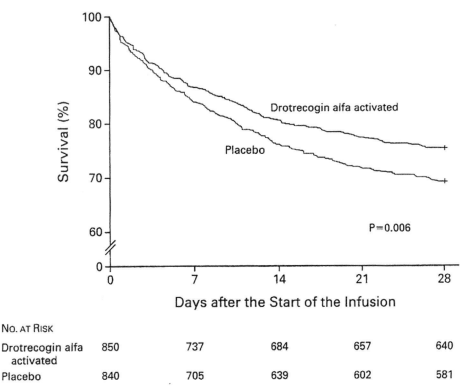

FIG. 6-22 Kaplan-Meier estimates of survival in the Drotrecogin alfa activated group (850 patients) versus the placebo group (840 patients). The survival benefit was measured as significant in the study group.
Source: Reproduced with permission from Bernard GR, Vincent J-L, Latere P-F, et al. Efficacy and safety of recombinant human activated protein C for severe sepsis. *N Engl J Med* 2001;344(10):699–709.

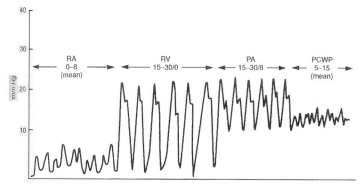

FIG. 6-23 Evolution of the pulmonary artery catheter waveform during the advancement from the right atrium to the pulmonary arterial branch (wedge position). The pressure of each chamber is also shown. RA—right atrium, RV—right ventricle, PA—pulmonary artery, PCWP—pulmonary capillary wedge pressure.
Source: Reproduced with permission from Bongard FS, Sue DY. Critical care monitoring. In: Bongard FS, Sue DY (eds.), *Current Critical Care Diagnosis and Treatment,* 1st ed. Stamford, CT: Appleton & Lange, 1994, 179.

Hotchkiss RS, Karl IE. Medical progress: the pathophysiology and treatment of sepsis. *N Engl J Med* 2003;348(2): 138–150.

Levi M, ten Cate H, van der Poll T. Endothelium: interface between coagulation and inflammation. *Crit Care Med* 2002;30(5):S220–S224.

ten Cate H. Pathophysiology of disseminated intravascular coagulation in sepsis. *Crit Care Med* 2000;28(9):S9–S12.

52. (C) Since its development in 1970, the pulmonary artery catheter, or the Swan-Ganz catheter, has remained an essential tool in the management of critically ill patients. This flexible, balloon-tipped, flow-directed catheter is inserted via a central vein (internal jugular or subclavian vein) and directed through the right heart to a branch of the pulmonary artery. As the catheter is advanced, its location is signaled by variations in the waveform and pressures (Fig. 6-23). At a catheter length of 50–55 cm, a pulmonary capillary wedge tracing is obtained. A more accurate PCWP is generated when the distal tip of the catheter lies in zone III of the lung, where the column of blood between the pulmonary artery and the left atrium remain uninterrupted (Fig. 6-24). In zones I and II, intermittent vascular collapse from surrounding high airway pressures interferes with the continuity of this column of blood. The pulmonary artery catheter directly measures cardiac output, pulmonary artery pressures, and the mixed-venous oxygen saturation. The PCWP, obtained when the balloon is inflated, approximates left atrial pressure and, therefore, left ventricular end diastolic pressure (LVEDP) and volume (LVEDV). The correlation of the PCWP and left atrial pressure is best at a pressure less than 25 mmHg; at a pressure greater than 25 mmHg, the LVEDP is

overestimated. The PCWP serves as a reliable indication of cardiac preload, based on the assumptions that the mitral valve is normal; no pulmonary vascular disease exists; the column of blood between the distal tip of the catheter in the pulmonary artery and the left atrium is intact; and that the LVEDP and LVEDV are directly related. In the absence of a left-to-right or a right-to-left shunt, cardiac output is accurately determined by a thermodilution technique. The oxygen saturation of blood within the pulmonary artery represents the mixed venous oxygen saturation (SvO_2), measured by reflectance spectrophotometry. The systemic utilization of oxygen—the

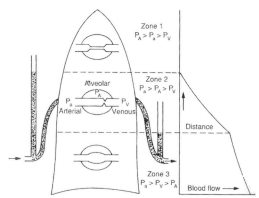

FIG. 6-24 In zone III of the lung, the column of blood between the pulmonary artery catheter tip and the left atrium is uninterrupted by collapse of the surrounding airways, allowing for a more accurate estimation of left ventricular end-diastolic volume and pressure P_a—arterial pressure, P_A—alveolar pressure, P_v—venous pressure.
Source: Reproduced with permission from Bongard FS, Sue DY. Critical care monitoring. In: Bongard FS, Sue DY (eds.), *Current Critical Care Diagnosis and Treatment.* Stamford, CT: Appleton & Lange, 1994, 180.

difference between oxygen delivery and its consumption in the periphery—is reflected by the SvO_2. In the case of a low SvO_2, the supply of oxygen may be deficient or, alternatively, the use of oxygen by the tissues may be increased. A septic patient, however, demonstrates an elevated SvO_2, resulting from a decrease in consumption of oxygen by the peripheral tissues.

Despite the widespread use of the pulmonary artery catheter, few studies have evaluated its role in the treatment of critically ill patients. No absolute indications for pulmonary artery catheter placement exist. Among the situations in which the catheter has been recommended for use include shock refractory to fluid resuscitation, oliguria despite adequate volume replacement, multiple organ failure, cardiac or major vascular surgery, multi system trauma, and complicated MI. A prospective cohort study of 5735 critically ill adult patients from Connors et al. (1996) revealed a significantly increased 30-day mortality associated with the use of a pulmonary artery catheter. The authors cited several possible explanations for this high mortality: the alteration in treatment prompted by the information from the catheter, an association of the use of the catheter with patients at high risk of death, or its complications. Pulmonary artery catheter-related complications occur either during its placement or utilization. The most common complication (50%) is a self-limited arrhythmia, evident on insertion of the catheter through the tricuspid and pulmonary valves. Other complications linked to catheter placement include pneumothorax, catheter knotting, right bundle branch block, tracheal laceration, innominate artery injury, pulmonary artery rupture, and bleeding. The routine use of the catheter is affiliated with air emboli, thromboemboli, infective endocarditis, sepsis, aseptic thrombotic endocarditis, and rupture of the chordae tendineae. These more serious complications transpire in less that 1 in 1000 insertions. Connors et al. (1996) recommended that further study of the value of the pulmonary artery catheter be pursued in light of their finding of an increased mortality. Sandham et al. (2003) undertook a randomized trial comparing goal-directed therapy guided by a pulmonary artery catheter with standard treatment not employing this tool. No significant difference was demonstrated in the mortality or 6-month survival rates among the two groups. The pulmonary artery catheter cohort did exhibit an increased incidence of pulmonary embolus (8 vs. 0%). In sum, the authors detected no benefit to therapy directed by a pulmonary artery catheter; however, the decision to use a pulmonary artery catheter must be tailored to the individual patient.

Bibliography

Bongard FS, Sue DY. Critical care monitoring. In: Bongard FS, Sue DY (eds.), *Current Critical Care Diagnosis & Treatment*, 1st ed. Stamford, CT: Appleton & Lange, 1994, 178–182.

Connors AF, et al. The effectiveness of right heart catheterization in the initial care of critically ill patients. *JAMA* 1996;276(11):889–897.

Manikon M, Grounds M, Rhodes A. The pulmonary artery catheter. *Clin Med* 2002;2(2):101–104.

Sandham JD, et al. A randomized, controlled trial of the use of pulmonary-artery catheters in high-risk surgical patients. *N Engl J Med* 2003;348(1):5–14.

53. **(B)** Controversy exists regarding the optimal goals of resuscitation in shock. Currently, resuscitation is directed toward the correction of blood pressure, heart rate, and urine output; however, studies have demonstrated that an oxygen deficit persists in many of these shock states despite the normalization of these traditional criteria. Often, the abnormalities in perfusion are realized only after increases in oxygen delivery result in pronounced elevations in oxygen consumption by the oxygen-deprived peripheral tissues. In a study of 381 trauma patients, adequately resuscitated based on the current goals, Claridge et al. (2000) demonstrated occult hypoperfusion in 263 cases, based on abnormal lactate levels (>2.4 mmol/L); in those patients with a serum lactate uncorrected by 12 hours after the trauma, the rate of infection and mortality were both increased. Fiddian-Green et al. attribute this continuous oxygen debt to misdistribution of the supply of blood and oxygen to certain tissues. In the case of the gastrointestinal tract, the occult hypoperfusion is further exacerbated by endogenous constriction of the splanchnic vessels as well as the relatively high oxygen demand by the stomach and intestine. Moreover, the gastrointestinal mucosa is especially deprived of oxygen, as compared to the adventitia, because of the shunting of blood directly from the arterioles to the venules within the mucosal vasculature. The poorly perfused gastrointestinal mucosa thus sustains ischemic damage and becomes penetrable, a source of translocated bacteria and toxins.

The gastrointestinal tract has been studied extensively as a portal by which occult hypoperfusion may be detected. Gastric tonometry has become the preferred method for identifying splanchnic hypoperfusion. In a series of 83 patients with circulatory failure, Maynard et al. (1993) demonstrated that gastric mucosal pH was the most reliable sign of inadequate tissue oxygenation, with the mean gastric pH of survivors and nonsurvivors differing significantly on admission (7.40 and 7.28, respectively). This minimally-invasive technique, using a balloon-tipped nasogastric tube, directly measures the partial pressure of carbon dioxide (PCO_2) in the mucosa of the stomach. Gastric tonometry relies on the principle that, at equilibrium, the PCO_2 of the mucosa and lumen of a hollow organ is equivalent. Following placement of a saline-filled silicone balloon, permeable to carbon dioxide, the saline equilibrates with the carbon dioxide of the mucosa, a process with a duration of approximately 60 minutes. Ultimately, the PCO_2 of the saline solution approximates that of the mucosa. The mucosal pH is then calculated using the Henderson-Hasselbach equation, with the bicarbonate level provided by an arterial blood gas. The normal mucosal pH ranges from 7.35 to 7.41. The PCO_2 obtained by tonometry correlates well with values determined directly, especially after including a correction factor for incomplete equilibration; however, the mucosal pH, under conditions of ischemia, varies depending on the method of measurement, direct or tonometric. Measurements are also confounded by the saline within the silicone balloon, in which CO_2 is unstable; Knichwitz et al. (1996) recommend the replacement of saline with a phosphate buffered solution to enhance the accuracy and reliability of the results. Air tonometry also serves as an adequate substitute for saline. The determination of gastric mucosal PCO_2 and pH is also limited by gastric acid secretion and intragastric feeding, both of whichhave unpredictable effects on these values. Groeneveld et al. suggest that gastric acid production be suppressed with histamine-2 (H_2) blockers or proton pump inhibitors. Moreover, intraduodenal feeding avoids difficulties with interpretation, as does stopping intragastric feeding 2 h prior to a measurement. The influence of systemic acid-base disorders on the determination of gastric mucosal PCO_2 is poorly elucidated. Also, systemic bicarbonate, the basis of the calculation of mucosal pH, has been found to be dissimilar to mucosal bicarbonate in low flow states. Additional sources of error include the contamination of the saline solution with residual fluids or bacteria, temperature fluctuations, blood gas analyzer bias, inadequate correction factors, and catheter deadspace. In a review of gastric tonometry, Benjamin and Oropello (1996) pose the question, "Does gastric tonometry work?" In response, these authors point to the mucosal PCO_2 as a potentially useful tool in patient management, with a currently unknown significance; however, they refute the correlation drawn between gastric hypercarbia, a common finding in low-flow states, and hypoxia. The authors suggest that further study of gastric oxygenation be performed to assess for tissue hypoxia.

Bibliography

Benjamin E, Oropello JM. Does gastric tonometry work? No. *Crit Care Clin* 1996;12(3):587–598.

Claridge JA, Crabtree T, Pelletier SJ, et al. Persistent occult hypoperfusion is associated with a significant increase in infection rate and mortality in major trauma patients. *J Trauma* 2000;48(1):8–14.

Fiddian-Green RG, Haglund U, Gutierrez G, Shoemaker WC. Goals for the resuscitation of shock. *Crit Care Med* 1993;21(2):S25–S31.

Groeneveld A, Johan B, Vervloet M, Kolkman JJ. Gastric tonometry in the fed or fasting state? *Crit Care Med* 1998;26(12):1937–1939.

Knichwitz, G, Kuhmann M, Brodner G, et al. Gastric tonometry: precision and reliability are improved by a phosphate buffered solution. *Crit Care Med* 1996;24(3):512–516.

Lee CC, Marill KA, Carter WA, Crupi RS. A current concept of trauma-induced multiorgan failure. *Ann Emerg Med* 2001;38(2):170–176.

Marino PL. *The ICU Book*, 2nd ed. Philadelphia, PA: Lippincott, Williams & Wilkins, 1998, 198–201.

Maynard N, Bihari D, Beale R, et al. Assessment of splanchnic oxygenation by gastric tonometry in patients with acute circulatory failure. *JAMA* 1993;270(10):1203–1210.

Taylor DE, Gutierrez G, Clark C, Hainley S. Measurement of gastric mucosal carbon dioxide tension by saline and air tonometry. *J of Crit Care* 1997;12(4):208–213.

CHAPTER 7

Biostatistics

Edward J. Brizendine

This is a review of basic statistical concepts. Statistical analysis has in general two parts to it, summarizing the data and hypothesis testing. Summarizing the data means describing the data to inform the reader of central tendency and variation. Summary data includes estimates of the mean, standard deviation, median, range, or proportions. Hypothesis testing includes comparing means and proportions and model building. Statistics is a science unto itself and should be performed for the most part by a statistician. The goal of this chapter is to present the more prevalent statistical concepts. The material presented here covers statistical concepts that every physician should be familiar with. With a growing emphasis on evidence-based medicine, a basic understanding of statistics is critical in order for the physician or researcher to make informed decision and conclusion from the paper he is reading.

The questions and answers are definition/conceptual based. No mathematical calculations are needed to answers the questions. The importance here is the understanding of statistical terms and concepts. The actual statistical calculations are best left to the statistician. It is the responsibility of the researcher to understand the numbers given to him so that he can properly interpret the results of his study.

The general references provided are geared toward the nonstatistician/physician. Any good introductory statistics or medical statistics book will cover these basic concepts.

Statisticians play an important role in the whole research process. If you are planning to conduct a research project, you should form a collaborative relationship with a statistician and involve him at the beginning of the project when the study objective is being defined. The statistician has the expertise and knowledge to help through the entire research process. He or she can and should be thought of as an expert in the research process.

Questions

1. Match the different types of data with their definitions.

   (A) categorical
   (B) ordinal
   (C) continuous

      I. data that can be any numeric value.
     II. data that have a finite number of categories.
    III. data that have a finite number of categories with an implied order.

2. Match the different summary statistics for continuous data with their definitions.

   (A) mean
   (B) median
   (C) mode

      I. the middle value when the data are ordered from smallest to largest
     II. the most frequently occurring value
    III. the arithmetic average of a set of numbers

3. Match the different summary statistics for categorical data with their definitions.

   (A) percent
   (B) rate
   (C) prevalence
   (D) incidence

      I. the proportion of cases at a given point in time
     II. the proportion of occurrences out of the total sample
    III. the proportion of occurrences over some measured time period
    IV. the proportion of new cases that occur within a specified time

4. Match each of these measures of variability with their definitions.

   (A) standard deviation
   (B) standard error
   (C) range
   (D) inter-quartile range (IQR)
   (E) confidence interval (CI)

      I. An interval expressing the uncertainty in an estimate
     II. The difference between the 25th and 75th percentiles
    III. A measure of the variability of a set of numbers
    IV. The difference between the maximum and minimum
     V. A measure of the variability of a statistic

5. Match these probabilities used with hypothesis testing with their definitions.

   (A) alpha (α)
   (B) beta (β)
   (C) power
   (D) P-value

      I. the observed significance level
     II. probability of a type I error
    III. 1 – probability of a type II error
    IV. probability of a type II error

6. Match each of these measures of association with their definitions.

   (A) relative risk (RR)
   (B) odds ratio (OR)
   (C) risk difference
   (D) sensitivity

(E) specificity

(F) Pearson correlation(r)

I. the ratio of the odds of disease between two groups

II. the ratio of the risks of disease between two groups

III. the probability of testing positive when the condition is present

IV. the strength of the linear association between two variables

V. the difference in the risk of disease between two groups

VI. the probability of testing negative when the condition is not present

7. A study is conducted to investigate the effectiveness of a new analgesic in relieving headache (HA) pain. A subject's headache intensity is recorded at baseline and subsequently at 15-minute intervals after treatment administration up to 1 hour. Headache intensity is measured using a 0–100 mm visual analog scale (VAS) with 0 representing no headache and 100 representing worst pain imaginable. The initial analysis consists of comparing various outcomes between the treatment group and the control group. For each outcome measure below select the most appropriate statistical test to use to analyze the data.

Outcome
I. HA intensity at 30 minutes
II. Percent of subjects with at least 50% reduction in HA intensity at 30 minutes
III. Time to complete HA relief. Subjects are observed for upto 2 hours

(A) Pearson's chi-square test

(B) Student's *t*-test

(C) Log rank test

8. For each study scenario select the most appropriate study design.

Study scenario
I. A survey on people's use and attitudes toward use of car seat belts
II. Comparing the effectiveness of two analgesics in relieving headache pain in patients presenting to the emergency department with severe headaches
III. Comparing pain intensity of instillation in two ophthalmic anesthetics where each subject gets both treatments
IV. Determining factors associated with skeletal fluorosis in sibling pairs (one sibling with skeletal fluorosis and one without)
V. Review of previously published papers on the effectiveness of hyperdynamic therapy for cerebral vasospasm

(A) randomized clinical trial

(B) metaanalysis

(C) case-control

(D) observational

(E) crossover

9. A study is conducted to investigate the effectiveness of a new analgesic in relieving HA pain. A subject's headache intensity is recorded at baseline and subsequently at 15 min intervals after treatment administration up to 1 h. Headache intensity is measured using a 0–100 mm VAS with 0 representing no headache and 100 representing worst pain imaginable. For each outcome measure below select the most appropriate statistical model to use to analyze the data.

Outcome	Factors
I. HA intensity at 30 minutes	HA intensity at baseline (mm VAS) Age (in years) BMI (kg/m^2)
II. Subject has at least 50% relief in HA intensity at 30 minutes	Treatment group (treatment/control) Gender History of severe headaches (yes/no)
III. Change in HA intensity at 30 minutes	Treatment group (treatment/control) Gender History of severe headaches (yes/no)
IV. Rate of change of HA intensity —measured at baseline and at 15, 30, 45, and 60 minutes	Treatment group (treatment/control) Gender History of severe headaches (yes/no)
V. Time to complete HA relief. Subjects are observed for all most 2 hours	Treatment group (treatment/control) Gender History of severe headaches (yes/no)

(A) analysis of variance (ANOVA)

(B) logistic regression

(C) linear regression

(D) proportional hazards regression

(E) repeated measures ANOVA

Answers and Explanations

1. **I (C), II, (A), III (B)** Examples of categorical data include gender (male/female), randomization group (treatment/control), and mortality (dead/alive). Likert-type scales (no pain, some pain, terrible pain) and the New York Heart Association classification of congestive heart failure are examples of ordinal data. Continuous data examples are age and body mass index (BMI). It is important to know the type of data that is being collected and/or presented. For instance, blood pressure can be captured as the actual systolic blood pressure in mmHg or it may be dichotomized into hypertensive or nonhypertensive. How the data is captured influences the summary measures and statistical tests that can be used. Certain statistical measures and tests can only be used on categorical data while other measures and tests can only be used on continuous data. While ordinal data has its own set of statistical techniques, it falls in between categorical and continuous data and as such, statistical techniques appropriate for either categorical or continuous data can be used.

2. **I (B), II (C), III (A)** These three measures are appropriate only for continuous and ordinal data. The mean is perhaps the most common measure of central tendency for continuous or ordinal data. It is found by adding all of the data values together and then dividing by the sample size. A limitation of using the mean is that it is very sensitive to extreme values—particularly when the sample size is small. For example, suppose the length of stay in days for 7 patients is as follows (1, 2, 2, 1, 30, 1, and 3). The mean of these values is 5.7 days. But most of the patients were in the hospital less than 3 days. Hence the mean in this case is not giving accurate information. It is overestimating the number of days a patient would expect to stay.

   The median is less sensitive to extreme values and is most often used when the data are left or right skewed. Data is said to be left or right skewed if when plotted it no longer has a nice bell shape curve. If the left (or right) tail is elongated, then the data is left (right) skewed. The median is found by ordering all of the data from smallest to largest and then finding the middle data value. It is balanced in that 50% of the observations are below the median and 50% are above. Since 50% of the data is less then the median, another name for the median is the 50th percentile. Other percentiles can also be found. For example, the 25th percentile is the data point where 25% of the data is below it. In the example of length of stay, the median is found to be 2 days. This is a more reasonable estimate of the true length of stay.

   The mode is the most frequently occurring value in a set of data. The mode has no real meaning with continuous data, but it can be used to smmarize ordinal and categorical data. In the length of stay example the mode is 1 day. The mode is a seldom-used summary statistic.

3. **I (C), II (A), III (B), IV (D)** Mathematically, percents and prevalences are defined the same way. They are the number of cases of interest divided by the total number of samples (times 100 to convert to a percent). They differ in semantics. For example, we never say the prevalence of females in a study is 45%; rather, we say the *percent* of females is 45%. Prevalence is used to define the proportion of cases in a population. Similarly, rates and incidences are mathematically similar but differ in how the terms are used. The key difference between percents/prevalences and rates/incidences is the inclusion of a time factor in the divisor.

   To further confuse the difference between prevalence and rates, we often use the term *rate* to express prevalence in a more convenient format. For instance, suppose the prevalence of a disease is 0.014% (i.e., 0.00014). We often report this prevalence or *rate* as of 14 out of 100,000. It is not a rate *per se* since there is not a defined time period in the denominator, but we use the term anyway—most often in epidemiology or population-based studies.

4. **I (E), II (D), III (A), IV (C), V (B)** The standard deviation and standard error are two terms that are often

confused. The standard deviation is a summary statistic (like the mean) used to describe the variability of continuous or ordinal data. Mathematically, it is the square root of the average squared deviation of each data point about the sample mean. The standard error, however, describes the variability of a statistic and can be thought of as being the standard deviation of a statistic. The standard error of a measure depends on the statistic and can often be cumbersome to calculate (even more difficult than the standard deviation!). It should be noted that even the standard deviation has a standard error.

The beauty of the range is its simplicity to calculate, as it is just the difference between the maximum and minimum values. However, it conveys little information about how the data are distributed. Since the interquartile range (IQR) describes the spread of the middle 50% of the data, it is usually more informative.

A CI can be estimated for any statistic. While the method used to determine each is quite different, they are all similar in that they are measures of the uncertainty in a parameter estimate. We usually report a 95% CI. When we say that we are 95% confident, we are commenting on the procedure that we used not on the specific interval calculated. That is, if we were to perform an experiment 100 times and estimate a 95% CI in each of these trials, 95% of these CIs would contain the true population parameter.

In presenting summary statistics to describe the data collected, both a measure of central tendency and its associated measure of variability should be presented. In general, if the mean is reported then the standard deviation or the standard error of the mean should be reported. If the median is reported, then the range or, preferably, the IQR should also be reported. For all statistical measures, a 95% CI should be reported.

5. **I (D), II (A), III (C), IV (B)** In statistical tests of hypotheses, we have a null hypothesis (H_0) and an alternative hypothesis (H_A). In general, we make the assumption in the null hypothesis of "no difference." For example, we assume the effects of two different treatments are the same. In the alternative hypothesis we believe that a difference exists (i.e., the two effects are different from each other). In hypothesis testing we always assume that the null hypothesis is true. We must then have overwhelming evidence to reject the null hypothesis to conclude that a difference exists. We get our evidence to reject or not reject by performing an appropriate statistical test and assessing the P-value obtained. We conclude a difference exists if this P-value is less than our predefined significance level α. In most

situations we define α of to be 0.05, although an α of 0.10 is often used in exploratory analyses.

A problem with hypothesis testing is that an incorrect conclusion can be reached. Hypothesis testing can be thought of in terms of a diagnostic test and is in fact conceptually equivalent. With any diagnostic test we can make an error—such as concluding that a patient has a disease when in fact they do not (i.e., a false positive). A type I error is made when we reject the null hypothesis when in fact the null hypothesis is true. A type II error occurs when we fail to reject the null hypothesis when we should. The sensitivity of a diagnostic test is the same as $(1 - \alpha)$ in hypothesis testing and specificity is the same as power $(1 - \beta)$.

A P-value that falls between 0.05 and 0.10 is often misinterpreted. Frequently an investigator desperately wants to show that a difference exists and so when he gets a P-value of 0.08 he says there is a 'trend' toward significance. In fact, he has often convinced himself from the beginning of the study that a difference exists and is seeking to prove his beliefs rather than on relying on what the data and statistical analyses tell him. This deficiency in hypothesis testing is one of the major reasons most medical journals now require investigators to report confidence intervals instead of (or in addition to) P-values.

The P-value can be viewed as the *observed* significance level. It is the probability of getting a more extreme result assuming under the null hypothesis that no difference exists. It is not the probability that the null hypothesis is true.

6. **I (B), II (A), III (D), IV (F), V (C), VI (E)** While the relative risk (RR) and risk difference can always be calculated, they are not always interpretable. Both are dependent on the prevalence of the disease. The odds ratio (OR), however, is always interpretable and, in cases where the disease prevalence is small, it is a good estimate of the RR.

The sensitivity and specificity are just two of many measures that are used to describe the characteristics of a diagnostic test. Other measures include the accuracy, the positive and negative predictive values, the positive and negative errors, the positive and negative likelihood ratios and the likelihood ratio. All of these measures estimate the error rates that are inherent in all diagnostic tests.

Statistically, correlation and association are not synonymous terms. These terms are often confused by study investigators much to the disdain of statisticians. The term *correlation* is often used when what is really meant is *association*. Correlation is a measure of the strength of the association between two variables.

It is a mathematically defined quantity. Association describes the nature of the relationship between two variables. For instance, an investigator may state that the objective of a study is to assess the *correlation* between use of a treatment and some outcome of interest, but what is really being assessed is the *association* between the treatment and outcome. Two variables that are highly correlated are associated with each other, but two variables that are associated with each other may not be correlated.

7. **I (B), II (A), III (C)** These basic tests are also called univariate tests of association. They are called univariate because the effect of one factor is being assessed on one outcome variable. They are usually performed first to identify factors that are associated with the outcome of interest or to compare demographic characteristics of the two groups. Once factors are identified a more sophisticated model can be developed that uses all of the factors in one model.

The Student's *t*-test is not always the most appropriate test to use when comparing continuous data. One of the underlying assumptions made with the Student's *t*-test is that the data follow a normal distribution. The other and more critical assumption that is made with the *t*-test is that the variances (i.e., the square of the standard deviation) between the two groups are equal. If these assumptions are violated as often is the case when the data is skewed, then the Wilcoxon rank-sum test should be used. The Wilcoxon rank-sum test (also called the Mann-Whitney *U*-test) is a nonparametric test. In nonparametric tests we relax many of the assumptions that we make in using the more common parametric tests. The Wilcoxon test is in essence comparing the medians of the two groups. It should be noted that there is no such thing as nonparametric data. Statistical tests are parametric or nonparametric, whole data are simply data.

The Pearson's chi-square is what is called a large-sample test. That is, it holds when there is a large sample size, but it may give spurious results when the sample size is small or when the outcome of interest has a small probability of occurring. In either of these cases, Fisher's exact test should be used. The Fisher's exact test is like a nonparametric test in that it makes no assumptions but the distribution of the data. Another test that can be used instead of Pearson's chi-square is the Z-test. The Z-test compares two proportions, but is only applicable when there is a large number of subjects in each group. The chi-square test and the Z-test are actually mathematically related to each other.

The log-rank test is a basic test used in survival analysis to compare the survival curves of two or more groups. When comparing survival times, a plot of the survival curves should be made. The Kaplan-Meier method is the most commonly used method of estimating survival curves. Along with estimates of the survival curves, estimates of the median survival times should also be reported. The log-rank test compares the survival curves and is not a direct comparison of median survival times.

While the *P*-value is traditionally reported in manuscripts, an estimate of the effect size (i.e., the difference between groups) is preferred by many medical journals. That is, instead of reporting the *P*-value from a *t*-test comparing two means, the difference in the group means should be estimated along with a 95% CI for the difference.

8. **I (D), II (A), III (E), IV (C), V (B)** All study designs have their own strengths and weaknesses. The appropriate design for a study depends on many factors, including the outcome of interest, availability of a patient population to sample, and investigator resources (time, money, and manpower). A study should not be criticized or dismissed based merely on its design if the design used is the most appropriate to meet the study objectives. While a prospective randomized clinical trial is considered the gold standard for study designs, in many research projects this type of study design is not feasible because of resource constraints or ethical concerns.

Knowing the study design is essential for statistical analysis and interpretation of the results. The correct statistical analysis is dependent on the study design. An investigator should consider the advantages and disadvantages of the study design when it is selected and a reader should also consider them when interpreting the results. Consulting with a statistician when planning the study design should be part of very investigator's plan of action. A good study design will yield a good study—whether or not the results obtained are what the investigator expects.

The strength of the results of a study is dictated by the study design and the stage of the research process. Usually new ideas or investigations start out as case studies. Case studies then lead to observational (exploratory) studies to see if there is evidence that what was seen in the case studies holds in a larger set of subjects. From an observational study, an investigator may generate a hypothesis which can then be tested with a randomized clinical trial. Once several clinical trials have been conducted and published, a metaanalysis can be performed to synthesize the results reported in each of these trials. A metaanalysis is considered to be the most definitive clinical research study since it combines the results of several trials—regardless of whether the results are "positive" or "negative." Hence it is just as important to report negative studies as it is to report positive studies. Both add to the knowledge base of researchers and are indispensable to the physician when making an informed decision on patient care.

9. **I (C), II (B), III (A), IV (E), V (D)** All statistical models have the same form. There is an outcome variable and we wish to explain the variability in this outcome as a function of independent factors. In fact, most statistical models come from a general class of statistical models called general linear models (GLMs). The key point to knowing which statistical model is most appropriate is to know the data type of the outcome variable.

Repeated measures analysis of variance (ANOVA) is used when an outcome measure is recorded at multiple time points on each subject. These repeated outcome measures are correlated with each other within a subject. This correlation of the outcome within a subject must be taken into account when modeling the outcome. It should be noted that the Student's paired *t*-test is really a simplified form of a repeated measures ANOVA using only two time points and no other factors in the model.

Proportional hazards regression is a statistical model used in analysis of survival data. Survival data occurs when the outcome of interest is the time to an event occurrence (e.g., time to death, time to reinfection, fistula patency, etc.). If the subject does not experience the event by the end of the study observation period, the subject's survival time is said to be censored. Proportional hazard models take into account this censoring of the data. If every subject experiences the event, then the time to event occurrence should be analyzed using an ANOVA model.

A regression analysis can be simple, multiple, or multivariate. A simple regression model means that there is one and only one independent factor. A multiple regression model means that there are two or more independent factors. A multivariate regression model means there are two or more dependent factors with one or more independent factors. The terms multiple and multivariate are often mistakenly interchanged, but statistically speaking they imply two very different models.

Bibliography

Campbell MJ, Machin D. *Medical Statistics: A Commonsense Approach*, 2nd ed. Chichester, England: John Wiley & Sons, 1993.

Gardner MJ, Altman DG. Statistics with confidence. *Br Med J*, 1990.

Katz DL. *Epidemiology, Biostatistics, and Preventive Medicine Review*. Philadelphia, PA: W.B. Saunders, 1997.

Norman GR, Streiner DL. *Biostatistics: The Bare Essentials*. St. Louis, MO: BC Decker, 1998.

CHAPTER 8

Fluids and Electrolytes

Sunil Gollapudi, Kevin W. Finkel, and Akinsansoye K. Dosekun

Questions

1. A 70-year-old patient underwent transurethral resection of the prostrate (TURP). An irrigating solution (1.5% glycine) was used to distend the urethra and to obtain a clear surgical field. Postoperatively, in the recovery area, he became agitated, began to vomit, and developed muscle twitching, bradyarrythmias, hypertension, and respiratory failure. What is the most likely cause of his symptoms?

   (A) hyperglycinemia
   (B) urosepsis
   (C) acute hyponatremia
   (D) hypoxia
   (E) hypertensive crisis

2. A 28-year-old male presents to the emergency room after falling while working in the yard. He also complains of feeling weak and dizzy when he stands up. His supine BP is 120/60 mmHg with a heart rate of 96 bpm. On standing he has a BP of 85/30 mmHg and a heart rate of 120 bpm. He states he was fine earlier in the day and drank fluids to try to avoid dehydration. The rest of his examination is unremarkable except for a small laceration on his right elbow. X-rays did not reveal a fracture. His laboratory findings are as follows:

Na^+	137	WBC	8.4
K^+	5.0	Hgb	16.2
Cl^-	101	Hct	48
HCO_3^-	28	Plts	345
BUN	45	Urine Na^+	10
Cr	1.2	Urine Cr	120

   Which of the following would not help support the diagnosis of volume depletion?

   (A) urine creatinine
   (B) blood urea nitrogen (BUN)/Cr ratio

   (C) urinary Na
   (D) Fractional excretion of Na

Questions 3 through 8 refer to the scenario below:
A 40-year-old woman with type 1 diabetes mellitus presents to the emergency room 3 days after developing a febrile illness with confusion, a systolic blood pressure of 90 mmHg, a regular heart rate of 120 bpm. Her examination reveals a purulent draining ulcer on the planter surface of her right foot and admitted to the surgery service. Her laboratory findings are as follows:

Na^+	120
K^+	7.5
Cl^-	86
HCO_3^-	10
BUN	40
Cr	1.3
Glucose	1000
Urine	ketones positive and 3+ proteinuria
ABG	7.27/17/95

3. A bladder catheter is placed and there is minimal urine output. What is the most appropriate intravenous fluid to administer at this time?

   (A) Ringer's lactate
   (B) 3% saline
   (C) 0.9% saline
   (D) 0.9% saline with 20 meq/L of KCl
   (E) D_5W with three ampules of $NaHCO_3$

4. What is the initial acid-base disorder on the patient's arrival to the emergency room?

   (A) metabolic acidosis
   (B) respiratory acidosis
   (C) metabolic acidosis and respiratory acidosis
   (D) metabolic acidosis and respiratory alkalosis
   (E) metabolic alkalosis and respiratory acidosis

5. What is the likely cause of the hyponatremia?

   (A) urinary salt wasting from diabetic kidney disease
   (B) syndrome of inappropriate ADH (SIADH)
   (C) hypovolemia
   (D) hyperlipidemia
   (E) dilutional

6. Which of the following would *least* likely explain the presence of hyperkalemia in this patient?

   (A) decreased distal urinary flow
   (B) metabolic acidosis
   (C) insulin deficiency
   (D) serum hyperosmolality

7. Which of the following does *not* lower serum K concentrations?

   (A) $CaCl_2$
   (B) albuterol
   (C) epinephrine
   (D) insulin
   (E) kayexalate

8. Which of the following is *least* effective in lowering the serum K concentration?

   (A) albuterol
   (B) hemodialysis
   (C) bicarbonate
   (D) insulin
   (E) kayexalate

Questions 9 through 11 refer to scenario below:
The patient from the previous scenario receives 5 L of intravenous 0.9% saline and an insulin drip. Her vital signs stabilize and her urine output increases to 50 mL/h. Her laboratory findings 4 h later are as follows:

Na^+	136
K^+	4.0
Cl^-	110
HCO_3^-	18
BUN	20
Cr	0.7
Glucose	300
PO_4^-	1.7
ABG	7.32/32/102

9. What is the patient's current acid-base disorder?

   (A) metabolic acidosis with anion gap (AG)
   (B) metabolic acidosis without AG
   (C) metabolic acidosis with respiratory acidosis

   (D) metabolic acidosis with respiratory alkalosis
   (E) metabolic acidosis and alkalosis with respiratory alkalosis (triple disorder)

10. What is the most likely cause of the acid-base disorder?

    (A) intravenous administration of sodium-chloride solution
    (B) loss of potential bicarbonate in the urine
    (C) diabetic diarrhea
    (D) low serum aldosterone levels associated with diabetic kidney disease
    (E) renal tubular acidosis (RTA)

11. What is the most appropriate intravenous fluid to administer at this point?

    (A) 0.45% saline
    (B) D_5W 0.45% saline
    (C) D_5W 0.45% saline with 20 meq KCl
    (D) D_5W 0.45% saline with 20 mM KPO_4
    (E) Ringer's lactate

12. Which of the following medications is mostly likely to cause hyponatremia?

    (A) furosemide
    (B) thiazide diuretic
    (C) lithium
    (D) demeclocyline
    (E) lovastatin

13. The patient is a 63-year-old man with end-stage liver failure (secondary to cryptogenic cirrhosis), ascites and hypotension; he is awaiting liver transplantation. He presents in the emergency room with severe decompensation of his liver failure, hepatic encephalopathy, septic shock, and anuric renal failure. There is evidence of disseminated intravascular coagulation. Continuous venovenous hemodialysis (CVVHD) is initiated using a citrate anticoagulation protocol. Twenty-four hours later his chemistries reveal the following:

Na^+	148 meq/L
K^+	3.6 meq/L
Cl^-	98 meq/L
HCO_3^-	16 meq/L
Calcium	17 mg/dL
Ionized calcium	3.8 mg/dL
Phosphate	2.1 mg/dL
Serum osmolality	318 mOsm/L
Serum albumin	1.4 g/dL

What is the most likely explanation of the serum calcium abnormalities?

(A) error in prescribed calcium replacement rates in the CVVHD order

(B) laboratory error

(C) severe hypophosphatemia resulting from excessive dialytic clearances

(D) severe liver failure resulting in the excess metabolism of citrate

(E) this is the typical picture of citrate toxicity

14. Which of the following is *not* an action of angiotensin II?

(A) aldosterone secretion

(B) sodium absorption

(C) efferent arteriolar constriction

(D) arterial dilation

(E) nephrosclerosis in the kidney

15. All of the following symptoms are seen with hypermagnesemia *except*:

(A) tachypnea

(B) depression of reflexes

(C) arrhythmias

(D) hypotension

(E) central nervous system depression

16. Which of the following is *not* a complication of hypophosphatemia?

(A) muscle weakness

(B) respiratory failure

(C) hemolysis

(D) seizures

(E) rhabdomyolysis

Questions 17 and 18 refer to the scenario below:
An 80-year-old man is admitted to hospital from his nursing home for severe obtundation and possibly dehydration. He is diabetic and on tube feeding. The day before admission, he was found on the floor in his room, semicomatose. His urine volume was 1.5L within the first 12 h. Some of his vitals and laboratory findings are as follows:

Blood pressure	128/60 mmHg
Na^+	170 meq/L
Cl^-	130 meq/L
Blood glucose	410 mg/dL
BUN	100 mg/dL
Creatinine	1.5 mg/dL
Serum osmolality	396 mOsm/L
Urine osmolality	408 mOsm/L

17. Which of the following statements is true?

(A) He has a simple central DI.

(B) He is very hyperchloremic and therefore acidotic.

(C) To be described as polyuric, he needs to make a minimum of 4.0 L per day of urine.

(D) He has an ongoing osmotic diuresis.

(E) His well-preserved blood pressure shows that he is not severely volume depleted.

18. Given that he weighs 80 kg, his estimated water deficit is

(A) 5 L

(B) 10 L

(C) 15 L

(D) 18 L

(E) cannot be calculated

19. You are caring for an 80-year-old man in the ICU with multiple injuries after a motor vehicle accident 2 weeks ago. He is currently receiving intravenous heparin for a recently diagnosed pulmonary embolism. The nurse calls you because the patient is hypotensive and unresponsive to boluses of normal saline. Electrolytes measured 24 h ago were normal and the Hb was 11.9. Laboratory findings at this time reveal the following:

Na^+	120
K^+	6.0
Cl^-	100
HCO_3^-	16
BUN	10
Cr	0.7
Glucose	110
Hb	11
ABG	pH 7.30; PCO_2 30; PO_2 100

What is the most likely diagnosis?

(A) gastrointestinal hemorrhage

(B) RTA

(C) sepsis

(D) Addisonian crisis

(E) Bartter's syndrome

20. Which of the following disorders is *not* associated with hypocalcemia?

(A) sarcoidosis

(B) vitamin D deficiency

(C) renal insufficiency

(D) hypoparathyroidism

(E) pancreatitis

21. A 50-year-old woman with chronic renal failure (baseline serum creatinine = 4.0), presents with diarrhea of 2 days duration. Her electrolyte panel reveals the following abnormalities:

Na^+	130 meq/L
Cl^-	102 meq/L
HCO_3^-	6 meq/L
Arterial pH	7.18

What is her acid-base abnormality and what is the clinical explanation for your diagnosis?

(A) severe high AG metabolic acidosis

(B) mixed metabolic acidosis and respiratory alkalosis

(C) mixed high AG metabolic acidosis and hyperchloremic metabolic acidosis

(D) severe hyperchloremic metabolic acidosis

(E) triple acid-base disorder

22. Which hormone is produced by the kidney?

(A) calcitonin

(B) erythropoietin

(C) 25 hydroxyvitamin D

(D) aldosterone

(E) antidiuretic hormone

23. You are caring for a 24-year-old man in the ICU with sepsis from a ruptured diverticular abscess. The patient has been treated for 1 week with aminoglycoside antibiotics and underwent an abdominal CT scan with contrast 2 days ago. The urine output has remained 50 mL/h and a pulmonary wedge pressure by Swan-Ganz catheter is 18. The serum creatinine has increased from 1.0 to 1.8 mg/dL.

Which of the following has been shown to be effective in improving acute renal failure in such patients?

(A) low-dose dopamine

(B) atrial natriuretic peptide (ANP)

(C) furosemide

(D) *N*-acetyl-cysteine (Mucomyst)

(E) none of the above

24. A 55-year-old male with benign prostatic hypertrophy is admitted to the urological service for acute renal failure. A Foley catheter is placed and 2 L of urine is initially drained. He has no other medical history and his baseline creatinine is 1. His initial laboratory findings are as follows:

Na^+	138
K^+	5.0
Cl^-	118
HCO_3^-	24
BUN	52
Cr	3.1

Which of the following abnormalities would not be expected to occur?

(A) hyponatremia

(B) hypernatremia

(C) hyperkalemia

(D) hypophosphatemia

(E) hypomagnesmia

25. You are caring for a man with bladder cancer who has undergone cystectomy with urinary drainage via an ileal conduit. Which of the following is *not* a complication of urinary diversions?

(A) metabolic acidosis

(B) urolithiasis

(C) cholelithiasis

(D) hyperkalemia

(E) adenocarcinoma

26. Hyperkalemia is associated with which disorder?

(A) type 1 distal RTA

(B) type 2 proximal RTA

(C) type 4 RTA

(D) Gitelman's syndrome

27. A 29-year-old male presents to your office after waking up the previous night with sudden right lower quadrant pain. He states that he vomited several times last night and has been unable to eat or drink. He feels weak and tired. He describes his pain as constant and nonradiating. He has no other past medical history. His vitals include a heart rate of 120 bpm, a BP of 94/56 mmHg, and a temperature of 100.7°F. Your physical examination is significant for guarding and a psoas sign. You suspect appendicitis and admit him to the hospital for an appendectomy. The patient's laboratory findings are the following:

Na^+	143	WBC	14.2
K^+	4	Hgb	15
Cl^-	101	HCT	46
HCO_3^-	23	Plts	250
BUN	38	Serum	305
Cr	1.0	osmolarity	
Ca^{2+}	9	ABG	pH 7.47; PCO_2 30;
Alb	4		PO_2 93

What acid-base disorder does this patient have?

(A) respiratory alkalosis

(B) respiratory alkalosis and metabolic acidosis

(C) respiratory alkalosis, metabolic acidosis, and metabolic alkalosis

(D) respiratory acidosis and metabolic alkalosis

28. A 65-year-old female has been found to have a infrarenal abdominal aortic aneurysm by ultrasound during an evaluation for renal insufficiency. She is scheduled for a CT scan with IV contrast. Her only other medical history is hypertension. Her creatinine cleareance is 57 mL/min with a creatinine of 1.2. Her list of medications is the following:

- furosemide: 20 mg PO qd
- ramapril: 10 mg PO qd
- asa: 81 mg PO qd
- atrovastatin: 10 mg PO qhs

What recommendation will increase the risk of contrast nephropathy?

(A) Hydration with normal saline 1 mL/kg/h for 12 h before and after CT

(B) Withdrawal of diuretic

(C) Acetylcysteine 600 mg PO bid for 2 days starting 1 day before the procedure

(D) Use of mannitol for forced diuresis

Questions 29 and 30 refer to the scenario below:
A 75-year-old man with diabetic kidney disease and chronic obstructive pulmonary disease (COPD) from tobacco use is in the surgical ICU following a motor vehicle accident that caused multiple injuries. The patient is mechanically ventilated and has developed multiple-organ dysfunction syndrome (MODS) from sepsis. His laboratory findings are as follows:

Na^+	144
K^+	4.6
Cl^-	110
HCO_3^-	14
BUN	50
Cr	3.5
ABG	pH 7.00; PCO_2 60; PO_2 95

29. What is the patient's acid-base disorder?

(A) AG metabolic acidosis

(B) non-AG metabolic acidosis

(C) respiratory acidosis

(D) AG and non-AG metabolic acidosis

(E) metabolic acidosis and respiratory acidosis

30. Which of the following treatments for metabolic acidosis will *not* worsen the patient's elevated PCO_2?

(A) bicarbonate

(B) citrate

(C) acetate

(D) lactate

(E) *N*-tromethamine (THAM)

31. Which ion channel does amiloride inhibit?

(A) sodium channel in the collecting tubule

(B) sodium-potassium-2 chloride channel in the thick ascending limb of the loop of Henle

(C) sodium-chloride channel in the distal convoluted tubule

(D) aquaporin 2 water channel in the collecting tubule

32. Which of the following molecules does not aid in the secretion of acids by the kidney?

(A) ammonia

(B) urea

(C) phosphate

(D) sulfate

Questions 33 and 34 refer to the scenario below:
A 44-year-old man, well-known to you with a duodenal ulcer presents with intractable vomiting for 3 days. His laboratory findings are given below:

Na^+	140 meq/L	Urine pH	7.0
K^+	1.8 meq/L	Urine Na^+	40 meq/L
Cl^-	80 meq/L	Urine K^+	80 meq/L
HCO_3^-	44 meq/L	Urine Cl^-	<10 meq/L
Arterial pH	7.50		
Arterial PCO_2	52 mmHg		

33. What is the acid-base disorder and how is his severe hypokalemia explained?

(A) metabolic alkalosis with massive K^+ losses in his vomitus

(B) respiratory acidosis resulting from muscle fatigue

(C) metabolic alkalosis from vomiting and hypokalemia from renal K^+ losses

(D) hypokalemia is the result of intracellular shifts secondary to the alkalemia

(E) hypokalemia is the result of inadequate oral intake

34. What further information can be obtained from an analysis of the urinary electrolytes?

   (A) The patient is definitely not volume depleted, as evidenced by his urine sodium concentration.

   (B) The high urine pH is most likely related to a urinary infection.

   (C) The high urine pH must be an error; the test should be repeated.

   (D) A severe tubular dysfunction is responsible for such potassium wasting in the presence of severe hypokalemia.

   (E) In the alkalotic patient, urinary chloride concentration is a more reliable indicator of volume status than urinary sodium concentration.

35. You admit a 69-year-old man for resection of squamous cell carcinoma of the lung. Laboratories demonstrate a serum calcium level of 16. Which of the following will *not* lower the calcium level?

   (A) gallium nitrate

   (B) calcitonin

   (C) furosemide

   (D) hydrochlorothiazide

   (E) bisphosphonates

36. Which of the following causes of acute renal failure is not associated with anuria (<50 mL per day urine output)?

   (A) obstruction

   (B) cortical necrosis

   (C) aortic dissection

   (D) glomerulonephritis

   (E) contrast nephropathy

37. You are caring for a 65-year-old woman who underwent repair of an abdominal aortic aneurysm 1 week ago. Her hospital course has been complicated by intermittent episodes of hypotension necessitating fluid resuscitation and vasopressors. Because of persistent fevers, she is receiving cephalosporin and aminoglycoside antibiotics. She received intravenous radiocontrast on the day prior to surgery. She has now developed decreasing urine output associated with a rising serum creatinine level. On examination, BP is 130/68 P110; heart and lung examination is normal; abdomen is mildly diffusely tender without rebound; hypoactive bowel sounds; lower extremities have a

nonraised, reddish rash with a reticular pattern. Laboratory findings are as follows:

BUN	60
Cr	4.5
WBC	15 (12% eosinophils)
ESR	115
Bili	0.8
LDH	150
AST/ALT	35/40
Amylase	900
U/A	10–20 RBC/Hpf

What is the most likely cause of the acute renal failure?

   (A) contrast nephropathy

   (B) ischemic acute tubular necrosis (ATN)

   (C) aminoglycoside nephrotoxicity

   (D) allergic interstitial nephritis from cephalosporin

   (E) cholesterol emboli syndrome

38. Magnesium is not absorbed in which segments of the nephron?

   (A) proximal convoluted tubule

   (B) thin ascending segment of loop of Henle

   (C) thick ascending segment of loop of Henle

   (D) distal convoluted tubule

39. A 40-year-old man with end-stage renal disease is admitted to hospital for elective A-V access surgery. His medications include calcium channel antagonists and ACE inhibitors for his high blood pressure, phosphate binders, a vitamin D analogue and multivitamins. His serum calcium and phosphate levels are 11.4 and 5.8 mg/dL, respectively. He complains of severe constipation since his surgery, and three doses of fleet phospho-soda are administered in the course of the night. His morning laboratory data reveal a life-threatening hyperphosphatemia (18 mg/dL). What is the appropriate measure to take?

   (A) intravenous injection of 1,25 dihydroxy vitamin D_3 (calcitriol)

   (B) intravenous infusion of alkali ($NaHCO_3$) to facilitate intracellular shift of phosphate

   (C) obtain a nephrology consultation and have emergent dialysis started (CVVHD, or conventional intermittent hemodialysis)

   (D) take a conservative approach and follow serial phosphate levels closely; do not give any further enemas

40. A patient with acute renal failure has a urine dipstick with 4+ blood but only 2–3 red blood cells (RBCs) per HPF on microscopic examination. What is the cause of renal failure?

(A) rhabomyolysis
(B) tumor lysis syndrome
(C) multiple myeloma
(D) vasculitis
(E) hemolytic-uremic syndrome (HUS)

41. During passage from the glomerular capillary to Bowman's space what structure does the glomerular filtrate *not* pass through?

(A) glomerular basement membrane
(B) glomerular capillary fenestrated endothelium
(C) Bowman's visceral epithelial cells
(D) vasa recta

42. You are called by a nurse about a 24-year-old male who was admitted to the intensive care unit after a motor vehicle accident 18 h ago. He was initially seen in the trauma room and found to have a compound fracture of right femur, several fractured ribs, multiple abrasions, and in a comatose state. A CT scan of his head was unremarkable at that time. His vital signs and fractures were stabilized and he was placed on a ventilator. The nurse has noticed 4 L of urine output in the last hour. This was a change from the previous 12 h when he had a total of 1 L of urine output. His intravenous fluid is 0.9% saline at 100 mL/h and he is currently on no scheduled medications. His vitals include a BP of 135/82 mmHg, pulse of 90/min, temperature of 99.2°F, and respirations of 16. The following laboratory tests are ordered:

Admitting labs		Current labs			
Na⁺	139	Na⁺	150	Serum osmolarity	313
K⁺	4	K⁺	4.5	Urine osmolarity	50
Cl⁻	105	Cl⁻	110		
HCO₃⁻	24	HCO₃⁻	27		
BUN	12	BUN	30		
Cr	0.9	Cr	1.0		
Glu	98	Glu	110		

What is the most likely diagnosis?

(A) osmotic diuresis
(B) adrenal insufficiency
(C) central DI
(D) nephrogenic DI
(E) cerebral salt wasting

43. What segment of the nephron is responsible for the majority of sodium absorption?

(A) proximal convoluted tubule
(B) loop of Henle
(C) distal convoluted tubule
(D) collecting tubule

44. You are caring for a 50-year-old man who is 3 years out from a cadaveric renal transplant for diabetic nephropathy. He had a single episode of vascular rejection 1 month after transplant, but otherwise has done well with a baseline serum Cr of 1.8 mg/dL. He is admitted to your service with increasing fatigue, dyspnea with exertion, and acute renal failure. His medications include cyclosporine, mycophenolate mofetil, prednisone, and nifedipine. On examination, he is pale and weak with a BP of 150/95 mmHg and a pulse of 110/min. He has a few scattered ecchymoses on his skin, but otherwise the examination is normal.

Laboratory values 3 months ago		Laboratory findings on admission	
Na⁺	142	Na⁺	144
K⁺	4.8	K⁺	6.7
Cl⁻	105	Cl⁻	110
HCO₃⁻	25	HCO₃⁻	17
BUN	30	BUN	68
Cr	1.8	Cr	5.8
LDH	150	LDH	650
Bili	0.7	Bili	2.9
Alb	3.9	Alb	3.5
AlkP	78	AlkP	80
WBC	8	WBC	14
Hb	11	Hb	5
Hct	33	Hct	15
Plts	221	Plts	45
U/A	trace pro	U/A	2+ protein
No cells			20–30 RBC/Hpf

Which of the following is the most appropriate step in the evaluation of your patient?

(A) schedule a renal biopsy
(B) give IV pulse steroids
(C) order a renal ultrasound
(S) obtain a right upper quadrant (RUQ) ultrasound
(E) review the peripheral smear looking for schiztocytes

Answers and Explanations

1. (C) A transurethral resection syndrome (TURS) has been reported in 1–7% of patients undergoing TURP. The syndrome is attributed to varying degrees of absorption of the irrigating fluid (300 mL to 4 L), via the exposed or open vascular bed of the prostate. The severity of the syndrome depends on the volume of solution absorbed as well as the nature of the irrigating solution. Amongst the currently used irrigating solutions are glycine (most common), mannitol, and sorbitol. Irrigation with glycine is associated with a parasthesia (prickling and burning sensation of the skin), transient blindness, hypertension and chest pain, nausea, vomiting, followed by signs of encephalopathy—confusion, apprehension, muscular twitching, and altered consciousness. Grand mal seizures, severe hypotension, bradyarrythmias, pulmonary edema, and cardiac arrest may supervene in the most severe cases. There is usually a severe hyponatremia, but other pathogenetic factors are thought to play a role in this syndrome, including volume overload and acute hypertension, the result of not only the volume of absorbed irrigating solution, but also of its hypertonicity, which will cause fluid shifts from intracellular to intravascular compartment.

The absorbed glycine is rapidly redistributed in all of the fluid compartments. In the cells, it is metabolized and free water is released so that hyponatremia is actually dilutional. Another product of glycine metabolism is ammonia, and this has been suggested to contribute to the encephalopathy. Finally, hyperkalemia results from the transcellular fluid shifts and may contribute to the arrythmias and hemodynamic instability in this syndrome.

Bibliography

Farber MD, Schmidt RJ, Bear RA, Narins RG. Management of fluid, electrolyte and acid base disorders in surgical patients. In: Narins RG, ed., *Maxwell and Kleeman's Clinical Disorders of Fluid and Electrolyte Metabolism*, 5th ed. New York: McGraw-Hill, 1993:1407–1463.

2. (A) The serum chemistries and urine indices are a result of compensatory mechanisms to maintain volume status. The indices reflect relative handling of sodium, urea, and creatinine in a volume depleted state. With volume depletion, there is an increase in the renin-angiotension-aldosterone system (RAAS) and the sympathetic nervous system leading to increased absorption of sodium along the nephron to increase volume status. The RAAS system generates angiotensen II which increases sodium absorption in the proximal tubule and promotes aldosterone secretion; aldosterone increases Na uptake in the collecting tubule. Sympathetic outflow to the kidney causes an increase in sodium absorption and renin release. Similarly urea is absorbed along the nephron. Urea absorption is enhanced by volume depletion by a decreased glomerular filtration rate (GFR) and antidiuretic hormone (ADH) release. Renal handling of creatinine begins with filtration through the glomerulus then excretion into the tubule along the nephron. There is some creatinine absorption, but this is minimal. The cumulative effects are a sodium avid state with low urine sodium and increased sodium and urea uptake relative to creatinine. These are manifested in a fractional excretion of Na <1%, low urine Na <20, and BUN/Cr >20 in patients with a volume depleted state, all of which are present in this patient. Since renal creatinine handling is not significantly altered by volume depletion it would not be helpful. It is important to note that other pathologic processes mimic these laboratory findings, requiring analysis of the entire patient to make diagnosis and not just laboratory data.

Bibliography

Blantz RC. Pathophysiology of pre-renal azotemia. *Kidney Int* 1998;53(2):512–523.

Miller TR, et al. Urinary diagnostic indices in acute renal failure: a prospective study. Ann Intern Med 1978; 89(1):47–50.

3. **(C)** The patient is volume depleted as evidenced by the vital signs and lack of urine output. The volume depletion is a result of poor oral intake combined with polyuria induced by glycosuria. Although such patients are usually total body K^+ depleted, K^+ should not be administered until the establishment of good urinary flow. Lactated Ringer's solution contains K^+, as well as unnecessary alkali. Hypertonic saline is not indicated in the treatment of hyponatremia associated with diabetic ketoacidosis (DKA).

Bibliography

Powers AC. Diabetes mellitus. In: Braunwald (ed.), *Harrison's Principles of Internal Medicine*, 15th ed. New York, NY: McGraw-Hill, 2001, 2116–2118.

4. **(D)** The low pH and low bicarbonate concentration indicates the patient has a metabolic acidosis. The appropriate respiratory response should be a fall in the PCO_2 of 1.25x the fall in bicarbonate, in this case 17.5. If the measured PCO_2 were 22.5, then the disorder would be a pure metabolic acidosis with respiratory compensation. It would be incorrect to call it a respiratory alkalosis since "-osis" implies a disorder rather than appropriate compensation. In this case, the PCO_2 of 17 is lower than mere compensation, so there is in fact a secondary disorder of respiratory alkalosis. In this patient, the metabolic acidosis is secondary to DKA and the patient is also hyperventilating because of ketosis and Kaussmaul breathing.

Bibliography

Finkel KW, DuBose TJ. Metabolic acidosis. In: DuBose TJ, Hamm L (eds.), *Acid-Base and Electrolyte Disorders: A Companion to Brenner & Rectors The Kidney*. Philadelphia, PA: W.B. Saunders, 2002, 56–57.

5. **(E)** Hyponatremia can develop in disorders associated with low, normal, or high serum osmolality. In severe hyperglycemia, the high serum osmolality draws water from the intracellular space into the serum and dilutes the serum sodium concentration. The serum sodium will fall approximately 2 meq/L for every 100 mg/dL rise in serum glucose concentration. In this case, correction of hyperglycemia alone will correct the sodium concentration. SIADH is associated with hyponatremia and a low serum osmolality. Hyperlipidemia at one time caused a false hyponatremia (pseudohyponatremia) because of measuring technique. Newer assays for serum sodium measurements have alleviated this problem. Renal salt wasting is a rare disorder not associated with diabetic nephropathy.

Bibliography

Finkel KW. Electrolyte abnormalities in the intensive care unit. In: DuBose TJ, Hamm L (eds.), *Acid-Base and Electrolyte Disorders: A Companion to Brenner & Rector's The Kidney*. Philadelphia, PA: W.B. Saunders, 2002, 348–350.

6. **(B)** Decreased distal urinary flow decreases renal excretion of potassium. Insulin deficiency allows potassium to leak out of cells. Serum hyperosmolality drags water out of cells along with intracellular potassium. The effect of metabolic acidosis on potassium shift is dependent on the type of acidosis. In mineral acidosis, such as infusion of HCl, chloride is restricted to the extracellular space, so that potassium must leave the cell as hydrogen ions enter in order to maintain electroneutrality. In organic acidoses, such as DKA or lactic acidosis, the anion accompanies hydrogen ion entering the cell so that potassium exchange is minimal. Although acidosis does contribute to the hyperkalemia, it is the least important of the choices.

Bibliography

Perez GO, Oster JR, Vaamonde CA. Serum potassium concentration in acidemic states. *Nephron* 1981;27:233–243.

7. **(A)** $CaCl_2$ stabilizes cardiac membrane potential in the face of hyperkalemia and is the drug of first choice in treating hyperkalemia associated with changes on the electrocardiogram (ECG); however, it does not lower the potassium concentration. The other choices lower the potassium concentration either by shifting potassium into cells or hastening its removal from the body.

Bibliography

Weiner ID, Wingo CS. Hyperkalemia. In: DuBose TJ, Hamm L (eds.), *Acid-Base and Electrolyte Disorders: A Companion to Brenner & Rector's The Kidney*. Philadelphia, PA: W.B. Saunders, 2002, 406–407.

8. **(C)** Kayexalate and dialysis both lower potassium levels by removing it from the body. Insulin and inhaled albuterol are highly effective in temporarily lowering potassium concentrations by driving it into the intracellular compartment. As described above, because of the minimal effect of organic acidosis on potassium concentrations, bicarbonate administration is the least effective means.

Bibliography

Allon M, Shanklin N. Effect of bicarbonate administration on plasma potassium in dialysis patients: interactions with insulin and albuterol. *Am J Kidney Dis* 1996;28:508–514.

9. **(B)** The pH and bicarbonate are both low indicating a metabolic acidosis. The AG is calculated to be 8, which is normal. The expected fall in PCO_2 is 1.25×6, or

approximately 8. Since the PCO_2 has fallen appropriately to 32, this is a pure non-AG metabolic acidosis with respiratory compensation.

10. **(B)** Although all of the listed conditions cause a non-AG metabolic acidosis, it is the loss of potential bicarbonate in the urine in the form of ketones that is the most likely explanation. In DKA, the production of ketones leads to the generation of hydrogen ions and the consumption of bicarbonate. In the presence of insulin, metabolism of ketones results in the regeneration of bicarbonate. Any ketones lost in the urine during the polyuria associated with glycosuria are no longer available for regeneration of bicarbonate. Administration of insulin will correct the AG acidosis as the ketones present in the serum are converted to bicarbonate. The resulting non-AG acidosis represents the "bicarbonate" lost in the urine as ketones. The non-AG acidosis will correct over 3–4 days by generation of new bicarbonate by the kidneys.

Bibliography

Adrogue HJ, Eknoyan G, Suki WK. Diabetic ketoacidosis: the role of the kidney in the acid-base homeostasis re-evaluated. *Kidney Int* 1984;25:591.

11. **(D)** Although the patient was initially hyperkalemic, it was the result of decreased distal urinary flow, hyperosmolality, and insulin deficiency. In fact this patient is likely total body potassium depleted as the result of urinary losses of potassium incurred by the osmotic diuresis induced by the glycosuria. It was only masked by the aforementioned factors. Once good urinary flow is established and treatment with hydration and insulin is initiated, patients are at risk of developing severe hypokalemia. Therefore, potassium should be added to the intravenous fluids. Once the glucose falls to 300 mg/dL, glucose is required to avoid hypoglycemia. In addition, this patient's serum phosphorous is borderline low. Patients with DKA are typically phosphate depleted which will be exacerbated by the infusion of insulin by driving phosphorous into cells. Therefore, to avoid the complications of hypophosphatemia, phosphate should also be provided.

Bibliography

Foster DW, McGarry JD. The metabolic derangements and treatment of diabetic ketoacidosis. *N Engl J Med* 1983;309:159.

12. **(B)** Thazide diuretics have been documented to cause hyponatremia. Proposed mechanisms for hyponatremia include (1) inhibition of dilution at the distal convoluted tubule leading to an increase in minimum urinary osmolarity, (2) a decrease in GFR resulting in less tubular fluid (i.e., free water) reaching the collecting tubule to be excreted, (3) a volume depleted state that increases ADH causing free water reabsorption, and (4) transcellular shifts of sodium to the intracellular space secondary to potassium losses. Loop diuretics (furosemide) have less frequently been documented to cause hyponatermia. Loop diuretics inhibit the Na-K-2CL transporter in the thick ascending limb in the loop of Henle which is involved in both the diluting and concentrating system. By altering the concentrating system, the medullar interstitium is diluted and free water absorption is decreased. Loop diuretics also act for short periods of time, limiting sodium loss. Lithium and demeclocyline are both known to cause diabetes insipidus (DI) leading to hypernatremia. Hyponatremia is not a common side effect of lovastatin.

Bibliography

Holtzman, et al. Nephrogenic diabetes insipidus: causes revealed. *Hosp Pract* 1994;29(3):89–93, 97–98, 103–104.

Mevacor (Lovastatin). In: Sifton DW (ed.), *Physicians Desk Reference*, 57th ed. Montvale, NJ: Thomson PDR, 2003, 2036–2040.

Spital A. Diuretic-induced hyponatremia. *Am J Nephrol* 1999;19:447–452.

13. **(E)** Citrate has been used as an anticoagulant (especially in blood banking and in plasmapheresis), for more than 50 years. More recently, it has been used in continuous renal replacement procedures, to anticoagulate the extracorporeal system (regional anticoagulation), and thereby minimize the risk of bleeding. Anticoagulation is achieved by the chelation of ionized calcium. Thus, there is a potential risk of ionized hypocalcemia. This is prevented by a calcium replacement infusion which is titrated to maintain ionized calcium at acceptable levels. Both the citrate/calcium complex and any extra citrate are either cleared by the dialysis filter, or metabolized in citrate-metabolizing tissues (liver and muscle), with the generation of bicarbonate. In patients with severe liver disease, there may occur, the accumulation of unmetabolized citrate, a hypercitric acidemia, severe ionized hypocalcemia, resulting from excessive calcium chelation, and a very large increase in the total calcium, the result of accumulation of the citrate/calcium complex. This complication should be anticipated in patients with severe liver dysfunction and close watch should be kept of the difference between total and ionized calcium, as well as the AG. It can be minimized or avoided by not using citrate anticoagulation in patients at risk, or using either much lower citrate infusion rates or lower concentrations of citrate for anticoagulation. Paradoxically, on cessation of, or

interruption of continuous dialysis, a severe total and ionized hypercalcemia tends to develop as a result of the delayed metabolism of the previously accumulated citrate/calcium complex.

Bibliography

Maria-Kriesche HU, Finkel KW, Gitomer JJ, Dubose T. Unsuspected severe hypocalcemia during continuous venovenous hemodialysis with regional citrate anticoagulation. *Am J Kidney Dis* 1999;33:1–4.

14. **(D)** Angiotensin II is generated through a cascade of enzymes. Angiotensinogen is synthesized in the liver. The presence of renin cleaves angiotensinogen to angiotensin I. Angiotensin I is cleaved further to obtain angiotensin II by angiotensin cleaving enzyme (ACE). ACE is synthesized in the lungs and released into the plasma. The effects of angiotensin II are mediated mainly through its two receptors, AT1 and AT2. The effects of AT1 and AT2 are generally antagonistic. The AT1 receptor is responsible for angiotensin II's effects on aldosterone secretion, arterial constriction, sodium reabsorption, glomerular efferent arteriolar constriction, nephrosclerosis in the kidney, and cardiac hypertrophy.

Bibliography

Unger T. Neurohormonal modulation in cardiovascular disease. *Am Heart J* 2000;(1 pt 2):S2–S8.

15. **(A)** Hypermagnesemia develops when magnesium intake exceeds excretion by the kidney. The most common cause of this is renal insufficiency, leading to decreased magnesium clearance. Other situations in which hypermagnesemia has been documented are during its use as a tocolytic in obstetrics, use of antacids that contain magnesium, and excess absorption from the sigmoid colon when magnesium is used as a cathartic. Hypermagnesemia affects neurons, neuromuscular junctions, and muscles to produce its effect. The symptoms are related to its concentration in the blood and range from hypotension to death. The treatment of hypermagnesemia usually involves withholding magnesium intake and allowing for excretion to occur through the kidneys. In the presence of life-threatening symptoms, hypermagnesemia can be antagonized with calcium. If renal insufficiency is significant enough that magnesium excretion is hindered then dialysis is the only option to decrease magnesium levels.

Bibliography

Van Hook JW. Endocrine crises. Hypermagnesemia. *Crit Care Clin* 1991;7(1):215–223.

16. **(D)** High-energy phosphate is needed by cells to provide adenosine triphosphate (ATP) for multiple functions. Lack of phosphate impairs muscle function and the ability of red cells to maintain cell membrane integrity. Therefore, common complications of hypophosphatemia include muscle weakness with rhabdomyolyis and respiratory failure, and hemolysis.

Bibliography

Bugg NC, Jones JA. Hypophosphatemia: pathophysiology, effects and management on the intensive care unit. *Anaesthesia* 1998;53:895–902.

17. **(D)** A urine output of 2.0 L per day can be described as polyuria. The urine osmolality of 408 mOsm/L is not consistent with a simple central DI. There is an ongoing osmotic diuresis which is attributable to hyperglycemia, glycosuria, and azotemia. A measurement of his urine urea concentration should reveal a high level. He is not necessarily acidotic; rather, his high serum chloride is simply in keeping with the need for electrical neutrality, given a sodium of 170 meq/L. He is likely to be severely volume depleted; this is camouflaged by a high serum osmolality, which helps to preserve intravascular fluid volume and therefore maintain a good blood pressure. This must be fully considered during treatment as too rapid a dilution of his serum back toward normal osmolality can cause a redistribution of body fluids that will result in severe hypovolemia and even possibly, shock.

Bibliography

Morrrison, L, Singer I. Hyperosmolal states. In: Narins RG, ed., *Maxwell and Kleeman's Clinical Disorders of Fluid and Electrolyte Metabolism*, 5th ed. New York: McGraw-Hill, 1993:617–658.

18. **(B)** Given a weight of 80 kg, his total body water is approximately 60% of this (48 L). If we presume that this has a sodium concentration of 170 meq/L, how much water will need to be added to dilute this down to 140 meq/L. If we assume that he has the same content of sodium, then the equation below should hold true: $170 \times 48 = 140 \times$ (new TBW).

Therefore, the new TBW $\times 170 = 48/140$. The difference of new TBW and current TBW is the free water deficit $= 170 \times 48/140 - 48$ L ~ 10 L.

Bibliography

Morrrison, L, Singer I. Hyperosmolal states. In: Narins RG, ed., *Maxwell and Kleeman's Clinical Disorders of Fluid and Electrolyte Metabolism*, 5th ed. New York: McGraw-Hill, 1993:617–658.

19. **(D)** The constellation of hypotension unresponsive to fluid resuscitation with hyponatremia, hyperkalemia, and a non-AG metabolic acidosis suggests Addisonian crisis. It is likely the result of heparin-induced adrenal

hemorrhage. Gastrointestinal bleeding is less likely given the stable Hb. It also would not explain the electrolyte disorder. This would also be true for sepsis and RTA. Bartter's syndrome causes a metabolic alkalosis.

Bibliography

Williams G, Dluhy R. Diseases of the adrenal cortex. In: Isselbacher, KJ (ed.), *Harrison's Principles of Internal Medicine*, 13th ed. New York, NY: McGraw-Hill, 1994, 1970–1973.

20. **(A)** Calcium homeostasis requires the kidney, the parathyroid gland, and vitamin D to maintain calcium levels. Failure of these mechanisms leads to hypocalcemia. Renal insufficiency leads to hypocalcemia by the development of hyperphosphatemia, resistance to parathyroid hormone (PTH) by bone, and decreased synthesis of vitamin D. Hyperphosphatemia, a result of decreased GFR, is believed to cause hypocalcemia by the binding calcium and depositing it into tissues. PTH is secreted by the parathyroid gland when decreased ionized calcium is present. PTH is responsible for increased synthesis of 1,25 vitamin D, increased absorption of calcium and phosphate wasting by the kidney, and increased activity of osteoclasts in bones all of which increase plasma calcium level. A deficiency in PTH by hypoparathyroidism or resistance of bone to PTH can lead to hypocalcemia. 1,25 Vitamin D, the most potent form of vitamin D, is result of series of enzymatic steps. The final step of synthesis occurs in the proximal tubules in the kidney. Vitamin D helps maintain calcium levels by increasing absorption of calcium from the GI tract and augments the effects of PTH on bone. Hypocalcemia from pancreatitis has been ascribed to the action of pancreatic lipase on omental and retroperitoneal fat, with the release of fatty acids that, in turn, bind calcium. Sarcoidosis, like other granulomatosis diseases, can produce excess quantities of vitamin D and can lead to a hypercalcemic state.

Bibliography

Bourke E, et al. Assessment of hypocalcemia and hypercalcemia. *Clin Lab Med* 1993;13(1):157–181.
Sharma OP. Hypercalcemia in granulomatous disorders: a clinical review. *Curr Opin Pulm Med* 2000;6(5):442–447.

21. **(C)** This case illustrates how much information is obtainable from a close examination of serum electrolytes alone. The patient has an AG of 22 and therefore a high AG acidosis. The increase in AG (from a normal of 10–12 meq/L) is 10 meq/L. If the acidosis were explained solely by the AG, then we should expect a diminution of bicarbonate of comparable degree; 8–12 meq/L. The HCO_3 should be in the range of 14–18 meq/L. Why, then, is the patient's HCO_3^- as low as 6 meq/L? This suggests that there is a mixed acid-base disorder, with an additional abnormality that lowers the bicarbonate level from the expected 14–18 meq/L to the actual 6 meq/L. This may be a respiratory alkalosis or a hyperchloremic metabolic acidosis. The pH of 7.18 suggests the diagnosis of mixed AG metabolic acidosis and hyperchloremic metabolic acidosis. This is in concordance with the clinical history, with chronic renal failure as a cause of the high AG, and diarrhea the cause of hyperchloremic acidosis.

Bibliography

Hamm L, Mixed acid-base disorders. In: Kokko and Tannen, *Fluids and Electrolyte*, 3rd ed. Philadelphia: W.B. Saunders, 1996:343–357.

22. **(B)** There are a variety of hormones synthesized in the kidney. Erythropoietin is made in the proximal cells of the kidney. It is deficient in patients with chronic kidney disease and leads to anemia. Fortunately, this hormone can be manufactured and its administration is a major advance in the management of renal insufficiency. Other hormones that are produced in the kidney include 1,25 vitamin D, renin, and prostaglandins. Calcitonin is produced in the thyroid gland and regulates calcium homeostasis. 25 Hydroxyvitamin D is synthesized from vitamin D_3 to 25 hydroxyvitamin D by 25 hydroxylase in the liver. Aldosterone is produced in the adrenal cortex and released in response to angiotensin II. The posterior pituitary is normal the site of synthesis of antidiuretic hormone and normally released in volume depletion or hypertonic states.

Bibliography

Leavey SF, et al. Endocrine abnormalities in chronic renal failure. *Endo Met Clin North Am* 2002;31(1):107–119.
Peart WS. The kidney as an endocrine organ. *Lancet* 1977;2:543–548.

23. **(E)** Low-dose dopamine, ANP, and furosemide are all effective in reversing acute renal failure in animal models. Although small trials and case series have also suggested benefits in clinical trials, large randomized controlled trials with these agents have shown none are effective in humans and their use should be abandoned. Although studies suggest Mucomyst may decrease the risk of acute renal failure from administration of radiocontrast in high-risk patients when given as prophylaxis, there is no evidence it ameliorates established acute renal failure.

Bibliography

Star R. Treatment of acute renal failure. *Kidney Int* 1998;54:1817–1831.

24. **(C)** Relief from an obstructive nephropathy results in a number of electrolyte and volume disturbances. Clinically this is manifested as postobstructive diuresis. The increase in urine output is caused by increase in volume status from obstruction, accumulation of solutes that generate an osmotic load (urea and the like), and possible retained natriuretic compounds. Obstruction also impairs ion channels which are responsible for the kidney's concentrating ability, sodium handling, and response to ADH which all lead to further loss of free water and sodium. This unregulated relative loss of free water to sodium determines whether hyponatremia or hypernatremia develops. Tubular functions that are responsible for potassium, phosphorus, and magnesium balance are also affected and results in their respective loss.

Bibliography

Curhan GC, et al. Urinary tract obstruction. In: Brenner (ed.), *Brenner & Rector's The Kidney*, 6th ed. Philadelphia, PA: W.B. Saunders, 2000, 1820–1844.

Klahr S, et al. Effects of obstruction on renal function. *Pediatr Nephrol* 1988;2(1):34–42.

25. **(D)** Reabsorption of urinary ammonium chloride by the intestinal segment causes a non-AG metabolic acidosis. Patients with urinary diversions have increased urinary calcium levels because metabolic acidosis causes dissolution of the skeleton. In addition, removal of the terminal ileum can lead to increased intestinal absorption of dietary oxalate. The resulting increased urinary calcium and oxalate levels can result in stone formation. With urinary diversions, there is an increased potential for the formation of gallstones, primarily related to ileal resection. Pigment stones are the predominant type. Ureterointestinal anastomosis such as ileal conduit, colon conduit, etc. are associated with a wide variety of cancers. The most commonly reported anastomosis associated with cancer is ureterosigmoidostomy. These cancers are usually diagnosed 10-20 years after surgery. Hypokalemia, rather than hyperkalemia is typically seen with urinary diversions.

Bibliography

Cruz D, Huot S. Metabolic complications of urinary diversions: an overview. *Am J Med* 1997;102:477–484.

McDougal WS. Metabolic complications of urinary intestinal diversion. *J Urol* 1992;147:1199–1208.

26. **(C)** The clinical distinction between the different RTA is based on the presence of hypokalemia or hyperkalemia, urinary pH, response to $NaHCO_3$, and serum aldosterone levels. Type 1 RTA is a disorder of the distal acidification process. It can be caused by a number of disorders including hydrogen ATPase dysfunction, a sodium channel abnormality in the parietal cell, or back diffusion of hydrogen. It usually manifests with hypokalemia, a urine pH >5.5, and no change in fractional excretion of HCO_3 with $NaHCO_3$ loading. Proximal acidification defect presents with type 2 RTA. This disorder is usually seen with disturbances of other proximal tubular functions like phosphaturia and aminoaciduria. Proximal RTA presents with hypokalemia, urine pH <5, and an increase in fractional excretion of HCO_3 to $NaHCO_3$ load. Type 4 is usually a deficiency of aldosterone or resistance to its presence. Aldosterone promotes hydrogen ion and potassium secretion by enhancing sodium absorption and the hydrogen ATPase activity. Hyperkalemia, urine pH <5, and a varying aldosterone level are the clinical features of type 4 RTA. Gitelman's syndrome presents with hypomagnesemia, hypokalemia, and metabolic alkalosis. It simulates activation of the thiazide sensitive sodium-chloride channel in the distal convoluted tubule.

Bibliography

Barakat A, et al. Gitelman's syndrome (familial hypokalemia-hypomagnesemia). *J Nephrol* 2001;14:43–47.

Soriano R. Renal tubular acidosis: the clinical entity. *J Am Soc Nephrol* 2002;13(8):2160–2170.

27. **(C)** Examination of his arterial blood gas (ABG) shows a respiratory alkalosis. The pH is elevated with a decrease in PCO_2. Typically in a simple acid-base disorder there would be compensation for the primary disorder. In a respiratory alkalosis, a compensatory metabolic acidemia is generated by the kidney depending on the duration of the primary disorder. Examination of this patient's electrolytes shows a normal HCO_3 as well as an elevated AG of 19 indicating metabolic acidosis. With an AG metabolic acidosis present, he must have a metabolic alkalosis in order to have a normal HCO_3; thus, a triple disorder (respiratory alkalosis, metabolic acidosis, and metabolic alkalosis). The etiology of this acid-base disorder can be understood from the patient's illness. Respiratory alkalosis occurs from an increase in respiratory drive with subsequent increase in minute ventilation and decreased PCO_2. The pain he is experiencing is mostly likely the cause of his respiratory alkalosis. Other reasons for respiratory alkalosis include anxiety, salisylate intoxication, CNS pathology, and primary pulmonary pathology. This patient also has an AG metabolic acidosis. An AG acidosis is caused by an acid after it disassociates leaving an unmeasured anion and a hydrogen ion that is buffered by HCO_3. His AG is probably a combination of lactic acidosis (hypoperfusion

and infection) and ketosis (starvation). Further testing would be needed to confirm this suspicion. To generate a metabolic alkalosis, hydrogen must be lost in excess of HCO_3 or HCO_3 must be added. This patient expressed vomiting as part of his disease course. Gastric fluid contains a significant concentration of hydrogen ions (a low pH) that is secreted from the parietal cells in the stomach which is normally reabsorbed in the small intestine. Vomiting leads to a loss of hydrogen and retention of bicarbonate leading to a metabolic alkalosis.

Bibliography

DuBose TD. Acid-Base Disorders. In: Brenner (ed.), *Brenner & Rector's The Kidney*, 6th ed. Philadelphia, PA: W.B. Saunders, 2000, 1820–1844.

28. **(D)** Contrast nephropathy is a multifactorial process. It is likely a combination of decreased blood flow resulting in ischemia to the medulla, the generation of reactive oxygen species leading to cellular injury, and atheroembolic phenomena. Contrast nephropathy usually manifests within 48 h. Hydration has been shown to decrease the risk of contrast nephropathy by increasing blood flow and possibly limiting the time that the tubular epithelium is exposed to contrast. In a recent study, normal saline has been shown to be superior to half normal saline in diminishing the risk. Furthermore, IV hydration is superior to oral liquid intake. Acetylcysteine is a free radial scavenger that has been used to minimize the risks of contrast nephropathy. In a recent study when acetylcysteine was added to hydration versus hydration alone there was a relative risk of 10% of developing contrast nephropathy. The use of diuretics and mannitol to minimize the risk of contrast nephropathy has been unsuccessful and may actually heighten the risk. Withholding furosemide and avoiding the use of mannitol are recommended.

Bibliography

Mintz E, et al. Radiocontrast-induced nephropathy and percutaneous coronary intervention: a review of preventive measures. *Expert Opin Pharmacother* 2003;4(5): 639–652.

Mueller C, et al. Prevention on contrast media-associated nephropathy: randomized comparison 2 hydration regimens in 1620 patients undergoing coronary angioplasty. *Arch Inter Med* 2002;162(3):329–336.

Solomon R, et al. Effects of saline, mannitol, and furosemide to prevent acute decreases in renal function induced by radiocontrast agents. *N Engl J Med* 1994;331: 1416–1420.

Tepel M, et al. Prevention of radiographic-contrast-agent-induced reductions in renal function by acetylcysteine. *N Engl J Med* 2000;343:180–184.

Trivedi HS, et al. A randomized prospective trial to assess the role of saline hydration on the development of contrast nephrotoxicity. *Nephron Clin Pract* 2003;93:c29–c34.

29. **(E)** The pH and bicarbonate are low so the patient has a metabolic acidosis. The AG is elevated. An appropriate respiratory response to the metabolic acidosis would be hyperventilation resulting in a low PCO_2. Since this patient's PCO_2 is high, there is also a respiratory acidosis.

30. **(E)** In order for bicarbonate to buffer a proton, water and CO_2 is produced and the lungs must exhale CO_2. Likewise, the byproduct of converting citrate, lactate, or acetate into bicarbonate is CO_2. Retained CO_2 in a patient with COPD or fixed ventilation will accumulate CO_2 and the acidosis will worsen. THAM, on the other hand, is both a CO_2 and proton pump. It corrects both metabolic acidosis and respiratory acidosis. Its side effects include hypoventilation, hyperkalemia, hyperglycemia, and vascular necrosis.

Bibliography

Adrogue H, Madias N. Management of life-threatening acid-base disorders. *N Engl J Med* 1998;338:26–33.

31. **(A)** Amiloride inhibits the sodium channel located on the tubular epithelial surface of the collecting tubule. It is involved in volume balance, potassium, and acid excretion. The channel allows sodium to move intracellularly from the tubule. This absorption produces a negative transcellular electrical gradient that aids in potassium and hydrogen ion secretion. An activating mutation of this sodium channel causes Liddle's syndrome. Liddle's syndrome is manifested by hypertension, hypokalemia, metabolic alkalosis, and suppression of the renin-angiotensin-aldosterone system. The manifestations of this syndrome can be treated with amiloride by blocking sodium absorption. The sodium-potassium-2 chloride channel and sodium-chloride channel are inhibited by forsemide and thiazide diuretics, respectively. Aquaporins are water channels that are located throughout the course of the nephron. Aquaporin 2 is one of these channels located in the collecting tubule. Under the influence of ADH binding to its V_2 receptor, the channel is translocated from intracellular vesicles to the epithelial membrane increasing water absorption. Inhibitors of V_2 receptor are under development and in clinical trials. They may become important for the treatment of hyponatremia.

Bibliography

Brater DC. Pharmacology of diuretics. *Am J Med Sci* 2000;319(1):38–50.

Cadnapaphornchai M, et al. Pathogenesis and management of hyponatremia. *Am J Med* 2000;109:688–692.

Schafet J. Abnormal regulation of ENaC: syndromes of salt retention and salt wasting in by the collecting duct. *Am J Physiol Renal Physiol* 2002;283:F221–F235.

32. **(B)** The kidney excretes 50 meq of hydrogen ions daily that is derived from metabolic processes. To meet the daily goal of acid secretion, titratable acids and ammonia are used since free hydrogen ion secretion is minimal. Phosphate and sulfate, derived from the metabolism of amino acids, are both titratable acids. Both molecules bind hydrogen that is secreted into the tubule and are excreted in the urine; however, they do not provide enough buffering capacity because of limited quantities. Ammonia provides a larger buffering capacity since it can be generated to meet demand. Ammonium is produced in the proximal tubules principally from the metabolism of glutamine. Ammonium enters the proximal tubule via a carrier transport protein where ammonia is then formed. Ammonia (NH_3) is freely permeable in cellular membranes since it carries no charge. Ammonia is trapped in the tubular lumen by the conversion to ammonium (NH_4^+) by combining ammonia with a secreted hydrogen ion a process called "diffusion trapping." Through a mechanism of ammonia absorption, ammonium uptake, and recycling by the thick ascending limb, an increased concentration of ammonia is established in the medullary interstitium. In the inner medullar collecting tubule, ammonia is converted to ammonium as it diffuses from the high interstitium concentration into the tubule and trapped by the acidification process and finally excreted in the urine. Through this trapping mechanism and titrable acids, the kidney is able to excrete the acid load. Urea is not involved is acid secretion, but plays a significant role in water handling.

Bibliography

Sands J. Regulation of renal urea transporters. *J Am Soc Nephrol* 1999;10:635–646.

Unwin R, et al. Urinary acidification and distal renal tubular acidosis. *J Nephrol* 2002;15(S5):S140–S150.

33. **(C)** The patient has a metabolic alkalosis related to profuse and prolonged vomiting. The same abnormality occurs commonly in surgical practice, as a result of prolonged nasogastric suction. In pathophysiologic reasoning, metabolic alkalosis is traditionally discussed in two phases. First is the generation of metabolic alkalosis. In this case, generation results from the loss of acid (protons) in the vomitus. For each proton that is secreted into the lumen of the stomach, a bicarbonate ion is added to the plasma. Normally that proton passes on to the duodenum and reacts with (we might say, it consumes) a bicarbonate ion from pancreatic secretion. With vomiting or nasogastric suction, however, the proton is lost to the body. Thus, loss of gastric juice, simultaneously results in a rise in serum bicarbonate concentration. There is some volume depletion and hemoconcentration to further accentuate the increase in bicarbonate concentration. Recall that there is a threshold of bicarbonate concentration above which, the reabsorptive capacity of the proximal tubule is surpassed, at which time bicarbonate begins to "spill" into the urine. This "spilled" bicarbonate, which is only poorly reabsorbable in the distal nephron, "drags" out cations (principally, Na^+ and K^+) with it, to maintain electrical neutrality. Gastric secretion has a potassium concentration comparable to plasma (4–5 meq/L only). The potassium losses that result in this patient's profound hypokalemia, occur at the kidney and are not the direct result of vomiting.

Bibliography

Sabatini S, Kurtzman NA. Metabolic alkalosis. In: Narins RG, ed., *Maxwell and Kleeman's Clinical Disorders of Fluid and Electrolyte Metabolism*, 5th ed. New York: McGraw-Hill, 1993:993–956.

34. **(E)** When there is the excretion of an anion in urine (a poorly reabsorbable anion such as bicarbonate, ketoanions, some drugs), electrical neutrality dictates that the anion must be accompanied by cations (usually sodium and potassium). Thus, sodium excretion does not reflect volume status in this situation, and the urinary chloride more accurately reflects volume status. Conversely, when there is the excretion of a cation such as ammonium (in a state of metabolic acidosis), the ammonium ion will drag out with it, anions such as chloride ions. The urinary chloride does not reflect volume status, rather it is the urine sodium that is a more reliable indicator of volume status.

The patient's high urine pH suggests that there is ongoing bicarbonaturia and that the patient is not in a state of equilibrium as yet. An alternative explanation is if the patient has been receiving bicarbonate or some other base, from an exogenous source. In this patient, he admitted to having ingested large amounts of "Tums" to alleviate his vomiting prior to hospitalization.

Bibliography

Sabatini S, Kurtzman NA. Metabolic alkalosis. In: Narins RG, ed., *Maxwell and Kleeman's Clinical Disorders of Fluid and Electrolyte Metabolism*, 5th ed. New York: McGraw-Hill, 1993:993–956.

Toto RD, Alpern RJ. Metabolic acid-base disorders. In: Kokko and Tannen, *Fluids and Electrolytes*, 3rd ed. Philadelphia: W.B. Saunders, 1996:201–266.

35. (D) Inhibition of bone resorption can be achieved with gallium nitrate, calcitonin, and bisphosphonates. Bisphosphonates are highly effective in inhibiting osteoclast activity in the bones. Action of onset is delayed for 3–4 days, so a more immediate acting agent is usually administered. Calcitonin is also a potent inhibitor of osteoclast activity. Its effect on serum calcium levels occurs within hours of administration, so it is often combined with bisphosphonates. Its effect is transient. Tachyphylaxis develops in 2–3 days. Lasix increases the renal excretion of calcium. Hydochlorothiazide, on the other hand, increases tubular reabsorption of calcium in the distal tubule and can cause hypercalcemia.

Bibliography

Mosekilde L, Eriksen E, Charles P. Hypercalcemia of malignancy: pathophysiology, diagnosis and treatment. *Crit Rev Oncol Hematol* 1991;11:1–27.

36. (E) Contrast nephropathy is usually a nonoliguric form of acute renal failure. Oliguria does occur, but frank anuria would be rare. On the other hand, complete bilateral renal obstruction, acute cortical necrosis associated with septic abortions, aortic dissection occluding the renal arteries, and severe acute glomerulonephritis are all associated with anuria.

Bibliography

Singri N, Ahya S, Levin M. Acute renal failure. *JAMA* 2003;289:747–751.

37. (E) Contrast nephropathy is defined as a rise in the serum creatinine within 48 h of contrast administration, so this is not the explanation. Ischemic ATN associated with her intermittent bouts of hypotension is a possibility, but it would not explain the peripheral eosinophilia, elevated amylase, or the lower extremity rash. Interstitial nephritis from the cephalosporin would cause renal failure, high eosinophil count, and a rash, but not the elevated amylase. All of the findings, however, are consistent with the diagnosis of cholesterol emboli syndrome. Often referred to as "pseudo-vasculitis," it develops days to weeks after an arterial vascular procedure. It causes renal failure, pancreatitis, intestinal ischemia, arthralgias, livedo reticularis, digital infarction, and cerebral infarction. Laboratory findings include high erythrocyte sedimentation rate (ESR) and eosinophil counts, and low complement levels. Therapy is supportive.

Bibliography

Modi K, Rao V. Atheroembolic renal disease. *J Am Soc Nephrol* 2001;12:1781–1787.

38. (B) Magnesium that is unbound to protein in plasma (~80%) is filtrated through the glomerulus. From there it is absorbed at different parts of the nephron, each with its own mechanism. In the proximal convoluted tubule, magnesium uptake is by bulk transport along with sodium and water absorption. The thick ascending limb is the major segment for magnesium absorption. Magnesium moves through a paracellular pathway driven by a potential gradient. This gradient is established by the Na-K-2Cl channel, inward rectifying potassium channel (ROMK), and the chloride channel on the basolateral membrane. The gradient is established by the electrical neutral absorption of Na, K, and Cl by the Na-K-2Cl channel. Some of the absorbed potassium reenters the tubule through the ROMK channel and chloride exits the cell into the basolateral space. The movement of potassium and chloride leads to a potential gradient that is positive in the lumen and negative in the basolateral space. Magnesium moves down this gradient to be absorbed. The remaining magnesium is taken up in the distal convoluted tubule. The mechanism of absorption in the distal convoluted tubule is not fully understood, but is connected to sodium and chloride absorption since it is inhibited by thiazide diuretics. The thin ascending segment on loop of Henle is not significantly involved in magnesium absorption.

Bibliography

Quamme G. Renal magnesium handling: new insights in understanding old problems. *Kidney Int* 1997;52:1180–1195.

39. (C) This case illustrates the danger of administration of fleet phospho-soda enemas to patients with end-stage renal disease. There is significant absorption of phosphate in the colon. Colonic disease with inflammation and poor colonic motility can result in even greater potential to absorb phosphate administered by this route. Because patients with end-stage renal disease are unable to excrete such absorbed phosphate, there is the potential for severe and sometimes, life-threatening hyperphosphatemia. Other possible sources of phosphate loads in these patients include poor dietary compliance with the phosphate-restricted diet, patients taking milk for the relief of dyspepsia, infants receiving cow's milk (which is richer in phosphate than human milk), blood transfusions, and patients receiving vitamin D or its analogs and tissue breakdown as in rhabdomyolysis or tumor lysis.

The most concerning consequences of severe hyperphosphatemia are

1. soft tissue (metastatic) calcifications, which can involve the skin, joints, blood vessels, heart, lungs, and kidneys.
2. hypocalcemia/tetany resulting from the reciprocal relationship of serum phosphate and calcium such that very high levels of phosphate are associated with low levels of calcium. The most appropriate intervention is dialysis; whether intermittent or continuous depends on the severity of the hyperphosphatemia and if it is expected to resolve rapidly or would require prolonged treatment.

Bibliography

Gennari FJ, ed. Diagnosis of acid-base disorders, in *Medical Management of Kidney and Electrolyte Disorders*. New York: Marcel Dekker, 2001:169–189.

40. **(A)** The urinary dipstick detects pigment present in both hemoglobin and myoglobin. If the microscopic examination of the urine demonstrates there are no RBCs present in the urine to account for the positive "blood," then myoglobin is present and the patient has rhabdomyolysis.

Bibliography

Zager R. Rhabdomyolysis and myohemoglobinuric acute renal failure. *Kidney Int* 1996;49:314–326.

41. **(D)** The structures that separate the glomerular capillary from Bowman's space are the glomerular capillary endothelium, basement membrane, and the Bowman's visceral epithelial cells called podocytes. These structures limit not only the formed elements of blood but also loss of protein in the filtrate. Proteins are limited to the capillary space by their size and electrical charge. The generation of filtrate is governed by Starling's forces, as in other capillary beds. The vasa recta is formed from the glomerular efferent arteriole and plays an important role in salt and water balance.

Bibliography

Pallone TL, et al. Physiology of the renal medullary microcirculation. *Am J Physiol Renal Physiol* 2003;284(2): F253–F266.

Tryggvason K, Wartiovaara J. Molecular basis of glomerular permselectivity. *Curr Opin Nephrol Hypertens* 2001; 10(4):543–549.

42. **(C)** The laboratory data can be consistent with either central or nephrogenic DI, but in this male patient with a recent motor vehicle accident who is in a comatose state, central DI is the most likely diagnosis. Generally, to differentiate between central and nephrogenic DI

a water deprivation test is performed, where desmopressin is given. An increase in urine osmolarity and decrease in urine output signifies central DI. Patients with a similar clinical picture have been described with pituitary stalk syndrome. The syndrome is usually seen in male patients in their 20s to 30s from motor vehicle accidents that are usually in a comatose state. The clinical picture has three phases. First there is a phase of the cessation of AVP secretion which occurs acutely and may have an onset from 5 h to 6 days. There is the acute onset of polyuria and hypernatremia. Close monitoring of serum electrolytes is needed to promptly diagnose this complication. Spontaneous recovery is frequent. Delayed diagnosis, on the other hand, can result in hypernatremic brain injury, hypovolemia, shock, and ischemic brain injury. The second phase (antidiuretic) is the result of AVP release from injured axons. This may occur within 3–12 days after injury and can result in life-threatening hyponatremia, especially as the patient is receiving large volumes of hypotonic fluid at the time for the treatment of the hypernatremia of the first phase.

There are important differential diagnoses of the second phase to be considered; however, hyponatremia may be the result of the development of SIADH. Hyponatremia may also be the result of high AVP levels, resulting from volume depletion secondary to the previous polyuria, or secondary to a cerebral salt wasting syndrome. Cerebral salt wasting is manifested by hyponatremia, volume depletion, and intracranial pathology. In the two latter cases, water or fluid restriction would be inappropriate measures to take. These patients also may have abnormalities of other pituitary hormones such as adrenocorticotropic hormone (ACTH) that leads to adrenal insufficiency that can minimize the first phase of hypernatremia or worsen the hyponatremia of the second phase. The third phase is the final phase of either complete recovery with return to normal posterior pituitary function, or of partial recovery (partial central DI), or no recovery (complete central DI). Spontaneous recovery is the more usual outcome. Osmotic diuresis from mannitol, glucose, and the like can lead to hypernatremia by loss of free water, but in this patient his urine osmolarity does not support this diagnosis.

Bibliography

Bichet DG. Nephrogenic and central DI. In Shrier RW, ed., *Diseases of the Kidney and Urinary Tract*. Baltimore: Lippincott, Williams & Wilkins, 2001:2549–2576.

Harrigan HR. Cerebral salt wasting syndrome. *Crit Care Clin* 2001;17(1):125–138.

Robinson AG, et al. Posterior pituitary gland. In: Larsen PR (ed.), *Williams Textbook of Endocrinology*, 10th ed. Philadelphia, PA: W.B. Saunders, 2003, 281–329.

43. **(A)** All of the tubular segments listed contribute to sodium absorption. Sodium absorption is the primary mechanism of volume regulation since water absorption generally follows sodium absorption. It is the proximal convoluted tubule that does the majority of absorption, about 65–75% of sodium. In a decreasing order, the loop of Henle, distal convoluted tubule, and collecting tubule contribute to 25, 10, and 0–5% of sodium absorption, respectively.

Bibliography

Andreoli TE. An overview of salt absorption by the nephron. *J Nephrol* 1999;12(S2):S3–S15.

44. **(E)** The patient has a hemolytic anemia (elevated LDH and bilirubin), thrombocytopenia, and renal failure. Therefore, the patient meets the criteria of HUS. The most important next step would be to obtain a peripheral smear to document the presence of schiztocytes. HUS is usually seen in children with bloody diarrhea associated with infection with verotoxin producing *E. coli* from undercooked meat; however, HUS is also seen in a variety of conditions including malignancy, scleroderma renal crises, bone marrow transplantation, and the administration of the immunosuppressants cyclosporine A and tacrolimus. In renal transplantation, cyclosporine associated HUS may develop in up to 10% of patients. Treatment is removal of the offending agent. Small case series suggest that plasma exchange may be helpful.

Bibliography

Zarifian A, Meleg-Smith S, O'Donovan R, et al. Cyclosporine-associated thrombotic microangiopathy in renal allografts. *Kidney Int* 1999;55:2457–2466.

CHAPTER 9

Intracranial and Spinal Trauma

Joshua Miller and John McGregor

Questions

1. A 23-year-old male presents to the emergency department after being involved in a motor vehicle accident. On physical examination, he opens his eyes to painful stimulation, he occasionally mumbles incomprehensible sounds, he localizes to painful stimulation with his right upper extremity, and he withdraws his left upper extremity to pain. His pupils are 4 mm bilaterally and reactive. What is this patient's Glasgow Coma Scale (GCS) score?

   (A) 7
   (B) 9
   (C) 8
   (D) 10

2. Cerebral perfusion pressure (CPP) is equal to

   (A) systolic blood pressure (SBP) – intracranial pressure (ICP)
   (B) diastolic blood pressure (DBP) –ICP
   (C) mean arterial pressure (MAP) + ICP
   (D) MAP –ICP

3. All of the following are classic signs of a basal skull fracture *except*:

   (A) dilated and nonreactive pupil
   (B) bilateral periorbital ecchymosis (Raccoon's eyes)
   (C) ecchymosis over mastoids (Battle's sign)
   (D) hemotympanum

4. Generally accepted criteria for elevating a depressed skull fracture in the operating room include all of the following *except*:

   (A) open fracture
   (B) coexistence of other traumatic lesion (i.e., hematoma) underlying fragment
   (C) dural tear with CSF leak
   (D) involvement of the anterior wall of the frontal sinus

5. Cardinal signs of intracranial hypertension include all of the following *except*:

   (A) flexor (decorticate) posturing
   (B) papilledema
   (C) aphasia
   (D) dilated and nonreactive pupil

6. A 42-year-old male presents to the emergency department as a level I trauma after being involved in a motor vehicle accident. On initial examination, the patient has a GCS of 7 (localizes to pain, no eye opening, and no verbal response). The patient has multiple injuries including a long bone fracture. The patient's vital signs are stable. You consult orthopedic surgery, and they want to take the patient to the operating room (OR) to repair his fracture. A CT scan of the head shows mild-to-moderate diffuse cerebral edema. What is the most appropriate course of action to take with this patient?

   (A) Allow the patient to go the OR immediately for repair of his fracture.
   (B) Consult neurosurgery to evaluate for placement of an ICP monitor prior to his going to the OR.
   (C) Consult neurosurgery to evaluate for placement of an ICP monitor after he returns from the OR.
   (D) Delay surgery indefinitely until the patient's neurologic status improves.

7. Initial routine measures for controlling ICP in a patient with a closed head injury include all of the following *except*:

   (A) hyperventilation
   (B) elevate head of bed to 30–45°
   (C) avoid hypotension
   (D) keep head midline

8. A 22-year-old female presents to the emergency department as a level II trauma after falling off a horse and hitting her head on the ground. She had brief loss of consciousness and is now oriented to name and place only. The patient has no apparent systemic injuries. A CT scan of the head shows mild generalized cerebral edema. What is the most appropriate intravenous fluid for this patient?

(A) Ringer's lactate
(B) 0.225% NS with 20 meq KCl
(C) 0.45% NS with 20 meq KCl
(D) 0.9% NS with 20 meq KCl

9. Late complications of traumatic brain injury may include all of the following *except*:

(A) seizures
(B) communicating hydrocephalus
(C) primary brain tumors
(D) memory impairment

10. A 24-year-old male is taken to the emergency department after being involved in a motor vehicle accident approximately 3 h ago. The patient was the unrestrained driver, and he cannot recall the accident. He complains of a left-sided headache, and you notice on physical examination that he has a palpable deformity over the left side of his skull and a boggy temporalis muscle. You order a CT scan of the head. The nurse calls you 20 min later to see the patient, because he has suddenly become unresponsive. A CT scan of the head is most likely to reveal what type of lesion?

(A) chronic subdural hematoma
(B) diffuse subarachnoid hemorrhage
(C) intraventricular hemorrhage
(D) epidural hematoma

11. What category of subdural hematoma appears isodense to brain on CT scans?

(A) acute
(B) subacute
(C) chronic
(D) none of these

12. A 19-year-old male presents to the emergency department after being shot in the head with a handgun. Appropriate initial steps in managing this patient include all of the following *except*:

(A) begin Solumedrol protocol
(B) control scalp bleeding
(C) elevate HOB to 30–45%
(D) give mannitol 1 g/kg bolus

13. A mother brings her 14-month-old son into the emergency department because he is difficult to arouse. The mother states that the infant accidentally fell off a changing table that is approximately 3 ft tall. On physical examination, you find that the infant has multiple bruises and bilateral retinal hemorrhages. Skull radiographs show a right frontal and a left parietal linear fracture. A CT scan of the head shows a left convexity chronic subdural hematoma. The most likely diagnosis is

(A) coagulopathy
(B) accidental trauma
(C) child abuse
(D) neglect

14. All of the following examination findings are consistent with a diagnosis of brain death *except*:

(A) dilated and nonreactive pupils
(B) absent oculocephalic reflex
(C) extensor (decerebrate) posturing
(D) absent gag reflex

15. Diffuse axonal injury (DAI) results from what type of force acting on the brain?

(A) direct impact
(B) axial loading
(C) linear acceleration
(D) rotational acceleration

Questions 16 through 20

MATCH the following CT scans with the appropriate diagnosis.

    (A) chronic subdural hematoma

    (B) subarachnoid hemorrhage

    (C) acute subdural hematoma

    (D) intracerebral hemorrhage

    (E) epidural hematoma

16. Figure 9-1

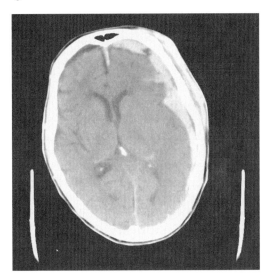

17. Figure 9-2

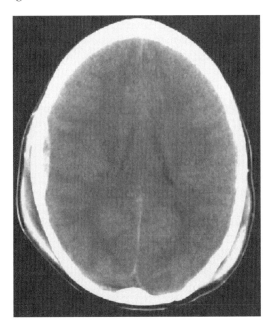

18. Figure 9-3

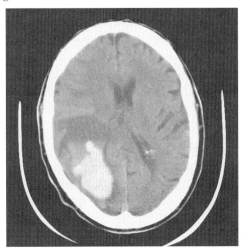

19. Figure 9-4

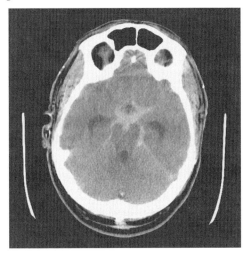

20. Figure 9-5

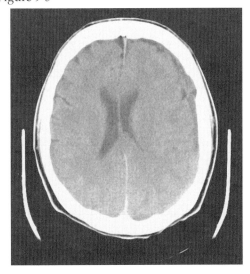

21. What percentage of patients who present with a major spinal injury will have a second spinal injury at another level?

    (A) 2%
    (B) 10%
    (C) 20%
    (D) 40%

22. A 20-year-old female presents to the emergency department as a level I trauma after being involved in an all terrain vehicle accident. She is unable to move her legs, has no sensation below her nipples, and she has a step-off deformity in her upper thoracic spine. Her only complaint is back pain, her initial vital signs are stable, and her abdominal examination is benign. Ten minutes later, her blood pressure suddenly falls to 75/35 mmHg. Her hemoglobin and hematocrit are within normal limits, and her blood pressure does not respond to boluses of intravenous fluids. The most likely cause of the hypotension is

    (A) spinal shock
    (B) myocardial infarction
    (C) hypovolemia
    (D) splenic laceration

23. The most appropriate treatment for hypotension related to spinal shock is

    (A) aggressive intravenous hydration
    (B) dopamine
    (C) trendelenberg position
    (D) phenylephrine

24. Appropriate steps in the initial management of a patient with a suspected spinal cord injury include all of the following *except*:

    (A) maintain on backboard until cervical spine is cleared
    (B) regulate temperature
    (C) place nasogastric tube to suction
    (D) place bladder catheter

25. Which of the following statements regarding a methylprednisolone protocol for the treatment of acute spinal cord injuries is true?

    (A) Most beneficial when started more than 8 h after time of injury.
    (B) The dose is a 2 g bolus followed by 350 mg/h for 23 h.

    (C) Should not be given to patients with a complete spinal cord injury.
    (D) Evidence suggesting harmful effects is more consistent than that supporting beneficial effects.

26. A 32-year-old male presents to the emergency department after being involved in a low velocity motor vehicle accident. He is wearing a cervical collar that was placed by emergency medical system personnel. He is awake, alert, oriented to name, place, and time, sober, and does not complain of neck pain. On physical examination, he has no cervical tenderness and no other significant injury. The most appropriate x-rays to order are

    (A) lateral cervical spine only
    (B) none
    (C) AP and lateral cervical spine
    (D) five views of the cervical spine

27. An inebriated 62-year-old male presents to the emergency department after a motor vehicle accident. He has ecchymosis and a small laceration on his forehead. His strength is 3/5 in his upper extremities and 4+/5 in his lower extremities. Sensation to pain and temperature is mildly decreased in his upper extremities, and he has urinary retention. The most likely diagnosis is

    (A) Brown-Sequard's syndrome
    (B) anterior cord syndrome
    (C) central cord syndrome
    (D) cervical herniated disc

28. All of the following are true statements regarding spinal cord injury without radiographic abnormality (SCIWORA) *except*:

    (A) higher incidence in children <9 years of age
    (B) radiographs including flexion/extension views are normal
    (C) immobilization for up to 3 months is often recommended
    (D) MRI studies are normal

29. Death related to an atlantooccipital dislocation is most often the result of

    (A) respiratory arrest
    (B) cardiac arrest
    (C) spinal shock
    (D) hemorrhagic shock

30. A fracture through the arches of the atlas, usually resulting from an axial load, is referred to as a

(A) Hangman's fracture

(B) odontoid fracture

(C) Jefferson fracture

(D) avulsion fracture

31. A fracture through the base of the odontoid is classified as

(A) type I

(B) type II

(C) type III

(D) type IV

32. How should locked or perched facets in the cervical spine be treated initially?

(A) open reduction and internal fixation

(B) closed reduction with cervical traction

(C) keep patient immobilized in cervical collar

(D) no treatment is needed

33. A clay-shoveler fracture is a fracture of what part of the vertebra?

(A) pedicle

(B) odontoid process

(C) body

(D) spinous process

34. A 20-year-old male presents to the hospital with a spine fracture and a complete spinal cord injury. Reasons to surgically stabilize the patient early include all of the following *except*:

(A) early mobilization

(B) psychological benefit

(C) improve neurologic function

(D) reduce comorbidities

35. Which of the following types of thoracolumbar spine fractures is considered unstable?

(A) burst fracture

(B) transverse process fracture

(C) articular process fracture

(D) spinous process fracture

36. According to the three column model of the spine, a seat-belt type fracture involves disruption of which columns?

(A) all three

(B) anterior and middle

(C) anterior and posterior

(D) middle and posterior

37. Indications for operating on gunshot wounds to the spine include all of the following *except*:

(A) persistent CSF leak

(B) neurologic deterioration

(C) compression of a nerve root

(D) operate on all cases

38. The overall mortality rate from deep venous thromboses in patients with spinal cord injuries is

(A) 1%

(B) 5%

(C) 10%

(D) 20%

Answers and Explanations

1. **(B)** The GCS is the most widely used scale for predicting outcome following head trauma. It was developed by Teasdale and Jennett as a practical means of assessing and categorizing a patient's level of arousal and neurologic function. The scale is divided into three categories: eye opening, best verbal response, and best motor response. Eye opening is rated on a scale of 1–4, verbal response is rated on a scale of 1–5, and motor response is rated on a scale of 1–6 (Table 9-1). Therefore, the lowest possible score is 3, and the highest possible score is 15. The patient in this question receives 2 points for opening his eyes to painful stimulation, 2 points for verbalizing incomprehensible sounds, and 5 points for localizing to stimulation since this represents his best motor response. Pupillary size and reactivity does not factor into the GCS score. Therefore, the patient's total score in this question is 9. A major disadvantage of using the GCS is that endotracheal intubation prevents the use of the best verbal response category. In such cases, the letter "t" follows the combined score of the remaining two categories. For example, if the above patient had been intubated,

then his score would have been 7t. When using the GCS, one must keep in mind that although it is an effective tool for rapidly assessing neurologic function and assisting with outcome predictions, it only shows general trends in the patient's status over time. It is not an accurate or valuable means of following a patient's specific clinical status, and it should not replace a thorough neurologic examination.

TABLE 9-1   Glasgow Coma Scale

Eye opening	
Spontaneous	4
To speech	3
To pain	2
No eye opening	1
Best verbal response	
Oriented and appropriate	5
Confused	4
Inappropriate words	3
Incomprehensible sounds	2
No verbal response	1
Best motor response	
Obeys commands	6
Localizes to pain	5
Withdraws to pain	4
Flexor (decorticate) posturing	3
Extensor (decerebrate) posturing	2
No motor response	1

2. **(D)** Cerebral blood flow remains relatively constant in the normal brain over a wide range of CPPs, a process that is termed autoregulation. When a patient suffers a severe head injury, however, this autoregulation may be disrupted. One study has suggested that approximately 50% of patients sustaining a severe head injury will have disrupted autoregulation. This causes cerebral blood flow to become dependent on CPP. Since CPP is equal to the difference between the ICP and the MAP, even small or transient drops in blood pressure could translate into decreased cerebral blood flow and lead to ischemia. Therefore, both hypotension and elevated ICP should be avoided in the head-injured patient. A problem arises in monitoring such patients since cerebral blood flow is difficult to measure. Fortunately, CPP may be obtained by simply knowing the blood pressure and ICP. Historically, most physicians taking care of patients with traumatic brain injuries focused on ICP alone. Several reports have now suggested that maintaining an adequate CPP is more important that controlling ICP alone. It is now believed that a CPP of >70 is associated with improved long-term outcome after severe head injury.

Bibliography

Bouma G, Muizelaar J. Cerebral blood flow, cerebral blood volume, and cerebrovascular reactivity after severe head injury. *J Neurotrauma* 1992;9:S333–S348.

Caron M, Kelly D, Shalmon E, et al. Intensive management of traumatic brain injury. In: Wilkins R, Rengachary S (eds.), *Neurosurgery*, 2nd ed. New York, NY: McGraw-Hill, 1996, 2706.

3. **(A)** Basal skull fractures are usually diagnosed by clinical signs. CT scan findings include linear lucencies through the skull base, pneumocephalus, and opacification of air sinuses. Clinical signs vary depending on the site of fracture. Anterior skull base fractures may cause anosmia, cerebrospinal fluid (CSF) rhinorrhea, and periorbital ecchymosis (raccoon's eyes). Middle fossa or temporal bone fractures may result in ecchymosis over the mastoids (Battle's sign, Fig. 9-6), hemotympanum, CSF otorrhea or rhinorrhea, and cranial nerve VII or VIII palsies. A dilated and nonreactive pupil is often the result of compression of cranial nerve III causing interruption of the sympathetic fibers traveling along this nerve. This is most often a sign of elevated ICP and not of a basal skull fracture, although related trauma to the orbit could result in a dilated and nonreactive pupil. Other consequences of basal skull fractures include optic nerve injury, abducens nerve injury, traumatic carotid artery aneurysms, carotid-cavernous fistulae, CSF fistulae, meningitis, and cerebral abscess.

Temporal bone fractures may be divided into two categories based on the relationship between the fracture line and the long axis of the petrous portion of the temporal bone. The longitudinal pattern, fracture is parallel to long axis of petrous bone, is more common (75–90% of all cases) than the transverse pattern, fracture is perpendicular to long axis of petrous bone (Figs. 9-7 and 9-8). Damage to cranial

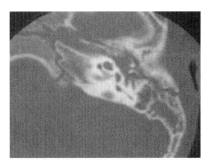

FIG. 9-7 CT scan showing a longitudinal temporal bone fracture.

nerves VII and VIII occur more frequently with transverse fractures, while longitudinal fractures are more likely to disrupt the ossicular chain and result in hearing loss. Treatment of basal skull fractures almost always involves expectant management, but surgery may be indicated to treat one of the secondary complications of these fractures.

Bibliography

Geisler F. Skull fractures. In: Wilkins R, Rengachary S (eds.), *Neurosurgery*, 2nd ed. New York, NY: McGraw-Hill, 1996, 2753–2754.

Greenberg M. *Handbook of Neurosurgery*, 4th ed., vol. 2. Lakeland, FL: Greenberg Graphics, 1997, 722.

4. **(D)** Depressed skull fractures are caused by a significant force being applied to a relatively small area of the head. The modality of choice for diagnosing depressed skull fractures is a CT scan of the head. Although recently disputed, generally accepted criteria for elevating a depressed skull fracture in the operating room include open depressed fractures, coexistence of an underlying traumatic lesion, dural tear with CSF leak, and cosmetic deformity. Depressed fractures that involve the frontal sinus represent a special category. Fractures involving the frontal sinus are divided into those that disrupt the anterior wall and those that disrupt the posterior wall. A fracture of the anterior wall

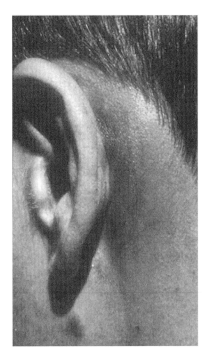

FIG. 9-6 Ecchymosis overlying the mastoid is known as Battle's sign. This is a sign of a basal skull fracture.

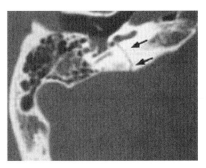

FIG. 9-8 CT scan showing a transverse temporal bone fracture (arrows).

of the frontal sinus would only require surgical repair if it caused a significant cosmetic deformity, and this could be done on an elective basis. A fracture through the posterior wall, however, is in a different category because communication between the sinus and brain increases the risk of developing meningitis or a cerebral abscess. Traditionally, the treatment of choice for fractures through the posterior wall of the frontal sinus involved removing the posterior wall, repairing any dural tear, removing all of the mucous membrane lining the sinus, and plugging the nasofrontal ducts (a process referred to commonly as *cranializing* the sinus). Removing every portion of the mucous membrane is necessary to prevent the formation of a mucocele. Recent studies, however, are proposing a more conservative approach to treating many types of depressed skull fractures, citing the improvements in diagnosis by CT scanning, antibiotic therapy, and rapid transfer to neurosurgical care.

Most practitioners caring for head-injured patients would consider an open depressed skull fracture to be an emergent situation secondary to the risk of intracranial infection. The goals of surgery are to remove contaminated material, debride devitalized tissue, and close the dura. Irrigation of the wound at bedside is often inadequate for thorough debridement. A recent study investigated the effects of delaying repair of open depressed fractures in seven male pediatric patients. The authors found that all patients suffered no ill effects, and the risk of intraoperative hypotension during the period of disrupted autoregulation and elevated ICP was avoided. More studies such as this one will be necessary, though, before a paradigm shift occurs in the management of open depressed skull fractures.

Bibliography

Avery N, Cheak T. Treatment of cranial vault fractures: recent trends toward a more conservative approach. *J Craniomaxillofac Trauma* 1998;4(3):42–48.

Curry D, Frim D. Delayed repair of open depressed skull fracture. *Pediatr Neurosurg* 1999;31(6):294–297.

5. **(C)** Intracranial hypertension may be defined as an ICP greater than 20 cmH$_2$O. Any process that increases the volume within the intracranial compartment may cause intracranial hypertension, such as hydrocephalus, cerebral edema, or a space occupying lesion. The most consistent and one of the only early signs of intracranial hypertension is papilledema. The other common signs of elevated ICP usually develop late and are related to brain herniation. There are four categories of brain herniation. These include cingulate (falcine) herniation, uncal herniation, central transtentorial herniation, and cerebellar tonsillar herniation.

Cingulate herniation results when an expanding mass in one of the cerebral hemispheres forces the cingulate gyrus under the falx cerebri. This may cause compression of the anterior cerebral arteries and internal cerebral veins leading to further ischemia of the herniating hemisphere. Uncal herniation is caused by an expanding lesion in a hemisphere that pushes the uncus and hippocampus over the edge of the tentorium cerebelli. The medial temporal lobe then compresses the posterior cerebral artery and oculomotor nerve lying within the ambient cistern, and continued herniation results in compression of the midbrain. The hallmarks of this type of herniation are a dilated, nonreactive pupil and contralateral hemiparesis. Of special note, a false localizing sign may occur if herniation causes grooving of the opposite cerebral peduncle against the tentorial edge (referred to as Kernohan's notch), resulting in ipsilateral hemiparesis. As uncal herniation progresses, distortion of the midbrain leads to decorticate and decerebrate posturing, coma, and midbrain hemorrhage leading to brain death. Similar patterns to this include central transtentorial and upward transtentorial herniation. Upward transtentorial herniation occurs when an expanding mass in the posterior fossa forces the cerebellum and lower brain stem up through the tentorial opening. The final category of brain herniation syndromes is cerebellar tonsillar herniation, which is usually the result of an expanding mass in the posterior fossa pushing its contents down through the foramen magnum.

A discussion of the signs of intracranial hypertension would not be complete without mentioning the triad of symptoms first described by Cushing in 1902. He noted that intracranial hypertension resulted in respiratory irregularity, bradycardia, and hypertension. These responses have been shown to be the result of damage to the medial pons, most likely the reticular formation, and to paramedian areas on the floor of the fourth ventricle. An additional common result of intracranial hypertension is pulmonary edema. This likely results from increased sympathetic tone which leads to left heart strain and pulmonary congestion. Aphasia is usually the result of ischemia or a focal mass lesion interfering with the temporo-parietal area of the dominant hemisphere. It is not regarded as a hallmark of intracranial hypertension.

Bibliography

Cohen D, Quest D. Increased intracranial pressure, brain herniation, and their control. In: Wilkins R, Rengachary S (eds.), *Neurosurgery*, 2nd ed. New York, NY: McGraw-Hill, 1996, 345–353.

Cushing H. Some experimental and clinical observations concerning states of increased intracranial tension. *Am J Med Sci* 1902;124:375–400.

6. **(B)** Although there is much debate regarding the precise indications for and benefit of ICP monitoring, several recent studies have suggested that an aggressive stance toward monitoring head-injured patients is associated with a reduced risk of mortality. In 2000, the American Association of Neurological Surgeons Joint Section on Neurotrauma and Critical Care in association with the Brain Trauma Foundation published guidelines relating to the indications for ICP monitoring. In this review, it was noted that ICP monitoring helps in the early detection of intracranial mass lesions, limits the indiscriminate use of therapies to control ICP that may be potentially harmful, helps in determining prognosis, and may improve outcome. Therefore, the Brain Trauma Foundation guidelines state that a comatose head-injured patient (GCS 3–8) with an abnormal CT scan should undergo ICP monitoring. Additionally, comatose head-injured patients with normal CT scans should undergo ICP monitoring if they have two or more of the following features at admission: age over 40, unilateral or bilateral motor posturing, or a SBP of less than 90 mmHg. A review of the Ontario Trauma Registry from 1989 to 1995 was completed to test the hypothesis that insertion of ICP monitors in patients with traumatic brain injuries is not associated with a decrease in the death rate. The conclusions were that monitor insertion rates varied widely from hospital to hospital and that, after controlling for injury scale and injury mechanism, insertion of an ICP monitor was associated with statistically significant decrease in the death rate among patients with severe traumatic brain injury. Finally, a retrospective review of data for consecutive patients with severe closed head injury (GCS ≤8) and long bone fracture admitted over an 8-month period in 34 academic trauma centers in the United States was completed. The purpose of this study was to examine variations in the care of patients with severe head injury, to determine the proportion of patients who received care according to the Brain Trauma Foundation guidelines, and to correlate the outcome from severe traumatic brain injury with the care received. The results revealed, in addition to considerable variation in the rates of ICP monitoring, that management at an aggressive center (defined as those placing ICP monitors in >50% of patients meeting the Brain Trauma Foundation criteria) was associated with a significant reduction in the risk of mortality. Another consideration regarding the patient in the above question is the anticipated use of intravenous fluids in the operating room under the situation of general anesthesia in which the neurologic examination is compromised. Worsening cerebral edema and secondary neurologic injury may progress unnoticed without the ability to monitor ICP and CPP. With all of these factors in mind, the most appropriate course of action is to consult neurosurgery to evaluate the patient for placement of an ICP monitor prior to his going to the operating room.

Bibliography

The Brain Trauma Foundation. The American Association of Neurological Surgeons. The Joint Section on Neurotrauma and Critical Care. Indications for intracranial pressure monitoring. *J Neurotrauma* 2000;17(6–7):479–491.

Lane P, Skoretz T, Doig G, et al. Intracranial pressure monitoring and outcomes after traumatic brain injury. *Can J Surg* 2000;43(6):406.

Bulger E, Nathens A, Rivara F, et al. Management of severe head injury: institutional variations in care and effect on outcome. *Crit Care Med* 2002;30(8):1870–1876.

7. **(A)** When a patient presents with a head injury, several initial routine measures may be instituted to help prevent intracranial hypertension. These include correct positioning of the patient, avoiding hypotension, controlling hypertension, light sedation, preventing hyperglycemia, and avoiding excessive hyperventilation. Correct positioning of the patient means elevating the head of the bed to 30–45° and keeping the head midline. Elevating the head of the bed even 30° has been shown to reduce ICP without reducing CPP or cerebral blood flow. Keeping the head midline prevents kinking of the jugular veins and subsequent reduced venous outflow which could lead to venous congestion and increased ICP. Hypotension is a predictor of poor outcome in a head-injured patient. Since autoregulation is likely disrupted, cerebral blood flow decreases as the blood pressure decreases. SBPs of less than 90 will result in inadequate perfusion of the brain. Likewise, hypertension must be controlled, because this may elevate ICP and increase the risk of hemorrhage. Light sedation is used to calm the head-injured patient. Caution should be used when administering sedatives, however, so that the patient is not too sedated to give a reliable neurologic examination. Another routine measure for controlling ICP is avoiding hyperglycemia since this aggravates cerebral edema and cell damage. With regards to ventilatory status, both hyperventilation and hypoventilation should be avoided. Hypoventilation will elevate PCO_2 causing vasodilation of cerebral vessels, increased intracranial blood volume, and elevated ICP.

Hyperventilation was once held as a first line defense against intracranial hypertension. Initiating hyperventilation prior to the appearance of signs of intracranial hypertension and prior to documenting the failure of other methods to reduce this has been associated with a worse outcome. Hyperventilation reduces ICP by reducing the PCO_2 which causes cerebral vasoconstriction and results in decreased cerebral blood volume. The danger arises in that this also reduces cerebral blood flow. In head-injured patients with disrupted autoregulation this may result in cerebral ischemia. Therefore, hyperventilation should not be used routinely in the first 24 h following head injury. The indications for hyperventilation include using it for brief periods when signs of intracranial hypertension appear prior to placement of an ICP monitor or after insertion of a monitor if there is a sudden increase in the ICP or there is acute neurologic deterioration. Hyperventilation may be used for longer periods if intracranial hypertension proves to be unresponsive to other aggressive measures. The appropriate goal for hyperventilation when initiated is a PCO_2 of 30–35. The PCO_2 should never drop below 25 as this carries a high risk of cerebral ischemia.

Bibliography

Feldman Z, Kanter M, Robertson C, et al. Effect of head elevation on intracranial pressure, cerebral perfusion pressure, and cerebral blood flow in head-injured patients. *J Neurosurg* 1992;76(2):207–211.

Greenberg M. *Handbook of Neurosurgery*, 4th ed., vol. 2. Lakeland, FL: Greenberg Graphics, 1997, 715–718.

8. **(D)** Management of intravenous fluids in head-injured patients is one area where trauma surgeons and neurosurgeons often disagree. Although reasons to convert to hypotonic solutions may develop, the initial choice for head-injured patients is isotonic solution. Hypotonic solutions should be avoided if possible, because they may impair cerebral compliance and worsen cerebral edema. With an intact blood-brain barrier, hypertonic solutions can establish an osmotic gradient that actually drives water out of the brain and into plasma. This is the principal method of action of mannitol, the most well-studied and proven osmotic diuretic for lowering ICP. In addition to mannitol, hypertonic saline has been shown in recent studies to lower ICP. A recent literature review concluded that hypertonic saline has favorable effects on both systemic hemodynamics and ICP. The most deleterious side effect of these agents is renal failure secondary to a hyperosmolar state and renal hypoperfusion. Therefore, urine output, serum osmolality, and serum sodium must be monitored closely when using hyper-

tonic agents. Other basic fluid management principles to keep in mind when treating a head-injured patient include the following: provide adequate resuscitation to avoid hypotension, maintain patient in euvolemia, and consider pressors over repeated fluid boluses.

Bibliography

Greenberg M. *Handbook of Neurosurgery*, 4th ed., vol. 2. Lakeland, FL: Greenberg Graphics, 1997, 715.

Qureshi A, Suarez J. Use of hypertonic saline solutions in treatment of cerebral edema and intracranial hypertension. *Crit Care Med* 2000;28(9):3301–3313.

9. **(C)** Well-documented late complications of head injury include seizures, communicating hydrocephalus, postconcussion syndrome, and varying degrees of intellectual impairment. Other documented late complications include hypogonadotropic hypogonadism and the deposition of amyloid proteins, which may be related to the development of Alzheimer's disease. Posttraumatic seizures are divided into early (occurring within 1 week of injury) and late (occurring after 1 week of injury) types. The incidence of early seizures ranges from 2.5 to 7% and the incidence of late seizures ranges from 5 to 7.1%. The risk of developing early posttraumatic seizures is related to the type of injury, with subdural and intracerebral hemorrhages being associated with the greatest risk. Approximately 25% of patients with early seizures will develop late seizures. Late seizures require around 8 weeks to develop. This seems to be related to the time it takes for the brain to develop an epileptogenic focus. The incidence of late seizures is directly proportional to the severity of the initial head injury. Although helpful in preventing early seizures in patients at high risk, prophylactic anticonvulsant administration does not reduce the frequency of late seizures.

Postconcussive syndrome is a constellation of symptoms that occurs after a minor head injury. The most common symptoms are headache, dizziness, and memory impairment. Other symptoms may include impaired concentration, anxiety, balance difficulties, tinnitus, loss of libido, impaired judgment, photophobia, and personality changes. In addition, one review notes that traumatic brain injury increases the risk for depression by a factor of 5–10, for psychotic disorders by a factor of 2–5, and for dementia by a factor of 4–5. The precise cause for these symptoms is often difficult to determine. Organic dysfunction, psychologic factors, and even secondary gain issues may contribute to a patient's symptomatology. As a recent Swedish study supports, there is no association between traumatic head injury and primary brain tumors.

Bibliography

Annegers J, Grabow J, Groover R, et al. Seizures after head trauma: a population study. *Neurology* 1980;30:683–689.

Greenberg M. *Handbook of Neurosurgery*, 4th ed., vol. 2. Lakeland, FL: Greenberg Graphics, 1997, 663–664, 739.

Gualtieri T, Cox D. The delayed neurobehavioral sequelae of traumatic brain injury. *Brain Injury* 1991;5(3):219–232.

Jennet B. *Epilepsy After Non-missile Head Injuries*, 2nd ed. Chicago, IL: Year Book, 1975.

Nygren C, Adami J, Ye W, et al. Primary brain tumors following traumatic brain injury a population-based cohort study in Sweden. *Cancer Causes Control* 2001;12(8):733–737.

Young B. Sequelae of head injury. In: Wilkins R, Rengachary S, (eds.), *Neurosurgery*, 2nd ed. New York, NY: McGraw-Hill, 1996, 2841–2843.

10. **(D)** Epidural hematomas comprise about 1% of all head trauma admissions. An epidural hematoma is defined as a blood clot that forms between the dura and the inner table of the skull. The classic presentation of an epidural hematoma, only occurring a minority of the time, is a young adult who has a brief loss of consciousness followed by a lucid interval for several hours. This is then followed by obtundation, contralateral hemiparesis, and ipsilateral pupillary dilation (signs of uncal herniation as described in question 5). Death may result from continued compression of the midbrain causing bradycardia and respiratory distress. Overall mortality from epidural hematomas ranges from 20 to 55%, with prompt diagnosis and treatment lowering this rate to 5 to 10%.

The most common location for an epidural hematoma is temporoparietal, and the most common cause is a tear in a branch of the middle meningeal artery. A temporoparietal skull fracture is the usual offending injury. Other sources of bleeding include meningeal veins and dural sinuses. The classic CT finding for an epidural hematoma is a biconvex, hyperdense area adjacent to the skull. The hematoma is usually limited to a small area of the skull and does not cross suture lines. Generally accepted indications for removing an epidural hematoma in the operating room include any symptomatic epidural or an acute asymptomatic epidural that is greater than 1 cm at its widest portion since these tend not to resorb. Additionally, the threshold for operating on pediatric patients is lower than for adults since children have less available intracranial space to accommodate a blood clot.

Bibliography

Greenberg M. *Handbook of Neurosurgery*, 4th ed., vol. 2. Lakeland, FL: Greenberg Graphics, 1997, 727–728.

11. **(B)** The brain is covered by the meninges which include pia (a thin membrane tightly adherent to the brain), arachnoid, and dura. A subdural hematoma is a hemorrhage that occurs between the dura and arachnoid membrane. Subdural hematomas may be divided radiographically into three categories: acute, subacute, and chronic. An acute subdural hematoma is seen within 3 days of the initial hemorrhage and appears hyperdense to brain on CT scans. A subacute subdural hematoma forms between 4 days and 3 weeks following the initial hemorrhage and appears isodense to brain on CT scans (Fig. 9–9). A chronic subdural hematoma may be seen after 3 weeks following the initial hemorrhage and appears hypodense to brain on CT scans. All categories of subdural

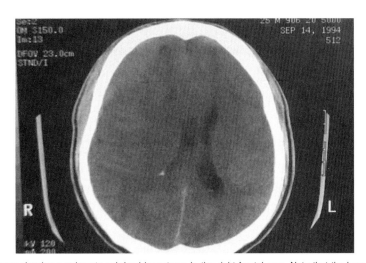

FIG. 9-9 CT scan showing a subacute subdural hematoma in the right frontal area. Note that the hemorrhage appears isodense to brain. Also note the midline shift from right to left.

hematomas usually appear as concave fluid collections that spread out over the convexity of the brain. Subdural hematomas may also occur along the tentorium cerebelli, along the interhemispheric fissure, and in the posterior fossa.

Clinically, a distinction is made between the acute and chronic categories of subdural hematomas, because these two categories differ so markedly in their presentation, treatment, and outcome. Subacute subdural hematomas are typically lumped into one of these categories based on the patient's presentation and symptoms. Acute subdural hematomas most often result from trauma and are commonly associated with a primary underlying brain injury. The actual hemorrhage may be the result of a parenchymal laceration or tearing of a vein that bridges the brain surface with the dura. The overall mortality with acute subdural hematomas is higher than with epidural hematomas and much higher than with chronic subdural hematomas, ranging from approximately 50 to 90%. Surgical evacuation of the hematoma should be considered for any symptomatic hematoma that is greater than 1 cm at its thickest point. Treatment of acute subdural hematomas involves making a large craniotomy to allow for removal of clotted blood over a large surface area of brain. Smaller subdural hematomas may be watched and will usually resorb over time. Time to surgery has been held as an important factor influencing mortality and functional survival, with evacuation within 4 h resulting in improved outcome.

On the other hand, chronic subdural hematomas typically occur in the elderly and are linked to trauma in only a minority of cases. Risk factors include coagulopathy, seizures, ventricular shunts, alcohol abuse, and any condition that increases the risk of falling. Symptoms of a chronic subdural hematoma may be mild, i.e., headache, lethargy, confusion, and diagnosis is often delayed. Treatment most commonly consists of drilling burr holes over the hematoma and irrigating the subdural space until it is clear. This is possible because the old blood has liquefied into a fluid with the appearance of motor oil. The outcome for patients following evacuation of a chronic subdural hematoma is generally good, although complications may include seizures or acute hemorrhage.

Bibliography

Greenberg M. *Handbook of Neurosurgery*, 4th ed., vol. 2. Lakeland, FL: Greenberg Graphics, 1997, 729–733.

12. **(A)** Gunshot wounds to the head represent the most lethal type of brain injury with two-thirds dying at the scene and ultimately resulting in death in greater than 90% of victims. Although previously held as the most critical determinant of tissue injury, projectile velocity has been shown to not be the primary factor related to wounding potential. According to recent literature, the major determinant of brain injury is the behavior of the projectile within the tissue such as its deformation, yaw, and fragmentation. These projectile characteristics result in varying degrees of primary and secondary brain injury. The impact of the projectile with the skull and its path through the brain results in primary injury that may include scalp laceration, skull fractures, tracking of debris into the brain, brain cavitation, and intracerebral hemorrhage (Fig. 9-10). A major goal of treating gunshot wounds to the head is

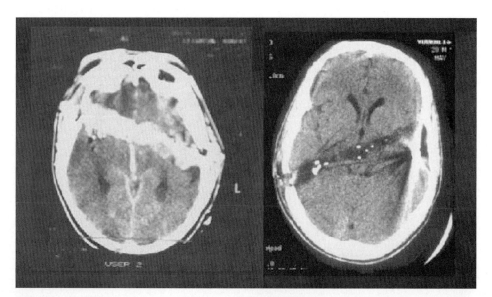

FIG. 9-10 Two CT scans showing gunshot wounds to the head. Note that the track of the bullet is filled with debris.

to prevent secondary injury which may include cerebral edema, intracranial hypertension, disseminated intravascular coagulopathy, seizures, cerebral abscess, and traumatic aneurysm.

Initial steps in the management of a patient with a gunshot wound to the head include cardiopulmonary resuscitation as needed, endotracheal intubation if airway is compromised, cervical spine precautions, control scalp bleeding, shave the scalp, and obtain a noncontrast CT scan of the brain. In addition, one must assume that the ICP is elevated in a patient with a gunshot wound to the head. Therefore, initial measures must be taken to control the patient's ICP. These steps are elevating the head of bed to 30–45%, keeping the head in midline position, administering a 1 gm/kg bolus of mannitol as blood pressure permits, and mild hyperventilation (PCO_2 = 35). The efficacy of steroids in penetrating head injuries is unsubstantiated and is therefore not recommended. Further medical management of this patient includes the use of prophylactic antibiotics, anticonvulsants, and antacids. Cerebral angiography is indicated in patients with a delayed hemorrhage or when the trajectory of the projectile is believed to involve named vessels or a dural venous sinus in a salvageable patient.

The most important prognostic indicator of outcome in patients with a gunshot wound to the head is the presenting GCS score. Additional risk factors for poor outcome are suicide attempts, intracranial hemorrhage, bullet traversing through ventricles or geographic center of brain, bihemispheric injury, and multilobar injury. One prospective study suggests a paradigm in which surgery is reserved for the following patients: those with a GCS score of 3–5 with a large extraaxial hematoma, those with a GCS score of 6–8 without bihemispheric, transventricular, or multilobar dominant hemisphere injury, and those with a GCS score of 9–15. In general, patients sustaining a gunshot wound to the head will either do relatively well or die.

Bibliography

Fackler M. Wound ballistics. A review of common misconceptions. *JAMA* 1988;259:2730–2736.

Grahm T, Williams F, Harrington T, et al. Civilian gunshot wounds to the head: a prospective study. *Neurosurgery* 1990;27:696–700.

Kaufman H. Civilian gunshot wounds to the head. *Neurosurgery* 1993;32:962–964.

Rosenberg W, Harsh G. Penetrating wounds of the head. In: Wilkins R, Rengachary S (eds.), *Neurosurgery*, 2nd ed. New York, NY: McGraw-Hill, 1996, 2813–2819.

The Brain Trauma Foundation. The use of mannitol in severe head injury. *J Neurotrauma* 1996;13(11):705–709.

13. **(C)** Homicide is the most frequent cause of death in children between the ages of 1 month and 1 year (17%). Common histories given by abusive caregivers include no known trauma, a presumed but unwitnessed fall, seizure, or respiratory arrest. Many studies have looked at the differences in injuries between abused children and children sustaining accidental injuries. In general, these studies have shown that abuse should be suspected when a child has retinal hemorrhages, bilateral chronic subdural hematomas if less than 2 years of age, multiple skull fractures, or skull fractures associated with intracranial injury. A recent retrospective review of cases further delineated several key differences between accidental and nonaccidental trauma in children. First of all, the mean age of the accident group in this study was 2.5 years while the mean age for the definite abuse group was 0.7 years. Distinctions in frequencies of various types of injuries included the following: subdural hematomas were found in 10% of the accident group and in 46% of the definite abuse group, subarachnoid hemorrhages were seen in 8% of the accident group and in 31% of the abuse group, retinal hemorrhages were documented in 2% of the accident group and in 33% of the abuse group, and associated cutaneous injuries were found in 16% of the accident group and in 50% of the definite abuse group. Although retinal hemorrhages are nearly pathognomonic for child abuse, these may also be seen following traumatic parturition, with benign subdural effusions in infants, and with acute high altitude sickness. In addition, mortality rates were 2% in the accident group and 13% in the definite abuse group. The increased mortality rate associated with abused children may often be related to a delay in seeking medical attention. Following an episode of abuse, the caregiver may place the unconscious child back in her crib or bed. Subsequently, the infant may develop cerebral edema and show signs of elevated ICP such as respiratory arrest or seizures. In other instances the child may not wake up for many hours. In either case, the child presents to the hospital too late to reverse the existing brain damage.

Radiographically, there appear to be certain skull fracture characteristics that suggest a diagnosis of abuse. Fracture characteristics seen more commonly in abused children are multiple or complex configuration, involvement of more than a single cranial bone, depressed fracture, wide or growing fracture, nonparietal fracture, and associated intracranial injury. Accidents typically cause single, narrow, linear fractures of the parietal bone without associated intracranial injury. With these differences in mind, a clinician will be better able to distinguish between accidental trauma and cases of abuse.

Bibliography

Greenberg M. *Handbook of Neurosurgery*, 4th ed., vol. 2. Lakeland, FL: Greenberg Graphics, 1997, 744–745.

Hobbs C. Skull fractures and the diagnosis of abuse. *Arch Dis Child* 1984;59(3):246–252.

Reece R, Sege R. Childhood head injuries: accident or inflicted? *Arch Pediatr Adolesc Med* 2000;154(1):11–15.

Waller A, Baker S, Szocka A. Childhood injury deaths: national analysis and geographic variations. *Am J Public Health* 1989;79:310–315.

14. **(C)** There are two reasons to declare that a patient is brain dead. The first is to allow for organ donation, and the second is to allow for removal of life support mechanisms once it is deemed that further medical treatment is futile. Most state governments and hospitals refer to the guidelines established by the President's Commission for the determination of brain death. For older children and adults, the physical examination must show absence of cerebral and brain stem function, no response to deep central pain, and absence of complicating conditions such as hypothermia or hypotension. Findings consistent with absence of brain stem function are dilated and nonreactive pupils, absent corneal reflexes, absent oculocephalic (doll's eyes) reflex, absent oculovestibular reflex, and absent oropharyngeal (gag) reflex. In addition to these, the apnea test is used to assess the function of the medulla. Brain death is confirmed if the patient has no spontaneous respirations after allowing the $PaCO_2$ to reach greater than 60 (hypercapnia of this degree will always produce spontaneous respirations in a patient with a functioning brain stem). If a patient has extensor (decerebrate) or flexor (decorticate) posturing in response to deep central pain, then information from the brain stem is still being transmitted down through the spinal cord which is incompatible with a diagnosis of brain death. Additionally, a patient should be free of any complicating condition that may simulate brain death. Such conditions include hypothermia, hypotension, intoxication, anoxia, immediate postresuscitation state, and patients emerging from a pentobarbital coma. Certain observation periods ranging from 6 to 24 h may also be warranted depending on the specific circumstances.

For children less than 5 years of age coma and apnea must coexist, and there must be absence of brainstem function on physical examination. Additional criteria include two examinations and two negative electroencephalograms (EEG) 48 h apart for children age 7 days to 2 months, two examinations and two negative EEGs 24 h apart for children age 2 months to 12 months, and an interval of 12 h between examinations and EEGs for children age 12 months to 5 years. Besides EEG, other confirmatory tests for diagnosing brain death include cerebral angiography and radionuclide blood flow studies. These studies may be helpful in patients with severe congestive heart failure or chronic obstructive pulmonary disease where the apnea test is invalid, in patients with severe facial trauma which would preclude cranial nerve testing, in patients coming out of a pentobarbital coma, and in allowing more expedient organ donation.

Bibliography

President's Commission for the study of ethical problems in medicine: guidelines for the determination of death. *JAMA* 1981;246:2184–2186.

Task force for the determination of brain death in children: guidelines for the determination of brain death in children. *Arch Neurol* 1987;44:587–588.

15. **(D)** DAI refers to a characteristic brain injury pattern. The patient presents with unconsciousness and a lack of a focal mass lesion on CT scanning (Fig. 9-11). Patients who suffer from DAI typically do not present with a lucid interval. Neuronal damage results from shearing of the axons that is caused by rotational acceleration forces. These same forces cause shearing of small blood vessels as well. Skull fractures are less common in patients with DAI than in those with a focal lesion. The rotational forces necessary to cause DAI most commonly occur in motor vehicle accidents. In motor vehicle accidents, the head makes contact

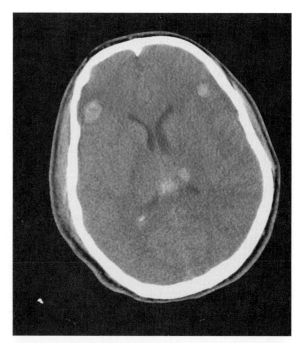

FIG. 9-11 CT scan showing diffuse axonal injury resulting from a motor vehicle accident. Note the multiple areas of hemorrhage within the brain.

with a relatively soft, broad surface such as a padded dashboard or energy-absorbing steering column resulting in a long period of acceleration within the skull. This longer period of acceleration translates into greater shearing and deformation of brain tissue.

There are three classic pathologic lesions seen in the brains of patients with DAI. The first is focal necrosis and/or hemorrhage in the corpus callosum. This may vary in size from microscopic to involving the entire corpus callosum. The second classic finding is hemorrhagic necrosis in the dorsolateral rostral pons. The third lesion is reactive axonal swelling from tearing of the axon, aka retraction balls. This is a microscopic finding that may develop as early as 3 h postinjury.

Direct impact forces cause injuries such as skull fracture, epidural hematomas, and coup contusions. These injuries are primarily the result of deformation of the skull. Linear acceleration forces are associated with subdural hematomas and contrecoup contusions. Differential movement between the skull and the brain causes tearing of bridging veins resulting in a subdural hematoma. In addition, brain movement away from the skull results in areas of low pressure creating sufficient tensile strain to produce a contrecoup contusion on the surface of the brain. Axial loading is associated with cervical spine fractures.

16. (C), 17. (E), 18. (D), 19. (B), 20. (A) Since subdural and epidural hematomas are discussed in other questions, the focus now will be on subarachnoid hemorrhage and intracerebral hemorrhage. A subarachnoid hemorrhage is defined as bleeding into the space between the pia and the arachnoid membranes. Trauma is the most common cause of a subarachnoid hemorrhage, and this occurs as a result of tearing of a superficial cortical vessel. The management and prognosis of a traumatic subarachnoid hemorrhage is far different than that of a spontaneous subarachnoid hemorrhage that is most often the result of a ruptured intracranial aneurysm (as shown in this question). On CT scan, a traumatic subarachnoid hemorrhage is typically less intense and is more often seen along the surface of the cerebral hemispheres or in the interhemispheric fissure rather than in the basal cisterns (as would be seen with a ruptured aneurysm). In addition, other related brain injuries such as cerebral contusions are more commonly seen with traumatic subarachnoid hemorrhages. Finally, the morbidity and mortality of a traumatic subarachnoid hemorrhage is much less than that of a subarachnoid hemorrhage related to a ruptured aneurysm. Spontaneous subarachnoid hemorrhages resulting from a ruptured aneurysm have a significant risk of vasospasm and hydrocephalus. Patients who present with a small amount of traumatic subarachnoid hemorrhage and are neurologically intact may be discharged safely to home after an overnight period of observation.

Although not as common, trauma may cause an intracerebral hemorrhage as well. This results from tearing of a blood vessel that lies within the brain parenchyma. These tend to occur in a lobar fashion (in cortex or subcortical white matter) rather than in the deeper basal ganglia region as seen in hemorrhages related to hypertension. It is important to remember that an intracerebral hemorrhage in a trauma patient may have preceded and led to the trauma rather than being the result of the trauma. Other important causes of lobar intracerebral hemorrhages to keep in mind are tumor, arteriovenous malformations, distal aneurysms that are adherent to the brain, and hemorrhagic transformation of an ischemic infarct. Intracerebral hemorrhages may need to be surgically evacuated if they are large and producing significant mass effect on surrounding brain.

The CT scan in Fig. 9-1 shows an acute subdural hematoma on the left. The blood is hyperintense to brain and is concave to brain. The CT scan in Fig. 9-2 shows an epidural hematoma on the right side. The blood is hyperintense to brain and is convex to brain. The CT scan in Fig. 9-3 shows an acute, right occipital lobar intracerebral hemorrhage. The CT scan in Fig. 9-4 shows a diffuse subarachnoid hemorrhage. Note that the blood is tracking within the cisternal spaces at the base of the brain. This was the result of a ruptured berry aneurysm. Also note the acute hypdrocephalus as evidenced by the enlarged temporal horns of the lateral ventricles. The CT scan in Fig. 9-5 shows a chronic subdural hematoma in the left frontal area. The blood is hypointense to brain.

Bibliography

Gennarelli T, Meaney D. Mechanisms of primary head injury. In: Wilkins R, Rengachary S (eds.), *Neurosurgery*, 2nd ed. New York, NY: McGraw-Hill, 1996, 2611–2621.

21. (C) One in five patients with a major spinal injury will have a second spine injury at another level. Most of these injuries will be to the cervical spine, and many of these patients will also have injuries to other systems. It is critical that patients suspected of having a spine injury have their entire spine immobilized during transport. Likewise, it is essential that the entire spine be examined when the patient is seen in the emergency department. Although the medical management of patients with spinal cord injuries has improved over time, the prognosis for functional recovery in patients with severe spinal cord injuries remains poor. The prognosis for functional recovery in these patients is directly related to the patient's neurologic condition at admission. In other words, a patient who presents with minimal weakness will have a very good chance of improving, while a patient who presents with no motor function will have almost no chance of improvement. Approximately 3% of patients with complete spinal cord injuries will show some sign of improvement within 24 h. If there is no improvement in 24 h, then it is almost certain that no recovery of function will occur. Therefore, it is important at the time of presentation to determine if a patient has a complete (no motor or sensory function below level of injury) or incomplete spinal cord injury. Additionally, patients with incomplete spinal cord injuries improve the greatest amount within the first year after injury, although improvement may continue for several years.

Bibliography

Greenberg M. *Handbook of Neurosurgery*, 4th ed., vol. 2. Lakeland, FL: Greenberg Graphics, 1997, 754.

22. **(A)** The term spinal shock may be used to describe two very different phenomena associated with spinal cord injury. The first type, as used in this question, refers to hypotension that commonly follows certain types of spinal cord injury. A cervical or high thoracic spinal cord injury may interrupt the sympathetic pathways to the body. This results in a loss of vascular tone in much of the body causing pooling of blood in the vascular system. Loss of muscle tone below the level of injury contributes to the hypotension as well. In the absence of any significant coexisting injury or worrisome examination findings, the most likely cause of the above-mentioned patient's hypotension is spinal shock. Of note, however, hypovolemia is the most common cause of hypotension in a trauma patient, and treatment should first be aimed at restoring euvolemia.

 The other way in which the term spinal shock is used is to describe the immediate, transient loss of all spinal reflexes below the level of spinal cord injury. This results in a flaccid paralysis that lasts approximately 2 weeks to 2 months. After this period of time, the patient will develop hyperreflexia and increased spasticity below the level of injury as the spinal cord damage becomes chronic in nature.

23. **(B)** Hypotension is a common finding in patients following acute spinal cord injury. As is the case with traumatic brain injury, hypotension may contribute to worsening neurologic function following spinal cord injury because of decreased perfusion to the spinal cord. Therefore, it is now recommended that hypotension (SBP <90) be avoided or corrected as soon as possible following spinal cord injury. In addition, maintaining a MAP of 85–90 for the first 7 days after acute spinal cord injury is recommended. Many clinicians even support invasive monitoring within an intensive care unit setting in the first 7 days following acute spinal cord injury because of the increased risk of cardiac and pulmonary disturbances in these patients. These practices are supported by investigators that have demonstrated improvements in neurologic outcome seemingly as a result of early, aggressive volume resuscitation and blood pressure augmentation alone. In regards to the treatment of hypotension in the face of acute spinal cord injury, pressors are recommended once volume resuscitation is completed since this counteracts the underlying physiologic disturbance, i.e., provides sympathetic tone. Dopamine is the agent of choice, because it has a lower incidence of reflex bradycardia than pure alpha agonist agents like phenylephrine. Intravenous fluids should be used to maintain a state of euvolemia, but these are usually inadequate to treat hypotension resulting from spinal shock. As such, there is a propensity to cause pulmonary edema if intravenous fluids alone are used for treating this disorder. Although it may be helpful in the initial resuscitation period, the Trendelenberg position should not be used as the definitive treatment for hypotension.

Bibliography

Hadley M, Walters B, et al. Section on Disorders of the Spine and Peripheral Nerves. The American Association of Neurological Surgeons and the Congress of Neurological Surgeons. Blood pressure management after acute spinal cord injury. Guidelines for the management of acute cervical spine and spinal cord injuries. *Neurosurgery* 2002;50(3):S58–S62.

Vale F, Burns J, Jackson A, et al. Combined medical and surgical treatment after acute spinal cord injury: results of a prospective pilot study to assess the merits of aggressive medical resuscitation and blood pressure management. *J Neurosurg* 1997;87:239–246.

24. **(A)** A patient presenting to the emergency department with an acute spinal cord injury will have several unique problems that should be addressed early in his/her management. First, the patient may present with poikilothermy (inability to regulate body temperature) as a result of vasomotor paralysis. Appropriate warming or cooling should be instituted early. Second, many patients with spinal cord injury will have paralytic ileus that may last for several days. Therefore, a

nasogastric tube should be placed to suction to prevent emesis and aspiration. Aspiration poses a significant risk to a patient with a cervical or high thoracic cord injury, because the paralyzed abdominal musculature is unable to develop a forceful cough. Third, many patients with spinal cord injury will have disrupted bowel and bladder function. These patients are at increased risk of developing severe bladder distension. This is especially important in patients who develop autonomic dysreflexia. This condition occurs in patients with spinal cord injury above the T6 level and is characterized by an exaggerated autonomic response (sympathetic usually dominates) secondary to a stimulus that is usually only mildly noxious. Common stimuli include bladder distension, fecal impaction, administration of enemas, skin infections, and urinary tract infections. The response to such stimuli may be severe hypertension, flushing, tachycardia, headache, hyperhidrosis, or diaphoresis. The hypertension resulting from this illness has been reported to have caused a fatal intracerebral hemorrhage. Therefore, it is very important to place a bladder catheter in patients with a spinal cord injury. Additional initial measures include rapid treatment of hypotension with pressors and maintaining adequate oxygenation. All patients with a suspected spinal cord injury should be immobilized on a backboard in the field. Patients should remain on the backboard, however, only while it is beneficial in assisting with patient transfers such as onto and off of the CT scanner. As soon as this period has passed, the backboard should be removed. It only takes a few hours on a backboard for a patient to develop pressure sores.

Bibliography

Greenberg M. *Handbook of Neurosurgery*, 4th ed., vol. 2. Lakeland, FL: Greenberg Graphics, 1997, 791–793.

25. **(D)** The use of methylprednisolone for treating patients with acute spinal cord injury remains one of the most controversial topics in trauma and neurosurgical literature. The most commonly cited guidelines for the use of methylprednisolone in spinal cord injury are derived from the second and third National Acute Spinal Cord Injury Studies (NASCIS). According to the results of NASCIS II, patients who were given a 30 mg/kg bolus of methylprednisolone in the first 15 min of the first hour followed by a 5.4 mg/kg/h infusion over the next 23 h had improvement in motor function and in sensation at the 6-month follow-up. Since this study included patients with complete and incomplete injuries, many clinicians use this regimen for both types of patients.

More recently, NASCIC III results showed benefits using a slightly altered regimen. In this study, patients could receive methylprednisolone for a total of 24 or 48 h. The results showed improvement in motor function for patients in both groups if treated within 3 h of injury and in the 48-h group if treatment began between 3 and 8 h postinjury. Therefore, the investigators recommended giving a 48-h methylprednisolone regimen to patients if administration of the drug began in the 3–8-h postinjury window and limiting the regimen to 24 h when the drug could be started within 3 h of injury. This study also noted the increased incidence of severe sepsis and severe pneumonia with the 48-h methylprednisolone treatment group. Several other studies have demonstrated an increased risk of gastrointestinal bleeding and poor wound healing with either of these regimens.

Along with many concerns regarding the harmful side effects of using high dose steroids, many investigators have questioned the significance of the NASCIS II and NASCIS III results. A thorough review of the published data on the use of methylprednisolone is provided in the recent American Association of Neurological Surgeons and Congress of Neurological Surgeons sponsored Guidelines for the Management of Acute Cervical Spine and Spinal Cord Injuries. After careful scientific review of the data, the authors of this publication note that there is insufficient evidence to support treatment standards or guidelines regarding the use of methylprednisolone in acute spinal cord injury. What they do conclude is that "treatment with methylprednisolone for either 24 or 48 h is recommended as an option in the treatment of patients with acute spinal cord injuries that should be undertaken only with the knowledge that the evidence suggesting harmful side effects is more consistent than any suggestion of clinical benefit." Until more successful therapies are developed, it is likely that most clinicians will continue to use methylprednisolone for the treatment of acute spinal cord injury in the hopes of obtaining some functional benefit in their patients. It is clear from this publication, however, that careful scrutiny must be given to deciding who should and who should not receive methylprednisolone because of its potentially harmful side effects.

Bibliography

Bracken M, Shepard M, Collins W, et al. A randomized, controlled trial of methylprednisolone or naloxone in the treatment of acute spinal cord injury: results of the second National Acute Spinal Cord Injury Study (NASCIS II). *N Engl J Med* 1990;322:1405–1411.

Bracken M, Shepard M, Holford T, et al. Administration of methylprednisolone for 24 or 48 h or tirilazad mesylate for 48 h in the treatment of acute spinal cord injury: results of the third National Acute Spinal Cord Injury Randomized Controlled Trial—NASCIS. *JAMA* 1997; 277:1597–1604.

26. **(B)** It is now standard care for emergency medical services (EMS) personnel to immobilize a patient's cervical spine with a collar following trauma. It is the physician's role to rule out spinal column or spinal cord injury in a patient before removing the cervical collar. In an effort to reduce expense and prevent unnecessary exposure to radiation, it is important to know which patients truly need to have plain radiographs of their cervical spine. One of the largest studies to address this issue looked at over 34,000 patients evaluated in 21 different emergency departments in the United States. Of the 576 patients who were deemed to have clinically significant injuries, two were originally assigned to the asymptomatic group (based on history and physical examination). Of these two patients, one developed paresthesias in an arm and underwent surgery. Therefore, the results showed that the negative predictive value of an asymptomatic examination was 99.9%. Several other well-developed investigations have had similar results. After reviewing numerous pertinent studies, the American Association of Neurological Surgeons and the Congress of Neurological Surgeons found the data convincing enough to publish a treatment standard. According to this standard, radiographic assessment of the cervical spine is not recommended in trauma patients who meet the following criteria: awake, alert, not intoxicated, without neck pain or tenderness, and without a significant distracting injury. The patient in this question meets these criteria and, therefore, needs no radiographs before clearing his cervical spine.

For those patients who are symptomatic or do not meet the above criteria, the same published guidelines recommend as a treatment standard obtaining a three view cervical spine series (AP, lateral, and odontoid views). In addition, supplemental CT scanning should be performed to further define suspicious areas or areas that are not well visualized on plain radiographs. Only treatment options are recommended for symptomatic patients who end up having normal x-rays and CT scans. Awake patients with neck pain or tenderness may have their cervical collars removed once they have either a normal and adequate dynamic flexion/extension series or a normal magnetic resonance imaging (MRI) study within 48 h on injury. Cervical collars on obtunded patients may be removed following the acquisition of a normal dynamic flexion/extension study performed under fluoroscopic guidance, after a normal MRI study obtained within 48 h of injury, or at the discretion of the treating physician. Of course, not every patient falls neatly into one of these categories. Much variation remains across hospitals and regions in the process used to clear cervical spines in trauma patients. Many hospitals will have algorithms for clearing cervical spines in place for physicians to reference.

Bibliography

Hadley M, Walters B, et al. Section on Disorders of the Spine and Peripheral Nerves. The American Association of Neurological Surgeons and the Congress of Neurological Surgeons. Blood pressure management after acute spinal cord injury. Guidelines for the management of acute cervical spine and spinal cord injuries. *Neurosurgery* 2002;50(3):S63–S72.

Hadley M, Walters B, et al. Section on Disorders of the Spine and Peripheral Nerves. The American Association of Neurological Surgeons and the Congress of Neurological Surgeons. Radiographic assessment of the cervical spine in asymptomatic trauma patients. Guidelines for the management of acute cervical spine and spinal cord injuries. *Neurosurgery* 2002;50(3): S30–S35.

Hoffman J, Mower W, Wolfson A, et al. Validity of a set of clinical criteria to rule out injury to the cervical spine in patients with blunt trauma: National Emergency X-Radiography Utilization Study Group. *N Engl J Med* 2000;343:94–99.

27. **(C)** The central cord syndrome is a common type of incomplete spinal cord injury. This syndrome usually results from hyperextension of the cervical spine such as when a person falls and hits his forehead or in a motor vehicle accident when a person's forehead strikes the windshield. It occurs most commonly in elderly patients who have preexisting cervical spinal spondylosis with a narrowed spinal canal. On hyperextension of the cervical spine, the spinal cord is compressed by bony spurs anteriorly or by buckling of the ligamentum flavum posteriorly. The arterial supply of the spinal cord is divided such that several radially oriented circumferential branches supply the outer white matter while a central anterior sulcal branch supplies the deep white and gray matter. This arrangement produces both a watershed area between the two arterial supplies and a greater susceptibility for disruption of blood flow into the central area of the spinal cord. As a result, blunt trauma to spinal cord is more likely to damage the central portion of the cord. Since the fibers in the corticospinal tract that supply the upper extremities are more medial than those supplying the lower extremities, this syndrome results in disproportionate weakness of the upper extremities.

Sensory loss is usually minimal and may occur in any distribution. Urinary retention is common, especially in more severe cases.

Another type of incomplete spinal cord injury is the Brown-Sequard's syndrome. This refers to hemisection of the cord. It is usually caused by penetrating trauma such as stab wounds, although it may also be caused by lateral cord compression. This syndrome or similar pattern is seen in 2–4% of traumatic spinal cord injuries. Clinically, the patient presents with ipsilateral paralysis (corticospinal tract) and loss of vibration and position sense (posterior columns) with contralateral loss of pain and temperature sensation (lateral spinothalamic tract). This syndrome carries a more favorable prognosis than the central cord syndrome.

The anterior cord syndrome is an infarction of the spinal cord in the territory supplied by the anterior spinal artery. This may result from anterior spinal artery occlusion or from anterior compression of the cord. The classic presentation is a patient who has no motor function below the level of the lesion, no pain and temperature sensation below the level of the lesion, and preservation of vibration and position sense. This occurs because the anterior spinal artery supplies the anterior two-third of the cord, thus sparing the posterior columns if this region becomes ischemic. The anterior cord syndrome is thought to carry the worst prognosis of the incomplete spinal cord injury syndromes with only 10–20% of patients ever recovering functional motor control.

Finally, a cervical herniated disc presents most commonly as a radiculopathy. The typical presentation is a patient who complains of pain and/or numbness down one arm in a specific nerve root distribution. Weakness of the muscles supplied by this nerve root may occur as well. On occasion, a herniated disc will be large enough to compress the spinal cord and cause a myelopathy. The hallmark of this entity is hyperreflexia with the presence of abnormal reflexes such as clonus, plantar extensor response, and Hoffman's sign. Pain, paresthesias, and weakness is variable with myelopathy. Rarely, a traumatic acute central disc herniation can cause an acute central cord syndrome as well.

Bibliography

Greenberg M. *Handbook of Neurosurgery*, 4th ed., vol. 2. Lakeland, FL: Greenberg Graphics, 1997, 764–766.

Roth E, Park T, Pang T, et al. Traumatic cervical Brown-Sequard and Brown-Sequard plus syndromes: the spectrum of presentations and outcomes. *Paraplegia* 1991; 29:582–589.

28. (D) The term SCIWORA was coined in 1982 by Pang and Wilberger to describe cases in which there were objective signs of myelopathy as a result of trauma with no evidence of fracture, subluxation, or instability on plain radiographs or tomography. Most physicians extend this definition to include patients with symptoms, as well as signs, of spinal cord injury. SCIWORA occurs more commonly in children younger than 9 years of age. In addition, younger children are more likely to have more severe injuries than older children. This is largely the result of younger children sustaining more upper cervical injuries than older children. In younger children, the maximal level of flexion occurs at C2/3 and C3/4. As a child ages, the maximal point of flexion migrates caudally to settle at the adult level of C5/6 around 8 years. This point helps explain the increased incidence of upper cervical spine injuries in young children, but how can such injuries occur without producing evidence of fracture or instability?

In addition to having a proportionately larger head and weaker neck muscles, children possess certain characteristics in their spine that make them more susceptible to excess intersegmental motion than an adult. First, children have a more horizontal orientation of their facet joints. Second, there is anterior wedging of the superior aspect of the vertebral bodies in children. Third, children have more elastic ligaments and joint capsules than adults. These characteristics allow for greater intersegmental instability without overt disruption of the ligaments, bones, or disc spaces. Spinal cord injury thus results from a transient compression of the spinal cord. The clinical presentation varies from transient paresthesias to complete spinal cord injury, and recurrent SCIWORA may occur as well (often after trauma of less magnitude than in original injury).

As alluded to earlier, the diagnosis of SCIWORA is made after all x-rays, including flexion/extension views, and tomograms are read as normal. An MRI scan, however, may be abnormal in a child diagnosed with SCIWORA. A MRI scan is helpful for detecting compressive lesions and for identifying transsection, hemorrhage, or edema within the cord. In addition, MRI is a valuable prognostic indicator of outcome with any visible injury to the cord signaling a worse prognosis than having no abnormality on MRI.

Treatment of SCIWORA is focused on preventing a recurrent spinal cord injury. Since spinal laxity with excessive motion is the cause of SCIWORA, immobilization of the spine is the mainstay of treatment. Although the time period of immobilization may vary depending on the patient's symptoms and MRI findings, many clinicians support a period of 12 weeks. Children with cervical injuries are often placed in a Guilford brace (harder to remove than a collar), and children with thoracic injuries are often placed in a thoracolumbosacral orthosis (TLSO). Limiting activity from contact sports for up to 6 months may be considered as well. In addition, many clinicians support the use of 24 h of methylprednisolone when initiated within 8 hours of the time of injury.

Bibliography

Grabb P, Albright A. Spinal cord injury without radiographic abnormality in children. In: Wilkins R, Rengachary S (eds.), *Neurosurgery*, 2nd ed. New York, NY: McGraw-Hill, 1996, 2867–2870.

Pang D, Wilberger J, Jr. Spinal cord injury without radiographic abnormalities in children. *J Neurosurg* 1982;57: 114–129.

Pang D, Pollack I. Spinal cord injury without radiographic abnormality in children the SCIWORA syndrome. *J Trauma* 1989;29:654–664.

29. (A) Traumatic atlantooccipital dislocation represents approximately 1% of patients who present to the emergency department with cervical spine injuries. Most of these injuries are related to a motor vehicle accident or a pedestrian versus automobile accident. Anatomically, the dislocation is most often the result of disruption of the tectorial membrane (continuation of posterior longitudinal ligament that connects dorsal surface of dens to ventral surface of basion) and the alar ligaments (connect lateral portions of dens to occipital condyles and lateral mass of atlas). Hyperextension may cause tearing of the tectorial membrane and lateral flexion may cause disruption of the alar ligaments. Hyperflexion may also produce this injury by causing separation of the posterior elements of the atlas and axis. Children are more susceptible to atlantooccipital dislocation than adults, because children have a more horizontal articulation between the skull and atlas and have less developed occipital condyles. Patients may present as neurologically intact or with spinal cord injury, cervical root injury, or brain stem injury. The most common cause of death in patients with atlantooccipital dislocation is respiratory arrest secondary to brain stem injury.

The diagnosis of atlantooccipital dislocation may be made with a lateral cervical spine x-ray (Fig. 9-12). Although there are many measurements used to diagnose this injury including the Power's ratio and x-line method, the American Association of Neurological Surgeons and the Congress of Neurological Surgeons recommend as an option using the basion-axial interval-basion-dental interval (BAI-BDI) method because of its increased sensitivity in diagnosing this injury. In this method, a displacement of

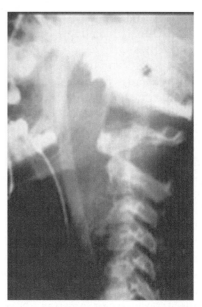

FIG. 9-12   Lateral cervical spine radiograph showing atlantooccipital dislocation. Note the increased distance between the base of the skull and the atlas.

more than +12 mm or more than –4 mm between the basion and the posterior axis line, or a displacement of more than 12 mm from the basion to the dens is considered diagnostic of a dislocation. Additionally, the presence of prevertebral soft tissue swelling should raise suspicion for this injury. CT and MRI imaging are recommended to further characterize the injury and assist with preoperative planning.

Treatment of atlantooccipital dislocations may vary depending on the type of dislocation. One group of investigators divided these dislocations into three types based on the direction of separation between the occiput and atlas: type I refers to anterior displacement of the occiput in relation to the atlas, type II refers to longitudinal distraction of the occiput away from the atlas, and type III refers to posterior displacement of the occiput in relation to the atlas. In this report, the authors suggest that light traction may be used for type I and type III injuries to realign the bones and decompress the spinal cord. Traction for type II dislocations is contraindicated, because a longitudinal force would only worsen the longitudinal distraction injury. Because of the high association of worsening neurologic condition and late instability with no treatment, cervical traction, and external immobilization alone, the American Association of Neurological Surgeons and the Congress of Neurological Surgeons recommend craniocervical fusion with internal fixation for patients with atlantooccipital dislocation.

Bibliography

Greenberg M. *Handbook of Neurosurgery*, 4th ed., vol. 2. Lakeland, FL: Greenberg Graphics, 1997, 767–768.

Harris J, Jr., Carson G, Wagner L, et al. Radiologic diagnosis of traumatic occipitovertebral dislocation: Part 2 Comparison of three methods of detecting occipitovertebral relationships on lateral radiographs of supine subjects. *Am J Radiol* 1994;162:887–892.

Lee C, Woodring J, Goldstein S, et al. Evaluation of traumatic atlantooccipital dislocations. *Am J Neuroradiol* 1987;8:19–26.

Powers B, Miller M, Kramer R, et al. Traumatic anterior atlanto-occipital dislocation. *Neurosurgery* 1979;4:12–17.

Traynelis V, Marano G, Dunker R, et al. Traumatic atlanto-occipital dislocation: case report. *J Neurosurg* 1986;65:863–870.

30. **(C)** Sir Geoffrey Jefferson reviewed several cases of atlas fractures in 1920 and characterized a burst fracture of the atlas ring (now known as a "Jefferson fracture"). An axial load to the head causes this type of fracture by forcing the occipital condyles down onto the lateral masses of the atlas. Enough force applied in this manner will result in fractures through the anterior and posterior arches of the atlas (Fig. 9-13). Treatment of atlas fractures varies depending on whether or not the fracture is considered to be stable. The critical structure providing stability to the atlas is the transverse atlantal ligament. There are several ways to determine radiographically if the transverse atlantal ligament is intact. First, the rules of Spence state that the transverse atlantal ligament is likely torn if the sum of the lateral mass displacement (LMD) of C1 over C2 on an AP x-ray is greater than 6.9 mm. Second, more recent studies have supported using an atlantodens interval of greater than 3 mm on a lateral x-ray to predict disruption of the transverse atlantal ligament. Finally, MRI is a sensitive indicator of transverse atlantal ligament injury. If the above criteria are not met and the fracture appears to be stable, then the American Association of Neurological Surgeons and the Congress of Neurological Surgeons recommend as a treatment option cervical immobilization alone. If the above criteria are met and the transverse atlantal ligament appears to be disrupted, then cervical immobilization alone or surgical fixation and fusion is recommended. Many surgeons support C1-C2 transarticular screw fixation with a posterior fusion for the treatment of unstable atlas fractures.

A Hangman's fracture is a fracture through the pars interarticularis of both pedicles of the axis that results in a traumatic spondylolisthesis (Fig. 9-14). The fracture was named after a similarity was noted between these fractures and those that occurred as a result of judicial hangings. The mechanism of injury is hyperextension and compression, often associated with a motor vehicle accident. Most patients with this fracture are neurologically intact and may be treated with cervical immobilization alone. Surgical stabilization may be considered for cases with severe angulation of C2 on C3, disruption of the C2-C3 disc space, or inability to establish or maintain alignment with external immobilization.

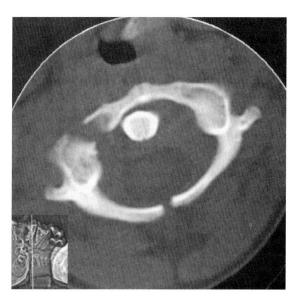

FIG. 9-13 CT showing fractures through the anterior and posterior arches of the atlas. This is known as a Jefferson fracture.

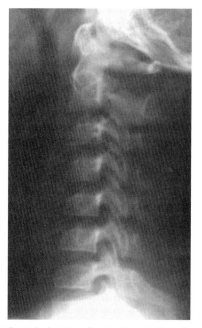

FIG. 9-14 Radiograph showing a fracture through the pedicles of C2, also known as a Hangman's fracture.

Bibliography

Hadley M, Walters B, et al. Section on Disorders of the Spine and Peripheral Nerves. The American Association of Neurological Surgeons and the Congress of Neurological Surgeons. Isolated fractures of the atlas in adults. Guidelines for the management of acute cervical spine and spinal cord injuries. *Neurosurgery* 2002;50(3):S120–S124.

Hadley M, Walters B, et al. Section on Disorders of the Spine and Peripheral Nerves. The American Association of Neurological Surgeons and the Congress of Neurological Surgeons. Isolated fractures of the axis in adults. Guidelines for the management of acute cervical spine and spinal cord injuries. *Neurosurgery* 2002;50(3):S125–S139.

Jefferson G. Fractures of the atlas vertebra: report of four cases and a review of those previously reported. *Br J Surg* 1920;7:407–422.

Spence K, Jr., Decker S, Sell K. Bursting atlantal fracture associated with rupture of the transverse ligament. *J Bone Joint Surg Am* 1970;52A: 543–549.

31. **(B)** Axis fractures account for about 17% of cervical spine fractures, and most of these are odontoid fractures. The mechanism of injury is usually flexion, and this is often associated with anterior subluxation of C1 on C2. Anderson and D'Alonzo developed a classification system in 1974 for odontoid fractures based on location of the fracture. Type I odontoid fractures involve the tip of the odontoid process, and they are the rarest type. These fractures are caused by an avulsion of the attachment of the alar ligament. Type II odontoid fractures involve the base of the odontoid process at the synchondrosis where the dens fuses with the body of C2 (Fig. 9–15). This is the most common type of odontoid fracture. Type III odontoid fractures are those that involve the base of the odontoid but extend into the body of C2. An addition to this classification system was made by Hadley et al. in 1988. They added a type IIA subtype fracture that represents a comminuted fracture through the base of the dens with associated free fragments of bone. In general, type II fractures are the least stable and have the highest nonunion rates. In addition, advanced age and dens displacement of >5 mm is associated with lower rates of fusion. After careful review of the literature, the current recommended guidelines in the neurosurgic literature are to consider surgical fixation and fusion for patients over the age of 50 years with type II odontoid fractures. Additionally, type II and type III fractures should be considered for surgical fixation is cases of dens displacement of 5 mm or greater, comminution of the fracture (type IIA), and inability to achieve or maintain alignment with external immobilization. Options for surgical treatment include posterior fusion with C1-C2 transarticular screw fixation and anterior odontoid screw fixation. The advantage

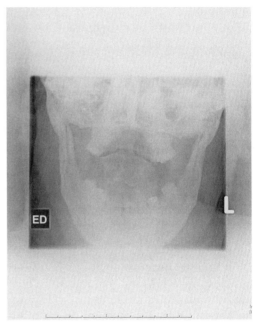

FIG. 9-15   Odontoid view cervical spine radiograph showing a type II fracture of the odontoid process.

of the latter procedure is that it provides greater preservation of cervical rotation. Other odontoid fractures may be successfully treated with halo brace immobilization.

Bibliography

Anderson L, D Alonzo R. Fractures of the odontoid process of the axis. *J Bone Joint Surg* 1974;56-A:1663–1674.

Hadley M, Browner C, Liu S, et al. New subtype of acute odontoid fractures (type IIA). *Neurosurgery* 1988;22: 67–71.

Hadley M, Browner C, Sonntag V. Axis fractures: a comprehensive review of management and treatment in 107 cases. *Neurosurgery* 1985;17:281–290.

32. **(B)** Severe flexion injuries of the cervical spine may cause unilateral or bilateral locked facets. Typically, unilateral locked facets result from flexion plus rotation injuries, and bilateral locked facets result from hyperflexion injuries. Anatomically, locked facets refer to the condition when the inferior articular facets of the upper dislocated vertebra slide forward over the superior facets of the vertebra below (Fig. 9-16). Bilateral locked facets are extremely unstable given the extensive amount of ligamentous injury involved. The forces applied in this type of injury rupture the posterior ligamentous complex, the joint capsules, the intervertebral disc, and, usually, the posterior and anterior longitudinal ligaments. In about 80% of these cases, the patients will present with complete spinal cord injuries. Nerve root injuries are common as well.

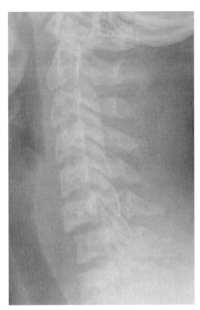

FIG. 9-16   Lateral cervical spine radiograph showing unilateral locked facets of C6 on C7.

Unilateral locked facets are more stable than bilateral, and these patients are usually neurologically intact. Patients in either of these groups should be treated initially with closed reduction using cervical traction. Once reduction of the cervical spine is achieved, patients may be stabilized by immobilization in a halo vest or by internal fixation and fusion. Surgical management is often preferred given the high incidence of unsatisfactory fusion when using a halo vest alone. Surgical management should be used if attempts at closed reduction are unsuccessful. MRI is helpful in evaluating for a herniated disc and determining the extent of damage to the spinal cord (Fig. 9-17). It is also useful for preoperative planning. Perched facets refer to facets that have just reached the point of locking without actually doing so. These injuries are treated in a similar manner to locked facets.

Bibliography

Hadley M, Fitzpatrick B, Sonntag V, et al. Facet fracture-dislocation injuries of the cervical spine. *Neurosurgery* 1992;31:661–666.

Sears W, Fazl M. Prediction of stability of cervical spine fracture managed in the halo vest and indications for surgical intervention. *J Neurosurg* 1990;72:426–432.

Sypert G, Arpin E. Management of lower cervical spinal instability. In: Wilkins R, Rengachary S (eds.), *Neurosurgery*, 2nd ed. New York, NY: McGraw-Hill, 1996, 2927–2937.

33. **(D)** A clay-shoveler fracture is an avulsion fracture of a spinous process that usually occurs at C6, C7, or T1 with C7 being the most common vertebra involved (Fig. 9-18). The mechanism of injury is flexion of the head combined with an opposing force of the posterior musculature attached to the spinous processes of the lower cervical and upper thoracic vertebra. This was originally described as occurring when clay stuck to the end of a shovel during the throwing phase causing the arms to be jerked upward. These fractures may also be caused by neck hyperflexion or by blunt trauma to the back of the neck. Patients presenting with these fractures are usually neurologically intact.

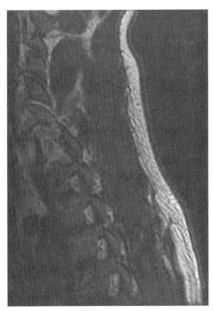

FIG. 9-17   MRI scan of the cervical and upper thoracic spine showing locked facets of C6 on C7.

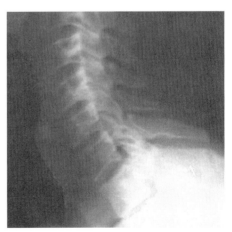

FIG. 9-18   Lateral cervical spine radiograph showing a clay-shoveler's fracture of T1.

These are stable fractures, and treatment involves placing the patient in a cervical collar for 6–8 weeks. Of course, clay-shoveler fractures may be associated with other cervical injuries. A CT scan is helpful to exclude other fractures, and flexion/extension radiographs are required to exclude significant ligamentous injury.

34. **(C)** Although the spine will usually fuse on its own in 8–12 weeks, this often requires the patient to remain on bed rest. Besides being difficult on the patient psychologically, prolonged bed rest carries a relatively high risk of several comorbidities such as deep venous thrombosis, pneumonia, pulmonary embolus, and decubitus ulcers. Early surgical fixation and fusion allows for early mobilization and expedites rehabilitation. It also helps prevent delayed kyphotic angulation deformity. Early surgery, however, does not improve neurologic function in a patient with a complete spinal cord injury.

    A difficult question to answer is when is the best time to operate on a patient who has an incomplete spinal cord injury. Although it may seem most appropriate to decompress and fixate the spine as quickly as possible, studies have shown that emergency surgery produces the greatest amount of neurological deterioration in patients with spinal cord injury. Other studies support the position that timing of surgery has no effect on neurologic function. Still others dispute the validity of these investigations and support emergent surgery for patients with incomplete spinal cord injury. Further research will be required before a consensus may be reached on this issue.

    Bibliography

    Benzel E, Larson S. Functional recovery after decompressive operation for thoracic and lumbar spine fractures. *Neurosurgery* 1986;19:772–778.

    Hall R. Clay-shoveller's fracture. *J Bone Joint Surg* 1940;22:63–75.

    Marshall L, Knowlton S, Garfin S, et al. Deterioration following spinal cord injury: a multicenter study. *J Neurosurg* 1987;66:400–404.

35. **(A)** Approximately two-thirds of all spine fractures occur at the thoracolumbar junction, and 70% of these present without neurologic injury. Many thoracolumbar fractures are considered minor injuries and are stable fractures. Fractures that fit into this category include transverse process, articular process, and spinous process fractures. Transverse process fractures may be associated with neurologic injury if they occur at T1 or T2 where the applied force might damage the brachial plexus or at L4 or L5 where the force might damage the lumbosacral plexus or the kidneys. Although no specific treatment of these fractures is

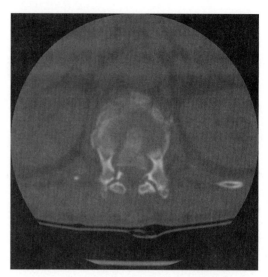

FIG. 9-19   CT scan of the lumbar spine showing a burst fracture of L1. Note the disruption of both the anterior and posterior portions of the vertebral body with retropulsion of bone into the spinal canal.

usually warranted, many clinicians will treat these fractures with a lumbar or thoracolumbar brace for several weeks.

A burst fracture, on the other hand, is considered an unstable fracture. It occurs as a result of an axial load that causes disruption of the anterior and posterior portions of the vertebral body (Fig. 9-19). These fractures usually occur between T10 and L2. Lateral x-ray will almost always show some degree of loss of posterior vertebral body height and retropulsion of bone into the spinal canal. An AP x-ray will demonstrate an increased interpeduncular distance. About half the patients presenting with a burst fracture will be neurologically intact. Burst fractures of thoracic vertebra tend to be more severe than fractures of the lumbar vertebra. Patients who present with no neurologic injury and have minor vertebral body disruption may be treated with a rigid thoracolumbar sacral orthosis (TLSO brace), but most burst fractures will require surgical decompression with stabilization.

Bibliography

Greenberg M. *Handbook of Neurosurgery*, 4th ed., vol. 2. Lakeland, FL: Greenberg Graphics, 1997, 784–787.

36. **(D)** In an attempt to define radiographic characteristics that would predict instability in thoracolumbar spine fractures, Denis created a three column model of the spine. According to this model, the anterior column includes the anterior half of the vertebral body and disc along with the anterior longitudinal ligament. The middle column is made up of the posterior half of

the vertebral body and disc as well as the posterior longitudinal ligament. The posterior column is comprised of the posterior bony complex (all structures posterior to the vertebral body) and the posterior ligamentous complex (interspinous and supraspinous ligaments, facet joint and capsule, and ligamentum flavum).

Using the three column model of the spine as a foundation, Denis proposed three degrees of instability associated with thoracolumbar fractures. Instability of the first degree, or mechanical instability, occurs when there is disruption of the anterior and posterior columns as in a severe compression fracture with distraction of the posterior elements or when there is disruption of the middle and posterior columns as in a seat-belt type fracture. A seat-belt fracture is caused by flexion as would occur when the spine is flexed over a lap belt. These fractures are considered mechanically unstable, because they are at risk for either further compression or angulation with increasing kyphotic deformity. External immobilization is usually adequate, although surgical stabilization may be required for severe cases. Although compression fractures that cause only anterior column disruption are usually considered stable, instability should be suspected if there are three or more compression fractures in a row or if there is greater than 50% loss of height of the vertebral body with angulation.

Instability of the second degree, or neurologic instability, occurs with burst fractures with no neurologic injury where there is disruption of the anterior and middle columns. These fractures are considered neurologically unstable, because there is a risk for further collapse of the vertebral body with further encroachment of free bone fragments into the spinal canal.

Instability of the third degree, or mechanical and neurologic instability, occurs with severe burst fractures with neurologic injury or with fracture-dislocations where there is disruption of all three columns. These fractures are at risk for further neurologic deterioration and deformity. Fractures with this degree of instability almost always require surgical reduction, decompression, and stabilization.

Bibliography

Denis F. The three column spine and its significance in the classification of acute thoracolumbar spinal injuries. *Spine* 1983;8:817–831.

37. **(D)** Most penetrating wounds of the spine in the United States of America today are caused by gunshot wounds. These are more common in urban areas where the rates of violent crimes are relatively high. Civilian gunshot wounds cause direct injury to the spinal cord by the bullet, whereas high velocity military weapons tend to cause more indirect damage from cavitation and shock waves. Although debated, surgery has been shown to have little effect on recovery for patients with spinal cord injury secondary to gunshot wounds to the spine. For this reason, the trend seems to be now to treat patients with gunshot wounds to the spine without surgery unless they have a specific indication to do so. One of the historically cited reasons for operating on all gunshot wounds to the spine was to prevent infection. This may likely remain pertinent with military gunshot wounds since these cause massive tissue injury. With the creation of new antibiotics, however, infections may be prevented in civilian gunshot wounds with adequate courses of antibiotics alone.

The more commonly accepted indications for operating on gunshot wounds to the spine include neurologic deterioration, compression of a nerve root, and persistent cerebrospinal fluid leak or fistula. In addition, there are a few late complications which may develop that require surgical treatment. First, an abscess could develop that requires surgical drainage, especially if there is compression of the spinal cord. Second, a syrinx may develop and be the cause of late neurologic deterioration. This could require a shunting procedure to alleviate the symptoms. Third, lead intoxication may result if the bullet is lodged in a disc space or joint capsule. The treatment for this would include removing the bullet fragment and administering a chelating agent. Finally, spinal deafferentation following spinal cord injury may result in intractable dysesthetic pain. Placement of a dorsal column stimulator or dorsal root entry zone lesioning may help in these cases.

38. **(C)** Patients with spinal cord injuries have a relatively high risk for developing deep venous thrombosis, especially with higher levels of injury. The overall mortality from deep venous thromboses in patients with spinal cord injury is approximately 10%. Death may result from pulmonary embolus or embolic stroke if the patient has a patent foramen ovale. Because of this risk, patients with spinal cord injury should be on some form of deep venous thrombosis prophylaxis. This may include passive lower extremity motion, pneumatic compression boots, and heparin delivered subcutaneously. Additionally, physicians caring for patients with spinal cord injuries should have a high index of suspicion and a low threshold for diagnosing and treating deep venous thromboses in these patients.

Bibliography

Greenberg M. *Handbook of Neurosurgery*, 4th ed., vol. 2. Lakeland, FL: Greenberg Graphics, 1997, 791.

CHAPTER 10

Abdominal and Chest Trauma

John D. Abad and Matthew W. Blanton

Questions

1. A 37-year-old unrestrained driver is involved in a motor vehicle accident where he is struck on the driver's side. The patient is brought to the emergency room (ER) by ambulance hemodynamically stable, complaining of left-sided abdominal pain. An abdominal CT is performed. Based on the CT (Fig. 10-1), what is the most appropriate management of this patient?

   (A) observe in the ER overnight and consider discharge to home in the morning if remains hemodynamically stable

   (B) observe in the intensive care unit (ICU) with serial hematocrits and monitoring physical examination for 48 h

   (C) take to interventional radiology for angiography and embolization

   (D) take to operating room for exploratory laparotomy

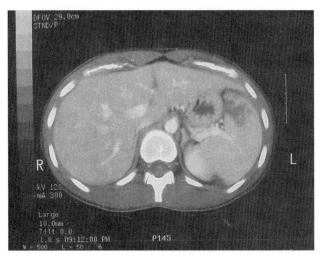

FIG. 10-1 CT depicting grade III spleen laceration.

2. A patient is taken to the operating room after a failed attempt at nonoperative management for a splenic laceration. The surgeon enters the peritoneum, packs all four quadrants, and notes on initial survey that there is active bleeding from the left upper quadrant. What is the first step in mobilizing the spleen?

   (A) divide the splenocolic ligament

   (B) clamp and tie off the short gastric vessels

   (C) mobilize the spleen and tail of the pancreas from lateral to medial

   (D) divide the splenorenal and splenophrenic ligaments

3. A 26-year-old male presents with vague abdominal pain in the shock room following a high velocity motor vehicle accident. Initially, reported as hemodynamically stable, while in ER, a blood pressure of 65/30 mmHg is recorded with a heart rate of 130 bpm. DPL is performed and is positive for >10 cc gross blood. The patient is taken to the operating room for immediate exploratory laparotomy. Upon entry into the peritoneum, massive hemorrhage is noted from the liver. What is the most appropriate next step?

   (A) partial hepatectomy

   (B) Pringle maneuver

   (C) direct suturing of any noticeable lacerations

   (D) pause to allow anesthesia to provide adequate resuscitation before further exploration

4. A 48-year-old restrained male passenger involved in a motor vehicle accident is transferred to ER. The patient is hemodynamically stable and complaining of vague abdominal pain. CT of the abdomen is performed (Fig. 10-2). Besides the liver injury, there is some fluid noted in the pelvis. Patient is admitted for close observation in the ICU. Approximately 24 h after admission, patient is complaining of increasing abdominal pain. The next morning he is noted to be hypotensive and acidotic with peritoneal signs on examination. What is the most likely diagnosis?

   (A) infected hepatic hematoma
   (B) missed bowel injury
   (C) liver hemorrhage
   (D) pulmonary embolus

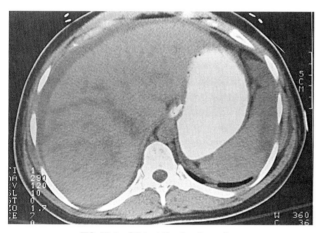

FIG. 10-2   CT depicting liver laceration.

5. A 41-year-old male is shot in the abdomen multiple times undergoes an extensive exploratory laparotomy with multiple bowel resections. Following surgery, he is taken to the ICU for further resuscitation. Which of the following signs would not be consistent with the development of an abdominal compartment syndrome (ACS)?

   (A) increasing peak airway pressures
   (B) increasing bladder pressures
   (C) decreasing cardiac output
   (D) decreasing PCO_2
   (E) decreasing urine output under 15 cc/h

6. A 65-year-old male who is involved in an all terrain vehicle (ATV) accident presents to the ER complaining of epigastric abdominal pain. Initial labs demonstrate an elevated amylase level. Abdominal CT is unremarkable. What is the most appropriate next step?

   (A) observation and repeat amylase level
   (B) exploratory laparotomy since increased morbidity and mortality with missed pancreatic injury
   (C) emergent endoscopic retrograde cholangiopancreatography (ERCP) to evaluate for pancreatic duct injury
   (D) check the intraperitoneal amylase level

7. A 21-year-old male with a stab wound to the abdomen presents to the ER in stable condition. On local wound exploration (Fig. 10-3), there is evidence of anterior fascia penetration. The patient is taken to the operating room for an exploratory laparotomy. A complete transection of the ascending colon with minimal contamination is identified. As a simple repair cannot be performed, the most appropriate surgical management would be:

   (A) ileostomy with Hartmann's pouch
   (B) colostomy with mucous fistula
   (C) debridement and ileocolostomy
   (D) debridement and colocolostomy
   (E) end ascending colostomy with long Hartman's pouch

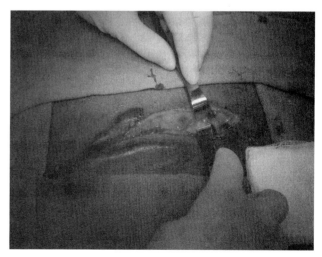

FIG. 10-3   Local abdominal wound exploration following a stab injury.

8. A 36-year-old female is ejected from a vehicle during an accident. She is found to have a pelvic fracture and hematuria. Cystogram is performed demonstrating the presence of an extraperitoneal bladder rupture. An indwelling bladder catheter is placed. After 14 days, a repeat cystogram identifies a persistent extraperitoneal leak. What is the most appropriate management?

(A) remove the bladder catheter and observe the patient

(B) leave the bladder catheter for 7–10 days longer and repeat cystogram

(C) cystoscopy to evaluate the extent of the rupture

(D) exploratory laparotomy and repair of extraperitoneal rupture

9. A 29-year-old male restrained passenger is brought to the ER in stable condition following a motor vehicle accident. He is admitted for observation following an abdominal CT demonstrating a moderate amount of free fluid in the pelvis. Within 48 h, patient develops worsening abdominal pain and undergoes exploratory laparotomy. A small bowel perforation is identified (Fig. 10-4). What is the following statements regarding small bowel injuries is *not* correct?

(A) thought to occur when bowel is crushed against spine

(B) frequently associated with lumbar spine fractures

(C) decreased incidence since the mandatory seat belt laws

(D) believed result of closed loop of bowel under high intraluminal pressure

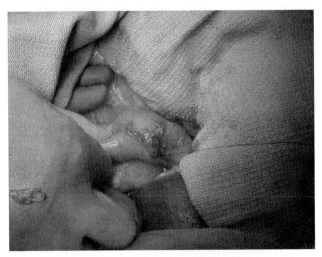

FIG. 10-4 Small bowel perforation following MVA.

10. An 18-year-old female unrestrained driver is involved in a head-on collision. Paramedics at the scene note extensive steering wheel and windshield damage. The patient is hemodynamically stable and complaining of head and abdominal pain. Head CT and abdominal CT are initially read as negative for acute injury. After observation overnight, the patient is discharged to home. Approximately 72 h later, the patient presents to the ER complaining of nausea and bilious emesis. Findings on repeat abdominal CT are consistent with duodenal hematoma. What is the most appropriate management?

(A) conservative management with nasogastric suction and total parenteral nutrition

(B) esophagogastroduodenoscopy to evaluate severity of duodenal injury

(C) exploratory laparotomy with evacuation of hematoma

(D) upper GI series with barium

(E) percutaneous drainage by interventional radiology

11. A 16-year old unrestrained driver is involved in a rollover head-on collision. Extensive damage to the vehicle and prolonged extrication time was noted. The patient was hemodynamically unstable upon extrication and was transported by air to level I trauma center. While in transport the patient became severely hypotensive, unresponsive, with impending respiratory distress. Which of the following is considered an immediate life-threatening injury in this patient?

(A) pneumothorax secondary to rib fractures

(B) aortic intimal tear

(C) diaphragm rupture

(D) tension pneumothorax

(E) myocardial contusion

12. An ER thoracotomy should *not* be performed in what setting?

    (A) a patient in shock with a penetrating anterior chest wound

    (B) a patient who sustained a penetrating chest wound and develops precipitous shock after endotracheal intubation and positive-pressure ventilation

    (C) a pulseless patient with a penetrating chest wound suspected to have a massive hemothorax

    (D) a patient arriving with no electrocardiogram (ECG) rhythm with known blunt trauma to the chest

    (E) C and D

13. An unrestrained 23-year-old male drag racer involved in high-speed motor vehicle accident presents to ER with intense pain in right chest. The primary survey demonstrates decreased breath sounds over the right hemithorax with noted paradoxical motion of the right chest wall during respiration (Fig. 10-5). The major pathologic sequela of this injury is

    (A) disruption of ventilation because of paradoxical motion of the chest wall

    (B) bleeding from disruption of intercostal vessels

    (C) underlying pulmonary contusion

    (D) pneumothorax

    (E) splinting from chest wall pain

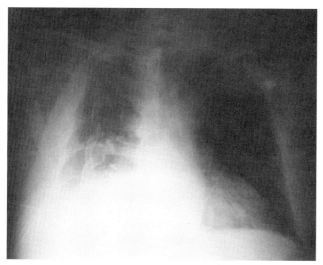

FIG. 10-5 Chest x-ray.

14. An unrestrained 45-year-old female involved in a rapid decelerating motor vehicle collision arrives hemodynamically stable. Paramedics noted a severely bent steering wheel. Initial primary survey reveals no abnormalities. A chest radiograph is performed, revealing a questionable widened mediastinum. There is a high index of suspicion of a possible thoracic aortic injury. The best method to diagnose this major vascular injury is

    (A) angiography

    (B) transesophageal echocardiography

    (C) CT scan chest

    (D) chest radiograph

    (E) transthoracic echocardiography

15. A 65-year-old male restrained driver involved in a high-speed motor vehicle accident suffered a severe blow to the epigastrium and presents to the emergency department with abdominal pain and shock out of proportion to the apparent injury. The patient is intubated at the scene and a nasogastric tube is placed on arrival. The primary survey reveals decreased left-sided breath sounds. After assuming proper endotracheal tube placement a chest tube is placed on the left side. Initial chest tube output is 50cc of blood, then particulate matter is noted inside the chest tube. The usual mechanism of this injury is

    (A) laceration of the esophagus by a portion of a fractured rib

    (B) inappropriate nasogastric tube placement

    (C) sudden deceleration resulting in shear stress to the esophagus

    (D) compression of the esophagus against the vertebral column

    (E) forceful compression of the stomach

16. A 30-year-old construction worker involved in a 25-ft fall struck the left side of his chest on a cement mixer. His primary survey is unremarkable. A chest radiograph reveals left-sided rib fractures with an associated left hemothorax. He has received a blood transfusion at the outside hospital and presents to your emergency department hemodynamically stable. The best therapy at this point is

    (A) observation for 24 h, then follow up in clinic in 1 week

    (B) exploratory thoracotomy and evacuation of the blood

    (C) angiography and embolization

    (D) large-bore chest tube placement to drain the hemothorax

    (E) ultrasound (FAST examination)

17. A restrained 52-year-old female involved in a high-speed motor vehicle accident has suffered blunt chest trauma. On arrival, primary survey reveals airway stridor and severe respiratory distress. A pneumothorax is suspected. Chest x-ray reveals massive pneumomediastinum. The patient is resuscitated and remains stable. Further evaluation of the chest radiograph reveals the right lung appearing to fall laterally and posteriorly away from the hilum. The next step in management should be

   (A) observation for 48 h
   (B) tube thoracostomy
   (C) immediate bronchoscopy
   (D) exploratory thoracotomy
   (E) place patient on humidified air

18. A 22-year-old male involved in an altercation suffered a penetrating gunshot wound to left anterior chest. At the scene the patient had a pulse, but started to hemodynamically decompensate prior to arrival in the trauma bay. On arrival immediate resuscitation is initiated. After rapid crystalloid infusion and blood transfusion the patient remains hemodynamically unstable. The next course of action is

   (A) emergent cardiac echocardiography
   (B) subxiphoid window then immediate transport to the operating room
   (C) ER thoracotomy then immediate transport to the operating room
   (D) ultrasound (FAST examination) then immediate transport to the operating room
   (E) immediate transfer to the operating room for thoracotomy and cardiorrhaphy

19. A 26-year-old male involved in a tree-cutting accident presents with blunt trauma to the thoracic outlet. Arteriography confirms a left subclavian artery injury. He is taken to the operating room where proximal control is obtained through an anterolateral thoracotomy while a separate supraclavicular incision provides distal control. In obtaining exposure, it is imperative to avoid injuring which nerve?

   (A) phrenic nerve
   (B) recurrent laryngeal nerve
   (C) median nerve
   (D) axillary nerve
   (E) vagus nerve

20. A 35-year-old female involved in a restrained motor vehicle accident presents to your emergency department with suspected multiple organ damage. After the patient is stabilized, a chest radiograph is performed revealing opacification of the left side of the patient's chest. A traumatic diaphragmatic injury is immediately suspected. The next step in management is

   (A) immediate exploratory laparotomy
   (B) delayed thoracotomy
   (C) video-assisted thoracoscopy
   (D) barium swallow
   (E) nasogastric tube insertion

Answers and Explanations

1. **(B)** Splenic injuries are extremely common in blunt abdominal trauma. The American Association for the Surgery of Trauma (AAST) developed a grading scale to describe these injuries (see Table 10-1) (Moore et al., 1995).

Based on the AAST grading scale, Fig. 10-1 is a grade III splenic laceration. The decision for nonoperative management is based mainly on two factors, hemodynamic stability and abdominal examination (Moore, Feliciano, and Mattox, 2004). Hemodynamically unstable patients involved in blunt abdominal trauma will require further diagnostic interventions, diagnostic peritoneal lavage (DPL), focused abdominal sonography for trauma (FAST) examination, or less commonly, operative exploration.

The stable blunt abdominal trauma patient should undergo CT to rule out any solid organ or hollow viscus organ damage. If there is evidence of active extravasation of contrast or "blush," the option of angiography with embolization by interventional radiologist is an appropriate treatment for active splenic bleeding in a hemodynamically stable patient. If there is no sign of bleeding, observing the patient with serial abdominal examinations and

hematocrit has demonstrated success rates in adults of 80% or higher (Trunkey, Hulka, and Mullins, 1997). It is recommended that adults with grade I splenic injuries may be observed on the floor; however, patients with grade II injuries or higher are best monitored in an ICU setting because of increased rates of delayed bleeding (Smith, Wengrovitz, and DeLong, 1992).

Bibliography

Moore EE, Cogbill TH, Jurkovich GJ, et al. Organ injury scaling: spleen and liver (1994 Edition). *J Trauma* 1995;38:323.

Moore E, Feliciano D, Mattox K. *Trauma* 2004;32:663–686..

Trunkey DD, Hulka F, Mullins RJ. Splenic trauma. In: Hiatt JR, Phillips EH, Morgenstern L (eds.), *Surgical Diseases of the Spleen*. New York, NY: Springer, 1997.

Smith JS, Wengrovitz MA, DeLong BS. Prospective validaton of criteria, including age, for safe, nonsurgical management of the ruptured spleen. *J Trauma* 1992;33:363.

2. **(D)** The mobilization of the spleen is performed in a stepwise approach to avoid further injury and provide improved visualization of the left hemidiaphragm, left kidney, and posterior distal pancreas and spleen.

TABLE 10-1   AAST Splenic Organ Injury Scale, 1994 Revision

Grade*	Injury description
I	Hematoma subcapsular, <10% surface area Laceration capsular tear, <1 cm parenchymal injury
II	Hematoma subcapsular, 10–50% surface area, <5 cm in diameter Laceration 1–3 cm parenchymal depth—does not involve trabecular vessels
III	Hematoma subcapsular, >50% surface area or expanding, ruptured or parenchymal hematoma Intraparenchymal hematoma >5 cm or expanding Laceration >3 cm parenchymal depth or involving trabecular vessels
IV	Laceration involving segmental or hilar vessels (>25% devascularization of spleen)
V	Laceration completely shattered spleen Vascular hilar vascular injury devascularizes spleen

*Advance one grade for multiple injuries, up to grade III.
Source: Reproduced with permission from Moore EE, Cogbill TH, Jurkovich GJ, et al. Organ injury scaling: spleen and liver (1994 Revision). *J Trauma* 1995;38:323–324.

The first step is to divide the splenorenal and splenophrenic ligaments initially by sharp dissection and continued with sharp and blunt dissection. Once these lateral attachments are divided, mobilizing the spleen and tail of the pancreas medially is the next step. The two structures should be moved as a unit to avoid any injuries to either structure. The next step is to clamp and tie off the short gastric vessels. Avoid dividing these vessels with only scissors or Bovie electrocautery because of the risk of delayed bleeding. The last step is to divide the splenocolic ligament. If bleeding is encountered during removal of the spleen, digital compression is preferred. Mass clamping of the hilum should be reserved for instances of extreme hemorrhage because of the increased risk for damage of the tail of the pancreas during this maneuver (Moore, Feliciano, and Mattox, 2004).

Bibliography

Moore E, Feliciano D, Mattox K. *Trauma*, Fifth Edition, 2004;32:663–686.

3. **(B)** Patients with hemodynamic instability and evidence of positive DPL require exploratory laparotomy. A positive DPL is described as aspiration of gross blood >10 mL or gastrointestinal (GI) contents, or lavage fluid with >100,000 RBC/mm^3 (for blunt trauma), >500 WBC/mm^3, or Gram's stain with bacteria present (Moore, Feliciano, and Mattox, 2004). The FAST examination is replacing DPL at some major trauma centers to determine hemoperitoneum. For grade III and higher liver injuries, the sensitivity of ultrasound has been reported as 98%

(Richards et al., 1999). Volumes of less than 400 mL are rarely visualized with current FAST examinations (Branney et al., 1997).

Exploratory laparotomy begins with the standard midline incision. The peritoneum is entered and hemoperitoneum is evacuated. Manual compression of the liver may be attempted. This maneuver is performed for prompt control of massive bleeding by placing both hands over the anterior surface of the liver and applying pressure. If there is an obvious source of major hemorrhage from the liver, the Pringle maneuver should be performed. The porta hepatis is clamped using either the finger or a noncrushing clamp. If significant bleeding persists, perihepatic packing should be considered. Less commonly, partial hepatectomy and veno-veno bypass are performed. If bleeding is controlled after the Pringle maneuver, direct suturing, as well as omental packing may be performed (Moore, Feliciano, and Mattox, 2004).

Bibliography

Moore E, Feliciano D, Mattox K. *Trauma* 2004;5(31)637–661.

Richards JR, McGahan JP, Pali MJ, et al. Sonographic detection of blunt hepatic trauma: hemoperitoneum and parenchymal patterns of injury. *J Trauma* 1999;47:1092.

Branney SW, Moore EE, Cantrill SV, et al. Ultrasound based key clinical pathway reduces the use of hospital resources for the evaluation of blunt abdominal trauma. *J Trauma* 1997;42:1086.

4. **(B)** Liver injuries are graded similarly to splenic injuries (Table 10-2) (Moore, Cogbill, and Jurkovich, 1995).

TABLE 10-2 AAST Hepatic Organ Injury Scale, 1994 Edition

Grade*	Injury description
I	Hematoma subcapular, nonexpanding, <10 cm surface area Laceration capsular tear, nonbleeding, <1 cm parenchymal depth
II	Hematoma subcapsular, nonexpanding, 10–50% surface area Intraparenchymal nonexpanding <10 cm diameter Laceration capsular tear, active bleeding; 1–3 cm parenchymal depth, <10 cm in length
III	Hematoma subcapsular, >50% surface area or expanding; ruptured supcapsular hematoma with active bleeding; intraparenchymal hematoma >10 cm or expanding Laceration >3 cm parenchymal depth
IV	Hematoma ruptured intraparenchymal hematoma with active bleeding Laceration parenchymal disruption involving 25–75% of hepatic lobe or 1–3 segments within a single lobe
V	Laceration parenchymal disruption involving >75% of hepatic lobe or >3 segments within a single lobe Vascular juxtahepatic venous injuries (i.e., retrohepatic vena cava/central major hepatic veins)
VI	Vascular hepatic avulsion

*Advance one grade for multiple injuries, up to grade III.
Source: Reproduced with permission from Moore EE, Cogbill TH, Jurkovich GJ, et al. Organ injury scaling: spleen and liver (1994 Revision). *J Trauma* 1995;38:323–324.

High-grade injury, large hemoperitoneum, and active extravasation are not contraindications for nonoperative management when the patient is otherwise hemodynamically stable; however, these factors increase the chances for failure during nonoperative management (Moore, Feliciano, and Mattox, 2004). The presence of fluid in the pelvis in the setting of solid organ injury requires observation. The fluid may be a result of the solid organ injury; however, a mesenteric or bowel injury may still exist. As a result, these injuries are occasionally missed. Other useful findings on abdominal CT include pneumoperitoneum, focal bowel wall thickening, mesenteric hematoma, mesenteric fat streaking, or extravasation of oral or intravenous contrast (Hagiwara et al., 1995). Surgeons should be suspicious of unexplained tachycardia, leukocytosis, hypotension, metabolic acidosis, and changes in the abdominal examination in patients managed nonoperatively for solid organ injuries.

Bibliography

Moore EE, Cogbill TH, Jurkovich GJ, et al. Organ injury scaling: spleen and liver (1994 Edition). *J Trauma* 1995;38:323.

Moore E, Feliciano D, Mattox K. *Trauma* 2004;5(31):637–661.

Hagiwara A, Yukioka, Satou M, et al. Early diagnosis of small intestine rupture from blunt abdominal trauma using computed tomography: significance of the streaky density within the mesentery. *J Trauma* 1995;38:630.

5. **(D)** ACS is the increase of intraabdominal pressure seen in a variety of clinical situations including abdominal trauma and severe sepsis. ACS leads to difficulties with ventilation, hypoxia, and renal failure (Moore, Feliciano, and Mattox, 2004). Leaving the fascia open prevents ACS in high-risk patients. These include patients with extensive intraabdominal injuries, prolonged surgical intervention, and massive resuscitation efforts. Placing catheters into the bladder, stomach, or inferior vena cava makes indirect measurements of intraabdominal pressures. Based on these measurements, recommendations regarding management have been proposed (see Table 10-3) (Meldrum, 1997).

TABLE 10-3 Grading of Abdominal Compartment Syndrome

Grade	Bladder pressure (mmHg)	Recommendation
I	10–15	Maintain normovolemia
II	16–25	Hypervolemic resuscitation
III	26–35	1p7Decompression
IV	>35	Decompression and reexploration

Once the abdomen is reopened and decompressed, many of the ventilation, cardiac, and renal findings of ACS quickly reverse. The further operative management of ACS may include several techniques. The simplest is placement of towel clips to close the skin along the midline incision, leaving the fascia open. Commonly, temporary silos and vacuum assisted wound closure devices are used (Fig. 10-6). Others include zippers, open packing, and meshes (Feliciano and Burch, 1991).

Bibliography

Moore E, Feliciano D, Mattox K. *Trauma* 2004;5(40):885–891.

Meldrum DR, Moore FA, Moore EE, et al. Prospective characterization and selective management of the abdominal compartment syndrome. *Am J Surg* 1997;174:667.

Feliciano DV, Burch JM. Towel clips, silos, and heroic forms of wound closure. In: Maull KI, Cleveland HC, Feliciano DV, et al. (eds.), *Advances in Trauma and Critical Care*, vol. 6. Chicago, IL: Year Book, 1991, 231.

6. **(A)** Hyperamylasemia is not a reliable marker for pancreatic injury; however, it does warrant further evaluation to exclude possible pancreatic damage. One study reported only 8% of patients involved in blunt abdominal trauma with elevated amylase levels had a pancreatic injury (White and Benfield, 1972). Another study demonstrated that only 40% of patients with a pancreatic injury had an elevated amylase level (Moretz et al., 1975). Also, elevated amylase levels have been documented frequently in patients with isolated head injuries where there is no evidence of abdominal trauma (Vitale et al., 1987).

Pancreatic injuries may present several days, weeks, or years following trauma. Therefore, elevated amylase levels following blunt abdominal trauma should be observed with serial amylase levels.

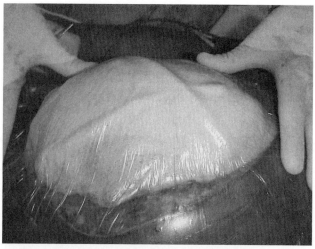

FIG. 10-6 Vacuum-assisted wound closure device.

Persistently elevated amylase levels or increasing abdominal pain should be evaluated with either abdominal CT, ERCP, or surgical exploration (Moore, Feliciano, and Mattox, 2004). Abdominal CT findings suspicious for pancreatic injury include parenchymal fracture or hematoma, fluid in the lesser sac, or retroperitoneal fluid or hematoma. Diagnosis by CT remains difficult. Some studies demonstrate up to 40% false-negative scans in patients with significant pancreatic injuries (Wilson and Moorehead, 1991). In hemodynamically stable patients, there have been reports of the successful utilization of ERCP to evaluate pancreatic duct injury. If a high suspicion of pancreatic injury remains, surgical exploration is warranted.

Bibliography

White P, Benfield J. Amylase in the management of pancreatic trauma. *Arch Surg* 1972;105:158.

Moretz J, et al. Significance of serum amylase level in evaluating pancreatic trauma. *Am J Surg* 1975;150:698.

Vitale G, et al. Analysis of hyperamylasemia in patients with severe head injury. *J Surg Res* 1987;43:226–233.

Moore E, Feliciano D, Mattox K. *Trauma* 2004;5(34):709–733.

Wilson R, Moorehead R. Current management of trauma to the pancreas. *Br J Surg* 1991;78(10):1196–1202.

7. **(C)** Multiple prospective, randomized studies have demonstrated that primary repairs following resection are as safe as routine diversion (Sasaki, Allaben, Golwala et al., 1995). There are two factors that several authors may view as relative contraindications to primary repair after resection. The first is those patients that received large amounts of transfusions because of massive hemorrhage (Stewart et al., 1994). These patients have increased visceral edema of the bowel that places added tension on the suture line and makes healing unpredictable. The second, and controversial factor, is the location of the colonic injury. Under emergent conditions, some authors believe that ileocolostomies are more secure repairs then colocolostomies (Miller et al., 2002). Therefore, injuries distal to the middle colic artery repaired with resection and primary repair may have a slightly higher risk for leaks than injuries proximal to the middle colic artery. In general, Hartmann's pouch is preferred over a mucous fistula for end colostomies because of the speed and fewer associated complications (Moore, Feliciano, and Mattox, 2004).

Bibliography

Sasaki LS, Allaben RD, Golwala, Mittal VK. Primary repair of colon injuries: a prospective randomized study. *J Trauma* 1995;89:895.

Stewart RM, Fabian TC, Croce MA, et al. Is resection with primary anastomosis following destructive colon wounds always safe? *Am J Surg* 1994;168:316.

Miller PR, Fabian TC, Croce MA, Magnotti LJ, et al. Improving outcomes following penetrating colon wounds. *Ann Surg* 2002.

Moore E, Feliciano D, Mattox K. *Trauma* 2004;5(35):735–752.

8. **(B)** Over 80% of patients with blunt bladder ruptures have associated pelvic fractures (Cass, 1984). Also, over 95% of bladder ruptures have gross hematuria on presentation (Carroll and McAninch, 1984). The diagnosis is made using stress cystography. The bladder is filled with 300–400 cc of contrast and a plain abdominal radiograph or abdominal CT is taken. The extravasation pattern determines whether the bladder rupture is intraperitoneal or extraperitoneal (Carroll and McAninch, 1983). The standard treatment for extraperitoneal bladder ruptures is catheter drainage for 10–14 days followed by repeat cystogram. On repeat cystogram, over 85% of extraperitoneal ruptures will have resolved. If there is evidence of a persistent extraperitoneal bladder rupture, then continued catheter drainage for an additional 7–10 days is recommended followed by repeat cystogram (Corriere and Sandler, 1986). After additional drainage, persistent extraperitoneal ruptures are rare, and CT or cystoscopy is performed to evaluate foreign bodies. With rare exception, intraperitoneal bladder perforations are uniformly repaired with operative management (Moore, Feliciano, and Mattox, 2004).

Bibliography

Cass AS. The multiple injured patient with bladder trauma. *J Trauma* 1984;24:731.

Carroll PR, McAninch JW. Major bladder trauma: mechanisms of injury and a unified method of diagnosis and repair. *J Urol* 1984;132:254.

Carroll PR, McAninch JW. Major bladder trauma: the accuracy of cystography. *J Urol* 1983;130:887.

Corriere JN Jr, Sandler CM. Management of the ruptured bladder: 7 years experience with 111 cases. *J Trauma* 1986;26:830.

Moore E, Feliciano D, Mattox K. *Trauma* 2004;5(38):809–848.

9. **(C)** Small bowel injuries secondary to blunt abdominal trauma are increasing in incidence because of high velocity motor vehicle accidents and mandatory seat belt laws (Moore, Feliciano, and Mattox, 2004). The "seat belt" syndrome is the complex of injuries, which includes lumbar fractures and small bowel injuries. Physical finding of ecchymoses along the anterior abdominal wall is referred to as the "seat belt sign" and may indicate underlying small bowel injuries (Appleby and Nagy, 1989).

The proposed mechanisms of injury include (1) crushing of bowel against spine, (2) tearing of bowel from mesentery by sudden deceleration, and (3) rupture of a closed loop of bowel under high intraluminal pressure (Guarino, Hassett, and Luchette, 1995).

Bibliography

Moore E, Feliciano D, Mattox K. *Trauma* 2004;5(33): 687–706.

Appleby JP, Nagy AG. Abdominal injuries associated with the use of seatbelts. *Am J Surg* 1989;157:457.

Guarino J, Hassett JM, Luchette FA. Small bowel injuries: mechanisms, patterns, and outcome. *J Trauma* 1995; 39: 1076–1080.

10. **(A)** Approximately one-third of duodenal hematomas present with signs of obstruction at least 48 h following blunt abdominal trauma. This is likely caused by fluid shifts causing expansion of the hematoma (Moore, Feliciano, and Mattox, 2004). Radiographic findings include the presence of retroperitoneal hematoma on abdominal CT and narrowing of the duodenum on upper GI radiograph. The management of duodenal hematomas is generally nonsurgical. Conservative management consisting of nasogastric suction and total parenteral nutrition is recommended until the obstruction resolves. Serial UGI studies should be performed at regular intervals of 5–7 days if obstruction is not resolving. If there is no resolution of symptoms by 2 weeks, surgical exploration with evacuation of hematoma may be appropriate to evaluate for pancreatic injury, duodenal perforation, or stricture (Touloukian, 1983). One study reviewing conservative management of duodenal hematomas reported an average hospitalization of 16 days (and 9 days of total parenteral nutrition) until resolution of symptoms (Czyrko et al., 1990).

Bibliography

Moore E, Feliciano D, Mattox K. *Trauma* 2004;5(34):709–734.

Touloukian R. Protocol for the nonoperative treatment of obstructing intramural duodenal hematoma. *Am J Surg* 1983;145:330–335.

Czyrko C, et al. Blunt abdominal trauma resulting in intestinal obstruction: when to operate? *J Trauma* 1990; 30(12):1567–1571.

11. **(D)** Injuries that interfere with breathing should be detected during the primary survey—they include tension pneumothorax, flail chest, open pneumothorax, and massive hemothorax. Tension pneumothorax caused by either penetrating or blunt trauma develops when air continuously enters pleural space from the lung, bronchi, trachea, or through the chest wall and cannot escape and causes the lung to collapse. Eventually, intrapleural pressure increases and causes shifting of the mediastinum which decreases venous return, and results in decreased cardiac output.

Clinically, a sense of impending death, marked by respiratory distress, deviated trachea, distended neck veins, unilateral absence of breath sounds, cyanosis, and hypotension may be seen. Diagnosis is generally clinical and not radiographic.

Treatment requires immediate decompression with a needle thorocentesis using a 14-gauge catheter over a needle inserted in the second intercostal space, midclavicular line. A rush of air escaping the catheter confirms diagnosis. This converts the tension component to a simple pneumothorax. Absence of rush of air suggests misdiagnosis or insertion of the needle into the wrong hemithorax. If the diagnosis of tension pneumothorax still seems likely, the initial catheter is left in the chest, and the opposite hemithorax is punctured. If no rush, the wrong diagnosis is likely, and cardiac tamponade should be considered. When the needle thorocentesis confirms the presence of tension pneumothorax, tube thorocostomy should follow to provide immediate definitive treatment.

Bibliography

Moore E, Feliciano D, Mattox K. *Trauma*, 5th ed. New York, NY: McGraw-Hill, 2004.

Mattox KL, et al. Emergency department treatment of chest injuries. *Emerg Med Clin North Am* 1984;2:783–797.

12. **(E)** The primary objectives of resuscitative thoracotomy are (a) release of percardial tamponade; (b) control of intrathoracic vascular or cardiac bleeding; (c) eliminate massive air embolism or bronchopleural fistula; (d) perform open cardiac massage; and (e) temporarily occlude the descending thoracic aorta. A left anterolateral thoracotomy incision is preferred. A right thoracotomy is reserved for hypotensive patients with penetrating injuries to the right chest in need of direct access to massive blood loss or air embolism. An ER thoracotomy is initiated at the level of fourth to fifth intercostal space with the proper level corresponding to inferior border of pectoralis major muscle. The incision is made through the intercostal muscle and parietal pleura is divided along superior margin of the rib. The rib retractor is inserted with the handle toward the axilla. Key resuscitative maneuvers are then initiated.

A pericardiotomy incision is made in the presence of cardiac tamponade and incised widely, anterior and parellel to the phrenic nerve. Blood clots are evacuated from the pericardium and cardiac bleeding sites should be controlled immediately with digital pressure on the surface of the ventricle and partially occluding vascular clamps placed on atrium or great vessels. In beating hearts, efforts at cardiorrhapy should be delayed until initial resuscitation measures have been completed. In the nonbeating heart, suturing should be performed prior to defibrillation. Temporary control of the bleeding can be accomplished with a skin-stapling device. Cardiac wounds are best repaired with 3-0 nonabsorbable horizontal mattress sutures in the operating room.

In cardiac arrest, bimanual internal massage of the heart should be instituted. If internal defibrillation does not restore vigorous cardiac activity, the descending thoracic aorta should be incompletely cross-clamped at the level inferior to the left pulmonary hilum to maximize coronary perfusion. Cardiopulmonary collapse from suspected intraabdominal hemorrhage should be temporized by occlusion of the descending thoracic aorta. Air embolism should be suspected in a patient with penetrating chest trauma who develops precipitous shock after endotracheal intubation and positive-pressure ventilation. Treatment involves pulmonary hilar cross-clamping, vigorous cardiac massage, along with aortic root and left ventricle air aspiration (Moore, Feliciano, and Mattox, 2004).

Trauma patients arriving in extremis with cardiopulmonary resuscitation (CPR) being initiated following blunt injury should undergo thoracotomy only if they show electrical cardiac activity on ECG, cardiac activity or pericardial effusion visualized via ultrasound. Patients exhibiting ECG cardiac activity or who have sustained penetrating thoracic wounds should undergo resuscitative thoracotomy (Cogbill et al., 1983).

Bibliography

Moore E, Feliciano D, Mattox K. Trauma, 5th ed. New York, NY: McGraw-Hill, 2004.

Cogbill JH, et al. Rationale for selective applications of emergency department thoracotomy in trauma. *J Trauma* 1983;23:453–460.

13. **(C)** A flail chest consists of segmental fractures of three or more adjacent ribs, or one or more rib fractures with associated costochondral separation or fracture of sternum (Fig. 10-5). This causes an unstable or floating segment of chest wall that moves paradoxically during respiration (ATLS, 1997). A pneumothorax or hemothorax may be present. A more significant injury, however, is associated with pulmonary contusion leading to hemorrhage and edema of the injured lung. A chest wall injury of this magnitude is also associated with significant pain, and respiratory efficiency is reduced.

Treatment is directed toward reversing hypoventilation caused by the pain, and hypoxia caused by the associated pulmonary contusion. Careful monitoring of ventilation and oxygenation is required,

and often time intubation and ventilatory support may be indicated in 20–40% of patients. Control of pain because of multiple rib fractures by using regional anesthetic techniques such as intercostal nerve block, insertion of intrapleural catheter, or insertion of an epidural catheter is important to improve respiratory mechanics. Rarely is physical stabilization of chest wall necessary (Moore, Feliciano, and Mattox, 2004).

Bibliography

Moore E, Feliciano D, Mattox K. *Trauma*, 5th ed. New York, NY: McGraw-Hill, 2004.

American College of Surgeons Committee on Trauma. *American Trauma Life Support*, 6th ed. Chicago, IL: American College of Surgeons, 1997.

14. **(A)** The thoracic aorta is particularly susceptible to injury from blunt trauma. These injuries usually involve proximal descending aorta (54–65% cases), but often involve other segments such as the ascending aorta or transverse aortic arch, and mid or distal descending thoracic aorta. The typical injury is seen when the mechanism of injury is rapid deceleration, resulting in differential forces on the proximal descending aorta between fixed and more mobile portions (Rogers et al., 1996). The most common site of injury is just beyond the ligamentum arteriosum. Blunt aortic injuries may be partial thickness, histologically similar to an intimal tear in aortic dissection, or full thickness and therefore equivalent to ruptured aortic aneurysm, which is contained by surrounding tissues (Williams et al., 1994).

The hallmark radiographic sign is a widened mediastinum seen on chest radiograph, related to advential hematoma. Other findings include obliteration of the aortic knob, deviation of the trachea to the right, depression of the left mainstem bronchus, obliteration of the space between the pulmonary artery and the aorta, widened paratracheal stripe, presence of a pleural or apical cap. When the initial chest x-ray demonstrates findings suggestive of a mediastinal hemotoma some clinicians require additional screening by CT scan to delineate changes seen on chest radiography and to substantiate a request for a diagnostic arteriogram. The gold standard for the diagnosis, however, remains arterial angiography. It allows precise localization of the injury and provides information regarding vascular anomalies and other factors that profoundly influence operative strategy (Moore, Feliciano, and Mattox, 2004). Transesophageal echocardiographic evaluation (TEE) contains numerous poorly visualized areas of the aorta, thus a negative TEE does not rule out an aortic injury (Horton et al., 2000).

Initial treatment involves permitting moderate hypotension (SBP 80–100 mmHg) and limiting fluid administration until operative control is achieved. Currently, it is difficult to make substantiated recommendations regarding the use of beta-blockers in patients with suspected or proven blunt aortic injury. While retrospective studies suggest that it is safe, no prospective studies have demonstrated either safety or efficacy of such treatment (Moore, Feliciano, and Mattox, 2004).

Bibliography

Rogers FB, Osler TM, Shackford SR. Aortic dissection after trauma: case report and review of the literature. *J Trauma* 1996;41:906.

Horton TG, Cohn SM, Heid MP, et al. Identification of trauma patients at risk of thoracic aortic tear by mechanism of injury. *J Trauma* 2000;48:1008–1014.

Williams JS, Graff JA, Uka JM, Steinig JP. Aortic injury in vehicular trauma. *Ann Thorac Surg* 1994;57:726.

Moore E, Feliciano D, Mattox K. *Trauma*, 5th ed. New York, NY: McGraw-Hill, 2004.

15. **(E)** Blunt esophageal trauma is uncommon but may result from a direct blow to the organ, usually in the neck, or from increased intraluminal pressures against a closed glottis causing a bursting-type injury (White et al., 1992). Intrathoracic esophageal injuries tend to occur just proximal to the esophagogastric junction on the left side where the esophagus has less protection by the pleural lining and heart. This injury is thought to be because of increased intraabdominal pressure transmitted to the stomach. The resulting mediastinitis and immediate or delayed rupture into the pleural space may be lethal if unrecognized (Glatterer et al., 1985).

For blunt trauma, determining which victims need further study for esophageal injury is a vexing task. Esophageal injury should be considered for any patient who (1) has a left pneumothorax or hemothorax or pleural effusion without a rib fracture, (2) has received a severe blow to the lower sternum or epigastrium and is in pain or shock out of proportion to the apparent injury, or (3) has particulate matter in the chest tube after the blood begins to clear. Presence of a pneumomediastinum also suggests the diagnosis (Moore, Feliciano, and Mattox, 2004).

Treatment entails placement of a tube thoracostomy for drainage. If output is suggestive of gastric contents or an injury is otherwise clinically suspected, a contrast study or an upper GI endoscopy is indicated to evaluate for the esophageal injury. Surgical repair entails local debridement, wide drainage, primary repair of the perforation, and buttressing with a pedicle flap for viable muscle (White et al., 1992).

Bibliography

Glatterer MS, Toon RS, Ellestad C, et al. Management of blunt and penetrating external esophageal trauma. *J Trauma* 1985;25:784–790.

Atter S, Hankins JR, Suter CM, et al. Esophageal perforation: a therapeutic challenge. *Ann Thorac Surg* 1990;50:45.

White RK, Morris DM. Diagnosis and management of esophageal perforation. *Am Surg* 1992;58:112.

Moore E, Feliciano D, Mattox K. *Trauma*, 5th ed. New York, NY: McGraw-Hill, 2004.

16. **(D)** Chest wall bleeding associated with rib fractures typically presents as a hemothorax or blood in the pleural space. The blood can come from any number of sources. Thoracic sources include the lung parenchyma, the chest wall including the intercostal or internal mammary arteries, or the heart and great vessels. They can also arise from intraabdominal organs, especially the liver and spleen, in the setting of a diaphragmatic laceration. In unstable patients following blunt or penetrating trauma, the diagnosis of hemothorax is usually suspected on the basis of the physical examination and confirmed on basis of a chest tube placement (Borlase et al., 1986).

A massive hemothorax is defined as presence of greater than 1 L of blood in the pleural space and is associated with systemic signs of shock. In hemodynamically stable patients the diagnosis is more commonly made on chest x-ray. It is estimated that 200–300 mL of blood must be present in the pleural space before a hemothorax can be detected on chest x-ray. Studies using ultrasound as part of the FAST examination have suggested this modality may be useful in identification of pleural fluid, but the sensitivity and specificity of ultrasonography for this indication is undetermined (Moore, Feliciano, and Mattox, 2004). In stable patients, the diagnosis of posterior fluid collections may also be made on truncal CT or cephalad cuts of an abdominal CT scan; however, CT scans are infrequently used in early management of penetrating chest trauma (Hauser et al., 2003).

The major goal in treatment of a hemothorax is to evacuate the pleural space completely. Expansion of the lung with apposition of parietal and viseral pleura decreases bleeding from the lung and other low-pressure sources and in most cases will result in the definitive control of bleeding. Overall, thoractomy to control bleeding is required in less than 10% of all chest trauma patients. The percentage is somewhat higher in penetrating trauma (Feliciano, 1992).

Bibliography

Hauser CJ, Visvikis G, Hinrichs C, et al. Prospective validation of CT screening of the thoracolumbar spine in trauma. *J Trauma* 2003;55:228.

Borlase B, Metcalf R, Moore E, et al. Penetrating wounds to the anterior chest. Analysis of thoracotomy and laparotomy. *Am J Surg* 1986;152:649.

Feliciano D. The diagnostic and therapeutic approach to chest trauma. *Semin Thorac Cardiovasc Surg* 1992;4:156.

Moore E, Feliciano D, Mattox K. *Trauma*, 5th ed. New York, NY: McGraw-Hill, 2004.

17. (B) Injury to the tracheobronchial tree is a rare but well-recognized complication of both penetrating and blunt chest trauma. Most victims die prior to emergency care from associated injuries to vital structures, hemorrhage, tension pneumothorax, or respiratory insufficiency from lack of adequate airway. The reported incidence of injury to the trachea or bronchus varies from 0.2 to 8%. Greater than 80% of tracheobronchial ruptures occur within 2.5 cm of the carina (Barmada et al., 1994).

The presentation of thoracic tracheobronchial injury depends on whether the injury is confined to the mediastinum or communicates with the pleural space. Thoracic tracheobronchial injuries confined to the mediastinum usually presents with massive pneumomediastinum. Injuries that do perforate into the pleural space usually create an ipsilateral pneumothorax. If the pneumothorax persists despite adequate placement of a chest tube and has a continuous air leak it is suggestive of a tracheobronchial injury and bronchopleural fistula. A pathognomonic radiographic feature termed "fallen lung sign," includes the affected lung falling away from the hilum, laterally and posteriorly, in contrast to the usual pneumothorax, which collapses toward the hilum (Moore, Feliciano, and Mattox, 2004).

Evaluation of a patient with a tracheobronchial injury involves immediate tube thoracostomy. If persistent atelectasis, collapse, or massive air leak is noted a bronchoscopy is the most reliable means of establishing the diagnosis and determining the site, nature, and extent of tracheobronchial disruption. Lesions selected for observation must involve less than one-third the circumference of the tracheobronchial tree with well-opposed edges, and no tissue loss. Tube thoracostomy must fully expand the lung and air leaks stop soon after insertion of the tube. There must be no associated injuries and no need for positive-pressure ventilation. Prophylactic antibiotics, humidified oxygen, voice rest, frequent suctioning, and close observation for sepsis and airway obstruction are required. If the aforementioned criteria are not met operative repair is warranted. Optimal repair includes adequate debridement of devitalized tissue, including cartilage, and a tension-free primary end-to-end anastomosis of clean tracheal or bronchial ends with a buttressed vascularized pedicle (Moore, Feliciano, and Mattox, 2004).

Bibliography

Barmada H, Gibbons JR. Tracheobronchial injury in blunt and penetrating chest trauma. *Chest* 1994;106:74.

Hancock BJ, Wiseman NE. Tracheobronchial injuries in children. *J Pediatr Surg* 1991;26:1316.

Flynn AE, Thomas AN, Schecter WP. Acute tracheobronchial injury. *J Trauma* 1989;29:1326.

Kaiser AC, O'Brian SM, Detterbeck FC. Blunt tracheobronchial injuries: treatment and outcomes. *Ann Thoracic Surg* 2001;71(6):2059.

Moore E, Feliciano D, Mattox K. *Trauma*, 5th ed. New York, NY: McGraw-Hill, 2004.

18. (B) The management of patients with a penetrating truncal wound begins with prompt transfer of the patient to the ER. Patients with a penetrating cardiac wound management begin with rapid initial assessment and attention to the primary survey. The subsequent management of these patients is determined by their hemodynamic stability. Stable patients or those who can be stabilized easily by rapid volume infusion may be investigated by the FAST examination. If positive for pericardial fluid, immediate transport to the operating room for sternotomy or thoracotomy is needed. Borderline stability or instability is an indication for ER thoracotomy and transport to the operating room (Rozycki et al., 1999).

The definitive treatment of cardiac injuries is cardiorrhapy through a thoracotomy or sternotomy. Surgical relief of the tamponade and repair of cardiac lacerations should be performed. Volume expansion, partial correction of acidosis, maintenance of coronary perfusion by heart massage, and avoidance of hypothermia are crucial to resuscitate the injured heart. A left anterior or anterolateral thoracotomy is the incision of choice, especially for an ER thoracotomy. A median sternotomy is a logical extension after a preliminary subxiphoid window. Once exposure is achieved the pericardium is opened anterior to the phrenic nerve and tamponade is relieved. The bleeding heart is controlled by digital occlusion and the laceration is sutured. For larger wounds, temporary closure to control hemorrhage is achieved by insertion of a Foley catheter into the wound with the balloon inflated and gentle traction is applied (Fig. 10-7). Definitive repair is undertaken in the operating room.

Bibliography

Mattox KL, VonKoch L, Beall AC Jr, et al. Logistic and technical considerations in the treatment of the wounded heart. *Circulation* 1975;52:210 (Moore, Feliciano, and Mattox, 2004).

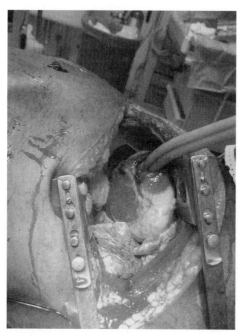

FIG. 10-7   Control of cardiac hemorrhage with an inflated foley catheter.

Mattox KL, Beall AC Jr, Jordan GL Jr, et al. Cardiorrhaphy in the emergency center. *J Thorac Cardiovasc Surg* 1974;68:886.

Rozycki GS, Schmidt JA, Ochsner MG, et al. The role of ultrasound in patients with possible penetrating cardiac wounds: a prospective multicenter study. *J Trauma* 1999;46:543.

Moore E, Feliciano D, Mattox K. *Trauma*, 5th ed. New York, NY: McGraw-Hill, 2004.

19. **(A)** Subclavian artery injuries can involve any combination of the following regions: intrathoracic, thoracic outlet, cervical (zone 1), and upper extremity injuries. Preoperative arteriography allows appropriate decisions to obtain adequate exposure and control. A cervical extension of a median sternotomy is employed for exposure of right-sided subclavian injuries. For left subclavian artery injuries, proximal control is obtained through a anterolateral thoracotomy (above the nipple, in second or third intercostal space), while a separate supraclavicular incision provides distal control (Pate et al., 1993). The formal "book thorocotomy" results in high incidence of postoperative neurologic complications and use should be limited. In obtaining exposure, it is imperative to avoid injuring the phrenic nerve (lies anterior to anterior scalene muscle) (Moore, Feliciano, and Mattox, 2004). Subclavian vascular trauma also has a high associated rate of brachial plexus injury. Vascular repair usually requires either later arteriorrhaphy or graft interposition. End-to-end anastomosis is unusual (Moore, Feliciano, and Mattox,

2004). An experimental, less invasive means of repair involves endovascular stenting. This is particularly attractive for patients with severe concomitant injuries who are unlikely to tolerate operative repair. Data regarding endovascular graft repairs in trauma patients, however, are limited (Patel et al., 1996).

Bibliography

Pate JW, Cole FH, Walker WA, Fabian TC. Penetrating injuries of the aortic and its branches. *Ann Thorac Surg* 1993;55:586.

Patel AV, Marin ML, Veith FJ, et al. Endovascular graft repair of penetrating subclavian artery injuries. *J Endovasc Surg* 1996;3:382.

Moore E, Feliciano D, Mattox K. *Trauma*, 5th ed. New York, NY: McGraw-Hill, 2004.

20. **(E)** A traumatic diaphragmatic rupture typically results from the rapid increase in intraabdominal pressure related to an episode of blunt trauma with subsequent rupture of the diaphragm. The diagnosis may be difficult in part because the force of injury is likely to result in multiple organ damage. A traumatic diaphragmatic rupture is more commonly diagnosed on the left side, and the stomach is the most common organ involved. Right diaphragmatic injuries are rarely diagnosed in the early postinjury period (Symbas et al., 1986). The liver often prevents herniation of other abdominal organs into the chest. The chest radiograph will often be missed initially if the film is misinterpreted as showing an elevated diaphragm, acute gastric dilatation, a loculated pneumohemothorax, or subpulmonary hematoma. Often times the chest radiograph will show opacification within the affected pleural cavity, air fluid levels, and mediastinal shift. If a laceration of the left diaphragm is suspected, a nasogastric tube should be inserted. If the nasogastric tube appears in the thoracic cavity on the chest film, the need for contrast studies is eliminated. An upper GI contrast study should be performed if the diagnosis is not clear. Treatment for acute cases usually involves exploratory laparotomy for reduction of the herniated contents, inspection for other intraabdominal injury, and diaphragm repair (Moore, Feliciano, and Mattox, 2004).

Bibliography

Symbas PN, Vlasis SE, Hatcher C. Blunt and penetrating diaphragmatic injuries with or without herniation or organs into the chest. *Ann Thorac Surg* 1986;42:158–162.

American College of Surgeons Committee on Trauma. *Advanced Trauma Life Support*, 6th ed. Chicago, IL: American College of Surgeons, 1997.

Moore E, Feliciano D, Mattox K. *Trauma*, 5th ed. New York, NY: McGraw-Hill, 2004.

CHAPTER 11

Burns

Madeline Zieger and John Coleman III

Questions

1. All of the following cell types are found in the epidermis *except*:

   (A) fibroblasts
   (B) Langerhans
   (C) keratinocytes
   (D) Merkel cells
   (E) melanocytes

2. Platelet microthrombus formation and vascular constriction occur in which of the zones of burn injury:

   (A) zone of hyperemia
   (B) zone of stasis
   (C) zone of coagulation
   (D) none of the above

3. All of the following are functions of cytokine activity after burn injury *except*:

   (A) anabolism
   (B) inflammation
   (C) immune response
   (D) hyper metabolism

4. An 11-month-old White female pulled a pot of hot grease off the stove and sustained burns to her chin, chest, and abdomen. On initial evaluation in the emergency room (ER), her wounds are noted to be dark red and dry in the central portion of the wound. This patient has most likely sustained a

   (A) superficial burn
   (B) superficial partial thickness burn
   (C) deep partial thickness burn
   (D) full thickness burn

5. All of the following are factors associated with burn wound edema *except*:

   (A) release of systemic and local cell mediators
   (B) increases in water and protein loss in the capillaries
   (C) occurs in burned and nonburned tissues
   (D) intravascular protein content

6. A 52-year-old male weighing 70 kg, sustained a 65% total body surface area (TBSA) burn. What are his fluid requirements?

   (A) 8000 cc in 24 h
   (B) 18,200 cc in 16 h
   (C) 12,800 cc in 24 h
   (D) 9100 cc in 8 h

7. A 10 kg male pulled a pot of hot water off the stove and sustained a 30% TBSA burn. What is his calculated fluid resuscitation?

   (A) 1200 cc in 24 h
   (B) 2200 cc in 24 h
   (C) 2000 cc in 24 h
   (D) 1500 cc in 24 h

8. Hypertonic saline resuscitation

   (A) reduces mortality in burn patients
   (B) requires careful monitoring of serum osmolarity and serum sodium
   (C) requires a serum sodium greater than 160 meq
   (D) increases the amount of tissue edema

9. A 12-year-old child rescued from a burning room may likely demonstrate all of the following components of smoke inhalation injury to the respiratory tree *except* for

   (A) hypersensitivity reaction
   (B) atelectasis
   (C) bronchorhea and mucus plugging
   (D) thermal burn of the subglottic larynx

10. All of the following are useful in obtaining a diagnosis of inhalation injury *except*:

    (A) chest x-ray
    (B) xenon-133 scan
    (C) bronchoscopy
    (D) physical signs

11. A 45-year-old previously healthy fireman sustains a 30% TBSA third degree burn and a severe inhalation injury while fighting a structural blaze. On postburn day 2 he experiences a cardiac arrest and is unable to be resuscitated. Autopsy evaluation of the lung may reveal all of the following *except*

    (A) bronchiolar fibrosis
    (B) bronchial mucus plugs
    (C) alveolar cell necrosis
    (D) bronchiolar vasodilatation

12. A 4-year-old girl sustains a 40% TBSA burn when trapped in her bedroom in a house fire. On postburn day 1 she develops respiratory insufficiency with a PO_2 of 65 and a PCO_2 of 59 on an FiO_2 of 100%. Which of the following interventions is most likely to be beneficial at this time?

    (A) tracheostomy
    (B) methyl prednisolone inhalation therapy
    (C) decreasing the crystalloid infusion and administering albumin
    (D) switching from volume controlled ventilation to pressure controlled ventilation

13. In a 45-year-old man with a 55% TBSA full thickness burn to the trunk, arms, neck and face, all of the following are indicators for escharotomy *except*:

    (A) interstitial tissue pressure in the forearm of 35 mmHg
    (B) gradual rise in mean airway pressures to 50 mmHg H_2O
    (C) increasing anion gap despite fluid resuscitation
    (D) loss of Doppler signals in the fingertips

14. In a 25-year-old patient with a 65% TBSA burn, the administration of phenobarbital in the first 24 h will have what dose response relationship?

    (A) higher than the uninjured state
    (B) lower than the uninjured state
    (C) equivalent to the uninjured state
    (D) hypersensitivity

15. A 3-year-old child with a 40% TBSA burn to the trunk, arms, scalp, and face is brought to the operating room in preparation for a tangential excision of the burn planned for approximately 20% TBSA. Which of the following measures are most important in assuring a safe procedure?

    (A) placement of a subclavian vein catheter
    (B) measurement of serum citrate level
    (C) circummandibular wire fixation of the endotracheal (ET) tube
    (D) transfusion of eight units of platelets and 250 cc of fresh frozen plasma in the preoperative period

16. A 30-year-old firefighter is 6 days postburn with a 55% TBSA burn to his bilateral legs, back, and a portion of his left arm. Prior to being burned, the patient was a marathon runner and weighed 75 kg. His pulse rate is 125 bpm, BP is 110/60 mmHg, T_{max} is 38.5°C, and urine output is 1 cc/kg/h. The most reliable assessment of his nutritional status at this time is

    (A) normal serum retinol-binding protein
    (B) indirect calorimetry with a calculated respiratory quotient (RQ) of less than 0.8
    (C) serum albumin of 2.5
    (D) prealbumin of 8

17. All of the following are true statements regarding burn hypermetabolism *except*:

    (A) The patient has a "resetting" of their homeostatic thermostat.
    (B) There is increased levels of circulating catecholamines.
    (C) Using an open dressing technique diminishes hypermetabolism.
    (D) There is protein catabolism from skeletal muscles.

18. Enteral feeding is preferred to parenteral feeding in the burn patient for which of the following reasons:

    (A) provision of carbohydrate calories
    (B) avoidance of gastric ileus
    (C) replacement of trace minerals
    (D) decrease in bacterial translocation from the gut
    (E) decreased risk of diarrhea

19. Deficiency of which of the following results in impaired collagen synthesis secondary to deficient hydroxylation of lysine and proline?

    (A) selenium
    (B) zinc
    (C) ascorbic acid
    (D) iron
    (E) vitamin E

20. Early anemia in the burn patient is frequently secondary to

    (A) idiopathic reaction to silver sulfadiazine (SSD)
    (B) decreased circulating erythropoeitin
    (C) depletion of bone marrow progenitor cells
    (D) increased erythrocyte fragility
    (E) microthrombus formation

21. A 42-year-old male who is 1 week S/P a 53% TBSA burn with inhalation injury. The patient has had two operative debridement procedures with grafting and currently has an increasing WBC count to 20, temperature spikes to 103°F, oliguria and hypotension. The most common source of sepsis in this patient is

    (A) invasive burn wound infection
    (B) urosepsis from indwelling catheters
    (C) pneumonia
    (D) bacteremia

22. The decrease in CO immediately following thermal injury is because of all of the following *except*:

    (A) decreased systemic vascular resistance
    (B) decreased venous return
    (C) decreased left ventricular distensibility
    (D) epinephrine release

23. Potential cadaver skin donors are serologically tested for all of the following *except*:

    (A) human immunodeficiency virus, type I and II
    (B) hepatitis B and C
    (C) type and cross-match
    (D) syphilis

24. All of the following are potential side effects of topical antimicrobials *except*:

    (A) SSD and leukopenia
    (B) mafenide and metabolic alkalosis
    (C) bacitracin and nephrotoxicity
    (D) nitrofurantoin and contact dermatitis

25. A 40-year-old electrical lineman is injured on a electric pole and is brought to the emergency department unconscious. He has an area on his left hand that is charred, evidence of thermal injury to the arm, and an exit wound on his right knee. Which of the following interventions is least appropriate in the emergency department?

    (A) escharotomy of the left arm
    (B) CT scan of the abdomen and pelvis
    (C) ET intubation
    (D) CT scan of the head and neck
    (E) measurement of serum creatinine phosphokinase levels

26. A 24-year-old petroleum worker presents with a burn to his leg approximately 6% TBSA when hydrofluoric acid spilled onto his clothing. In addition to irrigation of the wound with saline, what therapy is indicated?

    (A) irrigation with dilute sodium hydroxide (NaOH) solution
    (B) application of dimethyl sulfoxide (DMSO) to the wound area
    (C) local injection of calcium gluconate solution
    (D) systemic infusion of magnesium sulfate

27. Which of the following has not been implicated in the pathophysiology of frostbite?

    (A) microemboli in the arteriolar system
    (B) osmotic shifts in the intraextracellular interface
    (C) intracellular ice crystals
    (D) inhibition of the sodium-potassium pump

28. The site of injury in toxic epidermal necrolysis (TENS) and Stevens-Johnson syndrome (SJS) is

    (A) the Nikolsky body
    (B) the basement membrane of the epithelium
    (C) the dermoepidermal junction
    (D) the endoplasmic reticulum

29. Critical factors in the "take" of a skin autograft include all of the following *except*:

    (A) thickness of the graft
    (B) presence of elastin fibers in the graft
    (C) anastomosis of capillaries in the graft to capillaries in the bed
    (D) diffusion of metabolites in the graft cells to plasma of the wound bed

30. Which of the following skin substitutes does not originate, all or in part, from human tissue:

    (A) Transcyte
    (B) Integra
    (C) cultured epithelial autografts (CEA)
    (D) cadaver allograft

31. A 36-year-old male with a past medical history of insulin-dependent diabetes mellitus, sustained a 20% TBSA hot water scald burn to his abdomen, genitalia, and right leg. All of the following are referral criteria *except*:

    (A) 20% TBSA or greater
    (B) preexisting medical condition
    (C) scald burns
    (D) burns involving cosmetic or functional areas, i.e., face, joints, genitalia

Answers and Explanations

1. (A) The skin is the largest organ of the body and is composed of three distinct layers: the epidermis, the dermis, and the subcutaneous tissue. The epidermis is the most superficial layer and is composed of four separate layers ranging in thickness from 0.05 to 1 mm; the basal layer, stratum spinosum, the stratum granulosum, and the dead epidermis, the stratum corneum.

The basal layer is the innermost layer and contains mitotically active keratinocytes. Melanocytes are found within the basal layer and provide ultraviolet radiation protection. In the next layer, the stratum spinosum, the keratinocytes become more differentiated and are joined together by gap junctions that allow for cellular communication. The stratum granulosum is the most highly differentiated layer of the epidermis and it is where most keratin production occurs. Most superficial, the stratum corneum, the outside nonliving layer is composed of keratin providing the major barrier to the environment. Found scattered throughout the epidermis are Langerhans cells which are important in antigen-processing cells and Merkel cells which serve as touch receptors.

The epidermis and dermis are separated by the basement membrane zone. Anchoring fibrils connect these two layers. The dermis is separated by a superficial thin layer called the papillary dermis and a deep, dense layer called the reticular dermis. The primary cell of the dermis is the fibroblast that produces the collagen, elastic fibers, and ground substance that compose the bulk of the dermis. The papillary dermis contains collagen fibers laid out in a fine mesh. The reticular dermis has course collagen bundles that run in various directions. These bundles are embedded in the ground substance with elastic fibers. The collagen provides tensile strength and the elastic fibers provide elasticity to the skin. The ground substance is composed of proteoglycans, which bind water and provide for skin hydration. Inflammatory cells migrate through the ground substance beneath the dermis, a large plexus of arterioles

and venules called the subdermal plexus. This plexus further branches into superficial smaller vessels called the papillary plexus. The skin appendages, sebaceous glands, sweat glands, and hair follicles, all lie within the dermis.

The subcutaneous layer lies beneath the dermis. This layer contains fat cells that serve as an insulating layer for the body and supports blood vessels and nerves that travel into the dermis (Fig. 11-1).

Bibliography

Han H, Mustoe T. Strucure and function of skin. In: Eriksson E (ed.), *Plastic Surgery Indications, Operations, and Outcomes*, vol. 1. St. Louis, MO: Mosby, 2000, 23–36.

Okun M, Edelstein L, Fisher B. Normal histology of the skin. In: Okun M, Edelstein L, Fisher B (eds.), *Gross and Microscopic Pathology of the Skin*, 2nd ed. Canton, OH: Dermopathology Foundation Press, 1988, 9–73.

Watson K. Structure of the skin. In: Hall J (ed.), *Sauer's Manual of Skin Diseases*, 8th ed. Philadelphia, PA: Lippincott, Williams & Wilkins, 2000, 1–8.

2. (B) The depth of a burn wound is directly related to the temperature of the offending agent and the duration of contact of the agent with the skin. In 1953, Jackson published "The Diagnosis of the Depth of Burning" in the *British Journal of Surgery*. In this paper, Jackson describes three distinct zones of burn wound injury, the zones of coagulation, stasis, and hyperemia.

The zone of coagulation is the area that is in direct contact with the offending agent. In this zone, cellular proteins have denatured and coagulated, cellular necrosis has occurred and eschar is formed. This tissue has been irreparably damaged extending in both horizontal and vertical dimension.

The zone of stasis lies lateral and deep to the zone of coagulation. In this zone the cells are injured and dermal capillary stasis occurs. The damage in this region may progress to necrosis or may reverse and allow cellular recovery. There is a progression of

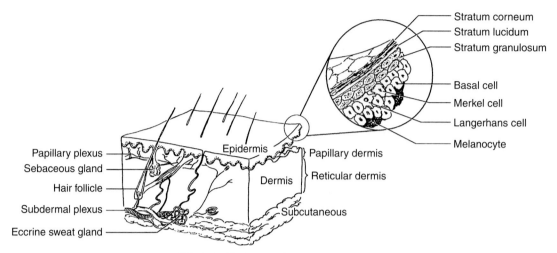

FIG. 11-1   The layers and structures of the skin.

microvascular changes that occur in this zone. Arteriole and venules dilate, slowing blood flow. Platelet, erythrocyte, and leukocyte aggregation occurs with eventual formation of microthrombi. Vascular constriction is compounded by endothelial edema with luminal narrowing and finally endothelial wall disruption and further edema formation. This stasis and edema formation inhibits already damaged cells from receiving the vital nutrients and oxygen they need to survive. If immediate interventions are not instituted, that is, preventing dehydration, minimizing inflammation and edema, and preventing infection, this zone will progress to coagulation and complete cell death.

The outermost zone is the zone of hyperemia. In this zone cellular injury is minimal, in part because of its distance from the offending agent. Vasodilation occurs in this region because of the inflammatory process. All cells in this region will recover unless infection, further dehydration, or edema occur (Fig. 11-2).

Bibliography

Garner W. Thermal burns. In: Achauer B (ed.), *Plastic Surgery Indications, Operations, and Outcomes*, vol. 1. St. Louis, MO: Mosby, 2000, 357–373.

Jackson D. The diagnosis of the depth of burning. *Br J Surg* 1953:40:588–589.

Williams W. Pathophysiology of the burn wound. In: Herndon D (ed.), *Total Burn Care*, 2nd ed. London: W.B. Saunders, 2002, 514–522.

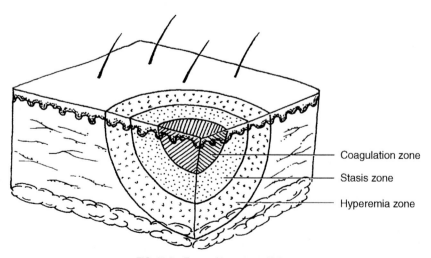

FIG. 11-2   Zones of burn wound injury.

3. (A) Cytokines are proteins that function as chemical messengers when secreted by cells, in particular by the reticulo-endothelial system and elsewhere. They play a major role in the systemic response to burn injury.

Cytokines such as tumor necrosis factor (TNF), interleukin (IL)-1, and IL-6 are produced locally at the site of the burn injury but are eventually spilled into the systemic circulation. TNF, produced primarily by macrophages and monocytes, plays an important role in the immunologic responses to burn injury. TNF stimulates the release of neutrophils from the bone marrow, neutrophil margination, and activation of macrophages to release oxidants. It stimulates an acute hepatic phase of protein synthesis, protein secretion, and enhances catabolic metabolism, and subsequent skeletal muscle breakdown. Systemically, it initiates antimicrobial defenses manifesting fever and activation of the coagulation cascade. TNF functions in burn wound inflammation by increasing vascular permeability and increasing the procoagulant activity of endothelial cells.

IL-1 is produced primarily by monocytes and macrophages. Some of the immune action of IL-1 include T-cell proliferation and neutrophil release from the bone marrow. IL-1 has metabolic actions which enhance catabolism, fever production, anemia, and increased endothelial permeability. IL-1 causes the liver to increase production of metalloproteins that bind to iron and zinc. Bacteria need these metalloproteins for cell growth.

IL-6 is produced by a variety of tissues and is released rapidly into circulation in response to injury or infection. IL-6 has the metabolic effects of stimulating hepatic acute phase proteins, such as C-reactive protein and of increasing B-cell proliferation and production of immunoglobulins. It also plays a role in fever production.

Bibliography

Heideman M, Bengtsson A. The immunologic response to thermal injury. *World J Surg* 1992;16:53–56.
Munster A. The immunological response and strategies for intervention. In: Herndon D (ed.), *Total Burn Care*, 2nd ed. London: W.B. Saunders, 2002, 316–330.
Sherwood E, Traber D. The systemic inflammatory response syndrome. In: Herndon D (ed.), *Total Burn Care*, 2nd ed. London: W.B. Saunders, 2002, 257–270.
Yonn Y, La Londe C, Demling R. The role of mediators in the response to thermal injury. *World J Surg* 1992;16:30–36.

4. (D) The superficial burn or first degree burn is usually red in appearance. The epidermis has been damaged and may exfoliate in approximately 7 days, but is usually healed underneath at the time of slough. An example of a superficial or first degree burn is a sun burn.

A partial thickness burn implies that damage has occurred to the dermis. These burns can be further subdivided into superficial or deep partial thickness burns. The superficial partial thickness burn extends into the papillary dermis. It is characterized by blister formation and on removal of the blister, the wound is noted to be pink and moist. The burn wound is extremely painful and will blanch easily when compressed. The hair follicles are intact and are difficult to remove. In a favorable environment these wounds will heal within a 2-week period. The injured area is reepithelialized by the epithelial cells lining the dermal appendages: hair follicles and sebaceous glands.

Deep partial thickness burns extend into the reticular dermis. These burns can be mottled and will likely form an eschar. Eschar is the product of coagulated proteins from the injured skin. The capillary refill of these wounds is slow and the hair follicles are usually not intact. These wounds may heal in greater than 3 weeks and will most likely produce an unfavorable scar if treated nonsurgically.

Full thickness burn injuries involve the entire thickness of skin. No dermal appendages are viable for reepithelialization. These wounds contain necrotic tissue and the eschar is usually dry and white or charred in appearance. These wounds may even be dark red in appearance as a result of intravascular coagulation but they do not blanch with pressure and are generally insensate.

The dermis of small children is proportionally thinner than that of adults and does not reach adult thickness until approximately age 5. The elderly, on the other hand, undergo dermal atrophy starting after age 50. It is therefore more likely that a scald burn will be deeper in the very young and elderly requiring surgical treatment, usually excision and skin grafting (Figs. 11-3 and 11-4).

Bibliography

Garner W. Thermal burns. In: Achauer B (ed.), *Plastic Surgery Indications, Operations, and Outcomes*, vol. 1. St. Louis, MO: Mosby, 2000, 357–373.
Heimbach D, Engrav L, Grube B, et al. Burn depth: a review. *World J Surg* 1992;16:10–15.
Williams W. Pathophysiology of the burn wound. In: Herndon D (ed.), *Total Burn Care*, 2nd ed. London: W.B. Saunders, 2002, 514–522.

5. (D) The pathophysiology of burn edema is multifactorial. The primary cause is the disruption of capillary membranes and the leakage of intravascular fluid into the extravascular space. This leakage occurs in both the burned and nonburned tissues because of the systemic circulation of vasoactive cytokines released from the

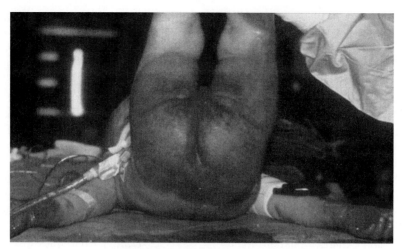

FIG. 11-3 Partial thickness scald burn.

burned area. The edema formation is biphasic in nature with an early rapid and late gradual phase. Maximal edema occurs by approximately 24 h.

In the early phase, burn edema is seen only in the burn wound. Histamine, a potent vasodilator which causes an increased separation in the capillary intracellular junction, is released from mast cells within the burned tissue and a rapid accumulation of water occurs within this tissue. Other vasoactive mediators are released from the damaged endothelium that promote in a more gradual propagation of the edema. These include substances such as kinins, prostaglandins, serotonin, and thromboxane.

The microvascular changes that occur with burn edema, apart from an increase in the separation of capillary intracellular junction, include changes in the capillary and interstitial pressures. The interstitial hydrostatic pressure increases, drawing fluid from the intravascular space into the interstitium by generating oncotic pressure. In addition, through leaking capillaries, protein-rich plasma enters the interstitium. The plasma colloid osmotic pressure is decreased and the interstitial colloid osmotic pressure is increased which further stimulates edema formation. Capillary pressure in the burned tissues significantly increases initially and slowly decreases over the next several hours.

Charles Baxter demonstrated that not only does edema formation occur within the interstitium but also within the cells. A decrease in cellular transmembrane potentials allows sodium to enter the cells and cellular water to increase. Despite knowledge of these capillary and inflammatory changes, a complete understanding of burn wound edema has yet to be obtained.

Bibliography

Baxter C. Fluid volume and electrolyte changes in the early post-burn period. *Clin Plast Surg* 1974;1:693–703.

Lund T. The 1999 Everett Idris Evans Memorial Lecture; edema generation following thermal injury: an update. *J Burn Care Rehabil* 1999;20:445–452.

Lund T, Onarheim H, Reed R. Pathogenesis of edema formation in burn injuries. *World J Surg* 1992;16:2–9.

Williams W. Pathophysiology of the burn wound. In: Herndon D (ed.), *Total Burn Care*, 2nd ed. London: W.B. Saunders, 2002, 514–522.

6. **(D)** The goal of fluid resuscitation of the burn victim is to preserve systemic tissue perfusion. This goal is made difficult because of the "capillary leak" that occurs in the burned and nonburned tissues. It is also known that plasma and blood volumes are decreased and extracellular fluid volume is increased. Peripheral vascular resistance is increased and cardiac output

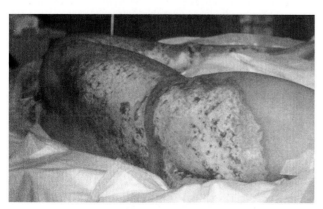

FIG. 11-4 Full thickness burn.

(CO) although initially decreased, over the ensuing 18–24 h, returns to or exceeds normal limits. Demling has experimentally shown that after 8 h postburn, the plasma protein content can be maintained. In other words, the "leak" will start to resolve.

There are numerous resuscitation formulas that have been described. The goal of each of these formulas is tissue perfusion. This perfusion can be verified by an adequate urine output of 0.5 cc/kg/h, reversal of acidosis, adequate mentation, and adequate filling pressures. These resuscitation formulas aim for adequate hydration with avoidance of over or under resuscitation.

The widely accepted Parkland formula is a lactated Ringer's solution of 4 cc/kg/% TBSA burn given over 24 h. One-half of the calculated volume is delivered in the first 8 h following the burn and the remainder is delivered over the ensuing 16 h. A lactated Ringer's solution is used because it is isotonic in nature and has a decreased chloride load that prevents hyperchloremic metabolic acidosis. Since colloid solutions are "leaked" from the capillaries creating increased osmotic pressure in the interstitium, crystalloid solutions are best for massive resuscitation. Another crystalloid resuscitation formula is the modified Brooke formula that uses a 2 cc/kg/% TBSA burn in the first 24 h.

Colloid resuscitation is another accepted form of resuscitation. Formulas such as Brooke and Evans use one-quarter to one-half of the resuscitation solution as colloid. Slater uses 2 L of lactated Ringer's and fresh frozen plasma at a rate of 75 cc/kg for the first 24 h. Other institutions initiate colloid after 8–12 h once the "capillary leak" has begun to resolve. Formulas using albumin, plasmanate, and low molecular weight dextran to fresh frozen plasma have all been described (Table 11-1).

TABLE 11-1   Formulas for Burn Resuscitation

Formula name	Formula	Solution
Parkland	4 cc/kg/% TBSA burn	Lactated Ringer's
Brooke	1.5 cc/kg/% TBSA burn	Lactated Ringer's
	0.5 cc/kg	Colloid
	2000 cc	D_5W
Evans	1.0 cc/kg/% TBSA burn	Normal saline
	1.0 cc/kg/% TBSA burn	Colloid
	2000 cc	D_5W
Slater	2 L/24 h	Lactated Ringer's
	75 cc/kg/24 h	Fresh frozen plasma

Adapted from: Warden G. Fluid resuscitation and early management. In: Herndon D (ed.), *Total Burn Care*, 2nd ed. London: W.B. Saunders; 2002:120–169.

Bibliography

American Burn Association. Burn shock resuscitation: initial management and overview. Practice guidelines for burn care. *J Burn Care Rehabil* 2001:27S–37S.

American Burn Association. Fluid resuscitation: colloid resuscitation. Practice guidelines for burn care. *J Burn Care Rehabil* 2001:38S–42S.

Morehouse J, Finkelstein J, Marano M, et al. Resuscitation of the thermally injured patient. *Crit Care Clin* 1992;8:355–365.

Warden G. Burn shock resuscitation. *World J Surg* 1992; 16:16–23.

Warden G. Fluid resuscitation and early management. In: Herndon D (ed.), *Total Burn Care*, 2nd ed. London: W.B. Saunders, 2002, 88–97.

7. **(B)** The burned child is not the equivalent of the burned adult. The child's resuscitation requires careful consideration to adequately meet their end-organs specific resuscitative needs. Merrell et al. in 1986 established that children need approximately 2 cc/kg/% more fluid resuscitation than adults with similar size burns. Merrell also noted that children require resuscitation for smaller body surface area burns than do adults.

Physiologically, children have a greater proportion of body surface area to weight than do adults. In addition, because of the larger surface area of their heads, the standard "Rule of Nines" chart does not accurately assess a child's burned surface area. Children have proportionately larger evaporative losses than adults because of their larger surface areas. Children less than 2 years of age have decreased glycogen stores and may therefore, become hypoglycemic easily. The child's heart is also less compliant and may be more prone to volume overload. A careful consideration of all these factors will mitigate over and under resuscitation.

Several resuscitative formulas have been devised for the pediatric patient. The simplest formula uses the Parkland formula of 4 cc/kg/% TBSA burned and adds the child's normal maintenance fluid. One-half of the total fluid volume indicated by the Parkland formula is infused over the first 8 h with the remainder over the ensuing 16 h and, in addition, an hourly maintenance fluid calculated by weight and age is delivered. The Parkland solution is lactated Ringer's and the maintenance fluid may be LR or, in children under 2 years, D_5LR.

The Shriner's Hospital in Galveston, TX uses a formula calculated using the child's body surface area. This formula is 5000 cc/m2 body surface area burned plus 2000 cc/body surface area over the first 24 h. One-half of this solution is given over the first 8 h and the remainder over the ensuing 16 h.

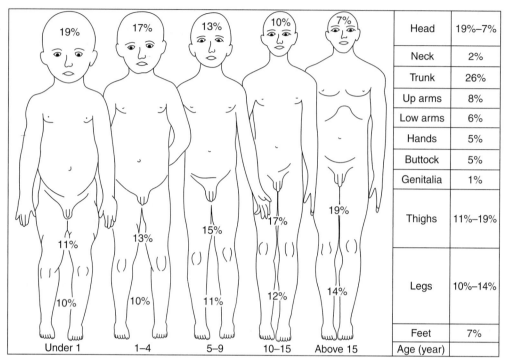

					Head	19%–7%
					Neck	2%
					Trunk	26%
					Up arms	8%
					Low arms	6%
					Hands	5%
					Buttock	5%
					Genitalia	1%
19%	17%	13%	10%	7%	Thighs	11%–19%
11%	13%	15%	17%	19%	Legs	10%–14%
10%	10%	11%	12%	14%	Feet	7%
Under 1	1–4	5–9	10–15	Above 15	Age (year)	

FIG. 11-5   Body surface area and age chart.

In children, resuscitation is titrated to maintain a urine output of 1–1.5 cc/kg/h. Acid-base balance, mentation, and vital signs are all monitored to aid in resuscitation (Fig. 11-5).

Bibliography

American Burn Association. Burn shock resuscitation: initial management and overview. Practice guidelines for burn care. *J Burn Care Rehabil* 2001:27S–37S.

Benjamin D, Herndon D. Special considerations of age: the pediatric burn patient. In: Herndon D (ed.), *Total Burn Care*, 2nd ed. London: W.B. Saunders, 2002, 427–438.

Merrell S, Saffle J, Sullivan J, et al. Fluid resuscitation in thermally injured children. *Am J Surg* 1986;152:664–669.

Sheridan R, Remensnyder J, Prelack K, et al. Treatment of the seriously burned infant. *J Burn Care Rehabil* 1998;19:115–118.

Warden G. Burn shock resuscitation. *World J Surg* 1992;16:16–23.

Warden G. Fluid resuscitation and early management. In: Herndon D (ed.), *Total Burn Care*, 2nd ed. London: W.B. Saunders, 2002, 88–97.

8. **(B)** The goal of fluid resuscitation of the burn patient is to infuse enough volume to maintain organ perfusion but limit the amount of edema that may cause progression of the burn injury and other negative systemic effects such as respiratory insufficency. This is, however, difficult because of the "capillary leak" that occurs in both the burned and nonburned tissues. This "leak" allows serum proteins to move into the interstitial space causing intravascular water to follow. Hypertonic saline resuscitation has been used for resuscitation of large burns and burns in children and the elderly since the amount of fluid given during early resuscitation is generally less.

Hypertonic saline resuscitation uses either normal saline or lactated Ringer's solution that is augmented by varying amounts of sodium bicarbonate. This solution produces a serum hypernatremia that in turn causes a serum hyperosmolarity. This hyperosmolarity increase the plasma oncotic pressure, therefore, less intravascular water is leaked into the interstitial space. The result is less tissue edema. The kidneys also produce more urine because of the concentrated serum that is filtered. Yoshioka et al. in 1980 reviewed 53 patients with greater than 30% TBSA burns. It was shown that patients treated with lactated Ringer's were given 4.8 cc/kg/% TBSA versus 2.2 cc/kg/% burn with hypertonic saline. Numerous studies, however, have not translated this decreased requirement to a decreased mortality with the use of hypertonic saline resuscitation.

Urine output will decrease if the patient's serum sodium increases to greater than 160 meq that may occur with too aggressive resuscitation. When this does happen, cerebral cortical shrinkage may occur with consequent hemorrhage. A vigorous correction of the hypernatremia may produce cerebral edema and even, death. Therefore, serial measurements of serum sodium and serum osmolarity must be obtained to avoid these complications.

Resuscitation should be based on urine output and end-organ perfusion. Hypertonic resuscitation is to be considered only during the first 24 h of resuscitation and if used, the patient must be carefully monitored to avoid serious complications.

Bibliography

American Burn Association. Burn shock resuscitation: initial management and overview. Practice guidelines for burn care. *J Burn Care Rehabil* 2001:27S–37S.

American Burn Association. Hypertonic fluid resuscitation. Practice guidelines for burn care. *J Burn Care Rehabil* 2001:38S–42S.

Warden G. Burn shock resuscitation. *World J Surg* 1992; 16:16–23.

Warden G. Fluid resuscitation and early management. In: Herndon D (ed.), *Total Burn Care*, 2nd ed. London: W.B. Saunders, 2002, 88–97.

9. **(D)** Inhalation injury is generally separated into three components. These components include carbon monoxide poisoning, injury above and injury below the glottis.

Carbon monoxide poisoning is a common cause of on-scene fire deaths. Carbon monoxide has a greater affinity than oxygen for the hemoglobin molecule and therefore, displaces oxygen. Measurement of the patient's carboxyhemoglobin level may give an assessment of the patient's exposure. Physically, the patient may demonstrate few signs and symptoms. A carboxyhemoglobin of 10 or less, has essentially no physical findings. Greater than 10, the patient may experience headache and mild confusion. At levels of 30–40, nausea and vomiting, confusion and dizziness develop. Greater than 40, cardiovascular and respiratory complications occur, including tachycardia or arrhythmias, increased or decreased respirations, obtundation, and even death.

The treatment for carbon monoxide poisoning is 100% oxygen. At lower carboxyhemoglobin levels, this can be delivered via nonrebreather facemask. If, however, the patient develops neurologic complications, i.e., obtundation, is unable to maintain his/her own airway, or is hypoxic, then intubation may be necessary. On 100% oxygen, the half-life of carboxyhemoglobin is 40 min. This short half-life may make it difficult to determine accurately the amount of carbon monoxide inhaled, since the 100% oxygen is routinely administered to patients as soon as they are extricated from the fire. So, the length of time that the patient has been treated with 100% oxygen must be considered when evaluating a patient's carboxyhemoglobin level.

Hyperbaric oxygen has been used to effectively treat carbon monoxide poisoning; however, because of the fact that this treatment is not readily available in most institutions and is cumbersome to use except in hemodynamically stable patients, it is not advisable at present to use in burn patients necessitating resuscitation.

Injuries above the glottis should be rapidly evaluated. The oropharynx has the ability to facilitate heat exchange because of its large surface area and good blood supply. The oropharynx, therefore can absorb a great amount of heat without permanent damage; however, edema develops rapidly and may cause temporary airway obstruction, especially in children. Facial and neck burns may also cause airway compromise, and patients with these injuries should be carefully considered for elective intubation if any signs of compromise become apparent. Even when initial evaluation demonstrates no edema, intubation may be prudent since resuscitation will result in significant tissue edema and possible upper airway obstruction.

Injury below the glottis can be divided into thermal injury or injury because of the inhalation of the byproducts of combustion. Thermal injury occurs when super heated air is inhaled, i.e., seam burns. This is a rare occurrence because of the tremendous heat exchange of the upper airways. The byproducts of combustion cause a chemical pneumonitis and an acute hypersensitivity reaction: bronchorhea and subsequent obstruction by mucus and atelectasis, the pathophysiology of which will be discussed in another question (Fig. 11-6).

Bibliography

Clark W. Smoke inhalation: diagnosis and treatment. *World J Surg* 1992;16:24–29.

Demling R. Smoke inhalation injury. *New Horiz* 1993;1:422–434.

Demling R, Chen C. Pulmonary function in the burn patient. *Semin Nephrol* 1993;13:371–381.

Ruddy R. Smoke inhalation injury. *Pediatr Clin North Am* 1994;41:317–336.

Traber D, Herndon D, Soejima K. The pathophysiology of inhalation injury. In: Herndon D (ed.), *Total Burn Care*, 2nd ed. London: W.B. Saunders, 2002, 221–231.

Weiss S, Lakshminarayan S. Acute inhalation injury. *Clin Chest Med* 1994;15:103–116.

10. **(A)** Lung injury is the leading cause of death in burn patients. Inhalation injury is the predominant cause of

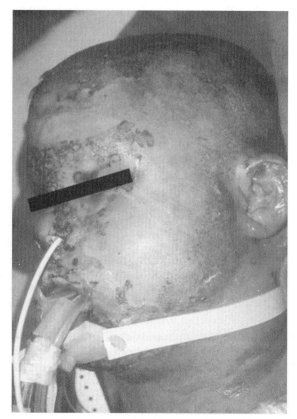

FIG. 11-6   Severe edema following facial burns.

lung injury. Inhalation injury has a reported mortality as high as 60%. Diagnosis and early treatment may help reduce the morbidity and mortality of this disease.

History and physical examination are key components to the diagnosis of inhalation injury. It is important to determine whether this injury occurred within an enclosed space; i.e., did the injury occur in a building, shed, or car? How long was the patient exposed to the smoke? Was the patient rescued unconscious or was the patient able to escape? Another important factor is the length of oxygen therapy prior to arrival to the emergency department. This will alter the amount of carboxyhemoglobin present in the patient's blood. A low carboxyhemoglobin level on arrival to the ER may be a function of time and oxygen treatment rather than a reflection of low exposure of the lung to chemical irritants. Determining the patient's past medical history is important for interpreting the patient's test results. Physical findings of facial burns, i.e., singed nasal hairs, soot in the nose or mouth, oral pharynx edema, hoarseness, stridor or wheezing all should alert the clinician to the possibility of inhalation injury.

Measurements of carboxyhemoglobin levels are helpful for indicating inhalation injury. Levels of 10 or greater are usually present. Truck drivers and heavy smokers may have elevated carboxyhemoglobin levels. Any patient with a suspicious history should be suspected of having an inhalation injury. Chest x-rays are not helpful in determining whether an inhalation injury has occurred. Most initial chest x-rays are normal in appearance or if abnormal, may be attributable to some other cause.

Xenon-133 scanning has been used to aid in the diagnosis of smoke inhalation. This scan shows areas of the lungs that are ventilated. Areas in the lung with small airway obstruction will be revealed; however, this test is not specific for inhalation injury and must be used to complement other diagnostic tests. Bronchoscopy is the current "gold standard" for the diagnosis of inhalation injury. This procedure allows for visualization of the upper airways and the tracheobronchial tree. Bronchoscopic findings of inhalation injury include erythema and/or edema of the airways, carbonaceous material, blistering, hemorrhage, and ulceration or necrosis of the mucosa; however, patients who are hypotensive or hypovolemic may not exhibit these findings initially until after resuscitation. Khoo et al. disputed this notion in their study in the *Journal of Trauma* in 1997. Their findings demonstrated that inhalation injury may be diagnosed within hours after injury regardless of the hemodynamic status of the patient. Furthermore, the absence of a cough reflex during bronchoscopy was found to be highly specific for inhalation injury.

Inhalation injury remains a leading cause of morbidity and mortality in the burn patients. High suspicion, accurate diagnosis, and prompt treatment of this injury are critical to early treatment (Figs. 11-7 and 11-8).

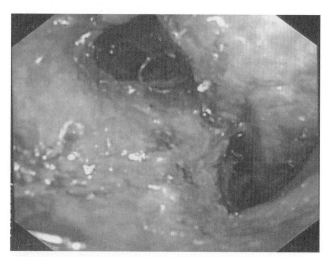

FIG. 11-7   Admission bronchoscopy for smoke inhalation.

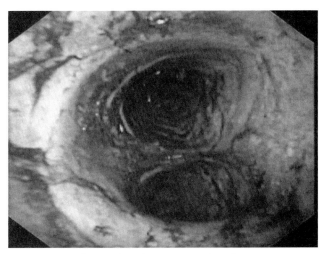

FIG. 11-8 Bronchoscopy on postburn day 3.

Bibliography

Clark W. Smoke inhalation: diagnosis and treatment. *World J Surg* 1992;16:24–29.

Fitzpatrick J, Cioffi W. Diagnosis and treatment of inhalation injury. In: Herndon D (ed.), *Total Burn Care*, 2nd ed. London: W.B. Saunders, 2002, 232–241.

Herndon D, Thompson P, Traber D. Pulmonary injury in burned patients. *Crit Care Clin* 1985;1:79–97.

Masanes M, Legendre C, Lioret N, et al. Using bronchoscopy and biopsy to diagnose early inhalation injury: macroscopic and histologic findings. *Chest* 1995;107: 1365–1369.

Peitzman A, Shire T III, Teixidor H, et al. Smoke inhalation injury: evaluation of radiographic manisfestations and pulmonary dysfunction. *J Trauma* 1989;29:1232–1238.

11. (A) Inhalation injury is devastating especially when combined with a cutaneous injury. Thompson et al. concluded in their study on *The Effect on Mortality of Inhalation Injury*, that inhalation injury is the most important determining factor for mortality in the in the burn injury regardless of TBSA or age of the patient. An understanding of the pathophysiology of inhalation injury is essential for optimizing the patient's therapy.

After significant smoke inhalation, the cilia cease to function and the epithelial cells immediately separate from the basement membrane. The local injury to the mucosa of the airway initiates the cascade of acute inflammation allowing plasma proteins to leak from the pulmonary microvasculature. Edema develops and is exacerbated by as much as 10-fold increase in blood flow to the lungs and tracheobronchial tree. Bronchoscopy may initially demonstrate evidence of edema and hyperemia. Diffuse exudate formation in the airway is noted with the protein leak and may result in bronchoconstriction and alveolar flooding. These exudates may congeal with neutrophils and cellular debris to form fibrin casts partially or fully obstructing the airways and providing excellent media for bacteria propagation. Neutrophil activation occurs within the alveoli and lung parenchyma stimulating proteolytic enzymes and oxygen-free radicals that further destroy the lung parenchyma and increase the microvascular permeability. Thus, further propagating edema formation, and decreasing gas exchange within the lungs. Surfactant is diminished which results in alveolar collapse and a decrease in lung compliance.

Permanent airway damage may occur with later fibrosis, airway stenosis, and granulomatous scar formation. The accumulation of mucus casts and spasm or fibrosis of the small airways result in obstruction, atelectasis, superinfection, and pneumonia. Patients usually succumb to infection with the inability of the patient to be ventilated despite aggressive measures.

Bibliography

Clark W, Nieman G. Smoke inhalation. *Burns* 1988;14: 473–494.

Demling R. Smoke inhalation injury. *New Horiz* 1993;1: 422–434.

Herndon D, Traber D. Pulmonary circulation and burns and trauma. *J Trauma* 1990;30:S41–S44.

Herndon D, Thompson PB, Traber D. Pulmonary injury in burned patients. *Crit Care Clin* 1985;1:79–96.

Ruddy R. Smoke inhalation injury. *Pediatr Clin North Am* 1994;41:317–336.

Thompson P, Herndon D, Traber D, Abston S. Effect on mortality of inhalation injury. *J Trauma* 1986;26:163–165.

Traber D, Herndon D, Soejima K. The pathophysiology of inhalation injury. In: Herndon D (ed.), *Total Burn Care*, 2nd ed. London: W.B. Saunders, 2002, 221–231.

Traber D, Linares H, Herndon D. The pathophysiology of inhalation injury—a review. *Burns* 1988;14:357–364.

12. (D) The treatment of smoke inhalation begins in the emergency department, if not on extraction from the fire. All patients with suspected inhalation injury should be placed on 100% oxygen. Appropriate diagnostic tests should be performed and any patient in obvious respiratory distress or with real or threatened upper airway obstruction should be intubated. The initial oxygen therapy will decrease the amount of carboxyhemoglobin within the patient's blood.

Fluid resuscitation in a patient with inhalation injury should not be kept at a minimum to reduce the amount of lung water. It has been shown that decreased fluid administration will not only produce hypovolemia and renal failure, but may promote an increase in extravascular lung water. The same consideration should be given to the patient with smoke inhalation and cutaneous burns. These patients can require up to 75% more fluid in the first 24 h than patients with cutaneous burns alone. Therefore, it is important to maintain the patient's urine output at approximately 0.5–1 cc/kg/h in an adult for proper maintenance of systemic perfusion.

Further therapy for smoke inhalation is essentially supportive. If the patient is intubated, the ventilation should be carefully modulated. FiO_2 and ventilator settings should produce an oxygen saturation of 93% or greater. All attempts should be made to limit peak airway pressures to less than 40 mmHg. High airway pressures decrease capillary blood flow to the mucosa eventually causing ischemia. Ischemia may be prevented by using the concept of permissive hypercapnea. Permissive hypercapnea allows for higher CO_2 levels and lowered pH levels, i.e., any PCO_2 that allows a pH of 7.2 or greater and an O_2 saturation of 85 or greater, in exchange for decreased airway pressures and decreased FiO_2, thereby reducing barotrauma to the lung and cumulative damage to the alveoli and decreasing oxygen toxicity. Many different modes of ventilation have been used to treat inhalation injury. Pressure controlled ventilation, volumetric diffusive respiration (VDR), and high frequency ventilation all have demonstrated some success in the reduction of barotrauma.

Antibiotics should only be given for documented infections to avoid the selection of multidrug resistant bacteria. Nebulized β_2-agonists can be given to relieve wheezing and bronchospasm. Steroids have not been proven to be of any benefit to the patient with inhalation injury. Aerosolized heparin has been used by some centers for relief of thickened secretions. Early tracheostomy has not been proven to reduce mortality but can aid in pulmonary toilet. Frequent suctioning, turning and chest physiotherapy all aid in the management of copious, often inspissated secretions.

Bibliography

Clark W. Smoke inhalation: diagnosis and treatment. *World J Surg* 1992;16:24–29.

Cioffi W, Rue L, Geaves T, McManus W, Mason A, Pruitt B. Prophylactic use of high-frequency percussive ventilation in patients with inhalation injury. *Ann Surg* 1991;213:575–582.

Fitzpatrick J, Cioffi W. Diagnosis and treatment of inhalation injury. In: Herndon D (ed.), *Total Burn Care*, 2nd ed. London: W.B. Saunders, 2002, 232–241.

Navar P, Saffle J, Warden G. Effect of inhalation injury on fluid resuscitation requirements after thermal injury. *Am J Surg* 1985;150:716–120.

Pruitt B, Cioffi W, Shimazu T, Ikeuchi H, Mason A. Evaluation and management of patients with inhalation injury. *J Trauma* 1990;30:S63–S68.

Ruddy R. Smoke inhalation injury. *Pediatr Clin North Am* 1994;41:317–336.

Tranbaugh R, Lewis F, Christensen J, Elings V. Lung water changes after thermal injury. *Ann Surg* 1980;192:479–490.

13. **(C)** Full thickness circumferential or near-circumferential burns of the extremities may cause vascular compromise to the affected extremity. This occurs because the burned skin with the subsequent interstitial edema is relatively inelastic. As tissue edema increases, especially in the first 24–48 h postburn, tissue pressures rise which may lead to further ischemia of the underlying tissue. The clinical manifestations of compartment syndrome, i.e., pain, pallor, paresthesias, paralysis, and pulselessness are not always easy to interpret in the burned extremity. Other methods must be used to determine whether a patient is at risk for tissue ischemia.

There are multiple means available for determining elevated tissue pressures. Clinical examination is not, however, always accurate. An absent pulse by palpation may represent difficulty with physical examination because of edema and eschar formation with adequate distal perfusion. Decreased sensorium because of analgesics may interfere with the evaluation of sensation. The most accurate and readily available method of evaluating impending tissue ischemia is to sequentially monitor Doppler flow to the affected extremity. The Doppler ultrasound will auscultate pulses that often cannot be palpated. This method is easy and reliable. An absent pulse by Doppler signals that an escharotomy should be performed. Another noninvasive method of assessing blood flow to an extremity is with infrared photoplethysmography. At any given moment in time the most reliable indicator is measurement of interstitial tissue pressure with a needle and fluid column or commercially available device such as a Stryker device. Pressures greater than 40 mmHg suggest tissue ischemia. An escharotomy should be performed if repeat pressures of 30 mmHg or greater are measured.

Escharotomies can be performed at either the bedside with intravenous sedation or in the operating room. The patient is placed in the anatomic position and longitudinal incisions are made in the midlateral or midmedial positions using either a knife or electrocautery. The incision is made through the inelastic burned skin, extending into the subcutaneous tissue. The midlateral surface should be incised first and perfusion reassessed. If perfusion is still diminished, then the midmedial portion of the burned extremity should be incised. Particular care must be exercised at joints and near superficial nerves. Occasionally, trunk escharotomies need to be performed because of circumferential full thickness

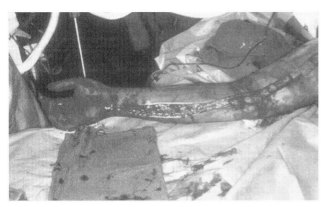

FIG. 11-9 Escharotomy to an arm.

trunk burns. These burns can interfere with chest excursion increasing the mean airway pressure necessary to expand the chest, especially in young children, and cause difficulties with ventilation. Escharotomies may be necessary on hands and fingers and rarely, the penis and neck.

Prophylactic escharotomies are performed in patients with circumferential or near-circumferential burned extremities and large body surface area burns. These patients will receive large volumes of fluid resuscitation with concomitant tissue edema formation (Fig. 11-9).

Bibliography

American Burn Association. Escharotomy. Practice guidelines for burn care. *J Burn Care Rehabil* 2001:53S–58S.

Garner W. Thermal burns. In: Achauer B (ed.), *Plastic Surgery Indications, Operations, and Outcomes*, vol. 1. St. Louis, MO: Mosby, 2000, 357–374.

Maylon J, Wellford W, Pruitt B. Circulatory changes following circumferential extremity burns evaluated by the ultrasonic flowmeter: an analysis of 60 thermally injured limbs. *J Trauma* 1971;11:763–770.

Mlcak R, Buffalo M. Pre-hospital management, transportation, and emergency care. In: Herndon D (ed.), *Total Burn Care*, 2nd ed. London: W.B. Saunders, 2002, 67–77.

Saffle J, Zeluff G, Warden G. Intramuscular pressure in the burned arm: measurement and response to escharotomy. *Am J Surg* 1980;140:825–831.

14. **(A)** The metabolic and circulatory changes that occur in the major burn patient can directly effect the distribution and effects of different pharmacologic agents. CO is initially diminished and there is decreased blood flow to the liver and kidneys because of the fluid and protein loss from the intravascular space. This intravascular redistribution will diminish metabolism and elimination of drugs through these organs. After 24–48 h, the patient has an increased CO and becomes hypermetabolic. This hypermetabolism increases the

blood flow to the kidneys and liver thereby, increasing drug distribution to the organs and metabolism and elimination. Drug clearance is impacted by the hepatic metabolism, renal excretion, and availability of binding proteins.

Muscle relaxants must be carefully assessed when used in burned patients. Succinylcholine, a commonly used muscle relaxant, when given to the burned patient, may cause hyperkalemia and even, death. Succinylcholine normally acts on the acetylcholine receptors at the neuromuscular junction. After burn injury, however, there is an increase in the number of acetylcholine receptors on the muscle cell membrane. When these receptors are depolarized by attachment of succinylcholine, a large amount of intracellular potassium is released, producing a dangerous hyperkalemia in the serum that may lead to cardiac arrythmia and even death. Burn patients also develop resistance to nondepolarizing muscle relaxants and therefore, require a higher dose to achieve effect.

Inhaled anesthetics are often necessary during operative burn procedures. Dose-dependent cardiovascular and peripheral vascular changes can occur that do not follow the usual dose relationships because of cardiotonic and vasoactive substances released by the burn injury. These include peripheral vasodilatation, decreased CO, and decreased mean arterial pressure. Nitrous oxide has the least cardiovascular effects. Ketamine is a useful intravenous agent because it has analgesic and dissociative amnestic properties with less respiratory depression than opiods and less cardiac effect than other agents. Opiods are good options for analgesia but burn patients will frequently develop tolerance to these agents and will require increasing dosages to obtain effect.

Bibliography

MacLennan N, Heimbach D, Cullen B. Anesthesia for the major thermal injury. *Anesthesiology* 1998;89:749–770.

Schaner P, Brown R, Kirksey T, Gunther R, Ritchey C, Gronert G. Succinylcholine-induced hyperkalemia in burned patients. *Anesth Analg* 1969;48:764–470.

Woodson L, Sherwood E, Morvant E, Peterson L. Anesthesia for burned patients. In: Herndon D (ed.), *Total Burn Care*, 2nd ed. London: W.B. Saunders, 2002, 183–206.

15. **(C)** The primary consideration for preparing the burn patient for an anesthetic is proper maintenance of the patient's airway. ET tubes, especially in patients with facial burns are difficult to secure. Adhesive tape does not adhere and umbilical tape can be unreliable. ET tube holders that secure the tube to an intraoral device

can make it difficult to treat facial burns topically or surgically. In patients with deciduous dentition, circummandibular wires or circum-alveolar wires through the pyriform aperture of the nose are useful. In patients with permanent dentition, wiring the ET tube to a tooth with at least two roots is an excellent method of maintenance. Proper positioning below the chords and above the carina must be confirmed prior to final wiring of the tube since displacement may be catastrophic.

Adequate intravenous access is essential for any burn procedure but more particularly for tangential excision and grafting since patients may lose from 25 to 250 cc of blood per body surface area (BSA) excised and grafted. The smaller grafting procedures can be performed with only peripheral access; however, larger procedures require large bore intravenous lines for rapid infusion of blood and fluids. Central lines are helpful for patient monitoring and the rapid infusion of fluid. Arterial catheters enable continuous monitoring of the patients blood pressure. Massive blood loss during these procedures can drop the patient's blood pressure precipitously.

Debridement and grafting procedures for the burned patient may require a large volume of blood transfused. Preoperatively, the size of the burned areas to be excised and whether the burn wound is infected help to determine the amount of blood to be available for surgery. Platelets and fresh frozen plasma may be necessary dependent on the patient's preoperative condition and the anticipated blood loss. Serial monitoring of the patient's hemoglobin, chemistries and coagulation profile is frequently necessary. Massive transfusions greater than 10 units of packed red cells can cause coagulopathies because of the depletion of clotting factors or thrombocytopenia. Citrate, used as an anticoagulant in blood storage, binds with calcium to prevent activation of the coagulation cascade. This may result in a drop in ionized calcium, which in turn, may result in cardiac abnormalities and hypotension. Frequent checks of these levels are important.

Thermoregulation of the burn patient in the operating room is very difficult. Evaporative losses, blood losses, the infusion of cool solutions or blood products and large body surface areas exposed will cause a rapid fall in the patient's body temperature. Every effort should be made to warm all solutions, warm the ambient room temperature, and use warming blankets and overhead heaters whenever possible. Cardiac dysfunction and coagulopathy can greatly complicate an already hazardous operation if the patient becomes hypothermic. Because of a child's large body surface area to volume ratio and

somewhat immature homeostatic mechanisms, small children are particularly vulnerable to hypothermia both in the operating room and in the burn unit.

Bibliography

Benjamin D, Herndon D. Special considerations of age: the pediatric patient. In: Herndon D (ed.), *Total Burn Care*, 2nd ed. London: W.B. Saunders, 2002, 427–438.

Lippman M, Myhre B. Hazards of massive transfusion. *J Am Assoc Nurse Anesth* 1975;43:269–277.

Woodson L, Sherwood E, Monvant E, Peterson L. Anesthesia for burned patients. In: Herndon D (ed.), *Total Burn Care*, 2nd ed. London: W.B. Saunders, 2002, 183–206.

16. **(D)** Accurate nutritional assessment of the burn patient is essential. The burn wound creates an acute stress state with marked catabolism and protein utilization. Inadequate nutritional support can lead to sepsis, immune dysfunction, and poor wound healing. Repeated assessments are imperative for patient survival.

There are several methods available for nutritional monitoring. Body weight is an important parameter to be measured in the burn patient and should be assessed in the ER and on arrival to the burn unit. Due to large fluctuations in body water from resuscitation, sepsis or decreased visceral protein synthesis, however, it is often an inaccurate measure of nutrition. Indirect calorimetry is the best available means to measure energy expenditure. Indirect calorimetry measures whole-body oxygen consumption and carbon dioxide production while the patient is at rest. The produced values are entered into the Weir equation and a resting energy expenditure (REE) is calculated. This value is then multiplied by a stress factor. A respiratory quotient (RQ) can be calculated using indirect calorimetry. An RQ less than 0.8 is consistent with fat and protein oxidation; therefore, underfeeding. A value of 0.8–0.95 suggests an appropriate mix of fat, protein, and carbohydrate oxidation. A RQ of greater than 1.0 is suggestive of overfeeding and a need to decrease caloric consumption; however, indirect calorimetry is operator and equipment dependent and the values maybe inaccurate because of mechanical dysfunction, operator error, or improper calibration.

Visceral proteins can be measured in the burned patient. Serum albumin, which has a half-life of 3 weeks, falls sharply after burn injury. Serum albumin levels can be falsely elevated by infusions of albumin and are not an accurate measure of nutritional status. Prealbumin has a short half-life of 2–3 days and is not affected by the infusion of albumin. Trends should be followed with a goal to achieve a normal prealbumin of 12 or greater. This is not a perfectly accurate measure, however, since large volume resuscitation and frequent operative procedures can lower these levels.

Nitrogen balance can be assessed by measuring 24-h urinary urea nitrogen thus estimating protein losses from burn wounds. It is not, however, a perfectly accurate yard stick for protein catabolism since there is also a significant protein exudation from the wound surface making total protein stores difficult to assess. Serum transferrin and retinol-binding protein are also markers of protein synthesis and are somewhat useful in trending nutritional status but are relatively nonspecific.

Bibliography

Curreri P. Assessing nutritional needs for the burned patient. *J Trauma* 1990;30:S20–S23.

Manelli J, Badett C, Botti G, Goldstein M, Bernini V, Bernard D. A reference standard for plasma proteins is required for nutritional assessment of adult burn patients. *Burns* 1998;24:337–345.

Saffle J, Hildreth M. Metabolic support of the burned patient. In: Herndon D (ed.), *Total Burn Care*, 2nd ed. London: W.B. Saunders, 2002, 271–287.

Saffle J, Medina E, Raymond J, Westenskow D, Kravitz M, Warden G. Use of indirect calorimetry in the nutritional management of burned patients. *J Trauma* 1985;25:32–39.

17. **(C)** Postburn hypermetabolism is not completely understood. There are a multitude of factors that may increase the metabolism of the burn patient. It is noted that burn patients have an elevated core and skin temperature. The "resetting" of their homeostatic thermostat causes the patient's metabolic rate to increase. The burn patient with a large body surface area injury has enormous fluid losses from evaporation that require energy of 0.6 cal/cc of water. In patients with large TBSA burns, this can require greater than 2000 cal per day. The use of dressings occlusive and otherwise on the burn wounds and increasing the ambient temperature of the patient rooms can prevent shivering which also uses a large amount of calories and mitigate fluid loss ameliorating these causes of hypermetabolism.

Hormonal changes influence burn hypermetabolism. Increased levels of circulating catecholamines, such as epinephrine, cortisol, and glucagons result in alterations in the metabolism of carbohydrates, lipids, and proteins. Although carbohydrate metabolism is increased significantly, glucose intolerance is commonly seen in burned patients probably because of increased circulating cortisol and glucagon. Serum insulin levels are increased with burn injury but not to the extent of gluconeogenesis. The endogenous carbohydrate stores are depleted so rapidly, that amino acids are released from muscle tissue for gluconeogenesis. In addition to muscle protein catabolism, proteolysis has been documented.

Lipid metabolism is also affected by the burn injury. There is an increase in lipolysis, which results in elevated serum free fatty acids. Free fatty acids are precursors for cytokines such as prostaglandins and thromboxanes. These cytokines influence immunosuppression and inflammation.

Endotoxin and infection are further factors that contribute to burn hypermetabolism. The excision of necrotic tissue and the treatment of infection may decrease hypermetabolism by removing a source of bacteria and their toxins as well as decreasing release of catabolic enzymes from neutrophils in the burn wound. Coverage of the burn wound with allograft that engrafts will improve the metabolic status of the patient diminishing the hypermetabolic state. Attaining complete healing of the burn wound, however, whether by grafting or reepithelialization, dramatically reduces hypermetabolism, catabolism, and allows for protein synthesis, although patients may remain relatively hypermetabolic for prolonged periods after healing.

Pharmacologic manipulations attempting to decrease the hypermetabolic and catabolic states have used β-blockade agents such as propranolol to lessen the effects of circulatory catecholamines on carbohydrate metabolism. Strict glucose control with insulin in diabetic patients may decrease protein catabolism and reduce rates of infection in ICU patients. Anabolic steroids such as oxandrolone may hasten protein synthesis and mitigate to some degree, the hypermetabolic state.

Bibliography

Baxter C. Metabolism and nutrition in burned patients. *Compr Ther* 1987;13:36–42.

Mayes T. Enteral nutrition for the burned patient. *Nutr Clin Pract* 1997;12:S43–S45.

Saffle J. What's new in general surgery: burns and metabolism. *J Am Coll Surg* 2003;196:267–285.

Spies M, Muller M, Herndon D. In: Herndon D (ed.), *Total Burn Care*, 2nd ed. London: W.B. Saunders, 2002, 363–381.

Van den Berghe G, Wouters P, Weekers F, et al. Intensive insulin therapy in critically ill patients. *N Engl J Med* 2001;345:1359–1367.

Waymack J, Herndon D. Nutritional support of the burned patient. *World J Surg* 1992;16:80–86.

Yu Y, Tompkins R, Ryan C, Young V. The metabolic basis of the increase in energy expenditure in severely burned patients. *J Parenter Enteral Nutr* 1999;23:160–168.

18. **(D)** There are many different formulas for nutritional repletion of the burned patient. The two most common are the Harris-Benedict formula and the

Curreri formula. The Harris-Benedict establishes the basal energy expenditure (BEE) of the patient and it is adjusted for stress by a factor of 1.2–2.0.

Harris-Benedict formula:

Men:

$$BEE = 66.5 + (13.8)(\text{weight in kg})$$
$$+ (5)(\text{height in cm}) - (6.76)(\text{age})$$

Women:

$$BEE = 65.5 + (9.6)(\text{weight in kg})$$
$$+ (1.85)(\text{height in cm}) - (4.68)(\text{age})$$

adjusted 1.2–2.0 for stress

This formula may be inaccurate because of the arbitrary stress factor. The Curreri formula uses weight and TBSA burned to calculate calories.

Curreri formula:

$$25(\text{weight in kg}) + (40)(\text{total body surface area burned})$$

This formula has a modification for elderly patients and a Curreri junior formula for pediatric patients; however, this formula tends to overestimate calories in small children and in adults with large body surface area burns.

The Galveston Revised formula uses the TBSA of the child and the body surface area burned to calculate the patient's nutritional needs.

Galveston Revised formula:

$$1800 \text{ kcal/m}^2 + 1300 \text{ kcal/m}^2 \text{ burn}$$

This formula is designed to provide adequate calories for wound healing and to help insure any growth changes the child may have are transient.

Carbohydrates are the principle source of non-protein calories based on calculated requirements and frequent nutritional monitoring. Lipids should be given in relatively small amounts. The composition of these lipids should include omega-3 free fatty acids, which are thought to improve immune response. Protein requirements are generally 1.5–2.0 g/kg per day in adults and up to 3.0 g/kg per day in children.

Large body surface area burn patients and patients who cannot eat should have a feeding tube placed to aid in nutritional support. Enteral feeds should always be used over parenteral feeding and should be initiated within 24 h postburn to decrease the incidence of gastric ileus; however, if gastric ileus does occur, placing the feeding tubes past the pylorus ensures that feeds are well tolerated and the risk of aspiration is decreased. Enteral feeds allow

the gut mucosa to remain intact, which may decrease gut-related sepsis. Parenteral nutrition is associated with elevated serum insulin levels, hypernatremia, hyperosmolarity, and line-related complications. Parenteral nutrition has been noted to have an adverse affect on immune function with an increase in TNF secretion. Therefore, if the gut can be used, enteral nutrition is the route of choice for burned patients.

Bibliography

Benjamin D, Herndon D. Special considerations of age: the pediatric burned patient. In: Herndon D (ed.), *Total Burn Care*, 2nd ed. London: W.B. Saunders, 2002, 427–438.

Khorram-Sefat R, Behrendt W, Heiden A, Hettich R. Long-term measurements of energy expenditure in severe burn injury. *World J Surg* 1999;23:115–122.

Mayes T, Gottschlich M, Khoury J, Warden G. Evaluation of predicted and measured requirements in burned children. *J Am Dietetic Assoc* 1996;96:24–29.

Raff T, Hartman B, Germann G. Early intragastric feeding of seriously burned and long-term ventilated patients: a review of 55 patients. *Burns* 1997;23:19–25.

Saffle J, Hildreth M. Metabolic support of the burned patient. In: Herndon D (ed.), *Total Burn Care*, 2nd ed. London: W.B. Saunders, 2002, 271–287.

Waymack J, Herndon D. Nutritional support of the burned patient. *World J Surg* 1992;16:80–86.

19. **(C)** The burn injury effects not only metabolism but also may cause alterations in several micronutrients that enhance wound healing or immunity. Some of the micronutrients that are regularly replaced are listed below.

- Vitamin A aids in wound healing and helps maintain epithelial integrity. Vitamin A functions as an antioxidant and has a positive effect on immune function.
- Vitamin C or ascorbic acid is an antioxidant and aids in the antibacterial function of the white blood cells (WBCs). Vitamin C is involved in the hydroxylation of proline and lysine, which is necessary for collagen synthesis. It is essential for wound healing and allows for tensile strength in wounds.
- Vitamin E serves as an antioxidant and aids in immune function. Vitamin E inhibits thromboxane and prostaglandin synthesis and stimulates fibroblasts.
- Zinc has an important role in wound healing. DNA and RNA replication, protein synthesis, and collagen formation are all influenced by zinc. Zinc is also important for immune function because it has a positive effect on lymphocyte function and cellular and humoral immunity.
- Selenium protects membrane lipids from free radical damage and is important in the function of lymphocytes.

- Iron is necessary for oxygen transport in the blood (hemoglobin) or muscles (myoglobin). Iron is a cofactor in many enzyme systems and is necessary for cell replication and DNA synthesis.

There are many other nutrients that are affected by the burn injury; however, these are the most commonly supplemented.

Bibliography

Gamliel Z, DeBiasse M, Demling R. Essential microminerals and their response to burn injury. *J Burn Care Rehabil* 1996;17:264–272.

Jeschke M. The hepatic response to a thermal injury. In: Herndon D (ed.), *Total Burn Care*, 2nd ed. London: W.B. Saunders, 2002, 288–299.

Mancoll J, Phillips J. Delayed wound healing. In: Eriksson E (ed.), *Plastic Surgery Indications, Operations, and Outcomes*, vol. 1. St. Louis, MO: Mosby, 2000, 65–78.

Saffle J, Hildreth M. Metabolic support of the burned patient. In: Herndon D (ed.), *Total Burn Care*, 2nd ed. London: W.B. Saunders, 2002, 271–287.

20. (D) Burn injuries greater than 15% TBSA can have a profound effect on red blood cell (RBC) production and the coagulation cascade of the burn patient. These major burn patients develop an anemia, which usually persists until their wounds are closed. There are various reasons for this loss. The burn patient can lose as much as 18% of his/her red cells in the first 24 h after a major burn injury. The RBC morphology may be changed and the cell membrane can become fragile making destruction easier. The patients undergo frequent blood draws and multiple surgical excisions and grafting, which further contribute to anemia. The burn patient has a decrease in the bone marrow production of red cells. There is an increase in circulating erythropoietin in these patients but the progenitor cells within the bone marrow do not respond appropriately. Therefore, red cell production is not increased to compensate for losses. Burn patients also have a decreased serum iron levels and total iron binding capacity which may further decrease erythropoiesis.

Platelets initially are consumed in large amounts because of microthrombi formation in the burn wounds. The platelets may be further decreased because of the large volume of fluid resuscitation; however, this thrombocytopenia is usually limited to the first week and will return to normal or supernormal levels during the ensuing weeks.

Coagulation protein levels are decreased during the first week following burn injury. This may be dilutional and partially because of the extravasation of plasma proteins to the interstitium. These levels return to normal in approximately 1 week.

WBCs are also affected by the burn injury. Initially, there is a period of leukocytosis that is because of acute volume loss and the release of white cells from the bone marrow. Leukopenia then follows because of massive resuscitation and leukocyte accumulation in the burn wound. Leukopenia may also be a drug-induced response to the application of SSD. The exact cause of this reaction is not understood and is usually self-limiting, lasting only several days.

Careful consideration of these hematologic changes is essential especially in preparation for operative procedures during the first postburn week.

Bibliography

Gabilonlo J. Coagulation and platelet changes after thermal injury in man. *Burns* 1981;7:370–377.

Deitch E, Sittig K. A serial study of the erythropoietic response to thermal injury. *Ann Surg* 1993;217:293–299.

Lawrence C, Atac B. Hematologic changes in massive burn injury. *Crit Care Med* 1992;20:1284–1288.

Shankar R, Amin C, Gamelli R. Hematologic, hematopoietic, and acute phase response. In: Herndon D (ed.), *Total Burn Care*, 2nd ed. London: W.B. Saunders, 2002, 331–346.

21. (C) Infection is the leading cause of morbidity and mortality in burn patients. In the immune compromised burn patient, host defenses can be quickly overcome, leading to sepsis and even death. Awareness of the potential sources of infection in the burn patient leads to prompt treatment and prevention of complications. A partial list of possible infectious sources is listed.

- *Wound infection.* The burn wound is always a potential source of systemic infection until complete healing is accomplished. Frequent clinical inspection of the wound itself and correlation with the clinical picture and quantitative tissue biopsy of suspicious lesions are necessary to alert the clinician to deterioration. Early excision of the burn wound and grafting with allograft or autograft can avert invasive wound infection. Full thickness burns should be excised to fascia unless they are very small since exposed fat is unlikely to granulate and serves as an excellent nutrient source for the numerous bacteria colonizing the burn wounds. All burns that have not yet been grafted or that have not healed primarily are heavily colonized with bacteria that reflect the ambient environment. Differentiation between colonization of the wound and invasive wound infection can usually be made clinically but quantitative cultures may also be useful. More than 100,000 bacteria/g of burned tissue constitute invasive infection. Burn wound sepsis must be treated with surgical excision not simply antibiotics.

- *Pneumonia.* Pneumonia is one of the most common infectious complications in the burn patient. These infections usually start as infections of the tracheobronchial tree and spread to the distal lung periphery. Factors that increase the patient's susceptibility to pneumonia are aspiration, inhalation injury, burn size, and the presence of an endo or nasal tracheal tube. Patients who have persistent fever without a known source should have a chest x-ray and sputum culture performed. A sputum culture with greater than 25 neutrophils and less than 10 epithelial cells is considered to be free of oral pharyngeal contamination.

- *Urosepsis.* Urinary tract infections (UTIs) are common sources of infection in the burn population because of the necessity of in-dwelling catheters to monitor systemic perfusion. Meticulous insertion and daily care of urinary catheters and removal as early as possible may decrease the incidence of urosepsis. The pathogenic organisms are frequently those seen in the burns.

- *Bacteremia.* Burn patients with significant body surface area involvement often require central venous access or intraarterial lines for monitoring. These catheters are frequent sources of infection because of their proximity to the burn wound, their "seeding" because of the necessity of frequent operative procedures such as burn wound debridements. These catheters should be meticulously placed and cared for and changed on a regular basis with the insertion site rotated routinely. Showers of bacteria from manipulation of these lines can cause rapid clinical deterioration and a picture of acute sepsis. Bacteremia can occur from any infected site including the wound. In patients with long hospitalizations or severe injury, endocarditis or valvulitis must be considered if a picture of recurrent bacteremia presents. Septic thrombophlebitis must also be considered and present and past intravenous sites carefully examined for the presence of pus.

- *Sinusitis.* Sinusitis is an often overlooked cause of infection in the burn patient. Obstruction of the drainage of the paranasal sinuses because of long-term nasal intubation with tracheal or gastric tubes causes overgrowth of bacteria and invasive infection. Because the patient is sedated, clinical signs and symptoms may be difficult to elicit. Patients with sinusitis may have purulent nasal drainage but the absence of this drainage does not preclude the infection. If suspected, x-rays or sinus CT scans are usually diagnostic. Surgical drainage may be necessary to obtain an accurate culture to guide antibiotic therapy. Removal of all nasal tubes, appropriate antibiotics instituted, and the use of nasal decongestants may be helpful.

- *Cholecystitis.* Cholecystitis, frequently acalculus, is a complication of critical illness, trauma, or major surgery. There are two proposed mechanisms. Ischemia of the gall bladder secondary to shock, sepsis, hypotension and systemic inflammatory mediators and biliary stasis resulting from opiod use, dysmotility, and volume depletion. Fever, abdominal pain and tenderness, leukocytosis, and elevated liver function tests (LFTs) are usual but since these signs and symptoms are relatively nonspecific and because many patients are heavily sedated and difficult to examine, a high index of suspicion should lead to the liberal use of abdominal ultrasound. Distended or thickened gall bladder wall, the presence of "sludge" or stones themselves or fluid around the gall bladder are all indicative of cholecystitis which will usually require cholecystectomy to prevent necrosis, perforation, or other intraabdominal catastrophe. Obviously, any other intraabdominal event such as appendicitis or diverticulitis may occur in the burn patient but these are considerably less frequent.

- *Antibiotic-associated colitis.* AAC may be caused by any antibiotic regardless of route of administration or length of therapy. The antibiotics alter the normal colonic flora and allowing the overgrowth of *Clostridium difficile* bacterium. The resulting diarrhea is profuse, watery, and foul smelling; diagnosis of the stool should be sent for leukocytes and *C. difficile* toxin. Complications include toxic megacolon and perforation. Although diarrhea is common in burn patients for many reasons, a high index of suspicion is necessary for AAC. Treatment includes antidiarrheals as appropriate as well as specific antibiotic therapy usually with oral metronidazole and vancomycin.

Bibliography

Fischer J, Nussbaum M, Chance W, Luchette F. Manifestations of gastrointestinal disease. In: Schwartz S (ed.), *Principles of Surgery*, 7th ed. New York, NY: McGraw Hill, 1999, 1075–1076.

Heggars J, Hawkins H, Edgar P, Villarreal C, Herndon D. Treatment of infection in burns. In: Herndon D (ed.), *Total Burn Care*, 2nd ed. London: W.B. Saunders, 2002, 120–169.

Pruitt B, McManus A. Opportunistic infections in severely burned patients. *Am J Med* 1984;76:146–154.

Schwartz S. Gallbladder and extrahepatic biliary system. In: Schwartz S (ed.), *Principles of Surgery*, 7th ed. New York, NY: McGraw Hill, 1999, 1437–1466.

22. (A) Thermal injury has a dramatic effect of decreasing the patient's CO during the first 8–12 h postburn, followed by a hyperdynamic state if therapy is adequate. The cause of the decrease in CO is multifactorial including decreased venous return secondary to the capillary leak and fluid sequestration in the extracellular space, an increase in systemic vascular resistance, and decreased left ventricular distensibility as demonstrated on echocardiogram. This diastolic dysfunction decreases the amount of blood pumped out with each heartbeat. There is considerable evidence suggesting a systemic increase in cytokines such as TNF-α and necrosis factor-kappa-β, serve as direct myocardial depressants that decrease contractility despite adequate intravascular volume replacement. A myocardial depressant factor has been described but not identified, although recent studies have shown that transient endotoxemia may play a role in myocardial dysfunction.

The systemic hormonal cascade triggered by trauma is dramatically present in any significant burn injury. Epinephrine is released immediately and gradually decreases. Norepinephrine peaks on day 2 and gradually decreases. Angiotensin II hormone is gradually elevated until it peaks on day 3. Vasopressin acts to increase vascular smooth muscle tone, increase systemic vascular resistance, and activating parasympathetic pathways of the heart. Vasopressin is immediately elevated and gradually diminishes over subsequent days. Atrial natriuretic peptide is initially decreased and begins to elevate by day 2. This was reported to be associated with an increased stroke volume, CO, and a decreased systemic vascular resistance.

Bibliography

Crum R, Dominic W, Hansbrough J, Shackford S, Brown M. Cardiovascular and neurohumoral responses following burn injury. *Arch Surg* 1990;125:1065–1069.

Hilton J, Marullo D. Effects of thermal trauma on cardiac force of contraction. *Burns* 1986;12:167–171.

Horton J, Baxter C, White D. Differences in cardiac responses to resuscitation from burn shock. *Surg Gynecol Obstet* 1989;168:201–213.

Jones S, de Silva K, Shankar R, Gamelli R. Significance of the adrenal and sympathetic response to burn injury. In: Herndon D (ed.), *Total Burn Care*, 2nd ed. London: W.B. Saunders, 2002, 347–362.

Kuwagata Y, Sugimoto H, Yoshioka T, et al. Left ventricular performance in patients with thermal injury or multiple trauma: a clinical study with echocardiography. *J Trauma* 1992;32:158–165.

Saffle J. What's new in general surgery: burns and metabolism. *J Am Coll Surg* 2003;196:267–285.

23. (C) Cadaver allograft (homograft) is an extremely useful method of temporary wound coverage for deep partial or full thickness burn wounds providing many of the benefits of autogenous skin for a period of time during which the patient's systemic conditions can be stabilized and the wound prepared for autografting. Since cadaver allograft will be engrafted and revascularized for short periods of time in the immunocompromised patient, allograft can replace the skin's important homeostatic mechanisms including fluid and electrolyte control, thermoregulation, reduction of energy expenditure, and protection from external insults such as bacteria, chemicals. If the allograft temporarily engrafts, it is likely that the wound will accept autograft and if limited donor sites are available, the allograft may be reapplied to allow donor sites to reepithelialize for reharvesting. Cadaver allograft can be used either fresh or frozen and engrafts better if used fresh although this is rarely possible.

Human cadaver skin that is slowly cooled increases cellular dehydration because of elevated extracellular electrolyte concentrations. Allograft that is rapidly cooled develops intracellular ice crystal formation that disturbs the cells. Cadaver allograft that is bathed in a cryoprotectant solution prior to placement into a controlled rate freezer offers the best possibility of skin viability. May and DeClements (1981) have shown that cryopreserved allograft stored in liquid nitrogen maintains 73.4% of the original viability. May and Wainwright have demonstrated that skin stored for 1 week at 4°C nutrient media retains near normal structure and can be rapidly revascularized. Skin stored at 4°C for 2–3 weeks in nutrient media demonstrates significant loss of vascular tracts, loss of intracellular cohesiveness, and significant cell death making the allograft less useful.

Donor human cadaver skin is not type and cross-matched or human leukocyte antigen (HLA) typed. Donor individuals are screened for medical, social, and sexual history, physical examination, autopsy findings, and laboratory findings. The donor is examined for risk of sexual disease, i.e., herpes, syphilis, condyloma, puncture marks such as needle tracts, tatoos, lymphadenopathy, oral thrush, Kaposi's sarcoma, hepatomegaly, and jaundice which exclude the use of cadaver allograft since it may serve as a vehicle for transmission of viruses or other infective agents that may survive preservation.

The present protocol for serologic testing of cadaver allograft includes the following:

- human immunodeficiency virus, type I and II (anti-HIV-1 and anti-HIV-2)

- hepatitis B surface antigen (HB_sA_g)
- antibodies to the hepatitis C virus (anti-HCV)
- antibodies to lumen T-lymphotropic virus type I and II (anti-HTLV-I and anti-HTLV-II)
- syphilis

Bibliography

Baxter C, Aggarwal S, Diller K. Cryopreservation of skin: a review. *Transplant Proc* 1985;17:112–119.

Fielding G, Pegg S. Homograft skin banking—current practices and future trends. *Aust N Z J Surg* 1988;58:153–156.

Konstantinow A, Muhlbauer W, Hartinger A, von Donnersmarck G. Skin banking: a simple method for cryopreservation of split-thickness skin and cultured human epidermal keratinocytes. *Ann Plastic Surg* 1991;26:89–96.

May SR, DeClement FA. Skin banking. Part III. Cadaveric allograft skin viability. *J Burn Care Rehabil* 1981;2:128–139.

May SR, Wainwright J. Integrated study of the structural and metabolic degeneration of skin during 4°C storage in nutrient medium. *Cryobiology* 1985;22:18–34.

McCauley R. The skin bank. In: Herndon D (ed.), *Total Burn Care*, 2nd ed. London: W.B. Saunders, 2002, 207–211.

Wall J, Kasprisin D (eds.), *American Association of Tissue Banks Standards for Tissue Banking*. Arlington, VA, 2001, 31–42.

Yang H, Jia X, Acker J, Lung G, McGann L. Routine assessment of viability in split-thickness skin. *J Burn Care Rehabil* 2000;21:99–104.

24. **(B)** Topical antimicrobials have been used as the first line burn wound treatment for many years. The advent of SSD has been one of the revolutionary advances in burn care but many other agents are useful and clear knowledge of their antibacterial spectrum and other characteristics is critical to appropriate care of the burn wound (Table 11-2).

    - SSD is at present the most frequently used topical agent in burn care. SSD is a broad-spectrum bactericidal agent that has action against both gram positive and negative bacteria, and to some degree, yeast. SSD is relatively painless to apply but has poor eschar penetration. Used twice a day, it is an effective topical therapy. Side effects include transient leukopenia, argyria that is a slate-gray or bluish discoloration of the skin or deeper tissues, interstitial nephritis, and rarely, methemoglobinemia.

    - Silver nitrate solution (0.25–0.5%) is a bacteriostatic solution with both gram-positive and gram-negative spectrum. Silver nitrate has poor eschar penetration and is painless to apply. This solution leaches sodium and chloride from the wound and must be kept continuously wet to avoid precipitation in the wound and mechanical interference with wound healing by epithelialization. Side effects include hyponatremia, hypochloremia, argyria, and methemoglobinemia. Silver nitrate solution is extremely labor intensive to use because of the need for frequent reapplication and its characteristic staining of the bed linens, floors and dressings a dark brown to black color. It is thus not a popular choice in most burn centers today although it was standard in the past.

    - Mafenide acetate (sulfamylon cream and 5% solution) is a broad-spectrum bacteriostatic topical antimicrobial with excellent eschar penetration. Sulfamylon is painful to apply especially in the cream form but is better tolerated by patients in solution or slurry. Side effects include being a potent cationic anhydrase inhibitor, especially when applied over a large surface area. This results in a hyperchloremic metabolic acidosis that may result in hyperventilation and respiratory alkalosis. Cutaneous hypersensitivity and pain on application are other known side effects.

TABLE 11-2   Commonly Used Topical Agents

	Bactericidal	Bacteriostatic	Pain	Gram + /Gram−	Eschar Penetration
SSD	+		−	g+/g−	Poor
Silver nitrate		+	−*	g+/g−	Poor
Sulfamylon		+	++	g+/g−	Excellent
Bacitracin		+	−	g+/g−	Poor
Bactroban (Mupirocin)	+		−	g+	Poor
Furacin	+		−	some g+/ Mostly g−	Poor
Betadine	+		−	g+/g−	Poor

* If kept moist

Adapted from: Heggars J, Hawkins H, Edgar P, Villareal C, Herndon D. In: Herndon D (ed.), *Total Burn Care*, 2nd ed. London: W.B. Saunders; 2002:109–119.

- Acticoat is a silver impregnated into a flexible sheet that is applied topically to the burn wound. Acticort uses body fluid and water to activate the bacteriostatic silver ions. The dressing theoretically is left in place up to 72 h making nursing care simpler and decreases pain for the patient. Side effects—no significant toxicity has been reported with this product.
- Bacitracin ointment is a broad-spectrum bacterial topical antimicrobial that is an adequate prophylactic agent but should not be used for controlling wound infections. Bacitracin is nontoxic to skin grafts and does not impede epithelialization of the wound as much as other topical antibacterial agents. Side effects include contact dermatitis that is very common with protracted use, nephrotoxicity, and ototoxicity when applied to large surface areas.
- Mupirocin (Bactroban cream—ointment) is a bactericidal topical antimicrobial useful against gram-positive organisms. Side effects include inhibition of wound healing.
- Nitrofurantoin (Furacin) is a bacteriocidal topical ointment that is effective against gram-negative organisms and some gram-positive organisms. Side effects include possible severe contact dermatitis and nephrotoxicity.
- Povidone iodine (Betadine) is a broad-spectrum bactericidal and fungicidal topical antimicrobial that is not efficacious against *Pseudomonas*. Side effects include renal dysfunction, thyroid dysfunction that is rare, and inactivation by the wound exudate.

Bibliography

Barret J, Herndon D. Wound care. In: Barret J, Herndon D (eds.), *Color Atlas of Burn Care*. London: W.B. Saunders, 2001, 5.25–5.38.

Carroughers G. Burn wound assessment and topical treatment. *Burn Care and Therapy*. St. Louis, MO: Mosby, 1998, 145–147.

Heggars J, Hawkins H, Edgar P, Villarreal C, Herndon D. In: Herndon D (ed.), *Total Burn Care*, 2nd ed. London: W.B. Saunders, 2002, 120–169.

Monafo W, Bessey P. Wound care. In: Herndon D (ed.), *Total Burn Care*, 2nd ed. London: W.B. Saunders, 2002, 109–119.

Trofino R. Basics of burn care. *Nursing Care of the Burn-Injured Patient*. Philadelphia, PA: FA Davis, 1991, 44–50.

25. (A) Electrical burns are devastating injuries that are frequently associated with additional trauma. The pathophysiology of electrical burns is related to the resistance of the contact point, the amperage involved, the time of contact, and the type of current. Electricity is converted into heat within the body. Joule's law is described as

$$P(\text{power} = \text{heat}) = I^2(\text{amperage})R(\text{resistance})$$

The areas of greatest resistance are the skin and bone; however, once the electricity overcomes the resistance of the skin, the body acts as a volume conductor of heat. The tissue destruction is highest when the current enters an area with a small cross-sectional diameter and tends to be dissipated when a larger surface is crossed. Maximal tissue destruction occurs in the areas adjacent to the contact spots and is decreased as distance from these points increases. Often, the electrical burn patient will have normal appearing skin with muscular tissue destruction beneath.

The acute care of the electrical burn patient requires an initial assessment of his/her cardiac status. Cardiac arrhythmia, in particular ventricular fibrillation, is the most common cause of death at the scene and occurs soon after the burn injury. An electrocardiogram (ECG) should be obtained in the emergency department because myocardial injury can occur similar to myocardial contusion. Cardiac markers and serial ECGs should be obtained if myocardial injury is suspected.

Acute muscle destruction in an electrical burn causes a release of myoglobin from the damaged cells. The myoglobin is then excreted in the urine; however, these pigments can cause acute renal failure by obstructing the renal tubules. The patient's intravenous fluid should be increased to maintain an increased urine output and these solutions alkalinized to prevent precipitation of these pigments in the renal tubule. The urine output should be maintained between 75 and 100 cc/h until the myoglobin is cleared. Mannitol may be used for a rapid osmotic diuresis.

The patient with an electrical injury is at significant risk of developing compartment syndrome. The damaged or necrotic muscle swells within the overlying fascia producing dangerously elevated tissue pressures. Serial measurements of compartment pressures are essential to avoid unnecessary muscle necrosis. If compartment syndrome is suspected, then prompt fasciotomies should be performed. All four compartments in the lower leg and two in the forearm should be released. Release of the thigh and upper arm compartments may be necessary. Serial measurements of serum creatinine kinase (CK) are essential in these patients. The CKs will continue to rise for 24–48 h; however, they should decrease thereafter. Any continued elevation requires a reevaluation of the patient for further muscle necrosis.

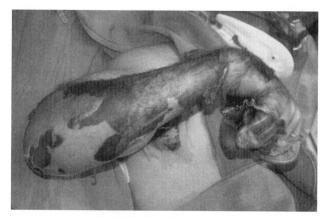

FIG. 11-10 Electrical burn to arm.

Electrical injuries are often associated with other forms of trauma. Patients with electrical injuries can sustain such strong tetanic muscle contractions that compression fractures may occur. These patients may also fall from heights or be thrown and sustain further trauma. Extensive evaluation of these patients in the emergency department is imperative (Fig. 11-10).

Bibliography

Hunt J, Mason A, Masterson T, Pruitt B. The pathophysiology of acute electrical injuries. *J Trauma* 1976;16:335–340.

McCauley R, Barret J. Electrical injuries. In: Achauer B (ed.), *Plastic Surgery Indications, Operations, and Outcomes*, vol. 1. St. Louis, MO: Mosby, 2000, 375–385.

Nichter L, Bryant C, Kenney J, Morgan R, Tribble C, Rodeheaver G, Edlich R. Injuries because of commercial electrical current. *J Burn Care Rehabil* 1984;5:124–137.

Purdue G, Hunt J. Electrical injuries. In: Herndon D (ed.), *Total Burn Care*, 2nd ed. London: W.B. Saunders, 2002, 455–460.

26. **(C)** Although chemical burns make up a small percentage of the burns treated at a burn center, prompt initial treatment is important to prevent severe tissue damage. Chemical burns vary in severity depending on the type of offending agent and its manner of reactivity, the concentration or strength of the agent, the quantity of the agent in contact with the tissue, the duration of exposure, and the amount of tissue penetration of the agent.

Like thermal burns, chemical burns cause protein denaturation that results in protein coagulation. The great majority of chemicals involved in burns are either acids or alkalis although solvents and hydrocarbons may also be occasionally involved. Acid chemicals cause a more "superficial" burn resulting in a coagulation necrosis. Alkali substances produce a liquefaction necrosis and tend to penetrate deeper into the tissues.

The initial treatment of all chemical burns begins with protection of the rescuer by avoiding contact with the offending agent. The patient's clothing should be immediately removed and copious irrigation with water begun. The water should be made to drain or flow away from the patient and thereby, diluting the concentration of the chemical and avoiding further injury by the dissolved chemical. Irrigation should continue for at least 30 min and ocular injuries should likewise be irrigated using Morgan irrigation catheters. Neutralizing agents should not be used because of the exothermic reactions these agents can produce when they come in contact with the offending agent. Hydrofluoric acid is an agent used commonly in petroleum production and glass etching and requires therapy in addition to irrigation. In addition to the coagulative necrosis caused by the low pH, the fluoride ion, once in contact with the cells, combines with the positively charged ions of calcium and magnesium acting as a metabolic poison. Until the fluoride ion is completely neutralized by calcium or magnesium, the acid will continue to penetrate deeper into the tissues and cause further protein denaturation. Local injections of calcium gluconate 10% solution with or without topical calcium gluconate gel are necessary in addition to irrigation. These treatments are used four to six times per day until the patient has relief from the significant pain that is the cardinal symptom. Because of the attendant coagulation and necrosis these wounds often require debridement and grafting as well.

Systemic toxicity may also occur with these chemical agents. Petroleum, formic acid, phenol, and nitrates cause systemic toxicity including pneumonitis, pulmonary edema, hemolysis, renal failure, and even, death. Resuscitation and wound debridement of these patients is identical to a thermal burn. An accurate identification of the offending agent is important for tailoring the appropriate therapy (Fig. 11-11).

Bibliography

Leonard L, Scheulen J, Munster A. Chemical burns: effects of prompt first aid. *J Trauma* 1982;22:420–423.

Moran KD, O'Reilly T, Munster A. Chemical burns: a ten-year experience. *Am Surg* 1987;53:652–653.

Mozingo D, Smith A, McManus W, Pruitt B, Mason A. Chemical burns. *J Trauma* 1988;28:642–647.

Sanford A, Herndon D. Chemical burns. In: Herndon D (ed.), *Total Burn Care*, 2nd ed. London: W.B. Saunders, 2002, 475–480.

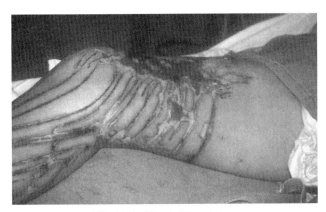

FIG. 11-11 Chemical burns to leg.

27. (D) Frostbite injury is a commonly seen injury in the burn unit in the northern states. Frostbite injury occurs because of a multitude of factors. There may be a peripheral vasoconstriction and decreased blood flow to the extremities because of a drop in core body temperature and the homeostatic response of mandatory heat for the viscera at the expense of the extremities. Impaired patient recognition of impending injury is often because of alcohol, drugs, or psychologic disorders. Other factors, such as homelessness, improper clothing, diabetes with neuropathy, and significant wind chill may predispose a patient to frostbite. After prolonged or rapid exposure to cold depending on the temperature, rapid intracellular ice formation causes cell death. At more gradual cooling rates, osmotic shifts produce cellular dehydration and eventual cell death. Further tissue ischemia occurs because of vasoconstriction of the microcirculation. After this initial vasoconstriction, the capillaries dilate for a short period of time and microemboli are formed because of the damage to the endothelium. Tissue edema leads to further vascular resistance and progression to thrombosis, ischemia, and tissue necrosis suggestive of reperfusion injury.

The severity of frostbite cannot be assessed until rewarming of the affected part is complete. In most cases, there is initial insensitivity, followed by significant pain and hyperesthesia. First degree frostbite demonstrates either erythema or pallor of the affected area but no blister formation. Second degree frostbite involves some dermal injury and the formation of "white" blisters. Third degree frostbite is a deeper injury that manifests with the formation of hemorrhagic blisters that evolve to eschar formation. Fourth degree injury involves muscle or bone.

The treatment of frostbite injury begins with rapid rewarming of the affected part with warm water and environment (40–42°C). White blisters are debrided and treated with aloe vera and hemorrhagic blisters are left intact. Extremities are elevated and aspirin or ibuprofen is administered. Antibiotics are used as necessary for the treatment of cellulitis. Other adjuncts to rewarming have been investigated including hyperbaric oxygen, intraarterial vasodilators and anticoagulants such as dextran, but none have been demonstrated conclusively to be effective. Surgical intervention is appropriate early for the treatment of infection or for wound closure of deeper injuries. Although observation is appropriate if there is no critical event indicating that surgery is necessary since areas that appear damaged may recover. Amputation of dry necrotic areas is generally performed after there is complete demarcation of the affected part (Figs. 11-12 and 11-13).

Bibliography

Morris S. Cold-induced injury: frostbite. In: Herndon D (ed.), *Total Burn Care*, 2nd ed. London: W.B. Saunders, 2002, 470–474.

Murphy J, Banwell P, Roberts A, McGrouther DA. Frostbite: pathogenesis and treatment. *J Trauma* 2000;48:171–178.

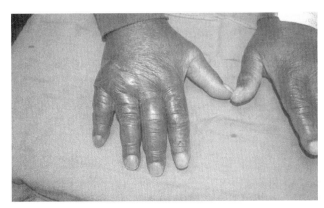

FIG. 11-12 Initial presentation of a frostbite injury.

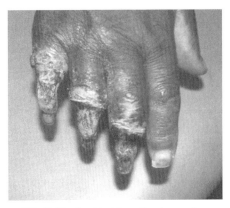

FIG. 11-13 Frostbite injury after demarcation.

Su C, Lohman R, Gottlieb L. Frostbite of the upper extremity. *Hand Clin* 2000;237–247.

28. **(C)** SJS and TENS are exfoliative skin disorders that are often treated in burn units. Stevens-Johnson syndrome generally involves an area of 10% TBSA or less. TENS affects an area of 30% or greater. The most common etiology is a rapid immune response to a foreign agent most frequently a drug (77.94%). Occasionally, SJS may be attributable to a viral or mycoplasmal infection but TENS is almost always drug related. The most common causative agents are antibiotics or anticonvulsants. The mortality of TENS can reach as high as 80% and usually occurs from sepsis.

These skin disorders are usually preceded by a prodromal phase, which includes fever and malaise. Skin tenderness and an erythematous rash follow this prodromal phase and are often suggestive of common viral infections with a viral exanthem. Next, however, large blisters develop in the erythematous area and epidermolysis follows. These blisters represent separation of the dermis and epidermis and the definitive diagnosis of these syndromes is the positive Nikolsky sign which manifests when light finger pressure causes the epidermis to desquamate in sheets. Mucosal involvement is common especially in the oropharynx, anal, and ocular mucosa. Diagnosis is confirmed by skin biopsy, which reveals a dermoepidermal separation with areas of epidermal detachment. Epidermal necrosis is seen with TENS. The pathophysiology is not clearly understood, but a hypersensitivity reaction or keratinocyte apoptosis have been postulated.

The treatment of SJS/TENS begins with the removal of the offending agent. The wounds in SJS/TENS are superficial and if treated conservatively, will heal spontaneously. The sloughed epidermis is debrided and a biologic or synthetic dressing is applied. This dressing will promote wound healing, decrease the risk of wound infection, and decrease pain and fluid losses. Topical antimicrobials may be used, such as bacitracin ointment, SSD cream, and Bactroban ointment, but special care must be taken not to use agents that contain components of the initial causative agent, e.g., sulfa in any systemic, topical or ophthalmic application. Intravenous fluids are administered to maintain adequate urine output and avoid renal failure. Nutritional support is initiated immediately to facilitate wound healing particularly when oral mucosal damage has occurred. Corticosteroids, especially with large body surface area involvement, are contraindicated and studies have shown an increased mortality with their use. Recently, studies have been published demonstrating some benefit to the administration of high-dose intravenous immunoglobulins with inhibition of skin slough and a survival rate of 88% at day 45. Further investigation of this treatment is ongoing.

Ocular involvement necessitates frequent ocular examinations by an ophthalmologist. Adhesions progressing to conjunctival scarring, keratoconjunctivitis sicca, ectropion, and symblepharon may occur. Oral mucosal involvement may extend into the esophagus causing severe dysphagia. Gastrointestinal mucosal slough may occur with massive hemorrhage. Pulmonary tree sloughing may also occur with resultant airway obstruction. Pneumonia is a frequent complication and pulmonary embolism has been reported. These patients should be in barrier isolation to decrease nosocomial infections. Sepsis is the most common cause of death in these patients although acute respiratory failure is occasionally seen when pulmonary mucosal involvement occurs.

Bibliography

Halebian P, Madden M, Finklestein J. Improved burn centre survival of patients with toxic epidermal necrolysis managed without corticosteroids. *Ann Surg* 1986;204: 503–512.

Halebian P, Shires G. Burn unit treatment of acute, severe exfoliating disorders. *Ann Rev Med* 1989;40:137–147.

Prins C, Kerdel F, Padilla S, et al. Treatment of toxic epidermal necrolysis with high-dose intravenous immunoglobulins. *Arch Dermatol* 2003;139:26–32.

Spies M, Hollyoak M, Muller M, Goodwin C, Herndon D. Exfoliative and necrotizing diseases of the skin. In: Herndon D (ed.), *Total Burn Care*, 2nd ed. London: W.B. Saunders, 2002, 492–500.

29. **(B)** A skin graft or skin autograft is the autologous transfer of dermis, epidermis, and component structures to another site on the organism after complete separation of the graft from its original site and blood supply. After transplantation occurs, the skin graft must adhere to the wound bed and become revascularized. This process is referred to as skin graft "take." There are three phases of skin graft take: plasmatic imbibition, inosculation, and revascularization.

Immediately after a skin graft is placed on a wound bed, a network of fibrin mesh is formed between the graft and the wound bed allowing for graft adherence and setting stage for the phase of graft nutrition that depends solely on diffusion. In the first 24 h, the graft imbibes plasma like a sponge passively from bed to cells in the graft both by passive osmotic gradient and cell membrane transport. During this time, the graft becomes edematous and increases 40–50% in weight. This action referred to as plasmatic imbibition, sustains the graft until revascularization occurs. The grafts are adherent but pale in appearance during this phase that persists from 12 to 36 h.

The next phase of graft take is inosculation. This term is used to describe the alignment or "kissing" of vessels from the wound bed with patent vessels remaining in the graft after harvest. There is controversy over whether the capillary buds project from the wound bed into the preexisting vessels or from new vessel formation by angiogenesis. This inosculation phase occurs from approximately 36 to 48 h and gradually replaces the phase of plasmatic imbibition as the method of nutrition.

Revascularization continues after grafting for approximately 3–7 days. Initially, all of the vessels are unidirectional into the graft. Over time, these vessels differentiate into afferent and efferent vessels and revascularization is complete. In this phase, the grafts appear pink and blanch with compression. Lymphatic flow is reestablished by postgraft day 5. Reinnervation of skin grafts depends on the graft thickness and the wound bed that the graft was placed on. The sensation to the graft is not normal; however, it does obtain some of the nervous characteristics of the adjacent skin and wound bed. The nerves grow into the skin graft from the wound base and periphery through the empty graft neurilemmal sheaths. Pain sensation returns first, followed by light touch and temperature. Reinnervation of the graft stops from 12 to 24 months. Split thickness skin grafts have a faster rate of reinnervation, though, full thickness grafts have a more complete reinnervation.

Full thickness skin grafts are grafts in which the full thickness of the skin, the epidermis, and the entire dermis, are taken. The donor site must be closed primarily, by split thickness skin grafting or by flap. Full thickness skin grafts are at greater jeopardy both because of the greater distance of diffusion in the phase of plasmatic imbibition and the slower rate of revascularization. These grafts have a greater primary contraction than do split thickness grafts. Primary contraction occurs immediately after the skin graft is harvested. This is because of the recoil of the dermal elastic fibers that are fully functional in the full thickness graft. Full thickness grafts have approximately 40% primary contraction and split thickness grafts have 10–20% primary contraction. Much of the primary contraction in full thickness grafts can be overcome by stretching the grafts to the edges of the defect. Secondary contraction occurs after the graft has been transplanted onto the wound bed. Secondary contraction occurs because of the stimulus of myofibroblasts most of which exist in the wound bed. By increasing the amount of dermal

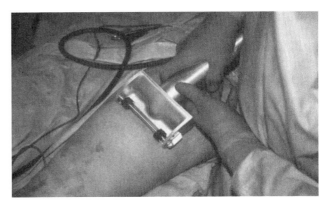

FIG. 11-14 Dermatome harvesting of a split thickness skin graft.

thickness transplanted, the myofibroblast function is suppressed and contraction is inhibited.

Full thickness skin grafts are used for areas where graft secondary contraction must be kept to a minimum, such as the face or hands. Full thickness grafts are limited by the amount of donor skin available without compromising function at the donor site. Split thickness skin grafts are used to cover large surfaces, may be reharvested multiple times and can be meshed to cover larger surfaces (Fig. 11-14).

Bibliography

Kelton P. Skin grafts. *SRPS* 1995;8:2–18.
Rudolph R, Ballantyne D. Skin grafts. In: McCarthy J (ed.), *Plastic Surgery*. Philadelphia, PA: W.B. Saunders, 1990, 221–274.
Skouge J. Split thickness skin grafting. *Skin Grafting*. New York, NY: Churchill Livingstone, 1991, 5–45.
Skouge J. Full thickness skin grafting. *Skin Grafting*. New York, NY: Churchill Livingstone, 1991, 47–63.
Vasconez H. Skin grafts. In: Cohen M (ed.), *Mastery of Plastic and Reconstructive Surgery*, vol. 1. Boston, MA: Little, Brown & Company, 1994, 45–55.

30. **(B)** There are many skin substitutes available for use in burn care, each with advantages and disadvantages. Skin substitutes can be divided into temporary or permanent agents. All skin substitutes attempt to restore the burn wound to a more homeostatic state to improve the patient's ability to heal and avoid systemic deterioration. Thus, they imitate the skins mechanisms and in some cases, structure.

Temporary

- *Allograft skin*. The "gold standard" for temporary biologic wound coverage is cadaver allograft or homograft, harvested in sheets, which can be used fresh or frozen and meshed or unmeshed. Temporary wound closure results, as well as decreased pain and fluid losses, though ultimately the homograft is rejected and sloughs off leaving an open wound.

- *Xenograft.* Xenografts are grafts from other species. Porcine graft is homogenized dermis of the pig, which provides temporary coverage for superficial wounds with no eschar. The xenograft provides pain relief and initially adheres to the wound bed but lifts off as the wound heals beneath. Xenograft may sometimes be used as a temporary biologic cover until the wound is amenable to autografting.

- *Transcyte.* Transcyte is an agent in which fibroblasts from neonatal foreskin are layered onto a silicone backing. The fibroblasts produce growth factors and collagen that decrease the inflammatory phase of wound healing. Transcyte is frozen and must be thawed prior to use. The product is clear which allows for easy visualization of the wound bed. Transcyte can be applied to partial to deep partial thickness burn wounds.

- *Biobrane.* Biobrane is a two-layered wholly synthetic product that has a nylon mesh for fibrovascular ingrowth and an outer silastic layer as a bacterial barrier. This product is useful for superficial partial thickness wounds that blanch easily and have been cleansed of all debris.

Permanent

- *CEA.* Cultured epithelial autografts are keratinocytes grown in tissue culture from a full thickness biopsy of the patient's unburned skin and applied to a backing that can be transferred to carry them to the wound. Trypsin is used to separate the epithelial cells, which then undergo multiple cell culturings. In 2–3 weeks, the cells have grown into sheets of undifferentiated cells that are then available for transplantation. CEA is used to cover large body surface area burns and the defect resulting from excision of large congenital nevi, where the donor site availability is limited or undesirable. Graft success rates are variable. This technique requires meticulous care to ensure reasonable adherence of the cells. These grafts are susceptible to infection with little tolerance to bacterial counts greater than 10^3. Skin grafts can tolerate bacterial counts up to 10^5 without graft loss. Histologic examinations of these grafts have revealed the basement membrane is intact at 2–3 weeks following grafting. The demonstration of rete ridges and other structures of normal dermis varies among authors from approximately 21 weeks to 3 years postgrafting. A "neodermis" was observed within 2–5 years postgrafting, where fine elastin filaments

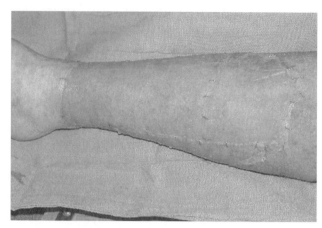

FIG. 11-15   Transcyte applied to arm burn.

were observed below the basement membrane and coarse fibers beneath that layer.

- *Integra.* Integra is a synthetic dermal replacement that is a bilaminar product. The inner layer, composed of bovine neodermis collagen in a scaffold of shark cartilage chondroitin-6-sulfate, allows for fibrovascular ingrowth. An outer silicone layer prevents evaporative loss and bacterial invasion. The neodermis revascularizes in 2–3 weeks and the silicone layer is removed and thin autografts are placed on the neodermis to achieve wound closure.

- *AlloDerm.* AlloDerm is an acellular nonantigenic cadaver dermal replacement. The product is freeze-dried and reconstituted prior to use. Once it is applied to the wound, a thin autograft is overlaid. This product is useful for grafting over joints and in burn reconstruction procedures (Figs. 11-15 through 11-17).

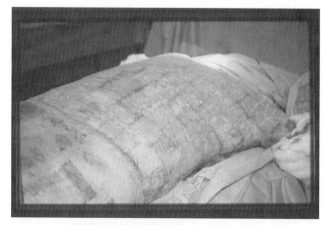

FIG. 11-16   CEA applied intraoperatively.

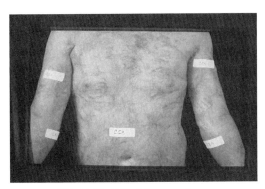

FIG. 11-17   CEA at 2-year postburn.

Bibliography

Carsin H, Ainaud P, LeBever H, et al. Cultured epithelial autografts in extensive burn coverage of severely traumatized patients: a five year single-center experience with 30 patients. *Burns* 2000;26:379–387.

Jones I, Currie L, Martin R. A guide to biological skin substitutes. *Br J Plast Surg* 2002;55:185–193.

Munster A. Cultured skin for massive burns. *Ann Surg* 1996;224:372–377.

Noordenbos J, Dore C, Hansbrough J. Safety and efficacy of transcyte for the treatment of partial-thickness burns. *J Burn Care Rehabil* 1999;20:275–281.

Putland M, Snelling C, Macdonald, et al. Histologic comparison of cultured epithelial autograft and meshed expanded split-thickness skin graft. *J Burn Care Rehabil* 1995;16:627–640.

Saffle J. What's new in general surgery: burns and metabolism. *J Am Coll Surg* 2003;196:267–285.

Sheridan R, Tompkins R. Alternative wound coverings. In: Herndon D (ed.), *Total Burn Care*, 2nd ed. London: W.B. Saunders, 2002, 212–218.

Wainwright D. Use of an acellular allograft dermal matrix (Alloderm) in the management of full-thickness burns. *Burns* 1995;21:243–248.

31. **(C)** On arrival to the emergency department, the burn patient should have their airway, breathing, and circulation assessed. The patient should be intubated if necessary and supplemental oxygen of 100% FiO_2 provided. Complete exposure of the patient should be performed and secondary surveys undertaken to assess the extent of injury and rule out associated trauma. Evaluations of circumferential burns to the limbs or thorax should be completed to assess the need for escharotomy. Arterial blood gas, carboxyhemoglobin levels, a complete blood count, serum electrolytes, glucose, blood urea nitrogen (BUN), and creatinine laboratory evaluations should be obtained for major burn patients. Chest x-ray and any other radiologic examinations are to be performed as deemed necessary.

A complete history should be completed with details of the accident of particular importance. The patient should have intravenous access established and Ringer's lactate solution infused per Parkland formula. An indwelling urinary catheter should be placed, a tetanus immunization given and gastric decompression with a nasogastric tube performed if necessary. The patient must be kept warm with warmed intravenous solutions and blankets. Transportation should be via ground or air depending on the stability of the patient and the travel distance.

There are established criteria for transferring patients to a burn center. These criteria include greater than 10% TBSA partial thickness burns, full thickness burns, burns involving specialty areas such as the face, perineum, genitalia, hands, feet and joints, chemical and electrical burns, and patients with inhalation injury. Patients with preexisting medical conditions that would adversely affect patient management should be transferred. Any patient with associated trauma, where the burn injury poses the greatest threat to the patient should also be transferred.

Bibliography

American Burn Association. *Advanced Burn Life Support Providers Manual.* Chicago, IL: American Burn Association, 2001.

Bueno R, Demling R. Management of burns in the multiple trauma patient. *Adv Trauma* 1989:165–78.

Mlcak R, Buffalo M. Pre-hospital management, transportation, and emergency care. In: Herndon D (ed.), *Total Burn Care*, 2nd ed. London: W.B. Saunders, 2002, 67–77.

Rosenkranz K, Sheridan R. Management of the burned trauma patient: balancing conflicting priorities. *Burns* 2002;28:665–669.

CHAPTER 12

Vascular Trauma

Charles E. Morrow Jr. and Satinderjit Singh Gill

Questions

1. A 33-year-old male is transported to your facility following a single stab wound to the anterior abdomen at the umbilicus. Initial vital signs are a blood pressure of 93/67 mmHg, pulse of 125 bpm, and respiratory rate of 28 breaths/min. Intraoperatively a large midline retroperitoneal hematoma is explored and transection of the superior mesenteric artery (SMA) is identified after division of the body of the pancreas. Operative management of the mesenteric artery is

   (A) ligation only if proximal arterial injury
   (B) ligation only if distal arterial injury
   (C) proximal arterial ligation with bypass graft from the infrarenal aorta
   (D) end-to-end anastomosis with polytetrafluoroethylene (PTFE) graft
   (E) end-to-end anastomosis with saphenous vein graft

2. Following a motor vehicle crash (MVC), a 23-year-old trauma patient undergoes a contrast enhanced CT scan of the abdomen which reveals a large right perinephric hematoma with associated contrast extravasation, failure of the right kidney to uptake contrast, and a normal appearing left kidney. The patient is hemodynamically stable and with no other intraabdominal injuries. Appropriate management of the right kidney is

   (A) admit for observation of residual renal function
   (B) retroperitoneal exploration
   (C) exploration through Gerota's fascia to exclude a parenchymal injury
   (D) radiologic vascular stent placement
   (E) nephrostomy tube and *n*-acetylcysteine

3. A 19-year-old male, involved in a motor vehicle crash, presents to the emergency department (ED). After initial evaluation he is hemodynamically stable and undergoes a contrast enhanced CT scan of the abdomen. He is found to have a severely damaged left kidney (grade V) and a normal appearing right kidney. Appropriate management of the injured kidney is

   (A) nephrostomy tube placement
   (B) renal artery bypass or graft
   (C) observation with exploration for hemodynamic instability
   (D) nephrectomy
   (E) renal artery stent

4. A 20-year-old male presents to the ED following a stabbing to the right lower abdomen. On exploration he has a 2 cm cecal laceration with gross contamination as well as a laceration to the right iliac vein. The best treatment option with regard to the iliac vein is

   (A) primary repair
   (B) ligation
   (C) repair with PTFE
   (D) extraanatomic bypass graft
   (E) repair with autogenous vein

5. Management options for suprarenal inferior vena cava (IVC) injuries include all *except*

   (A) ligation
   (B) lateral venorraphy
   (C) spiral saphenous vein graft
   (D) extraanatomic bypass
   (E) panel graft using saphenous vein

6. At abdominal exploration for penetrating trauma, a portal vein laceration is identified. The patient has gross hemoperitoneum, a transverse colostomy with gross spillage, and severe hypotension.

Management of the portal vein includes all *except*

(A) Pringle maneuver
(B) ligation portal vein
(C) lateral portal vein venorraphy
(D) end-to-end anastomosis
(E) portocaval shunt

7. Following blunt abdominal trauma, mandatory exploration is indicated for any nonexpanding hematoma identified on CT scan in which of the following areas:

(A) right perinephric
(B) midline inframesocolic
(C) lateral pelvic area
(D) retrohepatic
(E) left perinephric

8. Following a gunshot wound (GSW) to the lower extremity, sign and symptoms that mandate exploration include which of the following:

(A) history of significant hemorrhage at the scene although no longer actively bleeding
(B) deficit in anatomically related nerve
(C) hypotension
(D) small, stable, nonpulsitile hematoma
(E) palpable thrill

9. After being struck by a train, a 23-year-old male arrives to your ED hemodynamically stable with a severe injury to the lower extremity. Which injury would alone most indicate nonviability and warrant immediate amputation of the injured extremity?

(A) degloving of >50% skin from posterior aspect of the extremity
(B) open tib/fib, proximal femur, and talus fractures
(C) loss of >65% extensor muscles from proximal extremity
(D) lack of popliteal pulse
(E) complete disruption of the tibeal nerve

10. The earliest symptoms of compartment syndrome are because of tissue intolerance to hypoxia. Which structure is the most sensitive to hypoxia?

(A) skin
(B) bone

(C) nonmyelinated nerve
(D) myelinated nerve
(E) skeletal muscle

11. Which of the following is *not* correct regarding fasciotomy in the lower extremity for compartment syndrome?

(A) A four compartment fasciotomy may be performed using a single incision with or without a fibulectomy.
(B) A four compartment fasciotomy may be performed using anterolateral and posteromedial incisions
(C) Compartment syndrome involving the thigh may be treated by decompression of the quadriceps compartment only.
(D) The superficial branch of the peroneal nerve is especially vulnerable when extending the fascial incision proximally in the superficial posterior compartment.
(E) The most common cause of acute compartment syndrome in the lower extremity is a tibial fracture.

12. One day following fixation of a complex femur fracture sustained in a MVC, a 24-year-old male complaining of severe pain along the ipsilateral thigh. On examination he is hemodynamically stable with a pulse rate of 104 breaths/min, oxygen saturation of 94%, and blood pressure 140/78 mmHg. He has no urinary catheter and no recorded urine output. Laboratory studies at that time include a Hgb 8.1 (down from 12.3 preop), potassium 5.8 (from 3.4).

Appropriate next steps include all of the following *except*:

(A) urinary catheter
(B) compartment pressure measurement
(C) mannitol
(D) crystalloid infusion
(E) 2u packed red blood cells (PRBC) transfusion

13. In which of the following venous injuries is ligation *most* tolerated?

(A) infrarenal vena cava
(B) suprarenal vena cava
(C) common femoral vein
(D) opliteal vein
(E) innominate vein

14. Which statement is *true* regarding the incidence of contrast nephropathy (CN)?

    (A) The incidence in overall healthy patients is 5%.

    (B) The most important risk factor is dehydration.

    (C) In patients with a normal serum creatinine, contrast doses in excess of 200 mL of 300 mgI/mL solution is considered a significant risk factor.

    (D) Mannitol has been shown to decrease the risk of CN.

    (E) The most important prophylactic maneuver is hydration.

15. Three months following a MVC in which she suffered a grade III liver laceration, a 34-year-old female presents with hematemesis. She has no history of peptic ulcer disease and denies nonsteroidal anti-inflammatory drug (NSAID) use. Following initial stabilization, the next most appropriate step would be

    (A) upper endoscopy

    (B) contrast enhanced CT of the abdomen

    (C) abdominal ultrasonography (US)

    (D) admission for observation

    (E) angiography

16. Arterial injuries that can be safely ligated in the unstable trauma patient include all *except*:

    (A) SMA

    (B) radial artery

    (C) inferior mesenteric artery

    (D) internal iliac artery

    (E) celiac artery

17. Fasciotomy for extremity compartment syndrome should be performed at what compartment pressure?

    (A) 20 mmHg

    (B) 30 mmHg

    (C) 40 mmHg

    (D) 50 mmHg

    (E) none of the above

18. The most appropriate management of isolated radial artery injuries is

    (A) primary repair

    (B) ligation

    (C) repair with vein graft

    (D) repair with PTFE graft

    (E) all of the above

19. A 20-year-old male suffers a gunshot blast to the right neck. Initial workup reveals stable vital signs, an intact airway, and no active bleeding from the multiple small entrance sites visible along the right neck. As part of his workup, the arteriogram below is obtained (Figs. 12-1 and 12-2).

This arteriogram demonstrates

    (A) normal arteriogram with no evidence of injury

    (B) right internal jugular vein injury

    (C) right common carotid artery injury

    (D) right internal carotid artery injury

    (E) right external carotid artery injury

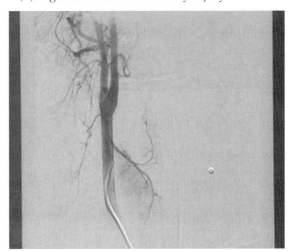

FIG. 12-1   Arteriogram

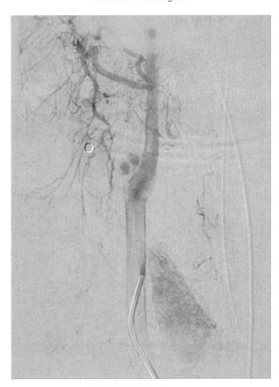

FIG. 12-2   Arteriogram

20. The patient described in Question 19 remains hemo-dynamically stable and with a Glasgow Coma Scale (GCS) of 15, the next step in the management of the patient is

   (A) tube thoracostomy in the emergency room (ER)
   (B) admission and observation alone
   (C) neck exploration
   (D) tracheobronchoscopy, esophagram, esophagoscopy, and observation
   (E) admission and anticoagulation therapy

21. A 22-year-old male presents to the ER after being struck in the neck with a baseball bat. Initial vitals include GCS 15, pulse rate 96 bpm, respiration rate 16 breaths/min, and SBP 125. An arteriogram is performed and reveals a right internal carotid artery dissection.

   Initial management includes all the following *except*:

   (A) cervical spine x-rays
   (B) heparin
   (C) neck exploration with repair
   (D) CT scan of the neck
   (E) tracheobronchoscopy

22. A left neck exploration is performed for a stab injury to the neck in an otherwise healthy male. The left internal jugular vein is found to be completely transected with significant bleeding and hemodynamic instability. No other vascular injury is identified. Appropriate management of the internal jugular vein is

   (A) primary repair
   (B) interposition saphenous vein graft
   (C) interposition with 6 mm PTFE
   (D) ligate the left internal jugular vein
   (E) external jugular vein transposition

23. A 33-year-old female was the unrestrained driver of a motor vehicle in a high-speed motor vehicle crash. EMS reported a significant steering wheel deformity. Primary and secondary surveys revealed a GCS of 15, pulse rate of 79 bpm, respiratory rate of 12 breaths/min, a blood pressure of 134/76 mmHg, a deformed left femur without open wound, and the upright chest x-ray (CXR) shown in Fig. 12-3.

   The next step in management of this patient is

   (A) x-ray of the left femur
   (B) admit and observe

   (C) cervical C-spine x-ray series
   (D) spiral CT scan of the chest
   (E) flat and upright abdominal x-ray

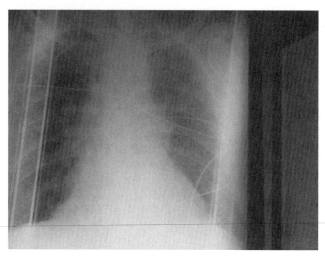

FIG. 12-3   Chest X-Ray

24. The previously described patient subsequently develops weakness in her right arm and hand. The following arteriogram was performed (Fig. 12-4).

   This arteriogram demonstrates

   (A) no injury
   (B) cardiac contusion
   (C) sternal fracture
   (D) aortic tear
   (E) innominate artery pseudoaneurysm

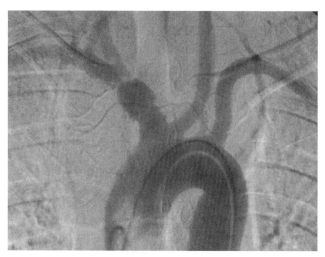

FIG. 12-4   Arteriogram

25. After arteriogram, the next step in the management of the patient described in Questions 23 and 24 is

    (A) anticoagulation with heparin, blood pressure control
    (B) repair of the injury via right anterolateral thoracotomy
    (C) repair of the injury via left anterolateral thoracotomy
    (D) repair of the injury via medianstinotomy
    (E) admission and observation

26. A 62-year-old male is brought to the ER after being involved in a motor vehicle collision. Vital signs include GCS 15, pulse rate 78 bpm, respiration rate 12 breaths/min, and blood pressure 195/110 mmHg. Radiologic workup includes the arteriogram shown below (Fig. 12-5). This study demonstrates

    (A) ascending aortic injury
    (B) descending aortic injury
    (C) normal study, no injury demonstrated
    (D) subclavian artery injury
    (E) pericardial tamponade

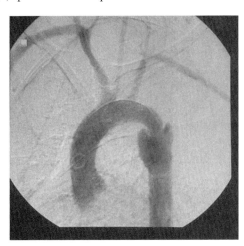

FIG. 12-5 Arteriogram

27. After stabilization and full workup, the patient in Question 26 is found to have no other significant injuries.

    The next step in management of this patient is

    (A) admit and observe on cardiac monitor
    (B) repair of the aortic tear
    (C) placement of a thoracic aortic stent
    (D) EGD and bronchoscopy
    (E) ER thoracotomy

28. A 22-year-old male presents into the ER after sustaining a stab wound to the left chest. The injury is 2 cm left of the sternum at the level of his nipple. Initial vital signs include a pulse rate 88 bpm, GCS 15, respiratory rate 12 breaths/min, and blood pressure 139/74 mmHg.

    Initial management of this patient should be

    (A) CXR
    (B) pericardiocentesis
    (C) left chest tube thoracostomy
    (D) esophagogram
    (E) echocardiogram

29. An arteriogram is performed on the patient described in Question 28 and an injury to the proximal left subclavian artery is identified. The patient remains hemodynamically stable.

    The next step in the management of this patient is

    (A) admit and observe
    (B) subclavian repair through a mediastinotomy
    (C) subclavian repair through a supraclavicular incision
    (D) subclavian repair through an anterolateral thoracotomy
    (E) explorative laparotomy

30. A 19-year-old male presents to the ED following a self-inflicted gunshot wound to the left shoulder. His initial vital signs are pulse rate 100 bpm, respiratory rate 12 breaths/min, blood pressure 122/83 mmHg, and a GCS 15.

   Physical examination reveals absent pulses in the left brachial, radial, and ulnar arteries. Neurologic examination of the left hand and arm reveals no gross motor or sensory deficit.

   Following complete examination, an arteriogram is obtained (Fig. 12-6).

   The arteriogram reveals an injury to the

   (A) left subclavian artery
   (B) left axillary artery
   (C) left brachial artery
   (D) left carotid artery
   (E) left internal mammary artery

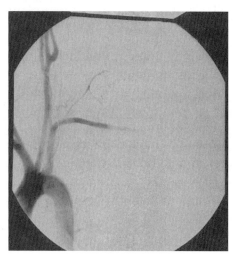

FIG. 12-6   Arteriogram

31. Management of the vascular injury described in Question 30 includes

   (A) admit for observation and anticoagulation
   (B) repair the axillary artery with PTFE
   (C) repair the axillary artery with reversed saphenous vein graft

(D) fracture stabilization with IM rodding
(E) temporary shunting of the vascular injury followed by fracture stabilization

32. A 27-year-old male is transported to the ED following a GSW to the left thigh. sustaining a gunshot wound to this left thigh. Physical examination reveals an entrance wound on the medial aspect of the left thigh and an exit wound on the lateral aspect of the left thigh. There is no pulse or Doppler signal in his left foot.

   The patient's arteriogram is shown in Fig. 12-7 and reveals

   (A) normal arteriogram
   (B) left common femoral artery injury
   (C) left profunda femoris artery injury
   (D) left superficial femoral artery injury
   (E) left external iliac artery injury

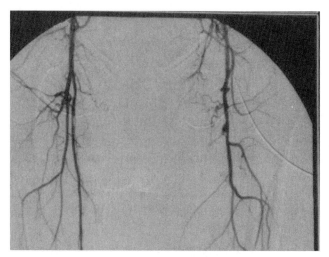

FIG. 12-7   Arteriogram

33. The next step in the management of the vascular injury presented in Question 32 is

   (A) admit and heparin anticoagulation
   (B) reversed saphenous vein interposition
   (C) PTFE graft interposition
   (D) immediate above knee amputation
   (E) reversed saphenous vein bypass graft

Answers and Explanations

1. (C) Injury to the SMA is suggested by a hematoma at the base of the transverse mesocolon. Supramesocolic retroperitoneal hematomas are best approached using a "Mattox" maneuver, medially rotating the left-sided abdominal viscera (left colon, spleen, tail of pancreas, fundus of stomach, and often left kidney). If the penetrating injury is actively bleeding, aortic compression should be applied for proximal control until the injury is identified.

Fullen et al. described four anatomic classes of SMA injury.

Zone I—Beneath the pancreas
Zone II—Beyond the pancreas at base of the transverse mesocolon (between the pancreaticoduodenal artery and the middle colic branches)
Zone III—Distal SMA, beyond the middle colic branches
Zone IV—Level of the enteric branches

In zone I, the pancreas is divided for control or medial rotation of the viscera to include the tail of the pancreas is performed.

Zones I and II should be treated with primary repair using lateral repair techniques or ligation with bypass grafting from the infrarenal aorta using vein or PTFE. Ligation alone in theory should be tolerated because of collateral flow; however, this is often not true because of concomitant shock and vasospasm. *In situ* grafting should be avoided because of the risk of pancreatic leakage postoperatively.

Zones III, IV must be repaired because of midgut ischemia with ligation.

Bibliography

Bongard F. Thoracic and abdominal vascular trauma. In: Rutherford RB (ed.), *Vascular Surgery*. Philadelphia, PA: W.B. Saunders, 2000.

Carrillo EH, et al. Abdominal vascular injuries. *J Trauma* 1997;43:164–171.

Feliciano DV. Management of traumatic retroperitoneal hematoma. *Ann Surg* 1990;211:109.

Feliciano DV. *Abdominal Vascular Injury*. In: Trunkey DD, Lewis FR (eds.), *Current Therapy of Trauma*. St. Louis, MO: Mosby, 1999.

Feliciano DV, Burch JM, Graham JM. Abdominal vascular injury. In: Feliciano DV, Moore EE, Mattox KL (eds.), *Trauma*. Stamford, CT: Appleton & Lange, 1996.

Fullen WD, Hunt J, Altemeier WA. The clinical spectrum of penetrating injury to the superior mesenteric arterial circulation. *J Trauma* 1972;12:656.

2. (B) Hemorrhage or hematoma in the lateral perirenal region often represents renal artery, vein, or parenchymal injury. Exploration of the kidney should be avoided if the preoperative workup includes a normal intravenous pyelogram (IVP), renal arteriogram, or contrasted CT of the involved kidney. If the hematoma is not rapidly expanding and there is no free intraperitoneal bleeding, vascular control of the renal artery may be obtained using vascular tapes in the midline at the base of the mesocolon. On the right this necessitates mobilization of the c-loop of the duodenum. If there is active bleeding from the renal parenchyma through a break in Gerota's fascia, no central renovascular control is necessary and the injury may be directly controlled through this laceration. Repair options include lateral arteriorrhaphy or end-to-end anastomosis if possible. Interposition grafts using either vein or PTFE are indicated only if there appears to be reasonable hope of renal salvage. In those patients with significant renovascular injuries, multiple intraabdominal injuries, or a long preoperative ischemic period, nephrectomy is likely a more reasonable choice.

Bibliography

Bongard F. Thoracic and abdominal vascular trauma. In: Rutherford RB (ed.), *Vascular Surgery*. Philadelphia, PA: W.B. Saunders, 2000.

Carroll PR, McAninch JW, Klosterman P, Greenblatt M. Reno-vascular trauma: risk assessment, surgical management, and outcome. *J Trauma* 1990;30:547.

Feliciano DV. Management of traumatic retroperitoneal hematoma. *Ann Surg* 1990;211:109.

Feliciano DV, Burch JM, Graham JM. *Abdominal Vascular Injury.* In: Feliciano DV, Moore EE, Mattox KL (eds.), *Trauma.* Stamford, CT: Appleton & Lange,1996.

Sclafani SJA. The diagnosis of bilateral renal artery injury by computed tomography. *J Trauma* 1986;26:295.

3. **(B)** Major renal injuries are uncommon following both blunt and penetrating trauma. These are often challenging cases because of the high rate of associated injuries. Attempts to revascularize severe renal injuries are often unsuccessful with subsequent impaired renal function, renal hypertension, or progressive renal failure. Many, though not all patients, suffering severe renal injuries will present in hemodynamic shock. Gross hematuria is seen in only 50% of all patients with up to 18% having no hematuria at all. Nearly 90% of patients will have associated injuries. In those with grade IV or V renal injuries, nearly three quarters will have associated abdominal injuries. Treatment options include observation, nephrectomy, primary vascular repair, and vascular repair using graft. Recent studies have shown that attempts at vascular repair in grade V injuries are not warranted and when attempted, are 15 times more likely to result in a poor outcome such as impaired renal function, renal failure, delayed nephrectomy, or new onset hypertension. In cases of grade V renal injuries with evidence of a normally functioning contralateral kidney, immediate nephrectomy should be performed (Table 12-1).

Bibliography

Goldblatt H, Lynch J, Hanzel RF. Studies on experimental hypertension. *J Exp Med* 1934;59:347–349.

TABLE 12-1   Renal Injury Scale

Grade		Description
I	Contusion	Microscopic or gross hematuria; normal urologic studies
	Hematoma	Subcapsular, nonexpanding without parenchymal laceration
II	Hematoma	Nonexpanding perirenal hematoma confined to renal retroperitoneum
	Laceration	<1.0 cm parenchymal depth of renal cortex without urinary extravasation
III	Laceration	>1.0 cm parenchymal depth of renal cortex with collecting system rupture or urinary extravasation
IV	Laceration	Parenchymal laceration extending through renal cortex medulla, and collecting system
	Vascular	Main renal artery/vein with contained hemorrhage
V	Laceration	Completely shattered kidney
	Vascular	Avulsion of renal hilum which devascularizes kidney

Knudson MM, Harrison PB, Hoyt DB, Shatz DV, Zietlow SP, Bergstein JM, Mario LA, McAninch JW. Outcome after major renovascular injuries: a Western Trauma Association multicenter report. *J Trauma* 2000;49:1116–1122.

Lock JS, Carraway RP, Hudson HC, Laws HL. Proper management of renal artery injury form blunt trauma. *South Med J* 1985;78:406–410.

Moore EE, Shackford SR, Patcher HL, et al. Organ injury scaling: spleen, liver, and kidney. *J Trauma* 1989;29:1664–1666.

Narrod JA, Moore EE, Posner M, Peterson NE. Nephrectomy following trauma-impact on patient outcome. *J Trauma* 1986;25:842–844.

Page IH. The production of persistent arterial hypertension by cellophane perinephritis. *JAMA* 1939;113:2046–2048.

Peterson NE. Complications of renal trauma. *Urol Clin North Am* 1989;16:221–235.

Stables DP, Fouche RF, DeVilliers JP, et al. Traumatic renal artery occlusion: 21 cases. *J Urol* 1976;115:229–233.

4. **(A)** Penetrating injuries that involve the iliac vessels commonly involve the overlying viscera. Cecum, ileum, sigmoid colon, ureters, bladder, and rectum are all at risk. Preferred exposure is via medial rotation of the cecum and ileum on the right and sigmoid colon on the left. Following proximal and distal control, repair of the external iliac artery is usually accomplished using 4.0–5.0 polypropylene via a lateral arteriorrhaphy. Resection with mobilization to allow end-to-end repair is possible for injuries less than 2 cm in length. Injuries to the iliac veins are approached in a similar fashion as arteries with proximal and distal control prior to exploration of the hematoma. Most injuries can be treated with primary repair via lateral venorrhaphy. If needed, the iliac vein may be ligated in young patients but should be avoided if possible. Since a large percentage will have associated gastrointestinal (GI) or genitourinary (GU) injuries, autogenous material should be used whenever possible although prosthetic grafts have been tried with success in certain groups.

Bibliography

Bongard F. Thoracic and abdominal vascular trauma. In: Rutherford RB (ed.), *Vascular Surgery.* Philadelphia, PA: W.B. Saunders, 2000.

Burch JM, Richardson RJ, Martin RR, et al. Penetrating iliac vascular injuries: recent experience with 233 consecutive patients. *J Trauma* 1989;30:1450.

Carillo EH, Spain DA, Wilson MA, et al. Alternatives in the management of penetrating injuries to the iliac vessels. *J Trauma* 1998;44:1024.

Landreneau RJ, Lewis DM, Snyder WH:.Complex iliac arterial trauma: autologous or prosthetic vascular repair? *Surgery* 1993;114:9.

5. **(A)** Overall, injuries to the suprarenal and retrohepatic vena cava carry a mortality rate of 33–67% because of associated injuries.

Exposure of the suprarenal cava can be achieved with a generous Kocher maneuver mobilizing the duodenum and ascending colon to the midline. Initial vascular control is accomplished with manual compression of the vena cava using sponge sticks, finger pressure, or with balloon occlusion.

Repair options are similar to that of the infrarenal vena cava although unlike the infrarenal cava, ligation of the suprarenal cava is discouraged because of its high mortality rate.

Options include lateral venorrhaphy as long as the diameter is not narrowed greater than 50%. Large defects are repaired with saphenous vein or panel grafts. Entire segment damage can be repaired with spiral vein grafts dependent on patient stability. Extraanatomic bypass is generally not done in the acute setting because of associated injuries.

In extreme cases where ligation is the only possible option, some suggest that temporary occlusion be done to evaluate the degree of venous hypertension and level of subsequent renal function. If urine output remains >0.5 mL/kg/h and IVC pressure <30 cm H_2O the suprarenal vena cava may be safely ligated.

Bibliography

Carrillo EH, et al. Abdominal vascular injuries. *J Trauma* 1997;43:164–171.

Feliciano DV. Abdominal vascular injury. In: Trunkey DD, Lewis FR (eds.), *Current Therapy of Trauma*. St. Louis, MO: Mosby, 1999.

Feliciano DV, Burch JM, Graham JM. Abdominal vascular injury. In: Feliciano DV, Moore EE, Mattox KL (eds.), *Trauma*. Stamford, CT: Appleton & Lange, 1996.

Ombrellaro MP, Freeman MB, Stevens SL, Diamond DL, Goldman MH. Predictors of survival after inferior vena cava injuries. *Am Surg* 1997;63:178–183.

Wilson RF, Dulchavsky S:.Abdominal vascular trauma. In: Wilson RF, Walt AJ (eds.), *Management of Trauma: Pitfalls and Practice*. Baltimore, MD: Williams & Wilkins, 1996.

6. **(E)** Exposure of the portal vein and porta hepatis structures is achieved by mobilizing the hepatic flexure and right colon. A Kocher maneuver for duodenal mobilization may also be required for added exposure. Injuries at the porta hepatis require dissection and mobilization of the common bile duct, cystic duct, hepatic artery and portal vein. Each must be thoroughly inspected for possible injury.

A Pringle maneuver (proximal placement of a noncrushing clamp across the common bile duct, portal vein, and hepatic artery) may be used to control bleeding.

Lateral venorrhaphy or end-to-end anastomosis should be performed whenever technically possible. Saphenous vein panel grafts may be required for

significant disruptions. Repair is preferred over ligation because of the high risk of hepatic necrosis associated with portal vein ligation.

When the patient is unstable and/or coagulopathic, portal vein ligation may be the only logical option and has been shown to be compatible with survival in several studies. When done, the resultant relative systemic hypovolemia must be treated with aggressive volume resuscitation during the first 2–3 postoperative days.

Bibliography

Bongard F. Thoracic and abdominal vascular trauma. In: Rutherford RB (ed), *Vascular Surgery*. Philadelphia, PA: W.B. Saunders, 2000.

Feliciano DV, Burch JM, Graham JM. Abdominal vascular injury. In: Feliciano DV, Moore EE, Mattox KL (eds.), *Trauma*. Stamford, CT: Appleton & Lange, 1996.

Graham JM, Mattox KL, Beall AC. Portal venous system injuries. *J Trauma* 1978;18:419.

Pachter HL, Drager S, Godfrey N, et al. Traumatic injuries of the portal vein. *Ann Surg* 1979;189:283.

Stone HH, Fabian TC, Turkleson ML. Wounds of the portal system. *World J Surg* 1982;6:335.

Wilson RF, Dulchavsky S. Abdominal vascular trauma. In: Wilson RF, Walt AJ (eds.), *Management of Trauma: Pitfalls and Practice*. Baltimore, MD: Williams & Wilkins, 1996.

7. **(B)** A midline (supramesocolic or inframesocolic) hematoma (zone I), regardless if because of blunt of penetrating trauma, requires exploration to evaluate the significant vascular structures located in this area. Exposure is best accomplished using the Mattox maneuver, medially rotating the left-sided abdominal viscera including the left colon, spleen, tail of pancreas, and gastric fundus. (The kidney may sometimes be included in this mobilization.) The infrarenal aorta is exposed by lifting the transverse colon onto the lower chest and eviscerating the midgut to the right. Exposure of the inferior vena cava is done by combining a Kocher maneuver for duodenal mobilization with elevation of the right colon to the midline. Hematomas in the lateral retroperitoneum (zone II) or perinephric region require exploration following penetrating injuries; however, in blunt trauma, a normal appearing kidney on preoperative contrast enhanced CT scan or a normal renal arteriogram does not mandate exploration as a significant vascular injury is unlikely. Lateral pelvic area (zone III) retroperitoneal hematomas from penetrating trauma should be explored through a midline retroperitoneal incision over the aortic bifurcation. In patients with blunt trauma, pelvic retroperitoneal hematoma found on CT or incidentally on celiotomy is not an indication for exploration unless it is ruptured, pulsitile, or associated

with an injury to the iliac vessels, male urethra, or bladder. Hematoma or hemorrhage in the porta hepatis should be explored using a Pringle maneuver for vascular control with complete dissection of the porta structures. A hematoma in the retrohepatic retroperitoneum is not explored unless it is rapidly expanding or has ruptured with ongoing hemorrhage. A stable hematoma can be managed by perihepatic packing and damage control laparotomy techniques.

Bibliography

Carrillo EH, et al. Abdominal vascular injuries. *J Trauma* 1997;43:164.

Feliciano DV. Management of traumatic retroperitoneal hematoma. *Ann Surg* 1990;211:109.

Feliciano DV. Abdominal vascular injury. In: Trunkey DD, Lewis FR (eds.), *Current Therapy of Trauma*. St. Louis, MO: Mosby, 1999.

Feliciano DV, Burch JM, Graham JM. Abdominal vascular injury. In: Feliciano DV, Moore EE, Mattox KL (eds.), *Trauma*. Stamford, CT: Appleton & Lange, 1996.

8. **(E)** Management of penetrating injuries with vascular trauma continues to be controversial with regard to mandatory exploration, workup, and observation with serial examination. Frykberg et al. (1991) have shown that the presence of "hard signs" in penetrating trauma mandate immediate exploration and that observation with serial examination in patients presenting with "soft signs" only can be safely done. Richardson et al. (1987) found that mandatory exploration for a mix of "hard " and "soft" signs (proximity, absent or decreased pulse, sensory/motor deficit, large/expanding hematoma, or bleeding) lead to a negative exploration in 42% of patients. While the management protocol should be based on resources and experience specific to individual institutions, most trauma surgeons agree that any "hard sign" is an indication for surgical exploration (Table 12-2).

Bibliography

Frykberg ER, Dennis JW, Bishop K, et al. The reliability of physical examination in the evaluation of penetrating extremity trauma for vascular injury: results at one year. *J Trauma* 1991;31:502.

Richardson JD, Vitale GC, Flint LM Jr. Penetrating arterial trauma. *Arch Surg* 1987;122:678.

Shackford SR, Rich NH. Peripheral vascular injury. In: Feliciano DV, Moore EE, Mattox KL (eds.), *Trauma*. Stamford, CT: Appleton & Lange, 1996.

9. **(E)** Many severely damaged limbs can now be salvaged when previously amputation was the only option. Despite advances in limb salvage, there remain many cases where primary amputation is the most reasonable choice (i.e., completion of a traumatic

TABLE 12-2   Physical Signs of Vascular Injury

Hard signs
- Active bleeding
- Distal pulse deficit
- Large, expanding, or pulsatile hematoma
- Distal ischemia
  - Pallor
  - Paresthesia
  - Paralysis
  - Pain
  - Pulselessness
  - Poikilothermia
- Palpable thrill
- Audible bruit

Soft signs
- History of moderate hemorrhage no longer present
- Injury in proximity to major vascular structure
- Diminished pulse
- Peripheral nerve deficit
- Small, stable, nonpulsatile hematoma
- Hypotension

amputation, irreparable major peripheral nerve damage, and/or severe crush injuries in combination with a prolonged ischemic time). Efforts to inappropriately preserve severely injured limbs can lead to significant morbidity as well as additional expensive hospital costs. In some situations, early amputation is preferred as it can greatly speed up the recovery and rehabilitation of the severely injured patient. The main indication for early amputation is loss of tissue viability and loss of limb function, both of which may be difficult to assess in the acute setting. As an aid to the clinical judgment needed to make this often-difficult decision, multiple scoring systems have been developed to predict the need for early amputation. One such system, the MESS (mangled extremity severity score) developed by Johansen has been shown in both prospective and retrospective studies to indicate the need for amputation with a score of 7 or higher. In general, when four out of five of the main structures are injured (skin, bone, muscle, vascular, nerve) with little or no nerve injury, salvage should be considered. If, however, the nerve injury is severe and there is little likelihood of function, immediate amputation is the most prudent treatment option (Table 12-3).

Bibliography

Bondurant FJ, Cotler HB, Buckle R, et al. The medical and economic impact of severely injured lower extremities. *J Trauma* 1988;28:1270.

Gregory RT, Gould RJ, Peclet M, et al. The mangled extremity score (MES): a severity grading system for multisystem injury of the extremity. *J Trauma* 1985;25:1147.

Hansen ST Jr. The type III-C tibial fracture: salvage or amputation. *J Bone Joint Surg* 1987;69-A:799.

TABLE 12-3   MES Score

A. Skeletal/soft tissue injury	
Low energy—stab	1
Intermediate energy—fracture	2
High energy—close range GSW, crush	3
Very high energy—addition of gross contamination to any above	4
B. Limb ischemia—double score if ischemia time >6 h	
Reduced/absent pulse, normal capillary refill	1
Pulseless, decreased capillary refill	2
Cool, paralyzed, insensate, numb	3
C. Shock	
SBP > 90 mmHg	0
Transient hypotension	1
Persistent hypotension	2
D. Age (year)	
<30	0
30–35	1
>50	2

Howe HR, Poole GV, Hansen KJ, et al. Salvage of lower extremities following combined orthopedic and vascular trauma: a predictive salvage index. *Am Surg* 1987;53:205.

Johansen K, Daines M, Howey T, et al. Objective criteria accurately predict amputation following lower extremity trauma. *J Trauma* 1990;30:568.

Lange RH, Bach AW, Hansen ST Jr, et al. Open tibial fractures with associated vascular injuries: prognosis for limb salvage. *J Trauma* 1985;25:203.

Pozo JL, Powell B, Andrews BG, et al. The timing of amputation for lower limb trauma. *J Bone Joint Surg* 1990; 72B:288.

Seiler JG, Richardson JD. Amputation after extremity injury. *Am J Surg* 1986;152:260.

Wilson RF, Georgiadis GM. Amputations after trauma. In: Wilson RF, Walt AJ (eds.), *Management of Trauma: Pitfalls and Practice*. Baltimore, MD: Williams & Wilkins, 1996.

10. **(C)** The earliest symptoms of compartment syndrome are neurologic because of the fact that nonmyelinated type C sensory fibers are most sensitive to oxygen deprivation. These nerve fibers carry fine touch and mediate symptoms such as paresthesias. Tissue intolerance to hypoxia increases from nonmyelinated to myelinated nerves, to skeletal muscle, to the most resistant, skin and bone.

Classically pain is described as out of proportion to the clinical findings and worsens despite appropriate care of the injury (i.e., fracture stabilization). Important neurologic symptoms are of distal motor and sensory dysfunction, characteristically weakness and numbness in the distribution of the affected nerve(s). Commonly the peroneal nerve in the lower extremity is affected leading to weakness on dorsiflexion and numbness in the first dorsal web space. The median nerve of the upper extremity is most often affected with weakness in wrist extension and numbness in the first webspace.

Bibliography

Haimovici H. Muscular, renal, and metabolic complications of acute arterial occlusions: myonephropathic-metabolic syndrome. *Surgery* 1979;85:461–468.

Johansen KH, Watson JC. Compartment syndrome: pathophysiology, recognition, and management. In: Rutherford RB (ed.), *Vascular Surgery*. Philadelphia, PA: W.B. Saunders, 2000.

Mabee JR, Bostwick TL. Pathophysiology and mechanisms of compartment syndrome. *Orthop Rev* 1993;22:175–181.

Matava MJ, Whitesides TE, Seiler JG, et al. Determination of the compartment pressure threshold of muscle ischemia in a canine model. *J Trauma* 1994;37:50–58.

Walker PM. Ischemia/reperfusion injury in skeletal muscle. *Ann Vasc Surg* 1991;5:399–402.

11. **(D)** The most common cause of extremity acute compartment syndrome in trauma patients is the tibial fracture. The lower extremity has four compartments bound by muscle fascia. To decompress the anterior and lateral compartments, a lateral incision between the tibial crest and fibula is made. A short transverse incision is then made through the leg fascia allowing access to the lateral intramuscular membrane which is then divided. The superficial branch of the peroneal nerve is especially vulnerable as the membrane is divided proximally as it lies posterior to this septum and must be avoided. The posterior compartments are exposed through a medial incision made 2 cm posterior to the posterior tibial crest. Care is taken to avoid the saphenous nerve and vein. A transverse incision through the enveloping fascia allows identification of the septum between the deep and superficial compartment

for division. Alternatively, all four compartments may be released through a single lateral incision with or without a fibulectomy.

Bibliography

Gulli B, Templeman D. Compartment syndrome of the lower extremity. *Orhtop Clin North Am* 1994;25:677.

Johansen KH, Watson JC. Compartment syndrome: pathophysiology, recognition, and management. In: Rutherford RB (ed.), *Vascular Surgery*. Philadelphia, PA: W.B. Saunders, 2000.

Owings JT, Kennedy JP, Blaisdell FW. Injuries to the extremities. In: Wilmore DW, et al. (eds.), *ACS Surgery: Principles & Practice*. New York, NY: WedMD, 2002.

12. **(E)** The key to treatment of compartment syndrome is early recognition. This requires a high index of suspicion whenever treating injuries historically at high risk for developing elevated compartment pressures. Classically compartment syndrome in trauma is seen following major extremity trauma such as crush injury, closed fractures, or with reperfusion following acute arterial injuries with a prolonged ischemic time. Once suspected, compartment pressures should be measured using commercially available devices or simple insertion of an intravenous (IV) catheter into the compartment with pressure transduction using standard monitoring equipment. Pressures greater than 30–40 mmHg are generally indications that fasciotomy should be performed emergently. Immediate complications of compartment syndrome result from muscle necrosis and include hyperkalemia, renal failure because of myoglobinuria, infection, and possibly limb loss.

The above patient is demonstrating signs of early compartment syndrome and must be treated aggressively. The patient's compartment pressures should be measured and if elevated the patient taken emergently for fasciotomy. A bladder catheter should be placed to allow frequent measurement of urine output. Urine dipstick analysis positive for hemaglobinuria but without microscopic RBCs identified is indicative of myoglobinuria. Myoglobinuria should be treated aggressively with fluid resuscitation using a crystalloid solution to maintain a urine output >100 mL/h. Alkalization of the urine to above pH 7.0 using sodium bicarbonate may help prevent crystallization of the myoglobin within the renal tubules. Mannitol has been shown to act as a free radical scavenger and may help prevent reperfusion injury. There is no indication to transfuse blood products in this patient based on the given information.

Bibliography

Buchbinder D, Karmody AM, Leather RP, et al. Hypertonic mannitol: its use in the prevention of revascularization syndrome after acute arterial ischemia. *Arch Surg* 1981;116:414.

Ditmars DM, Janevski PK, Contesti LA. Extremity trauma. In: Trunkey DD, Lewis FR (eds.), *Current Therapy of Trauma*. St. Louis, MO: Mosby, 1999.

Johansen KH, Watson JC. Compartment syndrome: pathophysiology, recognition, and management. In: Rutherford RB (ed.), *Vascular Surgery*. Philadelphia, PA: W.B. Saunders, 2000.

Perry MO, Shires GT III, Albert SA. Cellular changes with graded limb ischemia in reperfusion. *J Vasc Surg* 1984; 1:536.

Wilson RF, Georgiadis GM. Compartment syndrome. In Wilson RF, Walt AJ (eds.), *Management of Trauma: Pitfalls and Practice*. Baltimore, MD: Williams & Wilkins, 1996.

13. **(A)** Following extensive research by Rich and others, early misconceptions regarding the long-term effects of venous repair have been corrected. The previous approach of ligation of venous injuries often lead to venous hypertension and decreased outflow jeopardizing arterial repairs. Long-term effects included significant edema and venous insufficiency. A primary concern regarding venous repair was that the risk for pulmonary emboli increased significantly, especially if performed in the pelvis or lower extremity. Rich's work, however, showed this not to be the case. It is therefore now recommended that venous injuries be repaired if reasonably possible. Most repairs are made via lateral venorrhaphy or interposition vein grafts. Areas of questionable collateral flow, such as the innominate, common femoral, popliteal veins, and suprarenal vena cava, should always have repair attempted. Other venous injuries can be safely ligated should attempted repair be too dangerous because of the patients associated injuries.

Bibliography

Carrillo EH, et al. Abdominal vascular injuries. *J Trauma* 1997;43:164.

Feliciano DV, Burch JM, Graham JM. Abdominal vascular injury. In: Feliciano DV, Moore EE, Mattox KL (eds.), *Trauma*. Stamford, CT: Appleton & Lange, 1996.

Hardin WD, et al. Management of traumatic peripheral vein injuries. *Am J Surg* 1982;144:235–238.

Timberlake GA, et al. Venous injury: to repair or ligate, the dilemma. *J Vasc Surg* 1986;4:553–558.

Wilson RF, Dulchavsky S. Abdominal vascular trauma. In Wilson RF, Walt AJ (eds.), *Management of Trauma: Pitfalls and Practice*. Baltimore, MD: Williams & Wilkins, 1996.

Yelon JA, Scalea TM. Venous injuries of the lower extremities and pelvis: repair versus ligation. *J Trauma* 1992;33: 532–538.

14. **(E)** The mechanism for the pathogenesis of CN is complex, consisting of osmotic effects, direct tubular effects, as well as hemodynamic effects of the kidney.

Contrast medium (CM) is concentrated 100 times in the urine with a peak concentration of up to 2–500 mg/mL during the first 4-h period following administration of the dose. Consequently the osmotic load of the CM presented to the kidney is extremely high. CM exerts a low but significant chemical toxicity on several nephric enzyme systems, intracellular adenosine triphosphate (ATP), and isolated tubular cells. Finally the effect of CM on renal blood flow (RBF) is biphasic. A very brief increase in RBF is followed by a sustained decrease in RBF. This is unique to the kidney as CM induces vasodilatation in all other vascular beds.

IV administration of CM represents a very low risk for CN in otherwise healthy patients (<1%). The most important risk factors are decreased renal function followed by diabetes. The risk increases with the dose of CM. In patients with a normal serum creatinine, doses >300 mgI/mL are considered a risk factor. Adequate hydration is the most important preventive measure against CN. Controlled studies have failed to show an effect with prophylactic treatment with mannitol or furosemide while studies using *N*-acetylcysteine are inconclusive (Table 12-4).

Bibliography

Berg KJ. Nephrotoxicity related to contrast media. *Scand J Urol Nephrol* 2000;34:317–322.

Lautin EM, Freeman NJ, Schoenfeld AH, Bakal CW, Haramati N, Friedman AC, et al. Radiocontrast-associated renal dysfunction: incidence and risk factors. *Am J Roentgenol* 1991;157:49–58.

Solomon R, Werner C, Mann D, D'Elia J, Silva P. Effects of saline, mannitol, and furosemide on acute decreases in renal function induced by radiocontrast agents. *N Engl J Med* 1994;331:1416–1420.

TABLE 12-4   Contrast Nephropathy

Risk factors for contrast nephropathy
Preexisting reduced renal function
Diabetes mellitus
Vascular disease
Reduced ejection fraction
Dehydration
CHF
Intraarterial injection
High contrast dose
Repeated exposure over short period of time
Nephrotoxic drugs
High osmolar contrast media
Prevention of contrast nephropathy
Assess for risk factors
Prestudy serum creatinine
Alternative study in high-risk patients
IV hydration
Avoid mannitol, furosemide
Reduced contrast volume
5-day interval between contrast studies
Avoid hypovolemia, hypotension
Avoid nephrotoxic drugs
Prophylactic treatment with potential antidotes
Use low osmolar or iso-osmolar contrast media

15. **(E)** The popularity of observation for blunt liver trauma has lead to an increase in the incidence of hemobilia. Although still rare and often difficult to recognize, it should be included in the differential in any patient with GI bleeding following a liver injury. Hemobilia usually presents as jaundice, right upper quadrant pain, and/or GI bleeding although all three are present in only about 22% of patients. Following blunt liver trauma, arteries, veins, and bile ducts are often injured without rupture of the liver capsule. Healing in this area is inhibited by bile stasis as well as tissue necrosis as a result of the injury. This can subsequently erode into hepatic blood vessels resulting in bleeding into the biliary tree. Evaluation of a patient suspected of hemobilia depends on presentation as well as suspected etiology. Upper endoscopy may be attempted to demonstrate blood from the Ampula of Vater; however, as few as 12% are diagnostic and further studies are usually needed. Many patients with hemobilia and a history of blunt liver trauma will eventually have an abdominal CT performed as part of their diagnostic workup. Active bleeding or evidence of recent bleeding as demonstrated by pooling of CM, intraluminal clots, and biliary dilatation may be noted. Angiography is the definitive diagnostic study and identifies the vascular abnormality in over 90% of cases. Transarterial embolization is the treatment of choice for hemobilia. Studies have shown a success rate of 80–100% with a morbidity and mortality rate lower than that of surgery.

Bibliography

Green MHA, Duell RM, Johnson CD, et al. Haemobilia. *Br J Surg* 2001;88:773–786.

Krudy AG, Doppman JL, Bissonette MB, et al. Hemobilia: computed tomographic diagnosis. *Radiology* 1983;148:785–789.

Merrell SW, Schneider PD. Hemobilia—evolution of current diagnosis and treatment. *West J Med* 1991;155:621–625.

Samuels RS, Shriver M, Patel NH. Hemobilia after a gunshot injury to the liver. *Am J Roentgenol* 1996;166:1304.

Yoshida J, Donahue PE, Hyhus LM. Hemobilia: review of recent experience with a worldwide problem. *Am J Gastroenterol* 1987;82:448–453.

16. **(A)** Major abdominal vascular injuries are most often because of penetrating trauma. Frequently these

patients present in hypovolemic shock with multiple associated injuries. In theory, the proximal SMA could be ligated with bowel viability maintained through collateral circulation. In practice, however, the mortality rate from SMA injuries remains approximately 50%, most likely secondary to the profound hypovolemia these patients invariably suffer contributing to overall visceral ischemia as well as associated injuries. The mortality rate may be decreased to as low as 22% if definitive repair is performed. Injuries to the inferior mesenteric artery, on the other hand, can be safely ligated in the majority of patients without significant morbidity. The common iliac artery should be repaired whenever feasible. If ligated secondary to heavy contamination or severe instability, a four-compartment fasciotomy should be performed with an expected amputation rate as high as 50%. In the similar patient, the internal iliac artery may be safely ligated without significant sequela.

In patients with an intact SMA, the celiac artery may be safely ligated. Complete disruption of the celiac plexus should be treated with repair of the aortic injury then ligation of the individual celiac vessels. Without evidence of acute ischemia, either the radial or ulnar artery may be safely ligated with long-term patency of attempted repairs reported to be as low as 50%.

Bibliography

Aftabuddin M, et al. Management of isolated radial or ulnar arteries at the forearm. *J Trauma* 1995;38:149.

Burch JM, Richardson RJ, Martin RR, et al. Penetrating iliac vascular injuries: recent experience with 233 consecutive patients. *J Trauma* 1990;30:1450.

Carrillo EH, et al. Abdominal vascular injuries. *J Trauma* 1997;43:164.

Donahue TK, Strauch GO. Ligation as definitive management of injury to the superior mesenteric vein. *J Trauma* 1988;28:541.

Feliciano DV, Burch JM, Graham JM. Abdominal vascular injury. In: Feliciano DV, Moore EE, Mattox KL (eds.), *Trauma*, 3rd ed. Stamford, CT: Appleton & Lange, 1996, 615–632.

Gelberman RH, Blasingame JP, Fronek A, et al. Forearm arterial injuries. *J Hand Surg Am* 1979;4A:401.

Gelberman RH, Diego S, Nunley JA, et al. The results of radial and ulnar artery repair in the forearm. *J Bone Joint Surg Am* 1982;64A:383.

Lucas AE, Richardson JD, Flint LM, et al. Traumatic injury of the proximal superior mesenteric artery. *Ann Surg* 1981;193:30.

Pachter HL, Drager S, Godfrey N, et al. Traumatic injuries to the portal vein. *Ann Surg* 1979;189:383.

Salam AA, Stewart MT. New approach to wounds of the aortic bifurcation and inferior vena cava. *Surgery* 1985; 98:105.

Stone HH, Fabian TC, Turkleson ML. Wounds of the portal venous system. *World J Surg* 1982;6:335.

17. **(B)** Traditionally sustained compartment pressures greater than 30 mmHg have been considered the threshold for indication for compartment release. Such thresholds are dogmatic and notoriously lack sensitivity and specificity. More importantly, arterial perfusion pressure (mean arterial pressure – interstitial pressure) should be followed in evaluating for compartment syndrome. Many now recommend compartment release for a perfusion pressure 30 mmHg or less than the mean arterial pressure.

Bibliography

Johansen KH, Watson JC. Compartment syndrome: pathophysiology, recognition, and management. In: Rutherford BR (ed.), *Vascular Surgery*, 5th ed. Denver, CO: W.B. Saunders, 2000, 902–907.

Mabee JR, Bostwick TL. Pathophysiology and mechanisms of compartment syndrome. *Orthop Rev* 1993;22:175–181.

Matava MJ, Whitesides TE, Seiler JG, et al. Determination of the compartment pressure threshold of muscle ischemia in a canine model. *J Trauma* 1994;37:50–58.

Whitesides TE, Haney TC, Seiler JG, et al. Tissue pressure measurements as a determinant for the need of fasciotomy. *Clin Orthop* 1975;113:43–51.

18. **(B)** Laceration of the radial or ulnar artery is often clinically silent. Injuries to the ulnar artery are often accompanied by injuries to the ulnar nerve, which may be the only clinical finding. The ulnar artery is the predominant artery to the hand and should be repaired when feasible using interposition vein if a primary repair cannot be performed. The radial artery is the smaller of the two arteries that supply the hand. In the absence of obvious ischemia along its distribution, it may be ligated safely.

Bibliography

Ditmars DM, Janevski PK, Contesti LA. Upper extremity, hand, and peripheral nerve injuries. In: Trunkey DD, Lewis FR (eds.), *Current Therapy of Trauma*, 4th ed. St. Louis, MO: Mosby, 1999, 267–278.

Aftabuddin M, et al. Management of isolated radial or ulnar arteries at the forearm. *J Trauma* 1995;38:149.

19. **(D)** Penetrating neck trauma is a potentially complex entity and demands a thorough understanding of anatomy and treatment algorithms in order to avoid missed injuries. Essential to this is recognition of the three arbitrary zones of the neck.

Zone I—From clavicle to cricoid cartilage and includes the great vessels, lungs, trachea, esophagus, thoracic duct, spinal cord, and nerve trunks.
Zone II—From cricoid cartilage to the angle of the mandible and includes the common carotid arteries

and its branches, vertebral arteries, jugular veins, trachea, esophagus, spinal cord, and larynx.

Zone III—From angle of the mandible to the base of the skull and includes the pharynx, jugular veins, vertebral arteries, and distal internal carotid arteries.

In the hemodynamically *unstable* patient a neck exploration is mandatory regardless of the entrance site. In a hemodynamically *stable* patient most authors agree that penetrating injuries to zone I or III should be evaluated by arteriography, tracheobronchoscopy, esophagram, and esophagoscopy. Currently the management of zone II injuries is debated. Previously a mandatory neck exploration was recommended for all zone II injuries penetrating the platysma. This has been challenged and many authors now recommend arteriogram, tracheobronchoscopy, esophagram, and esophagoscopy.

This patient has a "blush" around the right common carotid artery bifurcation with careful examination revealing a laceration to the right internal carotid artery.

Bibliography
Ballard JL, McIntyre WB. Cervicothoracic vascular injuries. In: Rutherford RB (ed.), *Vascular Surgery*. Philadelphia, PA: W.B. Saunders, 2000.

Britt, LD, Peyser MB. Penetrating and blunt neck trauma. In: Mattox KL, Feliciano DV, Moore EE (eds.), *Trauma*, 4th ed. Stamford, CT: Appleton & Lange, 2000.

20. **(C)** For penetrating injuries to the carotid artery, level of consciousness is a key determinant for treatment decisions. This patient was described as hemodynamically stable with a normal level of consciousness. He should undergo right neck exploration and repair of the carotid artery injury. Because of the high incidence of associated injuries, tracheobronchoscopy and esophagoscopy should also be considered.

This injury is best approached through an anterior neck incision along the sternocleidomastoid muscle. Methods for arterial repair include primary repair, patch angioplasty, internal-to-external carotid artery transposition, and interposition grafting with saphenous vein or prosthetic conduit. Many authors advocate the use of shunts during the repair if the stump pressure is less than 60 mmHg or if there is minimal back bleeding. Unless there is an absolute contraindication (intracranial bleed, abdominal hemorrhage), systemic heparinization should be used.

Controversy exists regarding the appropriate management of similar patients with an associated neurologic defect. There are anecdotal reports of conversion of ischemic infarction to hemorrhagic infarction after revascularization. Carotid artery ligation is

reserved for those patients who sustain a carotid injury and present in a coma with no prograde flow in the internal carotid artery, uncontrollable hemorrhage, and when temporary shunt placement is technically impossible. In all other patients with neurologic deficit the outcome is better if repair is performed.

The final population is those patients with distal internal carotid artery (ICA) lesions. These are most often inaccessible and can be treated with ligation and anticoagulation.

Bibliography
Britt LD Peyser MB. Penetrating and blunt neck trauma. In: Mattox KL, Feliciano DV, Moore EE (eds.), *Trauma*, 4th ed. Stamford, CT: Appleton & Lange, 2000.

Ballard JL, McIntyre WB. Cervicothoracic vascular injuries. In: Rutherford RB (ed.), *Vascular Surgery*. Philadelphia, PA: W.B. Saunders, 2000.

21. **(C)** When compared to penetrating carotid artery injuries, blunt carotid injuries have a much poorer prognosis. A high index of suspicion allowing for early injury detection has been shown to improve outcomes.

Clinical features suggestive of blunt carotid injury include hematoma of the lateral neck, Horner's syndrome (ptosis, miosis, and anhidrosis), transient ischemic attacks, a lucid interval followed by decreased consciousness, and limb paresis in an alert patient. Despite or likely because of these somewhat nonspecific findings, many patients are not diagnosed until neurologic deficit occurs.

The patient as presented is hemodynamically stable, neurologically intact, with a right internal carotid artery dissection demonstrated by arteriogram. As with any other trauma patient, evaluating for possible associated injuries is essential therefore cervical spine x-rays should be obtained. Further workup for possible esophageal or tracheal injuries may necessitate CT scan or tracheobronchoscopy.

Because most carotid dissections extend intracranially, neck exploration is technically very difficult. Most authors recommend nonoperative management with 3–6 months of anticoagulation.

The carotid artery dissection should be followed routinely at 6–12 months interval as up to 30% may develop pseudoaneurysm. Pseudoaneurysm found in the acute setting should be treated with anticoagulation but subsequent ligation or excision and repair if surgically accessible.

Thrombosis of the carotid following blunt trauma is also treated with anticoagulation as operative management often leads to distal embolization.

Bibliography

Ballard JL, McIntyre WB. Cervicothoracic vascular injuries. In: Rutherford RB (ed.), *Vascular Surgery*. Philadelphia, PA: W.B. Saunders, 2000.

Britt LD, Peyser MB. Penetrating and blunt neck trauma. In: Mattox KL, Feliciano DV, Moore EE (eds.), *Trauma*, 4th ed. Stamford, CT: Appleton & Lange, 2000.

22. **(D)** The initial management of penetrating neck trauma is determined by hemodynamic stability. In the unstable patient, the diagnostic test of choice is immediate operative neck exploration. In the stable patient many vascular injuries may be diagnosed with duplex ultrasound studies, arteriogram, or even complete physical examination.

The operative approach is via an oblique incision along the anterior border of the sternocleidomastoid muscle. Bleeding from the internal jugular vein may be easily controlled with digital pressure while control of the injured vessel is obtained. If the lumen will not be compromised by more than 50%, a lateral venorrhaphy may be performed. If the vein has been transected primary repair will significantly compromise the lumen and an interposition graft should be performed.

In those patients who are hemodynamically unstable and have significant associated injuries, unilateral venous ligation is the treatment of choice.

Bibliography

Ballard JL, McIntyre WB. Cervicothoracic vascular injuries. In: Rutherford RB (ed.), *Vascular Surgery*. Philadelphia, PA: W.B. Saunders, 2000.

Britt, LD, Peyser MB. Penetrating and blunt neck trauma. In: Mattox KL, Feliciano DV, Moore EE (eds.), *Trauma*, 4th ed. Stamford, CT: Appleton & Lange, 2000.

Yelon JA, Scalea TM. Venous injuries of the lower extremities and pelvis: repair versus ligation. *J Trauma* 1992; 33:532.

23. **(D)** Mechanism of injury is a significant part of any trauma patient's history as it may suggest an increased risk for specific injuries. The history of a steering wheel deformity implies a significant deceleration force to the thoracic aorta and great vessels. This is further suggested by the supplied CXR, which demonstrates a widened mediastinum. The next step in evaluating this hemodynamically stable patient is spiral CT of the chest.

Blunt injury of the thoracic aorta and the intrathoracic great vessels is a complex and life-threatening entity. Shearing stress because of rapid deceleration leads to rupture of the aorta at sites of fixation. The most common site is the descending aorta at the level of the ligamentum arteriosum. Injuries of the great vessels occur but they are because of direct contact with the anterior chest wall.

There are clinical findings associated with traumatic rupture of the thoracic aorta and intrathoracic great vessel injury. These include flail chest, a fractured first or second rib, and pulse deficits in the upper extremity, hoarseness or voice changes without laryngeal injury, fractured sternum and history of high-speed deceleration. Any of these should increase your suspicion for a thoracic aortic disruption. Neurologic changes should initiate a search for intracranial injury, cervical carotid artery injury, and intrathoracic great vessel injury.

Radiographic findings associated with traumatic thoracic aortic tears include mediastinal widening (>8 cm on supine films), esophagus and tracheal deviation to the right, obliteration of the aortopulmonary window, apical cap, and obscuring of the aortic knob.

It should be noted that many authors argue the use of chest CT in this setting and would proceed directly to arteriogram. This, however, remains controversial as more and more institutions are using chest CT as a screening tool with arteriogram reserved for those patients with positive findings on CT. Benefits of performing a spiral CT of the chest include a negative predictive value of 99.9%.

Bibliography

Ballard JL, McIntyre WB. Cervicothoracic vascular injuries. In: Rutherford RB (ed.), *Vascular Surgery*. Philadelphia, PA: W.B. Saunders, 2000.

Mattox KL, Wall MJ, LeMaire SA. Injury to the thoracic great vessels. In: Mattox KL, Feliciano DV, Moore EE (eds.), *Trauma*, 4th ed. Stamford, CT: Appleton & Lange, 2000.

Pate JW, Fabian TC, Walker WA. Acute traumatic rupture of the aortic isthmus: repair with cardiopulmonary bypass. *Ann Thorac Surg* 1995;59:90–99.

24. **(E)** The diagnosis of thoracic aortic injury requires a high index of suspicion based on clinical findings and mechanisms of injury. Once suspected, the initial evaluation remains controversial although spiral CT is quickly becoming a widely accepted screening tool. Arteriogram remains the gold standard for diagnosis of aortic injury and if not the initial diagnostic test, is almost always used as a confirmatory study following a suspicious CT.

Aortic injuries are described using multiple classification systems, all based on anatomic features of the disruption. Involvement of the ascending aorta (DeBakey type I or II, Stanford type A) is the single most important anatomic determinant related to clinical behavior of the injury.

The supplied arteriogram demonstrates a normal aorta, left common carotid, and left subclavian artery.

Close evaluation of the innominate artery reveals a pseudoaneurysm extending beyond the bifurcation into the common carotid and subclavian arteries.

This patient's CT scan was used as a screening test and revealed blood in the mediastinum but was not diagnostic. The patient's progressive neurologic changes are explained by the extension of the pseudoaneurysm along the subclavian artery and subsequent vascular compromise.

Bibliography

Ballard JL, McIntyre WB. Cervicothoracic vascular injuries. In: Rutherford RB (ed.), *Vascular Surgery*. Philadelphia, PA: W.B. Saunders, 2000.

Mattox KL, Wall MJ, LeMaire SA. Injury to the thoracic great vessels. In: Mattox KL, Feliciano DV, Moore EE (eds.), *Trauma*, 4th ed. Stamford, CT: Appleton & Lange, 2000.

25. **(D)** With the diagnosis of an innominate pseudoaneurysm and neurologic changes, the patient requires appropriate preoperative evaluation for concomitant injuries, stabilization with aggressive blood pressure control, followed by surgical management of the pseudoaneurysm.

    The approach to the innominate artery is via a mediastinotomy. A partial occlusion clamp is then placed along the ascending aorta proximal to the pseudoaneurysm. A Dacron graft is then placed end-to-side on the ascending aorta. The mediastinotomy can be extended to the right neck or the medial head of the clavicle resected for increased exposure of the distal pseudoaneurysm. Temporary shunting should be used if the stump pressure in either the carotid or innominate arteries is less than 60 mmHg or there is not vigorous back bleeding. At this point, the pseudoaneurysm can then be resected and the aortic stump oversewn.

    In this case, a bifurcated graft was used for distal anastomosis to both the subclavian and common carotid arteries.

Bibliography

Ballard JL, McIntyre WB. Cervicothoracic vascular injuries. In: Rutherford RB (ed.), *Vascular Surgery*. Philadelphia, PA: W.B. Saunders, 2000.

Mattox KL, Wall MJ, LeMaire SA. Injury to the thoracic great vessels. In: Mattox KL, Feliciano DV, Moore EE (eds.), *Trauma*, 4th ed. Stamford, CT: Appleton & Lange, 2000.

26. **(B)** CT scan of the chest revealed blood in the mediastinum and what appeared to be an injury at the aortic isthmus. Arteriogram confirms this diagnosis and demonstrates an aortic tear just opposite the ligamentum arteriosum.

Injuries to the aortic isthmus are the most common cause of death because of aortic injury secondary to blunt thoracic trauma. In comparison to the remainder of the aorta, the aortic isthmus is inherently weak and acts as a point of fixation allowing for the transmission of deceleration forces onto the vessel wall. Those injuries that are contained within a mediastinal hematoma may survive to reach the hospital where they must be recognized early based on mechanism of injury.

After establishing the diagnosis of an aortic transection, the patient should be stabilized and concomitant injuries evaluated. One should closely monitor the cardiac rhythm, urine output, oxygen saturation, and blood pressure. Antihypertensives are often needed to maintain a systolic blood pressure less than 120 mmHg.

As in this case, based on CXR and mechanism of injury, a CT of the chest is often used as a screening tool; however, the arteriogram remains the gold standard for diagnosing aortic injuries.

Bibliography

Ballard JL, McIntyre WB. Cervicothoracic vascular injuries. In: Rutherford RB (ed.), *Vascular Surgery*. Philadelphia, PA: W.B. Saunders, 2000.

Mattox KL, Wall MJ, LeMaire SA. Injury to the thoracic great vessels. In: Mattox KL, Feliciano DV, Moore EE (eds.), *Trauma*, 4th ed. Stamford, CT: Appleton & Lange, 2000.

Pate JW, Fabian TC, Walker WA. Acute traumatic rupture of the aortic isthmus: repair with cardiopulmonary bypass. *Ann Thorac Surg* 1995;59:90–99.

27. **(B)** Although there are multiple approaches to the repair of an aortic isthmus injury, the primary concern is prevention of rupture prior to repair and then prevention of postoperative paraplegia secondary to spinal ischemia. Paraplegia develops with a rate of 2–20% in emergency situations.

    The injured aorta is approached through a left posterolateral thoracotomy in the fourth intercostals space with the patient in a right decubitus position. From this approach the aortic arch, left carotid, and left subclavian arteries can be controlled to allow repair of the injured segment. Only 20% of injuries can be repaired primarily with the remainder requiring prosthetic graft placement via one of several methods.

    The "clamp and sew" method is useful when the hematoma has ruptured and does not require bypass. Unfortunately the surgeon has less than 30 min of aortic cross clamp time in which to complete the repair and return blood flow, as this method offers no spinal protection. If the injury extends to the arch and ascending aorta this method is inadequate.

A second method uses cardiopulmonary bypass from the right atrium to the distal arterial bed. This allows repair of the aortic tear and any extension of the injury. It also provides cerebroperfusion through the intercostal arteries and protects the spinal cord from ischemia. In rare cases it can be converted to total cardiopulmonary bypass with cardiac arrest if necessary. Unfortunately this requires full anticoagulation and is contraindicated in patients with associated injuries at high risk for bleeding.

Another method uses left heart bypass from the left atrium to the femoral artery. A centrifugal pump is used which does not require an oxygenator or systemic anticoagulation. This method offers the spinal protection of cardiopulmonary bypass without the risks associated with anticoagulation.

The final method is the use of thoracic aortic stents. There are case reports and small retrospective reviews showing the efficacy of endovascular stents in trauma. More studies need to be performed to ensure its overall safety. The ability to dramatically decrease postoperative paraplegia and minimize the need for full anticoagulation are two factors that make this ant attractive treatment alternative.

Bibliography

Ballard JL, McIntyre WB. Cervicothoracic vascular injuries. In: Rutherford RB (ed.), *Vascular Surgery*. Philadelphia, PA: W.B. Saunders, 2000.

Mattox KL, Wall MJ, LeMaire SA. Injury to the thoracic great vessels. In: Mattox KL, Feliciano DV, Moore EE (eds.), *Trauma*, 4th ed. Stamford, CT: Appleton & Lange, 2000.

Pate JW, Fabian TC, Walker WA. Acute traumatic rupture of the aortic isthmus: repair with cardiopulmonary bypass. *Ann Thorac Surg* 1995;59:90–99.

28. **(C)** Many patients suffering penetrating trauma to the chest present initially as hemodynamically stable only to decompensate acutely. Such patients must be carefully evaluated with attention to subtle clinical findings that may be the only warning of impending instability. Standard advanced trauma life support (ATLS) protocols should be followed including evaluation for a patent airway and adequate respirations, as well as adequate vascular access with two large bore peripheral IVs.

The location of the injury will determine structures at risk. Abdominal injuries must be considered as the diaphragm can elevate to the level of the nipples anteriorly and the tip of the scapula posteriorly. With an injury between the areas bordered by the nipples laterally, the heart, lungs, aorta, great vessels, trachea, thoracic duct, phrenic nerve, and esophagus are all at risk of injury.

A CXR is essential to assess for pneumothorax, hemothorax, widened mediastinum, and pneumoperitoneum.

Tube thoracostomy is often needed because of respiratory compromise secondary to pneumothorax and/or hemothorax. A chest tube also allows for quantification of the bleeding into the chest and the presence of large air leaks suggestive of injury to the bronchial tree.

Acute pericardial effusion of <30 mL may cause pericardial tamponade. Echocardiogram is often useful in detecting small amounts of pericardial hemorrhage prior to the development of tamponade. Signs often present with cardiac tamponade include JVD, muffled heart sounds, narrowed pulse pressure, and pulsus paradoxis. Pericardiocentesis is a useful maneuver that may buy the time needed until a surgical team is assembled. Repeated aspiration may be needed; however, this should never delay operative intervention.

Esophagram may be indicated based on the clinical symptoms such as dysphagia or location of the injury (i.e., penetrating zone I or midline neck). This, however, is not done as part of the initial assessment.

Bibliography

Ballard JL, McIntyre WB. Cervicothoracic vascular injuries. In: Rutherford RB (ed.), *Vascular Surgery*. Philadelphia, PA: W.B. Saunders, 2000.

Mattox KL, Wall MJ, LeMaire SA. Injury to the thoracic great vessels. In: Mattox KL, Feliciano DV, Moore EE (eds.), *Trauma*, 4th ed. Stamford, CT: Appleton & Lange, 2000.

Trunkey D. *Vascular Trauma*. In: Lynne G (ed.), *Current Surgical Therapy*, 7th ed. St. Louis, MO: Mosby, 2001;1135–1139.

29. **(D)** Penetrating injuries to the great vessels are life-threatening emergencies. Although many will exsanguinate prior to arrival in the ER, others will present hemodynamically stable only to rapidly decompensate in the ED. Early diagnosis and prompt treatment is the key to decreased morbidity and mortality.

Additional injuries contribute significantly to overall morbidity of great vessel injuries and should be assessed at the time of the initial operation through direct visualization, bronchoscopy, and/or esophagoscopy of the lungs, heart, diaphragm, thoracic duct, trachea, and esophagus.

A mediasternotomy provides access to all of the great vessels with the exception of the proximal left subclavian artery. Injuries in the proximity of the proximal left subclavian artery are best approached through an anterolateral thoracotomy through the third or fourth interspace. If the vascular injury extends distally, a "trapdoor" incision (combining a limited sternotomy and a supraclavicular incision with resection of the medial clavicle) may be performed giving access to the distal left subclavian artery.

Once proximal and distal vascular control is obtained, small lacerations may be debrided and repaired primarily while larger defects require reverse saphenous vein or prosthetic material for graft.

Bibliography

Ballard JL, McIntyre WB. Cervicothoracic vascular injuries. In: Rutherford RB (ed.), *Vascular Surgery*. Philadelphia, PA: W.B. Saunders, 2000.

Mattox KL, Wall MJ, LeMaire SA. Injury to the thoracic great vessels. In: Mattox KL, Feliciano DV, Moore EE (eds.), *Trauma*, 4th ed. Stamford, CT: Appleton & Lange, 2000.

Trunkey D. Vascular trauma. In: Lynne G (ed.), *Current Surgical Therapy*. St. Louis, MO: Mosby, 2001;1135–1139.

30. **(B)** The left subclavian artery originates at the aortic arch. The subclavian artery then becomes the axillary artery as it crosses the lateral border of the first rib. The axillary artery then becomes the brachial artery at the lateral border of the teres major muscle.

In the axilla, the pectoralis minor muscle crosses anterior to the axillary artery, dividing the vessel into three segments. The first segment of the axillary artery is medial to the pectoralis minor muscle and lateral to the clavicle. It gives off only the supreme thoracic artery. The second segment lies beneath the pectoralis minor muscle and gives off the thoracoacromial and lateral thoracic arteries. The third segment of the axillary artery is lateral to the pectoralis minor muscle and gives rise to the subscapular and the anterior and posterior circumflex humeral arteries.

The vascular injury demonstrated on the arteriogram is the axillary artery. Along with a vascular injury there is also a humerus fracture at the same level.

Bibliography

Graham JM, Mattox KL, Feliciano DV, DeBakey. Vascular injuries of the axilla. *Ann Surg* 1982;195:232.

Ballard JL, McIntyre WB. Cervicothoracic vascular injuries. In: Rutherford RB (ed.), *Vascular Surgery*. Philadelphia, PA: W.B. Saunders, 2000.

Shackford SR, Rich NH. Peripheral vascular injury. In: Mattox KL, Feliciano DV, Moore EE (eds.), *Trauma*, 4th ed. Stamford, CT: Appleton & Lange, 2000.

31. **(C)** Recently, some authors have recommended non-operative management for a select group of patients suffering low velocity injuries, with a minimal intimal defect (<5 mm), a small pseudoaneurysm (<5 mm), intact distal circulation, and reliable patient compliance.

Failure to meet each of these criteria delegate the patient to required operative intervention.

Because of the risk of irreversible cellular damage, warm ischemia time should not exceed 6 h. Should extensive orthopedic manipulation at the site of the vascular injury be required, many now recommend temporary vascular shunting using a heparin bonded shunt in order to restore blood flow while the fracture is stabilized. Following fracture repair the vascular repair may then be performed without the risk of disruption by subsequent bone manipulation.

In the presented patient, the arteriogram reveals an axillary artery injury. Proximal control is obtained through an infraclavicular incision with extension into the anterior axilla for distal control. The pectoralis minor tendon may be divided for complete exposure of the middle section of the axillary artery. Once controlled both proximally and distally, the artery is then debrided at the injury site with primary repair if possible. For significant tissue loss or destruction, an interposition vein graft or prosthetic interposition graft can be performed.

Postoperatively the extremity is at risk for compartment syndrome and consideration should be given for a compartment release procedure at the time of the initial surgery based on the ischemia time.

Bibliography

Ballard JL, McIntyre WB. Cervicothoracic vascular injuries. In: Rutherford RB (ed.), *Vascular Surgery*. Philadelphia, PA: W.B. Saunders, 2000.

Graham JM, Mattox KL, Feliciano DV, DeBakey. Vascular injuries of the axilla. *Ann Surg* 1982;195:232.

Shackford SR, Rich NH. Peripheral vascular injury. In: Mattox KL, Feliciano DV, Moore EE (eds.), *Trauma*, 4th ed. Stamford, CT: Appleton & Lange, 2000.

32. **(D)** The external iliac artery becomes the common femoral artery as it passes beneath the inguinal ligament. In the leg the common femoral artery divides into the superficial femoral artery and the deep femoral (profunda femoris) arteries. The superficial femoral artery becomes the popliteal artery that then divides below the knee to form the posterior tibial, anterior tibial, and peroneal arteries. Significant collateral blood supply is found at the level of the knee through various geniculate branches from the profunda femoris, superficial femoral, and popliteal arteries. This collateral circulation may develop to supply the distal extremity in patients with chronic peripheral vascular disease but fails to provide sufficient blood flow in the acutely injured extremity.

The arteriogram presented demonstrates a lesion at the left superficial femoral artery.

Bibliography

Feliciano DV, et al. Management of vascular injuries in the lower extremities. *J Trauma* 1988;28:319.

Weaver FA, Hood DB, Yellin AE. Vascular injuries of the extremities. In: Rutherford RB (ed.), *Vascular Surgery*. Philadelphia, PA: W.B. Saunders, 2000.

33. **(B)** The initial approach to this injury is proximal control of the injured vessel to limit blood loss. This should be accomplished prior to aggressive volume resuscitation in an effort to restore a normal blood pressure.

Proximal control is best obtained in the inguinal region at the common femoral, profunda femoris, and superficial femoral arteries. Once proximal control is achieved, an incision is made over the injury along the medial aspect of the distal thigh. Devitalized muscle and tissue are often present and should be debrided prior to closure of the wound.

Once isolated, the superficial femoral artery should be sharply debrided. Thrombectomy is then performed using a balloon-tipped catheter and heparin solution both proximally and distally.

Primary anastomosis is often possible with minimal vessel destruction and with modest proximal and distal vessel immobilization. With significant tissue destruction, however, a reverse saphenous vein graft should be placed.

Postoperatively, the extremity is at high risk for compartment syndrome and consideration should be given for a compartment release procedure at the time of the initial surgery based on the length of the ischemia time.

Bibliography

Feliciano DV, et al. Management of vascular injuries in the lower extremities. *J Trauma* 1988;28:319.

Weaver FA, Hood DB, Yellin AE. Vascular injuries of the extremities. In: Rutherford RB (ed.), *Vascular Surgery*. Philadelphia, PA: W.B. Saunders, 2000.

CHAPTER 13

Pediatric Trauma
Kristine A.K. Lombardozzi and L.R. Scherer III
Questions

1. The care of pediatric trauma patients differs from the care of adult trauma patients for many reasons. Which of these statements accurately describes the differences between these two patient populations?

   (A) Children have a lower body surface area to weight ratio and therefore are less susceptible to hypothermia.
   (B) The pediatric skeletal system has areas of growth and remodeling which make bones less susceptible to injury.
   (C) Children have greater physiologic reserve than adults and do not manifest signs of shock until they have lost >45% of their blood volume.
   (D) Children's torsos are broad and shallow, providing greater protection of solid organs.
   (E) None of the above.

2. An understanding of anatomy is essential to the management of the pediatric airway. Which of these statements is true?

   (A) Tonsil and adenoid tissue rarely cause airway narrowing.
   (B) The larynx in a child is located more posteriorly than in adult airways.
   (C) The membranous portion of the child's trachea is thinner and is more easily damaged than in the adult.
   (D) A cuffed endotracheal tube is not required in young children because the arytenoid cartilage narrows enough to act as a functional cuff.
   (E) Children have a proportionally large occiput which causes neck extension and subsequent airway narrowing.

3. Emergent intubation of the traumatized child is performed using rapid sequence intubation (RSI). During RSI, one must be sure to

   (A) use an oral airway during preoxygenation in all cases
   (B) attempt nasotracheal intubation because it is easily performed in children
   (C) not give sedation, given children's propensity to hypotension after traumatic injury
   (D) give repeated doses of succinylcholine until the desired effect is achieved
   (E) use a noncuffed endotracheal tube in children less than 8 years of age.

4. An 8-year-old child, who has suffered massive facial and chest injuries in a motor vehicle crash, has undergone multiple unsuccessful attempts at intubation by an experienced physician. The child is now hypoxic with oxygen saturations in the 70s despite bag-mask ventilation. What should be the next step in his management?

   (A) surgical cricothyroidotomy
   (B) continued bag-mask ventilation with another attempt at intubation by another physician
   (C) nasotracheal intubation
   (D) emergency tracheostomy
   (E) place an orogastric tube and attempt intubation after the stomach is decompressed

5. The signs of hypovolemia in children differ from those of an adult because

   (A) a child will have minimal signs of shock with a blood loss of 20%
   (B) the presence of hypotension in a child suggests a blood loss of 30%
   (C) poor skin perfusion is not a reliable indicator of blood loss in children
   (D) a child's circulating blood volume is >100 cc/kg
   (E) a systolic blood pressure of 40 mmHg is appropriate in children less than 6 months of age.

6. A 10-month-old female presents after involvement in a motor vehicle crash. On initial examination, her heart rate is 220 bpm, her systolic blood pressure is 80 mmHg, she is difficult to arouse and her skin is cyanotic. The appropriate steps for resuscitation include

   (A) 10cc/kg bolus of warm saline solution
   (B) saline administration until her urine output is greater than 3 cc/kg/h.
   (C) a 20 cc/kg bolus of packed red blood cells (PRBCs) if her vital signs do not normalize after two saline boluses.
   (D) continued resuscitation until her heart rate is less than 100 bpm and her systolic blood pressure is greater than 110 mmHg.
   (E) consider operative intervention if she does not stabilize after receiving three saline boluses and two boluses of PRBCs

7. A 3-week-old child is involved in a motor vehicle crash. He was restrained in a car seat at the time of the crash. He is noted by paramedics to have a systolic blood pressure of 70 mmHg, a heart rate of 170 bpm, is awake and has a large scalp laceration as his only identifiable injury. Based on his pediatric trauma score (PTS), the paramedic decides to transport him to the local emergency department (ED). Which statement is true regarding the PTS and how it relates to this patient's care?

   (A) The PTS is based on the examination on arrival to the ED and therefore should not have been used to guide triage of this patient.
   (B) The PTS is based solely on the evaluation of the patient's airway, systolic blood pressure, and Glascow Coma Scale.
   (C) A score of +10 requires triage to the nearest trauma center.
   (D) The PTS is designed to estimate mortality based on severity of injury and is used to triage a patient to the appropriate hospital.
   (E) The PTS does not apply to children weighing less than 10 kg and therefore should not have been used to guide decision making for this patient.

8. An 8-year-old female arrives to the ED after being involved in a motor vehicle crash. The paramedics were unable to establish intravenous access prior to arrival. On arrival, her heart rate is 150 bpm and her systolic blood pressure is 70 mmHg. She appears lethargic. Which of the statements below is *correct*?

   (A) This patient is significantly hypovolemic and therefore should have central venous access.
   (B) If attempts at peripheral venous access are unsuccessful, this patient should have an intraosseous access placed.
   (C) A venous cutdown is no longer a useful means of establishing intravenous access and should not be attempted.
   (D) Central venous access is a rapid and safe means of obtaining intravenous access when peripheral access is not possible.
   (E) Subclavian central venous access should not be attempted in a hypovolemic child because difficulty in cannulating the vein and the subsequent risk of pneumothorax.

9. A 5-year-old child presents to the ED after being struck while riding his bicycle. Initial vitals are: heart rate 120 bpm, systolic blood pressure 100 mmHg, respiratory rate of 40 breaths/min, and oxygen saturations of 88% on a 100% nonrebreather face mask. On examination, he is crying vigorously, moving all extremities, has bruising to both upper quadrants of the abdomen and his abdomen is firm, distended, and extremely tender on palpation in both upper quadrants. As the trauma evaluation continues, what is the next step in his management?

   (A) placement of bilateral chest tubes
   (B) place a nasogastric tube (NG), repeat vital signs, and reexamine of the abdomen
   (C) prepare the patient for the operating room given the obvious signs of a duodenal injury
   (D) transport the patient to computed tomographic (CT) scan for imaging of his head and abdomen
   (E) none of the above

10. Which statement is correct regarding the most appropriate way to evaluate this child's abdomen for injury?

   (A) A focused abdominal sonogram for trauma (FAST) examination should be performed because the presence of free fluid would necessitate evaluation in the operating room.
   (B) A diagnostic peritoneal lavage (DPL) is the best evaluation because it would exclude a duodenal injury.
   (C) A CT scan should be used because it is very sensitive and specific for hollow viscus injury detection.

(D) A CT scan with intravenous (IV) contrast is the preferred imaging modality in hemodynamically unstable patients.

(E) A CT scan with IV contrast should be performed to best delineate solid organ injuries, free fluid, and any retroperitoneal abnormalities.

11. A 12-year-old female presents to the ED after being involved in a motor vehicle crash. She was a restrained front seat passenger in a vehicle struck on the passenger side. On arrival she is alert and hemodynamically stable. She complains of pain in her left shoulder and left lower chest. She demonstrates tenderness on palpation inferior to her left costal margin. Which of the following in not an appropriate part of her evaluation?

(A) obtain a chest radiograph to evaluate for thoracic injury

(B) obtain a radiograph of her left shoulder to evaluate for a bony injury

(C) evaluate her urine for hematuria

(D) admit her to the hospital, follow serial abdominal examinations and plan to perform a CT scan if she becomes hemodynamically unstable

(E) perform a CT scan of her abdomen

12. A CT scan of her abdomen was obtained (see Fig. 13-1). This is her only injury. What should be done during her hospitalization?

(A) admit her to the intensive care unit (ICU)

(B) take her to the operating room for splenectomy

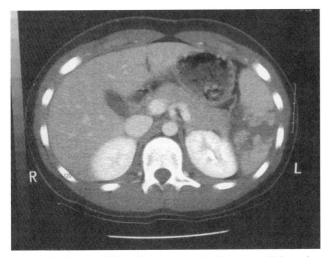

FIG. 13-1 Abdominal CT of 12-year-old female after motor vehicle crash.

(C) take her to the operating room for splenectomy if she requires transfusion of greater than 10 cc/kg of PRBCs for anemia

(D) follow her as an inpatient for at least 7 days to be certain this injury will not bleed

(E) perform a repeat CT scan of the abdomen before she is released to home

13. This child becomes hemodynamically unstable while being observed in the ICU. Her blood pressure was only transiently responsive to fluid boluses and she required transfusion of PRBCs. After receiving 4 units of PRBCs she is taken to the operating room. Which statement is false?

(A) Splenorraphy may be undertaken if the patient is hemodynamically stable and is adequately resuscitated.

(B) The use of horizontal or vertical mattress sutures, omental buttressing, argon beam coagulation, hemostatic agents, or the use of a mesh bag are all acceptable forms of splenic salvage in children.

(C) Total splenectomy should be performed for any injury greater than grade III because of the high risk for rebleeding from such injuries in children.

(D) Complete mobilization of the spleen is necessary for adequate inspection of the parenchyma for injury.

(E) If the patient has had excessive hemorrhage or continues to demonstrate physiologic signs of under resuscitation, splenectomy should be performed.

14. Overwhelming postsplenectomy sepsis

(A) occurs in greater than 10% of children who have undergone splenectomy for trauma

(B) has greater than 60% mortality

(C) occurs most often greater than 5 years after splenectomy

(D) can be prevented by the administration of vaccines against pneumococcus and *H. influenzae*.

(E) can initially present as a simple febrile illness

15. Which statement is true regarding pediatric gastric injuries?

    (A) Gastric injuries are less common in children than adults.

    (B) Gastric perforations from blunt trauma are usually found on the lesser curvature.

    (C) Gastric injuries should be suspected if the NG aspirate is blood tinged.

    (D) Gastric injuries in the prepyloric region should not be primarily repaired.

    (E) Traumatic gastric injuries can be conservatively managed if the patient has no peritoneal signs.

16. A 6-year-old female presents to the ED after being kicked by a horse. She has a heart rate of 120 bpm and a systolic blood pressure of 100 mmHg on arrival. She complains of pain in her right upper quadrant and has tenderness on palpation of that area. A CT scan of the abdomen is obtained (see Fig. 13-2). Which statement is true regarding her management?

    (A) All blunt hepatic injuries greater than grade II should be observed in the ICU for 48 h.

    (B) This patient should remain on bed rest until a follow up CT scan showing no worsening of the injury has been obtained.

    (C) The management of these injuries has not been prospectively evaluated and therefore their management cannot be standardized.

    (D) Children with grade IV injuries can return to normal activities in 3 months.

    (E) No routine postinjury imaging of these patients is indicated.

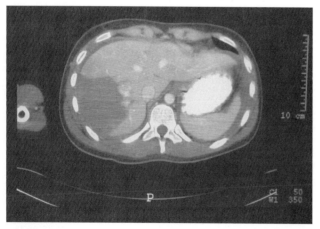

FIG. 13-2 Abdominal CT of 6-year-old female after suffering a horse kick to the abdomen.

17. Nonoperative management of blunt hepatic injuries can be made difficult by the occurrence of complications. Which statement is true regarding these complications?

    (A) Complications occur in 10% of cases.

    (B) These complications do not have significant morbidity associated with them.

    (C) Abscess, biloma, and hemobilia are known complications of blunt hepatic injury.

    (D) The complications from nonoperative management of blunt hepatic injuries differ greatly from those complications encountered after operative management.

    (E) Most of these complications require operative management.

18. Which statement is false regarding operative management of hepatic injuries?

    (A) If initial control of bleeding cannot be obtained with packing, measures such as the Pringle maneuver and mobilization of the liver with total vascular occlusion can be performed.

    (B) The use of an atrial-caval shunt is difficult to perform and usually unnecessary.

    (C) Expanding hematomas should be incised and the bleeding vessels should be directly ligated or cauterized.

    (D) Limited segmental debridement of devitalized tissue is safe but major resection should be avoided given its mortality rate of 25–30%.

    (E) If the patient is suspected of having a retrohepatic caval injury and bleeding has been controlled by packing, the packing should be left in the abdomen, the patient returned to the ICU for resuscitation and plans should be made for packing removal in 12 h.

19. A 10-year-old male presents to the ED after a motor vehicle crash. He was a backseat passenger restrained with a lap belt. He is hemodynamically normal and has no complaints of abdominal pain. This finding is noted on his physical examination (see Fig. 13-3). He has no complaints of pain on palpation of his abdomen. Which of the following statements are *incorrect*?

    (A) An abdominal CT scan should be obtained.

    (B) A DPL should be performed because CT scans are too insensitive to diagnose a hollow viscus injury.

(C) The patient should be admitted for observation and serial abdominal examinations.

(D) This patient is at risk for a lumbar spine fracture.

(E) None of the above.

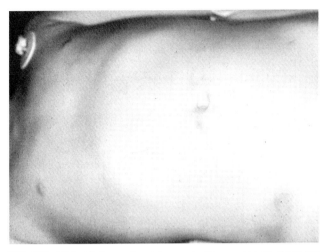

FIG. 13-3 Clinical finding on the abdomen of a 10-year-old male after motor vehicle crash.

20. A CT scan of the abdomen is obtained and demonstrates free fluid in the pelvis without solid organ injury. A hollow viscus injury is suspected. Which of the following statements is *incorrect* regarding this situation?

(A) Often, unexplained free fluid in the peritoneum is the only CT detected abnormality in cases of bowel injury.

(B) These injuries will become clinically apparent with serial abdominal examinations and physiologic monitoring within approximately 24 h.

(C) There has been no increase in mortality or morbidity with recognition and treatment of these injuries within 48 h.

(D) Usually small intestinal injuries can be managed with either primary repair or resection and primary anastomosis.

(E) Colonic injuries can be managed with primary repair or segmental resection with primary anastomosis, regardless of location, if there is no excessive contamination, other associated major injuries or ongoing physiologic derangement.

21. A 10-year-old male presents in the late evening with rectal bleeding. He states he fell from a ladder on the playground at school and landed onto concrete on his buttocks. On external examination there appears to be bruising and abrasions to the buttocks bilaterally. A rectal examination cannot be performed secondary to pain. Which of these statements is true?

(A) Rectal injuries are common after falls.

(B) An examination under anesthesia (EUA) should be performed.

(C) Injuries to the rectum below the internal sphincter should always be managed with diversion.

(D) A sexual assault examination is not needed given the mechanism of injury.

(E) Anoscopy should be performed in the ED after the administration of pain medication.

22. Regarding thoracic injuries in children, which of these statements is true?

(A) Less than 20% of children with a thoracic injury will have other organ system injuries.

(B) Thoracic injuries are the leading cause of traumatic deaths.

(C) Children will usually have rib fractures if they have sustained a significant thoracic injury.

(D) A pulmonary contusion is the most common thoracic injury.

(E) Tracheal injuries are less common in children than adults.

23. A 6-year-old child presents to the ED after being struck by a car. The initial trauma evaluation found bilateral pneumothoraces. Chest tubes were placed (see Fig. 13-4). A massive air leak is noted from the right chest tubes. Which of the following is true?

    (A) This injury occurs more commonly in adults than in children.

    (B) This patient should undergo esophagoscopy to best delineate this injury.

    (C) This injury will require operative management.

    (D) Children who suffer bilateral pulmonary contusions will require mechanical ventilatory support more often than an adult who suffers the same injury.

    (E) All of the above.

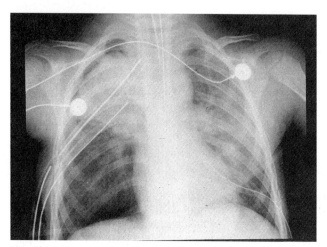

FIG. 13-4   Chest x-ray findings after chest tube placement in a 6-year-old female.

24. In which of these situations is ED thoracotomy appropriate?

    (A) A 5-year-old child, involved in a motor vehicle crash, who arrives in the ED asystolic.

    (B) An 8-year-old child, suffering from a gunshot wound to the chest, who arrives in the ED asystolic with fixed and dilated pupils. The paramedics estimate the time from injury to ED arrival was 15 min.

    (C) A 10-year-old child, involved in a motor vehicle crash, who arrives in the ED hypotensive and tachycardic. The child subsequently suffers a cardiopulmonary arrest. This does not improve despite pediatric advanced life support (PALS) algorithms and intubation. Bilateral chest tubes are placed and 1000 cc of blood is drained from the left chest.

    (D) ED thoracotomy is never appropriate in children.

    (E) A 4-year-old child, involved in a motor vehicle crash, arrives in the ED with an agonal cardiac rhythm, no blood pressure, and fixed and dilated pupils.

25. A 3-year-old child presents to the ED after being run over by a car (see Fig. 13-5). Which statement is *incorrect*?

    (A) Treatment consists of supportive care with head elevation.

    (B) This syndrome results from sudden compression of the abdomen or chest against a closed glottis.

    (C) Brain injuries are commonly associated with this syndrome and are usually the result of massive hemorrhage.

    (D) Cardiac injuries are rare with this injury type.

    (E) The physical findings are a result of capillary extravasation caused from transmission of pressure through the vena cava.

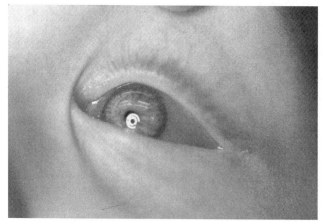

FIG. 13-5   Clinical finding in a 3-year-old after being run over by a car.

26. Which statement is true regarding pediatric fractures?

    (A) Children have a lower rate of fractures after trauma than the adult trauma population.

    (B) Fractures through the epiphyseal growth plate occur less commonly because the growth plate has not ossified and therefore can withstand applied forces without damage.

    (C) Fractures through the metaphysis may stimulate bone overgrowth causing limb lengthening.

(D) Osteomyelitis causes less damage in children than in adults.

(E) Early involvement of an orthopedic surgeon and long-term follow-up are unnecessary given children's greater capacity for healing.

27. A 14-year-old child presents after a bicycle crash. This finding is noted on physical examination (see Fig. 13-6). He was noted to have a "coiled spring" sign on an upper GI series. Which statement is false?

(A) Blunt trauma to the upper abdomen is the most common mechanism for this injury.

(B) This injury likely occurred secondary to compression against the vertebral column.

(C) This injury is caused by shearing force between submucosa and muscularis.

(D) This injury usually requires operative intervention.

(E) None of the above.

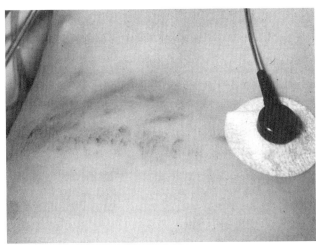

FIG. 13-6 Clinical finding on the abdomen of a 14-year-old after a bicycle crash.

28. Which statement is false regarding the management of duodenal injuries?

(A) In the absence of other injuries requiring operative intervention, duodenal hematomas can be managed nonoperatively with supportive care.

(B) Duodenal hematomas usually resolve within 7 days. If resolution has not occurred by this point consideration must be given to operative evacuation of the clot.

(C) If a duodenal hematoma is being explored and inspection of the submucosa finds it to be intact, the repair can be done by reapproximating the seromuscular layer.

(D) Simple lacerations, <50% of the duodenal circumference, can most often be managed with debridement and primary repair.

(E) More extensive injuries or those found after significant delay are best managed with duodenal diverticulization.

29. A 5-year-old female was pinned between the bumpers of two cars. This abdominal CT is obtained as part of her trauma evaluation (see Fig. 13-7). Which of the following statements is false?

(A) This injury is uncommon, occurring in less than 5% of all blunt trauma.

(B) CT scan is the most accurate radiologic test to evaluate for this injury.

(C) The key to decreased morbidity and mortality from this injury is prompt diagnosis and treatment.

(D) Nonoperative management should be used in this patient.

(E) Operative management should be undertaken is this case.

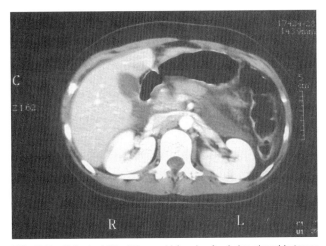

FIG. 13-7 Abdominal CT of 5-year-old female after being pinned between the bumpers of two cars.

30. Which of the following is true regarding pancreatic trauma and its complications?

   (A) Complications of pancreatic trauma include pancreatic pseudocyst, abscess, hemorrhage, and fistula.

   (B) Asymptomatic pseudocysts may be managed conservatively, as approximately 80% will spontaneously resolve.

   (C) Pseudocysts which do not spontaneously resolve can be managed with percutaneous drainage, if ductal disruption is identified.

   (D) If a pancreatic fistula is secondary to a major ductal disruption it will not respond to sphincterotomy and pancreatic duct stenting via endoscopic retrograde cholangiopancreatography (ERCP).

   (E) Overall mortality from pancreatic injuries is approximately 45%.

31. An 8–year-old male presents to the ED after an all-terrain vehicle crash. He is hemodynamically normal. He complains of left-sided abdominal pain and has gross hematuria on placement of his Foley catheter. A CT scan of his abdomen is obtained (see Fig. 13-8). Which of the following statements concerning this patient's injury and its management is *incorrect*?

   (A) This injury can be managed nonoperatively.

   (B) He should be placed on bedrest until his gross hematuria clears.

   (C) He may return to normal activities when his microscopic hematuria clears.

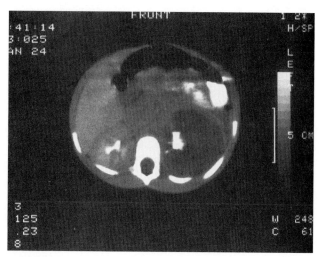

FIG. 13-8 Abdominal CT of 8-year-old male after an ATV crash.

   (D) Repeat CT scan prior to discharge may be employed to rule out significant urinary extravasation.

   (E) Most cases of urinary extravasation require operative intervention.

32. Concerning operative management of renal injuries, which of these statements is false?

   (A) Operative intervention is used for hemodynamically unstable patients, when renal vascular injury is suspected or when other injuries require abdominal exploration.

   (B) If renal vascular injury is suspected, early exploration of the hilar vessels is warranted as the warm ischemic time is limited in children.

   (C) Renal vein ligation can be tolerated on the right but ligation on the left will cause kidney loss.

   (D) If a perinephric hematoma is nonexpanding and either the CT or intravenous pyelogram (IVP) demonstrates intact renal function exploration of the hematoma is not required.

   (E) A repeat CT scan may be useful in the early postoperative period to evaluate the repairs and rule out significant urinary extravasation.

33. Childhood traumatic bladder injuries

   (A) occur less frequently than in the adult population because the bladder is protected by its anatomical position within the pelvis

   (B) have subtle physical examination findings, the most common of which is gross hematuria

   (C) are most accurately diagnosed by CT scan

   (D) are managed with 2 months of Foley catheter drainage when the injury location is extraperitoneal

   (E) are operatively managed with a single layered closure and Foley catheter drainage when the injury is located in an intraperitoneal location

34. In children with suspected or existing urethral injuries which of the following is *incorrect*?

   (A) Foley catheter placement should not be attempted and a retrograde urethrogram should be obtained.

   (B) Complications of posterior urethral injuries include impotence, incontinence, and stricture.

   (C) Urethral injuries are less common in girls.

(D) In both boys and girls, definitive diagnosis of urethral injury is done using urethroscopy.

(E) Pelvic fractures are the primary cause of urethral injuries.

35. A 3-year-old child presents to the ED via paramedics after being involved in a house fire. The child has areas of injury described as "white and leathery" circumferentially involving both legs and trunk. There are areas of injury described as "mildly pink and non-blistered" involving the face and neck and arms. Which of the following statements are *correct*?

(A) The estimated total body surface area (TBSA) involved with partial and/or full thickness burns is 54%.

(B) The body surface area of a child changes as they age. The head and neck having less surface area in children than in adults.

(C) The fluid requirements for resuscitation following burn injury is based on the TBSA involved with superficial, partial, and full thickness burns.

(D) Adult resuscitation formulas (i.e., Parkland formula) underestimate insensible fluid losses that result from the child's high surface area to weight ratio.

(E) Assessment of adequacy of resuscitation involves observing for decreasing heart rate, adequate blood pressure, clearing mental status, and urine output of 0.5 cc/kg/h.

36. What findings on history or physical examination should raise suspicions for child abuse?

(A) Inconsistencies between the reported mechanism of injury and the injuries sustained.

(B) A significant delay in presentation for medical evaluation.

(C) A history of frequent injury.

(D) A long bone fracture in a child under age 3.

(E) All of the above.

37. A 2-year-old child was found outside at 2 a.m. The ambient temperature was 10°F. The child was lying in a snow drift and was wearing a cotton tee shirt and diaper only. It is unclear how long the child had been outside. On arrival to the ED, the child is unresponsive and apneic. What initial evaluations and treatments should be performed?

(A) measurement of an oral temperature

(B) face mask oxygen supplementation

(C) boluses of room temperature fluids

(D) cardiopulmonary resuscitation (CPR)

(E) preparations for active rewarming

38. The child's initial core temperature was noted to be 28°C. What clinical findings can be expected?

(A) ventricular fibrillation

(B) significant dehydration

(C) osborn waves

(D) pulmonary edema

(E) all of the above

39. What is true regarding active rewarming?

(A) It should be initiated for a core temperature less than 35°C.

(B) It can be achieved with a forced air heating system (i.e., Bair Hugger).

(C) Rewarming rates of 1°C/min can be achieved on cardiopulmonary bypass (CPB).

(D) Recovery is universally poor if active rewarming is required.

(E) All of the above are true.

40. Which of the following is true regarding the ICU management of children?

(A) Impaired host defenses, invasive monitoring, exposure to multiple antibiotics and colonization with resistant microorganisms all contribute to make ICU patients susceptible to nosocomial infections.

(B) High frequency positive pressure ventilation, high-frequency jet ventilation, and high-frequency oscillation are new modes of ventilation that have been used in children with acute respiratory distress syndrome (ARDS).

(C) The goals of ventilatory strategies to minimize secondary lung injury are to limit high concentration oxygen use and to limit peak pressure and tidal volume by using pressure control, square wave ventilation, inspiratory/expiratory ratio manipulation, and positive expiratory end pressure (PEEP).

(D) During the postinjury phase of traumatic illness, the child experiences a hypermetabolic state. They exhibit an increase in oxidation of carbohydrates, fats, and proteins.

(E) All of the above.

Answers and Explanations

1. **(E)** There are many significant differences in anatomy of pediatric patients and their physiologic response to injury, when compared to adults. Children have a larger surface area to weight ratio (Brandt and Minifee, 1994). This, in combination with a lack of subcutaneous fat and increased metabolism make them more susceptible to hypothermia. The pediatric skeletal system is incompletely ossified and has areas of growth and remodeling which make bones more susceptible to injury (Ramenofsky and Gilchrist, 2000; Advanced Trauma Life Support for Physicians, 1997). A child's blood volume is approximately 70–80 mL/kg and therefore, a relatively small amount of blood loss can be physiologically significant (Ramenofsky and Gilchrist, 2000). Children have greater physiologic reserve than adults and do not manifest signs of shock until they have lost >25% of their blood volume (Ramenofsky and Gilchrist, 2000; Advanced Trauma Life Support for Physicians, 1997). A loss of >45% of their blood volume is required to see hypotension (Ramenofsky and Gilchrist, 2000; Advanced Trauma Life Support for Physicians, 1997). Children have a smaller body mass which means that any traumatic force will result in more damage per unit of body area (Advanced Trauma Life Support for Physicians, 1997). Multisystem injury occurs in >50% of cases of pediatric trauma (Ramenofsky and Gilchrist, 2000). Mechanism of injury differs significantly between adults and children (Brandt and Minifee, 1994). Penetrating trauma is less common and most injuries result from falls or the blunt force of a motor vehicle crash (Brandt and Minifee, 1994). Children's head sizes are proportionally larger and thus head injuries are more common in children than adults (Brandt and Minifee, 1994). Conversely, children's torsos are broad and shallow, leaving solid organs and the bladder less protected (Ramenofsky, 1998).

Bibliography

Advanced Trauma Life Support for Physicians. Chicago, IL: American College of Surgeons, 1997, 291–310.

Brandt ML, Minifee P. Pediatric complications. In: Mattox KL (ed.), *Complications of Trauma*. New York, NY: Churchill Livingstone, 1994, 173–181.

Ramenofsky ML. Infants and children as accident victims and their emergency management. In: O'Neill JA, Rowe MI, Grosfeld JL, et al. (eds.), *Pediatric Surgery*, 5th ed. St. Louis, MO: Mosby Year Book, 1998, 235–243.

Ramenofsky ML, Gilchrist BF. Initial hospital assessment and management of the trauma patient. In: Ashcroft KW (ed.), *Pediatric Surgery*, 3rd ed. Philadelphia, PA: W.B. Saunders, 2000, 159–190.

2. **(C)**

3. **(E)**

4. **(D)**

Explanations 2 through 4

The assessment of the airway is the first step in the initial assessment of an injured child. Proper assessment of the airway requires knowledge of its anatomy. The supraglottic area in the child is narrow secondary to the presence of a relatively large tongue, and tonsil and adenoid tissue (Ramenofsky and Gilchrist, 2000; Gerardi et al., 1996). The larynx is small and located high and anterior in the neck (Ramenofsky and Gilchrist, 2000; Gerardi et al., 1996). The trachea is about 5 cm long in an infant and grows to 7.5 cm by 18 months (Ramenofsky and Gilchrist, 2000). The growth of the trachea continues until the child is no longer gaining height (Ramenofsky and Gilchrist, 2000). The membranous portion of the trachea is thin and easily damaged (Ramenofsky and Gilchrist, 2000). The cricoid ring is the narrowest portion of the child's airway and serves as a functional cuff until the child is greater than 8–10 years of age (Ramenofsky and Gilchrist, 2000; Gerardi et al., 1996). The proportionally large occiput causes the child to have a slightly head-flexed position when supine making the airway even smaller (Ramenofsky and Gilchrist, 2000; Gerardi et al., 1996).

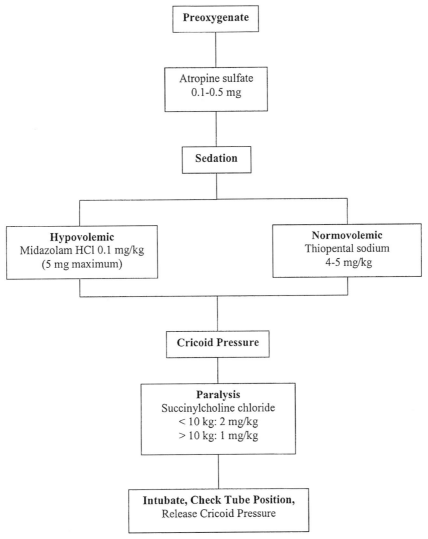

FIG. 13-9 Algorithm for rapid sequence intubation (RSI) for the pediatric patient. *Source:* Reproduced with permission from American College of Surgeons Committee on Trauma, Advanced Trauma Life Support for Doctors, Student Course Manual, 6th ed. Chicago, IL: American College of Surgeons, 1997, 297.

The first step in the management of the child's airway is to clear it. The small caliber of the child's supraglottic region makes it more prone to obstruction by secretions, blood, and foreign bodies. Once the airway is clear, supplemental oxygen should be administered. The child's head should be brought into a "sniffing" position to compensate for the large occiput and thus open the airway. Care must be taken to maintain cervical spine alignment throughout this maneuver. If this doesn't improve the child's airway patency, a jaw lift may be performed. An oral airway is tolerated only in an unconscious child. A nasopharyngeal airway may be tolerated in the awake child. If the airway cannot be adequately maintained at this point, preparations should be made for endotracheal intubation. The angle of the child's nasopharyngeal

region makes nasotracheal intubation difficult and more prone to complication. Its use is not recommended.

Emergent intubation is performed using RSI protocols. The use of a Broselow tape assists in weight estimations and drug dosing in the emergent setting. Each institution uses their own protocols for this process. This is the protocol set forth in advanced trauma life support (ATLS) (see Fig. 13-9) (Advanced Trauma Life Support for Physicians, 1997). In general, each protocol proceeds with the same steps. The child should be preoxygenated with 100% FiO_2. Children have a high metabolic rate causing them to desaturate at a rate faster than adults. Next, atropine is administered to prevent reflex bradycardia from laryngeal manipulation. For the head injured patient, the addition of bolus lidocaine and/or opioid administration is advocated at this point to prevent increases in intracranial pressure with intubation (Gerardi et al., 1996). Next, sedation is administered. The choice of appropriate medication to use is made by determining what injuries the child most likely has and whether the child is hypovolemic. Midazolam is the medication chosen most often for hypovolemic patients. Etomidate has gained wide acceptance as an alternative in this patient population (Gerardi et al., 1996; Snyder, 2000). Thiopental is advocated for use in the patient with an isolated head injury with no hemodynamic compromise. Once an adequate level of sedation has been achieved, the Sellick maneuver is used to maintain cricoid pressure. This is done to prevent aspiration of gastric contents. This is followed by administration of a paralytic medication. The choice of agents again depends on the clinical situation. Succinylcholine chloride, a depolarizing paralytic medication, is used most often. It has the shortest onset of action, 30 s, and shortest duration of clinical effect, 3–12 min (Gerardi et al., 1996). It has been reported to cause marked increase in bradycardia and asystole in infants and young children if a repeat dose is given (Gerardi et al., 1996). Repeat dosing is contraindicated. Vecuronium and rocuronium are alternative, nondepolarizing paralytic medications. Their onset of action is slower, 4 min and 60 s, respectively (Gerardi et al., 1996). Their duration of action is longer, 45 and 27 min, respectively (Gerardi et al., 1996). Once paralysis has been achieved, oral tracheal intubation is performed. Selection of endotracheal tube size can be calculated as

$$\frac{\text{Age in years} + 16}{4} = \text{endotracheal tube size}$$

or may be estimated by the size of the child's small finger or the diameter of the external nares (Ramenofsky and Gilchrist, 2000; Ramenofsky, 1998). A noncuffed tube should be used in children under the age of 8–10 (Ramenofsky and Gilchrist, 2000; Ramenofsky, 1998). The cricoid ring serves as a cuff in these children. The child's trachea is shorter than an adult and care must be taken to place the endotracheal tube above the carina. Correct placement should be confirmed with auscultation, end-tidal CO_2 monitor, and portable chest radiograph.

A surgical airway is rarely necessary in children (Advanced Trauma Life Support for Physicians, 1997). Surgical cricothyroidotomy is a safe option in children older than 11 years of age (Advanced Trauma Life Support for Physicians, 1997). In younger children, the small airway and short cricothyroid membrane create an increased risk for subsequent subglottic stenosis and vocal cord damage if a surgical cricothyroidotomy is performed (Brandt and Minifee, 1994). For children younger than this, formal tracheostomy is the procedure of choice (Brandt and Minifee, 1994). Needle cricothyroidotomy may be used in this younger patient population as a temporizing measure until a surgeon is available (Advanced Trauma Life Support for Physicians, 1997).

Appropriate oxygenation and ventilation are vital. Tidal volume should be 7–10 mL/kg (Brandt and Minifee, 1994; Ramenofsky, 1998). Respiratory rate should be appropriate to the age of the child. An infant needs 40–60 bpm while an older child only requires 20 bpm (Advanced Trauma Life Support for Physicians, 1997). Oxygenation can be monitored with a pulse oximeter and arterial blood gases. Adequacy of ventilation can be judged by chest excursion and can be adjusted based on arterial blood gases.

The placement of an orogastric tube may allow for easier ventilation by decreasing chest excursion compromise from gastric distention, it will not make subsequent attempts at intubation more successful.

Bibliography

Advanced Trauma Life Support for Physicians. Chicago, IL: American College of Surgeons, 1997, 291–310.

Brandt ML, Minifee P. Pediatric complications. In: Mattox KL (ed.), *Complications of Trauma*. New York, NY: Churchill Livingstone, 1994, 173–181.

Gerardi MJ, Sacchetti AD, Cantor RM, et al. Rapid sequence intubation of the pediatric patient. *Ann Emerg Med* 1996;28(1):55–74.

Ramenofsky ML. Infants and children as accident victims and their emergency management. In: O'Neill JA, Rowe MI, Grosfeld JL, et al. (eds.), *Pediatric Surgery*, 5th ed. St. Louis, MO: Mosby Year Book, 1998, 235–243.

Ramenofsky ML, Gilchrist BF. Initial hospital assessment and management of the trauma patient. In: Ashcroft KW (ed.), *Pediatric Surgery*, 3rd ed. Philadelphia, PA: W.B. Saunders, 2000, 159–190.

Snyder CL. Abdominal and genitourinary trauma. In: Ashcroft KW (ed.), *Pediatric Surgery*, 3rd ed. Philadelphia, PA: W.B. Saunders, 2000, 204–229.

5. **(A)**

6. **(E)**

Explanations 5 and 6

The signs of hypovolemia in a child may be subtle. A child has a greater physiologic reserve than an adult and therefore demonstrates only minimal signs of shock until >25% of their blood volume is lost (Advanced Trauma Life Support for Physicians, 1997).

TABLE 13-1   Systemic Responses to Blood Loss in the Pediatric Patient

System	<25% blood volume loss	25–45% blood volume loss	>45% blood volume loss
Cardiac	Weak, thready pulse; increased heart rate	increased heart rate	Hypotension, tachycardia to bradycardia
CNS	Lethargic, irritable, confused	Change in level of consciousness, dulled response to pain	Comatose
Skin	Cool, clammy	Cyanotic, decreased capillary refill, cold extremities	Pale, cold
Kidneys	Minimal decrease in urinary output; increased specific gravity	Minimal urine output	No urinary output

Source: Reproduced with permission from American College of Surgeons Committee on Trauma, *Advanced Trauma Life Support for Doctors, Student Course Manual*, 6th ed. Chicago, IL: American College of Surgeons, 1997, 297.

Given that a child's circulating blood volume is 80cc/kg, this magnitude of blood loss is approximately 20 cc/kg (Ramenofsky ML, Gilchrist, 2000; Ramenofsky, 1998). Tachycardia is the child's primary response to hypovolemia. Other signs include a narrowed pulse pressure, cool or mottled skin, decreased level of consciousness or decreased urine output (Advanced Trauma Life Support for Physicians, 1997). See Tables 13-1 and 13-2 for age-specific normal vital functions and systemic responses to blood loss (Advanced Trauma Life Support for Physicians, 1997). The presence of hypotension or bradycardia signal blood loss in excess of 45% of the child's circulating volume and severe shock for which the child is no longer able to compensate (Ramenofsky, 1998). Initial volume resuscitation is given as a bolus of 20 cc/kg (based on the goal of replacing 25% of the child's circulating volume) of warmed crystalloid solution. This may be repeated two times if appropriate hemodynamic response is not demonstrated or maintained. Response to fluid resuscitation is demonstrated by a decrease in heart rate, return of skin warmth and color, improving mental status, increased systolic blood pressure, and adequate urine output (1–2 cc/kg/h)

(Advanced Trauma Life Support for Physicians, 1997). If a third bolus is required, a 10 cc/kg bolus of PRBCs should be readied and used as the next bolus. If type-specific blood is not available, the child may initially be given O-negative blood. Efforts should be ongoing to identify the source of blood loss and control that hemorrhage. If the patient is still not maintaining an appropriate physiologic response after transfusion of PRBCs operative intervention is warranted (Tables 13-1 and 13-2).

Bibliography

Advanced Trauma Life Support for Physicians. Chicago, IL: American College of Surgeons, 1997, 291–310.

Brandt ML, Minifee P. Pediatric complications. In: Mattox KL (ed.), *Complications of Trauma*. New York, NY: Churchill Livingstone, 1994, 173–181.

Ramenofsky ML. infants and children as accident victims and their emergency management. In: O'Neill JA, Rowe MI, Grosfeld JL, et al. (eds.), *Pediatric Surgery*, 5th ed. St. Louis, MO: Mosby Year Book, 1998, 235–243.

Ramenofsky ML, Gilchrist BF. Initial hospital assessment and management of the trauma patient. In: Ashcroft KW (ed.), *Pediatric Surgery*, 3rd ed. Philadelphia, PA: W.B. Saunders, 2000, 159–190.

TABLE 13-2   Vital Functions

Age group	Weight (kg)	Heart rate (bpm)	Blood pressure (mmHg)	Respiratory rate	Urinary output (ml/kg/h)
Birth to 6 months	3–6	180–160	60–80	60	2
Infant	12	160	80	40	1.5
Preschool	16	120	90	30	1
Adolescent	35	100	100	20	0.5

Source: Reproduced with permission from American College of Surgeons Committee on Trauma, *Advanced Trauma Life Support for Doctors, Student Course Manual*, 6th ed. Chicago, IL: American College of Surgeons, 1997, 297.

TABLE 13-3 Pediatric Trauma Score

Component	+2	+1	−1
Size	>20 kg	10–20 kg	<10 kg
Airway	Normal	Maintainable	Unmaintainable
Systolic BP	>90 mmHg	50–90 mmHg	<50 mmHg
CNS	Awake	Obtunded/LOC	Coma/decerebrate
Skeletal	None	Closed fracture	Open/multiple fractures
Cutaneous	None	Minor	Major/penetrating

Source: Reproduced with permission from Tepas JJ, Ramenofsky ML, et al. The pediatric trauma score as a predictor of injury severity: an objective assessment. *J Trauma* 1988;28:425–429.

7. **(D)** The PTS is used to estimate mortality based on injury severity and is used as a triage tool to insure that patients are transported to a hospital offering the appropriate level of care (Tepas et al., 1998). Data from the National Pediatric Trauma Registry was analyzed using a multiple regression analysis and six factors were identified as being the most predictive of death and disability (Tepas et al., 1998). These factors were combined to create the PTS (see Table 13-3) (Tepas et al., 1998). The PTS ranges from +12 (minor injury) to −6 (fatal injury) (Tepas et al., 1998). The possibility of death increases significantly starting from a score of 8 and this is used as the critical triage point (Table 13-3) (Tepas et al., 1998).

Bibliography

Tepas JJ, Ramenofsky ML, et al. The pediatric trauma score as a predictor of injury severity: an objective assessment. *J Trauma* 1988;28:425–429.

8. **(D)** Establishment of intravenous access in children can be challenging. This is especially true in a hypovolemic child. Ideally venous access should be obtained through percutaneous peripheral route. If this is unsuccessful after two to three attempts, more invasive means of obtaining access should be attempted (Sanchez and Paidas, 1999). Depending on the skill of the physicians available options include intraosseous, venous cutdown, and central venous access. In children <6 years of age, intraosseous access is a fast and efficacious means of starting intravenous resuscitation. This can be performed on the proximal tibia or distal femur of an uninjured extremity. Fluids, blood, and medication are directly infused into the marrow cavity (Ramenofsky, 1998). This access should be used until suitable intravenous access has been established. Complications of intraosseous cannulation include fluid extravasation, cellulitis, and osteomyelitis (Brandt and Minifee, 1994; Ramenofsky, 1998; Sanchez

and Paidas, 1999). In experienced hands, venous cut down and central venous cannulation can both offer safe and rapid access to the intravenous system. The saphenous vein is in a constant location anterior to the medial maleolus at the ankle. Central venous access may be obtained at the femoral or subclavian veins.

Bibliography

Advanced Trauma Life Support for Physicians. Chicago, IL: American College of Surgeons, 1997, 291–310.

Brandt ML, Minifee P. Pediatric complications. In: Mattox KL (ed.), *Complications of Trauma*. New York, NY: Churchill Livingstone, 1994, 173–181.

Ramenofsky ML. Infants and children as accident victims and their emergency management. In: O'Neill JA, Rowe MI, Grosfeld JL, et al. (eds.), *Pediatric Surgery*, 5th ed. St. Louis, MO: Mosby Year Book, 1998, 235–243.

Ramenofsky ML, Gilchrist BF. Initial hospital assessment and management of the trauma patient. In: Ashcroft KW (ed.), *Pediatric Surgery*, 3rd ed. Philadelphia, PA: W.B. Saunders, 2000, 159–190.

Sanchez JI, Paidas CN. Childhood trauma: now and in the new millennium. *Surg Clin North Am* 1999;79:1503–1535.

9. **(B)**

10. **(E)**

Explanations 9 and 10

Thorough examination of a child's abdomen can be more difficult than in the adult patient. Therefore, it is important to proceed in an organized fashion to prevent missed injuries. A NG should be placed to decompress the stomach. Children can develop significant gastric distention from swallowing air while crying. This decompression not only enables a more accurate examination, but may even alleviate respiratory distress. Passage of a Foley catheter, when not contraindicated, will decompress the bladder and again enable an accurate examination. The child's abdomen should first be inspected for any contusions or abrasions. Next, the child's abdomen should be palpated to identify areas of tenderness, the presence of peritoneal signs or masses. This part of the examination may be difficult in children with painful lower chest or pelvic injuries. This examination should be repeated over time by the same examiner to obtain the most accurate assessment. Additional evaluation of the abdomen by CT scan, DPL, or FAST examination is most often required.

CT scan with intravenous contrast infusion is a quick and useful adjuvant imaging study. It is the preferred method for evaluating truncal trauma (Sanchez and Paidas, 1999; Eichelberger and Moront, 1998; Tepas, 2000). The presence and severity of solid organ injuries are readily assessed. The presence of abnormal fluid collections is easily demonstrated. The highlighting of the genitourinary system by the infused contrast aids in the detection of injuries to that organ system. Pneumoperitoneum, bowel wall thickening, or oral contrast extravasation are findings suggestive of intestinal perforation (Sanchez and Paidas, 1999); however, the CT scan's ability to detect hollow visceral injuries is low. The contraindication to CT scanning is hemodynamic instability.

DPL is rarely necessary; however, in the setting of a hemodynamically unstable child, a child with severe head injuries requiring emergent neurosurgic intervention or a child with suspected hollow visceral injury it can be used to rule out the presence of a significant intraabdominal injury (Sanchez and Paidas, 1999; Snyder, 2000). An open technique for lavage is most often used. After placement of both a NG tube and a Foley catheter, the child's abdomen is prepped and draped. A vertical skin incision is made below the umbilicus. (The exception to this is the child with a pelvic fracture where the DPL incision is made above the umbilicus to avoid entering a pelvic hematoma.) The fascia is identified and incised carefully. A DPL catheter is then gently inserted into the peritoneal cavity. The catheter is aspirated gently to assess for the presence of gross blood. If 10 cc of blood is aspirated, this test is considered positive. If the aspiration is negative, then a volume of 10 cc/kg of warmed lactated Ringer's is infused. When the infusion is complete, the infusate bag is placed in a dependent position and the effluent is collected back into the bag. The fluid is then sent to lab for evaluation. Criteria for a positive lavage in blunt trauma are the presence of greater than 100,000 red blood cells/mm^3 more than 500 white blood cells/mm^3, presence of enteric contents, bile or amylase (Advanced Trauma Life Support for Physicians). A positive examination is an indication for laparotomy. The results of the DPL in the hemodynamically stable patient need to be interpreted carefully to prevent nontherapeutic laparotomies. The DPL does not evaluate the retroperitoneum and therefore other diagnostic modalities should be employed if these injuries are suspected.

The use of the FAST examination is common in adult trauma patients. Its use in the pediatric population has not been well evaluated and appears to be limited (Sanchez and Paidas, 1999; Snyder, 2000). The presence of free intraperitoneal fluid is suggestive of organ injury and bleeding, but since most children with solid organ injuries are successfully managed nonoperatively this information is of limited application (Eichelberger and Moront, 1998). It appears that the greatest role for the FAST examination is in the hemodynamically unstable child (Sanchez and Paidas, 1999).

Bibliography

Advanced Trauma Life Support for Physicians. Chicago, IL: American College of Surgeons, 1997, 291–310.

Eichelberger MR, Moront M. Abdominal trauma. In: O'Neill JA, Rowe MI, Grosfeld JL, et al. (eds.), *Pediatric Surgery*, 5th ed. St. Louis, MO: Mosby Year Book, 1998, 261–284.

Sanchez JI, Paidas CN. Childhood trauma: now and in the new millennium. *Surg Clin North Am* 1999;79:1503–1535.

Snyder CL. Abdominal and genitourinary trauma. In: Ashcroft KW (ed.), *Pediatric Surgery*, 3rd ed. Philadelphia, PA: W.B. Saunders, 2000, 204–229.

Tepas JJ. Pediatric trauma. In: Mattox KL, Feliciano DV, Moore EE (eds.), *Trauma*, 4th ed. New York, NY: McGraw-Hill, 2000, 1075–1098.

11. (D)

12. (A)

13. (C)

14. (E)

Explanations 11 through 14

The spleen is a commonly injured organ after blunt trauma (Eichelberger, 1998). The child may complain of pain in the abdomen or referred pain in the left shoulder (Kehr's sign). Inspection of the abdomen may demonstrate bruising or abrasions in the left upper quadrant. Palpation may elicit localized or generalized abdominal tenderness. CT scan of the abdomen is the imaging test of choice in the evaluation of intraabdominal injuries. CT scan allows grading of splenic injuries, which in turn guides management. Splenic injuries are divided into five grades (see Table 13-4) (Moore, 1995).

The majority of splenic injuries, in children, can be successfully managed nonoperatively (Tepas, 2000). The decision for laparotomy for splenic injury is based on the child's hemodynamic status, not the grade of injury (Eichelberger, 1998). Nonoperative management is appropriate in a child who is hemodynamically stable, has no concomitant intraabdominal injuries, and has not required more than 40 cc/kg volume of blood replacement in 24 h (Eichelberger, 1998; Tepas, 2000). Nonoperative management has been standardized and prospectively evaluated in the pediatric trauma population (Stylianos, 2000; Stylianos, 2002). The data from these two papers outline guidelines for the nonoperative management of splenic injuries (see Table 13-5) (Stylianos, 2002). ICU admission is limited to those children with grade IV injuries secondary to their

TABLE 13-4   AAST Spleic Organ Injury Scale, 1994 Revision

Grade*		Injury description
I	Hematoma	Subcapsular, <10% surface area
	Laceration	Capsular tear, <1 cm parenchymal depth
II	Hematoma	Subcapsular, 10–50% surface area; intraparenchyma, <5 cm in diameter
	Laceration	1–3 cm parenchymal depth which does not involve a trabecular vessel
III	Hematoma	Subcapsular, >50% surface area or expanding; ruptured subcapsular or parenchymal hematoma Intraparenchymal hematoma >5 cm or expanding
	Laceration	>3 cm parenchymal depth or involving trabecular vessels
IV	Laceration	Laceration involving segmental or hilar vessels production major devascularization (>25% of spleen)
V	Laceration	Completely shattered spleen
	Vascular	Hilar injury which devascularizes the spleen

*Advance one grade for multiple injuries, up to grade III.
Source: Reproduced with permission from Moore EE, Cogbill TH, Jurkovich GJ, et al. Organ injury scaling: spleen and liver (1994 Revision). *J Trauma* 1995;38:323–324.

increased rate of transfusion and operation as compared to other injury grades (Stylianos, 2000). Total hospital stay and time to resumption of normal activities is adjusted according to injury grade (Stylianos, 2000). No follow-up imaging is recommended

TABLE 13-5   Guidelines for Resources Used in Children with Isolated Spleen or Liver Injury

	Grade I	Grade II	Grade III	Grade IV
ICU stay (day)	None	None	None	1
Hospital stay (day)	2	3	4	5
Predischarge imaging	None	None	None	None
Postdischarge imaging	None	None	None	None
Activity restriction (week)	3	4	5	6

(Stylianos, 2000). Their follow-up study evaluating compliance with these new guidelines found no compromise in patient safety (Stylianos, 2002).

Operative management is undertaken when the child is hemodynamically unstable, has required more than 40 cc/kg blood replacement, or has other intraabdominal injuries that require exploratory laparotomy. Mobilization of the spleen, by releasing all splenic attachments, is necessary for adequate inspection. The type of procedure to be performed on the injured spleen is dependent on the patient's hemodynamic status and his/her ability to withstand a longer operative period (Eichelberger, 1998). Splenorrhaphy may be undertaken in the hemodynamically stabilized, resuscitated patient. Techniques used include horizontal or vertical mattress sutures, omental buttressing, argon beam coagulation, use of hemostatic agents, the use of a mesh "bag" or "sling" (Eichelberger, 1998). Dissection of the hilar vessels may allow for selective ligation and/or subsequent partial splenectomy. Total splenectomy should be performed in those children with physiologic compromise or excessive hemorrhage in whom prolongation of operative time would be life-threatening (Eichelberger, 1998).

During splenectomy, care must be taken to avoid injury to the stomach and tail of the pancreas. As always, a thorough exploration of the abdomen must be undertaken to assess for any associated injuries. Once a child has undergone a total splenectomy, measures should be taken to prevent overwhelming postsplenectomy sepsis syndrome (OPSI). OPSI following splenectomy after trauma occurs in 1.5% of splenectomized children (Tepas, 2000). The mortality of OPSI is almost 50% (Sanchez and Paidas, 1999; Snyder, 2000; Tepas, 2000).

This risk of OPSI is greatest within the first 2 years after splenectomy and occurs most frequently in the first 5 years of life (Stafford, Blinman, and Nance, 2002; Tepas, 2000). To help prevent this, all splenectomized patients should receive vaccines against pneumococcus, *H. influenzae*, and meningococcus (Eichelberger, 1998). It is recommended that splenectomized children under the age of 5 should receive antibiotic prophylaxis with penicillin or ampicillin (Sanchez and Paidas, 1999). The need for continued prophylaxis in all splenectomized children is controversial (Sanchez and Paidas, 1999; Eichelberger, 1998). Decisions regarding prophylaxis beyond the age of 5 should be made on an individual basis (Eichelberger, 1998). Both the patient and the parents should be educated about OPSI. They should be instructed to be evaluated by a physician should the child experiences a febrile illness

(Eichelberger, 1998). Medic alert tags may also be helpful (Eichelberger, 1998).

Bibliography

Eichelberger MR, Moront M. Abdominal trauma. In: O'Neill JA, Rowe MI, Grosfeld JL, et al. (eds.), *Pediatric Surgery*, 5th ed. St. Louis, MO: Mosby Year Book, 1998, 261–284.

Moore EE, Cogbill TH, Jurkovich GJ, et al. Organ injury scaling: spleen and liver (1994 Revision). *J Trauma* 1995;38:323–324.

Sanchez JI, Paidas CN. Childhood trauma: now and in the new millennium. *Surg Clin North Am* 1999;79:1503–1535.

Snyder CL. Abdominal and genitourinary trauma. In: Ashcroft KW (ed.), *Pediatric Surgery*, 3rd ed. Philadelphia, PA: W.B. Saunders, 2000, 204–229.

Stafford PW, Blinman TA, Nance ML. Practical points in the evaluation and resuscitation of the injured child. *Surg Clin North Am* 2002;82:273–301.

Stylianos S. Evidence-based guidelines for resource utilization in children with isolated spleen or liver injury. *J Pediatr Surg* 2000;35(2):164–169.

Stylianos S. Compliance with evidence-based guidelines in children with isolated spleen or liver injury: a prospective study. *J Pediatr Surg* 2002;37(3):453–456.

Tepas JJ. Pediatric trauma. In: Mattox KL, Feliciano DV, Moore EE (eds.), *Trauma*, 4th ed. New York, NY: McGraw-Hill, 2000, 1075–1098.

15. **(C)** While infrequent, gastric injuries are more common in children than in adults (Brandt and Minifee, 1994; Snyder, 2000). Suspicion should increase if bloody gastric aspirate is found or if the NG tube is in an abnormal position on x-ray or CT scan (Snyder, 2000). Instillation of a small amount of air into the NG tube can allow for the finding of free air on x-ray or CT (Snyder, 2000). Gastric perforations are most commonly found near the greater curvature and are amenable to primary repair in a two layered closure (Snyder, 2000; Tepas, 2000). Gastric decompression should be maintained for several days postoperatively (Tepas, 2000).

Bibliography

Brandt ML, Minifee P. Pediatric complications. In: Mattox KL (ed.), *Complications of Trauma*. New York, NY: Churchill Livingstone, 1994, 173–181.

Snyder, CL. Abdominal and genitourinary trauma. In: Ashcroft KW (ed.), *Pediatric Surgery*, 3rd ed. Philadelphia, PA: W.B. Saunders, 2000, 204–229.

Tepas JJ. Pediatric trauma. In: Mattox KL, Feliciano DV, Moore EE (eds.), *Trauma*, 4th ed. New York, NY: McGraw-Hill, 2000, 1075–1098.

16. **(E)**

17. **(C)**

18. **(E)**

Explanations 16 through 18

The liver is injured as frequently as the spleen after blunt trauma in children (Eichelberger and Moront, 1998). The right lobe is injured more often than the left (Snyder, 2000). Liver injuries more often cause serious hemorrhage requiring operative intervention than splenic injuries (Eichelberger and Moront, 1998). Even so, most hepatic injuries can be successfully managed nonoperatively (Snyder, 2000; Tepas, 2000). The CT scan with intravenous contrast offers the best visualization of the anatomy of a hepatic injury (Snyder, 2000; Eichelberger and Moront, 1998). Hepatic injuries are graded by the organ injury grading scale (see Table 13-6) (Moore et al., 1995).

The same criteria for management that have been applied to patients with splenic injury are also applied

TABLE 13-6   AAST Hepatic Organ Injury Scale, 1994 Revision

Grade*		Injury description
I	Hematoma	Subcapsular, <10% surface area
	Laceration	Capsular tear, <1 cm parenchymal depth
II	Hematoma	Subcapsular, 10–50% surface area; intraparenchyma, <10 cm in diameter
	Laceration	1–3 cm parenchymal depth, <10 cm in length
III	Hematoma	Subcapsular, >50% surface area or expanding; ruptured subcapsular or parenchymal hematoma Intraparenchymal hematoma >10 cm or expanding
	Laceration	>3 cm parenchymal depth
IV	Laceration	Parenchymal disruption involving 25–75% of hepatic lobe or 1–3 Couinaud's segments within a single lobe
V	Laceration	Parenchymal disruption involving >75% of hepatic lobe or >3 Couinaud's segments within a single lobe
	Vascular	Juxtahepatic venous injuries
VI	Vascular	Hepatic avulsion

*Advance one grade for multiple injuries, up to grade III.
Source: Reproduced with permission from Moore EE, Cogbill TH, Jurkovich GJ, et al. Organ injury scaling: spleen and liver (1994 Revision). *J Trauma* 1995;38:323–324.

to those with hepatic injuries (Tepas, 2000). The decision to proceed with nonoperative management is based on hemodynamic stability, minimal blood replacement, and lack of other intraabdominal injuries that require operative intervention (Eichelberger and Moront, 1998; Tepas, 2000). Nonoperative management requires a secure diagnosis, the ability to monitor the child's hemodynamic status and an experienced surgeon. Nonoperative management of hepatic injuries does have known complications (in 25–70% of patients) some of which carry significant morbidity (Eichelberger and Moront, 1998; Tepas, 2000). These complications include hemobilia, biloma, abscess, and sepsis (Brandt and Minifee, 1994; Eichelberger and Moront, 1998).

Operative management is undertaken in the patients who are hemodynamically unstable, have required greater than 40 cc/kg blood replacement or have other identified intraabdominal injuries requiring operation (Snyder, 2000). Intravenous access should be obtained to allow crystalloid and blood infusion above the diaphragm. Access to the abdomen should be obtained through a generous midline incision. Initial control of bleeding may be obtained with packing. If needed, measures such as occlusion of the porta hepatis (Pringle maneuver) and mobilization of the liver with total vascular occlusion can be performed. The use of an atrial-caval shunt is difficult to perform and usually unnecessary (Eichelberger and Moront, 1998).

Once hemodynamic control is obtained specific injuries can be addressed. No intervention is needed for nonbleeding lacerations or nonexpanding subcapsular hematomas (Snyder, 2000; Eichelberger and Moront, 1998). Expanding hematomas should be incised and the bleeding vessels should be directly ligated or cauterized (Snyder, 2000; Eichelberger and Moront, 1998). Bleeding lacerations should be carefully explored, with extension of the laceration by finger fracture if needed, to identify and ligate bleeding vessels (Eichelberger and Moront, 1998). Postoperative drainage of larger lacerations may be needed. More severe wounds may require selective hepatic devascularization, such as right hepatic artery ligation, to definitively control bleeding (Snyder, 2000; Eichelberger and Moront, 1998). Limited segmental debridement of devitalized tissue is safe but major resection should be avoided given its mortality rate of 25–30% (Snyder, 2000; Eichelberger and Moront, 1998).

If the patient has sustained massive hepatic injury or is suspected of having a retrohepatic caval injury and bleeding has been controlled by packing, an alternative course of management is to leave the packing in the abdomen, return the patient to the ICU for resuscitation, warming and coagulopathy correction and plan for packing removal in 24–48 h (Eichelberger and Moront, 1998). The same complications that are found after nonoperative management are also complications of operative intervention. As with splenic injuries, nonoperative management of hepatic injuries has been standardized and prospectively evaluated in the pediatric trauma population (Stylianos, 2000, 2002) (see Table 13-6). ICU admission is limited to those children with grade VI injuries secondary to their increased rate of transfusion and operation as compared to other injury grades (Stylianos, 2000). Total hospital stay and time to resumption of normal activities is adjusted according to injury grade (Stylianos, 2000). No follow-up imaging is recommended (Stylianos, 2000).

Bibliography

Brandt ML, Minifee P. Pediatric complications. In: Mattox KL (ed.), *Complications of Trauma*. New York, NY: Churchill Livingstone, 1994, 173–181.

Eichelberger MR, Moront M. Abdominal trauma. In: O'Neill JA, Rowe MI, Grosfeld JL, et al. (eds.), *Pediatric Surgery*, 5th ed. St. Louis, MO: Mosby Year Book, 1998, 261–284.

Moore EE, Cogbill TH, Jurkovich GJ, et al. Organ injury scaling: spleen and liver (1994 Revision). *J Trauma* 1995;38:323–324.

Snyder CL. Abdominal and genitourinary trauma. In: Ashcroft KW (ed.), *Pediatric Surgery*, 3rd ed. Philadelphia, PA: W.B. Saunders, 2000, 204–229.

Stylianos S. Evidence-based guidelines for resource utilization in children with isolated spleen or liver injury. *J Pediatr Surg* 2000;35(2):164–169.

Stylianos S. Compliance with evidence-based guidelines in children with isolated spleen or liver injury: a prospective study. *J Pediatr Surg* 2002;37(3):453–456.

Tepas JJ. Pediatric trauma. In: Mattox KL, Feliciano DV, Moore EE (eds.), *Trauma*, 4th ed. New York, NY: McGraw-Hill, 2000, 1075–1098.

19. **(B)**

20. **(C)**

21. **(B)**

Explanations 19 through 21

Hollow viscus injuries occur in approximately 2–14% of those children who sustain blunt abdominal trauma (Stafford, Blinman, and Nance, 2002; Sanchez and Paidas, 1999; Tepas, 2000). The mechanisms which cause these injuries include burst or compressive force on a distended viscus, shear force near a point of fixation and crush or compression force against a solid surface (Snyder, 2000). A lap belt injury and the blunt force to the upper abdomen (i.e., bicycle handle) are common mechanisms for hollow viscus injury (Snyder, 2000). The lap belt injury complex includes abdominal wall contusion, hollow viscus injury, and vertebral fracture or dislocation (Chance fractures) (Snyder, 2000). The presence of abdominal wall bruising or seat belt ecchymosis should raise the index of suspicion for hollow viscus injury (Sanchez and Paidas, 1999; Snyder, 2000). Figure 13-3 demonstrates periumbilical bruising typical of that caused by a lap belt. Early physical examination may be normal or it may be difficult to evaluate secondary to abdominal wall tenderness (Snyder, 2000). Excessive pain or blood noted on rectal examination may signal a rectal injury (Eichelberger and Moront, 1998). CT scan is limited in its ability to detect these injuries.

While pneumoperitoneum, bowel wall thickening or enhancement, mesenteric hematoma or contrast extravasation are suggestive of bowel injury, these occur infrequently. Often, unexplained free fluid in the peritoneum is the only CT detected abnormality (Sanchez and Paidas, 1999; Snyder, 2000; Eichelberger and Moront, 1998). Figure 13-10 demonstrates bowel wall thickening and free peritoneal fluid. DPL may be a useful adjuvant study to evaluate free fluid with no solid organ injury (Stafford, Blinman, and Nance, 2002; Snyder, 2000; Eichelberger and Moront, 1998). These injuries will become clinically apparent over time with serial abdominal examinations and physiologic monitoring (Stafford, Blinman, and Nance, 2002).

Injuries that are intraperitoneal will usually present themselves, with peritoneal signs or significant ady-

namic ileus, within approximately 24 h (Eichelberger and Moront, 1998; Tepas, 2000); however, retroperitoneal injuries, duodenum or proximal jejunum, may not be evident for 3–4 days (Eichelberger and Moront, 1998). There has been no increase in mortality or morbidity with recognition and treatment of these injuries within 24 h (Stafford, Blinman, and Nance, 2002). Usually small intestinal injuries can be managed with either primary repair or resection and primary anastomosis. Regardless of location, colonic injuries can be managed with primary repair or segmental resection with primary anastomosis. Colostomy may be indicated if there is no excessive contamination, other associated major injuries or ongoing physiologic derangement (Snyder, 2000; Eichelberger and Moront, 1998).

Rectal injuries are uncommon in children (Snyder, 2000). They occur most often by impalement or nonaccidental trauma such as abuse (Snyder, 2000). Examination of these injuries must be undertaken under general anesthesia using anoscopy and sigmoidoscopy (Snyder, 2000; Eichelberger and Moront, 1998; Tepas, 2000). Significant disruption of the rectum or anal canal above the internal sphincter requires a diverting colostomy, debridement, and primary repair (Snyder, 2000; Eichelberger and Moront, 1998; Tepas, 2000). Drainage may also be required (Snyder, 2000; Eichelberger and Moront, 1998). Injuries below the internal sphincter can be managed by primary repair alone (Tepas, 2000). A thorough examination of the genitalia should accompany evaluation of a rectal injury (Brandt and Minifee, 1994). A physician experienced in sexual assault examination should be involved in the assessment of these children.

Bibliography

Brandt ML, Minifee P. Pediatric complications. In: Mattox KL (ed.), *Complications of Trauma*. New York, NY: Churchill Livingstone, 1994, 173–181.

Eichelberger MR, Moront M. Abdominal trauma. In: O'Neill JA, Rowe MI, Grosfeld JL, et al. (eds.), *Pediatric Surgery*, 5th ed. St. Louis, MO: Mosby Year Book, 1998, 261–284.

Sanchez JI, Paidas CN. Childhood trauma: now and in the new millennium. *Surg Clin North Am* 1999;79: 1503–1535.

Snyder CL. Abdominal and genitourinary trauma. In: Ashcroft KW (ed.), *Pediatric Surgery*, 3rd ed. Philadelphia, PA: W.B. Saunders, 2000, 204–229.

Stafford PW, Blinman TA, Nance ML. Practical points in the evaluation and resuscitation of the injured child. *Surg Clin North Am* 2002;82:273–301.

Tepas JJ. Pediatric trauma. In: Mattox KL, Feliciano DV, Moore EE (eds.), *Trauma*, 4th ed. New York, NY: McGraw-Hill, 2000, 1075–1098.

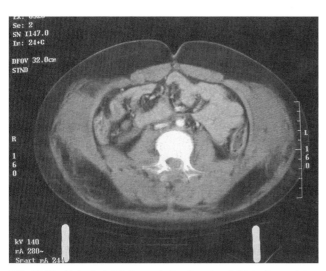

FIG. 13-10 Abdominal CT demonstrating bowel wall thickening and free peritoneal fluid.

22. (D)

23. (C)

24. (C)

Explanations 22 through 24

Thoracic injuries occur commonly after blunt trauma in children with a 25–29% incidence (Lofland, 2000). They are second only to head injures as cause of death in children after trauma (Sanchez and Paidas, 1999; Wessen, 1998). Isolated thoracic injuries are far less common in children (Sanchez and Paidas, 1999; Lofland, 2000). Two-thirds of children with thoracic trauma also have injuries to other organ systems (Advanced Trauma Life Support for Physicians, 1997). Compliant chest walls and substantial force result in significant injuries to the diaphragm, lungs, and mediastinum without overlying rib fractures (Sanchez and Paidas, 1999; Wessen, 1998; Lofland, 2000). There may also be few signs of injury on external examination (Sanchez and Paidas, 1999).

Unlike adults in whom rib fractures are the most common injury, pulmonary contusions are the most common blunt injury to the chest in children (Wessen, 1998). Other common injuries include pneumothorax and hemothorax (Wessen, 1998). Tracheobronchial injuries occur more often in children than adults (Wessen, 1998). Aortic injuries are less common in children (Tepas, 2000; Wessen, 1998). Life-threatening thoracic injuries, airway obstruction, tension pneumothorax, massive hemothorax, and cardiac tamponade should be identified and addressed during the primary survey (Stafford, Blinman, and Nance, 2002; Wessen, 1998). Open pneumothorax and massive flail chest are rare injuries in children (Tepas, 2000; Wessen, 1998).

Potentially life-threatening injuries, pulmonary contusion, myocardial contusion, aortic tear, ruptured diaphragm, tracheobronchial injury, and esophageal perforation should be identified during the secondary survey and addressed subsequently (Wessen, 1998). The diagnosis and management of most thoracic injuries are the same as in the adult patient (Stafford, Blinman, and Nance, 2002). Figure 13-9 depicts a child with bilateral chest tubes and bilateral pulmonary contusions. This figure in combination with the finding of a massive air leak is suggestive of a tracheobronchial injury. Bronchoscopy is the most reliable way to diagnose this injury (Wessen, 1998). Most airway injuries occur within 2.5 cm of the carina (Wessen, 1998).

Operative management of this injury is the same as that of the adult patient. The most common

injuries, pulmonary contusion, pneumothorax, and hemothorax can most often be managed with chest tube and nonoperative management (Sanchez and Paidas, 1999; Wessen, 1998). The mobility of the child's mediastinum makes them more likely to experience hemodynamic compromise from tension pneumothorax (Advanced Trauma Life Support for Physicians, 1997). Children require intubation and mechanical ventilation less often than adults for thoracic injuries and their overall prognosis is better than in the adult patient (Brandt and Minifee, 1994; Lofland, 2000).

Urgent operative thoracotomy may be indicated for massive air leak, cardiac tamponade, initial chest tube drainage >20 cc/kg or ongoing chest tube losses of >2 cc/kg/h for more than 2 h (Stafford, Blinman, and Nance, 2002). ED thoracotomy is employed in children when presenting after penetrating trauma with vital signs or with recent loss of vital signs or in blunt trauma with loss of vital signs during evaluation in the department (Sanchez and Paidas, 1999). Even with children's greater physiologic reserve, the salvage rate for ED thoracotomy for blunt trauma is very low (0–2%).

Bibliography

Advanced Trauma Life Support for Physicians. Chicago, IL: American College of Surgeons, 1997, 291–310.

Brandt ML, Minifee P. Pediatric complications. In: Mattox KL (ed.), *Complications of Trauma*. New York, NY: Churchill Livingstone, 1994, 173–181.

Lofland GK. Thoracic trauma in children. In: Ashcroft KW (ed.), *Pediatric Surgery*, 3rd ed. Philadelphia, PA: W.B. Saunders, 2000, 191–203.

Sanchez JI, Paidas CN. Childhood trauma: now and in the new millennium. *Surg Clin North Am* 1999;79:1503–1535.

Stafford PW, Blinman TA, Nance ML. Practical points in the evaluation and resuscitation of the injured child. *Surg Clin North Am* 2002;82:273–301.

Tepas JJ. Pediatric trauma. In: Mattox KL, Feliciano DV, Moore EE (eds.), *Trauma*, 4th ed. New York, NY: McGraw-Hill, 2000, 1075–1098.

Wessen DE. Thoracic injuries. In: O'Neill JA, Rowe MI, Grosfeld JL, et al. (eds.), *Pediatric Surgery*, 5th ed. St. Louis, MO: Mosby Year Book, 1998, 245–260.

25. (C) Traumatic asphyxia results from sudden compression of the chest and/or abdomen against a closed glottis. This is the type of force seen when a child is crushed or run over by a vehicle (Lofland, 2000). This compression causes an increase in intrathoracic pressure. Since the child's vena cava has no valves, this pressure is transmitted through all of the tributaries of the vena cava (Wessen, 1998; Lofland, 2000). Signs of this on physical examination include capillary rupture or petechia in the skin of the upper torso, head and neck, and sclera (Wessen, 1998; Lofland, 2000). Figure 13-5 illustrates typical conjunctival capillary rupture. The brain may also suffer injury from both hypoxia and capillary extravasation causing confusion and occasionally seizures (Wessen, 1998; Lofland, 2000). The patient may suffer from respiratory insufficiency and hemoptysis secondary to pulmonary contusion (Stafford, Blinman, and Nance, 2002; Wessen, 1998; Lofland, 2000). The extent of the chest wall trauma may be severe enough to cause respiratory failure (Wessen, 1998; Lofland, 2000). Cardiac injuries are rare (Stafford, Blinman, and Nance, 2002). The treatment is supportive care with elevation of the head of the bed, supplemental oxygen, and electrocardiogram (ECG) monitoring (Stafford, Blinman, and Nance, 2002; Wessen, 1998).

Bibliography

Lofland GK. Thoracic trauma in children. In: Ashcroft KW (ed.), *Pediatric Surgery*, 3rd ed. Philadelphia, PA: W.B. Saunders, 2000, 191–203.

Stafford PW, Blinman TA, Nance ML. Practical points in the evaluation and resuscitation of the injured child. *Surg Clin North Am* 2002;82:273–301.

Wessen DE. Thoracic injuries. In: O'Neill JA, Rowe MI, Grosfeld JL, et al. (eds.), *Pediatric Surgery*, 5th ed. St. Louis, MO: Mosby Year Book, 1998, 245–260.

26. **(C)** Children have a higher rate of fractures after trauma than the adult trauma population. A child's bones are incompletely ossified and have anatomically developing regions that respond differently to injury (Price, 2000). Fractures through the epiphyseal growth plate occur more commonly because the growth plate is a weak structure (Price, 2000). These fractures are classified by the Salter fracture classification. These fractures may cause subsequent growth deformities such as limb shortening (Brandt and Minifee, 1994). Fractures through the metaphysis may stimulate bone overgrowth causing limb lengthening (Brandt and Minifee, 1994). Some complications of fractures, such as osteomyelitis, are far more destructive in children than in adults (Brandt and Minifee, 1994). Since fractures in children differ in their management from those in the adult population, early involvement of an orthopedic surgeon and long-term follow-up are needed to optimize their outcomes.

Bibliography

Brandt ML, Minifee P. Pediatric complications. In: Mattox KL (ed.), *Complications of Trauma*. New York, NY: Churchill Livingstone, 1994, 173–181.

Price N. Pediatric orthopedic trauma. In: Ashcroft KW (ed.), *Pediatric Surgery*, 3rd ed. Philadelphia, PA: W.B. Saunders, 2000, 230–237.

27. **(D)**

28. **(B)**

Explanations 27 through 28

Blunt trauma to the upper abdomen is the most common mechanism for injury to both the duodenum and pancreas in children (Eichelberger and Moront, 1998; Tepas, 2000). Both are susceptible to injury from compression against the vertebral column (Eichelberger and Moront, 1998). Figure 13-6 demonstrates upper abdominal bruising which should raise suspicions for a duodenal or pancreatic injury. Diagnosis of blunt duodenal injury is difficult. Loss of the right psoas shadow (retroperitoneal fluid) or right perinephric air is suggestive of this injury (Snyder, 2000; Eichelberger and Moront, 1998). Figure 13-11 demonstrates duodenal wall thickening and pneumatosis. The use of water soluble oral contrast during CT scan can aid in identification of this injury (Eichelberger and Moront, 1998).

Injuries can range from intramural hematoma to rupture. Intramural duodenal hematomas are caused by shearing force between the submucosa and muscularis (Eichelberger and Moront, 1998; Tepas, 2000). The hematoma may be large enough to cause narrowing of the duodenal lumen and subsequent gastric outlet obstruction. The finding of a "coiled spring" sign on upper gastrointestinal radiographic studies is suggestive of a duodenal hematoma (Eichelberger and Moront, 1998; Tepas, 2000).

In the absence of other injuries requiring operative intervention, these hematomas can be managed nonoperatively with supportive care including total

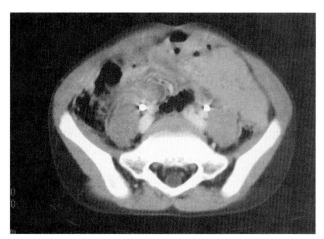

FIG. 13-11 Abdominal CT demonstrating duodenal wall thickening and pneumatosis.

parenteral nutrition (Snyder, 2000; Brandt and Minifee, 1994; Eichelberger and Moront, 1998; Tepas, 2000). They usually resolve within 3 weeks (Eichelberger and Moront, 1998; Tepas, 2000). If resolution has not occurred by this point consideration must be given to operative evacuation of the clot (Snyder, 2000). If the abdomen is being explored and a duodenal hematoma is encountered, evacuation of the hematoma may be considered (Brandt and Minifee, 1994; Eichelberger and Moront, 1998). Incising of the serosa and muscularis allows for clot evacuation and inspection of the submucosa. If the submucosa is intact the seromuscular layer may be reapproximated (Eichelberger and Moront, 1998).

Perforation of the duodenum can be managed with primary repair, repair with pyloric exclusion, and gastrojejunostomy or duodenal diverticulization (vagotomy, distal gastrectomy, and Billroth II reconstruction) depending on the type and severity of injury (Eichelberger and Moront, 1998). Simple lacerations, <50% of the duodenal circumference, can most often be managed with debridement and primary repair. More extensive injuries or those found after significant delay are best managed with repair, pyloric exclusion, and closed suction drainage (Snyder, 2000; Ladd et al., 2002). The pylorus will reopen within 2–3 weeks (Snyder, 2000; Ladd et al., 2002). Duodenal diverticulization is rarely necessary (Snyder, 2000).

Bibliography

Brandt ML, Minifee P. Pediatric complications. In: Mattox KL (ed.), *Complications of Trauma*. New York, NY: Churchill Livingstone, 1994, 173–181.

Eichelberger MR, Moront M. Abdominal trauma. In: O'Neill JA, Rowe MI, Grosfeld JL, et al. (eds.), *Pediatric Surgery*, 5th ed. St. Louis, MO: Mosby Year Book, 1998, 261–284.

Ladd AP, West KW, Rouse TM, et al. Surgical management of duodenal injuries in children. *Surgery* 2002;132(4): 748–753.

Snyder CL. Abdominal and genitourinary trauma. In: Ashcroft KW (ed.), *Pediatric Surgery*, 3rd ed. Philadelphia, PA: W.B. Saunders, 2000, 204–229.

Tepas JJ. Pediatric trauma. In: Mattox KL, Feliciano DV, Moore EE (eds.), *Trauma*, 4th ed. New York, NY: McGraw-Hill, 2000, 1075–1098.

29. (D)

30. (A)

Explanations 29 and 30

Pancreatic injuries in children are uncommon, occurring in less than 5% of all blunt traumas (Snyder, 2000). Blunt trauma is the most common cause of pancreatic injury in children (Brandt and Minifee, 1994; Eichelberger and Moront, 1998; Tepas, 2000). This injury may result from motor vehicle crash, handle bar injury or other direct blow to the upper abdomen (Brandt and Minifee, 1994; Eichelberger and Moront, 1998; Tepas, 2000). Associated injuries are common (Snyder, 2000). Patients may present with upper abdominal abrasions or contusion or they may demonstrate few external signs of injury (Stafford, Blinman, and Nance, 2002; Tepas, 2000).

The mechanism of injury should raise the index of suspicion for pancreatic injury (Brandt and Minifee, 1994). CT scan is the most accurate radiologic test to evaluate for this injury. CT scans with 3 mm cut are preferred (Eichelberger and Moront, 1998). Radiologic signs of an injury range from obvious (visible pancreatic transection), to subtle (a small amount of fluid in the lesser sac) to no signs of injury at all (Snyder, 2000). Figure 13-7 demonstrates the CT finding of pancreatic transection. Serial abdominal examinations are required to diagnose those injuries that are not readily apparent on initial evaluation. Initial amylase or lipase levels may be misleading (Snyder, 2000; Eichelberger and Moront, 1998). Looking at these levels over time (24–48 h) is more accurate in diagnosing significant injuries (Snyder, 2000; Tepas, 2000).

The key to decreased morbidity and mortality from this injury is prompt diagnosis and treatment (Tepas, 2000). Nonoperative management may be used in those patients who are found to have no major ductal disruption, no clinical deterioration, and no additional injuries requiring operative intervention (Tepas, 2000). Minor injuries such as contusions and minor lacerations make up >75% of pediatric pancreatic injuries (Snyder, 2000). Operative management should be undertaken when pancreatic transection is seen or clinical deterioration occurs during a period of observation (Brandt and Minifee, 1994). Operative management must include inspection and palpation of the entirety of the pancreas, adequate debridement of devitalized tissue, closure of any ductal injuries and drainage (Snyder, 2000; Eichelberger and Moront, 1998; Tepas, 2000).

Pancreatic transections to the left of the superior mesenteric vessels should be managed with distal pancreatectomy, without splenectomy if possible (Eichelberger and Moront, 1998; Tepas, 2000). Injuries to the head of the pancreas often are associated with duodenal injuries. In these severe injuries efforts should be made to conserve as much pancreatic tissue as possible (Snyder, 2000). Combined repairs with duodenal exclusion or Roux-en-Y drainage may be employed (Snyder, 2000;

Eichelberger and Moront, 1998). Major resections are rarely needed (Snyder, 2000). Children can tolerate resection of 75% of the pancreas and still progress normally in growth and development (Tepas, 2000).

Complications of pancreatic trauma include pancreatic pseudocyst, abscess, hemorrhage, and fistula. Asymptomatic pseudocysts may be managed conservatively (Snyder, 2000). Pancreatic pseudocysts will spontaneously resolve in approximately 50% of cases (Tepas, 2000). Of those which become symptomatic, the majority can be treated with percutaneous drainage (Snyder, 2000). Pseudocysts which do not spontaneously resolve can be managed with percutaneous drainage, if no ductal disruption is identified (Tepas, 2000). If the duct does communicate to the cyst, internal drainage should be used. Pancreatic fistulas which are not secondary to major ductal disruption will most often close with supportive care (Eichelberger and Moront, 1998). If the fistula is secondary to a major ductal disruption it may respond to sphincterotomy and pancreatic duct stenting via ERCP or it may require operative intervention. Overall mortality from pancreatic injuries is approximately 5–10% and is usually secondary to associated injuries (Snyder, 2000).

Bibliography

Brandt ML, Minifee P. Pediatric complications. In: Mattox KL (ed.), *Complications of Trauma*. New York, NY: Churchill Livingstone, 1994, 173–181.

Stafford PW, Blinman TA, Nance ML. Practical points in the evaluation and resuscitation of the injured child. *Surg Clin North Am* 2002;82:273–301.

Snyder CL. Abdominal and genitourinary trauma. In: Ashcroft KW (ed.), *Pediatric Surgery*, 3rd ed. Philadelphia, PA: W.B. Saunders, 2000, 204–229.

Eichelberger MR, Moront M. Abdominal trauma. In: O'Neill JA, Rowe MI, Grosfeld JL, et al. (eds.), *Pediatric Surgery*, 5th ed. St. Louis, MO: Mosby Year Book, 1998, 261–284.

Tepas JJ. Pediatric trauma. In: Mattox KL, Feliciano DV, Moore EE (eds.), *Trauma*, 4th ed. New York, NY: McGraw-Hill, 2000, 1075–1098.

31. (E)

32. (C)

Explanations 31 and 32

Children's kidneys are more susceptible to injuries because their pliable rib cage provides less protection, the kidneys are proportionally larger and are more mobile, there is a higher likelihood of undiagnosed congenital renal abnormalities that predispose to injury, Gerota's fascia is less developed and the abdominal musculature is weaker (Brandt and Minifee, 1994; Snyder, 2000; Tepas, 2000; Garcia and Sheldon, 1998). Most renal injuries in children are secondary to blunt trauma (Snyder, 2000; Garcia and Sheldon, 1998). The physical signs of renal injuries can be nonspecific. There may be bruising over the abdomen or flank. There may be flank or abdominal tenderness on palpation. Hematuria is the most common sign of a renal injury (Snyder, 2000); however, the magnitude of the hematuria does not correlate well with the degree of injury (Snyder, 2000; Garcia and Sheldon, 1998). Isolated microscopic hematuria after trauma is not an indication for complete genitourinary workup (Snyder, 2000; Tepas, 2000). Gross hematuria or microscopic hematuria in the face of shock, suspicious mechanism, or other associated injuries should be evaluated thoroughly (Snyder, 2000). CT scan is the initial radiologic evaluation of choice in the hemodynamically stable patient (Garcia and Sheldon, 1998). A single image IVP can be used in unstable patients to find whether there is flow to both kidneys (Tepas, 2000).

In the absence of suspected renal artery injury, hemodynamic instability or associated injuries requiring operative intervention, a nonoperative strategy is used (Snyder, 2000; Tepas, 2000). Most renal injuries in children are minor and can be managed this way. Patients are placed on bedrest until their gross hematuria clears and are instructed to return to normal activities only when their microscopic hematuria clears (Snyder, 2000). Repeat CT scan prior to discharge may be employed to rule out significant urinary extravasation. Most cases of urinary extravasation, in the absence of abscess, are managed expectantly with serial imaging studies.

Operative intervention is used for hemodynamically unstable patients, renal vascular injury, or when other injuries require abdominal exploration. If renal vascular injury is suspected, early exploration of the hilar vessels is warranted as the warm ischemic time is limited in children (Snyder, 2000). Most instances of main renal artery injury require nephrectomy because reconstruction is not possible (Snyder, 2000). Attempts should be made to repair renal vein injuries (Snyder, 2000). Renal vein ligation can be tolerated on the left if the adrenal and gonadal veins are intact but ligation on the right will cause kidney loss (Snyder, 2000).

When a perinepheric hematoma is encountered during abdominal exploration for other injuries two different management strategies can be employed. If the hematoma is nonexpanding and either the CT or IVP demonstrates intact renal function, exploration of the hematoma is not warranted (Snyder, 2000). If there is concern about lack of renal function or hematoma expansion, exploration is warranted. Prior to opening the hematoma control of the hilar vessels should be obtained (Snyder, 2000). Once opened, bleeding can be arrested, devitalized tissue may be debrided and any collecting system injury is closed (Snyder, 2000). A repeat CT scan may be useful in the early postoperative period to evaluate the repairs and rule out significant urinary extravasation (Snyder, 2000). Long-term follow-up of children who have suffered a major renal injury should be done at least yearly and include urinalysis, measurement of renal function, and blood pressure evaluation (Sanchez and Paidas, 1999; Snyder, 2000; Garcia and Sheldon, 1998). The incidence of posttraumatic hypertension in children is low (Sanchez and Paidas, 1999; Snyder, 2000; Garcia and Sheldon, 1998).

Bibliography

Brandt ML, Minifee P. Pediatric complications. In: Mattox KL (ed.), *Complications of Trauma*. New York, NY: Churchill Livingstone, 1994, 173–181.

Garcia V, Sheldon C. Genitourinary tract trauma. In: O'Neill JA, Rowe MI, Grosfeld JL, et al. (eds.), *Pediatric Surgery*, 5th ed. St. Louis, MO: Mosby Year Book, 1998, 285–302.

Sanchez JI, Paidas CN. Childhood trauma: now and in the new millennium. *Surg Clin North Am* 1999;79:1503–1535.

Snyder CL. Abdominal and genitourinary trauma. In: Ashcroft KW (ed.), *Pediatric Surgery*, 3rd ed. Philadelphia, PA: W.B. Saunders, 2000, 204–229.

Tepas JJ. Pediatric trauma. In: Mattox KL, Feliciano DV, Moore EE (eds.), *Trauma*, 4th ed. New York, NY: McGraw-Hill, 2000, 1075–1098.

33. **(B)** Bladder injuries are not common in children (Snyder, 2000). Like renal injuries, the majority result from blunt trauma (Snyder, 2000; Garcia and Sheldon, 1998). The child's bladder is less protected than the adult's because it lies in an intraabdominal position (Snyder, 2000; Garcia and Sheldon, 1998). When a bladder injury is found, injuries to other intraabdominal organs (50% of patients) and pelvic fractures (75–95% of bladder injuries have associated pelvic fractures) are common (Snyder, 2000; Garcia and Sheldon, 1998).

Physical examination findings in a patient with a bladder injury may be subtle or nonspecific. Gross hematuria is a common finding. Microscopic hematuria in a patient with a known pelvic fracture should undergo a work up to elucidate its source (Snyder, 2000). A CT scan is useful in identifying intraabdominal injuries, but is not the ideal study for detection of bladder injuries. A cystogram with a postvoid film is the best study (Snyder, 2000; Garcia and Sheldon, 1998). The finding of contrast extravasation is diagnostic of a bladder injury.

Bladder injuries may be intra- or extraperitoneal in location. Extraperitoneal injuries are managed conservatively with Foley catheter drainage (Snyder, 2000; Garcia and Sheldon, 1998). This catheter should remain in place for at least 10 days at which time a cystogram is performed to document healing (Garcia and Sheldon, 1998). The majority of injuries have healed by this point and the catheter may be removed (Garcia and Sheldon, 1998). For those injuries with ongoing extravasation at 10 days, expectant management with catheter drainage is continued as most will have documented healing by 3 weeks (Garcia and Sheldon, 1998).

Intraperitoneal injuries are managed operatively (Snyder, 2000; Garcia and Sheldon, 1998). Repair of intraperitoneal bladder injuries is most often done with a layered closure and placement of a suprapubic cystostomy tube (Snyder, 2000; Garcia and Sheldon, 1998). A cystogram is performed at 7–10 days to document healing.

Bibliography

Garcia V, Sheldon C. Genitourinary tract trauma. In: O'Neill JA, Rowe MI, Grosfeld JL, et al. (eds.), *Pediatric Surgery*, 5th ed. St. Louis, MO: Mosby Year Book, 1998, 285–302.

Snyder, CL. Abdominal and genitourinary trauma. In: Ashcroft KW (ed.), *Pediatric Surgery*, 3rd ed. Philadelphia, PA: W.B. Saunders, 2000, 204–229.

34. **(D)** Childhood urethral injuries are most often secondary to blunt trauma. Pelvic fractures are the primary cause (Garcia and Sheldon, 1998). A urethral injury should be suspected if there is a significant scrotal hematoma, gross hematuria, blood at the urethral meatus or a "boggy" or "high riding" prostate on initial physical examination (Snyder, 2000; Garcia and Sheldon, 1998). If this injury is suspected, Foley catheter placement should not be attempted and a retrograde urethrogram should be performed (Snyder, 2000; Garcia and Sheldon, 1998).

The anterior and posterior urethra are the most common injury classifications (Snyder, 2000). Anterior injuries result from straddle type injuries while posterior injuries occur from shearing at the junction of the membranous and prostatic urethra caused by pelvic fracture (Garcia and Sheldon, 1998). Minor anterior injuries, contusion or stretch injury, may be treated conservatively, without a catheter, if the injury is mild and the patient can void (Snyder, 2000; Garcia and Sheldon, 1998). If the anterior injury is moderate in severity or if the patient cannot void, a Foley catheter is the treatment of choice (Snyder, 2000). Suprapubic catheter placement and delayed repair may be needed for the most complex anterior injuries (Snyder, 2000; Garcia and Sheldon, 1998).

Minor posterior urethral injuries, like anterior injuries, can be managed conservatively if the patient is able to void (Snyder, 2000; Garcia and Sheldon, 1998). More severe injuries are managed by either primary suture repair or with suprapubic cystostomy tube placement and delayed (2 weeks to 9 months) repair (Snyder, 2000; Garcia and Sheldon, 1998). The choice of management strategy in this situation in controversial (Snyder, 2000; Garcia and Sheldon, 1998). Complications of posterior urethral injury include impotence, incontinence, and stricture (Snyder, 2000; Garcia and Sheldon, 1998). Impotence rates are approximately 30% (Snyder, 2000). The incidence of incontinence is 6% (Garcia and Sheldon, 1998). The incidence of both incontinence and impotence differs little when primary versus delayed repair is performed (Snyder, 2000; Garcia and Sheldon, 1998).

Strictures occurrences range from 23 to 96% (Snyder, 2000; Garcia and Sheldon, 1998). They are significantly more common after delayed urethral repair (Snyder, 2000; Garcia and Sheldon, 1998). Urethral injuries are uncommon in girls. When they do occur, they are usually associated with pelvic fratures (Garcia and Sheldon, 1998). Associated bladder and vaginal injuries are common (Garcia and Sheldon, 1998). This injury in girls is more difficult to diagnose as there is usually no difficulty in Foley placement (Garcia and Sheldon, 1998). A thorough examination of the perineum and vagina are mandatory in the setting of vaginal blood, vulvar hematoma, or gross hematuria (Garcia and Sheldon, 1998). Definitive diagnosis is obtained with urethoscope as urethrogram is unreliable in females (Garcia and Sheldon, 1998). Treatment of urethral injuries in girls ranges from catheter drainage to primary repair depending on the extent of injury and involvement of the bladder outlet.[2] Complications of urethral injuries in girls are common. Complications include stricture, incontinence, and fistula (Garcia and Sheldon, 1998).

Bibliography

Garcia V, Sheldon C. Genitourinary tract trauma. In: O'Neill JA, Rowe MI, Grosfeld JL, et al. (eds.), *Pediatric Surgery*, 5th ed. St. Louis, MO: Mosby Year Book, 1998, 285–302.

Snyder CL. Abdominal and genitourinary trauma. In: Ashcroft KW (ed.), *Pediatric Surgery*, 3rd ed. Philadelphia, PA: W.B. Saunders, 2000, 204–229.

35. **(D)** Burn mortality in children has decreased significantly in the last 50 years (Herndon and Pierre, 1998).

TABLE 13-7   Body Surface Area Changes with Age

	Head TBSA (%)	Trunk TBSA (%)	Arms TBSA (%)	Legs TBSA (%)
1–4 year olds	19	32	9.5	15
5–9 year olds	15	32	9.5	17
10–14 year olds	13	32	9.5	18
Adult	10	36	9	18

Improvements in resuscitation, nutritional support, and wound management have paved the way for this improved survival (Herndon and Pierre, 1998). The initial treatment and resuscitation of the burned child is very similar to that of the adult. Once the initial stabilization and ABCs have been addressed, the TBSA involved with partial and full thickness burns is measured. The body surface area of a child changes as the child ages (Herndon and Pierre, 1998). The head and neck have a larger surface area in children while the extremities have proportionally less surface area (Wolf and Herndon, 2000; Herndon and Pierre, 1998) (see Table 13-7).

The Berkow Chart for Estimation of Burn Size in Children gives a more detailed delineation of the TBSA changes and can be used for more specific calculations (Wolf and Herndon, 2000). The patient's fluid requirements are then calculated using one of the resuscitation formulas. The Parkland formula is the most commonly used formula for adults (Herndon and Pierre, 1998). This formula calculates the patient's fluid requirement to be 4 cc/kg of body weight/percentage TBSA burned. This is administered as a lactated Ringer's solution. Adult formulas, which are weight based, do not specifically address the issue of increased body surface area to weight ratio in children (Herndon and Pierre, 1998). This means that these formulas can underestimate insensible fluid losses from the child's open wounds (Herndon and Pierre, 1998). To counteract this, children's formulas, like the Shriners Burn Institute formula, calculate replacements based on TBSA and add additional maintenance fluids (Herndon and Pierre, 1998). This formula calculates the patient's fluid requirements to be 5000 cc/m^2 TBSA + 2000 cc/m^2 body surface area (Herndon and Pierre, 1998). Both formulas require that 50% of the volume requirements be given within the first 8 h after injury with the second 50% being given over the next 16 h. Assessment for adequacy of resuscitation involves observing for a decreasing heart rate, adequate blood pressure, clear mental status examination, and urine output >1–2 cc/kg/h. Adjustments in the volume of resuscitation fluid given can be made if these goals are not achieved. The management of circumferential burns is identical in children and adults (Table 13-7).

Bibliography

Herndon DN, Pierre EJ. Treatment of burns. In: O'Neill JA, Rowe MI, Grosfeld JL, et al. (eds.), *Pediatric Surgery*, 5th ed. St. Louis, MO: Mosby Year Book, 1998, 343–358.

Wolf SE, Herndon DN. Burns and radiation injuries. In: Mattox KL, Feliciano DV, Moore EE (eds.), *Trauma*, 4th ed. New York, NY: McGraw-Hill, 2000, 1137–1152.

36. **(E)** The syndrome of the abused child describes a child who has sustained multiple injuries, has bruises of varying ages, injury marks consistent with being caused by a specific object, subdural hematomas, and poor growth or development (Harris and Stylianos, 1998). These injuries or the failure to thrive were caused by the acts of a parent, guardian, or acquaintance of the child (Advanced Trauma Life Support for Physicians, 1997). Inconsistencies between the described mechanism of injury and the injuries themselves or a significant delay between the time of injury and the presentation for evaluation should raise suspicions that abuse has occurred (Advanced Trauma Life Support for Physicians, 1997; Harris and Stylianos, 1998). Injury patterns that include multiple subdural hematomas without associated external signs of trauma, retinal hemorrhages, perioral injuries, perforated viscera without preceding major blunt trauma, genital or perineal trauma, evidence of frequent injuries, long bone fractures in children under the age of 3, or burns of unusual shape or in unusual locations are suspicious and warrant extensive investigation (Advanced Trauma Life Support for Physicians, 1997).

Bibliography

Advanced Trauma Life Support for Physicians. Chicago, IL: American College of Surgeons, 1997, 291–310.

Harris BH, Stylianos S. Special considerations in trauma: child abuse and birth injuries. In: O'Neill JA, Rowe MI, Grosfeld JL, et al. (eds.), *Pediatric Surgery*, 5th ed. St. Louis, MO: Mosby Year Book, 1998, 359–365.

37. **(E)**

38. **(E)**

39. **(C)**

Explanations 37 through 39

Accidental hypothermia is defined as a core temperature below 35°C in a patient with an otherwise normal thermoregulatory system (Danzl, 2002; Gentilello, 2000). Children are more susceptible to hypothermia because of their high body surface area to weight ratio (Danzl, 2002). These patients may experience many cardiac, respiratory, renal, and metabolic complications related to the magnitude of their hypothermia. Cardiac complications include an initial tachycardia which is followed by progressive bradycardia as the core temperature approaches 28°C. Osborn (J) waves become evident on ECG at a core temperature <30°C (Danzl, 2002). Dysrhythmias are common as the core temperature decreases with ventricular fibrillation (VF) and asystole occurring when the core temperature falls below 25°C (Danzl, 2002). VF rarely responds to defibrillation below a core temperature of 30°C (Danzl, 2002).

Hypothermia causes diuresis (Danzl, 2002). This diuresis is more pronounced in intoxicated individuals and those who suffer cold water immersion (Danzl, 2002). Respiratory drive is stimulated by decreasing core temperature, initially. As hypothermia progresses, respiratory drive decreases, carbon dioxide is retained, secretions pool, pulmonary edema occurs and respiratory arrest follows (Danzl, 2002). For those patients with severe hypothermia (core temperature <30°C), some of these complications do not become apparent until rewarming is initiated (Gentilello, 2000). A further drop in core temperature, called the afterdrop, can be observed despite the initiation of external warming (Gentilello, 2000).

Initial assessment of the hypothermic patient should include a core temperature measurement. Care should be taken to use a measuring device capable of reading low temperatures. Oral temperatures are unreliable and while tympanic membrane temperatures equalizes with core temperature most rapidly, the reliability of these measuring devices at low temperatures is uncertain (Danzl, 2002). Therefore, rectal or esophageal temperatures should be followed.

Endotracheal intubation is warranted unless the degree of hypothermia is minimal enough to allow for spontaneous airway protection (Danzl, 2002). Patients should have intravenous or intraosseous access established. Boluses of warm (40–42°C) fluid should be given to initiate treatment of both the hypothermia and the associated dehydration (Danzl, 2002).

Cardiac monitoring should be followed. If the patient has no organized electrical activity, CPR should be initiated (Advanced Trauma Life Support for Physicians, 1997; Danzl, 2002). Any organized electrical activity is presumed to provide sufficient flow in the hypothermic patient (Advanced Trauma Life Support for Physicians, 1997; Gentilello, 2000).

The initiation of CPR could convert the organized rhythm into VF (Advanced Trauma Life Support for Physicians, 1997; Gentilello, 2000). CPR should be continued until organized electrical activity returns, CPB has been initiated, or a core temperature of at least 35°C has been achieved with failure of all resuscitative measures (American Heart Association, 2000). As arrhythmias are not responsive to defibrillation until a core temperature of 30°C, defibrillation should be attempted to a maximum of three times until sufficient warming has occurred (Danzl, 2002; American Heart Association, 2000).

Active rewarming is indicated in those patients with cardiac instability or core temperature <32°C (Danzl, 2002). Active rewarming can be done externally or internally (core rewarming). Techniques included in active external warming are forced air heating systems, hot water bottle application and radiant heating sources (Danzl, 2002). Active core rewarming techniques include administration of heated, humidified oxygen, peritoneal lavage, gastric or bladder lavage, thoracic lavage, and CPB (Danzl, 2002). These techniques warm at rates from 2°C/h with heated oxygen administration to 1°C/min on CPB (Danzl, 2002). Outcome after severe hypothermia is difficult to predict (Danzl, 2002). The rapidity of onset of hypothermia, the overall length of time spent hypothermic, and any preexisting medical problems all affect the patient's ability to recover from this insult (Gentilello, 2000).

Bibliography

Advanced Trauma Life Support for Physicians. Chicago, IL: American College of Surgeons, 1997, 291–310.

Danzl DF. Accidentalhypothermia. In: Marx JA, Hockberg RS, Walls Ron MW, et al. (eds.), *Rosen's Emergency Medicine*, 5th ed. St. Louis, MO: Mosby, 2002, 1979–1996.

Gentilello LM. Temperature-Associated Injuries and Syndromes. In: Mattox KL, Feliciano DV, Moore EE eds. Trauma, 4th ed. New York: McGraw-Hill; 2000:1153-1162.

American Heart Association in collaboration with International Liaison Committee on Resuscitation. Guidelines 2000 for Cardiopulmonary Resuscitation and Emergency Cardiovascular Care: International Consensus on Science. Part 3. Adult basic life support. *Circulation* 2000;102(Suppl I):1-22-1-59.

40. **(E)** The risk of nosocomial infection in ICUs is increasing. Impaired host defenses, invasive monitoring, exposure to multiple antibiotics and colonization with resistant microorganisms all contribute to make ICU patients more susceptible. Nosocomial pneumonia is the infection seen most frequently in ventilated trauma patients. Urinary tract and bloodstream infections are also common secondary to the use of invasive catheters. While respiratory failure is less common in children than in adults, ARDS remains a significant cause of morbidity and mortality in the pediatric trauma population. The goals of ventilatory strategies used in patients with ARDS are to minimize secondary lung injury, limit high concentration oxygen use and to limit peak pressure and tidal volume by using pressure control, square wave ventilation, inspiratory/expiratory ratio manipulation and PEEP. High-frequency positive pressure ventilation, high-frequency jet ventilation, and high-frequency oscillation are new modes of ventilation that have been used to better achieve those ventilatory goals in the more compromised patients. During the postinjury phase of traumatic illness, children can experience certain characteristic metabolic responses. They can develop a systemic inflammatory response, characterized by fever, tachycardia, tachypnea, and leukocytosis/leukocytopenia. They can exhibit an increase in oxidation of carbohydrates, fats, and proteins. They can also experience hyperglycemia resultant from the body's increased glucose production and the inability of insulin-dependent tissues to absorb glucose both of which are typical after significant trauma.

Bibliography

Scherer LR. Critical care of the severely injured child. *Surg Clin North Am* 2002;82:333–347.

CHAPTER 14

Head and Neck

Priya Krishna

Questions

1. All of these are intraoperative techniques during parotidectomy to locate the main trunk of the extracranial facial nerve *except:*

    (A) identification of the nerve at the stylomastoid foramen
    (B) location of the "tragal pointer"
    (C) retrograde tracking of the marginal mandibular nerve
    (D) retrograde tracking of the greater auricular nerve
    (E) identification of the temporoparotid fascia

2. All of these are part of the oral cavity *except*

    (A) floor of mouth
    (B) soft palate
    (C) base of tongue
    (D) upper gingivae
    (E) retromolar trigone

3. On delivery, a newborn has respiratory distress with evidence of cyanosis. During laryngoscopy for intubation, the anesthesiologist notes a pedunculated mass emanating from somewhere in the posterior naso- or oropharynx. The mass does not interfere with intubation but on further examination it appears to have hair on its ventral surface. Figure 14-1 shows the magnetic resonance imaging (MRI) obtained to evaluate the mass. The most likely diagnosis is

    (A) glioma
    (B) craniopharyngioma
    (C) teratoma
    (D) hemangioma
    (E) lymphangioma

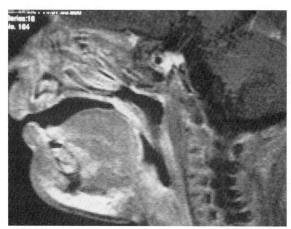

FIG. 14-1 T1-weighted sagittal MRI of head and neck with mass in oral cavity and nasopharynx.

4. A 7-year-old presents to your office a diagnosis of a right-sided neck mass. The mother states that the mass seems to fluctuate in size somewhat and drains clear fluid every time the child eats. On examination, you find a small pore anterior to the right SCM muscle and diagnose this as a branchial cleft cyst. This branchial cleft cyst is a (Fig. 14-2)

(A) type 1 branchial cleft cyst
(B) type 2 branchial cleft fistula
(C) type 2 branchial cleft cyst
(D) type 3 branchial cleft cyst
(E) type 4 branchial cleft cyst

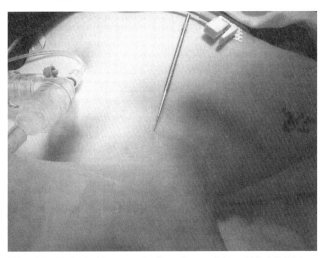

FIG. 14-2 Probe inside external orifice of second branchial cleft fistulous tract anterior to sternocleidomastoid muscle.

5. A 65-year-old man has an 8 mm squamous cell carcinoma (SCC) that involves the lateral half of the left ear canal. Occult spread of the tumor most likely would occur through

(A) a patent Huschke's foramen
(B) the tympanomastoid suture
(C) the tympanosquamosal suture
(D) Santorini's fissure
(E) the subepithelial space of the annulus

6. Which of the following is the most common nerve deficit after resection of a poststyloid compartment parapharyngeal neurilemmoma?

(A) ptosis
(B) painful shoulder syndrome
(C) deviation of tongue to the operated side
(D) voice change or hoarseness
(E) corneal exposure

7. A 58-year-old man undergoes a left-sided modified radical neck dissection (MRND) for an unknown primary. While dissecting inferiorly lateral to the carotid sheath, the operative field is suddenly inundated with a milky fluid. What structure was injured?

(A) cisterna chyli
(B) thoracic duct
(C) left IJV
(D) a cystic left thyroid lobe
(E) trachea

8. A 60-year-old man has a SCC involving the middle of the left true vocal cord. There is 3 mm supraglottic extension on the left and no reduction in cord mobility. The treatment that will best preserve voice quality is

(A) laser excision
(B) cordectomy
(C) primary radiation
(D) vertical hemilaryngectomy
(E) horizontal hemilaryngectomy.

9. A 56-year-old man with a 120 pack year smoking history and an alcohol abuse history presents with hoarseness for 1 year, progressive dysphagia over several months, and now stridor in a dependent position. His clinical examination is depicted in Fig. 14-3 and his CT scan is in Fig. 14-4. You decide to perform a tracheostomy for control of his airway and perform triple endoscopy with biopsies. The biopsy of the visible right true vocal cord reveals poorly differentiated invasive squamous cell carcinoma. Optimal management would include

(A) partial laryngectomy with bilateral neck dissections
(B) total laryngectomy with resection of the involved skin, bilateral neck dissections, and reconstruction of the defect
(C) concurrent chemorradiation
(D) total laryngectomy with resection of the involved skin, bilateral neck dissections, reconstruction of the defect followed by postoperative radiation therapy
(E) primary radiation therapy as single modality treatment

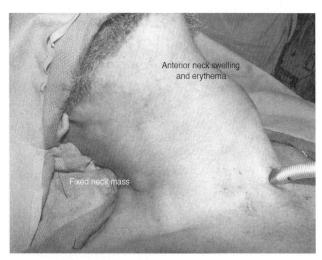

FIG. 14-3 Patient with advanced laryngeal cancer.

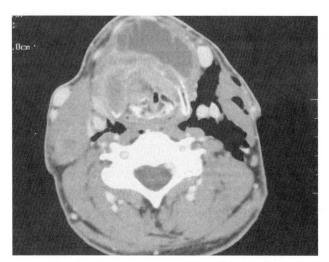

FIG. 14-4 CT scan with IV contrast of patient in Fig. 14-3.

10. A 2-year-old child swallows a short straight pin and is brought to the emergency room (ER) by his parents. On examination, he is alert and able to control his secretions (i.e., saliva). He has not experienced any respiratory distress and is afebrile. What is the appropriate course of action?

   (A) see the child in the clinic again in 10 days

   (B) perform endoscopy if the pin is found in the stomach or esophagus on x-ray

   (C) perform endoscopy whether or not a pin is seen on x-ray

   (D) admit the child for observation and daily abdominal plain films until the pin is passed in the stool

   (E) counsel the parents to strain the child's stool and feed him a high-roughage diet if the pin is radiographically identified in the stomach

11. A 14-year-old male is involved in a dirt bike accident in which he suffers a "clothesline" injury. On examination in the ER you see a 7 cm laceration in the anterior neck, subcutaneous emphysema, and a hematoma which does not appear to be expanding. He is unable to lay flat and has a muffled voice. On flexible laryngoscopy, you see diffuse but mild edema of the supraglottis and glottis, reduced vocal cord abduction, and bloody secretions in the subglottis. Initial management of this patient would involve

   (A) nasal intubation, laryngeal and cervical spine CT, exploration and repair with intraoperative tracheotomy

   (B) tracheostomy under local anesthesia, cervical spine series, endoscopy, exploration and repair

   (C) percutaneous tracheostomy, cervical spine series, exploration and repair with stenting

   (D) oral intubation, laryngeal and cervical spine CT, endoscopy, exploration and repair

   (E) tracheostomy under general anesthesia, CT of the larynx and cervical spine, endoscopy, exploration and repair with stenting over a T-tube

12. A 73-year-old woman suffers a fall after having a few drinks. She presents to the ER with right-sided periorbital ecchymosis and edema and has double vision on looking upward. She also complains of numbness of her right cheek and upper lip. Her CT is seen in Fig. 14-5. The *least* important reason for repairing the orbital floor is

   (A) radiographic evidence of extraocular muscle entrapment

   (B) double vision on upward gaze

   (C) enophthalmos from displaced periorbital fracture

   (D) gross displacement of orbital contents into the maxillary sinus

   (E) positive forced-duction test

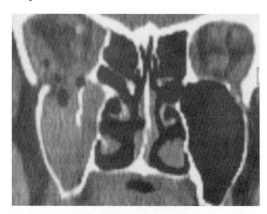

FIG. 14-5 Coronal fine of cut CT scan (bone window) with evidence of right blowout fracture.

13. A 40-year-old man presents 8 days after suffering a midfacial wound after facial trauma. The laceration was repaired by another physician who noted transection of the parotid duct but did not repair it. His facial nerve function is normal on examination. Your next step in management is

(A) perform a sialogram

(B) irradiate the parotid gland

(C) observe for complications

(D) explore the wound from an intraoral approach

(E) place a pressure dressing to prevent sialocele development

14. A 19-year-old woman presents to the ER with few days history of fever and pain in the submandibular region. She says that over the last several hours she has been having more trouble speaking with pain in her tongue and is afraid to lie down. On oral examination, you see that the floor of mouth is indurated and swollen and very tender. The patient has very poor dentition but you do not appreciate an abscess. Her submandibular and submental regions are also tender and indurated with some fluctuance. What entity in the differential diagnosis are you most worried about?

(A) Vincent's angina

(B) Bezold's abscess

(C) Ludwig's angina

(D) a retropharyngeal abscess

(E) submandibular and sublingual gland sialadenitis

15. Which of these tumors has the highest frequency of being bilateral?

(A) pleomorphic adenoma

(B) monomorphic adenoma

(C) Warthin's tumor

(D) cylindroma

(E) benign lymphoepithelial lesion

16. A 20-year-old man involved in an altercation presents to the ER with epistaxis and nasal airway obstruction. When inspecting his nose externally, you feel crepitus when moving the nasal bones and mild flattening of the dorsum; there is no active bleeding. On anterior rhinoscopy, you see an ecchymotic, swollen area on either side of the caudal septum (Fig. 14-6). The next step in management would be to

(A) reduce the nasal fracture externally and employ an external nasal splint

(B) place internal nasal splints to stabilize the fracture

(C) drain the septal hematoma

(D) place anterior nasal packing to treat the epistaxis

(E) get facial x-rays if they were not already performed

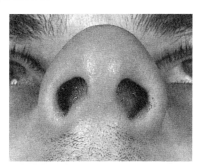

FIG. 14-6 Bilateral septal hematomas. (*Source:* Reprinted from Bull TR. *Color Atlas of ENT Diagnosis*, 3rd ed., plate 225, copyright, 1995, with permission from Elsevier).

17. A 50-year-old man has a 2-day history of headaches and of proptosis with failing vision in the right eye. Vision has been reduced to light perception only and the globe is displaced inferior and laterally. Rhinoscopy shows swelling in the middle meatus with some purulence. The next step in management would be to

(A) obtain a CT scan of the orbits and sinuses and immediate ethmoidectomy

(B) IV aqueous penicillin G, 2 million U every 4 h

(C) IV levaquin 500 mg every 24 h

(D) immediate exploration of the orbits

(E) oral dexamethasone, 4 mg daily for 1 week

18. A 24-year-old woman is assaulted by her boyfriend and has an anterior zone 1 stab injury to the neck. She has a midline moderate hematoma which is not expanding and is subcutaneous. She is also having hemoptysis of bright red blood but is hemodynamically stable and her voice is normal. An angiogram is performed which is negative for any major vascular injury. Intraoperatively, you note an anterior tracheal laceration across the first and second tracheal rings. The next step in evaluation would include inspection of the

(A) course of both recurrent nerves

(B) cricothyroid membrane and external branch of the superior laryngeal nerve

(C) posterior tracheal wall

(D) innominate artery

(E) brachiocephalic vein

19. A 46-year-old male is struck by a train and suffers a nonpenetrating temporal bone fracture. Immediately after the injury, his facial nerve function seems intact; however, the next day he has some facial nerve weakness that evolves into complete paralysis by the fourth day (see Figs. 14-7 and 14-8). You should

(A) obtain a high-resolution temporal bone CT to see if bony fragments are impinging on the facial nerve

(B) obtain electroneuronography (ENOG) to determine the need for surgical intervention

(C) proceed with immediate exploration of the facial nerve for decompression

(D) obtain a facial electromyogram (EMG) to determine the need for surgical intervention

(E) continue to observe the patient because the prognosis for recovery is good

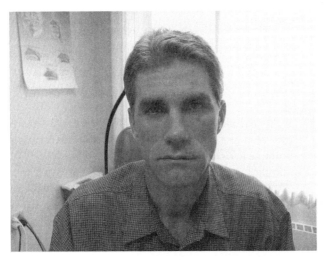

FIG. 14-7   Patient with history of blunt temporal bone trauma at rest.

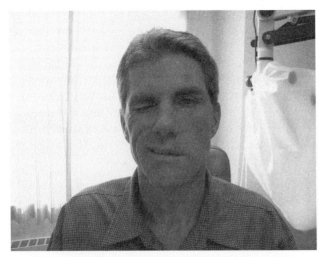

FIG. 14-8   Patient with gross facial asymmetry on maximum effort.

20. A 42-year-old man presents with a several month history of dental pain and progressive swelling of the anterior cheek. In addition he has had a 1-year history of nasal obstruction and epistaxis which was attributed to allergies. You see a gray ulcerative lesion in the left upper gingivobuccal sulcus which you biopsy. The biopsy indicates invasive squamous cell carcinoma. The patient's CT scan appears in Fig. 14-9. The indication to perform orbital exenteration in this case is

(A) invasion of periorbita

(B) erosion of the lamina papyracea

(C) invasion of orbital fat

(D) A and C

(E) all of the above

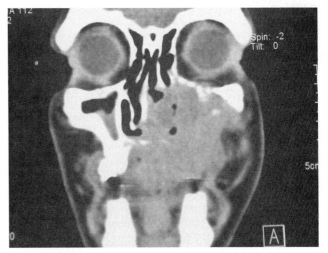

FIG. 14-9   Coronal CT scan with evidence of bony destruction of maxillary and possibly the orbit.

21. A 6-year-old boy on a bike collides with another individual on a motor bike. On presentation to the ER, after stabilization, the following CT is obtained (Fig. 14-10). What would make this a LeFort III fracture?

(A) presence of pyramidal fractures

(B) presence of naso-orbito-ethmoid fractures (NOE complex)

(C) presence of a unilateral horizontal maxillary fracture

(D) presence of a bilateral horizontal maxillary fracture

(E) craniofacial dysjunction

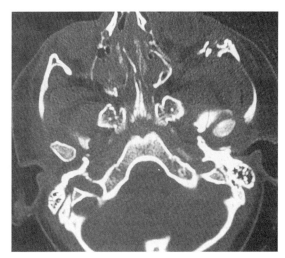

FIG. 14-10 Axial fine cut facial bone CT of patient in case 21. Seen is a midface comminuted fracture of ethmoid bones, septum, and fracture of the medial maxilla on the left.

22. A 60-year-old male with a history of hypertension and coronary artery disease presents to the ER with steady bleeding from the right nare. He is on aspirin 325 mg a day as well as Plavix; he had a percutaneous transluminal coronary angioplasty (PTCA) with stenting 5 years ago. You first examine him and are not sure where the bleeding is arising from so you place an anterior nasal pack. He has no bleeding until 20 min later, but then bleeds through your pack and is bleeding from his mouth. Your next step in management after careful reexamination is

    (A) place a new anterior pack and admit him for observation
    (B) place a posterior nasal pack and admit him for observation
    (C) place a posterior nasal pack and admit him to a monitored floor
    (D) schedule him for an internal maxillary artery ligation
    (E) schedule embolization with interventional radiology

23. A 47-year-old man is brought to the physician's office by his wife who is having difficulty sleeping because of her husband's extremely loud snoring. He does complain of headaches and daytime sleepiness as well as some irritability. On examination, his collar size is 18 in. and he is moderately obese. In addition you note a septal deviation to the right and an elongated redundant uvula and posterior pharyngeal mucosa. You obtain a polysomnogram because you suspect sleep apnea: the patient's RDI is 40 with a low saturation of 80%. Appropriate treatment options include all of the following *except*:

    (A) nasal continuous positive airway pressure (CPAP)
    (B) septoplasty with uvulopalatopharyngoplasty (UPPP)
    (C) encourage weight loss as the sole treatment
    (D) orthodontic devices in conjunction with CPAP
    (E) tracheostomy

24. A 46-year-old patient had respiratory failure from pneumonia and developed acute respiratory distress syndrome (ARDS). He remained on a ventilator for a prolonged period of time and ultimately underwent a tracheostomy at the level of tracheal ring 4. The patient is now in the rehabilitation unit of your hospital 2 weeks after his tracheostomy and you are called to see him about bright red blood around his tracheostomy site. The most common cause of this bleeding is

    (A) granulation tissue
    (B) erosion of the inferior thyroid artery
    (C) erosion of the innominate artery
    (D) tracheal chondritis
    (E) recurrence of pneumonia

25. A 75-year-old White farmer presents with a 3.0 cm ulcerated lesion of his lower lip. On examination you find that it involves the central portion of the lower lip. You perform a biopsy confirming squamous cell carcinoma. The optimal treatment of this patient would be

    (A) primary full-thickness excision
    (B) vermilionectomy and bilateral supraomohyoid neck dissections
    (C) radiation therapy
    (D) Mohs' micrographic surgery
    (E) full-thickness excision and bilateral supraomohyoid neck dissections

26. A 67-year-old patient presents with a ulcerating lesion of the cervical esophagus that does not directly involve the party wall between the esophagus and larynx. It does, however, extend into the thoracic esophagus for 2 cm. The patient is consented for a total laryngopharyngoesophagectomy. The best reconstructive option is

    (A) gastric pull-up
    (B) radial forearm free flap
    (C) pectoralis major myocutaneous tubed flap
    (D) jejunal free flap/transfer
    (E) cervical skin flaps

27. A 56-year-old woman with an 80-pack-year smoking history and who drinks a fifth of vodka every night presents to the ER with odynophagia and bleeding from her mouth. On examination of her oropharynx, you find a 3.5 cm exophytic lesion of the left tonsil with some extension into the anterior tonsillar pillar and soft palate (Fig. 14-11). After confirmation that this is SCC on triple endoscopy with biopsies, which of these would definitely *not* be an approach to removal of this lesion?

    (A) composite resection
    (B) suprahyoid pharyngotomy
    (C) subhyoid approach (lateral pharyngtotomy)
    (D) midline (anterior) mandibulotomy
    (E) transoral approach

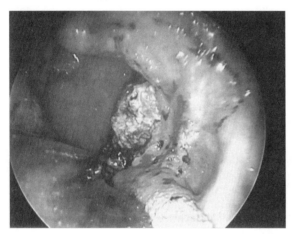

FIG. 14-11 Left tonsillar cancer with anterior tonsillar pillar and soft palate extension.

28. A 80-year-old woman who is a nursing home patient is brought to the hospital with a GI bleed. She ultimately undergoes a left hemicolectomy for diverticulosis and has a lengthy postoperative ileus. Postoperative day 5 she complains of a sour taste in her mouth and her right cheek feeling warm and very tender. You notice a swelling in the parotid area and that she is febrile at the time. All of the following would be part of the treatment of this disorder *except*:

    (A) IV antibiotics against *S. aureus*
    (B) heat application to the area over the parotid
    (C) IV hydration
    (D) lemon drops
    (E) cannulation of the right Stensen's duct with drainage

29. A 10-year-old girl presents with a solitary left-sided submandibular neck mass that has been present for a month. It is nontender and initially grew over the

course of 2-3 days and then has not grown further. The most likely etiology of this mass is

    (A) reactive lymph node
    (B) atypical mycobacterial infection
    (C) branchial cleft cyst
    (D) submandibular gland sialadenitis
    (E) lymphoma

30. What muscle defines the posterior limit of a modified radical or radical neck dissection?

    (A) levator scapulae
    (B) SCM
    (C) omohyoid
    (D) anterior scalene
    (E) trapezius

31. A 47-year-old man undergoes resection of a right lateral tongue and retromolar trigone SCC with a wide local resection with hemiglossectomy and modified neck dissection. There is a significant soft tissue deficit and you decide to use a pectoralis myocutaneous flap for reconstruction. All of these are potential complications of this flap *except*:

    (A) hematoma
    (B) infection
    (C) wound dehiscence
    (D) skin necrosis
    (E) thrombosis of the thoracodorsal artery

32. The most likely pathogen to be involved with supraglottitis (epiglottitis) is

    (A) *Streptoccocus pneumonia*
    (B) *H. influenzae*
    (C) influenza virus
    (D) parainfluenza virus
    (E) *S. aureus*

33. A 25-year-old male is thrown from his motorbike and his chin hits first against a concrete sidewalk. A panorex x-ray indicates a symphyseal fracture of the mandible. You note that he is unable to close his mouth at all. What other injury has the patient most likely suffered?

    (A) unilateral subcondylar/condylar fracture
    (B) bilateral subcondylar or condylar fractures
    (C) rupture of pterygoid muscle tendon attachments to pterygoid plates
    (D) a ramus fracture
    (E) a contralateral body fracture

34. What structure passes through the foramen ovale?

   (A) infraorbital nerve
   (B) V_3
   (C) meningeal artery
   (D) sphenopalatine artery
   (E) V_2

35. What study is used to monitor response to therapy for malignant otitis externa?

   (A) technetium-99 scan
   (B) gallium-67 scan
   (C) CT scan
   (D) MRI
   (E) culture

36. Nasopharyngeal carcinoma is associated most strongly with which virus?

   (A) CMV
   (B) varicella zoster
   (C) herpes simplex
   (D) Epstein-Barr virus (EBV)
   (E) human papilloma virus

37. The main difference between keloids and hypertrophic scars is

   (A) keloids are only found in dark skinned individuals
   (B) hypertrophic scars are only found in light skinned individuals
   (C) keloids extend beyond the confines of the original wound
   (D) hypertrophic scars extend beyond the confines of the original wound
   (E) keloids result from an overall increase in collagen

38. What is the term for a flap that is raised and pivoted into a defect along an arc in a curvilinear fashion?

   (A) rotation
   (B) island
   (C) transposition
   (D) hinge
   (E) random

39. Which of these histologic findings is considered pathognomonic for Hodgkin's lymphoma?

   (A) Mikulicz's cells
   (B) Charcot-Leyden crystals
   (C) Birbeck granules
   (D) Reed-Sternberg cells
   (E) physaliferous cells

40. Pott's puffy tumor is seen most commonly with which of these conditions?

   (A) otitis media
   (B) frontal sinus fracture
   (C) ethmoid sinusitis
   (D) bacterial pharyngitis
   (E) cervical spinal infection

Answers and Explanations

1. **(D)** Embryologically, the parotid gland develops as a unilobular structure from the first branchial pouch at 5.5 weeks. The facial nerve itself begins as the fascioacoustic primordium during the third week of gestation and by the eleventh week, most of its branching is complete. In young children (under age 3), the mastoid bone is poorly developed and the nerve courses much more superficially and caudally. The facial nerve is the most superficial structure to pass through the parotid gland, dividing it into superficial and deep lobes. The nerve first exits the skull base at the stylomastoid foramen and then courses anteriorly and somewhat inferiorly toward the posterior surface of the parotid gland. The pes anserinus (Fig. 14-12) is the point at which the facial nerve divides into its temporozygomatic and cervicofacial divisions within the substance of the parotid gland. Once the anterior border of the parotid is reached, the nerve will have divided into its five branches: temporal, zygomatic, buccal, marginal mandibular, and cervical (Fig. 14-13).

A superficial parotidectomy commences with a preauricular incision which then curves around the lobule of the ear to reach the mastoid and then extends into the neck past the angle of the jaw in a natural skin crease. Anterior and posterior skin flaps are developed but the temporoparotid or "heavy" fascia is left intact. The mastoid and posterior border of the sternocleidomastoid (SCM) are located. The gland is then separated by blunt dissection from the cartilage of the external auditory canal and the tragal pointer, and extension of this cartilage, is exposed. The main trunk of the facial nerve can then be identified approximately 1–1.5 cm deep and inferior as the temporoparotid fascia is divided. The tympanomastoid suture line is another landmark: the main trunk can be found 6–8 mm deep to the suture. Any of the branches if identified first peripherally can be followed retrograde to the main trunk or "pes." The full course of each branch should be followed to prevent a "flanking" injury. The greater auricular nerve is derived from cervical roots C2 and C3 and supplies sensation to the inferior part of the auricle as

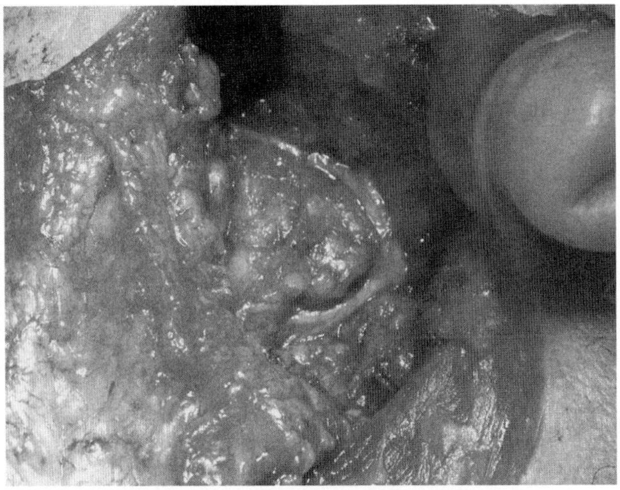

FIG. 14-12 Intraoperative photograph of the pes anserinus in the parotid gland.

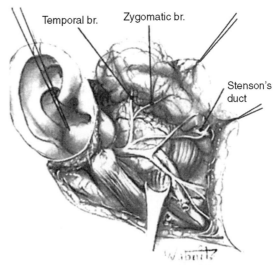

FIG. 14-13 Identification of the main trunk of the facial nerve and Stenson's duct. (*Source:* Reprinted from Lore JM Jr. *An Atlas of Head and Neck Surgery,* 3rd ed., p. 711, copyright 1988, with permission from Elsevier).

well as the neck and the area between the mastoid and angle of the mandible. Although it is one of the early structures encountered during parotidectomy, it is not used specifically as a landmark for the main trunk. A deep lobe or total parotidectomy would involve taking the portion of the parotid gland deep to the facial nerve requiring complete skeletonization of the nerve branches.

Bibliography

Carrasco VN, et al. Facial nerve paralysis. In: Lee KJ (ed.), *Essential Otolaryngology Head and Neck Surgery*, 8th ed. New York, NY: Mc-Graw Hill, 2003, 169–191.

Gosain AK. Surgical anatomy of the facial nerve. Surgery of the midface and nasolabial fold. *Clin Plast Surg.* 1995;22(2):241–249.

Hanna EY, Suen JY. Neoplasms of the salivary glands. In: Cummings CW, Fredrickson JM, Harker LA, et al. (eds.), *Otolaryngology Head & Neck Surgery*, 3rd ed., vol. 2. St. Louis, MO: Mosby, 1998, 1255–1302.

Lore JM Jr. *An Atlas of Head and Neck Surgery*, 3rd ed. Philadelphia, PA: WB Saunders, 1988, 708–712.

2. **(C)** The oral cavity is bounded by the vermilion border of the lips and the junction of the hard and soft palate and circumvallate papillae. It can be thought of having eight subunits: lips, buccal mucosa, floor of mouth, anterior two-thirds of the tongue (i.e., oral tongue), upper and lower alveolar ridges, hard palate, and retromolar trigone. The retromolar trigone is a triangular spaced area from the distal surface of the last molar tooth to the maxillary tuberosity. This area is important in cancer spread as the mucosa of the mandible is tightly adherent to the underlying periosteum and therefore a weak barrier to tumor extension. The vestibule is the area lateral to the alveolar ridges and the oral cavity proper the area medial to the teeth. The layers of the cheek itself from superficial to deep are as follows: skin, subcutaneous tissue, the buccinator muscle, the buccinator fat pad, the pharyngobuccal fascia, and the mucosa/lip complex. The salivary ducts traverse the mucosa to drain into the oral cavity. These include Stensen's duct of the parotid gland, the papilla of which is located lateral to the second molars; Wharton's duct of the submandibular gland which is found in the midline floor of mouth adjacent to the frenulum of the tongue; and ducts of Rivinius of the sublingual gland which drain into the floor of mouth or into Wharton's duct itself.

The vascular supply of the oral cavity is derived from several branches of the external carotid artery. These include the lingual artery which supplies the floor of mouth; the (internal) maxillary artery which transmits the descending palatine artery, ultimately dividing into the greater and lesser palatine arteries to supply the hard and soft palate, respectively, and the posterior, middle, and anterior superior alveolar arteries and nasopalatine artery which supply the upper alveolar ridge. The lesser palatine artery anastomoses posteriorly with a branch of the facial artery, the ascending palatine artery. The mandibular teeth and gingiva are vascularized by the inferior alveolar artery. Venous drainage of the palate is via the pterygoid plexus (hard palate) and pharyngeal plexus (soft palate) and tongue and floor of mouth via the lingual vein. Lymphatic drainage occurs via submandibular (hard palate, lateral tongue), deep jugular (most subunits), lateral pharyngeal, parotid and submental nodes (tip of tongue). The oral tongue does not have bilateral drainage whereas the base of tongue (posteriorone-third, part of the oropharynx) does have bilateral drainage. Hence, the answer is "**C**."

The embryology of the oral cavity and specifically the tongue is important in describing the innervation. The anterior two-thirds of the tongue are derived from ectoderm of the first and second branchial arches and the posterior one-third from endoderm between the second and third branchial arches. The anterior or oral tongue receives general sensation from V_3, a nerve of the first arch and special sensation (taste) from the chorda tympani, a branch of VII which is the second arch nerve. The base of tongue receives innervation from the glossopharyngeal nerve. The principle of referred otalgia from lesions or processes in the oral cavity is explained by lingual nerve (V_3) innervation, the lingual also supplying the external ear, external auditory canal, and tympanic membrane.

Bibliography

Eibling DE. The oral cavity, pharynx and esophagus. In: Lee KJ (ed.), *Essential Otolaryngology Head and Neck Surgery*, 8th ed. New York, NY: Mc-Graw Hill, 2003, 439–461.

Moore KL. *Clinically Oriented Anatomy*, 3rd ed. Baltimore, MD: Williams & Wilkins, 1992.

Lee KJ, Farrior JB. Embryology of clefts and pouches. In: Lee KJ (ed.), *Essential Otolaryngology Head and Neck Surgery*, 8th ed. New York, NY: Mc-Graw Hill, 2003, 232–247.

Levine PA, Hood RJ. Neoplasms of the oral cavity. In: Bailey BJ, et al. (eds.), *Head & Neck Surgery Otolaryngology*, 3rd ed., vol. 2. Philadelphia, PA: Lippincott, Williams & Wilkins, 2001, 1311–1326.

Lore JM Jr. *An Atlas of Head and Neck Surgery*, 3rd ed. Philadelphia, PA: WB Saunders, 1988, 708–712.

3. **(C)** The differential diagnosis for airway obstruction in the neonate is broad. The first group of disorders involves congenital anatomic anomalies. These may involve the nose, nasopharynx, and oropharynx and

include etiologies such as choanal atresia, pyriform aperture stenosis, and craniofacial anomalies such as the micrognathia and glossoptosis found in the Pierre-Robin sequence. Choanal atresia can be diagnosed at birth by the inability to pass an eight French catheter into the oropharynx. Other congenital anomalies in the nasopharynx would include nasopharyngeal cysts which can be intra- or extraadenoidal or branchial cleft in origin.

An important group of nasal masses is those of neuroectodermal origin. These include the glioma, encephalocele, and dermoid. Only the encephalocele is characterized by an ependyma-lined tract that communicates with the ventricles of the brain. The encephalocele can be characterized by a positive Furstenburg test. The Furstenburg test is performed by compression of the jugular veins which causes increased cerebrospinal fluid (CSF) pressure leading to enlargement of the encephalocele.

Anomalies of the larynx would include laryngomalacia, laryngeal webs, cysts, laryngoceles, subglottic stenosis, laryngeal atresia, or laryngeal clefts. Birth trauma can cause stretching of one or both recurrent laryngeal nerves although this is uncommon and only paralysis of both nerves would cause airway obstruction.

Neoplastic lesions are another important category. The first mass would be a hemangioma. Though these can be located anywhere in the upper aerodigestive tract, there is a propensity for the anterior subglottic region. Hemangiomas of the subglottis do not produce symptoms of stridor or airway obstruction at birth because they are small initially and several weeks after birth they begin a proliferative stage. Lymphangiomas are caused by failure of lymph spaces to link to the rest of the lymphatic system. They range in size from the lymphangioma simplex to the large multicystic cystic hygroma. These are more typically found in the neck. The craniopharyngioma is a tumor of the nasopharynx derived from Rathke's pouch elements. Rathke's pouch contains the ectoderm that becomes the anterior pituitary gland and the tumor itself contains well-differentitated epithelial elements. Just inferior to Rathke's pouch can be found Thornwaldt's cyst which is a remnant of the inferior notochord.

The teratoma is a benign mass originating from pleuripotential cells and occurs in 1 in 4000 births. It may be associated with other anomalies such as anencephaly and palatal fissures. Although some sources indicate a higher incidence in females, others note that the incidence is the same in the head and neck whereas in other parts of the body, teratomas

may still be more common in females. Sources for teratomas in the head and neck include orbital, nasal nasopharyngeal (nasal and nasopharyngeal comprising 50% of those in the head and neck), oral cavity, and neck. The teratoma is part of a spectrum of masses which includes the dermoid cyst, the teratoid cyst, and epignathi. The dermoid is the most common and has both epidermal and mesodermal elements and can have hair. The teratoid cyst and teratoma contain all three germ layers but the teratoma has much more cellular differentiation (and can exhibit hair growth as well). Epignathi also contain all three germ layers and are the most differentiated with complete organs and/or body parts.

Bibliography

Gagliano JR, Jafek BW. The pediatric airway. In: Jafek BW, Murrow BW (eds.), *ENT Secrets*, 2nd ed. Philadelphia, PA: Hanley & Belfus, 2001, 429–436.

Knudsen SJ, Bailey BJ. Midline nasal masses. In: Bailey BJ, et al. (eds.), *Head & Neck Surgery Otolaryngology*, 3rd ed., vol. 1. Philadelphia, PA: Lippincott, Williams & Wilkins, 2001, 309–320.

Lee KJ, Latorre RC. Highlights and pearls. In: Lee KJ (ed.), *Essential Otolaryngology Head and Neck Surgery*, 8th ed. New York, NY: Mc-Graw Hill, 2003, 1015–1093.

Wetmore RF, Potsic WP. Differential diagnosis of neck masses. In: Cummings CW, Fredrickson JM, Harker LA, et al. (eds.), *Otolaryngology Head & Neck Surgery: Pediatric*, 3rd ed. St. Louis, MO: Mosby, 1998, 248–261.

4. **(B)** The structures of the head and neck are derived from the branchial arches, grooves (clefts), or the pharyngeal pouches. The arches are mesodermal, the grooves are ectodermal, and the pouches endodermal in origin. Much of the development of the arches occurs in the first 8 weeks of embryonic life. Each of the arches is associated with a nerve, artery, and bar of cartilage whereas the pouches become glandular or are associated with the digestive tract. A cervical sinus develops where structures of each arch develop. Eventually the sinus is obliterated by the growth of the arch derivatives. When the sinus does not obliterate, a branchial arch anomaly exists. These anomalies come in three forms: a sinus, cyst, or fistula. The sinus has an opening in the mucosa of the foregut or skin and ends in the soft tissue of the neck. The fistula is a complete tract with an internal and external opening indicating persistence of both a groove and a pouch. The fistula can present as both intermittent swelling or with drainage. The cyst is formed from remnants of the grooves or sinuses. One source cites that branchial anomalies comprise approximately 17% of pediatric neck masses.

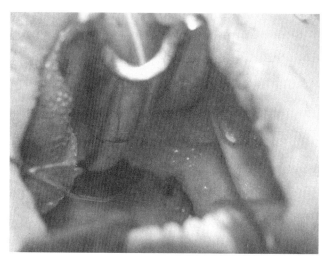

FIG. 14-14   Metal probe inserting into internal orifice of second branchial cleft fistula at base of right tonsillar fossa.

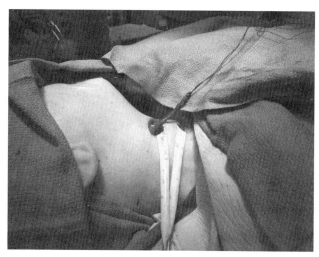

FIG. 14-15   Dissection of entire fistulous tract with "stair step" incision.

The path of the first arch anomaly starts at the external auditory canal and is divided into two types as described by Work. Type I is a duplication of the membranous canal alone and contains only ectodermal elements without cartilage or adnexa. It is found medial to the concha and may extend to the postauricular area and runs superior to the facial nerve, the nerve for the second branchial arch. Type II are the more common type and involve duplication of both the membranous and cartilaginous external auditory canal and can be intimately associated with the facial nerve and have a tract at the level of the mandible. These first arch anomalies should be differentiated from the preauricular pits or cysts which are inclusion cysts from fusion of the auricular hillocks (which are derivatives of the first and second arch) during development of the pinna. Surgical excision is the treatment of choice and if the parotid gland is involved with the tract, a superficial parotidectomy with facial nerve dissection may be required for complete removal.

The second branchial arch anomaly, which is the most common type of branchial arch defect, has a pathway that begins at the tonsillar bed (Fig. 14-14)—and if a complete fistulous tract—will open just anterior to the ipsilateral SCM muscle (Fig. 14-15). The tract passes between the internal and external carotid arteries and lies superficial to derivatives of the third arch. Second arch derivatives include all facial mimetic muscles, posterior belly of the digastric muscle, styloid muscle and lesser cornu and body of the hyoid bone. The anomalies can be delineated by ultrasound, contrast enhanced CT or MRI. Surgical excision, usually via two stair step incisions, is the treatment of choice.

The third branchial arch anomaly has a tract which extends from the pyriform sinus, runs deep to the bifurcation of the carotid and cranial nerve IX but superficial to cranial nerve XII, and opens (if a fistula) in the skin of the lower neck anterior to the SCM. The fourth arch anomaly has a similar course but loops around the subclavian on the right and around the arch of the aorta on the left.

Bibliography

Graney DO, Sie KY. Developmental anatomy. In: Cummings CW, Fredrickson JM, Harker LA, et al. (eds.), *Otolaryngology Head & Neck Surgery: Pediatric*, 3rd ed. St. Louis, MO: Mosby, 1998, 11–24.

Koopmann CF Jr. Congenital neck masses. In: Gates GA (ed.), *Current Therapy in Otolaryngology Head and Neck Surgery*, 6th ed. St. Louis, MO: Mosby, 1998, 299–301.

Lee KJ, Farrior JB. Embryology of clefts and pouches. In: Lee KJ (ed.), *Essential Otolaryngology Head and Neck Surgery*, 8th ed. New York, NY: Mc-Graw Hill, 2003, 232–247.

Pincus RL. Congenital neck masses and cysts. In: Bailey BJ, et al. (eds.), *Head & Neck Surgery Otolaryngology*, 3rd ed., vol. 1. Philadelphia, PA: Lippincott, Williams & Wilkins, 2001, 933–939.

Stanford M, Chan KH. Congenital malformations. In: Jafek BW, Murrow BW (eds.), *ENT Secrets*, 2nd ed. Philadelphia, PA: Hanley & Belfus, 2001, 444–447.

5. **(D)** The auricle develops from six hillocks, three from the first branchial arch and three from the second. Though the fusion of these hillocks should theoretically provide a barrier to tumor or infection spread, the areas of fusion can actually serve as conduits for spread. In addition to these fusion planes, there are two other important lymphatic communications that travel anteriorly from the auricle and external canal to

the glenoid fossa and parotid gland. These are Santorini's fissure(s) in the lateral cartilaginous canal and Huschke's foramen, an embryologic remnant that starts in the medial bony external canal. The other three answers (B, C, E) are natural fusion planes or bony dehiscences which may be more important in tumor spread in the bony or medial external canal. The external canal is one-third cartilaginous laterally and two-third bony in its medial portion; this is in contrast to the Eustachian tube which is two-thirds cartilaginous and one-third bony.

The most common malignant tumor of the pinna is basal cell carcinoma. These cancers appear as indurated nodules with classic "rolled" or raised edges and they tend to be locally invasive with rare metastatic behavior. The "H" zone of the face is a mask-like area including the periorbital skin, nose, upper lip, ears, and preauricular skin between the angle of the mandible and the temple. Basal cell carcinomas that occur in the "H" zone have a more aggressive behavior. The SCC comprises only 15% of malignancies of the pinna and ear canal but four-fifths of advanced tumors in the area. It is typically ulcerative and more deeply invasive. The development of both of these carcinomas is related to exposure to actinic radiation, specifically ultraviolet B rays (UVB). Sun protection factor (SPF) indicates the effectiveness of sunscreen against UVB specifically, i.e., a product with an SPF of 20 is interpreted as 20 h of sun exposure while sustaining the actinic damage of one unprotected hour of sun exposure. Other risk factors include Fitzpatrick type I or II skin (fair skin which burns easily), advanced age, male gender, freckling, and history of previous similar skin cancer.

The treatment of choice is excision, either via Mohs' micrographic surgery or wide local excision. Mohs' surgery maps the histologic border between normal tissue and the tumor along its entire circumference. If areas are positive on frozen section, then the affected quadrant is excised further. Mohs' methods have decreased the recurrence of both basal cell and squamous cell carcinomas, rates of which are 8 and 3%, respectively. Mohs' does have disadvantages, including lengthy operating times and associated higher costs, and the potential for missing skip or satellite lesions. Wide local excision of a tumor of the external canal would include one of several types of temporal bone resections. These involve a cortical mastoidectomy and frozen sections of mucosa of the mastoid and middle ear. If these are involved with tumor, then a subtotal temporal bone resection is performed. Depending on the extent of the tumor here, superficial parotidectomies, partial mandibulectomies, and/or neck dissections may

need to be performed. Staging of external auditory canal carcinoma can be easily summarized. Any lesion greater than a T1 requires postoperative adjunctive radiotherapy. More extensive T3 and T4 lesions still have a fairly poor 5-year survival of less than 50%.

Bibliography

Calhoun KH, Tan LKS. Skin cancer. In: Gates GA (ed.), *Current Therapy in Otolaryngology Head and Neck Surgery*, 6th ed. St. Louis, MO: Mosby, 1998, 213–216.

Kinney SE. Malignancies of the temporal bone: limited temporal bone resection. In: Brackmann DE, Shelton C, Arriaga MA (eds.), *Otologic Surgery*, 2nd ed. Philadelphia, PA: WB Saunders, 2001, 35–42.

Niparko JK, Swanson NA, Baker SR, et al. Local control of auricular, periauricular, and external canal cutaneous malignancies with Mohs surgery. *Laryngoscope* 1990;100:1047–1051.

Saunders JE, Medina JE. Ear and temporal bone. In: Close LG, Larson DL, Shah JP (eds.), *Essentials of Head and Neck Oncology*. New York, NY: Thieme, 1998, 135–145.

6. **(A)** The parapharyngeal space (PPS) can be thought of as an inverted pyramid. The boundaries of this space are the base of skull superiorly and the hyoid bone inferiorly. The space itself is deep to the pharyngeal mucosa and superficial to the carotid sheath and it communicates with the submandibular space. It can be divided into a prestyloid and poststyloid or retrostyloid space by the syloid muscles and a band of fascia from the tensor veli palatini. These spaces are important when discussing tumor pathology and surgical approaches. The prestyloid space contains fat, the mandibular branch of the facial nerve, the pterygoid venous plexus, whereas the poststyloid space contains cranial nerves IX–XII, the cervical sympathetic chain and the internal carotid artery and internal jugular vein (IJV).

The differential of masses in the PPS is large but can be broken into four categories: salivary gland tumors, neurogenic tumors, lymph node enlargement, or miscellaneous tumors. Patients can present with symptoms of airway obstruction from poststyloid masses, pain or cranial nerve palsies of nerves in the PPS. Patients can also present with a unilateral serous otitis media from Eustachian tube dysfunction. A CT scan and/or MRI would be the initial test(s) of choice to delineate between pre- and poststyloid masses. Findings for a prestyloid PPS mass would include displacement of PPS fat medially and posteriorly, displacement of the posterior belly of the digastric and styloid muscles more posteriorly and medially, and location medial to the medial pterygoid muscle. Findings for a poststyloid mass would

include location or extension posteriorly to the styloid process, lateral and anterior displacement of the posterior belly of the digastric and styloid muscles and usually displacement of the carotid sheath contents anteriorly.

The most common PPS masses are tumors of the salivary glands (40–60%), and of these, a benign pleomorphic adenoma is most frequent. Neurogenic tumors and paragangliomas are the second and third most common masses, respectively. The PPS is the second most common site in the head and neck for the location of a nerve sheath tumor, and the incidence of these is higher in females. Neurogenic tumors are slow growing and as described above, may present with obstructive symptoms because of medial displacement of the pharynx, tonsil, and soft palate. Neurilemmomas (schwannomas) are the most common PPS neurogenic tumor and the cervical sympathetic chain is the nerve most frequently involved. As a result, in resection of these tumors, a Horner's syndrome is the nerve deficit usually encountered. For all PPS tumors, however, (including prestyloid), a temporary paresis of the mandibular division of the facial nerve is the most common complication reported. Of paragangliomas, the carotid body tumor is the most common.

Resection of these tumors includes transcervical approaches with or without mandibulotomy, infratemporal approaches, transparotid and various combinations. The transcervical approach typically provides the best exposure for poststyloid PPS neurogenic tumors.

Bibliography

Keane WM. Tumors of the parapharygeal space. In: Gates GA (ed.), *Current Therapy in Otolaryngology Head and Neck Surgery*, 6th ed. St. Louis, MO: Mosby, 1998, 242–246.

Hamza A, et al. Neurilemmomas of the parapharyngeal space. *Arch Otolaryngol Head Neck Surg* 1997;123:622–626.

Gluckman JL. Parapharyngeal mass. In: Tami TA, et al. (eds.), *Otolaryngology: A Case Study Approach*. New York, NY: Thieme, 1998, 108–110.

Mafee MF. Nasopharynx, parapharyngeal space, and base of skull. In: Valvassori GE, Mafee MF, Carter BL. *Imaging of the Head and Neck*. New York, NY: Thieme, 1995, 332–365.

7. **(B)** The role of the neck dissection in the treatment of head and neck cancer is based on the principle that the presence of metastatic SCC to lymph nodes decreases survival by 50%. The percentage of positive nodes differs by the site of the primary (see Table 14-1). If a primary is known, then the chance of finding positive nodes will vary with the T stage of the tumor (AJCC criteria).

TABLE 14-1   Relationship Between Primary Site and a Clinically Negative Neck at Presentation and the Incidence of Occult Metastases

Primary site	% N$_0^*$	% Positive nodes in elective neck dissection[†]
Oral Cavity	50	23–34
Tongue	58	25
Floor of mouth	66	21
Gum		12
Retromolar	57	35
Oropharynx	34	31–35
Hypopharynx	29	17–55
Larynx		21–37
Glottic		16
Supraglottic	49	26

* Data derived from Lindberg R. Distribution of cervical lymph node metastases from squamous cell carcinoma of the upper respiratory and digestive tracts. *Cancer* 1972; 29: 1446–1449.

† Data derived from Shah IP. Patterns of cervical node metastases from squamous carcinomas of the upper aerodigestive tract. *Am J Surg* 1990; 160:405–409; Byers RM, Wolf PF, Ballantyne AJ. Rationale for elective modified neck dissection. *Head Neck Surg* 1988;10: 160–167.

Source: Reprinted from Gates HA, et al. *Current Therapy in Otolaryngolory—Head and Neck Surgery*, 6th ed., copyright 1998, with permission from Elsevier.

The workup of an unknown primary begins with a complete head and neck examination. Patients with unknown primary carcinomas present with an asymmetric neck mass, and up to two-thirds of the primaries are discovered on the initial examination. If the first examination fails to reveal a primary site, the examination should be repeated to concentrate on less visible areas of the upper aerodigestive tract independently. If this also is negative, a fine needle aspiration (FNA) biopsy is required. Immediate lymph node removal is contraindicated before a thorough search for the primary. If the FNA proves positive or suspicious, then radiologic imaging is recommended either via contrast enhanced CT or T2 weighted MRI scans. At this point, triple endoscopy with biopsies of the more typical areas for occult primaries would be undertaken: these include the nasopharynx, ipsilateral tonsil, base of tongue, and pyriform sinus. If still no primary is found, treatment of the neck, including possible neck dissection, is still required and surgery with or without postoperative radiation is the recommended treatment option (see Fig. 14-16).

This being said, there are several complications associated with neck dissections. Some are general to all surgery in general including bleeding, hematoma, and infection. Others are particular to the procedure itself: incisional complications, neural, and vascular complications. It is important to raise skin flaps in a subplatysmal plane to preserve blood supply to the

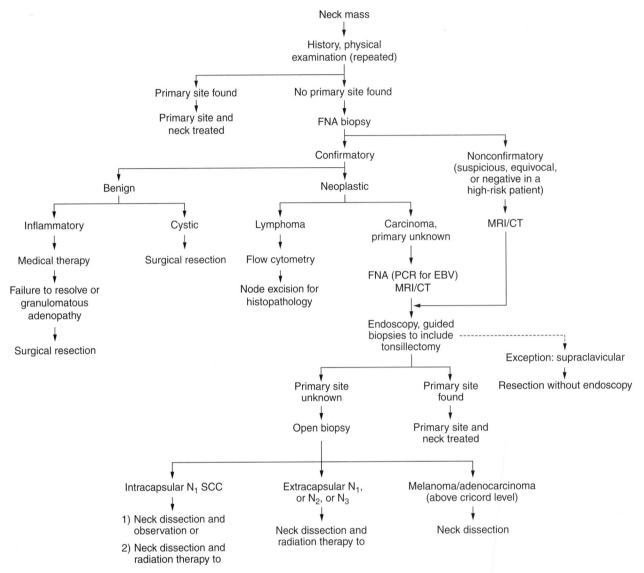

FIG. 14-16   Algorithm for workup of an unknown primary. (*Source:* Reprinted from Cummings CW, et al. *Otolaryngology—Head and Neck Surgery*, 3rd ed., 1686—1699, copyright 1998, with permission from Elsevier).

skin. The chance for flap necrosis increases if incisions are brought together at acute angles and no incision should run along the carotid artery. Neural complications are damage to mandibular branches of the trigeminal nerve (inferior alveolar nerve, lingual nerve), branches of the facial nerve (especially marginal mandibular), vagus nerve, spinal accessory nerve (SAN), and hypoglossal nerve. Vascular complications are those related to the IJV (facial/cerebral edema and blindness, especially when bilateral neck dissections are performed, as well as rupture of the jugular vein) and carotid artery. Not only is carotid artery rupture a concern; carotid body stimulation intraoperatively or bilateral carotid body denervation from bilateral neck dissections (which can cause apnea) are also serious concerns.

The incidence of chyle leak as a complication in neck dissection is 1–2% of cases. The thoracic duct transports fats as chylomicrons absorbed from the GI tract. Injury to the thoracic duct typically occurs in the left neck because of the thoracic duct emptying into the left subclavian vein near the junction of this structure and the IJV. To test for possible injury of the duct during surgery, positive airway pressure is required for greater than 30 s or more, and the operative field should be examined for milky or oily fluid in the region of the distal jugular stump. In the postoperative period, drains should be observed for any high output milky drainage. The presence of chylomicrons may not necessarily indicate a chylous fistula (or chyle leak). Normal triglyceride content of neck drainage is approximately 100 mg/dL.

Conservative treatment starts with continuous suction drainage and fluid replacement, and head of bed elevation. Fistulous output may reach 4 L a day. Nutrition should consist of medium chain triglycerides which are directly absorbed into the portal system and bypass the lymphatic system. This alone may obviate the need for total parenteral nutrition (TPN). Indications for surgical exploration would include output >600 mL per day as these fistulas do not respond to conservative measures. Chyle leak into the mediastinum if left unchecked may cause a chylothorax, with need for a thoracostomy tube.

Bibliography

Davidson BJ, Sessions RB. Cervical metastasis. In: Gates GA (ed.), *Current Therapy in Otolaryngology Head and Neck Surgery*, 6th ed. St. Louis, MO: Mosby, 1998, 291–295.

Bier-Laning CM. Surgical complications of the neck. In: Cummings CW, Fredrickson JM, Harker LA, et al. (eds.), *Otolaryngology Head & Neck Surgery*, 3rd ed., vol. 3. St. Louis, MO: Mosby, 1998, 1811–1820.

McGuirt WF Sr. Differential diagnosis of neck masses. In: Cummings CW, Fredrickson JM, Harker LA, et al. (eds.), *Otolaryngology Head & Neck Surgery*, 3rd ed. St. Louis, MO: Mosby, 1998, 1686–1699.

Medina JE. Neck dissection. In: Bailey BJ, et al. (eds.), *Head & Neck Surgery Otolaryngology*, 3rd ed., vol. 2 Philadelphia, PA: Lippincott, Williams & Wilkins, 2001, 1345–1366.

8. **(C)** Cancer of the larynx typically originates on the true vocal cord itself (in 75%), and it is this location where it has the best prognosis. This particular cancer is staged as a T_2 and we can assume N_0 (see Table 14-2). Early laryngeal carcinoma is usually treated with

TABLE 14-2   UICC (International Union Against Cancer) Staging of Laryngeal Carcinoma

Supraglottis	
T_1	Tumor limited to one subsite of supraglottis with normal vocal cord mobility
T_2	Tumor invades mucosa of more than one adjacent region outside the supraglottis (eg. mucosa of base of tongue, vallecula, medial wall of piriform sinus) without fixation of the larynx
T_3	Tumor limited to larynx with vocal cord fixation and/or invades any of the following: postcricoid area, pre-epiglottic tissue, deep base of tongue
T_4	Tumor invades through thyroid cartilage and/or extends into soft tissue of the neck, thyroid and/or esophagus
Glottis	
T_1	Tumor limited to vocal cord(s) (may involve anterior or posterior commisure) with normal mobility
T_{1a}	Tumor limited to one vocal cord
T_{1b}	Tumor involves both vocal cords
T_2	Tumor extends to supraglottis and/or subglottis and/or with impaired vocal cord mobility
T_3	Tumor limited to larynx with vocal cord fixation
T_4	Tumor invades through thyroid cartilage and/or extends to other tissue beyond the larynx—eg, trachea, soft tissue of the neck, thyroid, pharynx
Subglottis	
T_1	Tumor limited to subglottis
T_2	Tumor extends to vocal cord(s) with normal or impaired mobility
T_3	Tumor limited to larynx with vocal cord fixation
T_4	Tumor invades through cricoid or thyroid cartilage and/or extends into other tissue beyond the larynx—eg, trachea, soft tissue of the neck, thyroid, esophagus
N stage	
N_g	Regional lymph nodes cannot be assessed
N_0	No regional metastases
N_1	Metastases in a single ipsilateral lymph node, 3 cm or less in greatest dimension
N_{2a}	Metastases in a single ipsilateral lymph node, more than 3 cm but not more than 6 cm in greatest dimension
N_{2b}	Metastases in multiple ipsilateral lymph nodes, none more than 6 cm in greatest dimension
N_{2c}	Metastases in bilateral or contralateral lymph nodes, none more than 6 cm in greatest dimension
N_3	Metastases in a lymph node more than 6 cm in greatest dimension
M stage	
M_g	Distant metastases cannot be assessed
M_0	No distant metastases
M_1	Distant metastases

Source: Reprinted from Lee KJ et al. *Essential Otolaryngology—Head and Neck Surgery*, 8th ed., copyright 2003, with permission from McGraw-Hill.

one modality. Current treatment options include as radiation, transoral/endoscopic laser excision or cold knife excision or partial laryngeal surgeries. Historically, radiation therapy has been the treatment of choice for early glottic carcinoma because of the advantages of avoiding surgery and hospitalization and good voice quality. The voice never returns completely to normal, however. Endoscopic laser excision/cordectomy as it has been refined is now showing evidence of equivalent cure rates and nearly equivalent voice preservation. Single modality cure with radiation is approximately 85% with radiation and 90–95% with surgical salvage. If a cancer recurs after radiotherapy which is more of a concern when the cord displays decreased mobility (up to 50% recurrence), then radiation cannot be used again because the patient has already theoretically received a maximum lifetime dose. Also lesions involving the anterior commissure are not readily amenable to radiation as a primary treatment even when the lesions are in an early stage.

Early glottic carcinoma is diagnosed by the physical symptoms and signs. The patient typically complains of hoarseness and "globus" or a "lump in the throat" sensation. Some may even present with dysphagia. The history should be carefully sought for alcohol and tobacco abuse. The initial examination should involve careful listening of the acoustical features of the voice, assessment of swallowing and respiration during the examination, palpation and careful inspection of the oral cavity, oropharynx and hypopharynx by means of fiberoptic laryngoscopy. Careful palpation of the neck to rule out neck metastases is crucial. CT scan is important to check for any soft-tissue infiltration although this is less of an issue with early glottic carcinoma. The final stage is direct laryngoscopy with biopsies and mapping of the lesion.

The anatomy of the glottis lends early glottic carcinomas to have a good prognosis. This is chiefly because the glottis proper has very few lymphatics and cancers confined to the true vocal cords present with neck metastases in 5%. When the mobility of the cord is affected, this implies invasion of the thyroarytenoid muscle and probable involvement of the paraglottic space; the tumor then has wide access to other subsets of the larynx (Fig. 14-17).

Bibliography

Adams GJ. Malignant tumors of the larynx and hypopharynx. In: Cummings CW, Fredrickson JM, Harker LA, et al. (eds.), *Otolaryngology Head & Neck Surgery*, 3rd ed., vol. 3. St. Louis, MO: Mosby, 1998, 2130–2175.

Bailey BJ. Glottic carcinoma. In: Gates GA (ed.), *Current Therapy in Otolaryngology Head and Neck Surgery*, 6th ed. St. Louis, MO: Mosby, 1998, 281–285.

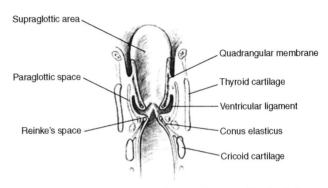

FIG. 14-17 Coronal view of larynx demonstrating natural barriers to tumor spread, the quadrangular membrane, and conus elasticus. (*Source:* Reprinted from Lee KJ et al. *Essential Otolaryngology—Head and Neck Surgery*, 8th ed., copyright 2003, with permission from McGraw-Hill).

Bailey BJ. Early glottic and supraglottic carcinoma: vertical partial laryngectomy and laryngoplasty. In: Bailey BJ, et al. (eds.), *Head & Neck Surgery Otolaryngology*, 3rd ed., vol. 2. Philadelphia, PA: Lippincott, Williams & Wilkins, 2001, 1469–1482.

Beasley NJP, Gullane PJ. Cancer of the larynx, paranasal sinuses and temporal bone. In: Lee KJ (ed.), *Essential Otolaryngology Head and Neck Surgery*, 8th ed. New York, NY: Mc-Graw Hill, 2003, 596–616.

Robbins KT (ed.), *Pocket Guide to Neck Dissection Classification and tnm Staging of Head and Neck Cancer: Subcommittee for Neck Dissection Terminology and Classification*. Alexandria, VA: AAO-HNS Foundation, 1991, 25.

9. **(D)** This patient demonstrates many of the features of advanced laryngeal carcinoma, stage IV. He has progressive compressive symptoms including dysphagia and airway obstruction. As evidenced by his physical examination (Fig. 14-3) and the CT scan, he has a destructive lesion of the glottis with a cartilage invasion anteriorly and a fixed lymph node. In addition, he has a low density area on the CT scan anteriorly indicating probable necrotic component or abscess in the tumor. This patient required a pretreatment tracheostomy which has been associated with increased stomal. This patient would not have been a candidate for this alone; however, with salvage neck dissections radiation could be an option. Radiation alone has local control with 50% and about half of these patients go onto salvage treatment. Induction chemotherapy followed by radiation therapy has led to a laryngeal preservation rate of 64%; however, there is an increased chance for local recurrence. The therapy of choice for this patient would be choice D. This would have the greatest chance for locoregional control in this patient, and with the destructive nature of the cancer, postoperative radiation treatment is a requirement. This patient would also need a subtotal thyroidectomy. In this

setting of advanced laryngeal cancer treated with surgery and radiation, the risk of hypothyroidism is 65%.

The nodal drainage for this cancer would be the upper and middle chains of the lateral jugular nodes including in the least levels II–IV. This patient would also require paratracheal nodal dissection (level VI) including the Delphian node. The anatomy of the larynx divides it into three parts: the supraglottis is the larynx above the ventricles, the glottis proper extends to 1 cm below the free edge of the true vocal cords and the subglottis is from this point to the lower border of the cricoid cartilage. The preepiglottic space is confined by the hyoepiglottic ligament and the mucosa of the vallecula on its superior border, anteriorly by the thyrohyoid ligaments and posteriorly by the thyroepiglottic ligament and epiglottis. The epiglottis itself has many fenestrations which can act as pathways for tumor spread into the preepiglottic space. The paraglottic space is actually a potential space external to the laryngeal inlet but medial to the thyroid cartilage with the quadrangular membrane superiorly and the conus elasticus inferiorly to this space. These membranes act as barriers to tumor spread and when violated, they lead to the paraglottic space allowing a tumor to become transglottic or local recurrence. To lessen this risk, the literature currently recommends definitive surgery within 48 h with removal of the stoma.

A partial laryngectomy would be precluded by the presence of subglottic extension to the cricoid, bilateral arytenoid involvement and cartilage invasion or spread to surrounding soft tissue (thus answer A would be incorrect). Current recommendations for primary radiation would be patients with T3 lesions with low tumor volume and patients who are reliable with follow-up.

Bibliography

Adams GJ. Malignant tumors of the larynx and hypopharynx. In: Cummings CW, Fredrickson JM, Harker LA, et al. (eds.), *Otolaryngology Head & Neck Surgery*, 3rd ed., vol. 3. St. Louis, MO: Mosby, 1998, 2130–2175.

Bailey BJ. Glottic carcinoma. In: Gates GA (ed.), *Current Therapy in Otolaryngology Head and Neck Surgery*, 6th ed. St. Louis, MO: Mosby, 1998, 281–285.

Beasley NJP, Gullane PJ. Cancer of the larynx, paranasal sinuses and temporal bone. In: Lee KJ (ed.), *Essential Otolaryngology Head and Neck Surgery*, 8th ed. New York, NY: Mc-Graw Hill, 2003, 596–616.

Robbins KT (ed.), *Pocket Guide to Neck Dissection Classification and tnm Staging of Head and Neck Cancer: Subcommittee for Neck Dissection Terminology and Classification*. Alexandria, VA: AAO-HNS Foundation, 1991, 12.

The Department of VA Laryngeal Cancer Study Group. Induction chemotherapy plus radiation compared with surgery plus radiation in patients with advance laryngeal cancer. *N Engl J Med* 1991;324(24):1585–1691.

10. **(E)** Young children make up the majority of patients suffering from foreign body aspiration: children under 3 account for between 70 and 80% of all foreign body aspirations. Children in this age group tend to explore with their mouths. Another factor is the lack of development of molars for grinding and lack of maturity of swallowing and airway protection processes. Boys outweigh girls by 2:1 in frequency. Whereas the most common airway foreign body is vegetable matter, esophageal foreign bodies are coins in 75% of cases. Others may include disc batteries, screws, tacks, nails, and other hardware items. Increasing in frequency are toy plastic parts.

The esophagus has four layers: the mucosa, submucosa, inner circular layer of muscle, and outer longitudinal layer of smooth muscle. The upper 5 cm are skeletal muscle, the upper midsection is an overlap of striated (skeletal) and smooth muscle, and the lower half is smooth muscle. The myenteric plexus of Auerbach is found within muscle layers and the submucosal plexus of Meissner is found in the submucosa. Both plexi are parasympathetic in innervation. The mucosa of the esophagus contains stratified squamous epithelium with poor absortion and low level secretory functions. Because there is no serosa, the esophagus is relatively more prone to perforation. There are four anatomic narrowings in the esophagus: the cricopharyngeus muscle, aortic crossing, left mainstem bronchus crossing, and the diaphragm.

The signs and symptoms of esophageal foreign body aspiration are dyspnea or airway distress, drooling, and dysphagia. The party wall between the anterior esophagus and posterior trachea is very compliant and if a large foreign body is engaged here it can compress the airway from behind. Any evidence of fever, tachycardia, tachypnea, and increasing pain should arouse suspicion for esophageal perforation and possible mediastinal emphysema or retropharyngeal abscess. The most common area for an esophageal foreign body to lodge is at the level of the cricopharyngeus or at C6. If it lodges elsewhere, investigation for another congenital anatomic disorder of the esophagus is warranted.

Typically, small sharp objects pass spontaneously and thus, this type of ingestion can be treated conservatively. Objects that require immediate removal include disc batteries or any ingestions with airway symptoms. Disc batteries can cause esophageal perforation within 8–12 h of ingestion, but if radiography reveal they have passed into the stomach, these

ingestions can be treated more conservatively. Coins less than 20 mm in diameter (dimes, pennies) can pass spontaneously. Other objects that are high risk for causing perforation are long straight pins, chicken and fish bones, and toothpicks.

Initial workup for any foreign body ingestion are posterior to anterior (PA) and lateral chest x-rays. As the majority of objects are coins, these are radiopaque and easy to spot on film. If there is still no evidence radiographically, then a very small sip of barium can be given to outline a possible nonradiopaque object. Barium esophagography is generally not used, however for several reasons, including the possible delay of an endoscopic procedure because of nullifying the nothing by mouth (NPO) status of the patient, increased difficulty of subsequent removal with barium, and possible barium aspiration with mediastinitis. The safest method of extraction of esophageal foreign bodies is a controlled situation with a protected airway under general anesthesia.

Bibliography

Byrne WJ. Foreign bodies, bezoars, and caustic ingestion. *Gastrointest Endosc Clin North Am* 1994;4(1):99–119.

Friedman EM. Caustic ingestion and foreign bodies in the aerodigestive tract. In: Bailey BJ, et al. (eds.), *Head & Neck Surgery Otolaryngology*, 3rd ed., vol. 1. Philadelphia, PA: Lippincott, Williams & Wilkins, 2001, 925–932.

Holinger LD. Foreign bodies of the airway and esophagus. In: Gates GA (ed.), *Current Therapy in Otolaryngology Head and Neck Surgery*, 6th ed. St. Louis, MO: Mosby, 1998, 470–474.

Murray AD, Mahoney EM, Holinger LD. Foreign bodies of the airway and esophagus. In: Cummings CW, Fredrickson JM, Harker LA, et al. (eds.), *Otolaryngology Head & Neck Surgery: Pediatric*, 3rd ed. St. Louis, MO: Mosby, 1998, 377–387.

11. **(B)** External laryngeal trauma is diagnosed on the basis of history and physical findings. A patient who presents with evidence of anterior neck trauma should be assumed to have upper airway trauma. This compounded with subcutaneous emphysema, voice changes, and orthopnea should arouse suspicion for disruption of the larynx or trachea. As in any trauma situation, the "ABCs" come first: airway, breathing and circulation. Although on fiberoptic examination this patient had "mild edema" it is presumable early after the trauma and the entire injury may have not evolved. There is potential for worsening of the edema and bleeding in the next 8–12 h. As a result, an awake tracheostomy is the best option. The addition of general anesthesia in this situation may cause laryngospasm and resultant complete airway obstruction.

In addition, "clothesline" injuries are high risk for being associated with laryngotracheal separation. Any situation in which this is considered precludes oral or nasal intubation as intubation may worsen the existing damage or convert a partial laryngotracheal or cricotracheal separation into a complete separation.

The pathophysiology behind blunt trauma to the larynx involves crushing of the laryngeal skeleton against the cervical spine. There is a shearing effect between the laryngeal ligaments, the thyroarytenoid (vocalis) muscle, and the perichondrium of the thyroid and cricoid cartilages. In addition arytenoid cartilage dislocation or subluxation and recurrent laryngeal nerve injury via traction or actual transection may occur. The result is mucosal tears, edema, and hematoma or hemorrhage. A "clothesline" injury can be associated with bilateral recurrent nerve damage. Any damage to the cricoid can be particularly devastating as it is the only complete ring of the airway and is the cornerstone of structural support for the larynx.

Some external laryngeal trauma can be treated conservatively with medical management. Conditions include: minor edema or hematomas with intact mucosa, single nondisplaced thyroid cartilage fractures, small lacerations without exposed cartilage. Medical management would include elevation of the head of bed with bedrest to reduce edema. Corticosteroids are probably only beneficial in the early postinjury period and antibiotics are used in the event of lacerations or mucosal tears as prophylaxis. Cool humidified air is important to prevent crust formation with tracheostomies and with mucosal tears. Voice rest is sometimes recommended to reduce edema or hematoma progression. Gastroesophageal reflux prevention is also important with either H2 blockers or proton-pump inhibitors. Any patient not meeting the criteria for conservative management proceeds to surgery. Frequently, the lacerations are used to explore the laryngeal framework and mucosa. Early intervention is advocated for less scarring and granulation tissue.

Discussion about surgical techniques is beyond the scope of this question; however, the reader is recommended to review the attached bibliography.

Bibliography

Bent JP, Silver JR, Porubsky ES. Acute laryngeal trauma: a review of 77 patients. *Otolaryngol Head Neck Surg* 1993;109:441–449.

Schaefer SD. Acute laryngeal trauma. In: Gates GA (ed.), *Current Therapy in Otolaryngology Head and Neck Surgery*, 6th ed. St. Louis, MO: Mosby, 1998, 456–460.

Schaefer SD. Laryngeal and esophageal trauma. In: Cummings CW, Fredrickson JM, Harker LA, et al. (eds.), *Otolaryngology Head & Neck Surgery*, 3rd ed., vol. 3. St. Louis, MO: Mosby, 1998, 2001–2012.

Schaefer SD, Stringer SP. Laryngeal trauma. In: Bailey BJ, et al. (eds.), *Head & Neck Surgery Otolaryngology*, 3rd ed., vol. 1. Philadelphia, PA: Lippincott, Williams & Wilkins, 2001, 741–749.

12. **(B)** This patient is presenting with a classic blowout fracture. The "blowout" refers to an outfracturing of the orbital floor and sometimes medial wall from a direct force to the eye which increases intraorbital pressure. The pressure is dissipated by the fracture of the floor. Characteristics of a missile injury to the globe with resulting blunt trauma include a diameter of <5 cm. Common objects are fists, hockey pucks, baseballs, and bottle corks. This can also occur with direct force to the eye from a fall as in this patient. The orbital fat and contents lose their support and fall into the maxillary sinus in varying amounts depending on the size of the bony defect. These are pure blowout fractures when only the floor is damaged; impure fractures involve the inferior orbital rim as well.

The physical findings of the orbital fracture include periorbital ecchymosis, numbness in the V_2 distribution, limited upward gaze with diplopia and enophthalmos. An important test to administer is the forced duction test which tests for inferior rectus muscle entrapment. If the patient is alert and there is no obvious evidence of globe injury, a small amount of topical tetracaine can be administered to the eye. The inferior rectus is then grasped through the conjunctiva on the inferior surface of the globe and the globe is passively moved through a range of motion. This is then compared to the nontraumatized eye to judge any limitation in movement; however, soft tissue swelling around the globe can also be associated with subjective diplopia and this will improve; this should be differentiated from true extraocular muscle entrapment. CT scans are the studies of choice and less reliance is placed on forced duction testing. The forced duction test is important after repair of an orbital floor fracture, however.

The orbit itself has a volume of 30 cc³. It is shaped as a four-sided pyramid. The superior wall or roof is formed by the orbital plate of the frontal bone and posteriorly by the lesser wing of the sphenoid bone. The optic canal is located in the posterior part of the roof, transmitting the optic nerve and its associated ophthalmic vein. The medial wall of the orbit is formed by the lamina papyracea of the ethmoid bone, as well as parts of the frontal, lacrimal, and sphenoid bones. The frontoethmoid suture contains the anterior ethmoid foramen, transmitting the anterior ethmoid

artery and nerve (off the ophthalmic artery) and the posterior ethmoid foramen (also off the ophthalmic artery) which transmits the posterior ethmoid artery and nerve. The inferior wall of the orbit or the floor is formed by the orbital surface of the maxilla with contributions from the palatine bone and zygomatic bone. The inferior orbital fissure is found between the floor and the lateral wall and transmits the maxillary nerve. The infraorbital foramen which is on the anterior surface of the maxilla is 1 cm below the rim of the orbit and this foramen houses the nerve of the same name. Contents of the orbit include the extraocular muscles, lacrimal gland, and globe.

The chief indication for immediate repair of an orbital floor fracture is a rapid onset of intraorbital hemorrhage with decreased visual acuity. This implies increased intraocular pressure with ischemia of the optic nerve. Other indications for repair though not immediate would be enophthalmos and muscle entrapment. The floor can be repaired with bone (calvarial or maxilla), cartilage from the septum or concha, and implants including Marlex, silastic, and titanium mesh. Although implants were frequently used for smaller defects, they are finding application with good results in larger floor fractures with comminution.

Bibliography

Moore KL. *Clinically Oriented Anatomy*, 3rd ed. Baltimore, MD: Williams & Wilkins, 1992.

Netter FH. *Atlas of Human Anatomy*. Summit, NJ: CIBA-GEIGY, 1989.

Rubin PAD, Shore JW, Yaremchuk MJ. Complex orbital fracture repair using rigid fixation of the internal orbital skeleton. *Ophthalmology* 1992;99(4):553–559.

Shumrick KA, Kersten RC. Orbital trauma. In: Tami TA, et al. (eds.), *Otolaryngology: A Case Study Approach*. New York, NY: Thieme, 1998, 278–282.

Stanley RB. Maxillary and periorbital fractures. In: Bailey BJ, et al. (eds.), *Head & Neck Surgery Otolaryngology*, 3rd ed., vol. 1. Philadelphia, PA: Lippincott, Williams & Wilkins, 2001, 777–792.

13. **(D)** Penetrating parotid gland injuries have the potential to involve both Stensen's duct (parotid duct) and the facial nerve. Wounds occurring posterior to the anterior masseter muscle may injure the duct. These injuries can carry with them several sequelae including sialoceles, fistulas, and infections.

Treatment of these injuries requires initially careful inspection of the wound and duct. If the duct cannot be identified externally then the duct should be explored intraorally. This may involve cannulation of the duct and if it is not readily found, the gland can be massaged to expel saliva and uncover the

duct orifice. Inspection ideally should be done in the operating room. If the duct itself is transected, then it should be debrided at the ends and repaired under magnification with 9–0 or 10–0 nonabsorbable sutures. Most of the current literature recommends repair over a 16 or 20 gauge silastic catheter or stent to prevent placing backwall sutures and to prevent stricture formation when left in place for up to 14 days. The catheter is either sutured to the orifice intraorally or brought out through the parenchyma externally. If the distal duct is injured significantly and there is adequate length of the proximal portion, this portion can be diverted to the buccal mucosa. Some surgeons have also employed vein grafts in this instance.

The other two injuries in this area would be trauma to the parotid gland parenchyma and facial nerve. The parenchymal injury can be treated conservatively by closing the capsule of the gland after judicious debridement. Pressure dressings may be applied to prevent saliva accumulation. Delayed treatment of parenchymal and ductal injuries is fraught with dissecting through granulation tissue. If a swelling develops postinjury, it can be aspirated and tested for amylase to prove parenchymal origin. A sialogram may be used in this instance as well. Persistent sialoceles or fistulas to the skin are treated with tympanic neurectomy, total parotidectomy, atropine or repeated aspiration, and pressure dressings. Facial nerve injuries occurring in a line anterior to an imaginary line between the lateral canthus and mental foramen do not need to be repaired because of abundant cross innervation between buccal, zygomatic, and mandibular branches. Proximal to this line, direct repair if feasible should be performed, and the ends of the nerve can be tested by electrical stimulation up to 3 weeks after the injury.

The parotid gland is the largest of the major salivary glands. It develops from the posterior embryologic ectodermal stomodeum which is the precursor of the oral cavity, first appearing in the sixth week. Cords develop from the stomodeum and canalize to become ducts with acini at the terminal portions. The capsule of the parotid gland develops late and therefore incorporates lymph nodes. Stensen's duct runs approximately 1 cm inferior and parallel to the zygoma and opens opposite the second molar tooth in the oral cavity, and the facial nerve is the most superficial structure passing through the gland, making it vulnerable to penetrating or blunt injury. The parotid gland consists almost entirely of serous cells, hence its secretion is watery, low in mucin but rich in enzymes, whereas that of the sublingual gland is opposite, being viscid and mucinous saliva also contains opsonins, leukotaxins, lysozymes, and IgA and is important in preventing infection in the oral cavity. Saliva also helps promote calcification of teeth.

Bibliography

Haller JR. Trauma. In: Cummings CW, Fredrickson JM, Harker LA, et al. (eds.), *Otolaryngology Head & Neck Surgery*, 3rd ed., vol. 2. St. Louis, MO: Mosby, 1998, 1247–1254.

Rice DH. Nonneoplastic diseases of the salivary glands. In: Bailey BJ, et al. (eds.), *Head & Neck Surgery Otolaryngology*, 3rd ed., vol. 1. Philadelphia, PA: Lippincott, Williams & Wilkins, 2001, 453–462.

Shemen LJ. Salivary glands: benign and malignant diseases. In: Lee KJ (ed.), *Essential Otolaryngology Head and Neck Surgery*, 8th ed. New York, NY: Mc-Graw Hill, 2003, 535–565.

14. **(C)** This scenario describes a neck space infection with abscess. Historically these types of infections were caused by pharyngeal or tonsillar infections with involvement of the PPC, but since the advent of antibiotics, these infections are treated early in their course. Most contemporary adult neck space abscesses are caused by odontogenic or salivary gland infections, although tonsillar and pharyngeal infections still account for the majority of pediatric neck space infections. Other etiologies include preexisting congenital anomalies (branchial cleft sinuses and the like), trauma, upper respiratory tract infections, iatrogenic causes, or spread from a superficial infection.

The neck spaces are divided by fascial layers. The most superficial fascia is the superficial cervical fascia beginning at the zygomatic process and extending into the thorax. It envelops the platysma muscle and muscles of facial expression and is rarely involved in serious neck space infections. The next deeper layer is the superficial layer of the deep cervical fascia which covers the strap muscles, trapezius, SCM, major salivary glands, and muscles of mastication (temporalis, masseter, and pterygoids). This superficial layer of the deep fascia or "investing fascia" splits around the superior surface of the manubrium to form the suprasternal space of burns. The middle layer of the deep cervical fascia is also known as the visceral fascia and is ensheathed around the pharynx, larynx, esophagus, trachea, thyroid and parathyroid glands, buccinator and constrictor muscles and the deeper strap muscles (sternohyoid, sternothyroid, thyrohyoid, and omohyoid). This layer runs from the base of skull to the mediastinum. The deep cervical fascia is also called the prevertebral fascia and covers the paraspinous muscles and cervical vertebrae and extends from the base of skull to the chest. The deep layer actually is comprised of two layers: the prevertebral layer proper and the alar layer which lies anterior to the prevertebral layer but posterior to the visceral middle layer. This layer also extends from base of skull to mediastinum. Just anterior to the alar layer is the retropharyngeal space and just posterior is the potential "danger" space which ends at the diaphragm. The carotid sheath which houses the common carotid artery, IJV, and vagus nerve has contributions from all three deep fascial layers (investing, visceral, and prevertebral). It is referred to as the "Lincoln Highway of the Neck."

Any of the layers listed above can be involved in neck space infections. The patient above is exhibiting signs of a submandibular space infection which has progressed. The majority of these are of odontogenic source, especially infections of the second and third molars because the roots of these teeth lie at (second molar) or below the mylohyoid line. The mylohyoid line separates the sublingual and submandibular spaces. If this infection goes untreated it rapidly progresses to a gangrenous cellulitis with brawny induration involving bilateral sublingual, submental (between anterior bellies of the digastric muscles and between the mylohyoid muscle and skin), and submandibular spaces. This infection does not spread through lymphatics, but rather direct involvement of fascial planes. The clinical presentation is marked by drooling, severe pain, trismus, dysphagia, and respiratory distress. Because of floor of mouth swelling and induration, the tongue is compressed against the palate, thereby obstructing the oral airway. Ludwig's angina is the deep neck space infection which is most associated with the need for tracheostomy.

The typical microorganisms involved are oral flora, such as *Peptostreptococcus*, *Streptococcus pyogenes*, *Fusobacterium* as well as *Bacteroides melaninogenicus* and *Staphylococcus aureus*. Penicillin remains the drug of choice but any antibiotic with a similar spectrum (i.e., clindamycin, first generation cephalosporins) is usually adequate. Most neck space infections in the abscess stage require surgical drainage.

Vincent's angina, also known as trench mouth, is an acute necrotizing ulcerative gingivitis secondary to a mixed anaerobic infection. Patients present with malodorous breath, drooling and gingival bleeding; penicillin and adequate oral hygiene are the treatments. Bezold's abscess refers to a postauricular abscess secondary to mastoiditis. A retropharyngeal abscess can also present with symptoms of dysphagia and odynophagia, snoring, noisy breathing and cervical adenopathy, but airway obstruction is less common. Retropharyngeal infections are more common in children as lymph nodes (which are the typical source) regress or atrophy by the age of 4 or 5.

Bibliography

Byrne MN, Lee KJ. Neck spaces and fascial planes. In: Lee KJ (ed.), *Essential Otolaryngology*, 8th ed. New York, NY: Mc-Graw Hill, 2003, 422–438.

Eibling DE. The oral cavity, pharynx and esophagus. In: Lee KJ (ed.), *Essential Otolaryngology Head and Neck Surgery*, 8th ed. New York, NY: Mc-Graw Hill, 2003, 439–461.

Endicott JN. Deep neck infection. In: Gates GA (ed.), *Current Therapy in Otolaryngology Head and Neck Surgery*, 6th ed. St. Louis, MO: Mosby, 1998, 295–298.

Har-El G, Aroesty JH, Shaha A, et al. Changing trends in deep neck abscesses: a retrospective study of 110 patients. *Oral Surg Oral Med Oral Pathol* 1994;77:446–450.

Kirse DJ, Roberson DW. Surgical management of retropharyngeal space infections in children. *Laryngoscope* 2001;111:1413–1422.

Scott BA, Stiernberg CM, Driscoll BP. Infections of the deep spaces of the neck. In: Bailey BJ, et al. (eds.), *Head & Neck Surgery Otolaryngology*, 3rd ed., vol. 1. Philadelphia, PA: Lippincott, Williams & Wilkins, 2001, 701–715.

15. **(C)** This pathology is characteristic of a Warthin's tumor (a.k.a., papillary cystadenoma lymphomatosum), the second most common type of benign neoplasm of the parotid gland; this tumor rarely is found in the other major or minor salivary glands. It represents approximately 6–10% of parotid gland tumors and in 10% of cases is bilateral. Several epidemiologic characteristics are singular to Warthin's: it is chiefly found in males between the fourth and seventh decades of life, those of White race, is more common in smokers and can be multifocal. The tumor may arise from either heterotopic salivary duct tissue or from glandular inclusions within lymph nodes; this is thought to be because the parotid, though the first salivary gland to develop, is the last to be encapsulated and incorporates lymphoid tissue. Papillary fronds with a double layer of oncocytic cells are seen, with the inner layer of cells having nuclei which face the basement membrane. These cells have a high density of mitochondria. Copious lymphoid tissue is associated with the tumor and this tissue is at the center of the papillary fronds. There are usually multiple cystic components as well that contain a brown mucinous material. On occasions, metaplastic squamous epithelium may be found which could lead to a misdiagnosis of SCC on FNA.

FNA for Warthin's tumors has a sensitivity of around 90%; however, there is a large false positive rate and therefore reliance on FNA should not be strong. The overall sensitivity of FNA in the diagnosis of salivary gland tumors is anywhere from 85 to 99%.

TABLE 14-3 Table of Types of Salivary Gland Tumors and Incidence

Tumor	Incidence (%)
Benign	
Pleomorphic adenoma	52
Warthin's tumor	5
Monomorphic adenoma	3.4
Oncocytoma	1.4
Malignant	
Mucoepidermoid	12.4
Acinic cell	6.4
Adenocarcinoma	6.2
Adenoid cystic	4.3
Malignant mixed	2.3
Squamous cell	1.6
Others	5
Total	100

Source: Reprinted from Lee KJ et al. *Essential Otolaryngology—Head and Neck Surgery,* 8th ed., copyright 2003, with permission from McGraw-Hill.

The most useful setting for FNA is when there is a suspicion for lymphoma. FNA indicating lymphoma would obviate the need for a superficial parotidectomy as a diagnostic procedure. The treatment of choice for Warthin's tumors is surgical excision.

The most common benign neoplasm of the salivary glands is the pleomorphic adenoma (Table 14-3) which arises from the intercalated duct cells and myoepithelial cells. This lesion contains both connective tissue and epithelial elements. When occurring in the minor salivary glands, they occur mostly in the hard and soft palate. When found in the parotid gland, 90% are superficial to the facial nerve. Microscopically, spindle and stellate cells in a myxoid stroma are seen, and frequently these tumors have fine extensions throughout the capsule of the gland; recurrence is common if only an enucleation rather than a complete superficial parotidectomy is performed. These can degenerate into the carcinoma ex pleomorphic adenoma in up to 25% of cases if the tumor has been present for several years.

In the pediatric population, the most common parotid mass is a hemangioma. Monomorphic adenomas also arise from ductal epithelium and usually occur in the parotid gland but have a more uniform appearance than a pleomorphic adenoma. Benign lymphoepithelial lesion is a term encompassing salivary conditions in Sjogren's disease, Mikulicz's disease, and chronic punctate sialadenitis. It may histologically be confused with lymphoma or even metastatic carcinoma but is a reactive process and not a neoplastic process. These lesions are more commonly found in middle aged women and can present as bilateral diffuse enlargement of the salivary or lacrimal glands.

Bibliography

Hanna EY, Suen JY. Neoplasms of Cummings CW, Fredrickson JM, ⌐. *Otolaryngology Head & Neck Surgery,* 3rd eu., t. Louis, MO: Mosby, 1998, 1255–1302.

Olsen KD, Lewis JE. Carcinoma ex pleomorphic adenoma: a clinicopathologic review. *Head Neck* 2001;23:705–712.

Raymond MR, Yoo JH, Heathcote JG, et al. Accuracy of fine-needle aspiration biopsy for Warthin's tumours. *J Otolaryngol* 2002;31(5):263–270.

Rice DH, Batsakis JG. *Surgical Pathology of the Head and Neck.* Philadelphia, PA: Lippincott, Williams & Wilkins, 2000.

Shemen LJ. Salivary glands: benign and malignant diseases. In: Lee KJ (ed.), *Essential Otolaryngology Head and Neck Surgery,* 8th ed. New York, NY: Mc-Graw Hill, 2003, 535–565.

Zbaren P, Schar C, Hotz MA, Loosli H. Value of fine-needle aspiration cytology of parotid gland masses. *Laryngoscope* 2001;111(11 Pt 1):1989–1992.

16. (**C**) A history of trauma to the nose with epistaxis should raise concern for a nasal fracture. Signs of crepitus of the nasal cartilaginous and bony framework and obvious external deformity are virtually pathognomic for a nasal fracture. The nasal bone is the most frequently fractured facial bone. Diagnosis rests on the physical examination especially after topical decongestion; x-rays have not been helpful in adding to diagnostic accuracy. In nearly 50% of cases, nasal x-rays may not reveal a fracture when one is actually present. Photographic documentation is important, however. A careful rhinoscopic examination should be performed as there are few injuries and/or complications associated with nasal trauma to the nose that require immediate repair or attention. One of these is the septal hematoma (Fig. 14-6).

A septal hematoma presents with nasal airway obstruction, usually bilaterally. Less often do patients with a septal hematoma present with epistaxis. The hematoma develops in the plane between the perichondrium of the septal cartilage and the cartilage itself. As the cartilage receives its blood supply from the perichondrium, the hematoma causes ischemic injury and eventually degeneration of the cartilaginous septum. A devastating cosmetic and functional consequence of this is the "saddle nose" deformity. Another complication is a septal abscess, usually caused by *S. aureus*, which can lead to cavernous sinus thrombosis because of valveless veins of the so called "danger triangle" of the face (bounded by the superior most aspect of the nasal dorsum and the lateral edges of the lips). The hematoma is drained with bilateral incisions called Killian incisions, 1 cm behind the caudal end of the septum.

These should be staggered to avoid causing septal perforation. Nasal packing or splints are used to coapt the septal mucoperichondrial flaps against the cartilage and the patient is placed on antistaphyloccocal antibiotics. Early hematomas can be aspirated but this situation is less common.

Other complications of nasal fractures include edema, ecchymosis, infection, and cerebrospinal fluid leak. CSF rhinorrhea implies a cribriform plate fracture. Small leaks are treated conservatively. Later complications may include fibrosis, contracture, airway obstruction and mucosal adhesions.

The nasal vestibule, the most anterior part of the nasal cavity is lined by stratified squamous epithelium which has sweat glands, sebaceous glands, and vibrissae. Respiratory epithelium (pseudostratified columnar ciliated epithelium) appears just beyond the epithelium. A very small area (1 cm^2) is occupied by the olfactory epithelium for smell. Small myelinated fibers pass through cribriform plate foramina to the olfactory bulb. The external nose has an arterial supply with contributions from both internal and external carotid arteries. Internal branches are minor; external branches are the superior labial artery, lateral nasal artery, angular artery. Venous drainage is from the anterior facial vein and anterior ophthalmic vein and both ultimately drain into the cavernous sinus.

The internal nasal and sinus arterial supply is from internal carotid branches (ophthalmic, anterior and posterior ethmoidal arteries, and supraorbital and supratrochlear arteries) and external carotid branches (sphenopalatine, descending palatine, greater palatine, pharyngeal and superior labial arteries). Venous drainage parallels the arteries and also empties into the cavernous sinus. Innervation is supplied by branches of V_1 and V_2. Thirty to fifty percent of airway resistance is found in the nasal cavities at the external and internal nasal valve and at the level of the inferior turbinates. Humidification of air occurs in the nasal cavity. Seventy to 80% of people have a nasal cycle with alternating vasoconstriction of the inferior turbinates.

Bibliography

Bailey BJ, Tan LKS. Fractures of the nasal and frontal sinuses. In: Bailey BJ, et al. (eds.), *Head & Neck Surgery Otolaryngology*, 3rd ed., vol. 1. Philadelphia, PA: Lippincott, Williams & Wilkins, 2001, 793–811.

Emanuel JM. Epistaxis. In: Cummings CW, Fredrickson JM, Harker LA, et al. (eds.), *Otolaryngology Head & Neck Surgery*, 3rd ed., vol. 2. St. Louis, MO: Mosby, 1998, 852–865.

Jafek BW, Dodson BT. Nasal obstruction. In: Bailey BJ, et al. (eds.), *Head & Neck Surgery Otolaryngology*, 3rd ed., vol. 1. Philadelphia, PA: Lippincott, Williams & Wilkins, 2001, 293–308.

Randall DA. The nose and paranasal sinuses. In: Lee KJ (ed.), *Essential Otolaryngology Head and Neck Surgery*, 8th ed. New York, NY: Mc-Graw Hill, 2003, 682–723.

17. **(A)** The most common complication of acute sinusitis necessitating immediate operative intervention involves the eye. All the sinuses can be culprits of orbital complications but the ethmoid is the most common because of its adjacency. The indication in this patient to operate immediately would be the visual acuity change as complications can lead to blindness. As the ethmoids are the culprit, decompressing the infection or abscess if present can be performed via the lamina papyracea, the medial wall of the orbit. Infections spread by direct extension and thrombophlebitis of ethmoidal veins. Other complications may include neurologic infections: subdural and epidural abscesses and meningitis.

Orbital complications are stratified by the Chandler classification system. Stage I is simply inflammatory edema or preseptal cellulitis (orbital septum of the eyelid) of the lids and extraocular muscles are not involved. Stage II indicates orbital cellulitis with edema of the contents of the orbit. The first two stages should be aggressively treated with medical therapy with antibiotics against *Streptoccocus pneumoniae* and *Haemophilus influenzae* to prevent progression to stage III. Stage III is the subperiosteal abscess which is beneath the periosteum of the lamina papyracea; the globe is displaced inferolaterally and vision is affected. Stage IV is an orbital abscess (Fig. 14-18) which is in the orbit itself; this is accompanied by ptosis, chemosis, and ophthalmoplegia with visual loss. Stage V is the most severe: cavernous sinus thrombosis. This stage can be fatal if not treated aggressively and is seen with bilateral eye

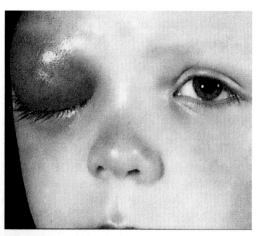

FIG. 14-18 Orbital cellulitis in a young child. (*Source:* Reprinted from Bull TR. *Color Atlas of ENT Diagnosis*, 3rd ed., plate 286, copyright 1995, with permission from Elsevier).

findings and meningismus. Aside from intravenous antibiotics and drainage of the abscess, some physicians choose to heparinize to minimize thrombosis. Later stages (III–V) are associated with polymicrobial infections with streptococci, staphylococci, *H. influenazae* and the anaerobes *Bacteroides, Peptostreptococcus,* and *Fusobacterium* to name a few.

Orbital complications are typically treated with an external approach rather than and endoscopic approach although the trend is changing. Since the ethmoid sinuses are the most frequently involved, at minimum, an external ethmoidectomy is performed with removal of a portion of the lamina papyracea.

Acute bacterial rhinosinusitis is diagnosed by the symptomatology of nasal congestion and rhinorrhea lasting for 7–14 days. Other symptoms include facial pain or dental pain, headache, fever and malaise. Anterior rhinoscopy may reveal unilateral or bilateral purulent drainage and tenderness on palpation of soft tissue over the sinuses. Various processes may lead to acute or chronic sinusitis. The first is obstruction of sinus ostia which can be caused by anatomic factors (septal deviation), edema from allergens or polyps. The second process is ciliary dysfunction either primary or acquired such as after a viral upper respiratiory infection (URI). The last is changes in mucus quality or quantity systemic factors may include steroid use, diabetes or immune compromise in general.

Nosocomial sinusitis may be caused by indwelling nasogastric catheters or nasotracheal intubation. A critically ill patient may present with a fever of unknown origin; acute rhinosinusitis should be given careful consideration, usually with an original or reconstructed coronal CT scan (optimal images for sinuses). These patients should be treated for gram-positive and gram-negative organisms. Culture can be obtained with maxillary sinus puncture and irrigation. Patients should improve within 48–72 h but treatment should last for a minimum of 10 days. For all acute sinusitis patients, topical and systemic decongestants can provide some symptom relief and facilitate oxygenation and drainage of us, but topical types should not be continued past 3 days to avoid rhinitis medicamentosa. Pain medicine and mucolytics can be given as needed.

Bibliography

Johnson JT, Ferguson BJ. Infection. In: Cummings CW, Fredrickson JM, Harker LA, et al. (eds.), *Otolaryngology Head & Neck Surgery*, 3rd ed., vol. 2. St. Louis, MO: Mosby, 1998, 1107–1118.

Manning SC. Orbital cellulitis and abscess. In: Gates GA (ed.), *Current Therapy in Otolaryngology Head and Neck Surgery*, 6th ed. St. Louis, MO: Mosby, 1998, 359–362.

Pinheiro AD, Facer GW, Kern EB. Rhinosinusitis; current concepts and management. In: Bailey BJ, et al. (eds.), *Head & Neck Surgery Otolaryngology*, 3rd ed., vol. 1. Philadelphia, PA: Lippincott, Williams & Wilkins, 2001, 345–357.

Vandenbussche T, De Moor S, Bachert C, Van Cauwenberge P. Value of antral puncture in the intensive care patient with fever of unknown origin. *Laryngoscope* 2000;110(10 Pt 1):1702–1706.

18. **(C)** This question illustrates principles in the workup of penetrating neck trauma. There are three horizontal zones in the neck which are used to describe penetrating neck injuries. Zone I comprises the root of the neck to the inferior border of the cricoid cartilage. Zone II is the most exposed and the largest zone in surface area, extending from the inferior cricoid border to the angle of the mandible. Zone III begins at the angle of the mandible and extends to the base of the skull. Zone II is the most frequently injured and the carotid is the most commonly injured artery in 6% of cases of penetrating neck trauma. The average mortality at level one trauma centers is from 3 to 6%.

Signs of significant vascular injury include shock, hematoma or hemorrhage, pulse and neurologic deficits, and bruits or thrills in the neck. Signs of laryngotracheal injury include hemoptysis, subcutaneous emphysema, dyspnea, stridor and hoarseness depending on the exact location of the injury. Esophageal or pharyngeal injury is associated with dysphagia or odynophagia, subcutaneous emphysema, and possibly hematemesis. This patient in the case study has evidence of vascular injury but is stable with negative angiography. Angiography is indicated in zone I injuries as up to one-third of patients can be asymptomatic on presentation and this is a difficult area to examine. Zone I injuries are also the most lethal especially when the carotid artery is involved. Any positive findings in the mediastinum may require thoracotomy for vascular control. Another aspect of the workup not mentioned here is evaluation of the esophagus; zone I esophageal injury complications may be insidious and result in mediastinitis. Use of both esophagoscopy and esophagography probably has the sensitivity and specificity approaching 100%.

Zone II injuries are easier to follow clinically. If any worrisome symptoms or signs develop or are present at initial evaluation such as evolving neurologic deficits, then a neck exploration is recommended. Otherwise serial examinations and careful observation are all that is necessary according to several recent papers. Zone III injuries are also difficult to examine and gain surgical exposure because of the mandible, but are the least common location for penetrating neck trauma. These injuries therefore require angiography although a few papers have refuted this concept.

Answers "D" and "E" can be ruled out on the basis of a negative arteriogram. Answers "A" and "B" can be ruled out because of the lack of voice changes or lack of mention of vocal cord mobility. A posterior tracheal wall injury should be sought because delay in diagnosis of this entity could lead to a tracheoesophageal (TEP) fistula. Other complications of penetrating neck trauma include airway obstruction, neck abscess, mediastinitis, vocal cord paresis or paralysis, and cervical spine osteomyelitis. Behind the carotid, the subclavian artery is the next most injured artery. Vertebral artery injuries are detected well with four-vessel angiography. The IJV is the most commonly injured vein, seen in 9% of cases of penetrating trauma. Mortality from this injury occurs less often because of hemorrhage compared to an air embolism.

Bibliography

AAO-HNS Foundation. *Home Study Course Symposium: Trauma and Critical Care Medicine.* Sections 3, Feb–March 1998 (p. 17) and Jan–Feb 2000 (p. 17).

Grewal H, Prakashchandra MR, Mukerji S, et al. Management of penetrating laryngotracheal injuries. *Head Neck* 1995;17:494–502.

Klyachkin M, Rohmiller M, Charash W, et al. Penetrating injuries of the neck: selective management evolving. *Am Surg* 1997;63(2):189–194.

Stewart MG. Penetrating face and neck trauma. In: Bailey BJ, et al. (eds.), *Head & Neck Surgery Otolaryngology*, 3rd ed., vol. 1. Philadelphia, PA: Lippincott, Williams & Wilkins, 2001, 813–821.

Villaret DB, Shumrick KA. Penetrating neck trauma. In: Tami TA, et al. (eds.), *Otolaryngology: A Case Study Approach.* New York, NY: Thieme, 1998. 297–300.

19. **(E)** Temporal bone fractures are usually associated with some type of blunt or closed head injury. Motor vehicle accidents rank first in causes, smaller numbers are caused by falls; however, gunshot wounds are beginning to make up a significant minority. Pediatric temporal bone fractures are associated more with males than females, presumably because of increased physical activities and sports. These fractures are diagnosed by physical findings but fine cut (1 mm) CT scans and/or MRI are essential to evaluate for facial nerve involvement.

Temporal bone fractures are divided into three types. Seventy to 90% are longitudinal fractures, named according to their plane relative to the petrous apex. Starting at the mastoid process or the posterior squamous temporal bone, they follow a path of least resistance to the petrous apex. These extend to the region of the foramina lacerum and ovale and pass through the external auditory canal. Longitudinal fractures are frequently associated with conductive hearing loss, either because of tympanic membrane trauma, hemotympanum or direct ossicular disruption. Also seen is bleeding from the ear canal. CSF otorrhea is possible if a fracture involves the tegmen tympani which is the roof of the middle ear and mastoid. In addition, the perigeniculate region of the facial nerve is at risk and can be involved in the fracture line. Facial paralysis is seen in 10–20% of cases.

Transverse temporal bone fractures are associated with severe occipital injuries. Because of their perpendicular course relative to the petrous apex these fractures involve the bony labyrinth and can cause profound sensorineural hearing loss with vertigo. Transverse fractures are associated with facial nerve injury in 50% of cases; the labyrinthine segment of the facial nerve can be injured. CSF otorrhea and meningitis can be caused by disruption of the otic capsule because the bone does not heal by callus (it is endochondral bone). Another type is the mixed type which involves both fracture planes. Recent sources feel that most temporal bone fractures are actually mixed. "Battle's sign" refers to ecchymosis over the mastoid portion of the temporal bone and can be seen in any fracture type.

Facial nerve paralysis in this setting occurring immediately after the injury requires surgical and immediate intervention. ENOG tests evoked summation potentials of the facial nerve and is the best method for determining remaining function in the case of a weakness or paresis; the weak side is compared to the normal side. A few patients are in an especially poor prognostic category with respect to return of facial nerve function. These are patients with obvious bony disruption of the facial canal on CT scan (defined as a diastasis in the facial canal of 1 mm or greater or a spicule of bone in the canal) with immediate paralysis, and facial nerve injuries associated with CSF otorrhea. Patients with immediate paralysis showing evidence of degeneration on ENOG with decrease in potentials to less than 10% of their normal side and those with no clinical recovery within 1 week should undergo facial nerve exploration and repair if needed. Patients who uniformly do well, however, are those with delayed paralysis that had normal function at the time of injury. These patients can be observed and function should return in between 6 months to a year. Proper eye care is important with artificial tears or moisture chambers. Steroids may be helpful in the acute situation.

Other complications requiring immediate intervention are brain herniation into the middle ear and massive bleeding from a laceration in the intratemporal carotid artery. Early intervention may be needed in ossicular disruption associated with stapes subluxation and vertigo because of a perilymphatic fistula.

The temporal bone has four parts: the mastoid, squamosa, tympanic, and petrous portions. The internal auditory canal lies midway across its surface and carries cranial nerves VII and VIII. The endolymphatic duct is found on the inferior and posterior face of the temporal bone. The vestibular aqueduct enters the temporal bone and travels to the vestibule's inferior surface. Several important structures enter the skull base via the temporal bone such as contents of the jugular foramen (cranial nerves IX, X, and XI), the internal carotid artery, and the hypoglossal nerve in its canal.

Bibliography

AAO-HNS Foundation. Home study course symposium: trauma and critical SP. Management of facial nerve injury due to temporal bone trauma. *Am J Otol* 1999;20:96–114.

Farrior JB, Lee KJ. Noninfectious disorders of the ear. In: Lee KJ (ed.), *Essential Otolaryngology Head and Neck Surgery*, 8th ed. New York, NY: Mc-Graw Hill, 2003, 512–534.

Kamerer DB, Thompson SW. Middle ear and temporal bone trauma. In: Bailey BJ, et al. (eds.), *Head & Neck Surgery Otolaryngology*, 3rd ed., vol. 1. Philadelphia, PA: Lippincott, Williams & Wilkins, 2001, 1773–1785.

Kim HJ, et al. Imaging studies of the temporal bone. In: Bailey BJ, et al. (eds.), *Head & Neck Surgery Otolaryngology*, 3rd ed., vol. 2. Philadelphia, PA: Lippincott, Williams & Wilkins, 2001, 1689–1710.

Pensak ML. Temporal bone fracture. In: Tami TA, et al. (eds.), *Otolaryngology: A Case Study Approach.* New York, NY: Thieme, 1998, 24–26.

20. **(D)** This patient presents with a typical scenario for maxillary sinus malignancy: unilateral facial pain, nasal obstruction, and epistaxis. When a tumor is advanced, the patient may present with visual impairment and proptosis from involvement of the orbit or cranial nerve palsies of CN II–VI. Epiphora is caused by involvement of the lacrimal duct in the anteromedial maxilla. Other symptoms include trismus and malocclusion with involvement of muscles of mastication. The most common histologic type of maxillary sinus carcinoma is squamous cell, followed by mucosal adenocarcinomas and minor salivary gland adenocarcinomas or adenoid cystic carcinomas. In several series, the maxillary sinus is the most common sinus affected by malignancy in approximately 60–80% of cases.

Several epidemiologic and environmental factors have been linked to the development of paranasal sinus malignancies. Nickel refiners have a significant risk of developing squamous cell and anaplastic types with a long latency before presentation. Adenocarcinoma is associated with ethmoid sinus exposure to chemicals used in hardwood manufacturing or carpentry, and smoking exists as an independent risk factor. Other agents may be radium dial paint, mustard gas, hydrocarbons and chrome pigment.

Diagnostic assessment begins with imaging via CT scan or MRI. CT scans provide very good bony detail in general and soft tissue detail in the retroorbital and orbital apex regions. The advantage of MRI is in differentiating between secretions in the sinuses or actual tumor mass, especially with gadolinium enhancement. Angiography is indicated in tumors involving the sphenoid sinuses or in consideration of preoperative embolization for vascular tumors. Biopsy can be done endoscopically or if actually in the palate or gingival, through sampling of these regions. Ohngren's line is an imaginary line from the medial canthus to the angle of the mandible. Tumors above the line have a poorer prognosis as they tend to spread superoposteriorily. Those below the line are more easily resected and have a better prognosis.

Treatment is typically combined modality as most paranasal sinus malignancies present at a late stage. If the cancer is found early, complete resection is the treatment of choice. For poor surgical candidates or lymphoid malignancies, radiation is the main treatment. The surgical options for all paranasal sinus tumors (benign or malignant) include: external ethmoidectomy, inferior medial maxillectomy, medial maxillectomy, radical maxillectomy, and craniofacial resection. The patient described in this question required a radical maxillectomy because of his advanced carcinoma. The radical maxillectomy involves removal of the hard palate, part of the zygoma body, anteromedial orbit, lateral nasal wall and maxillary sinus and initial exposure is provided via the lateral rhinotomy incision, Weber-Fergusson incision or modifications thereof (Fig. 14-19). Another approach is the midface degloving procedure.

The issue of controversy here is management of the orbit. Bony invasion (i.e., invasion of the lamina papyracea) in and of itself is not a contraindication to preservation of orbital contents; however, some papers do support orbital exenteration with radical maxillectomy in the event of periorbita or orbital fat invasion which was the indication in this case. The general trend, however, is to spare the orbit and radiate the area as more recent papers have not shown a survival advantage between orbital sparing and preserving procedures. Radiation can cause visual impairment independently, however. Overall 5-year survival rate is

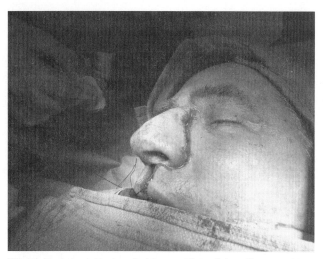

FIG. 14-19   Lateral rhinotomy incision used in medial maxillectomy with an infraorbital extension this would be called a Weber-Ferguson incision.

30%. Elective neck treatment is not warranted in most cases as only 5–10% of patients present with neck metastases; patients with neck metastases have a uniformly poor prognosis (Fig. 14-20).

Bibliography

Beasley NJP, Gullane PJ. Cancer of the larynx, paranasal sinuses and temporal bone. In: Lee KJ (ed.), *Essential Otolaryngology Head and Neck Surgery*, 8th ed. New York, NY: McGraw-Hill, 2003, 596–616.

Carrau RL, Myers EN. Neoplasms of the nose and paranasal sinuses. In: Bailey BJ, et al. (eds.), *Head & Neck Surgery Otolaryngology*, 3rd ed., vol. 2. Philadelphia, PA: Lippincott, Williams & Wilkins, 2001, 1247–1265.

Mount MR. Tumors of the nose and paranasal sinuses. In: Jafek BW, Murrow BW (eds.), *ENT Secrets*, 2nd ed. Philadelphia, PA: Hanley & Belfus, 2001, 275–279.

Villaret DB, Wilson KM. Maxillary sinus carcinoma. In: Tami TA, et al. (eds.), *Otolaryngology: A Case Study Approach*. New York, NY: Thieme, 1998, 101–104.

Weymuller EA Jr. Neoplasms. In: Cummings CW, Fredrickson JM, Harker LA, et al. (eds.), *Otolaryngology Head & Neck Surgery*, 3rd ed., vol. 2. St. Louis, MO: Mosby, 1998, 1118–1134.

21. **(E)** Statistics from the last decade indicate that trauma is the leading cause of death in children under the age of 14. Though approximately 15,000 children die from trauma related injuries every year, the proportion of facial injuries is low, at a maximum of 15%. Younger children are less likely to present with facial fractures because of their higher craniofacial ratio and less involvement with high-risk activities. Midface fractures in adults and children can be classified by the LeFort system. To understand midfacial fractures, the buttress system of the midface should be discussed.

The vertical buttresses of the face are the nasomaxillary, zygomaticomaxillary, and pterygomaxillary bony buttresses. These are important in maintenance of the vertical height of the face and must withstand the strong vertical masticatory forces. The horizontal buttresses of the face are important in facial width maintenance and bridging the vertical buttressed together but are weaker than the vertical buttresses. The components are the inferior orbital rims, greater wing of sphenoid, medial and lateral pterygoid plates, zygomatic process of the temporal bone and the maxillary alveolus and palate. LeFort or midface fractures in general are caused by anterior impact forces.

A LeFort I fracture indicates separation of the palate from the rest of the maxilla. The fracture line extends through the pterygoid plates, maxillary sinus, and the floor of the nose/pyriform aperture. A floating or mobile palate is a sign of this fracture and is demonstrated by being able to pull the entire palate forward while stabilizing the forehead with the other hand. A LeFort II fracture is also called pyramidal dysjunction. The palate and nose are separated from the cranium and the fracture line extends through the pterygoid plates, lateral and anterior maxillary walls, inferior orbital rims, medial orbital wall (lamina papyracea), nasofrontal suture, and the bony septum. The palate-nose complex are then mobile with respect to the rest of the face. A LeFort III fracture causes craniofacial dysjunction (answer E). All buttresses connecting the face to the skull are fractured, including the frontozygomatic suture. This classification does not take into account comminution of fractures which is a more critical finding.

Other symptoms or findings of midface fractures are epistaxis, airway obstruction and CSF rhinorrhea, and rarely blindness (2.2% in LeFort III) fractures. These fractures are contraindications to any type of nasogastric or nasotracheal intubation and even possibly orotracheal intubation because of the concern of penetration of the cranium and brain parenchyma. A tracheotomy should be considered in LeFort II and III fractures.

Treatment of midface fractures begins with appropriate imaging. Fine cut CT scans in axial and coronal (if possible) are performed as well as three-dimensional reconstructions if available. In children especially, simple LeFort I fractures are treated with MMF (maxillomandibular fixation, a.k.a., IMF), but those with gross displacement require open reduction with internal rigid fixation with plates and possibly MMF as well. LeFort II fractures are approached via gingivolabial sulcus incisions and a transconjunctival or subciliary incision. A coronal

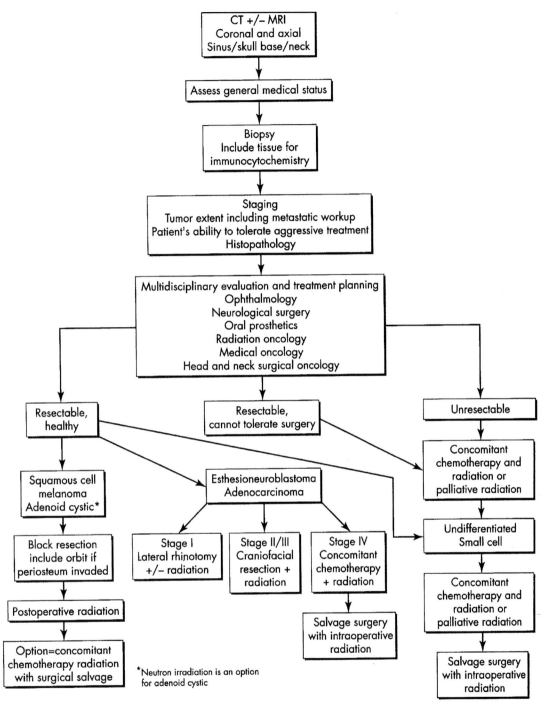

FIG. 14-20 Algorithm for diagnosis and management of paranasal sinus cancer. (*Source:* Reprinted from Cummings C, et al. *Otolaryngology—Head and Neck Surgery*, 3rd ed., copyright 1998, with permission from Elsevier).

incision is used for widest exposure. Principles of reduction of these fractures include rigid fixation and establishment of dental occlusion before proceeding to repair of the rest of the midface. There is controversy in whether plates should be removed in pediatric patients as some studies have demonstrated inhibition of facial growth with rigid fixation.

The nasoethmoid fracture is a unique midface fracture not incorporated into the LeFort system. It is a true orbital wall injury caused by impaction of frontal processes of the maxilla and nasal bones into the orbital space with comminution of ethmoid air cells and lateral displacement of the medial orbital walls. Classic findings of this fracture are nasal dorsum flattening and telecanthus, or widened intercanthal distance where the intercanthal distance is greater than the length of the palpebral fissure.

Bibliography

Dodson BT. Zygomatic, maxillary, and orbital fractures. In: Jafek BW, Murrow BW (eds.), *ENT Secrets*, 2nd ed. Philadelphia, PA: Hanley & Belfus, 2001, 415–421.

Senders CW. Pediatric facial trauma. In: Wetmore RF, et al. (eds.), *Pediatric Otolaryngology: Principles and Practice Pathways*. New York, NY: Thieme, 2000, 497–511.

Stanley RB Jr. Maxillofacial trauma. In: Cummings CW, Fredrickson JM, Harker LA, et al. (eds.), *Otolaryngology Head & Neck Surgery*, 3rd ed., vol. 1. St. Louis, MO: Mosby, 1998, 453–485.

Stanley RB Jr. Maxillary and periorbital fractures. In: Bailey BJ, et al. (eds.), *Head & Neck Surgery Otolaryngology*, 3rd ed., vol. 1. Philadelphia, PA: Lippincott, Williams & Wilkins, 2001, 777–792.

22. **(C)** Epistaxis or nosebleeding is one of the most common ear, nose and throat (ENT) emergencies. The role of the nose in humidification, filtration and warming of inspired air and its copious blood supply all put it at risk for bleeding. Epistaxis more commonly occurs in older individuals because of vessel wall aging with fibrosis and slower vasoconstriction and in the winter months because of cold, dry air exposure. Other risk factors include trauma (nose picking, most common in children), nasal sprays including nasal steroids, intranasal or sinus tumors, allergies, medications such as antiplatelet agents and anticoagulants, and anatomic deformities such as septal deviation. Systemic factors and diseases putting patients at epistaxis risk include hypertension, hereditary hemorrhagic telangiectasia (Osler-Weber-Rendu disease, an autosomal dominant disease with associated mucosal telangiectasias and pulmonary AVMs), von Willebrand disease, hemophilia, nutritional deficiencies, alcohol abuse with associated hepatic disease, and lymphoreticular disorders or malignancies.

Epistaxis most commonly occurs in the anterior portion of the nasal cavity, specifically the septum and the area known as Kiesselbach's plexus (in 90%). This area is particularly susceptible to trauma and drying effects. The first step in management of epistaxis is fluid resuscitation and control of life-threatening hemorrhage. This involves fluid replacement in patients with dehydration or hypovolemic shock. Special attention should be given to the patient with coronary ischemia history and a low hematocrit. One must then determine from which side the bleeding originates and whether the bleeding is anterior or posterior (Fig. 14-21). When a bleed is severe or profuse, endoscopy is difficult to use effectively.

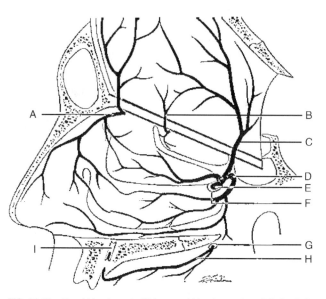

FIG. 14-21 Nasal blood supply. Major nasal blood vessels and their relative positions are depicted. Note that the nasal septum has been reflected superiorly. A, Anterior ethmoidal artery; B, Posterior ethmoidal artery; C, Posterior septal nasal artery; D, Lateral nasal artery; E, Sphenopalatine artery; F, Sphenopalatine foramen; G, Greater palatine foramen; H, Greater palatine artery; I, Incisive canal. (*Source:* Reprinted from Gates HA, et al. *Current therapy in Otolaryngology—Head and Neck Surgery*, 6th ed., copyright 1998, with permission from Elsevier).

The anterior bleed is treated with an anterior pack which traditionally is a 6 ft piece of Vaseline impregnated strip gauze which is the most secure. An antibacterial ointment is used to cover the gauze, and if this controls the bleeding, the patient is discharged with pain medication and antibiotic prophylaxis against *S. aureus* and sinus pathogens, with instructions to return in 3–5 days for pack removal. The two reasons an anterior pack fails are inadequate packing and a posterior bleed. Other methods of anterior packing are with expandable sponges, microfibrillar collagen slurries, or absorbable cellulose fiber packings. Small volume bleeds with obvious focal sources can be treated with silver nitrate chemical cauterization.

Posterior nasal packing carries significant morbidity. The traditional pack employed a Foley balloon catheter to tamponade posterior bleeding with an anterior gauze pack. There are now double balloon devices to serve the same purpose. These packs are left in place for days as well; however, because of the morbidity involved, patients must be admitted, typically to a monitored floor, for observation. Pain control is crucial to avoid blood pressure fluctuations. Pack insertion complications include nasovagal reflexes (a reflex bradycardia), hypovolemic shock, topical anesthetic, and vasocontrictor complications. Pack maintenance complications include hypoxia or hypoventilation because of nasal obstruction, respiratory obstruction, local infection, bacteremia or toxic shock syndrome, and inadequate oral intake. Major complications (including cardiorespiratory and septic complications) may occur in up to 20% of patients with posterior packs. Minor complications include hypesthesia, nasal necrosis with synechiae, sinusitis, hemotympanum, and oroantral fistula. Packs may actually exacerbate (OSA) symptoms.

When packing fails there are several surgical options for bleeding control. The first is the internal maxillary artery ligation, which takes care of bleeding from sphenopalatine sources. This is performed via a sublabial incision and approach to the artery through the posterior wall of the maxillary sinus. The second is the anterior ethmoid artery ligation which is performed via an external ethmoidectomy or "Lynch" incision. Endovascular embolization is used in selective cases where epistaxis recurs after surgery, in patients with unresectable sinonasal tumors; patients who are poor surgical candidates and those with life-threatening hemorrhage can also be considered. There are significant sequelae and moribidities associated with embolization, however, such as femoral artery injury or pseudoaneurysm, facial pain or paresis. There is a newer procedure called transnasal endoscopic sphenopalatine artery ligation which has less morbidity but there is little long-term data to advocate this as a sole approach. The last resort is the external carotid artery ligation.

Bibliography

Citardi MJ, Kuhn FA. Refractory posterior epistaxis. In: Gates GA (ed.), *Current Therapy in Otolaryngology Head and Neck Surgery*, 6th ed. St. Louis, MO: Mosby, 1998, 331–335.

Emanuel JM. Epistaxis. In: Cummings CW, Fredrickson JM, Harker LA, et al. (eds.), *Otolaryngology Head & Neck Surgery*, 3rd ed., vol. 2. St. Louis, MO: Mosby, 1998, 453–485.

Randall DA. The nose and paranasal sinuses. In: Lee KJ (ed.), *Essential Otolaryngology Head and Neck Surgery*, 8th ed. New York, NY: McGraw-Hill, 2003, 682–723.

Santos PM, Lepore ML. Epistaxis. In: Bailey BJ, et al. (eds.), *Head & Neck Surgery Otolaryngology*, 3rd ed., vol. 1. Philadelphia, PA: Lippincott, Williams & Wilkins, 2001, 415–428.

23. **(C)** In the United States, OSA has a prevalence of 4% in men and 2% in women. There are several systemic consequences to sleep apnea including hypertension, myocardial infarction, and stroke. Patients with sleep apnea have three to seven times the risk of having motor vehicle accidents. As a result of these statistics, sleep apnea is being diagnosed earlier and treated aggressively. There is a continuum of sleep disordered breathing which ranges from sleep apnea to the Pickwickian's syndrome. OSA is caused by an obstruction at any level of the upper airway above the glottis. The muscle relaxation occurring in the deeper stages of sleep occurs in the upper airway as well and patients predisposed to OSA have excess tissue in the upper airway, causing an airway collapse during inspiration. The patient is then awakened by desaturation, signaled as a snorting or gasping noise, and then resumes the pattern.

The RDI is the respiratory disturbance index which is obtained by polysomnography. An RDI of greater than 5 is abnormal. Apnea itself is defined as cessation of airflow for at least 10 s, and hypopneas are desaturations without complete cessation. The RDI is the number of apneas and hypopneas in 1 h. This measure allows stratification of patients into mild, moderate, and severe groups and treatment is thus tailored. Patients with sleep apnea can be identified by certain physical characteristics, including large neck circumference (>17 in.) with a short neck, redundant pharyngeal tissue or enlarged tonsils, a large base of tongue, elongated uvula and a retrognathic chin. Symptoms include daytime somnolence, headaches, mood changes, snoring.

An RDI of less than 15 is considered mild, that between 15 and 30 moderate, and above 30 severe. These are not absolute categories; however, because a patient with a lower RDI but significant desaturation (i.e., below 80) would be considered to have moderate apnea. The patient in this question clearly had severe apnea. The treatment of sleep apnea is multidimensional involving behavioral modifications, devices, and surgery. The first two options tend to apply to mild or moderate cases. Nasal CPAP is the most effective nonsurgical method but is very uncomfortable because of a tight fitting mask and the positive pressure. The CPAP can be used in conjunction with orthodontic devices or with nasal surgery (septoplasty and the like) to improve compliance. Weight loss is the chief behavioral modification but rarely works when used alone.

Surgical options are divided into phase I and phase II surgeries. Phase I surgeries address the primary site of obstruction which may be retropalatal or retroglossal or both, most likely both in the case of a severe apneic patient. Surgeries to the palate include uvulopalatopharyngoplasty (UP3), laser-assisted uvulopalatoplasty, radiofrequency ablation of the palate, cautery-assisted palate stiffening, chemical sclerosis of the palate, and coblation of the palate. UP3 is very effective in controlling snoring but only 50% or so for treatment of OSA. Surgeries that address the hypophayrnx include the genioglossus advancement or mortised genioplasty which also moves the hyoid bone anteriorly. Radiofrequency ablation of the tongue and partial midline glossectomy address the retroglossal area also. Phase II surgery is comprised of maxillomandibular advancement which is very effective in patients who require it; patients reach phase II when phase I procedures have failed. Finally, the tracheostomy is the most effective surgical option in any patient with severe apnea as it bypasses all areas of upper airway obstruction. Most patients avoid this option; it is usually reserved for patients who are severely debilitated by their sleep apnea.

Bibliography

Campana JP. Snoring and obstructive sleep apnea. In: Jafek BW, Murrow BW (eds.), *ENT Secrets*, 2nd ed. Philadelphia, PA: Hanley & Belfus, 2001, 200–207.

Goldberg AN. Obstructive sleep apnea: treatment algorithms. In: Friedman M (ed.), *Operative Techniques in Otolaryngology Head and Neck Surgery: Neck and Upper Airway Surgical Techniques: Update of Otolaryngology Surgical Techniques*. Philadelphia, PA: WB Saunders, 2002, vol. 13, no. 3, 225–230.

Piccirillo JF, Thawley SE. Sleep-disordered breathing. In: Cummings CW, Fredrickson JM, Harker LA, et al. (eds.), *Otolaryngology Head & Neck Surgery*, 3rd ed., vol. 2. St. Louis, MO: Mosby, 1998, 1546–1571.

Walker RP. Snoring and obstructive sleep apnea. In: Bailey BJ, et al. (eds.), *Head & Neck Surgery Otolaryngology*, 3rd ed., vol. 1. Philadelphia, PA: Lippincott, Williams & Wilkins, 2001, 579–597.

24. **(C)** Tracheotomies are performed to provide temporary openings in the trachea for longer term ventilation. Tracheostomies, on the other hand, are the permanent counterpart to the tracheotomy, because of the creation of a skin-lined tract to the trachea. There are four chief indications for tracheotomies or tracheostomies: to bypass mechanical obstruction in the upper airway, to bypass secretional obstructions in patients who cannot clear secretions, to help in maintaining respiration over a long duration, and to prevent aspiration of oral or gastric secretions.

Causes of mechanical obstruction include obstructive tumors or postradiation edema in the upper aerodigestive tract, inflammation of the larynx, trachea, tongue and the like (i.e., epiglottitis), congenital anomalies, laryngeal or tracheal trauma, maxillofacial trauma, bilateral vocal cord paralysis, foreign bodies, and OSA. Secretional blockage can be caused by poor cough effort from surgery, pneumonia, burns, or decreased mental status from coma. Alveolar hypoventilation of various causes may also lead to secretion retention.

Elective tracheotomies are performed in the operating room, and the patient's head is hyperextended with use of a shoulder roll (if there are no contraindications to hyperextension). An incision is made approximately 3–5 cm long midway between the cricoid and the sternal notch in a horizontal fashion down through the platysma. When strap muscles are seen, they are divided in the midline vertically and the thyroid isthmus is encountered and either retracted upward or divided sharply or via electrocautery. A cricoid hook attached to the inferior border of the cricoid is used to retract the entire framework upward while the pretracheal fascia is bluntly dissected away. At this point there are variations. Some surgeons remove a cartilage window at the second or third cartilage ring, but a large proportion still use the Bjork flap described first in 1960. The Bjork flap is an inferiorly-based flap of the anterior portion of a single ring sutured to the inferior skin margin. It is designed for ease of tube insertion especially in the event the patient is accidentally decannulated, so that no false passages are created.

The cricothyrotomy is preferable in an emergency situation because the cricothyroid membrane is much closer to the skin surface and less dissection is needed and less bleeding encountered. A short transverse stabbing incision is made directly over the cricothyroid membrane, while the thyroid cartilage is grasped with the other hand to stabilize the larynx. Once the subglottis is entered, the knife handle is inserted and rotated to open the wound, and then a tracheostomy tube is placed. The drawback with this surgical airway is that it must be converted within 3–5 days to avoid the long-term and inevitable sequela of subglottic stenosis. As an alternative, emergency tracheostomies can be done via vertical incision beginning at the level of the cricoid cartilage and extending 2.5–4 cm inferiorly.

The tracheotomy can help decrease the dead space in the tracheobronchial tree by 70–100 mL or by 10–50% depending on the patient. It also greatly reduces resistance to airflow and improved compliance and ventilation. It allows for swallowing without reflex apnea and good access for pulmonary hygiene measures as well as for humidification and direct administration of medications. It also decreases the power of the cough so secretions are not propelled into distal airways where they are harder to clear.

There are two categories of complications related to tracheotomies. Early or immediate complications are hemorrhage, apnea, pneumothorax, pneumomediastinum, subcutaneous emphysema, malpositioned tube, TEP fistula, high tracheotomy with cricoid damage, recurrent nerve paralysis, aerophagia, and aspiration. Delayed complications include delayed hemorrhage, TEP fistula after decannulation, tracheocutaneous fistula, tube displacement or cuff displacement, tracheomalacia, dysphagia, atelectasis or pneumonia, difficult decannulation, stomal healing problems, and tracheal stenosis. Delayed hemorrhage, as occurred in this patient, is usually because of erosion of a major blood vessel from pressure necrosis from the tube cuff or the tip of the tube itself. This is more a concern when a tracheotomy is placed low. The most common vessel involved is the innominate artery but inferior and superior thyroid arteries, aortic arch, common carotid, and even the innominate vein can be sources.

Bibliography

Friedman M, Ibrahim H. The difficult tracheotomy simplified. In: Friedman M (ed.), *Operative Techniques in Otolaryngology Head and Neck Surgery: Neck and Upper Airway Surgical Techniques: Update of Otolaryngology Surgical Techniques.* Philadelphia, PA: WB Saunders, 2002, vol. 13, no. 3, 215–218.

Weissler MC. Tracheotomy and intubation. In: Bailey BJ, et al. (eds.), *Head & Neck Surgery Otolaryngology*, 3rd ed., vol. 1. Philadelphia, PA: Lippincott, Williams & Wilkins, 2001, 677–689.

Weymuller EA Jr. Acute airway management. In: Cummings CW, Fredrickson JM, Harker LA, et al. (eds.), *Otolaryngology Head & Neck Surgery*, 3rd ed., vol. 3. St. Louis, MO: Mosby, 1998, 2368–2381.

Woo P, Yanagisawa E. The larynx. In: Lee KJ (ed.), *Essential Otolaryngology Head and Neck Surgery*, 8th ed. New York, NY: McGraw-Hill, 2003, 724–792.

25. **(E)** Lip cancer has an incidence of approximately 2 per 100,000. It is disproportionately found in the lower lip as compared to the upper lip as the upper lip tends to be shaded from actinic exposure. The most common histologic subtype is SCC in the lower lip, whereas in the skin of the upper lip, basal cell carcinoma is the most common histology. Within squamous cell cancers there are four growth patterns: exophytic, ulcerative, infiltrative, and verrucous. The exophytic is least common in the oral cavity as a whole except in the lip. It metastasizes later than the other patterns, but once advanced it takes on an infiltrative and/or ulcerative growth. The ulcerative type is the most common type in the oral cavity as a whole and may have a higher grade on presentation than the exophytic types. Infiltrative SCC presents as a mass or plaque covered by mucosa and extends deeply into surrounding tissues. Verrucous carcinoma has a predilection for elderly patients with poor oral hygiene or poorly fitting dentures and is more common in the buccal mucosa in patients with a history of snuff use or tobacco chewing. It has a fungating and warty appearance and does not invade deeply and rarely if at all metastasizes. Its advancing histologic margin pushes rather than invades deep tissue. Clinical behavior is worse in cancers that are higher grade, have evidence of neural invasion, are greater than 6 mm in thickness and grow in a disorganized infiltrative pattern.

Other types of lip cancer are the basal cell carcinoma which arises on the vermilion border rather than the vermilion itself. Minor salivary gland carcinomas arise in the minor salivary glands of the upper and lower lip. The most common histologies are adenoid cystic and mucoepidermoid carcinoma. Melanoma is rarely observed and is considered mucosal in origin when it arises directly from the vermilion from melanocytes normally found in the lip. Rare malignancies in the differential include Merkel cell carcinoma, microcystic adnexal carcinoma, malignant fibrous histiocytoma, and malignant granular cell tumors. One benign lesion that deserves mention is the keratoacanthoma which can mimic SCC. It occurs on the lip in 8% of cases and is seen in patients from the sixth decade upward. It has an initial rapid growth phase but then spontaneously regresses after several months. Inflammatory lesions such as syphilitic chancres, pyogenic granulomas (superficial polypoid masses that bleed easily), epidermal inclusion cysts, keratoses, and viral stomatitis should be ruled out also.

It is agreed that for early stage lesions (small T2 and T1) both surgery and radiation are equally effective. Five-year survival rates are about 90%. Advantages of surgery are rapidity of treatment, histologic evaluation, better overall cure in advanced lesions, and avoidance of radiation-induced morbidity to surrounding structures. The disadvantage is that surgery is invasive as compared to radiation and cosmesis is an issue in certain tumors. Radiation is delivered by brachytherapy implants, or external beam radiation via orthovoltage photon or electron beams. Radiation is low risk and is appropriate in those that are poor surgical candidates. It, however, takes an extended period of time to complete and surrounding tissues are subjected to radiation damage.

Surgical options include full-thickness excision in the shape of a V, W, or rectangle to help with closure. Superficial carcinomas can be excised with Mohs' micrographic excision. Eight to 10 mm of minimum normal tissue margin should be taken with the lesion. Marginal mandibulectomy (single cortex) may need to be incorporated in lesions encroaching the alveolar ridge or outer mandibular cortex and segmental mandibulectomy is needed for tumors invading the mandible. Elective neck dissection is only recommended in advanced stage tumors, those of high grade, and for recurrences. Lymph node basins that require removal are the intraparotid, submandibular and submental lymph nodes for cancer of the upper lip and submental and bilateral submandibular lymph nodes in the case of carcinoma of the lower lip involving the central one-third of the lip as well as the upper jugular group of lymph nodes. There is controversy as to whether modified or selective neck dissections should be performed. Combined surgery and adjuvant radiation is required in advance local disease as in the case of T4 lesions or those with positive lymph nodes after neck dissection. There are multiple methods of reconstruction of the upper and lower lips after surgical excision but these are beyond the scope of this question and the reader is encouraged to review the bibliography for further information.

Bibliography

Baker SE. Cancer of the lip. In: Gates GA (ed.), *Current Therapy in Otolaryngology Head and Neck Surgery*, 6th ed. St. Louis, MO: Mosby, 1998, 256–262.

DeLacure MD. Lip and oral cavity. In: Close LG, Larson DL, Shah JP (eds.), *Essentials of Head and Neck Oncology.* New York, NY: Thieme, 1998, 178–191.

Esclamado RM, Krause CJ. Lip cancer. In: Bailey BJ, et al. (eds.), *Head & Neck Surgery Otolaryngology*, 3rd ed., vol. 2. Philadelphia, PA: Lippincott, Williams & Wilkins, 2001, 1299–1309.

Sharma PK, Schuller DE, Baker SE. Malignant neoplasms of the oral cavity. In: Cummings CW, Fredrickson JM, Harker LA, et al. (eds.), *Otolaryngology Head & Neck Surgery*, 3rd ed., vol. 2. St. Louis, MO: Mosby, 1998, 1418–1462.

Zitsch RP, Renner GJ. *Carcinoma of the Lip. Self-Instructional Package*. Alexandria, VA: American Academy of Otolaryngology Head and Neck Surgery Foundation, 1996.

26. **(A)** There are several reconstructive options for a pharyngolaryngectomy defect but the appropriate choice depends on the size of the defect and tissues involved. The options available are free tissue transfer with a jejunal autograft, colon interposition or lateral thigh, a radial forearm fasciocutaneous flap, a pectoralis major myocutaneous flap, and a gastric pull-up procedure. In this patient, the gastric pull-up would be the procedure of choice as the defect and lesion involve the thoracic esophagus. It is also a useful procedure if a total esophagectomy is required for skip lesions in the esophagus (Fig. 14-22).

The chief advantage of the gastric pull-up is the need for a single anastomosis as opposed to multiple anastomoses. With a single anastomosis, there is less opportunity for stricture or fistula formation. The stomach is elevated up through the posterior mediastinum without the need for a thoracotomy by using blunt dissection. The stomach relies then on vascularity from the right gastric and gastroepiploic vessels while the left gastric, short gastrics, and left gastroepiploic origins are divided. A Kocher maneuver is used to mobilize the duodenum which allows for anastomosis as high as the nasopharynx if needed,

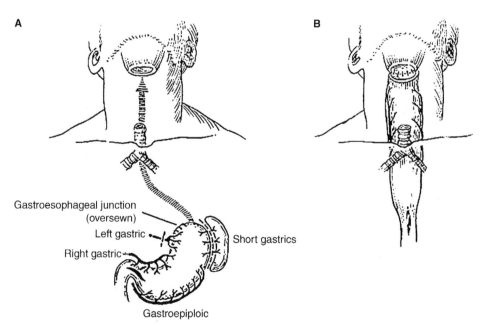

FIG. 14-22 Gastric pull-up. (*Source:* Reprinted from Cummings C, et al. *Otolaryngology—Head and Neck Surgery*, 3rd ed., copyright 1998, with permission from Elsevier).

and vagotomy and pyloroplasty is performed to help with gastric emptying. A jejunostomy tube is used for postoperative decompression. The gastric fundus is opened for the pharyngeal anastomosis.

There is a 5–15% mortality rate with gastric pull-up, which is its chief disadvantage. There is danger of ischemic necrosis if too high a defect is created. Because of mediastinal dissection there is possibility of pneumothorax and hemothorax; either of these complications can be treated effectively with thoracotomy tubes. There are several long-term GI complaints, including emesis, early satiety, and dumping. One-layer anastomoses and those that are hand-sewn have less chance of stricture. Fistulae that develop may heal spontaneously over 4–6 weeks in a previously nonirradiated patient; however, this healing may lead to stricture. An average of 10 days passes before oral alimentation is started. Speech rehabilitation with a TEP or tracheogastric puncture is possible, though the quality of speech reported in many studies is inferior to that of total laryngectomy with TEP.

The jejunal autograft allows reconstruction of almost any pharyngolaryngectomy defect but has the disadvantage of requiring two anastomoses. There is no special bowel prep needed and the segment harvested must be supplied by a single vascular arcade with adequate caliber vessels for microvascular anastomosis. It must be positioned in an isoperistaltic fashion and a small segment of bowel is partitioned and brought externally to serve as a monitor for flap viability. A barium swallow is performed at least a week after surgery to check for fistula or stricture. The main contraindications are ascites or chronic diseases of the jejunum. Colon interposition, which involves a segment of right colon based on the superior mesenteric artery, does not require microvascular techniques but is fraught with a high incidence of postoperative infection. Fistula when it occurs typically occurs at the superior anastomosis between the jejunum and pharynx; conversely, strictures tend to occur at the inferior anastomosis between the jejunum and esophagus (Fig. 14-23).

The radial forearm flap is used for selected hypopharyngeal and cervical esophageal defects. It is thin and pliable and can be tubed, has large vessels and is easier to harvest than other free tissue transfers. It has excellent speech and voice rehabilitation potential. The flap is based on the radial artery. An Allen's test should be done prior to harvest.

The pectoralis major myocutaneous flap is based on the thoracoacromial artery. It is very reliable with low donor site morbidity. There is more discussion on this in another question in this chapter.

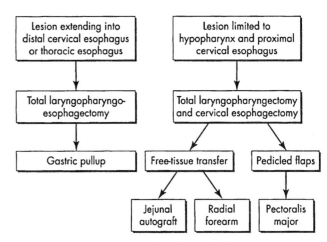

FIG. 14-23 Reconstructive options for cervical esophagectomy and laryngopharyngectomy defects. (*Source:* Reprinted from Cummings C, et al. *Otolaryngology—Head and Neck Surgery*, 3rd ed., copyright 1998, with permission from Elsevier).

Bibliography

Gleich L, Gluckman JL. Hypopharynx and cervical esophagus. In: Close LG, Larson DL, Shah JP (eds.), *Essentials of Head and Neck Oncology.* New York, NY: Thieme, 1998, 211–222.

Johnson JT. Cervical esophageal cancer. In: Bailey BJ, et al. (eds.), *Head & Neck Surgery Otolaryngology*, 3rd ed., vol. 2. Philadelphia, PA: Lippincott, Williams & Wilkins, 2001, 1459–1467.

Varvares MA, Cheney ML. Reconstruction of the hypopharynx and cervical esophagus. In: Cummings CW, Fredrickson JM, Harker LA, et al. (eds.), *Otolaryngology Head & Neck Surgery*, 3rd ed., vol. 3. St. Louis, MO: Mosby, 1998, 2242–2257.

27. **(E)** Oropharyngeal carcinomas are similar to malignancies of the upper aerodigestive tract. Greater than 90% are squamous cell carcinomas, and these are usually linked to a history of tobacco and alcohol use. Apart from the nonkeratinizing well or moderately differentiated squamous cell carcinoma, there are the spindle cell, verrucous, lymphoepithelioma, adenoid squamous, adenosquamous and basaloid squamous subtypes. The spindle cell subtype clinically behaves like the garden variety squamous cell carcinoma. The verrucous subtype is very exophytic and fungating and is a slow-growing tumor with rare metastases. The lymphoepithelioma occurs in a younger age group than the other subtypes and is less associated with the standard risk factors. The last three subtypes are highly aggressive with early spread to regional lymph nodes and distant sites but are fortunately rare. Other types of malignancies include lymphoma (mostly non-Hodgkin's), minor salivary gland tumors, mucosal melanoma and sarcomas.

Of all sites in the oropharynx, the anterior tonsillar pillar and tonsillar fossa are the most common location for tumors. The tonsil is frequently the primary site in the situation of the unknown primary. The oropharynx in general has a very rich lymphatic network with spread occurring in a progressive manner from level II, then III, then the retropharynx. Soft palate lesions have a high chance of bilateral nodal involvement if found close to midline (more than 40%). Base of tongue cancers are thought to have a better overall prognosis despite the fact they are found at a more advanced stage. Neck adenopathy may be the presenting symptom in approximately 30% of patients with oropharyngeal cancer.

With regards to treatment, early oropharyngeal cancers can be treated by radiation therapy or surgery as a sole modality. Tonsillar carcinomas are quite radiosensitive and 85% cure rates with primary radiation can be obtained with T1 cancers; however, any lesion that has extended beyond the anterior tonsillar pillar or to the base of tongue is not effectively treated by only external beam radiation and requires surgery as the primary modality. Radiation is then reserved for tumors with positive pathologic margins and aggressive behavior. Any lesion larger than T1 requires treatment of at least the ipsilateral neck; for N0 or N1 necks, surgery or radiation can be used alone depending on what method was used to treat the primary tumor. Postoperative radiation is recommended for the ipsilateral side with extracapsular nodal spread, N2 disease, and primaries greater than 3 cm in size (at least T2). If the neck is clinically involved or if the lesion is central or midline (more a concern with soft palate primaries), then both necks should be treated. Staging for oropharyngeal carcinomas is similar to that of oral cavity.

Several approaches to the oropharynx are available for resection of the primary tumor. The first is the transoral approach which has limited application in lesions only on the tonsillar pillar, tonsil fossa, or upper pharyngeal wall. Because an adequate 1–2 cm margin of normal tissue is needed beyond the primary for resection, exposure is limited and the presence of dentition, any trismus or the mandible itself further limit visualization, thus this would be the poorest choice for approach. The composite resection (a.k.a., Commando procedure) is used for large oropharyngeal cancers with gross mandibular invasion or when there is suspicion for mandibular invasion. A cheek flap is used and the lip is split in the midline and carried in the buccal sulcus posteriorly to give wide exposure. The mental nerve is sacrificed and ultimately a segment of mandible is removed in continuity with the primary. The transhyoid or suprahyoid pharyngoto-

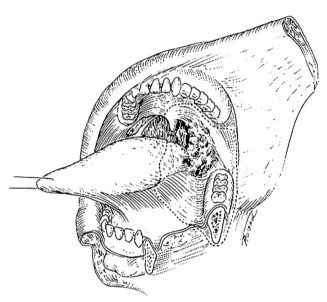

FIG. 14-24 Diagram of mandible split procedure and exposure to the tonsil and base of tongue region. (*Source:* Reprinted from Cummings C, et al. *Otolaryngology—Head and Neck Surgery*, 3rd ed., copyright 1998, with permission from Elsevier).

my preserves mandibular continuity and access to the tongue base area is via the neck. It can be extended laterally but superior exposure is not optimal. The lateral pharyngotomy involves entrance of the neck posterior to the thyroid ala on the contralateral side and is also used for smaller lesions of the tongue base and pharyngeal walls. The mandibulotomy, otherwise known as a mandibular swing, can be midline or lateral and provides excellent exposure to the entire oropharynx (Fig. 14-24). This approach would be a good choice in this patient.

Bibliography

Genden EM, Thawley SE, O'Leary MJ. Malignant neoplasms of the oropharynx. In: Cummings CW, Fredrickson JM, Harker LA, et al. (eds.), *Otolaryngology Head & Neck Surgery*, 3rd ed., vol. 2. St. Louis, MO: Mosby, 1998, 1463–1511.

Holsinger FC, Meyers JN. Carcinoma of the oral cavity and pharynx. In: Lee KJ (ed.), *Essential Otolaryngology Head and Neck Surgery*, 8th ed. New York, NY: McGraw-Hill, 2003, 566–595.

Parks R, Close LG. Oropharynx. In: Close LG, Larson DL, Shah JP (eds.), *Essentials of Head and Neck Oncology*. New York, NY: Thieme, 1998, 198–204.

Seikaly H, Rassekh CH. Oropharyngeal cancer. In: Bailey BJ, et al. (eds.), *Head & Neck Surgery Otolaryngology*, 3rd ed., vol. 2. Philadelphia, PA: Lippincott, Williams & Wilkins, 2001, 1427–1441.

Zeitels SM, Komisar A. *Surgical Management of Tumors of the Oropharynx. Self-Instructional Package.* Alexandria, VA: American Academy of Otolaryngology Head and Neck Surgery Foundation, 1997.

28. (E) This case is typical of acute bacterial parotitis or sialadenitis. This disorder occurs in individuals with dehydration from any cause. The dehydration may be a result of being NPO for an extended period of time or in the patient being in a relative state of anorexia after surgery and patients who have undergone abdominal procedures are at the most risk. Chronic and/or debilitating illnesses also may predispose a patient to development of acute parotitis such as in the case of a nursing home patient. Other causes may be radiation, chemotherapy or immunosuppression in general, medications with anticholinergic side effects, and Sjogren's disease. The incidence is reported at approximately 1 in 1–2000 operative procedures. Acute parotitis presents with symptoms of pain, erythema, and diffuse enlargement of the gland which is usually unilateral; gentle milking of Stensen's duct with manual pressure on the gland and intraorally causes purulent exudate to be expressed from the orifice.

The pathophysiology of acute parotitis is retrograde bacterial infection through Stensen's duct. Mucoid saliva which has a high molecular weight glycoprotein and sialic acid has superior bacteriostatic activity because of the ability to trap bacteria. Mucoid saliva also has a higher lysozyme and IgA concentration. As the parotid expresses predominantly serous saliva, it is at a relative disadvantage compared to the other salivary glands. Salivary stasis can occur with either decreased production, ductal stricture or calculi (stones). Poor oral hygiene also contributes to infection. When a patient is NPO, stimulation of salivary flow by mastication is not possible and food itself helps prevent bacterial aggregation by a detergent-like action. The primary bacterium responsible is *S. aureus*. Oral anaerobes including *Prevotella* and *Porphyromonas* species, *Fusobacterium* and *Peptostreptococcus*. Gram-negative organisms are found more frequently in hospitalized patients such as *Haemophilus* and *Pseudmonas*. Finally, mycobacteria (tuberculosis and atypical species) are more rare causes of acute bacterial parotitis.

The treatment of parotitis is both local and systemic. The patient must be adequately hydrated and if applicable, good oral hygiene measures should be observed. Warm compresses are used for comfort and to assist with drainage of pus from the duct. Sialogogues can also be used (lemon-drops or lemons themselves) to assist in stimulation of salivary flow. The most important arm of treatment is intravenous antibiotics preferably with antipenicillinase properties. An improvement should be seen within 24–48 h and if not then imaging with CT scan or ultrasound should be considered to look for an abscess. Sialography (imaging of the ducts with dye) is contraindicated because it has the potential to worsen the infection. An abscess requires surgical drainage which is performed by raising a standard cheek skin flap over the parotid capsule and make small stabs into the parenchyma of the gland in the direction of the facial nerve. The differential of parotitis is lymphoma, a mastoid abscess, cervical adenitis, external otitis-induced lymphangitis, buccal or masseteric space abscesses, and sebaceous or infected branchial cleft cysts. Complications are rare but include osteomyelitis, thrombophlebitis of the jugular vein, respiratory obstruction or septicemia, indicating the importance of early diagnosis and treatment. An algorithm for evaluation and treatment of salivary gland inflammation is given in Fig. 14-25.

Bibliography

Brook I. Acute bacterial suppurative parotitis: microbiology and management. *J Craniofac Surg* 2003;14(1):37–40.

Gayner SM, Kane WJ, McCaffrey TV. Infections of the salivary glands. In: Cummings CW, Fredrickson JM, Harker LA, et al. (eds.), *Otolaryngology Head & Neck Surgery*, 3rd ed., vol. 2. St. Louis, MO: Mosby, 1998, 1235–1246.

Rice DH. Nonneoplastic diseases of the salivary glands. In: Bailey BJ, et al. (eds.), *Head & Neck Surgery Otolaryngology*, 3rd ed., vol. 1. Philadelphia, PA: Lippincott, Williams & Wilkins, 2001, 453–461.

Shemen LJ. Salivary glands: benign and malignant diseases. In: Lee KJ (ed.), *Essential Otolaryngology Head and Neck Surgery*, 8th ed. New York, NY: McGraw-Hill, 2003, 535–565.

29. (A) The differential diagnosis for a neck mass in a child or adult is large, but can be organized in a few simple categories: congenital, inflammatory and infectious, neoplastic, traumatic, and idiopathic. The differential can also be narrowed down considering the location of the neck mass. One large series examined the etiologies of pediatric neck masses undergoing biopsy: approximately 55% were congenital and close to 30% were inflammatory and infectious. Eleven percent was found to be malignant. This is probably an underestimate of lesions that were actually infectious or inflammatory as a majority of these masses do not make it to biopsy because of clear histories supporting that etiology.

History should be elicited for any recent illness, trauma, travel exposure, pets, and constitutional symptoms such as fever and night sweats. The age of the patient is very important in considering the cause: children tend to have more inflammatory than congenital and adults tend to have more neoplastic

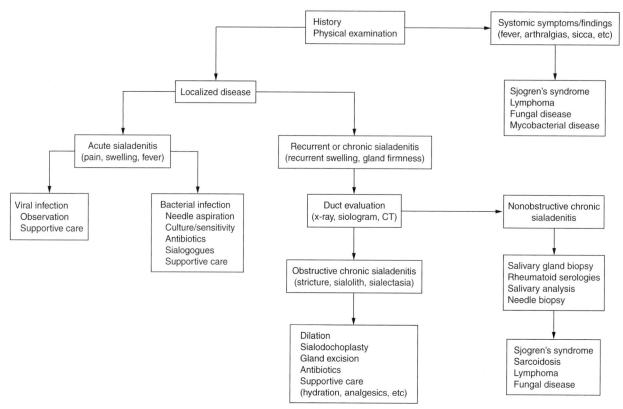

FIG. 14-25 Algorithm for management of acute and chronic sialadenitis. (*Source:* Reprinted from Cummings C, et al. *Otolaryngology—Head and Neck Surgery*, 3rd ed., copyright 1998, with permission from Elsevier).

processes overall. The location of the mass is another distinguishing characteristic (Table 14-4)—the various locations being the anterior triangle, posterior triangle, and midline neck. The most common midline lesion is the thyroglossal duct cyst, a remnant of the embryonic migration tract for the thyroid gland which starts at the base of tongue (foramen cecum). It is important to do a complete head and neck examination with careful inspection of all mucosal surfaces and not be distracted by the mass itself. The neck mass should be examined for fixation to surrounding structures, consistency (fluctuant, cystic, solid and the like), tenderness, and any associated skin changes overlying the mass. It should be noted whether the mass exhibits a bruit or thrill, signs which would indicate a vascular lesion. A flexible endoscopic examination may be necessary and consideration should be given to examining the axillary and inguinal lymph node groups.

If there is a low suspicion of malignancy, a lymph node can be observed for 2–4 weeks and a course of antibiotic therapy can be given to see if the mass or node responds. Laboratory tests such as the complete blood count (CBC) with differential help guide the diagnosis of an acute infectious or inflammatory

process. Atypical lymphocytes and heterophile antibody titers are associated with infectious mononucleosis. When suspicion for a mycobacterial infection exists, the patient should undergo skin testing with the purified protein derivative (PPD) test as well as a chest x-ray. Disseminated TB is associated with fixed posterior chain lymphadenopathy. Tests for cat-scratch bacillus (*Bartonella henselae*) include serology and the Warthin-Starry silver stain on histology. Serology is also used in ruling out other infectious disorders and agents including cytomegalovirus (CMV), toxoplasmosis, brucellosis, tularemia, histoplasmosis, and coccidiomycosis.

Imaging studies include ultrasound, CT scan, and MRI scan. Ultrasonography is very helpful especially in the pediatric patient as it is noninvasive and quick. It chiefly aids in distinguishing between solid and cystic masses and multiplicity of a mass. In the neonate, a disorder called fibromatosis colli (which is fibrosis of the SCM muscle with a mass-like effect), can be diagnosed. CT scans with intravenous contrast can show ring-enhancement around a low-attenuation area in the presence of necrosis (such as in a malignancy) or abscess, and the CT is very good at providing bony detail. MRI scans are useful in the

TABLE 14-4   Differential Diagnosis of Neck Mass by Location and Age Group

	Age, (y)	
0–15	**16–40**	**40+**
Causative group and location		
Congenital	Congenital	Neoplastic
Vascular lesion (AT)	Brachial cyst (AT)	Metastatic
Brachial cyst (AT)	Thyroglossal cyst (M)	Carcinoma
Thyroglossal cyst (M)	Dermoid	Thyroid
Dermoid (M)	Inflammatory adinitis	Inflammatory adinitis
Inflammatory adenitis	Viral (AT/PT)	Viral (AT/PT)
Bacterial (AT/PT)	Bacterial (AT/PT)	Bacterial (AT/PT)
Viral (AT/PT)	Granulomatous	Granulomatous
Granulomatous (PT/AT)	(PT/AT)	(PT/AT)
Neoplastic	Neoplastic	Neoplastic
Lymphoma (AT/PT)	Lymphoma (AT/PT)	Brachial cyst (AT)
Thyroid carcinoma (M)	Thyroid carcinoma (M)	Thyroglossal cyst (M)
Sarcoma (AT/PT)	Salivary (AT)	
	Metastatic (AT/PT)	
	Vascular (AT/PT)	
	Neurogenic (AT)	

*Descending order of frequency.

AT—Anterior triangle; *M*—Midline and anterior neck; *PT*—Posterior triangle.

Source: Reprinted from Cummings C, et al. *Otolaryngology—Head and Neck Surgery*, 3rd ed., copyright 1998, with permission from Elsevier.

setting of a vascular lesion and provide superior soft-tissue detail; however, these are difficult to perform in a pediatric patient without sedation because of the extended duration of acquisition. Thyroid scans and other nuclear medicine tests are rarely used unless there is high suspicion of ectopic thyroid tissue.

FNA has an important role in the evaluation of neck masses in adults and children. It can obviate need for an open cervical biopsy. If there is concern for a lymphoma and not enough tissue is obtained for flow cytometry, then an open biopsy is required. Other indications for a cervical lymph node or mass biopsy are a palpable node in a neonate that does not respond to therapy, any lymph node enlargement during therapy, supraclavicular or lower neck adenopathy (supraclavicular nodes having a 60% rate of malignancy in children) not responsive to therapy, adenopathy with constitutional symptoms and any firm or fixed nodes, especially in the posterior triangle that are greater than 1 cm and that are unresponsive to therapy.

Bibliography

Eusterman VD. Tumors of the oral cavity and pharynx. In: Jafek BW, Murrow BW (eds.), *ENT Secrets*, 2nd ed. Philadelphia, PA: Hanley & Belfus, 2001, 263–269.

Liu ES, Bernstein JM, Sculerati N, Wu HC. Fine needle aspiration biopsy of pediatric head and neck masses. *Int J Pediatr Otorhinolaryngol* 2001;60(2):135–140.

McGuirt WF Sr. Differential diagnosis of neck masses. In: Cummings CW, Fredrickson JM, Harker LA, et al. (eds.), *Otolaryngology Head & Neck Surgery*, 3rd ed., vol. 3. St. Louis, MO: Mosby, 1998, 1686–1699.

Myer CM. Head and neck neoplasms in children. In: Gates GA (ed.), *Current Therapy in Otolaryngology Head and Neck Surgery*, 6th ed. St. Louis, MO: Mosby, 1998, 493–496.

Wiatrak BJ. Clinical evaluation of the neck. In: Wetmore RF, et al. (eds.), *Pediatric Otolaryngology: Principles and Practice Pathways*. New York, NY: Thieme, 2000, 931–948.

30. **(E)** Although answers B–E are all encountered during the course of a neck dissection, the anterior border of the trapezius is traditionally the posterior limit of a modified radical or radical neck dissection. It can also define the limit of a selective neck dissection provided level V lymph nodes are part of the dissection.

The nomenclature of neck dissections has been an object of debate and has been difficult to standardize until more recently. The radical neck dissection is defined as removal of lymph node groups I through V as well as the SAN, IJV, and SCM muscle. MRND involve sparing of one or two of either the SAN, IJV, or SCM. A type I MRND removes levels I through V and the IJV and SCM (Fig. 14-26). A type II MRND removes these lymph node groups and only the IJV. A type III MRND preserves all three structures (aka functional neck dissection). Selective neck dissections refer to four different subtypes: the

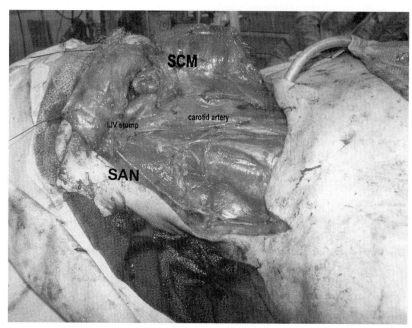

FIG. 14-26   Right modified radical neck dissection with preservation of spinal accessory nerve (SAN), sacrifice of internal jugular vein (IJV), and sternocleidomastoid muscle (SCM).

supraomohyoid, lateral, anterolateral, and postero-lateral neck dissections. The supraomohyoid neck dissections remove levels I–III and are recommended for oral cavity primaries with presumed occult neck metastases. Oropharyngeal primaries would require a lateral (II–IV) or anterolateral neck dissection (I–IV) depending on the approach. Hypopharyngeal and laryngeal primaries would in the least require a lateral neck dissection. Level V is rarely involved in the N_0 (no clinical adenopathy) neck, and may be involved in a N_+ (clinical adenopathy present) when the primary is hypopharyngeal or laryngeal. When a patient has clinical adenopathy, the indication is stronger for performance of an MRND. Usually the SAN can be preserved unless it is grossly involved by tumor. In a classic study by Lindberg in 1972, the incidence of nodal metastasis correlated with the size of the primary tumor in primaries of the anterior two-third tongue, floor of mouth, retromolar trigone and anterior tonsillar pillar, and soft palate. Primaries with sizes that did not correlate with the incidence of cervical metastasis were base of tongue, tonsillar fossa, supraglottic larynx, and hypopharynx.

An important anatomical point is identification of the SAN in the neck. The external jugular vein crosses the SCM in its upper half and about one fingerbreadth superiorly, the greater auricular nerve exits Erb's point to cross the outer surface of the muscle. Erb's point is located at the midpoint of the posterior border of the SCM. Also found at Erb's point are branches of the cervical plexus which cross the outer surface of the SCM to become anterior cutaneous nerves of the neck. The SAN is deep to the SCM and parallels the external jugular vein, and is at Erb's point just superior to the greater auricular nerve. It sends branches to the SCM and continues on to the trapezius muscle. CN XI has rootlets from the brainstem (cranial nerve origin) and the cervical plexus from C1 through C6. These rootlets course superiorly from the cervical spinal cord through the foramen magnum but then exit via the jugular foramen in conjunction with the brainstem component of CN XI as the SAN. A second location to find the nerve is two fingerbreadths superior to the clavicle at the anterior border of the trapezius muscle.

Bibliography

Andersen PE. Cervical metastases. In: Close LG, Larson DL, Shah JP (eds.), *Essentials of Head and Neck Oncology*. New York, NY: Thieme, 1998, 256–265.

Davidson BJ, Sessions RB. Cervical metastasis. In: Gates GA (ed.), *Current Therapy in Otolaryngology Head and Neck Surgery*, 6th ed. St. Louis, MO: Mosby, 1998, 291–295.

Lingeman RE. Surgical anatomy. In: Cummings CW, Fredrickson JM, Harker LA, et al. (eds.), *Otolaryngology Head & Neck Surgery*, 3rd ed., vol. 3. St. Louis, MO: Mosby, 1998, 1673–1685.

Medina JE. Neck dissection. In: Bailey BJ, et al. (eds.), *Head & Neck Surgery Otolaryngology*, 3rd ed., vol. 2. Philadelphia, PA: Lippincott, Williams & Wilkins, 2001, 1346–1366.

Robbins KT, et al. Neck dissection classification update. *Arch Otolaryngol Head Neck Surg* 2002;128:751–758.

31. **(E)** The pectoralis major myocutaneous flap is the most frequently used axial flap used in head and neck reconstruction. It is very well vascularized by perforating branches of the thoracoacromial artery which gives off the lateral thoracic artery. The thoracodorsal artery supplies the latissimus dorsi muscle and flap (hence answer E is incorrect). The pectoralis muscle origin is at the medial clavicle, costal cartilage and sternum, and the external oblique aponeurosis and it inserts into the intertubercular sulcus of the humerus. The flap is used as an island or pedicle flap but more frequently as an island flap. It can also be used as an osteomyocutaneous flap with a rib in some cases.

To raise the flap, a template is marked on the anterior chest wall beginning at the level of the nipple in order to have an appropriate length pedicle to reach the oral cavity. The incisions are made through the skin and subcutaneous tissue, and in a female patient, these are hidden in the inframammary crease if possible. The skin and subcutaneous tissue can be sutured to the fascia overlying the muscle to prevent shearing of the cutaneous blood supply. The muscle is incised and separated from its sternal attachments and removed from chest wall fascia. The neurovascular bundle location should be confirmed to avoid kinking or inadvertent damage while raising the flap. The medial and lateral pectoral nerves are divided. The flap is designed to be 6–8 cm wide but the skin portion can be extended beyond the insertion of the muscle; this however, creates a random pattern flap in that area that has a less durable vasculature. The flap is pivoted on itself and passed under an island of intact skin at or above the level of the clavicle. Care should be made to make this island compliant enough to avoid compressing the pedicle. The flap is then inset into the defect. It can be tubed either partially by tacking it posteriorly to the prevertebral fascia or tubed completely depending on the situation. The donor site is closed primarily.

The flap has advantages of low morbidity, reliability, bulk when needed, and ease of elevation without need for microvascular techniques in a single stage. There are a few disadvantages including excessive bulk depending on the design of the flap, and lack of movement and sensation. There is potential for complications. These complications include venous thrombosis and flap necrosis, wound dehiscence, postoperative hematoma, fistula formation, and very rarely infection. One study indicated that female gender, subtotal or total glossectomy defects, prior chemotherapy, bipedicling of flaps and systemic disease such as diabetes were all significant risk factors for flap necrosis.

Bibliography

Johnson JT, Meyers EN, Shestak K, Jones NF. *Reconstruction of the Oral Cavity. Self-Instructional Package*, 2nd ed. Alexandria, VA: American Academy of Otolaryngology-Head and Neck Surgery Foundation, 1994.

Mehta S, et al. Complications of the pectoralis major myocutaneous flap in the oral cavity: a prospective evaluation of 220 cases. *Plast Reconstr Surg* 1996;98(1):31–37.

Sultan M. Local and regional flaps. In: Close LG, Larson DL, Shah JP (eds.), *Essentials of Head and Neck Oncology*. New York, NY: Thieme, 1998, 330–342.

Varvares MA, Cheney ML. Reconstruction of the hypopharynx and cervical esophagus. In: Cummings CW, Fredrickson JM, Harker LA, et al. (eds.), *Otolaryngology Head & Neck Surgery*, 3rd ed., vol. 3. St. Louis, MO: Mosby, 1998, 2244–2257.

32. **(B)** Despite the advent and widespread use of the HIB vaccine, *H. influenzae* type b still remains the most common cause of epiglottitis. Historically, the disease was more common in children between ages 2 through 6; however, with vaccine use, the incidence in children has dropped from 3.5 in 100,000 to 0.6 in 100,000, whereas that in adults has remained the same or has risen slightly. Other bacteria that are found commonly include other types of *H. influenzae*, β-hemolytic streptococci, *Staphylococcus*, *Klebsiellae pneumoniae*, *Bacteroides melanogenicus*, and *Mycobacterium tuberculosis*. The presentation in children is fever, sore throat of a rapid onset with inspiratory stridor; adults will also complain of odynophagia. The key is the rapid onset of pain with a paucity of oropharyngeal findings (such as lack of evidence of acute tonsillitis or peritonsillar abscess). Children may have trouble handling secretions and may drool and patients in general may have a muffled or "hot potato" voice all related to edema of the epiglottis. Patients sit forward and upright in a "sniffing" position to relieve some of the respiratory obstruction.

Diagnosis is based chiefly on history and physical examination. Though a classic "thumbprint" sign of the epiglottis on lateral neck x-ray has been described in the setting of supraglottitis, the sensitivity of lateral neck films is on the order of 40% and the specificity around 75%. If there is any suspicion of this process, final diagnosis via laryngoscopy should be performed in a controlled setting in the operation room (OR). The epiglottis alone is affected in children by appearing beefy red and edematous, whereas in the adult, all supraglottic tissue is inflamed appearing and edematous and thus is referred to as supraglottitis. Attempts should be made to not arouse the patient or make them upset as this may precipitate complete airway obstruction. Oral intubation should be performed by the most skilled person available to avoid trauma and subsequent further reactive edema from the epiglottis. Preparations should be ready for tracheostomy if needed. Racemic epinephrine is not recommended because of a rebound effect after it has been absorbed.

The patient is left intubated for 48–72 h during which time the edema should have subsided. The patient is placed on broad spectrum antibiotics that especially have activity against *H. influenzae* and is kept in the intensive care unit (ICU). The patient should be extubated only after direct assessment of the airway via laryngoscopy and an endotracheal tube leak test to confirm edema resolution. Although steroids are sometimes employed to decrease edema, there is no definitive data to advocate their use. Despite the technological advances of the last two decades, the mortality rate is still 1.6% for adults.

Epiglottitis should be differentiated from two other respiratory disorders: viral croup and bacterial trachneitis. Viral croup is found in children less than 2 years and is associated with parainfluezae and respiratory syncytial viruses. The stridor is usually biphasic as the inflammation is subglottic compared to epiglottitis which has an associated inspiratory stridor. There is a characteristic "seal-barking" cough and patients usually do not have odynophagia. These patients are treated with humidity, inhaled steroids and racemic epinephrine as well as antibiotics to prevent superinfection. Bacterial tracheitis is usually a staphylococcal infection of the trachea that can occur at any age and patients present with an expiratory stridor and hoarseness. This is also a serious disorder and requires ICU care, bronchoscopy with suctioning, and IV antibiotics.

Bibliography

Gagliano JR, Jafek BW. The pediatric airway. In: Jafek BW, Murrow BW (eds.), *ENT Secrets*, 2nd ed. Philadelphia, PA: Hanley & Belfus, 2001, 429–436.

Nakamura H, et al. Acute epiglottitis: a review of 80 patients. *J Laryngol Otol* 2001;115(1):31–34.

Postma GN, Amin MR, Koufman JA. Laryngitis. In: Bailey BJ, et al. (eds.), *Head & Neck Surgery Otolaryngology*, 3rd ed., vol. 1. Philadelphia, PA: Lippincott, Williams & Wilkins, 2001, 599–605.

Sack JL, Brock CD. Identifying acute epiglottitis in adults: high degree of awareness, close monitoring are key. *Postgrad Med* 2002;112(1):81–82, 85–86.

Sie KCY. Infectious and inflammatory disorders of the trachea. In: Wetmore RF, et al. (eds.), *Pediatric Otolaryngology: Principles and Practice Pathways*. New York, NY: Thieme, 2000, 811–825.

33. **(B)** This patient has a classic "open-bite" deformity which is associated with a symphyseal fracture and a direct anterior midline or anteroinferior and midline force. The symphyseal fracture occurs anteriorly between the mandibular incisors (usually central). Condylar fractures in general involve the intracapsular condyle head in the temporomandibular joint or the neck which is known as the subcondylar region. The open bite occurs because of both anteromedial condyle displacement because of pull of the lateral pterygoid muscle and loss of the functional height of the ramus. The mandibular and maxillary molars then contact prematurely. It is important to note that the lateral pterygoid muscle is the only protractor (i.e., both depresses and protrudes) of the mandible. A deviation of the chin toward the fractured side is seen with a unilateral condyle fracture. Panorex plain films provide a panoramic view of the mandible and are the main imaging modality used in diagnosis; however, lateral or medial condyle displacement can be missed and a special x-ray called the Towne view should be requested if suspicion for a condyle fracture is present.

The most common place for a mandible fracture is the subcondylar area (36%) because of an inherent weakness. The next is the body (21%), followed by the angle (20%), parasymphysis (14%), ramus (3%), alveolar process (3%), coronoid process (2%), and symphysis (1%). The angle of the mandible is an especially vulnerable area when an impacted third molar is present. Diagnosis of a mandible fracture be made with the following constellation of signs and symptoms (though not all need be present): malocclusion, fragment mobility, trismus, deviation on opening to side of condyle fracture, hematoma in the floor of mouth, laceration of gingivae at fracture site, and possible anesthesia in the lower lip and chin (from inferior alveolar nerve trauma). All mandible fractures in tooth bearing areas are exposed by definition and therefore require antibiotics such as penicillin or clindamycin, with adequate coverage of oral flora.

Mandible fractures can be favorable or unfavorable in the vertical and horizontal axes. Favorable fractures occur in areas where native muscular forces act to pull the segments together; conversely, unfavorable fracture segments are distracted. Vertically unfavorable fractures are pulled apart in the horizontal direction and horizontally unfavorable fractures are pulled apart vertically. Body and symphyseal fractures are vertically unfavorable as the anterior segment is distracted toward the floor of mouth in the posterior-medial direction. Teeth in a fracture line can provide stability for reduction and stabilization; however, teeth should be removed if gross periodontal disease exists, if the tooth involved is carious, or if it prevents adequate stabilization. In body fractures, compression stresses occur inferiorly while tension forces act superiorly because of muscle pull. Both of these forces have to be addressed when repairing a fracture.

Techniques for treatment of mandibular fractures include closed reduction with arch bars (maxillo-mandibular fixation or MMF), acrylic splints, Ivy loops, or dentures with wiring in an edentulous patient. Techniques for open reduction and internal fixation include metal plates with screws, interosseous wires, and lag screws. Wiring and plates should be used with MMF to address superior border tension forces. With respect to condylar fractures, a nondisplaced unilateral fracture can be managed with a soft diet and close follow-up. Bilateral nondisplaced condyle fractures or a unilateral displaced fracture can be treated with MMF for 2–3 weeks for immobilization. Longer duration of MMF may cause TM joint ankylosis so all patients should receive physiotherapy. This is even more a concern in pediatric patients who heal rapidly and should undergo only a short period of immobilization. Open reduction of condyle or subcondylar fractures is used only in specific situations: the condyle is displaced into the middle cranial fossa, if only poor occlusion with closed techniques is achieved, if there is lateral extracapsular condyle displacement, and if there is a foreign body in the joint or region. Relative indications may include bilateral fractures in an edentulous patient when splinting cannot be performed or is not recommended for other reasons, if there are associated comminuted midface fractures and if the patient had significant malocclusion prior to the injury.

Bibliography

Aragon SB, Gardner KE. The mandibular fracture. In: Jafek BW, Murrow BW (eds.), *ENT Secrets*, 2nd ed. Philadelphia, PA: Hanley & Belfus, 2001, 408–414.

Clark WD, Simko EJ. Mandibular fracture. In: Gates GA (ed.), *Current Therapy in Otolaryngology Head and Neck Surgery*, 6th ed. St. Louis, MO: Mosby, 1998, 150–152.

Leach JL, Newcomer MT. Mandibular fractures. In: Bailey BJ, et al. (eds.), *Head & Neck Surgery Otolaryngology*, 3rd ed., vol. 1. Philadelphia, PA: Lippincott, Williams & Wilkins, 2001, 765–774.

Stanley RB. Maxillofacial trauma. In: Cummings CW, Fredrickson JM, Harker LA, et al. (eds.), *Otolaryngology Head & Neck Surgery*, 3rd ed., vol. 1. St. Louis, MO: Mosby, 1998, 453–485.

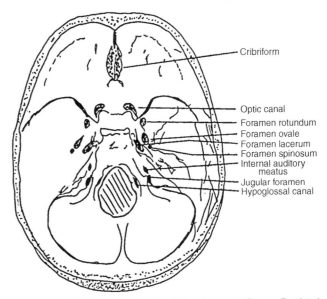

FIG. 14-27 Skull base foramina from internal aspect. (*Source:* Reprinted from Lee, et al. *Essential Otolaryngology Head and Neck Surgery*, 8th ed., copyright 2003, with permission from McGraw-Hill).

34. **(B)** The skull base is a complex anatomical region which houses multiple vital structures. Any disease process in this region has the potential to affect the function of the various contents of the skull base foramina. The skull base can be simplified by separating it into an anterior, middle, and posterior cranial fossa (Fig. 14-27).

The anterior cranial fossa (ACF) is the most shallow. The main component is the frontal bone and the floor is chiefly composed of the orbital plates of the frontal bone and ends at the anterior border of the greater wing of sphenoid. The fovea ethmoidalis is the portion of the ethmoid sinuses that forms part of the ACF floor. The main foramina of the ACF are those in the cribriform plate which transmit the olfactory nerve axons. Other important foramina are those for the anterior and posterior ethmoidal neurovascular bundles. The optic nerve is located 5–6 mm behind the posterior ethmoidal artery. A vestigial foramen cecum is seen between the crista galli and frontal crest and in 1% it is open and transmits a nasal emissary vein.

The middle cranial fossa is formed by the greater wing and body of the sphenoid bone, the squamous part of the temporal bone, and a portion of the petrous temporal bone. The foramina from anterior to posterior are: optic canals, superior orbital fissures, foramen rotundum, foramen ovale, foramen spinosum, foramen lacerum, and the hiatus of the greater petrosal nerve. The contents of the optic canal are the optic nerve, ophthalmic artery, and the central retinal artery. The contents of the superior orbital fissures are cranial nerves III, IV, V_1 branches (frontal, lacrimal, and nasociliary), VI, sympathetic fibers, the superior and inferior ophthalmic veins and orbital branch of the middle meningeal artery. The foramen rotundum carries V_2 and the foramen ovale transmits V_3, an accessory meningeal artery, small petrosal nerve, and an emissary vein. The foramen spinosum carries the middle meningeal artery and vein and lymphatics as well as a meningeal branch of V_3. The foramen lacerum carries the internal carotid artery and its accompanying sympathetic and venous plexi. The hiatus of the greater petrosal nerve carries the greater petrosal nerve and a petrosal branch of the middle meningeal artery.

The posterior cranial fossa has five foramina. The foramen magnum carries the medulla, meninges, vertebral arteries, spinal roots of XI, dural veins, and anterior and posterior spinal arteries. The jugular foramen has three compartments. The anterior compartment houses the inferior petrosal sinus. The middle compartment contains cranial nerves IX, X, and XI and the posterior compartment transmits the IJV, meningeal branches from the occipital and ascending phyangeal arteries and the nodes of Krause (lymph nodes). The hypoglossal canal carries cranial nerve XII and the condylar canal carries an emissary vein. Finally the mastoid foramen carries a mastoid emissary vein and a meningeal branch of the occipital artery.

Bibliography

Constantino PD, Janecka IP. Cranial-base surgery. In: Bailey BJ, et al. (eds.), *Head & Neck Surgery Otolaryngology*, 3rd ed., vol. 2. Philadelphia, PA: Lippincott, Williams & Wilkins, 2001, 1575–1596.

Lee KJ, Latorre RC. Highlights and pearls. In: Lee KJ (ed.), *Essential Otolaryngology Head and Neck Surgery*, 8th ed. New York, NY: McGraw-Hill, 2003, 1015–1093.

Moore KL. *Clinically Oriented Anatomy*, 3rd ed. Baltimore, MD: Williams & Wilkins, 1992.

35. **(B)** Malignant otitis externa (or necrotizing otitis externa, NOE) does not refer to a neoplastic process but rather a potentially life-threatening infectious external ear infection. Though newer antibiotics have somewhat decreased the incidence, there are certain patient groups at risk. These at-risk groups are the elderly, diabetics, and the immunocompromised. In fact, up to 80% of cases are found in diabetics. NOE is associated with a skull base osteomyelitis which is the source of its lethal nature.

Diagnosis rests on a few key symptoms and signs. These include a persistent and severe otalgia that has lasted for more than 1 month, purulent otorrhea with granulation tissue for several weeks,

immunocompromised because of age, diabetes or other condition and a lower cranial neuropathy of nerves VII, IX, X, or XI. The granulation tissue is seen at the posteroinferior aspect of the external auditory canal at the tympanomastoid suture line. The granulation tissue seen in an AIDS patient is less exuberant but suspicion should be maintained, as these patients are usually severely immunocompromised. Granulation tissue can be seen in severe otitis externa when there is a tympanic membrane perforation. SCC can present in a similar fashion, so biopsies should be considered. Other entities in the differential diagnosis include glomus jugulare tumor, cholesteatoma, nasopharyngeal carcinoma, meningeal carcinoma, Hans-Schuller-Christian disease, eosinophilic granuloma, Wegener's granulomatosis, and clival chordoma.

Pseudomonas aeruginosa is the causative organism in a majority of cases, although cases of *S. aureus*, *Klebsiella*, and *Proteus* sp. have been reported, and fungal or other unusual organisms have been isolated from AIDS and bone marrow transplant patients. CT scan of the temporal bone with IV contrast is the usual first imaging modality. It provides excellent bony detail and can outline extension of disease and specific location. It is very poor at monitoring response to therapy; however, because remineralization of the osteomyelitic bone must occur for changes to be detected by CT, and sometimes this may not take place. A nuclear medicine study, the technetium-99m bone scan, is performed when clinical suspicion is high but the CT scan is negative for disease. The scan highlights areas of increased osteoblastic activity whether it is because of bone destruction or bone repair. It may remain positive, however, for 9 months after the initial infection. The gallium-67 scan is important in monitoring NOE and its resolution. Gallium-67 citrate is incorporated into macrophages and reticular endothelial cells as a Ga-67 lactoferrin complex. It indicates an active infection but is not as accurate in locating the entire extent of the osteomyelitis. The Ga-67 scan reverts to normal, however, when resolution progresses. Sequential scanning is recommended. Newer modalities which may become the standard of care but that are still somewhat experimental are Indium-111 wbc planar scinitigraphy and Ga-67 SPECT scanning.

Treatment formerly involved aggressive surgical debridement. The danger of aggressive surgical debridement is possible exposure of more of the skull base to the active infection. Current standard of care is intravenous antipseudomonal antibiotic therapy with judicious surgical debridement of granulation tissue and sequestered bone. Initially, the ear may need to be debrided via otomicroscopic examination daily until the granulation tissue has subsided. Some sources also recommend topical otic drops. The patient may be discharged from the hospital once the otalgia resolves or otorrhea decreases and granulation tissue shrinks. The erythrocyte sedimentation rate (ESR) can also be followed to monitor therapy as sometimes the white blood cell count is normal. It cannot be overemphasized that if the patient is diabetic, strict control of the blood glucose must be maintained. Severe infections may respond to hyperbaric oxygen therapy but HBO is not widely available. Mortality rates are still high, reported at up to 60%.

Bibliography

Buchman CA, Levine JD, Balkany TJ. Infections of the ear. In: Lee KJ (ed.), *Essential Otolaryngology Head and Neck Surgery,*. 8th ed. New York, NY: McGraw-Hill, 2003, 462–511.

Linstrom CJ, Lucente FE, Joseph EM. Infections of the external ear. In: Bailey BJ, et al. (eds.), *Head & Neck Surgery Otolaryngology*, 3rd ed., vol. 2. Philadelphia, PA: Lippincott, Williams & Wilkins, 2001, 1711–1724.

Paramsothy M, Khanijow V, Ong TO. Use of gallium-67 in the assessment of response to antibiotic therapy in malignant otitis externa—a case report. *Singapore Med J* 1997;38(8):347–349.

Strunk CL. Necrotizing otitis externa. In: Gates GA (ed.), *Current Therapy in Otolaryngology Head and Neck Surgery*, 6th ed. St. Louis, MO: Mosby, 1998, 8–9.

36. **(D)** Nasopharyngeal carcinomas (NPC) and lymphomas are the two most common malignant neoplasms of the nasopharynx with NPC accounting for approximately 90% of the total. In children, a group in which NPC is rare, the differential of a nasopharyngeal mass should include embryonal rhabdomyosarcoma, neuroblastoma, non-Hodgkin lymphoma, and juvenile nasopharyngeal angiofibroma. Though uncommon in the United States, it makes up nearly 20% of cancers in China.

The etiology of NPC has been linked to genetic susceptibility at the HLA-A2, HLA-B-SIN 2, HLA Bw46, and B17 loci. In addition, the EBV has shown a close association with NPC. This is evidenced by the fact that sera containing IgA antibodies to the EBV viral capsid antigen and early antigen diffuse component help in the diagnosis of occult disease but are less helpful in detection of recurrent or persistent disease. Clonal EBV DNA has been found in premalignant lesions. EBV is a double-stranded DNA virus that is in the herpesvirus family; it causes a persistent and chronic infection especially in B lymphocytes and the latent membrane protein of the virus may be the inciting agent in carcinogenesis. Antibody-dependent cellular cytotoxicity titers are followed to monitor the clinical course of the disease with lower titers being significantly associated with progression and higher death rates. The amplification of the c-erbB-3 gene is also associated with poor prognosis and this gene may be involved in carcinogenesis. Other possible contributors to the pathogenesis are polycyclic hydrocarbons, nitrosamine ingestion, and poor nasal hygiene or chronic rhinosinusitis.

NPC is stratified according to the World Health Organization classification system. WHO 1 carcinomas exhibit large amounts of keratin production and are similar to other head and neck squamous cell carcinomas. WHO type II NPC is a nonkeratinizing or transitional cell carcinoma and it may contain papillary excrescences. WHO type III NPC is the undifferentiated or anaplastic form, formerly known as lymphoepithelioma or Schminke tumors; this is the most common form of NPC, and anti-EBV titers are seen more closely with types II and III, suggesting a different pathogenesis of type I from the other types.

NPC most often presents as an asymptomatic neck mass (60%) at the level of the angle of the mandible because of cervical metastases. Bilateral mets can also occur as lymphatics communicate across the midline via retropharyngeal nodes. Other symptoms include ear fullness, plugging, and hearing loss from Eustachian tube blockage, epistaxis, nasal obstruction, headache or otalgia, and weight loss. The most common cranial nerve deficits on presentation are VI and V via the foramina ovale and rotundum causing diplopia and pain or paresthesias of the lower two-thirds of the face; this is seen in less than 10% of patients on presentation. Treatment is chiefly radiation though combination modality treatment has shown promising results with use of chemotherapy. Surgery is used in radiation failure or tumor recurrence situations. Five-year survival is 70–80% with current chemoradiation protocols.

The nasopharynx is a trapezoid-shaped area bounded by the base of skull at the sphenoid and occipital bones. It is posterior to the nasal choanae and anterior to the prevertebral fascia and bodies of C1 and C2. The lateral wall contains the Eustachian tube and the fossa of Rosenmuller which is where most NPCs are thought to originate. It is formed by the pharyngobasilar fascia and superior constrictor muscles. This wall provides little barrier to tumor spread. The posterior wall merges with the roof of the nasopharynx at the skull base and the inferior limit is the soft palate in a raised position. In the neonate, nasopharyngeal epithelium is respiratory epithelium. Over time, the epithelium changes to a stratified squamous epithelium and this is thought to be because of metaplasia. There are remnants of the pseudostratified columnar (respiratory) epithelium in the lateral nasopharyngeal wall. The area where this epithelium meets the stratified squamous epithelium is bridged by transitional epithelium which contains globular or cuboidal cells. There are also scattered lymphoid tissue and minor salivary glands found in the nasopharyngeal mucous membrane.

Bibliography

Holsinger FC, Meyers JN. Carcinoma of the oral cavity and pharynx. In: Lee KJ (ed.), *Essential Otolaryngology Head and Neck Surgery*, 8th ed. New York, NY: McGraw-Hill, 2003, 566–595.

Neel HB III, Fee WE. Benign and malignant tumors of the nasopharynx. In: Cummings CW, Fredrickson JM, Harker LA, et al. (eds.), *Otolaryngology Head & Neck Surgery*, 3rd ed., vol. 2. St. Louis, MO: Mosby, 1998, 1512–1526.

Wei WI. Carcinoma of the nasopharynx. In: Gates GA (ed.), *Current Therapy in Otolaryngology Head and Neck Surgery*, 6th ed. St. Louis, MO: Mosby, 1998, 251–256.

Witte MC, Neel HB III. Nasopharyngeal cancer. In: Bailey BJ, et al. (eds.), *Head & Neck Surgery Otolaryngology*, 3rd ed., vol. 2. Philadelphia, PA: Lippincott, Williams & Wilkins, 2001, 1413–1426.

37. **(C)** Though the true etiology behind keloids and hypertrophic scars is unknown, both processes are associated with an overall increase in the quantity of collagen synthesized by wound fibroblasts. The definition of a keloid is an overgrowth of thick fibrous scar tissue that extends beyond the confines of the original wound, while the hypertrophic scar stays within the margins. Dark-skinned persons are at risk for developing both hypertrophic scars and keloids, though hypertrophic scars are more often seen in light-skinned persons. Hypertrophic scars usually develop soon after an injury whereas keloids may develop up to a year after the original wound was created. The fibroblasts in keloids contain elevated levels of TGF-β1 and TGF-β2 as compared to those in hypertrophic scars. Abnormal scars rarely develop in thin skin areas such as the eyelids.

Many treatments have evolved to deal with hypertrophic scars and keloids. Hypertrophic scars do have the potential to regress and flatten whereas keloids do not. Treatment options include intralesional steroids, cryotherapy, radiation, pressure dressings, silicone gel sheeting, and either CO_2 or pulsed dye laser therapy. Intralesional 5-fluorouracil and interferon have been investigated and interferon in particular has provided very promising results.

Normal wound healing can be divided into four phases. The phases in chronologic order are: coagulation, inflammation, proliferation, and maturation or remodeling. Coagulation is the first step in wound healing because hemostasis must be achieved. This is mediated chiefly by platelets that aggregate in response to exposed extravascular collagen. The platelets release numerous substances such as adenosine diphosphate (ADP), which with calcium, promotes further platelet aggregation and vasoactive catecholamines and serotonin. The serum and platelet α-granules contain fibrinogen, fibronectin, thrombospondin and von Willebrand factor and the granules also release platelet-derived growth factor, transforming growth factors α and β. The coagulation cascade begins and ultimately a fibrin plug is created to which fibroblastes, leukocytes, and keratinocytes migrate.

The inflammatory phase begins in conjunction with the coagulation phase. Via diapedesis, leukocytes leave the vasculature. Initially, neutrophils predominate in the first 1–2 days. This population then shifts to a predominantly monocyte or macrophage cell. Macrophages are extremely crucial to this phase of wound healing and may be the most important cell in wound healing. The macrophage has a pivotal role as it is the primary source of cytokines that stimulate fibroblast proliferation, collagen production, and neovascularization. Macrophages phagocytose any dead tissue and bacteria and remodel the matrix via collagenases and elastases. Lymphocytes release macrophage migration inhibition factor to keep the macrophages in the wound. This phase lasts for 2–4 days.

The proliferation stage marks development of the extracellular matrix which was started in the inflammatory stage. The matrix contains collagen, hyaluronic acid, fibronectin, and chondroitin sulfate. Epithelial cells are also stimulated to cover the wound and granulation tissue is formed. Myofibroblasts in the granulation tissue help contract the wound. With increasing oxygen tension because of new blood vessels, further fibroblast proliferation is inhibited but collagen production is stimulated. This process begins at approximately 48–72 h after the injury and continues for 2–4 weeks.

Finally the maturation phase is the longest phase and may take up to 2 years. An equilibrium between collagen formation and lysis is created. Collagen is also laid down in a more organized and cross-linked fashion across stress lines. Type III collagen is immature collagen and is elevated for 3–4 days before type I collagen levels increase. The presence of mostly type I collagen indicates a mature scar. Ultimately, damaged skin after healing only reaches 80% of its original strength.

Bibliography

Brown MT. Wound healing. In: Cummings CW, Fredrickson JM, Harker LA, et al. (eds.), *Otolaryngology Head & Neck Surgery*, 3rd ed., vol. 1. St. Louis, MO: Mosby, 1998, 187–196.

Lawrence WT. Wound healing biology and its application to wound management. In: O'Leary JP (ed.), *The Physiologic Basis of Surgery*, 2nd ed. Baltimore, MD: Williams & Wilkins, 1996, 188–140.

Roska DC, Jafek BW. Wound healing and dehiscence. In: Jafek BW, Murrow BW (eds.), *ENT Secrets*, 2nd ed. Philadelphia, PA: Hanley & Belfus, 2001, 536–539.

Terris DJ. Dynamics of wound healing. In: Bailey BJ, et al. (eds.), *Head & Neck Surgery Otolaryngology*, 3rd ed., vol. 1. Philadelphia, PA: Lippincott, Williams & Wilkins, 2001, 175–188.

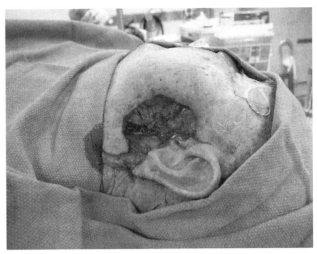

FIG. 14-28 Defect after removal of preauricular squamous cell carcinoma and superficial parotidectomy.

38. **(A)** Local flaps are designed immediately next to or near the location of a cutaneous defect. There are several ways to classify local flaps: by blood supply, shape, location, or method of transfer. Most local flaps are based on a random pattern blood supply from unnamed arteries in the subdermal plexus. In contrast, larger regional flaps use axial pattern blood supply dependent on larger named arteries. Two general types of local skin flaps in terms of the method of transfer are those that rotate around a fixed point to reach a defect and those that are advanced into a defect. The first group can be referred to as pivotal flaps and these are the rotation, transposition, and interpolated (island) flaps. The second group, or advancement flaps, are shaped linearly and are stretched into the defect after appropriate relaxing incisions. Examples are the rectangular monopedicled or bipedicled flaps and the V-Y advancement flap.

The rotation flap has a curvilinear shape and is best designed for triangular defects. It rotates in an arc, and a back cut or Z-plasty may be done to address redundant tissue at the base. Vascularity is dependable because of the broad base. The flap should be based inferiorly to restrict flap edema and assist with lymphatic drainage. A special type of rotation flap is the rhomboid flap which is used frequently in the head and neck for which at least four designs can be created to repair the defect. The rotation flap is helpful in repairing medial cheek defects and large rotational flaps are helpful in repairing large posterior and upper neck defects (Figs. 14-28 and 14-29). The transposition flap is a pivotal flap that has a linear axis but can be designed like a rotational flap in that one border is a border of the defect. It has the advantage though of being able to be designed further away from the defect with an axis independent of the linear axis. Optimum skin for closure can be selected this way. The interpolated flap has a base located away from the defect and is also based on a linear axis. It is passed either over or under a complete bridge of skin.

The advancement flap is based on sliding of donor tissue in a straight line without any lateral movement. Bipedicled advancement flaps are useful in lip and forehead defects. Burow's triangles are excised from the base to avoid a dog-ear deformity at the base of the donor site. The V-Y advancement involves pushing the donor skin into the defect by a primary straight line closure of the donor site. It is useful in treating contracted scars that distort critical aesthetic areas such as the vermilion border or eyelid. It is widely used in the repair of cleft lip-nasal deformities to lengthen the columella. A hinge flap is designed either linearly or curvilinearly and the pedicle is based on one margin of the defect. The flap is turned on to the defect like a page in a book, but a second graft is required for the exposed deep surface that is now external. It is used primarily in

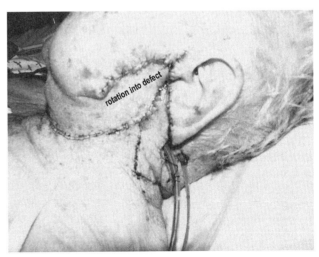

FIG. 14-29 Closure of defect with a cervicofacial rotation flap.

full-thickness nasal defects and in replacing internal nasal lining.

Bibliography

Baker SR. Reconstruction of facial defects. In: Cummings CW, Fredrickson JM, Harker LA, et al. (eds.), *Otolaryngology Head & Neck Surgery*, 3rd ed., vol. 1. St. Louis, MO: Mosby, 1998, 527–559.

Clevens RA, Baker SR. Conceptual considerations in head & neck reconstruction: defect analysis and options for reconstruction. *Otolaryngol Clin North Am* 1997;30(4):495–517.

Shumrick KA, Campbell AC. Local skin flaps: anatomy, physiology and general types. In: Bailey BJ, et al. (eds.), *Head & Neck Surgery Otolaryngology*, 3rd ed., vol. 2. Philadelphia, PA: Lippincott, Williams & Wilkins, 2001, 2035–2044.

Winslow CP, Lepore ML. In: Jafek BW, Murrow BW (eds.), *ENT Secrets*, 2nd ed. Philadelphia, PA: Hanley & Belfus, 2001, 331–339.

Summers BK, Siegle RJ. Facial cutaneous reconstructive surgery: facial flaps. *J Am Acad Dermatol* 1993; 29(6):917–941; quiz 942–944.

39. **(D)** Diagnosis of Hodgkin's disease rests on the pathologic finding of the Reed Sternberg cells, which are multinucleated giant cells. The disease presents in the head and neck as cervical and supraclavicular lymphadenopathy and rarely at extranodal sites such as the spleen (<10%). It has a male predilection, can be familial, and usually occurs in adolescents or young adults. There may be a relationship to Epstein-Barr viral infection. Four histologic types are recognized: these are lymphocyte predominant, nodular sclerosis, mixed cellularity, and lymphocyte depletion. Nodular sclerosis is the most common type encountered. The lymphocyte-depleted variety can be confused with non-Hodgkin's lymphoma (NHL) and is rarely seen in children.

Staging is the most critical prognostic indicator and is done by examination and imaging, and less often with staging laparotomy. The Ann Arbor system's stage I refers a single lymph node and stage II to multiple lymph nodes on the same side of the diaphragm or one extranodal site on the same side of the diaphragm. Stage III refers to both supra- and infradiaphragmatic nodal or extranodal involvement and the spleen. Stage IV disease is disseminated with one or more than one extranodal site. Group A indicates no symptoms whereas B refers to presence of constitutional symptoms such as fever, night sweats, and weight loss greater than 10% of body weight. This staging refers to NHL as well. Treatment usually involves combined chemoradiation except in the early stages where radiation can be used as a single modality.

NHL is five times more common in the head and neck and is the second most common head and neck malignancy. It has two peaks of incidence, one in individuals in the fifth and sixth decade of life and one in the 2–12-year-old pediatric population. There is still a male predilection and in the pediatric population, NHL is highly aggressive and poorly differentiated. It presents as asymptomatic cervical and supraclavicular adenopathy, similar to Hodgkin's. Waldeyer's ring can be involved which is in contrast to Hodgkin's disease in which this area is rarely affected. NHL is frequently extranodal. HIV infection and other causes of immunocompromise are significant risk factors for development of NHL. These lymphomas usually have B-cell lineage though T-cell lymphomas are seen as well. NHL is classified according to the Working Formulation althought the World Health Organization has more recently proposed a new scheme. The nodes are described as follicular or diffuse and low, intermediate or high-grade. Most head and neck lymphomas are intermediate grade with the diffuse large cell as the most common subtype. Burkitt's lymphoma is a high-grade NHL and is very commmon in Africa. It is also an EBV associated tumor and exhibits an extremely rapid growth rate with early involvement of the CNS. The pathogenesis derives from a chromosomal translocation on 8q24 involving the c-*myc* oncogene to an immunoglobulin receptor subunit on chromosomes 2, 14, or 22. Lymphomas of the salivary gland are associated with Sjogren's disease and are known as MALTomas (mucosal-associated lymphoid tissue). They are B-cell lymphomas with a slow growth rate. Therapy for NHL is tailored for the patient's age, stage, symptoms, and curative potential. Early disease is treated with radiation whereas intermediate and high grade need combined chemoradiation with treatment of the CNS when indicated. Bone marrow transplant may be an option for high-grade disease if response to conventional treatment is suboptimal.

Mikulicz cells are seen in rhinoscleroma, a granulomatous and sometimes destructive nasal infection caused by *Klebsiella rhinoscleromatis*. Birbeck granules are organelles in the nuclear cytoplasm of Langerhans' cells and are seen in histiocytosis X syndromes. Charcot-Leyden crystals are byproducts of dead eosinophils seen in allergic mucin. Physaliferous cells are foamy cells with a "soap-bubble" appearance seen in chordoma.

Bibliography

Bent JP, III, Hebert RL, Smith RJH. Pediatric neck neoplasms. In: Wetmore RF, et al. (eds.), *Pediatric Otolaryngology: Principles and Practice Pathways*. New York, NY: Thieme, 2000, 993–1019.

Kraut EH. Lymphomas. In: Cummings CW, Frederickson JM, Harker LA, et al. (eds.), *Otolaryngology Head & Neck Surgery*, 3rd ed., vol. 3. St. Louis, MO: Mosby, 1998, 1758–1763.

Nathu M, et al. Non-Hodgkin's lymphoma of the head and neck: a 30-year experience at the University of Florida. *Head Neck* 1999;21(3):247–254.

Sie KYC. Pediatric otolaryngology. In: Lee KJ (ed.), *Essential Otolaryngology Head and Neck Surgery*, 8th ed. New York, NY: McGraw-Hill, 2003, 811–861.

Yuen AR, Jacobs C. Lymphomas of the head and neck. In: Bailey BJ, et al. (eds.), *Head & Neck Surgery Otolaryngology*, 3rd ed., vol. 2. Philadelphia, PA: Lippincott, Williams & Wilkins, 2001, 1377–1384.

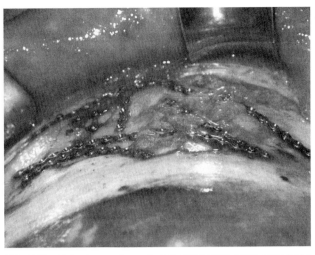

FIG. 14-30 Plate closure of comminuted anterior table fracture that had a displaced posterior fracture. Fat obliteration was used after complete mucosal removal.

40. **(B)** Pott's puffy tumor is a term used to describe a soft tissue swelling because of a subperiosteal abscess over the region of the frontal sinus. This occurs when the anterior table of the frontal sinus is involved in an osteomyelitic process which is usually because of a sinusitis but may be a result of a mucocele from a fracture. The offending organism in many cases is *S. aureus*. A malignancy of the frontal sinus, though exceedingly rare, should be considered in the differential. The pathophysiologic of development of a mucocele with subsequent osteomyelitis is an obstructed frontal sinus outflow tract. This occurs by thrombophlebitis of the diploic veins of the frontal bone or via direct extension.

The treatment of frontal sinus fractures depends on which table(s) of bone are fractured and the degree of displacement or comminution. Nondisplaced noncomminuted anterior table fractures can usually be observed unless CT scan shows persistent opacification, in which case endoscopic exploration or trephination of the sinus may be warranted. Displaced anterior table fractures produce obvious cosmetic deformity and can be reduced with low profile miniplates and preservation of as much native bone as possible. Nondisplaced posterior table fractures that do not cause CSF leaks can be observed with antibiotic treatment. Indications for exploration are the same as for anterior table nondisplaced fractures. Displaced posterior table fractures require surgical exploration and repair. This is because of CSF leakage and possible frontal sinus outflow tract involvement. If there is not much bone loss and no involvement of the outflow tract, these fractures can be reduced. If there is concern of injury to the duct, then a frontal sinus obliteration procedure using abdominal fat and removing all sinus mucosa is advocated (Fig. 14-30). This is in order to prevent any spread of infection from the nasal cavity. This procedure is also used to remove all mucosa in the setting of a frontal sinus osteomyelitis after the acute infection has resolved to prevent development of a mucocele. Endoscopic approaches more recently have been successful.

Mucoceles can develop several years after the initial fracture, the average being 7.5 years. Other complications of frontal sinus fractures include sinusitis, headache, forehead numbness (from supraorbital or supratrochlear nerve trauma), meningitis, brain abscess, cosmetic deformity, and diplopia and eye pulsations in the event of a carotid-cavernous fistula. Other intracranial complications of sinusitis in general include meningitis, epidural, subdural and intracerebral abscesses, and superior sagittal sinus thrombosis as well as Pott's puffy tumor. Pott's abscess is an eponym to describe tuberculosis of the spine and the other answer choices are merely distractors.

Bibliography

Bailey BJ, Tan LKS. Fractures of the nasal and frontal sinuses. In: Bailey BJ, et al. (eds.), *Head & Neck Surgery Otolaryngology*, 3rd ed., vol. 1. Philadelphia, PA: Lippincott, Williams & Wilkins, 2001, 793–811.

Deutsch E, Hevron I, Eilon A. Pott's puffy tumor treated by endoscopic frontal sinusotomy. *Rhinology* 2000;38(4): 177–180.

Johnson JT, Ferguson BT. Infection. In: Cummings CW, Fredrickson JM, Harker LA, et al. (eds.), *Otolaryngology Head & Neck Surgery*, 3rd ed., vol. 2. St. Louis, MO: Mosby, 1998, 1107–1118.

Rao AK, Campana J. Deep space neck infections. In: Jafek BW, Murrow BW (eds.), *ENT Secrets*, 2nd ed. Philadelphia, PA: Hanley & Belfus, 2001, 194–199.

Richter G, Jafek BW, Lewark TM. Sinusitis. In: Jafek BW, Murrow BW (eds.), *ENT Secrets*, 2nd ed. Philadelphia, PA: Hanley & Belfus, 2001, 131–139.

CHAPTER 15

Breast Surgery

Christa R. Balanoff and Larry Micon

Questions

1. The long thoracic nerve

   (A) innervates the latissimus dorsi muscle
   (B) arises from the posterior cord of the brachial plexus
   (C) is located deep to the axillary artery and vein, then travels superficial to the deep fascia of the serratus anterior muscle
   (D) is also called the internal respiratory nerve of Bell
   (E) has minimal significant sequelae if damaged during axillary dissection

2. Axillary lymph nodes are classified according to the relationship with the

   (A) axillary vein
   (B) pectoralis major muscle
   (C) pectoralis minor muscle
   (D) latissimus dorsi muscle
   (E) serratus anterior muscle

3. All are important features of a patient's initial assessment and are known risk factors for breast cancer *except*:

   (A) family history of breast cancer
   (B) age of menarche (regular cycles starting < 13 years old)
   (C) history of atypical hyperplasia
   (D) radiation exposure as a teenager
   (E) history of ductal adenosis

4. All are part of the Gail model calculation of 5-year and lifetime breast cancer risk *except*:

   (A) race
   (B) age of first menses
   (C) age of first live birth/full-term pregnancy
   (D) age at menopause
   (E) number of first degree relatives with breast cancer

5. Epidermal growth factor receptors (EGFR)

   (A) are autocrine factors
   (B) have no known mitogenic activity
   (C) are related to acquired tamoxifen resistance
   (D) have not been shown to have any response to estrogen
   (E) have no known role in apoptosis

6. BRCA2

   (A) is associated with a 50% risk of breast cancer
   (B) is not associated with an increased of male breast cancer
   (C) is thought to play a role in DNA damage response pathways
   (D) is a cystosolic protein
   (E) is associated with a 40% lifetime risk of ovarian cancer

7. Li-Fraumeni's syndrome is associated with all of the following *except*:

   (A) early onset breast cancer
   (B) p53 mutation
   (C) leukemia
   (D) chromosome 13 mutation
   (E) sarcoma

8. Oral contraceptive use is associated with

   (A) an increase incidence of breast cancer in current users
   (B) an increased incidence of ovarian cancer
   (C) an increased incidence of endometrial cancer
   (D) an increased incidence in overall breast cancer risk
   (E) an increased incidence of breast cancer if other risk factors are also present

9. A 40-year-old woman arrives at your office stating that she has a 1-month history of a palpable right breast lump. On physical examination, you are able to palpate a 1 cm mobile, firm nodule at the 2 o'clock position. Your diagnostic test of choice for this newly found breast mass is a(n)

   (A) mammogram
   (B) ultrasound
   (C) excisional biopsy
   (D) incisional biopsy
   (E) none of the above

10. The limitations of mammography include

   (A) 10–15% false negative rate
   (B) 10% false positive rate
   (C) difficulty visualizing tumors in the tail of Spence
   (D) all of the above.
   (E) none of the above

11. Characteristics of a malignant lesions on an ultrasound include all of the following *except*:

   (A) irregular borders
   (B) asymmetry
   (C) posterior enhancement
   (D) poorly circumscribed
   (E) high acoustic attenuation

12. Breast magnetic resonance imaging (MRI)

   (A) is useful as a screening tool
   (B) accurately differentiates tumor recurrence and postsurgical scar formation
   (C) should not be used if the patient has a breast implant
   (D) allows easy tissue procurement for pathologic diagnosis
   (E) is very specific for detecting malignant lesions

13. Breast cellulitis found in a lactating patient

   (A) is best treated with incision and drainage in the operating room
   (B) is reason for the infant to stop breast-feeding
   (C) that develops into an abscess is diagnosed by fever, leukocytosis, and a fluctuant mass
   (D) is treated by antibiotics, warm packs, and emptying the breast
   (E) involves multiple organisms

14. The most common cause of bloody nipple discharge is

   (A) carcinoma
   (B) fibrocystic disease
   (C) intraductal papilloma
   (D) ductal ectasia
   (E) trauma

15. Phyllodes tumors

   (A) present in postmenopausal women
   (B) are often malignant
   (C) require mastectomy because of their high recurrence rate
   (D) tend to recur
   (E) are responsive to hormonal manipulation

16. A 22-year-old college senior presents to your clinic stating that she has recently found a new breast mass. She reports that this initially caused discomfort but has since resolved. She has no nipple discharge or other complaints.
   You do an ultrasound in the office and find the following (Fig. 15-1):
   Your recommendations to her are

   (A) partial mastectomy with sentinel node biopsy
   (B) total mastectomy with sentinel node biopsy followed by immediate reconstruction

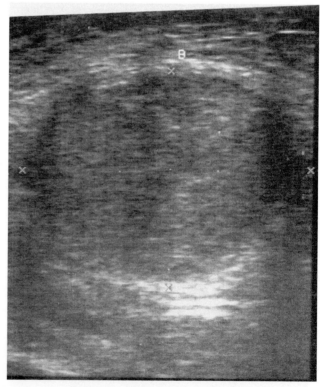

FIG. 15-1   Ultrasound—22-year-old female

(C) core needle biopsy (CNB)

(D) needle localized excisional biopsy

(E) close followup

17. The most common etiology of senescent gynecomastia is

(A) cirrhosis

(B) testicular tumor

(C) renal disease

(D) idiopathic causes

(E) drug induced

18. A 67-year-old male arrives at your office with a 1-month history of right breast pain, most subareolar. He now is able to palpate a mass. He denies any nipple discharge or skin changes.
Your next step is

(A) clinical breast examination and office ultrasound

(B) mammogram

(C) measure estrogen and testosterone levels

(D) ask the patient to stop all medications

(E) give reassurance that this is not cancer and see him back in 6 months to 1 year for a repeat examination

19. A 34-year-old lady is referred to your office for evaluation of breast pain. She describes the pain as burning, occasionally sharp in nature. It is mostly located in the subareolar area and seems to be fairly well localized. When asked when the pain occurs, she states that it is always present and is very troublesome to her. On physical examination, she has dense glandular tissue throughout both breasts, but no discrete nodules.
Your working diagnosis at this point is

(A) cyclical breast pain

(B) noncyclical breast pain

(C) cancer

(D) psychosomatic pain

(E) Tietze's syndrome

20. Your next step in management is

(A) reassurance

(B) start a diuretic

(C) refer her to a psychologist

(D) give a steroid injection

(E) perform a surgical excision of the painful area

21. Tamoxifen

(A) is an estrogen receptor (ER) agonist

(B) is an ER antagonist

(C) has been shown to decrease the incidence of recurrent breast cancer by 47%

(D) has been shown to decrease the risk of future breast cancer by 49% in high-risk patients

(E) all of the above

22. Following a needle localized excisional biopsy for microcalcifications, pathology is found to be fibrocystic changes associated with sclerosing adenosis and ductal hyperplasia. There is no atypia noted; however, the report also states that there is LCIS present. You discuss with your patient

(A) that she needs at a partial mastectomy followed by radiation therapy

(B) that she would benefit from a mirror biopsy because this disease is bilateral

(C) that she has a future cancer risk of 1% per year

(D) that there is no known therapy to help her reduce her risk and she should have close follow-up

(E) that bi-yearly mammograms would be the best way to detect further LCIS

23. A 62-year-old female comes to your office following a stereotactic CNB. The lesion was initially seen on mammogram and ultrasound demonstrated a solid nodule. Pathology shows this area to be an intracystic papillary carcinoma (IPC). You counsel her that

(A) this in an invasive cancer and she should undergo a partial or total mastectomy with a sentinel node biopsy

(B) this tumor is frequently very aggressive

(C) radiation therapy should follow surgical therapy

(D) she likely has associated DCIS or invasive cancer

(E) she likely would not benefit from antiestrogen therapy

24. A 63-year-old lady comes to your office for her routine yearly examination. She has been reading on the Internet about estrogen causing breast cancer. She wants to know what you think and if she should stop her estrogen replacement therapy. You counsel her that

(A) she should stop immediately because estrogen has been linked breast cancer

(B) the risk of breast cancer seems to be increased if she is taking combination estrogen/progesterone replacement therapy

(C) benefits of hormonal replacement therapy include decreased osteoporosis, improved lipid profiles, and decreased cardiovascular disease

(D) cons of hormonal replacement therapy include increased risk of deep venous thrombosis, stroke incidence, and increased metastatic disease if she does develop breast cancer

(E) that the optimal duration of hormonal therapy is 3 years or less

25. With respect to inherited breast cancer, which of the following are true?

(A) Most newly-diagnosed breast cancers in women are related to either BRCA-1 or BRCA-2 positivity.

(B) Early age of onset, multiple primary tumors, and bilateral cancers are typical in inherited breast cancer.

(C) The lifetime risk of developing breast cancer if carrying a BRCA-1 or BRCA-2 gene mutation is approximately 50%.

(D) Patients carrying the BRCA-1 or BRCA-2 gene should have a prophylactic bilateral mastectomy before the age of 25 if possible.

(E) Careful surveillance with monthly breast self-examination, annual physician physical examination, and total breast ultrasound will minimize risk associated with a strong pedigree of inherited breast cancers.

26. A 40-year-old woman presents with a 2 cm mass in her right breast first detected by mammography (Fig. 15-2). Radiographic core biopsy of the lesion is selected for diagnosis and reveals infiltrating ductal carcinoma. She has no palpable axillary lymph nodes. Appropriate therapy for the patient would include

(A) partial mastectomy (lumpectomy)

(B) sentinel lymph node biopsy

(C) consideration of adjuvant chemotherapy

(D) radiation therapy

(E) all of the above

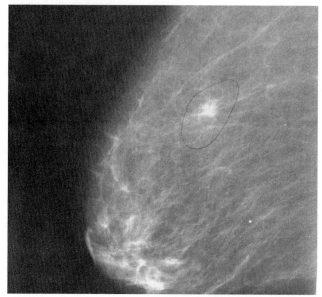

FIG. 15-2 Mammogram showing an irregular, speculated mass in the right breast. Core biopsy reveals invasive ductal carcinoma.

27. A sentinel lymph node biopsy in the patient described above reveals metastatic carcinoma. There is no evidence of distant metastases on further investigation. Her stage by the American Joint Committee on Cancer (AJCC) TNM staging system is

(A) I

(B) II

(C) III

(D) IV

(E) V

28. A 65-year-old female presents with a large (5 cm) mass in her right breast with overlying ulceration of the skin. She is noted to have several enlarged, mobile axillary lymph nodes on examination. She is subjected to a core biopsy which confirms the impression of invasive ductal carcinoma of the breast. Her management should begin with

(A) mastectomy

(B) sentinel lymph node biopsy

(C) systemic chemo or hormonal therapy

(D) radiation therapy

(O) alternative therapy

29. Which of the following are true with respect to sentinel lymph node biopsy?

(A) Localization of the sentinel node is successful in approximately 75% of cases.

(B) Misses isolated micrometastases in nonsentinel nodes in 20% of cases.

(C) It is unnecessary in patients with primary tumors less than 1 cm (T1a), as the rate of metastases is less than 1%.

(D) The time from injection to accumulation of dye in the sentinel node is longer for the radioactive tracer than isosulfan (Lymphazurin) dye.

(E) When properly performed should yield a single sentinel lymph node.

30. Appropriate management of a patient with a positive sentinel node (involved with metastases) might include

(A) axillary lymph node dissection

(B) axillary radiation therapy

(C) systemic chemotherapy

(D) observation only

(E) A, B, or C

31. All of the following is true about Cystosarcoma phyllodes of the breast *except*:

(A) is the most common primary breast sarcoma

(B) treatment is local excision with margin of normal tissue

(C) only 10% are malignant

(D) lymph node dissection is not indicated

(E) in the male patient the prognosis is worse

32. Which of the following is false regarding lobular carcinoma *in situ*?

(A) It is a marker for increased risk of breast cancer.

(B) Mirror image breast biopsy is indicated.

(C) Subsequent invasive cancer is more often ductal in origin.

(D) Treatment is close observation versus bilateral prophylactic mastectomy.

(E) Prognosis is solely related to the development of subsequent cancer.

33. Which of the following statements is incorrect regarding ductal carcinoma *in situ*?

(A) Breast-conservation therapy should be done for localized disease, particularly of the noncomedo variety.

(B) Axillary lymph node dissection is not necessary.

(C) The most common clinical presentation is a palpable mass.

(D) After breast-conserving surgery, radiotherapy is administered in tangential fields to the whole breast.

(E) There is no role for chemotherapy in the treatment of ductal carcinoma *in situ* (DCIS).

34. A 45-year-old male presents with a 2 cm, painless subareolar mass of his left breast, with nipple retraction. Physical examination reveals no lymph node involvement. A fine needle biopsy of the mass is performed and reveals infiltrating ductal carcinoma with positive hormone receptors. Further workup reveals no evidence of metastatic disease. What is the most appropriate treatment plan?

(A) hormone therapy with tamoxifen

(B) wide local excision with sentinel lymph node biopsy

(C) segmental mastectomy

(D) modified radical mastectomy

(E) radical mastectomy

35. A 29-year-old White female, in her second trimester of pregnancy, presents with a stage II breast lesion. The lesion is visualized on ultrasound and there is no evidence of metastatic or lymph node disease. Which of the following is the most appropriate treatment option?

(A) routine ultrasound examination, followed by postpartum lumpectomy, axillary dissection, chemotherapy and irradiation

(B) lumpectomy and axillary dissection, followed by postpartum chemotherapy and irradiation

(C) lumpectomy and axillary dissection, followed by immediate chemotherapy and postpartum irradiation

(D) lumpectomy and axillary dissection, followed by immediate chemotherapy and irradiation

(E) termination of pregnancy, lumpectomy, axillary dissection, chemotherapy and irradiation

36. A 22-year-old White female, in her ninth week of pregnancy, presents with a painless lump of her left breast. Physical examination reveals both breasts to be fibrous and dense. A 2 cm lesion is palpated in the left breast. No nipple discharge is noted and there are no palpable lymph nodes of either axilla. Which of the following imaging studies should be used first to evaluate the lesion?

(A) ultrasound

(B) single view mammogram

(C) two view mammogram

(D) MRI

Answers and Explanations

1. (C) The long thoracic nerve, or the external respiratory nerve of Bell, arises from the fifth, sixth, and seventh cervical nerves and passes deep to the axillary artery and vein, staying close to the chest wall. It innervates the serratus anterior muscle. This muscle is important in stabilizing the scapula on the thorax. Injury to the long thoracic nerve results in a winged scapula. This can lead to significant morbidity.

The thoracodorsal nerve arises from the posterior cord of the brachial plexus and passes beneath the axillary vein. It runs in the posterior axilla and through the areolar tissue containing the lymph nodes. It innervates the latissimus dorsi muscle. Loss or injury of the thoracodorsal nerve results in weakness of extension, internal rotation, and adduction of the humerus. This can be well tolerated by most patients.

Bibliography

Osbourne M. Breast anatomy and development. In: Harris JR, Lippman ME, Morrow M, et al. (eds.), *Diseases of the Breast*, 2nd ed. Philadelphia, PA: Lippincott, Williams & Wilkins, 2000, 6–9.

Spratt J, Donegan W, Tobin G. Gross anatomy of the breast. In: Donegan W, Sprattt J (eds.), *Cancer of the Breast*, 5th ed. St. Louis, MO: W.B. Saunders, 2002, 32–37.

2. (C) The axillary lymph nodes are classified according to their relationship with the pectoralis minor muscle.

Level I: lateral to the pectoralis minor
Level II: posterior to the pectoralis minor
Level III: medial to the pectoralis minor

Rotter's nodes, or interpectoral nodes, are anterior to the pectoralis minor muscle.

Axillary lymph node status is one of the most important prognostic indicators for breast cancer. The likelihood of node positive disease is directly related to the size of the tumor, not other tumor markers (estrogen/progesterone receptors, Her-2-neu status) (Tables 15-1 and 15-2).

TABLE 15-1 Axillary Nodes and Tumor Size

Tumor size (cm)	Chance of node positive disease (%)
0.1–0.5	11
0.6–1.0	15
1.1–1.3	25
1.4–1.6	34
1.7–2.0	43

Lymph node status also gives an indication about overall survival.

Subsequent therapy is often based on the status of the lymph nodes. If the patient has lymph node positive disease, chemotherapy should be strongly considered.

Bibliography

Osbourne M. Breast anatomy and development. In: Harris JR, Lippman ME, Morrow M, ct al. (eds.), *Diseases of the Breast*, 2nd ed. Philadelphia, PA: Lippincott, Williams & Wilkins, 2000, 4–6.

Spratt J, Donegan W, Tobin G. Gross anatomy of the breast. In: Donegan W, Sprattt J (eds.), *Cancer of the Breast*, 5th ed. St. Louis, MO: W.B. Saunders, 2002, 39–43.

3. (E) There are many known risk factors for breast cancer. The most important risk factor is being female. There is a 100:1 ratio of female breast cancers as compared to male breast cancers. Through recent research, two important genes have been localized that appear

TABLE 15-2 Axillary Nodes and Survival Rates (*5-Year Survival Rates*)

Tumor size (cm)	0 lymph nodes (%)	1–3 LN (%)	>4 LN (%)
<2	96.3	89.4	66
2-5	89.4	79.9	58.7
>5	82.2	73	42.5

to play a role in breast cancer. These are BRCA1 and BRCA2. BRCA1 is located on chromosome 17 and is also linked to ovarian, prostate, and possibly colon cancer. BRCA2 is located on chromosome 13 and is linked to male breast cancer, a lesser rate of ovarian cancer, and possibly prostate and colon cancer. Having one of the genes confers a 60–80% lifetime risk of developing breast cancer; however, only 5–10% of all breast cancer cases are genetically driven.

Other important risk factors include estrogen exposure (early menarche, late menopause, nulliparity, first full-term pregnancy after 31 years of age), radiation exposure when younger than 30 years old (i.e., as treatment for Hodgkin's lymphoma), and a prior history of breast cancer (0.5–1% risk per year). Also, some forms of benign breast disease place the patient at increased risk for developing breast cancer in the future. This includes atypical hyperplasia (four to five times the risk) and lobular carcinoma *in situ* (LCIS) (8–10 times the risk). Benign papillomas, adenomas, ductal ectasia, cysts and the like do not increase a patient's risk significantly.

Bibliography

Briton L, Lacey J, Devesa S. Epidemiology of breast cancer. In: Donegan W, Spratt J (eds.), *Cancer of the Breast*, 5th ed. St. Louis, MO: W.B. Saunders, 2002, 115–123.

Willett WC, et al. Epidemiology and nongenetic causes of breast cancer. In: Harris JR, Lippman ME, Morrow M, et al. (eds.), *Diseases of the Breast*, 2nd ed. Philadelphia, PA: Lippincott, Williams & Wilkins, 2000, 175–220.

4. **(D)** The Gail model is a statistical model based on data from the Breast Cancer Detection Demonstration Project. By using known risk factors (race, age, age at first menses, age at first live birth, number of first degree relatives with breast cancer, number of previous biopsies—including benign ones, number of biopsies with atypical hyperplasia), the program derives an age-specific risk. A risk greater than 1.7% at 5 years deserves further addressing and the patient should be appropriately counseled regarding her increased risk. Tamoxifen has now been shown to decrease the 5-year and lifetime risks in these patients by almost 50%. This is based on the NSABP-P1 study data. Further studies are ongoing to examine the role of other estrogen blocking drugs, such as Evista (STAR trial).

Bibliography

Allain D, Gilligan M, Redlich P. Genetics and genetic counseling for breast cancer. In: Donegan W, Spratt J (eds.), *Cancer of the Breast*, 5th ed. St. Louis, MO: W.B. Saunders, 2002, 256–257.

Isaacs C. Evaluations and management of women with a strong family history of breast cancer. In: Harris JR, Lippman ME, Morrow M, et al. (eds.), *Diseases of the Breast*, 2nd ed. Philadelphia, PA: Lippincott, Williams & Wilkins, 2000, 238–239.

5. **(C)** EGFR are transmembrane tyrosine kinase receptors. The family includes HER-1 (EGFR), HER-2, HER-3, and HER-4. This group of growth factor receptors is also known as c-erb-b2, c-erb-b3, and c-erb-b4. c-erb-b2 (Her-2-*neu*) is over-expressed in 20–30% of breast cancer cases. Also included in this family of receptors is transforming growth factor-alpha (TGF-α). They act in a paracrine manner during the proliferative stages of ductal development. Breast tissue is known to respond to estrogen via EGFR. EGFR can regulate apoptosis of epithelial cells. Breast cancer cells that express HER-2 have an increased expression of Bcl-2 and Bcl-xl. This is associated with resistance to tamoxifen-induced apoptosis. Recent advances in tyrosine kinase inhibitors have proven to be beneficial in the treatment of tamoxifen resistance secondary to EGFR upregulation.

When EGFR is activated, tyrosine kinase activity is induced. This in turn leads to autophosphorylation and subsequent intracellular activity. This includes mitogen activated protein (MAP) kinase family. Next, nuclear transcription factors are activated.

EGFR is now being used as a prognostic indicator and to guide treatment. c-erb-b2 appears to correlate to early transition to ductal invasive disease and high mitotic rates. In addition, tumors that are c-erb-b2 positive appear to be less responsive to 5-flurouracil (5-FU), methotrexate, cyclophosphamide, and tamoxifen. When tumors become tamoxifen resistance, if is felt to be secondary to the upregulation of epidermal growth factors.

Bibliography

Chang M, Liu H, Jordan V. Hormonal and growth factors. In: Donegan W, Spratt J (eds.), *Cancer of the Breast*, 5th ed. St. Louis, MO: W.B. Saunders, 2002, 429–433.

Dickson R. Autocrine and paracrine growth factors in the normal and neoplastic breast. In: Harris JR, Lippman ME, Morrow M, et al. (eds.), *Diseases of the Breast*, 2nd ed. Philadelphia, PA: Lippincott, Williams & Wilkins, 2000, 282–289.

6. **(C)** BRCA2 is a breast cancer susceptibility gene that has been localized to chromosome 13q12-13. It is a nuclear protein. The function of BRCA2 is similar to BRCA1 in that it plays a role in the DNA damage response pathways. BRCA2 is associated with a 60–85% lifetime risk of breast cancer in female carriers. Males that carry the BRCA2 gene have a 6% lifetime risk of developing breast cancer. This is 100 times the general population risk. The lifetime risk of ovarian cancer is 10–20%. BRCA2 mutations are also associated

with an increased risk of melanoma, colon, prostate, pancreatic, biliary, and stomach cancers. Patients who develop breast cancer tend to be slightly older than those patients with BRCA1. The tumors also tend to be less aggressive than those associated with BRCA1. BRCA2 tumors are more like sporadic tumors.

BRCA1 is located on chromosome 17q21. It is also a nuclear protein that plays a role in the DNA damage response pathways. It is thought to affect transcription factors, and can enhance p53 transactivation. The lifetime risk of breast cancer for female carriers is 60–80% and the risk of ovarian cancer is 20–40%. The breast and ovarian cancers linked to BRCA1 tend to be unstable and aggressive. In addition, BRCA1 is also a factor in prostate cancer and possible colon cancer.

Bibliography

Allain D, Gilligan M, Redlich P. Genetics and genetic counseling for breast cancer. In: Donegan W, Sprattt J (eds.), *Cancer of the Breast*, 5th ed. St. Louis, MO: W.B. Saunders, 2002, 251–253.

Beenken S, Bland K. Breast cancer: cellular, biochemical, and molecular biomarkers. In: Cameron J (ed.), *Current Surgical Therapy*, 7th ed. St. Louis, MO: Mosby, 2001, 697–698.

DeMichele A. Inherited genetic factors. In: Harris JR, Lippman ME, Morrow M, et al. (eds.), *Diseases of the Breast*, 2nd ed. Philadelphia, PA: Lippincott, Williams & Wilkins, 2000, 224–230.

7. **(D)** Li-Fraumeni's syndrome is an autosomal dominate disease that was first documented in families whose children had sarcomas. Relatives were also found to have an increased number of early onset breast cancer, leukemia, osteosarcoma, brain tumors, and adrenocortical tumors. It is estimated that 45% of women with this mutation will develop breast cancer before the age of 60. Over 75% of these women develop breast cancer between the ages of 22 and 45 years. Interestingly, the affected males do not appear to have an increased risk of breast cancer. The genetic defect only accounts for 1% of all breast cancers. It is associated with a p53 mutation located on chromosome 17.

TP53 is a tumor suppressor gene located on chromosome 17q13. This gene is responsible for a multifunctional DNA damage response protein. When TP53 undergoes mutation, it functions as an inhibitor of p53. Unmutated p53 is a nuclear protein that affects DNA damage response proteins also. p53 normally acts to block the cell cycle at the G1-S phase, to induce apoptosis, and to allow induction of differentiation. This all in turn slows cellular growth and allows for DNA repair. Inhibition or loss of p53 function may lead to cellular instability.

Bibliography

Allain D, Gilligan M, Redlich P. Genetics and genetic counseling for breast cancer. In: Donegan W, Sprattt J (eds.), *Cancer of the Breast*, 5th ed. St. Louis, MO: W.B. Saunders, 2002, 253–254.

Dickson R. Oncogenes, suppressor genes, and signal transduction. In: Harris JR, Lippman ME, Morrow M, et al. (eds.), *Diseases of the Breast*, 2nd ed. Philadelphia, PA: Lippincott, Williams & Wilkins, 2000, 292–294.

Isaacs C. Evaluation and management of women with a strong family history of breast cancer. In: Harris JR, Lippman ME, Morrow M, et al. (eds.), *Diseases of the Breast*, 2nd ed. Philadelphia, PA: Lippincott, Williams & Wilkins, 2000, 242–243.

8. **(A)** Oral contraceptive use results in a decrease incidence of both endometrial and ovarian cancers. The effect on breast cancer has been studied extensively. The results are conflicting, but most do not show any increased risk. The largest study pooled 54 studies and examined 53,297 patients with breast cancer and 100,239 patients without breast cancer. No increased risk of breast cancer was found in those that had ever used oral contraceptives. This study is flawed in that they enrolled and evaluated women who "ever used" oral contraception. This includes both long- and short-term usage. In the most recent study, 4575 women were enrolled. They were aged 35–64 years. They evaluated women who are current users, recent past users, long-term past users, and never used. They concluded that current and recent users were at a small increased risk of breast cancer (RR = 1.24, 95% CI 1.15–1.33). The effect was not sustained, however, after 10 years of discontinued use.

Bibliography

Marchbanks P, McDonald J, et al. Oral contraceptives and the risk of breast cancer. *N Engl J Med* 2002;26: 2025–2032.

Willett W. Epidemiology and nongenetic causes of breast cancer. In: Harris JR, Lippman ME, Morrow M, et al. (eds.), *Diseases of the Breast*, 2nd ed. Philadelphia, PA: Lippincott, Williams & Wilkins, 2000, 187–189.

9. **(B)** The diagnostic test of choice for a newly found breast mass is an ultrasound. This will tell you if the mass is cystic or solid. If it is cystic, the mass can be aspirated and then followed at 6 weeks with a repeat ultrasound. This will rule out recurrence. If the cyst has recurred, the mass should be excised. The mass/cyst should also be excised if the initial aspirate is bloody.

If the mass is found to be solid, a core needle biopsy (CNB) should be performed. If the pathology is benign, is should be excised with narrow margins at a later date. If it is malignant, a bilateral mammogram should be obtained to rule out other nonpalpable pathology that will need to be addressed. Appropriate loco-regional therapy can then be discussed.

A CNB is preferred over a fine needle aspirate. A CNB gives a histologic diagnosis whereas a fine needle aspiration (FNA) only gives a cytologic diagnosis. An FNA cannot differentiate between invasive and *in situ* disease. In addition, an experienced cytopathologist is needed to interpret FNA data.

Ultrasound is not an effective screening modality for breast cancer. It is unreliable at detecting microcalcifications and early stage breast cancer. Ultrasound should be used to differentiate solid from cystic lesions, as a primary modality in patients less than 25 years old with a palpable abnormality, and to evaluate mammographically occult palpable masses. It is also useful in evaluating silicone implant rupture and detecting an underlying abscess in a patient with mastitis.

Bibliography

Kern K. Diagnostic options in symptomatic breast disease. In: Cameron J (ed.), *Current Surgical Therapy*, 7th ed. St. Louis, MO: Mosby, 2001, 680–681.

Kopans D. Imaging analysis of breast lesions. In: Harris JR, Lippman ME, Morrow M, et al. (eds.), *Diseases of the Breast*, 2nd ed. Philadelphia, PA: Lippincott, Williams & Wilkins, 2000, 135–137.

Mahoney M. Breast imaging: mammography, sonography, and emerging technology. In: Donegan W, Sprattt J (eds.), *Cancer of the Breast*, 5th ed. St. Louis, MO: W.B. Saunders, 2002, 298–304.

10. **(D)** There is a 10–15% false negative rate of current mammography. In women 40–49 years old, nearly 25% of invasive breast cancers are not visualized. This drops to 10% for women 50–59 years old. Almost 10% of patients who have routine screening mammography are asked to return for additional studies. This is to better clarify the abnormality. The additional studies may include additional mammographic views or ultrasounds, or it may require invasive studies such as a biopsy. Mammograms in general are less sensitive in younger women with dense breast tissue. Breast implants may also obscure a mammographic evaluation. Routine mammography has a difficult time visualizing lesions deep against the chest wall, lateral in the tail of breast, or inferior in the inframammary fold.

Bibliography

Kopans D. Imaging analysis of breast lesions. In: Harris JR, Lippman ME, Morrow M, et al. (eds.), *Diseases of the Breast*, 2nd ed. Philadelphia, PA: Lippincott, Williams & Wilkins, 2000, 128–134.

11. **(C)** Malignant lesions seen on ultrasound tend to have irregular or spiculated borders, are poorly circumscribed, asymmetric, and hypoechoic. They have a high acoustic attenuation that leads to posterior shadowing. The accuracy of characterizing a malignant lesion on ultrasound is 80% of T1 lesions, 93% for T2 lesions, and 100% for T3 lesions. This gives an overall accuracy of 88.9%

Benign lesions tend to have smooth borders, are well circumscribed, symmetric, and hypo/iso/anechoic. They may have posterior enhancement with apparent bilateral shadowing—this is especially true of cysts (Fig. 15-3).

Solid benign lesions tend to have smooth borders, are well circumscribed, and hypoechoic. They tend to be wider than taller (Fig. 15-4).

Bibliography

Kopans D. Imaging analysis of breast lesions. In: Harris JR, Lippman ME, Morrow M, et al (eds.), *Diseases of the Breast*, 2nd ed. Philadelphia, PA: Lippincott, Williams & Wilkins, 2000, 134–137.

Mahoney M. Breast imaging: mammography, sonography, and emerging technologies. In: Donegan W, Spratt J (eds.), *Cancer of the Breast*, 5th ed. St. Louis, MO: W.B. Saunders, 2002, 298–304.

Smith S, Osburne M. Screening for breast cancer. In: Cameron J (ed.), *Current Surgical Therapy*, 7th ed. St. Louis, MO: Mosby, 2001, 694–695.

12. **(B)** Currently, breast MRI is too expensive to be considered a useful screening tool. In addition, although

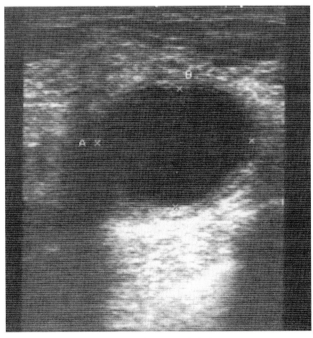

FIG. 15-3 Benign cystic lesion

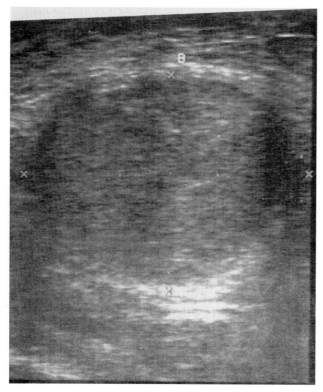

FIG. 15-4   Benign solid lesion

it is very sensitive, it is not specific. Some studies have shown specificity to be as low as 30%. If a lesion is found on MRI, but not seen on mammogram or ultrasound and is not palpable, tissue procurement becomes a problem. At this time, MRI guided biopsy or needle placement for excisional biopsy is not available. Despite these limitations, MRI is gaining clinical value. Gadolinium is used to aid enhancement. Dedicated breast coils are used and both breasts are imaged at the same time. Most examinations can be completed within 30 min. Invasive cancers do demonstrate enhancement; however, *in situ* cancers may not enhance. Current approved indications for breast MRI are (1) tumor staging to determine extent of diseases, (2) differentiating scar tissue from cancer recurrence, (3) evaluating axillary metastasis of unknown origin. MRI is the best way to evaluate implant rupture.

Bibliography

Kopans D. Imaging analysis of breast lesions. In: Harris JR, Lippman ME, Morrow M, et al. (eds.), *Diseases of the Breast*, 2nd ed. Philadelphia, PA: Lippincott, Williams & Wilkins, 2000, 137–142.

Mahoney M. Breast imaging: mammography, sonography, and emerging technologies. In: Donegan W, Sprattt J (eds.), *Cancer of the Breast*, 5th ed. St. Louis, MO: W.B. Saunders, 2002, 305–306.

13. **(D)** Cellulitis associated with lactation is caused by gram-positive cocci. It is best treated by oral antibiotics, warm packs, and keeping the breast emptied. The infant does not need to be weaned and can continue to breast-feed without any ill-effect.

    If an abscess does form, it should be drained in the operating room, usually under a general anesthetic. At this point, the infant should be weaned. An abscess should be suspected based on fever, leukocytosis, and point tenderness. A fluctuant mass does not usually develop because of the diffuse fibrous septa.

    Breast infections found in the nonlactating patient are usually caused by multiple organisms. They are often recurrent and are associated with periductal mastitis or ductal ectasia. Acutely, the infections should be treated with antibiotics and drainage. If the infection is chronic and relapsing, the acute infection needs to be treated with antibiotics and the subareolar duct system should be excised.

Bibliography

Dixon JM. Management of disorders of the ductal system and infections. In: Harris JR, Lippman ME, Morrow M, et al. (eds.), *Diseases of the Breast*, 2nd ed. Philadelphia, PA: Lippincott, Williams & Wilkins, 2000, 52–54.

14. **(C)** The most common cause of bloody nipple discharge is an intraductal papilloma. This is a benign condition. Intraductal papillomas occur in the major lactiferous ducts. The patient is usually 30–50 years old. The papilloma is typically attached to the wall of the duct by a small stalk; however, it may also be sessile. Isolated intraductal papillomas are not premalignant. Multiple papillomas do appear to have an increased risk of future cancer. This seems to be related to the degree of atypical hyperplasia associated with them.

    Malignant nipple discharge is characterized by being unilateral, spontaneous, and bloody. Occasionally the discharge may also be yellow, green, or even clear. There is often an associated mass or asymmetry. Twenty percent of nipple discharge in older women is associated with ductal carcinoma *in situ* (DCIS). As some bloody nipple discharge may be malignant, the etiology must be evaluated and this often means excision of the affected ductal system. The chance of an underlying cancer rises as the patient's age increases.

    Fibrocystic disease may also cause nipple discharge; however, this is usually green or yellow/brown in color. It is not bloody.

    Galactorrhea manifests as bilateral milky discharge not associated with pregnancy or lactation. Numerous drugs can cause milky nipple discharge, including psychotropic agents. Prolactin levels should be obtained and if elevated, evaluation for a pituitary tumor should be done.

Bibliography

Dixon JM. Management of disorders of the ductal system and infections. In: Harris JR, Lippman ME, Morrow M, et al. (eds.), *Diseases of the Breast*, 2nd ed. Philadelphia, PA: Lippincott, Williams & Wilkins, 2000, 47–50.

Donegan W. Diagnosis of breast cancer. In: Donegan W, Sprattt J (eds.), *Cancer of the Breast*, 5th ed. St. Louis, MO: W.B. Saunders, 2002, 318–319.

Donegan W. Diagnosis of breast cancer. In: Donegan W, Sprattt J (eds.), *Cancer of the Breast*, 5th ed. St. Louis, MO: W.B. Saunders, 2002, 341–342.

Kern K. Diagnostic options in symptomatic breast disease. In: Cameron J (ed.), *Current Surgical Therapy*, 7th ed. St. Louis, MO: Mosby, 2001, 683–684.

Schnitt S. Pathology of benign breast disorders. In: Harris JR, Lippman ME, Morrow M, et al. (eds.), *Diseases of the Breast*, 2nd ed. Philadelphia, PA: Lippincott, Williams & Wilkins, 2000, 83–85.

15. (D) Phyllodes tumors, also known as cystosarcoma phyllodes, are stromal tumors. They are well circumscribed and do not have a true capsule. The cut surface of one of these tumors tends to be mucoid. There are numerous small projections that make surgical enucleation difficult.

Phyllodes tend to occur in an older population than fibroadenomas (FAs). FAs are also stromal tumors, and it is thought that phyllodes may arise from these benign tumors. Phyllodes tend to occur in the fourth decade of life. Most of these tumors present as painless masses that are round and smooth. On mammogram and ultrasound they are similar in appearance to FAs—smooth, solid, multilobulated margins. There may also be fluid within the mass on ultrasound, suggesting phyllodes over FA.

Seventy-five percent of phyllodes tumors are benign. Similar to other stromal tumors, malignancy is difficult to establish and is based on histologic appearance. Stromal overgrowth is now considered the most important predictor of aggressive behavior. Other characteristics that are considered are cellular atypia, mitotic activity, and tumor margins.

Phyllodes tend to recur regardless of benign or malignant status. The reported incidence is 20–25% of recurrence. Current recommendations for initial surgical treatment of theses tumors are wide local excision with a 2–3 cm margin. This can usually be done without requiring a mastectomy and is based on tumor to breast mass ratio. Usually if the tumor recurs, a total mastectomy is required; however, some women may be able to tolerate a reexcision without poor cosmesis. Less than 5% of all phyllodes tumors metastasize. Regional lymph node metastasis

is rare and an axillary dissection is not warranted. Radiation therapy is also not indicated because this is not a multifocal disease like ductal breast cancer. The tumors are only weakly radiosensitive; however, radiation therapy may offer some palliation for recurrent disease. Hormonal manipulation is not beneficial for these patients. This is felt to represent the mixed epithelial (positive receptors) and stromal (no receptors) components.

Bibliography

Donegan W. Sarcomas of the breast. In: Donegan W, Sprattt J (eds.), *Cancer of the Breast*, 5th ed. St. Louis, MO: W.B. Saunders, 2002, 918–923.

Petrek J. Phyllodes tumor. In: Harris JR, Lippman ME, Morrow M, et al. (eds.), *Diseases of the Breast*, 2nd ed. Philadelphia, PA: Lippincott, Williams & Wilkins, 2000, 669–675.

Wood W. Benign breast disease. In: Cameron J (ed.), *Current Surgical Therapy*, 7th ed. St. Louis, MO: Mosby, 2001, 691.

16. (C) Given her age and the mass's typical appearance on ultrasound, this is most likely an FA. Any new breast mass deserves serious evaluation and workup to exclude malignancy. Therefore, close follow-up of a new mass would not be justified. This may lead to a delay in diagnosis of a cancer, especially in the young patient. Proceeding with mastectomy, either partial or total, is not appropriate without tissue diagnosis first. A needle localized excisional biopsy is not required as this is a palpable mass. The best methods of diagnosing this mass are either CNB, which may be done under ultrasound guidance to ensure adequate and proper sampling, or an excisional biopsy. Fine needle aspiration is also an option if you have an experienced cytopathologist available.

FAs can present at any age but are most common in young women, aged 16–24. The masses are typically described as rubbery and mobile. On ultrasound, they are hypoechoic, solid masses with smooth margins. There may be posterior enhancement. Microscopically, FA have both epithelial and stromal component. Fifteen to sixty percent of FAs are thought to spontaneously resolve; however, because many of these women are subjected to repeat and frequent mammogram and ultrasound, as well as needle biopsies, you will find that many of the women who first opted for observation will proceed with excisional biopsy at some point.

Transformation of an FA to invasive cancer is a rare event; however, recent studies show that a subgroup of women may be a higher risk of future cancer. This group includes women with a "complex fibroadenoma"—FAs that contain cysts >3 mm, apocrine changes, adenosis, and epithelial calcifications—

as well as women with a family history of breast cancer, and women who displayed parenchymal proliferation adjacent to the FA.

Bibliography

Clare S. Management of the palpable breast mass. In: Harris JR, Lippman ME, Morrow M, et al (eds.), *Diseases of the Breast*, 2nd ed. Philadelphia, PA: Lippincott, Williams & Wilkins, 2000, 38–41.

Donegan W. Common benign conditions of the breast. In: Donegan W, Sprattt J (eds.), *Cancer of the Breast*, 5th ed. St. Louis, MO: W.B. Saunders, 2002, 71–73.

Wood W. Benign breast disease. In: Cameron J (ed.), *Current Surgical Therapy*, 7th ed. St. Louis, MO: Mosby, 2001, 691.

17. **(D)** Gynecomastia is the benign proliferation of breast glandular tissue in males. This tends to occur in infancy, at puberty, and in old age.

Gynecomastia results from an imbalance of the normal hormonal milieu or a change in breast tissue sensitivity to estrogen. The testes secrete 95% of the total body testosterone and only 15% of the circulating estradiol. The vast majority of circulating estradiol is from the peripheral conversion of testosterone and adrenal steroids via the aromatase enzyme. Most of the hormones are bound to sex-hormone binding globulin (SHBG), a protein formed in the liver. SHBG has a higher affinity for androgens than estrogen. An imbalance in any of these pathways may results in an increase of free estrogen as compared to bound estrogen (Fig. 15-5).

TABLE 15-3   Gynecomastia—Drug-induced Causes

Increased estrogen	Decreased testosterone	Unknown
Steroids	Cimetidine	Lasix
Heroin	Diazepam	Isoniazid
Digoxin	Ketoconazole	Theophylline
Cannabis	Phenytoin	Tricyclics
	Spironolactone	Verapamil
	Chemotherapy	Amiodarone
		Clonidine
		Captopril
		Nifedipine
		Amiloride
		Phenothiazine
		Reglan
		Omeprazole

The potential causes of gynecomastia are numerous. In young men, a testicular lesion must be excluded. In the neonate, the etiology is often a response to circulating material estrogens. Despite the long list, about two-thirds of patients have idiopathic gynecomastia (25%), pubertal gynecomastia (25%), or drug induced (10–20%) (Tables 15-3 and 15-4).

Bibliography

Braunstein G. Management of gynecomastia. In: Harris JR, Lippman ME, Morrow M, et al. (eds.), *Diseases of the Breast*, 2nd ed. Philadelphia, PA: Lippincott, Williams & Wilkins, 2000, 67–73.

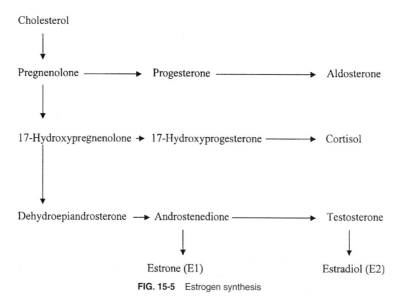

FIG. 15-5   Estrogen synthesis

TABLE 15-4   Gynecomastia—Misc Etiologies

Increased estrogen	Decreased androgen
Increased Secretion	Decreased production
Gonadal	Gonadal
Testicular tumors (teratomas, seminomas)	Viral orchitis
	Testicular trauma
	Testicular irradiation
	Hydrocele, varicocele
	Spermatocele
	Bilateral cryptorchidism
	Congenital anorchidism
Nongonadal	Nongonadal
Lung cancer	Chromosomal defect
Liver cancer	Renal disease
Adrenocortical disease	Aging
Increased aromatization	Peripheral resistance
Adrenal disease	Testicular feminization
Liver disease	
Thyrotoxicosis	

Donegan W. Common benign conditions of the breast. In: Donegan W, Sprattt J (eds.), *Cancer of the Breast*, 5th ed. St. Louis, MO: W.B. Saunders, 2002, 85–89.

Webster D. The male breast. In: Hughes L, Mansel R, Webster D (eds.), *Benign Disorders and Diseases of the Breast: Concepts and Clinical Management*, 2nd ed. London: W.B. Saunders, 2000, 202–226.

18. **(A)** As with any new breast mass, a serious evaluation and workup is indicated. Male breast cancer is present in 1:100,000 men. A clinical breast examination can be very helpful in differentiating a clinical cancer from gynecomastia. Examination should be done with the patient in the supine position. His arms should be raised, with his hands behind his head. With the examiners fingers on either side of the nipple/reolar complex, a firm disc of tissue can be appreciated when the fingers are gently brought together. The disc of tissue is concentric with the nipple. Cancers, on the other hand, tend to be eccentric and hard. An ultrasound can also quickly identify a solid lesion. If a solid mass is found, a CNB can be done quickly and a diagnosis delivered. A mammogram is secondary to evaluate any other possible breast pathology.

Once the diagnosis of gynecomastia is made, an evaluation for the etiology of the hormonal imbalance should be sought. This includes obtaining a history of renal or liver disease, hyperthyroidism, malnutrition, and reviewing a current list of medications. Physical examination should also be done to evaluate for a testicular mass. Additional blood tests that may be helpful include β-HCG, luteinizing hormone, testosterone, and estradiol.

Male breast cancer is estimated to occur in 1:100,000 men. It accounts for about 1% of all new breast cancers. The median age of diagnosis is 65–67 years old. Risk factors for male breast cancer include relative estrogen excess or testosterone deficiency, Klinefelter's syndrome, BRCA2, liver disease, and possibly gynecomastia. Men usually present with a mass. Invasive ductal carcinoma accounts for 85% of the cancers. Treatment is a modified radical mastectomy. Survival statistics are similar stage for stage when compared to their female counterparts. Men, in general, are diagnosed at a later stage and this accounts for the apparent increased mortality rates.

Bibliography

Braunstein G. Management of gynecomastia. In: Harris JR, Lippman ME, Morrow M, et al. (eds.), *Diseases of the Breast*, 2nd ed. Philadelphia, PA: Lippincott, Williams & Wilkins, 2000, 67–73.

Donegan W. Common benign conditions of the breast. In: Donegan W, Sprattt J (eds.), *Cancer of the Breast*, 5th ed. St. Louis, MO: W.B. Saunders, 2002, 85–89.

Gradishar W. Male breast cancer. In: Harris JR, Lippman ME, Morrow M, et al. (eds.), *Diseases of the Breast*, 2nd ed. Philadelphia, PA: Lippincott, Williams & Wilkins, 2000, 661–665.

Winchester D. Male breast cancer. In: Cameron J (ed.), *Current Surgical Therapy*, 7th ed. St. Louis, MO: Mosby, 2001, 732–734.

Winchester D. Male breast cancer. In: Donegan W, Sprattt J (eds.), *Cancer of the Breast*, 5th ed. St. Louis, MO: W.B. Saunders, 2002, 951–956.

19. **(B)**

20. **(A)**

Explanations 19 and 20

Mastalgia, or breast pain, is a common complaint and a common reason for referral to a breast center. Evaluation of breast pain should include a thorough history and examination. With a good history, you can begin to categorize the pain. Typical types of mastalgia can be described as cyclical pronounced, noncyclical, trauma, musculoskeletal/chest wall, and miscellaneous uncommon cause.

Cyclical pronounced pain is the most common. It is related to the menstrual cycle, especially ovulation. The average age is 34 years. Patients complain of "heaviness" and "tenderness." Nodularity is common, especially in the upper outer quadrants. This also tends to fluctuate with the menstrual cycle. The pain is often in the upper outer quadrant, may be bilateral, and can radiate down the arm.

Noncyclical mastalgia is not related to the menstrual cycle. The average age of the patient is again 34 years old. The pain is different from cyclical pain in that is more localized and described as a "burning" or "pulling." Nodularity is typically less pronounced, but it is present in greater than 50% of the patients.

Musculoskeletal pain is usually unilateral. It is often either lateral chest wall pain or costochondral junction pain (Tietze's syndrome). Pain can be generally reproduced. Treatment includes local injection of anesthetic and steroids.

Trauma can many times be localized to a previous biopsy site. The etiology of this pain is uncertain but may be related to postsurgical/procedural infection or hematoma, or to placing the incision across Langer's lines.

An uncommon cause of mastalgia is cancer. Literature reports a 7–24% frequency of breast pain as a symptom of operable breast cancer. In a study of 232 patients with mastalgia, only one patient (0.5%) had cancer. The pain associated with a cancer is generally unilateral, persistent, and stable in its position.

The idea that mastalgia is psychosomatic can be traced back to Sir Astley Cooper in 1829; however, recent studies have shown no greater tendency toward mental illness in this population over other patients.

The management of mastalgia patients starts with excluding cancer and giving reassurance. This is the most successful treatment. For refractory pain, it is important to classify the type of pain, as this will affect future therapies. A pain chart is helpful.

For refractory cyclical pain, evening primrose oil (EPO) is a safe first option. This contains essential fatty acids and is believed to correct a deficiency that may lead to mastalgia. Side effects are rare. Second line therapy is danazol. This drug is limited by its side effects (weight gain, acne, hirsutism, and amenorrhea). Third line treatment is bromocriptine and is also limited by its side effects, especially nausea and vomiting. The most efficacious of these medications is danazol.

Noncyclical breast pain is less responsive to medications. Efficacy in descending order is danazol, bromocriptine, and EPO. In select instances, steroid and local anesthetic injections have proven beneficial.

Musculoskeletal pain and Tietze's syndrome can be treated with steroid/local anesthetic injections.

Surgery is a last resort option and in most cases, segmental resection of the breast is not sufficient. Mastectomy is required. Even with complete removal of the offending breast tissue, pain is persistent in 50% of the patients. In addition, complications may occur with the mastectomy and/or reconstruction that may result in additional pain.

Bibliography

Fentiman I. Management of breast pain. In: Harris JR, Lippman ME, Morrow M, et al. (eds.), *Diseases of the Breast*, 2nd ed. Philadelphia, PA: Lippincott, Williams & Wilkins, 2000, 57–61.

21. **(E)** Tamoxifen, a selective estrogen receptor (ER) agonist antagonist, first came into the market in the 1970s. It is a well-studied drug. The antagonist effects of tamoxifen are related to its competitive binding of the estrogen receptor, especially in breast tissue. This results in a reduced transcription of estrogen related proteins and effective blockade of cell cycle in G1. This in turn then translates to ineffective tumor growth.

Tamoxifen has apparent estrogen agonist effects on the endometrial lining, as shown by the increase in endometrial cancer found in women being treated with the drug. This risk is about 1%. The cancers are usually found in stage I and are very treatable. In addition, there is an increased risk of venous embolic phenomena that is related to the estrogen agonist effects. Tamoxifen also increases bone density and improves lipid profiles—both related to ER agonist activity. The major side effects that women complain about while taking tamoxifen are hot flashes and sleep disturbances—similar to menopausal symptoms attributed to decreased estrogen.

A landmark study for tamoxifen was the NSABP-14 trial. This evaluated 2644 patients with ER positive tumors that were also lymph node negative. These women were randomized to receive 5 years of tamoxifen versus a placebo. They found that for the ER positive cancer patients, both pre- and postmenopausal, 5 years of treatment with tamoxifen was associated with a 47% reduction in disease recurrence and a 26% improvement in overall mortality (Table 15-5).

These results lead to the NSABP-P1 trial. Over 13,000 high-risk women (Gail model >1.7% 5-year risk) were randomized to receive tamoxifen versus placebo for 5 years. The women in the tamoxifen arm had a 49% reduction in the risk of future cancer compared to the women in the placebo arm (Table 15-6).

Bibliography

Fisher B, Costantino JP, Wickerham DL, et al. Tamoxifen for prevention of breast cancer: report of the National Surgical Adjuvant Breast and Bowel Project P-1 Study. *J Natl Cancer Inst* 1998;90:1371–1388.

TABLE 15-5   NSABP-14 Results*

	7-year follow-up	Disease-free survival (%)	Recurrence-free survival (%)
Placebo	579	82	94
Tamoxifen	593	78 $P = 0.03$	92 $P = 0.07$

* No benefit of additional tamoxifen over 5 years of therapy. The decrease in DFS and RFS may be attributable to the agonist effects of tamoxifen.

TABLE 15-6   NSABP-P1 Results

	Breast cancer incidence	
Tamoxifen	89 new cases	49% reduction
		$P = <0.00001$
Placebo	175 new cases	

Fisher B, Kignam J, Bryant J, Wolmark N. Five versus more than five years of tamoxifen for lymph node-negative breast cancer: updated findings of the National Surgical Adjuvant Breast and Bowel Project B-14 randomized trial. *J Natl Cancer Inst* 2001;93:684–690.

Jordan VC. Chemoprevention. In: Harris JR, Lippman ME, Morrow M, et al. (eds.), *Diseases of the Breast*, 2nd ed. Philadelphia, PA: Lippincott, Williams & Wilkins, 2000, 266–267.

Kardinal C. Hormonal and endocrine therapy of breast cancer. In: Donegan W, Sprattt J (eds.), *Cancer of the Breast*, 5th ed. St. Louis, MO: W.B. Saunders, 2002, 709–718.

22. **(C)** LCIS is a noninvasive disease in the lobules or terminal ducts. Foote and Stewart first described it in 1941. The true incidence of LCIS in unknown as it is not detectable on routine screening measures, i.e., mammography or clinical breast examination. It is an incidental pathologic finding. LCIS is not seen macroscopically. Microscopically, it is often a solid proliferation of small cells with distinct borders and uniform, small nuclei. The cells often distend the lobules and terminal ducts.

Currently, LCIS is felt to be a risk factor for the future development of breast cancer. It is known from previous studies that a majority of women with LCIS do not develop cancer; when they do develop cancer, it is often infiltrating ductal. The risk is bilateral. The risk of future cancer is 1% per year indefinitely.

Therapy for LCIS is tamoxifen. Tamoxifen can decrease the risk of breast cancer by almost 50%. If there are contraindications to tamoxifen therapy, or if the patient is unable or unwilling to comply with close follow-up, bilateral prophylactic mastectomy with or without reconstruction is also an option.

There is no indication for reexcision, standard chemotherapy, radiation therapy, or mirror biopsies.

Bibliography

Morrow M. Lobular carcinoma in situ. In: Harris JR, Lippman ME, Morrow M, et al. (eds.), *Diseases of the Breast*, 2nd ed. Philadelphia, PA: Lippincott, Williams & Wilkins, 2000, 377–381.

Schell S, Copeland E. In situ carcinoma of the breast: ductal and lobular cell origin. In: Cameron J (ed.), *Current Surgical Therapy*, 7th ed. St. Louis, MO: Mosby, 2001, 725–727.

23. **(D)** Intracystic papillary carcinoma (IPC) is a noninvasive cancer. It represents 0.5–1% of all breast cancers. The mean age of diagnosis is 68 years. Eighty percent of patients have a palpable mass and 15% have nipple discharge. IPC is generally a low-grade carcinoma. It has high ER positivity. Often, DCIS or invasive cancers are found associated with the IPC (DCIS 46%, invasive cancer 38%). Because of this, FNA and CNB are not adequate in establishing a final diagnosis. Excisional biopsy is required. An analysis done at MD Anderson reviewed 40 patients who had IPC. No standard treatment was defined. In general, they found that associated risk of spread (metastasis) and subsequent mortality was related to the invasive component. In addition, they found that radiation therapy did not affect outcome.

Their conclusions were that IPC has an excellent prognosis. There is a low probability of axillary node involvement, and axillary node dissection is not warranted. Partial mastectomy appears to be adequate treatment. Radiation therapy is controversial. Additional treatment must be tailored to the associated pathology, i.e., DCIS or invasive breast cancer.

Bibliography

Damiani S, Eusebi V. Gross and microscopic pathology. In: Donegan W, Sprattt J (eds.), *Cancer of the Breast*, 5th ed. St. Louis, MO: W.B. Saunders, 2002, 354–355.

24. **(B)** Hormonal replacement therapy has become a hot topic in the past few years. This can be closely related to the results of the Heart and Estrogen Replacement Studies (HERS I and HERS II) and to the Women's Health Initiative (WHI) results. These studies were both published in *JAMA* in early July 2002.

The HERS I and II studies examined 2763 postmenopausal women with known cardiac disease. The initial study was conducted over 4.1 years, and the follow-up study was continued for a total of 6.8 years. The women were randomized to receive estrogen/progesterone or placebo. The results focused initially on the cardiovascular effects. Overall, they found no long-term cardiovascular benefits. In fact, the relative risk in the first year of therapy was statistically higher in the hormone group. Additional effects were further examined in the follow-up study. This showed that there is a two- to threefold increase in deep vein thrombosis (DVT) and pulmonary embolism in the hormonal group (5.9 vs. 2.8 per 1000 person years, $P = 0.003$). There is a threefold increase in biliary disease in the hormone treated group (19.1 vs. 6.2 per 1000 person years, $P = 0.002$). Hip fractures were also elevated in the hormone treated group; however, this was not significant. In addition, there was also an increase in breast cancer for the hormone treated group, but this was not significant (5.9 vs. 4.7 per 1000 person years, $P = 0.26$).

The WHI was published a week later in *JAMA*; 16,608 postmenopausal women were enrolled in the study. The women were randomized to receive either estrogen/progesterone or placebo for the duration of the study. The study was stopped after 5.2 years when an arbitrarily set risk/benefit ratio outcome was surpassed in regards to breast cancer. The study outcomes for the hormone treated group showed a twofold increase of DVT; a reduced incidence of hip fractures (10 vs. 15 per 10,000 person years); no significant increase in coronary heart disease (37 vs. 30 per 10,000 person years, $P = 0.5$). The study reported a 26% increase in breast cancer in the women treated with the combination estrogen/progesterone therapy (38 vs. 30 per 10,000 person years). Although this was only nominally significant, if you extrapolate this to the number of women who develop breast cancer every year, the number is quite large. Interestingly, the increase is 15% if the patient takes hormone replacement therapy (HRT) for less than 5 years and jumps to 53% if the treatment is longer than 5 years.

Recent studies show that bone metastasis are actually decreased in patients who develop breast cancer and are taking HRT. This may be related to the normalization of bone metabolism secondary to estrogen.

There are many theories but the exact mechanism of estrogen and breast cancer has yet to be elucidated. The theories can be divided into direct and indirect influences. The direct mechanisms include induction of enzymes and proteins in nucleic acid synthesis, the activation of oncogenes, and the excess stimulation of an organ that is normally under its control. The indirect theories relate mostly to the production of growth factors.

Aromatase promotors vary their expression in different tissues. Promotor I.4 is found in normal breast tissue, whereas promotor II and I.3 are found in breast cancer. The latter two promotors are more active and result in an increase of aromatase mRNA. This may then contribute to growth of breast cancer in an autocrine or paracrine manner. In this manner, the aromatase gene may act as an oncogene. Another oncogene important in breast cancer is p53. With loss of this suppressor gene, there is failure to down regulate the ER or failure to suppress the division of cells expressing estrogen receptors.

The metabolites of estrogen also have differing estrogenic strengths. 4-Hydroxyestrone and 16α-hydroxyestradiol are estrogenic and thought to be carcinogenic. The 2-hydroxy and 4-hydroxy metabolites are further converted to anticarcinogenic methoxylated metabolites. Thus, depending on which pathway the breakdown of estrogen takes, there may be an increase or decrease in estrogen stimulation activity (Fig. 15-6).

Cumulative estrogen exposure has also been shown to be important in breast cancer risk. Using bone density studies and mammographic breast density, lifetime cumulative estrogen exposure can be estimated. Patients in the highest quartile of both subgroups have increased breast cancer risk.

Current recommendations of HRT are first and foremost to tailor the therapy for each individual woman. HRT is no longer indicated for treating or preventing cardiovascular disease. It is appropriate in the treatment of vasomotor symptoms associated with menopause. The duration of therapy should be less than 5 years. It is important to realize that the above studies do not apply to surgically menopausal women. In addition, they only examined combination estrogen/progesterone therapy; the role of unopposed estrogen is not known.

Bibliography

Willett W. Epidemiology and nongenetic causes of breast cancer. In: Harris JR, Lippman ME, Morrow M, et al. (eds.), *Diseases of the Breast*, 2nd ed. Philadelphia, PA: Lippincott, Williams & Wilkins, 2000, 189–191.

Rossouw J, Anderson G, et al. Risks and benefits of estrogen plus progestin in healthy postmenopausal women: principal results from the women's health initiative randomized controlled trial. *J Am Med Assoc* 2002;3:321–333.

Hulley G, et al. Cardiovascular disease outcomes during 6.8 years of hormone therapy: heart and estrogen/progestin replacement study follow-up (HERSII). *J Am Med Assoc* 2002;1:49–57.

Hulley G, et al. Noncardiovascular disease outcomes during 6.8 years of hormone therapy: heart and estrogen/progestin replacement study follow-up (HERSII). *J Am Med Assoc* 2002;1:58–66.

Clemons M, Goss P. Estrogen and the risk of breast cancer. *N Engl J Med* 2001;4:276–285.

25. **(B)** The overwhelming majority of newly diagnosed breast cancers are sporadic. Approximately 5% are felt related to BRCA-1 or BRCA-2 mutations. Hereditary breast cancers are more likely to occur at younger age, involve both sides or include multiple organs (especially ovary) than sporadic cases. Inheritance pattern is autosomal dominant with variable penetrance. Lifetime breast cancer risk associated with BRCA-1 or BRCA-2 is estimated to be 85%. Management options thus include screening with self-examination, mammography, and even breast magnetic resonance imaging (MRI) beginning at age 25. Though controversial, bilateral prophylactic mastectomy, chemoprevention with tamoxifen or aromatase inhibitors, and

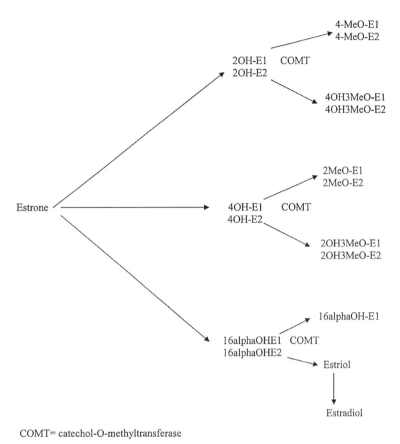

COMT= catechol-O-methyltransferase

FIG. 15-6   Estrogen breakdown

contralateral prophylactic mastectomy when managing ipsilateral breast cancer should be considered.

Bibliography

Easton DF. Breast and ovarian cancer incidence in BRCA1 mutation carriers. *Am J Hum Genet* 1995;56:265.

Ford D, Easton DF. The genetics of breast and ovarian cancer. *Br J Cancer* 1995;72:805.

Kriege M, Brekelmans C, Boetes C, et al. Efficacy of MRI and mammography for breast cancer screening in women with a familial or genetic predisposition. *N Engl J Med* 2004;351: 427–436.

Lynch HT, Marcus JM, Lynch JF, et al. Breast cancer genetics. *The Breast: Comprehensive Management of Benign and Malignant Disorders*, 3rd ed. St. Louis, MO: W.B. Saunders, 2004, 380–392.

Scheuer L. Outcome of preventive surgery and screening for breast and ovarian cancer in BRCA mutation carriers. *J Clin Oncol* 2002;20:1260.

26. **(E)** The initial surgical management of clinically localized breast cancer must address the primary cancer in the breast and sample axillary lymph nodes for staging.

This may be accomplished by partial mastectomy with sentinel lymph node biopsy, partial mastectomy with axillary lymph node dissection, or modified radical mastectomy. Alternative means of primary tumor therapy including laser, radiofrequency, or cryablation are under investigation but not clinically applicable at present. As multicentricity of breast cancers is relatively high (approximately 25%) and excised tumors may return, there is a significant risk of ipsilateral recurrence of cancer following a partial mastectomy. This risk can be significantly reduced by complete removal of the primary tumor to clear margins and the addition of postoperative radiotherapy. Radiation has reduced the incidence of ipsilateral recurrence following partial mastectomy from 39 to 14% after 20 years of follow-up in the NSABP B-04 trial. Thus, radiation therapy should generally be considered essential in the breast-conserving treatment of cancer.

Systemic chemotherapy is generally considered useful in the management of breast cancer when the reduction of recurrence risk is at least 3% or more over

5 years. This assessment of recurrence risk depends on review of known prognostic factors. Most patients with involved axillary lymph nodes and those with node-negative disease but primary tumors over 2 cm in diameter should be considered for systemic therapy.

Bibliography

Dowlatshahi K, Singletary SE, Staren E. Image-guided ablation of breast tumors. *Contemp Surg* 2002;58:61–71.

Fisher B, Anderson S, Bryant J, et al. Twenty year follow up of a randomized trial comparing total mastectomy, lumpectomy, and lumpectomy plus irradiation for the treatment of invasive breast cancer. *N Engl J Med* 2002; 347:1233–1240.

Gump FE. The extent and distribution of cancer in breasts with palpable primary tumors. *Ann Surg* 1986;204:384.

Lippman ME, Hayes DF. Adjuvant therapy for all patients with breast cancer? *J Natl Cancer Inst* 2001;93:80.

Singletary SE. Systemic treatment after sentinel lymph node biopsy in breast cancer: who, what and why? *J Am Coll Surg* 2001;192:220–228.

27. **(B)** Currently, the most widely used description of breast cancer staging is the TNM system. This has been popularized by the AJCC, sponsored by the American Cancer Society and the American College of Surgeons. The system demands an assessment of the primary tumor, regional lymph nodes, and any distant metastasis. Defining various groups of TNM stages with similar prognoses allows appropriate consensus treatment recommendations. Further, the system aids the design, conduct, and analysis of clinical trials. The AJCC TNM Clinical Staging System is as follows:

1. Primary tumor (T)

   - Tx: primary tumor cannot be assessed
   - T0: no primary tumor
   - Tis: carcinoma *in situ*
   - T1: tumor ≤ 2 cm.
   - T2: tumor > 2 cm. but ≤ 5 cm.
   - T3: tumor > 5 cm.
   - T4: tumor with extension to chest wall, skin edema or ulceration or inflammatory carcinoma

2. Regional lymph nodes (N)

   - Nx: regional lymph nodes cannot be assessed
   - N0: no regional lymph node metastasis
   - N1: metastases to mobile axillary lymph nodes
   - N2: metastases to fixed, matted or clinically apparent axillary lymph nodes or internal mammary nodes
   - N3: metastases to axillary and infraclavicular lymph nodes, clinically apparent internal mammary nodes or supraclavicular lymph nodes

3. Distant metastasis

   - Mx: distant metastasis cannot be assessed
   - M0: no distant metastasis
   - M1: distant metastasis

4. Stage grouping

   - Stage 0: TisN0M0
   - Stage 1: T1N0M0
   - Stage 2A: T0N1M0, T1N1M0, T2N0M0
   - Stage 2B: T2N1M0, T3N0M0
   - Stage 3A: T0N2M0, T1N2M0, T2N2M0, T3N1M0, T3N2M0
   - Stage 3B: T4N0M0, T4N1M0, T4N2M0
   - Stage 3C: AnyTN3M0
   - Stage 4: AnyT AnyN M1

Used with the permission of the American Joint Committee on Cancer (AJCC), Chicago, Illinois. The original source for this material is the *AJCC Cancer Staging Manual, Sixth Edition* (2002) published by Springer-Verlag New York, www.springer-ny.com.

Bibliography

Beahrs O, Hensen D, Hutter R. American Joint Committee on Cancer. *Manual for Staging Breast Cancer*, 6th ed. Philadelphia, PA: JB Lippincott, 2002.

Iglehart JD, Kaelin CM. Diseases of the breast. *Sabiston Textbook of Surgery*, 17th ed. Philadelphia, PA: Elsevier, 2004, 893–895.

28. **(C)** Advanced breast cancer poses a serious threat to life by means of systemic disease. Even if micrometastases are undetectable by diagnostic testing, the high rate of distant treatment failure suggests their presence. Therefore, after confirming the diagnosis, therapy is usually initiated with systemic treatment. Chemotherapy followed by surgery has been demonstrated to yield improved local control and survival. Thus, initial treatment of stage 3 and stage 4 breast cancer including inflammatory cancer is by systemic chemotherapy.

Bibliography

Brito RA. Long term results of combined modality therapy for locally advanced breast cancer with ipsilateral supraclavicular metastases: The University of Texas M.D. Anderson Cancer Center Experience. *J Clin Oncol* 2001;19:628.

Hortobagyi GN, Ames FC, Buzdar AU. Management of stage III primary breast cancer with primary chemotherapy, surgery, and radiation therapy. *Cancer* 1988;62:2507–2513.

Hunt KK, Ames FC, Singletary SE. Locally advanced non-inflammatory breast cancer. *Surg Clin North Am* 1996;76: 393–397.

29. **(D)** Sentinel lymph node biopsy has emerged as a safe and accurate approach to assessing axillary lymph nodes for metastases from breast cancer. The successful identification of one or more sentinel lymph nodes is reported to be between 85 and 100%. Sensitivity and specificity for the procedure is 90–100%, as compared to completion axillary lymph node dissection. A serious reservation has been the possibility of skip metastases involving nonsentinel lymph nodes (or false negative sentinel node), but this has been demonstrated to occur in less than 10% of patients. Several series have revealed positive sentinel nodes in T1 tumors (less than 2 cm), ranging from 5 to 44%. Multiple sentinel lymph nodes are common, with an average yield of two to three nodes. The technique of sentinel node biopsy involves injection of dye in either a subareolar or peritumoral location. The dye used is either radiocolloid or 1% isosulfan blue. The optimal interval from injection to identification of the sentinel node in surgery is approximately 2 h for the radioisotope, as opposed to 5 min for the isosulfan blue.

Bibliography

Derossis AM, Fey J, Yeung H, et al. A trend analysis of the relative value of blue dye and isotope localization in 2000 consecutive cases of sentinel node biopsy for breast cancer. *J Am Coll Surg* 2001;193:473–478.

Grube BJ, Giuliano AE. Lymphatic mapping and sentinel lymphadenectomy for breast cancer. *The Breast: Comprehensive Management of Benign and Malignant Disorders*, 3rd ed. St. Louis, MO: W.B. Saunders, 2004, 1041–1061.

Tuttle TM, Zogakis TG, Dunst CM, et al. A review of technical aspects of sentinel lymph node identification for breast cancer. *J Am Coll Surg* 2002;195:261–267.

Veronesi U, Pahanelli G, Viale G, et al. A randomized comparison of sentinel node biopsy with routine axillary dissection in breast cancer. *N Engl J Med* 2003;349:546–553.

30. **(E)** The optimal management of the axilla following a positive sentinel lymph node biopsy is an area of controversy. Axillary lymph node metastases imply systemic disease and should be treated with systemic therapy to improve long-term survival. The effect of such systemic therapy on axillary recurrence rate is controversial. Axillary recurrence of cancer has been variably reported, ranging 5–21% if no further locoregional treatment is rendered. Both axillary dissection and radiation have been effective at reducing the recurrence risk to less than 5%.

Bibliography

Guenther JM, Hansen NM, DiFronzo LA, et al. Axillary dissection is not required for all patients with breast cancer and positive sentinel nodes. *Arch Surg* 2003;138:52–56.

Iglehart JD, Kaelin CM. Diseases of the breast. *Sabiston Textbook of Surgery*, 17th ed. Philadelphia, PA: Elsevier, 2004, 904–905.

Singletary SE. Systemic treatment after sentinel lymph node biopsy in breast cancer: who, what and why? *J Am Coll Surg* 2001;192:220–228.

Wolff AC, Stearns V, Davidson NE. Adjuvant systemic therapy of breast cancer. *The Breast: Comprehensive Management of Benign and Malignant Disorders*, 3rd ed. St. Louis, MO: W.B. Saunders, 2004, 1193–1195.

31. **(E)** Cystosarcoma phyllodes is the most common neoplasm of nonepithelial origin in the breast. Phyllodes tumors of the breast may present as benign, borderline, or malignant tumors that grossly have an appearance similar to fibroadenomas, often initially resulting in misdiagnosis prior to histopathologic review. Moreover, the benign and malignant forms can be difficult to differentiate, as histologically the two may be identical except for differences in proliferative activity. When this is the case identification is based solely on cellular mitotic activity. However, sarcomatous elements are present in overwhelmingly malignant tumors simplifying their identification.

Controversy has surrounded proper treatment, especially since there are benign, malignant, and borderline forms. They can be any size, but frequently are large with a median size of 5 cm. Minimal treatment of small tumors should include local excision with at least a 2 cm margin of normal tissue. Enucleated tumors, often misdiagnosed as fibroadenomas, are inadequately treated and should undergo reexcision to remove all the surrounding breast tissue and scar to obtain clearly adequate tissue margins. Large tumors should be treated by total mastectomy, although axillary dissection is generally not indicated.

Phyllodes tumor is an exclusive tumor of the female breast.

Bibliography

Iglehart JD, Kaelin CM. Diseases of the breast. *Sabiston Textbook of Surgery*, 17th ed. Philadelphia, PA: Elsevier, 2004, 904–905.

Solorzano CC, Ahearne PM, Leach SD, et al. Invasive breast cancer. In: Feig BW, Berger DH, Fuhrman GM (eds.), *The M.D. Anderson Surgical Oncology Handbook*, 3rd ed., 2003, 14–40.

32. **(B)** The histologic picture consists of many clusters of epithelial cells forming islands of neoplastic cells but maintaining a lobular architecture. It occurs more often in premenopausal women and does not form a palpable mass. It is most commonly found as an incidental finding on biopsy, as it does not have any mammographic findings.

Lobular carcinoma *in situ* carries a risk of developing into an invasive ductal carcinoma in 10–35% of patients over a period of 15–20 years.

Because the risk of subsequent breast cancer is almost the same for both breasts, mirror image biopsies of the opposite breast are not indicated.

Histologic examinations are generally favorable and deaths are unusual in women with appropriate medical care. Any treatment of *in situ* carcinoma is aimed at preventing invasive disease.

Treatment options include close observation or pharmacologic prophylaxis. A 5-year course of tamoxifen has been shown to reduce the relative risk of invasive cancer by 56% in women with LCIS. Surgical options such as bilateral mastectomy or breast-conserving surgery are considered only in special circumstances in which the patient may have multiple risk factors.

Bibliography

Meric F, Robinson EK, Hunt KK. Noninvasive breast cancer. In: Feig BW, Berger DH, Fuhrman GM (eds.), *The M.D. Anderson Surgical Oncology Handbook*, 3rd ed., 2003, 1–13.

Schell SR, Copeland III EM. In situ carcinoma of the breast: ductal and lobular cell origin. In: Cameron JL (ed.), *Current Surgical Therapy*, 7th ed., 2001, 722–726.

33. **(C)** Ductal carcinoma *in situ* of the breast consists of the clonal proliferation of cells that appear malignant and that accumulate within the lumens of the mammary duct. There is no evidence of invasion beyond the epithelial basement membrane into the adjacent breast stroma. This lesion, which is a precursor to invasive ductal carcinoma, is frequently diagnosed on screening mammography. The incidence of DCIS is increasing, and, because of screening mammography, the disease is diagnosed in an increasing proportion of asymptomatic patients. The most common clinical presentation is that of calcifications on mammography. Approximately 47,000 cases of DCIS will be diagnosed this year. DCIS accounts for nearly 20% of all breast cancers detected by screening (1 case of DCIS detected per 1300 screening mammograms) in North America. DCIS will evolve into an invasive ductal carcinoma in approximately 30–50% of the patients over 10 years.

The options for surgical treatment include simple mastectomy or breast-conserving surgery. After breast-conserving surgery, radiotherapy is administered in tangential fields to the whole breast. According to the results of NSABP-B17, breast-conserving therapy is an effective option in the management of DCIS. The use of radiotherapy after lumpectomy significantly decreases the rate of recurrence. The presence of comedo necrosis and surgical margin involvement are the most commonly used predictors of the likelihood of recurrence. If relapse occurs after breast-conserving therapy, the chance of an invasive component is approximately 50%. The risk for in-breast recurrence at 5 years after breast-conserving therapy is approximately 8%.

There is no role for chemotherapy in the treatment of DCIS. Neither dissection of axillary lymph nodes nor mapping of sentinel lymph nodes is routinely warranted in patients with DCIS, owing to the very low incidence of axillary metastases. Intense surveillance needs to be maintained for a patient's lifetime.

Bibliography

Burstein HJ, Polyak K, Wong JS, Lester SC, Kaelin CM. Ductal carcinoma in situ of the breast. *N Engl J Med* 2004; 350(14):1430–1441.

Meric F, Robinson EK, Hunt KK. Noninvasive breast cancer. In: Feig BW, Berger DH, Fuhrman GM (eds.), *The M.D. Anderson Surgical Oncology Handbook*, 3rd ed., 2003, 1–13.

Schell SR, Copeland III EM. In situ carcinoma of the breast: ductal and lobular cell origin. In: Cameron JL (ed.), *Current Surgical Therapy*, 7th ed., 2001, 722–726.

34. **(D)** Male breast carcinoma remains a rare cause of cancer in men, accounting for less than 1% of cases of cancer in men. The incidence of this disease has remained stable, at approximately 1400–2000 new cases per year over the past several decades. The average age at diagnosis is 68 years, which is older than the age of diagnosis seen in women.

At 10%, the proportion of noninvasive carcinomas in men is much higher than that of women. This is likely due to the ease of detection of smaller breast lesions in the comparatively smaller quantity of tissue seen in the male breast. The most common histologic subtype of invasive carcinomas remains invasive ductal carcinoma. This accounts for more than 80% of all invasive breast lesions in men. All subtypes of invasive carcinoma found in women have been reported in men. Nearly all of the noninvasive lesions in men are DCIS, but unlike females, DCIS in males is almost always low-to-intermediate grade and in more than 75% it is of the papillary subtype. The lack of terminal lobules in the male breast results in minimal incidence of lobular carcinoma *in situ* and invasive lobular carcinoma. Review of reported literature has shown a higher incidence of hormone receptors than in women. Approximately 74% of male breast lesions are shown to be progesterone receptor positive and 81% are found to be estrogen receptor positive.

Significant prognostic indicators in men include lymph node status, tumor size, histologic grade, and hormone receptor status. The most indicative negative prognostic indicator in male breast cancer remains lymph node status. Staging and survival outcomes are similar to those found in women.

The most common presenting sign in men with breast lesions is a painless subareolar mass (50–97%). Other common presenting signs and symptoms include nipple retraction (10–51%), local pain (4–20%), and nipple ulceration (4–17%). Male patients who present with a breast lesion should undergo a thorough physical examination to evaluate for multiple lesions, contralateral disease, and lymph node involvement. Carcinomas can be differentiated of mammogram by their irregular boarder and spiculated margins, but the diagnostic use of mammograms remains limited in men because of the paucity of tissue in the male breast. All lesions should have a fine needle aspiration performed to evaluate tumor histology and hormone status.

Treatment of patients with nonmetastatic disease involves removal of all breast tissue and lymph node dissection. The local recurrence and survival rates are similar between radical mastectomy and modified radical mastectomy, as such, the recommended treatment is the less morbid modified radical mastectomy. The small quantity of male breast tissue and the need for lymph node dissection in invasive disease limits the use of breast-conservation therapy.

Adjuvant chemotherapy and radiation therapy in male invasive breast cancer remains unclear. The low incidence of the disease makes it difficult to determine which patients would have increased risk of recurrence and benefit from adjuvant therapy. Most centers use the same guidelines in men as they do for women and recommend adjuvant chemotherapy if lymph nodes are involved or if the tumor is greater than 1 cm and radiation therapy for tumors that are T3 or T4 or if >4 lymph nodes are involved. All male patients with hormone receptor positive lesions benefit with adjuvant tamoxifen treatment for 5 years.

For metastatic disease of hormone receptor positive lesions the mainstay of treatment is hormonal therapy. First line treatment is tamoxifen. If there is evidence of disease progression, second line hormonal agents can be added including aminoglutethimide, progestins, antiandrogens, GnRH agonists, steroid, or androgens. Chemotherapy is recommended for receptor negative metastatic lesions.

Bibliography

Dickerson R, Lippman ME. Pathogenesis of breast cancer. In: Harris J, Lippman ME, Morrow M, et al. (eds.), *Disease of the Breast*, 2nd ed., vol. 200. Philadelphia, PA: Lippincott, Williams & Wilkins, 281–302.

Giordano SH, Buzdar AU, Hortobagyi GN. Breast cancer in men. *Ann Intern Med* 2002;137:678–687.

Winchester DJ. Male breast cancer. In: Cameron JL (ed.), *Current Surgical Therapy*, 7th ed., 2001, 732–734.

Winchester DJ. Male breast cancer: a multi-institutional challenge. *Cancer* 1998;83:399–402.

35. (C)

36. (A)

Explanations 35 and 36

After cervical, breast cancer remains the second most common malignancy encountered in pregnancy. During pregnancy, breast cancer most commonly presents as a painless mass, in up to 95% of patients. The differential diagnosis of breast lesions during pregnancy includes cancer, lactating ademona, fibroadenoma, cystic disease, lobular hyperplasia, galactocele, abscess, and lipoma. Eighty percent of all breast masses found during pregnancy are benign.

The interpretation of diagnostic tests and physical examination becomes difficult during pregnancy as breast weight and firmness increase. Ultrasound remains the best first imaging choice of the pregnancy patient and can differentiate between cystic and solid masses. Mammographic evaluation during pregnancy is a comparatively benign radiographic test, exposing the fetus to only 0.0004 Gy. Interpretation is often difficult with the density changes of the pregnant breast, as a result there is a high false negative rate. MRI may prove to be a useful imaging tool in the pregnant patient, but currently the risks and benefits are undetermined. Radiographs and bone scan imagings searching for metastatic disease in pregnant patients without symptoms or laboratory abnormalities remains low yield.

Biopsy is essential in the evaluation of breast lesions in the pregnant patient. It can be done by core or fine needle aspiration, as most patients present with palpable, painless masses. The pathologist must be made aware of the patient's pregnancy and trimester to avoid misdiagnosis secondary to breast changes. Lactation must be stopped prior to the biopsy to avoid milk fistulas. This can be done with ice packs and breast bindings.

The histology of breast cancer in pregnancy parallels that of the nonpregnant female. There is a higher incidence of lymph node metastases and lower incidence of positive hormone receptor status. The cause of this is multifactorial and may include delay in diagnosis, breast cancer at a younger age, breast hypervascularity and physiologic changes associated with pregnancy (hormone level, down regulation of hormone receptors, and immunosuppressed state).

Treatment of breast cancer in the pregnant patients involves a thorough understanding of the risks involved with each treatment modalitity, in each trimester of pregnancy. The clinician must also comprehend the consequences of delaying treatment. Surgery remains the mainstay of treatment. The risks of surgery involve preterm labor, spontaneous abortion, and congenital abnormalities. Surgery can be performed safely at any stage of pregnancy. Adjuvant therapy with irradiation and chemotherapy are conclusively linked to birth defects. The teratogenicity and increased likelihood of newborn malignancy with irradiation is cumulative dose dependent and it is contraindicated during any part of the pregnancy. Chemotherapy has the greatest teratogenic risk during the first trimester and is recommended for use only after 12 weeks.

The treatment of stage I and II lesions during the first trimester should be treated with modified radical mastectomy, as it eliminates the need for postoperative chemotherapy or irradiation, neither of which should be offered in the first trimester.

Patients with stage I and II lesions presenting in the second and third trimester can again be offered modified radical mastectomy. Another option would be to offer breast-conservation therapy, followed immediately by chemotherapy and postpartum radiation therapy. There is no benefit survival or recurrence difference between modified radical mastectomy and breast-conservation therapy in the pregnant patient.

Prognosis of breast cancer in pregnant patients in early stages (I and II) is similar to age-matched nonpregnant patients. Decreased survival is noted in pregnant patients in later stages. Patients should be advised to avoid pregnancy for 2 years following treatment for stage I and II cancers, 5 years for stage III, and to avoid childbearing for stage IV. Women should also avoid breastfeeding during chemotherapy.

Termination of pregnancy has not been shown to increase maternal survival.

Bibliography

Byrd BJ, Bayer D, Robertson J. Treatment of breast tumors associated with pregnancy or lactation. *Ann Surg* 1962;155:940–947.

Lishner M. Cancer in pregnancy. *Ann Oncol* 2003;14 (Suppl 3): 31–36.

Solorzano CC, Ahearne PM, Leach SD, et al. Invasive breast cancer. In: Feig BW, Berger DH, Fuhrman GM (eds.), *The M.D. Anderson Surgical Oncology* Handbook, 3rd ed., 2003, 14–40.

Woo JC, Yu T, Hurd TC. Breast cancer in pregnancy. *Arch Surg* 2003;138:91–98.

CHAPTER 16

Thyroid and Parathyroid

Amit D. Tevar and Dinesh P. Tevar

Questions

1. Fine needle aspiration (FNA) cytology of a thyroid Hurthle cell neoplasm will most likely show which of the following reports?

   (A) nondiagnostic/unsatisfactory
   (B) benign nonneoplastic
   (C) inconclusive
   (D) malignant

2. Which of the following is the most accurate statement concerning the accuracy of FNA in thyroid nodules?

   (A) false positive rate of 5%
   (B) false negative rate of 15%
   (C) use of ultrasound can decrease the rate of unsatisfactory results
   (D) FNA findings classified as inconclusive have a malignancy rate of 15%
   (E) FNA diagnosis of follicular neoplasm without atypia is malignant in 20%

3. Which of the following ultrasound findings are most suggestive of malignancy in a 55-year-old male with risk factors and a nonpalpable thyroid lesion?

   (A) anechoic
   (B) hypoechoic
   (C) hyperechoic

4. A 35-year-old female presents with a painless midline mass above the hyoid bone for the past 4 months. She denies any history of neck radiation or previous surgery. The mass is 2 × 2 cm on physical examination and elevates on deglutination. What is the most common malignancy associated with this condition?

   (A) follicular
   (B) Hurthle cell
   (C) papillary
   (D) medullary
   (E) anaplastic

5. A motivational speaker has a right lobe thyroidectomy for papillary carcinoma. Postoperatively he notices that he is no longer able to project his voice. The ligation of which vessel resulted in his nerve injury?

   (A) inferior thyroid artery
   (B) superior thyroid artery
   (C) inferior thyroid vein
   (D) middle thyroid vein
   (E) middle thyroid artery

6. Which of the following is the most common postoperative complication seen in thyroid surgery?

   (A) recurrent laryngeal nerve injury
   (B) superior laryngeal nerve injury
   (C) transient hypoparathyroidism
   (D) permanent hypoparathyroidism
   (E) airway obstruction

7. Which of the following is *not* a manifestation or associated condition with Graves hyperthyroidism?

   (A) diffuse goiter
   (B) ophthalmopathy
   (C) localized dermopathy
   (D) diffuse arthropathy
   (E) Addison's disease

8. Which of the following statements about iodine-131 is false?

   (A) It is trapped and organified by the thyroid gland.
   (B) It may destroy residual occult microscopic foci of papillary and follicular malignancies.
   (C) There is no increase incidence of malignancy associated with radiation exposure.
   (D) It can safely be used in pregnancy.
   (E) It is *not* trapped in thyroid metastases and lymphoma.

9. A 45-year-old female presents with a 2 cm nodule of the upper pole of the left lobe of the thyroid gland. There are no palpable lymph nodes and no other lesions are found during ultrasound evaluation. FNA show this to be a well-differentiated papillary carcinoma. What is the most appropriate treatment?

(A) total thyroidectomy
(B) total thyroidectomy with postoperative iodine-131 therapy
(C) lobectomy with 1 cm margins
(D) lobectomy with postoperative iodine-131 therapy
(E) lobectomy with ultrasound examination of the contralateral lobe
(F) observation with interval ultrasound examination and thyroglobulin measurement

10. A 35-year-old woman is found to have a solitary, painless 3 cm thyroid lesion. FNA finds this to be a follicular lesion. What is the most appropriate step in the management of this patient?

(A) total thyroidectomy with iodine-131 therapy
(B) magnetic resonance imaging of the lesion
(C) ipsilateral thyroid lobectomy
(D) open excisional biopsy with permanent section pathology
(E) ultrasound examination of the contralateral lobe

11. A 20-year-old marfanoid male with bilateral thyroid tender lesions has evidence of submucosal neuromas, diarrhea, and facial flushing. A FNA of the nodules is performed. What measurement on the FNA sample would aid in making the diagnosis?

(A) calcitonin
(B) vanillylmandelic acid (VMA)
(C) carcinoembryonic antigen
(D) A and C
(E) all of the above

12. The patient described above has FNA which demonstrates medullary thyroid carcinoma. Which is the recommended treatment after the possibility of pheochromocytoma is definitely excluded?

(A) ipsilateral thyroid lobectomy with ultrasound examination of the contralateral lobe
(B) total thyroidectomy with postoperative iodine-131 treatment

(C) total thyroidectomy with postoperative calcitonin monitoring
(D) total thyroidectomy with postoperative chemoradition therapy
(E) excisional biopsy with permanent pathology examination

13. Which of the following is the most common site of origin for isolated metastatic lesions to the thyroid?

(A) kidney
(B) breast
(C) colon
(D) soft tissue
(E) lung

14. A 31-year-old female develops sudden onset of neck pain radiating to the jaw with a temperature of 40°C after recovering from a "sore throat." Thyroid function test are normal and the white blood cell count is 22,000. There are no areas of fluctuance found on physical examination. What is the most appropriate form of treatment?

(A) total thyroidectomy
(B) operative incision and drainage of the infected segment
(C) intravenous antibiotics
(D) high dose immunosuppressants

15. A 56-year-old female is found to have symptoms of hypothyroidism with a painless, enlarged, firm, rubbery thyroid gland. FNA shows diffuse infiltration of the gland with lymphocytes and plasma cells. Which of the following best describes her condition?

(A) Hashimoto's thyroiditis
(B) acute suppurative thyroiditis
(C) Riedel's thyroiditis
(D) painless thyroiditis
(E) subacute de Quervain thyroiditis

16. Which of the following medications do *not* result in increased thyroxine binding globulin levels?

(A) tamoxifen
(B) lithium
(C) heroin
(D) mitotane
(E) estrogen

17. A 27-year-old female with a history of insulin-dependent diabetes mellitus develops symptoms of hyperthyroidism 3 months after delivery of her first child. Three months later she develops symptoms of hypothyroidism that persist. A small, nontender, firm goiter is present. What is the best method of treatment for her disease?

    (A) iodine-131 treatment
    (B) total thyroidectomy
    (C) FNA
    (D) thyroid hormone replacement
    (E) high dose steroids

18. Where does the arterial supply to the superior and inferior parathyroids originate from?

    (A) superior thyroid artery
    (B) inferior thyroid artery
    (C) external carotid artery
    (D) internal carotid artery
    (E) common carotid artery

19. Which of the following organs is *not* directly acted on by parathyroid hormone (PTH) to increase calcium levels?

    (A) small bowel
    (B) kidney
    (C) bone

20. A 45-year-old female without history of previous hospitalization or significant medical history presents to her primary care physician with complaints of headache, lethargy, and constipation. Electrocardiogram findings show shortened QT interval and a widened T wave. Which of the following is the most likely etiology of her disease?

    (A) vitamin D toxicity
    (B) malignancy
    (C) primary hyperparathyroidism
    (D) sarcoidosis
    (E) secondary hyperparathyroidism

21. Which of the following is *not* an acceptable treatment for hypercalcemia?

    (A) intravenous hydration
    (B) furosemide
    (C) thiazide
    (D) biphosphonate
    (E) calcitonin

22. A 33-year-old female has had elevated serum calcium levels since birth. Further evaluation demonstrates a normal PTH and hypocalciuria. She denies any symptoms. What would be the most appropriate treatment?

    (A) 3 1/2 parathyroidectomy
    (B) technetium-99m sestamibi scintigraphy
    (C) biphosphonate
    (D) observation
    (E) single adenoma parathyroidectomy

23. A 47-year-old female develops symptoms of hypercalcemia and further workup demonstrates her to have primary hyperparathyroidism. Surgical treatment shows the following gross and permanent histologic sections (Figs. 16-1 and 16-2). What is the most likely etiology of her disease?

    (A) single adenoma
    (B) double adenoma
    (C) hyperplasia
    (D) carcinoma

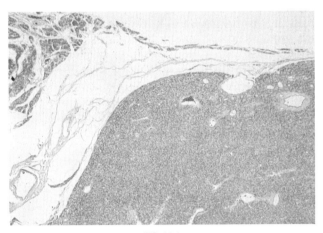

FIG. 16-1

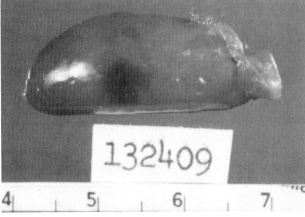

FIG. 16-2

24. A 55-year-old woman with primary hyperparathy-roidism is noted to have an asymptomatic kidney stone noted on an abdominal radiograph. What is the next step in her management?

(A) cystoscopy

(B) serum oxalate measurement

(C) parathyroid localization studies

(D) bilateral neck exploration

(E) observation

25. A patient with primary hyperparathyroidism under-goes surgical exploration. A single irregularly enlarged parathyroid gland is found that invades into sur-rounding tissue. The specimen histology is shown in Fig. 16-3. What is the most appropriate surgical resection?

(A) single parathyroidectomy, with visual inspection of the other three glands

(B) subtotal parathyroidectomy

(C) gland resection, with ipsilateral thyroid lobectomy

(D) total parathyroidectomy with reimplantation

(E) no surgical resection

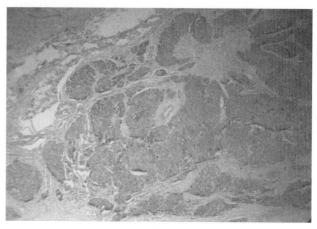

FIG. 16-3

26. Surgical exploration for a patient with primary hyper-parathyroidism reveals all four glands to be enlarged. What is the most appropriate way to manage this?

(A) closure with localization study

(B) incision biopsy of all glands

(C) subtotal parathyroidectomy

(D) excision of the largest enlarged gland

(E) selective venous PTH sampling

Answers and Explanations

1. **(C)** FNA has revolutionized the diagnosis of thyroid nodules. It remains an economic and elementary diagnostic tool that can be performed in the office by the surgeon who would perform the resection if needed.

   The procedure can be performed in the office setting. Strict aseptic technique must be used. A 25 gauge needle is then placed into the nodule, approaching it from a medial to lateral direction while grasping the lesion with the nondominant hand. Once the mass is entered, the needle is moved in an up and down fashion. The aspirate is immediately placed on a cytology specimen slide and fixed with the pathologist's choice of fixative. Three specimens are usually obtained for a single nodule.

   Several results can be obtained. The nondiagnostic specimen occurs in 10–20% of FNA specimens. It is reported when few follicular or colloid cells are seen. The FNA should be repeated. After three failed attempts at FNA with nondiagnostic specimens, surgical excisional biopsy should be performed.

   Nodular goiter, thyroiditis, and colloid cyst when adequately biopsied with appropriate cellular content can be identified as benign lesions of FNA. Inconclusive specimen is the classification that is given when epithelial cells are the most dominate cell type found in the specimen. The inconclusive classification is the finding most often seen with follicular and Hurthle cell neoplasms. There must be evidence of capsular, vascular, or lymphatic invasion to make the diagnosis of Hurthle or follicular cancers, which usually cannot be determined with FNA cytology. Twenty percent of all biopsy specimens are classified as inconclusive.

   The classification of malignant is given to approximately 5% of specimens which are conclusively identified as neoplastic lesions with corresponding cell type. These cell types include papillary, anaplastic, medullary, lymphoma, and metastatic.

Bibliography

The Papanicolau Society of Cytopathology Task Force on Standards of Practice: Guidelines of the Papanicolau Society of Cytopathology for the examination of fine needle aspiration specimens from thyroid nodules. *Mod Pathol* 1996;9:710–715.

Kukora JS, Sack MJ, Weiss NM. Thyroid nodule. In: Cameron JL (ed.), *Current Surgical Therapy*, 7th ed. St. Louis, MO: Mosby, 2001, 636–642.

2. **(C)** FNA has become the mainstay for the diagnosis of thyroid nodules. It remains a technically simple procedure with a high yield of information and minimal complications. The specimens do require immediate fixation and the diagnostic yield is dependent on the experience of the cytopathologist.

   The false negative rates with FNA range from 1% to 10% and the false positive rates are approximately 2%. The four classifications of biopsy specimens are nondiagnostic, benign, inconclusive, and malignant. Diagnosis of follicular malignancy remains difficult because of the need for histologic evidence of vascular, lymphatic, or capsular invasion for unequivocal classification. Unfortunately, this cannot be reliably determined on FNA. In those specimens without atypia, the rate of follicular malignancy is 6.8%. Of the patients with the classification of suspicious or inconclusive, the rate of malignancy is 40–45%.

   Ultrasound is being used as an adjunct to FNA. In comparison with palpable FNA, ultrasound guided FNA has an overall sensitivity (89.8%) and specificity (86.7%) improvement that is not statistically significant. It has been shown to decrease the number of nondiagnostic samples.

Bibliography

Amrikachi M, Ramzy I, Rubenfeld S, et al. Accuracy of fine needle aspiration of thyroid. *Arch Pathol Lab Med* 2001;125:484–488.

Goldstein RE, Netterville JL, Burkey B, et al. Implications of follicular neoplasms, atypia, and lesions suspicious for malignancy diagnosed by fine needle aspiration of thyroid nodules. *Ann Surg* 2002;235:656–664.

Ogawa Y, Kato Y, Ikeda K, et al. The value of ultrasound guided fine needle aspiration cytology for thyroid nodules: an assessment of its diagnostic potentials and pitfalls. *Surg Today* 2001;31:97–101.

Roman SA. Endocrine tumors: evaluation of the thyroid nodule. *Curr Opin Oncol* 2003;15:66–70.

3. **(B)** Ultrasound is a commonly used modality that employs sound waves to image thyroid nodules. It is a simple, operator-dependent, noninvasive test that can reliably visualize thyroid lesions and can be performed in the office setting. Greater than 20% of patients evaluated with ultrasound in high resolution (5–10 MHz) with a palpable lesion will have a second lesion 1 cm or less in size discovered. On the other hand, 10% of patients with a palpable lesion will have no nodule seen on ultrasound examination. It can reliably differentiate solid (hyperechoic) from cystic (anechoic) lesions, but it lacks the ability to distinguish malignant from benign growths.

Malignant lesions are generally found on ultrasound to be hypoechoic in 63% of patients. When the finding of a hypoechoic lesion is combined with microcalcifications, irregular borders and tall shape, the sensitivity for malignancy increases to 93.8%, specificity of 66%, and an accuracy of 74.8% in nonpalpable lesions. Vascular evaluation with color flow Doppler ultrasound has been found to be predictive of malignancy when there is the presence of nodule vascular spots.

Cysts are a common finding that are readily diagnosed with ultrasound. The finding of an anechoic, well-circumscribed lesion with smooth walls is usually a finding with benign simple cysts.

Hyperechoic lesions are associated with solid nodules and 96% are found to be benign.

Ultrasound may aide in localization and examination of nodules, but the determination of malignancy is still best made with FNA or excisional biopsy.

Bibliography

Marquesee E, Benson CB, Frates MC, et al. Usefulness of ultrasonography in the management of nodular thyroid disease. *Ann Intern Med* 2000;133:696–700.

Roman SA. Endocrine tumors: evaluation of the thyroid nodule. *Curr Opin Oncol* 2003;15:66–70.

Udelsman R. Thyroid gland. In: Greenfield LJ, Mulholland MW, Oldham KT, et al. (eds.), *Surgery: Scientific Principles and Practice.* Philadelphia, PA: Lippincott, Williams & Wilkins, 2001, 1261–1284.

4. **(C)** The patient described above has the classic findings associated with a thyroglossal duct cyst. This lesion results from an incomplete involution of the epithelial cells from during the embryologic path of the thyroid from the floor of the mouth to the low anterior neck. The cysts are generally lined with squamous epithelium and most often present in childhood.

It is estimated that 7% of the population have thyroglossal duct remnants. A majority present in early childhood as a painless midline neck mass with infection or drainage from a fistula. Often the mass will elevate when the tongue is extruded. After early childhood the remainder present in the second and third decade. A majority (60%) of cysts are located between the thyroid gland and the hyoid bone. Other less common locations include suprahyoidal (24%), suprasternal (13%), and intralingual (1%). Histologically most cysts are lined with squamous epithelium, respiratory epithelium, or a combination of both. Ectopic thyroid tissue is rarely found in cyst walls.

There is a small chance of developing a carcinoma from a thyroglossal duct cyst. Papillary carcinoma is the cell type that is found in an overwhelming majority of cysts with malignancy. Although it is the most common type, papillary carcinoma is found in only 1.6% of patients with duct excisions. Nevertheless, the risk of malignancy does mandate that prompt surgical excision be carried out for these patients.

The Sistrunk procedure, which was first described in 1920, is still the recommended procedure. It involves complete cyst excision in continuity with the involved portion of the hyoid bone. The procedure has proved to have minimal morbidity. Recurrence is involved with inadequate excision of the tract.

Bibliography

Ewing CA, Kornblut A, Greeley C, et al. Presentation of thyroglossal duct cysts in adults. *Eur Arch Otorhinolaryngol* 1999;256:136–138.

Katz AD, Hachigian M. Thyroglossal duct cyst. A thirty year experience with emphasis on occurrence in older patients. *Am J Surg* 1988;155:741–743.

Lubben B, Alberty J, Lang-Roth R, et al. Thyroglossal duct cyst causing intralaryngeal obstruction. *Otolaryng Head Neck* 2001;125:426–427.

Udelsman R. Thyroid gland. In: Greenfield LJ, Mulholland MW, Oldham KT, et al. (eds.), *Surgery: Scientific Principles and Practice.* Philadelphia, PA: Lippincott, Williams & Wilkins, 2001, 1261–1284.

5. **(B)** The symptoms described above occur after injury to the external branch of the superior laryngeal nerve. This is most commonly injured during the mobilization of the superior pedicle (Fig. 16-4).

A thorough understanding of the vascular and nervous anatomy of the thyroid is of paramount

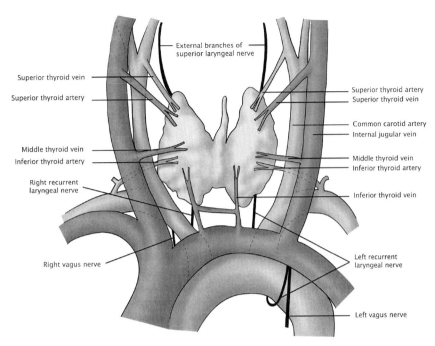

FIG. 16-4 Thyroid anatomy

importance to avoid unnecessary morbidity with surgery. The arterial vascular anatomy involves a superior thyroid artery, which is the first branch of the external carotid artery and an inferior thyroid artery which travels posterior to the carotid, originating from the thyrocervical trunk. The venous drainage of the thyroid is divided into superior, middle, and inferior portions, all of which drain into the internal jugular vein.

The relationships and functions of the nerves in proximity to the thyroid gland are also important in avoiding injuries during thyroidectomy. The recurrent laryngeal nerve originates from the vagus and provides motor function to all muscles of the larynx with exception of the cricothyroid muscle. On the right it passes behind the subclavian artery and travels in the tracheal esophageal groove lateral and deep to the carotid sheath. On the left it passes around the aorta at the level of the ligamentum arteriosum and again travels cephalad to the thyroid in the tracheal esophageal groove.

The superior laryngeal nerves also originate from the vagus nerve and divide into internal and external branches. The internal superior laryngeal nerve provides mostly sensory function, while the external superior laryngeal nerve provides motor function to the cricothyroid muscle.

The recurrent laryngeal nerve is intimately associated with the inferior thyroid artery, while the external branch of the superior laryngeal nerve is most commonly in proximity to the superior thyroid artery and vein. It is during this mobilization of the superior pedicle that most injuries to the external superior laryngeal nerve occur.

Injury to the recurrent laryngeal nerve can remain largely asymptomatic if unilateral. This injury may often result in altered voice with the vocal cord immobility. Bilateral recurrent nerve injury is more dramatic with bilateral cord immobility and loss of airway. Injury to the superior external laryngeal results in the inability to attain and sustain high pitched notes and the loss of ability to project one's voice.

Bibliography

Mansberger AR Jr, Wei JP. Surgical embryology and anatomy of the thyroid and parathyroid gland. *Surg Clin North Am* 1993;73:727.

Udelsman R. Thyroid gland. In: Greenfield LJ, Mulholland MW, Oldham KT, et al. (eds.), *Surgery: Scientific Principles and Practice*. Philadelphia, PA: Lippincott, Williams & Wilkins, 2001, 1261–1284.

6. **(C)** Thyroid surgery is routinely performed at high volume centers with minimal morbidity and mortality. Nerve injuries are uncommon, but intensely discussed complications. Recurrent laryngeal nerve injury occurs in less than 1% of all thyroidectomy patients. The recurrent laryngeal nerves originate from the vagus and course around the aorta (left) and subclavian (right) arteries before traveling posterior to

the carotid sheath to the thyroid in the trachealesophageal groove. Unilateral injuries are associated with ipsilateral vocal cord paralysis and hoarseness of the voice, while bilateral cord injuries lead to loss of airway. Postoperatively these patients will present with stridor mandating an emergent intubation. Subsequent failure of extubation requires permanent tracheostomy. Recurrent laryngeal stretch or crush injuries may resolve after 12 months. Injuries present after 1 year may need Teflon injection into the paralyzed cord. Suspected recurrent laryngeal cord injuries are best diagnosed with fiberoptic examination or indirect laryngoscopy.

Superior laryngeal nerve injury which may present as a change in the pitch of voice or inability to reach sustained high notes is more difficult to diagnose. The best method of diagnosis is laryngeal videostroboscopy and spectrographic analysis. This permits early diagnosis and treatment with speech rehabilitation.

Airway obstruction is seen in those with the rare complication of bilateral recurrent laryngeal nerve injury and with postoperative hematoma. Hematoma occurs secondary to hemorrhage deep to the strap muscles and patients present with stridor followed closely by complete loss of the airway. This diagnosis should be made at the bedside and warrants immediate treatment. The incision and deep layers should be emergently opened at the bedside. Simultaneously an operative suite should be prepared for further exploration, ligation of bleeding site, and closure. Evacuation of the hematoma will result in immediate opening of the airway. If airway compromise still exists after bedside evacuation, immediate intubation or emergent tracheostomy should be performed.

The most common complication of thyroid surgery remains transient hypoparathyroidism, occurring in 6.9–46% of patients. Mild asymptomatic hypocalcemia does not require calcium supplementation. In patients with severe disturbances or symptoms of hypocalcemia, intravenous supplementation should be implemented and patients should be released with an oral calcium regimen until the hypoparathyroidism resolves. In 2% of patients, permanent hypocalcemia requires permanent calcium and vitamin D supplementation to avoid the long-term complications of hypocalcemia. Factors that have been shown to increase the incidence of hypoparathyroidism after thyroidectomy include: extended thyroid resection, central ligation of the inferior thyroid artery versus peripheral ligation, and lack of specialized training for surgeons performing high-risk thyroid procedures.

Bibliography

Aluffi P, Policarpo M, Cherovac C, et al. Post-thyroidectomy superior laryngeal nerve injury. *Eur Arch Otorhinolaryngol* 2001;258:451–454.

Efron G. Thyroid cancer. In: Cameron JL (ed.), *Current Surgical Therapy*, 7th ed. St. Louis, MO: Mosby, 2001, 645–652.

Thomusch O, Machens A, Sekulla C, et al. The impact of surgical technique on postoperative hypoparathyroidism in bilateral thyroid surgery: a multivariate analysis of 5846 consecutive patients. *Surgery* 2003;133:180–185.

7. **(D)** Graves disease is characterized by autoimmunity by thyroid-stimulating antibodies that results in activation of thyrotropin receptors leading to unregulated hyperthyroidism. Graves disease is the most common autoimmune disease in the United States. The peak age of incidence is between 40 and 60 years and is exceedingly rare in children.

The clinical manifestations specific to Graves disease include diffuse goiter, exophthalmos, dermopathy, and lymphoid hyperplasia. Common diseases associated with Graves are diabetes mellitus, Addison's disease, vitiligo, pernicious anemia, myasthenia gravis, alopecia areata, and other autoimmune diseases. Patients will often present with signs and symptoms of hyperthyroidism.

Diagnosis of Graves disease begins through the finding of hyperthyroidism with an elevated free thyroxine level and a low serum thyrotropin. The differential of hyperthyroidism includes Graves disease, toxic nodular goiter, thyroiditis, gestational hyperthyroidism, carcinoma, struma ovarii, Albright's syndrome, and iatrogenic hyperthyroidism. To differentiate, there must be clinical signs of Graves such as diffuse goiter, exophthalmos and the like. When the diagnosis is uncertain, a radionuclide scan may be used to show diffuse goiter supportive of Graves. Thyrotropin-receptor antibodies may also be measured in serum.

Treatment of Graves disease can be accomplished through antithyroid drugs, radioactive iodine, or subtotal or near-total thyroidectomy. The three drugs most commonly used are carbimazole, methimazole, and propylthiouracil. Each inhibits the synthesis of thyroid hormone by blocking thyroid peroxidase. Medication takes 2–4 weeks before initial improvement of symptoms. After discontinuation of drugs, 60–70% will see a recurrence. Propylthiouracil may be used in pregnant patients.

Radioactive iodine is the most common treatment in the United States. It takes 4–8 weeks before results are seen in most patients. This treatment is contraindicated in pregnant patients. The main side effect of radioactive iodine treatment is hypothyroidism.

Subtotal or near-total thyroidectomy is an effective and expensive method of treatment. It is the preferred method of treatment of those patients with a large goiter or with a second thyroid lesion. Euthyroid state must be obtained prior to surgery with a thyroid peroxidase inhibitor and iodide is given 7 days prior to surgery.

Bibliography

Weetman AP. Graves' disease. *N Engl J Med* 2000; 342: 1236–1248.

8. **(D)** Most patients who have undergone total thyroidectomy are recommended to have ablative iodine-131 therapy. This has been shown to decrease local recurrence and improve long-term survival. Iodine-131 is easily trapped and organified by the thyroid gland as well as in well-differentiated thyroid malignancies. In the setting of total thyroidectomy for well-differentiated lesions, iodine-131 allow for ablation of residual thyroid tissue to allow for the use of thyroglobulin to monitor for recurrence. It has also been shown to ablate microscopic foci of residual carcinoma resulting in a decrease in local recurrence. Well-differentiated papillary and follicular lesions actively trap iodine-131. Hurthle cells have decreased trapping and there is iodine-131 resistance in medullary, anaplastic, lymphoma, nonthyroidal metastases, and other poorly differentiated lesions.

Iodine-131 therapy may be performed 4–6 weeks after thyroidectomy with no interim thyroid replacement. It can also be performed 8–12 weeks after surgery with thyroid replacement discontinued prior to treatment. Triiodothyronine (T3) should be discontinued 14 days before treatment and thyroxine (T4) 4 weeks prior. Thyroid-stimulating hormone (TSH) must be greater than 30 mU/L to facilitate adequate uptake.

A total body scan is performed and if any iodine-131 is noted on scan than a treatment dose is given. A repeat scan is then performed 4–7 days later and thyroid replacement restarted. Another iodine-131 ablation scan should be performed 6 months later.

Complete ablation allows for the use of thyroglobulin to monitor for recurrence. Iodine-131 therapy is used extensively for the treatment of Grave's disease and there has not been a proven radiation-induced malignancy risk. Therapeutic and diagnostic scans are contraindicated in pregnancy.

Bibliography

Harris PE. The management of thyroid cancer in adults: a review of new guidelines. *Clin Med* 2002;2:144–146.

Schlumberger MJ. Papillary and follicular thyroid carcinoma. *N Engl J Med* 1998;338:297–306.

Udelsman R. Thyroid gland. In: Greenfield LJ, Mulholland MW, Oldham KT, et al. (eds.), *Surgery: Scientific Principles and Practice.* Philadelphia, PA: Lippincott, Williams & Wilkins, 2001, 1261–1284.

9. **(B)** Thyroid nodules are fairly common, occurring in 5–10% of the population. A majority of these lesions are benign. Thyroid carcinomas makeup less than 1% of all cancers. Papillary and follicular lesions occur most often in adults between 45 and 50 years of age and are two times more frequent in women.

In areas of iodine deficiency, follicular carcinoma predominates in contrast to the papillary predominance in areas with iodine supplementation. Radiation exposure has shown to cause an increase in the incidence of papillary lesions. The risk of development of malignancies is greatest when radiation exposure is obtained during childhood. The latency between exposure and presentation is greatest at 20 years. Tumors in those patients with radiation exposure have higher rates of multicentricity and recurrence. There is no increase in risk after exposure to iodine-131.

Papillary lesions have classic histologic findings of overlapping nuclei with ground glass appearance and longitudinal grooves (Fig. 16-5).

On gross pathologic examination, the tumor is multicentric in 20–80% of patients and bilateral in approximately 60–85%. Cancer spread is generally through lymphatic channels (Fig. 16-6).

There remains some controversy concerning the extent of thyroid resection required for long-term control. Most recommend total thyroidectomy for almost all patients with lesions greater than 1 cm and those with previous radiation exposure. This is supported

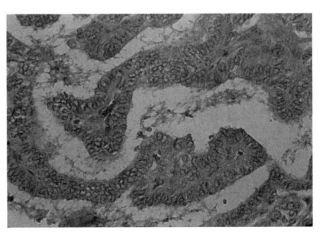

FIG. 16-5 Thyroid papillary lesion

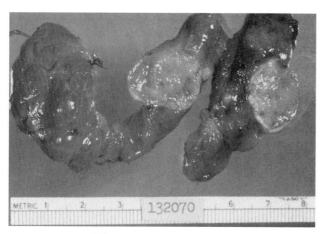

FIG. 16-6 Thyroid papillary lesion

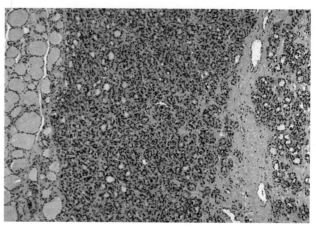

FIG. 16-7 Thyroid follicular carcinoma

by the high rate of contralateral lobe involvement and the ability to use iodine-131 treatment and thyroglobulin monitoring. Recurrence rates after total thyroidectomy are 8% versus 22% in those with lobectomy. In those with lesions less than 1 cm, no evidence of multicentricity and no radiation exposure, lobectomy is adequate.

Lymphatic invasion is microscopically present in 80% of patients with papillary lesions and grossly present in 35%. There is no relationship between presence of nodal spread and long-term survival. Ipsilateral neck dissection and central neck dissection with evidence of palpable nodal spread may decrease the incidence of local recurrence. There is no indication for prophylactic lymph node dissection.

Survival is 95% at 20 years with well-differentiated lesions appropriately treated.

Bibliography

Sherman SI. Thyroid carcinoma. *Lancet* 2003;361:501–511.
Harris PE. The management of thyroid cancer in adults: a review of new guidelines. *Clin Med* 2002;2:144–146.
Schlumberger MJ. Papillary and follicular thyroid carcinoma. *N Engl J Med* 1998;338:297–306.

10. **(C)** Follicular cancer of the thyroid makes up approximately 10% of the thyroid malignancies and is most commonly associated with iodine deficiency. This lesion is more common in females and occurs at a median age of 50 years.

    The classic histologic findings seen with these lesions are follicular changes, without the nuclear changes seen with papillary cancer (Fig. 16-7).

    The diagnostic dilemma of differentiating follicular cancer from benign follicular adenoma is not one that can be solved with FNA. The diagnosis of follicular cancer is made on permanent section with evidence of capsular, vascular, or lymphatic invasion.

This diagnosis can also be made intraoperatively with obvious invasion into thyroid arterial or venous supply or surrounding structures.

Unlike papillary carcinoma, follicular cancer is less likely to be multicentric. It spreads mostly hematogenously to the lung and bone. The treatment options are based on the diagnosis of follicular cancer versus the benign follicular adenoma. Once patients have the diagnosis of a follicular lesion based on FNA they should proceed with an ipsilateral thyroid lobectomy, since 20% are found to harbor malignancy on final pathologic examination. Intraoperative frozen section has not been shown to be helpful. Those who are found to have invasive follicular carcinoma should have a completion thyroidectomy, followed by iodine-131 therapy.

Patients that need total thyroidectomy as the primary procedure are those with gross lymph node spread, distant metastases, age greater that 50 years, history of head and neck radiation, patients that do not desire a second procedure and those with lesions greater than 4 cm. Patients with lesions greater that 4 cm have been shown to have a 50–80% malignancy rate. Patients do not require prophylactic lymph node dissection.

Prognosis is worse than papillary carcinoma with 20-year survival of 70% with appropriate treatment. Patients with age less than 40 years have a significantly better long-term survival that those older than 40 years.

Bibliography

Efron G. Thyroid cancer. In: Cameron JL (ed.), *Current Surgical Therapy*, 7th ed. St. Louis, MO: Mosby, 2001, 645–652.
Harris PE. The management of thyroid cancer in adults: a review of new guidelines. *Clin Med* 2002;2:144–146.

Schlumberger MJ. Papillary and follicular thyroid carcinoma. *N Engl J Med* 1998;338:297–306.

Sherman SI. Thyroid carcinoma. *Lancet* 2003;361:501–511.

11. **(D)** The patient described above has features suggestive of hereditary medullary carcinoma with inherited multiple endocrine neoplasia (MEN) 2B syndrome features. Medullary thyroid carcinoma originates from the parafollicular C cells and is responsible for 5% of all thyroid malignancies. Sporadic medullary carcinoma occurs in 80% of patients, while the remainder is involved with an inherited MEN syndrome.

This syndrome originates from mutations in the *RET* protooncogene and has an very high penetrance (90–95%). MEN 2A (Sipple's syndrome) consists of medullary carcinoma of the thyroid, pheochromocytoma, and hyperparathyroidism and MEN 2B (Sizemore's syndrome) consists of medullary thyroid cancer, pheochromocytoma, submucosal neuromas, and marfanoid habitus.

Patients generally present with a painful mass with palpable lymphadenopathy in 20%. Other symptoms arise from this aggressive tumor growth into surrounding structures (trachea, esophagus and the like) and release of calcitonin and adrenocorticotropic hormone lead to facial flushing and diarrhea.

Pathologic diagnosis can be obtained with FNA. The pathologic features of medullary carcinoma include C-cell hyperplasia, presence of amyloid, and specimen staining for the presence of calcitonin and carcinoembryonic antigen (Figs. 16-8 and 16-9).

Sporadic disease is most prevalent in the fifth and sixth decade and has a slight female preponderance. Familial disease is inherited in an autosomal dominant fashion. *RET* protooncogene mutations are detectable in 98% of affected patients warranting genetic screening at an early age for family members.

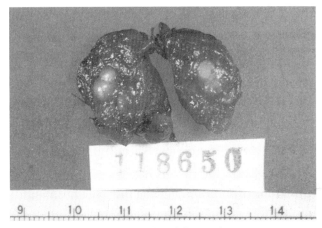

FIG. 16-9   Thyroid medullary carcinoma

12. **(C)** Sporadic disease is found in 80% of patients with medullary thyroid carcinoma. This remains a locally aggressive cancer and greater than 75% of patients with palpable lesions have evidence of lymph node spread. In those with suspected sporadic disease, exclusion of pheochromocytoma and parathyroid disease must be performed before proceeding to surgery. The treatment of choice for sporadic and inherited disease is total thyroidectomy with central lymph node dissection. Ipsilateral modified neck dissection should be performed if there is neck disease, positive findings during central neck dissection or tumor size greater than 1 cm.

In children with inherited disease, detected through genetic testing, prophylactic thyroidectomy should be performed. For MEN 2A total thyroidectomy should be done by 6 years of age and for MEN 2B by 2 years. The prophylactic total thyroidectomy should have a concurrent central neck dissection performed with ipsilateral modified neck dissection if positive.

Postoperatively, patients will benefit from thyroid hormone replacement after total thyroidectomy. There is no role for postoperative iodine-131 therapy. Chemotherapy has not been shown to be useful, but radiation therapy has been shown to decrease local recurrence in high-risk patients.

After a period of 8–12 weeks if serum calcitonin and carcinoembryonic antigen levels are within normal limits, they can be used as sensitive markers for recurrence or metastases. Somatostatin may be used for the treatment of facial flushing and diarrhea.

Bibliography

Efron G. Thyroid cancer. In: Cameron JL (ed.), *Current Surgical Therapy*, 7th ed. St. Louis, MO: Mosby, 2001, 645–652.

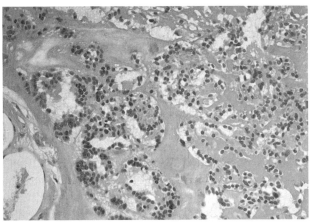

FIG. 16-8   Thyroid medullary carcinoma

Harris PE. The management of thyroid cancer in adults: a review of new guidelines. *Clin Med* 2002;2:144–146.

Sherman SI. Thyroid carcinoma. *Lancet* 2003;361:501–511.

Udelsman R. Thyroid gland. In: Greenfield LJ, Mulholland MW, Oldham KT, et al. (eds.), *Surgery: Scientific Principles and Practice.* Philadelphia, PA: Lippincott, Williams & Wilkins, 2001, 1261–1284.

13. **(A)** Patients that die from malignancy have a 1.9–24.2% incidence of thyroid metastatic lesions. Breast, lung, and renal malignancy all have been noted to have isolated spread to the thyroid. Renal cell carcinoma is the most common and is responsible for 50% of isolated thyroid metastases.

The treatment for patients with isolated metastatic lesions should take into account the prognosis of the primary lesion. Surgical management centers around complete surgical excision of the lesion.

Bibliography

Udelsman R. Thyroid gland. In: Greenfield LJ, Mulholland MW, Oldham KT, et al. (eds.), *Surgery: Scientific Principles and Practice.* Philadelphia, PA: Lippincott, Williams & Wilkins, 2001, 1261–1284.

14. **(C)** Acute suppurative thyroiditis remains a rare finding because of the thyroid's excellent blood supply and lymphatic drainage routes and resultant ability to resist infection in the nonimmunocompromised host.

The infection of the thyroid gland seen with acute suppurative thyroiditis is most often caused by gram-positive infection of the gland. *Staphylococcus aureus* is the most common organism seen, although *Streptococcus pyogenes, Streptococcus pneumoniae,* and *Haemophilus influenzae* are also frequently found on culture. Fungal infection has also been seen in the immunosuppressed host.

The infection usually follows an upper respiratory tract infection, trauma to the neck or thyroid, or recent surgery. Patients usually present with anterior neck pain and tenderness with fever, pharyngitis, and dermal erythema. Pain is usually worsened with swallowing and can radiate to the jaw and ear. It is paramount that the examining physician carefully searches for evidence of abscess cavities, which are often present.

Infection that has persisted for some time will lead to systemic signs of infection including tachycardia and hypotension. Leukocytosis and elevated erythrocyte sedimentation rate (ESR) are commonly seen. TSH, T4, and T3 are typically normal. Ultrasound is the best method for examining the thyroid gland for abscess collections. Radioactive iodine scanning is another method to determine the presence of abscess collections which appear as cold spots.

Further studies are usually unnecessary, although FNA is a useful method of obtaining samples for the identification of the causative organism.

Once the diagnosis is confirmed and the organism is identified, the treatment is appropriate antibiotic therapy. If abscess cavities do exist, they require operative drainage.

Bibliography

Arici C, Clark OH. Thyroiditis. In: Cameron JL (ed.), *Current Surgical Therapy,* 7th ed. St. Louis, MO: Mosby, 2001, 645–652.

Elorza JL, Echenique-Elizonda M. Acute suppurative thyroiditis. *J Am Coll Surg* 2002;195:729–730.

Hamburger JI. The various presentations of thyroiditis. Diagnostic considerations. *Ann Intern Med* 1986; 104:219–224.

15. **(A)** The patient above has the classic findings of Hashimoto's thyroiditis. This disease is also referred to as autoimmune-chronic lymphocytic thyroiditis, chronic progressive thyroiditis, and struma lymphomatosa. The disease stems from the destruction of thyroid cells by antibody-mediated immune processes impairing the thyroid's ability to organify trapped iodine. Initially there is a transient elevation of thyroxine (T3) and triiodothyronine (T4) that is released into circulation from damaged cells. The destruction of the cells leads to an eventual hypothyroid state and without the inhibition to TSH, a goiter develops.

This disease is the most common cause of hypothyroidism in the United States and in areas of adequate iodine intake. It most commonly affects women between the ages of 30 and 50 years. There is some degree of family susceptibility.

The most common presenting symptoms are those of hypothyroidism and include fatigue, constipation, weight gain, cold intolerance, menstrual irregularities, depression, hair loss, and so on. Other possible causes of hypothyroidism that should be considered are thyroidectomy, radiation injury, iodine deficiency, drugs, thyroid infiltrative disease, and hypothalamic disease. Patients will typically have an enlarged, firm, rubbery thyroid gland on examination.

The diagnostic laboratory findings that will be seen with hypothyroidism are an elevated TSH level with low total T4 and free T4 levels. T3 measurements are not useful in the diagnosis of hypothyroidism. Thyroid antimicrosomal and antithyroglobulin autoanitbodies are very sensitive tests to delineate the cause of hypothyroidism as Hashimoto's thyroiditis. Imaging studies are not necessary in the diagnosis of Hashimoto's thyroiditis, but FNA should be performed on any dominant nodule to

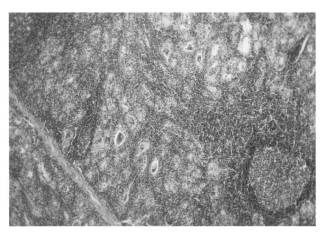

FIG. 16-10   Hashimoto's thyroiditis

exclude the presence of lymphoma, which has a slightly higher incidence in those with this disease. The histologic findings seen in Hashimoto's thyroiditis are diffuse plasma cell and lymphocytic infiltration, extensive fibrosis, and gland destruction (Fig. 16-10).

Treatment is thyroid replacement with small doses. This results in a decrease of goiter size and resolution of hypothyroid signs and symptoms. Thyroidectomy is indicated for suspicion of malignancy, lymphoma, cosmetically unsightly goiters, and for goiters that cause compressive symptoms.

Bibliography

Arici C, Clark OH. Thyroiditis. In: Cameron JL (ed.), *Current Surgical Therapy*, 7th ed. St. Louis, MO: Mosby, 2001, 645–652.

Canaris GJ, Manowitz NR, Mayor G. The Colorado thyroid disease prevalence study. *Arch Intern Med* 2000; 160:526–534.

Kon YC, DeGroot LJ. Painful Hashimoto's thyroiditis as an indicator for thyroidectomy: clinical characteristics and outcome in seven patients. *J Clin Endocrinol Metab* 2003;88:2667–2672.

16. **(B)** There are multiple drug interactions that result in hyperthyroid and hypothyroid states. The mechanism of action causing these changes is altering TSH secretion, thyroid hormone secretion, thyroid hormone absorption, serum transport (thyroxine binding globulin levels), displacing from protein binding sites and altering metabolism.

Drugs that commonly decrease thyroid hormone production are methimazole, propylthiouracil, lithium and iodide containing compounds. Lithium blocks the synthesis and secretion of the hormone. Long-term use leads to goiter formation in 50% of patients and hypothyroid symptoms in 20%. Iodide given as a supplement in contrast, amiodarone (75 mg/tablet), douches, and topical antiseptic agents can all cause hypothyroidism, especially in those with autoimmune thyroiditis and those with partial thyroidectomy.

Medications that decrease TSH secretion are dopamine, glucocorticoids, and octreotide. Those that decrease T4 absorption include colestipol, cholestyramine, aluminum hydroxide, ferrous sulfate, and sucralfate.

The T4 and T3 in serum is 99% bound to thyroxine binding globulin, transthyretin, and albumin. The 1% of unbound hormone is the only active hormone and therefore changes in the binding proteins have major effects on the euthyroid state.

Commonly used drugs that increase serum TBG concentration are estrogens, tamoxifen, heroin, methadone, mitotane, and fluorouracil. Those that decrease levels are androgens, anabolic steroids, nicotinic acid, and glucocorticoids.

Bibliography

Surks MI, Sievert R. Drugs and thyroid function. *N Engl J Med* 1995;333:1688–1694.

17. **(D)** The patient described above has the classic findings of postpartum painless thyroiditis. This disease is characterized by lymphocytic inflammation of the thyroid after pregnancy. It occurs 1–3 months after delivery, in up to 10% of all women. It is more prevalent in women with known history of autoimmune disorders.

The classic pattern of thyroid hormone levels and their correlating signs and symptoms begins with a thyrotoxicosis. This usually is first seen 1–6 months after delivery and lasts for up to 2 months. This is followed by a hypothyroid phase which lasts between 4 and 6 months. A majority (80%) of women will return to a euthyroid state within a year of delivery. A small fraction of women develop a persistent hypothyroid state. This happens most commonly in multiparous women or those with a history of abortion.

Patients will generally first present with symptoms and signs of hypothyroidism or hyperthyroidism. Careful physical examination shows a firm, nontender goiter. Autoimmune serum tests including the thyroid peroxidase antibody and thyroglobulin antibody are usually positive. Twenty-four hours later, an iodine-123 uptake scan may be useful to distinguish painless postpartum thyroiditis (low uptake) from Graves' disease (high uptake).

Treatment is usually not necessary for either the thyrotoxicosis or hypothyroid phases of the disease. If the patient does have a persistent hypothyroid state, replacement therapy is indicated. Treatment

should be discontinued after 6–9 months to determine if the patient has returned to a euthyroid state.

Bibliography

Pearce EN, Farwell AP, Braverman LE. Thyroiditis. *N Engl J Med* 2003;348:2646–2655.

18. **(B)** The anatomy of the parathyroid gland is variable and a thorough understanding of the embryological and adult anatomy can be an indispensable tool in locating the glands during difficult preservations or resections.

The usual pattern for parathyroid glands is two superior parathyroid glands and two inferior thyroid glands. Each gland weighs 30–50 mg, with the inferior parathyroids being slightly larger. The glands are normally oval and flat, but change into a more globular state when abnormal. In the newborn, glands are usually gray and transparent, while in the adult they are red-brown to yellow in color.

The superior glands arise from the fourth pharyngeal pouch with the lateral thyroid. Their location is more predictable and is on the posterior surface of the upper pole where the recurrent laryngeal nerve enters the larynx.

The inferior gland is slightly larger and arises from the third pharyngeal pouch. This gland is more variable and since it migrates with the thymus, it can be found from the pharynx to the mediastinum. Occasionally the parathyroid gland will be found completely embedded in the body of the thyroid.

The arterial supply to the superior and inferior parathyroid gland is most commonly from the inferior thyroid artery. The venous outflow is to the inferior, middle, and superior thyroid veins.

Bibliography

Doherty GM. Parathyroid glands. In: Greenfield LJ, Mulholland MW, Oldham KT, et al. (eds.), *Surgery: Scientific Principles and Practice.* Philadelphia, PA: Lippincott, Williams & Wilkins, 2001, 1284–1302.

Doherty GM, Wells SA. Parathyroid glands. In: Townsend CM, Beauchamp RD, Evers BM, Mattox KL (eds.), *Sabiston Textbook of Surgery: The Biological Basis of Modern Surgical Practice*, 16th ed. Philadelphia, PA: WB Saunders, 2001, 629–645.

19. **(A)** PTH is principally responsible for the regulation of calcium. Calcitonin and vitamin D also play an important role in calcium homeostasis. Under normal physiologic circumstances PTH is released in response to hypocalcemia. The hormone is released from parathyroid glands as a larger pre-proparathyroid hormone which is cleaved into the active 84 amino acid PTH form.

The PTH's direct effects on the kidney include decreasing the clearance of calcium and increasing the excretion of renal phosphate. This process begins with the cholecalciferol (vitamin D_3) being produced by the effect of sunlight on 7-dehydrocholesterol in the skin. Cholecalciferol is then hydroxylated to calcifediol (25-hydroxyvitamin D). This is then further hydroxylated to its active form of calcitrol (1,25-dihydroxyvitamin D). This activated form results in a greater absorption of calcium and phosphate from the intestine. PTH directly increases the hydroxylation of calcifediol to calcitrol.

The effects of PTH also extend to the skeletal system where almost all of the bodily stores of calcium are contained. It acts to promote osteoclast function, while inhibiting osteoblast function, resulting in significant calcium release.

Bibliography

Doherty GM. Parathyroid glands. In: Greenfield LJ, Mulholland MW, Oldham KT, et al. (eds.), *Surgery: Scientific Principles and Practice.* Philadelphia, PA: Lippincott, Williams & Wilkins, 2001, 1284–1302.

Doherty GM, Wells SA. Parathyroid glands. In: Townsend CM, Beauchamp RD, Evers BM, Mattox KL (eds.), *Sabiston Textbook of Surgery: The Biological Basis of Modern Surgical Practice*, 16th ed. Philadelphia, PA: WB Saunders, 2001, 629–645.

20. **(C)** Hypercalcemia occurs in the general outpatient population in 0.1–0.5% of the population. The most common etiology of this is primary hyperparathyroidism. In the inpatient population, 5% will have evidence of hypercalcemia and approximately 66% will be found to have a malignancy which is responsible for the abnormality. The most likely malignancies noted with hypercalcemia are lung carcinoma, breast carcinoma, squamous cell carcinoma of the head and neck, or renal cell cancer.

The signs and symptoms of hypercalcemia involve almost every organ system. Neurologic symptoms are subtle and nonspecific and include lethargy, confusion, headache, depression, paranoia, muscle weakness, hyporeflexia, incontinence, memory loss, and ataxia. Gastrointestinal symptoms that may be seen are constipation, anorexia, nausea, polydipsia, weight loss, pancreatitis, and nonspecific abdominal pain. The electrocardiogram findings are shortening of the QT interval and widening of the T wave. When calcium levels reach an extreme, bradycardia and complete heart block can be seen.

Although malignancy and hyperparathyroidism are the most likely causes, others that must be considered are vitamin D intoxication, thiazide diuretics, hyperthyroidism, milk-alkali syndrome, sarcoidosis,

familial hypocalciuric hypercalcemia, Paget's disease, lithium treatment, Addisonian crisis, and chronic immobilization.

Bibliography

Doherty GM. Parathyroid glands. In: Greenfield LJ, Mulholland MW, Oldham KT, et al. (eds.), *Surgery: Scientific Principles and Practice.* Philadelphia, PA: Lippincott, Williams & Wilkins, 2001, 1284–1302.

21. **(C)** The treatment for symptomatic hypercalcemia begins with inpatient admission for continuous cardiac monitoring. Any medication that may increase calcium levels should be discontinued. This includes vitamin D supplements and thiazide diuretics. Any dietary calcium (dairy products) should also be stopped.

The foundation of treatment is intravenous rehydration. A normal or half normal saline solution is appropriate. Care should be taken to avoid pulmonary edema in those with a fragile cardiac function. Urine output should be maintained at 100 mL/h and after adequately rehydrated, patients may be given furosemide, which increases renal calcium excretion. Intravenous hydration and furosemide will generally correct symptoms and bring calcium levels to normal in those patients with hyperparathyroidism as the cause of their hypercalcemia.

Malignant hypercalcemia may be more difficult to manage and may require the use of disodium etridronate or other biphosphonates. These agents work by inhibiting the action of osteoclast activity.

Calcitonin is another agent that can be used to lower calcium levels. It is a comparatively poor hypercalcemic treatment agent, but has a short time to action and minimal adverse effect profile. Mithramycin is also effective and high dose steroids work well for sarcoid patients with hypercalcemic symptoms.

A final method of removing calcium is acute hemodialysis.

Bibliography

Doherty GM. Parathyroid glands. In: Greenfield LJ, Mulholland MW, Oldham KT, et al. (eds.), *Surgery: Scientific Principles and Practice.* Philadelphia, PA: Lippincott, Williams & Wilkins, 2001, 1284–1302.

Doherty GM, Wells SA. Parathyroid glands. In: Townsend CM, Beauchamp RD, Evers BM, Mattox KL (eds.), *Sabiston Textbook of Surgery: The Biological Basis of Modern Surgical Practice*, 16th ed. Philadelphia, PA: WB Saunders, 2001, 629–645.

22. **(D)** The patient described above has familial hypocalciuric hypercalcemia disease. This is an autosomal dominant disease that expresses itself as an error in the calcium-sensing receptor. This causes the baseline or normal serum calcium level to be higher than normal. These patients are always asymptomatic and key laboratory abnormalities include hypercalcemia, hypocalciuria, and normal to slightly elevated PTH levels.

The diagnosis of familial hypocalciuric hypercalcemia can be done with the measurement of urine calcium levels that are lowered in these patients. It is paramount to exclude this diagnosis in all patients with high serum calcium.

The treatment of this disease is strictly observational. Patients do not require surgery or further workup.

Bibliography

Doherty GM. Parathyroid glands. In: Greenfield LJ, Mulholland MW, Oldham KT, et al. (eds.), *Surgery: Scientific Principles and Practice.* Philadelphia, PA: Lippincott, Williams & Wilkins, 2001, 1284–1302.

23. **(A)** Primary hyperparathyroidism is defined as the excess production of PTH, resulting in hypercalcemia. This is still the most common cause of hypercalcemia in patients not in the hospital. It occurs most commonly in women and the elderly.

The systemic manifestations of primary hyperparathyroidism are usually noticed by the systemic manifestations of hypercalcemia, rather than detection of enlarged or abnormal parathyroid glands. The exception to this is with the diagnosis of parathyroid carcinoma, which will frequently have palpable glands. The finding of a palpable lesion in the anterior neck in a patient with hyperparathyroidism will most likely be found to be a thyroid lesion.

Laboratory tests will be able to reliably diagnose primary hyperparathyroidism. An elevated PTH level is a necessary value in making the diagnosis, although this alone does not confirm the diagnosis. Elevated calcium levels confirm the diagnosis. In those patients with pH or albumin fluctuations, ionized calcium levels are useful in determining an accurate calcium level. Patients should have a normal creatinine and low phosphate level to exclude secondary hyperparathyroidism. All patients with hypercalcemia should have urine calcium levels measured to rule out familial hypocalciuric hypercalcemia disease. This distinction is paramount in making sure that patients with this disease do *not* undergo parathyroidectomy, which is not indicated.

The most common etiology of primary hyperparathyroidism is a single adenoma, which is found in 76% of patients. The next most common etiology is diffuse hyperplasia, which is seen in 18%. Multiple adenoma is seen in 6% and parathyroid carcinoma is rarely a cause.

The classic histologic findings of parathyroid adenoma include a compressed rim of parathyroid tissue compressed by proliferating chief cells.

Bibliography

Doherty GM. Parathyroid glands. In: Greenfield LJ, Mulholland MW, Oldham KT, et al. (eds.), *Surgery: Scientific Principles and Practice.* Philadelphia, PA: Lippincott, Williams & Wilkins, 2001, 1284–1302.

Lowney JK, Weber B, Johnson S, et al. Minimal incision parathyroidectomy: cure, cosmesis and cost. *World J Surg* 2000;24:1442–1445.

Udelsman R. Primary hyperparathyroidism. In: Cameron JL (ed.), *Current Surgical Therapy*, 7th ed. St. Louis, MO: Mosby, 2001, 662–667.

24. (D) The indications for surgical intervention in the asymptomatic patient with hyperparathyroidism were first set at the National Institutes of Health Consensus Development Conference in 1990. The indications for surgical intervention include

1. markedly elevated serum calcium
2. history of life-threatening episode of hypercalcemia
3. reduced creatinine clearance
4. presence of one or more kidney stones detected by abdominal radiograph
5. elevated 24-h urinary calcium excretion
6. reduced bone mass
7. medical surveillance is unsuitable

Once the decision for surgical management has been made, the need for localization studies should be assessed. Employing full neck exploration, under general anesthesia, an experienced surgeon will be able to identify all four parathyroid glands and successfully cure the disease in 95% of patients. This has made the need for preoperative localization studies a costly and controversial area of debate. The more frequent use of minimally invasive techniques for parathyroid surgery may bring about more frequent preoperative localization.

The most sensitive and commonly employed localization study is technetium-99m sestamibi scintigraphy. This is imaged with single photon emission computed tomography and can pick up abnormal parathyroid tissue in 75–80% of patients. It is limited in patients with smaller adenomas.

Bibliography

Doherty GM. Parathyroid glands. In: Greenfield LJ, Mulholland MW, Oldham KT, et al. (eds.), *Surgery: Scientific Principles and Practice.* Philadelphia, PA: Lippincott, Williams & Wilkins, 2001, 1284–1302.

Udelsman R. Primary hyperparathyroidism. In: Cameron JL (ed.), *Current Surgical Therapy*, 7th ed. St. Louis, MO: Mosby, 2001, 662–667.

25. (C) The slide above demonstrates parathyroid carcinoma, which is a rare (<1%), but possible cause of primary hyperparathyroidism.

The population of patients with carcinoma is younger and more symptomatic than those with other more common causes of primary hyperparathyroidism.

The diagnosis is made unequivocal with evidence of invasion into surrounding structures. Parathyroid carcinoma is resistant to chemotherapy or radiation therapy, therefore complete surgical resection is the only option for long-term cure.

The more appropriate resection would include a radical parathyroidectomy of the affected gland, regional lymph node resection, and ipsilateral thyroid lobectomy. Recurrences should be treated with resection.

Bibliography

Doherty GM. Parathyroid glands. In: Greenfield LJ, Mulholland MW, Oldham KT, et al. (eds.), *Surgery: Scientific Principles and Practice.* Philadelphia, PA: Lippincott, Williams & Wilkins, 2001, 1284–1302.

Udelsman R. Primary hyperparathyroidism. In: Cameron JL (ed.), *Current Surgical Therapy*, 7th ed. St. Louis, MO: Mosby, 2001, 662–667.

26. (C) Surgical exploration for primary hyperparathyroidism starts with a Kocher incision. The thyroid lobes are carefully rotated in a medial fashion and the inferior thyroid artery and the recurrent laryngeal nerve are identified. The superior glands remain more constant and are usually found on the dorsal surface on the upper half of the thyroid. The inferior glands are more variable in location. If the inferior glands are not visualized after initially inspecting the region where the thyrothymic ligament attaches to the lower pole, the thymus must be pulled up and inspected. It is crucial for a successful exploration that all four glands are visualized and inspected.

The operation for a single adenoma, with the remainder of the glands visualized and normal, is a single parathyroidectomy. This results in a near 100% cure. In the case of multiple gland enlargement and the remaining visualized and normal, a 90% cure rate has been reported with parathyroidectomy of only the enlarged glands.

Primary hyperparathyroidism caused by hyperplasia of all four glands can be treated with either subtotal (3 1/2) parathyroidectomy or total parathyroidectomy and immediate heterotropic transplant in the nondominant arm. It is vital to leave approximately 40 mg of tissue.

In the event that three normal glands are identified, but the fourth parathyroid cannot be found, the upper pole should be completely mobilized and the entire dorsal surface must be palpated, as well as the retrolaryngeal, retrotracheal, and posterior mediastinal spaces. If it is a lower parathyroid that is not found, the thymus must be retracted into the field and examined. It is not recommended to extend the incision, or proceed with a sternotomy at this point. Instead the visualized glands are biopsied, the wound is closed, localization studies are obtained, and the patient is reexplored at a later date.

Bibliography

Doherty GM. Parathyroid glands. In: Greenfield LJ, Mulholland MW, Oldham KT, et al. (eds.), *Surgery: Scientific Principles and Practice.* Philadelphia, PA: Lippincott, Williams & Wilkins, 2001, 1284–1302.

Udelsman R. Primary hyperparathyroidism. In: Cameron JL (ed.), *Current Surgical Therapy,* 7th ed. St. Louis, MO: Mosby, 2001, 662–667.

Histologic and gross pathologic images provided by Frank W Fitch, MD, Ph.D., Department of Pathology, The University of Chicago.

This chapter is dedicated to the memory of my father, Dinesh P. Tevar. He possessed a passionate love of surgery that few ever know and is remembered by his peers, patients and family as a compassionate and gifted sureon with an unparalleled generosity of spirit. As an extraordinary mentor, he taught me integrity and professionalism, all the while demonstrating his unmistakable personal humility, wry humor and charm. He is deeply missed.

CHAPTER 17

Adrenal Gland

Chad Wiesenauer and C. Max Schmidt

Questions

1. A computed tomography (CT) scan is obtained on a 60-year-old patient to diagnose acute diverticulitis. In addition to sigmoid colon findings consistent with diverticulitis, he is found to have a 2 cm homogeneous left adrenal mass, as seen in Fig. 17-1. Which of the following is true concerning the further workup of the adrenal mass?

   (A) Because of the risk of pheochromocytoma, this lesion should never be biopsied.
   (B) Given the patient's age, this is likely a metastatic lesion from a nonadrenal primary.
   (C) Normal serum aldosterone, in the face of normokalemia and normal blood pressure, essentially rules out functional aldosteronoma.
   (D) Normal plasma cortisol level essentially rules out cortisol-producing adrenocortical adenoma.

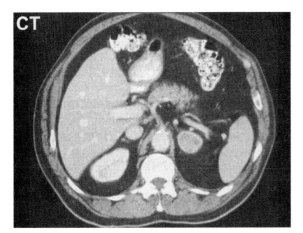

FIG. 17-1 CT scan of a left-sided, benign adrenal adenoma

2. In the above patient, you have demonstrated that this is a nonfunctional adrenal mass, and you have no suspicion of this being metastatic. Which of the following is the best choice of management?

   (A) biopsy via fine needle aspiration
   (B) laparoscopic adrenalectomy
   (C) repeat imaging with CT scan in 3 month's time
   (D) transabdominal adrenalectomy with exploration of the contralateral adrenal gland for occult tumor

3. A 22-year-old lady with hypertension refractory to medical management is referred to you after a CT scan was obtained that demonstrates a 3 cm mass in the right adrenal gland. The initial diagnostic test of choice is

   (A) measurement of catecholamines, metanephrines, and vanillylmandelic acid in a 24-h urine collection
   (B) MRI
   (C) measurement of catecholamines and metanephrines in a morning serum sample
   (D) high-dose dexamethasone suppression test

4. Perioperative and operative management of pheochromocytoma include all *except* which one of the following?

   (A) use of a long-acting alpha-adrenergic antagonist preoperatively
   (B) laparoscopic removal is not acceptable because of the need to adequately explore both adrenal glands
   (C) ligation of the adrenal vein(s) before the adrenal artery(ies)
   (D) surgical debulking is indicated even if the pheochromocytoma is deemed unresectable on exploration

5. You have been asked to see a full-term infant born yesterday with ambiguous genitalia. There is a small urethral phallus, apparent hypertrophy of a clittoris, and near fusion of the labioscrotal folds. The neonatalogist tells you that this child has elevated 17-hydroxyprogesterone. Which of the following is false?

   (A) This will likely require adrenal surgery.
   (B) The sex in this patient is usually female (two X chromosomes).
   (C) Serum levels of cortisol will be lower than normal.
   (D) If the sex is female, then ovaries and uterus will likely develop normally.

6. Which of the following is false concerning adrenal tumors that secrete androgens?

   (A) These tumors often go unnoticed in the postpubertal male until signs and symptoms of tumor enlargement or metastasis occurs.
   (B) It is likely a benign tumor.
   (C) Surgical resection is the mainstay of treatment.
   (D) Levels of DHEA in the plasma will likely be elevated.

7. Which of the following is true regarding anatomy of the adrenal glands?

   (A) Venous drainage of the right adrenal gland is predominantly into the right renal vein.
   (B) Both adrenal glands receive significant blood supply from branches of the superior mesenteric artery.
   (C) Venous drainage of both adrenal glands is directly into the inferior vena cava.
   (D) Both adrenal glands receive significant blood supply from their corresponding renal arteries.

8. In which one of the following patients is laparoscopic adrenalectomy contraindicated?

   (A) A 40-year-old male with a 7 cm homogeneous, well-defined, nonfunctional adrenal mass with previous surgical history of open cholecystectomy.
   (B) A 20-year-old female with a 3 cm well-defined mass in the right adrenal gland with episodes of hypertension, whose father died of thyroid carcinoma and apparently had also undergone adrenalectomy at a young age.

   (C) A 60-year-old female with back pain and a poorly-defined, 7 cm right adrenal mass, and a history of modified radical mastectomy 3 years previously to remove invasive ductal carcinoma.
   (D) A 30-year-old male with a 5 cm smooth-bordered right adrenal mass with a 3-month history of diastolic hypertension and elevated serum aldosterone.

9. Which of the following is false concerning laparoscopic adrenalectomy?

   (A) It is associated with a lower hospital cost compared to open adrenalectomy.
   (B) It is an acceptable technique to remove small hereditary pheochromocytoma.
   (C) It is associated with shorter operating room time.
   (D) It is associated with a reduced rate of perioperative blood transfusions.

10. A 55-year-old male undergoes workup for recent onset of diastolic hypertension, polyuria, and fatigue. The diagnosis of hyperaldosteronism is considered. The diagnostic test(s) of choice is(are) which of the following?

    (A) CT scan with special attention to the adrenal glands and kidneys
    (B) low-dose dexamethasone suppression test
    (C) magnetic resonance image of the abdomen
    (D) serum potassium and aldosterone levels

11. You have diagnosed hyperaldosteronism in the above patient. You obtain a CT scan which shows bilateral adrenal nodules or bilateral adrenal hyperplasia. Your next step in the management of this patient should be

    (A) MRI
    (B) bilateral adrenalectomy
    (C) selective adrenal venous sampling
    (D) medical therapy with spironolactone, triamterene, or amiloride

12. Which of the following is true concerning primary hyperaldosteronism?

    (A) Bilateral hyperplasia of the zona glomerulosa is about twice as likely as either adrenal adenoma or adrenal carcinoma to be responsible for primary hyperaldosteronism.
    (B) Unilateral adrenalectomy is usually curative for bilateral hyperplasia.

(C) All patients are hypokalemic.

(D) These patients often present with metabolic alkalosis.

13. Each of the following pairs of steroid product with its adrenal site of production is correct *except*:

(A) aldosterone in the zona fasciculata

(B) cortisol in the zona fasciculata

(C) cortisol in the zona reticularis

(D) DHEA in the zona reticularis

14. Which of the following is false concerning adrenal physiology?

(A) The enzyme 17-alphahydroxylase is necessary to produce both cortisol and the adrenal androgen DHEA.

(B) Steroid hormones exert their local effects so quickly because they bind directly to cell membrane receptors.

(C) Cholesterol can be either synthesized by the adrenal cortex or extracted from the plasma.

(D) Cholesterol is the ultimate precursor of cortisol, aldosterone, and DHEA.

15. The effects of the steroid hormone cortisol include all of the following *except*:

(A) It curtails the inflammatory response by inhibiting the migration of monocytes and neutrophils.

(B) It promotes hyperglycemia by both antogonizing glucose uptake peripherally and by stimulating hepatic gluconeogenesis.

(C) It sustains positive nitrogen balance by increasing amino acid delivery to the liver and by increasing peripheral protein synthesis.

(D) It retards wound healing by impairing collagen formation and fibroblast activity.

16. Which of the following stimuli to adrenal aldosterone secretion is the weakest?

(A) Longstanding unilateral renal artery stenosis that restricts blood supply by 80%

(B) Acute hemorrhage from a gunshot wound to the chest in which 30% of total blood volume is lost

(C) A rise in serum potassium from 4.0 to 4.3 meq/L

(D) A pituitary adenoma that secretes ACTH, with serum ACTH levels twice normal

17. Which of the following is true regarding adrenal production of androgens?

(A) Production of adrenal DHEA is primarily under control of luteinizing hormone (LH) and follicle stimulating hormone (FSH).

(B) DHEA is converted to estrogen peripherally.

(C) The presence of adrenal androgens in the developing fetus influences development of male genitalia.

(D) In adults, excessive adrenal production of androgens is most likely secondary to an enzyme deficiency.

18. A 35-year-old male patient presents with signs and symptoms consistent with Cushing's syndrome. A low-dose dexamethasone suppression test shows no significant suppression of serum cortisol. Measurement of serum ACTH level demonstrates profoundly low levels of ACTH. A CT scan shows a 4 cm, well-circumscribed mass in the right adrenal gland. The best choice for further therapy is which one of the following?

(A) laparoscopic or open right adrenalectomy

(B) suppression of cortisol production with aminoglutethimide

(C) CT scan of the head to delineate pituitary anatomy

(D) CT-guided biopsy of the right adrenal mass

19. Which statement best describes the role of exogenous steroids in the perioperative period in the above patient?

(A) There is no role for exogenous steroids in the above patient.

(B) Exogenous steroids are indicated only if there is suspicion of an additional contralateral adrenal tumor.

(C) Almost all patients undergoing surgery for this disease will require perioperative exogenous steroids.

(D) The high-dose dexamethasone suppression test will determine whether this patient needs perioperative exogenous steroids.

20. A 35-year-old male patient presents with signs and symptoms consistent with Cushing's syndrome. A low-dose dexamethasone suppression test shows no significant suppression of serum cortisol. Measurement of serum ACTH demonstrates a higher-than-normal level. A high-dose dexamethasone suppression test reveals only partial suppression of serum cortisol levels. The next step should be which of the following?

    (A) MRI of the head
    (B) CT scan of the chest and abdomen
    (C) bilateral adrenalectomy and lifelong exogenous steroid administration
    (D) transsphenoidal resection of pituitary gland

21. A 35-year-old male patient presents with signs and symptoms consistent with Cushing's syndrome. A low-dose dexamethasone suppression test shows no significant suppression of serum cortisol. Measurement of serum ACTH demonstrates a higher-than-normal level. High-dose dexamethasone suppression test reveals no suppression of serum ACTH. Which of the following is not likely to be indicated?

    (A) CT scan of the abdomen and chest
    (B) medical adrenalectomy if deemed inoperable

    (C) administration of exogenous steroids to suppress ACTH production
    (D) surgical debulking if deemed unresectable

22. Among the following, the test of choice to diagnose Cushing's syndrome (hypercortisolism) is

    (A) 24-h urine-free cortisol
    (B) plasma ACTH level
    (C) CRH test
    (D) high-dose dexamethasone suppression test

23. Among the following, the test of choice to diagnose adrenal insufficiency is

    (A) ACTH stimulation test
    (B) low-dose stimulation test
    (C) plasma ACTH level
    (D) random serum cortisol level

24. Any of these tests can be used to differentiate between a pituitary or ectopic source of ACTH excess *except*

    (A) high-dose dexamethasone suppression test
    (B) inferior petrosal venous sampling
    (C) ACTH stimulation test
    (D) CRH test

Answers and Explanations

1. **(C)**

2. **(C)**

Explanations 1 and 2

Adrenal incidentalomas have been reported to occur in up to 5% of CT scans obtained for unrelated reasons. The frequency becomes higher as age of the patient increases. Up to 90% of these are nonfunctioning cortical adenomas. Cortical adenomas are usually small and homogeneous, with a smooth, encapsulated margin on CT scan. They usually do not enhance with intravenous contrast, and are usually low-attenuation lesions (less than 10 Hounsfield units) when intravenous contrast is not used. The most important step once an adrenal incidentaloma is discovered is to rule out causes other than nonfunctioning cortical adenoma.

Adrenocortical carcinomas are rare tumors. Half of them are functional, producing either Cushing's syndrome or virilization, or both. Plasma dehydro-epiandrosterone (DHEA), a marker of androgen excess, is touted by some as a marker for adrenocortical carcinoma, but there is considerable overlap between levels found in malignant and benign adrenocortical lesions. Most of these malignant tumors are larger than 6 cm in size when discovered. They are inhomogeneous masses with irregular borders that enhance with intravenous contrast. For example, see Fig. 17-2 of a left-sided adrenal carcinoma. Surgery is the only possible cure for this rare entity.

The most important tumor to exclude in the case of adrenal incidentaloma is pheochromocytoma. These are tumors of the chromaffin cells of the adrenal medulla. Pheochromocytomas are also relatively rare tumors, unless there is a patient or family history of its predisposing syndromes: von Recklinghausen's neurofibromatosis, von Hippel-Lindau's disease, and multiple endocrine neoplasia (MEN) syndromes 2A and 2B. All patients with an adrenal mass need to be biochemically tested for pheochromocytoma, which

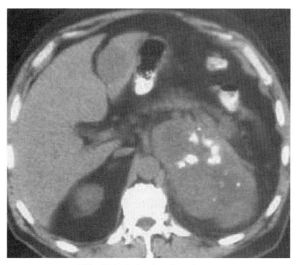

FIG. 17-2 Left adrenal carcinoma

consists of 24-h urine collection for catecholamines and metanephrines.

The risk of an adrenal incidentaloma being metastatic rises precipitously when an extraadrenal malignancy is diagnosed. Primary tumors that tend to metastasize to the adrenals include breast, lung, renal cell, melanoma, and lymphomatous cancers. In a patient with known extraadrenal malignancy and adrenal mass, this mass can be assumed to be metastatic. In a patient with a history of extraadrenal malignancy, but who is deemed disease-free, the finding of an adrenal mass warrants fine needle aspiration biopsy. This should never be done until the possibility of pheochromocytoma is excluded.

Functional cortical adenomas can be essentially ruled out with serum biochemical tests. Functional aldosteronomas usually cause hypertension, hypokalemia, weakness, and polyuria. Laboratory abnormalities include elevated serum aldosterone, hypokalemia, and suppressed renin activity. In a patient without hypertension and with normal serum potassium, functional aldosterona is extremely unlikely. Functional cortisol-producing adenomas usually cause Cushing's syndrome: weight gain, hypertension, easy bruisability, diabetes mellitus, and centripetal obesity ("buffalo hump" and "moon face"). Because the total amount of daily cortisol secreted in these patients can be normal, 24-h urine collection for cortisol may be normal, and this test is insensitive. Random serum tests for cortisol are also insensitive, as these patients lose the normal diurnal variation in cortisol secretion. The test of choice to diagnose functional cortisol-producing adenoma is the low-dose dexamethasone suppression test. Patients with functional cortisol-producing adenoma will fail to suppress plasma cortisol level after low dose of dexamethasone. Further testing in the form of plasma adrenocorticotropic hormone (ACTH) level is then necessary to exclude a pituitary source. A hormonally active adenoma is an indication for adrenalectomy.

Once the entities of functional adenoma, metastatic lesion, pheochromocytoma, and carcinoma are ruled out, it is assumed that this is a nonfunctional adenoma. Because of the increased risk of malignancy with increased size, it is recommended that adrenalectomy be performed for lesions 4 or 5 cm in diameter or larger, or if there is suggestion of atypical features on CT or magnetic resonance imaging (MRI). If the mass is less than 4–5 cm in diameter and its appearance is benign on imaging, repeat imaging should be performed at 3 and 12 months. Growth of the lesion on repeat imaging warrants surgical resection. If the lesion is stable in size at 12 months, no further imaging is necessary.

Bibliography

Moley JF, Brunt LM. Adrenal incidentaloma. In: Cameron JL, *Current Surgical Therapy*, 7th ed. St. Louis, MO: Mosby, 2001, 632–635.

Moley JF, Wells SA. Pituitary and adrenal glands. In: Townsend CM, Beauchamp RD, Evers BM, et al. (eds.), *Sabiston Textbook of Surgery*, 16th ed.. Philadelphia, PA: WB Saunders, 2001, 674, 678, 688.

3. (A)

4. (B)

Explanations 3 and 4

There are multiple adrenal causes of surgically correctable hypertension, including functional aldosteronoma, cortisol-producing adenoma, and pheochromocytoma. Regardless of which one, if any, this patient has, it is imperative to rule out pheochromocytoma early, and the test of choice is 24-h urine col-

lection for catecholamines (epinephrine, norepinephrine, and dopamine), metanephrines (metanephrine and normetanephrine), and vanillylmandelic acid. If all three are measured, there is virtually 100% sensitivity for pheochromocytoma.

Pheochromocytoma is a catecholamine-secreting tumor of the adrenal medulla chromaffin cells. Pheochromocytomas can also be extraadrenal, occurring in sympathetic ganglia, most often the organ of Zuckerkandl. They are rare tumors unless there exists a predisposing hereditary setting: MEN type 2A or 2B, von Recklinghausen's neurofibromatosis, and von Hippel-Lindau's disease. Often cited is the "rule of tens": pheochromocytomas are bilateral in 10%, extraadrenal in 10%, familial in 10%, malignant in 10%, and occur in children in 10%. Symptoms include palpitations, anxiety, headaches, and flushing. Hypertension is often present, paroxysmal in some and sustained in others. As stated above, the diagnosis is made with urine testing for increased products of the pheochromocytoma. Imaging studies to confirm the adrenal or extraadrenal mass include CT and MRI, including down to the aortic bifurcation to examine the organ of Zuckerkandl. 131 Iodine-metaiodobenzylduanidine (MIBG) scanning is also available, and although less sensitive than MRI or CT, it is useful in detecting small and/or extraadrenal pheochromocytomas. MIBG scanning is often indicated in patients at higher risk for multiple or extraadrenal tumors, such as those with MEN syndrome.

Surgical resection is indicated for pheochromocytoma. Preoperative medical management includes control of hypertension, alpha-adrenergic blockade to prevent hypertensive crisis intraoperatively, and maintenance of adequate fluid resuscitation. Phenoxybenzamine is the alpha-adrenergic antagonist of choice, and is usually begun 1 week before surgery. Dose is titrated to the point of postural hypotension. If tachycardia occurs, beta-adrenergic blockade is indicated, but only after sufficient alpha-adrenergic antagonism is confirmed. A beta-adrenergic antagonist administered to a patient with pheochromocytoma can result in unopposed alpha-adrenergic effects of the tumor products, precipitating hypertensive crisis. There are several surgical approaches to pheochromocytoma. Laparoscopic adrenalectomy is acceptable if the tumor appears benign and is 8 cm or less in diameter. Modern imaging techniques are sensitive enough to preclude routine exploration of the contralateral adrenal gland. Transabdominal open adrenalectomy is excellent for exploration of bilateral or extraadrenal tumors if necessary. Large, malignant tumors may best be approached via a thoracoabdominal approach. The posterior retroperitoneal approach is less morbid than the transabdominal approach, but exposure is limited, reserving this procedure for smaller tumors.

Management of pheochromocytoma in patients with MEN syndrome is controversial. Thirty to 40% of these patients, regardless of type (2A or 2B) develop pheochromocytoma. Some surgeons perform bilateral adrenalectomy for unilateral pheochromocytoma in order to avoid the approximately 30% chance of developing a metachronous lesion in this contralateral gland in the future. This does result in a 10–30% chance of Addisonian crisis afterward, so other surgeons choose to perform unilateral adrenalectomy with close follow-up. For bilateral pheochromocytomas on presentation, the standard operation is bilateral adrenalectomy, although some surgeons offer total adrenalectomy on one side with cortical-sparing adrenalectomy on the other.

Malignant pheochromocytoma is diagnosed by demonstrating invasion of local structures or by proving metastasis. Therapy is surgical adrenalectomy and resection of metastases, with debulking. Radiation therapy may ameliorate pain from bone metastases. MIBG can be attempted as ablative therapy, and there exist chemotherapy protocols. Five-year survival has been reported to be from 36 to 60%.

Bibliography

Kebebew E, Duh Q. Pheochromocytoma. In: Cameron JL, *Current Surgical Therapy*, 7th ed. St. Louis, MO: Mosby, 2001, 624–630.

Moley JF, Wells SA. Pituitary and adrenal glands. In: Townsend CM, Beauchamp RD, Evers BM, et al. (eds.), *Sabiston Textbook of Surgery*, 16th ed. Philadelphia, PA: WB Saunders, 2001, 684–688.

Newsome HH. Adrenal glands. In: Greenfield LJ, Mulholland MW, Oldham KT, Zelenock GB, Lillemoe KD (eds.), *Surgery: Scientific Principles and Practice*, 3rd ed. Philadelphia, PA: Lippincott, Williams & Wilkins, 2001, 1318.

5. **(A)** This infant most likely has congenital adrenal hyperplasia, which often presents itself as ambiguous genitalia in the newborn infant. The enzymatic defect in the steroidogenesis pathway causes a decrease in cortisol secretion, with consequent increased ACTH production, which acts in a vicious cycle to further drive the production of other steroids in the pathway other than cortisol. These excess adrenal androgens are converted peripherally to testosterone.

The most common enzymatic deficiency is 21-hydroxylase deficiency, responsible for more than 90% of the congenital adrenal hyperplasias. In this deficiency, progesterone and 17-hydroxyprogesterone cannot be converted into 11-deoxycortisol and 11-deoxycorticosterone, respectively. There is therefore decreased production of both aldosterone and cortisol. In complete absence of 21-hydroxylase, there is androgen excess, salt-wasting in the urine, diarrhea, hypovolemia, hyponatremia, hyperkalemia, and hyperpigmentation. Partial absence of the enzyme presents only as virilization, and may not present itself until later in childhood. The high levels of ACTH are able to force production of cortisol and aldosterone into near-normal range. Virilization of the female fetus produces female pseudohermaphroditism: clitoral hypertrophy, labioscrotal fold fusion, and a urogenital sinus that appears as a phallic urethra. The ovaries, fallopian tubes, and uterus are not affected by androgens, and thus develop normally. In fact, medical control of the endocrine defect and surgical correction of the external genital abnormalities may allow these females to bear children. Virilization of the male fetus may not be detected unless the enzyme deficiency is complete, and thus salt-wasting is present. Partial deficiency in male infants may go undiagnosed until precocious puberty occurs. Diagnosis is easily confirmed by measuring the elevated plasma 17-hydroxyprogesterone. Treatment of this disorder consists of glucocorticoid and mineralocorticoid replacement. In the case of the female pseudohermaphrodite, the external genitalia are surgically modified to be female.

The second most common is 11-beta-hydroxylase deficiency. Without this enzyme, 11-deoxycorticosterone and 11-deoxycortisol cannot be converted to corticosterone or cortisol. In contrast to 21-hydroxylase deficiency, the mineralocorticoid 11-deoxycorticosterone is produced, and in fact is overproduced as the decreased level of cortisol causes excess ACTH production. This overproduction of a mineralocorticoid causes hypokalemia and hypertension. 11-Beta-hydroxylase deficiency also causes androgen excess, and thus virilization. Diagnosis is performed by measuring elevated 17-hydroxyprogesterone (as in 21-hydroxylase deficiency), and treatment is similar: replacement of glucocorticoids and surgical correction of ambiguous genitalia in female infants.

3-Beta-hydroxydehydrogenase deficiency reduces levels of glucocorticoids, mineralocorticoids, and androgens, shunting steroidogenesis to the production of 17-hydroxypregnenolone and DHEA, a weak androgen. Female infants show virilization, whereas male infants show incomplete virilization. These infants rarely survive because of profound saltwasting.

17-Hydroxylase deficiency results in decreased production of cortisol and androgens, with a concomitant overproduction of mineralocorticoids.

Affected patients thus present with hypertension and hypokalemia. Treatment is with corticosteroid and androgen replacement.

Bibliography

Moley JF, Wells SA. Pituitary and adrenal glands. In: Townsend CM, Beauchamp RD, Evers BM, et al. (eds.), *Sabiston Textbook of Surgery*, 16th ed. Philadelphia, PA: WB Saunders, 2001, 674, 680.

Newsome HH. Adrenal glands. In: Greenfield LJ, Mulholland MW, Oldham KT, Zelenock GB, Lillemoe KD (eds.), *Surgery: Scientific Principles and Practice*, 3rd ed. Philadelphia, PA: Lippincott, Williams & Wilkins, 2001, 1313.

6. **(B)** Adrenal neoplasms that overproduce androgen are almost always carcinomas. In children, they present as clitoral enlargement and pubic hair formation in girls and as hirsutism, enlarged penis, and small testes in boys. In adults, women present with hirsutism and other masculinizing features, and men often go unnoticed until the disease progresses to local tumor enlargement symptoms or metastasis. These tumors secrete very large amounts of the weak androgen DHEA, which can be detected in the serum or in the urine as a 17-ketosteroid. Surgical resection is warranted. Malignancy is best determined by local invasion or distant metastases. Aminoglutethimide or mitotane may help ameliorate symptoms in patients with metastases or unresectable adrenal disease.

Bibliography

Moley JF, Wells SA. Pituitary and adrenal glands. In: Townsend CM, Beauchamp RD, Evers BM, et al. (eds.), *Sabiston Textbook of Surgery*, 16th ed. Philadelphia, PA: WB Saunders, 2001, 679–680.

Newsome HH. Adrenal glands. In: Greenfield LJ, Mulholland MW, Oldham KT, Zelenock GB, Lillemoe KD (eds.), *Surgery: Scientific Principles and Practice*, 3rd ed. Philadelphia, PA: Lippincott, Williams & Wilkins, 2001, 1313.

7. **(D)** There are normally three main adrenal arteries to each gland. The superior adrenal artery is a branch from the inferior phrenic artery. The middle adrenal artery comes directly from the aorta on each side. The inferior adrenal artery arises from each glands corresponding renal artery. The venous drainage is predominantly via one central vein. This vein drains into the vena cava on the right, and into the left renal vein on the left.

Bibliography

Clemente C. *Anatomy. A Regional Atlas of the Human Body*, 3rd ed. Malvern, PA: Lea & Febiger, 1987, 322–323.

Newsome HH. Adrenal glands. In: Greenfield LJ, Mulholland MW, Oldham KT, Zelenock GB, Lillemoe KD (eds.), *Surgery: Scientific Principles and Practice*, 3rd

ed. Philadelphia, PA: Lippincott, Williams & Wilkins, 2001, 1307.

8. **(C)**

9. **(C)**

Explanations 6 and 7

Laparoscopic adrenalectomy can be considered in any patient who does not have one of the following contraindications:

> Adrenocortical carcinoma larger than 5–6 cm
> Malignant pheochromocytoma
> Invasive adrenal mass
> Adrenal mass diameter larger than 8–10 cm
> Contraindication to laparoscopy

The only patient in the above question that portrays one of these contraindications is the 60-year-old lady with a likely invasive adrenal mass (which has a very high likelihood of being metastatic breast cancer). It is currently recommended that likely invasive adrenal tumors and malignant tumors larger than 5–6 cm in diameter be approached surgically with an open approach. Pheochromocytomas can be removed laparoscopically if deemed benign on preoperative imaging. In fact, the laparoscopic approach may result in less hemodynamic instability than in open adrenalectomy. Although adrenal masses larger than 8–10 cm have been successfully resected, this size has been suggested by some authors to serve as a threshold for using one of the open adrenalectomy techniques.

In comparison to any of the open approaches to adrenalectomy, laparoscopic adrenalectomy has been proven to result in decreased postoperative analgesic use, shorter postoperative ileus time, faster rehabilitation times, less use of postoperative blood transfusions, and overall lower hospital costs. Laparoscopic adrenalectomy does require more operating time than the open techniques.

Bibliography

Brunt LM. Laparoscopic adrenalectomy. In: Cameron JL. *Current Surgical Therapy*, 7th ed. St. Louis, MO: Mosby, 2001, 1460–1466.

Moley JF, Wells SA. Pituitary and adrenal glands. In: Townsend CM, Beauchamp RD, Evers BM, et al. (eds.), *Sabiston Textbook of Surgery*, 16th ed. Philadelphia, PA: WB Saunders, 2001, 690–691.

10. **(D)**

11. **(C)**

12. **(D)**

Explanations 10 through 12

Aldosterone excess can be primary or secondary. Secondary hyperaldosteronism is caused by stimulation of the renin-angiotensin-aldosterone system, such as in renal artery stenosis, congestive heart failure, and normal pregnancy. Primary hyperaldosteronism occurs when aldosterone secretion by the adrenal gland becomes autonomous. In approximately two-thirds of cases, this is because of an aldosterone-producing adenoma, and in approximately one-third of cases is because of bilateral adrenal hyperplasia (often idiopathic in nature). In less than 1% of cases aldosterone hypersecretion is because of adrenal carcinoma. Most patients afflicted with primary aldosteronism have some degree of diastolic hypertension because of sodium retention, and many (80%) have hypokalemia. Other signs and symptoms are secondary to potassium depletion and include muscle weakness, fatigue, polyuria, polydipsia, hyperglycemia, metabolic alkalosis, and impaired insulin secretion. Edema is characteristically absent. The test of choice in a hypertensive patient is demonstration of hypokalemia and elevated serum or urine aldosterone. Demonstration of urine potassium excretion greater than 30 meq per day is also used, as is demonstration of low plasma renin activity. Confirmation of the diagnosis can be performed by the saline infusion test, in which patients who have followed a low-sodium diet for 3 days are then infused with 2 L of normal saline over 4 h. A 24-h urine collection is then tested for aldosterone, and if the aldosterone level is more than 14 µg, the diagnosis of primary hyperaldosteronism is secured. In patients with congestive heart failure that would not tolerate the fluid infusion, the captopril test can be performed. In this test, the angiotensin-converting enzyme inhibitor captopril is used to lower angiotensin II levels instead of saline volume loading, and if plasma or urine aldosterone remains supranormal, the diagnosis is confirmed. Once primary hyperaldosteronism is diagnosed, the distinction between adrenal adenoma and bilateral adrenal hyperplasia must be made. CT is an excellent test to determine this. Confusion arises only as in the above patient, in whom CT imaging has shown bilateral adrenal nodules, which could actually be bilateral hyperplasia. In this instance, bilateral adrenal venous sampling is used. Another test that may discern between the two diagnoses is serum measurement of an aldosterone precursor, 18-hydroxycorticosterone. For unknown reasons, this steroid is increased in adenomas but normal in bilateral adrenal hyperplasia. There is also a test that distinguishes between bilateral hyperplasia and adenoma that involves measuring plasma renin and aldosterone levels in both recumbent and upright positions. Finally, the NP-59 nuclear scintigraph

scan can distinguish between aldosterone-producing adenomas and bilateral hyperplasia. The reason that the distinction between adenoma and bilateral hyperplasia must be made is that treatment is completely different for each. The treatment of choice for adenoma is surgical resection. Preoperative preparation of the patient includes spironolactone and potassium administration in order to replete potassium stores and correct any alkalosis. Because aldosterone-secreting adenomas are characteristically small and very rarely malignant, these tumors are ideally suited to a laparoscopic approach in most cases. The treatment of choice for bilateral adrenal hyperplasia is medical, and consists of spironolactone, triamterene, or amiloride. In patients with bilateral hyperplasia, surgical unilateral adrenalectomy will improve symptoms in only 20–30% of patients, and these patients usually behave as unilateral adenomas on testing for 18-hydroxycorticosterone. In the uncommon case of bilateral adrenal adenomas, medical therapy to control hypertension should be given, as this is usually much easier to do than treating adrenal insufficiency after bilateral adrenalectomy. Bilateral adrenalectomy is indicated if the hypertension associated with bilateral adrenal hyperplasia or bilateral adenomas is refractory to medical therapy.

Bibliography

Moley JF, Wells SA. Pituitary and adrenal glands. In: Townsend CM, Beauchamp RD, Evers BM, et al. (eds.), *Sabiston Textbook of Surgery*, 16th ed. Philadelphia, PA: WB Saunders, 2001, 677–679.

Newsome HH. Adrenal glands. In: Greenfield LJ, Mulholland MW, Oldham KT, Zelenock GB, Lillemoe KD (eds.), *Surgery: Scientific Principles and Practice*, 3rd ed. Philadelphia, PA: Lippincott, Williams & Wilkins, 2001, 1313–1314, 1317–1321.

13. (A)

14. (B)

Explanations 13 and 14

The adrenocortical hormones are all synthesized from cholesterol, which is either synthesized from within the adrenal cortex or is extracted directly from the plasma. The cholesterol is transformed into delta-5-pregnenolone inside the mitochondria, and this molecule, which serves as the precursor for all of the adrenal steroid hormones, enters the smooth endoplasmic reticulum and is diverted into one of many possible pathways. The different zones of the adrenal cortex (zona glomerulosa, fasciculata, and reticularis) each have differing combinations and amounts of the enzymes necessary to form the adrenocortical steroids. All mineralocorticoids are synthesized within the zona glomerulosa. The glucocorticoids and the adrenal androgens are synthesized within both the zona fasciculata and the zona reticularis.

The steroid hormones pass through the cell membrane and bind directly to cytosolic receptors. This steroid-receptor complex then translocates into the nucleus and binds to the DNA itself, affecting transcription of DNA. This chain of events is why the final physiologic effects of steroid hormones are delayed more than an hour after release into the bloodstream or after intravenous administration. This is in direct contrast to the products of the adrenal medulla—the catecholamines. The catecholamines dopamine, norepinephrine, and epinephrine bind to specific cell membrane receptors that are coupled to their effector proteins via G proteins, which allows for very fast actions once the catecholamine reaches its receptor.

The plasma half-life of cortisol is approximately 90 min, and it is the liver that transforms cortisol into its inactive metabolites, which are eventually secreted in the urine and can be detected as 17-hydroxycorticosteroids. The plasma half-life of aldosterone is approximately 15 min, it is again the liver that inactivates this steroid. DHEA is the major sex steroid secreted from the adrenal glands. DHEA is a weak androgen, and most of its virilizing effect is because of peripheral conversion to the more powerful androgen testosterone. It is important to remember that DHEA secretion is not regulated by the gonadotropins, as is testicular production of testosterone, but instead by ACTH.

Bibliography

Moley JF, Wells SA. Pituitary and adrenal glands. In: Townsend CM, Beauchamp RD, Evers BM, et al. (eds.), *Sabiston Textbook of Surgery*, 16th ed. Philadelphia, PA: WB Saunders, 2001, 672–674, 683–684.

Newsome HH. Adrenal glands. In: Greenfield LJ, Mulholland MW, Oldham KT, Zelenock GB, Lillemoe KD (eds.), *Surgery: Scientific Principles and Practice*, 3rd ed. Philadelphia, PA: Lippincott, Williams & Wilkins, 2001, 1317.

15. **(C)** The adrenal glucocorticoid cortisol has many effects on human physiology. It stimulates the release of glucagon, stimulates hepatic gluconeogenesis, and antagonizes insulin-stimulated glucose uptake in peripheral cells, all of which contribute to hyperglycemia. It decreases peripheral protein synthesis and amino acid uptake in order to increase the delivery of amino acids back to the liver for gluconeogenesis. Cortisol also stimulates peripheral lipolysis. The net effect of these metabolic regulatory functions is a catabolic state peripherally (skin, muscle, adipocytes and the like) in order to provide glucose energy for the liver and brain. Cortisol stimulates angiotensinogen release, decreases capillary permeability, and inhibits the vasodilatory prostaglandin I_2, all in an effort to maintain adequate intravascular volume. Cortisol inhibits lymphocyte activation, suppresses interleukin-2 production, prevents neutrophil and monocyte migration, inhibits histamine release by mast cells, and prevents T-cell activation of B cells. These actions are responsible for cortisol's profound anti-inflammatory effect, which is increased greatly at higher doses at which cortisol directly inhibits B-cell activation and proliferation. Cortisol negatively affects wound healing by impairing fibroblast activity, which reduces wound tensile strength and delays epithelialization, and also by inhibiting osteoblast activity. Common side effects of hypercortisolism include proximal muscle weakness, insulin-resistant diabetes mellitus, truncal obesity ("buffalo hump" and "moon faces"), and psychologic disturbances.

Bibliography

Moley JF, Wells SA. Pituitary and adrenal glands. In: Townsend CM, Beauchamp RD, Evers BM, et al. (eds.), *Sabiston Textbook of Surgery*, 16th ed. Philadelphia, PA: WB Saunders, 2001, 672.

Newsome HH. Adrenal glands. In: Greenfield LJ, Mulholland MW, Oldham KT, Zelenock GB, Lillemoe KD (eds.), *Surgery: Scientific Principles and Practice*, 3rd ed. Philadelphia, PA: Lippincott, Williams & Wilkins, 2001, 1312.

16. **(D)** The major stimuli to aldosterone secretion are the renin-angiotensin system and the serum potassium concentration. Significant renal artery stenosis causes release of renin from the kidney's juxtaglomerular cells, thus invoking the renin-angiotensin system, resulting in a significantly higher release of adrenal aldosterone than normal. Acute hemorrhage with corresponding acute intravascular volume depletion also invokes the renin-angiotensin system by decreasing bloodflow to the kidneys. Adrenal secretion of aldosterone is most strongly controlled by the plasma concentration of potassium. An increase in plasma potassium concentration by only 0.1 meq/L will increase adrenal aldosterone secretion by more than 30%. Decreases in plasma potassium concentration have the converse effect: lowering plasma potassium concentration severely restricts the ability of the adrenal gland to secrete aldosterone. ACTH has a relatively mild effect as far as increasing adrenal aldosterone secretion.

Bibliography

Moley JF, Wells SA. Pituitary and adrenal glands. In: Townsend CM, Beauchamp RD, Evers BM, et al. (eds.), *Sabiston Textbook of Surgery*, 16th ed. Philadelphia, PA: WB Saunders, 2001, 672.

17. (C) The predominant sex steroid produced by the adrenal glands is DHEA, which is a relatively weak androgen compared to testosterone, produced mainly by the gonads. DHEA exerts its androgen effects after conversion to testosterone, occurring only peripherally. Unlike gonadal testosterone, the stimulation of DHEA release from the adrenal glands is by ACTH, not the gonadotropins LH and FSH. Adrenal androgens are very important in fetal development, as they promote development of male external genitalia, male ductal structures (vas deferens, epididymis, seminal vesicles), and male prostate. If androgens are not circulating in the fetal blood stream, female genitalia result. Excessive adrenal production of androgens in adults is likely because of carcinoma. Any enzyme deficiency responsible for excessive adrenal androgen production would almost certainly have been detected shortly after birth, or at the time of puberty. (Androgen overproduction in male children may be overlooked until precocious puberty ensues.) Regardless of whether the patient with excessive adrenal androgen production is a child or adult, it is important to maintain a very high suspicion for an adrenocortical carcinoma.

Bibliography

Moley JF, Wells SA. Pituitary and adrenal glands. In: Townsend CM, Beauchamp RD, Evers BM, et al. (eds.), *Sabiston Textbook of Surgery*, 16th ed. Philadelphia, PA: WB Saunders, 2001, 674.

Newsome HH. Adrenal glands. In: Greenfield LJ, Mulholland MW, Oldham KT, Zelenock GB, Lillemoe KD (eds.), *Surgery: Scientific Principles and Practice*, 3rd ed. Philadelphia, PA: Lippincott, Williams & Wilkins, 2001, 1313, 1316–1317.

18. (A)

19. (C)

Explanations 18 and 19

The clinical picture of Cushing's syndrome (hypercortisolism) should prompt the physician to test for elevated production of cortisol. Determining plasma cortisol levels is often not useful because of the episodic nature of cortisol secretion. The most sensitive and specific screening test is determination of a 24-h urine free cortisol. This test will demonstrate hypercortisolism. If equivocal, hypercortisolism can be confirmed by the low-dose dexamethasone suppression test. In this test, the patient is administered 1–2 mg of oral dexamethasone at night and then cortisol level is measured the next morning by checking plasma cortisol, urine-free cortisol, or urinary 17-hydroxycorticosteroids. In normal individuals, this amount of synthetic glucocorticoid (dexamethasone) is able to suppress cortisol levels to less than half the normal value (less than 5 μg/dL), but in individuals with hypercortisolism it will not be as significantly suppressed, as in the above patient. Once Cushing's syndrome is diagnosed, the cause must be sought. The best initial test is to determine the amount of plasma ACTH, which in the normal human is between 10 and 100 pg/mL. Suppression of ACTH to levels below 5 pg/mL is nearly diagnostic of an adrenocortical neoplasm (high levels of cortisol profoundly suppress ACTH production from the pituitary gland).

Biochemical testing has thus essentially diagnosed the cause of hypercortisolism, and the CT scan has localized the adrenocortical neoplasm in the above patient. The CT scan also suggests benign disease (well-circumscribed, size less than 5 cm, no apparent extraadrenal disease). Since this is a functional adrenocortical tumor, the therapy of choice is surgical adrenalectomy. Unless this patient cannot withstand surgical intervention, medical suppression of the adrenal gland with a drug such as aminoglutethimide or metyrapone is contraindicated. Medical suppression may be indicated if surgery must be delayed for whatever reason, but neither of these drugs will prevent growth of the neoplasm. Biopsy of the adrenal mass is not indicated—this will not add any information that will change management of this patient. Imaging of the pituitary gland is not indicated because the finding of a low ACTH level has ruled out a pituitary source of hypercortisolism. Choice of laparoscopic versus open adrenalectomy is up to the surgeon caring for this patient; this patient as presented has no contraindication to laparoscopic removal of an adrenal gland.

Prophylactic preoperative administration of glucocorticoids should be performed if adrenalectomy is contemplated or if there is suspicion of adrenal suppression. This patient presents with both—one assumes that the contralateral, "normal" adrenal gland is suppressed because of a profoundly low ACTH status. One regimen for steroid administration is 100 mg of hydrocortisone (or equivalent dose of another glucocorticoid) preoperatively and then every 6 h for the first 48 h postoperatively. This dose can be halved every 2–3 days if everything proceeds well, but depending on how long hypercortisolism has been present, the pituitary-adrenal axis can remain suppressed for up to 2 years. The duration of replacement steroid therapy can be guided by the ACTH stimulation test, in which ACTH is administered intravenously and plasma cortisol and aldosterone are measured. In patients with adequate adrenal function, both plasma cortisol and aldosterone will rise appropriately.

Bibliography

Bakerman S. *ABC's of Interpretive Laboratory Data*, 3rd ed. Myrtle Beach, SC: Interpretive Laboratory Data, 1994, 18, 21, 198–199.

Brennan MF. Adrenocortical tumors. In: Cameron JL, *Current Surgical Therapy*, 7th ed. St. Louis, MO: Mosby, 2001, 620–623.

Moley JF, Wells SA. Pituitary and adrenal glands. In: Townsend CM, Beauchamp RD, Evers BM, et al. (eds.), *Sabiston Textbook of Surgery*, 16th ed. Philadelphia, PA: WB Saunders, 2001, 674–677.

Newsome HH. Adrenal glands. In: Greenfield LJ, Mulholland MW, Oldham KT, Zelenock GB, Lillemoe KD (eds.), *Surgery: Scientific Principles and Practice*, 3rd ed. Philadelphia, PA: Lippincott, Williams & Wilkins, 2001, 1315–1316, 1320–1321.

20. **(A)** In this patient with Cushing's syndrome, biochemical testing reveals elevated ACTH. Patients with pituitary neoplasms secreting ACTH (Cushing's disease) have serum values of ACTH over the upper limits of normal (100 pg/mL), and often much higher than this. In order to further delineate the source of this exogenous ACTH, the high-dose dexamethasone suppression test is performed. In this test, 2 mg of dexamethasone is given orally every 6 h for 2–3 days. In the morning following the last day, cortisol level is checked as either serum cortisol, urine-free cortisol, or urinary 17-hydroxycorticosteroids. In Cushing's disease (pituitary neoplasm), cortisol level will be suppressed by at least 50% ("partial suppression"). Ectopic tumors that produce ACTH will not show any suppression with the high-dose dexamethasone suppression test, and neither will adrenal tumors.

Another test useful in diagnosing Cushing's disease is the corticotropin-releasing hormone (CRH) test. In this test, CRH is administered intravenously and then plasma levels of ACTH and cortisol are drawn for 3 h afterward. In normal individuals, there is a moderate increase in both ACTH and cortisol. In individuals with pituitary neoplasms, this increase is accentuated. In individuals with either ectopic ACTH-producing tumors or adrenocortical tumors, there is no response to CRH administration.

At this point the diagnosis rests on either pituitary neoplasm or ectopic tumor that produces ACTH. Because pituitary adenoma is much more likely in this young patient, the next best test is MRI of the head to search for a pituitary adenoma. MRI for this purpose reaches 100% sensitivity, whereas CT scanning of the head approaches only half that sensitivity. Once diagnosed by imaging, the therapy of choice is transsphenoidal resection of the pituitary tumor. If inoperable or unsuccessful, irradiation and medical adrenalectomy are alternatives.

Bibliography

Bakerman S. *ABC's of Interpretive Laboratory Data*, 3rd ed. Myrtle Beach, SC: Interpretive Laboratory Data, 1994, 18, 20, 198–199.

Moley JF, Wells SA. Pituitary and adrenal glands. In: Townsend CM, Beauchamp RD, Evers BM, et al. (eds.), *Sabiston Textbook of Surgery*, 16th ed. Philadelphia, PA: WB Saunders, 2001, 674–677.

Newsome HH. Adrenal glands. In: Greenfield LJ, Mulholland MW, Oldham KT, Zelenock GB, Lillemoe KD (eds.), *Surgery: Scientific Principles and Practice*, 3rd ed. Philadelphia, PA: Lippincott, Williams & Wilkins, 2001, 1315–1316, 1320–1321.

21. **(C)** The absence of suppression after high-dose dexamethasone suppression testing coupled with an elevated serum ACTH in this patient with Cushing's syndrome points to an ectopic tumor that produces ACTH. The most likely sources are small cell carcinoma of the lung and bronchial carcinoid, although there are many other less-common sources from the abdomen. Diagnosis is hopefully made by CT scanning. Surgical removal of the tumor is indicated, and debulking is indicated if deemed unresectable. Medical adrenalectomy is an option, with drugs such as aminoglutethimide or metyrapone. Bilateral adrenalectomy may be indicated if hypercortisolism cannot be controlled medically or if imaging techniques fail to discover the ectopic source. Giving the patient with an ectopic ACTH-producing tumor exogenous steroids would not help—the pituitary gland is already suppressed.

Bibliography

Bakerman S. *ABC's of Interpretive Laboratory Data*, 3rd ed. Myrtle Beach, SC: Interpretive Laboratory Data, 1994, 18, 198–199.

Moley JF, Wells SA. Pituitary and adrenal glands. In: Townsend CM, Beauchamp RD, Evers BM, et al. (eds.), *Sabiston Textbook of Surgery*, 16th ed. Philadelphia, PA: WB Saunders, 2001, 674–677.

Newsome HH. Adrenal glands. In: Greenfield LJ, Mulholland MW, Oldham KT, Zelenock GB, Lillemoe KD (eds.), *Surgery: Scientific Principles and Practice*, 3rd ed. Philadelphia, PA: Lippincott, Williams & Wilkins, 2001, 1315–1316, 1320–1321.

22. **(A)**

23. **(A)**

24. **(C)**

Explanations 22 through 24

The most sensitive and specific test to determine hypercortisolism is the 24-h urine-free cortisol test. This avoids the episodic nature of cortisol secretion. ACTH level can be elevated, suppressed, or normal in hypercortisolism. The CRH test is a test used to differentiate between a pituitary cause for hypercortisolism and other causes. The high-dose dexamethasone test separates a pituitary source of hypercortisolism from an ectopic source of ACTH.

The ACTH stimulation test is used to determine the function of the adrenal gland(s), and is the test of choice to diagnose adrenal insufficiency. The low-dose dexamethasone suppression test is used to diagnose hypercortisolism. Although plasma ACTH level will most likely be elevated in adrenal insufficiency, this test is not specific for this condition. Random serum cortisol levels are quite variable because of the episodic nature of cortisol secretion, and thus this test is not sensitive enough for diagnosing adrenal insufficiency.

Several tests are available to aid in differentiating between a pituitary neoplasm and an ectopic source of ACTH as the cause of hypercortisolism. These include MRI of the head and CT scanning of the chest and abdomen, neither of which is listed in the above question. Inferior petrosal sinus sampling for ACTH is an invasive but very useful test to diagnose pituitary neoplasm as the source of elevated ACTH. As described previously, both the high-dose dexamethasone suppression test and the CRH test can be used to help differentiate between pituitary and ectopic sources of ACTH. The ACTH stimulation test is not useful in making this distinction.

Bibliography

Bakerman S. *ABC's of Interpretive Laboratory Data*, 3rd ed. Myrtle Beach, SC: Interpretive Laboratory Data, 1994, 18, 20, 198–199.

Efron DT, Fishel R, Barbul A. Endocrine changes with critical illness. In: Cameron JL, *Current Surgical Therapy*, 7th ed. St. Louis, MO: Mosby, 2001, 1338–1339.

Moley JF, Wells SA. Pituitary and adrenal glands. In: Townsend CM, Beauchamp RD, Evers BM, et al. (eds.), *Sabiston Textbook of Surgery*, 16th ed. Philadelphia, PA: WB Saunders, 2001, 674–676.

Newsome HH. Adrenal glands. In: Greenfield LJ, Mulholland MW, Oldham KT, Zelenock GB, Lillemoe KD (eds.), *Surgery: Scientific Principles and Practice*, 3rd ed. Philadelphia, PA: Lippincott, Williams & Wilkins, 2001, 1315–1316.

CHAPTER 18

Pituitary

Richard B. Rodgers and Julius M. Goodman

Questions

1. Which statement about pituitary microadenomas is true?

   (A) by definition are less than 10 mm in size

   (B) best seen on coronal T2 gadolinium enhanced MR scans

   (C) rarely found at autopsy in asymptomatic individuals

   (D) approximately 15% will enlarge to macroadenomas

2. A 19-year-old newly married woman has had amenorrhea for 9 months. Her prolactin level is 80 ng/mL (normal 5–20 ng/mL). She does not have galactorrhea. She brought a recent MRI with her (Fig. 18-1). After other causes of hyperprolactinemia have been ruled out, the best advice for this patient would be

   (A) begin medical treatment with dopamine agonists

   (B) begin medical treatment and avoid birth control pills

   (C) withhold medical treatment until pregnancy is desired

   (D) transsphenoidal resection of the lesion

3. A 30-year-old surgeon has noted painless loss of vision for several weeks. On examination he has a dense bitemporal hemianopsia, marked decreased visual acuity, and difficulty reading color plates. In retrospect he has been gaining a considerable amount of weight and has noted a decrease in libido. An emergency MR scan is shown in Fig. 18-2. Before proceeding with definitive treatment, the most important diagnostic test he needs is

   (A) a serum cortisol level

   (B) thyroid function studies

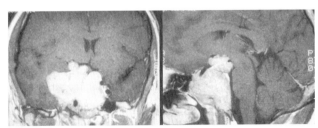

FIG. 18-2

   (C) a prolactin level

   (D) cerebral angiography

4. A 27-year-old man developed signs and symptoms of fulminant Cushing's syndrome over 3 months. He has central obesity, hypertension, and glucose intolerance. He is likely to have all of the following signs, which are fairly specific for Cushing's syndrome, *except*:

   (A) enlarged supraclavicular fat pads

   (B) purple stria

   (C) proximal neuropathy

   (D) ecchymosis

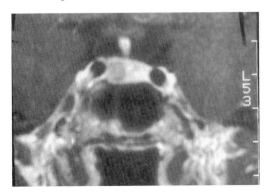

FIG. 18-1   Coronal MR scan (T-1 with contrast)

5. If the above patient presents with a normal MR scan of the sella with and without contrast enhancement, the most likely etiology of his Cushing's is

    (A) adrenal tumor
    (B) lung carcinoid
    (C) lung adenocarcinoma
    (D) pituitary tumor

6. The best laboratory test to establish the presence of pathologic hypercortisolism in the above patient suspected of having Cushing's is

    (A) AM serum cortisol
    (B) AM ACTH level
    (C) 24-h urine-free cortisol
    (D) 2-day low-dose dexamethasone suppression test

7. After the presence of hypercortisolism is demonstrated in this patient, tests need to be performed to establish whether the hypercortisolism is ACTH dependent or independent. All of the following would be consistent with ACTH-*dependent* Cushing's *except*:

    (A) no response of ACTH to CRH (corticotropin releasing hormone
    (B) an elevated random ACTH level
    (C) a normal random ACTH level
    (D) a low random ACTH level

8. The laboratory test results on the above patient are consistent with ACTH-dependent Cushing's disease. The *best* test for distinguishing pituitary versus ectopic secretion of excess corticotropin would be

    (A) high-dose dexamethasone suppression test
    (B) high resolution CT scan of the chest
    (C) CRH stimulation test
    (D) selective inferior petrosal sinus sampling

9. All of the laboratory tests in the above patient eventually lead to the diagnosis of pituitary Cushing's disease. An MRI of the pituitary is normal. A transsphenoidal procedure is performed and no tumor is found. The entire gland has been explored, and the right half of the gland has been removed, based on the lateralization of the petrosal sinus sampling; however, the patient's Cushing's disease is not cured. All of the following would be reasonable options *except*:

    (A) reexploration via the transsphenoidal approach
    (B) restudy to look for ectopic source
    (C) radiosurgery of the residual pituitary tissue
    (D) bilateral laparoscopic adrenalectomy

10. A 47-year-old woman with Cushing's syndrome who is in the process of evaluation presents to the emergency room (ER) with sudden onset of back pain and paraparesis with a T9 sensory level. The most likely diagnosis is

    (A) an osteoporotic vertebral compression fracture with spinal cord injury
    (B) thoracic disk herniation
    (C) epidural lipomatosis
    (D) spontaneous spinal epidural hematoma

11. A painful thoracic compression fracture secondary to the osteoporosis that accompanies Cushing's disease is best treated by

    (A) prolonged bed rest and narcotics
    (B) methylmethacrylate injection
    (C) endoscopic transthoracic stabilization
    (D) bracing and medical therapy for osteoporosis

12. The *best* laboratory test to confirm the clinical impression of acromegaly is

    (A) any growth hormone (GH) level above 5 ng/mL
    (B) a GH level of 25 ng/mL
    (C) failure of GH to suppress with 75 mg glucose
    (D) an elevated somatomedin C (insulin-like growth factor 1, IGF-1) level

13. An acromegalic patient is at increased risk for all of the following *except*:

    (A) sleep apnea
    (B) cardiomyopathy
    (C) coronary artery disease
    (D) carcinoma of the colon

14. A 68-year-old male presents with clinical and laboratory acromegaly. His vision is normal. An MRI demonstrates a sellar tumor invading the left cavernous sinus (Fig. 18-3). The patient's prolactin and GH levels are 10 times normal. The IGF-1 level is three times the upper limit of normal. The *best* treatment for this patient would be

    (A) transsphenoidal excision
    (B) radiosurgery
    (C) long-acting octreotide
    (D) bromocriptine

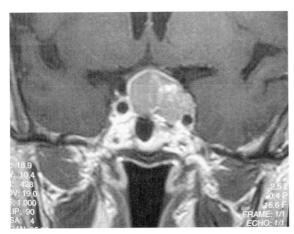

FIG. 18-3 Coronal MR (T-1 with contrast) demonstrating pituitary macroadenoma extending into the left cavernous sinus that is secreting excess growth hormone, causing acromegaly.

15. When abdominal surgery is contemplated in a patient with acromegaly, the following anesthetic technique is most useful:

(A) awake fiberoptic intubation

(B) extra long rigid laryngoscope

(C) blind nasal intubation

(D) larger than usual endotracheal tube

16. A newly diagnosed acromegalic with adult onset diabetes mellitus presents in the ER with chest pain. He is treated with tissue plasminogen activator (TPA) for suspected myocardial ischemia. The following morning he has a severe retroorbital headache and is unable to look up, down, or in with the right globe and there is ptosis of the right lid. The most likely cause is

(A) diabetic oculomotor neuropathy

(B) temporal lobe hematoma

(C) posterior communicating artery aneurysm

(D) pituitary apoplexy

Answers and Explanations

1. **(A)** By definition a pituitary microadenoma is a pituitary tumor less than 10 mm in size. The lesion is best visualized in a coronal T-1 magnetic resonance imaging (MRI) of the pituitary with gadolinium enhancement. The spinal fluid is black and outlines the optic chiasm, pituitary stalk, and the diaphragm sella. The pituitary gland, stalk, and cavernous sinuses enhance with contrast. Microadenomas usually enhance less than the normal pituitary and therefore can be easily visualized as an area of hypointensity. The cavernous sinuses are on either side of the sella. In a scan of good quality the third, fourth, and first and second divisions of the fifth nerve can be seen as black dots in the enhanced cavernous sinuses. The carotid arteries appear as black flow voids. The pituitary stalk may be shifted to the opposite side and the diaphragm sella on the side of the lesion may be slightly elevated. T2 MR images by convention are not performed with gadolinium. Microadenomas are common and can be seen in 20% of autopsy pituitary specimens and in routine MRIs of the brain in asymptomatic people. It is rare for microadenomas to grow into macroadenomas. In order for a pituitary adenoma to cause compression of the optic chiasm, it needs to grow at least 1 cm above the top of the sella. Microadenomas can secrete hormones (endocrine active adenoma), the most common being prolactin, but most microadenomas are not endocrinologically active.

Bibliography

Krist A, Husain M. Pathology of sellar and parasellar tumors. In: Krisht A, Tindall G (eds.), *Pituitary Disorders: Comprehensive Management*. Baltimore, MD: Lippincott, Williams & Wilkins, 1999, 99–119.

Litt A, Kricheff I. Magnetic resonance imaging of pituitary tumors. In: Cooper P (ed.), *Neurosurgical Topics: Contemporary Diagnosis and Management of Pituitary Adenomas*. Park Ridge, IL: American Association of Neurological Surgeons, 1990, 1–20.

2. **(A)** The MRI in Fig. 18-1 demonstrates a microadenoma on the right side of the sella. The elevated prolactin level makes it likely, but not certain, that the microadenoma is secreting prolactin. Because the microadenoma may be incidental, other causes of hyperprolactinemia must be ruled out, including primary hypothyroidism, liver and kidney disease, chronic chest wall or breast stimulation, other structural lesions in the area of the hypothalamus and a variety of drugs (phenothiazines, tricyclic antidepressants, calcium channel blockers, cimetidine, and fluoxetine). Prolactin is secreted by the normal pituitary in both in men and women. Unlike most other pituitary hormones, secretion of prolactin is primarily under inhibitory control by dopamine, which reaches the pituitary from secretory cells in the hypothalamus via the portal blood in the pituitary stalk. Increased prolactin will cause decreased estrogen production, which in turn can result in amenorrhea or oligomenorrhea and in both men and women, galactorrhea, decreased libido, and infertility. A late effect may be osteoporosis secondary to low estrogen or testosterone levels. Consequently, hyperprolactinemia should be treated in the above patient. About 80% of microadenomas will respond to therapy with dopamine agonists, such as bromocriptine or cabergoline. Most endocrinologists would recommend initial treatment with a dopamine agonist, which is effective in lowering prolactin in over 80% of prolactinomas. If the medication fails to reduce the prolactin level, there is an excellent chance that removal of the lesion by transsphenoidal surgery would restore normal endocrine function and fertility. It is safe to take birth control pills while receiving dopamine agonist therapy. A pregnancy test on this patient would also be appropriate. Dopamine agonists are not associated with increased birth defects, but in the United States it is customary to stop them as soon as pregnancy is achieved.

3. **(C)** This patient (see Fig. 18-2) should have an emergency prolactin level drawn. While waiting for the level to return, he should be started on steroids and

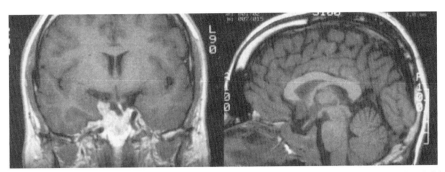

FIG. 18-4 Coronal and sagittal MR scans (T-1 with contrast) after treatment with bromocriptine, demonstrating shrinkage of giant pituitary macroadenoma.

specific treatment with dopamine agonist therapy. Within hours of starting bromocriptine, this patient's vision began to subjectively improve as the tumor began to soften. A very high percentage of prolactinomas will shrink with medical therapy over a period of weeks to months. It is necessary to continue medical therapy, perhaps indefinitely, as these tumors may enlarge again when medication is stopped. This patient's prolactin level dropped from 15,000 to 21 ng/mL on dopamine agonist therapy, and he has normal vision and a partially empty sella (Fig. 18-4). In large lesions, when the skull base has been eroded, the patient must be warned that there is a possibility of spontaneous cerebral spinal fluid rhinorrhea. It is common for patients with hyperprolactinemia to gain weight.

Bibliography

Frankel R, Tindall G. Prolactinomas. In: Krisht A, Tindall G (eds.), *Pituitary Disorders: Comprehensive Management.* Baltimore, MD: Lippincott, Williams & Wilkins, 1999, 199–207.

Katznelson L, Klibanski A. Hyperprolactinemia: physiology and clinical approach. In: Krisht A, Tindall G (eds.), *Pituitary Disorders: Comprehensive Management.* Baltimore, MD: Lippincott, Williams & Wilkins, 1999, 189–198.

Molitch M. Prolactinoma. In: Melemed S (ed.), *The Pituitary.* Cambridge: Blackwell Science, 1995, 443–447.

4. **(C)** Primary Cushing's syndrome occurs when there is excess secretion of cortisone by the adrenal glands. The symptoms usually begin insidiously, but occasionally the signs and symptoms can come on very rapidly. Women are more frequently involved than men. Most patients present in the third to the fifth decade of life, but the disorder can occur in childhood and adolescents. Central weight gain is the hallmark of the disorder and sometimes can be quite spectacular; however, some patients only gain a slight amount, but their body fat is redistributed around their abdomen. The skin is thin and stretched and purple stria and easy bruising are suggestive of the diagnosis. Many patients with Cushing's have proximal weakness in the legs, but the weakness is because of a proximal *myopathy* rather than a *neuropathy*. Hypertension and glucose intolerance are common. Other features of Cushing's may include a moon facies secondary to deposition of fat around the ears and cheeks, fat enlargement in the supraclavicular areas and posterior neck (buffalo hump), acne and facial hirsutism. Unfortunately there are no signs or symptoms of Cushing's syndrome to absolutely establish the diagnosis without a series of supportive laboratory tests.

5. **(D)** Endogenous Cushing's syndrome can be divided into ACTH *dependent* and ACTH *independent* types. Adrenocortical stimulating hormone (ACTH)-dependent Cushing's is the most common type (80%). The pathologic hypercortisolism results from excess secretion of ACTH by a pituitary tumor or an ectopic tumor. In 85% of cases hypersecretion by a pituitary tumor is the cause. The pituitary tumor may be so small (less than 5 mm) that it cannot be visualized on an MR of the sella in half the cases. The term Cushing's *disease* implies that a pituitary adenoma or rarely pituitary hyperplasia is the source of excess secretion of ACTH. Therefore, most patients with Cushing's syndrome presenting to a primary care physician will have a pituitary tumor. In about 15% of ACTH-dependent Cushing's syndrome ACTH is secreted by an ectopic tumor, such as an oat cell carcinoma of the lung, a bronchial or thymic carcinoid, a medullary thyroid carcinoma, or an islet cell tumor of the pancreas.

    ACTH-independent Cushing's usually results from either an adrenal adenoma or carcinoma that autonomously produces excess cortisol. Micro or macronodular adrenal hyperplasia is a rare cause. Only about 15% of Cushing's syndrome will have an adrenal etiology.

6. **(C)** The first step in diagnosing Cushing's syndrome is demonstrating endogenous hypercortisolism. This is a very important and sometimes difficult step, because there are many individuals that are obese, hypertensive, glucose intolerant, and have other physical characteristics such as acne and hirsutism that may overlap with Cushing's syndrome. Probably the most reliable test is the measurement of 24-h urine-free cortisol. This test has a sensitivity of 95% in diagnosing Cushing's syndrome and only a 1% false positive rate. The overnight 1 mg dexamethasone suppression test is very specific for Cushing's, but not very sensitive because of false positive rates of 12–30%. False negative tests in conditions that increase dexamethasone metabolism can also occur. When first evaluating a patient with suspected Cushing's disease, other diseases that result in hypercortisolemia must also be considered, including alcoholism and depression. Most surgeons will rely on the consultation of an experienced endocrinologist to arrive at the diagnosis.

7. **(A)** A normal or elevated ACTH level usually assures that the patient has ACTH-dependent Cushing's. Cortisol from an adrenal tumor would, by negative feedback, suppress CRH and ACTH secretion and the blood ACTH level would be low or hardly detectable; however, a random low ACTH can occur with an ACTH secreting pituitary tumor because secretion of ACTH is pulsatile. In the presence of a low ACTH value, the CRH stimulation test should be performed. ACTH secreting tumors (pituitary or ectopic) will respond to stimulation by CRH and the peripheral ACTH level will rise. In the presence of excess cortisol secreted by an adrenal tumor, the suppressed pituitary corticotropin cells will not respond to stimulation with CRH.

8. **(D)** The dexamethasone suppression test is based on the fact that the glucocorticoid can suppress secretion of ACTH in pituitary and ectopic tumors secreting ACTH by negative feedback. However, pituitary tumors are more sensitive to the doses of dexamethasone used in the high-dose dexamethasone suppression test and ACTH levels will drop much lower than will levels from an ectopic source; however, the test lacks sensitivity and specificity. The best method to distinguish between pituitary and ectopic secretion of excess ACTH is via inferior petrosal sinus sampling. The procedure is performed by cannulating the inferior petrosal sinuses bilaterally and measuring ACTH levels simultaneously from the sinuses and peripheral blood at baseline and after the administration of CRH. In pituitary Cushing's there will be a significant elevation of ACTH in the sinus blood as opposed to the peripheral blood. (This test cannot be used to diagnose Cushing's because a normal person will also have elevated levels in the petrosal sinuses, particularly with ACTH stimulation.) If a pituitary tumor is not visible on MRI, petrosal sinus sampling can sometimes lateralize the tumor in the gland, which can be very helpful during transsphenoidal surgery.

9. **(D)** Transsphenoidal surgery may fail to cure presumed pituitary Cushing's in as many 15–20% of cases, even in the most experienced hands. Reexploration will occasionally reveal a missed tumor. Before this is undertaken, it wise to restudy the patient to be sure an ectopic source was not overlooked. Radiosurgery of the sella (the entire dose of radiation in one session) or conventional irradiation using stereotactic planning but delivering the dose in fractions, is a reasonable option. It may take 2 years to achieve a response, during which time the patient is treated medically, usually with ketoconazole. This is an antifungal drug that inhibits some steroidogenic enzymes involved in the synthesis of cortisol. There are numerous side effects, including liver toxicity, nausea and vomiting, gynecomastia, and inhibition androgen synthesis. In an older patient total hypophysectomy would be an option, but most neurosurgeons would want to avoid this in a young individual.

Bilateral adrenalectomy, even though it can now be done laparoscopically, is usually a last resort option. The operation leaves the patient completely dependent on exogenous steroid replacement with the risk of an Addisonian crisis in the event of poor compliance. In addition there is a 10% risk of developing Nelson's syndrome, which is the continued growth of a missed pituitary adenoma, even after many quiescent years, with compression of adjacent cranial structures and extremely high ACTH levels. These patients often develop hyperpigmentation of their skin secondary to melanin stimulating hormone (MSH) cross-reactivity with high levels of ACTH. The lesion is difficult to control and patients may die as a result of an expanding and spreading mass. If adrenalectomy is selected, most surgeons and endocrinologists would probably recommend prophylactic pituitary irradiation around the time of the adrenalectomy.

Bibliography

Graham K, Samuels M. Cushing's disease. In: Krisht A, Tindall G (eds.), *Pituitary Disorders: Comprehensive Management.* Baltimore, MD: Lippincott, Williams & Wilkins, 1999, 209–224.

O'Riordain D, Farley D, Young W, et al. Long term outcome of bilateral adrenalectomy in patients with Cushing's syndrome. *Surgery* 1994;116:1088–1094.

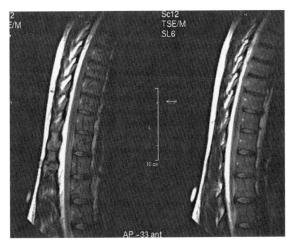

FIG. 18-5 Sagittal T-1 image with contrast, demonstrating excess fat (epidural lipomatosis) posterior to the spinal cord.

10. **(C)** It would be unusual for an osteoporotic compression fracture to cause spinal cord compression. In Cushing's syndrome of any cause there is deposition of excess adipose tissue around visceral organs, the retroperitoneal space, and in the epidural space in both the lumbar and spinal canal (epidural lipomatosis). Occasionally there will be infarction and swelling of the fat with spinal cord compression. Iatrogenic Cushing's is implicated more often than endogenous Cushing's, and it has even been reported in a pulmonary ectopic ACTH secreting tumor. The syndrome has also has been described in obese individuals that do not have Cushing's syndrome. The diagnosis is made by spinal MRI (Figs. 18-5 and 18-6), which reveals extensive epidural fat. The treatment is by laminectomy.

Bibliography

Haddad S, Hitchon P, Godersky J. Idiopathic and glucocorticoid-induced spinal and epidural lipomatosis. *J Neurosurg* 1991;74:38–42.

11. **(B)** Vertebroplasty has revolutionized the management of osteoporotic compression fractures. Injection of methylmethacrylate into the vertebral body via a needle introduced through the pedicle is safe and effective in giving almost immediate relief of pain. Figure 18-7a shows an MRI of a patient with two painful compression fractures. Figure 18-7b is a lateral plain radiograph after transpedicular vertebroplasty at both levels. The patient had almost complete relief of pain immediately postprocedure.

Bibliography

Amar A, Larsen D, Esnaashari N, et al. Percutaneous transpedicular polymethylmethacrylate vertebroplasty for the treatment of spinal compression fractures. *Neurosurgery* 2001;49:1115.

12. **(D)** A random measure of GH is not helpful in the diagnosis of acromegaly because GH is secreted in a pulsatile fashion. Depending on when the blood sample is taken, an acromegalic may have a normal level and person without acromegaly may have a significantly elevated level. Failure of GH to suppress to near zero following 75 gm of glucose is helpful to determine cure after pituitary surgery. The action of GH is mediated through the liver by the production of

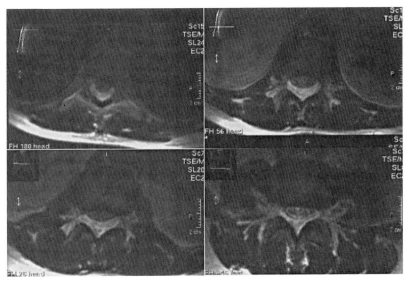

FIG. 18-6 Coronal T-1 images with contrast, demonstrating excess fat (epidural lipomatosis) posterior to the spinal cord.

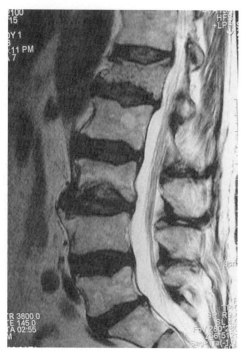

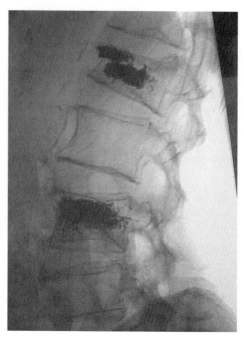

FIG. 18-7b

FIG. 18-7a   Lateral film of the lumbar spine, demonstrating osteoporotic fractures of L2 and L4 vertebral bodies before (*a*) and after (*b*) vertebroplasty with methylmethacrylate.

somatomedin C (IGF-1). This protein reflects overall GH activity and is the best measure of excess GH production in acromegaly.

13. **(C)** Acromegaly results from excess secretion of GH from the pituitary gland. When present in childhood, before closure of the epiphyseal plates, gigantism may result. In adults, acromegaly results in skeletal overgrowth (prognathism, frontal bossing, teeth separation), soft tissue swelling (macroglossia, large hands and feet, increased heel pad and scalp thickness), glucose intolerance (25% of cases), hypertension, intractable headache, and, if there is a macroadenoma, compression of the optic nerves and chiasm. Even though some of these clinically obvious manifestations make for a grotesque appearance, the more worrisome effects of acromegaly are premature cardiac death from cardiomyopathy and serious sleep apnea from the soft tissue changes in the upper airway. There is also an increased incidence of malignancy, particularly colon cancer. This risk for colon cancer may persist after biochemical cure of acromegaly and requires indefinite follow-up.

14. **(C)** It is unlikely that transsphenoidal surgery will cure this patient's acromegaly since the cavernous sinus is full of tumor. Also, it is hard to get a biochemical cure when the initial GH level is very high.

Since this patient's visual acuity and visual fields are normal, there is no urgency to decompress the optic chiasm and nerves. An attempt to remove tumor from the cavernous sinus will probably not be completely successful in returning GH levels to normal and there would be significant risk to the cranial nerves. Even though the prolactin level is elevated, which may occur in 20% of acromegalics, the chance of improving the acromegaly with a dopamine agonist such as bromocriptine is low. Radiosurgery should be considered, but the effects may not be evident for 2 or more years. In the meantime there is a reasonable chance that octreotide, a somatostatin analog, can lower the GH hormone levels to normal. The medication is now available in a parenteral long-acting form that only needs to be given monthly.

15. **(A)** Intubation of an acromegalic patient can be extremely difficult. It may be hard to get a large enough properly fitting face mask, and even with an oral airway and jaw thrust, it may not be possible to ventilate the patient after induction of anesthesia. There may be marked sleep apnea with the induction of anesthesia. Because of soft tissue changes, it may not be possible to visualize the vocal cords. A smaller than predicted endotracheal tube may be necessary because of glottis narrowing. A blind nasal intubation is extremely difficult. The safest way to intubate an acromegalic is awake with fiberoptic laryngoscope.

Postoperatively the patient must be watched carefully for airway obstruction.

Bibliography

Thapar K, Laws E. Growth hormone-secreting tumors: operative management. In: Krisht A, Tindall G (eds.), *Pituitary Disorders: Comprehensive Management.* Baltimore, MD: Lippincott, Williams & Wilkins, 1999, 243–258.

Vance, M. Growth hormone secreting adenomas. In: Krisht A, Tindall G (eds.), *Pituitary Disorders: Comprehensive Management.* Baltimore, MD: Lippincott, Williams & Wilkins, 1999, 235–242.

16. **(D)** This patient most likely had pituitary apoplexy. Anticoagulation of any type can precipitate spontaneous hemorrhage into a pituitary tumor. The hemorrhage can result in visual loss if the tumor is adjacent to the optic chiasm. In cases where the tumor is entirely intrasellar, pressure is exerted against one or both cavernous sinuses, which form the lateral boundaries of the sella. The third, fourth, and first and second divisions of the fifth cranial nerves pass through the cavernous sinus. A combination of unilateral or bilateral palsies of these cranial nerves can result from pituitary apoplexy. Occasionally apoplexy can result from spontaneous infarction of a pituitary tumor rather than hemorrhage. Treatment involves transsphenoidal decompression and treatment of

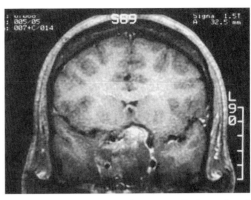

FIG. 18-8 Coronal MR (T-1 with contrast) demonstrating hemorrhage following treatment with IV TPA for a suspected MI.

hypopituitarism, particularly hypocortisolemia. Figure 18-8 is an MRI of a similar patient with pituitary apoplexy, revealing acute spontaneous hemorrhage (hypodense on T1 weighted image) into a previously diagnosed tumor.

Bibliography

Krisht A, Vaphiades M, Husain M. Pituitary apoplexy. In: Krisht A, Tindall G (eds.), *Pituitary Disorders: Comprehensive Management.* Baltimore, MD: Lippincott, Williams & Wilkins, 1999, 295–303.

CHAPTER 19

Multiple Endocrine Neoplasia

Earl Gage and Thomas Broadie

Questions

1. The gene involved in the pathogenesis of multiple endocrine neoplasia (MEN) 2 syndromes is

   (A) menin
   (B) RET
   (C) APC
   (D) p53
   (E) none of the above

2. The chromosome carrying the gene associated with MEN 1 is

   (A) chromosome 14
   (B) chromosome 13
   (C) chromosome 12
   (D) chromosome 11
   (E) chromosome 10

3. The most common clinical manifestation of MEN 1 is

   (A) hypoglycemia
   (B) renal stones
   (C) galactorrhea
   (D) osteoporosis
   (E) peptic ulcer disease

4. The most common endocrinologic manifestation of MEN 1 is

   (A) hyperinsulinemia
   (B) hyperprolactinemia
   (C) hypercalcemia
   (D) hypergastrinemia
   (E) hyperglucagonemia

5. A 35-year-old with recently diagnosed HPT also gives a history of poorly controlled gastroesophageal reflux disease and chronic diarrhea. Fasting serum gastrin is 150 pg/mL. To confirm your diagnosis, what additional test is essential?

   (A) *Helicobacter pylori* probe
   (B) gastric acid secretion test
   (C) esophageal manometry
   (D) esophagogastroduodenoscopy (EGD)
   (E) secretin test

6. MEN-associated gastrinomas are most frequently found in what anatomic location?

   (A) head of the pancreas
   (B) tail of the pancreas
   (C) gastric antrum
   (D) duodenum
   (E) jejunum

7. A 40-year-old man has recently been diagnosed with sporadic HPT. Compared to MEN 1-associated HPT, this patient's disease is most likely to involve

   (A) a single parathyroid gland
   (B) all four parathyroid glands
   (C) the thyroid gland
   (D) the pituitary gland
   (E) none of the above

8. A 50-year-old man with a recently diagnosed gastrinoma is noted to have a serum calcium of 12.5 mg/dL. A serum PTH level is drawn and found to be elevated. Although proton pump inhibitors have been prescribed, the patient has persistent reflux symptoms. The next most appropriate step in managing this patients reflux symptoms would be

   (A) total parathyroidectomy with autotransplantation
   (B) sestamibi scan
   (C) addition of an H2 blocker
   (D) distal pancreatectomy
   (E) highly selective vagotomy

9. All of the following may be included in standard screening protocols for MEN 1 *except*:

   (A) identification of specific MEN 1 mutations in germline DNA
   (B) serial measurements of ionized calcium, parathyroid hormone and prolactin every 3 years in first degree relatives of MEN 1 patients who have negative or inconclusive genetic tests
   (C) tumor DNA analysis for MEN 1 somatic mutations
   (D) selected yearly biochemical and imaging tests in patients carrying MEN 1 mutations(E) all of the above may be included in screening protocols

10. In MEN 1, the most common pancreaticoduodenal tumors are

    (A) gastrinomas
    (B) nonfunctioning tumors
    (C) insulinomas
    (D) somatostatinomas
    (E) VIPomas

11. A male patient with the most common type of pituitary neoplasm in MEN 1 would be most likely to present with which of the following clinical findings:

    (A) galactorrhea
    (B) hypogonadism
    (C) abdominal striae
    (D) hyperthyroidism
    (E) acral enlargement

12. Medullary thyroid cancer associated with MEN 2 syndromes

    (A) is more aggressive in MEN 2B than 2A
    (B) is more aggressive in MEN 2A than 2B
    (C) is most often bilateral
    (D) is most often unilateral
    (E) A and C
    (F) A and D
    (G) B and C
    (H) B and D

13. Medullary thyroid cancer accounts for what percent of all thyroid malignancies?

    (A) 5–10
    (B) 15–20
    (C) 25–30
    (D) 35–40
    (E) 45–50

14. What percent of MTCs are familial?

    (A) 10
    (B) 20
    (C) 40
    (D) 60
    (E) 80

15. A 22-year-old woman is being evaluated for a multinodular thyroid noted on physical examination by her primary physician. She also gives a recent history of "terrible headaches" and anxiety. She is noted to have a serum calcitonin level of 1400 pg/mL after standard administration of calcium gluconate and pentagastrin. Which of the following is the most important laboratory test to perform prior to any surgical intervention?

    (A) serum calcium
    (B) serum parathyroid hormone level
    (C) 24-h urine catecholamines
    (D) serum thyroid stimulating hormone (TSH) and free T4 levels
    (E) serum phosphorous

16. All of the following statements are true of MTC *except*:

    (A) there is no effective adjuvant therapy for MTC
    (B) MTC in MEN 2A tends to have an indolent course
    (C) direct DNA testing is the most sensitive means of screening kindred of those with the MEN 2-associated MTC
    (D) laparoscopy is an effective means of evaluating for liver metastases in MTC
    (E) Kindred of patients with MEN-associated MTC should undergo screening with regular radionuclide scanning

17. Nonendocrine manifestations of MEN 2B include all of the following *except*:

    (A) pectus excavatum
    (B) megacolon
    (C) hypertrophied corneal nerves
    (D) lisch nodules
    (E) mucosal neuromas

18. A 45-year-old man with a history of MTC underwent total thyroidectomy 4 years ago. He now presents with poorly controlled hypertension, severe paroxysmal headaches and palpitations. Urinary catecholamines are elevated and MR of the abdomen is performed as shown in Fig. 19-1.

    Which of the following medications must be administered prior to surgical intervention?

    (A) esmolol

    (B) sodium nitroprusside

    (C) isoproterenol

    (D) phenoxybenzamine

    (E) calcium gluconate

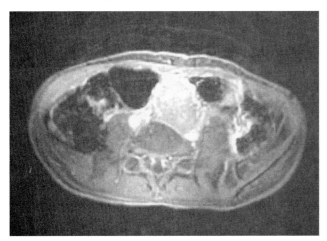

FIG. 19-1   MRI of the abdomen.

19. A 24-year-old woman presents to her physician complaining of intermittent fatigue, confusion, and diaphoresis. She states that these symptoms are especially prominent on waking in the morning but seem to get better after she has her usual glass of orange juice. Routine laboratory workup reveals hypercalcemia, an elevated PTH level, and no other abnormalities. A monitored 24-h fast reproduces her symptoms. At that time, she is additionally noted to have an inappropriately high serum insulin level and a corresponding blood glucose of 48 mg/dL. For the majority of cases, the most appropriate surgical management for the hypoglycemia is

    (A) pancreaticoduodenectomy

    (B) total pancreatectomy

    (C) distal pancreatectomy with enucleation of grossly visible tumor in the head of the pancreas

    (D) simple enucleation of grossly visible tumor

    (E) no surgery is indicated

20. A 37-year-old nonpregnant woman presents to her primary care doctor complaining of milky discharge from both breasts. Initial workup reveals an elevated prolactin level as well as elevated serum calcium and serum parathyroid hormone levels. The patient is currently asymptomatic with regard to her hypercalcemia. MRI of the brain is shown in Fig. 19-2.

    The most appropriate initial therapy for this problem is

    (A) bromocriptine therapy

    (B) transphenoidal resection

    (C) carbidopa/levodopa therapy

    (D) octreotide therapy

    (E) radiation therapy

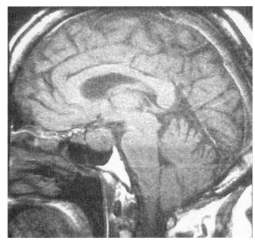

FIG. 19-2   MRI of the brain.

Answers and Explanations

1. **(B)** MEN 2 syndromes are characterized by the presence of medullary thyroid cancer (MTC) and pheochromocytomas. The MEN 2A variant is further characterized by hyperparathyroidism (HPT). MEN 2B, on the other hand, is notable for mucosal and musculoskeletal abnormalities which include neuromas of the mouth and lips, "marfanoid" habitus, and ganglioneuromatosis of the bowel myenteric and submucosal plexus. Additional abnormalities associated with MEN 2B include congenital hip dislocation, pes cavus, pectus excavatum, and kyphosis. Both MEN 2 syndromes are inherited in an autosomal dominant fashion with nearly 100% penetrance but varying degrees of expressivity. Mutations in the RET protooncogene, which maps to chromosome 10, have been identified in individuals with MEN 2 syndromes. This gene encodes a receptor tyrosine kinase important in transmembrane signal transduction.

MEN 2A variants are characterized by mutations in one of five codons which specify highly conserved cysteine residues in the extracellular domain (Fig. 19-3).

In the normal RET gene, two cysteine residues are juxtaposed and a resultant disulfide bond is formed. When the RET gene is mutated such that one of these cysteine residue is replaced, the free remaining cysteine residue is available to form a disulfide bond with a cysteine residue of a neighboring receptor. When this aberrant disulfide bond is formed, dimerizing the two receptors, the result is a constitutively activated tyrosine kinase and unopposed signal transduction (Fig. 19-4).

In contrast to MEN 2A, MEN 2B variants are characterized by a single point mutation in the catalytic domain of the RET gene product. This mutation, specifying replacement of a methionine with a

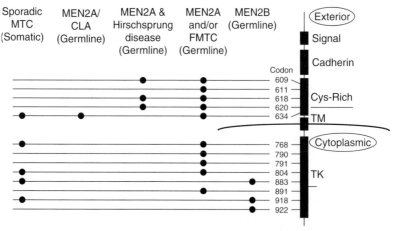

FIG. 19-3 RET mutations in MEN 2 and sporadic MTC. Adapted from Gagel RF, Marx SJ: Multiple endocrine neoplasia. In Larsen PR, Kronenberg HM, Shlomo M, Polonsky KS (eds): *Williams Textbook of Endocrinology, 10th ed*. Philadelphia, PA: WB Saunders, 2003, p. 1741. With permission of Elsevier Science.

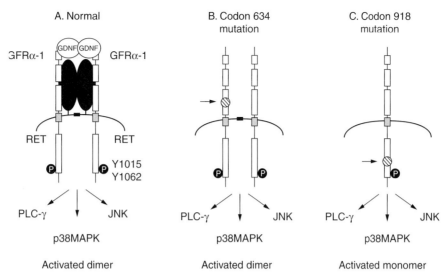

A. Normal   B. Codon 634 mutation   C. Codon 918 mutation

FIG. 19-4 RET mutations in the cysteine-rich extracellular domain lead to dimerization and constitutive activation while mutations in the intracellular domain result in changed substrate specificity. Adapted from Gagel RF, Marx SJ: Multiple endocrine neoplasia. In Larsen PR, Kronenberg HM, Shlomo M, Polonsky KS (eds): *Williams Textbook of Endocrinology, 10th ed.* Philadelphia, PA: WB Saunders, 2003, p. 1742. With permission of Elsevier Science.

threonine residue at the tyrosine kinase domain, occurs most frequently at codon 918 and results in changed substrate specificity.

In both MEN 2 syndromes, there seems to be a strong correlation between disease phenotype and mutation at a specific codon. This seems to be especially true with regard to prediction of pheochromocytomas and HPT and may offer clinicians valuable information in disease treatment and surveillance among kindred of MEN 2 patients.

Bibliography

Eng C, Clayton D, Schuffenecker I, Lenoir G, et al. The relationship between specific RET proto-oncogene mutations and disease phenotype in multiple endocrine neoplasia type 2: international RET mutation consortium analysis. *J Am Med Assoc* 1996;276(19):1575–1579.

Larsen PR, Kronenberg HM, Melmed S, Polonsky KS (eds.), *Williams Textbook of Endocrinology,* 10th ed. Philadelphia, PA: WB Saunders, 2003, 51–52, 1741–1742.

Townsend CM (ed.), *Sabiston Textbook of Surgery: The Biological Basis of Modern Surgical Practice,* 16th ed. Philadelphia, PA: WB Saunders, 2001, 697–707.

Yip L, Cote GJ, Shapiro SE, Ayers GD, et al. Multiple endocrine neoplasia type 2: evaluation of the genotype-phenotype relationship. *Arch Surg* 2003:138(4);409–416.

2. **(D)** MEN 1 is characterized by the presence of HPT, adenomas of the anterior pituitary, and neuroendocrine tumors (NETs) of the pancreas and duodenum. Clinically overt disease is usually picked up between the third and fifth decade; however, laboratory abnormalities are frequently apparent much earlier.

Like MEN 2 syndromes, MEN 1 is inherited in an autosomal dominant fashion. The gene responsible for MEN 1 has been mapped to chromosome 11 and codes for a 610 amino acid protein called menin which consists of 10 exons, only nine of which are translated during creation of an mRNA transcript. The gene product is ubiquitously expressed in many tissues, most notably thymus, thyroid, and pancreas. Although recognized for its importance in the pathogenesis of MEN 1, the precise function of the menin protein is not well understood and is an area of active research. Although the precise location and type of mutation varies from patient to patient, it appears that nearly all result in a truncated protein.

In contrast to RET, which requires only a single mutated gene in order to produce MEN 2 syndromes, menin follows the so-called "two hit" hypothesis of tumorogenesis, requiring both an inherited faulty copy of the gene as well as a second somatic mutation in order to produce disease. This suggests a role for menin as a tumor supressor gene, likely coding for a nuclear protein. The second hit in approximately 90% of MEN patients involves chromosomal deletions at the 11q13 locus; however, some studies have shown other somatic mutations in the remaining MEN 1 patients, even in the absence of 11q13 deletions.

Bibliography

Chandrasekharappa SC, Guru SC, Manickam P, Olufemi SE, et al. Positional cloning of the gene for multiple endocrine neoplasia-type 1. *Science* 1997:276(5311);404–407.

Norton JA, Bollinger RR, Chang AE, Lowry SF, Muvlihill SJ, Pass HI, Thompson RW (eds.), *Surgery: Basic Science and Clinical Evidence.* New York, NY: Springer-Verlag, 2000, 955–966.

Pannett AA, Thakker RV. Somatic mutations in MEN type 1 tumors, consistent with the Knudsen "two-hit" hypothesis. *J Clin Endocrinol Metab* 2001:86(9);4371–4374.

Skogseid B. Multiple endocrine neoplasia type 1. *Br J Surg* 2003:90(4);383–385.

Townsend CM (ed.), *Sabiston Textbook of Surgery: The Biological Basis of Modern Surgical Practice,* 16th ed. Philadelphia, PA: WB Saunders, 2001, 697–707.

3. **(E)** The clinical expression of MEN 1 usually does not occur until the third or fourth decade of life, although endocrinologic manifestations (e.g., asymptomatic hypercalcemia) may be picked up earlier on routine lab examination or during workup for another problem. In fact, some studies have shown biochemical abnormalities occurring as early as 14–18 years of age, suggesting there may be a delay of nearly 20 years from the development of tumors and their clinical manifestations. Although HPT does occur in nearly 100% of MEN 1 patients, it is frequently asymptomatic. For this reason, the most commonly encountered clinical complaint of MEN 1 patients on initial presentation is peptic ulcer disease attributable to gastrinoma.

Since peptic ulcer disease is so common, it is important to define some guidelines for diagnosing the very specific entity of MEN 1 since clearly not all of the patients presenting with peptic ulcer disease have MEN. A Consensus Statement on diagnosis and therapy of MEN types 1 and 2 from an international group of clinical endocrinologists suggested the following definition. MEN 1 is a case of at least two of the three classic MEN 1 features (i.e., pituitary adenoma, HPT, and NETs of the pancreas or duodenum). The diagnosis of familial MEN 1 further requires at least one MEN 1 case and at least one first degree relative having one of the three classic tumors.

MEN 1 patients with gastrinoma frequently have malignant disease, and approximately 50% have metastatic disease at the time of diagnosis. Metastatic gastrinoma is not an infrequent cause of death among these patients.

All the other possible answers represent other clinical manifestations of MEN 1. Hypoglycemia may result from an insulinoma, accounting for nearly a quarter of MEN 1-associated pancreaticoduodenal tumors. Nephrolithiasis and osteoporosis are both common manifestations of symptomatic HPT. Galactorrhea may suggest the presence of a prolactin secreting pituitary adenoma.

Bibliography

Abeloff MD, Armitage JO, Lichter AS, Niederhuber JE. *Clinical Oncology,* 2nd ed. Philadelphia, PA: Churchill Livingstone, 2000, 1377–1379.

Brandi ML, Gagel RF, Angeli A, Bilezikian JP, et al. Guidelines for diagnosis and therapy of MEN type 1 and type 2. *J Clin Endocrinol Metab* 2001:86(12);5658–5671.

Townsend CM (ed.), *Sabiston Textbook of Surgery: The Biological Basis of Modern Surgical Practice,* 16th ed. Philadelphia, PA: WB Saunders, 2001, 697–707.

4. **(C)** As noted previously, MEN 1 frequently presents between the third and fifth decade of life with men and women equally affected. Individuals of different ethnic and racial backgrounds are also equally affected. Incidence ranges from 1/10,000 to 1/100,000. Among those with MEN 1, nearly 100% are diagnosed with HPT by 50 years of age, making this the most common endocrine manifestation of MEN 1. Histologically, these patients develop multiglandular parathyroid hyperplasia (Fig. 19-5).

HPT is characterized by hypercalcemia with an inappropriately elevated serum parathyroid hormone level and is most often asymptomatic at the time of diagnosis. Laboratory abnormalities obtained while working up other complaints thus can provide the first clues to the diagnosis. For instance, since HPT and gastrinoma often present together, incidental note may be made of hypercalcemia while working the patient up for symptoms attributable to the gastrinoma. When symptomatic HPT is the presenting problem, patients most often present with complaints comparable to those of patients with sporadic HPT. These include nephrolithiasis, weakness, fatigue, myalgias, arthralgias, or mental disturbances.

HPT associated with MEN 1 is typically multiglandular, involving all four glands. This stands in contrast to sporadic primary HPT which is

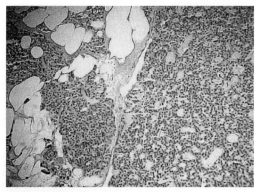

FIG. 19-5   Histologic representation of parathyroid hyperplasia.

most frequently uniglandular. Preoperative imaging has little role in the diagnosis or surgical treatment of MEN-associated HPT since all four glands should be visualized at neck exploration. The surgical procedure of choice is a matter of controversy. Some surgeons advocate subtotal parathyroidectomy, leaving behind a remnant of parathyroid tissue. Others prefer total parathyroidectomy with autotransplantation of a portion of parathyroid tissue to the forearm. The latter procedure may preclude the morbidity associated with reexploration of the neck should the patient manifest persistent or recurrent HPT requiring surgical intervention. In both procedures, a near-total thymectomy is also performed in order to remove any potential ectopic parathyroid tissue. Additionally, since both of the above-mentioned procedures carry a risk of postoperative hypoparathyroidism, some advocate cryopreservation of resected parathyroid tissue in anticipation of a future need for autotransplantation.

Bibliography

Brandi ML, Gagel RF, Angeli A, Bilezikian JP, et al. Guidelines for diagnosis and therapy of MEN type 1 and type 2. *J Clin Endocrinol Metab* 2001;86(12);5658–5671.

Chandrasekharappa SC, Guru SC, Manickam P, Olufemi SE, et al. Positional cloning of the gene for multiple endocrine neoplasia type 1. *Science* 1997;276(5311);404–407.

Goldman L, Bennett JC (eds.), *Cecil Textbook of Medicine*, 21st ed. Philadelphia, PA: WB Saunders, 2000, 1402–1403.

Larsen PR, Kronenberg HM, Melmed S, Polonsky KS (eds.), *Williams Textbook of Endocrinology*, 10th ed. Philadelphia, PA: WB Saunders, 2003, 1292–1294.

5. **(E)** In a patient with diagnosed HPT and refractory reflux disease, the diagnosis of MEN 1 with associated gastrinoma must be considered. Developing in 30–80% of MEN 1 patients, NETs of the pancreas and duodenum constitute the second most common manifestation of MEN 1 after HPT. The majority of these tumors are nonfunctioning. Among functional tumors, the two most common are gastrinoma and insulinoma. Among MEN 1 patients with functional neuroendocrine pancreaticoduodenal tumors, approximately 47% have gastrinomas and 12% have insulinomas. Other rare functional NETs include VIPomas and somatostatinomas. As noted in earlier discussions, patients may actually present with symptomatic NETs (e.g., gastric ulcers, reflux and so on) with laboratory evidence of HPT discovered incidentally during the workup.

Patients with gastrinoma typically present with the Zollinger-Ellison's syndrome. The most common manifestations include epigastric pain and reflux esophagitis because of increased gastric acid secretion.

Also noteworthy is the presence of a secretory diarrhea in many patients with gastrinoma, and in some patients, this may be the only symptom. This latter finding is a result of gastric acid hypersecretion which leads to destruction of pancreatic enzymes and mucosal injury.

Patients with suspected gastrinoma should have a serum gastrin level drawn. Fasting serum gastrin levels greater than 100 pg/mL are concerning for gastrinoma and should prompt a secretin test to confirm the diagnosis. Serum gastrin levels >1000 pg/mL are virtually diagnostic. The secretin test is performed by measuring serum gastrin levels after administration of 2 U/kg of secretin IV. A positive secretin test is confirmed by an increase in serum gastrin to at least 200 pg/mL above the basal value.

MEN 1-associated gastrinomas are malignant in a majority of cases with a tendency to metastasize to liver, lymphatics, and bone. Liver metastases, developing in 23% of MEN 1-associated gastrinomas, are the most concerning clinical finding and may ultimately lead to death in a subset of this patient population with aggressive tumor growth. Initial therapy in all gastrinomas is directed toward control of gastric acid hypersecretion with proton pump inhibitors. Additionally, surgical management of any associated HPT is an important initial step in the management of gastrinoma since correction of hypercalcemia aids in control of gastric acid hypersecretion.

Unfortunately, gastrinomas are rarely amenable to curative resection since they are typically multifocal and frequently extrapancreatic. Extrapancreatic tumors are found most frequently within the duodenal wall with more than 90% of duodenal gastrinomas occurring in the first or second portions of the duodenum. MEN-associated gastrinomas may also be found within peripancreatic lymph nodes. The multifocal nature of MEN 1-associated gastrinomas stands in contrast to sporadic gastrinomas which are more likely to be solitary tumors. For these reasons, curative surgical resection is most frequently undertaken in sporadic ZEs. Surgical management of gastrinomas in MEN 1 patients with a goal of cure is more controversial. Some advocate resection for cure while others argue for wide local excision only as a palliative debulking procedure or in an attempt to limit ongoing metastatic spread.

Bibliography

Fathia G, Venzon DJ, Ojeaburu JV, Showkat B, et al. Prospective study of the natural history of gastrinoma in patients with MEN 1: definition of an aggressive and a nonaggressive form. *J Clin Endocrinol Metab* 2001;86(11); 5282–5293.

Feldman M, Tschumy WO, Friedman LS, Sleisinger MH (eds.), *Sleisinger and Fordtran's Gastrointestinal and Liver Disease: Pathophysiology, Dignosis, Management*, 7th ed. Philadelphia, PA: WB Saunders, 2002, 782–792.

Marx S, Spiegel AM, Skarulis MC, Doppman JL, et al. Multiple endocrine neoplasia type 1: clinical and genetic topics. *Ann Intern Med* 1998:129(6);484–494.

Townsend CM (ed.), *Sabiston Textbook of Surgery: The Biological Basis of Modern Surgical Practice*, 16th ed. Philadelphia, PA: WB Saunders, 2001, 697–707.

6. **(D)** The majority of gastrinomas occur within the so-called gastrinoma triangle. This space is bounded by the confluence of the cystic and common hepatic ducts superiorly, the junction of the head and neck of the pancreas medially, and by the junction of the second and third portions of the duodenum inferiorly (Fig. 19-6).

Both sporadic and MEN-associated gastrinomas occur most frequently within the pancreas and duodenum. Although there seems to be an equal number occurring in each of these two locales when all gastrinomas are considered, evidence suggests MEN-associated disease has a predilection for the duodenum with upward of 80% being found in the duodenal wall. When occurring within the duodenal wall, gastrinomas are found most frequently within the first and second portions of the duodenum. Gastrinomas have also been found in the peripancreatic lymph nodes as well as in ectopic locations such as ovary, liver, common bile duct, and gastric pylorus.

As noted in previous discussions, MEN-associated gastrinomas tend to be multifocal making curative resection difficult and a matter of controversy.

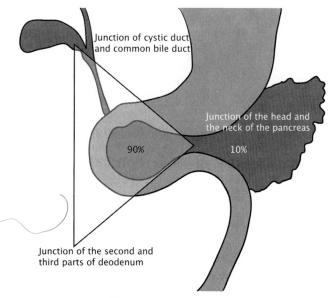

FIG. 19-6   Gastrinoma triangle.

Bibliography

Feldman M, Tschumy WO, Friedman LS, Sleisenger MH (eds.), *Sleisenger and Fordtran's Gastrointestinal and Liver Disease: Pathophysiology, Dignosis, Management*, 7th ed. Philadelphia, PA: WB Saunders, 2002, 782–792.

Jensen RT. Management of the Zollinger-Ellison syndrome in patients with multiple endocrine neoplasia type 1. *J Intern Med* 1998;243(6):477–488.

Norton JA, Doppman JL, Jensen RT. Curative resection in Zollinger-Ellison syndrome: results of a 10-year prospective study. *Ann Surg* 1992;215(1):8–18.

Stabile BE, Morrow DJ, Passaro E. The gastrinoma triangle: operative implications. *Am J Surg* 1984;147(1):25–31.

Thompson NW, Vinik AI, Eckhauser FE. Microgastrinomas of the duodenum: a cause of failed operations for the Zollinger-Ellison syndrome. *Ann Surg* 1989;209(4):396–404.

7. **(A)** Sporadic primary HPT is genetically distinct from its MEN-associated counterpart. One of the ways in which these two entities differ is in the number of glands involved. Whereas MEN-associated disease tends to produce diffuse multiglandular parathyroid involvement, sporadic primary HPT tends to involve only a single gland. Additionally, patients with HPT associated with MEN tend to have age-associated increases in levels of parathyroid hormone notable for a marked acceleration in patients over 40 years of age. Interestingly, in these patients, the concomitant elevation in calcium and decrease in serum phosphate were more mild than in patients with sporadic HPT.

The difference in number of glands involved in sporadic versus MEN-associated disease has important implications for surgical management of patients with primary HPT. In MEN-associated HPT, most surgeons advocate exploration with identification of all four glands. The specifics of which procedure to perform in MEN-associated disease, however, are controversial. Some surgeons advocate total parathyroidectomy with autotransplantation while others prefer subtotal or 3½ gland parathyroidectomy. In any event, it is agreed that unilateral or minimally invasive procedures which do not allow identification of all four glands are not appropriate for MEN-related disease.

In contrast, surgical therapy for sporadic adenomas may be directed at removal of the single adenomatous gland. Historically, this has been accomplished by bilateral exploration with visual identification of all four glands, removal of the enlarged one, and biopsy of one other to confirm histologically the uniglandular nature of the process. More recently a more limited exploration directed by sestamibi scanning has come into vogue. Sestamibi scanning using ^{99m}Tc sestamibi, which is taken up by parathyroid tissue, will localize 70–80% of enlarged and hyperfunctional parathyroid glands. Such localization may then allow dissection of a limited area of the neck directed by a gamma probe. If that scanning does not reliably differentiate uniglandular from multiglandular disease, parathyroid hormone levels must be assessed intraoperatively in a rigorous fashion to assure surgical correction of the disease. Failure of intraoperative parathyroid hormone test (PTH) levels to fall both into the normal range and also to levels less than one-half of preoperative levels mandates conversion of the limited approach to the traditional bilateral exploration.

Bibliography

Howe JR. Minimally invasive parathyroid surgery. *Surg Clin North Am* 2000;80(5):1399–1426.

Katai M. Primary hyperparathyroidism in patients with multiple endocrine neoplasia type 1: comparison with sporadic hyperparathyroidism. *Horm Metab Res* 2001;33(8):499–503.

Townsend CM (ed.), *Sabiston Textbook of Surgery: The Biological Basis of Modern Surgical Practice*, 16th ed. Philadelphia, PA: WB Saunders, 2001, 629–645, 697–707.

8. **(A)** The majority of gastrinomas are sporadic and account for approximately 75% of all patients with the Zollinger-Ellison's syndrome; however, nearly one-fourth of patients with gastrinomas have an associated MEN 1 syndrome. HPT is the most common endocrine abnormality in patients with MEN 1. Present in virtually all MEN 1 patients by 50 years of age, this endocrinopathy leads to elevated serum calcium in the setting of an inappropriately elevated parathyroid hormone level. NETs of the pancreas and duodenum, with gastrinomas being the most common, develop in 30–80% of MEN 1 patients. The third type of endocrinopathy associated with MEN 1 is anterior pituitary adenoma, developing in 15–50% of MEN 1 patients. Prolactinomas constitute the most frequent type of pituitary neoplasm in this setting.

This patient has both a gastrinoma and a laboratory diagnosis of HPT, strongly suggesting a diagnosis of MEN 1. When these two endocrinopathies coexist, the hypercalcemia of HPT actually can lead to increased gastrin secretion. This, in turn, may make management of symptoms associated with gastrinoma more difficult. For this reason, surgical treatment of HPT is advocated as part of the initial treatment of gastrinoma. If normocalcemia can be achieved, gastrin secretion decreases, basal acid output diminishes and the symptoms of marginally controlled reflux frequently improve. At times, the doses of PPIs or H2 blockers required to achieve control of reflux symptoms can be scaled back, as well.

Although there is some controversy among parathyroid surgeons regarding which procedure to perform for MEN-associated HPT, the most appropriate option listed above would be total parathyroidectomy with autotransplantation. This procedure is performed through a cervical neck incision. A bilateral neck exploration is done with identification and removal of all four parathyroid glands. A transcervical thymectomy is also performed in an attempt to remove any ectopic parathyroid tissue.

Bibliography

Brandi ML, Gagel RF, Angeli A, Bilezikian JP, et al. Guidelines for diagnosis and therapy of MEN type 1 and type 2. *J Clin Endocrinol Metab* 2001;86(12);5658–5671.

Norton JA, Cornelius MJ, Doppman JL. Effect of parathyroidectomy in patients with hyperparathyroidism and multiple endocrine neoplasia type 1. *Surgery* 1987; 102(6):958–966.

Norton JA, Bollinger RR, Chang AE, Lowry SF, Muvlihill SJ, Pass HI, Thompson RW (eds.), *Surgery: Basic Science and Clinical Evidence*. New York, NY: Springer-Verlag, 2000, 955–966.

9. **(C)** As noted previously, the gene responsible for MEN 1 is located on chromosome 11q13 and codes for a protein called menin. Although the precise function of menin is poorly understood, this 610 amino acid protein is thought to play a role in cell growth and proliferation via interaction with the transcription factor JunD.

Since identification of the gene associated with MEN 1, attention has been directed toward genetic testing and screening which might allow earlier identification and treatment of patients with the disease. Identification has been made possible through direct DNA sequencing techniques and haplotype analysis in connection with biochemical and imaging tests.

Patients presenting with sporadic MEN 1 or kindred with suspected or proven MEN 1 should first have genetic sequencing studies performed on peripheral blood samples in an attempt to identify germline MEN 1 mutations. When these studies fail to identify germline mutations but clinical suspicion is high for an inherited MEN 1 syndrome, the next step in genetic testing is haplotype analysis or genetic linkage analysis around the 11q13 locus. These studies require 7–10 affected family members for statistical significance and are therefore more difficult to perform in small kindreds or when germline mutations are newly acquired.

When genetic testing reveals definite or probable MEN 1 mutations, yearly biochemical screening is recommended beginning as early as 5 years of age.

Although no formal protocol has been developed, biochemical testing might include measurements of serum calcium, parathyroid hormone levels, prolactin levels as well as measurements of other substances secreted by MEN 1-associated tumors as clinically indicated (e.g., adrenocorticotropic hormone or ACTH, growth hormone and the like). Selective use of imaging modalities every 3–5 years should also be undertaken. In contrast, when genetic testing is inconclusive, first degree relatives of MEN 1 patients should undergo only serial biochemical testing every 3 years. This testing should include ionized calcium, PTH, and prolactin values.

Tumor DNA analysis for MEN 1 mutations is not warranted since MEN 1 somatic mutations are found in many sporadic endocrine tumors, among them sporadic parathyroid adenomas, gastrinomas, insulinomas, and bronchial carcinoids. This fact makes differentiation between germline mutations and purely acquired somatic mutations difficult if not impossible.

Bibliography

Brandi ML, Gagel RF, Angeli A, Bilezikian JP, et al. Guidelines for diagnosis and therapy of MEN type 1 and type 2. *J Clin Endocrinol Metab* 2001:86(12);5658–5671.

Marx S, Spiegel AM, Skarulis MC, Doppman JL, et al. Multiple endocrine neoplasia type 1: clinical and genetic topics. *Ann Intern Med* 1998:129(6);484–494.

Townsend CM (ed.), *Sabiston Textbook of Surgery: The Biological Basis of Modern Surgical Practice*, 16th ed. Philadelphia, PA: WB Saunders, 2001, 697–707.

10. **(B)** NETs of the pancreas and duodenum are the second most common endocrinopathy associated with MEN type 1, occurring in anywhere from 30 to 80% of all patients with this syndrome. Gastrinomas, accounting for 47% of MEN associated, functional pancreaticoduodenal tumors, lead to hypergastrinemia and the Zollinger-Ellison's syndrome; however, the most common type of NET seems to be a nonfunctioning or pancreatic polypeptide secreting adenoma. When present, these adenomas produce symptoms by exerting mass effect on surrounding structures. This stands in contrast to the functioning adenomas (e.g., gastrinoma or insulinoma) which may produce symptoms by hormone oversecretion. Nonfunctioning tumors may be detected with assays for pancreatic polypeptide.

Other common types of NETs of the pancreas and duodenum in MEN include gastrinoma and insulinoma. These two tumors account for the majority of functional enteropancreatic NETs in MEN 1, comprising 47 and 12% of functional tumors, respectively. These tumors, when present, tend to be multifocal. MEN-associated gastrinoma also tends to be somewhat aggressive with upward of 15–50% metastasizing to the liver by the time of diagnosis.

Functional NETs which secrete vasoactive intestinal peptide (VIP), glucagon, or somatostatin are decidedly less common although they have been described.

Bibliography

Marx S, Spiegel AM, Skarulis MC, Doppman JL, et al. Multiple endocrine neoplasia type 1: clinical and genetic topics. *Ann Intern Med* 1998;129(6):484–494.

Mutch MG. Pancreatic polypeptide is a useful plasma marker for radiographically evident pancreatic islet cell tumors in patients with multiple endocrine neoplasia type 1. *Surgery* 1997;122(6):1012–1019.

Norton JA, Bollinger RR, Chang AE, Lowry SF, Muvlihill SJ, Pass HI, Thompson RW (eds.), *Surgery: Basic Science and Clinical Evidence*. New York, NY: Springer-Verlag, 2000, 955–966.

Townsend CM (ed.), *Sabiston Textbook of Surgery: The Biological Basis of Modern Surgical Practice*, 16th ed. Philadelphia, PA: WB Saunders, 2001, 629–645, 697–707.

11. **(B)** Pituitary neoplasms are the third most frequent type of tumor associated with MEN 1, affecting 15–50% of patients with the disease. In roughly 25% of sporadic MEN 1 patients, pituitary disease may be the presenting endocrinopathy. Overall prevalence in MEN 1 ranges from 10 to 60%. The most common type of functional pituitary adenoma is a prolactinoma, accounting for approximately 62% of MEN 1-associated pituitary adenomas. The next most common type of pituitary adenoma is growth hormone secreting, accounting for around 10% pituitary adenomas. Other types included ACTH-producing tumors and "cosecreting" adenomas which release multiple substances. Pituitary adenomas may also become symptomatic owing to mass effects, in particular compression of the optic chiasm which may cause visual field defects. Finally, in rare cases, an enlarging pituitary adenoma may cause hypopituitarism by compression of the adjacent normal gland.

According to one multicenter study, the mean age of patients diagnosed with MEN 1-associated pituitary disease was 38 years old with 25% of patients diagnosed by age 26. There was a near 2:1 female predominance noted as well. The vast majority (85%) are macroadenomas. MEN 1-associated pituitary adenomas are associated with mutation of a tumor suppressor gene called *menin* located at chromosome location 11q13. This is in contradistinction to sporadic pituitary adenomas which do not appear to share the same mechanism of tumorigenesis.

Males and females with prolactinomas may present in very different ways despite a common pathology. Women who have prolactinomas typically present with amenorrhea or galactorrhea. In contrast, men with prolactin secreting tumors typically present with hypogonadism.

Although patients with ACTH secreting tumors may present with cushingoid symptomatology such as centripetal fat distribution, abdominal striae and hypertension, ACTH secreting tumors are far more rare than prolactinomas. Acral enlargement, a characteristic of growth hormone oversecretion in an adult patient, may occur in growth hormone secreting pituitary tumors; however, these tumors account for somewhere near 10% of MEN 1-associated pituitary adenomas and rank second behind prolactinoma in terms of frequency.

Bibliography

Goldman L, Bennett JC (eds.), *Cecil Textbook of Medicine*, 21st ed. Philadelphia, PA: WB Saunders, 2000, 1210–1212.

Larsen PR, Kronenberg HM, Melmed S, Polonsky KS (eds.), *Williams Textbook of Endocrinology*, 10th ed. Philadelphia, PA: WB Saunders, 2003, 184–185.

Townsend CM (ed.), *Sabiston Textbook of Surgery: The Biological Basis of Modern Surgical Practice*, 16th ed. Philadelphia, PA: WB Saunders, 2001, 629–645, 697–707.

Verges B, Boureille F, Goudet P, Murat A, et al. Pituitary disease in MEN type 1: data from the France-Belgium MEN 1 multicenter study. *J Clin Endocrinol Metab* 2002:87(2);457–465.

12. **(E)** MTC is a tumor of the parafollicular cells of the thyroid gland which secrete calcitonin. Accounting for 10% of all thyroid malignancies, MTC is a feature common to both MEN 2 syndromes with a penetrance of greater than 90%. Although, sporadic MTC accounts for somewhere near 80% of all MTC cases, familial forms, as in MEN 2 syndromes, are a significant source of morbidity and mortality among this patient population. MTC is generally the first manifestation of MEN 2 and the major cause of death of those with these syndromes.

In contrast to sporadic MTC, where the tumors tend to be unilateral and unifocal, MEN 2-associated MTC tends to be bilateral and multifocal. Furthermore, whereas onset of sporadic disease tends to occur in the fifth and sixth decades of life, hereditary MTC tends to occur much earlier. This seems to be especially true in MEN 2B where disease may be diagnosed as early as 2 years of age, with metastasis already having occurred in upward of 70% of patients at the time of diagnosis.

This difference in clinical behavior, with MEN 2B being far more aggressive, can likely be attributed to differing mutations in the RET protein, a tyrosine kinase that regulates cell growth. In fact, although MEN 2 syndromes, as well as the closely related familial medullary thyroid cancer (FMTC), all share a mutated RET protooncogene in their pathogenesis; the location of this mutation within the protein can vary from syndrome to syndrome. For example, in MEN 2A, mutations most often affect one of five cysteine residues at codons 609, 611, 618, 620, or 634. These codons correlate to portions of the extracellular domain of the RET protooncogene, and mutations likely alter ligand binding. In MEN 2B, however, mutations involving a methionine residue at codon 918, which corresponds to a portion of the intracellular domain, have been most commonly implicated. This mutation may alter the catalytic domain. In any event, current research continues to affirm that the different behaviors of MTC in either MEN 2 syndrome can be understood in terms of the different mutations involved.

Total thyroidectomy is recommended for all patients with any hereditary MTC in light of its propensity for multifocality and bilateral gland involvement. Furthermore, early, elective total thyroidectomy is advocated in the treatment of MEN 2 patients diagnosed by genetic screening before gross disease is evident. Surgery between the ages of 5 and 10 years is recommended in patients carrying MEN 2A mutations. Earlier surgery is advocated for patients found to have the MEN 2B mutation owing to its more aggressive nature. Among patients found to have mutations consistent with MEN 2B, surgery is advocated during the first year of life. Total thyroidectomy should also include a central compartment node dissection.

In cases of recurrent or inoperable disease, external beam radiation therapy has been used in an attempt to control local disease. Doxorubicin-based chemotherapy has also been employed in treating more widespread disease; however, neither radiation nor chemotherapy have yielded very promising results. Early detection and complete surgical excision of tumor tissue remains the only hope for long-term survival.

Bibliography

Cummings CW, Fredrickson JM, Harker LA, Krause CJ, et al. (eds.), *Otolaryngology: Head and Neck Surgery*, 3rd ed. St Louis, MO: Mosby, 1998, 2508–2509.

Heshmati HM, Gharib H, van Heerden JA, Sizemore GW. Advances and controversies in the diagnosis and management of medullary thyroid carcinoma: review. *Am J Med* 1997:103(1);60–69.

Townsend CM (ed.), *Sabiston Textbook of Surgery: The Biological Basis of Modern Surgical Practice*, 16th ed. Philadelphia, PA: WB Saunders, 2001, 697–707.

Utiger RD. Medullary thyroid carcinoma, genes and the prevention of cancer. *N Engl J Med* 1994:331(13);870–871.

Wella SA Jr, Franz C. Medullary carcinoma of the thyroid. *World J Surg* 2000;24(8):952–956.

Yip L, Cote GJ, Shapiro SE, Ayers GD, et al. Multiple endocrine neoplasia type 2: evaluation of the genotype and phenotype relationship. *Arch Surg* 2003:138(4); 409–416.

13. **(A)** Thyroid cancer is relatively rare, accounting for only 1% of all newly diagnosed cancers yearly in the United States; however, thyroid malignancy accounts for over 90% of all endocrine tumors. Papillary thyroid cancers account for approximately 80% of all thyroid malignancies, its incidence peaking in the third or fourth decades. Follicular thyroid cancer accounts for approximately 10% of all thyroid malignancies and has a slightly older age of onset. MTC accounts for an additional 7–10% of all thyroid malignancies, has a slight female predominance and is familial 20% of the time, as in MEN 2 syndromes and FMTC (Fig. 19-7).

MTC involves calcitonin-producing parafollicular or C cells. In sporadic cases, it tends to be unilateral with a later age of onset. In a familial setting, multiglandular involvement and multifocality is the rule. Overt malignancy is preceded by C-cell hyperplasia which may be detectable histopathologically in the absence of gross or palpable disease. Unfortunately, these tumors have a tendency toward early metastasis with positive cervical nodes confirmed in cases where the primary tumor is as small as 1.5 cm.

MTCs may secrete a variety of substances, including calcitonin, serotonin, ACTH, carcinoembryonic antigen (CEA), histmaninase, and VIP. The most common of these is calcitonin, and elevated serum values once were the mainstay of diagnosis. With the advent of genetic screening for RET gene mutations, the role of serum calcitonin measurements

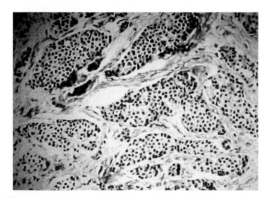

FIG. 19-7   Histologic representation of medullary thyroid carcinoma.

has largely been relegated to one of monitoring patients for recurrent disease.

A special mention should be made regarding thyroid nodules. Thyroid nodules are very common in the general population and may be present in upward of 50–60% of otherwise asymptomatic patients. When palpable, these nodules can be very concerning to patients and many clinicians, as well; however, the vast majority of thyroid nodules are benign. In fact, only 10% of nodules are subsequently found to be malignant. Risk factors increasing the likelihood that a palpable nodule may be malignant include history of radiation exposure (especially as a child), age extremes, male gender (especially over age 60), family history, previous thyroid disease, and physical examination findings suggesting malignancy, such as lymphadenopathy.

Bibliography

Cummings CW, Fredrickson JM, Harker LA, Krause CJ, et al. (eds.), *Otolaryngology: Head and Neck Surgery*, 3rd ed. St Louis, MO: Mosby, 1998, 2480–2518.

Engelbach M, Gîrges R, Forst T, PfÅtzner A, et al. Improved diagnostic methods in the follow-up of medullary thyroid carcinoma by highly specific calcitonin measurements. *J Clin Endocrinol Metab* 2000:85(5);1890–1894.

Heshmati HM, Gharib H, van Heerden JA, Sizemore GW. Advances and controversies in the diagnosis and management of medullary thyroid carcinoma: review. *Am J Med* 1997:103(1);60–69.

14. **(B)** MTC accounts for nearly 10% of all thyroid malignancies. Although sporadic in 80% of cases, MTC may be inherited in as many as 20% of those affected. Inherited cases include those associated with MEN 2A and 2B, which have been described above, as well as FMTC. MEN 2A is the most common setting in which inherited MTC occurs. FMTC is least common when considering inherited MTCs.

FMTC is defined by the presence of kindreds with at least four members having MTC but not having any of the other classic findings associated with the MEN 2 syndromes. Like MEN 2 syndromes, FMTC is associated with germline mutations in the RET protooncogene. FMTC behaves more like MEN 2A than 2B, having a more indolent course. This is likely attributable to the similarities in the causative mutations which typically involve the cysteine-rich extracellular domain. Additional mutations at codon 768, which codes for a portion of the intracellular domain have also been observed in patients with FMTC; however, like MTC in both of the MEN 2 syndromes, diagnosis of the disease requires early, elective total thyroidectomy with central compartment node dissection. Although the specific timing of surgery is a matter of debate among surgeons, the general consensus seems to be elective removal at the age of 5 years in FMTC. The same recommendation applies to MEN 2A as noted previously.

Since MTC is the most frequent cause of death among patients with MEN 2 syndromes or FMTC, early diagnosis and treatment is paramount. This is accomplished most easily in inherited MTC by genetic screening of the family members of patients confirmed to have MTC. When predisposing germline mutations in the RET gene are detected, total thyroidectomy is recommended.

When MEN 2 syndromes are suspected, it is essential to rule out the simultaneous presence of a pheochromocytoma by assessing urine catecholamines. Pheochromocytoma may be present in up to 24% of MEN 2 patients at the time their thyroid disease is diagnosed. If pheochromocytoma is discovered, adrenalectomy should be performed first, followed by thyroidectomy 1–2 weeks later.

Bibliography

Heshmati HM, Gharib H, van Heerden JA, Sizemore GW. Advances and controversies in the diagnosis and management of medullary thyroid carcinoma: review. *Am J Med* 1997:103(1);60–69.

Townsend CM (ed.), *Sabiston Textbook of Surgery: The Biological Basis of Modern Surgical Practice*, 16th ed. Philadelphia, PA: WB Saunders, 2001, 697–707.

Yip L, Cote GJ, Shapiro SE, Ayers GD, et al. Multiple endocrine neoplasia type 2: evaluation of the genotype and phenotype relationship. *Arch Surg* 2003:138(4);409–416.

15. **(C)** The multinodular thyroid in the setting of an extremely elevated serum calcitonin is virtually diagnostic for MTC. Although one cannot be certain based on the above clinical information whether that thyroid malignancy is sporadic or familial, the presence of severe headaches and anxiety occurring with MTC should arouse suspicion that there may be a synchronous pheochromocytoma. Pheochromocytoma may be present in up to 24% of MEN 2 patients at the time their thyroid disease is diagnosed. Undiagnosed pheochromocytomas present significant difficulties for the anesthesiologist, and patients will require α-blockade in the weeks leading up to surgery in an effort to minimize anesthetic risks and facilitate intraoperative blood pressure control. For this reason, 24-h urine catecholamines must be checked prior to surgery so that an occult pheochromocytoma is not missed. If catecholamine values are abnormally elevated, computed tomography (CT) scan or magnetic resonance imaging (MRI) are usually confirmatory.

If a pheochromocytoma is identified in this patient, removal of the pheochromocytoma becomes the operative priority with subsequent total thyroidectomy 1–2 weeks later. Pheochromocytomas in MEN 2 syndromes may be unilateral or bilateral and are characterized by hyperplastic chromaffin tissue. Although chromaffin cells frequently invade the adrenal capsule, metastasis is rare. When the pheochromocytoma involves both adrenal glands, then bilateral adrenalectomy is the rule.

However, in cases of unilateral pheochromocytoma, whether to perform unilateral or bilateral adrenalectomy is a matter of controversy. Unilateral laparoscopic adrenalectomy is advocated by most surgeons in cases where the contralateral gland is radiographically normal. This approach allows preservation of adrenal function from the contralateral gland, thus minimizing the risk of postoperative adrenal insufficiency. While this approach is most reasonable in patients with unilateral, sporadic disease, MEN 2 syndromes frequently go on to develop disease in the contralateral gland. In fact, upward of 50% of MEN patients presenting with unilateral tumors eventually develop bilateral disease. Therefore, in an attempt to preserve cortical function in MEN patients who either do have or may go on to have bilateral disease, some endocrine surgeons advocate cortical sparing adrenalectomy. In theory, this approach allows for the possibility of cortical preservation even when bilateral pheochormocytomas are resected. Although not practiced widely, early data seem encouraging.

Bibliography

Brandi ML, Gagel RF, Angeli A, Bilezikian JP, et al. Guidelines for diagnosis and therapy of MEN type 1 and type 2. *J Clin Endocrinol Metab* 2001:86(12);5658–5671.

Larsen PR, Kronenberg HM, Melmed S, Polonsky KS (eds.), *Williams Textbook of Endocrinology*, 10th ed. Philadelphia, PA: WB Saunders, 2003, 1733–1737.

Townsend CM (ed.), *Sabiston Textbook of Surgery: The Biological Basis of Modern Surgical Practice*, 16th ed. Philadelphia, PA: WB Saunders, 2001, 697–707.

16. **(E)** As has been noted in previous discussions, MTC accounts for nearly 10% of all thyroid malignancies and is inherited in as many as 20% of those affected. Inherited cases include those associated with MEN 2 syndromes and FMTC. MEN 2A and FMTC have a more indolent course than MEN 2B which often affects the very young and is frequently diagnosed at an advanced stage except in cases where rigorous familial screening is undertaken. Since chemotherapeutic regimens and external bean radiation have proved disappointing, efforts have been redoubled to screen for inherited MTC among kindred of those diagnosed with these tumors. Although monitoring serum calcitonin

and radionuclide scanning have been used in the past for surveillance among kindred with MTC, especially in confirmed cases of inherited disease, these modalities have largely been supplanted by genetic screening for mutations in the RET protooncogene. This technique is now considered the most sensitive means of screening for MTC in kindred of patients diagnosed with inherited MTC.

When a patient is diagnosed with MTC, genetic screening for a mutant RET gene should be undertaken. If the patient does, in fact, have a defective gene, RET screening in all first degree relatives is then recommended. Germline mutations affecting codon 634 are most often associated with MEN 2A syndromes. Codons 768 and 891 are aberrant in FMTC. Codon 918 is the culprit most often in MEN 2B.

All family members with RET mutations predisposing them to MTC should undergo total thyroidectomy as soon as they are able to tolerate the procedure. Infants born to families known to have the predisposing RET mutation should undergo screening at birth. When the MEN 2B RET mutation is identified, total thyroidectomy should be done as soon as possible and is generally advocated prior to 2 years of age. If the MEN 2A or FMTC RET mutations are identified, surgery may generally be deferred until the child is 5 years old, although this is a matter of controversy.

Bibliography

Clayman GL, El-Baradie TS. Medullary thyroid cancer. *Otolarygol Clin North Am* 2003:36(1);91–105.

Cummings CW, Fredrickson JM, Harker LA, Krause CJ, et al. (eds.), *Otolaryngology: Head and Neck Surgery*, 3rd ed. St Louis, MO: Mosby, 1998, 2504–2509.

Heshmati HM, Gharib H, van Heerden JA, Sizemore GW. Advances and controversies in the diagnosis and management of medullary thyroid carcinoma: review. *Am J Med* 1997:103(1);60–69.

Townsend CM (ed.), *Sabiston Textbook of Surgery: the Biological Basis of Modern Surgical Practice*, 16th ed. Philadelphia, PA: WB Saunders, 2001, 697–707.

17. **(D)** The MEN 2 syndromes, as discussed previously, are notable for the presence of MTC and pheochromocytomas. In addition to these endocrinopathies, MEN 2B is further distinguished by nonendocrine features including marfanoid body habitus, mucosal neuromas, ganglioneuromas, and skeletal abnormalities. Although MEN 2B is an autosomal dominant trait, many cases appear to represent new mutations.

The mucosal neuromas most often occur on the oral mucosa, lips, and tongue. These neuromas are almost invariably present by 10 years of age and occasionally at birth. These neuromas may also involve the corneal nerves. Notable for an increase in both size and number of nerves, these corneal neuromas are visible by slit lamp ophthalmologic examination. Ganglioneuromatoses of the gastrointestinal (GI) tract are also frequent, affecting predominantly the large and small bowel. Occasionally, the esophagus may also by involved. These GI ganglioneuromas often lead to GI dysmotility, problems with chronic constipation and even megacolon. In some instances, bowel obstruction may also result. The skeletal abnormalities associated with MEN 2B are multiple and include a tall, slender Marfanoid habitus, pectus excavatum, kyphosis, pes planus or cavus, and congenital hip dislocation. In contrast to true Marfanoids, MEN 2B patients do not typically develop aortic arch disease or ectopia lentis.

Since mucosal neuromas and habitus may be the first clinical presentation of MEN 2B, physicians need to be alert to these traits. This is important because these characteristic phenotypic features may presage the discovery of MTC which, in MEN 2B in particular, is very aggressive. Since MTC is the most frequent cause of death among MEN 2 patients and since early diagnosis and surgical removal provides the only hope of cure, recognition of mucosal neuromas, therefore, should prompt a workup for MTC including measurement of serum calcitonin and genetic screening for the RET mutation. The most common RET germline mutation in MEN 2B involves codon 918 which affects the tyrosine kinase domain.

Bibliography

Goldman L, Bennet JC (eds.), *Cecil Textbook of Medicine*, 21st ed. Philadelphia, PA: WB Saunders, 2000, 1407.

Larsen PR, Kronenberg HM, Melmed S, Polonsky KS (eds.), *Williams Textbook of Endocrinology*, 10th ed. Philadelphia, PA: WB Saunders, 2003, 1739.

Ledger GA, Khosla S, Lindor NM, Thibodeau SN, et al. Genetic testing in the diagnosis and management of multiple endocrine neoplasia type II. *Ann Intern Med* 1995:122(2);118–124.

Townsend CM (ed.), *Sabiston Textbook of Surgery: The Biological Basis of Modern Surgical Practice*, 16th ed. Philadelphia, PA: WB Saunders, 2001, 697–707.

18. **(D)** Anyone undergoing surgery for MTC should undergo screening for pheochromocytoma. This clinical scenario does not specify whether such an evaluation was undertaken. Nevertheless, this patient presents with complaints and findings which suggest he has a pheochromocytoma, especially in light of his history of MTC. Resection of the mass is now needed.

Pheochromocytomas are rare catecholamine secreting tumors that most frequently occur in the adrenal medulla; however, they also may arise in any sympathetic ganglia. In this case, the patient's mass occurs in the pelvis, abutting a lumbar vertebra. Pheochromocytomas have also been noted in such diverse places as the right atrium, spleen, broad ligament of the ovary, and in the organ of Zuckerkandl. The organ of Zuckerkandl, located at the aortic bifurcation, is the most common extraadrenal site. Extraadrenal tumors secrete norepinephrine only since they lack the enzyme ethanolamine-N-methyl transferase. This is in contradistinction to adrenal tumors which secrete both norepinephrine and epinephrine.

Although rare in the general population, these tumors are found with greater frequency in patients who have predisposing conditions, such as MEN 2 syndromes, von Recklinghausen's disease, and von Hippel-Lindau's disease. Inherited pheochromocytoma syndromes account for 10% of all pheochromocytomas and are frequently bilateral.

Typical symptoms include hypertension, profuse sweating, headaches and palpitations. Although the most common clinical finding is hypertension when all pheochromocytomas are considered, severe hypertension may not be a prominent finding in MEN 2 patients since these patients are diagnosed earlier in the course of their disease because of screening. When suspected clinically, 24-h urine catecholamines should be measured. The normal value for total urine catecholamines is 100 mg/24 h. Values two to three times greater are typical of patients having a pheochromocytoma. CT scanning and MRI are most often used for tumor localization although 3-iodobenzylguanidine (MIBG) scanning and octreotide scanning may also be used.

Patients with pheochromocytomas are particularly subject to intraoperative hypertension resulting from tumor manipulation and the subsequent release of excessive catecholamines. In severe cases, this hypertension may lead to stroke or death. Therefore, every effort should be made to optimize these patients prior to surgery. This optimization includes alpha-adrenergic blockade with either prazosin or phenozybenzamine as well as volume resuscitation to compensate for the vasodilatory effects of alpha blockade. Effective therapy is achieved with good blood pressure control and mild postural hypotension. Patients using phenozybenzamine usually require doses in the range of 60–250 mg per day. When patients experience persistent tachycardia on this alpha blockade regimen, beta blockade with propranolol is recommended. Preoperative alpha blockade is generally required for a minimum of 10–14 days prior to surgery. When intraoperative hypertension occurs, nitroprusside is generally the agent of choice for blood pressure control.

Bibliography

Larsen PR, Kronenberg HM, Melmed S, Polonsky KS (eds.), *Williams Textbook of Endocrinology*, 10th ed. Philadelphia, PA: WB Saunders, 2003, 555–562.

Miller RD (ed.), *Anesthesia*, 5th ed. Philadelphia, PA: Churchill Livingstone, 2000, 924–925.

Townsend CM (ed.), *Sabiston Textbook of Surgery: The Biological Basis of Modern Surgical Practice*, 16th ed. Philadelphia, PA: WB Saunders, 2001, 684–688, 697–707.

19. **(C)** As noted in previous discussions, NETs of the pancreas and duodenum constitute the second most common endocrine abnormality associated with MEN 1. Although gastrinomas are the most common type of functional pancreaticoduodenal tumor, accounting for anywhere from 50 to 70% of functional, MEN-associated NETs, insulinomas constitute the second most common type of functional tumor. When present, these tumors produce symptoms of neuroglycopenia during fasting. These symptoms include anxiety, tremor, confusion, sweating, seizure, and syncope and are frequently most prominent in the morning. Also significant in making the diagnosis is a remarkable improvement or resolution of the symptoms after administration of glucose. Since these tumors are rare, exogenous insulin administration should be excluded as an alternative diagnosis. This can be done by careful history as well as measurement of serum C-peptide and proinsulin levels. Proinsulin is a natural precursor to endogenous insulin and should be elevated when oversecretion of endogenous insulin occurs. C-peptide, a cleavage product of endogenous insulin production, should be elevated as well. If proinsulin and C-peptide levels are normal, this finding may suggest exogenous administration of insulin. Some also advocate measurement of serum sulfonylureas to rule out oral hypoglycemic abuse.

Initial management of insulinomas is directed at controlling hypoglycemia. This is first attempted with diet and medications. Frequent meals are advocated with small snacks between normal meals and at bedtime. Additionally, complex carbohydrates, such as those found in potatoes, bread, and rice are preferable to simple carbohydrates since the former are digested more slowly, leading to more consistent blood glucose levels. Medical therapy with diazoxide or octreotide has also been used with some success in managing hypoglycemia. Diazoxide works by both inhibiting insulin release from pancreatic beta cells and enhancing glycogenolysis. Octreotide works by interactions with somatostatin receptors on the tumor, decreasing insulin secretion. Although medical therapy has been used with some success over the long term in small numbers of patients, its primary role is in controlling hypoglycemia in anticipation of a definitive surgical procedure.

Surgical removal of insulinomas is frequently challenging since these tumors are notoriously difficult to localize. This is in part because of their small size. Ninety percent of MEN 1-associated insulinomas are also multifocal, in contrast to sporadic insulinomas which are multifocal only 10% of the time. In fact, historically as many as 20–60% of insulinomas could not be visualized preoperatively and as many as 20% could not be visualized during exploration even when excellent exposure of the pancreas was achieved. Standard preoperative imaging modalities, such as CT, MRI, and ultrasound, though frequently used, are often inadequate, correctly localizing only 10–30%. Among more invasive imaging techniques, abdominal angiography is perhaps most sensitive, localizing up to 60% of tumors. Portal venous sampling now offers the best method for preoperative localization of insulinomas and may be successful in up to 80% of cases. When intraoperative imaging is an option, intraoperative ultrasound (IOUS) is the most effective modality, identifying anywhere from 80 to 90% of tumors. This modality is widely advocated now as a standard part of any abdominal exploration for insulinoma.

Surgical exploration is typically performed through either a midline laparotomy or bilateral subcostal incisions depending on surgeon's preference. An extensive Kocher maneuver is performed and the pancreas is mobilized by dividing the gastrocolic ligament and opening the posterior peritoneal lining of the lesser sac. Although sporadic insulinomas are frequently benign and amenable to simple enucleation, this is not the case for MEN 1-associated tumors which are often multifocal, involving all parts of the pancreas. Therefore, a more extensive procedure is warranted in treating MEN 1-associated disease. Although total pancreatectomy was once advocated in the treatment of MEN 1 pancreatic tumors, more recent trends have been toward less aggressive procedures. Most surgeons now favor enucleation of gross disease in the head of the pancreas combined with distal subtotal pancreatectomy.

Bibliography

Brandi ML, Gagel RF, Angeli A, Bilezikian JP, et al. Guidelines for diagnosis and therapy of MEN type 1 and type 2. *J Clin Endocrinol Metab* 2001:86(12);5658–5671.

Demeure MJ, Klonoff DC, Karam JH, Clark OH. Insulinomas associated with multiple endocrine neoplasia type 1, the need for a different surgical approach. *Surgery* 1991:110(6);998–1004.

Feldman M, Friedman LS, Sleisenger MH (eds.), *Sleisenger and Fordtrans Gastrointestinal and Liver Disease: Pathophysiology, Diagnosis, Management*, 7th ed. Philadelphia, PA: WB Saunders, 2002, 993–994, 1005.

Huai JC, Zhang W, Niu HO, Su ZX, et al. Localization and surgical treatment of pancreatic insulinomas guided by intraoperative ultrasound. *Am J Surg* 1998:175(1);18–21.

Lo CY, Lam KY, Fan ST. Surgical strategy for insulinomas in multiple endocrine neoplasia type 1. *Am J Surg* 1998:175(4);305–307.

Norton JA, Bollinger RR, Chang AE, Lowry SF, et al. *Surgery: Basic Science and Clinical Evidence.* New York, NY: Springer-Verlag, 2000, 956–958.

Townsend CM (ed.), *Sabiston Textbook of Surgery: The Biological Basis of Modern Surgical Practice*, 16th ed. Philadelphia, PA: WB Saunders, 2001, 652–653, 697–707.

20. **(A)** Pituitary adenomas occur in anywhere from 15 to 50% of MEN 1 patients with a significantly higher frequency in women than men by nearly 2:1 in some studies. The mean age of onset is approximately 38 years with 25% diagnosed by 26 years of age and as many as 75% diagnosed by the fifth decade. The most common type of functional pituitary adenoma among both MEN and non-MEN patients is prolactinoma. Among MEN 1 patients, prolactinomas account for upward of 62% of all functional pituitary adenomas. The next most common are growth hormone secreting adenomas (9%), followed by ACTH secreting tumors (4%). Additionally, a small percentage of pituitary adenomas may secrete multiple substances.

In terms of tumor size, approximately 85% of pituitary tumors occurring in MEN 1 patients are macroadenomas, defined as tumors measuring at least 1 cm in diameter. This stands in contrast to non-MEN tumors where macroadenomas occur in approximately 42% of patients. This is clinically significant since macroadenomas are far more likely to cause neurologic symptoms from compression of surrounding structures than microadenomas which measure less than 1 cm. Symptoms may also result, naturally, from hormone oversecretion. When prolactinoma is the diagnosis, the oversecretion of prolactin most often results in hypogonadism in men and amenorrhea or galactorrhea in women. Galactorrhea was the presenting complaint of the patient in this particular clinical vignette.

Treatment of prolactinomas has generally involved medical treatment with dopamine agonists, such as bromocriptine, and/or transphenoidal surgical resection. Clinical research has shown that microadenomas typically respond well to transphenoidal resection, as measured by normalization of serum prolactin levels; however, treatment with a dopamine agonist has also been shown to induce normalization of prolactin levels and tumor shrinkage in many of these patients, as well. Therefore, patients with microadenomas are frequently offered either surgery or medical treatment.

When patients have macroadenomas, most surgeons and endocrinologists recommend medical management with a dopamine agonist such as bromocriptine as first line treatment. This recommendation is based on lower observed rates of prolactin normalization following surgery for macroadenomas compared to microadenomas (32% vs. 71%). Furthermore, transphenoidal or craniotomy resection of macroadenomas is associated with increased morbidity and is currently deemed to pose more risk to the patient than is justified by the anticipated rate of postoperative hormone normalization. Therefore, for this patient who has galactorrhea and a pituitary macroadenoma by MRI, bromocriptine is the preferred initial treatment. If this line of treatment fails, surgical resection does remain an option with or without external beam radiation for any residual disease.

Bibliography

Abeloff MD, Armitage JO, Lichter AS, Niederhuber JE, et al. (eds.), *Clinical Oncology*, 2nd ed. Philadelphia, PA: Churchill Livingstone, 2000, 1171–1174.

Gsponger J, De Tribolet N, Deruaz JP, Janzer R, et al. Diagnosis, treatment and outcome of pituitary tumors and other abnormal intrasellar masses: a retrospective analysis of 353 patients. *Medicine* 1999:78(4);236–269.

O'Brien T, O'Riordan DS, Gharib H, Scheithauer BW, et al. Results of treatment of pituitary disease in multiple endocrine neoplasia, type 1. *Neurosurgery* 1996:39(2); 273–279.

Verges B, Boureille F, Goudet P, Murat A, et al. Pituitary disease in MEN type 1: data from the France-Belgium MEN 1 multicenter study. *J Clin Endocrinol Metab* 2002:87(2);457–465.

Townsend CM (ed.), *Sabiston Textbook of Surgery: The Biological Basis of Modern Surgical Practice*, 16th ed. Philadelphia, PA: WB Saunders, 2001, 697–707, 1527–1528.

CHAPTER 20

Gastrointestinal Physiology

Robert Vire

Questions

1. Which of the following statements regarding innervation of the gastrointestinal (GI) tract is true?

   (A) Sympathetic innervation has a primarily excitatory effect on the GI tract.
   (B) Parasympathetic innervation is supplied solely by the vagus nerve and its branches.
   (C) The enteric nervous system is composed of a serosal plexus and submucosal plexus.
   (D) Local reflex activity occurs in the enteric nervous system in the absence of any sympathetic or parasympathetic innervation.
   (E) Most sympathetic fibers terminate in the mucosa.

2. Which of the following is true with regard to esophageal anatomy?

   (A) It consists of a mucosal, submucosal, and serosal layer.
   (B) It travels to the right of the aorta below the carina.
   (C) It receives parasympathetic innervation via the cervical and thoracic parasympathetic chains.
   (D) It has a segmental arterial supply.
   (E) The lower esophageal sphincter (LES) is a well-defined anatomical sphincter

3. Which of the following is *not* a component of the normal swallowing mechanism?

   (A) elevation of the soft palate
   (B) anterosuperior movement of the hyoid bone
   (C) initiation of a peristaltic wave down the esophageal body
   (D) vagally mediated contraction of the smooth muscle of the upper esophageal sphincter (UES)
   (E) coordination of the swallowing mechanism by the swallowing center in the medulla

4. Regarding the esophageal phase of swallowing, which is correct?

   (A) The vagus nerve innervates both skeletal and smooth muscle.
   (B) There is a clear line of demarcation between the skeletal muscle of the upper one-third of the esophagus and the smooth muscle of the lower two-thirds.
   (C) Atropine stimulates esophageal motility.
   (D) The force generated by esophageal peristalsis is approximately 3–5 kg.
   (E) Relaxation of the LES coincides with passage of the food bolus into the distal esophagus.

5. An important barrier to esophageal mucosal injury from gastric secretions is the prevention of reflux by the LES. Factors important for preventing reflux include all of the following *except*:

   (A) the resting pressure of the LES
   (B) the overall length of the LES
   (C) the length of LES exposed to intraabdominal pressure
   (D) increased LES pressure in response to gastric distension
   (E) an intact angle of His

6. Which of the following has been shown to increase LES pressure?

   (A) cholecystokinin (CCK)
   (B) ethanol
   (C) estrogen
   (D) theophylline
   (E) motilin

7. Vomiting is a reflex behavior best characterized by which of the following?

   (A) It is caused by relatively few stimuli.
   (B) The vomiting center, located in the pons, acts to coordinate the vomiting reflex.
   (C) Vomiting is accompanied by reverse peristalsis of the esophagus.
   (D) The chemoreceptor trigger zone is located on the floor of the fourth ventricle and can elicit vomiting following exposure to some blood-borne substances.
   (E) Failure of the LES to relax is the most notable motor difference between retching and vomiting.

8. Which of the following statements regarding gastric anatomy is correct?

   (A) The greater curvature requires blood flow from either the right or left gastroepiploic artery to remain viable.
   (B) Vagal nerve fibers to the stomach are predominately efferent.
   (C) Sympathetic afferent nerve fibers synapse in the celiac plexus, leading to referred pain.
   (D) The right vagus nerve gives off a hepatic branch before traveling along the lesser curvature.
   (E) Most of the lymphatic drainage for the stomach passes through celiac nodes.

9. Which of the following best characterizes the electrolyte and acid/base disturbances seen with protracted vomiting?

	Plasma pH	Urine pH	Plasma chloride	Plasma potassium
(A)	Alkalosis	Alkauria	Hypochloremia	Hypokalemia
(B)	Alkalosis	Aciduria	Hypochloremia	Hypokalemia
(C)	Alkalosis	Adicuria	Hyperchloremia	Hypokalemia
(D)	Alkalosis	Aciduria	Hyperchloremia	Hyperkalemia
(E)	Alkalosis	Alkauria	Hyperchloremia	Hyperkalemia

10. Gastric protein digestion is notable for

   (A) secretion of pepsinogen by parietal cells
   (B) leading to malnutrition if impaired
   (C) conversion of pepsinogen to pepsin by pepsinogenase
   (D) cessation of pepsin activity when it encounters the alkaline environment of the duodenum
   (E) cleavage of terminal peptide bonds by pepsin

11. All of the following affect gastrin release *except*:

   (A) antral acidification
   (B) antral alkalization
   (C) carbohydrates in the antrum
   (D) gastric distension
   (E) somatostatin release

12. A patient has been prescribed famotidine to treat a peptic ulcer. At which location in the parietal cell does famotidine act (Fig. 20-1)?

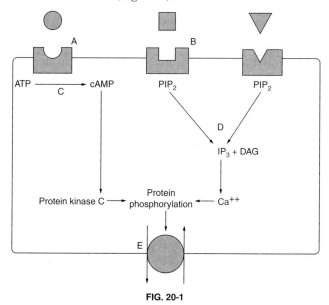

FIG. 20-1

13. Truncal vagotomy causes an increased rate of gastric emptying of liquids by

   (A) increasing the rate of the gastric "pacemaker"
   (B) destroying the receptive relaxation reflex in the proximal stomach
   (C) decreasing resting pyloric tone
   (D) increasing the amplitude of gastric contractions
   (E) eliminating the potentiating effect of cholinergic input on somatostatin release

14. Carbohydrate digestion and absorption is characterized by

   (A) digestion of starch by brush border enzymes
   (B) transportation of glucose, galactose, and fructose across the luminal membrane by an active transport system
   (C) increased activity of brush border enzymes in the jejunum relative to the ileum

(D) initiation of digestion in the duodenum by amylase secreted from the pancreas

(E) decreased osmotic effect as starch is digested into oligosaccharides

15. Lingual lipase and pancreatic lipase both

(A) are inactivated in an acidic environment

(B) cleave triglycerides primarily into monoglycerides and fatty acids

(C) make use of a coenzyme

(D) are secreted in active form

(E) are activated by trypsin

16. Cholecystokinin

(A) relaxes the sphincter of Oddi

(B) inhibits gastric acid secretion

(C) inhibits gallbladder contractions

(D) causes mesenteric vasodilation

(E) inhibits pancreatic exocrine secretions

17. The intestines play an important role in calcium metabolism. Which of the following patients might be expected to have impaired calcium absorption?

(A) a patient taking penicillin for otitis media

(B) a patient with gastric hypersecretion

(C) a patient with colon cancer

(D) a patient taking cholestyramine

(E) a hyperparathyroid patient

18. Which of the following statements regarding vitamin D is correct?

(A) It undergoes 25-hydroxylation in the kidney and 1-hydroxylation in the liver.

(B) An adequate dietary intake of foods naturally rich in vitamin D is necessary for proper calcium metabolism.

(C) Vitamin D is water soluble and absorption is enhanced after ionization in an alkaline environment.

(D) Vitamin D has its most important effect on calcium metabolism by increasing intestinal absorption.

(E) Vitamin D deficiency results in the clinical disease state of beriberi.

19. Which of the following individuals is least likely to have a folate deficiency?

(A) a patient with microcytic anemia

(B) a strict vegetarian

(C) an alcoholic

(D) an epileptic on phenytoin

(E) a patient with Crohn's disease

20. Which of the following individuals is least likely to have a B_{12} (cobolamin) deficiency?

(A) a patient with macrocytic anemia

(B) a strict vegetarian

(C) a patient with atrophic gastritis

(D) a patient with chronic pancreatitis

(E) an epileptic on phenytoin

21. A patient has undergone an ileal resection. Which of the following conditions would he be least likely to develop?

(A) alopecia

(B) megaloblastic anemia

(C) nephrolithiasis

(D) steatorrhea

(E) cholelithiasis

22. Which of the following dietary adjustments could be made to help treat a patient with a chylothorax?

(A) removal of all galactose from the diet

(B) use of medium chain triglycerides (MCTs) as the only source of fat

(C) use of long chain triglycerides as the only source of fat

(D) use of aromatic amino acids as the only source of protein

(E) a gluten-free diet

23. Which of the following peptides is matched to its correct effect?

(A) Secretin acts to increase pancreatic endocrine secretions.

(B) Motilin plays an important role in digestion by increasing enteric motility during a meal.

(C) Somatostatin works in concert with CCK to increase pancreatic exocrine secretions.

(D) Gastric inhibitory peptide (GIP) inhibits acid production and insulin release.

(E) Bombesin acts to stimulate GI motility.

24. Small intestinal motility is characterized by which of the following?

    (A) A "pacemaker potential" which is responsible for initiating peristaltic contractions
    (B) both peristaltic and segmental contractions
    (C) a mean transit time through the small intestine of 24 h
    (D) increasing motility more distally in the bowel
    (E) a migrating motor complex (MMC) that serves to facilitate the digestion of consumed protein

25. Host defense mechanisms in the gut include both immunologic and nonimmunologic components. One important agent is IgA. Which of the following statements regarding IgA in the intestines is correct?

    (A) It is produced in quantities second only to IgG.
    (B) It is released by B cells in the follicle of Peyer's patches.
    (C) It is secreted as a monomer bound to a glycoprotein which facilitates transepithelial migration.
    (D) Antigen-specific IgA production to antigens first encountered in the gut can be found in other secretory tissues, and can even be transferred via breast milk.
    (E) IgA incapacitates bacteria by binding them and promoting phagocytosis.

26. What is the primary fuel source of enterocytes?

    (A) glucose
    (B) glutamine
    (C) ketones
    (D) MCTs
    (E) arginine

27. What portion of the colon absorbs the majority of fluid?

    (A) ascending colon
    (B) transverse colon
    (C) descending colon
    (D) sigmoid colon
    (E) rectum

28. Which of the following is the primary energy source for colonocytes?

    (A) glutamine
    (B) short chain fatty acids
    (C) glucose
    (D) MCTs
    (E) alanine

29. Which of the following statements regarding the defecatory mechanism is correct?

    (A) There is voluntary control of the internal anal sphincter.
    (B) Passage of feces into the rectal vault results in reflex contraction of the internal anal sphincter.
    (C) Squatting aids in defecation by straightening the anorectal angle.
    (D) The external anal sphincter is composed of smooth muscle.
    (E) In the setting of normal innervation and musculature, incontinence is rare even with rectal volumes greater than 600 cc.

30. The concentration of which electrolyte in pancreatic secretions increases as the rate of secretion increases?

    (A) sodium
    (B) potassium
    (C) chloride
    (D) bicarbonate
    (E) calcium

31. Islets of Langerhans

    (A) account for 30% of pancreatic mass
    (B) are composed chiefly of alpha cells
    (C) secret bicarbonate into the duodenum via the pancreatic duct
    (D) have varying cellular compositions depending on their location within the pancreas
    (E) are found in lesser numbers in the liver

32. The caudate lobe of the liver corresponds to which hepatic segment?

    (A) I
    (B) II
    (C) III
    (D) IV
    (E) V

33. Regarding normal human bile

    (A) cholesterol is the most prevalent lipid
    (B) deoxycholic acid is the most prevalent bile acid
    (C) lethicin is the most prevalent phospholipid
    (D) micelles with a higher bile acid concentration are able to solubilize more cholesterol
    (E) lecithin-rich micelles form a sphere shape

34. With regard to the enterohepatic circulation, which of the following is a true statement?

    (A) The primary means of replenishing the bile acid pool is by enteric absorption from dietary sources.
    (B) The level of bile acids in the serum undergoes a postprandial increase.
    (C) The highest concentration of bile acids in the body is found in hepatic bile.
    (D) Most of the bile acids that leave the body do so in the urine.
    (E) Chenodeoxycholic acid is metabolized to ursodeoxycholic acid in the liver before being secreted.

35. A 43-year-old woman has had a cholecystectomy. Compared to a 43-year-old woman who has not had a cholecystectomy?

    (A) Her fasting levels of bile acids in the serum are lower.
    (B) The proportion of bile acids extracted by the liver is increased.
    (C) Her bile acids are predominantly stored in the liver.
    (D) She would have a relative increase in the number of secondary bile acids.
    (E) Her serum bilirubin level would be elevated.

36. In which state on the phase diagram below (Fig. 20-2) would cholesterol gallstone formation be least likely to occur?

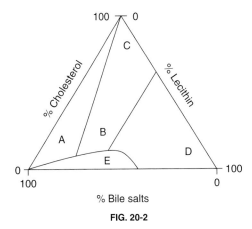

FIG. 20-2

37. Which of the following statements concerning the hepatic acinus is correct?

    (A) Zone 1 hepatocytes are the first to regenerate.
    (B) Bilirubin is absorbed primarily in zone 2.
    (C) Zone 3 hepatocytes are furthest from the hepatic venules.
    (D) Solutes that enter hepatocytes by simple diffusion are absorbed mainly in zone 3.
    (E) The sinusoidal endothelium is characterized by tight junctions with numerous carrier proteins for facilitated diffusion.

38. Which of the following statements regarding hepatic carbohydrate metabolism is correct?

    (A) Insulin facilitates gluconeogenesis.
    (B) Insulin promotes glucose uptake by hepatocytes.
    (C) Glucose storage as fat is more energy efficient than as glycogen.
    (D) Alanine is converted to glucose by deamination to ribose, which is then phosphorylated and enters the phosphogluconate pathway.
    (E) Glucose is the primary fuel source of hepatocytes.

Answers and Explanations

1. **(D)** Innervation of the GI tract can be broadly divided into three categories: sympathetic, parasympathetic, and enteric. Sympathetic innervation is chiefly inhibitory, resulting in decreased motility and secretions, although sympathetic stimulation does increase contraction of the muscularis mucosa and certain sphincters. These nerve fibers are typically adrenergic fibers arising from prevertebral and paravertebral plexuses. Few fibers terminate on muscle itself, instead exercising an inhibitory effect by terminating in the submucosal and myenteric plexuses and inhibiting synaptic transmission. Sympathetic fibers also cause vasoconstriction of blood vessels and provide innervation to glandular structures.

   The vagus nerve and its branches supply parasympathetic innervation to the preponderance of the GI tract. The distal colon, however, receives parasympathetic innervation from the hypogastric plexus. Like sympathetic fibers, parasympathetic fibers mainly terminate in the submucosal and myenteric plexuses. Unlike sympathetic fibers, they have a stimulatory effect on GI motility and secretions.

   The enteric nervous system is composed primarily of the submucosal plexus (Meissner's plexus) and the myenteric plexus (Auerbach's plexus). These plexuses consist of ganglia connected by unmyelinated fibers. Other, less well-defined, plexuses also contribute to the enteric nervous system. The enteric nervous system is influenced by sympathetic and parasympathetic innervation, but consists of a rich pathway of afferent and efferent nerves such that much of the activity of the gut, including local reflex activity, continues even in the absence of any extrinsic input.

   ### Bibliography

   Kutchai HC. Gastrointestinal motility. In: Berne RM, Levy MN (eds.), *Physiology*, 2nd ed. St Louis, MO: CV Mosby, 1988, 649–652.

2. **(D)** The esophagus is notable for containing a mucosal, submucosal, and external muscular layer, but no serosa. The cervical esophagus begins below the cricopharyngeus muscle, extending for about 5 cm from C6 to T1 at which point it becomes the thoracic esophagus. Important adjacent structures include the trachea and larynx anteriorly, the carotid sheath laterally, and the recurrent laryngeal nerve in the tracheoesophageal groove.

   The thoracic esophagus travels to the right of the descending aorta in close approximation to the posterior wall of the trachea. At the level of the tracheal bifurcation, it passes to the left of the aorta and then passes through the diaphragmatic hiatus into the abdomen. Other important considerations include a close association with the azygos vein on the right, and the relation with the thoracic duct, which travels posterior and to the right of the distal esophagus before migrating to the left of the esophagus at approximately the level of the fifth thoracic vertebra.

   The abdominal esophagus begins when the esophagus enters the abdomen through the diaphragmatic hiatus. The hiatus is formed by the left and right diaphragmatic crura. The abdominal esophagus is surrounded by the phrenoesophageal ligament, which arises from the subdiaphragmatic fascia. There is no anatomically definable LES, as it is a functional rather than anatomic sphincter.

   The blood supply to the esophagus is segmental. At various points, the esophagus is supplied by the inferior thyroid artery, bronchial arteries, direct branches from the aorta, left gastric artery, and inferior phrenic arteries. The venous drainage is similarly segmental. Lymphatic drainage from the esophagus begins with a rich submucosal lymphatic network that drains into periesophageal lymph nodes. In the proximal two-thirds of the esophagus, this drainage is usually cephalad, but drainage from the distal one-third is bidirectional. This rich lymphatic network is important to understanding the ease with which malignancy may spread longitudinally along the esophagus.

Innervation to the esophagus is primarily from the vagus nerve and its branches. Both the left and right recurrent laryngeal nerves supply the cricopharyngeus and cervical esophagus. The left recurrent laryngeal nerve also supplies the proximal thoracic esophagus, as do branches from both the right and left vagus, before they branch to form the esophageal plexus, which supplies the distal thoracic esophagus. Sympathetic fibers reach the esophagus from the cervical and thoracic sympathetic chain by way of the cervical and thoracic sympathetic ganglia. Visceral sensory fibers follow both sympathetic and vagal fibers to the first three segments of the thoracic spinal cord.

Bibliography

Orringer MB. Tumors, injuries, and miscellaneous conditions of the esophagus. In: Greenfield L (ed.), *Surgery: Scientific Principles and Practice*, 3rd ed. Philadelphia, PA: Lippincott, Williams & Wilkins, 2001, 692–693.

Peters JH, Demeester TR. Esophagus: anatomy, physiology, and gastroesophageal reflux disease. In: Greenfield L (ed.), *Surgery: Scientific Principles and Practice*, 3rd ed. Philadelphia, PA: Lippincott, Williams & Wilkins, 2001, 667–669.

3. **(D)** Swallowing is a complex activity that is not yet fully understood. The pharyngeal phase of swallowing begins when food is pushed posteriorly from the oral cavity into the oropharynx and hypopharynx by the tongue. At the same time, the soft palate elevates, pulled by the levator levi palatini and tensor veli palatini muscles, to prevent passage of the food bolus into the nasopharynx and to allow for the creation of positive pressure in the oropharynx. The hyoid bone moves upward and anteriorly, bringing the epiglottis under the tongue, and elevating the larynx, allowing for opening of the retrolaryngeal space. As well, the larynx closes at the level of the epiglottis.

As the tongue moves back and the posterior pharyngeal constrictors contract, hypopharygneal pressure rises to 60 mmHg. As the cricopharyngeus relaxes, this pressure gradient between the hypopharynx and the thoracic esophagus serves, in conjunction with the peristaltic contractions of the pharyngeal constrictors, to propel the food bolus into the esophagus. The UES then closes to prevent retrograde passage of food. Initially, the pressure of the UES will reach twice the resting pressure, but will return to normal with further progression of the food bolus. The muscles of the UES and upper third of the esophagus are striated muscles, and receive innervation from the vagus nerve and its recurrent larygneal branches. The whole act of swallowing is coordinated by the swallowing center, located in the medulla, which acts

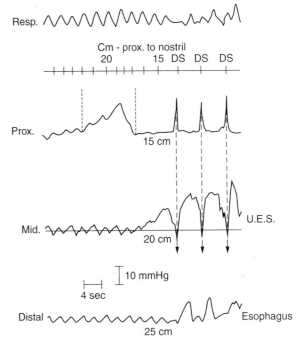

Upper esophageal sphincter-normal

FIG. 20-3 Demonstration of manometry of a normal upper esophageal sphincter. The diagram demonstrates relaxation of the upper esophageal sphincter in response to pharyngeal contractions, allowing for the passage of a food bolus. This is followed immediately by contraction of the upper esophageal sphincter to prevent retrograde passage. (Reprinted with permission from Sabiston DC, *Surgery: The Biological Basis of Modern Surgical Practice*, 15th ed., 1997, The Netherlands: Elsevier Science.)

through cranial nerves V, VII, X, XI, and XII, as wells as motor nerves C1–3 to control the swallowing mechanism. It works in conjunction with areas of the brainstem devoted to respiration to smoothly transform the pharynx from a respiratory to gustatory conduit (Fig. 20-3).

Bibliography

Chung DH, Evers MB. The digestive system. In: O'Leary JP (ed.), *The Physiologic Basis of Surgery*, 3rd ed. Philadelphia, PA: Lippincott, Williams & Wilkins, 2002, 464–465.

Peters JH, Demeester TR. Esophagus: anatomy, physiology, and gastroesophageal reflux disease. In: Greenfield L (ed.), *Surgery: Scientific Principles and Practice*, 3rd ed. Philadelphia, PA: Lippincott, Williams & Wilkins, 2001, 663–665.

Waters PF, Demeester TR. Foregut motor disorders and their surgical management. *Med Clin North Am* 1981; 65:1235–1241.

4. **(A)** The esophageal phase of swallowing is initialized by the pharyngeal phase, as the UES relaxes in a reflex mediated by the swallowing center. The peristaltic wave begun in the pharynx continues down the esophagus,

reaching pressures of 30–120 mmHg and traveling at 2–4 cm/s. At any one point, the rise and fall of the peristaltic range may last for 3–5 s; however, the propulsive force of the esophagus is weak, reaching only 5–10 g. The striated muscles of the upper third of the esophagus receive innervation from the vagus and its recurrent laryngeal branches. The smooth muscle derives innervation from the vagus via cholinergic fibers synapsing on the myenteric plexus—therefore, atropine impairs esophageal motility. There is a gradual transition from striated to smooth muscle that occurs over the middle third of the esophagus. The LES, which is tonically contracted, relaxes coincidentally with the pharyngeal phase of swallowing. Tonicity of the LES is increased by alpha-andrenergic neurotransmitters, beta blockers, or increased vagal tone.

Bibliography

Chung DH, Evers MB. The digestive system. In: O'Leary JP (ed.), *The Physiologic Basis of Surgery*, 3rd ed. Philadelphia, PA: Lippincott, Williams & Wilkins, 2002, 465–467.

Peters JH, Demeester TR. Esophagus: anatomy, physiology, and gastroesophageal reflux disease. In: Greenfield L (ed.), *Surgery: Scientific Principles and Practice*, 3rd ed. Philadelphia, PA: Lippincott, Williams & Wilkins, 2001, 663–665.

Waters PF, Demeester TR. Foregut motor disorders and their surgical management. *Med Clin North Am* 1981; 65:1235–1241.

5. **(D)** The LES cannot be defined anatomically, but can be detected manometrically by an increase in pressure above the gastric baseline as the probe is withdrawn into the esophagus. There are two situations in a normal subject when this high pressure zone is absent: (1) when the stomach is distended to allow for a belch and (2) during swallowing. The three most important characteristics for determining the efficacy of the LES in preventing reflux are its resting pressure, overall length, and length exposed to intraabdominal pressure. The resting pressure and overall length act in concert. A shorter zone of high pressure requires a higher resting pressure to prevent reflux and vice versa. The length of sphincter in the abdomen is also important, as high intraabdominal pressure can overcome the resting pressure of the LES if this pressure is applied only to the stomach and not also to a significant portion of the LES. As mentioned previously, the LES relaxes with gastric distension to allow belching. Even without this reflex, gastric distention works to lower the resistance of the LES by pulling on the terminal esophagus, in effect incorporating it into the fundus. This then shortens the length of the LES, particularly the component exposed to intraabdominal pressure. Patients with a normal angle of His are more resistant to this process, as measured by a higher intragastric pressure required to overcome the sphincter, than are patients with a hiatal hernia.

Bibliography

Peters JH, Demeester TR. Esophagus: anatomy, physiology, and gastroesophageal reflux disease. In: Greenfield L (ed.), *Surgery: Scientific Principles and Practice*, 3rd ed. Philadelphia, PA: Lippincott, Williams & Wilkins, 2001, 667–669.

6. **(E)** A wide array of substances have been demonstrated to affect the resting pressure of the LES. Alpha-adrenergic innervation increases the LES pressure and beta-adrenergic stimulation decreases it. Hormones that have been shown to increase LES pressure include gastrin, motilin, bombesin, beta-enkephalins, and substance P. Those that have been shown to decrease it include CCK, estrogen, glucagons, progesterone, somatostatin, secretin, and vasoactive intestinal peptide (VIP). Medications which increase LES pressure are antacids, cholinergics, alpha-adrenergic agonists, and metoclopramide. Medications which lower LES pressure include anticholinergics, barbiturates, calcium-channel blockers, caffeine, diazepam, dopamine, meperidine, and theophylline. Dietary factors which decrease LES tone include peppermint, chocolate, ethanol, caffeine, and fat.

Bibliography

Peters JH, Demeester TR. Esophagus: anatomy, physiology, and gastroesophageal reflux disease. In: Greenfield L (ed.), *Surgery: Scientific Principles and Practice*, 3rd ed. Philadelphia, PA: Lippincott, Williams & Wilkins, 2001, 665.

7. **(D)** Vomiting is defined as expulsion of gastric and sometimes enteric contents via the oral cavity. There are a large number of stimuli which may precipitate vomiting. Once initiated, however, the reflex is the same. Retrograde peristalsis occurs in the small intestines. This, combined with pyloric and gastric relaxation results in the enteric contents being pushed into the stomach. The pylorus then contracts as gastric distension acts via a reflex mechanism to cause relaxation of the LES. The abdominal wall muscles then contract, causing an increase in the intraabdominal pressure, which forces the gastric contents into the esophagus. The UES relaxes, allowing continued passage of the vomitus out through the oral cavity. Occurring concomitantly with the GI events, inspiration against a closed glottis occurs, which decreases the intrathoracic pressure and aids the passage of gastric contents into the esophagus. Closure of the glottis, along with approximation of the vocal cords and anterior movement of the

larynx serves to prevent aspiration. The chief difference between retching and vomiting is that in the case of retching, the UES does not relax, preventing passage of gastric contents into the pharynx. The reflex of vomiting is controlled by the vomiting center, which is located in the medulla. A wide variety of stimuli can elicit vomiting, including gastric or duodenal distension, dizziness, pharyngeal stimulation, injury to the genitourinary system, and exposure to emetics, which may act by stimulating gastric or duodenal receptors, or may act directly on the central nervous system by stimulating the chemoreceptor trigger zones located in the floor of the fourth ventricle.

Bibliography

Kutchai HC. Gastrointestinal motility. In: Berne RM, Levy MN (eds.), *Physiology*, 2nd ed. St. Louis: CV Mosby, 1988, 671–672.

8. **(E)** Grossly, the stomach can be divided into four regions. These are the cardia, which is just distal to the gastroesophageal junction, the fundus, which lies to the left and cephalad to the gastroesophageal junction, the antrum, which runs from the incinsura angularis on the lesser curvature to the pylorus, and the body, which lies between the cardia and the antrum. The stomach is bordered by a number of other structures, including the esophagus, diaphragm, duodenum, liver, spleen, pancreas, left kidney and adrenal gland, aorta, omentum, and the transverse colon and its mesentery.

The vascular supply to the stomach is rich and characterized by anastamotic channels such that preservation of only one major vessel is necessary for gastric viability. The major vessels to supply the stomach are the left gastric artery from the celiac trunk, the right gastric artery coming off the hepatic artery, the short gastric arteries and left gastroepiploic artery, both of which originate from the splenic artery, and the right gastroepiploic artery, which branches off the gastroduodenal artery. Venous drainage parallels the arterial supply. The lymphatic drainage also grossly approximates the arterial supply. Lymph flow from the proximal stomach drains into the superior gastric nodes. The greater curvature is drained by pancreatic and splenic nodes proximally, while distally it is drained by subpyloric and omental nodes. The lesser curvature drains into suprapyloric nodes. Eventually, all of these nodal groups drain into celiac nodes. In practice, however, the lymphatic network is characterized by numerous areas of communication, both within and outside of the stomach wall. Clinically, this can result in spread of disease beyond regional nodal groups.

The left and right vagus nerves form a plexus above the diaphragm before passing through the esophageal hiatus. The left vagus nerve then passes anteriorly over the stomach and runs along the lesser curvature after sending off a branch to the liver. The right vagus rotates posteriorly to join the celiac plexus and innervates the posterior gastric wall. Ninety percent of vagal fibers are afferent, but they provide no sensation of pain. Sympathetic innervation is supplied from T5 to T10 spinal segments which travel in the splanchnic nerves to the celiac plexus. There, they synapse with secondary sympathetic nerves which innervate the stomach. Afferent sympathetic nerves travel without synapsing from the stomach to the spinal cord and are responsible for sensations of pain.

Bibliography

Mulholland MW. Gastric anatomy and physiology. In: Greenfield L (ed.), *Surgery: Scientific Principles and Practice*, 3rd ed. Philadelphia, PA: Lippincott, Williams & Wilkins, 2001, 737–739.

9. **(B)** Gastric secretions are rich in hydrogen ions, potassium, and chloride. As these ions are lost to the body with vomiting, a resultant hypokalemic, hypochloremic, metabolic alkalosis results. The body compensates by decreasing the respiratory rate and increasing renal bicarbonate secretion in an attempt to normalize the acid/base balance. With protracted vomiting, however, a paradoxical aciduria occurs. The patient becomes dehydrated secondary to sodium and fluid losses in the vomitus, stimulating the renin-angiotensin-aldosterone axis to preserve sodium. This results in sodium retention in the kidney with a reciprocal loss of potassium and hydrogen ions.

Bibliography

Fischer JE, Nussbaum MS, Chance WT, Luchetta F. Manifestations of gastrointestinal disease. In: Schwartz SI (ed.), *Principles of Surgery*, 7th ed. New York, NY: McGraw-Hill, 1999, 1049–1050.

10. **(D)** Unlike carbohydrates, digestion of proteins does not begin until the food bolus reaches the stomach. Pepsin is the end product of the proenzyme pepsinogen, which is secreted by chief cells and converted to pepsin by hydrocholoric acid. Pepsinogen production is stimulated by food in the stomach and low gastric pH. Once converted into the active form of pepsin, the enzyme works as an endopeptidase by disrupting peptide bonds involving aromatic amino acids. Pepsin is inactivated by the alkaline milieu of the duodenum. At this point, proteases produced by the pancreas continue protein digestion. Because of the presence of

pancreatic proteases, pepsin is not a necessary component of protein digestion in the normal state, becoming essential only if pancreatic function is abnormal. Pancreatic proteases may be endopeptidases, sush as trypsin or chymotrypsin, or exopeptidases, such as carboxypeptidases A and B. They are secreted as proenzymes, and trypsinogen is activated by enterokinase, with trypsin then activating the other proteases. Proteases cleave proteins into tripeptides, dipeptides, or amino acids, all of which can be absorbed by enterocytes, usually involving sodium-mediated transport. Once in the cytosol, further enzymes digest tri- and dipeptides to single amino acids before they are released into the portal blood.

Bibliography

Chung DH, Evers MB. The digestive system. In: O'Leary JP (ed.), *The Physiologic Basis of Surgery*, 3rd ed. Philadelphia, PA: Lippincott, Williams & Wilkins, 2002, 475.

11. **(C)** The primary factors stimulating gastrin release are vagal stimulation, food in the antrum, and gastric distension. Both polypeptides and amino acids result in increased gastrin release—fats and carbohydrates have no effect. Gastric distension increases gastrin release via cholinergic pathways. Prolonged alkalinization (>8 h) will increase gastrin release, while acute alkalinization does not directly cause release of gastrin, but does potentiate the release by other stimuli. The primary inhibitor of gastrin release is antral acidification (pH <2.5). Increased acid in the antrum results in somatostatin release from antral D cells, which then inhibits gastrin release. Indeed, a reciprocal inhibitory relationship exists between gastrin and somatostatin, such that the release of one inhibits the release of the other.

Bibliography

Chung DH, Evers MB. The digestive system. In: O'Leary JP (ed.), *The Physiologic Basis of Surgery*, 3rd ed. Philadelphia, PA: Lippincott, Williams & Wilkins, 2002, 470–471.

Debas HT. Physiology of gastric secretion and emptying. In: Miller TA (ed.), *Physiologic Basis of Modern Surgical Care*. St. Louis, MO: CV Mosby, 1988, 285.

12. **(A)** The three main stimulants to acid production by the parietal cells are histamine, gastrin, and acetylcholine. The main inhibitors are somatostatin and prostaglandins. Adrenergic stimulation acts indirectly to up regulate somatostatin production and down regulate gastrin production. Histamine is released by mast cells located in the lamina propria and diffuses to the mucosa. Histamine receptors are located on the basal membrane of the parietal cell and are classified as H2 receptors.

When stimulated by the binding of histamine, they activate adenylate cyclase, which catalyzes the conversion of adenosine triphosphate (ATP) to cyclic adenosine monophosphate (cAMP). This, in turn, leads to activation of protein kinase C, which causes further protein phosphorylation, ultimately leading to stimulation of the proton pump. H2 blockers, such as famotidine, act to impede gastric acid secretion by competitively binding to the receptors, which provides reversible inhibition of histamine-mediated gastric acid production.

Cholinergic stimulation and gastrin act through a similar pathway to increase acid production. Whether they act through identical pathways is unknown. What is known is that both rely on increases in intracellular calcium. This is accomplished by catalyzing the conversion of phosphatidylinositol-4,5 bisphosphate (PIP_2) into inositol triphosphate (IP_3) and diacylglycerol (DAG). IP_3 causes release of intracellular calcium stores from the endoplasmic reticulum, leading to stimulation of a protein kinase (not protein kinase C) with subsequent protein phosphorlyation and proton pump activation. The proton pump is a membrane-bound H^+-K^+ ATPase which exchanges cytoplasmic H^+ for luminal K^+. To maintain a ready supply of K^+ on the luminal side of the plasma membrane, luminal K^+ is repleted from intracellular stores. With activation of the H^+-K^+ ATPase, OH^- is produced, which is then converted to HCO_3^- by carbonic anhydrase. HCO_3^- is in turn exchanged for Cl^- at the basal membrane. Chloride ions then diffuse across the canalicular membrane into the lumen. In sum, then, the proton pump results in net movement of H^+ and Cl^- into the lumen and HCO_3^- into the interstitial space (Fig. 20-4).

Bibliography

Mason GR, Kahrilu PJ, Otterson MF, et al. The digestive system. In: O'Leary JP (ed.), *The Physiologic Basis of Surgery*, 2nd ed. Baltimore, MD: Williams & Wilkins, 1996, 416–418.

Mulholland MW. Gastric anatomy and physiology. In: Greenfield L (ed.), *Surgery: Scientific Principles and Practice*, 3rd ed. Philadelphia, PA: Lippincott, Williams & Wilkins, 2001, 744–746.

13. **(B)** When considering gastric motility, the stomach can be broken down into two regions—the proximal one-third and distal two-thirds. These regions do not correspond to any gross anatomic distinctions, but serve differing roles in the gastric handling of a food bolus. The proximal one-third of the stomach has no pacemaker potential or action potentials. Because of this, there is no peristaltic contraction, only prolonged, tonic contractions which serve to increase the intraluminal pressure of the proximal stomach. By contrast,

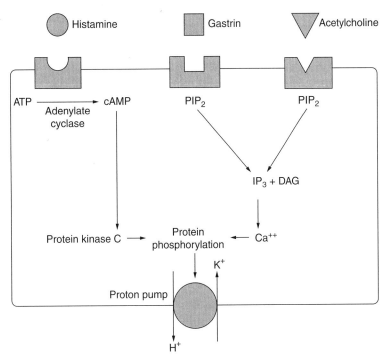

FIG. 20-4 The parietal cell and stimulants of gastric acid secretion.

the distal two-thirds of the stomach has a pacemaker located approximately one-third of the way along the greater curvature. Pacesetter potentials, or electrical control activity (ECA), cause partial depolarizations that occur at a rate of 3/min. By themselves, they do not stimulate a contraction, but must be coupled with an action potential to cause smooth muscle contractions. When contractions occur, they spread more rapidly along the greater curvature so that the peristaltic wave reaches the pylorus in a coordinated fashion from all parts of the stomach. The pylorus typically tightens before the peristaltic wave arrives, resulting in a backwash of gastric contents. The repeated churning aids in the digestion of foodstuffs and causes solid food particles to be broken down into smaller particles until they are small enough to pass through the pylorus, typically less than 1 mm. For liquids, however, the rate determining factor in gastric emptying is the pressure gradient between the stomach and the duodenum. Vagotomy, either truncal or proximal, causes a loss of receptive relaxation. This causes an increase in intragastric pressure and leads to an increased emptying rate of liquids.

Bibliography

Chung DH, Evers MB. The digestive system. In: O'Leary JP (ed.), *The Physiologic Basis of Surgery*, 3rd ed. Philadelphia, PA: Lippincott, Williams & Wilkins, 2002, 481–482.

Mulholland MW. Gastric anatomy and physiology. In: Greenfield L (ed.), *Surgery: Scientific Principles and Practice*, 3rd ed. Philadelphia, PA: Lippincott, Williams & Wilkins, 2001, 744–746.

14. **(C)** Ingested carbohydrates can be broadly thought of as simple sugars, such as glucose or fructose, disaccharides, such as sucrose or lactose, starches, such as amylose, and undigestible fibers such as cellulose. Digestion of carbohydrates is initiated in the mouth by salivary amylase. Salivary amylase is inactivated in the stomach when the gastric pH is reduced to less than 4.0. Before inactivation, however, amylase hydrolyzes starch into maltose, maltotriose, and alpha-limit dextrins, by cleaving internal alpha-glycosidic bonds. Fibers such as cellulose are indigestible because their beta-glycosidic bonds are not hydrolyzed by amylase, or any other human enteric enzyme. Amylase secreted by the pancreas completes the hydrolysis of starch, usually by the time the proximal jejunum is reached. These oligosaccharides, along with such dietary disaccharides as lactose, are digested by the brush border enzymes to form glucose, galactose, and fructose. Deficiency of brush border enzymes, as seen with lactase deficiency in lactose intolerance, can result in cramping and diarrhea secondary to the osmotic burden of the unabsorbed sugars. The activity of the brush border enzymes is greatest in the duodenum and jejunum, with

markedly less activity in the ileum. Once carbohydrates are broken down into monosaccharides, they are absorbed by the enterocytes. Fructose absorption occurs primarily via facilitated diffusion. This differs from the transport of glucose and galactose, which are transported into the enterocyte via an active transport system which couples their movement to that of sodium. They are then transported out of the enterocyte into the interstitial space via a sodium-independent carrier. The osmotic value of one molecule of starch is equal to that of one molecule of maltose or glucose. Therefore, as starch is digested, the osmotic effect is increased; however, under normal circumstances, the absorptive mechanisms along the brush border work very rapidly, preventing massive fluid shifts into the luminal space.

Bibliography

Chung DH, Evers MB. The digestive system. In: O'Leary JP (ed.), *The Physiologic Basis of Surgery*, 3rd ed. Philadelphia, PA: Lippincott, Williams & Wilkins, 2002, 472–475.

Simeone DM. Anatomy and physiology of the small intestine. In: Greenfield L (ed.), *Surgery: Scientific Principles and Practice*, 3rd ed. Philadelphia, PA: Lippincott, Williams & Wilkins, 2001, 793–794.

15. **(D)** The initial step in lipid metabolism is the breakdown of triglycerides, which are the main component of dietary fat. Two of the enzymes involved in this process are lingual and pancreatic lipase. Both enzymes are secreted in active form, and remain active even in an acidic environment. Lingual lipase is active from a pH of 2.2–6.0, and while pancreatic lipase is most active at an alkaline pH of 8.0, it is not inactivated until the pH is less than 3.0. Lingual lipase acts to hydrolyze the ester linkages in the 1 and 3 positions of the triglyceride molecule, and its actions result in free fatty acids and diglycerides. Pancreatic lipase acts to hydrolyze triglycerides primarily into free fatty acids and monoglycerides. Pancreatic lipase must first, however, gain access to the glyceride moiety of the triglyceride. This is accomplished through the actions of colipase, a coenzyme secreted by the pancreas as the proenzyme procolipase, before being activated by trypsin. Colipase binds to lipase and causes a structural transformation which enables lipase to successfully compete with bile salts for access to the glyceride moiety. Lingual lipase does not use a coenzyme.

Other enzymes important to lipid digestion are also secreted by the pancreas. Phospholipase A_2 acts to catalyze phospholipids into lysophospholipids and free fatty acids. Both bile salts and calcium are required for this hydrolysis, and phospholipase A_2 acts on both dietary and biliary phospholipids. It is secreted as a proenzyme and requires activation by trypsin. Another pancreatic enzyme important for lipid digestion is cholesterol esterase. This enzyme acts to hydrolyze a variety of lipid ester linkages, including cholesterol, vitamins A, D, C, and E, as well as the ester linkages found in triglycerides. Like phospholipase A_2, its activity is dependent on bile salts. On the completion of enzymatic digestion, dietary lipids have been metabolized into free fatty acids, 2-monoglycerides, and phospholipids.

Enzymatic digestion can be impaired by a number of conditions, leading to fat malabsorption and resultant diarrhea. These include pancreatic insufficiency, although only 10–15% of normal pancreatic exocrine function is needed for adequate lipid digestion, hypersecretion of gastric hydrochloric acid to the point that lipase is persistently inactivated, and failure of enterohepatic circulation such that enzymatic activity is impaired by the resulting bile salt deficiency.

Bibliography

Mason GR, Kahrilu PJ, Otterson MF, et al. The digestive system. In: O'Leary JP (ed.), *The Physiologic Basis of Surgery*, 2nd ed. Baltimore, MD: Williams & Wilkins, 1996, 426–428.

16. **(A)** A variety of peptides serve to act in an endocrine, paracrine, or autocrine manner to regulate the complex interrelationships between the stomach, small bowel, gallbladder, and pancreas. One such peptide is CCK, which is found in the central nervous system, as well as in the GI tract. In the gut, CCK is found in I cells of the duodenum and jejunum. Its release is stimulated by fatty acids and peptides in the duodenal lumen. When released, it acts to up regulate small intestinal digestion. It aids in micelle formation by stimulating the gallbladder to contract, while at the same time relaxing the sphincter of Oddi, leading to increased bile secretion. Along with secretin, it acts to increase pancreatic bicarbonate and exocrine secretions, neutralizing gastric acid in the duodenum and assisting with protein digestion. Finally, while CCK increases small intestinal motility, it acts to inhibit gastric emptying, ensuring that the small intestinal digestive mechanisms do not become overwhelmed.

Bibliography

Chung DH, Evers MB. The digestive system. In: O'Leary JP (ed.), *The Physiologic Basis of Surgery*, 3rd ed. Philadelphia, PA: Lippincott, Williams & Wilkins, 2002, 457–461.

17. **(D)** The recommended daily intake of calcium is 1000 mg. In order to absorb this, a number of hormonal,

enteric, and physiologic factors must work in concert to allow for calcium absorption. Vitamin D acts to facilitate calcium absorption by up regulating various calcium-specific transport proteins. Parathyroid hormone acts indirectly to increase calcium absorption by stimulating the hydroxylation of 25-OH vitamin D in the kidney, resulting in the metabolically active 1,25 $(OH)_2$ vitamin D. This active transport is necessary when low intraluminal concentrations of calcium are present, but passive absorption can be observed if the intraluminal concentration rises to high levels. Calcium must be ionized as a soluble salt to be absorbed.

Gastric acid would theoretically enhance calcium absorption by causing the dissociation of food calcium compounds and dissolving insoluble salts. In practice, however, gastric acid has been demonstrated to have no significant effect. Intraluminal factors which do enhance calcium absorption are bile acids, amino acids, and certain medications such as penicillin and chloramphenicol, which act to form more soluble calcium complexes. Sugars also act to enhance calcium absorption by altering fluid transport.

But while some substances result in more soluble calcium complexes, factors such as fatty acids or cholestyramine bind to calcium and form relatively insoluble complexes, impairing absorption. Of course, a healthy mucosal surface is necessary for adequate calcium absorption and conditions such as Crohn's disease, celiac sprue, or intestinal bypass will inhibit calcium absorption. Primary biliary cirrhosis has also been implicated in decreased calcium absorption, as have a variety of other factors, including glucocorticoids, thyroxine, thiazides, and aging, either by direct effects on the intestine or secondary to alterations in vitamin D metabolism. Conversely, growth hormone, estrogens, prolactin, and sarcoidosis increase calcium absorption.

Bibliography

Sellin JH. Physiology of digestion and absorption. In: Miller TA (ed.), *Physiologic Basis of Modern Surgical Care.* St. Louis, MO: CV Mosby, 1988, 338–339.

18. **(D)** Vitamin D (calciferol) is an inactive compound absorbed in the intestines or formed from sterol precursors by ultraviolet radiation in the skin. It undergoes activation to its most biologically active form, $1,25(OH)_2$ vitamin D by successive 25-hydroxylation in the liver and 1-hydroxylation in the kidney. Thus, a breakdown at any one of these steps can produce vitamin D deficiency, although an increase in peripheral bioconversion of sterols to vitamin D can compensate for decreased intestinal absorption, or vice versa; however, barring adequate compensation, either lack of sunlight or intestinal malabsorption can result in vitamin D deficiency, which results in rickets in children and osteomalacia in adults. Of note, much of the vitamin D ingested is found in foods that are not naturally rich in vitamin D, but are instead fortified, such as milk. Vitamin D is fat soluble and therefore dependent on micelle formation for absorption. It has also been demonstrated to undergo enterohepatic circulation. Interestingly, while hepatic 25-hydroxylation is necessary for bioactivation, liver disease does not correlate well with vitamin D deficiency, although significant disruption in calcium metabolism may be seen with primary biliary cirrhosis.

Bibliography

Sellin JH. Physiology of digestion and absorption. In: Miller TA (ed.), *Physiologic Basis of Modern Surgical Care.* St. Louis, MO: CV Mosby, 1988, 338–339.

19. **(B)** Folate is an important vitamin and megaloblastic anemia can result when stores are deficient. Folate is found primarily in green leafy vegetables. Because body stores are low (5–20 mg), either inadequate dietary intake or impaired intestinal absorption can readily lead to deficiency. People who might have inadequate intake include alcoholics and those without a well-rounded diet, such as the elderly on tea and toast diets or those who eat primarily junk food. Besides inadequate dietary intake, folate deficiency can also result from inadequate intestinal absorption, as is seen in disease states such as celiac sprue and inflammatory bowel disease. Phenytoin and methotrexate have been implicated in folate deficiency. Sulfasalazine, as well, can contribute to folate deficiency, exacerbating the malabsorption already seen in patients with inflammatory bowel disease.

When ingested, folate is generally bound to a polyglutamate chain which is broken down by brush border enzymes to form a monoglutamate folate, which can be absorbed, and free amino acids. The rate limiting step is absorption of folate across the mucosa which can happen passively at high luminal concentrations, but under most conditions is dependent on carrier-mediated facilitated diffusion. Folate is then released into the blood and is stored primarily in the liver, where it is found chiefly in the polyglutamate form. As a monoglutamate, it can undergo enterohepatic circulation.

Bibliography

Sellin JH. Physiology of digestion and absorption. In: Miller TA (ed.), *Physiologic Basis of Modern Surgical Care.* St. Louis, MO: CV Mosby, 1988, 339.

20. **(E)** Vitamin B_{12} (cobalamin) is an essential cofactor in the hematopoietic process and its deficiency is associated

with megaloblastic anemia. Ingested sources of B_{12} are necessary, and it is found only in animal sources such as meat and dairy foods. Unlike folate, there are adequate stores of B_{12} to meet the body's needs for several years. It has a fairly complex pattern of absorption, beginning with being freed from food complexes in the acidic environment of the stomach. It then binds to R proteins from the saliva and stomach before being carried into the small bowel. In the small bowel, the R proteins are degraded by pancreatic proteases, allowing for the binding of B_{12} to intrinsic factor. Because this step is necessary for vitamin B_{12} absorption, patients with pancreatic exocrine insuffiency may develop B_{12} deficieincy. Intrinsic factor is produced in the stomach by parietal cells and has binding sites for both B_{12} and an ileal receptor. Because patients with atrophic gastritis, or those who have undergone gastric resection, may have decreased or absent intrinsic factor production, these conditions may also lead to B_{12} deficiency. The B_{12}-intrinsic factor complex is resistant to proteolysis and travels down the intestine to the terminal ileum where intrinsic factor binds to the ileal cells and B_{12} is absorbed. Clearly, patients who have undergone ileal resection will therefore be prone to B_{12} deficiency. Other conditions associated with B_{12} deficiency include Zollinger-Ellison's syndrome and bacterial overgrowth.

Bibliography

Sellin JH. Physiology of Digestion and Absorption. In: Miller TA, ed. *Physiologic Basis of Modern Surgical Care*. St. Louis, MO: CV Mosby, 1988, 339–340.

21. **(A)** Up to 50% of the small bowel may be resected with expectation of normal GI function; however, because of specialized absorptive or secretory properties, the duodenum, proximal jejunum, and distal ileum must be spared. Because it is the sole or primary absorptive site for a range of substances found in the gut, resection of the distal ileum can result in an array of deficiency states. Loss of the distal ileum results in decreased bile salt absorption, and the losses often exceed the capacity of the liver to produce new bile salts, reducing the total bile salt pool. This has two adverse effects. First, it results in lithogenic bile and formation of cholesterol gallstones. Second, there is a decreased ability to form micelles, and fat absorption is therefore impeded, resulting in steatorrhea, which is then worsened by the osmotic diarrhea caused by excessive bile salts in the colon. This dearth of bile salts also results in impaired absorption of the fat soluble vitamins A, D, E, and K. Fat malabsorption results in the formation of insoluble calcium salts formed from the binding of calcium to fatty acids. This serves to decrease the intraluminal calcium concentration such that oxalate, which normally precipitates as an insoluble calcium salt, is

free to pass into the colon in soluble form, where it is then absorbed. Increased oxalate absorption leads to hyperoxaluria and the formation of kidney stones. Finally, vitamin B_{12} is absorbed in the distal ileum, and the deficiency thereof results in megaloblastic anemia.

Bibliography

Magnuson DK. Neonatal and pediatric physiology. In: Greenfield L (ed.), *Surgery: Scientific Principles and Practice*, 3rd ed. Philadelphia, PA: Lippincott, Williams & Wilkins, 2001, 1928.

Seal AM. Derangements in intestinal function secondary to previous surgery. In: Miller TA (ed.), *Physiologic Basis of Modern Surgical Care*. St. Louis, MO: CV Mosby, 1988, 395–396.

22. **(B)** Following digestion into monoglycerides and fatty acids in the intestinal lumen, lipid breakdown products are absorbed and the process is reversed in the enterocyte, resulting in reformation of triglycerides. The triglycerides are then formed into chylomicrons, which are large spheres consisting of a hydrophobic core covered by phospholipids and apolipoproteins. The chylomicron then exits the enterocyte across the basolateral membrane and is taken up by the intestinal lymphatic system, as chylomicrons are too large to fit through the capillary junctions and enter the portal venous system. Chylomicrons travel through the lymphatics to the cisterna chyle and thoracic duct before entering the systemic circulation. Medium chain fatty acids, however, secondary to their increased polarity, are to some degree water soluble and can therefore be directly absorbed without the need for bile salt facilitated solubilization into micelles. Similarly, once in the enterocyte, they can be transported into the portal venous system as fatty acids without undergoing reassembly into triglycerides. They are thus able to bypass the lymphatic system and decrease the effluent seen in cases of chylothorax.

Bibliography

Davidson NO, Magun AM, Glickman RM. Enterocyte lipid absorption and secretion. In: Schultz SG, Field M, Frizell RA, Rauner BB (eds.), *Handbook of Physiology. Section 6: The Gastrointestinal System. Volume IV: Intestinal Absorption and Secretion.* Bethesda, MD: American Physiologic Society, 1991, 506.

Sellin JH. Physiology of digestion and absorption. In: Miller TA (ed.), *Physiologic Basis of Modern Surgical Care*. St. Louis, MO: CV Mosby, 1988, 333–334.

23. **(E)** A variety of peptides serve to act in an endocrine, paracrine, or autocrine manner to regulate the complex interrelationships between the stomach, small bowel, gallbladder, and pancreas. These include secretin, which is found in the S cells of the duodenum and jejunum

and is released in response to duodenal fat, acid, or bile salts. It acts with CCK to increase pancreatic secretions rich in bicarbonate. It has a feedback mechanism such that its release is inhibited when the duodenal pH rises above 4.5. Secretin is notable for causing an unexpected increase in gastrin release and gastric acid production when applied exogenously to a patient with Zollinger-Ellison's syndrome.

Somatostatin is a widely distributed peptide, found in both the central and peripheral nervous systems, as well as in the GI tract. Somatostatin acts like a global brake on the GI system, decreasing motility, as well as gastric, enteric, and pancreatic secretions. GIP is found in the K cells of the duodenum. It acts as a true hormone to inhibit gastric acid secretion and stimulate insulin release. Its own release is stimulated by intraluminal amino acids, glucose, and fatty acids.

Motilin is found throughout the small intestine, but is present in higher concentrations more proximally. It is released during fasting, and has an important role in gut motility, serving some role in the initiation of migrating motor complexes. Its release is inhibited by somatostatin, secretin, pancreatic polypeptides, and intraluminal fat. Neurotensin is another peptide found in the central nervous system as well as the gut. In the GI tract, it is located predominantly in the ileum. It is released in response to luminal fatty acids and acts to inhibit gastric acid secretion and intestinal motility while stimulating pancreatic exocrine secretions and causing mesenteric vasodilation. Other peptides of note include peptide YY, which is found in the distal ileum and colon, released in response to intraluminal fat, and acts to inhibit gastric emptying and acid production, as well as pancreatic exocrine secretions, and bombesin, which stimulates GI motility and secretions.

Bibliography
Chung DH, Evers MB. The digestive system. In: O'Leary JP (ed.), *The Physiologic Basis of Surgery*, 3rd ed. Philadelphia, PA: Lippincott, Williams & Wilkins, 2002, 457–461.

24. **(B)** The normal resting potential of human enterocytes is −50 to −70 mV. Depolarizations called pacemaker potentials occur at regular intervals but do not cause muscular contractions. Instead, additional neural or chemical stimuli are needed to exceed the excitation threshold and cause an action potential. Thus, while the pacemaker potential is necessary for a contraction to occur, and is thus able to regulate the rate of contractions, it does not itself initiate peristaltic contractions. In the duodenum, these depolarizations occur 11–13 times/min, while they slow to 8–10 times/min in the ileum. Once a contraction occurs, it can be either a peristaltic contraction or a segmental one. Segmental contractions occur as circular muscle acts to churn

intestinal contents and cause mixing of the food bolus and exposure to the luminal mucosa. Peristaltic contractions, however, are the result of contractions of longitudinal muscle and serve to propel intestinal contents distally by a combination of proximal contraction and distal relaxation. These contractions serve to propel the intestinal contents fairly briskly, with a mean transit time through the intestines of just under 4 h. This transit time is shortened by meals high in glucose and lengthened by meals high in fat. The MMC is mediated by motilin. It occurs during the fasting state and serves to clear the intestines of residual material. When present, it cycles every 9–12 min, beginning in the proximal bowel and progressing distally to the terminal ileum. There are four phases. Phase I is a quiescent phase. During phase II, irregular, intermittent contractions occur. In phase III, the intestines exhibit regular, high amplitude contractions, before progressing to phase IV which, like phase II, has irregular, intermittent contractions. The MMC moves at a rate of 4–6 cm/min in the proximal small bowel and 1–2 cm/min more distally. Control for the MMC rests in the enteric nervous system and is destroyed with enteric resection. While extrinsic innervation can modulate the MMC, it continues to occur even after total extrinsic denervation.

Bibliography
Chung DH, Evers MB. The digestive system. In: O'Leary JP (ed.), *The Physiologic Basis of Surgery*, 3rd ed. Philadelphia, PA: Lippincott, Williams & Wilkins, 2002, 482–484.

Simeone DM. Anatomy and physiology of the small intestine. In: Greenfield L (ed.), *Surgery: Scientific Principles and Practice*, 3rd ed. Philadelphia, PA: Lippincott, Williams & Wilkins, 2001, 791–792.

25. **(D)** Host defense mechanisms in the gut include both immunologic and nonimmunologic components. Some of the nonimmunologic processes include hydrochloric acid secretion by the stomach, and mucus production, which serves to entrap bacteria. Peristalsis acts to clear the gut of harmful agents, while various enzymes lyse bacteria and toxins. The rapid turnover of epithelial cells seen in the intestines serves to slough infected cells and prevent deeper penetration of harmful organisms, and competition from endogenous, nonpathogenic organisms prevents harmful bacteria from colonizing the gut. Peyer's patches are large collections of lymphoid follicles with intervening interfollicular areas which are rich in T cells. A specialized epithelium composed of membrane cells (M cells) covers the Peyer's patch and acts as an antigen presenter by transporting particles from the intestinal lumen and delivering them to the underlying immune cells.

B cells mature in the germinal centers of the follicles in response to antigen under the regulation of T cells in the interfollicular areas. But while B cell maturation occurs in Peyer' patches, immunoglobulin secretion does not occur until they migrate to the lamina propria. The vast majority of B cells (80–90%) here produce IgA. Unlike in the serum, IgA in mucosal tissue exists as a dimer, connected by a J chain and linked to a transmembrane glycoprotein secretory component which facilitates transmembrane migration. Unlike other antibodies, IgA inhibits bacterial activity not by initiating the complement cascade or opsonization, but by binding to the offending agent and promoting entrapment within the mucin layer, as well as by directly impeding bacterial activity by binding to external bacterial effector mechanisms such as fimbriae. Exposure to antigens in the gut will lead to antigen-specific IgA secretion in other mucosal tissues as well. Following stimulation in the Peyer's patch, mature B cells migrate to mesenteric lymph nodes before eventually entering the systemic circulation via the thoracic duct. From there, they localize to other mucosa-associated lymphoid tissue. In this way, IgA can be secreted into breast milk and impart antigen-specific immunity to the GI tract of an infant.

Bibliography

Simeone DM. Anatomy and physiology of the small intestine. In: Greenfield L (ed.), *Surgery: Scientific Principles and Practice*, 3rd ed. Philadelphia, PA: Lippincott, Williams & Wilkins, 2001, 808–811.

26. **(B)** Glutamine is the chief fuel source of enterocytes. It is absorbed either from the gut lumen or from the arterial circulation. Glutamine is formed in peripheral tissues from glutamate and ammonia by the actions of glutamine synthetase. In the enterocyte, glutamine is broken down into glutamate and ammonia. Glutamate enters the tricarboxylic acid cycle while the ammonia is taken up in the portal circulation and delivered to the liver where it is used to form urea. About 50% of the ammonia in the portal circulation comes from glutamine metabolism, with the remainder coming as a result of bacterial metabolism.

Bibliography

Kolton WA, Pappas TN. Anatomy and physiology of the small intestine. In: Greenfield L (ed.), *Surgery: Scientific Principles and Practice*, 2nd ed. Philadelphia, PA: Lippincott, Williams & Wilkins, 1997, 816–817.

27. **(A)** Water composes approximately 90% of small intestinal contents that pass into the colon. The colon will absorb roughly 90% of this water before passing the remainder in the stool. The majority of water absorption occurs in the right colon as a passive response to an osmotic gradient established via the active transport of sodium, powered by the Na^+-K^+-ATPase on the basolateral membrane of colonic epithelial cells. The electrochemical gradient thus created also allows for passive passage of K^+ into the colonic lumen. The colon is also a site of chloride absorption with reciprocal excretion of bicarbonate.

Bibliography

Sweeney JF. Colonic anatomy and physiology. In: Greenfield L (ed.), *Surgery: Scientific Principles and Practice*, 3rd ed. Philadelphia, PA: Lippincott, Williams & Wilkins, 2001, 1066–1067.

28. **(B)** Colonocytes are unable to actively absorb glucose or amino acids; however, bacteria in the colonic lumen metabolize carbohydrates and proteins into short chain fatty acids, principally acetate, propionate, and butyrate. In fact, these short chain fatty acids are the predominant anions in the colon. Short chain fatty acids appear to be absorbed both by passive means and by carrier-mediated transport. Short chain fatty acids account for 7–10% of all the calories absorbed, and serve as the primary fuel source for colonocytes.

Bibliography

Montrose MH, Keely SJ, Barrett KE. Electrolyte secretion and absorption: small intestine and colon. In: Yamada T (ed.), *Textbook of Gastroenterology*, 3rd ed. Philadelphia, PA: Lippincott, Williams & Wilkins, 1999, 334–335.

29. **(C)** The defecatory mechanism begins with the passage of a fecal bolus into the rectum. Rectal distension is transmitted via parasympathetic mechanoreceptors; however, the rectosphincteric reflex is mediated by the myenteric plexus, and results in relaxation of the internal anal sphincter as the rectum contracts. At this time, voluntary contraction of the striated muscle of the external anal sphincter can forestall defecation; however, at rectal volumes exceeding 400 cc, incontinence can commonly occur, even in the setting of normal innervation and musculature. Once a socially acceptable situation is reached, a squatting position is assumed, which serves to straighten the anorectal junction, facilitating the passage of fecal material. The anorectal junction is further straightened by relaxation of the pelvic musculature, particularly the puborectalis muscle. A Valsalva maneuver is performed as the external anal sphincter relaxes, allowing passage of the stool out through the anus.

Bibliography

Chung DH, Evers MB. The digestive system. In: O'Leary JP (ed.), *The Physiologic Basis of Surgery*, 3rd ed.

Philadelphia, PA: Lippincott, Williams & Wilkins, 2002, 485–486.

Sweeney JF. Colonic anatomy and physiology. In: Greenfield L (ed.), *Surgery: Scientific Principles and Practice*, 3rd ed. Philadelphia, PA: Lippincott, Williams & Wilkins, 2001, 1067–1068.

30. **(D)** Pancreatic secretions consist of water and electrolytes secreted by centroacinar and intercalated duct cells and digestive enzymes from acinar cells. The secretions are alkalotic, and the concentration of bicarbonate increases from 20 mmol/L in the resting state to 150 mmol/L under conditions of maximal secretion. As bicarbonate concentration increases, there is a concomitant decrease in the chloride concentration such that the total concentration of the two anions remains constant and equal to their combined concentration in the plasma. The acinar cells secrete three main categories of enzymes—lipases, amylases, and proteases. The lipases secreted by the pancreas include pancreatic lipase, phospholipases A and B, and cholesterol esterase, which act to hydrolyze lipids. Amylase hydrolyzes carbohydrates into monosaccharides and disaccharides and α-limit dextrins. Proteases act to digest protein and are notable for being secreted into the intestinal lumen in inactive, proenzyme form. One of these proenzymes, trypsinogen, is activated either by an acidic environment or by the enteric enzyme enterokinase into its active form, trypsin. Trypsin then activates the other proteases. Pancreatic secretion can by increased by a variety of stimuli. Vagal stimulation increases both bicarbonate and enzymatic secretion. Secretin results in an increase in bicarbonate and fluid secretion but has little effect on enzyme secretion. VIP has similar effects but with less potency. CCK, as well as bombesin and gastrin to a lesser degree, is a strong stimulator of enzyme secretion, while having little effect on bicarbonate or fluid secretion (Table 20-1).

Bibliography

Brunicandi FC, Fisher WE. Pancreatic anatomy and physiology. In: Greenfield L (ed.), *Surgery: Scientific Principles and Practice*, 3rd ed. Philadelphia, PA: Lippincott, Williams & Wilkins, 2001, 855–857.

Kauffman GL. Pancreatic exocrine function. In: Miller TA (ed.), *Physiologic Basis of Modern Surgical Care*. St. Louis, MO: CV Mosby, 1988, 453–460.

31. **(D)** The pancreas can functionally be divided into the exocrine and endocrine pancreas. Structurally, this correlates with the acinar cells and ductal network for the exocrine pancreas, and the islets of Langerhans for the endocrine pancreas. The islets of Langerhans contribute little to pancreatic mass, accounting for only 2% of its weight. Within the islets of Langerhans

TABLE 20-1 Factors Affecting Pancreatic Secretion*

Stimulus	Enzyme production	Bicarbonate/volume production
Vagus	↑	↑
Secretin	–	↑
VIP	–	↑
CCK	↑	–
Gastrin	↑	–
Bombesin	↑	–
PP	↓	↓
Somatostatin	↓	↓
Glucagon	↓	↓
Sham feeding	↑	↓
Duodenal acid	–	↑
Fatty acids	↑	↑
Amino acids	↑	–

*Bicarbonate and total volume show concomitant increases or decreases. Production of enzymes may be independent from that of bicarbonate.

can be found alpha cells which secrete glucagon, beta cells which produce insulin, delta cells which manufacture somatostatin, and pancreatic polypeptide cells, which, not surprisingly produce pancreatic polypeptide. Beta cells are the most predominant cell type; they are located centrally within the islet and account for 70% of the mass of the endocrine pancreas. The other cell types account for a smaller percentage of the endocrine pancreas mass, with pancreatic polypeptide cells accounting for 15%, alpha cells for 10%, and delta cells for 5%.

Islets have varying compositions depending on their location within the pancreas. While beta and delta cells are relatively uniform in their distribution, alpha cells are found in greater predominance in the body and tail, while pancreatic polypeptide cells are more plentiful in the uncinate process. The acinar cells and ducts account for 80% of pancreatic mass. Acinar cells produce the enzymes necessary for digestion. Centroacinar cells secrete fluid and bicarbonate. Together, these cells form a structural unit called an acinus. The cells in an acinus secrete their products into an acinar lumen which drains into intercalated ducts, which in turn drain into interlobular ducts. The interlobular ducts eventually coalesce into the main pancreatic duct which carries the products of pancreatic exocrine production into the duodenum (Fig. 20-5, Table 20-2).

Bibliography

Brunicardi FC, Fisher WE. Pancreatic anatomy. In: Greenfield L (ed.), *Surgery: Scientific Principles and Practice*, 3rd ed. Philadelphia, PA: Lippincott, Williams & Wilkins, 2001, 853–854.

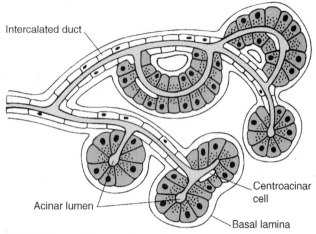

FIG. 20-5 Pancreatic acinus. Acinar cells secrete enzymes and centroacinar cells secrete water and bicarbonate into the acinar lumen. The acinar lumen in turn drains into intercalated ducts and eventually into the main pancreatic duct. (Reprinted with permission from Bockman DE, Histology and fine structure. In: Beger HG, Warshaw AC, Buechler MW, et al. (eds.), *The Pancreas*. Malden, MA: Blackwell Science, 1998.)

32. (A) The French nomenclature for hepatic anatomy, described by Couinaud, is now widely accepted. It divides the liver into four sectors based on vertical planes, termed scissura, created by the hepatic veins. Each sector can then be divided into two segments based on their portal venous supply. The chief benefit of this system is the accurate location of lesions and the ability to perform resections of less than a complete lobe while minimizing blood loss and maximizing hepatic function. Segment I corresponds to the caudate lobe. The caudate lobe is unique in that it often receives portal blood from both the left and right side, and it drains directly into the inferior vena cava. Collectively, segments II–IV comprise the left lobe of the liver, and segments V–VIII the right. The blood supply to the liver is supplied by the hepatic artery and portal vein. Classically, the common hepatic artery arises from the celiac trunk and becomes the proper

hepatic artery after giving off the gastroduodenal artery. It then bifurcates into the right hand left hepatic arteries. The cystic artery arises from the right hepatic artery. Variations are common; however, most frequently either a replaced right hepatic artery arising from the superior mesenteric artery, or a replaced left hepatic artery coming off the left gastric artery. The hepatic artery provides approximately 50% of the inflow to the liver, as well as approximately 75% of its oxygen. The portal vein is formed by the merging of the splenic vein and superior mesenteric vein behind the pancreas. It courses posteriorly in the hepatoduodenal ligament before draining into the liver in a manner parallel with the arterial supply.

Bibliography

Byrd DR. Hepatobiliary anatomy. In: Greenfield L (ed.), *Surgery: Scientific Principles and Practice*, 3rd ed. Philadelphia, PA: Lippincott, Williams & Wilkins, 2001, 916–920.

33. (C) Bile is a solution composed chiefly of water, which accounts for about 85% of its volume. Because cholesterol is nonpolar and insoluble in water, and because bile acids and phospholipids are amphipathic, these lipids form micelles in solution. Cholesterol aggregates centrally in association with the nonpolar aspects of the bile acids and phospholipids. The polar, hydrophilic aspects of these molecules are found on the periphery, in contact with the aqueous environment. When rich in bile salts, the micelles form into a sphere shape, but when rich in lecithin, they form disk-shaped micelles, which tend to be larger and are capable of solubilizing more cholesterol. The main lipid component in bile are the bile acids, with the two main primary bile acids, cholic acid and chenodeoxycholic acid accounting for about 80% of all bile acids. Phospholipids, of which lecithin is the most prevalent, account for about 20% of all lipids. Cholesterol is the least prevalent lipid, accounting for less than 10%. In addition to lipids, bile contains smaller amounts of proteins, chiefly albumin, and various electrolytes. The concentration of the main electrolytes approximates that of plasma. Of course, bilirubin is also present in bile, almost exclusively in conjugated form.

Bibliography

Cabral DJ, Small DM. Physical chemistry of bile. In: Schultz SG, Forte JG, Rauner BB (eds.), *Handbook of Physiology, Section 6, Volume III: Salivary, Gastric, Pancreatic, and Hepatobiliary Secretion*. Bethesda, MD: American Physiologic Society, 1989, 651–653.

McFadden DW, Gadacz TR. Calculous disease of the gallbladder and common bile duct. In: Miller TA (ed.), *Physiologic Basis of Modern Surgical Care*. St. Louis, MO: CV Mosby, 1988, 431–433.

TABLE 20-2   A Comparison of the Various Cells Comprising the Islets of Langerhans with a Review of Their Endocrine Products, the Percent of Pancreatic Endocrine Mass They Contribute, and Their Predominant Location within the Pancreas

Cell	Product	% of Endocrine Mass	Location
α-cells	Glucagon	10	Body and tail
β-cells	Insulin	70	Uniform
δ-cells	Somatostatin	5	Uniform
Pancreatic polypeptide cells	Pancreatic polypeptide	15	Uncinate process

Sharp KW, Chapman WC, Potts JR, et al. Liver, biliary tract, and pancreas. In: O'Leary JP (ed.), *The Physiologic Basis of Surgery*, 3rd ed. Philadelphia, PA: Lippincott, Williams & Wilkins, 2002, 497–498.

34. **(B)** Understanding of the enterohepatic circulation of bile acids began with Moritz Schiff in 1855 who observed an increased rate of bile secretion in dogs in proportion to the amount of exogenous bile instilled into their small intestines. New bile acids are typically added to the pool by conversion of cholesterol to one of the two primary bile acids, either chenodeoxycholic acid or cholic acid. The concentration of bile acids in hepatocytes is low (<50 μmol), as active secretion prevents the accumulation of bile acids. Hepatic bile, on the other hand, is quite concentrated (20,000–40,000 μmol). This bile either flows freely into the duodenum, or, if the sphincter of Oddi is contracted, will flow into the gallbladder. Once in the gallbladder, water is absorbed from the bile across the mucosa, resulting in the highest concentration of bile acids (50,000–200,000 μmol).

    With the release of CCK in response to a meal, the gallbladder contracts and the sphincter of Oddi relaxes, causing flow of the bile into the small intestine. A small amount of bile acids will be passively absorbed in the proximal intestine, but most will proceed distally. Chenodeoxycholic acid and cholic acid may undergo transformation into ursodeoxycholic acid and deoxycholic acid, respectively, by enteric bacteria. Most of these bile acids, both primary and secondary, will be actively absorbed in the terminal ileum. A small percentage of bile acids will pass into the colon. Some of these will be reabsorbed and the rest will be lost to the body in the feces. This accounts for almost all of the loss of bile acids. The bile acids absorbed by the terminal ileum will pass back to the liver bound to albumin in portal blood, where they will be extracted by hepatocytes. The percentage of bile acids extracted remains relatively constant, as the capacity for bile acid extraction greatly exceeds the typical bile acid load seen by the liver.

    Thus, as enterohepatic circulation of bile acids is increased by a meal, a greater absolute number of bile acids will bypass the liver and enter the systemic circulation, resulting in a postprandial increase in the serum bile acid level. Bile acids in the systemic circulation can be excreted in the urine, but urine losses are negligible for three main reasons. First, the hepatic extraction of bile acids from portal venous blood is extremely efficient. Second, most bile acids in the blood are protein bound, and third, bile acids are reabsorbed by the renal tubules (Fig. 20-6).

    Bibliography

    Hofmann AF. Enterohepatic circulation of bile acids. In: Schultz SG, Forte JG, Rauner BB (eds.), *Handbook of Physiology, Section 6, Volume III: Salivary, Gastric, Pancreatic, and Hepatobiliary Secretion.* Bethesda, MD: American Physiologic Society, 1989, 567–574.

35. **(D)** For patients with a normal gallbladder in the fasting state, over half of the bile acid pool will be stored in the gallbladder. Alterations in function or surgical removal of the gallbladder, therefore, cause changes in characteristics of the bile acid pool. After cholecystectomy, bile passes directly into the intestines, which

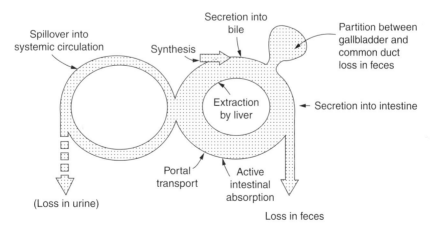

FIG. 20-6 Enterohepatic circulation. The majority of bile acids remain in a circulating pool between the liver, gallbladder, and intestines. Some bile acids are lost via the feces, and a small percentage of bile acids which enter the systemic circulation are lost in the urine. Nonetheless, this enteric reuptake of bile acids is extremely efficient, and those bile acids which are lost are replaced by hepatic synthesis. (Reprinted with permission from Hofmann AF, Enterohepatic circulation of bile acids. In: Schultz SG, Forte JG, Rauner BB (eds.), *Handbook of Physiology, Section 6, Volume III: Salivary, Gastric, Pancreatic, and Hepatobiliary Secretion.* Bethesda, MD: American Physiologic Society, 1989, 567–574.)

essentially serves as the storage reservoir for bile salts; however, this is not a static process, and distal passage of the bile acids results in absorption in the terminal ileum and an increase in enterohepatic cycling. This, in turn, results in slight elevations in the fasting serum bile acid levels, as the percentage of bile acids extracted by the liver remains constant. Because a greater proportion of bile acids are located enterically, they are more exposed to bacterial biotransformation and a relative increase in secondary bile acids is seen, although patients who have undergone cholecystectomy have a smaller total pool of bile acids. In patients with celiac sprue, conversely, CCK release is impaired and the gallbladder does not effectively contract in response to a meal. This results in a large number of bile acids being sequestered in the gallbladder, and leads to a greatly enlarged bile acid pool.

Bibliography

Hofmann AF. Enterohepatic circulation of bile acids. In: Schultz SG, Forte JG, Rauner BB (eds.), *Handbook of Physiology, Section 6, Volume III: Salivary, Gastric, Pancreatic, and Hepatobiliary Secretion.* Bethesda, MD: American Physiologic Society, 1989, 586.

36. **(E)** Cholesterol is insoluble in water and thus in bile relies on the formation of micelles with bile salts and phospholipids, chiefly lecithin, to maintain solubility. The relationship of these three lipids and the effect of their relative concentrations on cholesterol solubility can be expressed in a phase diagram. In Figure 20-2 phase E represents a state where the lipids in bile are contained in mixed micelles of bile salt, phospholipid, and cholesterol, in equilibrium with free bile acids. In this state, all of the cholesterol is solubilized. In all the other states, cholesterol is supersaturated. In the area denoted by the letter A, the lipids exist as cholesterol crystals and mixed micelles. In the area denoted by the letter D, the lipids are found in mixed micelles and in liquid crystals composed of phospholipids and cholesterol. In the area denoted by B and C, all three phases exist—micelles, cholesterol crystals, and liquid crystals. The proposed model of cholesterol gallstone formation is one in which cholesterol supersaturation leads to microcrystal precipitation, followed by the formation of macrocrystal cholesterol stones. The phase diagram reflects the relationship of bile acids, lecithin, and cholesterol at a given total lipid content. As the percentage of lipids in the bile decreases, cholesterol becomes relatively less soluble, and the area denoted by the letter E becomes smaller. Interestingly, *in vivo*, many individuals with supersaturated bile do not demonstrate cholesterol precipitation, a state referred to as metastable bile. It is unclear if individuals who do have stones have a lithogenic factor in

their bile which encourages precipitation, or if individuals who do not form stones have a factor which stabilizes the bile in its metastable state.

Bibliography

Cabral DJ, Small DM. Physical chemistry of bile. In: Schultz SG, Forte JG, Rauner BB (eds.), *Handbook of Physiology, Section 6, Volume III: Salivary, Gastric, Pancreatic, and Hepatobiliary Secretion.* Bethesda, MD: American Physiologic Society, 1989, 649–655.

McFadden DW, Gadacz TR. Calculous disease of the gallbladder and common bile duct. In: Miller TA (ed.), *Physiologic Basis of Modern Surgical Care.* St. Louis, MO: CV Mosby, 1988, 433–435.

Sharp KW, Chapman WC, Potts JR, et al. Liver, biliary tract, and pancreas. In: O'Leary JP (ed.), *The Physiologic Basis of Surgery*, 3rd ed. Philadelphia, PA: Lippincott, Williams & Wilkins, 2002, 498–499.

37. **(A)** The acinus is a diamond-shaped mass which composes the smallest functional unit of the liver. Its apices are the hepatic venules and its axis is defined by the terminal braches of the portal vein and hepatic artery, in conjunction with the bile ductules. The hepatocytes within the acinus are further subdivided based on their proximity to the portal venules. Those hepatocytes closest to the venules are in zone 1, those at an intermediate distance in zone 2, and those hepatocytes furthest from the portal venules, and thus closest to the hepatic venules, are termed zone 3 hepatocytes. Obviously, zone 1 hepatocytes, being closest to the terminal portal venule, receive the best blood supply and are therefore the last cells to die, the first to regenerate, and are in general more resistant to toxic insults than zone 3 hepatocytes. They are also the first cells exposed to solutes which are taken up by simple diffusion and therefore most such solutes enter zone 1 hepatocytes. Zones 1 and 2 are also the site of uptake of most solutes which require receptor-mediated endocystosis, while albumin-bound solutes, such as bilirubin, are taken up in all three zones. The endothelium of the hepatic sinusoids is characterized by large fenestrations which allow for the passage of relatively large particles into contact with the hepatocytes.

Bibliography

Raper SE. Hepatic physiology. In: Greenfield L (ed.), *Surgery: Scientific Principles and Practice*, 3rd ed. Philadelphia, PA: Lippincott, Williams & Wilkins, 2001, 727–728.

38. **(B)** One of the chief functions of the liver is maintaining a steady concentration of glucose in the blood. Glucose, fructose, and galactose are the three mononsaccharides which are the endpoint of intestinal carbohydrate digestion. Both fructose and galactose are

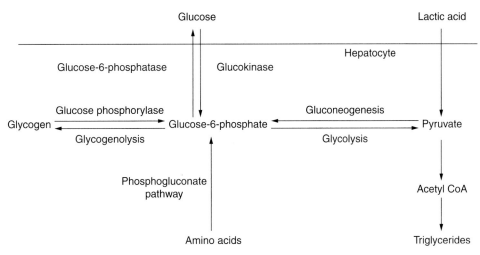

FIG. 20-7   A schematic of the hepatic metabolism of carbohydrates.

capable of enzymatic conversion to glucose. These hexoses are carried in portal blood to the liver. The rate of glucose uptake by the hepatocyte is greatly increased by insulin. Phosphorylated glucose does not leave the hepatocyte and the cleavage of the phosphate group by glucose-6-phosphatase is necessary for glucose release. Glycogenesis is favored after feeding, as insulin reduces cAMP levels. Glucokinase facilitates the phosphorylation of glucose to glucose-6-phosphate (G6P). G6P will then be converted to glucose-1-phosphate and ultimately to glycogen. As the hepatic glycogen capacity is reached, excess glucose is converted to fat by the glycolytic pathway. Phosphofructokinase, induced by insulin, facilitates the conversion of fructose-6-phosphate to fructose-1,6-bisphosphate, the rate limiting step of glycolysis. One molecule of glucose will yield two molecules of pyruvate, which will then undergo conversion to acetyl-CoA, which then acts as the building block for triglyceride synthesis. The conversion of glucose into triglycerides is fairly efficient, with about 85% of the energy retained. The efficiency of glucose storage as glycogen, however, is a remarkable 97%. In the fasting state, when blood glucose levels fall, glucagon is released and insulin secretion diminishes. This favors glycogenolysis and gluconeogenesis. Glucagon acts to increase intracellular levels of cAMP, which activates phosphorylase A, the enzyme responsible for liberating glucose molecules from

glycogen. Glucose can then be released from the hepatocyte into the systemic circulation after cleavage of the phosphate group by glucose-6-phosphatase. When hepatic glycogen stores are exhausted, some amino acids, glycerol, or lactate can serve as substrates for glucose production. This process is simplest for alanine, which can be converted to pyruvic acid by deamination, and then undergoes conversion to glucose by a reversal of the glycolytic pathway. Other amino acids are converted to three to five carbon sugars and undergo subsequent conversion to glucose via the phosphogluconate pathway. About 40% of amino acids in the body cannot be converted into glucose. Interestingly, while the liver is central to glucose metabolism, it derives most of its energy from ketoacid oxidation (Fig. 20-7).

Bibliography

Lipid metabolism. In: Guyton AC, Hall JE (eds.), *Textbook of Medical Physiology*, 9th ed. Philadelphia, PA: WB Saunders, 1996, 869–870.

Metabolism of carbohydrates and formation of adenosine triphosphate. In: Guyton AC, Hall JE (eds.), *Textbook of Medical Physiology*, 9th ed. Philadelphia, PA: WB Saunders, 1996, 855–864.

Raper SE. Hepatic physiology. In: Greenfield L (ed.), *Surgery: Scientific Principles and Practice*, 3rd ed. Philadelphia, PA: Lippincott, Williams & Wilkins, 2001, 933–935.

CHAPTER 21

Esophagus

Ben M. Tsai and Kenneth A. Kesler

Questions

1. A 33-year-old female arrives to the emergency department following a suspected suicide attempt in which she swallowed an unknown cleaning solution. The patient is obtunded and unable to provide any history. Vital signs are as follows: temperature 98.6°F, BP 136/88 mmHg, HR 114 bpm, RR 32 breaths/min. On examination, she is drooling from the mouth and there are visible burns in the oropharynx and crepitus in the neck and upper chest. All of the following are appropriate *except*:

   (A) endotracheal intubation
   (B) administer broad-spectrum intravenous antibiotics
   (C) perform endoscopy
   (D) administer intravenous corticosteroids
   (E) prepare for operative intervention

2. For the surgical treatment of gastroesophageal reflux disease (GERD), which of the following treatment-condition pairs is most likely to fail?

   (A) Nissen fundoplication for scleroderma
   (B) Toupet fundoplication for peptic stricture
   (C) Belsey Mark IV fundoplication for low-amplitude peristalsis
   (D) Collis gastroplasty with Nissen fundoplication for short esophagus
   (E) Dor fundoplication for achalasia

3. Which of the following statements is false?

   (A) The esophageal mucosal epithelium normally consists of squamous cells.
   (B) The right vagus nerve is located anterior to the esophagus, whereas the left vagus nerve is posterior to the esophagus.
   (C) The upper third of the esophagus consists of striated muscle and the lower two-thirds consists of smooth muscle.

   (D) The esophageal muscle is made of an outer longitudinal muscle layer overlying an inner circular muscle layer.
   (E) The embryonic esophagus forms from the primitive foregut.

4. A 63-year-old White male complains of a 6-month history of dysphagia and 30-lb weight loss. His primary care physician suspects esophageal carcinoma and refers the patient to you. The barium esophagogram obtained is shown in Fig. 21-1. What treatment should you recommend to this patient?

   (A) pneumatic dilation
   (B) diverticulectomy
   (C) endoscopic stapled division
   (D) cervical esophagomyotomy
   (E) esophagectomy

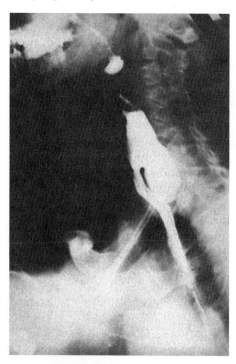

FIG. 21-1 Barium esophagogram.

5. A 52-year-old female complains of heartburn that has been worsening in recent months. She has been self-medicating with over-the-counter agents with only mild relief in symptoms. She undergoes esophagoscopy which reveals moderate to severe esophagitis. Which of the following medications is most effective for healing the esophagus?

(A) Drug A binds the proton pump in gastric parietal cells and inhibits gastric acid production.

(B) Drug B antagonizes histamine-2(H2)-receptors to inhibit stimulation of acid secretion.

(C) Drug C dopamine antagonist that promotes motility.

(D) Drug D neutralizes gastric acidity and stimulates prostaglandin activity.

(E) Drug E anticholinergic agent that decreases esophageal contractions and saliva production.

6. A 44-year-old female with achalasia is treated with oral nitrates but experiences significant side effects and is switched to calcium antagonists. There is mild improvement in symptoms during the first several months but she now complains of regurgitation and weight loss. What surgical option(s) should be considered in this patient?

(A) fundoplication

(B) laparoscopic esophagomyotomy

(C) esophagectomy

(D) myotomy and fundoplication

(E) none of the above

7. Approximately 24 h after an uneventful transhiatal esophagectomy with a cervical esophagogastric anastomosis for esophageal carcinoma, the patient develops respiratory distress requiring emergent intubation. The postintubation chest radiograph shows an infiltrate in the right middle lobe. What is the likely etiology of this complication?

(A) phrenic nerve injury

(B) tracheal laceration

(C) gastric outlet obstruction

(D) esophagogastric anastomotic leak

(E) recurrent laryngeal nerve injury

8. A 76-year-old female with a 12-month history of dysphagia is admitted to the hospital for pneumonia. A barium esophagogram shows a tracheoesophageal fistula (TEF). Endoscopic biopsies at this site reveal squamous cell carcinoma. What is the preferred treatment?

(A) esophagectomy

(B) cervical esophagostomy and gastric tube placement

(C) esophageal stent placement

(D) radiation therapy

(E) chemoradiation followed by esophagectomy

9. The gastroesophageal junction is located above the diaphragmatic hiatus in which type(s) of hiatal hernia?

(A) type I and II

(B) type I and III

(C) type II and III

(D) type I, II, and III

(E) type II only

10. A 49-year-old female with Barrett's esophagus undergoes routine surveillance esophagoscopy. Random biopsies reveal low-grade dysplasia. Which of the following recommendations should you make to this patient?

(A) no change in treatment is required with continued routine endoscopic surveillance in 2–3 years

(B) Nissen fundoplication to eliminate the need for future endoscopic surveillance

(C) repeat endoscopic surveillance in several months time regardless of choice of therapy

(D) increase the dose of PPIs to allow regression of the dysplastic epithelium

(E) esophagectomy because of the risk of invasive adenocarcinoma

11. A 42-year-old business executive presents with occasional symptoms of intense chest pain during swallowing. An electrocardiogram was unremarkable; however, a barium swallow was obtained during these symptoms and is shown in Fig. 21-2. All of the following regarding this abnormality are true *except*:

(A) Patients typically have high underlying psychologic stress levels.

(B) An aggressive trial of medical management should be the first line of therapy.

(C) Manometry is usually diagnostic.

(D) Barium esophagogram may appear normal.

(E) A Heller myotomy relieves symptoms in most patients.

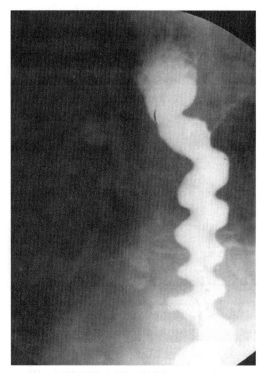

FIG. 21-2   Barium esophagogram.

12. Which of the following studies is the most accurate method for evaluating regional lymph node involvement in esophageal cancer?

   (A) barium esophagogram
   (B) endoscopic ultrasound
   (C) computed tomography (CT)
   (D) positron emission tomography (PET)
   (E) magnetic resonance imaging (MRI)

13. A 40-year-old female complains of a 3-month history of dysphagia. The barium swallow and endoscopic ultrasound obtained are shown in Figs. 21-3 and 21-4. What is the likely etiology of the patient's symptoms?

   (A) sqaumous cell carcinoma
   (B) congenital duplication cyst
   (C) fibrovascular polyp
   (D) leiomyoma
   (E) benign stricture

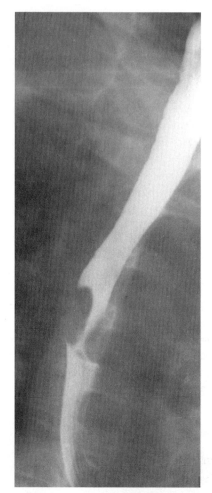

FIG. 21-3   Barium esophagogram.

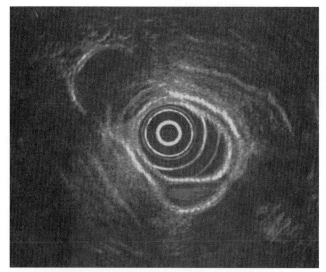

FIG. 21-4   Endoscopic esophageal ultrasound (EUS). (Reprinted with permission from Cameron JL (ed.), *Current Surgical Therapy*, 7th ed. The Netherlands: Elsevier, 2001, 53.)

14. Which of the following statements is *true*?

    (A) The majority of esophageal carcinomas in the United States are squamous cell carcinomas.

    (B) There are no identified risk factors for esophageal carcinoma.

    (C) The incidence of squamous cell carcinoma of the esophagus has risen dramatically as a result of gastroesophageal reflux and Barrett's metaplasia.

    (D) Esophageal adenocarcinoma occurs more frequently in females than in males.

    (E) Black males have an increased risk of developing squamous cell carcinoma of the esophagus.

15. A 54-year-old male complains of dysphagia and a sticking sensation in his chest after meals. He also experiences regurgitation of undigested food and has lost 10 lbs in the last 2 months. A barium esophagogram is obtained and is shown in Fig. 21-5. Which of the following should be considered in the differential diagnosis?

    (A) malignancy
    (B) achalasia

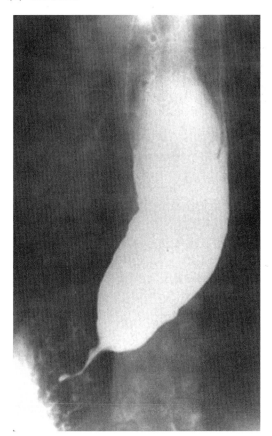

FIG. 21-5 Barium esophagogram.

(C) Chagas disease
(D) stricture
(E) all of the above

16. Which of the following tests are used to guide management of GERD?

    (A) endoscopy
    (B) gastric scintigraphy
    (C) manometry
    (D) esophageal pH monitor
    (E) all of the above

17. Starting with the innermost structure, what is the correct order of the layers of the esophageal wall?

    (A) epithelium, muscularis propria, muscularis mucosa, submucosa, periesophageal tissue

    (B) epithelium, submucosa, muscularis propria, muscularis mucosa, lamina propria

    (C) epithelium, lamina propria, muscularis mucosa, submucosa, muscularis propria

    (D) mucosa, submucosa, muscularis mucosa, muscularis propria, periesophageal tissue

    (E) mucosa, muscularis propria, lamina propria, submucosa, muscularis mucosa

18. Which of the following statements regarding GERD is true?

    (A) The LES must be permanently defective for GERD to occur.

    (B) The presence of pepsin in refluxed gastric juice potentiates the injurious effects of gastric acid on esophageal mucosa.

    (C) The reflux of duodenal juice tends to neutralize acidic gastric juice and therefore causes less injury to the esophageal mucosa than gastric content reflux alone.

    (D) Patients with normal LES pressures will not develop clinically significant reflux.

    (E) The presence of *Helicobacter pylori* is associated with GERD.

19. A 59-year-old male with a several month history of dysphagia is diagnosed with adenocarcinoma of the distal esophagus. An endoscopic ultrasound shows the tumor to invade periesophageal tissue but not adjacent structures. CT scans of the chest and abdomen show no distant metastasis. The patient is otherwise healthy. Which of the following treatments provide the best chance for long-term survival?

(A) chemotherapy followed by surgery

(B) chemoradiation alone

(C) chemoradiation followed by surgery

(D) surgery alone

(E) chemoradiation after surgery

20. A 68-year-old female reports a 3-year history of dysphagia and epigastric pain. She has been hospitalized twice in the last year for aspiration pneumonia. Her primary physician orders the barium esophagogram shown in Fig. 21-6. What treatment will provide the best long-term improvement in this patient's symptoms?

(A) pneumatic esophageal dilation

(B) hiatal hernia repair and fundoplication

(C) diverticulopexy or diverticulectomy

(D) diverticulectomy and myotomy

(E) esophagectomy

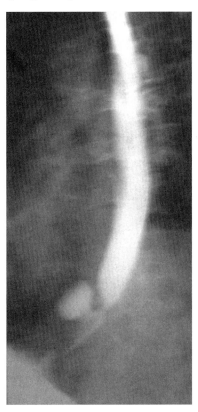

FIG. 21-6 Barium esophagogram.

21. All of the following promote LES relaxation *except*:

(A) atropine

(B) nitric oxide

(C) cholecystokinin (CCK)

(D) gastric distention

(E) pharyngeal stimulation

22. A 38-year-old male complains of dysphagia and regurgitation. A CT scan is obtained and is shown in Fig. 21-7 An endoscopic esophageal ultrasound is subsequently performed which demonstrates a submucosal cystic mass with normal overlying mucosa. All of the following are true *except*:

(A) Endoscopic biopsy is normally diagnostic.

(B) Occurs most frequently in infants and young children.

(C) The lining may consist of ciliated columnar epithelium.

(D) Potential complications include compression of adjacent structures, ulceration, hemorrhage, and infection.

(E) Surgical resection is indicated in most cases.

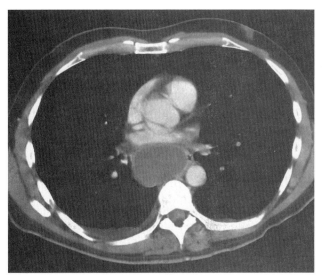

FIG. 21-7 Computed tomography (CT) of the chest.

23. The advantages of a transhiatal esophagectomy compared to a transthoracic approach with an intrathoracic anastomosis include all of the following *except*:

(A) avoiding a thoracotomy incision

(B) decreased operative mortality

(C) decreased mortality with an anastomotic leak

(D) decreased incidence of postoperative gastroesophageal reflux

(E) decreased risk of pulmonary complications

24. Which of the following patients is least likely to benefit from antireflux surgery?

  (A) A 36-year-old male with no improvement in reflux symptoms after a 6-week course of H2-receptor antagonist therapy.

  (B) A 52-year-old female with a 10-year history of GERD and Barrett's metaplasia.

  (C) A 44-year-old male taking PPIs for 5 years with linear ulceration in the distal esophagus.

  (D) A 41-year-old female whose reflux symptoms are well controlled on escalating doses of PPIs.

  (E) A 49-year-old male with asthma and a 10-year history of reflux whose symptoms are well controlled with PPIs.

25. A 24-year-old female swallowed drain cleaning solution containing concentrated lye. Which of the following complications is she most likely to experience several weeks after the injury?

  (A) TEF

  (B) esophageal stricture

  (C) esophageal carcinoma

  (D) hiatal hernia

  (E) esophageal perforation

26. An otherwise healthy 56-year-old male complains of dysphagia and intermittent chest pain over the last several months. A cardiac workup, including electrocardiogram and treadmill stress test, is unremarkable. Esophageal manometry is performed with the resulting tracing depicted in Fig. 21-8. What is the diagnosis?

  (A) achalasia

  (B) DES

  (C) nutcracker esophagus

  (D) hypertensive lower esophageal sphincter

  (E) inadequate esophageal motility

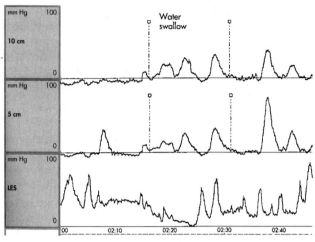

FIG. 21-8 Esophageal manometry tracing. (Reprinted with permission from Cameron JL (ed.), *Current Surgical Therapy*, 7th ed. The Netherlands: Elsevier, 2001, 21.)

27. Which of the following protects esophageal mucosa against acid-induced injury?

  (A) high pressure zone in the distal esophagus

  (B) esophageal peristalsis and gravity

  (C) swallowed saliva

  (D) submucosal gland secretions

  (E) all of the above

28. A 74-year-old male complains of postprandial fullness and bloating over the past 9 months. He presents to the emergency department with epigastric pain and dry retching. Attempts to pass a nasogastric tube are unsuccessful. A barium esophagogram is obtained and is shown in Fig. 21-9. Which of the following regarding this abnormality is false?

  (A) Surgery is urgently indicated because of the risk of obstruction, bleeding, and particularly strangulation.

  (B) Laparoscopic repair is equally safe and effective compared to open repair.

  (C) Fundoplication is not necessary once the primary abnormality is repaired.

  (D) Gastroesophageal reflux is commonly associated with this disorder.

  (E) Respiratory complications are frequently associated with this abnormality.

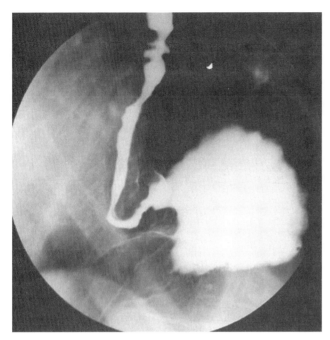

FIG. 21-9   Barium esophagogram.

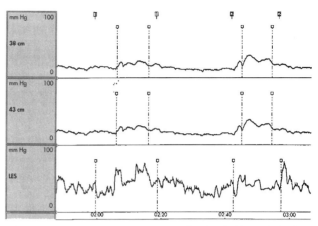

FIG. 21-10   Esophageal manometry tracing. (Reprinted with permission from Cameron JL (ed.), Current Surgical Therapy, 7th ed. The Netherlands: Elsevier, 2001, 22.)

29. A 42-year-old male reports a 6-month history of dysphagia. The esophageal manometry tracing obtained is shown in Fig. 21-10. Which treatment provides the best long-term clinical response?

(A) nifedipine

(B) isosorbide dinitrate

(C) atenolol

(D) pneumatic dilation

(E) botulinum toxin injection

30. All of the following supply blood to the esophagus *except*:

(A) inferior thyroid artery

(B) left gastric artery

(C) bronchial arteries

(D) inferior phrenic artery

(E) internal thoracic artery

31. A 79-year-old male with dysphagia and 30-lb weight loss over the last 6 months is diagnosed with adenocarcinoma of the distal esophagus. Chest and abdominal CT scans are demonstrated in Fig. 21-11. Which of the following is *least likely* to benefit this patient?

(A) radiation therapy

(B) endoscopic stenting

(C) laser therapy

(D) photodynamic therapy

(E) esophagectomy

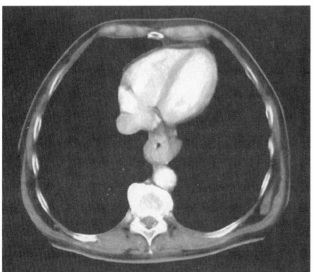
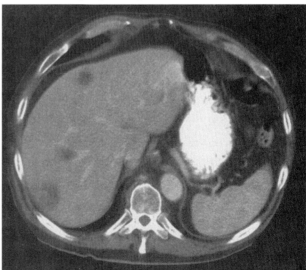

FIG. 21-11   Computed tomography (CT) of the chest and abdomen.

32. A 58-year-old male with a history of GERD undergoes routine esophagogastroscopy. The endoscopist notes salmon-pink mucosa extending 2 cm above the gastroesophageal junction. Biopsies of this area reveal columnar epithelium-containing goblet cells. Which of the following is true regarding this patient?

    (A) Because the abnormality extends only 2 cm above the gastroesophageal junction, the risk of adenocarcinoma is not increased.
    (B) Reflux of duodenal contents (i.e., bile) into the esophagus is protective against the development of this abnormality.
    (C) The presence of gastric-type columnar cells and intestinal-type columnar cells has equal risk of progressing to adenocarcinoma.
    (D) The presence of *H. pylori* gastritis increases the risk of developing this abnormality.
    (E) The presence of goblet cells increases the risk of dysplasia and subsequent adenocarcinoma.

33. Which of the following statements regarding self-expanding metallic stents is false?

    (A) Placement of a self-expanding metallic stent does not preclude the patient from undergoing further treatment with radiation or chemotherapy.
    (B) Complications following placement of self-expanding metallic stents include esophageal perforation and gastroesophageal reflux.
    (C) Most self-expanding metallic stents cannot be removed or repositioned after deployment.
    (D) Self-expanding metallic stents can be stacked on end to treat longer obstructive lesions.
    (E) Self-expanding metallic stents are contraindicated in malignant tracheoesophageal or bronchoesophageal fistula because of the increased risk of perforation.

34. Regarding GERD and scleroderma, which of the following statements is false?

    (A) Decreased LES pressures may play a role.
    (B) Complications include Barrett's esophagus, esophagitis, and stricture.
    (C) Prokinetic drugs provide no benefit.
    (D) PPIs are used in first-line therapy.
    (E) The primary abnormality is a motility disorder.

DIRECTIONS (Questions 35 and 36): For each of the following questions, choose the BEST ANSWER from the lettered set listed below. Each answer may be used once, more than once, or not at all.

Questions 35 and 36

    (A) stage IIA
    (B) stage IIB
    (C) stage III
    (D) stage IVA
    (E) stage IVB

35. A 68-year-old White male presents with a biopsy-proven esophageal squamous cell carcinoma. On transesophageal ultrasound, the tumor is seen to invade periesophageal tissue but not adjacent structures. There is no lymph node involvement and no evidence of distant metastases by chest and abdominal CT scans. What is the stage of this patient's esophageal carcinoma?

36. A 78-year-old male with dysphagia and a 30-lb weight loss undergoes endoscopic esophageal ultrasound for evaluation of adenocarcinoma of the distal esophagus. The tumor invades muscularis propria but not periesophageal tissue. There is an enlarged lymph node measuring 2.2 cm around the celiac axis, which is biopsied by FNA with EUS guidance and cytology is positive for adenocarcinoma. CT scans of the chest and abdomen and PET scan show no evidence of distant metastasis. What is the stage?

DIRECTIONS (Questions 37 through 40): For each of the following questions, choose the BEST ANSWER from the lettered set listed below. Each answer may be used once, more than once, or not at all.

Questions 37 through 40

    (A) nonoperative management
    (B) primary repair with local tissue reinforcement
    (C) esophagectomy with immediate reconstruction
    (D) proximal and distal diversion, jejunostomy feeding tube
    (E) proximal diversion, esophagectomy, jejunostomy tube, delayed reconstruction

37. A 65-year-old male with a history of cervical spine fracture developed osteomyelitis and underwent a C6 corpectomy 24 h ago. He now has subcutaneous emphysema in the neck and upper chest, and a CT scan is shown in Fig. 21-12. He is afebrile and hemodynamically stable. What is the appropriate treatment?

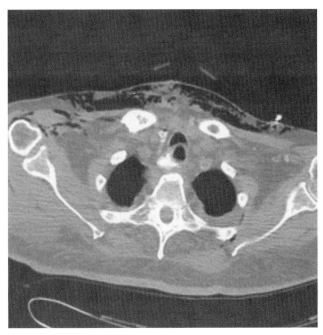

FIG. 21-12 Computed tomography (CT) of the chest.

38. A 76-year-old male with congestive heart failure and an ejection fraction of 20% presents with a 3-day history of forceful vomiting, epigastric pain, and fevers. He is tachycardic and has a leukocytosis of 18,000 WBC/mm^3. The abdominal CT obtained is shown in Fig. 21-13. What is the appropriate treatment?

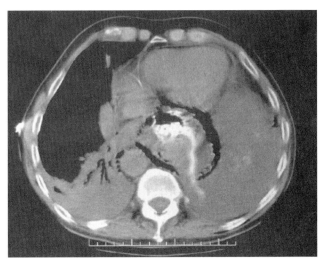

FIG. 21-13 Computed tomography (CT) of the abdomen.

39. An otherwise healthy 53-year-old female with Barrett's metaplasia underwent an esophagogastroscopy 2 days ago and biopsies showed high-grade dysplasia in the distal esophagus. She presents to the emergency room complaining of epigastric pain, fever, and dysphagia. The abdominal CT obtained is shown in Fig. 21-14. What is the preferred treatment?

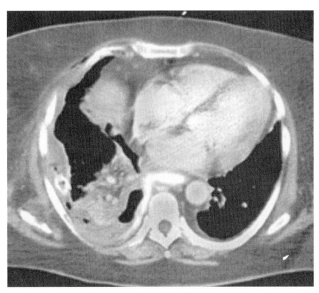

FIG. 21-14 Computed tomography (CT) of the abdomen.

40. A 58-year-old female underwent a general anesthetic for an elective surgical procedure 3 days ago. The endotracheal intubation was very difficult. She presents complaining of dysphagia and neck pain. Her vital signs are as follows: temperature 97.8°F, HR 86 bpm, RR 14 breaths/min, BP 128/68 mmHg; she has a white blood cell count within normal limits. A barium esophagogram is obtained and is shown in Fig. 21-15. What is the appropriate treatment?

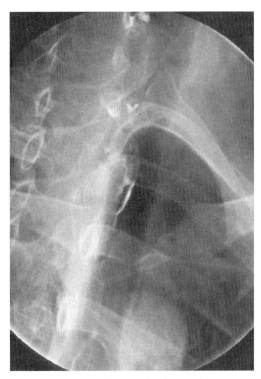

FIG. 21-15 Delayed images of barium esophagogram.

Answers and Explanations

1. **(D)** The presentation of the patient described should raise suspicion for ingestion of a caustic substance. Household agents capable of producing caustic injuries include detergents, bleaches, drain cleaners, and ammonia products. Lye substances, which cause a liquefactive necrosis, generally result in deeper penetration and tissue injury than acid agents, which cause coagulative necrosis. It is helpful to ascertain the nature of the product ingested, as this may determine the distribution and severity of injury, however, will rarely affect subsequent management.

Following ingestion of a caustic agent, destruction of the superficial epithelium occurs and necrosis may extend into mucosa and muscularis. The injured tissue is invaded by bacteria and leuokocytes. Between the second and fifth days, the necrotic tissue forms a cast and sloughs. Following this phase, granulation tissue forms at the periphery of injury as tissue repair begins. Collagen deposition continues for several months. Scar contraction begins following the second week and frequently results in esophageal shortening and stricture formation.

The acute clinical course is marked by oral burning pain, dysphagia, drooling, and emesis. Pulmonary symptoms may occur with aspiration of caustic material. With severe injuries, visceral perforation may occur along with septicemia, mediastinitis, hemorrhage, and possibly death. Initial treatment should follow the usual guidelines of managing trauma patients. The airway should be assessed with the recognition that laryngeal inflammation and edema may progress rapidly to airway obstruction. Oropharyngeal intubation is appropriate in anticipation of this event. The circulatory status should also be addressed and resuscitation with intravenous fluids begun. Broad-spectrum antibiotics are warranted if perforation is suspected. A nasogastric tube may be placed under fluoroscopy to drain gastric contents.

Any evidence of perforation as demonstrated by physical examination or radiographic studies mandates surgical exploration. Subcutaneous emphysema, fever, hypotension, and peritonitis may be signs of perforation. Esophagography with water-soluble contrast may be performed when perforation is suspected. Endoscopy provides the best means of assessing the severity of injury in the absence of perforation. Patients with gastric injuries or linear esophageal burns require hospital observation for possible transmural extension of these injuries. Patients in whom endoscopy demonstrates near-circumferential esophageal burns are at risk for strictures, which may occur any time after the second week. Corticosteroids have been used in the past as prophylactic therapy against stricture formation, but clinical trials have shown no benefit from steroid administration.

Bibliography

Hugh TB, Kelly MD. Corrosive ingestion and the surgeon. *J Am Coll Surg* 1999;189:508–522.

Kikendall JW. Caustic ingestion injuries. *Gastroenterol Clin North Am* 1991;20:847–857.

Zwischenberger JB, Alpard SK, Orringer MB. Esophagus. In: Townsend CM, Beauchamp DR, Evers MB, et al. (eds.), *Sabiston Textbook of Surgery: The Biological Basis of Modern Surgical Practice*, 16th ed. Philadelphia, PA: W.B. Saunders, 2001, 717–719.

2. **(A)** The surgical treatment of GERD has evolved greatly since Rudolf Nissen in 1956 first described the 360-degree fundoplication that bears his name. The principle behind surgical treatment is the restoration of the mechanical barrier between the stomach and distal esophagus. In this regard, the original Nissen fundoplication successfully created an anatomic flap valve and increased lower esophageal sphincter (LES) pressure to prevent reflux; however, side effects were frequent and included bloating, dysphagia, early satiety, and inability to vomit. Partial fundoplications were then suggested as alternatives to Nissen's procedure. These procedures left a portion of esophagus uncovered to decrease LES pressures and provide less

outflow resistance. Examples of partial fundoplications include the original Toupet (180-degree posterior wrap), Thal (90-degree anterior patch), and Dor (180-degree anterior wrap). Although these procedures decreased the incidence of dysphagia and bloating, the resistance to reflux was also reduced.

As surgical treatment of gastroesophageal reflux became more common, several special situations deserved recognition. The most common postoperative complaint following antireflux surgery is dysphagia. It is also becoming apparent that patients with motility abnormalities who undergo a 360-degree fundoplication will inevitably have postoperative dysphagia. Therefore, manometry should be performed prior to antireflux surgery to identify patients with motility disorders who would likely benefit from a partial fundoplication. When peristalsis is absent, impaired, or of low magnitude, the Belsey Mark IV 270-degree transthoracic fundoplication is an excellent choice. Partial fundoplications performed using laparoscopic techniques may also be considered in these cases. In the setting of achalasia, a Heller myotomy in conjunction with a partial fundoplication, such as the Dor 180-degree anterior wrap, is appropriate.

A basic principle in antireflux surgery is to create a tension-free fundoplication below the diaphragm crus. A fundoplication is destined to fail if esophageal length is insufficient to allow a tension-free repair. This is most common in long-standing reflux disease in which chronic inflammation results in fibrotic shortening of the esophagus. Other conditions associated with short esophagus include caustic ingestion, paraesophageal hernia, scleroderma, and Crohn's disease. In these situations, mobilization of the mediastinal esophagus may provide sufficient length for the fundoplication. Occasionally, a Collis gastroplasty, in which neoesophagus is formed from stapled division of the gastric fundus, is required to provide additional esophageal length.

Of the choices above, the Nissen procedure performed for GERD associated with scleroderma is most likely to fail because of absence of contractility in the distal esophagus. A partial fundoplication would surgically treat the reflux disease while minimizing the incidence of postoperative dysphagia as compared to a complete fundoplication in these cases. In addition, esophageal shortening is frequently found in patients with scleroderma, which may necessitate a gastroplasty procedure.

Bibliography

DeMeester TR, Hagen JA. Transthoracic antireflux procedures. In: Baker RJ, Fischer JE (eds.), *Mastery of Surgery*, 4th ed. Philadelphia, PA: Lippincott, Williams & Wilkins, 2001, 748–763.

Hinder RA, Klingler PJ, Perdikis G, et al. Management of the failed antireflux operation. *Surg Clin North Am* 1997; 77:1083–1098.

Horvath KD, Swanstrom LL, Jobe BA. The short esophagus: pathophysiology, incidence, presentation, and treatment in the era of laparoscopic antireflux surgery. *Ann Surg* 2000;232:630–640.

Stein HJ, DeMeester TR. Who benefits from antireflux surgery? *World J Surg* 1992;16:313–319.

Swanstrom LL. Partial fundoplications for GERD: indications and current status. *J Clin Gastroenterol* 1999;29: 127–132.

3. **(B)** At approximately 3 weeks gestation, fusion of septa arising from the primitive foregut results in formation of the esophagus and upper trachea. The esophagus elongates and is structurally formed by 5–6 weeks gestation, but the epithelial lining continues to develop. The initial epithelium is stratified columnar in type which is covered by ciliated columnar cells at 8 weeks gestation. At 5 months gestation, stratified squamous epithelium replaces the ciliated columnar layer. The muscular layers develop along a similar time-line as the epithelium. The inner circular muscle layer develops at 6 weeks gestation and the outer longitudinal layer forms by 9 weeks gestation. The muscularis propria consists entirely of smooth muscle initially with striated muscle gradually developing in the upper third. By 5 months gestation, the upper third of the esophagus is striated muscle and the lower two-thirds smooth muscle, which is the normal ratio at birth. The position of the vagus nerves on the esophagus results from unequal growth of the greater curve of the stomach relative to the lesser curve so that the left vagus nerve is positioned anterior to the esophagus and the right nerve posteriorly.

Bibliography

Albertucci M, Russell SS. Anatomy of the esophagus. In: Baker RJ, Fischer JE (eds.), *Mastery of Surgery*, 4th ed. Philadelphia, PA: Lippincott, Williams & Wilkins, 2001, 741–747.

Patti MG, Gantert W, Way LW. Surgery of the esophagus, anatomy and physiology. *Surg Clin North Am* 1997;77: 959–970.

Zwischenberger JB, Alpard SK, Orringer MB. Esophagus. In: Townsend CM, Beauchamp DR, Evers MB, et al. (eds.), *Sabiston Textbook of Surgery: The Biological Basis of Modern Surgical Practice*, 16th ed. Philadelphia, PA: W.B. Saunders, 2001, 709–711.

4. **(D)** The barium esophagogram is diagnostic for a pharyngoesophageal, or Zenker's, diverticulum. This is a false diverticulum that occurs at the transition between the oblique fibers of the thyropharyngeus muscle and the horizontal fibers of the cricopharyngeus muscle. Zenker and von Zeimssen first summarized

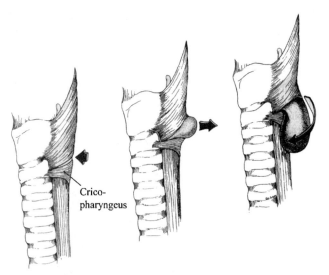

27 cases of pharyngoesophageal diverticula in 1877 and suggested that these pouches resulted from forces acting within the esophageal lumen against an area of resistance. Killian in 1907 identified this area of weakness as the space between the inferior pharyngeal constrictor muscles and the cricopharyngeus muscle. Zenker's diverticulum occurs predominantly in the seventh and eighth decades of life, and more often in men than women. The etiology of pharyngoesophageal diverticula is thought to be related to incoordination in the swallowing mechanism and upper esophageal sphincter dysfunction. These abnormalities raise the intraluminal pressure and cause herniation of mucosa and submucosa through the area of potential weakness near the junction of pharynx and esophagus (Fig. 21-16).

Symptoms are highly characteristic and include dysphagia, regurgitation of undigested food, gurgling noises with swallowing, retrosternal pain, and respiratory obstruction. The most serious complication is respiratory infection as a result of aspiration. A history of dysphagia and weight loss may raise suspicion of malignancy, but a barium esophagogram which is diagnostic for a Zenker's diverticulum with no other abnormalities essentially excludes this possibility. A concomitant sliding hiatal hernia is not an uncommon finding on esophagogram. Upper gastrointestinal (UGI) endoscopy, while possible if performed carefully, is usually not necessary to confirm the diagnosis and may risk perforation at the diverticulum site.

Other than observation of small, asymptomatic diverticula, there is no effective medical therapy. Surgical therapy is indicated in symptomatic patients as untreated diverticula will continue to progress in size and potentially result in pulmonary morbidity. Simple resection of the pouch with primary closure was one of the early approaches to pharyngoesophageal diverticula; however, the underlying motor dysfunction was not addressed with this technique and the persistent functional obstruction resulted in suture line disruptions. The most important component of surgical therapy is an esophagomyotomy. This involves dissection to the base of the diverticulum and division of the cricopharyngeus muscle fibers in a vertical direction. Because most pouches are directed posteriorly or to the left, the procedure is usually performed through a left cervical incision and may include resection of the pouch, especially those larger than 3–4 cm. Diverticulopexy, which involves anchoring the pouch to the posterior pharyngeal wall or prevertebral fascia, performed concurrently with myotomy is another option. Endoscopic stapling of the wall separating the diverticular and esophageal lumens has been used with some success. To date however, endoscopic techniques have been shown to be less effective at providing symptomatic relief compared to open myotomy. Esophagectomy is not indicated for Zenker's diverticulum without evidence of malignancy.

Bibliography

Ellis FH. Pharyngoesophageal (Zenker's) diverticulum. *Adv Surg* 1995;28:171–189.

Gutschow CA, Hamoir M, Rombaux P, et al. Management of pharyngoesophageal (Zenker's) diverticulum: which technique? *Ann Thorac Surg* 2002;74:1677–1683.

Orringer MB. Tumors, injuries, and miscellaneous conditions of the esophagus. In: Greenfield LJ, Mulholland MW, Oldham KT, et al. (eds.), *Surgery: Scientific Principles and Practice*, 3rd ed. Philadelphia, PA: Lippincott, Williams & Wilkins, 2001, 724–726.

Zwischenberger JB, Alpard SK, Orringer MB. Esophagus. In: Townsend CM, Beauchamp DR, Evers MB, et al. (eds.), *Sabiston Textbook of Surgery: The Biological Basis of Modern Surgical Practice*, 16th ed. Philadelphia, PA: W.B. Saunders, 2001, 715–716.

5. **(A)** The initial treatment of gastroesophageal reflux disease is nonoperative and includes behavioral modification as well as pharmacotherapy. Behavior modification includes avoiding fatty foods, alcohol, cigarette smoking, substituting frequent smaller meals for large meals, and avoiding eating for several hours before lying down. The mainstay of medical therapy, however, is with antisecretory drugs that help reduce symptoms of GERD, promote healing of esophageal epithelium, and prevent recurrence and complications of GERD.

Many patients initiate therapy on their own early in the course of disease with over-the-counter medications such as antacids or histamine-2-receptor antagonists. Antacids work by neutralizing acidic gastric juices, thus increasing intragastric pH. This results in a more neutral pH when gastric reflux does occur, and the conversion of pepsinogen to pepsin, which has been demonstrated to intensify the severity of esophageal injury, is reduced at a pH greater than 4.0. Antacids also stimulate the release of gastrin and prostaglandins, which protect esophageal mucosa. Antacids provide quick relief of symptoms, but their duration of action is short and they must be administered several times a day. Moreover, antacids do not affect acid secretion. Adverse reactions of antacids are usually mild and consist of gastrointestinal disturbances. Calcium- and aluminum-containing antacids can cause constipation, while magnesium salts can cause diarrhea. Antacids may also interact with many other drugs, altering their rate or extent of absorption, and therefore should be taken at least 2 h before or after other medications.

Histamine-2-receptor antagonists competitively inhibit histamine at H2-receptors, resulting in reduced gastric acid secretion. They also reduce gastrin-induced acid and pepsin release. H2-receptor antagonists have relatively few and minor side effects including headache, dizziness, diarrhea, and rash. Drug interactions are most common with cimetidine, which inhibits cytochrome P-450 enzymes involved with drug metabolism. Metabolism of drugs such as warfarin, tricyclic antidepressants, and theophylline are inhibited by cimetidine.

Proton pump inhibitors (PPIs) are the agent of choice with severe GERD or the presence of esophageal mucosal damage. PPIs such as omeprazole bind irreversibly and noncompetitively to the H^+/K^+-adenosine triphosphatase pump, thereby inhibiting acid secretion. These drugs are the most effective inhibitors of acid secretion because they block the final pathway for acid release. They are longer-acting than alternative medications and usually only require once-a-day dosing. PPIs have been demonstrated to be more effective than H2-receptor antagonists at providing symptomatic relief and allowing healing of reflux-induced esophagitis. The most common side effects reported with PPIs include nausea, diarrhea, constipation, abdominal pain, headache, and dizziness.

Promotility drugs may also play a role in the treatment of GERD. Metoclopramide is a dopamine antagonist that promotes motility by increasing LES tone and increasing peristalsis in the stomach and small bowel. Adverse effects include extrapyramidal symptoms, anxiety, depression, hallucinations, and tardive dyskinesia. Because of the side effect profile and the effectiveness of alternative medications, metoclopramide is not commonly employed in the treatment of GERD. Anticholinergic agents that impair esophageal contractions and reduce saliva production can exacerbate gastroesophageal reflux. Alternative medications should be considered in patients with reflux symptoms.

Bibliography

Eubanks TR, Pellegrini CA. Hiatal hernia and gastroesophageal reflux disease. In: Townsend CM, Beauchamp DR, Evers MB, et al. (eds.), *Sabiston Textbook of Surgery: The Biological Basis of Modern Surgical Practice*, 16th ed. Philadelphia, PA: W.B. Saunders, 2001, 755–760.

Peters JH, Demeester TR. Esophagus: anatomy, physiology, and gastroesophageal reflux disease. In: Greenfield LJ, Mulholland MW, Oldham KT, et al. (eds.), *Surgery: Scientific Principles and Practice*, 3rd ed. Philadelphia, PA: Lippincott, Williams & Wilkins, 2001, 676.

Vivian EM, Thompson MA. Pharmacologic strategies for treating gastroesophageal reflux disease. *Clin Ther* 2000; 22:654–672.

6. **(D)** The initial treatment of achalasia is usually nonoperative and may include pharmacologic therapy, esophageal dilation, or botulinum toxin injections into the lower esophageal sphincter. Nitrates and calcium-channel blockers have been shown to decrease LES pressure, but adverse effects of these medications and the development of tolerance lead to ultimate failure of pharmacologic management. Botulinum toxin injections into the LES and esophageal dilation can improve dysphagia in some patients, but the duration of relief is variable and repeated treatments are often required.

Esophageal myotomy remains the gold standard of therapy for achalasia and is indicated when conservative management fails or in younger patients who are more likely to benefit from the long-term effects of surgical treatment. Heller originally described myotomy of the lower esophageal sphincter. This approach has been modified and can now be performed laparoscopically. Myotomy involves division of the circular and longitudinal muscles of the lower esophagus. The procedure can be performed through transthoracic and transabdominal approaches. The length of myotomy and the need for a concomitant antireflux procedure remain controversial. Some studies have shown transabdominal myotomy with fundoplication to have the lowest incidence of postoperative gastroesophageal reflux. If a fundoplication is performed, a subtotal wrap is recommended to minimize postoperative dysphagia in these patients who have an underlying motility disorder.

Esophagectomy is reserved for end-stage achalasia, which is identified by progressive dilatation and marked tortuosity of the esophagus. Resection of the diseased esophagus is the only treatment for this irreversible condition. Reconstruction can be with gastric transposition or a colonic conduit.

Bibliography

Adler DG, Romero Y. Primary esophageal motility disorders. *Mayo Clin Proc* 2001;76:195–200.

Anselmino M, Perdikis G, Hinder RA, et al. Heller myotomy is superior to dilatation for the treatment of early achalasia. *Arch Surg* 1997;132:233–240.

Banbury MK, Rice TW, Goldblum JR, et al. Esophagectomy with gastric reconstruction for achalasia. *J Thorac Cardiovasc Surg* 1999;117:1077–1085.

Finley RJ, Clifton JC, Stewart KC, et al. Laparoscopic Heller myotomy improves esophageal emptying and the symptoms of achalasia. *Arch Surg* 2001;136:892–896.

Vogt D, Curet M, Pitcher D, et al. Successful treatment of esophageal achalasia with laparoscopic Heller myotomy and Toupet fundoplication. *Am J Surg* 1997;174:709–714.

7. **(E)** Dissection in the left tracheoesophageal groove may result in recurrent laryngeal nerve neuropraxia or even permanent paresis. Accordingly, caution should be undertaken to avoid retraction injury to prevent neuropraxia during this dissection and cervical esophagogastric anastomosis. Injury to the recurrent nerve results in vocal cord incompetence and a propensity to aspirate. Patients who manifest postoperative hoarseness should be evaluated with laryngoscopy. If recurrent nerve injury is suspected, either vocal cord injection or phonoplastic surgery are indicated to minimize the risk of aspiration prior to beginning oral feeding.

A tracheal laceration is a rare complication and is usually identified intraoperatively when large amounts of air begin escaping through the operative field or when the anesthesiologist notices a sharp decrease in ventilatory pressure. If tracheal injury is not recognized intraoperatively, it may present in the early postoperative period with persistent air leak through chest tubes or subcutaneous emphysema in the face and neck. Bronchoscopic examination will reveal the injury.

Gastric atony and/or gastric outlet obstruction can contribute to postoperative aspiration following esophagectomy; however, with vocal cord competence it is less likely to cause aspiration. Phrenic nerve injury is extremely rare after esophagectomy and is identified by an elevated hemidiaphram on chest radiograph. A cervical esophagogastric anastomotic leak may present with fevers and leukocytosis. It is usually noticed several days postoperatively, however, and should be well controlled through drains placed at the time of surgery and, therefore, not affect the lungs.

Orringer et al. (1999) report a large series of patients with transhiatal esophagectomy, of which recurrent laryngeal nerve injury occurred in 7% of patients, anastomotic leak in 13%, and tracheal injury in less than 1%. In separate reviews by Gandhi and Katariya, the rates of recurrent laryngeal nerve injury and anastomotic leak following transhiatal esophagectomy are reported at 9 and 12% (Gandhi) and 11 and 15% (Katariya), respectively.

Bibliography

Gandhi SK, Naunheim KS. Complications of transhiatal esophagectomy. *Chest Surg Clin North Am* 1997; 7:601–610.

Hulscher JBF, ter Hofstede E, Kloek J, et al. Injury to the major airways during subtotal esophagectomy: incidence, management, and sequelae. *J Thorac Cardiovasc Surg* 2000;120:1093–1096.

Katariya K, Harvey JC, Pina E, et al. Complications of transhiatal esophagectomy. *J Surg Oncol* 1994;57:157–163.

Orringer MB, Marshall B, Iannettoni, MD. Transhiatal esophagectomy: clinical experience and refinements. *Ann Surg* 1999;230;392–400.

8. **(C)** The prognosis of malignant TEF secondary to esophageal carcinoma is extremely poor. Most patients die within 3 months from pulmonary complications. The disease is typically inoperable because of extensive mediastinal invasion. When surgical resection is possible, esophagectomy with enteric interposition for palliation restores swallowing ability; however, there is little justification for performing a noncurative procedure with relatively high associated morbidity and mortality. Esophageal intubation, especially with self-expanding metallic stents, provides the best means of palliation by preventing recurrent aspiration and restoring swallowing ability. Esophageal stents are preferred over alternative palliative therapies because they provide immediate relief of dysphagia. The stents are placed by endoscopy under fluoroscopic guidance and occlude the esophageal side of the fistula so that oral intake can be resumed without the risk of aspiration. Self-expanding stents maintain luminal patency when subsequent therapies, such as radiation and/or chemotherapy, result in tumor shrinkage. Potential complications of stent placement include infection, tumor ingrowth at the ends, and stent migration.

Radiation with or without chemotherapy offers little curative potential in unresectable esophageal cancer. It may provide some symptomatic relief of dysphagia but usually requires 1–2 months before this effect is appreciated. Neither radiation nor chemotherapy contributes to closure of TEFs, which will continue to cause significant morbidity and mortality. The therapies themselves can cause life-threatening complications as well as increase the risks of concurrent stent placement by compromising tissue viability in proximity of the tumor. Cervical esophagostomy with gastric tube placement would divert secretions away from the TEF and decrease the risk of aspiration, but would not allow the patient to eat normally and, therefore, is not optimal palliation.

Bibliography

De Palma GD, Galloro G, Sivero L, et al. Self-expanding metal stents for palliation of inoperable carcinoma of the esophagus and gastroesophageal junction. *Am J Gastroenterol* 1995;90:2140–2142.

Orringer MB. Tumors, injuries, and miscellaneous conditions of the esophagus. In: Greenfield LJ, Mulholland MW, Oldham KT, et al. (eds.), *Surgery: Scientific Principles and Practice*, 3rd ed. Philadelphia, PA: Lippincott, Williams & Wilkins, 2001, 731–732.

Spivak H, Katariya K, Lo AY, et al. Malignant tracheoesophageal fistula: use of esophageal endoprosthesis. *J Surg Oncol* 1996;63:65–70.

Weigel TL, Frumiento C, Gaumintz E. Endoluminal palliation for dysphagia secondary to esophageal carcinoma. *Surg Clin North Am* 202;82:747–761.

9. **(B)** There are three types of hiatal hernias. In type I hernias, the gastroesophageal junction is displaced superior to the hiatus. This is also known as a sliding hiatal hernia because the gastric cardia migrates back and forth between the posterior mediastinum and the peritoneal cavity. Type I hernias are the most common of the three and are often associated with gastroesophageal reflux. Paraesophageal hernias usually refer to type II and III hernias. A true paraesophageal hernia (type II) is characterized by an upward displacement of the gastric fundus with a normally positioned gastroesophageal junction. More common, however, is the type III hernia where the gastroesophageal junction is displaced above the diaphragm along with all or part of the stomach. The exact cause of paraesophageal hernias is unknown, but it is thought to be related to the structural deterioration of the phrenoesophageal membrane and becomes more prevalent with advancing age. The phrenoesophageal membrane is stretched over time with repeated movement of the esophagus during swallowing and as intraabdominal pressures are exerted against the membrane (Fig. 21-17).

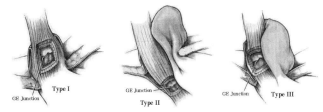

FIG. 21-17 The three types of hiatal hernia. (Reprinted with permission from Townsend CM, Beauchamp DR, Evers MB, et al. (eds.), *Sabiston Textbook of Surgery: The Biological Basis of Modern Surgical Practice*, 16th ed. The Netherlands: Elsevier, 2001, 756.)

Bibliography

Eubanks TR, Pellegrini CA. Hiatal hernia and gastroesophageal reflux disease. In: Townsend CM, Beauchamp DR, Evers MB, et al. (eds.), *Sabiston Textbook of Surgery: The Biological Basis of Modern Surgical Practice*, 16th ed. Philadelphia, PA: W.B. Saunders, 2001, 756–766.

Hashemi M, Sillin LF, Peters JH. Current concepts in the management of paraesophageal hiatal hernia. *J Clin Gastroenterol* 1999;29:8–13.

Oddsdottir M. Paraesophageal hernia. *Surg Clin North Am* 2000;80:1243–1252.

10. **(C)** Barrett's esophagus is the most serious complication of GERD. Approximately 10% of patients with GERD will have Barrett's metaplasia, which is defined as the presence of columnar metaplasia extending 3 cm or greater into the esophagus or specialized intestinal-type metaplasia of any length. Nondysplastic Barrett's epithelium has been estimated to progress to dysplasia at a rate of 5–10% per year, with adenocarcinoma developing in 1% of cases per year. If there is no dysplasia present, medical therapy with PPIs should be continued with routine endoscopic surveillance every 2–3 years. Although PPIs reduce the volume of gastric acid reflux, it does not entirely eliminate gastric and duodenal reflux. Columnar metaplasia may continue to occur. Some authors advocate the use of surgical antireflux procedures to restore LES function. Despite effective antireflux surgery, the incidence of adenocarcinoma in patients with Barrett's esophagus has not decreased. As a result, routine endoscopic surveillance is required in all patients with Barrett's esophagus.

Once dysplasia is identified on histology specimens, management should be tailored according to the severity of dysplasia. If the specimens are indeterminate for dysplasia, high-dose PPIs should be instituted to resolve any inflammation, and a repeat biopsy should be performed in 3–6 months. If repeat biopsy is still indeterminate for dysplasia, then the patient should be treated as if low-grade dysplasia were present. The presence of low-grade dysplasia should raise concern because it represents progression of a disease process that eventually leads to adeno-carcinoma. Low-grade dysplasia may be treated with aggressive medical therapy or antireflux surgery and repeat biopsy every 6 months.

Most authors agree that the presence of high-grade dysplasia is an indication to perform esophagectomy. Studies have shown that 30–40% of patients with high-grade dysplasia who undergo esophagectomy pathologically demonstrate invasive adenocarcinoma in the resected specimens despite negative findings on repeat endoscopy and endoscopic ultrasound. Reid et al. (1992) estimated the progression from high-grade dysplasia to invasive adenocarcinoma to occur at a mean duration of 14 months. Prior to performing esophagectomy for high-grade dysplasia, histologic findings should be confirmed by two experienced pathologists. Any discordance in opinion should be addressed with repeat biopsies.

Bibliography

Bremner CG, Bremner RM. Barrett's esophagus. *Surg Clin North Am* 1997;77:1115–1137.

McDonald ML, Trastek VF, Allen MS, et al. Barrett's esophagus: does an antireflux procedure reduce the need for endoscopic surveillance? *J Thorac Cardiovasc Surg* 1996; 111:1135–1140.

Peters JH, Demeester TR. Esophagus: anatomy, physiology, and gastroesophageal reflux disease. In: Greenfield LJ, Mulholland MW, Oldham KT, et al. (eds.), *Surgery: Scientific Principles and Practice*, 3rd ed. Philadelphia, PA: Lippincott, Williams & Wilkins, 2001, 671–675.

Reid BJ, Blount PL, Ruben CE, et al. Flow-cytometric and histologic progression to malignancy in Barrett's esophagus. *Gastroenterology* 1992;102:1212–1219.

Zaninotto G, Parenti AR, Ruol A, et al. Oesophageal resection for high-grade dysplasia in Barrett's oesophagus. *Br J Surg* 2000;87:1102–1105.

11. (E) The barium esophagogram shows disruption of peristalsis with tertiary activity producing segmentation of the esophagus, typical of diffuse esophageal spasm (DES). DES is characterized by normal peristalsis intermittently interrupted by simultaneous contractions. The disorder is uncommon and its cause unknown. Some evidence suggests a defect in neural inhibition along the esophageal body. Esophageal spasm has been linked to GERD and stressful events. Chest pain and dysphagia, the most common presenting symptoms, are usually intermittent which may make establishing a diagnosis of DES challenging.

The classic finding of the "corkscrew" or "rosary-bead" appearance of the esophageal body may be seen during a barium swallow study; however, the absence of these findings on barium swallow does not eliminate the possibility of DES, particularly if the patient is asymptomatic during the study. Conversely,

symptoms of chest pain do not always correlate with spastic activity. Esophageal manometry is usually diagnostic for DES and helps distinguish it from other esophageal motility disorders. Diagnostic criteria include simultaneous contractions in the esophageal body in greater than 30% (but less than 100%) of wet swallows and mean simultaneous contraction amplitude greater than 30 mmHg. Other criteria less consistently found include repetitive contractions (greater than three peaks), prolonged duration (greater than 6 s) of contractions, and abnormalities of LES relaxation. If manometry shows all contractions to be simultaneous, with associated impaired LES relaxation, then the diagnosis of achalasia should be considered.

Initial treatment of DES should be medical. Reassurance that the patient's symptoms are not cardiac-related is often beneficial. Nitrates and calcium-channel blockers can decrease high-amplitude contractions, thereby relieving symptoms of chest pain, but results are variable and long-term efficacy has not been adequately assessed. The incidence of psychiatric disorders such as anxiety, depression, and somatization is increased in patients with spastic disorders of the esophagus. Accordingly, psychotropic drugs such as trazodone and imipramine have shown some success in symptom relief. Botulinum toxin injections and pneumatic dilation have also shown some clinical response, but the duration of effect is variable.

Esophageal myotomy should be reserved for patients in whom medical therapy has failed. The results of surgery are not as predictable with DES as compared to achalasia. Myotomy decreases the intensity of esophageal contractions, but the frequency of contractions is often unaffected and symptoms occasionally persist despite surgery. Myotomy may also result in a hypocontractile esophagus, which can result in dysphagia. When surgery is contemplated, a long myotomy from the aortic arch to the LES is the procedure of choice.

Bibliography

Adler DG, Romero Y. Primary esophageal motility disorders. *Mayo Clin Proc* 2001;76:195–200.

Prakash C, Clouse RE. Esophageal motor disorders. *Curr Opin Gastroenterol* 2002;18:454–463.

Richter JE. Oesophageal motility disorders. *Lancet* 2001;358: 823–828.

Spechler SJ, Castell DO. Classification of oesophageal motility abnormalities. *Gut* 2001;49:145–151.

12. (B) Endoscopic ultrasound is the procedure of choice for evaluating primary tumor depth, regional nodal disease, and involvement of adjacent structures. The accuracy of lymph node staging ranges from 50 to

88% based on endoscopic ultrasonographic (EUS) characteristics such as lymph node size, shape, border characteristics, and central echogenicity. EUS can also accurately identify suspicious lymph nodes in the celiac axis and disease in the left liver lobe, both of which are considered distant metastases. EUS with fine-needle aspiration (FNA) under real-time guidance is usually recommended to cytologically document the presence of metastatic disease in suspicious appearing lymph nodes, particularly when the presence of distant metastases will change therapy.

CT scanning of the chest and abdomen may also detect regional and nonregional lymph node metastases, but assessment of T and N stage with CT is not as accurate as compared to EUS. Invasion of surrounding mediastinal structures may also be suggested by CT scan; however, operative exploration is not infrequently required to confirm unresectability. CT scanning is relied on to determine the presence of metastatic disease with 85–90% accuracy.

PET is a relatively new modality in the evaluation of esophageal cancer. It uses a radiolabeled glucose analog 18-F-fluoro-deoxy-D-glucose (FDG) which is taken up by neoplastic cells because of the increased expression of glucose transport enzymes in the cell membranes. As this is not specific for neoplastic processes, false-positives may be seen in areas of inflammation. Although lacking complete specificity, PET is very sensitive in identifying sites of tumor activity and is useful in the evaluation of metastatic disease. Flamen et al. (2000) reported 95% sensitivity of PET in identifying primary tumor in esophageal cancer and 82% accuracy of identifying stage IV disease. Unfortunately, PET is not as sensitive in assessing lymph node involvement. Flamen et al. (2000) reported a significantly lower sensitivity compared to endoscopic ultrasound, 33% versus 81%, respectively, which is attributed to the inability of separating 18-FDG uptake in the primary tumor from uptake in surrounding lymph nodes. PET is also not reliable for predicting primary tumor depth (T stage). Other disadvantages include high cost and lack of availability compared to conventional staging modalities. The routine use of PET for staging esophageal cancer requires further evaluation.

MRI is not routinely used for staging esophageal carcinoma. In select cases, MRI can accurately detect T4 disease with direct tumor extension into adjacent organs such as the aorta or trachea, but the relatively high cost and lack of significant imaging improvement as compared to conventional CT scans limit its use for this disease.

Video-assisted thoracoscopy (VATS) and laparoscopy are highly accurate methods of evaluating nodal disease in esophageal carcinoma. The disadvantages of these procedures include the need for general anesthesia, the costs and risks associated with surgery, and recovery which may delay neoadjuvant chemoradiation therapy. As a result, VATS and laparoscopy are infrequently used in the initial evaluation of esophageal cancer.

Bibliography

Flamen P, Lerut A, van Cutsem E, et al. Utility of positron emission tomography for the staging of patients with potentially operable esophageal carcinoma. *J Clin Oncol* 2000;18:3202–3210.

Kato H, Kuwano H, Nakajima M, et al. Comparison between positron emission tomography and computed tomography in the use of the assessment of esophageal carcinoma. *Cancer* 2002;94:921–928.

Luketich JD, Schauer P, Landreneau R, et al. Minimally invasive surgical staging is superior to endoscopic ultrasound in detecting lymph node metastases in esophageal cancer. *J Thorac Cardiovasc Surg* 1997;114:817–823.

Orringer MB. Tumors, injuries, and miscellaneous conditions of the esophagus. In: Greenfield LJ, Mulholland MW, Oldham KT, et al. (eds.), *Surgery: Scientific Principles and Practice*, 3rd ed. Philadelphia, PA: Lippincott, Williams & Wilkins, 2001, 701–702.

Van Dam J. Endosonographic evaluation of the patient with esophageal cancer. *Chest* 1997;112:184S–190S.

13. **(D)** The barium esophagogram demonstrates an extrinsic mass with a smooth surface. The endoscopic ultrasound shows a hypoechoic mass with smooth margins in the muscularis propria. Both studies are consistent with leiomyoma. Leiomyomas are smooth muscle tumors of the muscularis propria and account for 70% of benign esophageal tumors. They typically occur in patients between 20 and 50 years of age and occur with equal frequency in males and females. Most leiomyomas are located in the middle or distal thirds of the esophagus. Tumors less than 5 cm are rarely symptomatic and are usually found incidentally during UGI endoscopy or contrast studies obtained for nonrelated symptoms. Symptomatic leiomyomas may present with dysphagia or retrosternal pain. Leiomyomas have a characteristic appearance on barium esophagogram, typically showing a concave submucosal defect with sharp borders. Esophagoscopy is indicated to exclude malignancy or other occult pathology, but attempts at direct biopsy are typically not diagnostic as these tumors are located beneath the submucosal layer. Cells for cytologic analysis can be obtained with FNA under EUS guidance if the diagnosis based on contrast studies and EUS findings is in question.

Asymptomatic leiomyomas can be managed conservatively, since their growth rate is slow and malignant degeneration is rare. Symptomatic leiomyomas or those larger than 5 cm should be resected. The conventional approach is through a thoracotomy incision or upper midline laparotomy for very distal tumors. After splitting of the overlying muscle layers, a plane can be found between tumor and mucosa. The leiomyoma is an encapsulated mass that is relatively avascular and can be easily enucleated while preserving the submucosal layer. The split muscle edges should then be reapproximated. The procedure has been performed successfully withVATS, which has the advantage of reduced postoperative pain.

Bibliography

Bonavina L, Segalin A, Rosati R, et al. Surgical therapy of esophageal leiomyoma. *J Am Coll Surg* 1995;181:257–262.

Orringer MB. Tumors, injuries, and miscellaneous conditions of the esophagus. In: Greenfield LJ, Mulholland MW, Oldham KT, et al. (eds.), *Surgery: Scientific Principles and Practice*, 3rd ed. Philadelphia, PA: Lippincott, Williams & Wilkins, 2001, 693–694.

Rice TW. Esophageal tumors. In: Cameron JL (ed.), *Current Surgical Therapy*, 7th ed. St. Louis, MO: Mosby, 2001, 51–57.

Zwischenberger JB, Alpard SK, Orringer MB. Esophagus. In: Townsend CM, Beauchamp DR, Evers MB, et al. (eds.), *Sabiston Textbook of Surgery: The Biological Basis of Modern Surgical Practice*, 16th ed. Philadelphia, PA: W.B. Saunders, 2001, 727–731.

14. **(E)** Esophageal cancer represents 4% of newly diagnosed cancers in the United States. It occurs most commonly in the seventh decade of life and is 1.5–3 times more common in men than in women. The cause of esophageal carcinoma is unknown, but is thought to be related to mucosal injury from prolonged exposure to noxious stimuli. Alcohol consumption and cigarette smoking have been shown to be risk factors for squamous cell carcinoma. The histology of esophageal carcinoma can be seen as a progression from dysplastic cells to carcinoma *in situ*, which is limited to the mucosa. Once carcinoma extends beyond the basement membrane, early invasive carcinoma is present.

Worldwide, squamous cell carcinoma accounts for approximately 95% of esophageal cancer. Squamous cell carcinoma had been the predominant form of esophageal cancer in the United States until recently, when the incidence of adenocarcinoma doubled in the 1990s. Adenocarcinoma is now the most common type of esophageal carcinoma in the United States. This shift has been attributed to gastroesophageal reflux and secondary columnar metaplasia seen with Barrett's disease. In the United States, Black males have a greater risk of developing squamous cell carcinoma, whereas White males have a greater risk of adenocarcinoma.

Bibliography

El-Serag HB. The epidemic of esophageal adenocarcinoma. *Gastroenterol Clin North Am* 2002;31:421–440.

Orringer MB. Tumors, injuries, and miscellaneous conditions of the esophagus. In: Greenfield LJ, Mulholland MW, Oldham KT, et al. (eds.), *Surgery: Scientific Principles and Practice*, 3rd ed. Philadelphia, PA: Lippincott, Williams & Wilkins, 2001, 696–698.

Zwischenberger JB, Alpard SK, Orringer MB. Esophagus. In: Townsend CM, Beauchamp DR, Evers MB, et al. (eds.), *Sabiston Textbook of Surgery: The Biological Basis of Modern Surgical Practice*, 16th ed. Philadelphia, PA: W.B. Saunders, 2001, 731–733.

15. **(E)** The barium esophagogram shows a dilated proximal esophagus with bird-beak tapering. These findings are suggestive of achalasia or an achalasia-like motility disorder. Achalasia is an esophageal motility disorder characterized by inadequate LES relaxation and aperistalsis of the esophageal body. The etiology is unknown but is theorized to be related to the degeneration of inhibitory neurons that affect relaxation of esophageal smooth muscle. These parasympathetic ganglion cells reside in the myenteric plexus between the longitudinal and circular muscle layers of the esophagus. The smooth muscle of the LES is normally contracted at rest and relaxes when stimulated by inhibitory neurons, as occurs with swallowing. In achalasia, resting LES pressures may be increased and diminished relaxation of the LES is seen with swallowing. Loss of inhibitory neurons also affects normal peristalsis in the esophageal body.

Although the etiology of achalasia is unknown, infection with the parasite *Trypanosoma cruzi* (Chagas disease) seen in Central and South America causes loss of intramural ganglion cells and results in aperistalsis with inadequate LES relaxation, producing a motor abnormality identical to primary achalasia. Malignancies at the gastroesophageal junction can cause a pseudoachalasia that has the same radiographic and manometric findings as primary achalasia. In addition, strictures of the distal esophagus can cause proximal esophageal dilatation, but would be differentiated from achalasia on the basis of endoscopic and manometric findings.

As with other esophageal motility disorders, achalasia typically produces symptoms of chest pain and dysphagia. Patients may complain of a sticking sensation in the chest after swallowing and may drink large volumes of water to force food into the stomach. As the disease progresses, regurgitation of undigested food may occur and the risk of aspiration increases. Weight loss may also be seen and may raise the concern of malignancy.

Manometry is required for diagnosis. Classic manometric findings include an elevated resting LES pressure, lack of peristalsis, and incomplete relaxation of the LES with swallows. These findings are highly reproducible, unlike other esophageal motility disorders. Radiographic studies typically include a barium esophagogram, which shows a dilated proximal esophagus with tapering "bird-beak" appearance in the distal esophagus. Retained food may be seen in portions of the esophagus as well as air-fluid levels in the distal esophagus. Endoscopy is useful for ruling out malignancy as well as benign conditions such as strictures or stromal tumors that can mimic achalasia.

Bibliography

Adler DG, Romero Y. Primary esophageal motility disorders. *Mayo Clin Proc* 2001;76:195–200.

Dent J, Holloway RH. Esophageal motility and reflux testing. *Gastroenterol Clin North Am* 1996;25:51–73.

Prakash C, Clouse RE. Esophageal motor disorders. *Curr Opin Gastroenterol* 2002;18:454–463.

Spechler SJ, Castell DO. Classification of oesophageal motility abnormalities. *Gut* 2001;49:145–151.

Zwischenberger JB, Alpard SK, Orringer MB. Esophagus. In: Townsend CM, Beauchamp DR, Evers MB, et al. (eds.), *Sabiston Textbook of Surgery: The Biological Basis of Modern Surgical Practice*, 16th ed. Philadelphia, PA: W.B. Saunders, 2001, 720–722.

16. (E) Diagnostic testing is essential in planning the management of GERD. The gold standard for diagnosing reflux is the 24-h pH probe. Electrodes that measure fluctuation in pH are placed in the esophagus. Over the course of 24 h, the patient notes specific times that he or she experiences reflux symptoms. Reflux is calculated as the total percent of time the pH is below 4. Abnormal reflux occurs when the pH is less than 4 more than 1% of the time in the proximal esophagus, and more than 4% of the time in the distal esophagus. Correlation between the patient's symptoms and drops in pH are also taken into account when interpreting the study.

Manometry evaluates the function of the esophageal body and lower esophageal sphincter. Esophageal body function is evaluated by placing several channels along the esophageal body and peristaltic activity is measured at each channel with swallowing. Patients should normally have greater than 80% of peristaltic activity transmitted to each channel with swallows. The amplitude of the peri-

staltic wave can also be measured with normal values greater than 30 mmHg. Patients demonstrating compromised peristalsis by manometry are likely to experience dysphagia following a 360-degree fundoplication. A partial fundoplication should be considered in these cases.

Endoscopy is important in the workup of gastroesophageal reflux because it excludes other pathology and evaluates the severity of esophageal injury. Mucosal changes can be directly visualized and biopsies obtained to evaluate for metaplasia or dysplasia; however, endoscopy is not sensitive for diagnosing gastroesophageal reflux because many patients may not have obvious mucosal changes. Gastric scintigraphy helps identify patients with delayed gastric emptying which may contribute to gastroesophageal reflux. A gastric emptying procedure may benefit these patients.

Bibliography

DeMeester TR. Gastroesophageal reflux disease. In: Cameron JL (ed.), *Current Surgical Therapy*, 7th ed. St. Louis, MO: Mosby, 2001, 30–37.

Eubanks TR, Pellegrini CA. Hiatal hernia and gastroesophageal reflux disease. In: Townsend CM, Beauchamp DR, Evers MB, et al. (eds.), *Sabiston Textbook of Surgery: The Biological Basis of Modern Surgical Practice*, 16th ed. Philadelphia, PA: W.B. Saunders, 2001, 757–759.

Patti MG, Diener U, Tamburini A, et al. Role of esophageal function tests in the diagnosis of gastroesophageal reflux disease. *Dig Dis Sci* 2001;46:597–602.

17. (C) The esophagus consists of three layers, the mucosa, submucosa, and muscularis propria. The mucosa consists of a squamous epithelium, lamina propria, and muscularis mucosa. The epithelium, the innermost layer, is made of nonkeratinizing sqaumous cells. The squamous epithelium ends abruptly in the distal 1–2 cm of esophagus where the junctional columnar epithelium of the gastric cardia begins. This transition point, known as the "Z-line," is readily apparent on endoscopy as small projections of red gastric epithelium extend upward into the pink-white squamous epithelium. Beneath the epithelium lies the lamina propria, which is a loose matrix of collagen and elastic fibers and contains lymphatics. Surrounding the lamina propria is the muscularis mucosa, which contains mainly longitudinal muscle fibers (Fig. 21-18).

The submucosa consists of loose connective tissue containing blood vessels, nerve fibers including Meissner's plexus, lymphatics, and submucosal glands. The submucosa contains elastic and fibrous tissue and is the strongest layer of the esophageal wall. The muscularis propria consists of an inner circular layer and an outer longitudinal layer. This muscle

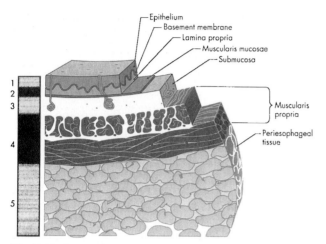

FIG. 21-18 Layers of the esophageal wall and endoscopic esophageal ultrasound (EUS). (Reprinted with permission from Cameron JL (ed.), *Current Surgical Therapy*, 7th ed. The Netherlands: Elsevier, 2001, 52.)

layer provides the propulsive force for swallowing. The myenteric, or Auerbach's, plexus is located between the circular and longitudinal muscle layers. On endoscopic ultrasound four distinct layers, superficial mucosa, deep mucosa, submucosa, and muscularis propria, can be visualized. The periesophageal tissue can be seen as a fifth layer on EUS.

Bibliography

Albertucci M, Russell SS. Anatomy of the esophagus. In: Baker RJ, Fischer JE (eds.), *Mastery of Surgery*, 4th ed. Philadelphia, PA: Lippincott, Williams & Wilkins, 2001, 741–747.

Patti MG, Gantert W, Way LW. Surgery of the esophagus, anatomy and physiology. *Surg Clin North Am* 1997;77: 959–970.

Rice TW. Esophageal tumors. In: Cameron JL (ed.), *Current Surgical Therapy*, 7th ed. St. Louis, MO: Mosby, 2001, 51–52.

18. **(B)** Everyone experiences some degree of symptomatology from transient reflux of gastric contents into the esophagus. Yet not everyone develops clinically significant GERD because of defense mechanisms which protect the esophageal mucosa from acid-induced injury including esophageal motor activity, gravity, and buffering secretions from saliva and submucosal glands. Reflux develops when these defense mechanisms are impaired, such as in esophageal motility disorders. The most common cause of GERD, however, is a defective lower esophageal sphincter. LES competence depends on baseline sphincter pressure, overall length, and length exposed to intraabdominal positive pressure. The LES does not have to be permanently defective for GERD to occur. Transient relaxation of the LES may be the cause of early gas-

troesophageal reflux. The sequelae of esophageal mucosal injury include esophagitis, stricture, and Barrett's metaplasia. The development of these complications is usually related to a defective LES.

The components of refluxed gastric juice include gastric acid and pepsin as well as biliary and pancreatic secretions from duodenal contents. Gastric acid alone causes minimal damage to the esophageal mucosa. The presence of pepsin in the acidic environment of refluxed gastric juice appears to be the major injurious agent. The addition of duodenal contents in refluxed juice results in a more alkaline environment. In this setting, bile acids and the pancreatic enzyme trypsin play a significant role in mucosal injury.

The significance of *H. pylori* in the development of peptic ulcer disease has been well documented. *H. pylori* does not potentiate the development of GERD and in fact, may have a protective effect in esophageal disease. The presence of *H. pylori* strains with the cytotoxin associated gene A (cagA+) has an inverse association with esophagitis, Barrett's epithelium, and adenocarcinoma of the distal esophagus.

Bibliography

Buttar NS, Falk GW. Pathogenesis of gastroesophageal reflux and Barrett esophagus. *Mayo Clin Proc* 2001;76: 226–234.

Mittal RK, Balaban DH. Mechanisms of disease: the esophagogastric junction. *N Engl J Med* 1997;336:924–932.

Peters JH, Demeester TR. Esophagus: anatomy, physiology, and gastroesophageal reflux disease. In: Greenfield LJ, Mulholland MW, Oldham KT, et al. (eds.), *Surgery: Scientific Principles and Practice*, 3rd ed. Philadelphia, PA: Lippincott, Williams & Wilkins, 2001, 667–671.

Warburton-Timms VJ, Charlett A, Valori RM, et al. The significance of cagA+ *H. pylori* in reflux oesophagitis. *Gut* 2001;49:341–346.

19. **(C)** Despite advances in surgical techniques and adjuvant therapies, esophageal cancer remains an aggressive disease with poor prognosis. Surgery has been the mainstay of treatment; however, 5-year survival following surgery alone for locally advanced disease ranges between 20 and 25%. The unacceptably poor outcomes with surgery alone prompted investigation into additional therapies.

Neoadjuvant chemotherapy alone has not conclusively shown any survival advantages. A large multicenter phase III study in the United States randomizing patients to chemotherapy followed by surgery compared to surgery alone demonstrated no survival advantage to preoperative chemotherapy. A similar phase III study completed in Europe, however, demonstrated survival advantage to preoperative chemotherapy. Some oncologists and radiation therapists believe that definitive chemoradiation therapy without surgery is optimal; however, this is based on data from earlier studies on patients with mainly squamous cell carcinoma histology. Postoperative chemotherapy or radiation therapy is difficult to administer; moreover, it has never been shown to improve survival.

To date, the most promising treatment regimen consists of preoperative chemotherapy and radiation therapy followed by surgery. The premise behind induction chemoradiation is that the tumor may be downstaged with chemoradiation, increasing the likelihood of a complete resection with tumor-free margins. In addition, micrometastases would be treated with preoperative chemoradiation. Unfortunately, there have been no large-scale prospective, randomized trials comparing induction chemoradiation followed by surgery versus surgery alone. Single institution studies have demonstrated mixed results as to the benefit of preoperative chemoradiation therapy. It is believed, however, that the subset of patients, estimated to range between 20 and 30%, who demonstrate a complete pathologic response following neoadjuvant chemoradiation therapy have a superior prognosis over patients who do not demonstrate a complete response. Moreover, neoadjuvant chemoradiation therapy in otherwise healthy patients has not been shown to significantly increase operative risks. In this regard, patients with good performance status probably should be offered preoperative chemoradiation therapy prior to esophagectomy.

Bibliography

Bhogaraju A, Hanna N, Brooks J, et al. Survival and disease recurrence for esophageal cancer patients achieving pathologic complete response (pCR) at surgery after neoadjuvant chemoradiation. *Proc Am Soc Clin Oncol* 2002; abstract #582:146a.

Clark P. Surgical resection with or without pre-operative chemotherapy in oesophageal cancer: an updated analysis of a randomised controlled trial conducted by the UK medical research council upper GI tract cancer group. *Proc Am Soc Clin Oncol* 2001; abstract #502:126a.

Kelsen DP, Ginsberg R, Pajak T, et al. Preoperative chemotherapy followed by operation versus operation alone for patients with localized esophageal cancers: a U.S. national intergroup study. *N Engl J Med* 1998;339: 1979–1984.

Urba SG, Orringer MB, Turrisi A, et al. Randomized trial of preoperative chemoradiation versus surgery alone in patients with locoregional esophageal carcinoma. *J Clin Oncol* 2001;19:305–313.

Urschel JD, Vasan HB, Blewett CJ. A meta-analysis of randomized controlled trials that compared neoadjuvant chemotherapy and surgery to surgery alone for respectable esophageal cancer. *Am J Surg* 2002; 183: 274–279.

Walsh T, Noonan N, Hollywood D, et al. A comparison of multimodal therapy and surgery for esophageal adenocarcinoma. *N Engl J Med* 1996;335:462–467.

20. (D) The barium esophagogram shows an epiphrenic, or lower, esophageal diverticulum. Epiphrenic diverticula, which occur in the distal 10 cm of the esophagus, are the most common type of esophageal diverticula. They are usually false diverticula that result from pulsion forces leading to mucosal herniation at an area of focal weakness in the esophageal wall.

There is an increasing amount of evidence to suggest a link between esophageal diverticula and motility disorders. In fact, findings of epiphrenic diverticula should raise suspicion of an underlying motility disorder and manometry should be performed. Achalasia is the most common esophageal motility disorder; however, diverticula occur in less than 5% of achalasia patients. DES is less prevalent than achalasia, but pulsion diverticula occur more frequently in these patients.

Small and asymptomatic diverticula may be observed. Symptomatic or large diverticula warrant operative intervention. Symptoms of dysphagia, regurgitation of undigested food, and even aspiration are primarily felt to be a result of the underlying motility disorder with a lesser contribution from the diverticulum itself. The most important component of any surgical treatment is, therefore, esophagomyotomy. Myotomy treats the underlying motor disorder and prevents recurrence or suture line disruption following diverticulectomy. Addition of an antireflux procedure is controversial, but should be included when myotomy is performed transabdominally.

Bibliography

Benacci JC, Deschamps C, Trastek VF, et al. Epiphrenic diverticulum: results of surgical treatment. *Ann Thorac Surg* 1993;55:1109–1113.

Nehra D, Lord RV, DeMeester TR, et al. Physiologic basis for the treatment of epiphrenic diverticulum. *Ann Surg* 2002;235:346–354.

Streitz JM Jr, Glick ME, Ellis FH. Selective use of myotomy for treatment of epiphrenic diverticula. *Arch Surg* 1992; 127:585–587.

Thomas ML, Anthony AA, Fosh BG, et al. Oesophageal diverticula. *Br J Surg* 2001;88:629–642.

21. (A) The LES has been the focus of intense research because of its role in gastroesophageal reflux and esophageal motility disorders. The LES is a zone of high pressure in the area of the diaphragmatic hiatus that extends over an axial distance of 2–3 cm. This zone maintains a pressure higher than intragastric pressure with inspiration and expiration, but the pressure drops significantly in response to swallow-induced peristalsis. LES tone and relaxation are controlled by central and peripheral mechanisms. Neural control of the LES involves cholinergic and noncholinergic inhibitory pathways. Contraction of the crural diaphragm increases LES pressure, whereas gastric distention, esophageal distention, pharyngeal and laryngeal inhibitory reflexes stimulate pathways resulting in LES relaxation.

Nitric oxide plays an important role in the relaxation of the lower esophageal sphincter. Studies in animals and humans have shown that blocking nitric oxide production with a NO synthase inhibitor reduces LES relaxation. CCK has also been shown to increase the rate of LES relaxation. Intravenous infusion of a CCK antagonist into healthy human volunteers resulted in a significant reduction in LES relaxation following oral feeding. Atropine, on the other hand, inhibits LES relaxation as demonstrated by esophageal manometry. Atropine has been shown to reduce the incidence of gastroesophageal reflux when assessed by esophageal pH monitoring in patients receiving postprandial atropine infusions.

Bibliography

Gawrieh S, Shaker R. Peripheral mechanisms affecting the lower esophageal sphincter tone. *Gastroenterol Clin North Am* 2002;31:S21–S33.

Mittal RK, Balaban DH. Mechanisms of disease: the esophagogastric junction. *N Engl J Med* 1997;336:924–932.

Peters JH, Demeester TR. Esophagus: anatomy, physiology, and gastroesophageal reflux disease. In: Greenfield LJ, Mulholland MW, Oldham KT, et al. (eds.), *Surgery: Scientific Principles and Practice*, 3rd ed. Philadelphia, PA: Lippincott, Williams & Wilkins, 2001, 665.

22. **(A)** Esophageal duplication cysts are rare congenital anomalies of the foregut, accounting for 0.5–2.5% of all esophageal tumors. Most duplications are discovered in infants and children, although 25–30% are found in the adult population. Duplication cysts result from developmental errors in the fifth to eighth weeks of embryonic life. During this time, the primitive foregut divides into dorsal and ventral segments. The dorsal segment elongates to form the esophagus and the ventral portion develops into the tracheobronchial tree. Vacuoles which form in the foregut during the solid-tube stage of development normally coalesce to form the esophageal lumen. It is theorized that failure of the vacuoles to coalesce results in formation of a duplication cyst. Esophageal cysts are lined by ciliated epithelium that may be columnar, squamous, or pseudostratified. Bronchogenic cysts are similarly lined by ciliated columnar epithelium and may contain cartilage. It is often difficult to differentiate bronchogenic cysts from esophageal cysts because of their close embryologic relationship. Many authors thus refer to these lesions collectively as foregut cysts.

Most duplication cysts are asymptomatic and are discovered incidentally while evaluating the esophagus for other pathology. When symptoms do occur, they typically include dysphagia, regurgitation, anorexia, chest pain, wheezing, and cough. Chest radiograph may show a posterior mediastinal mass. Barium esophagogram frequently demonstrates a filling defect in the esophagus with smooth edges. Endoscopic examination reveals a submucosal lesion with normal overlying mucosa, which may suggest a diagnosis of the more common leiomyoma. Biopsy should not be performed because it will not penetrate the submucosal location of the mass and may complicate future surgical intervention. Evaluation of duplication cysts with CT provides useful information about the size, location, and relationship to adjacent structures. The most accurate diagnostic modality, however, is endoscopic ultrasonography. EUS can distinguish cystic lesions from solid masses and shows the relationship to the esophageal wall. Moreover, EUS can differentiate bronchogenic from esophageal duplication cysts, which may not be apparent by CT imaging and can, therefore, be helpful with surgical planning.

Once the diagnosis of esophageal duplication cyst is established, surgical resection is usually indicated because of the potential for serious complications. These complications include compression of surrounding structures, ulceration with subsequent hemorrhage, suppurative infection, and rupture. Early attempts at treatment included marsupialization of the cyst and needle aspiration, but recurrences have been reported following incomplete surgical removal. Since most cysts are located in the right posterior mediastinum, cyst excision is conventionally performed through a posterolateral thoracotomy. Both vagus nerves should be identified and preserved. Similar to surgery for esophageal leiomyomas, extramucosal dissection can usually be performed with the mucosa left intact. The muscle edges should be reapproximated following cyst excision to prevent formation of a pseudodiverticulum. Thoracoscopic resection has recently been demonstrated to be as safe and effective as open surgery in select cases.

Bibliography

Cioffi U, Bonavina L, Matilde D, et al. Presentation and surgical management of bronchogenic and esophageal duplication cysts in adults. *Chest* 1998;113:1492–1496.

Nobuhara KK, Yara CG, La Quaglia, et al. Bronchogenic cysts and esophageal duplications: common origins and treatment. *J Pediatr Surg* 1997;32:1408–1413.

Van Dam J, Rice TW, Sivak MV. Endoscopic ultrasonography and endoscopically guided needle aspiration for the diagnosis of upper gastrointestinal tract foregut cysts. *Am J Gastroenterol* 1992;87:762–765.

Whitaker JA, Deffenbaugh LD, Cooke AR. Esophageal duplication cyst. *Am J Gastroenterol* 1980;73:329–332.

23. **(B)** Surgical resection provides the best means of palliation and provides a potential for cure for localized esophageal carcinoma. There are several options for surgical resection which can be broadly divided into transthoracic and transhiatal approaches. The transthoracic approach can be performed through a single thoracoabdominal incision or separate thoracic and abdominal incisions. The tumor-containing portion of esophagus, proximal stomach, and regional lymph nodes are resected and an intrathoracic esophagogastric anastomosis is usually performed. With the transhiatal approach, the entire intrathoracic esophagus is bluntly dissected through upper midline abdominal and neck incisions, thus avoiding a thoracotomy. The stomach is anastomosed to the cervical esophagus above the level of the clavicles.

Both transhiatal and transthoracic approaches have advantages and disadvantages. The most feared complication of a transthoracic procedure with an intrathoracic anastomosis is anastomotic leak. Although this complication is rare in most series, when leak does occur, it is associated with higher morbidity and mortality than leaks which occur in the neck. A leak in a cervical anastomosis can usually be managed conservatively with open drainage to establish a controlled fistula. On the other hand, intrathoracic leaks often require operative intervention, which may include takedown of the anastomosis and diversion through an esophagostomy. The risk of intrathoracic leak can be minimized for transthoracic approaches that involve initial right thoracotomy followed by abdominal and neck incisions by performing a cervical esophagogastric anastomosis or the so-called "3-Port" approach. This approach is mandatory for cancers that involve the mid-to-upper esophagus which are adjacent to the membranous wall of the trachea.

Another disadvantage of the transthoracic approach is the need for both thoracic and abdominal incisions, which may increase postoperative pain and, therefore, result in more respiratory complications. In addition, the incidence of gastroesophageal reflux may be increased, particularly when performed through a single left thoracoabdominal incision. The disadvantages of the transhiatal approach are limited exposure through the diaphragmatic hiatus resulting in potential life-threatening injuries to mediastinal structures. In addition, lack of a mediastinal lymph node dissection may result in an incomplete resection of gross disease and early recurrence.

A recent randomized trial comparing extended transthoracic to transhiatal resections for adenocarcinoma in the mid-to-distal esophagus found a lower morbidity in transhiatal esophagectomy as compared to transthoracic resection, but there was no significant difference in operative mortality. As both approaches have potential limitations and neither has conclusively been demonstrated superior, the specific approach used should be based on tumor location, tumor extent, and finally surgeon preference.

Bibliography

Bousamra M, Haasler GB, Parviz M. A decade of experience with transthoracic and transhiatal esophagectomy. *Am J Surg* 2002;183:162–167.

Boyle MJ, Franceschi D, Livingstone AS. Transhiatal versus transthoracic esophagectomy: complication and survival rates. *Am Surg* 1999;65:1137–1141.

Hulscher JBF, van Sandick JW, de Boer AGEM, et al. Extended transthoracic resection compared with limited transhiatal resection for adenocarcinoma of the esophagus. *N Engl J Med* 2002;347:1662–1669.

Orringer MB. Tumors, injuries, and miscellaneous conditions of the esophagus. In: Greenfield LJ, Mulholland MW, Oldham KT, et al. (eds.), *Surgery: Scientific Principles and Practice*, 3rd ed. Philadelphia, PA: Lippincott, Williams & Wilkins, 2001, 705–710.

Zwischenberger JB, Alpard SK, Orringer MB. Esophagus. In: Townsend CM, Beauchamp DR, Evers MB, et al. (eds.), *Sabiston Textbook of Surgery: The Biological Basis of Modern Surgical Practice*, 16th ed. Philadelphia, PA: W.B. Saunders, 2001, 739–742.

24. **(A)** Many patients with GERD can be successfully managed with medical therapy alone. Antireflux surgery is indicated when medical therapy has failed (usually determined by several months of high-dose PPIs or escalating doses of PPIs), with objectively documented severe reflux, when complications of GERD occur, and in patients who favor a single intervention rather than long-term pharmacologic therapy (e.g., young patients or those with financial considerations). Severe reflux can be objectively documented with a 24-h esophageal pH study, LES incompetence by manometry, or with mucosal changes on endoscopic examination. Complications of GERD include erosive esophagitis, stricture, and Barrett's esophagus. Patients with these abnormalities should undergo fundoplication. In general, patients whose remaining life expectance exceeds 10 years may avoid costly

long-term drug therapy by undergoing antireflux surgery.

The development of a stricture represents failure of medical therapy and is an indication for antireflux surgery. A malignant etiology must be excluded prior to surgery and dilation may be appropriate. Manometry is especially important in this setting as impaired peristalsis necessitates consideration of a partial fundoplication. With Barrett's metaplasia, antireflux surgery can arrest progression of disease and allow healing of ulceration, although it does not prevent subsequent development of adenocarcinoma. If biopsies show high-grade dysplasia or *in situ* carcinoma, resection should be performed.

A significant proportion of patients with GERD have concomitant respiratory disease such as asthma. The etiology of respiratory symptoms may be related to aspiration of gastric contents or bronchoconstriction in response to acid in the esophagus. Medical therapy of GERD in asthmatic patients improves respiratory symptoms in 25–50% of patients, but fewer than 15% have an objective improvement in pulmonary function. Antireflux surgery, on the other hand, improves respiratory symptoms in nearly 90% of children and 70% of adults and is, thus, the preferred therapy for patients with asthma and GERD.

Bibliography

Bowrey DJ, Peters JH, DeMeester TR. Gastroesophageal reflux disease in asthma: effects of medical and surgical antireflux therapy on asthma control. *Ann Surg* 2000; 231:161–172.

Peters JH, Demeester TR. Esophagus: anatomy, physiology, and gastroesophageal reflux disease. In: Greenfield LJ, Mulholland MW, Oldham KT, et al. (eds.), *Surgery: Scientific Principles and Practice*, 3rd ed. Philadelphia, PA: Lippincott, Williams & Wilkins, 2001, 675–677.

Stein HJ, DeMeester TR. Who benefits from antireflux surgery? *World J Surg* 1992;16:313–319.

25. **(B)** Ingestion of caustic substances has both immediate and long-term effects on the gastrointestinal tract. Caustic injuries occur most commonly in young children who accidentally swallow these substances and adults who attempt suicide. Corrosive agents include acids, alkalis, bleach, and detergents. Of these, alkalis are most damaging because they produce a liquefactive necrosis which results in deeper tissue penetration. Acids, on the other hand, cause a coagulative necrosis which limits tissue penetration. Hydrofluoric acid is an exception because it produces liquefactive injury similar to alkalis.

Following the ingestion of either acid or alkali, there is reflex pyloric spasm which prevents passage of the corrosive agent into the duodenum; however, gastric contraction also occurs which results in regurgitation of the substance back into the esophagus. Meanwhile, the esophagus is vigorously contracting against a closed cricopharyngeus to propel the substance into the stomach. This seesaw activity lasts approximately 3–5 min, after which esophagogastric atony occurs and the substance passes into the duodenum.

Esophageal injury continues for 24–48 h following exposure to caustic agents. It is during this time that esophageal wall necrosis and subsequent perforation may occur. Inflammatory cells infiltrate the submucosa in the first few days after injury. Granulation tissue forms over sloughing necrotic tissue approximately 10 days postinjury. By the third week, fibroblastic proliferation is present. The fibrosis that occurs results in stricture formation, which represents the most common complication following caustic injury to the esophagus. The amount of fibrosis that occurs is related to the severity of the initial injury. Full-thickness burns or circumferential ulcerations of the esophagus, accordingly, have the highest potential for stricture formation.

Because of the high incidence of stricture formation following severe caustic esophageal injury, prophylactic measures have been attempted. Unfortunately, most if not all of these therapies have little proven benefit in preventing strictures. Corticosteroids, esophageal stenting, prophylactic bougienage, and esophageal rest using nasoenteric feeding or parental nutrition have been previously used to prevent stricture formation, but there is little evidence to suggest any benefits. Vigilant anticipation, including patient counseling regarding the possibility of stricture development and reporting any symptoms of dysphagia for early intervention with dilatation, is perhaps the best means of managing this late complication.

Another potential consequence of esophageal caustic injury is TEF formation. TEF usually present within the first few weeks after injury, however, is less common than simple stricture formation. Symptoms include progressive pneumonia, choking, coughing with feedings, or aspiration of bile-stained mucus from the airway. Hiatal hernia is a late complication that usually occurs many years after caustic injury as a presumed result of esophageal foreshortening. Another long-term complication of esophageal scarring because of caustic injury is malignant degeneration. The incidence of esophageal carcinoma is 1000-fold greater after caustic injury than in the general population.

Bibliography

Hugh TB, Kelly MD. Corrosive injection and the surgeon. *J Am Coll Surg* 1999;189:508–522.

Kikendall JW. Caustic ingestion injuries. *Gastroenterol Clin North Am* 1991;20:847–857.

Zwischenberger JB, Alpard SK, Orringer MB. Esophagus. In: Townsend CM, Beauchamp DR, Evers MB, et al. (eds.), *Sabiston Textbook of Surgery: The Biological Basis of Modern Surgical Practice*, 16th ed. Philadelphia, PA: W.B. Saunders, 2001, 717–719.

26. **(B)** Esophageal motility disorders, or esophageal spasm syndromes, typically include DES, nutcracker esophagus, hypertensive lower esophageal sphincter, and inadequate esophageal motility. Patients with motility disorders usually complain of chest pain and dysphagia. Once cardiac and nonesophageal causes have been ruled out, esophageal disorders may be evaluated. The conventional methods of evaluating the esophagus may not be of value in diagnosing motility disorders because symptoms are often intermittent in nature. A barium esophagogram, endoscopy, and even manometry can appear normal unless they are performed during symptoms. Esophageal manometry remains the gold standard for evaluating motility disorders, however.

The manometry tracing in a normal patient shows a basal pressure of approximately 20 mmHg. LES pressure is normally 15–25 mmHg and relaxes with swallowing. Following the swallow, peristalsis progresses from the proximal esophagus through the esophageal body and eventually to the distal esophagus and LES. The LES remains open or relaxed until the peristaltic wave progresses to the LES. The mean amplitude of the distal peristaltic wave is 30–100 mmHg and duration is from 2 to 6 s. Under normal conditions there are few (usually less than 10%) simultaneous contractions, no repetitive contractions, and waveforms are monophasic after swallows (Fig. 21-19).

The manometry tracing in the above patient, however, shows simultaneous contractions with wet swallows as well as multiple, spontaneous contractions that are prolonged in duration. These are typical manometric findings of DES. Other possible findings include intermittent normal peristalsis, multiple peaks, and contractions of increased amplitude.

Nutcracker esophagus is a hypermotility disorder characterized by extremely high-amplitude contractions (greater than 180 mmHg) and prolonged duration of contractions (greater than 6 s). Peristaltic progression is usually normal. Hypertensive LES is defined by resting LES pressures greater than 45 mmHg with normal LES relaxation. Esophageal peristalsis is generally normal. In inadequate esophageal motility, lower

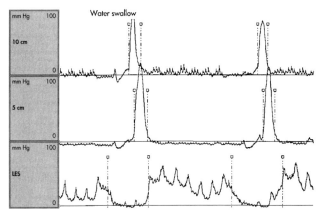

FIG. 21-19 Esophageal manometry tracing in a normal patient. (Reprinted with permission from Cameron JL (ed.), *Current Surgical Therapy*, 7th ed. The Netherlands: Elsevier, 2001, 20.)

esophageal pressure and relaxation are normal, but there is decreased amplitude or absent peristalsis following swallows. The manometric findings in achalasia include a baseline elevation of the LES pressure, generally greater than 45 mmHg. Unlike hypertensive lower esophageal sphincter, relaxation of the LES is diminished or absent, however. Peristalsis along the esophageal body is also abnormal in achalasia.

Bibliography

Adler DG, Romero Y. Primary esophageal motility disorders. *Mayo Clin Proc* 2001;76:195–200.

Dent J, Holloway RH. Esophageal motility and reflux testing. *Gastroenterol Clin North Am* 1996;25:51–73.

Moesinger R, Crowley M, Ravitch W, et al. Esophageal spasm syndromes. In: Cameron JL (ed.), *Current Surgical Therapy*, 7th ed. St. Louis, MO: Mosby, 2001, 19–25.

Prakash C, Clouse RE. Esophageal motor disorders. *Curr Opin Gastroenterol* 2002;18:454–463.

Spechler SJ, Castell DO. Classification of oesophageal motility abnormalities. *Gut* 2001;49:145–151.

27. **(E)** The main barrier to reflux of gastric contents into the esophagus is the lower esophageal sphincter. The sphincter mechanism is not an anatomically distinct structure, but is formed from the intrinsic smooth muscle of the distal esophagus and the skeletal muscle of the crural diaphragm. The LES normally has a resting baseline pressure greater than the baseline pressure of the stomach. When this high pressure zone is compromised, reflux of gastric contents occurs. The tonic resistance of the LES is a function of both its pressure and the overall length over which this pressure is exerted. The shorter the length, the higher the pressure must be to maintain sufficient resistance for the sphincter to be competent. Thus, an abnormally short length of high pressure zone can lead to significant

reflux even with normal LES pressures. For example, gastric distention causes the sphincter length to shorten, thus decreasing the pressure threshold for reflux to occur. This accounts for postprandial symptoms seen early in the course of disease. Transient increases in intraabdominal pressure may also overcome LES pressure and result in reflux.

Transient relaxation of the LES occurs in everyone, but not everyone develops clinically significant reflux because of the existence of other defense mechanisms. Gravity and esophageal peristalsis play a large role in limiting the contact time between gastric contents and the esophageal mucosa. Salivary gland secretions help buffer the acidic contents of gastric reflux and secretions from esophageal submucosal glands also provide additional buffering to restore neutral pH in the esophageal lumen. Esophageal submucosal glands secrete mucus that contains a high concentration of bicarbonate, and secretory activity occurs in response to acidification of the esophageal lumen.

Bibliography

Long JD, Orlando RC. Esophageal submucosal glands: structure and function. *Am J Gastroenterol* 1999; 94:2818–2824.

Mittal RK, Balaban DH. Mechanisms of disease: the esophagogastric junction. *N Engl J Med* 1997;336:924–932.

Peters JH, Demeester TR. Esophagus: anatomy, physiology, and gastroesophageal reflux disease. In: Greenfield LJ, Mulholland MW, Oldham KT, et al. (eds.), *Surgery: Scientific Principles and Practice*, 3rd ed. Philadelphia, PA: Lippincott, Williams & Wilkins, 2001, 667–671.

28. **(C)** The barium esophagogram demonstrates a type III paraesophageal hernia, where both gastric cardia as well as the gastroesophageal junction are displaced above the diaphragmatic hiatus. As a paraesophageal hernia develops, the stomach commonly rotates around its longitudinal axis so that the anterior and posterior walls of the gastric body are transposed. A volvulus may develop with upward displacement of the cardia.

Many patients with paraesophageal hernia may be asymptomatic or complain of mild symptoms such as postprandial fullness, bloating, epigastric or substernal discomfort, and nausea. Symptoms of gastroesophageal reflux are commonly associated with paraesophageal hernia. Complications may result from gastric incarceration, pulmonary compromise from decreased lung expansion or aspiration, and bleeding from mechanical or ischemic gastric ulcerations. The risk of complications justifies surgical repair in most cases of paraesophageal hernia. Certainly if gastric incarceration is suspected, then emergent surgery is indicated. Barium swallow is diagnostic and chest roentgenogram occasionally shows an air-fluid level behind the cardiac silhouette.

Once identified, paraesophageal hernias should be surgically repaired. This can be performed through a transabdominal or transthoracic approach, and laparoscopic repair has recently been shown to be equally effective and safe compared to open repair. Surgical repair consists of hernia reduction, crural closure, and fundoplication. The need for fundoplication is controversial, but many authors advocate its inclusion for several reasons. Sixty to seventy percent of patients with paraesophageal hernia have increased esophageal exposure to gastric acid based on 24-h pH monitoring. It is also difficult to adequately assess the presence of GERD in all patients with paraesophageal hernia, especially those presenting on an emergent basis. Finally, dissection at the gastroesophageal junction may lead to postoperative reflux.

Bibliography

Edye MB, Canin-Endres J, Gattorno F, et al. Durability of laparoscopic repair of paraesophageal hernia. *Ann Surg* 1998;228:528–535.

Eubanks TR, Pellegrini CA. Hiatal hernia and gastroesophageal reflux disease. In: Townsend CM, Beauchamp DR, Evers MB, et al. (eds.), *Sabiston Textbook of Surgery: The Biological Basis of Modern Surgical Practice*, 16th ed. Philadelphia, PA: W.B. Saunders, 2001, 756.

Hashemi M, Sillin LF, Peters JH. Current concepts in the management of paraesophageal hiatal hernia. *J Clin Gastroenterol* 1999;29:8–13.

Oddsdottir M. Paraesophageal hernia. *Surg Clin North Am* 2000;80:1243–1252.

29. **(D)** The esophageal manometry tracing shows incomplete relaxation of the LES with wet swallows as well as abnormal esophageal body peristalsis. These findings are consistent with achalasia. Achalasia is an uncommon disorder of esophageal motility involving destruction of the myenteric plexus leading to esophageal body aperistalsis and incomplete LES relaxation. As the disease progresses, functional obstruction of the esophagus occurs, which can be seen on barium esophagogram as a dilated esophagus with bird-beak tapering and air-fluid levels in the distal esophagus. Endoscopy is useful to exclude other disorders such as malignancy. Left untreated, achalasia may result in a massively dilated, tortuous esophagus with irreversible esophageal damage.

Esophageal dilation provides the best long-term response and has been the mainstay of nonoperative therapy. Endoscopic dilation is performed with a balloon dilator that stretches the LES to a diameter of 30–40 mm, which disrupts the hypertonic muscles of the LES. Fifty to ninety percent of patients have good to excellent symptom improvement using the newer pneumatic balloon dilators. The main risk of balloon dilation is esophageal perforation, with reported rates ranging from 2 to 6%.

Botulinum A toxin has recently received attention for its potential role in the treatment of neuromuscular disorders of the gastrointestinal tract. For achalasia, diluted botulinum toxin is injected into each quadrant of the lower esophageal sphincter. It binds to presynaptic cholinergic nerve terminals and inhibits the release of acetylcholine. This counteracts the impaired LES relaxation that results from unopposed acetylcholine excitation of esophageal smooth muscle that occurs in achalasia. Cumulative data show that botulinum toxin is initially effective in 85% of patients, but symptom recurrence is reported in more than 50% of patients at 6 months. The most common side effect is chest pain and adverse reactions such as swelling and rash have been observed. Several series have shown better long-term efficacy with pneumatic dilation compared to botulinum toxin injection.

Pharmacologic treatment is often used as first-line therapy for achalasia. Calcium-channel blockers have a relaxing effect on vascular and gastrointestinal smooth muscle. Nifedipine has specifically been shown to significantly decrease LES pressure as well as the amplitude of aperistaltic contractions in the esophageal body. Ten to 20 milligrams of nifedipine results in immediate improvement of symptoms in some patients, but sustained benefit occurs relatively infrequently. Side effects such as peripheral edema, hypotension, and flushing are not uncommon. Nitrates also have a relaxing effect on gastrointestinal smooth muscle. Isosorbide dinitrate reduces LES pressure, but the effect is short-lived and side effects are more frequently encountered than with calcium antagonists. Beta-blockers such as atenolol have never been demonstrated to improve achalasia symptomatology. Pharmacologic therapy should be limited to the treatment of early disease, patients who refuse pneumatic dilation, patients who are not candidates for surgery, or patients in whom botulinum toxin injections fail.

Bibliography

Tack J, Janssens J, Vantrappen G. Non-surgical treatment of achalasia. *Hepatogastroenterology* 1991;38:493–497.

Vaezi MF, Richter JE. Current therapies for achalasia. *J Clin Gastroenterol* 1998;27:21–35.

Vaezi MF, Richter JE, Wilcox M, et al. One-year follow-up: pneumatic dilatation more effective than botulinum toxin. *Gastroenterology* 1997;112:A318.

West RL, Hirsch DP, Bartelsman JFWM, et al. Long term results of pneumatic dilation in achalasia followed for more than 5 years. *Am J Gastroenterol* 2002;97:1346–1351.

30. **(E)** The distribution of arterial blood supply to the esophagus is segmental based on embryologic development. The cervical esophagus receives its blood supply from branches of the inferior thyroid artery. The bronchial arteries supply the upper portion of the thoracic esophagus and the midthoracic esophagus is supplied by vessels directly originating from the descending thoracic aorta. The lower thoracic and intraabdominal esophagus is nourished by branches of the left gastric and inferior phrenic arteries. There is often a communicating vessel between the inferior phrenic and left gastric arteries, commonly referred to as Belsey's artery. Branches from these arteries run within the muscularis propria and give rise to branches that course within the submucosa. There are extensive anastomoses, which accounts for the rarity of esophageal infarction. Mobilization of the distal esophagus must be approached with extreme caution to avoid injury to the arterial branches originating from the left gastric and inferior phrenic systems. This is especially important with left thora- cotomy approaches as these vessels may retract beneath the diaphragm before they are adequately controlled (Fig. 21-20).

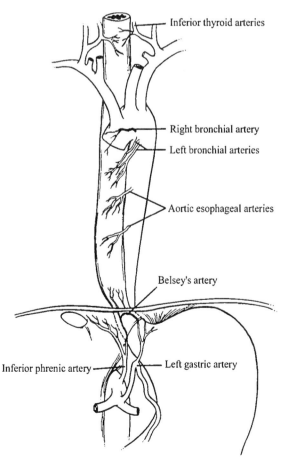

FIG. 21-20 Blood supply to esophagus.

Venous drainage of the esophagus occurs through an extensive submucosal venous plexus. The submucosal plexus communicates through perforating branches with longitudinally oriented veins on the outer esophageal surface. Branches from the upper two-thirds of the esophagus lead into the inferior thyroid vein and azygous system with eventual drainage into the superior vena cava. The lower esophagus drains into the left gastric veins and short gastric veins, which are part of the portal venous system. The caval and portal systems thus communicate through the submucosal veins. Portal hypertension may lead to dilation of the submucosal plexus, which is commonly referred to as esophageal varices.

Bibliography

Albertucci M, Russell SS. Anatomy of the esophagus. In: Baker RJ, Fischer JE (eds.), *Mastery of Surgery*, 4th ed. Philadelphia, PA: Lippincott, Williams & Wilkins, 2001, 744–745.

Patti MG, Gantert W, Way LW. Surgery of the esophagus, anatomy and physiology. *Surg Clin North Am* 1997; 77:959–970.

Peters JH, Demeester TR. Esophagus: anatomy, physiology, and gastroesophageal reflux disease. In: Greenfield LJ, Mulholland MW, Oldham KT, et al. (eds.), *Surgery: Scientific Principles and Practice*, 3rd ed. Philadelphia, PA: Lippincott, Williams & Wilkins, 2001, 660.

31. (E) The esophageal tumor present in the chest CT has evidence of multiple hepatic metastases on the abdominal CT. This equates to unresectable stage IVb disease and any treatment will be palliative with an expected survival of only 3–6 months. Although surgical resection can be used for palliation of malignant dysphagia, the morbidity and mortality associated with surgery make it a less than ideal option. Radiation therapy can be administered externally or via an endoluminal catheter (brachytherapy) and may provide some relief of dysphagia. One to two months may be required for appreciable symptom improvement and potential complications include radiation-induced esophagitis with persistent dyspagia. Of note, chemoradiation therapy usually provides the better long-term palliation as compared to radiation therapy alone, but would be poorly tolerated in a patient nearly 80 years of age with significant weight loss.

Endoscopic intubation and stenting provide excellent relief of dysphagia. Plastic stents were commonly used prior to 1990 with mixed results. The internal diameters were usually less than 12 mm and they required initial dilation of the malignant stricture to accommodate the large external diameters. Over the past decade, self-expanding metallic stents have become available for palliation of unresectable esophageal tumors. They are easier to insert, have larger internal diameters, and are less likely to cause perforation than the older plastic stents. They can expand as the tumor shrinks with concurrent use of other therapies, and silicone coatings prevent tumor ingrowth. Self-expanding metal stents provide excellent relief of malignant dysphagia and are the treatment of choice for malignant TEF. Complications include bleeding, perforation, and distal migration. Care must be taken to avoid placement of stents across the gastroesophageal junction as this may lead to gastroesophageal reflux.

Laser therapy, particularly the neodymium:yttrium-aluminum-garnet (Nd:YAG) laser, uses laser energy to vaporize tissue under endoscopic visualization. Multiple sessions are often required for restoration of comfortable swallowing. Successful relief of dysphagia has been reported in 69–83% of cases. Laser therapy may be combined with other treatments such as stenting and/or radiotherapy to provide palliation. Complications include perforation, bleeding, and formation of TEFs.

Photodynamic therapy is a recent development that uses a photosensitive compound that is activated by laser energy at a specific wavelenght, thus generating cytotoxic singlet oxygen causing cell death. Malignant cells selectively retain the photosensitive agent hematoporphyrin, which is given intravenously 48–72 h prior to endoscopic application of laser energy. Once activated, the singlet oxygen generated kills neoplastic cells resulting in tumor slough. The depth of tissue injury is usually between 2 and 5 mm and multiple sessions may be required to achieve an adequate clinical response. The most common complication is photosensitizer-induced skin injury, which occurs when patients are exposed to radiant heat such as sunlight or strong fluorescent lighting within 30 days of treatment.

Bibliography

Adler DG, Baron TH. Endoscopic palliation of malignant dysphagia. *Mayo Clin Proc* 2001;76:731–738.

Cordero JA Jr, Moores DWO. Use of esophageal stents. In: Cameron JL (ed.), *Current Surgical Therapy*, 7th ed. St. Louis, MO: Mosby, 2001, 57–62.

Orringer MB. Tumors, injuries, and miscellaneous conditions of the esophagus. In: Greenfield LJ, Mulholland MW, Oldham KT, et al. (eds.), *Surgery: Scientific Principles and Practice*, 3rd ed. Philadelphia, PA: Lippincott, Williams & Wilkins, 2001, 704–705.

Weigel TL, Frumiento C, Gaumintz E. Endoluminal palliation for dysphagia secondary to esophageal carcinoma. *Surg Clin North Am* 202;82:747–761.

32. (E) It has been estimated that approximately 10% of patients with GERD will develop Barrett's metaplasia. Barrett's esophagus has traditionally been defined as the presence of columnar mucosa extending at least 3 cm into the esophagus. Recent studies have shown that specialized intestinal-type epithelium has the potential to degenerate into dysplasia and subsequently adenocarcinoma, which may occur in segments of columnar mucosa shorter than 3 cm. The progression to Barrett's esophagus begins at the gastroesophageal junction, where repetitive exposure of distal esophageal squamous mucosa to gastric acid results in metaplasic conversion to gastric-type epithelium. As the severity of reflux increases, the length of columnar metaplasia increases and intestinal metaplasia may develop. Current evidence supports the role of duodenal contents in the pathogenesis of Barrett's metaplasia. Studies have shown that esophageal bile acid exposure is increased in patients with Barrett's esophagus, and bile acid gastritis is associated with an increased incidence of Barrett's metaplasia.

The diagnosis of Barrett's esophagus is made on endoscopy and biopsy. Endoscopically, columnar mucosa has a salmon-pink appearance, in contrast to the pearly white appearance of squamous epithelium. Barrett's is suspected when this salmon-pink columnar mucosa extends, often with flame-shaped projections into the white squamous epithelium, above the gastroesophageal junction. Histologic examination may show gastric fundic-type epithelium, gastric junctional-type epithelium, or specialized columnar epithelium that has a villiform surface and contains goblet cells. The presence of goblet cells differentiates specialized columnar cells from normal columnar cells and is the hallmark of intestinal metaplasia.

The role of *H. pylori* in gastritis and peptic ulcer disease has been well documented. Several authors reported an inverse relationship of *H. pylori* with the development of reflux esophagitis, Barrett's esophagus, dysplasia, and adenocarcinoma. In particular, they speculate that the cagA+ strain of *H. pylori* is associated with a lower incidence of esophageal mucosal disease.

Bibliography

Bremner CG, Bremner RM. Barrett's esophagus. *Surg Clin North Am* 1997;77:1115–1137.

Buttar NS, Falk GW. Pathogenesis of gastroesophageal reflux and Barrett esophagus. *Mayo Clin Proc* 2001;76: 226–234.

Dixon MF, Neville PM, Mapstone NP, et al. Bile reflux gastritis and Barrett's oesophagus: further evidence of a role for duodenogastro-oesophageal reflux? *Gut* 2001;49: 359–363.

Oksanen A, Sipponen P, Karttunen R, et al. Inflammation and intestinal metaplasia at the squamocolumnar junction in young patients with or without *Helicobacter pylori* infection. *Gut* 2003;52:194–198.

33. (E) Esophageal intubation with self-expanding metallic stents is an effective palliative measure for obstructing esophageal carcinoma. For inoperable or unresectable tumors, stenting can bridge the obstruction to allow esophageal patency and restore swallowing. Its main advantage over other palliative treatment options is the immediate relief of symptoms once deployed, whereas radiation and laser therapy may take several weeks or multiple treatments before significant relief is achieved. Esophageal stenting is the procedure of choice for malignant TEF.

Expandable metal stents are currently approved by the Food and Drug Administration for palliation of esophageal obstruction related to malignancies and for TEFs, but not for benign diseases. There are several types and sizes available and the choice of stent must be tailored to the patient and to tumor characteristics. The stents can be placed into narrow strictures because they are loaded on a small-diameter delivery applicator, although dilation is occasionally performed prior to stent placement. The newest generations of self-expanding metallic stents have an internal diameter of 17–22 mm and can be stacked on end to treat very long lesions. Care must be exercised, however, when the tumor involves the proximal esophagus because of the proximity with the airway. Stent placement across the gastroesophageal junction may also result in reflux and regurgitation. Placement of a self-expanding metallic stent does not preclude subsequent radiation and/or chemotherapy and the stents can expand to remain in place following response to other therapies. Some stents are coated with silicone polymer to prevent tumor ingrowth through the metal interstices.

Stent placement should be performed by an experienced endoscopist with fluoroscopic guidance. After assessment of tumor length, an appropriate stent size may be selected by adding 4–6 cm to tumor length. A guidewire is placed through the malignant stricture and a stent delivery applicator is passed over the guidewire. Dilation of the stricture may be required prior to stent placement if the luminal diameter is less than 6 mm. Stent position can be adjusted during the early stages of deployment using radiopaque markings on the stent. Most stents cannot be removed or repositioned after final deployment.

Complications are relatively rare with expandable metal stents. There is a risk of perforation during endoscopic placement of the stents, but this risk is small with the expandable metal stents that can be positioned over a small-diameter applicator. There is also less dilation required compared to that needed for placement of older plastic stents. The most common cause of failure of metallic stents is tumor ingrowth at either end of the stent or through the metal mesh. Bleeding, infection, and stent migration are other potential complications of metallic stents.

Bibliography

Cordero JA Jr, Moores DWO. Use of esophageal stents. In: Cameron JL (ed.), *Current Surgical Therapy*, 7th ed. St. Louis, MO: Mosby, 2001, 57–62.

Kaneko K, Ito H, Konishi K, et al. Implantation of self-expanding metallic stent for patients with malignant stricture after failure of definitive chemoradiotherapy for T3 or T4 esophageal squamous cell carcinomas. *Hepatogastroenterology* 2002;49:699–705.

Weigel TL, Frumiento C, Gaumintz E. Endoluminal palliation for dysphagia secondary to esophageal carcinoma. *Surg Clin North Am* 202;82:747–761.

Zwischenberger JB, Alpard SK, Orringer MB. Esophagus. In: Townsend CM, Beauchamp DR, Evers MB, et al. (eds.), *Sabiston Textbook of Surgery: The Biological Basis of Modern Surgical Practice*, 16th ed. Philadelphia, PA: W.B. Saunders, 2001, 737–738.

34. **(C)** Scleroderma or progressive systemic sclerosis is a systemic disease characterized by excessive deposition of collagen and other matrix elements in skin and other organ systems. Clinically significant gastrointestinal involvement occurs in approximately 50% of all patients with systemic sclerosis. In addition, many scleroderma patients without GI symptoms have subclinical involvement, which is documented by abnormalities on esophageal motility testing.

It is hypothesized that gastrointestinal involvement by scleroderma is secondary to either vascular ischemia or primary nerve damage. Neural dysfunction may result from arteriolar changes in the vasa nervorum or by compression of nerve fibers by collagen deposition. Vascular changes mainly involve the small arteries, which demonstrate a mononuclear inflammatory response. Subsequent fibroblastic changes induce severe sclerosis of the intima of the small arteries and interstitium. The vascular and neurogenic changes result in smooth muscle atrophy, which is the basis for the clinical features of scleroderma. Muscle function is diminished but capable of responding early in the disease process, during which time treatment with prokinetic drugs may be beneficial. As the disease progresses, muscle fibrosis occurs and muscle function is permanently lost.

The esophagus is the most frequently involved gastrointestinal organ in scleroderma. The primary manifestation of esophageal involvement in scleroderma is GERD. Several mechanisms contribute to the development of reflux. Decreased LES pressure results in an increased frequency of reflux and impaired peristalsis prevents clearance of refluxed material back into the stomach. Furthermore, many patients with scleroderma have a coexistent sicca syndrome and, therefore, have reduced acid-neutralizing capacity of swallowed saliva. Current evidence suggests that disordered motility is the primary abnormality contributing to GERD in scleroderma.

GERD in scleroderma patients is more likely to result in complications such as erosive esophagitis, Barrett's esophagus, and strictures. Manometric findings of low LES pressures and low-amplitude peristalsis have been found to correlate with the development of esophagitis. Endoscopy should be routinely performed in scleroderma patients with reflux to evaluate for Barrett's metaplasia. Although 24-h ambulatory pH testing is highly sensitive in the diagnosis of GERD, it is not necessary when there is documented abnormal manometry or endoscopic findings.

Treatment of GERD in patients with scleroderma is similar to treatment of patients without scleroderma. First-line therapy consists of behavioral modification and antisecretory drugs and/or prokinetic agents. Prokinetic agents are beneficial earlier in the disease process, prior to muscle fibrosis. If medical therapy fails, antireflux surgery may be considered. Although usually extremely effective in the treatment of GERD, results of antireflux surgery in scleroderma patients are not as promising. The esophageal motor dysfunction makes it challenging to create a wrap that is sufficient to prevent reflux, yet not too tight to cause dysphagia. Furthermore, chronic inflammation and fibrosis often result in esophageal shortening, which may necessitate an esophageal lengthening procedure.

Bibliography

Bassotti G, Battaglia E, Debernardi V, et al. Esophageal dysfunction in scleroderma: relationship with disease subsets. *Arthritis Rheum* 1997;40:2252–2259.

Ling TC, Johnston BT. Esophageal investigations in connective tissue disease: which tests are most appropriate? *J Clin Gastroenterol* 2001;32:33–36.

Rose S, Young MA, Reynolds JC. Gastrointestinal manifestations of scleroderma. *Gastroenterol Clin North Am* 1998;27:563–594.

Sjogren RW. Gastrointestinal motility disorders in scleroderma. *Arthritis Rheum* 1994;37:1265–1282.

35. **(A)**

36. **(D)**

Explanations 35 and 36

Esophageal carcinoma is staged with the TNM classification as defined by the American Joint Committee on Cancer (Table 21-1). Because the behavior of esophageal cancer and treatment depends on the anatomic location, the esophagus is divided into four anatomic regions for classification and staging. These four divisions are (1) cervical, from the lower border of the cricoid cartilage to the thoracic inlet; (2) upper thoracic, from the thoracic inlet to the level of the tracheal bifurcation; (3) middle thoracic, from the tracheal bifurcation to the distal esophagus just above the esophagogastric junction; and (4) lower thoracic and abdominal, which includes the intraabdominal portion of the esophagus and esophagogastric junction.

Esophageal cancer exhibits aggressive behavior, initially spreading along the extensive submucosal lymphatic channels and then frequently involving regional lymph nodes. More distant lymph node involvement, such as cervical or celiac nodes, is currently considered metastatic disease. The primary

TABLE 21-1 TNM Classification for Esophageal Carcinoma

Primary tumor (T)

TX	Primary tumor cannot be assessed
T0	No evidence of primary tumor
Tis	Carcinoma *in situ*
T1	Tumor invades lamina propria or submucosa
T2	Tumor invades muscularis propria
T3	Tumor invades adventitia
T4	Tumor invades adjacent structures

Regional lymph nodes (N)

NX	Regional lymph nodes cannot be assessed
N0	No regional lymph node metastasis
N1	Regional lymph node metastasis

Distant metastasis (M)

MX	Distant metastasis cannot be assessed
M0	No distant metastasis
M1	Distant metastasis
M1a	Metastasis in celiac or cervical lymph nodes
M1b	Other distant metastasis

State 0	Tis	N0	M0
Stage I	T1	N0	M0
Stage IIA	T2	N0	M0
	T3	N0	M0
Stage IIB	T1	N1	M0
	T2	N1	M0
Stage III	T3	N1	M0
	T4	Any N	M0
Stage IV	Any T	Any N	M1
Stage IVA	Any T	Any N	M1a
Stage IVB	Any T	Any N	M1b

Source. Used with the permission of the American Joint Committee on Cancer (AJCC), Chicago, Illinois. The original source for this material is the *AJCC Cancer Staging Manual*, 6th ed. New York, NY: Springer-Verlag, 2002; www.springer-ny.com.

tumor may directly extend into adjacent structures such as the aorta, trachea, diaphragm, and lung (T4). The most common sites for distant metastases are the liver, lung, and pleura (Fig. 21-21). The first patient described above has clinical T3N0M0 disease, which is stage IIa. The second patient has T2 disease since the tumor only infiltrates the muscularis propria; however, the presence of celiac lymph node involvement in a patient with a distal esophageal (not GE junction) carcinoma is considered distant metastasis. This latter patient would be considered to have biopsy-proven stage IVA disease. Controversy exists as to the curability of stage IVA disease. Christie et al. (1999) showed that although there was a statistically significant survival difference between M1A and M1B disease (median 11 months vs. 5 months), the increased survival time was consumed by treatment and recovery periods. These authors, therefore, believed that surgery did not provide a significant survival advantage.

Bibliography

Christie NA, Rice TW, DeCamp MM, et al. M1A/M1B esophageal carcinoma: clinical relevance. *J Thorac Cardiovasc Surg* 1999;118:900–907.

Greene FL, Page DL, Fleming ID, et al. (eds.). *AJCC Cancer Staging Manual*, 6th ed. New York, NY: Springer-Verlag, 2002, 91–95.

Rice TW. Esophageal tumors. In: Cameron JL (ed.), *Current Surgical Therapy*, 7th ed. St. Louis, MO: Mosby, 2001, 51–57.

37. (B)

38. (D)

39. (E)

40. (A)

Explanations 37 through 40

Esophageal perforation is commonly a life-threatening emergency. Successful management relies on prompt recognition and initiation of treatment. Delay in diagnosis results in increased morbidity, mortality, and can affect the choice of therapy. The majority of perforations (60%) are iatrogenic following endoscopy, esophageal dilatations, difficult endotracheal intubations, and other forms of instrumentation. Trauma accounts for approximately 20% of esophageal perforations and spontaneous rupture for another 15%. Symptoms vary according to the location of perforation, size of the perforation, and time duration since injury. Cervical perforations may present with neck pain, dysphagia, and odynophyagia. Palpation of the

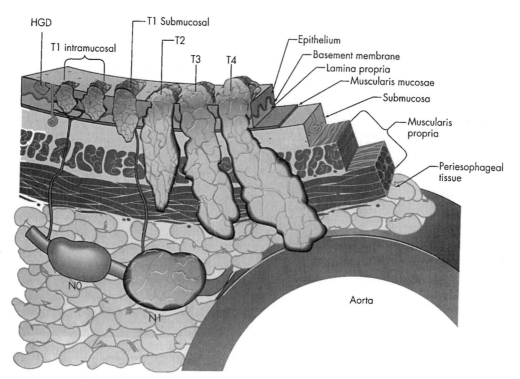

FIG. 21-21 Esophageal carcinoma invasion. (Reprinted with permission from Cameron JL (ed.), *Current Surgical Therapy*, 7th ed. The Netherlands: Elsevier, 2001, 55.)

neck may reveal crepitus. Thoracic perforations may present with substernal or epigastric pain as well as dysphagia. Abdominal perforations usually present with epigastric pain radiating to the back or left shoulder with signs of peritoneal irritation. Without treatment, frank sepsis and respiratory failure may develop.

The plain chest radiograph may appear normal early after esophageal perforation. Radiographic findings suggestive of perforation, however, include pneumomediastinum, subcutaneous emphysema, pleural effusion, and hydropneumothorax. The diagnostic study of choice in any patient suspected of having an esophageal perforation is a contrast radiograph of the esophagus. A water-soluble contrast esophagogram followed by barium, if necessary, is diagnostic in 90% of patients. CT scan of the chest and upper abdomen with oral contrast is also being used with more frequency. The site of perforation can often be defined on chest CT, as well as any areas of mediastinal and/or pleural space fluid collections which require drainage.

Treatment of esophageal perforation should be tailored to each individual patient. Factors to consider include the location of perforation, the extent of tissue necrosis, time interval since injury, and the presence of underlying esophageal disease. If an esophageal per-

foration is suspected, immediate treatment should begin with cessation of all oral intake, intravenous fluid resuscitation, gastric decompression, and broad-spectrum antibiotic therapy to cover both aerobic and anaerobic organisms.

In the stable patient with mild symptoms and a well-contained leak on esophagogram, nonoperative management can be successful. Patients meeting these criteria can be managed with cessation of oral intake, total parenteral nutrition, and antibiotics. A repeat esophagogram is performed in 7–14 days. Oral intake may be resumed following resolution and/or stabilization of the leak. Signs of clinical deterioration with conservative management should prompt surgical intervention.

In the absence of underlying esophageal pathology such as malignancy, primary repair with drainage of the contaminated area should be initially considered. This option is best suited for patients with early presentation demonstrating hemodynamic stability and minimal contamination. Primary repair is performed by exposing the entire length of mucosal injury, debriding any nonviable tissue, and closing the defect in two layers. The submucosal layer can frequently be stapled followed by interrupted suture closure of the muscular wall. The suture line can then be reinforced with a flap of parietal pleura, intercostal muscle, or gastric fundus. When perforation is associated with underlying esophageal disease, any pathology causing distal obstruction must be addressed to prevent breakdown of a primary repair. In the setting of achalasia, a distal esophagomyotomy on the side opposite of the perforation should be performed in addition to primary repair and partial gastric fundoplication buttress of the perforation site.

Although primary repair has traditionally been limited to perforations presenting within 24 h, several studies have shown that successful primary repair is possible with later presentations. Zumbro et al. (2002) reported acceptable outcomes in patients with delayed presentations who were treated with primary reinforced repair. Wang et al. (1996) divided patients into three groups depending on the time interval between perforation and primary repair. The incidence of postoperative leak and morbidity was increased in groups with delayed presentation, but the overall mortality was not statistically different between the groups. In select patients presenting after 24 h from the time of perforation with hemodynamic stability and viable esophageal tissues, primary closure with local tissue coverage and adequate drainage appears to be preferable to both diversion and esophagectomy.

Perforations accompanied by esophageal malignancy or severe contamination are best treated with esophageal resection. Proximal drainage through a cervical esophagostomy (so-called "spit fistula") and a feeding tube are appropriate in anticipation of a delayed reconstruction. In the setting of hemodynamic instability or frank sepsis, the patient may not tolerate a lengthy procedure. In this situation, esophageal exclusion with proximal and distal diversion including pleural space and mediastinal drainage is preferred. Consideration can also be given to T-tube drainage in these challenging cases.

Bibliography

Orringer MB. Tumors, injuries, and miscellaneous conditions of the esophagus. In: Greenfield LJ, Mulholland MW, Oldham KT, et al. (eds.), *Surgery: Scientific Principles and Practice*, 3rd ed. Philadelphia, PA:Lippincott, Williams & Wilkins, 2001, 717–722.

Wang N, Razzouk AJ, Safavi A, et al. Delayed primary repair of intrathoracic esophageal perforation: is it safe? *J Thorac Cardiovasc Surg* 1996;111:114–122.

Younes Z, Johnson DA. The spectrum of spontaneous and iatrogenous esophageal injury. *J Clin Gastroenterol* 1999; 29:306–317.

Zumbro GL, Anstadt MP, Mawulawde K, et al. Surgical management of esophageal perforation: role of esophageal conservation in delayed perforation. *Am Surg* 2002;68: 36–40.

Zwischenberger JB, Alpard SK, Orringer MB. Esophagus. In: Townsend CM, Beauchamp DR, Evers MB, et al. (eds.), *Sabiston Textbook of Surgery: The Biological Basis of Modern Surgical Practice*, 16th ed. Philadelphia, PA: W.B. Saunders, 2001, 723–727.

CHAPTER 22

Stomach

Chad Wiesenauer and C. Max Schmidt

Questions

1. Which one of the following statements concerning vascular anatomy of the stomach is most accurate?

    (A) The left gastric artery mainly supplies the greater curvature of the stomach.

    (B) Occlusion of the left gastroepiploic and left gastric arteries is likely to result in clinically significant gastric ischemia.

    (C) Bleeding gastric ulcer is often the result of the ulcer's erosion posteriorly into the gastroduodenal artery.

    (D) Both the short gastric arteries and the left gastroepiploic artery arise from the splenic artery in the majority of patients.

2. All of the following are true concerning innervation of the stomach *except*:

    (A) Parasympathetic innervation of the liver is through the left vagus nerve.

    (B) Sensation of gastric pain occurs through both vagus nerves, right and left.

    (C) Only approximately 10% of the vagal trunk fibers are motor or secretory efferents, leaving the remaining 90% vagal fibers as afferent back to the central nervous system.

    (D) The left vagal trunk winds around the esophagus and rests close to the anterior surface of the esophagus after exiting the esophageal hiatus.

3. Which of the following best describes the effects that parietal cell vagotomy, also called highly selective or proximal gastric vagotomy, would cause in a previously normal stomach (no other procedure is performed in addition to the vagotomy)?

    (A) Both liquids and solids would empty significantly faster.

    (B) Both liquids and solids would empty significantly slower.

    (C) Liquids would empty significantly faster, whereas the emptying rate of solids would not change significantly.

    (D) Solids would empty significantly faster, whereas the emptying rate of liquids would not change significantly.

4. Which of the following statements concerning gastric acid secretion is false?

    (A) Truncal vagotomy, when performed successfully, will annihilate the cephalic phase of gastric acid secretion.

    (B) The peptide hormone gastrin is the most important mediator of gastric acid secretion in the gastric phase.

    (C) Histamine is a stimulator of acid secretion in parietal cells.

    (D) Parietal cells do not have receptors for somatostatin.

5. Which of the following statements concerning gastrin is most accurate?

    (A) Gastrin in high levels has been shown to cause gastric mucosal hypertrophy.

    (B) Glucose in a meal is one of the most potent stimulators of gastrin release.

    (C) Gastrin-secreting cells (G cells) are found only in the gastric antrum and pylorus.

    (D) Regular administration of antacids will suppress gastrin release as long as pH is kept consistently above 5.0.

    (E) Omeprazole, a proton pump inhibitor, can completely suppress gastrin secretion if taken regularly.

6. Which of the following events is not a step essential to the parietal cell's production of acid?

   (A) entry of one K^+ ion into the parietal cell for every H^+ released into the stomach lumen
   (B) hydrolysis of adenosine triphosphate (ATP) into adenosine diphosphate (ADP) and inorganic phosphate
   (C) inhibition of carbonic anhydrase
   (D) exchange of HCO_3^- for Cl^- at the basolateral membrane

7. Which of the following statements concerning *Helicobacter pylori* is most accurate?

   (A) *H. pylori* organisms bind only to gastric-type epithelium.
   (B) The majority of persons living in developed countries harbor *H. pylori* in their stomachs.
   (C) *H. pylori* organisms directly stimulate G cells to secrete gastrin, thereby increasing acid secretion.
   (D) Despite cure of *H. pylori* infection in patients with healed duodenal ulcer disease, over 25% will have a recurrence of ulcer disease.

8. Which one of the following statements concerning the use of sucralfate to treat gastric or duodenal ulcer disease is false?

   (A) Sucralfate is unsafe for the treatment of ulcer disease in the pregnant patient.
   (B) Sucralfate stimulates the production of mucus, prostaglandin E2, and bicarbonate.
   (C) Sucralfate, when given alone at a dose of 1 g four times daily, can achieve ulcer healing rates equivalent to the rates achieved by H2-receptor antagonists alone.
   (D) Sucralfate polymerizes in an acidic environment, allowing it to adhere to gastric or duodenal mucosa.

9. Please choose the least appropriate combination of diagnostic test for *H. pylori* and clinical situation.

   (A) Performing the urea breath test to detect the presence of *H. pylori* in a 28-year-old otherwise healthy male after undergoing 12 weeks of therapy with omeprazole, clarithromycin, and amoxicillin for biopsy-proven infection.
   (B) Performing antral mucosal biopsy and subsequent histologic examination for *H. pylori* organisms in a 63-year-old lady with a finding of diffuse gastritis while undergoing endoscopy for epigastric pain.

   (C) Performing endoscopy and antral mucosal biopsy, with subsequent histologic examination for *H. pylori* organisms, in a 35-year-old lady who had a "normal" endoscopy 2 weeks ago in which biopsies were not taken.
   (D) Performing repeat endoscopy with antral mucosal biopsy, with subsequent histologic examination and bacterial culture for sensitivity, in 28-year-old otherwise healthy male who has persistent *H. pylori* infection as detected by urea breath test, after 8 weeks of therapy with omeprazole, clarithromycin, and amoxicillin.

10. A 31-year-old man presents to the emergency room with nausea and vomiting, with two bouts of hematemesis, of approximately 24-h duration. He is currently in stable condition. His past medical history is significant for a previous admission 2 months ago for hematemesis, which resolved after endoscopic coagulation. He has been diagnosed by endoscopy with a duodenal ulcer twice within the past 2 years, and twice has failed medical therapy because of noncompliance with triple therapy (omeprazole, clarithromycin, amoxicillin). Endoscopy at this admission reveals no active bleeding and an inability to pass the endoscope past the edematous pylorus. The most appropriate therapy for this patient is as follows:

    (A) urgent surgical exploration of the upper abdomen with vagotomy and pyloroplasty to relieve this patient's pyloric obstruction
    (B) seven-day trial of nasogastric suction and intravenous H2-receptor antagonists
    (C) supportive care, including intravenous H2-receptor antagonists, for 24 h, then elective vagotomy and antrectomy
    (D) gastric lavage with at least 10 L of ice cold saline

11. Which of the following statements is most accurate concerning the three most commonly performed duodenal ulcer surgeries, parietal cell vagotomy, truncal vagotomy and pyloroplasty, and truncal vagotomy and antrectomy?

    (A) Parietal cell vagotomy has the lowest ulcer recurrence rate among the three.
    (B) Truncal vagotomy and antrectomy is technically the least demanding and is the quickest to perform in an emergency situation.

(C) Parietal cell vagotomy is associated with the lowest occurrence of postoperative dumping syndrome.

(D) All three procedures involve severing the celiac and hepatic divisions of the vagus nerves.

12. A 65-year-old man with past medical history significant only for diabetes mellitus, controlled by strict diet, and rheumatoid arthritis, for which he takes indomethacin, presents to his primary care physician with a several month history of slowly worsening, vague epigastric pain. Referral to an endoscopist reveals mild antral gastritis and a shallow 2 cm ulcer at the lesser curvature. The remainder of the endoscopic examination was unremarkable. Which of the following is least important in the care of this patient?

(A) endoscopic biopsies of the ulcer margin

(B) medical therapy to eradicate *H. pylori* after histologic analysis of antral biopsies demonstrate the organism

(C) referral to a surgeon, who will perform elective parietal cell vagotomy

(D) cessation of indomethacin

13. The above-mentioned patient is not referred to a surgeon, but instead is prescribed a 2-week regimen of triple drug therapy (omeprazole, clarithromycin, and amoxicillin) after histologic analysis proved infection with *H. pylori*. He also discontinued his indomethacin. The pathologist's report concerning the two biopsies of the ulcer reads "necrotic tissue with prominent lymphocytic infiltration." After completing the triple drug therapy, the patient is pain free. Six months later, the patient is seen at follow-up and complains of the same epigastric pain. Urea breath test reveals that he is no longer infected with *H. pylori*. He is again referred for endoscopy, which reveals a shallow 4 cm ulcer at the lesser curvature. Three biopsies are taken off the ulcer margins. The pathology report reads "gastric epithelium with possibly dysplastic features—cannot rule out malignancy." The next most appropriate step is

(A) repeat endoscopy with more ulcer margin biopsies

(B) distal gastrectomy, including entire ulcer with 4 cm margins

(C) distal gastrectomy, including entire ulcer with 4 cm margins, and truncal vagotomy

(D) parietal cell vagotomy and ulcer excision with 6 cm margins

14. A 21-year-old female college student presents to the local emergency room complaining of severe epigastric pain. This pain started suddenly about 2 h ago, while studying for her final exam in chemistry that will occur in 2 days. She states that it is the worst pain she has ever experienced, and it is not getting any better. She has no past medical history, and has not seen a doctor since she was 16. She has taken oral contraceptive pills for 5 years, and occasionally uses regular strength Tylenol for a headache. On your physical examination, she has a rigid abdomen and avoids movement. An upright chest radiograph ordered before you saw her shows a thin stripe of free air under the right hemidiaphragm. Your next step should be

(A) analgesia with intravenous narcotics and observation for 6 h

(B) computed tomography (CT) of the abdomen with PO and intravenous contrast

(C) left lateral decubitus radiograph to confirm your suspicion

(D) preparation of the patient for urgent surgery

15. Regardless of what step you chose in the previous question, it is now 6 h later and the patient is under a general anesthetic in your operating room. You perform an abdominal exploration through a vertical upper midline abdominal incision, and find a 2 mm hole in the anterior portion of the second portion of the duodenum. There is minimal inflammation, and very scant soiling of the peritoneum with intestinal fluid. Which of the following statements is most appropriate?

(A) This problem could not have been adequately diagnosed and treated laparoscopically.

(B) The procedure of choice is suture closure of the duodenal perforation and suturing a well-vascularized portion of omentum over the repair.

(C) Because of the small size of perforation and minimal contamination, this patient probably should have undergone observation.

(D) The procedure of choice is a suture closure of the duodenal perforation and suturing a well-vascularized portion of omentum over the repair, plus parietal cell vagotomy.

16. A 44-year-old male automotive industry worker has been a resident of the surgical intensive care unit since sustaining second and third degree burns to approximately 45% of his body 4 days ago—including his chest, face, and both arms. He remains ventilated and sedated, and is receiving tube feeds via a transoral duodenal feeding tube that has been shown to cross the pylorus on radiograph. He has undergone debridement with xenograft (porcine) skin grafting over his chest the day before, and remains in stable condition. He received four units of blood during and immediately after surgery. This morning, while performing regular nasogastric check for gastric reflux of tube feeds, the nurse notices a small amount of blood in the nasogastric return. A serum hemoglobin value was checked and returns 12.5, not significantly different from his post-transfusion hemoglobin yesterday evening. Now, 6 h later, the nurse reports copious amounts of blood from the nasogastric tube. The patient's stomach is lavaged with 6 L of warm saline via the nasogastric tube, and there does not appear to be any return of blood afterward. Which of the following is not an important step in this patient's management at this point?

(A) arrangement for urgent endoscopic examination

(B) procurement of 4 units of typed and crossmatched packed red blood cells

(C) intravenous vasopressin, 0.4 units/min, continued for 48 h

(D) laboratory evaluation of coagulation by measuring prothrombin time, activated partial thromboplastin time, and platelet count

17. Within 1 h of the stomach lavage, the nasogastric tube again returns copious, bright red blood. Coagulation tests return from the lab and are within normal limits. The stomach is again lavaged with warm saline to prepare for endoscopy, which reveals multiple bleeding points from the fundus and proximal body. The bleeding is too profuse to be managed endoscopically, despite several attempts of coagulation and epinephrine injection. The patient becomes mildly hypotensive and tachycardic, and his arterial oxygen saturation has fallen somewhat. A successful attempt at resuscitation is made with transfusion of 4 units of packed red blood cells, and the patient is currently normotensive and only slightly tachycardic (110 bpm). The most appropriate next step would be

(A) selective cannulation of the left gastric artery via interventional radiology techniques, with continuous infusion of vasopressin into the left gastric artery for 48 h

(B) surgical gastrotomy and oversewing of the bleeding gastric ulcers

(C) surgical devascularization of the stomach by ligating the left and right gastric and gastroepiploic arteries

(D) tamponade of the gastric ulcers with a Sengstaken-Blakemore tube

18. A 67-year-old male patient undergoes upper endoscopy as part of a workup for fecal occult hemoglobin. The only finding of this examination is a bulge, approximately 4 cm in diameter and only slightly protuberant, with a small, central dimple, on the anterior body of the stomach. Four biopsies are taken from different areas of this bulge. Pathologic examination of biopsy specimens reveals only normal gastric mucosa. A CT scan of the abdomen is obtained to better define this abnormality, and it reveals a discreet, 5 cm by 5 cm mass that appears to be entirely within the wall of the stomach body anteriorly (Fig. 22-1). There is no apparent lymphadenopathy. The patient undergoes elective abdominal exploration, and a distal gastrectomy with inclusion of the mass with 2 cm margins is performed with gastroduodenotomy. Pathologic histologic analysis reveals "interlacing bundles of elongated cells with spindle-shaped nuclei." Which of the following statements is true regarding this tumor?

(A) Enucleation would have been the preferred surgical therapy.

(B) Surgery would have been appropriately abandoned if abdominal exploration revealed three 0.5 cm liver metastases, proven by frozen section.

(C) Five-year survival for all presentations is greater than 80%.

(D) This tumor is relatively resistant to radiation therapy.

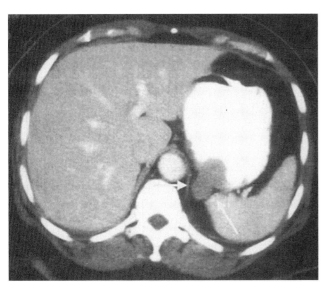

FIG. 22-1 Computed tomography scan of a lesion of the stomach.

pentagastrin reveals no black color within 10 min of instillation. Histologic examination of the biopsy specimens reveals intestinal metaplasia of gastric glands, a paucity of parietal cells, and an increase in the number of mucin cells usually seen. Which one of the following statements about this patient and his condition is false?

(A) There may be improvement in his symptoms and endoscopic findings on regularly taking cholestyramine.

(B) If unresponsive to medical therapy, his symptoms may be ameliorated by a Roux-en-Y procedure.

(C) Demonstration of gastric reflux on a nuclear medicine HIDA scan is pathognomonic of this condition.

(D) Performance of a parietal cell vagotomy would have been less likely to result in this particular complication.

19. A 55-year-old male patient, in whom you performed truncal vagotomy and antrectomy with gastroduodenostomy (Billroth I) because of recalcitrant duodenal ulcer disease 3 years ago, now presents with worsening epigastric pain. The pain is burning and almost always present, sometimes worsening with food. He has lost an estimated 30 lb and his primary care physician is no longer willing to prescribe narcotics for pain control until he is further evaluated. He has nausea but no episodes of vomiting. Of the following investigations, which one is the most important?

(A) measurement of serum gastrin level

(B) endoscopy with instillation of Congo red dye

(C) nuclear medicine ^{99m}Tc hepatic iminodiacetic acid (HIDA) scan

(D) trial of omeprazole (proton pump inhibitor) for 2 weeks

20. The patient undergoes upper endoscopy. Findings include mucosal erythema and friability throughout the remaining stomach, three small ulcers near the gastroduodenal anastomotic line with signs of recent hemorrhage, and a small pool of bile in the dependent stomach. Biopsies are taken of several sites of the stomach. Instillation of Congo red dye and intravenous

21. A 62-year-old man undergoes upper endoscopy for a suspected duodenal ulcer. He is found to not have any duodenal or gastric ulcer disease, and the only abnormal finding is mild antral gastritis. Three biopsies are taken of the antrum. On examination of the biopsy specimens, the pathologist's report reads "numerous spiral-shaped gram-negative organisms, presumably *H. pylori*, and multiple pockets of submucosal lymphoid tissue—cannot rule out low-grade lymphoma." The patient is referred to you for further management. The most appropriate therapy at this point is

(A) two-week regimen of clarithromycin and amoxicillin, followed by repeat endoscopic evaluation with deep antral biopsies 1 month after completion

(B) combined chemotherapy and radiation therapy

(C) generous antrectomy with frozen section evaluation of surgical margins

(D) parietal cell vagotomy, followed by repeat endoscopic evaluation with deep antral biopsies 1 month later

22. A 72-year-old man undergoes upper gastrointestinal barium study because of complaints of dull epigastric pain, nausea, vomiting, and weight loss. Upper endoscopy reveals a diffusely thickened stomach lining and biopsy shows high-grade lymphoma. A CT scan of the abdomen reveals a thickened stomach almost globally (Fig. 22-2). There is questionable perigastric lymph node involvement, but no apparent hepatic or splenic abnormalities. Which of the following statements concerning this patient and his disease is *incorrect*?

   (A) Immediate workup should include CT scan of the chest and pelvis, plus bone marrow biopsy.

   (B) On laparotomy, splenectomy is not indicated unless the spleen is grossly abnormal.

   (C) After subtotal gastrectomy, a microscopically positive margin at the duodenum warrants partial duodenectomy.

   (D) Most physicians recommend surgery as primary therapy if disease is limited to the stomach.

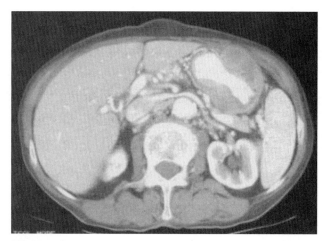

FIG. 22-2 Computed tomography scan of a patient with a gastric lesion.

23. A 45-year-old female patient is seen in your office for a 1 month follow-up visit after you performed omental patching, truncal vagotomy, and pyloroplasty to treat her perforated duodenal ulcer. She no longer has the burning epigastric pain that she experienced before her surgery, but complains to you of bloating and severe abdominal cramps soon after meals, followed by profuse diarrhea, sweating, and dizziness. These symptoms appeared shortly after she recovered from surgery, and have not gotten appreciably better in the month since surgery. She asks you for your advice about ameliorating this problem. You can correctly tell her all of the following *except*:

   (A) In most patients, these symptoms will improve significantly with minor modification of diet.

   (B) She should separate the ingestion of liquids from solids.

   (C) Regular administration of cholestyramine will likely prevent most of her symptoms.

   (D) None of the surgical treatments of this condition is uniformly successful.

24. You have just begun an open abdominal exploration on a 68-year-old Asian American man with biopsy-proven gastric adenocarcinoma. Previous endoscopy revealed a diffusely thickened area of mucosa about 10 cm in diameter at the body of the stomach without ulceration. CT revealed a thickened body wall and perigastric lymphadenopathy or tumor involvement. The spleen, pancreas, and liver appear normal. Endoscopic ultrasound revealed full involvement of the stomach wall with tumor. Which of the following statements about this patient and his disease is not true?

   (A) If superficial liver metatstases are found, this patient will likely achieve better palliation with symptom-directed endoscopic therapy than with gastric resection.

   (B) If the spleen is grossly normal, prophylactic removal of the spleen is not indicated in this patient.

   (C) If curative gastric resection is intended, a 6 cm margin of microscopically tumor-free, normal tissue is adequate.

   (D) Removing lymph nodes along the hepatoduodenal ligament, the root of the mesentery and the retropancreatic space is likely to improve survival in this patient.

25. Which of the following statements regarding gastric adenocarcinoma is true?

   (A) Premalignant conditions include infection with *H. pylori*, hyperplastic gastric polyps, chronic gastritis, and chronic alcohol abuse.

   (B) Mortality associated with total gastrectomy for gastric cancer is less than 10%.

   (C) Patients with metastatic gastric cancer are better served by surgical bypass because endoscopic techniques are not effective at relieving obstructive symptoms.

   (D) Japanese endoscopic screening programs have not been shown to improve survival for patients with gastric cancer.

26. Three days ago you performed a laparoscopic Roux-en-Y gastric bypass procedure on a 32-year-old male with a body mass index (BMI) of 45 kg/m². This patient has type II (adult onset) diabetes mellitus requiring insulin administration, degenerative joint disease in his knees, and echocardiographic evidence of moderate left ventricular dysfunction. He was administered prophylactic, intravenous cefoxitin at initiation of the procedure and 8 h after. During the night of postoperative day 2, he became progressively short of breath and is now receiving continuous positive airway pressure (CPAP) at 10 mmHg. His oxygen saturations improved from 85% on room air to 95% on 10 mmHg. You have just been informed that he now has a temperature of 38.8°C and his heart rate is 130 bpm. Physical examination of the chest reveals mild basilar crackles, and abdominal examination reveals mild discomfort with palpation. CT examination of the abdomen reveals atelectasis in the lung bases, but no apparent abdominal abnormalities. After CT scanning, the patient complains of abdominal pain and refuses to eat. On examination his abdomen is slightly more tender. Of the following, the best course of action would be

  (A) remove existing intravenous lines, culture the tips, draw blood cultures from a new line, check urine cultures, and start empiric cefoxitin

  (B) place a transoral intestinal feeding tube and slowly start administering tube feeds once the tip is confirmed to have crossed the pylorus

  (C) take this patient back to the operating room for open abdominal exploration

  (D) check arterial oxygen content, and intubate the patient if his PaO_2 is less than 60 mmHg

27. All of the following statements concerning surgical approaches to morbid obesity are true *except*:

  (A) Correction of morbid obesity improves insulin dependence, echocardiographic cardiac ventricular dysfunctions, and hypertension in over half of patients.

  (B) It is recommended that a Roux-en-Y gastric bypass incorporate a longer Roux limb (>60 cm) to enhance weight loss in patients with a BMI > 50 kg/m².

  (C) Roux-en-Y gastric bypass procedures result in more mean excess weight loss (MEWL) than either vertical banded gastroplasty (VBGP) or partial biliopancreatic division.

  (D) Menstruating women are at risk for iron-deficiency anemia after a Roux-en-Y gastric bypass.

28. Which of the following lesions is likely (greater than 50% chance) to fail medical and endoscopic therapy and require surgical intervention, assuming that the patient is hemodynamically stable and has not required blood transfusion?

  (A) An exposed, 4 mm pulsating vessel visualized endoscopically on the lesser curvature of the proximal stomach, in a 35-year-old man with no significant past medical history who presents with his first ever episode of hematemesis.

  (B) Two 2 cm linear tears, slowly oozing blood, seen in the mucosa of the lesser curvature approximately 1 cm distal from the gastroesophageal junction in a 45-year-old chronic alcohol abuser who presents with approximately 12 h of retching, vomiting, and hematemesis.

  (C) At least 10 small, slowly oozing mucosal erosions found diffusely in the body and antrum of a 66-year-old woman who has taken sulindac for osteoarthritis for the past 10 years, and presents after her first ever bout of hematemesis.

  (D) None of the above—all three patients' gastric lesions are likely to resolve after endoscopic and medical treatment.

29. Which of the following medical regimens against *H. pylori* is least likely to eradicate the organism?

  (A) omeprazole, clarithromycin, and metronidazole for 14 days

  (B) bismuth, omeprazole, metronidazole, and tetracycline for 14 days

  (C) ranitidine bismuth citrate, amoxicillin, and clarithromycin for 14 days

  (D) lansoprazole and amoxicillin for 14 days

Answers and Explanations

1. **(D)** The stomach is a very well-perfused organ, being supplied by several arteries and possessing a rich collateral network of both intramural and extramural arteries. Most of the blood supply is derived from the celiac trunk. The lesser curvature of the stomach is perfused superiorly by the left gastric artery, a direct branch off of the celiac artery, and inferiorly by the right gastric artery, a branch from either the hepatic artery (another direct branch off of the celiac) or more distally from the gastroduodenal artery. The greater curvature is perfused by the splenic artery (a branch off of the celiac) via its short gastric and left gastroepiploic artery branches. The left gastroepiploic in most individuals makes a direct collateralization with the right gastroepiploic artery, forming an arcade along the greater curvature. The right gastroepiploic artery derives from the gastroduodenal artery, ultimately from the celiac trunk via the hepatic artery, but it also receives oxygenated blood from the superior mesenteric artery via the pancreaticoduodenal arcade. Because of the extensive system of arterial collateralization, the stomach can be adequately perfused by only one primary artery. This often permits the surgeon to ligate all but one artery, including the hepatic artery, without significant risk to completely devascularizing the stomach. In fact, it is routine to ligate the left gastric and the left gastroepiploic arteries when using the stomach to replace a resected esophagus, leaving the right gastoepiploic artery as the main vessel to perfuse the mobilized stomach in the chest, with a smaller contribution by the right gastric artery.

Massive hemorrhage secondary to duodenal ulcer is often the result of erosion into the gastroduodenal artery, because of its position directly posterior to the first portion of the duodenum. Erosion of a gastric ulcer into the gastroduodenal artery is not common.

Bibliography

Cheung LY, Delcore R. Stomach. In: Townsend CM, Beauchamp RD, Evers BM, et al. (eds.), *Sabiston Textbook of Surgery*, 16th ed. Philadelphia, PA: W.B. Saunders, 2001, 837–838.

Clemente C. *Anatomy. A Regional Atlas of the Human Body*, 3rd ed. Malvern, PA: Lea & Febiger, 1987, 265–272.

Law S, Wong J. Esophagogastrectomy for carcinoma of the esophagus and gastric cardia, and the esophageal anastomosis. In: Baker RJ, Fischer JE (eds.), *Mastery of Surgery*, 4th ed. Philadelphia, PA: Lippincott, Williams & Wilkins, 2001, 813–827.

Mulholland, M. Gastric anatomy and physiology. In: Greenfield LJ, Mulholland MW, Oldham KT, Zelenock GB, Lillemoe KD (eds.), *Surgery: Scientific Principles and Practice*, 3rd ed. Philadelphia, PA: Lippincott, Williams & Wilkins, 2001, 737.

2. **(B)** There is both sympathetic and parasympathetic innervation to and from the stomach. The parasympathetic innervation occurs by way of the right and left vagus nerves. A distal esophageal plexus gives rise to these distinct right and left trunks, which descend the thorax alongside the esophagus and exit with it through the esophageal hiatus. The two vagal trunks rotate in a clockwise manner (looking cephalad to caudad), so that the left vagus nerve rests closely applied to the anterior portion of the gastroesophageal junction, whereas the right vagus rests somewhere between the esophagus and the anterior aorta, posterior to the gastroesophageal junction. The left vagus nerve gives off a hepatic division before branching to innervate the anterior gastric wall. This hepatic division passes through the lesser omentum to provide parasympathetic innervation to the liver and biliary tract. The right vagus nerve gives off a celiac division, which passes into the celiac plexus, and then innervates the posterior gastric wall. Only 10% of the total vagal fibers are motor or secretory efferents. The majority of vagal fibers transmit gastrointestinal information back to the central nervous system. The sympathetic innervation is derived from spinal segments T5 through T10. Preganglionic efferent fibers from the spine synapse within the right and left celiac ganglia to postganglionic fibers that then enter the stomach

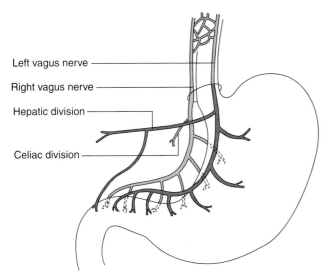

Left vagus nerve

Right vagus nerve

Hepatic division

Celiac division

FIG. 22-3 Vagal innervation of the stomach. Reproduced with permission from Greenfield LJ, Mulholland MW, Oldham KT, Zelenock GB, Lillemoe KD (eds.), *Surgery: Scientific Principles and Practice*, 3rd ed. Philadelphia, PA: Lippincott, Williams & Wilkins, 2001, 738–739.

alongside the vasculature. Afferent fibers from the stomach to the central nervous system pass without synapse from the stomach wall to the dorsal spinal roots. It is within these afferent sympathetic fibers that pain stimuli are transmitted back to the central nervous system (Fig. 22-3).

Bibliography

Cheung LY, Delcore R. Stomach. In: Townsend CM, Beauchamp RD, Evers BM, et al. (eds.), *Sabiston Textbook of Surgery*, 16th ed. Philadelphia, PA: W.B. Saunders, 2001, 838–839.

Mulholland, M. Gastric anatomy and physiology. In: Greenfield LJ, Mulholland MW, Oldham KT, Zelenock GB, Lillemoe KD (eds.), *Surgery: Scientific Principles and Practice*, 3rd ed. Philadelphia, PA: Lippincott, Williams & Wilkins, 2001, 738–739.

3. **(C)** Understanding the physiology of gastric emptying may help one to understand the appearance of postoperative side effects. When a meal enters the stomach, the fundus and body undergo a vagally-mediated receptive relaxation. This allows the normally collapsed stomach to expand, preventing intragastric pressure from rising greatly as it becomes filled with the meal. Liquids in the stomach are forced to empty primarily by increased intragastric pressure, normally created by low-amplitude tonic contractions of the fundus. The increased pressure gradient between the stomach and the lower pressure duodenum forces the liquids across the pylorus and out of the stomach. After parietal cell vagotomy, there is no

receptive relaxation, and intragastric pressure increases with the entry of the meal, whether liquid or solid. The relatively high intragastric pressure in this vagally denervated stomach forces liquids out at a greater rate than in the normal stomach. The emptying of solids is more dependent on the distal stomach. Strong ring contractions start in the midbody of the stomach and proceed toward the pylorus, propelling gastric contents against a closed pylorus. The pylorus closes 2–3 s before the arrival of the antral contraction ring. Continued pulsion and retropulsion mixes the solids with the liquids, and the antral contractions grind the solids into small particles. Solid particles that are 1 mm or smaller can then pass across the pylorus, along with liquids; larger particles do not normally pass. Since a properly performed parietal cell vagotomy leaves the vagal innervation to the distal stomach intact, the emptying of solids is unaffected.

Bibliography

Cheung LY, Delcore R. Stomach. In: Townsend CM, Beauchamp RD, Evers BM, et al. (eds.), *Sabiston Textbook of Surgery*, 16th ed. Philadelphia, PA: W.B. Saunders, 2001, 839–840.

Mulholland, M. Gastric anatomy and physiology. In: Greenfield LJ, Mulholland MW, Oldham KT, Zelenock GB, Lillemoe KD (eds.), *Surgery: Scientific Principles and Practice*, 3rd ed. Philadelphia, PA: Lippincott, Williams & Wilkins, 2001, 750.

4. **(D)** The regulation of gastric acid secretion is complex and involves several mediators. Parietal cells, responsible for secreting acid into the stomach lumen, are stimulated to produce acid by gastrin, histamine, and acetylcholine. Before food ever reaches the stomach, the sight, smell, or thought of food can stimulate gastric acid secretion. In this first phase of acid stimulation, the cephalic phase, vagal stimulation of the parietal cell causes it to secrete acid by releasing acetylcholine from nerve endings at or near the parietal cell's acetylcholine receptor. Because this phase is entirely dependent on vagal nerve transmission, a truncal vagotomy will prevent any effect on parietal cells, and the cephalic phase will be abolished. The second phase of acid stimulation, the gastric phase, begins once food enters the stomach. Both the presence of partially hydrolyzed food and the distension of the stomach stimulate the G cells of the antrum, pylorus, and duodenum to release gastrin. Gastrin is responsible for over 90% of meal-stimulated acid secretion. Enterochromaffin-like (ECL) cells and mast cells of the stomach also have receptors for gastrin. Gastrin stimulates them to release histamine, another potent stimulator of parietal cell acid secretion. Less is known about the third and final phase of acid stimulation, the

intestinal phase, in which small amounts of gastric juices are secreted in response to food entering the duodenum. In addition to stimulation of gastric acid secretion, there are mechanisms to inhibit the parietal cell from secreting acid. The vagus nerve, in addition to stimulating gastric acid secretion, has been shown to inhibit gastrin release also, thereby indirectly inhibiting parietal cell acid secretion. In addition to stimulatory receptors for gastrin, histamine, and acetylcholine, the parietal cell also has receptors for prostaglandin E2 and somatostatin, which when occupied cause inhibition of acid secretion. The most important inhibitor of acid secretion is actually a negative feedback mechanism in which gastrin-producing G cells are suppressed as the antral mucosa is exposed to acid. Gastrin production stops completely when the pH falls below 2.0, thus taking away the major stimulus for parietal cells to secrete acid.

Bibliography

Cheung LY, Delcore R. Stomach. In: Townsend CM, Beauchamp RD, Evers BM, et al. (eds.), *Sabiston Textbook of Surgery*, 16th ed. Philadelphia, PA: W.B. Saunders, 2001, 840–841.

Mulholland M. Gastric anatomy and physiology. In: Greenfield LJ, Mulholland MW, Oldham KT, Zelenock GB, Lillemoe KD (eds.), *Surgery: Scientific Principles and Practice*, 3rd ed. Philadelphia, PA: Lippincott, Williams & Wilkins, 2001, 744–747.

5. **(A)** The peptide hormone gastrin is very important in gastric physiology. Parietal cells, responsible for secreting acid into the stomach lumen, are stimulated to produce acid by gastrin, histamine, and acetylcholine. Gastrin is released from the G cells of the antrum, pylorus, and duodenum, and reaches the fundal parietal cells by way of the systemic circulation. The entrance of the meal into the stomach is the most important stimulus for gastrin release. Small peptides and amino acids are the most important stimulants; fat and glucose do not contribute to the release of gastrin. Gastric distension also stimulates gastrin release by activating cholinergic neurons that directly stimulate the G cells. Vagal cholinergic activity can also inhibit G cells, as shown by the hypergastrinemia that occurs after vagotomy. Gastrin release is subject to feedback inhibition, so that when the antral pH falls below 3.0, gastric release is suppressed, completely ceasing at pH below 2.0.

Gastric mucosa has been shown to hypertrophy when exposed to persistently high levels of gastrin, as seen in the Zollinger-Ellison's syndrome. This has not been shown to occur after either truncal or parietal cell vagotomy. The proton pump inhibitor drugs prevent the parietal cell from secreting acid. They do not suppress gastrin's release, and in fact often contribute to hypergastrinemia by raising the intraluminal pH of the stomach.

Bibliography

Cheung LY, Delcore R. Stomach. In: Townsend CM, Beauchamp RD, Evers BM, et al. (eds.), *Sabiston Textbook of Surgery*, 16th ed. Philadelphia, PA: W.B. Saunders, 2001, 840–841.

Mulholland M. Gastric anatomy and physiology. In: Greenfield LJ, Mulholland MW, Oldham KT, Zelenock GB, Lillemoe KD (eds.), *Surgery: Scientific Principles and Practice*, 3rd ed. Philadelphia, PA: Lippincott, Williams & Wilkins, 2001, 742–743.

6. **(C)** Acid production by the parietal cell ultimately occurs via a specialized ion transport system called the proton pump. This membrane-bound protein resides in the secretory canaliculus, so that H^+ ions released enter the stomach lumen. The proton pump is so named because it transports one H^+ ion (proton) into the lumen of the secretory canaliculus as it simultaneously transports one K^+ ion into the cell. The energy to drive this exchange against a very large electrical gradient comes from the hydrolysis of ATP into ADP and phosphate. In order to keep an ample supply of K^+ ion near the proton pump but on the luminal side, the parietal cell allows K^+ ions from the cytosol to diffuse across the cell membrane. Chloride ions also diffuse across the cell membrane from the cytosol to the lumen of the canaliculus. For every one H^+ ion transported into the lumen, there is an accompanying Cl^- ion to maintain electroneutrality. The supply of chloride ions comes from an exchange of Cl^- for HCO_3^- ions at the basolateral membrane. The bicarbonate (HCO_3^-) is produced by the enzyme carbonic anhydrase, which takes carbon dioxide and combines it with the excess OH^- ions (produced by the proton pump) to form HCO_3^-.

Bibliography

Mulholland M. Gastric anatomy and physiology. In: Greenfield LJ, Mulholland MW, Oldham KT, Zelenock GB, Lillemoe KD (eds.), *Surgery: Scientific Principles and Practice*, 3rd ed. Philadelphia, PA: Lippincott, Williams & Wilkins, 2001, 745–746.

7. **(A)** *H. pylori* is a gram-negative spiral bacterium whose natural habitat is the human stomach. It lives within an extracellular mucus layer, on the surface of gastric mucosa or gastric-type epithelium, such as gastric metaplasia in the duodenum, Barrett's esophagus, or Meckel's diverticulum. It produces large amounts of urease. *H. pylori* infection causes significant inflammatory responses that result in mucosal injury and possibly ulceration. Both basal and peak

acid output are increased in ulcer patients harboring *H. pylori*, and levels return to normal after eradication by antimicrobials. These abnormalities are likely because of *H. pylori*-induced hypergastrinemia. *H. pylori* infection indirectly activates mucosal inflammatory cells to release cytokines that stimulate gastrin release from the G cells.

The relation between infection with *H. pylori* and ulceration of the stomach and duodenum is quite strong. Several points reinforce this statement: (1) considering the combined data from more than 20 prospective studies, 94% of patients with duodenal ulcer and 84% of patients with gastric ulcer had *H. pylori* identified by endoscopic biopsy; (2) gastric metaplasia is very common around areas of duodenal ulceration, and *H. pylori* binds only to gastric-type epithelium (gastric metaplasia is a nonspecific response of the duodenal mucosa to injury); (3) antimicrobial eradication of *H. pylori* is just as effective in healing ulcers as are histamine type 2 (H2)-receptor antagonists; and (4) relapse of duodenal ulcer disease after antimicrobial therapy for *H. pylori* is preceded by reinfection of gastric mucosa with *H. pylori*. The incidence of *H. pylori* infection in the healthy person, in developed countries, is approximately 20%, and this increases with age. It is important to note that only a small fraction of these persons (about 1% per year) go on to develop ulcer disease, suggesting that other factors besides infection with *H. pylori* are important in ulcer disease.

Bibliography

Cheung LY, Delcore R. Stomach. In: Townsend CM, Beauchamp RD, Evers BM, et al. (eds.), *Sabiston Textbook of Surgery*, 16th ed. Philadelphia, PA: W.B. Saunders, 2001, 844–845.

Mulholland, M. Gastric anatomy and physiology. In: Greenfield LJ, Mulholland MW, Oldham KT, Zelenock GB, Lillemoe KD (eds.), *Surgery: Scientific Principles and Practice*, 3rd ed. Philadelphia, PA: Lippincott, Williams & Wilkins, 2001, 751–752.

8. **(A)** Sucralfate is the aluminum salt of sulfated sucrose. Sucralfate polymerizes in the acid milieu of the stomach and adheres to the mucosa and to any ulcer base. It stimulates the production of protective gastric mucus, prostaglandin E2, and bicarbonate. Sucralfate binds bile salts and inhibits the digestive action of pepsin. Sucralfate stimulates the proliferation of healthy epithelium at the margin of an ulcer. There is virtually no systemic absorption of sucralfate, and therefore sucralfate is safe for use in the pregnant patient. If taken correctly—1 g by mouth four times daily—sucralfate has been shown to be just as effective as ranitidine (an H2-receptor antagonist) at healing ulcer.

Bibliography

Lykkegaard Nielsen MC, Vagn Nielsen O, Moesgaard F. Ulcer healing after treatment with sucralfate emulsion or ranitidine: randomized controlled study in peptic ulcer disease. *J Clin Gastroenterol* 1998:10:377.

Mulholland, M. Gastric anatomy and physiology. In: Greenfield LJ, Mulholland MW, Oldham KT, Zelenock GB, Lillemoe KD (eds.), *Surgery: Scientific Principles and Practice*, 3rd ed. Philadelphia, PA: Lippincott, Williams & Wilkins, 2001, 756.

9. **(C)** There are many methods used commonly today to diagnose infection with *H. pylori*. The standard remains mucosal biopsy with histologic examination of the biopsy specimen for the organisms, with a reported sensitivity of 100% and specificity of 73%. There also exist rapid urease tests in which the biopsy specimen can be tested for the presence of urease activity, a characteristic of *H. pylori*. The "CLO test" (*Campylobacter*-like organism test) is an example of such a method. The rapid urease tests have been reported to have nearly 100% sensitivity and specificity. Culture of the biopsy specimen is not routinely performed because the organism is difficult to isolate in routine laboratories; however, if information is needed about the organism's antimicrobial sensitivity and resistance, culture of biopsy specimens for *H. pylori* should be performed by an experienced laboratory. In addition to tests on mucosal specimens, there exist two noninvasive methods to detect the organism. Serologic testing is available and is the method of choice as an initial screening test unless endoscopy is indicated for reasons other than diagnosis of *H. pylori*. These tests are quick, easy to perform, and relatively inexpensive, with a sensitivity of 85 and 79% specificity. Another noninvasive test is the urea breath test, in which urease activity is detected in the patient's inhaled breath after ingesting C^{14}- or C^{15}-labeled urea. This test has a reported sensitivity of 94 and 100% specificity. The breath test is the preferred method for diagnosing persistent infection after medical treatment.

In scenario A, the urea breath test is the method of choice to determine effectiveness of therapy. In scenario B, since the patient is already undergoing endoscopy for other reasons and gastritis has been observed, mucosal biopsy with either histologic examination or rapid urease test is certainly indicated. In scenario D, bacterial culture with subsequent determination of antimicrobial resistance and sensitivity is crucial to determine how to best treat this infection. In scenario C, the test of choice is the serologic test or possibly the urea breath test. The risks and cost of endoscopy are not justified to diagnose *H. pylori* when other, noninvasive tests are available.

Bibliography

Cheung LY, Delcore R. Stomach. In: Townsend CM, Beauchamp RD, Evers BM, et al. (eds.), *Sabiston Textbook of Surgery*, 16th ed. Philadelphia, PA: W.B. Saunders, 2001, 846.

Chua TS, Fock KM, Teo EK, et al. Validation of 13C-urea breath test for the diagnosis of *Helicobacter pylori* infection in the Singapore population. *Singapore Med J* 2002;43 (8):408–411.

Del Valle J, Cohen H, Laine L, et al. Acid peptic disorders. In: Yamada T, Alpers DH, Laine L, et al. (eds.), *Textbook of Gastroenterology*, 3rd ed. Philadelphia, PA: Lippincott, Williams & Williams, 1999, 1397–1400.

Mahachai V, Tangkijvanich P, Wannachai N, et al. Serodiagnosis of *Helicobacter pylori* infection by immunoblot assay. *Asian Pac J Allergy Immunol* 2000; 18(1):63–67.

10. **(B)** If left untreated, 10% of patients with duodenal ulcer will develop obstruction. Pyloric obstruction is indeed one of the four indications for operation on patients with duodenal ulcer: obstruction, hemorrhage, perforation, and intractability. Conservative therapy should, however, be attempted if possible. It is recommended that patients presenting with pyloric obstruction because of a swollen and inflamed pyloric channel, be admitted to the hospital and treated with nasogastric suction and intravenous H2-receptor antagonists for at least 7 days. Most patients' obstructions will clear within 1 week. If the obstruction has not cleared within 1 week with conservative therapy, then surgery is indicated. The procedure of choice in this situation is vagotomy, to definitively treat this patient's ulcer diathesis, and antrectomy. If conservative therapy is successful, there is still a chance that the patient will develop pyloric scarring and subsequent obstruction, even if the ulcer itself heals. Assuming that endoscopic biopsy excludes malignancy in this situation, the benign stricture can be dilated endoscopically in many cases, although the majority of these patients' symptoms will recur, requiring repeat dilations or surgical correction.

Lavaging the stomach with ice cold saline is not helpful in this patient with pyloric obstruction. It is also likely a poor choice in the patient with bleeding ulcer, because the cold fluid in the body's core can further cool an already cold and possibly coagulopathic patient.

Bibliography

Cheung LY, Delcore R. Stomach. In: Townsend CM, Beauchamp RD, Evers BM, et al. (eds.), *Sabiston Textbook of Surgery*, 16th ed. Philadelphia, PA: W.B. Saunders, 2001, 851.

Fisher WE, Brunicardi FC. Duodenal ulcer. In: Cameron JL (ed.), *Current Surgical Therapy*, 7th ed. St. Louis, MO: Mosby, 2001, 80–83.

Mulholland M. Duodenal ulcer. In: Greenfield LJ, Mulholland MW, Oldham KT, Zelenock GB, Lillemoe KD (eds.), *Surgery: Scientific Principles and Practice*, 3rd ed. Philadelphia, PA: Lippincott, Williams & Wilkins, 2001, 762.

11. **(C)** In the modern era of ulcer surgery, the old standard of subtotal gastrectomy has become quite rare, leaving the three most common procedures performed today: parietal cell vagotomy (also called proximal gastric vagotomy or highly selective vagotomy), truncal vagotomy and drainage, and truncal vagotomy and antrectomy. In truncal vagotomy, the vagus nerve trunks are divided as they lie along the intraabdominal esophagus, just above (proximal to) the branches of the hepatic (anterior vagus) and celiac (posterior vagus) divisions. To combat the gastric atony caused by vagotomy, the pyloric mechanism must be bypassed or destroyed, allowing the stomach to drain freely. This can be achieved by gastroduodenostomy (Billroth I) or gastrojejunostomy (Billroth II) bypass, or more frequently by pyloroplasty. The most commonly performed pyloroplasty is the Heineke-Mikulicz, but the slightly more elaborate Finney and Jaboulay pyloroplasties should be available in the ulcer surgeon's armamentarium in the case that there exists an extensively scarred or otherwise deformed duodenal bulb. One advantage of the truncal vagotomy and drainage procedure is that it is technically the least demanding of the three commonly performed procedures, and can therefore be performed quickly. The ideal application of this procedure is the patient with bleeding duodenal ulcer who will undergo an incision across the pylorus in order to oversew the bleeding vessel. Mortality of truncal vagotomy and drainage is midway between the other procedures at 0.5–1%. Ulcer recurrence rate is comparable to or slightly less than that of parietal cell vagotomy at 10%. The initial postoperative incidence of dumping is 10%, and this remains severe in 1%.

Truncal vagotomy and antrectomy obviously adds a distal gastric resection to the severing of the vagal trunks at the esophagus. A method of reconstruction of gastric and intestinal continuity must be chosen with this procedure, usually either gastroduodenostomy (Billroth I) or gastrojejunostomy (Billroth II). The preferred reconstruction for benign disease is gastroduodenostomy, avoiding the myriad of potential complications with gastrojejunostomy: duodenal stump leak, afferent loop obstruction, an additional suture or staple line, and so on; however, if extensive inflammation or deformity of the pylorus prevents the safe performance of a gastroduodenostomy, the gastrojejunostomy is a good alternative. The ulcer recurrence rate of the the truncal vagotomy and antrectomy is by far the lowest of the three procedures at 1–2%, but its mortality rate is the highest at 1–2%, hence its infrequent use relative to truncal vagotomy and drainage and parietal cell vagotomy. The dumping syndrome occurs in 10–15% of patients postoperatively, with 1–2% of patients exhibiting severe symptoms. Incidence of postoperative diarrhea is similar to that of truncal vagotomy and drainage (20–25%), with about 1–2% complaining of disabling diarrhea. Truncal vagotomy and antrectomy is the procedure of choice for treating prepyloric ulcers, because this type of ulcer does not respond as well to either parietal cell vagotomy or truncal vagotomy and drainage.

Parietal cell vagotomy is currently the most frequently performed elective surgery for duodenal ulcer disease worldwide. It is accomplished by disconnecting the nerves of Latarjet from the lesser curvature starting from a point 5 cm proximal to the gastroesophageal junction down to a point approximately 7 cm proximal to the pylorus. Division of these nerves should disconnect the parietal cell mass from the parasympathetic system. The hepatic and celiac divisions of the vagus trunks are not severed. Also spared are two or three branches of the each trunk to the pylorus and antrum ("the crow's foot"), thus preventing the need for drainage procedure. It is important to look for and sever the "criminal nerve" (Grassi's nerve), a branch of the posterior vagal trunk that branches high from the trunk and innervates the posterior fundus. Ulcer recurrence rates with parietal cell vagotomy are the highest among the three commonly performed procedures at 10–15%, but mortality is essentially nonexistent and occurrence of dumping and diarrhea are much lower than the truncal vagotomy procedures. As mentioned before, prepyloric ulcers do not respond as well to parietal cell vagotomy as do duodenal ulcers.

Bibliography

Cheung LY, Delcore R. Stomach. In: Townsend CM, Beauchamp RD, Evers BM, et al. (eds.), *Sabiston Textbook of Surgery*, 16th ed. Philadelphia, PA: W.B. Saunders, 2001, 848–850.

Mulholland, M. Duodenal ulcer. In: Greenfield LJ, Mulholland MW, Oldham KT, Zelenock GB, Lillemoe KD (eds.), *Surgery: Scientific Principles and Practice*, 3rd ed. Philadelphia, PA: Lippincott, Williams & Wilkins, 2001, 762.

12. (C)

13. (B)

Explanations 12 and 13

This patient has a gastric ulcer. In the general population, gastric ulcers occur at about one-third the frequency of duodenal ulcers. Similar to duodenal ulcers, gastric ulcers are associated with *H. pylori* colonization in 85–90% of patients. There is a classification system that groups benign gastric ulcers into five groups, according to their location and acid secretory status. Operative treatment strategy can also be generalized for each type.

Type I gastric ulcers usually occur along the lesser curvature. These ulcers are not associated with gastric acid hypersecretion, and in fact many patients with this type of gastric ulcer have low acid output. Type I ulcers are the most common type of benign gastric ulcer, occurring in about half of all patients with gastric ulcer. The elective procedure of choice is distal gastrectomy with inclusion of the ulcer. Reconstruction with a gastroduodenal anastomosis (Billroth I) is preferred, but a gastrojejunostomy (Billroth II) can be performed if the situation warrants it. Vagotomy is not routinely performed, as these ulcers are not associated with acid hypersecretion. Exceptions that might necessitate a vagotomy include a Billroth II anastomosis (an ulcerogenic procedure) and the absolute need to continue chronic use of nonsteroidal anti-inflammatory drugs (NSAIDs).

Type II gastric ulcer is a combination of two ulcers, one ulcer in the body of the stomach and another in the duodenum. The ulcer in the body often occurs on the lesser curvature, as in type I. These patients are often acid hypersecretors.

Type III gastric ulcer is a prepyloric ulcer, occurring within 3 cm of the pylorus. Like duodenal ulcers, these ulcers are often associated with acid hypersecretion. The elective procedure of choice for both type II and type III is truncal vagotomy and antrectomy with inclusion of the ulcer. Parietal cell vagotomy with ulcer excision in these types of gastric ulcers results in unacceptably high ulcer recurrence rates.

Type IV gastric ulcer occurs high on the lesser curvature, at or near the gastroesophageal junction. Similar to type I gastric ulcers, these ulcers are not associated with acid hypersecretion. Elective resection of these ulcers can be challenging. If the ulcer is more than 2 cm distal to the gastroesophageal junction, a distal gastrectomy can be performed with a vertical extension along the lesser curvature to include the ulcer. If the ulcer is closer to the gastroesophageal junction, a near-total gastrectomy may be considered with Roux-en-Y jejunal anastomosis. This procedure is associated with significant morbidity and mortality. If too risky to resect the ulcer, then an alternative is truncal vagotomy and antrectomy, leaving the ulcer intact and biopsying it. It is important to adequately exclude malignancy.

Type V gastric ulcer is an ulcer in any location of the stomach as a result of chronic use of NSAIDs, including aspirin. These patients often initially present with hemorrhage or perforation, warranting emergency surgical treatment. Obviously, therapy of type V gastric ulcer involves discontinuation of the offending agent.

Of course, most benign gastric ulcers are not treated initially with surgery. It is important to eradicate infection with *H. pylori*, and also to suppress acid hypersecretion if the type of ulcer warrants it. Antisecretory therapy is usually given for 12 weeks, with an additional 12 weeks if not completely successful at healing the gastric ulcer. One must be quite sure that malignancy has been adequately ruled out before attempting this additional 12 weeks of conservative therapy. Indications for elective operative intervention include failure of the gastric ulcer to heal after adequate medical therapy, a recurrence of gastric ulcer after an initial successful management, and an inability to exclude malignancy of the ulcer. Any ulcer larger than 3 cm should be suspected of harboring malignancy, and should undergo early operative excision.

In the clinical vignette, this gentleman was appropriately treated for an apparently benign, type I gastric ulcer, assuming that the endoscopic biopsies were considered adequate by the endoscopist and pathologist to eliminate the chance of malignant disease. Surgical management before a trial of medical therapy and cessation of NSAIDs is not the standard of care. At representation 6 months later, the physicians have demonstrated that he is *H. pylori*-free and he is no longer taking NSAIDs. The finding on endoscopy that the ulcer is now 4 cm in diameter is worrisome for malignancy, as is the finding of dysplasia on histologic examination of ulcer margin biopsies. At this point, surgery is indicated not only because of the increase in the ulcer size after adequate medical therapy, but because malignant disease cannot be excluded. The appropriate elective operation is distal gastrectomy with inclusion of the ulcer. There is no indication for an acid-suppressing procedure in this situation.

Bibliography

Cheung LY, Delcore R. Stomach. In: Townsend CM, Beauchamp RD, Evers BM, et al. (eds.), *Sabiston Textbook of Surgery*, 16th ed. Philadelphia, PA: W.B. Saunders, 2001, 844.

Conter RL, Kauffman GL Jr. Benign gastric ulcer and stress gastritis. In: Cameron JL (ed.), *Current Surgical Therapy*, 7th ed. St. Louis, MO: Mosby, 2001, 77–70.

Mulholland M. Duodenal ulcer. In: Greenfield LJ, Mulholland MW, Oldham KT, Zelenock GB, Lillemoe KD (eds.), *Surgery: Scientific Principles and Practice*, 3rd ed. Philadelphia, PA: Lippincott, Williams & Wilkins, 2001, 762–763.

14. **(D)**

15. **(B)**

Explanations 14 and 15

This patient has a duodenal perforation. The lifetime risk of perforation in an untreated duodenal ulcer is 10%, and perforation can occur without any preceding symptoms of duodenal ulcer (epigastric pain, bleeding). The classic presentation is an acute onset of severe pain, followed by immediate signs of peritonitis as gastric and duodenal fluids irritate the peritoneum. The diagnostic procedure of choice is an upright chest radiograph or left lateral decubitus radiograph, which will show free air in approximately 80% of patients with perforation. An upper gastrointestinal contrast study (performed with water-soluble contrast) may demonstrate the perforation if the diagnosis is still in question after negative chest or decubitus radiographs. Perforation of a duodenal ulcer is a strong indication for urgent surgical management. Delaying surgical treatment for more than 12 h after presentation results in increased complication rates, increased hospital stay, and increased mortality. Therefore, observation with intravenous narcotics is contraindicated in the acutely perforated patient described above. (There are reports of nonoperative management in patients several days after perforation, with contrast radiographic evidence of perforation closure.)

The surgical procedure of choice is suture oversewing of the perforation and placement of a well-vascularized portion of omentum over that suture line. The omentum can be fixed by separate sutures or by using the tails of the previously placed sutures to fix the omentum in place. The decision to add an antiacid procedure depends both on the presentation of the patient and on his or her ulcer history. If the patient has no history of ulcer disease, as in the patient described above, there is no indication to perform an antiacid procedure. In this situation, oversewing and omental patch is adequate treatment of the perforation, and proper diagnosis and medical therapy of ulcer disease can be performed once the patient recovers from surgery. This is also true of the patient with NSAID-induced ulcer perforation, in which cessation of the offending agent should be adequate therapy. If the patient does have a significant history of ulcer disease, then a definitive antiacid procedure should be performed, provided that three criteria are met: (1) there is no preoperative shock, (2) the perforation occurred less than 48 h previous to surgery, and (3) life-threatening medical problems do not coexist. If any of these criteria are not met, the definitive antiacid procedure should be omitted.

In the hands of an experienced laparoscopist, duodenal perforation can be effectively diagnosed, sutured and patched with omentum by laparoscopic techniques. In addition, acid-reducing procedures can be performed by surgeons with advanced laparoscopic skills.

Bibliography

Boey J, Wong J, Ong GB. A prospective study of operative risk factors in perforated duodenal ulcers. *Ann Surg* 1982;195(3):265–269.

Cheung LY, Delcore R. Stomach. In: Townsend CM, Beauchamp RD, Evers BM, et al. (eds.), *Sabiston Textbook of Surgery*, 16th ed. Philadelphia, PA: W.B. Saunders, 2001, 851.

Conter RL, Kauffman GL Jr. Benign gastric ulcer and stress gastritis. In: Cameron JL (ed.), *Current Surgical Therapy*, 7th ed. St. Louis, MO: Mosby, 2001, 82.

Mulholland M. Duodenal ulcer. In: Greenfield LJ, Mulholland MW, Oldham KT, Zelenock GB, Lillemoe KD (eds.), *Surgery: Scientific Principles and Practice*, 3rd ed. Philadelphia, PA: Lippincott, Williams & Wilkins, 2001, 761–762.

Svanes C, Lie RT, Svanes K, et al. Adverse effects of delayed treatment for perforated peptic ulcer. *Ann Surg* 1994;220 (2):168–175.

16. (C)

17. (A)

Explanations 16 and 17

Stress gastritis occurs most often in patients who have sustained severe burns, trauma, hemorrhagic shock, sepsis, or respiratory failure, and therefore is not uncommon in surgical intensive care units. The ulcers are usually multiple and superficial, occurring most frequently in the fundus. They start to occur within as little as 12 h after the injury or insult. The exact mechanisms responsible for stress gastritis are as yet unknown, but most experts agree that mucosal ischemia is the common denominator. The diagnosis is often suspected on detection of blood from nasogastric aspirates or an otherwise unexplained drop in hematocrit.

The initial treatment step should be lavage of the stomach with saline. This serves to fragment blood clots, prevent gastric distension, and wash out harmful bile salts and pancreatic juices that may have refluxed into the stomach. There is disagreement on the temperature of the lavage solution. Chilled saline was traditionally used, probably in an attempt to constrict vessels, but some investigators are opposed to using cold solutions in a central body cavity for fear of lowering the temperature in an already sick, potentially coagulopathic patient. The majority of bleeding gastritis will cease after this relatively simple management.

Regardless of whether the bleeding arrests or not, the next logical step is endoscopy, to both diagnose the problem and assess severity, and also to definitively treat the gastric erosions with a number of techniques, including heater probe, injection of epinephrine, and laser or electrocoagulation. At this point in the management, coagulation parameters should be checked and corrected if necessary. It would also be prudent to arrange for readily available blood products for the critically ill patient. Lavage of the stomach before endoscopy is an important step, serving to wash out gastric contents and blood to enable adequate visualization. Endoscopy is effective in permanent hemostasis in over 90% of patients with stress gastritis, but may fail if there is profuse bleeding or many ulcerations. In this situation, endoscopy is abandoned and the patient taken to the interventional radiology suite. If the left gastric artery can be selectively cannulated, a continuous infusion of vasopressin for up to 72 h is likely to effectively stop the bleeding. An alternative to continuous vasopressin is embolization of the left gastric artery. If interventional radiology techniques are either unsuccessful or unavailable, then surgery is warranted to stop the bleeding.

There exist no prospective clinical trials that determine what surgical procedure is best to perform. Long gastrotomy with oversewing of ulcers, with or without truncal vagotomy and either pyloroplasty or antrectomy, depending on the stability of the patient, is likely the least morbid operation, but any combination of these has a significant risk of recurrent hemorrhage. More aggressive procedures trade higher morbidity and mortality for lower recurrence rates, and include subtotal gastrectomy and gastric devascularization (ligation of right and left gastric arteries plus gastroepiploic arteries). If bleeding is diffuse or a previous attempt at surgical hemostasis has failed, total gastrectomy may be the only option.

Because more than 50% of patients at risk for stress gastritis will develop it, prophylaxis is the key. The "no acid-no ulcer" dictum has some truth in stress gastritis, because it appears that acid production is necessary for its development. It has been shown that maintaining gastric pH above 3.5 is effective prophylaxis against gastritis. How best to achieve this is still a subject of debate. Antacids, intravenous H2-receptor antagonists and sucralfate have all shown ability to prevent stress gastritis in the critically ill patient with essentially equal efficacy. Some investigators prefer the use of sucralfate, because acid-reducing agents may increase the risk of nosocomial pneumonia by favoring growth of gram-negative organisms in the more neutral stomach environment. Data supporting or rejecting this are mixed in the literature.

The Sengstaken-Blakemore tube is a transoral, dual-balloon device used to tamponade bleeding esophageal varices, and has no role in the treatment of gastric ulcers.

Bibliography

Cheung LY, Delcore R. Stomach. In: Townsend CM, Beauchamp RD, Evers BM, et al. (eds.), *Sabiston Textbook of Surgery*, 16th ed. Philadelphia, PA: W.B. Saunders, 2001, 854–855.

Conter RL, Kauffman GL Jr. Benign gastric ulcer and stress gastritis. In: Cameron JL (ed.), *Current Surgical Therapy*, 7th ed. St. Louis, MO: Mosby, 2001, 79–80.

Mulholland M. Duodenal ulcer. In: Greenfield LJ, Mulholland MW, Oldham KT, Zelenock GB, Lillemoe KD (eds.), *Surgery: Scientific Principles and Practice*, 3rd ed. Philadelphia, PA: Lippincott, Williams & Wilkins, 2001, 764–766.

18. **(D)** Gastrointestinal stromal tumors (GISTs) can appear anywhere in the digestive tract, from esophagus to colon, but are most frequently found in the stomach. These were originally called leiomyoma or leiomyosarcoma, reflecting the belief that they were of smooth muscle tumor origin. More recent studies and more elaborate immunohistochemical analyses have shown that there are multiple possible origins of the cells comprising GISTs, including Schwann cells, enteric glial cells, perineural cells, and intestinal pacemaker cells. They can be asymptomatic and found incidentally, or can present with symptoms such as bleeding, obstruction, nonspecific pain, or palpable mass. Bleeding occurs most frequently in larger GISTs, when the overlying mucosa ulcerates.

On endoscopy, they are usually described as an extrinsic bulge, possibly with umbilication or ulceration of the overlying mucosa. Routine endoscopic biopsies are likely to reveal only normal gastric mucosa, and even intentionally deep biopsies have only a 50% diagnostic yield. Upper gastrointestinal contrast studies often show only an extrinsic mass

with intact or ulcerated overlying mucosa. Abdominal CT can better define the total size of the mass and determine if there is any extragastric extension. CT-guided biopsy can often be performed, but seldom contributes to the preoperative management because biopsy—whether CT-guided or endoscopic—rarely is able to determine benign versus malignant disease. In fact, there is no consensus on what defines benign versus malignant GIST. One proposed method involves number of mitotic figures per high-powered field on light microscopy, with benign being defined as <5 mitotic figures, intermediate as 6–10 mitotic figures, and malignant as >10 mitotic figures.

Unfortunately, there are reports of metastases occurring after complete resection of GISTs with no mitotic figures. If a gastric GIST is discovered incidentally on laparotomy, it should be excised with a margin of 2–3 cm of normal gastric tissue. This is also the procedure to be performed if the diagnosis is known or suspected preoperatively. Because of the uncertainty of malignancy, these should never be enucleated. Lymphadenectomy is not indicated, as these tumors most often metastasize hematogenously. Distant metastases are discovered at presentation in less than 20% of patients. If metastases are discovered, and the primary GIST can be safely removed, that primary should be excised to prevent complications of bleeding and obstruction. Radiation has not proved beneficial in these tumors, and chemotherapy, although there are some reports of response, has not shown any increase in survival. Survival is reported to be 53% at 5 years for gastric GISTs. When asymptomatic tumors are diagnosed preoperatively, they should undergo surgical excision if they are greater than 3 cm in any dimension, but it is unclear how best to treat smaller, asymptomatic GISTs.

Bibliography

Cheung LY, Delcore R. Stomach. In: Townsend CM, Beauchamp RD, Evers BM, et al. (eds.), *Sabiston Textbook of Surgery*, 16th ed. Philadelphia, PA: W.B. Saunders, 2001, 867–869.

Lillemoe KD, Efron DT. In: Cameron JL (ed.), *Current Surgical Therapy*, 7th ed. St. Louis, MO: Mosby, 2001, 112–117.

19. **(B)**

20. **(C)**

Explanations 19 and 20

There are multiple etiologies to epigastric pain after surgery to correct ulcer disease, including but not limited to gastric outlet obstruction, pancreatico-biliary origins, gastroesophageal reflux, recurrent ulcer because of retained antrum or Zollinger-Ellison's syndrome, and alkaline reflux gastritis. This patient has alkaline reflux gastritis. The reflux of duodenal contents occurs to some extent in normal persons, and often becomes worse when the pylorus is either destroyed or bypassed. It is most commonly seen after a gastrojejunostomy (Billroth II) anastomosis, but it can become symptomatic even in the unoperated patient. Symptoms commonly include constant, burning epigastric pain that is made worse with eating; nausea; and vomiting of bitter, bilious material. The vomiting does not relieve the pain, as seen in the afferent loop syndrome. The combination of acid, bile, and pancreatic juices is well known to produce gastric mucosal injury. Bile acids themselves erode the protective mucosal barrier when they are allowed to remain in content with gastric mucosa for extended times.

Diagnosis of alkaline reflux gastritis should be made by excluding all other causes. A nuclear medicine gastric emptying study can demonstrate gastric outlet obstruction if present. Serum testing for gastrin levels will rule out Zollinger-Ellison's syndrome. The most useful test is upper endoscopy. This can effectively diagnose gastroesophageal reflux, can detect recurrent ulceration, can biopsy for *H. pylori* colonization, and can directly visualize the enterogastric reflux of bile into the stomach. Stomachs seriously affected by alkaline reflux gastritis will reveal a friable, erythematous mucosa. Histologic examination of damaged gastric mucosa will reveal intestinal metaplasia of gastric glands, a loss of parietal cells, and an increase in the density of mucin cells. Further confirmation of the diagnosis of alkaline reflux can be made with a HIDA scan, in which the radiolabeled ^{99m}Tc HIDA is injected intravenously and then secreted in the bile. An external scintigraphy device can quantitate how much of the bile is refluxed into the stomach. This test is not pathognomonic, however, because even normal persons demonstrate some bile reflux.

Medical therapy for alkaline reflux gastritis should include acid reduction if necessary, and eradication of *H. pylori* if necessary. Bile-absorbing agents like cholestyramine are often useful, as are promotility agents such as erythromycin. If medical therapy fails, then surgical correction is warranted. Many procedures have been attempted and are still performed to correct alkaline reflux, but the most commonly performed today is Roux-en-Y diversion of the alkaline stream away from the stomach. This reconstruction is inherently ulcerogenic, so if an acid-reducing procedure was not originally performed, a truncal vagotomy and antrectomy should be strongly considered in addition. Also, at least 10–15% of patients suffer from delayed gastric emptying after Roux-en-Y procedure, so a preoperative nuclear medicine gastric emptying study is useful to identify those patients who have significant preexisting problems. In these patients, serious consideration should be given to extensively resecting the remaining stomach. An alternative procedure to the standard Roux-en-Y involves converting the original procedure to a gastroduodenostomy (Billroth I). Then, the common bile duct is disconnected from the duodenum and reanastomosed to a newly-created Roux-en-Y limb, diverting the alkaline bile at least 45–60 cm from the stomach. Results with this technique have been good, with better gastric emptying compared to standard Roux-en-Y.

Congo red is a topical indicator dye that turns black when exposed to a pH less than 3.0. When instilled endoscopically, gastric mucosa that has acid-secreting capability will turn visibly black within 5 min of intravenous pentagastrin injection, thus identifying any gastric mucosa that is vagally innervated.

Parietal cell vagotomy, because it does not destroy or bypass the pylorus, has almost no incidence of alkaline reflux gastritis postoperatively.

Bibliography

Cheung LY, Delcore R. Stomach. In: Townsend CM, Beauchamp RD, Evers BM, et al. (eds.), *Sabiston Textbook of Surgery*, 16th ed. Philadelphia, PA: W.B. Saunders, 2001, 853–854.

Madura JA. Primary bile reflux gastritis: which treatment is better, Roux-en-Y or biliary diversion? *Am Surg* 2000; 66(5):417–423.

Madura JA. Postgastrectomy problems: remedial operations and therapy. In: Cameron JL (ed.), *Current Surgical Therapy*, 7th ed. St. Louis, MO: Mosby, 2001, 89–93.

Madura JA, Grosfeld JL. Biliary diversion: a new method to prevent enterogastric reflux and reverse the roux stasis syndrome. *Arch Surg* 1997;132(3):245–249.

Mulholland M. Duodenal ulcer. In: Greenfield LJ, Mulholland MW, Oldham KT, Zelenock GB, Lillemoe KD (eds.), *Surgery: Scientific Principles and Practice*, 3rd ed. Philadelphia, PA: Lippincott, Williams & Wilkins, 2001, 764.

21. (A)

22. (C)

Explanations 21 and 22

Malignant lymphoma is the second most common malignant tumor of the stomach at 1–5% of all gastric malignancies. Most gastric lymphomas, however, are actually secondary to systemic lymphomatous disease.

Gastric involvement occurs in at least 17% of patients with systemic lymphoma (50% at necropsy). A major predisposing factor to primary gastric lymphoma is mucosa-associated lymphomatous tissue (MALT). The gastric submucosa does not normally contain lymphoid tissue. These small Peyer's patch-like lymphoid aggregates are believed to occur in response to chronic infection with *H. pylori*, and in fact *H. pylori* infection occurs in more than 90% of patients with primary gastric lymphoma. The importance of this association is demonstrated by the fact that antibiotic eradication of *H. pylori* results in complete regression of MALT in 70–100% of cases, and some early low-grade gastric lymphomas also completely regress with only antibiotic therapy.

Symptoms of lymphoma are nonspecific and include nausea, vomiting, vague epigastric pain, weight loss, and possible bleeding and obstruction. Diagnosis can be suspected by CT scan of the abdomen or upper gastro intestinal contrast study, but endoscopy is considered essential. The appearance of MALT may be completely normal. Higher-grade lymphomas often appear as thickened mucosa with stellate ulcerations, most often in the antrum. Because overlying mucosa is often normal, deep biopsies are necessary. Treatment of MALT should be an initial trial of antibiotic eradication of *H. pylori*. If a higher-grade lymphoma is suspected, initial workup should include a search for systemic lymphomatous disease, because the treatment of systemic disease should include combination of chemo- and radiation therapy. Primary surgical therapy is often curative if the disease is limited to the submucosa of the stomach. Frozen section analysis of the margins is essential, because gastric lymphoma spreads by submucosal and direct extension. Splenectomy is not necessary unless there is direct extension involvement or the organ is grossly abnormal. Postoperative radiation is recommended only for residual disease. It is so effective that resection margins found to be microscopically positive do not predict local recurrence if radiation is administered postoperatively. In fact, if duodenal or esophageal extension is discovered on gastric resection, it is best to not perform extensive resections of these organs and to instead administer postoperative radiation. Although some physicians recommend chemotherapy and radiation as primary therapy to gastric lymphoma, most studies have shown that surgically resected patients fare better then those treated with chemo- and radiation therapy.

Bibliography

Cheung LY, Delcore R. Stomach. In: Townsend CM, Beauchamp RD, Evers BM, et al. (eds.), *Sabiston Textbook of Surgery*, 16th ed. Philadelphia, PA: W.B. Saunders, 2001, 865–867.

Mulholland M. Gastric neoplasms. In: Greenfield LJ, Mulholland MW, Oldham KT, Zelenock GB, Lillemoe KD (eds.), *Surgery: Scientific Principles and Practice*, 3rd ed. Philadelphia, PA: Lippincott, Williams & Wilkins, 2001, 782–783.

Palmer Smith J. Adenocarcinoma and other tumors of the stomach. In: Wolfe MM (ed.), *Therapy of Digestive Disorders*. Philadelphia, PA: W.B. Saunders, 2000, 200–201.

Pierie JEN, Ott MJ. Gastric cancer. In: Cameron JL (ed.), *Current Surgical Therapy*, 7th ed. St. Louis, MO: Mosby, 2001, 110.

23. **(C)** The dumping syndrome occurs to some extent after any gastric operation, with a very wide range of occurrence depending on the extent and type of procedure. Parietal cell vagotomy has only a 1% occurrence, whereas dumping occurs in over half of partial gastrectomy patients. The Billroth II reconstruction results in a higher incidence than the Billroth I. There are two distinct forms of dumping, early and late. Early dumping usually occurs within 30 min of a meal. Gastrointestinal symptoms include fullness, nausea, vomiting, abdominal cramps, bloating, and diarrhea. Vasomotor symptoms include diaphoresis, weakness, dizziness, flushing, paplitations, blurry vision, and tachycardia. It is believed that destruction of the stomach's reservoir capacity results in the rapid delivery of hyperosmolar contents into the duodenum, and extracellular fluid shifts into the intestinal lumen to restore isotonicity. This causes an acute decrease in intravascular volume, and this is the supposed cause of the vasomotor symptoms. Humoral substances such as serotonin, neurotensin, and vasoactive intestinal peptide may also contribute to the vasomotor substances. Late dumping occurs less frequently than early dumping. Vasomotor symptoms of diaphoresis, tachycardia, weakness, and drowsiness follow a meal by 1–3 h. It is believed that late dumping is caused by an exuberant outpouring of enteroglucagon in response to the rapid delivery of carbohydrates to the small intestine, causing an excessive secretion of insulin from the pancreas. The resultant hypoglycemia is responsible for the symptoms of late dumping.

The good news is that only 1% of patients who experience dumping of either kind will not improve with the passage of time and small changes in diet. Dietary management includes the separation of liquids and solids, decreasing liquid intake with meals, decreasing the amount of carbohydrates in meals, and avoiding extra salt. Octreotide, administered subcutaneously before meals, has been shown to improve dumping symptoms. This effect likely both because the somatostatin analogue octreotide acts as a splanchnic pressor and because it acts to inhibit intestinal transit time, peak insulin release, and the release of several intestinal vasoactive peptides. In the small number of patients failing dietary and medical management, several operations have been proposed to ameliorate dumping syndrome. Unfortunately, none has proved satisfactory. The most widely used procedure is Roux-en-Y gastrojejunostomy, but there is insufficient evidence to recommend it as the standard of care. Alternatives include reversal of pyloroplasty and placement of isoperistaltic or reversed (antiperistaltic) segments of jejunum between the gastric remnant and the duodenum in an effort to slow intestinal transit.

Cholestyramine, a bile acid chelator, has not been shown to be effective in ameliorating the symptoms of dumping syndrome.

Bibliography

Cheung LY, Delcore R. Stomach. In: Townsend CM, Beauchamp RD, Evers BM, et al. (eds.), *Sabiston Textbook of Surgery*, 16th ed. Philadelphia, PA: W.B. Saunders, 2001, 852–853.

Fisher WE, Brunicardi FC. Duodenal ulcer. In: Cameron JL (ed.), *Current Surgical Therapy*, 7th ed. St. Louis, MO: Mosby, 2001, 84.

Madura JA. Postgastrectomy problems: remedial operations and therapy. In: Cameron JL (ed.), *Current Surgical Therapy*, 7th ed. St. Louis, MO: Mosby, 2001, 89–90.

Mulholland M. Duodenal ulcer. In: Greenfield LJ, Mulholland MW, Oldham KT, Zelenock GB, Lillemoe KD (eds.), *Surgery: Scientific Principles and Practice*, 3rd ed. Philadelphia, PA: Lippincott, Williams & Wilkins, 2001, 764.

24. (D)

25. (B)

Explanations 24 and 25

Gastric adenocarcinoma represents more than 90% of gastric malignancies. The incidence in the United States has been declining for many decades, but remains quite high in such geographically and ethnicly diverse countries as Japan, Costa Rica, Romania, Portugal, and Chile. Several predisposing factors have been identified, including infection with *H. pylori* (threefold risk of developing gastric adenocarcinoma), presence of adenomatous gastric polyps, and chronic gastritis. Gastric polyps of the hyperplastic type are benign, and do not predispose to gastric cancer, but adenomatous gastric polyps can follow the same progression as their colonic counterparts and become dysplastic, carcinoma *in situ*, and finally invasive gastric

adenocarcinoma. Chronic alcohol intake has not shown a correlation with gastric adenocarcinoma.

Although the incidence of gastric adenocarcinoma correlates with diets high in nitrates, nitrites, and salt, there is no convincing evidence that any dietary component predisposes to gastric adenocarcinoma. Gastric adenocarcinoma is difficult to detect in early stages because of a paucity of symptoms. Later stages tend to cause complaints such as constant pain, anorexia, weight loss, nausea, and possibly occult blood loss. In Japan, where the incidence of gastric cancer is very high, screening endoscopy programs have led to improved survival in the 0.12% of screened patients identified because of discovery of cancers at earlier stage. Although screening is not economically justifiable in the United States, endoscopy is the diagnostic procedure of choice because of the ability to biopsy lesions (98% accuracy). Upper gastrointestinal contrast study with both air and barium is also useful, with 90% accuracy in diagnosis (Figs. 22-4 and 22-5).

There are two distinct types of gastric adenocarcinoma, intestinal and diffuse. In the intestinal type the malignant cells form glands. This type tends to metastasize hematogenously. The intestinal type is most commonly seen in those patients with a predisposing factor for gastric adenocarcinoma (geography, gastritis, and so on). The diffuse type is characterized by loosely adherent cells that do not form glands. This type spreads lymphatically and often presents with intraperitoneal metastases. The prognosis for diffuse type is worse than for intestinal.

The two surgical procedures most commonly performed for gastric adenocarcinoma are distal

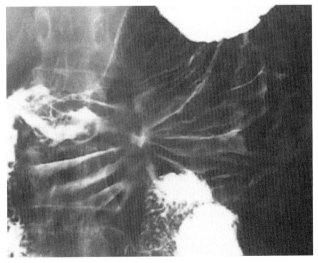

FIG. 22-4 Barium upper gastrointestinal study demonstrating a polypoid type of gastric adenocarcinoma.

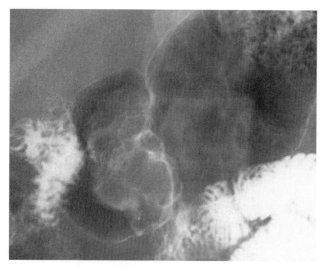

FIG. 22-5   Barium upper gastrointestinal study demonstrating an ulcerative gastric adenocarcinoma.

subtotal gastrectomy for distal cancers and total gastrectomy for large or more proximal cancers. Very proximal cancers warrant esophagogastrectomy in order to achieve the mandatory 6 cm margin of normal tissue. This margin is necessary because of the ability of gastric adenocarcinoma, especially the diffuse type seen more commonly in the United States, to spread intramurally via the extensive lymphatic network of the stomach. Microscopic evidence of residual tumor at the margins portends a very high rate of recurrence and poor survival.

Although in the past total gastrectomy has carried with it a prohibitively high mortality, with good nutritional support current mortality is reported at 3–7% in gastric cancer patients. Unless grossly involved, neither removal of the spleen nor the pancreatic tail has demonstrated improved survival. As for extent of node dissection, controversy still exists. In Western countries, most patients with apparently node-negative gastric cancer undergo resection with dissection of only the perigastric lymph nodes. This extent of node dissection is defined as D1 in the Japanese gastric cancer (JGC) nomenclature, the most widely used system today although the Union Internationale Contre le Cancer does offer a TNM classification. In Japan, gastric cancers with no evidence of lymph node metastasis routinely undergo more extensive dissections of lymph nodes: D2, D3, or D4. Japanese and German studies have shown that these more extensive node dissections improve survival. Other studies have not shown an increase in survival or have shown an increase in operative mortality with more extensive node dissections.

A relatively recent, retrospective study from the Memorial Sloan-Kettering Cancer Center has shown that D2 resection shows improved survival only in advanced T stage (T3), node-negative gastric cancers. Some authors consider "early" gastric cancer a different entity. Early gastric cancer is defined as confined to the mucosa or submucosa. If a patient has early gastric cancer that is defined to the mucosa, local resection with a negative margin is all that is necessary to achieve greater than 95% 10-year survival in lesions less than 3 cm in diameter. If a small (<3 cm) early gastric cancer does penetrate the submucosa or present with lymph node metastasis, studies have shown a clear survival benefit to D2 node dissection over D1 (80% 10-year survival with D2, 55% with D1). Unfortunately, without a screening program such as in Japan, only 10–15% of gastric adenocarcinomas present as early gastric cancer in the United States.

Laparoscopy can be very useful, in that 25% of patients will have small metastatic deposits on the liver, omentum or peritoneal surfaces and can avoid an extensive procedure. Palliation of metastatic gastric adenocarcinoma is most often best achieved with chemotherapy and radiation, with a mean life expectancy of 3–9 months. Endoscopic fulguration is effective in quelling the complication of hemorrhage and obstruction in more than 80% of patients. If surgical palliation is deemed necessary, resection is preferred to bypass, which provides relief of dysphagia in less than half of patients. Chemotherapy with or without radiation has shown only modest response rates, with no increase in survival, in gastric adenocarcinoma. Postoperative adjuvant chemo- and radiation therapy has recently shown a 28% survival benefit (5-fluorouracil, leucovorin, 4500 cGy external beam radiation). Overall survival for gastric cancer remains poor: 20% at 5 years.

Bibliography

Cheung LY, Delcore R. Stomach. In: Townsend CM, Beauchamp RD, Evers BM, et al. (eds.), *Sabiston Textbook of Surgery*, 16th ed. Philadelphia, PA: W.B. Saunders, 2001, 855–872.

Harrison LE, Karpeh MS, Brennan MF. Extended lymphadenectomy is associated with a survival benefit for node-negative gastric cancer. *J Gastrointest Surg* 1998; 2(2):126–131.

Hayashi H, Ochiai T, Suzuki T, et al. Superiority of a new UICC-TNM staging system for gastric carcinoma (comment). *Surgery* 2000;127(2):127–128.

Mulholland M. Gastric neoplasms. In: Greenfield LJ, Mulholland MW, Oldham KT, Zelenock GB, Lillemoe KD (eds.), *Surgery: Scientific Principles and Practice*, 3rd ed. Philadelphia, PA: Lippincott, Williams & Wilkins, 2001, 774–782.

Pierie JEN, Ott MJ. Gastric cancer. In: Cameron JL (ed.), *Current Surgical Therapy*, 7th ed. St. Louis, MO: Mosby, 2001, 105–112.

Roder JD, Bonenkamp JJ, Craven J, et al. Lymphadenectomy for gastric cancer in clinical trials: update. *World J Surg* 1995;19(4):546–553.

Smith JW, Shiu MH, Kelsey L. Morbidity of radical lymphadenectomy in the curative resection of gastric carcinoma. *Arch Surg* 1991;126(12):1469–1473.

Sowa M. Early gastric cancer. In: Wanebo HJ (ed.), *Surgery for Gastrointestinal Cancer: A Multidisciplinary Approach.* Philadelphia, PA: Lippincott,-Raven, 1997, 335.

26. (C)

27. (C)

Explanations 26 and 27

Morbid obesity is defined as either being 100 lb. over ideal body weight or having a BMI greater than $35 \, \text{kg/m}^2$. (BMI is a person's weight in kilograms over his or her height in meters, squared.) Persons who are morbidly obese have a significantly earlier mortality for a variety of obesity-related reasons, including increased incidences of coronary artery disease, peripheral and pulmonary hypertension, impaired cardiac ventricular function, diabetes mellitus, obesity hypoventilation, sleep apnea, hypercoagulability, necrotizing pancreatitis, necrotizing panniculitis, diverticulitis, and idiopathic intracranial hypertension (pseudotumor cerebri). Morbid obesity also places a person at higher risk for developing cancer of the colon, prostate, breast, and uterus. There also exist the numerous physical or psychologic disabilities incurred by the obese patient.

Correction of morbid obesity has been shown to improve several of these maladies. Eighty percent of type II diabetes patients no longer require insulin, 66–75% of hypertensive patients are normotensive, almost all ventricular dysfunctions resolve, and nearly 100% of cases of pseudotumor cerebri resolve. In 1992, the NIH Technology Assessment Conference concluded that dietary management of severe obesity could not provide evidence of long-term efficacy, with or without behavior modification.

In order to be considered for surgical correction of morbid obesity, one must have a BMI $>40 \, \text{kg/m}^2$, or a BMI $>35 \, \text{kg/m}^2$ with a significant comorbidity. Preoperative evaluation involves complete psychologic, nutritional, and medical evaluation. There are several techniques of so-called bariatric surgery.

The vertical or horizontal banded gastroplasty (VBGP or HBGP) involves partitioning the stomach with multiple staple rows in either a horizontal or vertical line. A polypropylene mesh or silastic ring is wrapped around the newly-partitioned proximal stomach to restrict food entry. Some surgeons prefer the vertical approach to avoid takedown of the short gastric vessels and to avoid damage to the spleen. Some also cut the stomach between the staple lines and suture-reinforce the cut edges, to prevent the possibility of failure because of staple line breakdown. Banded gastroplasty is a restrictive procedure, in that it restricts the amount of food that can be comfortably eaten at one meal.

In gastric bypass, a staple line is used to partition the stomach into two separate compartments: a small pouch along the lesser curvature, capable of holding approximately 15 mL, and the remainder of the stomach. Again, some surgeons prefer to completely separate the gastric pouch from the distal remainder by cutting between staple lines. Then, a portion of jejunum is brought up as a Roux limb and anastomosed to the small gastric pouch. The gastric bypass procedure is therefore partly restrictive and partly malabsorptive. The length of the Roux limb is usually 45–60 cm in length, but can be up to 150 cm if the patient is "superobese" (BMI $>50 \, \text{kg/m}^2$), resulting in more malabsorption as the meal has less exposure to bile and pancreatic juices.

The mean expected weight loss (MEWL) of gastric bypass averages about 60% at 5 years, significantly higher than that of VBGP, 40–50% at 5 years. With this better MEWL comes a higher complication rate considering stomal ulcers, stomal stenosis, vitamin B_{12} deficiency and iron deficiency. The percentage of patients undergoing gastric bypass that either regain lost weight or never achieve significant weight loss is reported to be 10–15%. A third procedure commonly performed is the partial biliopancreatic diversion (BPD). This procedure involves (1) subtotal gastrectomy, (2) anastomosis of the distal 250 cm of small intestine to the stomach remnant, and (3) anastomosis of the proximal small intestine to a point 50 cm from the terminal ileum. This creates a common tract of only 50 cm in which the meal is exposed to bile and pancreatic juices.

The BPD results in the largest MEWL of all procedures still performed, with greater than 75% sustained MEWL in a large Italian series. This partially restrictive, partially malabsorptive procedure commonly results in profound fat malabsorption (with concomitant malabsorption of vitamins A, D, E, and K) and has a higher incidence of nutritional deficiencies than either VBGP or Roux-en-Y gastric bypass. Bariatric procedures are also being performed laparoscopically, the most commonly performed procedures being the Roux-en-Y gastric bypass, and the adjustable silicone gastric band, with a subcutaneous balloon port for band constriction adjustment.

A dreaded complication of any procedure for morbid obesity is gastric leak and ensuing peritonitis. In obese patients this is often very difficult to diagnose, as in the patient presented. Abdominal tenderness may be significantly less obvious than in a thin patient. If suspected, upper gastrointestinal contrast study with water-soluble contrast is a good confirmatory test, but in a febrile, tachycardic, hypoxic patient with increasing abdominal tenderness, surgical exploration should not be delayed. The responsible anastomosis should be repaired, and drainage of that area performed. Other, less acute problems include stomal ulcer or stenosis, which usually respond to H2-receptor antagonists or endoscopic dilation, respectively, gallstones because of rapid weight loss, and various vitamin and mineral deficiencies. Vitamin B_{12} levels should be checked yearly, and replacement begun if appropriate. Iron-deficiency anemia is more common in menstruating women, and may be recalcitrant to oral iron supplementation because iron requires acidification to be absorbed in the duodenum and jejunum; iron dextran injections may become necessary. Operative mortality for bariatric surgery is approximately 0.5%.

Bibliography

Skroubis G, Sakellaropoulos G, Pouggouras K, et al. Comparison of nutritional deficiencies after Roux-en-Y gastric bypass and after biliopancreatic diversion with Roux-en-Y gastric bypass. *Obes Surg* 2002;12(4):551–556.

Sugerman HL. Morbid obesity. In: Greenfield LJ, Mulholland MW, Oldham KT, Zelenock GB, Lillemoe KD (eds.), *Surgery: Scientific Principles and Practice*, 3rd ed. Philadelphia, PA: Lippincott, Williams & Wilkins, 2001, 767–774.

Wise MW, Martin LF, O'Leary JP. Morbid obesity. In: Cameron JL (ed.), *Current Surgical Therapy*, 7th ed. St. Louis, MO: Mosby, 2001, 98–105.

28. **(D)** Diculafoy's lesion is the presence of arteries of consistently large caliber in the submucosa. These most often occur in the proximal stomach, although they have been described throughout the gastrointestinal tract. This occurs as a result of lack of the normally-occurring arterial arborization once they reach the submucosa, hence the alternate name "caliber-persistent artery." These become symptomatic if the artery compresses the overlying mucosa, leading to erosion of the arterial wall and rupture. Massive hemorrhage results, and this is the usual presenting symptom. Treatment follows that of all gastric bleeding, with resuscitation of the patient and gastric lavage, then

endoscopic examination. Many of these have stopped bleeding by the time endoscopy if performed, but if there is persistent hemorrhage, endoscopic therapy via heater probe, laser coagulator, injection, or band ligator is able to permanently stop bleeding in more than 90% of cases.

Mallory-Weiss tears are linear mucosal tears at or just below the gastroesophageal junction, usually at the lesser curvature. These were classically described as the source of profuse bleeding after a bout of retching or vomiting, but they are often found in association with other gastric pathologies, such as gastritis, ulcer, and hiatal hernia. Over 90% of bleeding tears cease after resuscitation and gastric lavage. On endoscopy, if there is active bleeding or a visible vessel, therapy is indicated via heater probe, laser coagulator, injection, or band ligator. Endoscopic therapy is highly effective even in patients with varices secondary to portal hypertension, who have a higher incidence of Mallory-Weiss tears than the general population.

Gastric ulcers secondary to chronic NSAID use, sometimes called type V gastric ulcers, almost always respond to resuscitation, withdrawal of the offending agent, and administration of acid-reducing medications such as H2-receptor antagonists. Endoscopic therapy may be indicated if bleeding persists after gastric lavage and supportive care. Embolization via interventional radiology techniques would be the next step in recalcitrant bleeding. Surgical therapy is occasionally needed if profuse bleeding persists, or certainly if a perforation occurs.

Bibliography

Cheung LY, Delcore R. Stomach. In: Townsend CM, Beauchamp RD, Evers BM, et al. (eds.), *Sabiston Textbook of Surgery*, 16th ed. Philadelphia, PA: W.B. Saunders, 2001, 871.

Conter RL, Kauffman GL Jr. Benign gastric ulcer and stress gastritis. In: Cameron JL (ed.), *Current Surgical Therapy*, 7th ed. St. Louis, MO: Mosby, 2001, 77–80.

Lichtenstein DR. Nonvariceal upper gastrointestinal hemorrhage. In: Wolfe MM, Cohen S, Davis GL, et al. (eds.), *Therapy of Digestive Disorders*. Philadelphia, PA: W.B. Saunders, 2000, 145–146.

Mehta S, Kauffman GL Jr. Mallory-Weiss syndrome. In: Cameron JL (ed.), *Current Surgical Therapy*, 7th ed. St. Louis, MO: Mosby, 2001, 94–97.

Schmulewitz MD, Baillie J. Dieulafoy lesions: a review of 6 years experience at a tertiary referral center. *Am J Gastroenterol* 2000;96(6):1688–1694.

29. **(D)** There are several pharmaceutical agents used in the medical treatment of ulcer disease. Some act as acid reduction agents, some as antibiotics, and some

perform both functions. Proton pump inhibitors, such as omeprazole and lansoprazole, selectively inhibit the H^+, K^+-ATPase of parietal cells, the enzyme that is the last step in producing luminal acid. If enough drug is administered, a state of anacidity can be produced. Proton pump inhibitors are ineffective at eradicating *H. pylori* infections as single agents, but act synergistically with antibiotics: the growth and survival of *H. pylori* is pH dependent, with slower growth rates at higher pH. Histamine 2-receptor antagonists (famotidine, ranitidine, cimetidine, and nizatidine) reduce acid secretion by blocking activation of the histamine receptor of parietal cells. This not only prevents histamine from stimulating acid secretion, but also reduces the effects of acetylcholine and gastrin on the remaining types of receptors. H2-receptor blockers significantly decrease acid production, but will not by themselves eradicate of *H. pylori*. Bismuth compounds exhibit antimicrobial activity against several bacteria, including *H. pylori*, by an unclear mechanism. They are also synergistic with other antibiotics. Importantly, there have been no reported instances of *H. pylori* resistance to bismuth compounds. Bismuth compounds in their most commonly administered forms—bismuth subsalicylate (Pepto Bismol) and colloidal bismuth subcitrate—are poorly absorbed, and therefore must act locally against *H. pylori* in the gastric lumen. Ranitidine bismuth citrate is a compound that combines the effects of an H2-receptor antagonist and a bismuth compound, and has found an important place in the armamentarium against *H. pylori*. The imidazoles, such as metronidazole and tinidazole, exhibit activity against *H. pylori* by damaging bacterial DNA. They are absorbed systemically and then transported to the gastric juice. Mutations can occur that allow *H. pylori* strains to prevent activation of imidazoles, rendering these strains resistant to this genre of antimicrobials. Macrolides, like clarithromycin and erythromycin, show activity against *H. pylori* by binding to the 50S ribosomal subunit, preventing protein synthesis. Like imidazoles, they are absorbed systemically and then transported to the gastric mucosa. Macrolides show greater antimicrobial efficacy at higher pH, explaining their improved efficacy when combined with an acid reduction agent. Of all antimicrobials, clarithromycin is the most effective single agent against *H. pylori* organisms, with eradication rates of 40% when used alone. This reinforces why multiple agent regimens are greatly preferred to single agent regimens. Resistance to macrolides occurs when strains of *H. pylori* develop mutated ribosomal subunits that no longer strongly bind these agents. Amoxicillin, a penicillin, is probably second only to clarithromycin in efficacy against *H. pylori*. Amoxicillin acts by preventing cell wall cross-linking. It probably acts against *H. pylori* both locally and systemically. *H. pylori* resistance to amoxicillin is very rare. Like the macrolides, amoxicillin shows increased efficacy at higher pH. Tetracycline inhibits protein synthesis by binding the 30S ribosomal subunit, and has shown good efficacy against *H. pylori*. Sucralfate probably exerts its antimicrobial action indirectly by promoting gastric mucus production. It is unclear if sucralfate is bactericidal or not, but it improves the minimum inhibitory concentration (MIC) of almost all antibiotics used against *H. pylori*.

In the question above, all of the combinations have proven at least 90% effective and are recommended in the attempt to eradicate *H. pylori* infection except for lansoprazole plus amoxicillin. All of the currently used proton pump inhibitors demonstrate comparable acid-suppressing ability, but even with the synergism between a proton pump inhibitor and most antibiotics, eradication rates higher than 70% have not been achieved when single antibiotics have been used. All currently recommended regimens involve some form of acid suppression and at least two antibiotics, and eradication rates have been shown to be approximately 90% or greater.

Bibliography

Cheung LY, Delcore R. Stomach. In: Townsend CM, Beauchamp RD, Evers BM, et al. (eds.), *Sabiston Textbook of Surgery*, 16th ed. Philadelphia, PA: W.B. Saunders, 2001, 847.

Fennerty MB. Treatment of *Helicobacter pylori* infection. In: Wolfe MM, Cohen S, Davis GL, et al. (eds.), *Therapy of Digestive Disorders*. Philadelphia, PA: W.B. Saunders, 2000, 81–95.

Mulholland M. Duodenal ulcer. In: Greenfield LJ, Mulholland MW, Oldham KT, Zelenock GB, Lillemoe KD (eds.), *Surgery: Scientific Principles and Practice*, 3rd ed. Philadelphia, PA: Lippincott, Williams & Wilkins, 2001, 753–756.

Sachs G. Molecular targets in the therapy of acid-related disease. In: Wolfe MM, Cohen S, Davis GL, et al. (eds.), *Therapy of Digestive Disorders*. Philadelphia, PA: W.B. Saunders, 2000, 67–74.

CHAPTER 23

Small Bowel

Jennifer Choi, Carol Palachko, and Larry Micon

Questions

1. Which of the following is not true of cholecystokinin (CCK)?

   (A) Its release stimulates pancreatic acinar cell secretion, pancreatic growth, and insulin release.

   (B) It is released by the small bowel in response to contact with carbohydrates.

   (C) Its release stimulates gallbladder contraction and sphincter of Oddi relaxation.

   (D) It is released by the small bowel in response to contact with tryptophan and phenylalanine.

2. A 45-year-old female with previous history of a TAH-BSO 2 years prior presents to the emergency department with an 18-h history of nausea, vomiting, and crampy abdominal pain. She denies fever or continuous abdominal pain. Which of the following is not true regarding her natural barrier mechanisms preventing bacterial translocation in this clinical scenario?

   (A) The GI tract has an abundance of lymphoid and myeloid cells that are located in Peyer's patches, in the lamina propria, and within the epithelium. Seventy percent of immunoglobulin (IgG, IgM, IgE, and IgA) producing cells are in the gut.

   (B) The nonimmunologic defenses of the gut include epithelial tight junctions, endogenous bacteria, mucin production, gastric acid, proteolytic enzymes, and peristalsis.

   (C) IgA acts by augmenting cell-mediated opsonization, antigen presentation, and overall destruction of the offending microorganism.

   (D) Secretory IgA prevents colonization of bacteria in the small bowel by prohibiting their adherence to the epithelial surface; it also prevents absorption of antigens and neutralizes bacterial toxins.

3. Regarding the epidemiology of Crohn's disease (CD), which of the following is *correct*?

   (A) The incidence in females is equal to the incidence in males.

   (B) The incidence of American whites is much greater than the incidence in American or African blacks.

   (C) CD affects rural dwellers more often than urban dwellers.

   (D) A family history of Crohn's is not important for first-degree relatives.

4. A 22-year-old female complains of daily sharp abdominal pain, weight loss totaling 7 lb in the past 6 weeks, and four to six bowel movements per day for the past several weeks. Upper GI endoscopy is negative for any disease. Which of the following findings on colonoscopic examination differentiate CD from UC?

   (A) There are ulcerated lesions in the distal sigmoid colon followed by a patch of normal colon and then more ulcers near the splenic flexure. The rectum appears to be spared.

   (B) The patient has two perianal fistulas.

   (C) On biopsy of a distal lesion, the ulcer is transmural.

   (D) Her lesions have improved since starting prednisone.

5. A 19-year-old army recruit presents to the emergency department with a 24-h history of right lower quadrant pain, fever to 100.5°F, anorexia, and two loose stools. He was taken to surgery for the presumptive diagnosis of appendicitis; however, the appendix looked completely normal while the terminal ileum was quite inflamed. What procedure should be performed?

   (A) appendectomy
   (B) ileocecectomy with ileostomy
   (C) full abdominal exploration to evaluate for further obvious lesions and colonoscopy prior to discharge
   (D) None. The patient should be closed and request immediate medical discharge from the army as he now must battle CD

6. Indications for surgical management of CD include

   (A) postoperative enterocutaneous fistulas (ECFs)
   (B) duodenal obstruction
   (C) small bowel obstruction that has not improved with conservative management
   (D) child with secondary growth retardation related to CD
   (E) all of the above

7. A 48-year-old female with HIV complains of severe right lower quadrant pain. A CT scan has been ordered after labs demonstrated a white blood cell (WBC) count 1.3, normal H/H, and normal electrolyte profile. Which of the following diseases in the differential diagnosis does not match its treatment?

   (A) cytomegalovirus (CMV) enteritis: ganciclovir
   (B) tuberculus fistulas: surgical resection and primary anastomosis
   (C) *Clostridium difficile*: vancomycin
   (D) *Salmonella/Shigella*: ciprofloxacin

8. Which treatment for CD is useful in maintaining remission?

   (A) prednisone
   (B) infliximab
   (C) azathioprine
   (D) interleukin (IL)-10 analogs

9. Which clinical scenario should be managed operatively immediately after appropriate resuscitation has taken place?

   (A) Sixty-eight-year-old male with metastatic pancreatic cancer who presents with 18 h of nausea, vomiting, and crampy abdominal pain. His abdominal x-rays demonstrate multiple air fluid levels and stair-stepping pattern.
   (B) Sixty-eight-year-old female postoperative day 5 status post colostomy takedown and reanastomosis with nausea, vomiting, and abdominal distension. Her abdominal x-rays demonstrate multiple air fluid levels and stair-stepping pattern.
   (C) Sixty-eight-year-old male status post prostatectomy and radiation therapy 6 years ago for prostate cancer, now with 24-h history of nausea, vomiting, and dull abdominal pain. His abdominal x-rays demonstrate multiple air fluid levels and stair-stepping pattern.
   (D) Sixty-eight-year-old female status postcolostomy takedown and reanastomosis 1 year ago with 24-h history of nausea, feculent vomiting, fever to 100.2°F, and persistent abdominal pain. Her abdominal x-rays demonstrate multiple air fluid levels and stair-stepping pattern.

10. A 62-year-old man with a history of chronic obstructive pulmonary disease (COPD) because of 35 years of heavy smoking presented to the emergency department with nausea, occasional nonbilious vomiting, loose stools, and nonspecific abdominal pain. On examination his abdomen was distended but soft and, mildly tender to deep palpation. An acute abdominal series is suspicious for pneumatosis intestinalis (PI); a CT was obtained which confirmed this finding but also demonstrated air within the falciform ligament. There was no free intraperitoneal air and no portal venous air. What is the next most appropriate step?

   (A) fluid resuscitation, Foley catheter placement, and NG tube
   (B) call the OR to add on an emergent exploratory laparotomy
   (C) admit for observation and a brief period of bowel rest and COPD management
   (D) broad-spectrum intravenous antibiotics

11. Which of these does not prevent fistula closure?

   (A) high output fistula (>500 cc per day)
   (B) radiation enteritis
   (C) active IBD of fistulized segment

(D) fistula tract <2.5 cm in length

(E) all of these prevent fistula closure

12. The most common presentation of Meckel's diverticulum in an adult is

(A) GI bleed

(B) intussuception

(C) Littre's hernia

(D) diverticulitis

13. Superior mesenteric artery (SMA) syndrome is not associated with which of the following?

(A) scoliosis

(B) placement of a body cast

(C) anorexia nervosa

(D) Abdominal aortic aneurysm

(E) rapid weight gain

14. The preferred treatment of SMA syndrome is

(A) Bilroth II

(B) duodenojejunostomy

(C) SMA bypass

(D) correction of scoliosis

15. A 25-year-old prisoner with schizophrenia presents to the emergency department two-and-a-half hours after he was seen ingesting a razor blade. An abdominal x-ray indeed demonstrates a razor blade in the patient's mid abdomen (Fig. 23-1). His abdominal examination is benign, and his WBC count is 8000. The next most appropriate step would be

(A) give milk of magnesia to speed excretion of the razor blade

(B) call the OR to prepare for an urgent exploratory laparotomy

(C) admit the patient for serial x-rays and serial abdominal examinations

(D) consult GI to retrieve the razor blade by enteroscopy

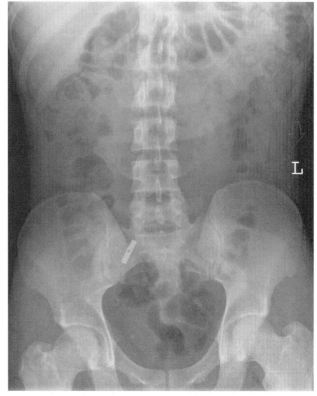

FIG. 23-1   25-year-old prisoner with schizophrenia who repeatedly ingests razor blades.

16. The percentage of cardiac output received by the small bowel at rest is

(A) 10–15%

(B) 20–25%

(C) 30–35%

(D) 45–50%

17. In operating for mesenteric ischemia from any source, the best method for assessing bowel viability is

(A) Doppler ultrasound

(B) oximetry

(C) fluoroscein

(D) second look surgery

18. Which is not true of the obstruction seen in Figs. 23-2 through 23-4?

    (A) It is the cause of nearly a quarter of nonstrangulated obstructions in the elderly.

    (B) The gallbladder and fistula tract must be dealt with at the time of laparotomy if the gallstone is impacted in the terminal ileum.

    (C) The gallbladder and fistula tract must be dealt with at the time of laparotomy if the gallstone is impacted in the gastric outlet.

    (D) If the gallstone is impacted in the colon, the stone should be excised and a colostomy created.

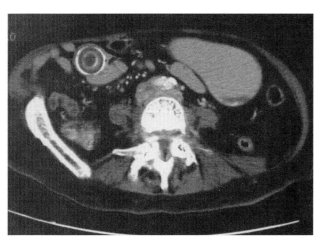

FIG. 23-2   Gallstone ileus on CT scan

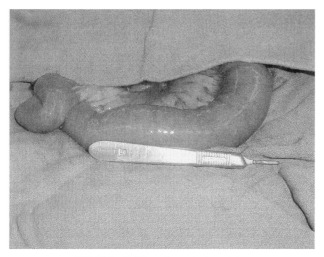

FIG. 23-3   Gallstone ileus prior to excision

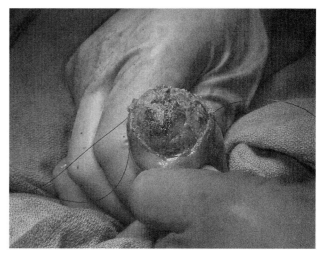

FIG. 23-4   Gallstone ileus after enterotomy

19. Which of the following is not true of intussusception in adults?

    (A) Intussusception is frequently caused by benign small bowel tumors.

    (B) Intussusception is frequently caused by primary malignant small bowel tumors.

    (C) Intussusception occurs episodically in Peutz-Jegher's associated hamartomas.

    (D) Reduction of intussusception in adults should not be attempted by air or contrast enema.

20. The most useful radiologic examination for small bowel tumors is

    (A) upper GI with small bowel follow through

    (B) enterocolysis

    (C) abdomen and pelvis CT scan

    (D) esophagoduodenoscopy

21. Which of the following is not true of malignant small bowel neoplasms?

    (A) Small bowel adenocarcinoma comprises 50% of small bowel malignancies. Treatment is directed primarily toward palliation. Chemoradiation is generally unhelpful.

    (B) Small bowel sarcomas comprise 20% of small bowel malignancies. They spread via hematogenous spread to liver and lung as well as by local invasion. Postoperative radiation therapy improves overall survival according to some studies.

(C) Primary small bowel lymphomas (PSBL) comprise 10–15% of small bowel malignancies. Presenting symptoms are fever, weight loss, and night sweats. Surgical resection with chemoradiation offers the best chance at survival.

(D) Foregut carcinoid tumors arise in the appendix and ileum with malignancy more common in ileal lesions. Frequently, presenting symptoms are those of longstanding abdominal pain, weight loss, and diarrhea.

22. Which of the following is not true of carcinoid tumors or malignant carcinoid syndrome?

(A) Symptomatic carcinoid tumors frequently present as do other small bowel tumors with weight loss, abdominal pain, and diarrhea, but many are found incidentally during unrelated laparotomies.

(B) Classic symptoms of malignant carcinoid syndrome include flushing, diarrhea, right heart valvular lesions, and asthma. It occurs in patients with near replacement of their livers with metastatic carcinoid tumor. Symptoms can be controlled somewhat with octreotide.

(C) Multiple methods of diagnosing carcinoid tumor exists including 24-h urine for 5-hydroxyindoleacetic acid (5-HIAA), plasma concentration of chromograffin A, and scintigraphic localization with ^{111}In-labeled pentetreotide.

(D) Resection of localized carcinoid tumors result in survival near 100%; however, only limited resection or intestinal bypass is indicated for patients with widely metastatic disease.

23. Which of the following adenomas cannot be managed endoscopically?

(A) a 3 cm pedunculated adenoma in the second segment of the duodenum

(B) a 3 cm Brunner's gland adenoma in the second segment of the duodenum

(C) a 3 cm villous adenoma in the second segment of the duodenum

(D) all of the above can be managed endoscopically

24. A 52-year-old male with a longstanding history of nausea and nonspecific abdominal pain was admitted twice with pancreatitis. He had no history of alcohol use, cholelithiasis, or hypertriglyceridemia. Endoscopic retrograde cholangiopancreatography (ERCP) was performed which revealed a moderate duodenal diverticulum approximately 1 cm from the ampulla. What is the most appropriate next step in management?

(A) pancreaticoduodenectomy

(B) sphincterotomy and stent placement

(C) choledochoduodenostomy

(D) extensive Kocher maneuver with duodenectomy

25. Which of the following cell types is considered the most likely candidate as the cell of origin for gastrointestinal stromal tumor (GIST)?

(A) interstitial cells of Cajal (ICCs)

(B) Kulchitsky cells

(C) myofibroblasts

(D) G cells

(E) Paneth cells

26. A 57-year-old male presents with symptoms consistent with an intermittent partial small bowel obstruction despite having no previous history of abdominal surgery. Workup includes a CT scan of the abdomen which demonstrates a midsmall bowel obstruction with adjacent soft tissue mass. He undergoes laparotomy and is found to have a partially obstructing solid neoplasm approximately 5 cm in diameter involving the wall of the distal jejunum. A small bowel resection is performed with complete tumor excision. Final pathology reveals a GIST, spindle-cell type. He has an uneventful recovery from this procedure and is discharged home. If this patient goes on to develop recurrent disease, which of the following is most likely to occur:

(A) lymph node metastasis

(B) lung metastasis

(C) liver metastasis

(D) diffuse small bowel metastasis

(E) carcinomatosis

27. The patient in the previous question returns 3 years later with local recurrence and multiple liver metastases. His disease is not surgically resectable and he is started on imatinib mesylate, a chemotherapeutic agent recently approved for the treatment of advanced GIST. What is imatinib mesylate's mechanism of action?

(A) crosslinks DNA through alkylation

(B) inhibits a tyrosine kinase receptor

(C) inhibits ribonucleotide reductase

(D) inhibits mitosis by binding microtubules

(E) inhibits topoisomerase II

28. An otherwise healthy 28-year-old female undergoes open appendectomy for perforated appendicitis. On the morning of the third postoperative day she complains of nausea and abdominal distension. She denies passage of stool or flatus since surgery. Supine and upright abdominal films demonstrate gas throughout the small bowel and colon consistent with ileus. Her present medications include oxycodone and ibuprofen. Recent laboratory values include WBC 11,000 mm^3, Hgb 13.0 g/dL, Na 134 mmol/L, K 4.0 mmol/L, Cl 109 mmol/L, HCO$_3$ 26 mmol/L, Cr 0.9 mg/dl. Which of the following is not a likely contributing factor to her ileus?

    (A) intraabdominal inflammation
    (B) narcotic pain medication
    (C) hyponatremia
    (D) nonsteroidal anti-inflammatory drug (NSAID) use
    (E) postlaparotomy status

29. Which of the following procedures is most likely to produce the shortest period of postoperative ileus?

    (A) laparotomy with sigmoid colectomy
    (B) laparoscopic sigmoid colectomy
    (C) exploratory laparotomy with lysis of adhesions, no enterotomy
    (D) exploratory laparotomy with lysis of adhesions, small bowel resection with primary anastomosis
    (E) none of the above, duration of ileus should be approximately the same for these procedures

30. Which of the following treatments have been proven to reduce duration of postoperative ileus in the clinical setting?

    (A) NG intubation
    (B) early ambulation/mobilization after surgery
    (C) erythromycin administration
    (D) naloxone administration
    (E) epidural local anesthetics in place of systemic narcotics for postoperative pain control

31. Intraabdominal adhesions following abdominal surgery have been associated with all of the following *except*:

    (A) small bowel obstruction
    (B) infertility
    (C) chronic pelvic pain
    (D) intestinal malabsorption
    (E) increased risk for enterotomy on subsequent laparotomy

32. Which of the following has been shown to be an important factor in the pathophysiology of adhesion formation following mesothelial trauma in the abdomen?

    (A) low levels of fibrin
    (B) high concentration of plasminogen-activating inhibitor type 1 (PAI-1)
    (C) protein C deficiency
    (D) high levels of urokinase-type plasminogen activator (uPA)
    (E) abnormal platelet activation

33. All of the following are true regarding radiation enteritis *except*:

    (A) Chronic radiation enteritis is believed to be the result of obliterative vasculitis with subsequent ischemia and full-thickness bowel wall fibrosis.
    (B) Acute radiation enteritis can be subclinical and when symptoms do occur the process is generally self-limited, resolving within 2–6 weeks after treatment.
    (C) The degree of chronic radiation enteritis is a function of the rate and duration of time over which the dose is applied rather than the total dose of radiation.
    (D) Symptoms of chronic radiation enteritis are related to abnormal intestinal transit.
    (E) The average onset of chronic radiation enteritis is between 2 and 3 years after radiation exposure.

34. A 64-year-old female undergoes surgical resection of an invasive rectal carcinoma. She is otherwise healthy, weighs 56 kg, and her previous surgical history includes appendectomy as a young adult. Postoperatively she is treated with 5-fluorouracil (5-FU) and pelvic radiotherapy. She receives a total dose of 5000 cGy of radiation in fractions of 200 cGy per day. Which of the following factors does not predispose this patient to the development of chronic radiation enteritis?

    (A) body habitus
    (B) previous appendectomy
    (C) adminstration of 5-FU
    (D) fractionation of radiation dose
    (E) total radiation dose over 4000 cGy

35. A patient with a T3 low rectal carcinoma is scheduled to undergo abdominoperineal resection and is likely to require postoperative pelvic radiotherapy. Which of following procedures performed at the time of initial operation have shown evidence to reduce the likelihood of radiation enteritis with postoperative radiotherapy?

(A) absorbable mesh sling

(B) omental hammock

(C) omentopexy

(D) pelvic tissue expander

(E) all of the above

36. A 75-year-old male with a history of diabetes mellitus type 2 and colon cancer status post right hemicolectomy 10 years ago presents with a small bowel obstruction and undergoes an uncomplicated laparotomy with small bowel resection for intestinal adhesions. On postoperative day 7 his incision is noted to be mildly cellulitic with purulent discharge from the superior aspect. The following day he is found to have copious bile-colored fluid draining from this site. Diagnostic workup includes a fistulogram and CT of the abdomen. These studies reveal a small bowel fistula with a 2 cm tract from the proximal jejunum to the skin. There is no intraabdominal leak or abscess, but there is evidence of a partial distal small bowel obstruction beyond the fistula. Conservative management with nothing per mouth, TPN, fluid and electrolyte replacement, and wound care is initiated. Over the course of the next several days, fistula output is 600–700 mL per day. Laboratory values include WBC count 9500/mm³, Hgb 12 g/dL, Na 137 mmol/L, K 3.9 mmol/L, and albumin 3.1 g/dL.

Which of the following factors do not either decrease the likelihood of spontaneous fistula closure or increase mortality associated with the fistula for this patient?

(A) history of previous colon cancer

(B) distal small bowel obstruction

(C) short fistula tract

(D) high fistula output

(E) albumin <3.5 g/dL

37. A 48-year-old male presents with severe upper abdominal pain of over 48 h duration and has diffuse peritoneal signs on examination. He is taken for laparotomy where he is found to have a perforated ulcer located in the second portion of the duodenum with gross intraabdominal contamination. An omental patch repair is performed and a drain is left in place. In the subsequent recovery period the drain begins putting out bilious fluid consistent with enteric contents. Further workup reveals development of a lateral duodenal fistula from the site of attempted repair. Conservative management is attempted, but after 6 weeks the fistula continues to drain over 500 mL per day. Which of the following techniques is most appropriate for surgical repair of this patient's enterocutaneous fistula?

(A) bowel resection with primary anastomosis

(B) debridement with two-layered primary closure of bowel wall

(C) injection of fibrin glue through the drain to occlude the fistula tract

(D) pancreaticoduodenectomy

(E) internal drainage via a Roux-en-Y duodenojejunostomy

38. All of the following are true regarding octreotide and its use in the treatment of ECFs *except*:

(A) Octreotide is an analog of native somatostatin with a longer elimination half-life.

(B) Pharmacologic effects of octreotide include reduction of GI, biliary, and pancreatic secretions as well as decreased intestinal motility.

(C) Clinical studies suggest that octreotide significantly decreases fistula output in patients with persistent ECFs.

(D) Clinical studies suggest that octreotide significantly increases the rate of spontaneous closure of ECFs.

(E) Possible side effects of octreotide administration include mild hyperglycemia and pain at the site of injection.

39. Which of the following is true regarding small bowel carcinoid tumors?

(A) Most are biochemically atypical tumors lacking the enzyme dopa decarboxylase.

(B) They are the most common GI carcinoid tumors.

(C) Regional lymph node involvement is common in tumors less than 1 cm in size.

(D) Diagnosis is frequently made in patients prior to surgery.

(E) Among carcinoid tumors, they are associated with the lowest rate of second primary malignancies.

40. A 36-year-old mildly mentally retarded male presents with a 3-day history of nausea, vomiting, crampy abdominal pain, and abdominal distension. He also reports a 10 lb weight loss over the past 2 months. Past medical history is otherwise unremarkable. Past surgical history includes laparoscopic cholecystectomy 10 years ago. Abdominal plain films reveal multiple dilated small bowel loops with a paucity of colonic air consistent with a partial mechanical small bowel obstruction. Conservative management with NPO status, NG decompression, and intravenous fluid hydration fail to resolve the obstruction and he is taken to the OR for exploratory laparotomy. At operation he is found to have multiple sychronous small bowel tumors located in the ileum with extension into the mesentery. Several enlarged lymph nodes are also noted. Wide resection of these tumors is performed including the involved mesentery and lymph nodes. The liver is palpated and no lesions are identified. Postoperative recovery is uncomplicated. Final pathology reveals carcinoid tumor with lymph node metastasis. What other tests or studies should be performed in this patient for staging purposes?

    (A) EGD
    (B) liver function tests
    (C) cardiac catheterization
    (D) head CT
    (E) hepatic ultrasound

41. A patient undergoes proximal gastric vagotomy (PGV) (highly selective vagotomy) for an intractable duodenal peptic ulcer. Which can be said regarding postvagotomy syndromes following this technique?

    (A) Dumping syndrome occurs with greater incidence in these patients than those who undergo truncal vagotomy with pyloroplasty.
    (B) Dumping syndrome can often be managed by diet modification including taking liquids 30 min before meals and adding concentrated carbohydrates to meals.
    (C) If postvagotomy diarrhea occurs, it tends to persist and become more severe.
    (D) Alkaline reflux gastritis can occur in up to 10% of patients.
    (E) The incidence of dysphagia is higher with PGV than truncal vagotomy.

42. A 68-year-old male presents to his primary care physician complaining of a 3-week history of upper abdominal pain, nausea, and epigastric distension occurring shortly after eating most meals. The pain is sudden in onset, crampy, localized to the right upper quadrant, nonradiating, and always postprandial. Frequently his symptoms are relieved after he vomits bilious fluid without food. In the past few weeks he has limited his food intake and has lost 10 lbs. He denies any jaundice, change in bowel movements, or urinary symptoms. His past medical history is significant for insulin-dependent diabetes mellitus and hypertension. His past surgical history includes Billroth II gastrectomy for peptic ulcer disease 25 years ago. He is not a smoker and rarely drinks alcohol. His medications include insulin and metoprolol.

What the most likely etiology of this patient's symptoms?

    (A) gallstone pancreatitis
    (B) recurrent gastric ulcer
    (C) afferent loop syndrome
    (D) choledocholithiasis
    (E) alkaline reflux gastritis

43. Which of the following statements regarding PSBL is not true?

    (A) They are generally associated with a poorer prognosis than primary gastric lymphomas.
    (B) Most are high-grade B cell lymphomas.
    (C) Most arise in the proximal jejunum.
    (D) Adjuvant chemotherapy after surgery is not indicated for completely resected, low-grade tumors.
    (E) None of the above is true.

44. PSBL in adults has been associated with which of the following?

    (A) celiac sprue
    (B) irritable bowel syndrome
    (C) synchonous small bowel adenocarcinoma
    (D) herpes zoster infection
    (E) female sex

45. A 76-year-old female with HTN, history of tobacco use, and peripheral vascular disease presents to her primary care physician complaining of intermittent epigastric abdominal pain and nausea. She states that her symptoms started 4 months ago and have been increasing in severity. The abdominal pain is dull and "gnawing," starts approximately 30 min after meals, and lasts 2–4 h. The pain is sometimes accompanied by nausea. She denies vomiting, diarrhea, hematochezia, and melena. She has gotten to the point that she fears eating and has lost 18 lbs. since her symptoms began. She has no significant past surgical history

except right carotid endarterectomy. Abdominal examination is unremarkable. Routine laboratory studies are normal except for hypoalbuminemia. Gallbladder ultrasound, EGD, and colonoscopy are normal. All of the following are true regarding the most likely diagnosis *except*:

(A) Weight loss occurs because of severe malabsorption.

(B) Greater than 95% of cases are secondary to atherosclerosis.

(C) The incidence is higher in women than in men.

(D) Mesenteric duplex ultrasound is a helpful screening tool in symptomatic patients.

(E) This condition is a risk factor for acute mesenteric ischemia.

46. Which of the following fulfills the imaging criteria for diagnosis of chronic mesenteric ischemia?

(A) celiac axis and SMA without significant stenosis, 100% occlusion of IMA

(B) 30% stenosis of celiac axis, 20% stenosis of both SMA and IMA

(C) 75% stenosis of celiac axis and SMA, IMA without significant stenosis

(D) A and C

(E) all of the above

47. The patient in Question 45 is found to have high-grade atheriosclerotic lesions involving both her celiac artery and SMA. She is taken electively for antegrade prosthetic bypass grafting of both vessels. Which of the following is *not* considered to be a potential advantage of the antegrade approach versus the retrograde approach for this procedure?

(A) avoids direct contact with the bowel

(B) decreased possibility of graft kinking

(C) inflow comes from the less frequently diseased supraceliac aorta

(D) shorter graft length with direct in-line flow

(E) significantly better long-term patency rates in prospective trials

48. A 57-year-old homeless male presents to the emergency department complaining of sudden onset, severe, epigastric pain which began approximately 8 h ago. The pain is constant, does not radiate, and is worse with

movement. He denies any other symptoms. On physical examination his abdomen is distended, tympanic to percussion, and diffusely tender with evidence of peritoneal irritation. Vital signs are stable. Acute abdominal series is significant for free air under the diaphragm. Laboratory studies are unremarkable with the exception of WBC count of 17,000/mm^3, and differential including 90% neutrophils. On further questioning, the patient reports a history of episodic vague upper abdominal pain in the past. He takes no medications, although he has used over-the-counter antacid tablets intermittently. He is taken to the OR for exploratory laparotomy where he is found to have a perforated duodenal ulcer involving the anterior aspect of the first portion of the duodenum. There is minimal intraperitoneal soilage. Which of the following is true regarding the further surgical and medical management of this patient's disease?

(A) The ulcer must be biopsied because of the risk for underlying malignancy.

(B) The patient will not require *H. pylori* testing or treatment based on the ulcer's location.

(C) Even if the surgeon is technically experienced, a laparoscopic approach to this problem is contraindicated.

(D) The procedure of choice is antrectomy with truncal vagotomy.

(E) The patient does not require further workup for an underlying hypersecretory disorder.

49. *H. pylori* produces hypersecretion of gastric acid in patients who develop *H. pylori*-related duodenal ulcers. What is a proposed mechanism for development of increased gastric acid secretion by this bacterium?

(A) attenuation of somatostatin release from antral D cells

(B) direct stimulation of gastrin receptor on parietal cells

(C) direct stimulation of proton pump on parietal cells

(D) blockage of somatostatin receptors on parietal cells

(E) bacterial enzymatic degradation of local prostaglandins

50. All of the following are true regarding small bowel resection and the development of short bowel syndrome *except*:

(A) Remaining small bowel can adapt after massive bowel resection by enterocyte hyperplasia and lengthening of villi.

(B) If nutrition is maintained only parenterally, no intestinal adaptation will occur.

(C) Large ileal resections are better tolerated than large jejunal resections.

(D) Resection of the ileocecal valve decreases intestinal absorption by increasing transit time and promoting development of small bowel bacterial overgrowth.

(E) Proximal small bowel resections can lead to deficiencies in iron, calcium, and folate.

Answers and Explanations

1. **(B)** CCK is produced in endocrine I cells in the first two-thirds of the small intestine. A significant amount is also produced in the brain but its function there has not been thoroughly studied. A small amount also exists in the enteric neurons. Multiple forms of CCK circulate but the most frequently studied form contains 33 amino acid residues. Others have also been studied and contain 8, 39, 58, and 83 residues; however, their basic functions appear to be the same. Its release is stimulated by amino acids and by small peptides. Long chain triglycerides and fatty acids also stimulate its secretion. Carbohydrates do not stimulate the release of any CCK. Trypsin and bile acids inhibit its release.

CCK functions similarly to gastrin because of its identical carboxyl terminal end. It acts to stimulate contraction of the gallbladder, to stimulate pancreatic acinar cell secretion of zymogens, and to slow gastric emptying by affecting muscular contraction of the pylorus. These function to improve overall digestion and absorption of key nutrients. CCK has a trophic effect on small bowel mucosa and on pancreas cells; it may also play role in intestinal motility and insulin release. Finally, CCK acts to produce a sense of satiety when released by fat and protein.

Measurement of CCK levels is not routinely performed as it is difficult to identify it separately from gastrin; however, the need for this assay is unknown as CCK producing tumors are seemingly quite uncommon.

Bibliography

Evers BM. Small bowel. In: Townsend CM, Beauchamp RD, Evers BM, et al. (eds.), *Sabiston Textbook of Surgery*, 16th ed. Philadelphia, PA: W.B. Saunders, 2001, 879.

Miller LJ. Gastrointestinal hormones and receptors. In: Yamada T, Alpers DH, Kaplowitz N, et al. (eds.), *Textbook of Gastroenterology*, 4th ed. Philadelphia, PA: Lippincott, Williams & Wilkins, 2003, 62–64.

Simeone DM. Anatomy and physiology of the small intestine. In: Greenfield L, Mulholland M, Oldham K, et al. (eds.), *Surgery: Scientific Principles and Practice*, 3rd ed. Philadelphia, PA: Lippincott, Williams & Wilkins, 2001, 797–798.

2. **(C)** The gut has a very complex array of defense mechanisms to protect it against constant pathogens. Its first line of defense is nonimmunologic barriers; these include gastric acid and proteolytic enzymes which directly degrade pathogens, the inhibition of bacterial growth by a mucinous coat on the epithelial cells, the spatial inhibition of exogenous bacteria by the presence of native bacteria, epithelial tight junctions preventing invasion of the epithelium by pathogens, and peristalsis to prevent stagnation of pathogens or carcinogens on the gut mucosa.

The immunologic barriers are vast. Gut-associated lymphoid tissue comprises a major division of the body's immune system with approximately 70% of all immunoglobulin production occurring here. Intraepithelial lymphocytes (IELs) live between gut epithelial cells in the crypts of the villi and primarily serve as cytolytic T cells during illness with a high CD8 expression; however, during health they serve to secrete cytokines such as interferon-gamma (IFN-γ.) Another function of IELs during health is that of immunosurveillance, insuring against abnormal epithelial cells and inducing apoptosis in them. The lamina propria houses a number of unaggregated lymphoid cells including B and T cells, presumably migrants from Peyer's patches, macrophages, neutrophils, eosinophils, and mast cells. The lamina propria B cells and plasma cells are the primary producers of IgA.

The lamina propria also is home to Peyer's patches, lymphoid nodules without capsules comprised primarily of B and T cells. These are found on the antimesenteric border of the ileum. Peyer's patches are covered by microfold cells (M cells). These cells allow the lymphoid cells selective exposure to intraluminal antigens by transporting endocytosed antigens transcellularly to the Peyer's patches. Once these cells are "educated" they travel to other areas of the lymph system.

Gut plasma cells produce a significant amount of IgA which confers great protection for the intestinal tract. IgA occurs in monomeric and polymeric forms; 50% of gut IgA is polymeric with its monomers connected by a J chain. The IgA and J chain are produced in the plasma cell and transported to the cell border to interact and complex with the epithelial polymeric immunoglobulin receptor (pIgR). This complex is endocytosed and transported to the epithelial surface to be secreted as sIgA. Secretory IgA prevents the mucosa against bacterial adherence and colonization. It neutralizes bacterial toxins and viral activity, and prohibits absorption of intraluminal antigens. Unlike other immunoglobulins, however, it does *not* activate complement or cell-mediated opsonization.

Bibliography

Blumberg RS, Stenson WF. The immune system and gastrointestinal inflammation. In: Yamada T, Alpers DH, Kaplowitz N, et al. (eds.), *Textbook of Gastroenterology*, 4th ed. Philadelphia, PA: Lippincott, Williams & Wilkins, 2003, 127–130.

Evers BM. Small bowel. In: Townsend CM, Beauchamp RD, Evers BM, et al. (eds.), *Sabiston Textbook of Surgery*, 16th ed. Philadelphia, PA: W.B. Saunders, 2001, 881–882.

Simeone DM. Anatomy and physiology of the small intestine. In: Greenfield L, Mulholland M, Oldham K, et al. (eds.), *Surgery: Scientific Principles and Practice*, 3rd ed. Philadelphia, PA: Lippincott, Williams & Wilkins, 2001, 795–797.

3. **(A)** The overall incidence of CD is three to seven new cases per year per 100,000 people and a prevalence of 80–120 per 100,000. It is more common in Europe and North America and has been rarely seen Asia or South America; however, Crohn's occurs in those moving to endemic areas at the same rate as normally seen for that area, suggesting an environmental contribution to its development. CD has a bimodal pattern of onset with the first peak seen in the second and third decade and a smaller peak in the sixth decade. CD is more common in urban areas than rural areas. This was observed even in a 1950s British study of CD when Scottish towns were noted to have less than half of the incidence as London.

CD similarly affects men and women although early studies suggested a predilection for women. American blacks and whites are afflicted equally, but the incidence is very low among African blacks. Jews of European decent are at significantly higher risk than similar age and gender matched Americans and Europeans. Smokers have double the risk of non-smokers, but smoking seems to confer some degree of protection against ulcerative colitis (UC). First-degree relatives of Crohn's patients are at 13-fold greater risk while siblings carry a risk increased by 30-fold.

Bibliography

Evers BM. Small bowel. In: Townsend CM, Beauchamp RD, Evers BM, et al. (eds.), *Sabiston Textbook of Surgery*, 16th ed. Philadelphia, PA: W.B. Saunders, 2001, 888.

Kirsener JB. Etiologic concepts of inflammatory bowel disease: past, present, future. In: Michelassi F, Milsom JW (eds.), *Operative Strategies in Inflammatory Bowel Disease*. New York, NY: Springer, 1999, 7–8.

Michelassi F, Hurst RD. Crohn's disease. In: Greenfield L, Mulholland M, Oldham K, et al. (eds.), *Surgery: Scientific Principles and Practice*, 3rd ed. Philadelphia, PA: Lippincott, Williams & Wilkins, 2001, 813.

4. **(C)** This patient's presentation is typical for that of inflammatory bowel disease (IBD), both CD and UC. Periods of colicky, sharp abdominal pain, diarrhea, weight loss, and malaise alternate with periods of normalcy, but overtime the symptomatic times become more frequent and prolonged. Diagnosis of IBD is made using endoscopy along with careful history and physical examination with possible computed tomography (CT) scan and barium studies.

In early diagnosis of IBD, distinguishing between CD and UC can be difficult, but time will allow a nearly undisputable diagnosis. UC typically affects the rectum and distal colon first in a continuous fashion, with diffuse erythema and edema accompanied by frequent crypt abscesses and loss of mucin production. On pathologic exam, the crypt base demonstrates a loss of goblet cells and basal plasmacytosis, and the lamina propria is infiltrated by inflammatory cells. It usually is limited to the colon. The anus is usually spared. However, early UC may defy these generalizations and initially spare the rectum; backwash ileitis and spared areas may also be present, and the anus can have superficial ulcers that act like perianal fistulas.

CD typically presents with aphthous ulcers, lesions a few millimeters in diameter surrounded by thickened edematous mucosa, that can involve any part of the GI tract; however, the rectum is usually spared. The ulcers traverse perpendicular to the mucosal plain. They are multiple foci of ulcers with intervening normal mucosa, known as skip lesions. The ulcers can form crossing linear tracts demonstrating the cobblestoning seen on barium examination. Anal involvement includes deep perianal fissures, fistulas, and abscess that result in severe limitations in defecation. Pathologic examination of endoscopically obtained biopsies demonstrates transmural involvement containing all types of acute and chronic inflammatory cells, rather than the predominance of plasma cells noted in UC.

Bibliography

Evers BM. Small bowel. In: Townsend CM, Beauchamp RD, Evers BM, et al. (eds.), *Sabiston Textbook of Surgery*, 16th ed. Philadelphia, PA: W.B. Saunders, 2001, 888–892.

Finkelstein SD, Sasatomi E, Regueiro M. Pathologic features of early inflammatory bowel disease. *Gastroenterol Clin North Am* 2002;31:133–145.

Rubesin SE, Scotiniotis I, Birnbaum BA, et al. Radiologic and endoscopic diagnosis of Crohn's disease. *Surg Clin North Am* 2001;81:39–70.

Stenson WF, Korzenik J. Inflammatory bowel disease. In: Yamada T, Alpers D, Kaplowitz N, et al. (eds.), *Textbook of Gastroenterology*, 4th ed. Philadelphia, PA: Lippincott, Williams & Wilkins, 2003, 1713–1714.

5. **(A)** This patient has acute ileitis. This may or may not be related to Crohn's (and most often is not related to CD). The correct procedure in this case is appendectomy only. Although the appendix appears normal on direct examination, the right lower quadrant wound or the laparoscopic wounds that the patient already has would be confusing in the future. There is no indication for an ileocecectomy as this is an infectious process and will heal with antibiotics. If this is in fact an initial presentation of CD, additional therapy will be required but will heal without surgery.

Acute ileitis presents with right lower quadrant pain, fever, and anorexia much the same as acute appendicitis. It is often caused by *Campylobacter* or *Yersinia* species. These can be cultured from the appendix and from the patient's stool. In one study of patients with signs and symptoms of acute appendicitis, nine patients had only thickened terminal ileum on ultrasound. Five of these proceeded to surgery in spite of these results. All nine had positive cultures of *C. jejuni*, and all recovered easily with no progression to CD. There were no adverse events from the appendectomies. Similarly, a study of 138 normal appendices excised for presumed appendicitis yielded positive cultures for *C. jejuni* and *Y. enterocolitoca*. At the time of surgery, the appendix appeared normal, but 62% of these culture positive patients had terminal ileitis or mesenteric adenitis. There were no pathologic cultures of *C. jejuni* or *Y. enterocolitoca* isolated from 326 normal appendices excised during gynecologic surgeries. Although acute terminal ileitis can present as appendicitis and appear to be early Crohn's, the majority are of infectious etiologies.

Bibliography

Evers BM. Small bowel. In: Townsend CM, Beauchamp RD, Evers BM, et al. (eds.), *Sabiston Textbook of Surgery*, 16th ed. Philadelphia, PA: W.B. Saunders, 2001, 893.

Puylaert JB, Lalisang RI, van der Werf SD, et al. *Campylobacter ileocolitis* mimicking appendicitis: differentiation with graded-compression US. *Radiology* 1988; 166:737–740.

Van Noyen R, Selderslaghs R, Bakaert J, et al. Causative role of *Yersinia* and other enteric pathogens in the appendicular syndrome. *Eur J Clin Microb Infect* 1991; 9: 735–741.

6. **(E)** Unfortunately surgery cannot cure CD, but it does address Crohn's complications and provide palliation of symptoms; approximately 80% of patients with CD require surgery at some point. The most common operations performed are intestinal resections, stricturoplasties, and intestinal bypasses. The most common indications for surgery are failure of medical therapy, intestinal obstruction, enteric fistulae, growth retardation, abscess formation, and cancer. The primary strategy in operating for CD must be to operate only on the complicating segment of bowel. Resection must not extend to all areas that are grossly diseased, but must be limited to the area of abscess, fistula, or obstruction.

ECFs most frequently occur postoperatively either immediately or even after significant delay (Fig. 23-5). They rarely occur spontaneously and rarely affect a clean unscarred abdominal wall. A trial of TPN and bowel rest is legitimate and will be effective if the drainage is limited and the CD well controlled medically; but most others require surgery especially in the face of CD unresponsive to medical therapy. Excision of the fistula tract and the diseased segment of bowel with reanastomosis is the preferred procedure.

Duodenal CD causing obstruction or severe symptoms frequently requires intestinal bypass for management. Fewer than 2% of patients with CD have duodenal disease, but 30% of these require surgery at some point. Intestinal bypass was once a mainstay of surgical therapy of all CD, but complications such as bacterial overgrowth and cancer in the excluded segment caused limitation of this technique to the one area where it was effective and relatively complication-free: the duodenum. Frequently vagotomy is also performed with the gastrojejunal bypass to reduce the potential for jejunal ulcers after the bypass.

Patients with intestinal obstruction related to CD flare should be managed initially with intensive medical therapy, bowel rest, nutritional support, and nasogastric (NG) suction. This will often be adequate for initial management of the obstruction and allow the intestinal tract to undergo further radiographic evaluation. When high- or mid-grade obstructions are present, surgery is indicated with the preference of operating after the acute exacerbation of CD has subsided. The presence of multiple or single strictures, the presence of abscesses and/or fistulas, and the patient's prior operative history determine the necessary

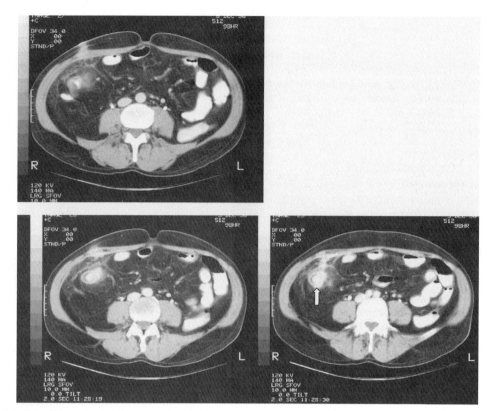

FIG. 23-5   Enterocutaneous fistula in patient with Crohn's disease of distal ileum. (Courtesy of Hal Kipfer M.D. and Indiana University Radiology Teaching files)

operation. Intestinal resection should be minimized given the severe morbidity resulting from short bowel syndrome. Stricturoplasty has been an excellent choice for conservation of intestinal length, but concerns exist about the potential for cancer in the remaining segment of bowel. This technique has been employed only in the previous two decades, so the final analysis is yet to come.

Growth retardation has been a consistent finding in children diagnosed with CD and has even been noticed prior to the onset of intestinal symptoms. Most children resume appropriate growth rates after surgical resection of diseased segments and occasionally experience and growth spurt following surgery; however, over time these children remain slightly smaller than the average American as adults. Using this as a sole indication for surgery has not been studied, but most children with CD do require surgery and do experience this benefit. When the growth retardation is severe, some authors do advocate surgery but do not recommend an exact length or criteria for intestinal resection. The cause of the slowed growth is attributed to increased metabolic rate, loss of protein and nutrients, growth hormone deficiency, and lack of appropriate response to growth hormone.

Bibliography

Becker JM. Surgical therapy for ulcerative colitis and Crohn's disease. *Gastroenterol Clin North Am* 1999; 28: 371–390.

Dokucu AI, Samacki S, Michel JL, et al. Indications and results of surgery in patients with Crohn's disease with onset under 10 years of age: a series of 18 patients. *Eur J Pediatr Surg* 2002;12:180–185.

Evers BM. Small bowel. In: Townsend CM, Beauchamp RD, Evers BM, et al. (eds.), *Sabiston Textbook of Surgery*, 16th ed. Philadelphia, PA: W.B. Saunders, 2001, 893–895.

Ferguson A, Sedgwick DM. Juvenile onset inflammatory bowel disease: height and body mass index in adult life. *Br Med J* 1994;308:1259–1263.

Michelassi F. Indications for surgical treatment in ulcerative colitis and Crohn's disease. In: Michelassi F, Milsom JW (eds.), *Operative Strategies in Inflammatory Bowel Disease*. New York, NY: Springer, 1999, 150–153.

Michelassi F. Surgical treatment of fistulas. In: Michelassi F, Milsom JW (eds.), *Operative Strategies in Inflammatory Bowel Disease*. New York, NY: Springer, 1999, 357–358.

Michelassi F, Hurst RD. Crohn's disease. In: Greenfield L, Mulholland M, Oldham K, et al. (eds.), *Surgery: Scientific Principles and Practice*, 3rd ed. Philadelphia, PA: Lippincott, Williams & Wilkins, 2001, 820–822.

Wolff BG, Nyam DC. Bypass procedures. In: Michelassi F, Milsom JW (eds.), *Operative Strategies in Inflammatory Bowel Disease*. New York, NY: Springer, 1999, 268–269.

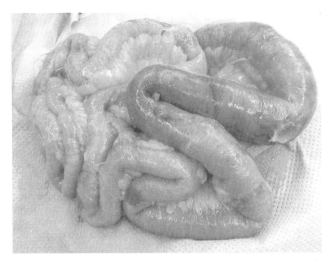

FIG. 23-6 Aspergillous enteritis in patient with AIDs, and example of neutropenic enteritis

7. **(B)** Patients who are severely immunosuppressed as a result of HIV/AIDS, chemotherapy or a solid organ transplant are subject to a host of GI diseases which are nonexistent or extremely limited in the immunocompetent (Fig. 23-6). CMV enteritis, GI tuberculosis, *Shigella*, and *Salmonella* are only a few of these opportunistic pathogens that occasionally masquerade as an acute abdomen as the patients demonstrate fever, severe abdominal pain, anorexia, and occasionally diarrhea with each of these.

CMV enteritis most frequently attacks the distal ileum and right colon, but it can occur anywhere along the GI tract. Hemorrhagic ulcerated lesions are typically seen at endoscopy. The diagnosis is made by culture or by seeing the characteristic nuclear inclusions (the "owl's eye") on cytology. Treatment consists of either ganciclovir or foscarnet. Both of these drugs are viridostatic, so complete elimination of the virus can be difficult.

GI mycobacterial disease also afflicts the severely immunocompromised. This includes *Mycobacterium avium* (MAC) and *Mycobacterium tuberculosis*. GI manifestations of MAC insinuate systemically disseminated disease. Tuberculosis affects the ileum and cecum, and demonstrating the organism in tissue confirms the diagnosis. It can sometimes cause fistulas, obstructions, and free perforation. Surgery is indicated for the latter two, but fistulas often resolve with typical multidrug tuberculosis therapy. MAC treatment is not as clearly delineated, but amikacin, clarithromycin, and ciprofloxacin have been used with some success.

Campylobacter jejuni, *Salmonella*, and *Shigella* cause blood-tinged diarrhea, weight loss, fever, and crampy abdominal pain that sometimes mimics an acute abdomen. Stool culture is diagnostic. They are all associated with high rates of bacteremia in this population. Treatment consists of fluoroquinolones, with ciprofloxacin providing the best coverage.

Clostridium difficile is quite common in HIV/AIDS patients because of the frequent hospitalization and use of antibiotics, but it is not considered opportunistic. Symptoms are similar to the immunocompetent: watery diarrhea, fever, abdominal pain, and leukocytosis. Severity of illness is also similar in both populations. Treatment with metronidazole and/or vancomycin is effective.

Bibliography

Evers BM. Small bowel. In: Townsend CM, Beauchamp RD, Evers BM, et al. (eds.), *Sabiston Textbook of Surgery*, 16th ed. Philadelphia, PA: W.B. Saunders, 2001, 896–897.

Smith PD, Janoff EN. Gastrointestinal complications of the acquired immunodeficiency syndrome. In: Yamada T, Alpers D, Kaplowitz N, et al. (eds.), *Textbook of Gastroenterology*, 4th ed. Philadelphia, PA: Lippincott, Williams & Wilkins, 2003, 2567–2579.

8. **(C)** The medical therapy of CD is one fraught with frustration on many fronts because of the side effects of many of the effective drugs and the limited choices of drugs that are effective. Of the choices above, all are regularly used in the treatment of CD except IL-10 which is currently under study. IL-10 has potential as a CD treatment because is suppresses IL-2 and IFN-γ production by Th-1 lymphocytes which mediate CD. Early studies have shown mixed results, so it is not yet available as a routine treatment of CD.

Steroids play a key role in the treatment of CD in bringing about a remission. Steroids are effective enterally and parenterally. They are effective in preventing or suppressing the inflammatory response in both early stages of inflammation (vascular permeability, vasodilatation, and neutrophil invasion) and the late stages of inflammation (vascular proliferation, collagen deposition, and activation of fibroblasts). However, in addition to their multiple side effects, corticosteroids do not bring about mucosal healing, and they are not effective in maintaining remission. Unfortunately there are no good studies elucidating the best dosing strategies or timing of the steroid taper. Most determine the taper based on symptomatic improvements; this frequently does not correlate with endoscopic improvements. The majority of patients can be weaned from steroids after remission has been achieved, but about 25% will require lifetime steroids as they have symptomatic flares each time the steroids are discontinued, in spite of combination therapy with 5-aminosalicylic acid (5-ASA), 6-mercaptupurine, methotrexate, or cyclosporine.

Infliximab, a mouse-human chimeric IgG antibody against tumor necrosis factor alpha (TNF-α), has been effective in inducing remission and in treating fistulas. Clinical benefits of remission and decreased fistula drainage can be maintained with the infusion of infliximab every 8 weeks. The fistulas, once closed, remain closed for approximately 12 weeks, and then usually require definitive treatment. Unfortunately, toxicity increases with increased number of infliximab infusions. Some develop human antichimeric antibodies and sustain acute and delayed hypersensitivity reactions. Infliximab has also been associated with varicella zoster, *Candida* esophagitis, and tuberculosis. Also patients can develop intestinal strictures as a result of rapid healing of ulcers. Once again, the optimal timing of infliximab treatment has not been studied, so much remains to be learned about this treatment.

The most useful agent for maintaining remission for CD at this time is azathioprine. Azathioprine and its metabolite 6-mercaptopurine (6-MP) block lymphocyte proliferation, activation, and efficacy. Their efficacy is not realized until 3–4 months after treatment has begun; therefore it is started concurrently with steroids and then continued well beyond the steroid taper. Azathioprine then is continued indefinitely; relapse rate in patients on this regimen remains about 30%, while 75% of those not taking the drug relapse. Leukopenia and pancreatitis are its primary toxicities; both resolve once the drug is stopped. Other maintenance drugs include various 5-ASA preparations (most effective in ileal and colonic CD), methotrexate, and cyclosporine. Tacrolimus is currently under study.

Bibliography

Harrison J, Hanauer SB. Medical treatment of Crohn's disease. *Gastroenterol Clin North Am* 2002;31:167–184.

Stenson WF, Korzenik J. Inflammatory bowel disease. In: Yamada T, Alpers D, Kaplowitz N, et al. (eds.), *Textbook of Gastroenterology*, 4th ed. Philadelphia, PA: Lippincott, Williams & Wilkins, 2003, 1726–1740.

9. **(D)** Small bowel obstructions are caused by intestinal adhesive disease in 60–80% of cases (Fig. 23-7). Other causes include hernia, volvulus, carcinoma, intussusception, CD, and radiation enteritis. Although all abdominal surgeries cause adhesions, those resulting in obstruction most frequently occur after pelvic procedures such as appendectomies, abdominal hysterectomies, and abdominopelvic resections. Adhesive obstructions occur in 5% of patients with previous laparotomies; however, most of these resolve with conservative management.

Patients present with varying degrees of nausea, vomiting, abdominal distension, and abdominal pain; these symptoms are more acute and severe in closed loop obstructions and strangulating obstructions. Patients with strangulation frequently demonstrate peritonitis and systemic signs of illness: fever, tachycardia, leukocytosis, and decreased urine output. These patients require emergent operation *after adequate resuscitation* and correction of electrolyte abnormalities for

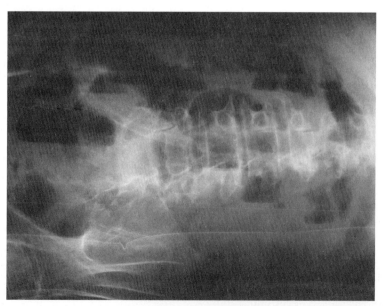

FIG. 23-7   Left lateral decubitus abdominal X ray demonstrating small bowel obstruction

relief of the obstruction as mortality significantly increases with delay of surgery.

Obstructions in the early postoperative period should be managed conservatively with bowel rest, NG decompression, and fluid resuscitation. These are often partial obstructions, so conservative management can be continued up to 2 weeks. Enterocolysis may be helpful in demonstrating the cause and degree of obstruction when these are persistent. Abdominal radiographs are rarely helpful as most have a similar appearance to postoperative ileus. If the early postoperative obstruction is complete or if systemic symptoms ensue, it must be managed surgically as other complete obstructions are managed. Symptoms that evolve over a short period of time carry a mortality of 15%.

Obstruction resulting from recurrent cancer and peritoneal studding is a special situation. One-third of these patients actually have adhesive disease and can be palliated or even cured with surgery. However, an extended opportunity for resolution of the obstruction with conservative management is warranted in the case of recurrent malignancy to spare the patient an additional laparotomy. Some advocate the use of the long intestinal decompression tube to attempt to decompress nearer the site of obstruction. Systemic symptoms, as before, warrant immediate surgery if the patient agrees. Malignant obstruction can be treated with intestinal bypass. If carcinomatosis is encountered, tube gastrostomy may prove palliative to avoid frequent NG intubation.

Radiation enteritis also presents a difficult situation. These obstructions also will frequently resolve with conservative management. If surgery is necessary, it carries a significant morbidity as suturing bowel scarred by chronic inflammation can result in fistulas, abscesses, and anastomotic leaks.

Bibliography

Evers BM. Small bowel. In: Townsend CM, Beauchamp RD, Evers BM, et al. (eds.), *Sabiston Textbook of Surgery*, 16th ed. Philadelphia, PA: W.B. Saunders, 2001, 882–888.

Maglinte D, Kelvin F, Rowe M. Small bowel obstruction: optimizing radiologic investigation and nonsurgical management. *Radiology* 2001;218: 39–46.

Pickelman J. Small bowel obstruction. In: Cameron J (ed.), *Current Surgical Therapy*, 7th ed. St. Louis, MO: Mosby, 2001, 122–128.

Soybel D. Ileus and bowel obstruction. In: Greenfield L, Mulholland M, Oldham K, et al. (eds.), *Surgery: Scientific Principles and Practice*, 3rd ed. Philadelphia, PA: Lippincott, Williams & Wilkins, 2001, 798–812.

10. **(C)** This patient indeed has PI or air within the wall of the bowel (Fig. 23-8); however, this is not a diagnosis in itself, so its significance and prognosis depends on the underlying cause. This finding has a wide range of possible causes and potential outcomes. PI can be primary, usually occurring in the distal large bowel, or secondary, more commonly occurring in the small bowel. Secondary PI can be associated with iatrogenic injury from endoscopy or invasive radiologic examination, autoimmune or infectious diseases,

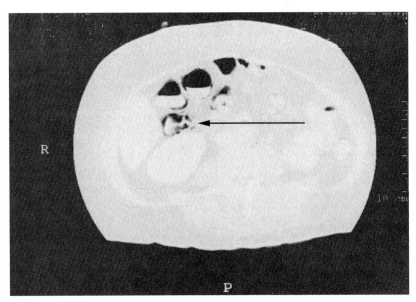

FIG. 23-8 Pneumatosis intestinalis on CT with lung windows. (Courtesy of Hal Kipfer, M.D. and Indiana University Radiology Teaching files)

ischemia, scleroderma, chemotherapy, trauma, or COPD among others. Presenting complaints include diarrhea, abdominal pain and distension, vomiting, weight loss, and hematochezia. Physical examination may demonstrate abdominal distension or mass. If pneumoperitoneum results from PI, it is usually sterile, the examination remains benign, and no surgical treatment is required unless signs of peritonitis are present.

PI appears as frequent cysts on radiologic examination occurring from the esophagus to the anus and can also occur in the mesentery, the omentum, and the falciform ligament. The cysts usually occur in the subserosa near the mesenteric border and in the submucosa. They can be a few millimeters to several centimeters in size and can involve very small or very lengthy segments of bowel. Pneumoperitoneum frequently is seen as well. Portal venous gas is most frequently associated with ischemia and is indicative of more urgent need for surgical intervention.

The cysts contain pressurized gas from three possible sources: intraluminal GI gas, pulmonary gas, or gas produced by bacteria. Many theories exist as to the source and the method of intramural gas. Many contend that the gas became intramural as a result of severe COPD with alveolar rupture and dissection from the mediastinum to the retroperitoneum by way of the great vessels through the mesentery and into the serosa. The mechanical theory purports that mucosal defects allow pressurized gas, as in endoscopy, trauma, or obstruction, to dissect into the bowel wall. The bacterial theory postulates that gas forming organisms invade the wall of the mucosa especially during times of immunosuppression or neutropenia allowing cysts to form; however, each of these theories is significantly flawed. In the pulmonary theory, many patients do not have any evidence of pneumomediastinum, pneumothorax, or pneumoretroperitoneum. The mechanical theory does not explain the high hydrogen content of the cyst gas compared with air or usual intestinal gas. And the bacterial theory does not explain the sterile pneumoperitoneum that exists when the cysts rupture.

Treatment is based on the underlying problem. Ischemia, acidosis, fever, peritonitis, leukocytosis, and clinical decline clearly necessitate intervention; however, frequently PI can be treated with minimal intervention if the treatment is based on the cause of the PI. Treatments noted in the literature include oxygen therapy maintaining a PaO_2 greater than 250 mmHg with supplemental oxygen, long-term metronidazole therapy, a short-term of bowel rest and observation, or high dose steroids as in the cases

concurrent with systemic lupus erythematosus (SLE). Overall, PI can be managed expectantly except in the case of ischemia.

Bibliography

Evers BM. Small bowel. In: Townsend CM, Beauchamp RD, Evers BM, et al. (eds.), *Sabiston Textbook of Surgery*, 16th ed. Philadelphia, PA: W.B. Saunders, 2001, 911.

Boerner M, Fried D, Warshauer D, et al. Pneumatosis intestinalis: two case reports and a retrospective review of the literature. *Dig Dis Sci* 1996;41:2272–2285.

St. Peter S, Abbas M, Kelly K. The spectrum of pneumatosis intestinalis. *Arch Surg* 2003;138: 68–75.

11. **(E)** ECFs are often disheartening postoperative complications as they often result from iatrogenic injuries. They can be caused by technical errors such as missed enterotomies, anastomotic tension, or compromised blood supply at the anastomosis resulting in its breakdown. Erosion into the bowel by foreign bodies such as suction catheters or nearby abscesses can also cause ECFs. Spontaneous ECFs result from CD, neoplasms, or radiation injury.

Once a fistula is recognized, one must consider the likelihood for spontaneous closure. Fistulas that are produce <500 cc per day are three times more likely to close than high output fistulas producing >500 cc per day. Fistulas that are more than 2.5 cm in length increase the likelihood of closure over shorter tracts because these are less likely to epithelialize to the skin and cause more resistance to flow. Patients with distal obstruction, active CD, foreign body, large abdominal wall defect, or involved neoplasm are unlikely to close fistulas spontaneously. Finally, patients who are malnourished (albumin <2.5, transferring <200) or septic are unlikely to resolve fistulas with conservative management.

ECFs should be considered in postoperative patients with fever and an erythematous wound. Once the wound is opened, the drainage of bilious of feculent contents confirm the diagnosis. Occasionally, ECFs present with overt peritonitis and sepsis. In either case, treatment begins with fluid and electrolyte resuscitation and broad-spectrum antibiotics. In the event of ongoing sepsis and clinical decline, emergent operation is indicated with resection of the fistulized segment of small bowel and primary end-to-end anastomosis. If the abdomen is overcome with contamination such that the diseased segment cannot be clearly delineated, a proximal stoma or intestinal bypass is indicated. This avoids resecting a lengthy segment of bowel and causing short bowel syndrome.

If the patient is clinically stable, conservative management can begin with broad-spectrum antibiotics, total parenteral nutrition (TPN), and CT scan to evaluate the position of the fistula. CT guided placement of percutaneous drains may be needed to control an enteric leak. A fistulogram may be needed to assess the length of the ECF tract and its exact location in the bowel. An enterostomal therapist should become involved to assist devising a method to keep enteric contents from causing skin breakdown. Pharmacologic agents can also be employed to decrease fistula drainage such as H2 blockers to decrease gastric acid output and octreotide to decrease bilious and pancreatic output. The use of octreotide has not been definitively shown to improve the rate of spontaneous closure in spite of decreasing fistula output. Maintaining adequate nutrition is imperative in fistula management to improve the likelihood for spontaneous closure or to improve outcome should surgery be needed. Some carefully selected ECF patients may receive enteral nutrition, but bowel rest and TPN should be the mainstay in early fistula management.

If an ECF is to close spontaneously, >90% close within the first month of treatment; however, if surgical management is required, one must carefully plan this difficult operation using contrast studies of the fistula and GI tract. Also nutritional status must be optimized. Delayed repair is advocated by some, waiting up to 4 months for repair because of optimal remodeling of intestinal adhesions. Fistulectomy with primary end-to-end anastomosis is the preferred surgical treatment, and one must carefully avoid additional enterotomies that would predispose to future ECFs.

Bibliography

Denham D, Fabri P. Enterocutaneous fistula. In: Cameron J (ed.), *Current Surgical Therapy*, 7th ed. St. Louis, MO: Mosby, 2001, 156–161.

Evers BM. Small bowel. In: Townsend CM, Beauchamp RD, Evers BM, et al. (eds.), *Sabiston Textbook of Surgery*, 16th ed. Philadelphia, PA: W.B. Saunders, 2001, 909–910.

12. **(A)** Meckel's diverticulum (Fig. 23-9) is the most common congenital abnormality of the GI tract. Frequently we remember it for its rule of 2's: present in 2% of the population, symptomatic in 2%, twice as common in males than females, within 2 ft of the ileocecal valve, approximately 2 in. in length and present with one of two complications: bleeding or obstruction. A Meckel's diverticulum is a remnant of the vitelline duct which initially served to connect the primitive gut to the fetal yolk sac. It usually obliterates by the seventh to eighth week of gestation. The remnant may endure as a fibrous band connecting the ileum to the umbilicus, as a fistulous tract to the umbilicus, or as a

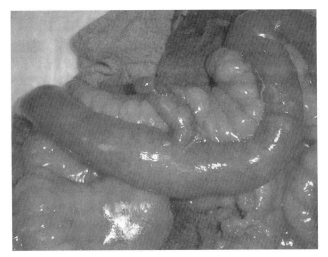

FIG. 23-9 Meckel's diverticulum

true diverticulum containing all layers of the small bowel wall. The vitelline duct contains pluripotent cells; therefore, the cells of the Meckel's diverticulum are those of small intestinal mucosa 50% of the time while gastric mucosa and pancreas cells are present 50% of the time. Rarely, colonic mucosa is present.

Complicated Meckel's diverticula most frequently contain gastric mucosa. These cells produce gastric acid and result in ileal ulcers that eventually bleed. Adults present with painless melena in this case while children generally present with bright red blood per rectum. Hemorrhage is the most common complication occurring in 30–50% of Meckel's complications. Obstruction can result by a number of mechanisms: intussusception, volvulus, or strangulation related to the fibrous band attached to the umbilicus, or rarely a Littre's hernia which is the incarceration of the Meckel's diverticulum in an inguinal hernia. Diverticulitis accounts for 10–20% of presentations. This should be considered in patients with right lower quadrant pain and a normal appendix at exploration.

Diagnosis of Meckel's is difficult, so high clinical suspicion is necessary. Technetium-99 can be used to identify normal and ectopic gastric mucosa; this is occasionally helpful, especially in children, but false negatives occur in the face of H2 blockers and proton-pump inhibitors. Arteriography is useful if brisk bleeding is occurring.

Treatment of Meckel's diverticula centers on resection. There has been significant debate over the treatment of incidentally found Meckel's diverticula. Most studies show incidental resection to be safe when not associated with CD or peritonitis unrelated to the diverticulum. This is especially true since resection no longer involves opening the bowel when stapling devices are used. In the cases of symptomatic Meckel's diverticula, diverticulectomy is rarely sufficient. Rather, segmental ileal resection with anastomosis is indicated especially when this is suspected as a source of bleeding. Barium or air enema can be used to reduce intussuscepted Meckel's, but surgery is still required to remove this as a lead point.

Bibliography

Evers BM. Small bowel. In: Townsend CM, Beauchamp RD, Evers BM, et al. (eds.), *Sabiston Textbook of Surgery*, 16th ed. Philadelphia, PA: W.B. Saunders, 2001, 907–908.

Matsagas M, Fatouros M, Koulouras B. Incidence, complications, and management of Meckel's diverticulum. *Arch Surg* 1995;130:143–146.

Rubin D. Small intestine: anatomy and structural abnormalities. In: Yamada T, Alpers DH, Kaplowitz N, et al. (eds.), *Textbook of Gastroenterology*, 4th ed. Philadelphia, PA: Lippincott, Williams & Wilkins, 2003, 1473–1474.

13. (E)

14. (B)

Explanations 13 and 14

SMA syndrome, also known as cast syndrome, chronic duodenal ileus or Wilkie's syndrome is a rare cause of duodenal obstruction. The third portion of the duodenum is compressed by the SMA as it branches from the aorta and passes over the duodenum at a sharp angle. The SMA typically has a 45 degree angle to the aorta, but in SMA syndrome the angle is decreased to 6-25 degrees. The aortomesenteric distance has also been found to be shorter. The increased acuity of this angle is associated with a period of rapid weight loss in adults, including eating disorders, burns, or neoplasms or a period of rapid growth in children; these result in decreased retroperitoneal or mesenteric fat. Other associated conditions include severe scoliosis, body casts that increase spinal lordosis, and large abdominal aortic aneurysms. Symptoms of SMA syndrome are somewhat vague. Postprandial epigastric pain, abdominal distension, nausea, and vomiting partially digested food are common presenting complaints. Patients may have some symptomatic relief in a knee to chest position. CT scan will demonstrate the acute angle of the superior mesenteric artery. Barium upper GI series show the abrupt obstruction of the third portion of the duodenum with some relief of the obstruction in the left lateral decubitus position (Fig. 23-10). Arteriography adds little to CT scan, but the acute angle can also be seen in the lateral view. Endoscopy demonstrates retained food in the stomach and a dilated duodenum with extrinsic compression easily noted at its third segment.

Treatment of SMA syndrome includes a trial of medical therapy where the patient takes multiple small feedings or a liquid diet. Some patients benefit from lying in the left lateral decubitus position or in the prone position after the meal. If this results in weight gain, the symptoms gradually subside. Also removal of the body cast can result in cure of the syndrome. If conservative management fails, surgical therapy is necessary. This includes resection of the obstructing aneurysm or treatment of scoliosis with a longer trial of medical therapy. The mainstay of

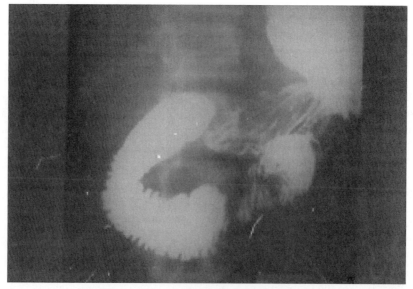

FIG. 23-10   Duodenal C sweep with significant proximal dilatation due to obstruction by the SMA.

surgical management is bypass of the third portion of the duodenum with a duodenojejunostomy. This is reportedly successful 90% of the time. Lysis of the ligament of Treitz also frees the obstruction and has been done laparoscopically.

Bibliography

Baltazar U, Dunn J, Floresguerra C, et al. Superior mesenteric artery syndrome: an uncommon cause of intestinal obstruction. *South Med J* 2000;93:606–608.

Evers BM. Small bowel. In: Townsend CM, Beauchamp RD, Evers BM, et al. (eds.), *Sabiston Textbook of Surgery*, 16th ed. Philadelphia, PA: W.B. Saunders, 2001, 913–914.

Raufman J. Stomach: anatomy and structural abnormalities. In Yamada T, Alpers DH, Kaplowitz N, et al. (eds.), *Textbook of Gastroenterology*, 4th ed. Philadelphia, PA: Lippincott, Williams & Wilkins, 2003, 1290.

Richardson W, Surowiec W. Laparoscopic repair of superior mesenteric artery syndrome. *Am J Surg* 2001; 181: 377–378.

Sostek M, Fine SN, Harris TL. Duodenal obstruction by abdominal aortic aneurysm: brief clinical observations. *Am J Med* 1993;94:220–221.

15. **(C)** Both children and adults ingest foreign objects accidentally, as a result of mental illness, for secondary gain, or in an effort to smuggle illicit drugs. Frequently ingested objects include paper clips, razor blades, safety pins, chicken bones, coins, toys, and batteries. Seventy-five percent of impactions occur in the esophagus. If this is the case, endoscopy is indicated for removal. Surgery would be necessary only if endoscopy was unsuccessful as in the case of a large object that could not be snared easily. Endoscopy is indicated emergently for sharp objects or batteries in the esophagus, or if the patient has airway compromise. If the foreign objects progress to the stomach, endoscopic removal is indicated if the foreign body is larger than 5 cm by 2 cm or if it is sharp; otherwise, serial films can be obtained with observation for up to 3 weeks or the patient experiences symptoms.

Most foreign bodies will pass without difficulty. The razor blade in the patient referred to in the question remained lodged at the ileocecal valve for less than 36 h and passed without requiring surgery. Serial examinations and serial abdominal films can be used to follow the passage of even sharp objects; however, the patient must be monitored carefully for any signs of peritonitis, fever, or leukocytosis at which time, emergent laparotomy is required. Laparotomy is also indicated for small bowel obstruction because of the presence of the foreign objects. Cathartic agents are absolutely contraindicated with ingestion of sharp object because of the increased risk of perforation.

Two special cases must be discussed when discussing foreign bodies: battery ingestion and "body packers." In the case of disk batteries, leakage of their alkaline compounds can result in corrosion of esophageal, gastric, or intestinal mucosa. They can also lead to pressure necrosis or low-voltage burns. Batteries must be removed immediately if lodged in the esophagus; they can be monitored for up to 48 h in the stomach in the asymptomatic patient but should be endoscopically removed after this time. Serial films should insure the ongoing progression of the battery through the GI tract if the battery is in the small intestine on presentation. Surgery should commence with any abdominal symptoms or leukocytosis or if the battery has remained stagnant for 48 h as the battery may have corroded into the bowel eventually leading to perforation.

"Body packers" are those who ingest small plastic bags of illicit drugs (usually cocaine or heroin) for smuggling. These can frequently result in severe small bowel obstruction or drug overdose should the packing material break down. Physical examination is typical for small bowel obstruction, but x-ray demonstrates small dense packets surrounded by crescents of air (called the "double condom sign"). The bowel obstruction is managed conservatively with NG decompression, fluid resuscitation, and bowel rest. Surgery is indicated if the bowel appears to be compromised or if the patient shows signs of drug overdose. This is especially necessary in the case of cocaine smuggling because of its life-threatening consequences. Laparotomy may be complicated by the need for multiple enterotomies to extract each bag individually as they become adherent to the bowel mucosa.

Bibliography

Evers BM. Small bowel. In: Townsend CM, Beauchamp RD, Evers BM, et al. (eds.), *Sabiston Textbook of Surgery*, 16th ed. Philadelphia, PA: W.B. Saunders, 2001, 907–908.

Faigel D. Miscellaneous diseases of the esophagus: systemic, dermatologic disease, foreign bodies and physical injury. In: Yamada T, Alpers D, Kaplowitz N, et al. (eds.), *Textbook of Gastroenterology*, 4th ed. Philadelphia, PA: Lippincott, Williams & Wilkins, 2003, 1262.

Greenberg R, Greenberg Y, Kaplan O. "Body Packer" syndrome: characteristics and treatment—case report and review. *Eur J Surg* 2000;166:89–91.

Rabine J, Nostrant T. Miscellaneous diseases of the stomach. In: Yamada T, Alpers D, Kaplowitz N, et al. (eds.), *Textbook of Gastroenterology*, 4th ed. Philadelphia, PA: Lippincott, Williams & Wilkins, 2003, 1460.

16. **(A)** At rest the small bowel receives 10–15% of a patient's cardiac output. This increases to up to 50% during digestion. Of the CO received 70–90% goes to mucosa and submucosa while remainder goes to the muscularis. Ischemic injury can therefore be caused by

a number of conditions causing reduced cardiac output such as bleeding, myocardial infarction, pericardial tamponade, and hypovolemic states. This is often referred to as nonocclusive mesenteric ischemia (NOMI). Initial treatment should be focused on restoring cardiac output by addressing the underlying cause; enteral feeding should also be discontinued to lower the cardiac output requirement by the small bowel. Reperfusion injury of some degree will likely occur depending on the period of insult; this will result in edema and subsequent mucosal sloughing with hemorrhage and possible loss of intestinal epithelial integrity.

Another cause of mesenteric ischemia includes mesenteric arterial embolus or thrombus causing acute disruption in splanchnic flow. This is especially true in patients with known arrhythmias or severe atherosclerotic disease. Acute disruption can also result from drugs such as cyclosporine that prohibit release of local vasodilators. Finally, reflex splanchnic arterial vasospasm occurs with venous thrombosis (as in patients with portal hypertension or hypercoagulable state) and with digitalis toxicity that may result in mesenteric ischemia. Approximately 20% of cases of mesenteric ischemia are due to NOMI, 50% from arterial embolization, 25% from arterial thrombosis, and 5% from venous thrombosis.

Bibliography

Gelabert H. Mesenteric vascular disease of the small bowel. In: Cameron J (ed.), *Current Surgical Therapy*, 7th ed. St. Louis, MO: Mosby, 2001, 149–156.

Patel CV, Durham R. ICU management. In: Longo WE, Peterson GJ (eds.), *Intestinal Ischemia Disorders: Pathophysiology and Management*. St. Louis, MO: Quality Medical Publishing, 1999, 51–53.

Turnage RH, Myers SI. Pathophysiology. In: Longo WE, Peterson GJ (eds.), *Intestinal Ischemia Disorders: Pathophysiology and Management*. St. Louis, MO: Quality Medical Publishing, 1999, 17–19.

17. **(D)** Once mesenteric ischemia has been diagnosed, mesenteric blood flow must be optimized. Adequate hydration, cardiac output optimization, and revascularization accomplish this goal. The next step is determination of viable bowel to determine margins for resection. Many options exist to accomplish this goal including clinical judgment, Doppler ultrasound, oximetry, fluorescein, myoelectric activity, and second look surgery. The best method to be assured remaining bowel is viable is in fact second look surgery, but all methods will be discussed in detail.

Using clinical judgment alone is 90% accurate in assessing bowel viability. Bowel that peristalses, bleeds at its cut edge, and is pink in color is indeed viable.

Unfortunately, we are not as accurate in assessing potentially salvageable bowel. Using clinical judgment alone can lead to significantly greater resection than necessary.

Doppler ultrasound is an easily accessible tool to assess viability. Early studies reported that bowel was viable within one centimeter of the last Doppler signal obtained at the bowel wall, making it very accurate in assessing viable bowel. Once again, the problem arises in judging bowel that can be salvaged. It cannot determine microvascular circulation nor can it accurately detect flow on the antimesenteric side of the bowel.

Fluorescein can be given intraoperatively (15 mg/kg or 1 gm IV) and used to assess bowel under a Wood's lamp. Viable bowel becomes fluorescent yellow quickly while nonviable bowel has no or patchy or delayed fluorescence. This method has been shown to be more accurate than clinical judgment or Doppler. Unfortunately, fluorescein dye can only be used once in a 24–48-hour period, and some people have allergic reactions to the dye. Fluorescein dye test is the second best option to second look surgery.

Oximetry, similar to the usual pulse oximetry, requires a probe to assess venous saturations of oxygen in the intestinal wall. Although the concept is familiar, it requires special equipment in the operating room to be accurate. Myoelectric activity measurements are based on the changes in electrical slow-wave patterns in the intestine during periods of ischemia. The most recent method uses a computer algorithm to combine electromyography (EMG) readings with evoked contractile response (ECR) to determine viability. This is quite accurate in animal models, but remains impractical in the OR setting.

Second look surgery is indeed the best option to prevent resection of potentially viable bowel in the cases where extensive areas of small bowel are compromised by embolus, venous thrombosis, or NOMI. This should be planned at the time of initial operation to take place within 12–48 h of the initial operation.

Bibliography

Belkin M, Whittemore AD, Donaldson MC, et al. Peripheral arterial occlusive disease. In: Townsend CM, Beauchamp RD, Evers BM, et al. (eds.), *Sabiston Textbook of Surgery*, 16th ed. Philadelphia, PA: W.B. Saunders, 2001, 1398–1401.

Langsfeld M, Marek J, Tullis M. Assessment of intestinal viability. In: Longo WE, Peterson GJ (eds.), *Intestinal Ischemia Disorders: Pathophysiology and Management*. St. Louis, MO: Quality Medical Publishing, 1999, 75–89.

Zelenek GB. Visceral occlusive disease. In: Greenfield L, Mulholland M, Oldham K, et al. (eds.), *Surgery: Scientific Principles and Practice*, 3rd ed. Philadelphia, PA: Lippincott, Williams & Wilkins, 2001, 1700–1702.

18. **(B)** Gallstone ileus has a reported incidence of 6 in 1000 cases of small bowel obstruction; however, it is the source of nearly 25% of nonstrangulated small bowel obstructions in the elderly with a 4:1 predominance in females. Gallstone ileus occurs as a result of a biliary enteric fistula. These develop when the inflammation associated with cholecystitis causes erosion of the gallbladder into an adjacent hollow viscus, most commonly duodenum, hepatic flexure of the colon, stomach, or jejunum. The stones then empty into the viscus and travel downstream. The ileus results as stones greater than 2.5 cm in size become impacted at the terminal ileum, the sigmoid colon, or the gastric outlet. Gallstone impaction at the gastric outlet is referred to as Bouveret's syndrome. The fistula generally heals once the gallbladder has decompressed.

Patients present with usual signs of small bowel obstruction (SBO): abdominal pain, nausea, vomiting, and abdominal distension; however, symptoms may vary based on the site of impaction. Patients occasionally have a history of episodic, right upper quadrant postprandial abdominal pain which may predate presentation by weeks, months, or even years. On presentation, the usual workup, including detailed history and physical examination, chemistries, complete blood count, and acute abdominal series, should be done. The abdominal plain films can be diagnostic of gallstone ileus with Rigler's triad: dilated small bowel loops, air in the biliary tree, and an ectopic gallstone. Also this diagnosis should be strongly suspected in an elderly female presenting with SBO with no prior history of surgery and no apparent hernia. If the diagnosis remains in question, CT scan (Fig. 23-2) or contrasted upper GI study is diagnostic.

Treatment commences by addressing the SBO: fluid resuscitation, correction of electrolyte abnormalities, and NG tube placement. Broad-spectrum antibiotics should also be given. At laparotomy, the abdomen should be thoroughly explored. If the stone is lodged in the terminal ileum, it can be milked distally through the ileocecal valve to the colon and allowed to be expelled via the feces; it can be milked proximally to an area of bowel that is not edematous and excised via enterotomy which is then primarily closed. It may require excision at the point of impaction which is then closed primarily, taking great care to avoid spillage of enteric contents (Fig. 23-4). If the stone is impacted in the colon, the stone should be excised via colostomy and an ostomy created. In either case, the fistula and the gallbladder may be left alone as fewer than 10% require reoperation for cholecystectomy. In addition, mortality is significantly higher when the fistula and gallbladder are excised.

The treatment for Bouveret's syndrome is significantly different. The gastric outlet obstruction must be relieved. If possible, this may be accomplished endoscopically. If surgery is required, the stone should be removed and the gallbladder and fistula excised with concurrent cholangiography. A Roux-en-Y may be required to repair the fistula.

Bibliography

Lee S, Ko C. Gallstones. In: Yamada T, Alpers DH, Kaplowitz N, et al. (eds.), *Textbook of Gastroenterology*, 4th ed. Philadelphia, PA: Lippincott, Williams & Wilkins, 2003, 2188–2189.

Levi D, Levi J. Gallstone ileus. In: Cameron J (ed.), *Current Surgical Therapy*, 7th ed. St. Louis, MO: Mosby, 2001, 472–474.

Maglinte D, Herlinger H. Plain film radiography of the small bowel. In: Maglinte D, Herlinger H, Birnbaum B (eds.), *Clinical Imaging of the Small Intestine*, 2nd ed. New York, NY: Springer, 1998, 62–65.

19. **(B)** Intussusceptions in adults cause approximately 1% of all small bowel obstructions. They are the cause of only 5% of all intussusceptions. Unlike pediatric intussusceptions, they all must be managed operatively as more than 95% have related pathology, most commonly a mass but adhesions have also been implicated in up to 48% in one cohort. Air or barium contrast reduction is not an option for management in adults. Diagnoses of intussusceptions are frequently made intraoperatively as patients present with signs and symptoms consistent with small bowel obstruction; as a result, many patients have only plain x-rays preoperatively. Of patients who do undergo additional workup, CT scan is the most sensitive study for preoperative diagnosis. A "target lesion" noted on CT demonstrates thickened edematous bowel surrounding decompressed bowel. Occasionally a mass is also identified on CT.

Intussusceptions require a lead point to occur. This is a mass lesion in more than half of cases. Benign lesions such as adenomas, lipomas, hamartomas, and neurofibromas most commonly serve as the lead point because they are asymmetric on the bowel and frequently pedunculated. Primary malignancies such as adenocarcinoma rarely cause intussusceptions because they are circumferential; however, small bowel metastases, such as malignant melanoma metastases, also can lead to intussusceptions.

Patients with Peutz-Jeguers's syndrome frequently experience intermittent abdominal pain resulting from intussusceptions that essentially come and go. Peutz-Jeguers's syndrome is an autosomal dominant genetic disease associated with GI hamartomas primarily involving the jejunum and ileum (but may also involve the stomach and the rectum), melanotic pigmentations of the face, buccal mucosa, palms of hands and soles of feet, and an increased risk of cancer of the ovaries, breast, and pancreas. When these patients present with intussusception or hemorrhage, resection should certainly be limited to the implicated short segment of bowel as extensive resections do not result in cure and can be quite morbid.

Bibliography

Azar T, Berger D. Adult intussusception. *Ann Surg* 1997; 226:134–138.

Bresalier RS, Ben-Menachem T. Tumors of the small intestine. In: Yamada T, Alpers DH, Kaplowitz N, et al. (eds.), *Textbook of Gastroenterology*, 4th ed. Philadelphia, PA: Lippincott, Williams & Wilkins, 2003, 1645.

Evers BM. Small bowel. In: Townsend CM, Beauchamp RD, Evers BM, et al. (eds.), *Sabiston Textbook of Surgery*, 16th ed. Philadelphia, PA: W.B. Saunders, 2001, 899.

Pickelman J. Small bowel obstruction. In: Cameron J (ed.), *Current Surgical Therapy*, 7th ed. St. Louis, MO: Mosby, 2001, 127.

20. **(B)** The most useful radiologic examination for small bowel tumors is enterocolysis (Fig. 23-11). This is a contrasted examination using a combination of methylcellulose with barium to distend the small bowel uniformly while preserving peristalsis. This is so successful over traditional small bowel follow through because the bowel can be fully distended.

The study does require sedation and passage of a thin nasointestinal tube which can be easily performed by those with expertise. Up to 90% of tumors can be identified by enterocolysis while small bowel follow through identifies 35%. Abdominal and pelvis CT is very poor in detecting small bowel lesions. Its use lies primarily in evaluation of metastatic disease. If, on presentation with small bowel obstruction, the small bowel is thicker than 1.5 cm or a mesenteric mass is demonstrated with CT scan, one must be suspicious for tumor. CT can be combined with enterocolysis in some centers thereby giving a much more comprehensive abdominal examination with a single study. Ultrasound has not been routinely effective in diagnosing small bowel neoplasms.

Esophagoduodenoscopy is not a radiologic evaluation; however, it is beneficial in evaluating for tumors of the duodenum and has essentially replaced upper GI barium studies for this purpose. Some advocate enteroscopy to evaluate the remaining small bowel for tumors, but generally only the proximal 2–3 ft can be evaluated by this means.

Bibliography

Evers BM. Small bowel. In: Townsend CM, Beauchamp RD, Evers BM, et al. (eds.), *Sabiston Textbook of Surgery*, 16th ed. Philadelphia, PA: W.B. Saunders, 2001, 898.

Maglinte DDT, Bender GN, Heitkamp DE, Lappas JC, Kelvin FM. Multidetector-row helical CT enterocolysis. *Radiol Clin North Am* 2003;41:254–257.

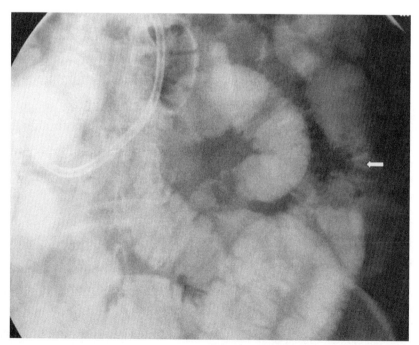

FIG. 23-11 This small bowel enterocolysis demonstrates a filling defect in the small intestine as would be seen with benign small bowel tumors.

Schrieber ML, Bass BL. Small intestinal neoplasms. In: Greenfield L, Mulholland M, Oldham K, et al. (eds.), *Surgery: Scientific Principles and Practice*, 3rd ed. Philadelphia, PA: Lippincott, Williams & Wilkins, 2001, 833–834.

21. (C) Primary small bowel malignancies share a few common threads: they present with nonspecific complaints such as longstanding nonspecific abdominal pain, weight loss, and diarrhea from partial obstructions, and they all generally present with advanced disease. Surgery is the mainstay for treatment, but overall survival is poor.

Adenocarcinomas comprise 50% of primary small bowel tumors. They are most common in the duodenum and proximal jejunum as are their benign counterparts, adenomas. The majority of duodenal tumors are polypoid while those in the jejunum and ileum have an annular configuration much like colonic adenocarcinoma. In addition to the symptoms previously discussed, duodenal adenocarcinoma may also present with obstructive jaundice or pancreatitis. Treatment relies on wide surgical resection of the tumor and regional lymph nodes; however, only 50% of patients present with resectable lesions, so surgery is frequently only palliative. Chemotherapy and radiation offer no benefit.

PSBL make up only 5% of lymphomas but comprise 20–30% of small bowel malignancies. Once again, presentation is indolent longstanding abdominal pain, weight loss, and diarrhea. Constitutional symptoms that are commonly seen with other lymphomas are not present in patients with small bowel lymphoma. Perforation, although quite rare, is a more common presentation than with adenocarcinoma. Treatment is surgical in patients with PSBL; however, laparotomy is only diagnostic in patients with a diffuse variant called immunoproliferative small intestinal disease. In both types, chemotherapy has some benefit, but it is not curative. Radiation is added occasionally with minimal success.

Small bowel tumors, also called GI stromal tumors, occasionally present with massive hemorrhage in addition to the usual presentation. They arise in the jejunum and the ileum in the fifth and sixth decades, more commonly in males. They also are treated with resection, but 5-year survival ranges from 20–80% depending on tumor grade. Some studies have shown modest survival benefit with adjuvant chemotherapy and radiation therapy, but this requires additional study for confirmation.

Bibliography

Bresalier RS, Ben-Menachem T. Tumors of the small intestine. In: Yamada T, Alpers D, Kaplowitz N, et al. (eds.), *Textbook of Gastroenterology*, 4th ed. Philadelphia, PA: Lippincott, Williams & Wilkins, 2003, 1643–1657.

Campbell K. Small bowel tumors. Cameron J (ed.), *Current Surgical Therapy*, 7th ed. St. Louis, MO: Mosby, 2001, 141–144.

Evers BM. Small bowel. In: Townsend CM, Beauchamp RD, Evers BM, et al. (eds.), *Sabiston Textbook of Surgery*, 16th ed. Philadelphia, PA: W.B. Saunders, 2001, 899–901.

Schrieber ML, Bass BL. Small intestinal neoplasms. In: Greenfield L, Mulholland M, Oldham K, et al. (eds.), *Surgery: Scientific Principles and Practice*, 3rd ed. Philadelphia, PA: Lippincott, Williams & Wilkins, 2001, 836–843.

22. (D) Carcinoid tumors are slow growing tumors found in the pulmonary tree and the GI tract. They arise from enterochromaffin cells in the crypts of Lieberkuhn and are characterized by their secretion of various humorally active peptides; these include serotonin, dopamine, histamine, substance P, neuropeptide K, and prostaglandins among others. GI carcinoids primarily occur in the appendix (45%), ileum (30%), and rectum (15%). Most are asymptomatic and discovered at an unrelated laparotomy; however, symptomatic carcinoids present in much the same way as other small bowel tumors: abdominal pain and weight loss. They can also present with obstructive symptoms from intermittent intussusception or from foreshortening of the mesentery by a reactive fibrosis resulting in kinking the small bowel. Five-year survival for patients with localized disease is 65% and 36% in patients with metastases.

Malignant carcinoid syndrome occurs in less than 10% of patients with carcinoid tumors. It happens when the liver is nearly completely replaced by metastases. Ovarian and retroperitoneal carcinoids also produce carcinoid syndrome without liver mets. Symptoms characterizing the syndrome include cutaneous flushing, diarrhea, right-sided cardiac lesions, asthma, and hepatomegaly. Cardiac lesions such as tricuspid insufficiency or stenosis and pulmonary stenosis may be a result of large amounts of serotonin produced by the hepatic lesions; however, they don't improve as other symptoms do when serotonin production is pharmacologically decreased.

Diagnosis of carcinoid tumors can be accomplished by multiple methods. Twenty-four-hour urine collection for 5-HIAA (a metabolite of serotonin) is highly specific for serotonin producing tumors. Plasma concentrations of chromogranin A are elevated in 80% of patients with carcinoid tumors regardless of the primary peptide produced. Barium x-ray demonstrates filling defects, while CT evaluates for metastases (Figs. 23-12 and 23-13). Most carcinoids have somatostatin receptors making scintigraphy with ^{111}In-pentetreotide valuable in assessing extent and locality of carcinoids.

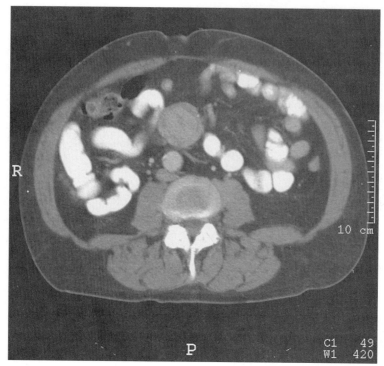

FIG. 23-12   Large carcinoid tumor in small bowel mesentery in patient with carcinoid syndrome. (Courtesy of Hal Kipfer, MD and Indiana University Radiology Teaching files)

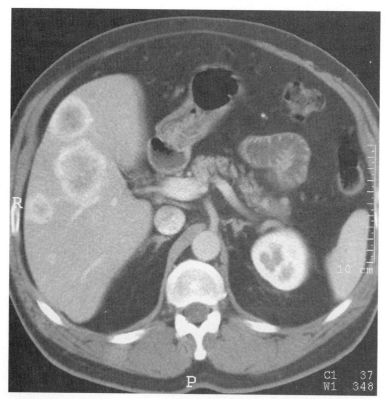

FIG. 23-13   Metastatic carcinoid tumor in patient with carcinoid syndrome. (Courtesy of Hal Kipfer, MD and Indiana University Radiology Teaching files)

Wide surgical resection of the tumors and associated nodes is required for cure. Carcinoid crisis characterized by hypotension, bronchospasm, flushing, and tachycardia can result from anesthetic induction. This is best countered by IV octreotide drip, antihistamine, and steroids. In patients with widespread tumor, surgical debulking including hepatic resection is very important in symptomatic relief; this often increases survival as well since carcinoid is a very slow growing tumor. Hepatic artery embolization is similarly useful in patients who are not surgical candidates. Symptomatic medical therapy centers on 5-hydroxytryptamine receptor antagonists such as ondansetron and 5-hydroxytryptamine release inhibitors such as octreotide and its analogs; these are effective in reducing the symptoms of carcinoid syndrome. Cytotoxic chemotherapy has had very limited success; radiation therapy is useful in palliation for bone and central nervous system (CNS) metastases.

Bibliography

Caplin ME, Buscombe JR, Hilson AJ, et al. Carcinoid tumour. *Lancet* 1998;352:799–805.

Evers BM. Small bowel. In: Townsend CM, Beauchamp RD, Evers BM, et al. (eds.), *Sabiston Textbook of Surgery*, 16th ed. Philadelphia, PA: W.B. Saunders, 2001, 901–904.

Kulke MH, Mayer RJ. Medical progress: carcinoid tumors. *N Engl J Med* 1999;340:858–868.

Schrieber ML, Bass BL. Small intestinal neoplasms. In: Greenfield L, Mulholland M, Oldham K, et al. (eds.), *Surgery: Scientific Principles and Practice*, 3rd ed. Philadelphia, PA: Lippincott, Williams & Wilkins, 2001, 839–841.

23. **(C)** Duodenal tubulovillous and villous adenomas frequently occur at the papilla. This is especially true for patients with inherited colonic polyposis syndromes. These have a high malignant potential with 30% of those greater than 3 cm having foci of invasive disease. These may be excised endoscopically when smaller than 3 cm, but the recurrence rate is approximately 25%; of these 40% are malignant recurrences. Patients, therefore, are best served with a surgical resection. Pancreaticoduodenectomy is indicated in patients with large villous adenomas near the papilla (Figs. 23-14 and 23-15). A Brunner's gland adenoma results from glandular hyperplasia of Brunner's glands normally found throughout the duodenal submucosa. These glands secrete alkaline substances and bicarbonate which serves to neutralize gastric acid. These adenomas have negligible malignant potential and can be manage at any size with local resection surgically or endoscopically to prevent obstruction or intussusception.

Simple tubular pedunculated adenomas (those with narrow, well-defined stalks) can be managed

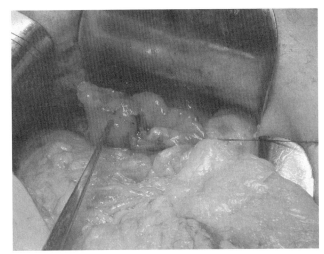

FIG. 23-14   Benign duodenal neoplasm in situ

endoscopically as they also have minimal malignant potential. The exception to this rule is in the case of a true surgical emergency such as intussusception or massive hemorrhage.

Bibliography

Bresalier RS, Ben-Menachem T. Tumors of the small intestine. In: Yamada T, Alpers DH, Kaplowitz N, et al. (eds.), *Textbook of Gastroenterology*, 4th ed. Philadelphia, PA: Lippincott, Williams & Wilkins, 2003, 1647–1649.

Campbell KA. Small bowel tumors. In: Cameron J (ed.), *Current Surgical Therapy*, 7th ed. St. Louis, MO: Mosby, 2001, 139–141.

Schreiber ML, Bass BL. Small intestinal neoplasms. In: Greenfield L, Mulholland M, Oldham K, et al. (eds.), *Surgery: Scientific Principles and Practice*, 3rd ed. Philadelphia, PA: Lippincott, Williams & Wilkins, 2001, 833–835.

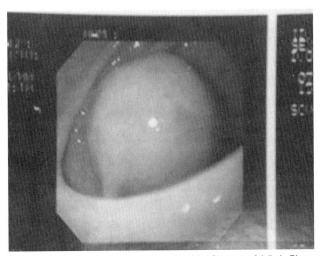

FIG. 23-15   Benign duodenal neoplasm on EGD (Courtesy of Julia LeBlanc, MD)

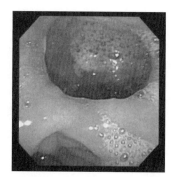

FIG. 23-16   Duodenal diverticulum on EGD. (Courtesy of Julia LeBlanc, MD)

24. **(B)** Duodenal diverticular disease is relatively common, but very few are clinically significant. In a similar fashion to other diverticula, duodenal diverticula occur as true diverticula, which are usually congenital, and false diverticula, which are usually acquired and rarely occur before the age of 40 (Fig. 23-16). Their overall prevalence ranges up to 25% in both autopsy studies and ERCP studies. Seventy-five percent occur within 2–3 cm of the ampulla of Vater, called juxtapapillary diverticula (JPD) or contain the ampulla, called intradiverticular papilla (IDP). These diverticuli result from the relative decrease in number of muscle fibers in the periampullary region along with more frequent migrating motor complexes and increased contraction pressure in the duodenum.

Complications of duodenal diverticula include pancreatitis, cholangitis, hemorrhage, perforation, and blind loop syndrome. Presenting symptoms include early satiety, nausea, epigastric pain radiating to the back, vomiting, and melena. Hemorrhage results from inflammation and eventual erosion into a branch of the SMA. Blind loop syndrome occurs when diverticular contents are static leading to bacterial overgrowth, malabsorption, steatorrhea, and eventual megaloblastic anemia. Perforation is quite rare. Pancreaticobiliary complications are most common. Pancreatitis may result from sphincter dysfunction because of the proximity of the ampulla to the diverticulum or from compression on the pancreatic duct by a diverticulum distended with food.

Diagnosis is frequently made by esophagogastroduodenoscopy (EGD) or ERCP. Barium studies can also be used but are much less sensitive and specific. Symptomatic duodenal diverticula are best treated conservatively with ERCP sphincterotomy and stent placement. Care must be taken to prevent iatrogenic perforation or hemorrhage in these cases. Surgery should generally be avoided because of its high rate of pancreaticobiliary complications and associated morbidity. Asymptomatic, incidental duodenal diverticula are an absolute contraindication to surgery.

If surgery must be undertaken due to unsatisfactory symptom control, several options exist and must be tailored to the patient. Diverticulectomy with or without transduodenal sphincterotomy is an option for anterior diverticula and posterior diverticula when a wide Kocher maneuver is performed. The diverticula is excised and the duodenum is closed in two layers in a direction that will not stricture the duodenum. This is an especially good option for hemorrhaging or perforated diverticula. Roux-en-Y duodenojejunostomy is used to exclude the diverticulum from the food stream thereby preventing stasis and subsequent pancreatitis. Bile may also be diverted with a choledochojejunostomy at the same time.

Bibliography

Evers BM. Small bowel. In: Townsend CM, Beauchamp RD, Evers BM, et al. (eds.), *Sabiston Textbook of Surgery*, 16th ed. Philadelphia, PA: W.B. Saunders, 2001, 905–906.

Lobo D, Balfour T, Iftikar S, et al. Periampullary diverticula and pancreaticobiliary disease. *Br J Surg* 1999;86:588–597.

Uthoff S, Galandiuk S. Diverticular disease of the small bowel. In: Cameron J (ed.), *Current Surgical Therapy*, 7th ed. St. Louis, MO: Mosby, 2001, 145–147.

25. **(A)** GISTs are uncommon mesenchymal neoplasms arising predominantly in the GI tract. They were initially believed to be smooth muscle neoplasms but advances in immunohistochemistry and electron microscopy have shown them to be distinctly separate tumors from leiomyomas and leiomyosarcomas. Current research has provided evidence that GISTs may arise from the ICCs. The ICCs function as pacemaker cells for the GI tract and are located around the myenteric plexus and muscularis propria. Evidence supporting ICCs' role as a cell of origin has been presented in recent literature. To begin with, ICCs demonstrate characteristics of both smooth muscle and neural cells which correlate with the spectrum of GIST. These tumors can have myoid (70%), neural (20%), or mixed (10%) attributes. Secondly, markers that have been most useful in identifying GIST from other tumors of the GI tract are highly expressed in ICCs. GISTs express Kit protein (CD117/c-kit) nearly uniformly and c-kit protoonocogene mutations are believed to play a major role in GIST tumorigenesis. ICCs and mast cells are the only two cell types that reside in the GI tract wall and normally express Kit protein. CD34, a hematopoietic stem cell antigen, is also highly expressed in GIST (70–80%) and constitutively found on ICCs. Finally, GISTs show predilection for certain anatomic regions of the GI tract most heavily populated with ICCs. ICCs are most common in the stomach and small intestine, with lower numbers in the esophagus and rectum. The distribution of GIST is as follows: 60–70% stomach,

20–25% small intestine, 5% colon and rectum, <5% esophagus. Evidence against ICCs as a cell of origin is the occasional GIST which develops in a non-GI location. GISTs have been found in the retroperitoneum, omentum, and peritoneum, all of which have no known population of ICCs.

Kulchitsky cells are enterochromaffin cells found in small intestinal crypts of Lieberkuhn. They are the cells of origin for carcinoids of the small bowel.

Myofibroblasts are fibroblast cells with predominance of actin and myosin filaments within the cytoplasm. They play an important role in wound contraction during the healing process.

G cells are gastrin-producing cells located in the upper GI tract. They can give rise to gastrinoma (Zollinger-Ellison's syndrome).

Paneth cells are another cell type found lining the crypts of Lieberkuhn of the small intestine. They secrete lysoyzme, tumor necrosis factor, and cryptidins.

Bibliography

Demetri GD. Identification and treatment of chemoresistant inoperable or metastatic GIST: experience with the selective tyrosine kinase inhibitor imatinib mesylate (STI571). *Eur J Cancer* 2002;38(Suppl. 5):S52–S59.

Evers BM, Townsend CM, Thompson JC. Small intestine. In: Swartz SI, Shires GT, Spencer FC (eds.), *Principles of Surgery*, 7th ed. New York, NY: McGraw-Hill, 1999, 1217–1263.

Graadt van Roggen JF, van Velthuysen ML, Hogendoorn PC. The histopathologic differential diagnosis of gastrointestinal stromal tumors. *J Clin Pathol* 2001;54:96–102.

Miettinen M, Lasota J. Gastrointestinal stromal tumors: definition, clinical, histological, and immunohistochemical, and molecular genetic features and differential diagnosis. *Virchows Arch* 2001;438:1–12.

Miettinen M, Majidi M, Lasota J. Pathology and diagnostic criteria of gastrointestinal stromal tumors (GISTs): a review. *Eur J Cancer* 2002;38(Suppl. 5):S39–S51.

Miettinen M, Monihan JM, Sarlomo-Rikala M, et al. Gastrointestinal stromal tumors/smooth muscle tumors (GISTs) primary in the omentum and mesentery: clinicopathologic and immunohistochemical study of 26 cases. *Am J Surg Pathol* 1999;23:1109–1118.

Sicar K, Hewlett BR, Huizinga JD, et al. Interstitial cells of Cajal as precursors for gastrointestinal stromal tumors. *Am J Surg Pathol* 1999;23:377–389.

26. **(C)** GIST represents 2–3% of all GI neoplasms and typically presents in adulthood, with a peak incidence in the fifth and sixth decades. No consistent sex difference has been observed. Clinical signs and symptoms tend to be nonspecific and may vary by tumor location. The most common symptoms include nausea/vomiting, abdominal pain, and GI bleeding. Very rarely GIST may be associated with a tumor syndrome. Carney's triad includes gastric GIST, paraganglioma, and pulmonary chondroma. GISTs are also occasionally associated with neurofibromatosis type 1 syndrome. Grossly, GISTs vary greatly in size and in morphologic appearance. The tumor is usually well circumscribed and can be found in a submucosal, intramural, or subserosal location. Depending on the degree of hemorrhage or necrosis, the tumor may vary from completely solid to partially cystic.

Up to 30% of GISTs will demonstrate malignant behavior, and recurrence is common.

Histopathologic features associated with malignant tumor behavior and poor prognosis include large tumor size, especially >5 cm, and high mitotic activity, generally >5 mitoses per 50 high-powered fields.

Locoregional infiltration or frank metastasis at presentation, incomplete surgical resection, and male sex are additional poor prognostic indicators. Median survival is less than 2 years for patients who present with metastatic or surgically unresectable disease; however, overall 5-year survival for GIST may be greater than 70%. This correlates with the long clinical course of these tumors, many of which tend to recur years after initial surgery. Notably, survival has not been shown to be affected by primary tumor location.

The most common site of metastasis for GISTs is the liver. Diffuse intraabdominal spread is also commonly seen. Unlike most soft tissue sarcomas, lymph node metatstasis is rare. A study of 200 patients with GIST who presented to Memorial Sloan-Kettering Cancer Center between 1982 and 1998 demonstrated that two-thirds of patients with metastatic disease had hepatic metastases, and that 53% of these patients had disease isolated to the liver. Lymph node involvement was only seen in 6% of patients. In this study, 40% of patients who presented with primary disease developed recurrence.

Bibliography

Dei Tos A. The reappraisal of gastrointestinal stromal tumors: from Stout to the KIT revolution. *Virchows Arch* 2003;442(5):421–428.

DeMatteo R, Lewis J, Leung D, et al. Two hundred gastrointestinal stromal tumors: recurrence patterns and prognostic factors for survival. *Ann Surg* 2000; 231(1): 51–58.

Demetri GD. Identification and treatment of chemoresistant inoperable or metastatic GIST: experience with the selective tyrosine kinase inhibitor imatinib mesylate (STI571). *Eur J Cancer* 2002;38(Suppl. 5):S52–S59.

Graadt van Roggen J, van Velthuysen M, Hogendoorn P. The histopathological differential diagnosis of gastrointestinal stromal tumors. *J Clin Pathol* 2001;54(2):96–102.

Miettinen M, Majidi M, Lasota J. Pathology and diagnostic criteria of gastrointestinal stromal tumors (GISTs): a review. *Eur J Cancer* 2002;38(Suppl. 5):S39–S51.

Plaat B, Hollema H, Molenaar W, et al. Soft tissue leiomyosarcomas and malignant gastrointestinal stromal tumors: differences in clinical outcome and expression of multidrug
resistance proteins. *J Clin Oncol* 2000; 18(8): 3211–3220.

27. **(B)** Imatinib mesylate is an orally-administered competitive inhibitor of the tyrosine kinase associated with
Kit protein. Kit protein (stem cell factor receptor) has an
intracellular domain with tyrosine kinase activity
responsible for cell signaling. In GIST, it is believed
that there is ligand-independent activation of the Kit
protein tyrosine kinase because of a gain-of-function
mutation. Imatinib blocks adenosine triphosphate
(ATP) binding which prevents substrate phosphorylation and therefore signal transduction. The drug has
activity both against wild-type Kit protein and also Kit
protein with gain-of-function mutations seen in GIST.

Limited experience with conventional chemotherapeutic agents and radiation for GIST has shown no
substantial benefit for these tumors. Imatinib, on the
other hand, appears to induce a sustained response in
>50% of patients with advanced GIST. A multicenter,
randomized clinical trial of imatinib included 147
patients with advanced unresectable or metastatic
GIST. This trial showed a partial response in 54%, stable disease in 28%, and 14% had no response with a
median followup of 41 weeks. Estimated 1-year survival was 88%. These results have been supported by
a smaller European trial of 36 patients of whom 53%
had partial response and 36% had stable disease.

The approved dosage of imatinib in the United
States is 400 or 600 mg once daily. The most common
side effect is edema, generally involving the face or
legs. GI side effects are frequent as well and include
nausea, vomiting, and diarrhea. GI bleeding may
also be seen in up to 5% of patients, possibly secondary to rapid anticancer effect on the tumors.

Alkylating agents such as cyclophosphamide add
alkyl groups to DNA which causes cross-linkage.

Hydroxyurea inhibits ribonucleotide reductase
which normally converts ribonucleotides into deoxy-
ribonucleotides.

Vinca alkaloids (vincristine and vinblastine) bind
tubulin and inhibit microtubule assembly. Paclitaxel
and docetaxel stabilize formed microtubules and prevent their disassembly. Both actions prevent completion of mitosis.

Anthracyclines such as doxorubicin inhibit topoisomerase II which normally repairs breaks in DNA.

Bibliography

Croom K, Perry C. Imatinib mesylate in the treatment of gastrointestinal stromal tumors. *Drugs* 2003;63(5): 513–522.

Demetri GD. Identification and treatment of chemoresistant
inoperable or metastatic GIST: experience with the selective tyrosine kinase inhibitor imatinib mesylate (STI571).
Eur J Cancer 2002;38(Suppl. 5):S52–S59.
Graadt van Roggen J, van Velthuysen M, Hogendoorn P.
The histopathological differential diagnosis of gastroin-
testinal stromal tumors. *J Clin Pathol* 2001;54(2):96–102.
Miettinen M, Majidi M, Lasota J. Pathology and diagnostic
criteria of gastrointestinal stromal tumors (GISTs): a
review. *Eur J Cancer* 2002;38(Suppl. 5):S39–S51.
Silberman S, Joensuu H. Overview of issues related to ima-
tinib therapy of advanced gastrointestinal stromal tumors:
a discussion among the experts. *Eur J Cancer* 2002; 38
(Suppl. 5):S66–S69.
Slapak C, Kufe D. Prinicples of cancer therapy. In: Fauci
A, Braunwald E, Isselbacher K, et al. (eds.), *Harrison's
Principles of Internal Medicine*, 14th ed. New York, NY:
McGraw-Hill, 1998, 530–531.

28. **(D)** Ileus after abdominal surgery is believed to be
caused by loss of the normal intinsic electromotor function of the GI tract. Although electrical and motor
activity can be demonstrated to continue to occur
immediately after operation, coordinated motility of
the intestine is temporarily distrupted. Motility resumes
over the course of hours to days, dependent on the site
along the GI tract. Normal activity returns within 24 h
in the small intestine, between 24 and 48 h in the stomach, and between 48 and 72 h in the colon after abdominal surgery. In general, ileus has resolved by 4–5 days
following laparotomy in the majority of patients.
Normal motility of the stomach and small bowel
varies over the fed and fasted states. In the fasted state
there is a cyclic fluctuation in motor activity termed
the migrating motor complex (MMC) which occurs
in three phases. The MMC starts in the stomach and
progresses through the small intestine over approximately 2 h. Along this course the three phases of the
MMC occur, phase I is a period of inactivity lasting
60–75 min, phase II is a period of increasing coordinated bowel contractions lasting up to 60 min, and
phase III is a period of maximal contractions occurring
for 5–10 min. This cyclic activity continues until it is
interupted by a meal. In the fed state, contractions
occur throughout the small intestine, spreading caudally at variable distances. The colon does not demonstrate MMCs but colonic motility also varies with the
fed and fasted states. Colonic activity is increased after
meals and fluctuates during periods of fasting.
Contractions vary along the length of the large intestine. The right colon has retrograde contractions to
increase absorption of water. Left colon contractions
move distally to expel stool.

In postoperative ileus the MMC is abnormal with
less phase II activity and increased phase III activity.

Fed phase contractions are also abnormal. In the colon, tone is increased initially and then progressively declines as ileus resolves. Dysfunction of the autonomic nervous system is likely the most important factor contributing to postoperative ileus. Sympathetic hyperactivity inhibits intestinal motility and it has been demonstrated that splanchnicectomy significantly decreases postoperative ileus. Production of inflammatory mediators like nitric oxide and prostaglandins, and altered release of GI hormones like motilin and calcitonin gene-related peptide may also contribute to the postoperative environment which causes ileus. For example, plasma motilin levels are decreased postoperatively and return to normal with resolution of ileus.

Multiple factors have been associated with GI ileus other than operative trauma. The patient in the above question has several factors besides her operation which may be contributing to her ileus. Narcotics such as oxycodone are known to decrease GI motility and prolong postoperative ileus. Hyponatremia, as well as other electrolyte disturbances can lead to ileus. Continued intraabdominal inflammation, specifically possible development of an intraabdominal abcess or wound infection, could lead to prolonged ileus in this patient with a history of acute appendicitis. NSAID use, however, has not been associated with development of ileus and in fact may aid in its resolution. NSAIDs have been proven to decrease the amount of narcotic pain medication given to postoperative patients and have resulted in improved GI motility in most studies.

Bibliography

Christensen J. Intestinal motor physiology. In: Feldman M, Scharschmidt B, Sleisenger M, et al. (eds.), *Sleisenger and Fordtran's Gastrointestinal and Liver Disease*. Philadelphia, PA: W.B. Saunders, 1998, 1437–1450.

Holte K, Kehlet H. Postoperative ileus: a preventable event. *Br J Surg* 2000;87(11):1480–1493.

Livingston E, Passaro E. Postoperative ileus. *Dig Dis Sci* 1990;35(1):121–132.

Luckey A, Livingston E, Tache Y. Mechanisms and treatment of postoperative ileus. *Arch Surg* 2003;138(2): 206–214.

Miedema B, Johnson J. Methods for decreasing postoperative gut dysmotility. *Lancet* 2003;4:365–372.

Turnage R, Bergen P. Intestinal obstruction and ileus. In: Feldman M, Scharschmidt B, Sleisenger M, et al. (eds.), *Sleisenger and Fordtran's Gastrointestinal and Liver Disease*. Philadelphia, PA: W.B. Saunders, 1998, 1799–1810.

29. **(B)** Small studies have shown that neither duration nor type of abdominal operation influence length of postoperative ileus when only considering open procedures. In a study of 13 patients undergoing a range of operations from exploratory laparotomy to more complex intraabdominal procedures including total gastrectomy, colon resection, and pancreaticojejunostomy, electrodes were placed in the ascending and descending colon and their signals recorded postoperatively. Organized electrical activity returned by the third or fourth postoperative day regardless of the type or duration of procedure. A similar study performed in primates, and using both electrodes and force transducers throughout the GI tract, also demonstrated that the duration of ileus was independent of site, duration, or extent of operation. Additionally, another study performed in humans, using passage of radioopaque pellets rather than electrical activity to monitor return of GI function, also could find no direct relationship between length of abdominal surgical procedure and duration of postoperative ileus. This study included 36 patients, 8 of whom underwent extraabdominal procedures. Overall, length of time before passage of flatus was only significantly greater in the intraabdominal surgery group compared to the extraabdominal surgery group. There also appeared to be an increased length of time before passage of flatus in the 2 patients who underwent colectomy compared to other types of procedures; however, the authors did not discuss the significance of this data. The findings of these small studies contradict the often commonly held belief among surgeons that ileus is related to the length of the procedure and amount of dissection or bowel manipulation which occurs. This remains a difficult area to study because the postoperative management of patients can differ greatly based on the type of abdominal procedure that they undergo, and many factors may contribute to ileus beside postoperative status.

Clearer in the literature is that laparoscopic procedures lead to shorter duration of postoperative ileus compared to open procedures. Many studies have examined laparoscopic colon resection and found a significantly shorter length of ileus and length of hospitalization compared to open colon resections for the same indications. In general there is a 1–2 days reduction in time to return of GI function for laparoscopic colectomy. Animal models have also supported these clinical studies. Similiarly, the laparoscopic technique has been proven to reduce ileus time for many other procedures. Laparoscopic appendectomy, adrenalectomy, and bowel resection have all been compared to their open counterparts in studies examining duration of ileus and hospitalization. In each case, the laparoscopic group tends to have significantly shorter duration of ileus and reduced hospital stays in comparison to traditional open surgery. Interestingly, many of these studies also compared length of operation between these groups. In general, most laparoscopic procedures have longer operative times than open procedures. This is further evidence that the length of the operation does not correlate with the duration of postoperative ileus. Finally, many authors propose that the laparoscopic technique causes less ileus than open surgery because it decreases intraabdominal trauma and bowel manipulation. While although this might be true, the results of the studies of open operations discussed earlier do not support the assumption that less dissection or bowel manipulation led to shorter ileus times. It is therefore likely that there are other factors associated with the laparoscopic technique which promote less postoperative ileus. Some factors that have been mentioned in the literature include reduced size of wound (decreased peritoneal trauma), reduced need for postoperative analgesia, and earlier resumption of oral feeding.

Bibliography

Aldrighetti L, Giacomelli M, Calori G, et al. Impact of minimally invasive surgery on adrenalectomy for incidental tumors: comparison with laparotomic technique. *Int Surg* 1997;82(2):160–164.

Chen H, Wexner S, Iroatulam A, et al. Laparoscopic colectomy compares favorably with colectomy by laparotomy for reduction of postoperative ileus. *Dis Colon Rectum* 2000;43(1):61–65.

Condon R, Frantzides C, Cowles V, et al. Resolution of postoperative ileus in humans. *Ann Surg* 1986;203(5):574–581.

Graber J, Schulte W, Condon R, et al. Relationship of duration of postoperative ileus to extent and site of operative dissection. *Surgery* 1982;92(1):87–92.

Maxwell-Armstrong C, Robinson M, Scholefield J. Laparoscopic colorectal cancer surgery. *Am J Surg* 2000;179(6):500–507.

Msika S, Iannelli A, Deroide G, et al. Can laparoscopy reduce hospital stay in the treatment of Crohn's disease? *Dis Colon Rectum* 2001;44(11):1661–1666.

Richards W, Watson D, Lynch G, et al. A review of the results of laparoscopic versus open appendectomy. *Surg Gynecol Obstet* 1993;177(5):473–480.

Tittel A, Schippers E, Anurov M, et al. Shorter postoperative atony after laparoscopic-assisted colonic resection? An animal study. *Surg Endosc* 2001;15(5):508–512.

Wilson J. Postoperative motility of the large intestine in man. *Gut* 1975;16:689–692.

30. (E) Ileus inevitably occurs after abdominal operation and methods to reduce its duration are a subject of ongoing investigation. One area of focus has been opioid analgesics because these drugs are known to cause GI ileus and are almost uniformly used in postoperative care. Reducing the amount of narcotic medication, especially by supplementation with NSAID analgesics, has been shown to decrease postoperative ileus.

Additionally, the route of administration of narcotic medication is important. Some studies have shown a significant improvement in bowel function when narcotic pain control was delivered by the epidural route versus systemic intravenous administration. Greater differences have been seen in studies comparing epidural local anesthetics like bupivacaine with systemic narcotics. Multiple groups have found thoracic epidural administration of local anesthetics to be superior to systemic opioids for reduction of postoperative ileus without compromise of pain control.

Despite their widespread use in postoperative patients, NG tubes clearly have no effect on duration of postoperative ileus as supported by multiple randomized clinical trials. They may, however, provide symptomatic relief to selected patients and should be used at the decretion of the clinician for this purpose. Their use should be weighed against the known possible complications of NG intubation, including fever, atelectasis, and pneumonia.

No studies have shown a benefit for early mobilization after surgery for return of GI function. In a study of healthy volunteers, exercise did not affect colonic motility.

Erythromycin is a macrolide antibiotic known to bind to the motilin receptor on GI smooth muscle. Despite this action, a randomized control trial showed no effect of erythromycin on duration of ileus. Likewise, naloxone, morphine receptor antagonist, has been studied but has shown to have no effect on postoperative ileus.

Other treatments that have shown promise for decreasing ileus but need further study include early refeeding following surgery, gum chewing, and abdominal massage. Early enteral feedings may theoretically decrease ileus by stimulating motility and secretion of intestinal hormones. Some studies have demonstrated earlier return of GI function with early enteral feedings; however, one recent study found early feeding to also be associated with impairment of pulmonary function and mobilization in the postoperative period. Postoperative gum chewing may stimulate return of bowel function by a similar mechanism and was examined in one randomized control trial of 19 patients undergoing elective laparoscopic colectomy for colon cancer. This trial demonstrated earlier return of flatus and earlier defecation in the gum-chewing group compared to controls. The effect of abdominal massage was examined in another study of patients undergoing colectomy. In this randomized trial the time to return to flatus was significantly decreased in the group undergoing active massage by 1.8 days compared to controls.

Bibliography

Asao T, Kuwano H, Nakamura J, et al. Gum chewing enhances recovery from postoperative ileus after laparoscopic colectomy. *J Am Coll Surg* 2002;195(1):30–32.

Holte K, Kehlet H. Postoperative ileus: a preventable event. *Br J Surg* 2000;87(11):1480–1493.

Le Blanc-Louvry I, Costaglioli B, Boulon C, et al. Does mechanical massage of the abdominal wall after colectomy reduce postoperative pain and shorten duration of ileus? Results of a randomized study. *J Gastrointest Surg* 2002;6(1):43–49.

Liu S, Carpenter R, Mackey D, et al. Effects of perioperative analgesic technique on rate of recovery after colon surgery. *Anesthesiology* 1995;83(4):757–765.

Luckey A, Livingston E, Tache Y, et al. Mechanisms and treatment of postoperative ileus. *Arch Surg* 2003; 138(2):206–214.

Miedema B, Johnson J. Methods for decreasing postoperative gut dysmotility. *Lancet* 2003;4:365–372.

Stewart B, Woods R, Collopy B, et al. Early feeding after elective open colorectal resections: a prospective randomized trial. *Aust N Z J Surg* 1997;68(2):125–128.

31. **(D)** Following laparotomy, up to 95% of patients will develop adhesions. Although the majority of patients will not develop any clinical consequences from adhesion formation, there are significant morbidities associated with their development. In a retrospective study using the Scottish National Health Service database, 5.7% of all readmissions following abdominal or pelvic surgery over 10 years were found to be related to adhesions. Mid- and hind-gut procedures had the highest number of adhesion-related readmissions, and most admissions occurred in the first year after surgery.

Intraabdominal adhesions are the leading cause for small bowel obstruction in the industrialized world. Up to 80% of admissions for small bowel obstruction are secondary to postoperative adhesions. Types of procedures most commonly associated with adhesions-related small bowel obstruction are gynecologic operations, appendectomy, and small bowel operations. Overall, patients who undergo any abdominal procedure have a 5% incidence of developing adhesion-related intestinal obstruction. Obstruction may occur at any time following laparotomy; however, in 17–29% of patients who develop postoperative obstruction, it occurs within the first month after surgery. In terms of location, obstructions from adhesions tend to occur at the level of the ileum, possibly because of its greater mobility within the abdomen.

Intraabdominal adhesions account for up to 20% of secondary infertility in women. Adhesions in the pelvis can cause infertility by blocking the fallopian tubes or interfering in ovum transfer from the ovary to the tubes. The risk of infertility is probably related to the degree of peritoneal trauma and severity of the ensuing adhesions. In a retrospective study of women with tubal infertility, a history of appendectomy with appendiceal rupture significantly increased the risk of infertility while the history of simple appendectomy without rupture did not. It is also believed that pelvic and abdominal adhesions can cause chronic pain. Theoretically, adhesions may cause pain by putting tension on the sensitive parietal peritoneum. Histologic study has also shown the presence of sensory nerve fibers within abdominal adhesions. Pain symptoms and degree of adhesions do not correlate well; however, most studies in the gynecologic literature show at least short-term improvement in pain following laparoscopic lysis of adhesions.

Patients with adhesions from previous laparotomy who undergo reoperation have an increased rate of inadvertent enterotomy. A study of 270 of such patients showed a 19% incidence of bowel injury. In this group, increased age and more than three prior laparotomies were independent predictors of greater risk of enterotomy.

Intestinal malabsorption is not associated with the presence intraabdominal adhesions.

Bibliography

Ellis H, Moran B, Thompson J, et al. Adhesion-related hospital readmissions after abdominal and pelvic surgery: a retrospective cohort study. *Lancet* 1999;353:1476–1480.

Evers B, Townsend C, Thompson J. Small intestine. In: Schwartz S, Shires G, Spencer F, et al. (eds.), *Principles of Surgery*, 7th ed. New York, NY: McGraw-Hill, 1999, 1217–1263.

Letterie G. Pelvic adhesive disease. In: Letterie G (ed.), *Structural Abnormalities and Reproductive Failure: Effective Techniques for Diagnosis and Management*. Oxford: Blackwell Science, 1998, 475–501.

Monk B, Berman M, Montz F. Adhesions after extensive gynecologic surgery: clinical significance, etiology, and prevention. *Am J Obstet Gynecol* 1994;170(5):1396–1403.

Reijnen M, Bleichrodt R, van Goor H. Pathophysiology of intra-abdominal adhesion and abscess formation, and the effect of hyaluronan. *Br J Surg* 2003;90:533–541.

Strickler R. Factors influencing infertility. In: Keye W, Chang R, Rebar R, et al. (eds.), *Infertility: Evaluation and Treatment*. Philadelphia, PA: W.B. Saunders, 1995, 8–18.

Sulaiman H, Gabella G, Davis C, et al. Presence and distribution of sensory nerve fibers in human peritoneal adhesions. *Ann Surg* 2001;234(2):256–261.

van der Krabben A, Dijkstra F, Nieuwenhuijzen M, et al. Morbidity and mortality of inadvertent enterotomy during adhesiotomy. *Br J Surg* 2000;87(4):467–471.

32. **(B)** Adhesion formation is the result of a shift toward the coagulation system and away from fibrinolysis within the peritoneal cavity following trauma and inflammation. The coagulation cascade results in deposition of

fibrin that can then act as scaffolding for ingrowth of fibroblasts and collagen deposition. The fibrinolytic system is also activated and results in the production of plasmin that degrades fibrin and counters adhesion formation; however, the equilibrium is overall shifted toward coagulation and fibrin deposition, and this seems primarily related to inhibition of fibrinolysis. Tissue-type plasminogen activator (tPA) is the main activator of plasminogen to plasmin within the intraabdominal cavity and has been found to be decreased after peritoneal trauma. It is suspected that low levels of tPA are secondary to elevated PAI-1. PAI-1 is the main inhibitor of tPA and high concentrations have been found in adhesions and within the peritoneum of patients with extensive adhesions.

Another activator of plasminogen, uPA, has lower activity than tPA, and is not believed to play as important a role in fibrinolysis within the abdominal cavity. Sulaiman et al. (2002) showed that tPA-deficient mice developed permanent intraabdominal adhesions more readily following surgical trauma than did uPA-deficient and wild-type mice; however, if high levels of uPA were present in the abdominal cavity this would theoretically favor the fibrinolytic system and the breakdown of fibrin deposits. Likewise, low levels of fibrin would not favor the development of adhesions. Protein C deficiency and abnormal platelet activation play no known role in the development of adhesions following abdominal surgery.

Understanding the pathogenesis of adhesion formation has been the basis for methods to prevent adhesion formation in the clinical setting. These methods fall into three main categories: surgical techniques, mechanical barriers, and intraperitoneal liquids. Although there are no randomized control trials in humans, the practice of minimal tissue handling, good hemostasis, thorough irrigation, minimization of foreign material, and prevention of electrocautery injury, are all techniques historically used by surgeons to decrease adhesion formation. These techniques are based on the assumption that minimization of the initial injury will lead to less inflammation and subsequently less scar formation. Mechanical barriers have been studied with the idea that they can prevent the traumatized peritoneal surface from contacting and developing adhesions to other areas. Three barriers which have shown efficacy include oxidized regenerated cellulose (Interceed), expanded polytetrafluoroethylene (Gore-tex Surgical Membrane), and hyaluronan-carboxymethylcellulose membrane (Seprafilm). Last, instillation of a variety of intraperitoneal liquids, either to act as barriers or to effect certain aspects of the pathogenesis of adhesion formation, have been studied and have met some success.

Hyaluronan solutions have shown promise in decreasing adhesions as they not only act as a barrier, but also have demonstrated evidence of improving healing of injured peritoneal surfaces. Plasminogen activators such as uPA and tPA have both been studied in animals and tPA has been shown to be consistently effective in adhesion prevention. Little work has been done in human subjects, however, and the possible risk of hemorrhage, especially after major surgery, has been a deterrent to pursuing these agents in the clinical setting.

Bibliography

Hellebrekers B, Trimbos-Kemper T, Trimbos J, et al. Use of fibrinolytic agentes in the prevention of postoperative adhesion formation. *Fertil Steril* 2000;74(2):203–212.

Johns A. Evidence-based prevention of post-operative adhesions. *Hum Reprod Update* 2001;7(6):577–579.

Monk B, Berman M, Montz F. Adhesions after extensive gynecologic surgery: clinical significance, etiology, and prevention. *Am J Obstet Gynecol* 1994;170(5):1396–1403.

Reijnen M, Bleichrodt R, van Goor H. Pathophysiology of intra-abdominal adhesion and abscess formation, and the effect of hyaluronan. *Br J Surg* 2003;90:533–541.

Suliaman H, Dawson L, Laurent G, et al. Role of plasminogen activators in peritoneal adhesion formation. *Biochem Soc Trans* 2002;30(2):126–131.

33. **(C)** It is the degree of acute radiation enteritis that is a function of the rate and duration of time over which the radiation dose is applied. Chronic radiation enteritis is dependent only on the total dose of radiation given. Doses below 4000 cGy only rarely cause bowel injury, above this there is a linear relationship between dose and incidence of GI damage. The immediate effects of radiation on the GI mucosa cause acute radiation enteritis. Symptoms include nausea, vomiting, diarrhea, abdominal pain, and anorexia, but this phase may also be asymptomatic. Histopathologic features include mucosal sloughing, shortening of villi, and prominent inflammatory infiltrate. This phase requires only supportive treatment and will resolve within several weeks of completion of radiation therapy.

Chronic radiation enteritis is thought to be an indirect transmural injury caused by progressive obliterative vasculitis. This vasculitis results in ischemia and fibrosis of the entire bowel wall. Normal intestinal transit is disturbed by these changes and may cause symptoms including intermittent diarrhea and constipation as well as abdominal pain. Long-term complications of chronic radiation enteritis include intestinal fistulas, perforation, and bowel obstruction. Histopathologic features include ulcerations that may penetrate the muscularis, vascular sclerosis, intestinal wall fibrosis, and lymph congestion. This phase of radiation injury is progressive, and although the average onset is within 2–3 years after radiation exposure, it may have a latency period up to 30 years. Conservative treatment for symptomatic patients without complications includes diet modifications, nutritional supplementation, anti-inflammatory drugs, and sometimes treatment of bacterial overgrowth and bile acid malabsorption. Treatment frequently requires surgical resection for those patients who present with obstruction, fistula, or perforation. Of those who undergo surgery, up to half develop further symptoms, and in one study, 39% went on to experience new complications not associated with their initial lesion. Multiple resections may lead to short gut syndrome and the need for long-term TPN. Results in this case are not favorable as these patients have a demonstrated 5-year survival of only 36–54%. Alternative surgical methods may be appropriate for these special cases, such as bypass procedures or diversion. Stricturoplasty has also recently been described and proven successful in a small group of selected patients.

Bibliography

Dietz D, Remzi F, Fazio V. Strictureplasty for obstructing small-bowel lesions in diffuse radiation enteritis—successful outcome in five patients. *Dis Colon Rectum* 2001;44(12):1772–1777.

Hauer-Jensen M. Late radiation injury of the small intestine clinical, pathophysiologic and radiobiologic aspects. A review. *Acta Oncol* 1990;29(4):401–415.

Rodier J. Radiation enteropathy—incidence, aetiology, risk factors, pathology and symptoms. *Tumori* 1995;81 (Suppl.):122–125.

Sher M, Bauer J. Radiation-induced enteropathy. *Am J Gastroenterol* 1990;85(2):121–128.

Waddell B, Rodriguez-Bigas M, Lee R, et al. Prevention of chronic radiation enteritis. *J Am Coll Surg* 1999;189(6): 611–624.

34. (D) Thin patients, the elderly, and women are all at slightly increased risk for radiation enteritis secondary to having a larger amount of small bowel located in the pelvis and less subcutaneous tissue. Radiation injury is dependent on the volume of bowel irradiated. Patients who have previously undergone abdominal surgery are at increased risk for radiation enteritis because of fixation of small bowel within the field of radiation from surgical adhesions. Techniques such as prone positioning, bladder distension, and abdominal-wall compression, used to reduce the amount of bowel within the radiation field are less effective in those patients with prior laparotomy. Combined chemotherapy with radiation treatment is also a risk factor for the development of radiation enteritis.

In terms of the radiation dose itself, it is the total dose which determines the degree of long-term bowel injury. Doses below 4000 cGy only rarely result in GI damage. Incidence of injury increases in a linear relationship to total radiation dose, with up to a 36% incidence at 7000 cGy reported in some series. Dose fractionation does not affect development of chronic injury; however, the effects of acute radiation enteritis are increased by a greater number of fractions.

Other factors that may increase the risk of radiation enteritis include vascular disease or low-flow states as in heart failure, and possibly rectal surgery itself secondary to development of more adhesions from this type of operation.

Bibliography

Hauer-Jensen M. Late radiation injury of the small intestine clinical, pathophysiologic and radiobiologic aspects. A review. *Acta Oncol* 1990;29(4):401–415.

Midis G, Feig B. Cancer of the colon, rectum, and anus. In: Feig B, Berger D, Fuhrman G (eds.), *The M.D. Anderson Surgical Oncology Handbook*, 2nd ed. Philadelphia, PA: Lippincott, Williams & Wilkins, 1999, 178–222.

O'Brien P, Jenrette J. Radiation enteritis. *Am Surg* 1987;9: 501–504.

Rodier J. Radiation enteropathy—incidence, aetiology, risk factors, pathology and symptoms. *Tumori* 1995;81 (Suppl.):122–125.

Sher M, Bauer J. Radiation-induced enteropathy. *Am J Gastroenterol* 1990;85(2):121–128.

Waddell B, Rodriguez-Bigas M, Lee R, et al. Prevention of chronic radiation enteritis. *J Am Coll Surg* 1999;189(6): 611–624.

35. (E) A number of different procedures have been used for abdominopelvic partitioning when radiotherapy to the pelvis is anticipated following surgical resection of a tumor. The term reperitonealization refers to suturing the patient's anterolateral peritoneum and posterior retroperitoneal tissues together to prevent the bowel from sliding inferiorly into the pelvis. A study by Chen et al. (1992) examined using the peritoneum as well as the posterior rectus sheath to exclude the small bowel in a series of 17 patients with rectal cancer who subsequently underwent radiation therapy. In this study there was a 12% incidence of complications related to radiation enteritis within 1 year, which is not significantly less than the incidence among patients who do not undergo abdominopelvic partitioning procedures. Studies that have evaluated the use of the omentum for partitioning have met with more success. Multiple techniques exist for using the omentum and include omental transposition flap, omental envelope or omentopexy, and omental hammock. For the omental transposition flap an omental pedicle is created based on the left gastroepiploic vessels and is sutured into the pelvis, displacing the bowel. A retrospective study of 24 patients undergoing this procedure reported improved tolerance for radiation therapy but gave limited supporting data. Omental envelope or omentopexy, where the omentum is sutured to the posterior abdominal wall above the pelvic inlet, had no small bowel complications after 38 months in a series of 43 patients with rectal cancer who underwent the procedure. Omental hammock is a technique in which an omental flap is created and sutured circumferentially to the abdominal wall above the pelvis. Choi and Lee (1995) used this technique in rectal cancer patients in a nonrandomized prospective study and demonstrated significantly less radiation injury in the omental hammock group compared to controls.

Although the patient's native tissues would be the ideal choice to exclude the bowel from the radiation field, they are not always sufficient, especially in those patients who have had previous abdominal surgery. The absorbable mesh sling has been studied extensively and consists of using a Dexon or Vicryl mesh to exclude the small bowel from the pelvis in a manner similar to those described for the omentum. Several retrospective studies and one large multiinstitutional series have demonstrated lower incidence of radiation injury in colorectal and gynecologic cancer patients using this technique for abdominopelvic partitioning. Although mesh placement can increase operative time and lead to slightly prolonged postoperative ileus, complications related to mesh placement have been uncommon. Pelvic tissue expanders have also been examined as a way to protect the small bowel from radiation injury. These saline-filled devices are placed at the time of surgery and then surgically removed following pelvic radiotherapy. Although studies have shown an improvement in radiation injury using tissue expanders, they have also documented complications including infection and fistula development which may make them a less attractive choice compared to the previously mentioned techniques.

Bibliography

Chen J, ChangChien C, Wang J, et al. Pelvic peritoneal reconstruction to prevent radiation enteritis in rectal carcinoma. *Dis Colon Rectum* 1992;35:897–901.

Choi H, Lee H. Effect of omental pedicle hammock in protection against radiation-induced enteropathy in patients with rectal cancer. *Dis Colon Rectum* 1995;38: 276–280.

O'Leary D. Use of the greater omentum in colorectal surgery. *Dis Colon Rectum* 1999;42(4):533–539.

Waddell B, Rodriguez-Bigas M, Lee R, et al. Prevention of chronic radiation enteritis. *J Am Coll Surg* 1999;189(6): 611–624.

36. **(A)** Although cancer arising at the site of fistula formation can impair healing and decreases spontaneous closure rates, the patient's history of cancer does not put him at increased risk for complications from this fistula as there is no evidence given that he has developed recurrent disease. Beside malignant infiltration there are a number of other characteristics of entercutaneous fistulas that are associated with low rates of spontaneous closure. These include high fistula output, end fistula defect, defects larger than 1 cm at their origin, distal bowel obstruction, short fistula tracts, epithelization of the tract, presence of a foreign body, associated abscess or sepsis, and fistulas in the setting of large abdominal wall defects.

High output fistulas are generally defined as those fistulas with >500 mL of discharge per 24 h. Proximally located fistulas tend to be high output because of the large volume of secretions in the upper GI tract and less time for absorption at that level. High fistula output has been clearly correlated with decreased spontaneous fistula closure. A study published by Sitges-Serra et al. (1982) examined 75 consecutive patients between 1975 and 1980 who presented with postoperative enterocutaneous fistula and demonstrated a 6% mortality and 97% spontaneous closure rate for patients with low output fistulas (<1000 mL/48 h) versus a 32% mortality and only 54% spontaneous closure rate for patients with high output fistulas (>1000 mL/48 h).

The size of the fistula and amount of disruption of the bowel wall also affect ability for spontaneous healing. If greater than 50% of the bowel circumference is involved in the fistula, or if there has been a complete loss of intestinal continuity (end fistula), spontaneous closure will never occur. Likewise, bowel wall defects greater than 1 cm at their origin have decreased healing rates and when they do heal successfully often lead to severe bowel stricturing. Bowel obstruction distal to the fistula, regardless of cause, results in complete diversion of enteric contents through the proximal fistula and prevents healing in a manner similar to large fistula defects. Mortality is also increased in these patients and reoperation is almost always required.

Characteristics of the fistula tract itself also influence spontaneous closure. Tracts which are <2.5 cm long rarely close on their own. Longer tracts have greater resistance to flow, and therefore a greater chance for spontaneous closure. Foreign bodies within the tract, for example mesh or suture, will prevent healing. Additionally, spontaneous closure of the fistula is impossible once epithelialization of the tract has occurred.

Fistulas are often associated with intraabdominal abscesses and patients can develop frank sepsis from infection. Both of these conditions greatly increase mortality and inhibit spontaneous fistula closure. Appropriate treatment of abscesses with drainage and sepsis with antibiotics and supportive measures can reduce these factors and promote healing.

Fistulas associated with large abdominal wall defects have extremely poor prognosis. In the study by Sitges-Serra et al. (1982), there was only one spontaneous closure out of 10 patients who presented with fistulas draining through large abdominal wall defects and this group had the highest mortality with the majority of deaths because of sepsis. In a NIH series of cancer patients who developed ECFs after operation there were no spontaneous fistula resolutions and mortality was 100% in the subgroup with fistulas associated with large abdominal wall defects.

Malnutrition is believed to predispose patients to fistula formation because of poor wound healing at sites of bowel injury or anastomosis. Hypoalbuminemia (albumin <3.5 g/dL) has been associated with increased fistula-related mortality in patients who develop postoperative ECFs. The effect of hypoalbuminemia on spontaneous fistula closure rates is not as clear and requires more study.

Bibliography

Chamberlain R, Kaufman H, Danforth D. Enterocutaneous fistula in cancer patients: etiology, management, outcome, and impact on further treatment. *Am Surg* 1998;64:1204–1211.

Evers B, Townsend C, Thompson J. Small intestine. In: Schwartz S, Shires G, Spencer F, et al. (eds.), *Principles of Surgery*, 7th ed. New York, NY: McGraw-Hill, 1999, 1217–1263.

Rubelowsky J, Machiedo G. Reoperative versus conservative management for gastrointestinal fistulas. *Surg Clin North Am* 1991;71:147–157.

Sitges-Serra A, Jaurrieta E, Sitges-Creus A. Management of postoperative enterocutaneous fistulas: the roles of parenteral nutrition and surgery. *Br J Surg* 1982; 69(3): 147–150.

Spiliotis J, Briand D, Gouttebel M, et al. Treatment of fistulas of the gastrointestinal tract with total parenteral nutrition and octreotide in patients with carcinoma. *Surg Gynecol Obstet* 1993;176(6):575–580.

37. **(E)** Duodenal fistulas pose a more complex problem than fistulas arising more distally in the GI tract because of the anatomy of the region they arise in. The appropriate surgical approach to ECFs involving the jejunum, ileum, or colon involves resection of the involved portion of intestine and a primary anastomosis to restore continuity. Although simple resection is sometimes feasible in the first and fourth portions of the duodenum, it is not possible in the midduodenum because of the anatomic relationships of the pancreas and bile ducts.

Because of their proximal location, duodenal fistulas tend to be high output and have enzyme-rich secretions capable of digesting surrounding tissues. These characteristics lead to increased morbidity and mortality rates for duodenal fistulas compared to fistulas arising in the distal GI tract. Rossi et al. (1986) reported a mean fistula output of over 800 mL per day, a mortality rate of 33%, and an operative rate of 50% in a series of 18 patients with entercutaneous duodenal fistulas. A study by Malangoni et al. (1981) of 14 patients with lateral duodenal fistulas had only one fistula-related death (7% mortality) but 10 patients required operative fistula repair.

Management of duodenal fistulas with a simple layered closure has a high incidence of recurrence except when a serosal patch is used. In this technique, the duodenorrhaphy is reinforced with a piece of serosa from the jejunum. Serosal patching decreases tension on the duodenal suture line which needs to be able to withstand pressures of at least 35 mmHg. A disadvantage of closure with a serosal patch is possible lumenal narrowing as the patch must be sutured to healthy duodenal wall. Although pancreaticoduodenectomy (Whipple procedure) has been advocated by some for the treatment of duodenal fistulas in patients with severe tissue destruction, alternative techniques with lower morbidity are better suited for the simple entercutaneous fistula.

Treatment of fistulas with less invasive techniques like fibrin glue is drawing more attention in the recent literature. Success has generally been limited to low output fistulas and further study is needed. Hwang and Chen (1996) performed a small randomized trial of percutaneous fibrin glue injection which included 13 patients with ECFs with outputs less than 20 mL per day. The fibrin glue group had significantly shorter mean healing time than controls (4 days vs. 13 days), and there were no adverse reactions to the treatment. Alternatively, using an endoscopic technique of fibrin injection, a group from Greece examined seven patients with high output (>200 mL per day) gastroduodenal fistulas and obtained healing in all patients, although most required multiple injections before closure. Other case studies found in the literature include the use of prolamine injection, gelfoam injection, and occluding spring emboli for fistula obliteration. Although percutaneous fibrin glue injection could be attempted on the patient described in the question, there is currently no available data to support its use in the patient with a high output duodenal fistula.

A Roux-en-Y duodenojejunostomy is the best choice among the procedures presented in the above question. The technique provides internal drainage and decompression of the duodenum rather than simple patching the fistula defect, and it does not distort the normal anatomic position of the duodenum. Ashall described successful repair of five duodenal fistulas, two of these high output, with a Roux-en-Y technique in 1986, and others have demonstrated success with the procedure for both duodenal and pancreatic fistulas.

Bibliography

Ashall G. Closure of upper gastrointestinal fistulas using a Roux-En-Y technique. *JR Coll Surg Edinb* 1986; 31(3): 151–155.

Bianchi A, Solduga C, Ubach M. Percutaneous obliteration of a chronic duodenal fistula. *Br J Surg* 1988;75:572.

Eleftheriadis E, Tzartinoglou E, Kotzampassi K, et al. Early endoscopic fibrin sealing of high-output postoperative enterocutaneous fistulas. *Acta Chir Scand* 1990; 156(9): 625–628.

Hwang T, Chen M. Short note: randomized trial of fibrin tissue glue for low output enterocutaneous fistula. *Br J Surg* 1996;83(1):112.

Khairy G, Al-Saigh A, Trincano N, et al. Percutaneous obliteration of duodenal fistula. *J RColl Surg Edinb* 2000; 45(5): 342–344.

Malangoni M, Madura J, Jesseph J. Management of lateral duodenal fistulas: a study of fourteen cases. *Surgery* 1981;90(4):645–651.

Padillo F, Regueiro J, Canis M, et al. Percutaneous management of a high-output duodenal fistula after pancrease transplantation using occluding coiled embolus and fibrin sealant. *Transplant Proc* 1999;31:1715–1716.

Rossi J, Sollenberger L, Rege R, et al. External duodenal fistula. *Arch Surg* 1986;121:908–912.

38. (D) Octreotide is an octopeptide analog of somatostatin. Both octreotide and somatostatin have significant inhibitory effects on the GI tract including decreased GI hormone release, decreased GI, biliary, and pancreatic secretions, decreased nutrient absorption, decreased GI transit, and decreased hepatic and splanchnic blood flow. Preliminary studies of somatostatin in the treatment of GI fistulas demonstrated reduction in fistula output and improved closure rates. This prompted investigation of octreotide, primarily because administration of octeotide is simpler than somatostatin. Unlike its parent compound which requires continuous intravenous infusion, octreotide has a longer half-life and good absorption which permits intermittent subcutaneous injection. Octreotide is

also associated with a lower incidence of hyperglycemia than somatostatin because of octreotide's higher specificity for inhibition of growth hormone and glucagon than for insulin. Side effects other than mild hyperglycemia are generally minimal and include pain or burning with injection, mild GI symptoms like nausea, vomiting, bloating, and diarrhea, and increased rate of cholelithiasis. Octreotide has also been associated with development of tachyphylaxis, and some authors suggest that its use for greater than 1 week is unnecessary.

Numerous clinical studies evaluating the effects of octreotide in the treatment of ECFs have been published; however, a concensus has not yet been reached regarding its overall efficacy. The majority of these studies have been case series. Well-designed, prospective, randomized trials on the subject are lacking; however, some general conclusions can be established based on the available evidence. In a review by Martineau et al. (1996), seven studies of octreotide in the treatment of ECFs were examined. Five of the seven studies demonstrated reduction in mean fistula output in patients treated with octreotide. The remaining two trials found no significant difference in fistula output reduction between octreotide treated patients and patients receiving placebo. Both of these studies were prospective, randomized control trials, but one was of small sample size and the other focused on treatment of fistulas at initial diagnosis rather than persistent, established fistulas. In this second study by Sancho et al. (1995), patients were started on TPN and octreotide or placebo simultaneously, within 7 days of fistula onset. Most other studies examined the effect of starting octreotide when a fistula persisted despite established treatment with TPN. Two other studies published since the review by Martineau also support reduction of fistula output by octreotide. A retrospective study of 39 patients with ECFs either treated with TPN alone or TPN with octreotide demonstrated a 50% mean reduction in fistula output in the octreotide group. A second retrospective study compared a group of patients with high output fistulas (>200 mL per day) treated with octreotide with a control group matched for patient and fistula characteristics, and found fistula output to be reduced 85% within the first 3 days of treatment with octreotide.

All of the above-mentioned studies also evaluated the effect of octreotide on spontaneous closure rates and mortality. Although a few trials have reported increased spontaneous fistula closure in octreotide treated groups, most do not support this finding. In general, closure rates are the same in patients treated with TPN alone or TPN with octreotide. Mortality rates also do not seem significantly affected by the use of octreotide in fistula management.

A definitive answer for octreotides role in management of ECFs will never be found unless sought by large multicenter prospective randomized control trials. Presently, studies have suggested that octreotide treatment decreases fistula output and may make fistulas more manageable. It is best suited for patients in whom a fistula has persisted despite initiation of conservative therapy with TPN.

Bibliography

Alivizatos V, Felekis D, Zorbalas A. Evaluation of the effectiveness of octreotide in the conservative treatment of postoperative enterocutaneous fistulas. *Hepatogastroenterology* 2002;49(46):1010–1012.

Alvarez C, McFadden D, Reber H. Complicated enterocutaneous fistulas: failure of octreotide to improve healing. *World J Surg* 2000;24(5):533–538.

Falconi M, Sartori N, Caldiron E, et al. Management of digestive tract fistulas. *Digestion* 1999;60(Suppl. 3):51–58.

Martineau P, Shwed J, Denis R. Is octreotide a new hope for enterocutaneous and external pancreatic fistulas closure? *Am J Surg* 1996;172(4):386–395.

Sancho J, di Costanzo J, Nubiola P, et al. Randomized double-blind placebo-controlled trial of early octreotide in patients with postoperative enterocutaneous fistula. *Br J Surg* 1995;82(5):638–641.

39. **(C)** Carcinoid tumors are classified as neuroendocrine neoplasms and arise from enterochromaffin cells. Overall prevalence is between 0.5 and 2 per 100,000 based on autopsy studies. Carcinoid tumors are classified as foregut, midgut, or hindgut in origin. Over 90% of carcinoid tumors arise in the GI tract. They account for 13–34% of all small bowel tumors. Other locations for carcinoid tumors include the lungs, thymus, and ovaries. The most common site of carcinoid tumor is the appendix, comprising up to 36% of cases. Twenty-five percent arise in the small bowel, making this the second most common site. Rectal carcinoids are third most common, and colonic carcinoids are relatively rare. Among small bowel carcinoids, most arise in the ileum. The mean age at diagnosis for small bowel carcinoids is 65 years.

Carcinoid tumors produce a large number of gastrointestinal neuroendocrine peptides and amines. Among these, serotonin is the principal biologically active compound and primarily responsible for development of the carcinoid syndrome which may accompany the presence of a tumor. Carcinoid tumors are characterized by being either biochemically typical or atypical based on their production of serotonin. Typical carcinoid tumors have dopa decarboxylase which converts 5-hydroxytryptophan (5-HPT) into serotonin (5-HT). Further metabolism of 5-HT results in 5-HIAA which is excreted in the urine. Atypical tumors lack dopa decarboxylase, leading to elevated circulatory levels of 5-HPT. The kidney does convert some of this 5-HPT into 5-HT. The end result is high levels of 5-HPT and 5-HT in the urine, but low or normal levels of 5-HIAA. Most small bowel carcinoids are biochemically typical.

Clinical manifestations of small bowel carcinoid include abdominal pain, symptoms of bowel obstruction, and carcinoid syndrome. Classic symptoms of carcinoid syndrome are flushing, diarrhea, bronchospasm, edema, right-sided valvular heart disease (tricuspid regurgitation and pulmonary stenosis), and pellagra. Development of the carcinoid syndrome requires delivery of tumor products into the systemic circulation, generally from hepatic or distant metastasis. Because GI symptoms are nonspecific and only 5–7% of patients with a small bowel carcinoid present with carcinoid syndrome, very few cases are diagnosed prior to surgery. Laboratory studies which may be obtained when a carcinoid is suspected include urinary 5-HIAA, urinary 5-HT, and platelet 5-HT levels. In a series of 75 patients with carcinoid tumors, 84% had an elevation in at least one of these levels. Chromogranin A level may also have a role in both diagnosis and followup of carcinoids. Chromogranin A is a glycoprotein expressed by these tumors and has a sensitivity of over 80%. If these studies are normal and a patient is still suspected to have carcinoid syndrome, provocative testing with pentagastrin may be used. Pentagastrin administration causes release of serotonin and substance P, resulting in flushing in nearly 100% of patients with carcinoid syndrome.

Small bowel carcinoids are frequently multicentric on presentation. Although most arise in the distal ileum, care must be taken to thoroughly explore the entire abdomen to identify multiple lesions on laparotomy. A study of patients presenting with multiple ileal carcinoid tumors found that these patients tend to be younger, have a higher risk of developing carcinoid syndrome, and have an overall poorer prognosis than patients with solitary lesions. Small bowel carcinoids also often present with metastatic disease. The most common sites are regional lymph nodes and the liver. In one comprehensive study, 25% of patients had local disease, 39% had regional metastasis, and 31% had distant metastasis on presentation. Tumor size is unreliable for prediction of metastatic spread. Up to 45% of tumors less than 1 cm in diameter already have local lymph node involvement. Metastasis has been reported in patients with tumors as small as 0.5 cm in diameter.

A number of radiographic modalities may be used to confirm the diagnosis of small bowel carcinoid and localize multiple primary or metastatic lesions. Because >80% of these tumors express somatostatin receptors, the somatostatin analog octreotide can be radiolabeled and used in scintigraphy to identify lesions. Similarly, ^{131}I-MIBG (metaiodobenzylguanididine) is a radiolabeled catecholamine analog which is selectively taken up by serotonin producing tumors and can be used to localize carcinoids. Ultrasound evaluation is best for evaluation of hepatic metastases. CT and magnetic resonance imaging (MRI) can identify both hepatic lesions and lymph node involvement.

Significant prognostic factors associated with midgut carcinoids include site (small bowel carcinoids have worse prognosis than appendiceal), depth of invasion, size of tumor(s), presence of metastasis to lymph nodes and liver, and circumstances of detection (incidentally found tumors have better prognosis). Five-year survival for small bowel carcinoids is up to 75% for patients with only local disease, 60% for patients with regional disease, but falls to less than 38% with presence of distant metastasis.

GI carcinoid tumors are associated with a high rate of second primary malignancies. Small bowel carcinoids appear to have the highest incidence of these related tumors. In a review by Habal et al. (2000), the rate of second primary malignancies was 29–52% in small bowel carcinoids, 13–32% in appendiceal carcinoids, and 5–32% in rectal carcinoids. The GI tract is the most common site of these secondary malignancies and adenocarcinoma is the most common histology. In general the second malignancy is more aggressive than the carcinoid tumor and the cause of most mortality among these patients. The underlying etiology for second primary malignancies in patients with carcinoid is not known but may be related to the production of a multitude of growth factors from the carcinoid tumor itself.

Bibliography

Box J, Watne A, Lucas G. Small bowel carcinoid: review of a single institution experience and review of the literature. *Am Surg* 1996;62(4):280–286.

de Vries H, Verschueren R, Willemse P, et al. Diagnostic, surgical, and medical aspect of the midgut carcinoids. *Cancer Treat Rev* 2002;28(1):11–25.

Habal N, Sims C, Bilchik A. Gastrointestinal carcinoid tumors and second primary malignancies. *J Surg Oncol* 2000;75:301–306.

Kulke M, Mayer R. Medical progress: carcinoid tumors. *N Engl J Med* 1999;340(11):858–868.

Kuwada S. Carcinoid tumors. *Semin Gastrointest Dis* 2000;11(3):157–161.

Oberg K. Carcinoid tumors: current concepts in diagnosis and treatment. *Oncologist* 1998;3:339–345.

Pasieka J, McKinnon J, Kinnear S, et al. Carcinoid syndrome symposium on treatment modalities for gastrointestinal carcinoid tumours: symposium summary. *Can J Surg* 2001;44(1):25–32.

Woods H, Phil D, Bax N, et al. Small bowel carcinoid tumors. *World J Surg* 1985;9(6):921–929.

Yantiss R, Farraye F, Rosenberg A. Solitary versus multiple carcinoid tumors of the ileum: a clinical and pathologic review of 68 cases. *Am J Surg Pathol* 2003;27(6):811–817.

40. **(E)** Hepatic ultrasound is the best answer choice for the above question because the liver must be completely evaluated to determine extent of disease. There is a clear correlation between tumor spread and survival, as noted in the previous discussion. The liver is by far the most common site of metastasis beyond regional lymph nodes. In this patient who has recently undergone laparotomy with thorough intraabdominal examination, hepatic ultrasound would probably suffice to rule out liver involvement. Alternatively a dual phase abdominal CT or abdominal MRI study could also be used to evaluate the liver and potentially localize previously undetected lesions in the abdomen. It should be noted, however, that CT has a low sensitivity for detecting primary carcinoid tumors and probably has greatest value in preoperative evaluation to determine extent of tumor spread, including hepatic and lymph node involvement. It has also been reported that although conventional radiographic studies may miss primary tumors preoperatively, these lesions are generally palpable at the time of operation.

Some authors also advocate the use of radiolabeled octreotide scintigraphy postoperatively and when recurrence is suspected. This study is most helpful in patients with elevated 5-HIAA levels which correlate with tumor somatostatin receptor expression. The octreotide scan localizes both primaries and metastatic deposits, and appears superior to CT for diagnosis of extraabdominal metastasis. It may also help predict tumor responsiveness to somatostatin analog treatment.

Abnormalities in liver function tests are not a reliable indicator of metastatic involvement of the liver by carcinoid. In the setting of diffuse hepatic metastasis, serum alkaline phosphatase may be normal.

EGD is not necessary in the patient with a small bowel carcinoid unless they present with GI bleeding and a source must be localized. Foregut carcinoids tend to be distinct tumors from small bowel carcinoids both biochemically and in their clinical history. A review of the literature produced no reports of gastric carcinoids presenting with small bowel carcinoids. As described previously, small bowel carcinoids are associated with second primary malignancies, the majority of which are discovered concurrently with the carcinoid. Although carcinomas of the stomach have been reported in series of second primary tumors in carcinoids, they are not common. EGD should probably be reserved for patients with a history of carcinoid and symptoms attributable to the upper GI tract.

Head CT is not indicated for patients with small bowel carcinoid unless neurologic symptoms warrant an investigation. Brain metastasis can occur in carcinoid tumors but is a rare, late occurrence. It is typically related to a pulmonary source. In one series of 219 carcinoid patients, 11 developed brain metastasis, of these, 5 patients had primary bronchial carcinoids and 5 had carcinoids metastatic to the lung.

Carcinoid heart disease occurs in approximately 50% of patients with carcinoid syndrome. It is generally a late occurrence, believed to be secondary to prolonged exposure to high levels of serotonin. The most common lesions are tricuspid regurgitation and pulmonary stenosis. The left side of the heart is rarely affected. Patients with carcinoid heart disease frequently complain of dyspnea and often have discernible heart murmurs on presentation. Electrocardiogram (ECG) and chest x-rays tend to be nonspecific in these patients. Echocardiogram is considered the diagnostic technique of choice for carcinoid heart syndrome. The patient described in the above question presents with no complaints attributable to carcinoid syndrome or carcinoid heart disease and therefore needs no cardiac evaluation. If the patient did have complaints or heart murmur, the best test would be an echocardiogram.

Bibliography

Botero M, Fuchs R, Paulus D, et al. Carcinoid heart disease: a case report and literature review. *J Clin Anesth* 2002; 14(1):57–63.

Box J, Watne A, Lucas G. Small bowel carcinoid: review of a single institution experience and review of the literature. *Am Surg* 1996;62(4):280–286.

de Vries H, Verschueren R, Willemse P, et al. Diagnostic, surgical, and medical aspect of the midgut carcinoids. *Cancer Treat Rev* 2002;28(1):11–25.

Habal N, Sims C, Bilchik A. Gastrointestinal carcinoid tumors and second primary malignancies. *J Surg Oncol* 2000;75:301–306.

Nida T, Hall W, Glantz M, et al. Metastatic carcinoid tumor to the orbit and brain. *Neurosurgery* 1992;31(5):949–952.

Oberg K. Carcinoid tumors: current concepts in diagnosis and treatment. *Oncologist* 1998;3:339–345.

Pasieka J, McKinnon J, Kinnear S, et al. Carcinoid syndrome symposium on treatment modalities for gastrointestinal carcinoid tumours: symposium summary. *Can J Surg* 2001;44(1):25–32.

41. **(E)** PGV has almost completely replaced truncal vagotomy with drainage or partial gastrectomy for the surgical treatment of peptic ulcer disease in this era of H2 blockers and proton-pump inhibitors. Although postvagotomy syndromes may still occur with PGV and the rate of ulcer recurrence is higher, the overall complication rate is significantly lower than these earlier techniques and recurrent ulceration generally responds well to medical treatment.

Postvagotomy GI complications include dumping syndrome, postprandial fullness, postvagotomy diarrhea, gastroesophageal reflux, alkaline reflux, delayed gastric emptying, and dysphagia.

Dumping syndrome is a group of GI and/or vasomotor symptoms which follow meal consumption. There are two types of dumping syndrome—early and late. Early dumping syndrome occurs within 15–30 min after a meal and consists of abdominal cramps, bloating, nausea/vomiting, explosive diarrhea, flushing, dizziness, diaphoresis, and palpitations. Late dumping syndrome occurs 2–4 h after a meal and consists only of the vasomotor symptoms. Both types of dumping syndrome are believed to be related to delivery of hyperosmolar contents into the small bowel causing fluid shifts and production of vasoactive substances and GI hormones. The incidence of dumping syndrome is significantly less after PGV compared to procedures that compromise the pylorus. Many patients will initially have complaints of dumping syndrome after gastric surgery but most will have symptom resolution by 4–5 months postprocedure. The medical management of dumping syndrome is primarily diet modification. Decreasing meal size, increasing meal frequency, avoiding concentrated carbohydrates, and taking liquids 30 min after meals all help minimize symptoms. Pharmacologic therapy with octreotide has also had some success. Surgical intervention is rarely necessary.

Postvagotomy diarrhea is a common side effect of all gastric surgery. For most patients, diarrhea is mild and self-limited, usually improving over the first 12 months after surgery. The incidence is highest in patients who have undergone truncal vagotomy. It is thought to be secondary to disruption of vagal innervation of the small intestine and biliary system.

Reflux of biliary juices into the stomach occurs when the pylorus no longer protects the stomach from retrograde flow. Symptoms of alkaline reflux gastritis include burning epigastric pain that is not relieved by eating, and bilious emesis, often containing food. Biliary reflux is rare post-PGV, occurring between 0 and 2% of the time. It is most common in following Billroth II. Medical treatment includes cholestyramine and sucralfate; however, full relief is usually not attained. The most common surgical intervention is Roux-en-Y gastrojejunostomy which generally has good results.

Interestingly, dysphagia is one complication that has a higher incidence in PGV versus other gastric procedures. Rates vary among series, but at least two studies clearly demonstrated a significantly higher rate of dysphagia in PGV than truncal vagotomy with pyloroplasty. It was also noted in these studies that dysphagia tended to be transient in nature and required no particular therapy for those patients affected.

Bibliography

Bar-Natan M, Larson G, Stephens G, et al. Delayed gastric emptying after gastric surgery. *Am J Surg* 1996; 172(2): 24–28.

Donahue P, Bombeck T, Condon R, et al. Proximal gastric vagotomy versus selective vagotomy with antrectomy: results of a prospective, randomized clinical trial after four to twelve years. *Surgery* 1984;96(4):585–590.

Eagon J, Miedema B, Kelly K. Postgastrectomy syndromes. *Surg Clin North Am* 1992;72(2):445–465.

Fischer J, Fegelman E, Johannigman J. Surgical complications. In: Schwartz S, Shires G, Spencer F, et al. (eds.), *Principles of Surgery*, 7th ed. New York, NY: McGraw-Hill, 1999, 441–483.

Fraser A, Brunt P, Matheson N. A comparison of highly selective vagotomy with truncal vagotomy and pyloroplasty—one surgeon's results after 5 years. *Br J Surg* 1983;70(8):485–488.

Leduc J, Meban S. Dysphagia following vagotomy. *Can J Surg* 1985;28(6):537–538.

Tytgat G, Offerhaus G, Mulder C, et al. Consequences of gastric surgery for benign conditions: an overview. *Hepatogastroenterology* 1988;35:271–278.

42. (C) Because partial gastrectomies are now rarely performed for ulcer disease, afferent loop syndrome is a complication infrequently encountered. Classically it occurs after Billroth II procedure; however, it may also be seen following pancreaticoduodenectomy and rarely after technical problems with Roux-en-Y gastrojejunostomy. The afferent limb of the Billroth II includes the duodenal stump and jejunum proximal to the gastric anastomosis. The syndrome presents in either acute or chronic form. In the acute form, there is a complete obstruction of this limb, causing sudden, unrelenting pain, nausea, nonbilious emesis, and sometimes an abdominal mass. As pressure in the limb increases, necrosis of the bowel wall and duodenal stump leakage can occur. The obstruction can occur from volvulus, herniation, or kinking at the anastomosis. Acute afferent loop syndrome is a surgical emergency and requires prompt intervention. The extent of operation performed depends on the amount of pressure necrosis which has occurred.

Chronic afferent loop syndrome results from partial obstruction of the afferent limb with intermittent decompression of the obstruction into the stomach. Besides the reasons for the acute obstruction, chronic obstruction can also be caused by extrinsic compression from adhesions or inflammatory processes, stricture at the anastomosis, or intussusception. Following gastric resection for gastric cancer, the most common cause of afferent loop syndrome is recurrent tumor. The patient described in the question demonstrates the classic presentation of chronic afferent loop syndrome. These patients have right upper quadrant pain and distension following meals as stimulated secretions from the biliary tract and pancreas build up behind the obstruction. Then the closed loop may empty suddenly into the stomach producing bilious vomiting. By this point the food from the meal has usually passed into the distal jejunum so that the emesis rarely contains food remnants. The diagnostic procedure of choice is endoscopy. CT scan and abdominal ultrasound often demonstrate characteristic findings but these may not be recognized as the syndrome is uncommon. CT scan often shows a fluid-filled tube-like structure, frequently containing air bubbles, which is located in the right upper abdomen. Treatment for chronic afferent loop syndrome has historically been surgical, with conversion of the Billroth II into a Roux-en-Y gastrojejunostomy. More recently, decompression of the afferent loop using either percutaneous transhepatic biliary or duodenal drainage or percutaneous tube enterostomy has been attempted as palliation for cancer patients who are no longer surgical candidates. All of these procedures have met with some success in reducing symptoms for this subgroup of patients.

The diagnosis of afferent loop syndrome is most difficult to distinguish from alkaline reflux gastritis. Both are postgastrectomy syndromes that result in bilious emesis. The major differences are that the onset of pain from alkaline reflux is not associated with meals and not relieved by vomiting, and that the emesis from alkaline reflux typically includes ingested food.

Recurrent ulcer disease at the site of anastomosis with resultant inflammation can lead to development of afferent loop syndrome but recurrent gastric ulcer itself would not lead to the symptoms described in this patient. Likewise, this patient's symptoms are not typical of gallstone pancreatitis or choledocholithiasis.

Bibliography

Eagon J, Miedema B, Kelly K. Postgastrectomy syndromes. *Surg Clin North Am* 1992;72(2):445–465.

Fischer J, Fegelman E, Johannigman J. Surgical complications. In: Schwartz S, Shires G, Spencer F, et al. (eds.), *Principles of Surgery*, 7th ed. New York, NY: McGraw-Hill, 1999, 441–483.

Gayer G, Barsuk D, Hertz M, et al. CT diagnosis of afferent loop syndrome. *Clin Radiol* 2002;57(9):835–839.

Lee K, Liu T, Wu C, et al. Non-surgical treatment for afferent loop syndrome in recurrent gastric cancer complicated by peritoneal carcinomatosis: percutaneous transhepatic duodenal drainage followed by 24-hour infusion of high-dose fluorouracil and leucovorin. *Ann Oncol* 2002;13:1151–1155.

Kim Y, Han J, Lee K, et al. Palliative percutaneous tube enterostomy in afferent-loop syndrome presenting as jaundice: clinical effectiveness. *J Vasc Interv Radiol* 2002;13(8):845–849.

Powell D, Bivins B, Bell R, et al. Technical complications of Roux-en-Y gastrojejunostomy. *Arch Surg* 1983; 118(8): 922–925.44.

43. (C) Overall, the GI tract is the most common extranodal location for non-Hodgkin's lymphoma. Within the GI tract, most frequently involved sites in order from highest to lowest in the Western world are the stomach, small bowel, and colon. Lymphoma is the third most common primary small bowel malignancy following adenocarcinoma and carcinoid. To put these figures in perspective, the small bowel is the site of less than 5% of all GI malignancies, making small bowel lymphoma a very rare tumor. The jejunum is the second most common location for PSBL to arise, most occur in the ileum, and the least are found in the duodenum. This distribution corresponds with the prevalence of lymphoid tissue along the GI tract, with the ileum having the densest concentration of lymphoid follicles.

Small bowel lymphoma is believed to arise in the Peyer's patches located in the submucosa of the bowel wall. Tumor can then extend either toward the mucosa or the serosa. This can lead to lesions which are polypoid, circumferential, ulcerative, or externally compressive on the bowel lumen. The most common symptoms of small bowel lymphoma in the Western world are abdominal pain, anorexia, weight loss, bowel obstruction, and abdominal mass. PSBL is generally not diagnosed prior to laparotomy. Endoscopy is only diagnostic for a small percentage of small bowel lymphomas. CT scan and ultrasound examination may reveal suspicious findings but are not sensitive enough for diagnosis. Enterolysis is probably the most sensitive radiographic study for detecting these lesions, but of course does not provide a tissue diagnosis. Finally, positron emission tomography (PET) scanning has shown promise but cannot completely distinguish between oncologically active lesions and inflammatory processes. Additionally, once the diagnosis of a PSBL is suspected, systemic disease with GI involvement must be ruled out. Primary disease is confirmed by absence of lymphoma on physical examination (no lymphadenopathy or hepatosplenomegaly), on chest x-ray or chest CT, on peripheral blood smear, and on bone marrow biopsy.

Surgery is first line therapy for all PSBL. Wide resection of all visible disease, including regional mesenteric lymph nodes, is the procedure of choice. Frozen section should be used to confirm negative margins. Complete resection is only possible in 30–40% of patients. If disease is too extensive for complete resection, tumor debulking should be performed.

The majority of PSBL are B-cell in origin. Histologically, they are classified as high, intermediate, and low grade. Most studies have demonstrated that high-grade lesions have the greatest prevalence. There is a clear difference in prognosis between high-grade and low-grade small bowel lymphoma. As a result, most authors recommend postoperative multidrug chemotherapy for all high- and intermediate-grade lesions, even if complete resection is achieved. Only completely resected, low-grade lesions are treated with surgery alone.

Other prognostic factors for primary lymphomas throughout the GI tract include site, number of lesions, presence of perforation, and residual disease. PSBL tend to have a poorer prognosis than gastric or colon primary lymphomas. This difference is probably because small bowel lesions are less symptomatic and are discovered at a more advanced stage. Patients who present with multiple primary tumors also have poor prognosis. Although most PSBL present at solitary lesions, up to 25% of patients may have multiple primaries at diagnosis. Patients who present with bowel perforation and undergo emergency laparotomy have poorer prognosis than those whose lesions are discovered incidentally. Presence of perforation correlates to degree of bowel wall involvement and is a marker of more advanced disease. Finally, those patients in whom complete resection is not possible, or in whom residual disease is left behind, have a poor prognosis.

Bibliography

Domizio P, Owen R, Shepherd N, et al. Primary lymphoma of the small intestine. *Am J Surg Pathol* 1993; 17(5): 429–442.

Gospodarowicz M, Sutcliffe S, Clark R, et al. Outcome analysis of localized gastrointestinal lymphoma treated with surgery and postoperative irradiation. *Int J Radiat Oncol Biol Phys* 1990;19(6):1351–1355.

Haber D, Mayer R. Primary gastrointestinal lymphoma. *Semin Oncol* 1988;15(2):154–169.

Neugut A, Jacobson J, Suh S, et al. The epidemiology of cancer of the small bowel. *Cancer Epidemiol Biomarkers Prev* 1998;7:243–251.

ReMine S, Braasch J. Gastric and small bowel lymphoma. *Surg Clin North Am* 1986;66(4):713–722.

Robinson E, Cusack J, Tyler D. Small-bowel malignancies and carcinoid tumors. In: Feig B, Berger D, Fuhrman G (eds.), *The M.D. Anderson Surgical Oncology Handbook*, 2nd ed. Philadephia, PA: Lippincott, Williams & Wilkins, 1999, 161–177.

Tedeschi L, Romanelli A, Dallavalle G, et al. Stages I and II non-Hodgkin's lymphoma of the gastrointestinal tract: A retrospective analysis of 79 patients and review of the literature. *J Clin Gastroenterol* 1994;18(2):99–104.

Ullerich H, Franzius C, Domagk D, et al. ^{18}F-Fluorodeoxyglucose PET in a patient with primary small bowel lymphoma: the only sensitive method of imaging. *Am J Gastroenterol* 2001;96(8):2497–2498.

44. **(A)** An association between celiac sprue and the development of PSBL has been established in a number of studies. Celiac sprue, also known as gluten-induced enteropathy, is a disease characterized by small bowel mucosal changes, malabsorption, and association with gluten, a component of wheat. The etiology of the disease in unknown but genetic, immunologic, and environmental factors probably all play a role. Celiac sprue is more common in women and sometimes demonstrates a dominant inheritance pattern with incomplete penetrance. Symptoms include diarrhea, bloating, abdominal pain, and weight loss. Pathologic changes are greatest in the proximal jejunum and include blunting of villi, lymphoid infiltration of the submucosa, change in cell shape from columnar to cuboid, and sometimes mucosal ulceration. Diagnosis requires the presence of typical symptoms that resolve after initiation of a strict gluten-free diet, evidence of malabsorption on clinical tests, and the exclusion of other causes of malabsorption. Characteristic small bowel biopsy is also diagnostic. The only treatment is strict adherence to a gluten-free diet.

The development of PSBL in the setting of celiac sprue most often occurs years after sprue diagnosis; however, there is a certain group of patients who are asymptomatic and not diagnosed with sprue until the discovery of lymphoma. Therefore, the evidence is not clear whether adherence to a gluten-free diet reduces the risk of lymphoma. In a study by Domizio et al. (1993), out of 115 patients with small bowel lymphoma, 13 had documented celiac sprue with a range of 2–23 years before diagnosis of lymphoma. Six other patients had histologic evidence of celiac sprue on pathologic evaluation of their specimens, three of these were asymptomatic and three others had a history of malabsorption. Finally, one patient developed celiac sprue after the diagnosis of lymphoma. There does seem to be a correlation to patient's age and the development of lymphoma in sprue. Celiac sprue patients over the age of 50 have a 10% risk of developing lymphoma as opposed to younger celiac sprue patients whose risk is closer to 3%. The risk of clinically undetected lymphoma may be even higher in these patients according to autopsy series. Diagnosis of lymphoma in the setting of celiac sprue may be difficult as symptoms of both diseases can be similar; however, suspicion of lymphoma should be raised in sprue patients who were previously well controlled and then relapse, or patients whose symptoms worsen without apparent cause.

Unlike the majority of PSBL, those associated with celiac sprue are T-cell in origin. Histologically, they do not differ from small bowel T-cell lymphoma in patients without celiac sprue. The site of lymphoma also differs in these patients as most lesions occur in the proximal small bowel. This corresponds to the site of maximum histologic change in celiac sprue. Because of the rarity of the malignancy, consensus regarding prognostic differences between patients with celiac sprue-related lymphoma and nonsprue-related disease has not been reached.

Development of PSBL has also been associated with a number of other conditions. These include other malabsorptive diseases, inflammatory bowel disease, and immunologic disorders. Malabsorptive diseases other than celiac sprue include idiopathic steatorrhea and dermatitis herpetiformis. The inflammatory bowel disease most commonly associated with development of small bowel lymphoma is CD. Incidence and prognosis of lymphoma in the setting of CD has not been well defined in the current literature. Many immunologic disorders have been linked to GI lymphoma, including AIDS, autoimmune disorders, and congenital immune deficiencies. Iatrogenic dysfunction of the immune system in organ transplant recipients is also associated with a higher incidence of lymphoma development. In both AIDS patients and organ transplant patients, lymphomas tend to be aggressive, involve extranodal sites like the GI tract, demonstrate B-cell origin, and frequently have evidence of Epstein-Barr virus infection.

Irritable bowel syndrome and herpes zoster infection have no association with the development of lymphoma. Although there have been reports of gastric adenocarcinoma and gastric lymphoma occurring simultaneously in the same patient, there is no evidence that this sort of event occurs in the small bowel with any frequency. Finally, female sex is not associated with an increased incidence of small bowel lymphoma. In fact, most series show a slightly higher rate in males for both small bowel lymphoma and for small bowel malignancy in general.

Bibliography

Domizio P, Owen R, Shepherd N, et al. Primary lymphoma of the small intestine. *Am J Surg Pathol* 1993; 17(5): 429–442.

Greenberger N, Isselbacher K. Disorders of absorption. In: Fauci A, Braunwald E, Isselbacher K, et al. (eds.), *Harrison's Principles of Internal Medicine*, 14th ed. New York, NY: McGraw-Hill, 1998, 1628–1630.

Haber D, Mayer R. Primary gastrointestinal lymphoma. *Semin Oncol* 1988;15(2):154–169.

Neugut A, Jacobson J, Suh S, et al. The epidemiology of cancer of the small bowel. *Cancer Epidemiol Biomarkers Prev* 1998;7:243–251.

O'Boyle C, Kerin M, Feeley K, Given H. Primary small intestinal tumours: increased incidence of lymphoma and improved survival. *Ann R Coll Surg Engl* 1998; 80: 332–334.

Rubesin S, Gilchrist A, Bronner M, et al. Non-Hodgkin lymphoma of the small intestine. *Radiographics* 1990; 10: 985–998.

45. (A) Chronic mesenteric ischemia is caused by atherosclerosis in more than 95% of cases. Other rare causes include hypercoagulable states, vasculitides, fibromuscular dysplasia, mesenteric artery dissection, external compression, and congenital vascular defects. Although atherosclerosis of the mesenteric vessels is common on autopsy, the development of chronic mesenteric ischemia is uncommon. This discrepancy is explained by the typically slow progression of arterial stenosis with development of collateral vessels. The mean age of diagnosis is 60 years, and there is a slightly higher incidence in women than men. Most patients with chronic mesenteric ischemia have evidence of vascular disease elsewhere as well. Forty percent have coronary artery disease, 40% have peripheral vascular disease, 15% have renal artery disease, and the incidence of cerebrovascular disease is also increased in this patient population. Chronic mesenteric ischemia has the same risk factors as does atherosclerosis anywhere in the body; however, hypercholesterolemia may be absent in these patients secondary to malnutrition. The most common risk factor for chronic mesenteric ischemia is smoking.

Symptoms of chronic mesenteric ischemia commonly include postprandial abdominal pain, fear of eating, and weight loss. Diarrhea, nausea and vomiting, and constipation are less common symptoms. Abdominal pain is the most consistent symptom and typically occurs 15–60 min after a meal and lasts several hours. It is generally described as midabdominal, achy or crampy in quality, and worsening in severity as the disease progresses. Some patients will naturally reduce the size of their meals, which may at least initially decrease their symptoms. In most cases, abdominal pain eventually leads the patient to avoid eating and lose weight. Average weight loss is around 10 kg. This weight loss correlates well with the severity of symptoms. Although some degree of malabsorption occurs with chronic mesenteric ischemia, malabsorption does not account for the majority of weight loss in these patients. On physical examination, abdominal tenderness is nonlocalized and mild, an abdominal bruit may be appreciated, and evidence of peripheral vascular disease is often present.

Diagnosis of chronic mesenteric ischemia has been discussed in detail in the comment for Question 47, but briefly, it requires ruling out other causes for abdominal pain and documenting significant mesenteric stenosis in a symptomatic patient. Mesenteric duplex ultrasound is a good screening test for symptomatic patients before progressing to angiography. It is inexpensive, noninvasive, and has a sensitivity of 87% for celiac stenosis and 92% for SMA stenosis. Disadvantages are that it requires expertise to both perform and interpret, and the inferior mesenteric artery is visualized less than 50% of the time. The diagnosis of chronic mesenteric ischemia requires at least two-vessel stenosis, and most patients with chronic mesenteric ischemia have significant stenosis involving the celiac axis and/or SMA. Therefore, patients without disease visualized on ultrasound can usually be ruled out for chronic mesenteric ischemia, and those patients with significant disease on ultrasound should be followed up with angiography.

Chronic mesenteric ischemia puts a patient at risk for acute mesenteric ischemia. Up to 80% of patients presenting with acute mesenteric ischemia from thrombosis may have had previous symptoms consistent with chronic ischemia. It has also been estimated that 20–50% of acute mesenteric ischemia secondary to thrombosis occurs in the setting of preexisting mesenteric stenosis. Therefore, the treatment for the patient who has documented symptomatic mesenteric stenosis is a revascularization procedure.

Bibliography

Cappell M. Intestinal (mesenteric) vasculopathy II: ischemic colitis and chronic mesenteric ischemia. *Gastroenterol Clin North Am* 1998;27(4):827–860.

Cunningham C, Reilly L, Stoney R. Chronic visceral ischemia. *Surg Clin North Am* 1992;72(1):231–244.

Kazmers A. Operative management of chronic mesenteric ischemia. *Ann Vasc Surg* 1998;12(3):299–308.

Thomas J, Blake K, Pierce G, et al. The clinical course of asymptomatic mesenteric arterial stenosis. *J Vasc Surg* 1998;27(5):840–844.

46. **(C)** Diagnosis of chronic mesenteric ischemia has three requirements. The patient must have symptoms consistent with the disease, other causes of abdominal pain and weight loss must be excluded, and moderate-to-high-grade stenosis must be demonstrated in at least two mesenteric arteries.

First, the patient must have a clinical presentation consistent with the disease. The symptoms of chronic mesenteric ischemia have already been discussed in Question 45. Occasionally an asymptomatic patient will incidentally be found to have significant mesenteric artery stenosis on aortogram. Those patients who go on to require aortic reconstruction generally have their mesenteric stenosis corrected at the time of aortic surgery; however, optimal management of the subgroup of asymptomatic patients who have mesenteric stenosis and do not require aortic surgery is not known. A study by Thomas et al. (1998) examined 60 asymptomatic patients with significant patterns of mesenteric stenosis and found that only four patients went on to develop mesenteric ischemia. All four of these patients had three-vessel mesenteric artery disease. Thomas et al. (1998) concluded that asymptomatic patients with one- or two-vessel disease should have close follow-up, but those with three-vessel disease should be considered for mesenteric artery reconstruction.

The second criterion for diagnosis of chronic mesenteric ischemia is exclusion of other causes of abdominal pain and weight loss. Patients typically undergo an extensive workup before the diagnosis is made. Laboratory studies tend to be nonspecific, and may include anemia, hypoalbuminemia, hypoproteinemia, and leukopenia. Malabsorption tests including fecal fat and D-xylose may also be abnormal. Common diagnostic tests performed include abdominal ultrasound and EGD. These exclude other causes of upper abdominal pain originating from gastroduodenal, hepatic, or biliary sources. EGD may on occasion demonstrate gastroduodenal ischemic ulcers. Colonoscopy should also be performed if there are symptoms concerning for lower tract disease, but is rarely helpful in diagnosis of chronic mesenteric ischemia. CT is also a good choice for further evaluation of causes for abdominal pain; however, it is not the best choice for demonstrating mesenteric artery disease.

Last, demonstration of significant two-vessel mesenteric stenosis must be made to complete the diagnosis. Often symptomatic patients are now screened for mesenteric stenosis with duplex ultrasound as discussed in the previous question. If stenosis of one or more arteries is suspected on ultrasound, the patient should next undergo mesenteric angiography to demonstrate the extent of the disease and possibly confirm the diagnosis. A diagnosis of chronic mesenteric ischemia can be made if angiography shows moderate (50–74%) to high (75–99%) grade stenosis or occlusion in at least two mesenteric arteries. In up to 90% of cases, significant disease of both the celiac axis and SMA will be discovered. Half of these patients will also have IMA disease. Rarely a patient may be found to have symptomatic single-vessel occlusion because of poor development of collaterals. This is only seen in occlusion of the celiac axis or SMA. The clinician should be cautious in the diagnosis of chronic mesenteric ischemia in those patients with only single-vessel occlusion because of the rarity of its occurrence. Visualization of mesenteric artery stenosis is best on the lateral angiographic projection, whereas collateral vessels are best evaluated by the anteroposterior view. The arteriogram then provides the required map for planning mesenteric artery reconstruction. Contrast-enhanced (CE)-MRA is a newer technique that has had excellent results in identifying mesenteric artery stenosis and may be an alternative to angiography. Diameters of stenotic arteries correlate between MRA and angiography, and several studies have demonstated sensitivities and specificities as high as 100% for CE-MRA detection of mesenteric stenosis.

Bibliography

Cappell M. Intestinal (mesenteric) vasculopathy II: ischemic colitis and chronic mesenteric ischemia. *Gastroenterol Clin North Am* 1998;27(4):827–860.

Cunningham C, Reilly L, Stoney R. Chronic visceral ischemia. *Surg Clin North Am* 1992;72(1):231–244.

Kazmers A. Operative management of chronic mesenteric ischemia. *Ann Vasc Surg* 1998;12(3):299–308.

Laissy J, Trillaud H, Douek P. MR angiography: noninvasive vascular imaging of the abdomen. *Abdom Imaging* 2002;27(5):488–506.

Thomas J, Blake K, Pierce G, et al. The clinical course of asymptomatic mesenteric arterial stenosis. *J Vasc Surg* 1998;27(5):840–844.

47. **(E)** Currently the preferred method of mesenteric arterial reconstruction by most authors is antegrade bypass grafting. A number of possible advantages of the antegrade approach have been described in the literature; however, studies which examine patency rates have not shown a difference between the two techniques.

Bypass grafting, either antegrade or retrograde, represents one type of therapy for chronic mesenteric ischemia. In the antegrade procedure, a graft is constructed from the supraceliac aorta to the distal mesenteric vessel(s). Anastomosis to the celiac trunk is generally performed in an end-to-side fashion whereas the anstomosis to the SMA is usually done with an end-to-end technique. If the surgeon decides to bypass the IMA as well, this is performed as an infrarenal aorto-IMA bypass. In retrograde celiac artery bypass grafting, the proximal anastomosis is from the iliac artery and the graft brought up to create and end-to-side distal anastomosis on the celiac artery bifurcation (either iliosplenic or iliohepatic bypass). The SMA may also be approached using this technique, creating an iliomesenteric artery bypass. For either method of bypass grafting, prosthetic material like Dacron is typically used, as autogenous vein has not demonstrated the advantage in mesenteric grafting that it holds in extremity bypasses. However, autogenous vein is recommended in situations in which there is intraabdominal contamination or infection. Potential advantages of the antegrade bypass approach include avoidance of graft contact with bowel, less potential for graft kinking when the bowel is replaced back in anatomic position, and shorter graft with a straight line in-flow from the aorta. Additionally, the supraceliac aorta, compared with the infrarenal aorta and iliac arteries, has less propensity for development of atherosclerotic disease and therefore may serve as a better proximal anastomotic site. Despite recognition of these potential advantages to antegrade bypass, retrospective studies of patency rates and long-term recurrence have shown no difference between the two methods. Mesenteric bypass grafting in general is associated with an 80–90% long-term success rate. Currently most authors prefer the antegrade approach for primary mesenteric artery reconstruction, but recommend the retrograde approach for repeat mesenteric bypass in which a second antegrade approach would be technically difficult.

Other therapies for chronic mesenteric ischemia include mesenteric endartertectomy, mesenteric artery reimplantation, and percutaneous mesenteric angioplasty and stenting. Mesenteric endarterectomy was one of the earliest procedures attempted for mesenteric ischemia. A transaortic approach which allows removal of both the aortic plaque and disease within the proximal mesenteric vessel is preferred, as it has been shown to have improved patency rates over a more limited, local approach to the vessel. Overall long-term patency rates are equivalent for transoartic endarterectomy and bypass grafting. Bypass grafting is generally preferred, however, because endarterectomy is a more technically demanding and time-consuming procedure. Mesenteric artery reimplantation is performed by directly anastomosing the disease-free distal mesenteric artery to the aorta. Although patency rates remain

similar, this method is also infrequently used secondary to its technical difficulty, especially at the celiac axis. Percutaneous mesenteric angioplasty and stenting are options which have been used for patients with short segment disease who are not good surgical candidates. A recent review of the literature and retrospective analysis found an increased incidence of recurrent symptoms in patients treated with angioplasty and stenting compared to surgery. Based on their findings they recommended an endovascular approach only for those patients who have unacceptable risk for surgical revascularization.

Bibliography

Cappell M. Intestinal (mesenteric) vasculopathy II: ischemic colitis and chronic mesenteric ischemia. *Gastroenterol Clin North Am* 1998;27(4):827–860.

Cho J, Carr J, Jacobsen G, et al. Long-term outcome after mesenteric artery reconstruction: a 37-year experience. *J Vasc Surg* 2002;35(3):453–460.

Cunningham C, Reilly L, Stoney R. Chronic visceral ischemia. *Surg Clin North Am* 1992;72(1):231–244.

Kasirajan K, O'Hara P, Gray B, et al. Chronic mesenteric ischemia: open surgery versus percutaneous angioplasty and stenting. *J Vasc Surg* 2001;33(1):63–71.

Kazmers A. Operative management of chronic mesenteric ischemia. *Ann Vasc Surg* 1998;12(3):299–308.

Kuestner L, Murray S, Stoney R. Transaortic renal and visceral endarterectomy. *Ann Vasc Surg* 1995;9(3):302–310.

Leke M, Hood D, Rowe V, et al. Technical consideration in the management of chronic mesenteric ischemia. *Am Surg* 2002;68(12):1088–1092.

Moawad J, McKinsey J, Wyble C, et al. Current results of surgical therapy for chronic mesenteric ischemia. *Arch Surg* 1997;132(6):613–618.

48. **(E)** Peptic ulcer disease is the development of ulceration through the mucosa in areas exposed to gastric secretions because of imbalance between acid secretion and mucosal defenses. The duodenum is the most common site of peptic ulcer formation. The vast majority of peptic ulcers arise in the setting of either *Helicobacter pylori* infection or NSAID use. In a small percent of patients, other etiologic factors including Zollinger-Ellison's syndrome may play a role. Complications of duodenal ulcers include hemorrhage, perforation, penetration into adjacent structures, and obstruction. Perforation is the second most common complication following hemorrhage, but is an uncommon event in peptic ulcer disease overall.

Symptoms of duodenal ulcer perforation result from peritonitis secondary to intraabdominal spillage of luminal contents. The patient develops severe, usually generalized, abdominal pain, which worsens over time and with movement. Paralytic ileus may accompany peritonitis and result in nausea, vomiting, and decreased passage of flatus. Abdominal examination will reveal marked tenderness, guarding, possible rebound tenderness, and often decreased bowel sounds and distension. Signs of shock may accompany late presentation of perforation. Laboratory studies are nonspecific but frequently reveal leukocytosis. Serum amylase may be slightly increased from peritoneal absorption of leaked pancreatic secretions. Pneumoperitoneum is present in 75% of perforations and can usually be demonstrated on abdominal plain films. In general, the patient who presents with peritoneal signs should undergo exploratory laparotomy, regardless if pneumoperitoneum is noted on x-rays. In the patient without peritoneal signs but suspected perforation and normal plain films, a water-soluble contrast study should be performed. There has been recent interest in the literature regarding self-sealing of duodenal ulcer perforations. Almost half of perforated duodenal ulcers may have already sealed by the time the patient presents to the hospital, although many of these patients still present with peritoneal signs. Donovan et al. (1998) proposed an alternative therapeutic plan to surgery based on a patient's current *H. pylori* status, prior *H. pylori* treatment, and initial gastroduodenogram results. Although supported by historic studies of self-sealing ulcers and the authors' own experience, few controlled trials of nonoperative treatment of perforated duodenal ulcers exist, thus the nonoperative approach is not accepted by most surgeons except possibly for highly selected cases.

H. pylori status should be determined in the setting of peptic ulcer perforation because the infection rate is high for these patients. Some have reported infection rate up to 80% in this group when excluding patients using NSAIDs. If *H. pylori* is not treated in the setting of duodenal ulcer, there is an 80% ulcer recurrence rate compared to only 10% recurrence if *H. pylori* is successfully eradicated. Risk factors for *H. pylori* infection include low socioeconomic status, crowded living conditions, poor sanitation and water supply, and possibly low intake of antioxidant micronutrients. This patient's homeless status, coupled with denial of NSAID use, further supports investigation for *H. pylori* as an etiology for ulcer disease. Diagnostic tests for *H. pylori* are divided into nonendoscopic tests and endoscopic tests. Nonendoscopic tests include serum antibody tests (including ELISA), urea breath or blood tests, and the fecal antigen test. Endoscopic tests include the rapid urease test, histologic evaluation, and culture. In the case of the patient who presents with acute perforation and undergoes laparotomy, nonendoscopic testing should be completed after

operation to establish a diagnosis. Antibody tests are widely available and accurate; however, they may remain positive even after successful eradication therapy and therefore cannot confirm active infection. Urea tests and fecal antigen testing identify patients with active infections, and both have sensitivity and specificity greater than 90%; however, these tests may be falsely negative in those patients taking proton-pump inhibitors, bismuth compounds, or antibiotics.

Multiple regimens of three and four drug combination therapy have been used successfully in eradication of *H. pylori*. Combinations generally include two antibiotics with a proton-pump inhibitor or H2 blocker. After treatment, followup testing should be done to confirm *H. pylori* eradication.

Average operative mortality is 5% for perforated duodenal ulcer. Mortality increases for the elderly, patients with multiple comorbidities, and for delay in presentation. Once perforation is suspected, NG decompression, broad-spectrum antibiotic coverage, and intravenous fluid resuscitation should be started immediately. Controversies in surgical repair involve use of nonoperative management, if a definitive ulcer operation should be performed, and application of the laparoscopic approach. Nonoperative management was already briefly discussed. In the one large randomized trial evaluating nonoperative management versus emergency surgery the authors found no difference in morbidity or mortality rates between the two groups; however, the length of hospitalization was significantly longer for the nonoperative group, and elderly patients had more frequent failure of nonoperative treatment.

Most surgeons favor simple closure of perforated duodenal ulcers with omental patch and peritoneal lavage. This is clearly the preferred procedure in the case of delayed presentation, signs of shock, or for patients with less than 3 months of symptoms attributable to peptic ulcer. Management of patients who present early with no systemic signs and with a longer history of ulcer disease is more controversial. Some surgeons would argue that this group of patients might benefit from a definitive ulcer procedure at the time of surgery. Because of the high rate of complications following procedures used in the past for ulcer disease, including antrectomy or truncal vagotomy with pyloroplasty, most surgeons who advocate a definitive procedure in this setting would propose highly selective vagotomy to be the best choice. HSV with simple ulcer closure carries with it up to 14% risk of ulcer recurrence, but has fewer complications than other ulcer procedures. A drawback to the use of HSV in the emergency setting is the longer operative time and need for expertise in the technique. A recent survey of 697 United Kingdom surgeons found that over 50% would "never" include any type of vagotomy, over 40% would "occasionally" include a vagotomy, and less than 3% would "usually" or "always" include a vagotomy in an operation for perforated duodenal ulcer. In general it appears that most surgeons would not attempt a definitive ulcer operation in the emergency setting of perforation, especially in a patient who possibly has a significant treatable risk factor like *H. pylori* infection, and who has not been receiving antisecretory drugs or *H. pylori*-directed antibiotic therapy. Finally, studies that have examined the role of the laparoscopy in duodenal perforation repair have found no difference in morbidity or mortality between laparoscopic and open approaches. Operative time is significantly longer for the laparoscopic approach, and postoperative pain medication requirements seem to be significantly less for the patients who undergo laparoscopic repair. One study demonstrated that conversion to an open procedure is much higher for patients who initially present in shock or have delayed presentation. Therefore, the presence of these conditions may be one contraindication to the laparoscopic approach.

This patient does not require further testing for Zollinger-Ellison's syndrome. Less than 1% of duodenal ulcers are associated with this condition caused by hypersecretion of gastrin. Factors that would warrant an investigation are multiple ulcers, ulcers of the jejunum, ulcers refractory to adequate medical therapy, and recurrent ulcer after a surgical procedure for ulcer disease. Finally, this patient does not require ulcer biopsy. Duodenal ulcers are not associated with an increased risk of malignancy. Gastric ulcers on the other hand are associated with increased risk of gastric cancer and should routinely be biopsied. The relative risk of gastric cancer in gastric ulcer disease is 1.8.

Bibliography

Ashley S, Evoy D, Daly J. Stomach. In: Schwartz S, Shires G, Spencer F, et al. (eds.), *Principles of Surgery*, 7th ed. New York, NY: McGraw-Hill, 1999, 1181–1215.

Chey W, Scheiman J. Peptic ulcer disease. In: Friedman S, McQuaid K, Grendell J (eds.), *Current Diagnosis and Treatment in Gastroenterology*, 2nd ed. New York, NY: Lange Medical Books/McGraw-Hill, 2003.

Donovan A, Berne T, Donovan J. Perforated duodenal ulcer: an alternative therapeutic plan. *Arch Surg* 1998;133(11):1166–1171.

Gilliam A, Speake W, Lobo D, et al. Current practice of emergency vagotomy and *Helicobacter pylori* eradication for complicated peptic ulcer in the United Kingdom. *Br J Surg* 2003;90(1):88–90.

Go M. What are the host factors that place an individual at risk for *Helicobacter pylori*-associated disease? *Gastroenterology* 1997;113:S15–S20.

Katkhouda N, Mavor E, Mason R, et al. Laparoscopic repair of perforated duodenal ulcers: outcome and efficacy in 30 consecutive patients. *Arch Surg* 1999; 134: 845–850.

Kauffman G. Duodenal ulcer disease: treatment by surgery, antibiotics, or both. *Adv Surg* 2000;34:121–135.

Millat B, Fingerhut A, Borie F. Surgical treatment of complicated duodenal ulcers: controlled trials. *World J Surg* 2000;24(3):299–306.

Verhulst M, Hopman W, Peters W, et al. Effects of *Helicobacter pylori* on endocrine and exocrine mucosal functions in the upper gastrointestinal tract. *Scand J Gastroenterol* 2000;232(Suppl.):21–31.

49. **(A)** *H. pylori* is a causative agent for peptic ulcer disease. Up to 50% of the world's population is probably colonized by the bacterium, and most people who are infected develop chronic gastritis. Only a fraction of these individuals go on to manifest the clinical entities associated with infection, including peptic ulcer disease. As there is a spectrum of clinical manifestations and many patients remain asymptomatic, it is likely that host and environmental factors influence the bacteria's effect on the GI system. Besides direct and immune-mediated epithelial damage, *H. pylori* also influences the GI milieu by affecting GI hormone and gastric acid secretion. In the portion of *H. pylori*-infected patients who develop duodenal ulcers there is an overall elevation in gastric acid secretion. The mechanism at play in this increase in acid production is not known with complete certainty, but a number of studies have supported the one popular theory. That theory is that *H. pylori* decreases the release of somatostatin from D cells located in the gastric antrum. With less inhibition by somatostatin, gastrin levels rise and cause more acid secretion. Gastrin acts both directly by stimulating acid release from parietal cells, and indirectly by stimulating histamine release from enterochromaffin-like (ECL) cells.

Studies have demonstrated consistently elevated plasma gastrin level in patients with *H. pylori* infection, and normalization of plasma gastrin level after eradication of *H. pylori* infection. Evidence to support somatostatin's role in elevating gastrin levels in *H. pylori* infection include the presence of smaller numbers of antral D cells in infected patients, smaller and less dense secretory granules in antral D cells in infected patients, decreased expression of somatostatin in infected gastric mucosa, decreased plasma somatostatin levels in *H. pylori*-infected patients, and normalization of all the above after eradication therapy. Alternative explanations for elevated gastrin levels in *H. pylori* infection include indirect gastrin stimulation through gastric alkalization, direct stimulation of gastrin release by bacterially-produced ammonium ions, and inflammatory mediator-induced gastrin release. Most of these explanations have minimal data to support them. Additionally, another proposed mechanism for increased gastric acid secretion in *H. pylori*-infected patients, not related to elevated gastrin levels, is bacterial production of N-α-methylhistamine. This bacterial compound acts as a histamine receptor agonist and may cause acid secretion through stimulation of histamine receptors on parietal cells. Overall, decreased somatostatin levels seem to have the most supportive data in the literature; however, the exact mechanism by which *H. pylori* decreases somatostatin remains unknown. Some have proposed it is simply because of an overall reduction in antral D cell mass secondary to chronic antral inflammation. Finally, not only are gastrin levels elevated in *H. pylori* patients with duodenal ulcers, but these patients may also have an increased acid response to gastrin. One group reported that *H. pylori*-infected patients who develop duodenal ulcers have a six-times greater acid response than control subjects do.

Interestingly, although the group of *H. pylori*-infected patients who develop duodenal ulcers has high gastric acid secretion, other *H. pylori*-infected patients may have low acid secretion and develop different clinical manifestations. *H. pylori*-infected patients with atrophic gastritis and gastric ulcers generally have low levels of gastric acid secretion. It is not presently known why individuals with the same infection may have different patterns of acid secretion, but it may reflect the portion of the stomach most affected by gastritis. Patients with duodenal ulcer tend to have only antral gastritis, sparing parietal cells in the body and fundus responsible for acid secretion. Patients with atrophic gastritis have a pangastritis, possibly limiting mucosal ability to secrete normal amounts of acid.

Answers B, C, and D all are mechanisms that would theoretically increase gastric acid secretion; however, none of these have been proposed to mediate *H. pylori*'s action. Answer E would not lead to increased acid secretion. Local prostaglandins do play a role in mucosal protection from acid secretion though, and blockage of their formation by NSAIDs is the mechanism by which these drugs predispose to ulcer formation.

Bibliography

Bechi P, Bacci S, Cianchi F, et al. Impairment of gastric secretion modulation in duodenal ulcer and in long-term PPI treatment. *Dig Dis Sci* 2001;46(9):1952–1959.

Graham D. *Helicobacter pylori* infection in the pathogenesis of duodenal ulcer and gastric cancer: a model. *Gastroenterology* 1997;113(6):1983–1991.

Kauffman G. Chapter 5: Duodenal ulcer disease: treatment by surgery, antibiotics, or both. *Adv Surg* 2000; 34: 121–135.

Mihaljevic S, Katicic M, Karner I, et al. The influence of *Helicobacter pylori* infection on gastrin and somatostatin values present in serum. *Hepatogastroenterology* 2000;47: 1482–1484.

Miltuinovic A, Todorovic V, Milosavljevic T, et al. Somatostatin and D cells in patients with gastritis in the course of *Helicobacter pylori* eradication: a six-month, follow-up study. *Eur J Gastroenterol Hepatol* 2003; 15(7): 755–766.

Park S, Lee H, Kim J, et al. Effect of *Helicobacter pylori* infection on antral gastrin and somatostatin cells and on serum gastrin concentrations. *Korean JIntern Med* 1999; 14(1):15–20.

Peura D. The report of the digestive health initiative[SM] international update conference on *Helicobacter pylori*. *Gastroenterology* 1997;113:S4–S8.

50. **(C)** Short bowel syndrome occurs when bowel resection leaves a patient with inadequate absorptive surface area to support nutrition. Clinically it is manifested by diarrhea, malnutrition, and fluid and electrolyte loss. In adults, such massive bowel resection is usually the result of intestinal ischemia from vascular compromise or volvulus. Multiple smaller bowel resections may also lead to short bowel syndrome in the case of CD, malignancy, or radiation injury. In children, necrotizing enterocolitis and intestinal atresia are the most common causes of short bowel syndrome. Defining an amount of bowel loss that is required for development of short bowel syndrome is difficult. There is variation among individuals, and the portion of the small bowel removed is also a factor. In general, some degree of short bowel syndrome will occur when less than 25–30% or <200 cm of small bowel remains following resection; however, loss of only the distal ileum and ileocecal valve can cause significant malabsorption despite preservation of bowel length. Likewise, the presence or absence of an intact contiguous colon also significantly influences the degree of malabsorption. Studies have shown that in the absence of a functional colon, at least 100 cm of small bowel must be preserved to prevent long-term dependence on TPN, whereas in the presence of a functional colon, only 60 cm of small bowel is required to prevent TPN dependence.

Following a significant resection of small bowel, the remaining small bowel undergoes adaptation to compensate for the loss in absorptive surface area. Villi lengthen and increase in diameter, and enterocytes increase in number. These changes effectively increase the remaining surface area. This process may continue for 1–2 years; however, adaptation will only occur in the presence of continued enteral nutrition. If only parenteral nutrition is provided, mucosal atrophy takes place. Stimulation of multiple GI hormones and growth factors by enteral feeding is the likely mechanism by which intestinal adaptation occurs.

Because small bowel function varies along its length, resection of different portions of the small bowel results in different clinical manifestations. The proximal small bowel is the primary digestive and absorptive site for most nutrients, as well as being responsible for absorption of iron, calcium, and folate. Proximal bowel resections result in at least temporary malabsorption, but generally can be compensated for by distal bowel adaptation. The ileum has a greater capacity to compensate for loss of absorptive function than the jejunum, therefore jejunal resection is generally better tolerated than ileal resection. The ileum normally plays a smaller role in nutrient absorption, but is responsible for the absorption of bile acids and vitamin B_{12}. Additionally, the ileum has a slower transit time, acting as a "brake" for digestion. Lost of the ileum and its "braking" function can reduce absorption by decreasing contact time between luminal contents and the absorptive mucosal surface. Additionally, absorption of bile acids and vitamin B_{12} cannot be replaced by the jejunum. Loss of bile acid reabsorption can increase diarrhea by direct injury to colonic cells, as well as stimulation of CCK release that in turn increases bowel motility. With severe impairment of the enterohepatic circulation, steatorrhea also occurs. Finally, the ileocecal valve functions to slow transit time and prevent reflux of colon contents into the small bowel. Therefore, loss of the ileocecal valve results in malabsorption from increased transit, as well as bacterial overgrowth in the small intestine. Bacterial overgrowth can further compromise absorption by competing with enterocytes for nutrients and causing mucosal injury.

Primary treatment of short bowel syndrome is aggressive fluid and electrolyte replacement, control of diarrhea, and initiation of TPN. As soon as enteral nutrition can be tolerated it must be started to promote intestinal adaptation. TPN may be weaned off gradually as enteric feedings advanced. Feedings should be isoosmolar and small volume at first, with progressive increase in volume and caloric content. Oral intake should be attempted; however, patients who do not tolerate oral feeds, or patients with very short bowel (<60 cm), may need to be continued on a tube-fed formula diet. The distribution and ideal form of nutrients is somewhat different for the patient with short bowel syndrome compared to the patient with a complete GI tract. Simple carbohydrates may create an osmotic fluid load which is intolerable for the patient with short bowel syndrome. Complex carbohydrates are good stimulators for intestinal adaptation and can be converted to short chain fatty acids and absorbed efficiently by the colon. Carbohydrates should still comprise the greatest percentage of daily calories, but simple carbohydrates and hyperosmolar formulas should be avoided. Proteins do not contribute greatly to osmotic load, and are generally well tolerated in short bowel syndrome. Although some clinicians promote the use of amino acid formulas for ease of digestion, there is no definitive proof that nitrogen absorption is improved by using such elemental diets. Finally, lipids, although they also do not produce a great osmotic load, generally are not digested effectively because of impaired bile acid physiology. In the past, low-fat diets have been promoted for short bowel syndrome; however, more recently there has been a trend to move away from fat restriction to prevent loss of possible nutritional benefits of dietary fat in this group of patients. Supplementation of vitamins and minerals must also be considered in the patient with short bowel syndrome. The fat-soluble vitamins A, D, and E are commonly deficient secondary to impaired fat absorption. Vitamin K, although a fat-soluble vitamin, is infrequently decreased except in patients without a functional colon because it is synthesized by colonic bacteria. Of the water-soluble vitamins, vitamin B_{12} must be supplemented in those patients with >60 cm of distal ileum resected. Important minerals that may be depleted in short bowel patients include magnesium, calcium, iron, zinc, and selenium.

Bibliography

American Gastroenterological Association. AGA technical review on short bowel syndrome and intestinal transplantation. *Gastroenterology* 2003;124:1111–1134.

Evers B, Townsend C, Thompson J. Small intestine. In: Schwartz S, Shires G, Spencer F, et al. (eds.), *Principles of Surgery*, 7th ed. New York, NY: McGraw-Hill, 1999, 1217–1263.

Scolapio J. Treatment of short-bowel syndrome. *Curr Opin Clin Nutr Metab Care* 2001;4:557–560.

Sundaram A, Koutkia P, Apovian C. Nutritional management of short bowel syndrome in adults. *J Clin Gastroenterol* 2002;34(3):207–220.

Thompson J. Surgical aspects of the short-bowel syndrome. *Am J Surg* 1995;170:532–536.

Vanderhoof J, Langnas A. Short-bowel syndrome in children and adults. *Gastroenterology* 1997;113:1767–1778.

CHAPTER 24

The Colon

Richard S. Mangus and Charles Morrison

Questions

1. Which of the following statements regarding the epidemiology of colonic diverticular disease is *correct*?

    (A) Approximately 10% of United States adults less than age 30 are affected.

    (B) Approximately 30% of United States adults older than age 80 are affected.

    (C) Fifty to seventy-five percent of persons with diverticulosis will manifest symptoms at some time in their life.

    (D) Incidence of diverticular disease is significantly higher in countries with a high-fiber diet.

    (E) In the Western world, the sigmoid colon is the predominant location of colonic diverticula.

2. Which of the following statements regarding colonic diverticulosis is *true*?

    (A) Diverticula are primarily located in the transverse colon.

    (B) The rectum is virtually never the site of diverticula.

    (C) The pathogenesis of diverticulosis has been associated with hyperactive colonic motility and high fecal volume.

    (D) No identifiable etiology for diverticulosis has been described at the cellular level.

    (E) In a patient undergoing sigmoid colon resection for apparent isolated sigmoid diverticulitis, the recurrence rate for diverticulitis approaches 90%.

3. Which of the following statements regarding diverticular disease of the colon is *true*?

    (A) According to the Law of LaPlace, the intraluminal pressure is directly proportional to the radius of the lumen.

    (B) True diverticula involve all layers of the colon wall and are most commonly found in the cecum.

    (C) The lifetime recurrence rate of diverticulitis after the first attack managed conservatively is 80%.

    (D) Less than 1% of persons with diverticula develop diverticula-associated bleeding.

    (E) False diverticula develop at sites of previous partial-thickness colonic ischemia.

4. Which of the following is *not* an indication for emergent surgery in diverticular disease of the colon?

    (A) free perforation/diffuse peritonitis

    (B) recurrence during observation period immediately after major episode of inflammatory diverticular disease

    (C) persistent massive hemorrhage

    (D) failed medical therapy in hospitalized patient

    (E) fistula formation

5. Each of the following is a contraindication to primary anastomosis after resection for diverticular disease *except*:

    (A) severe malnutrition

    (B) immunosuppression

    (C) questionable viability of bowel (severe edema/ischemia)

    (D) diverticular fistula

    (E) unprepared bowel

6. According to the Hinche classification for diverticular disease of the colon, which of the following statements is *correct*?

    (A) Antibiotics are not indicated for stage I disease.

    (B) Operative exploration is required for stage IV only.

    (C) All stages but stage I involve colonic wall perforation.

    (D) Stage I disease requires only observation.

    (E) Computed tomography (CT)-guided drainage is sometimes useful in stage I disease.

7. All of the following statements regarding colonic physiology are true *except*:

   (A) The primary fuel for colonocytes is butyric acid.

   (B) Following abdominal surgery, the colon is the last segment of the gastrointestinal (GI) tract to have resumption of motility.

   (C) The primary substrates absorbed in the colon include water and electrolytes.

   (D) Within the contiguous GI tract, the concentration of bicarbonate is highest in the colon.

   (E) The colon is the site of greatest water absorption in the GI tract.

8. Which of the following regarding inflammatory bowel disease is *true*?

   (A) Bloody diarrhea is more common in Crohn's disease than ulcerative colitis.

   (B) Associated extraintestinal disease is less common in ulcerative colitis than in Crohn's disease.

   (C) Crohn's disease frequently involves the entire colon.

   (D) Crohn's is more commonly associated with primary sclerosing cholangitis than is ulcerative colitis.

   (E) Surgical intervention for ulcerative colitis is limited to management of complications of the primary disease process.

9. Which of the following is *not* an indication for surgical intervention in ulcerative colitis?

   (A) intractable bloody diarrhea

   (B) perforation

   (C) toxic colitis

   (D) diagnosis of ulcerative colitis for more than 5 years

   (E) poorly controlled extraintestinal manifestations

10. Which of the following is generally *not* an acceptable surgical option for management of ulcerative colitis?

   (A) lifelong conservative observation with biannual colonoscopy

   (B) total proctocolectomy with ileostomy

   (C) total proctocolectomy with continent ileostomy (Kock pouch)

   (D) total abdominal colectomy with ileo-rectal anastomosis

   (E) total proctocolectomy with "J"-pouch anastomosis

11. All of the following are associated with an increased risk of perforation in acute colonic pseudoobstruction (Ogilvie's syndrome) *except*:

   (A) older age

   (B) increasing cecal diameter

   (C) delay in decompression

   (D) diabetes mellitus

   (E) chronic ischemia

12. Regarding acute colonic pseudoobstruction (Ogilvie's syndrome), each of the following is correct *except*:

   (A) This condition is defined as the radiographic appearance of a large bowel obstruction without mechanical etiology.

   (B) The best pharmacologic treatment is neostigmine, which leads to rapid decompression in a significant number of adults after a single infusion.

   (C) Ogilvie's syndrome is associated with a number of neurologic disorders, including Alzheimer's and Parkinson's disease and elderly dementia.

   (D) Most cases of this disease are idiopathic in etiology.

   (E) The proximal and transverse portions of the colon tend to be more involved than the left or sigmoid colon.

13. Which of the following statements regarding toxic megacolon is *not* true?

   (A) Toxic megacolon is more often seen in ulcerative colitis than Crohn's disease.

   (B) Associated clinical findings include fever, tachycardia, and leukocytosis.

   (C) Anemia is rarely seen in patients with toxic megacolon.

   (D) Radiographic evidence of toxic megacolon includes the absence of haustral pattern of the colon and a colon greater than 6 cm in diameter.

   (E) If there is no response to aggressive resuscitation and antibiotic therapy after 24–48 h, the patient should undergo a total colectomy with ileostomy.

14. All of the following statements regarding *C. difficile* are true *except*:

(A) Ten percent of hospitalized patients have gut colonization with *C. difficile*.

(B) *C. difficile* may colonize the upper and lower GI tract, but symptomatic infection appears to be isolated only to the colon.

(C) Pseudomembranous colitis is caused by transmural translocation of *C. difficile* bacteria with irritation of the muscularis propria.

(D) The first treatment option for pseudomembranous colitis should be oral metronidazole.

(E) Oral cholestyramine can be useful in controlling the effects of *C. difficile* by intraluminal binding of clostridial toxin.

15. Regarding volvulus of the sigmoid colon, each of the following is true *except*:

(A) Likely results from redundant sigmoid colon with an elongated narrow mesocolon.

(B) Eighty to ninety percent of colonic volvulus cases in the United States involve the sigmoid colon.

(C) There appears to be a congenital predisposition to sigmoid volvulus.

(D) Diagnostic x-ray for sigmoid volvulus shows a dilated loop of colon which points toward the right upper quadrant.

(E) Diagnostic barium enema for sigmoid volvulus shows a "bird's beak" deformity.

16. Which of the statements regarding cecal volvulus is *not* true?

(A) Cecal volvulus accounts for 10% of cases of colonic volvulus.

(B) Cecal vovulus is thought to have a congenital etiology related to incomplete peritoneal fixation of the right colon.

(C) Radiographic evidence of a cecal volvulus includes a large, dilated loop of colon with the loop of colon pointing to the left upper quadrant of the abdomen.

(D) Definitive treatment for cecal volvulus includes a right hemicolectomy.

(E) Reduction of the cecal volvulus with fixation of the cecum to the abdominal wall provides a similar outcome to segmental resection.

17. All of the statements are true regarding lower gastrointestinal hemorrhage (LGIH) *except*:

(A) The most common cause of a lower GI bleed in adults younger than age 60 is colonic diverticula.

(B) The most common cause of a lower GI bleed in adults older than age 60 is colonic diverticula.

(C) Lower GI bleeding because of arteriovenous malformations is much more common in older rather than younger persons.

(D) The most common cause of a LGIH in a child is inflammatory bowel disease.

(E) Massive LGIH is generally defined as an acute requirement for more than 6 unit of blood.

18. All of the following statements regarding large bowel obstruction are true *except*:

(A) The most common cause of colonic obstruction in adults is diverticulitis.

(B) The ileocecal valve is incompetent in 10–20% of people.

(C) Approximately 15% of intestinal obstructions occur in the large bowel.

(D) The most common site of large bowel obstruction is the sigmoid colon.

(E) Cecal perforation carries a 40% mortality rate.

19. Which of the following statements regarding colovesical fistula is *true*?

(A) It occurs with a 3:1 ratio of women to men.

(B) This complication occurs in 15% of cases of diverticulitis.

(C) The most common presenting complaint is pneumaturia.

(D) During repair, if the fistula tract is not apparent after takedown of the colon, it can safely be assumed that the fistula has closed.

(E) Colovesical fistulas frequently close spontaneously and repair may occasionally be deferred depending on the underlying pathology and the patient's health.

20. Which of the following statements related to ischemic colitis is *true*?

   (A) A common precipitating event is suprarenal abdominal aortic aneurysm.
   (B) Physical examination often demonstrates severe abdominal pain with guarding and peritoneal signs.
   (C) Diagnostic test of choice is endoscopy to visualize the colonic mucosa.
   (D) Overall mortality for a single episode of ischemic colitis is 10%
   (E) Common etiologies of colonic ischemia in the elderly include pancreatitis, lupus, and sickle cell crisis.

21. Regarding colonic polyps, each of the following is an unfavorable factor for endoscopic resection *except*:

   (A) polyp size >2 cm
   (B) margin less than 3 mm
   (C) poorly differentiated on histologic examination
   (D) presence of lymphovascular invasion
   (E) carcinoma invading the submucosa

22. According to the Haggitt classification for polyps, which of the following statements is *not* true?

   (A) A level 0 polyp refers to noninvasive carcinoma *in situ*.
   (B) All level IV polyps must be treated with segmental resection.
   (C) Endoscopic excision is adequate treatment for level I and level II polyps.
   (D) A wide-based sessile polyp with carcinoma at the tip of the polyp *only* is considered a level III polyp.
   (E) Carcinoma from a level I polyp invades the muscularis mucosa but remains contained within the head of the polyp.

23. Regarding colon cancer, which of the following is *not* true?

   (A) Colon cancer is the second most common cause of cancer death.
   (B) Loss of heterozygosity in malignant transformation involves both tumor suppressor gene inactivation and oncogene activation.
   (C) Risk factors for colon cancer include a family history of colon cancer, the presence of multiple colonic adenomas and a history of ulcerative colitis.

   (D) Isolated liver metastases from colon cancer should be treated emergently with both chemotherapy and radiation therapy.
   (E) Of all patients diagnosed with colon cancer, 10% have pulmonary metastases at the time of diagnosis.

24. Each of the following is a genetic mutation linked to colorectal cancer *except*:

   (A) adenomatous polyposis coli (APC)
   (B) CAG triplicate repeat sequence
   (C) K-ras
   (D) DCC/p53
   (E) hMLH1/hMSH2

25. According to the tumor, node, metastasis (TNM) staging for colon cancer, which of the following is *true*?

   (A) All perforated colon cancers are considered T4.
   (B) N2 refers to involvement of greater than one regional lymph node.
   (C) T5 grade involves direct carcinoma invasion into adjacent solid organs.
   (D) MX indicates metastatic disease involvement of more than one additional organ system (e.g., liver, lung, brain).
   (E) Five-year survival for stage I colon cancer is approximately 75%.

26. Each of the following is associated with a familial polyposis syndrome *except*:

   (A) Gardner's syndrome
   (B) Turcot's syndrome
   (C) MEN type IIb
   (D) Peutz-Jeghers' syndrome
   (E) juvenile polyposis syndrome

27. A patient presents with osteomas of the mandible, multiple lipomas and sebaceous cysts, a history of multiple dental abnormalities, and an apparent fibrotic retroperitoneal mass on CT scan obtained for abdominal pain. The next step in management of this patient is

   (A) colonoscopy
   (B) abdominal exploration with biopsy of retroperitoneal mass
   (C) bone marrow biopsy
   (D) 24-h urine calcium level
   (E) positron emission tomography (PET) scan of the chest, abdomen, and pelvis

28. All of the following are true regarding FAP syndrome *except:*

(A) All patients will eventually develop colon cancer.

(B) Polyps >1 cm in these patients carry a 50% risk of carcinoma.

(C) Ninety percent of these patients manifest polyps by age 10.

(D) Medical treatment with sulindac/celebrex decreases the number and size of polyps.

(E) Sulindac and tamoxifen have been shown to be effective in the treatment of desmoid tumors.

29. Regarding HNPCC, which of the following statements is *true*?

(A) autosomal recessive inheritance pattern

(B) mutation in tumor oncogene

(C) accounts for 25% of cases of colon cancer

(D) according to the Amsterdam criteria, diagnosis requires at least three familial generations diagnosed with colon cancer

(E) all female patients should be offered prophylactic hysterectomy/oopherectomy

30. In patients with HNPCC, each of the following is true *except:*

(A) Lynch I refers to those HNPCC patients affected by colon cancer only.

(B) Lynch II refers to those HNPCC patients affected by colon cancer and inflammatory bowel disease.

(C) Screening colonoscopy in HNPCC patients should begin between ages 20 and 25 or 5 years earlier than the earliest age of detection of colon cancer in affected family members.

(D) Treatment for HNPCC includes subtotal colectomy.

(E) Extracolonic cancers associated with HNPCC include sites in the GI tract, urinary tract, gynecologic organs, breast, and pancreas.

31. Each of the following is true regarding the surgical management of colon cancer *except:*

(A) Perioperative mortality in patients with perforated colon cancer approaches 90%.

(B) In addition to adequate margins, resection should include *en bloc* resection of draining lymphatics.

(C) Almost 90% of patients with colorectal cancer have tumors which are amenable to some form of resection.

(D) Patients presenting with an obstructing colon cancer have an in-hospital mortality rate of 15%.

(E) Direct extension of colon and rectal cancer to adjacent organs necessitates *en bloc* resection of those organs.

32. A previously healthy 22-year-old male college football player presents to your emergency department 24 h after the homecoming football game with complaints of severe left lower quadrant abdominal pain, fever of 102°F, nausea and vomiting. Laboratory findings include a WBC count of 16,300 with 7% bands. On physical examination his abdomen is soft, but he has marked tenderness in the left lower quadrant.

Which of the following is the most appropriate diagnostic study in this patient?

(A) CT abdomen and pelvis

(B) barium enema

(C) abdominal ultrasound

(D) colonoscopy

(E) laparoscopy

33. The best management plan for this patient is

(A) immediate surgical intervention

(B) intravenous antibiotics and observation

(C) intravenous antibiotics and a period of observation, with resection and primary anastamosis prior to hospital discharge

(D) intravenous antibiotics and observation, with subsequent elective resection of the diseased segment after recovery

(E) intravenous antibiotics and observation, with surgical intervention considered if a second episode of diverticulitis occurs

34. A 72-year-old female is hospitalized in the burn unit after sustaining 17% total body surface area (TBSA) flash burns in an explosion of methane fumes from a pile of manure. She undergoes uneventful excision and grafting of her burn wounds, but postoperatively develops significant abdominal distension and obstipation. Plain films reveal markedly dilated small bowel and colon, with a cecal diameter of 9 cm. Appropriate management at this time involves

    (A) urgent surgical intervention with resection and diverting ostomy
    (B) NG decompression, limitation of narcotic use, serial abdominal radiographs
    (C) colonoscopic decompression
    (D) intravenous neostigmine
    (E) placement of a rectal tube

35. An 92-year-old Black male presents to the local VA hospital from the nursing home where he resides with new onset of abdominal distension, constipation, nausea, and vomiting. On physical examination he has a distended abdomen, but no evidence of peritonitis. Abdominal radiograph is obtained (see Fig. 24-1).

    Regarding this patient's condition, which of the following statements is *true*?

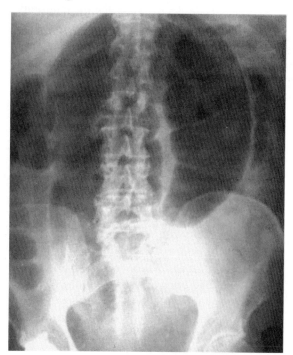

FIG. 24-1 Abdominal radiograph

(A) A gastrograffin enema is required to confirm the diagnosis.
(B) Colonoscopic decompression is unlikely to be successful, and may be dangerous.
(C) The recurrence rate may be as high as 90%.
(D) The patient should undergo emergent exploration and resection.

36. Which of the following is *not* an indication for urgent surgery in patients with ulcerative colitis?

    (A) ongoing hemorrhage
    (B) toxic megacolon
    (C) failure of maximal medical management
    (D) colonic perforation
    (E) all are indications for urgent surgery

37. Which of the following is the best diagnostic tool for ischemic colitis?

    (A) CT
    (B) colonoscopy
    (C) mesenteric angiography
    (D) plain abdominal radiographs
    (E) magnetic resonance imaging (MRI)

38. A 73-year-old male presents to your emergency department complaining of a large amount of bright red blood per rectum. He is moderately tachycardic, but otherwise is hemodynamically stable.

    Which of the following statements regarding the management of this patient is *false*?

    (A) Anoscopy followed by proctoscopy should be performed to exclude localized anorectal disease as the cause of hemorrhage.
    (B) Before surgical intervention is considered, he must undergo esophagogastroduodenoscopy (EGD).
    (C) He should undergo colonoscopy if clinically stable.
    (D) A positive tagged RBC scan should prompt segmental surgical resection.
    (E) None of the above.

Answers and Explanations

1. **(E)** Only 1–2% of United States adults age 30 and younger have diverticulosis, but this increases to >50% by age 80 and approximately 67% in persons older than 85. Only 10–25% of United States adults with diverticulosis will manifest symptoms, most commonly left lower quadrant pain and fever. Diverticulosis is relatively rare in countries in which a major portion of the diet consists of high-fiber foods. Diverticula occur primarily in the sigmoid colon in the Western world (Fig. 24–2).

Bibliography

Cima RR, Young-Fadok TM. New developments in diverticular disease. [Review] *Curr Gastroenterol Rep* 2001;3(5):420–424.

Morris CR, Harvey IM, Stebbings WS, et al. Epidemiology of perforated colonic diverticular disease. [Review] *Postgrad Med J* 2002;78(925):654–658.

Rolandelli RH, Roslyn JJ. In: Townsend CM, et al (ed.), *Sabiston Textbook of Surgery*, 16th ed. Philadelphia: W.B. Saunders; 2002, 944–947.

Welton ML, Varma RG, Amerhauser A. In: Norton JA, Barie PS, Bollinger RR et al (eds.), *Surgery: Basic Science and Clinical Evidence*. New York: Springer; 2000, 687–694.

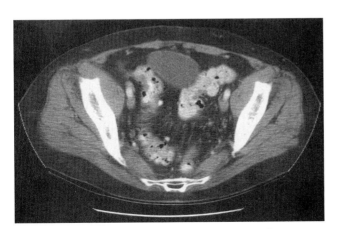

FIG. 24-2 Sigmoid diverticulosis on computed tomography scan.

2. **(B)** Colonic diverticula form primarily in the sigmoid colon and descending colon. The rectum is very rarely involved. The pathophysiology of this disease is related to decreased colonic motility and low overall fecal volume. The colonic wall musculature is shortened and thickened compared to those patients with a normal colon. These patients may have defective collagen and have been found to have an increased number of elastin fibers in the bowel wall. Treatment of sigmoid diverticulitis with sigmoid colectomy is very effective, resulting in an overall lifetime recurrence rate of only 20–25%.

Bibliography

Ludeman L, Shepherd NA. What is diverticular colitis? [Review] *Pathology* 2002;34(6):568.

Rolandelli RH, Roslyn JJ. In: Townsend CM, et al (ed.), *Sabiston Textbook of Surgery*, 16th ed. Philadelphia: W.B. Saunders; 2002, 944–947.

Simpson J, Scholefield JH, Spiller RC. Pathogenesis of colonic diverticula. [Review] *Br J Surg* 2002;89(5):546–554.

Stollman NH, Raskin JB. Diverticular disease of the colon. [Review] *J Clin Gastroenterol* 1999;29(3):241–252.

Welton ML, Varma RG, Amerhauser A. In: Norton JA, Barie PS, Bollinger RR et al (eds.), *Surgery: Basic Science and Clinical Evidence*. New York: Springer; 2000, 687–694.

3. **(B)** According to the Law of LaPlace, the intraluminal pressure is inversely proportional to the radius of the lumen while the wall tension is directly proportional to the pressure (pressure = tension/radius). True diverticula do involve all layers of the colon wall. True diverticula are most commonly found in the cecum and are more common among Asians. The lifetime recurrence rate of diverticulitis managed nonoperatively is only 30% after the first episode, 50% after two episodes, and 80% after the third attack. False diverticula account for the large majority of total colonic diverticula and are thought to form because of herniation of colonic mucosa through the muscularis in areas of penetration of vasa rectum.

Bibliography

Jani N, Finkelstein S, Blumberg D, et al. Segmental colitis associated with diverticulosis. [Review] Segmental colitis associated with diverticulosis. [Review] *Dig Dis Sci* 2002;47(5):1175–1181.

Rolandelli RH, Roslyn JJ. In: Townsend CM, et al (ed.), *Sabiston Textbook of Surgery*, 16th ed. Philadelphia: W.B. Saunders; 2002, 944–947.

Simpson J, Scholefield JH, Spiller RC. Origin of symptoms in diverticular disease. [Review] *Br J Surg* 2003;90(8): 899–908.

Welton ML, Varma RG, Amerhauser A. In: Norton JA, Barie PS, Bollinger RR et al (eds.), *Surgery: Basic Science and Clinical Evidence*. New York: Springer; 2000, 687–694.

4. **(E)** Emergent surgery is indicated in cases of perforated diverticulitis in which there is frank peritonitis, persistent massive hemorrhage or persistent fever or leukocytosis in the hospitalized patient. Colonic fistula formation can generally be managed on an elective basis. Recurrent diverticulitis can be managed with conservative antibiotic therapy, though emergent surgery may be necessary if the recurrence occurs immediately after a previous episode (Figs. 24-3 through 24-5).

Bibliography

Elsakr R, Johnson DA, Younes Z, et al. Antimicrobial treatment of intra-abdominal infections. [Review] *Dig Dis* 1998;16(1):47–60.

Fischer, JE. In: Baker RJ, Fischer JE (eds.), *Mastery of Surgery*, 4th ed. Philadelphia: Lippincott, Williams & Wilkins; 2001, 1524–1537.

Rolandelli RH, Roslyn JJ. In: Townsend CM, et al (ed.), *Sabiston Textbook of Surgery*, 16th ed. Philadelphia: W.B. Saunders; 2002, 944–947.

Welton ML, Varma RG, Amerhauser A. In: Norton JA, Barie PS, Bollinger RR et al (eds.), *Surgery: Basic Science and Clinical Evidence*. New York: Springer; 2000, 687–694.

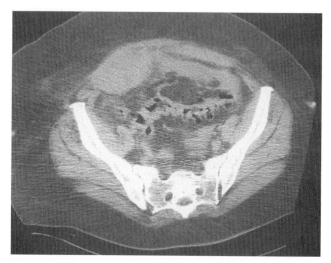

FIG. 24-4 Acute diverticulitis of the sigmoid colon.

Young-Fadok TM, Roberts PL, Spencer MP, et al. Colonic diverticular disease. [Review] *Curr Prob Surg* 2000; 37(7): 457–514.

5. **(D)** Diverticular fistula is not considered a contraindication to primary anastomosis after colon resection as long as there is minimal contamination with well-prepared bowel. Absolute contraindications to anastomosis include severe malnutrition, immunosuppression, compromised bowel, and severe anemia or massive blood loss. Relative contraindications include the presence of a chronic abscess cavity, moderate anemia, immunosuppression or malnutrition, unprepared bowel, and technical difficulty with the anastomosis.

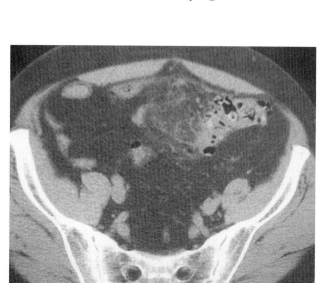

FIG. 24-3 Acute diverticulitis of the sigmoid colon.

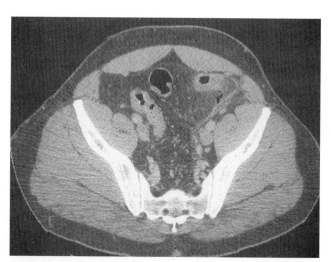

FIG. 24-5 Acute diverticulitis of the sigmoid colon with perforation (extraluminal air).

Bibliography

Fischer, JE. In: Baker RJ, Fischer JE (eds.), *Mastery of Surgery*, 4th ed. Philadelphia: Lippincott, Williams & Wilkins; 2001, 1497–1506.

Rolandelli RH, Roslyn JJ. In: Townsend CM, et al (ed.), *Sabiston Textbook of Surgery*, 16th ed. Philadelphia: W.B. Saunders; 2002, 944–947.

Scott-Conner CEH. In: Scott-Conner CEH (ed.), *Chassin's Operative Strategy in General Surgery*, 3rd ed. New York: Springer; 2002, 506–509.

Welton ML, Varma RG, Amerhauser A. In: Norton JA, Barie PS, Bollinger RR et al (eds.), *Surgery: Basic Science and Clinical Evidence*. New York: Springer; 2000, 687–694.

Wolff BG, Devine RM. Surgical management of diverticulitis. [Review] *Am Surg* 2000;66(2):153–156.

6. (C) According to the Hinche classification for diverticular disease, stage I involves only pericolic inflammation and can be managed with antibiotics with future elective resection. Stage II is characterized by the presence of a focal abscess and can often be managed by CT-guided drainage of the abscess cavity and future elective resection. Stages III and IV both involve diffuse peritonitis. The peritonitis in stage III is a diffuse purulent peritonitis, while that in stage IV includes the presence of gross fecal spillage. Both stage III and stage IV require operative exploration, voluminous irrigation, and a Hartman's procedure (Fig. 24-6).

Bibliography

Rolandelli RH, Roslyn JJ. In: Townsend CM, et al (ed.), *Sabiston Textbook of Surgery*, 16th ed. Philadelphia: W.B. Saunders; 2002, 944–947.

Simpson J, Spiller R. Colonic diverticular disease. [Review] *Clin Evid* 2002;7:398–405.

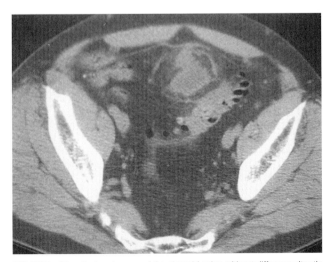

FIG. 24-6 Diverticular abscess of the sigmoid colon without diffuse peritontis (Hinche classification stage II).

Welton ML, Varma RG, Amerhauser A. In: Norton JA, Barie PS, Bollinger RR et al (eds.), *Surgery: Basic Science and Clinical Evidence*. New York: Springer; 2000, 687–694.

Wolff BG, Devine RM. Surgical management of diverticulitis. [Review] *Am Surg* 2000;66(2):153–156.

7. (E) The primary fuel source for the colon is free fatty acids, especially butyric acid. Following abdominal surgery under general anesthesia, GI motility is first seen in the small bowel, followed by the stomach and then the colon. The colon has two primary functions; storage of stool and absorption of water and electrolytes. Because of the electrolyte exchange that occurs with water resorption in the colon, a high concentration of bicarbonate results. The colon secretes potassium and bicarbonate in exchange for chloride (and water) absorption. Therefore, with profuse diarrhea a large volume of bicarbonate can be quickly lost from the colon and the patient can develop a relative acidosis (with hypokalemia). Though the primary function of the colon is water retention, the majority of water resorption occurs in the small bowel.

Bibliography

Kodner IJ, Fry RD, Fleshman JW, et al. In: Schwartz SI, Spencer FC (eds.), *Schwartz: Principles of Surgery*, 7th ed. New York: McGraw-Hill; 1999, 1271–1274.

Kunzelmann K, Mall M. Electrolyte transport in the mammalian colon: mechanisms and implications for disease. [Review] *Physiol Rev* 2002;82(1):245–289.

Pryde SE, Duncan SH, Hold GL, et al. The microbiology of butyrate formation in the human colon. [Review] *FEMS Microbiol Lett* 2002;217(2):133–139.

Priebe MG, Vonk RJ, Sun X, et al. The physiology of colonic metabolism. Possibilities for pre- and probiotics. [Review] *Eur J Nutr* 2002;41(S1):2–10.

Rolandelli RH, Roslyn JJ. In: Townsend CM, et al (ed.), *Sabiston Textbook of Surgery*, 16th ed. Philadelphia: W.B. Saunders; 2002, 931–934.

Welton ML, Varma RG, Amerhauser A. In: Norton JA, Barie PS, Bollinger RR et al (eds.), *Surgery: Basic Science and Clinical Evidence*. New York: Springer; 2000, 671–672.

Warth R, Bleich M. K$^+$ channels and colonic function. [Review] *Rev Physiol Biochem Pharmacol* 2000;140:1–62.

8. (B) Bloody diarrhea is a more common feature of ulcerative colitis than of Crohn's disease. Extraintestinal disease is more commonly associated with Crohn's disease and includes pyoderma gangrenosum, erythema nodosum multiforme, iritis, stomatitis, ankylosing spondylitis, and primary sclerosing cholangitis. Ulcerative colitis frequently involves the entire colon while total colonic involvement is very rare in Crohn's disease. Though both Crohn's disease and ulcerative colitis are associated with an increased risk of primary sclerosing cholangitis, this association is much stronger for ulcerative colitis. Management of Crohn's disease is generally confined to management of complications related to the primary disease, whereas preemptive surgery is commonly used in the management of ulcerative colitis.

Bibliography

Fischer, JE. In: Baker RJ, Fischer JE (eds.), *Mastery of Surgery*, 4th ed. Philadelphia: Lippincott, Williams & Wilkins; 2001, 1538–1547.

Guy TS, Williams NN, Rosato EF. Crohn's disease of the colon. [Review] *Surg Clin North Am* 2001;81(1):159–168.

Pare P. Management of fistulas in patients with Crohn's disease: antibiotic to antibody. [Review] *Can J Gastroenterol* 2001;15(11):751–756.

Rolandelli RH, Roslyn JJ. In: Townsend CM, et al (ed.), *Sabiston Textbook of Surgery*, 16th ed. Philadelphia: W.B. Saunders; 2002, 950–955.

Welton ML, Varma RG, Amerhauser A. In: Norton JA, Barie PS, Bollinger RR et al (eds.), *Surgery: Basic Science and Clinical Evidence*. New York: Springer; 2000, 672–686.

9. **(D)** Indications for surgical intervention in ulcerative colitis include intractable symptoms, perforation, toxic colitis, increasing cancer risk, hemorrhage, fulminating disease, and poorly controlled extraintestinal manifestations. The cancer risk after initial diagnosis is approximately 5–7% during the first 5–7 years, but increases to 40% at 20 years postdiagnosis. Therefore, surgical intervention is commonly recommended beginning approximately 10 years after initial diagnosis.

Bibliography

Campbell S, Ghosh S. Ulcerative colitis and colon cancer: strategies for cancer prevention. [Review] *Dig Dis* 2002;20(1):38–48.

Eaden JA, Mayberry JF. Colorectal cancer complicating ulcerative colitis: a review. [Review] *Am J Gastroenterol* 2000;95(10):2710–2719.

Fischer, JE. In: Baker RJ, Fischer JE (eds.), *Mastery of Surgery*, 4th ed. Philadelphia: Lippincott, Williams & Wilkins; 2001, 1538–1547.

Itzkowitz S. Colon carcinogenesis in inflammatory bowel disease: applying molecular genetics to clinical practice. *J Clin Gastroenterol* 2003;36(5S):S70–S74.

Kodner IJ, Fry RD, Fleshman JW, et al. In: Schwartz SI, Spencer FC (eds.), *Schwartz: Principles of Surgery*, 7th ed. New York: McGraw-Hill; 1999, 1311–1328.

Rolandelli RH, Roslyn JJ. In: Townsend CM, et al (ed.), *Sabiston Textbook of Surgery*, 16th ed. Philadelphia: W.B. Saunders; 2002, 944–947.

Welton ML, Varma RG, Amerhauser A. In: Norton JA, Barie PS, Bollinger RR et al (eds.), *Surgery: Basic Science and Clinical Evidence*. New York: Springer; 2000, 672–686.

10. **(A)** Given the extremely high risk of colon cancer in patient with ulcerative colitis, total colectomy with some form of reconstruction is eventually recommended for all patients. All of the listed surgical interventions are reasonable approaches and each may be appropriate in the proper clinical scenario. Lifelong conservative management with observation only is inadequate therapy.

Bibliography

Fischer, JE. In: Baker RJ, Fischer JE (eds.), *Mastery of Surgery*, 4th ed. Philadelphia, PA: Lippincott, Williams & Wilkins; 2001, 1538–1547 and 1507–1517.

Rolandelli RH, Roslyn JJ. In: Townsend CM, et al (ed.), *Sabiston Textbook of Surgery*, 16th ed. Philadelphia: W.B. Saunders; 2002, 944–947.

Scott-Conner CEH. In: Scott-Conner CEH (ed.), *Chassin's Operative Strategy in General Surgery*, 3rd ed. New York: Springer; 2002, 361–379 and 474–483.

Welton ML, Varma RG, Amerhauser A. In: Norton JA, Barie PS, Bollinger RR et al (eds.), *Surgery: Basic Science and Clinical Evidence*. New York: Springer; 2000, 672–686.

Wexner SD, Alabaz O. Anastomotic integrity and function: role of the colonic J-pouch. [Review] *Semin Surg Oncol* 1998;15(2):91–100.

11. **(D)** Acute colonic pseudoobstruction is a syndrome of massive dilation of the colon without mechanical obstruction that develops in hospitalized patients with serious underlying medical and surgical conditions. Increasing age, cecal diameter, delay in decompression, and status of the bowel significantly influence mortality, which is approximately 40% when ischemia or perforation is present. Evaluation of the markedly distended colon in the intensive care unit setting involves excluding mechanical obstruction and other causes of toxic megacolon such as *Clostridium difficile* infection, and assessing for signs of ischemia and perforation. The risk of colonic perforation in acute colonic pseudoobstruction increases when cecal diameter exceeds 12 cm and when the distention has been present for greater than 6 days. Appropriate management includes supportive therapy and selective use of neostigmine and colonoscopy for decompression. Early recognition and management are critical in minimizing complications.

Bibliography

Eaker EY. Update on acute colonic pseudo-obstruction. [Review] *Curr Gastroenterol Rep* 2001;3(5):433–436.

Eisen GM, Baron TH, Dominitz JA, et al. Acute colonic pseudo-obstruction. [Guidelines] *Gastrointest Endosc* 2002;56(6):789–792.

Rolandelli RH, Roslyn JJ. In: Townsend CM, et al (ed.), *Sabiston Textbook of Surgery*, 16th ed. Philadelphia: W.B. Saunders; 2002, 948.

Saunders MD, Kimmey MB. Colonic pseudo-obstruction: the dilated colon in the ICU. [Review] *Semin Gastrointest Dis* 2003;14(1):20–27.

12. (D) Only a few cases of Ogilvie's have been considered idiopathic in origin. Most cases of this disease process have identifiable etiologies such as peritonitis, electrolyte derangements, neurologic disorders, and pharmacologic side effect. The vast majority of these patients have been found to have the overt clinical picture of the syndrome in association with a wide array of clinical conditions. The diagnosis of the condition is through radiographic evidence of colonic obstruction without identifiable mechanical etiology. Neostigmine has been shown to have good efficacy in resolution of this process after only a single administration of the drug. The pathophysiologic process of acute colonic pseudoobstruction is thought to involve an early motor disturbance followed by complete cessation of peristalsis and entrapment of a large volume of gas in the proximal and transverse colon.

Bibliography
Krogh K, Christensen P, Laurberg S. Colorectal symptoms in patients with neurological diseases. [Review] *Acta Neurol Scand* 2001;103(6):335–343.

Loftus CG, Harewood GC, Baron TH. Assessment of predictors of response to neostigmine for acute colonic pseudo-obstruction. *Am J Gastroenterol* 2002;97 (12): 3118–3122.

Pham TN, Cosman BC, Chu P, et al. Radiographic changes after colonoscopic decompression for acute pseudo-obstruction. *Dis Colon Rectum* 1999;42(12):1586–1591.

Rolandelli RH, Roslyn JJ. In: Townsend CM, et al (ed.), *Sabiston Textbook of Surgery*, 16th ed. Philadelphia: W.B. Saunders; 2002, 948.

van der Spoel JI, Oudemans-van Straaten HM, Stoutenbeek CP, et al. Neostigmine resolves critical illness-related colonic ileus in intensive care patients with multiple organ failure- a prospective, double-blind, placebo-controlled trial. *Intensive Care Med* 2001;27(5):822–827.

13. (C) Toxic megacolon is rarely seen in Crohn's disease but is a frequent complication of ulcerative colitis. Patients with toxic megacolon will appear septic with fever, tachycardia, and leukocytosis being frequently noted signs. Toxic megacolon is often associated with chronic colonic or systemic pathology and these patients will often have significant anemia. Many patients require transfusion primary to surgery. Commonly noted radiographic abnormalities include a dilated colon with the absence of haustral markings. Toxic megacolon is a potentially life-threatening illness and the surgeon should follow only a short course of conservative management before intervening surgically.

Bibliography
Imbriaco M, Balthazar EJ. Toxic megacolon: role of CT in evaluation and detection of complications. *Clin Imaging* 2001;25(5):349–354.

Fischer, JE. In: Baker RJ, Fischer JE (eds.), *Mastery of Surgery*, 4th ed. Philadelphia: Lippincott, Williams & Wilkins; 2001, 1497–1506.

Sheth SG, LaMont JT. Toxic megacolon. [Review] *Lancet* 1998;351:509–513.

14. (C) *C. difficile* colonization is present in 3% of the general population and 10% of hospitalized patients. It is the major known etiology of nosocomial antibiotic-associated colitis. Colonization with this bacteria may be present throughout the GI tract, but symptoms appear to be isolated to the colon where the toxin is readily absorbed. Pseudomembranous colitis develops when *C. difficile* produces a number of toxins, including both an enterotoxin and a cytotoxin. Though the bacteria stays intraluminal, these toxics are absorbed causing the development of elevated plaques or confluent pseudomembranes. Oral cholestyramine binds these toxins, thereby minimizing its effects. The primary treatment should be oral metronidazole because it is as effective as oral vancomycin or intravenous metronidazole, but much less expensive.

Bibliography
Kyne L, Farrell RJ, Kelly CP. *Clostridium difficile*. [Review] *Gastroenterol Clin North Am* 2001;30(3):753–757.

Malnick SD, Zimhony O. Treatment of *Clostridium difficile*-associated diarrhea. [Review] *Ann Pharmacother* 2002; 36(11):1767–1175.

Moyenuddin M, Williamson JC, Ohl CA. *Clostridium difficile*-associated diarrhea: current strategies for diagnosis and therapy. [Review] *Curr Gastroenterol Rep* 2002;4 (4):279–286.

Rolandelli RH, Roslyn JJ. In: Townsend CM, et al (ed.), *Sabiston Textbook of Surgery*, 16th ed. Philadelphia: W.B. Saunders; 2002, 217 and 387.

Welton ML, Varma RG, Amerhauser A. In: Norton JA, Barie PS, Bollinger RR et al (eds.), *Surgery: Basic Science and Clinical Evidence*. New York: Springer; 2000, 694–695.

15. (C) The development of sigmoid volvulus is associated with an elongated narrow mesocolon attached to a redundant sigmoid colon, which allows the elongated portion to rotate and twist on a narrow base. The most common site of colonic volvulus is the sigmoid colon because of its inherent redundancy. The development of sigmoid volvulus is thought to be acquired, unlike cecal volvulus which is more likely congenital in etiology. Sigmoid volvulus is more common in older, institutionalized patients with neurologic disorders or with chronic constipation. Radiologic imaging characteristic of sigmoid volvulus includes a dilated loop of colon pointing to the right upper quadrant and barium enema showing a "bird's beak" deformity (Fig. 24-7).

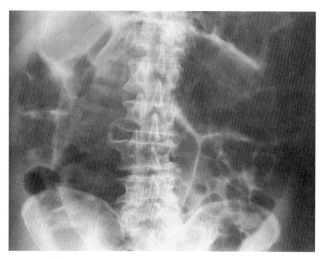

FIG. 24-7 Radiograph demonstrating sigmoid volvulus.

Bibliography

Cappell MS, Friedel D. The role of sigmoidoscopy and colonoscopy in the diagnosis and management of lower gastrointestinal disorders: endoscopic findings, therapy and complications. *Med Clin North Am* 2002; 86(6): 1253–1288.

Kodner IJ, Fry RD, Fleshman JW, et al. In: Schwartz SI, Spencer FC (eds.), *Schwartz: Principles of Surgery*, 7th ed. New York: McGraw-Hill; 1999, 1275–1276.

Madiba TE, Thomson SR. The management of sigmoid volvulus. [Review] *J R Coll Surg Edinb* 2000;45(2):74–80.

Rolandelli RH, Roslyn JJ. In: Townsend CM, et al (ed.), *Sabiston Textbook of Surgery*, 16th ed. Philadelphia: W.B. Saunders; 2002, 947–950.

Salas S, Angel CA, Salas N, et al. Sigmoid volvulus in children and adolescents. [Review] *J Am Coll Surg* 2000; 190(6):717–723.

Welton ML, Varma RG, Amerhauser A. In: Norton JA, Barie PS, Bollinger RR et al (eds.), *Surgery: Basic Science and Clinical Evidence*. New York: Springer; 2000, 698–700.

16. **(E)** While sigmoid volvulus accounts for >80% of colonic volvulus cases, cecal volvulus is relatively rare, accounting for 10% of cases. Sigmoid volvulus is felt to be "acquired" through accumulation of risk factors while cecal volvulus is considered "congenital" because of individual anatomic variation. Both sigmoid and cecal volvulus demonstrate a large, dilated loop of colon on plain radiograph. The loop "points" to the left upper quadrant of the abdomen with a cecal volvulus and to the right upper quadrant with a sigmoid volvulus. While cecopexy has been well described and does have some success, the definitive treatment for cecal volvulus is right hemicolectomy with primary anastomosis in the appropriate setting with resection, ileostomy, and mucous fistula in the presence of perforation or peritonitis.

Bibliography

Kodner IJ, Fry RD, Fleshman JW, et al. In: Schwartz SI, Spencer FC (eds.), *Schwartz: Principles of Surgery*, 7th ed. New York: McGraw-Hill; 1999, 1276–1277.

Madiba TE, Thomson SR. The management of cecal volvulus. [Review] *Dis Colon Rectum* 2002;45(2):264–267.

Rolandelli RH, Roslyn JJ. In: Townsend CM, et al (ed.), *Sabiston Textbook of Surgery*, 16th ed. Philadelphia: W.B. Saunders; 2002, 947.

Welton ML, Varma RG, Amerhauser A. In: Norton JA, Barie PS, Bollinger RR et al (eds.), *Surgery: Basic Science and Clinical Evidence*. New York: Springer; 2000, 698–700.

17. **(D)** LGIH is defined as bleeding beyond the ligament of Treitz. Determination must be made between the small bowel and the colon as the etiology of the hemorrhage. The most common cause of LGIH in all adults is colonic diverticula. In adults younger than age 60, the next most common causes are cancer and inflammatory bowel disease. In adults older than age 60, the next most common causes are arteriovenous malformations and cancer. Among children, the most common cause of lower GI hemorrhage is a Meckel's diverticulum, followed by inflammatory bowel disease and colonic polyps. Other common etiologies include hemorrhoidal bleeding and ischemic colitis. Blood loss requiring transfusion of more than 6 units of blood within a 24-h period is considered "massive" bleeding and should prompt a mesenteric arteriogram or operative exploration.

Bibliography

Enns R. Acute lower gastrointestinal bleeding. *Can J Gastroenterol* 2001;15(8):509–516 and 517–521.

Kodner IJ, Fry RD, Fleshman JW, et al. In: Schwartz SI, Spencer FC (eds.), *Schwartz: Principles of Surgery*, 7th ed. New York: McGraw-Hill; 1999, 1282–1284.

Lingenfelser T, Ell C. Lower gastrointestinal bleeding. [Review] *Best Pract Res Clin Gastroenterol* 2001; 15(1): 135–153.

Rolandelli RH, Roslyn JJ. In: Townsend CM, et al (ed.), *Sabiston Textbook of Surgery*, 16th ed. Philadelphia: W.B. Saunders; 2002, 829–832.

Zuckerman GR, Prakash C. Acute lower intestinal bleeding; etiology, therapy and outcomes. *Gastrointest Endosc* 1999;49(2):228–238.

18. **(A)** Approximately 15% of all bowel obstructions occur in the large intestine. The most common site of obstruction is the sigmoid colon, the right colon being much less likely to cause obstruction given its wider diameter. The most common cause of colonic obstruction in the adult is colon cancer which accounts for approximately 60–70%. The next most common etiologies include diverticulitis (20%) and volvulus (5%). Adhesive bands, the most common etiology of obstruction in the small bowel almost never cause

colonic obstruction. The ileocecal valve is incompetent in 10–20% of persons, allowing colonic decompression in these individuals, which can be protective against perforation in cases of distal colon obstruction. The overall mortality rate for colonic obstruction is 20%, with the rate being 40% in the event of cecal perforation. The higher mortality rate is likely associated with a completely obstructing cancer of the left or sigmoid colon causing a closed loop obstruction in combination with a competent ileocecal valve.

Bibliography

Bauer AJ, Schwarz NT, Moore BA, et al. Ileus in critical illness: mechanisms and management. [Review] *Curr Opin Crit Care* 2002;47(5):1175–1181.

Dervenis C, Delis S, Filippou D, et al. Intestinal obstruction and perforation—the role of the surgeon. [Review] *Dig Dis* 2003;21(1):68–76.

19. (E) Colovesical fistula is the most common type of fistulous communication between the bladder and the GI tract. This complication is felt to be less common in women because of the presence of the uterus and adnexa and has a 3:1 ratio of men to women. Though diverticulitis is the most common cause of colovesical fistula, this complication occurs in only 2% of cases of colonic diverticulitis. Though pneumaturia is a dramatic presenting complaint and almost always indicates colovesical fistula, refractory urinary tract infection is a more common presenting complaint. Repair of colovesical fistula is by excision of the mass *en bloc* for cancer and by blunt dissection for diverticulitis. If the fistula tract into the bladder is not obvious after takedown of the colon, the bladder should be distended with fluid containing methylene blue. The tract can then be oversewn. If a fistula closes spontaneously, which it may do in up to 50% of patients with diverticulitis, requirements for resection depend on the nature of the underlying colon disease.

Bibliography

Jarrett TW, Vaughan ED. Accuracy of computerized tomography in the diagnosis of colovesical fistula secondary to diverticular disease. *J Urol* 1995;153(1):44–46.

Kodner IJ, Fry RD, Fleshman JW, et al. In: Schwartz SI, Spencer FC (eds.), *Schwartz: Principles of Surgery*, 7th ed. New York: McGraw-Hill; 1999, 1280–1281.

Larsen A, Bjerklund-Johansen TE, Solheim BM, et al. Diagnosis and treatment of enterovesical fistula. *Eur Urol* 1996;29(3):318–321.

Pontari MA, McMillen MA, Garvey RH, et al. Diagnosis and treatment of enterovesical fistulae. *Am Surg* 1992; 58(4):258–263.

Rolandelli RH, Roslyn JJ. In: Townsend CM, et al (ed.), *Sabiston Textbook of Surgery*, 16th ed. Philadelphia: W.B. Saunders; 2002, 946.

20. (C) Ischemic colitis is caused by both occlusive and nonocclusive mechanisms. A common precipitating event is reconstruction of the infrarenal abdominal aorta with interruption of the blood supply from the inferior mesenteric artery. Physical examination findings classically include "pain out of proportion to exam," characterized by a complaint of severe pain but a relatively benign physical examination. Though many diagnostic tests can be suggestive of ischemia, the best test is endoscopy for its ability to directly visualize ischemic changes in the colonic mucosa. The mucosa is found to be edematous, hemorrhagic, friable, and sometimes ulcerated. Because patients with severe ischemia often have multiple other medical problems, the overall mortality rate approaches 50%. Most cases of bowel ischemia in the elderly are associated with vascular disease or vascular thrombi. Cases in younger individuals can result from systemic lupus erythematosus, sickle cell crisis, pancreatitis, diabetes mellitus, or an underlying coagulopathy.

Bibliography

Cappell MS. Intestinal (mesenteric) vasculopathy. II. Ischemic colitis and chronic mesenteric ischemia. [Review] *Gastroenterol Clin North Am* 1998;27(4):827–860.

Fischer, JE. In: Baker RJ, Fischer JE (eds.), *Mastery of Surgery*, 4th ed. Philadelphia: Lippincott, Williams & Wilkins; 2001, 2077.

Green BT, Branch MS. Ischemic colitis in a young adult during sickle cell crisis: case report and review. [Review] *Gastrointest Endosc* 2003;57(4):605–607.

Greenwald DA, Brandt LJ. Colonic ischemia. [Review] *J Clin Gastroenterol* 1998;27(2):122–128.

Hourmand-Ollivier I, Bouin M, Saloux E, et al. Cardiac sources of embolism should be routinely screened in ischemic colitis. *Am J Gastroenterol* 2003;98(7):1573–1577.

Kodner IJ, Fry RD, Fleshman JW, et al. In: Schwartz SI, Spencer FC (eds.), *Schwartz: Principles of Surgery*, 7th ed. New York: McGraw-Hill; 1999, 1284–1285.

MacDonald PH. Ischaemic colitis. [Review] *Best Pract Res Clin Gastroenterol* 2002;16(1):51–61.

Richardson SC, Willis J, Wong RC. Ischemic colitis, systemic lupus erythematosus, and the lupus anticoagulant: case report and review. [Review] *Gastrointest Endosc* 2003;57(2):257–260.

21. (E) Colonic polyps are categorized as either neoplastic or nonneoplastic. Most nonneoplastic polyps can be safely observed with endoscopic biopsy and surveillance. Neoplastic polyps have the potential for malignant transformation following the adenoma to carcinoma sequence. Polyps are seen as being tubular, tubulovillous, or villous with an increasing risk of carcinoma in moving from a more tubular to a more villous character. Most colonic polyps can be excised and definitively treated endoscopically. Factors which are unfavorable for endoscopic excision include a margin less than 3–5 cm, poor histologic differentiation, and lymphovascular invasion. Invasion of the submucosa is not considered an unfavorable factor for endoscopic excision.

Bibliography

Blumberg D, Ramanathan RK. Treatment of colon and rectal cancer. [Review] *J Clin Gastroenterol* 2002;34(1): 15–26.

Burgart LJ. Colorectal polyps and other precursor lesions. Need for an expanded view. [Review] *Gastroenterol Clin North Am* 2002;31(4):959–970.

Liangpunsakul S, Rex DK. Colon tumors and colonoscopy. [Review] *Endoscopy* 2002;34(11):875–881.

Masaki T, Mori T, Matsuoka H, et al. Colonoscopic treatment of colon cancers. [Review] *Surg Oncol Clin North Am* 2001;10(3):693–708.

Rolandelli RH, Roslyn JJ. In: Townsend CM, et al (ed.), *Sabiston Textbook of Surgery*, 16th ed. Philadelphia: W.B. Saunders; 2002, 957–958.

Welton ML, Varma RG, Amerhauser A. In: Norton JA, Barie PS, Bollinger RR et al (eds.), *Surgery: Basic Science and Clinical Evidence*. New York: Springer; 2000, 699–710.

22. **(D)** The Haggitt classification for colonic polyps is used to characterize polyps for treatment purposes. Level 0 polyps refer to carcinoma *in situ* and are considered noninvasive. They can be treated with excision only. Level I polyps contain carcinoma which invades the muscularis mucosa into the submucosa, but remains contained within the head of the polyp. Level II polyps contain carcinoma which invades the junction between the stalk and the adenoma itself. Both level I and level II polyps can generally be adequately treated with endoscopic excision. Level III polyps invade the stalk. These can occasionally be excised endoscopically depending on the margin obtained. The carcinoma in a level IV polyp invades the submucosa of the bowel but remains above the muscularis propria. Wide-based sessile polyps with any carcinoma are also considered level IV. All level IV polyps require segmental resection (Figs. 24-8 and 24-9).

Bibliography

Inoue H. Endoscopic mucosal resection for the entire gastrointestinal mucosal lesions. [Review] *Gastrointest Endosc Clin North Am* 2001;11(3):459–478.

Kodner IJ, Fry RD, Fleshman JW, et al. In: Schwartz SI, Spencer FC (eds.), *Schwartz: Principles of Surgery*, 7th ed. New York: McGraw-Hill; 1999, 1342–1346.

Kronborg O. Colon polyps and cancer. [Review] *Endoscopy* 2002;34(1):69–72.

Schulmann K, Reiser M, Schmiegel W. Colon cancer and polyps. [Review] *Best Pract Res Clin Gastroenterol* 2002; 16(1):91–114.

Waye JD. Endoscopic mucosal resection of colon polyps. [Review] *Gastrointest Endosc Clin North Am* 2001;11(3): 537–548.

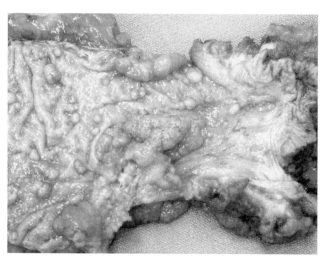

FIG. 24-8   Colonic polyposis

23. **(D)** Colon cancer is the fourth most common type of cancer in the United States and accounts for the second most cancer deaths after lung cancer. Development of colon cancer is thought to involve malignant transformation of colonic polyps (adenoma to carcinoma sequence). There is a definite genetic predisposition to colon cancer. Though many persons are thought to have a heterozygous status for important cancer-related genes, loss of heterozygosity is related to both tumor suppressor gene inactivation and oncogene activation. Isolated liver metastases from colon cancer will often decrease in size during chemotherapy and the residual tumor can then be excised surgically at a later date. Radiation therapy of liver metastases is not beneficial. Pulmonary metastases from colon cancer are present in 10% of patients at the time of their diagnosis;

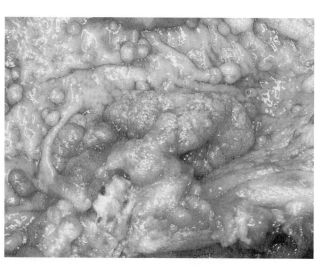

FIG. 24-9   Colonic polyposis

1% of all patients have a solitary lung nodule that is amenable to resection.

Bibliography

Adam R, Avisar E, Ariche E, et al. Five-year survival following hepatic resection after neoadjuvant therapy for nonresectable colorectal liver metastases. *Ann Surg Oncol* 2001;8(4):347–353.

Fraker DL, Soulen M. Regional therapy of hepatic metastases. *Hematol Oncol Clin North Am* 2002;16:947–967.

Giovannucci E. Modifiable risk factors for colon cancer. *Gastroenterol Clin North Am* 2002;31(4):925–943.

Headrick JR, Miller DL, Nagorney DM, et al. Surgical treatment of hepatic and pulmonary metastases from colon cancer. *Ann Thorac Surg* 2001;71:975–980.

Inoue M, Kotake Y, Nakagawa K, et al. Surgery for pulmonary metastases from colorectal carcinoma. *Ann Thorac Surg* 2000;70:380–383.

Kodner IJ, Fry RD, Fleshman JW, et al. In: Schwartz SI, Spencer FC (eds.), *Schwartz: Principles of Surgery*, 7th ed. New York: McGraw-Hill; 1999, 1346–1352.

Shoup MC, Nissan A, Dangelica MI, et al. Randomized clinical trials in colon cancer. [Review] *Surg Oncol Clin North Am* 2002;11(1):133–148.

Ueno H, Mochizuki H, Hatsuse K, et al. Indicators for treatment strategies of colorectal liver metastases. *Ann Surg* 2000;231:59–66.

Wu JS, Fazio VW. Colon cancer. [Review] *Dis Colon Rectum* 2000;43(11):1473–1486.

24. **(B)** APC is a tumor suppressor gene on chromosome 5. Loss of this gene is associated with familial adenomatous polyposis (FAP). This gene is autosomal dominant with 100% penetrance. CAG triplicate repeat sequence is related to certain neurodegenerative disorders but is not known to be related to colon cancer. K-ras is an oncogene having increased activity in patients with colon cancer. hMLH1/hMSH2 refers to a mismatch repair gene in which mutation leads to DNA instability. This gene is associated with hereditary nonpolyposis colon cancer (HNPCC).

Bibliography

Grady WM. Genetic testing for high-risk colon cancer patients. [Review] *Gastroenterology* 2003; 124(6): 1574–1594.

Grady WM, Markowitz SD. Hereditary colon cancer genes. [Review] *Methods Mol Biol* 2003;222:59–83.

Jiricny J, Marra G. DNA repair defects in colon cancer. [Review] *Curr Opin Genet Dev* 2003;13(1):61–69.

Lynch JP, Hoops TC. The genetic pathogenesis of colorectal cancer. [Review] *Hematol Oncol Clin North Am* 2002;16(4):775–810.

Neibergs HL, Hein DW, Spratt JS. Genetic profiling of colon cancer. [Review] *J Surg Oncol* 2002;80(4):204–213.

Markowitz S. DNA repair defects inactivate tumor suppressor genes and induce hereditary and sporadic colon cancers. [Review] *J Clin Oncol* 2000;18(21S):75S–80S.

Oving IM, Clevers HC. Molecular causes of colon cancer. [Review] *Eur J Clin Invest* 2002;32(6):448–457.

Peltomaki P. Deficient DNA mismatch repair: a common etiologic factor for colon cancer. [Review] *Hum Mol Genet* 2001;10(7):735–740.

Robbins DH, Itzkowitz SH. The molecular and genetic basis of colon cancer. [Review] *Med Clin North Am* 2002; 86(6):1467–1495.

Wu GD. A nuclear receptor to prevent colon cancer. [Review] *N Engl J Med* 2000;342(9):651–653.

25. **(A)** According to the TNM staging system for colorectal cancer, T1 tumors invade the submucosa, T2 tumors invade the muscularis propria, T3 tumors invade into the subserosa or pericolic tissue, and T4 tumors perforate the visceral peritoneum or directly invade other organs or structures. T5 tumors are not defined in the system. N0 classification refers to involvement of no regional lymph nodes, N1 involves one to three regional lymph nodes, N2 involves four or more regional lymph nodes, and N3 refers to any nodal involvement along a major, named vascular trunk. MX indicates that the presence of metastases cannot be adequately assessed. M0 refers to no distant metastases and M1 refers to the presence of any distant metastases. Stage I colon cancer has a 5-year survival rate of greater than 90%.

Bibliography

Bernick PE, Wong WD. Staging: what makes sense? Can the pathologist help? [Review] *Surg Oncol Clin North Am* 2000;9(4):703–720.

Green FL, Cera SM. Colon cancer: do we need a staging system? *Adv Surg* 2003;37:171–178.

Koch TR. Re-evaluation of colon cancer staging—stricture presence reflects advanced disease? [Review] *Am J Gastroenterol* 2002;97(3):759.

Rolandelli RH, Roslyn JJ. In: Townsend CM, et al (ed.), *Sabiston Textbook of Surgery*, 16th ed. Philadelphia: W.B. Saunders; 2002, 961–965.

Kodner IJ, Fry RD, Fleshman JW, et al. In: Schwartz SI, Spencer FC (eds.), *Schwartz: Principles of Surgery*, 7th ed. New York: McGraw-Hill; 1999, 1350–1351.

26. **(C)** Gardner's syndrome has a colonic manifestation similar to FAP with the addition of multiple extracolonic manifestations. Turcot's syndrome is characterized by the presence of colonic polyps and brain tumors. The brain tumors in this population generally occur in the first two decades of life. MEN type IIb is associated with medullary thyroid carcinoma, pheochromocytoma, multiple mucosal neuromas, and a marfanoid body habitus. It is not thought to be related to colonic polyposis. Peutz-Jeghers' syndrome is manifest through an autosomal dominant transmission resulting in multiple hamartomas throughout the GI tract;

melana in buccal mucosa, face, hands and feet; and signs including GI hemorrhage, obstruction, and mucocutaneous hyperpigmentation. Juvenile polyposis also has an autosomal dominant transmission and is a source of GI hemorrhage in the pediatric population. The peak age of symptoms in juvenile polyposis is 5–6 years when patients may experience abdominal pain, diarrhea, mucous discharge, and bleeding.

Bibliography

Agnifili A, Verzaro R, Gola P, et al. Juvenile polyposis: case report and assessment of the neoplastic risk in 271 patients reported in the literature. [Review] *Dig Surg* 1999;16(2):161–166.

Boardman LA. Heritable colorectal cancer syndromes: recognition and preventive management. [Review] *Gastroenterol Clin North Am* 2002;31(4):1107–1131.

Bronner MP. Gastrointestinal inherited polyposis syndromes. [Review] *Mod Pathol* 2003;16(4):359–365.

Hyer W. Polyposis syndromes: pediatric implications. [Review] *Gastrointest Endosc Clin North Am* 2001; 11(4): 659–682.

Jarvinen HJ. Genetic testing for polyposis: practical and ethical aspects. [Review] *Gut* 2003;52(S2):19–22.

McGarrity TJ, Kulin HE, Zaino RJ. Peutz-Jeghers syndrome. [Review] *Am J Gastroenterol* 2000;95(3):596–604.

Rolandelli RH, Roslyn JJ. In: Townsend CM, et al (ed.), *Sabiston Textbook of Surgery*, 16th ed. Philadelphia: W.B. Saunders; 2002, 958–961.

Thorson AG, Faria J. Familial adenomatous polyposis, hereditary nonpolyposis colon cancer, and familial risk: what are the implications for the surgeon? [Review] *Surg Oncol Clin North Am* 2000;9(4):683–697.

Wirtzfeld DA, Petrelli NJ, Rodriguez-Bigas MA. Hamartomatous polyposis syndromes: molecular genetics, neoplastic risk, and surveillance recommendations. [Review] *Ann Surg Oncol* 2001;8(4):319–327.

27. (A) FAP syndrome is categorized as Gardner's syndrome when the intestinal findings are accompanied by certain benign extraintestinal growths, particularly osteomas, epidermoid cysts, desmoid tumors, and congenital hypertrophy of the retinal pigment epithelium. These growths may precede the development of the polyposis syndrome. Presentation with these signs, therefore, necessitates colonoscopy to evaluate for colonic polyposis. The presence of a retroperitoneal desmoid tumor may require biopsy, but this could likely be accomplished percutaneously. The other choices above would not lead to an appropriate diagnosis.

Bibliography

Buch B, Noffke C, de Kock S. Gardner's syndrome—the importance of early diagnosis: a case report and a review. [Review] *SADJ* 2001;56(5):242–245.

Griffioen G, Bus PJ, Vasen HF, et al. Extracolonic manifestations of familial adenomatous polyposis: desmoid tumors and upper gastrointestinal adenomas and carcinomas. [Review] *Scand J Gastoenterol* 1998;225:85–91.

King JE, Dozois RR, Lindor NM, et al. Care of patients and their families with familial adenomatous polyposis. [Review] *Mayo Clin Proc* 2000;75(1):57–67.

Parks ET, Caldemeyer KS, Mirowski GW. Gardner syndrome. *J Am Acad Dermatol* 2001;45(6):940–942.

Vasen HF. Clinical diagnosis and management of hereditary colorectal cancer syndromes. [Review] *J Clin Oncol* 2000;18(21S):81S–92S.

Wehrli BM, Weiss SW, Yandow S, et al. Garner-associated fibromas in young patients: a distinct fibrous lesion that identifies unsuspected Gardner syndrome and risk for fibromatosis. *Am J Surg Pathol* 2001;25(5):645–651.

28. (C) FAP is related to the loss of the tumor suppressor gene APC located on the long arm of chromosome 5. The APC gene mutation appears to be an early event in carcinogenesis, and, in combination with other mutational events, leads to colon cancer. This genetic mutation is autosomal dominant with 100% penetrance and all patients will develop colon cancer by the third decade of life, if not treated. FAP is characterized by the presence of 100s to 1000s of 5–10 mm polyps throughout the colon. Polyps more than 1 cm in diameter carry a 50% risk of carcinoma. By age 10, 15% of FAP patients will manifest colonic polyps and this increases to 75% by age 20 and 90% by age 30. Extracolonic symptoms are frequently seen and have been discussed previously as Gardner's syndrome. Medical treatment of FAP is possible and sulindac and celebrex have been shown to decrease the number and size of colonic polyps. Sulindac and tamoxifen may also be effective in the treatment of desmoid growths. Surgical treatment of FAP includes total proctocolectomy with ileostomy or placement of an ileoanal or ileal pouch anastomosis.

Bibliography

Beech D, Pontius A, Muni N, et al. Familial adenomatous polyposis: a case report and review of the literature. [Review] *J Natl Med Assoc* 2001;93(6):208–213.

Chan TA. Non-steroidal anti-inflammatory drugs, apoptosis, and colon cancer chemoprevention. [Review] *Lancet Oncol* 2002;3(3):166–174.

Lal G, Gallinger S. Familial adenomatous polyposis. [Review] *Semin Surg Oncol* 2000;18(4):314–323.

Moslein G, Pistorius S, Saeger HD, et al. Preventive surgery for colon cancer in familial adenomatous polyposis and hereditary nonpolyposis colorectal cancer syndrome. *Langenbecks Arch Surg* 2003;388(1):9–16.

North GL. Celecoxib as adjunctive therapy for treatment of colorectal cancer. [Review] *Ann Pharmacol* 2001;35(12): 1638–1643.

Okai T, Yamaguchi Y, Sakai J, et al. Complete regression of colonic adenomas after treatment with sulindac in Gardner's syndrome: a 4-year follow-up. *J Gastroenterol* 2001;36(11):778–782.

29. **(E)** HNPCC is a genetic-linked autosomal dominant disorder with almost complete penetrance. The associated genetic defect is a mutation in hMLH1/hMSH2 which is a mismatch repair gene. Mutation in this gene leads to DNA instability and predisposes to cancer. HNPCC accounts for approximately 5% of colorectal cancer cases annually in the United States. This disease is diagnosed clinically according to the Amsterdam criteria: at least three relatives with colorectal cancer (at least one must be first-degree relative), at least two successive generations affected, and colorectal cancer diagnosed before age 50 in at least one of the relatives. HNPCC patients have a high risk of other cancers and close surveillance is crucial in long-term management. Female patients are at particular risk of gynecologic malignancies and should be offered prophylactic hysterectomy and oopherectomy (Figs. 24-10 and 24-11).

Bibliography

Allen BA, Terdiman JP. Hereditary polyposis syndromes and hereditary non-polyposis colorectal cancer. [Review] *Best Pract Res Clin Gastroenterol* 2003;17(2):237–258.

Cao Y, Pieretti M, Marshall J, et al. Challenge in the differentiation between attenuated familial adenomatous polyposis and hereditary nonpolyposis colorectal cancer: case report with review of the literature. [Review] *Am J Gastroenterol* 2002;97(7):1822–1827.

Frank TS, Critchfield GC. Hereditary risk of women's cancers. [Review] *Best Pract Res Clin Obstet Gynecol* 2002;16(5):703–713.

Giardiello FM, Brensinger JD, Petersen GM. AGA technical review on hereditary colorectal cancer and genetic testing. [Review] *Gastroenterology* 2001;121(1):198–213.

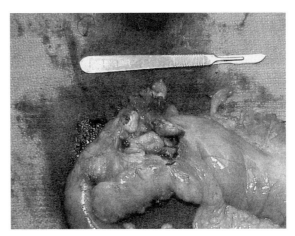

FIG. 24-11 HNPCC patient with synchronous lesions of the colon and duodenum.

Jass JR. Familial colorectal cancer: pathology and molecular characteristics. [Review] *Lancer Oncol* 2000;1:220–226.

Kennedy EP, Hamilton SR. Genetics of colorectal cancer. [Review] *Semin Surg Oncol* 1998;15(2):126–130.

Lynch HT, de la Chapelle A. Hereditary colorectal cancer. [Review] *N Engl J Med* 2003;348(10):919–932.

Lynch HT, Lynch JF. Hereditary nonpolyposis colorectal cancer. [Review] *Semin Surg Oncol* 2000;18(4):305–313.

Muller A, Fishel R. Mismatch repair and the hereditary non-polyposis colorectal cancer syndrome (HNPCC). [Review] *Cancer Invest* 2002;20(1):102–9.

Muller HH, Heinimann K, Dobbie Z. Genetics of hereditary colon cancer—a basis for prevention? [Review] *Eur J Cancer* 2000;36(10):1215–1223.

Soravia C, Berk T, Cohen Z. Genetic testing and surgical decision making in hereditary colorectal cancer. [Review] *Int J Colorectal Dis* 2000;15(1):21–28.

30. **(B)** Lynch syndrome type I includes all patients with HNPCC without any additional diagnosis of cancer (no other noncolon site). Lynch syndrome type II includes HNPCC patients with cancer diagnosed at an additional noncolon site. HNPCC patients are at high risk of colon cancer and should have close surveillance. Routine colonoscopy should begin in the second decade of life or 5 years earlier than the age of detection within the kindred. Definitive treatment for HNPCC includes subtotal colectomy given the high risk of synchronous colonic tumors. Cancers seen in Lynch syndrome type II, in addition to colon cancer, include noncolon GI tumors, urinary tract tumors, uterine and ovarian cancer, breast cancer, and pancreatic cancer.

Bibliography

Anwar S, Hall C, White J, et al. Hereditary non-polyposis colorectal cancer: an updated review. [Review] *Eur J Surg Oncol* 2000;26(7):635–645.

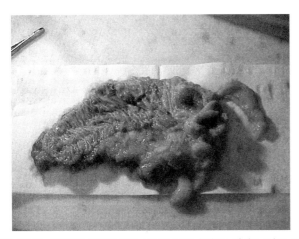

FIG. 24-10 HNPCC patient with synchronous lesions of the colon and duodenum.

Chung DC, Rustgi AK. The hereditary nonpolyposis colorectal cancer syndrome: genetics and clinical implications. [Review] *Ann Intern Med* 2003;138(7):560–570.

Hampel H, Peltomaki P. Hereditary colorectal cancer: risk assessment and management. [Review] *Clin Genet* 2000;58(2):89–97.

Jass JR. Pathology of hereditary nonpolyposis colorectal cancer. [Review] *Ann N Y Acad Sci* 2000;910:62–73.

Lawes DA, SenGupta SB, Boulos PB. Pathogenesis and clinical management of hereditary nonpolyposis colorectal cancer. [Review] *Br J Surg* 2002;89(11):1357–1369.

Moslein G, Krause-Paulus R, Hegger R, et al. Clinical aspects of hereditary nonpolyposis colorectal cancer. [Review] *Ann N Y Acad Sci* 2000;910:75–83.

Peterson KA, DiSario JA. Secondary prevention: screening and surveillance of persons at average and high risk for colorectal cancer. [Review] *Hematol Oncol Clin North Am* 2002;16(4):841–865.

Rolandelli RH, Roslyn JJ. In: Townsend CM, et al (ed.), *Sabiston Textbook of Surgery*, 16th ed. Philadelphia: W.B. Saunders; 2002, 961.

Scaife CL, Rodriguez-Bigas MA. Lynch syndrome: implications for the surgeon. [Review] *Clin Colorectal Cancer* 2003;3(2):92–98.

31. **(A)** Surgical management of colon cancer requires strict adherence to the oncologic principles of surgery including adequate colonic margins, resection of associated lymphatic drainage, resection of associated fascial layers and care with handling of the specimen. Carcinoma of the colon and rectum spreads by six modalities: intramucosal extension, direct invasion of adjacent structures, lymphatic spread, hematologic spread, intraperitoneal spread, and anastomotic implantation. Each of these mechanisms must be addressed in the preoperative, intraoperative, and postoperative care of these patients. Patients presenting with advanced stages of colorectal cancer have a significantly worse prognosis than those patients with early diagnosis. Perioperative mortality in patients with perforated colon cancer approaches 30% and those with obstructing colon cancer have in-hospital mortality of 15% after initial presentation. Most colon cancers require resection, either for cure or for local control of the disease. Direct extension into adjacent fascia, vascular or nervous tissue, or solid organs requires *en bloc* resection of the colon with those involved structures because the adhesions usually contain tumor cells. Although most patients do not require extensive resections for colon cancer, these resections should not be avoided as the size of the primary lesion is not associated with the risk of regional metastasis. Statistically, the finding of direct extension of colon cancer to adjacent tissue does not carry a significantly worse prognosis than finding involvement of regional lymph nodes (Figs. 24-12 and 24-13).

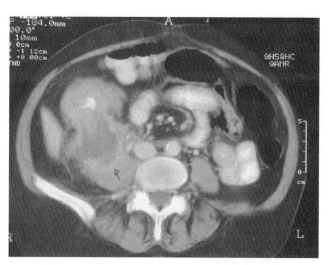

FIG. 24-12   Perforated colon cancer in the ascending colon.

Bibliography

Canter RJ, Williams NN. Surgical treatment of colon and rectal cancer. [Review] *Hematol Oncol Clin North Am* 2002;16(4):907–926.

Colquhoun PH, Wexner SD. Surgical management of colon cancer. [Review] *Curr Gastroenterol Rep* 2002; 4(5):414–419.

Kodner IJ, Fry RD, Fleshman JW, et al. In: Schwartz SI, Spencer FC (eds.), *Schwartz: Principles of Surgery*, 7th ed. New York: McGraw-Hill; 1999, 1348–1350.

Longo WE, Virgo KS, Johnson FE, et al. Risk factors for morbidity and mortality after colectomy for colon cancer. *Dis Colon Rectum* 2000;43:83–91.

Mitry E, Barthod F, Penna C, et al. Surgery for colon and rectal cancer. [Review] *Best Pract Res Clin Gastroenterol* 2002;16(2):253–265.

Obrand DI, Gordon PH. Incidence and patterns of recurrence following curative resection for colorectal carcinoma. *Dis Colon Rectum* 1997;40:15–24.

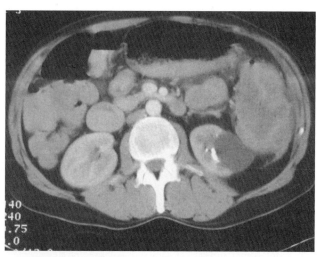

FIG. 24-13   Perforated colon cancer near the splenic flecture.

Taylor WE, Donohue JH, Gunderson LL, et al. The Mayo Clinic experience with multimodality treatment of locally advanced or recurrent colon cancer. *Ann Surg Oncol* 2002;9(2):177–185.

Welton ML, Varma RG, Amerhauser A. In: Norton JA, Barie PS, Bollinger RR et al (eds.), *Surgery: Basic Science and Clinical Evidence*. New York: Springer; 2000, 710–722.

32. **(A)** This patient has acute uncomplicated diverticulitis. This disease is characterized by localized diverticular perforation without abscess formation, free perforation, or bleeding. The majority of patients present with left lower quadrant pain, fever, and leukocytosis, making diverticulitis principally a clinical diagnosis. Diagnostic dilemmas do occur, however, and a wide differential including bowel perforation or obstruction, appendicitis, inflammatory bowel disease, and ischemic colitis must be considered. An imaging study is indicated when the clinical picture is not clear, or to help guide future therapy.

Endoscopy is contraindicated in the setting of acute diverticulitis because the insufflation required can disturb the tenuous seal containing the diverticular perforation and result in the conversion to free perforation and a need for more urgent surgical intervention with substantially higher morbidity and mortality. Endoscopy can be useful after the acute episode has resolved to evaluate for other distal pathologic processes.

Barium enema is also contraindicated in the acute setting for reasons similar to those described above. It is a very important part of the preparation for elective resection after recovery, as it accurately describes the extent of involvement and severity of disease, including strictures that may develop after acute diverticulitis.

Laparoscopy has been described as a highly sensitive diagnostic modality; however, its invasive nature precludes its routine use for this purpose.

Both CT and ultrasound can accurately diagnose diverticulitis. CT has a sensitivity of up to 95% and specificity of 72%. Both modalities can also identify abscesses, making it possible for patients to have early drainage of these collections. CT is generally more available in most institutions and is substantially less operator-dependent. CT findings such as presence of an abscess, extraluminal contrast or air strongly suggest that conservative treatment with antibiotics will not be successful.

33. **(D)** This patient has uncomplicated diverticulitis. In many cases, this disorder can be successfully treated as an outpatient with oral antibiotics. Such a regimen would not be appropriate for this patient because of his inability to tolerate a diet. Appropriate antibiotic therapy provides for coverage of usual colonic flora and is successful in resolving the acute episode at least 70% of the time. As the patient improves, he can be rapidly transitioned to oral antibiotics and discharged to home. If improvement does not occur within 3–4 days, and imaging does not reveal an abscess which is amenable to percutaneous drainage, immediate surgical treatment should be considered. Primary anastamosis can be considered in this situation, depending on the degree of local inflammation. Resection and Hartman's procedure is the preferred approach if any doubt exists as to the quality of the bowel or the degree of inflammation in the peritoneal cavity.

Overall, recurrent episodes of diverticulitis can be expected to occur in approximately 25% of patients, with the majority of those who develop a second episode continuing on to a third if elective resection is not performed. This has led to the recommendation that in most patients, resection of the diseased segment of colon be performed after a second bout of uncomplicated diverticulitis. Preoperative preparation should include imaging to determine the extent of disease so that an appropriate resection and primary anastamosis can be planned. A laparoscopic approach to these resections has become increasingly popular.

This patient differs from the typical victim of acute diverticulitis by his young age. Diverticulitis in patients less than 40 years of age is characterized by a course that is typically more virulent than in the older population. Recurrence rates after a single episode of uncomplicated diverticulitis are extremely high. Medical treatment of the initial episode is just as likely to be successful, but elective resection is recommended after a single episode of diverticulitis in these patients.

34. **(B)** This patient's findings and clinical scenario are most consistent with acute colonic pseudoobstruction (ACPO), also known as Ogilvie's syndrome. This condition is defined by signs, symptoms, and radiographic findings of colonic obstruction without a mechanical cause. It can be seen in a wide variety of medical conditions, but the postoperative state is perhaps the most common and most relevant to surgical practice. Autonomic imbalances, either sympathetic excess or parasympathetic deficiency are believed to be responsible.

The clinical scenario described above is typical of ACPO. In addition, patients may complain of abdominal pain, nausea, and vomiting. A water-soluble contrast enema should be performed to rule out an actual distal colonic obstruction, and can be therapeutic if the cause is simply postoperative constipation.

Cecal diameters of greater than 12 cm are associated with a high risk of perforation, and diameters of 9 cm or greater merit close observation. Subject to LaPlace's law, the cecum—with its inherently larger diameter—is the site where perforation typically occurs if treatment is not promptly undertaken.

Surgical intervention is reserved for perforation or patients who fail to respond to less invasive treatments, or if progression to ischemic necrosis and perforation has occurred. Perforation carries a mortality rate as high as 50%.

The initial approach is typically conservative management consisting of NG decompression, correction of any electrolyte disturbances, limitation of narcotic medications, and close monitoring of progress with serial abdominal radiographs. Many patients will improve with these measures only. If they fail to do so within 24–48 h, or if their cecal diameter continues to increase to 12 cm or greater, intervention should be pursued.

There are two viable approaches to intervention if conservative management fails. The first is colonoscopic decompression. This must be undertaken with great care and minimal insufflation of gas, and the endoscope should be passed at least to the hepatic flexure to ensure adequate decompression of the cecum. Rectal tubes can be placed at this time as well, but they are often ineffective. Colonoscopy is highly effective, but recurrence rates are up to 15%.

Another approach is pharmacologic in nature. Neostigmine, a powerful parasympathetic agonist, can produce a rapid and dramatic return of colonic motility. Results are usually dramatic and durable, and begin from 30 s to 10 min after administration. Life-threatening bradycardia can result, however, so this drug should be administered with cardiac monitoring and with atropine available at the bedside.

This patient has not yet undergone a trial of conservative therapy, and shows no signs of impending perforation.

35. **(C)** This patient has sigmoid volvulus. This disease is typically found in elderly Black males, who are often institutionalized or have chronic medical conditions. As a result, their presentation with these symptoms raises substantial concern for obstruction because of malignancy or other serious intraabdominal pathology. Fortunately, the abdominal radiograph is usually pathognomonic, revealing a large loop of colon pointing toward the right upper quadrant. A gastrograffin enema will show a "bird's beak" deformity, but is not usually required to make the diagnosis. Indications for emergent surgery include hematochezia, peritonitis, or

free intraperitoneal air. In the absence of these findings, sigmoidoscopy—either rigid or flexible—should be performed. This confirms the diagnosis and allows for an assessment of the viability of the colonic mucosa in the affected segment. It is also therapeutic in approximately 85% of cases, as the volvulus is reduced by the endoscope. Gastrograffin enema will also occasionally reduce the volvulus. If successful reduction is achieved and the colonic mucosa appears viable the patient can undergo bowel preparation prior sigmoid resection at this hospital admission. Sigmoid sparing procedures such as colopexy and mesosigmoidoplasty have a high rate of recurrence, and conservative management alone has a recurrence rate of 30–90%, making resection the only viable option.

If the volvulus cannot be reduced by gastrograffin or sigmoidoscopy, or if ischemia is encountered with the endoscope, emergent resection is required. In this setting, or the setting of hematochezia, peritonitis or free air, a Hartman's procedure should be performed, as the risk of a primary anastamosis in this setting would be unacceptable.

This patient does not display any findings indicating a need for emergent surgery.

36. **(C)** It is important to distinguish patients in need of urgent surgery for management of their ulcerative colitis from those who can tolerate elective workup and bowel preparation. The morbidity of urgent surgery is substantially higher, and outcomes are generally seen as less desirable by patients. The procedure of choice in urgent surgical therapy is subtotal colectomy with end ileostomy. Proctocolectomy carries an unacceptably high surgical risk in these patients because of the addition of an extensive pelvic resection to the already substantial abdominal procedure, and is of little benefit as the rectal stump can almost always be managed medically. The definitive reconstructive procedure—proctocolectomy with ileal pouch and pouch anal anastamosis—must be deferred until recovery from this initial operation.

Bleeding requiring transfusion occasionally develops despite maximal medical therapy. This almost never amounts to massive lower GI hemorrhage resulting in life-threatening hemorrhagic shock; however, once a reasonable transfusion threshold of 4–6 units of packed red blood cells (RBCs) has been reached it is safe to conclude that the hemorrhage will not resolve, and surgical intervention should be undertaken.

Toxic megacolon is present when the transverse colon measures more than 8 cm in diameter and signs and symptoms such as abdominal tenderness, fever, leukocytosis, acidosis, and tachycardia are present. This condition should initially be managed with aggressive medical therapy and serial abdominal radiographs. If improvement is not evident within 1–3 days subtotal colectomy and ileostomy should be performed.

The development of free perforation of the colon is a clear indication for emergent surgery. Morbidity and mortality in this setting is much higher even than for patients with other indications for urgent surgery.

Fulminating acute ulcerative colitis—initial presentation with the disease that is not responsive to medical therapy—is a fourth indication for urgent surgery.

Failure of maximal medical therapy to control symptoms or the development of unacceptable side effects of medical therapy with 5-ASA, antibiotics, immunosuppressive agents, and steroids is an indication to pursue elective bowel preparation and definitive surgery unless the patient develops one of the conditions described above. Other indications for elective surgery include development of dysplasia or colorectal carcinoma, or growth retardation in children with the disease.

37. **(B)** Colonic ischemia is a commonly encountered problem which is associated with a wide variety of predisposing and inciting factors. In general, clinical factors which predispose to ischemic colitis fall into three major categories: arterial compromise, venous compromise, and vasospasm. The clinical presentations vary from transient abdominal pain indicative of mild ischemia after cardiopulmonary bypass to frank perforation as a result of transmural ischemia because of overdistension caused by obstruction or *C. difficile* colitis.

Initial management prior to definitive diagnostic evaluation includes adequate resuscitation and optimization of hemodynamics with avoidance of vasopressors. Following these measures make an assessment of overall patient stability and search for evidence of peritoneal signs. Patients with peritoneal signs or evidence of clinical instability which could be attributed to colonic ischemia should be taken urgently to the operating room for exploration. Hemodynamically stable patients can undergo further evaluation to make a definitive diagnosis and assess the extent of disease involvement.

Plain radiographs are typically obtained early in the evaluation, and can provide valuable information, especially in excluding other potential etiologies. Findings of pneumatosis or of portal venous gas are indicative of gangrenous ischemia, and suggest a poor prognosis.

CT provides substantially more information, allowing accurate identification of which segments

of the colon are most affected. Ischemic colitis appears principally as areas of thickened bowel or stricture. CT is becoming increasingly popular as a diagnostic tool for ischemic colitis.

MRI offers the theoretical opportunity to both image the bowel and perform arteriography simultaneously; however, practical application is limited by the complexity of the scan, time, and the logistical difficulties of any MRI.

Arteriography is of little benefit acutely in ischemic colitis. Patients at risk for ischemic colitis often have multiple atheromatous lesions in the mesenteric vasculature which may or may not be of any clinical relevance.

Flexible sigmoidoscopy and colonoscopy are the diagnostic tool of choice for definitively identifying ischemic colitis. In the hands of an experienced practitioner using minimal insufflation, colonoscopy is both safe and effective. Endoscopy is highly sensitive because it allows direct visualization of the mucosa—the first layer affected by ischemia. Serial endoscopy allows for identification of worsening disease, making it possible to pursue surgical intervention before substantial clinical deterioration occurs.

38. **(D)** LGIH is defined as persistent gross bleeding from the rectum, with or without hemodynamic instability and hemorrhagic shock. This patient has early signs of hemodynamic instability, so aggressive resuscitation must be undertaken prior to engaging in any diagnostic studies. Anoproctosigmoidoscopy is the next step in his evaluation and management. Occasionally, localized and treatable lesions of the anus may be responsible for the hemorrhage. In hemodynamically stable patients, the next step would be to pursue colonoscopy. This study can identify active bleeding or stigmata of recent bleeding in up to 90% of patients. Endoscopic hemostasis can be attempted, although the success rate varies with the type of lesion (angiodysplasias have 85–90% success rate).

In stable patients, EGD can be deferred until after colonoscopy, but it remains an essential part of the evaluation, and with 5–15% of LGIH caused by upper GI bleed, it must be performed before surgical intervention is considered.

Tagged RBC scan allows for identification of the source of bleeding down to 0.1 mL/min; however, localization of these findings is somewhat vague, making segmental surgical resection based on bleeding scan alone a risky proposition. Findings should be correlated with a mesenteric arteriogram or the endoscopist should label the area with dye while performing the colonoscopy.

Questions 32 through 38

Bibliography

Efron J, Wexner SD. In: Cameron JL (ed.), *Current Surgical Therapy*, 7th ed. St. Louis: Mosby; 2001, 235–246.

Fischer, JE. In: Baker RJ, Fischer JE (eds.), *Mastery of Surgery*, 4th ed. Philadelphia: Lippincott, Williams & Wilkins; 2001, 1524–1537.

Hull TL, Fazio VW. In: Baker RJ, Fischer JE (eds.), *Mastery of Surgery*, 4th ed. Philadelphia: Lippincott, Williams & Wilkins; 2001, 1497–1506.

Kaufman HS. In: Cameron JL (ed.), *Current Surgical Therapy*, 7th ed. St. Louis: Mosby; 2001, 229–234.

Rolandelli R, Roslyn J. In: Beauchamp R, Evers D, Mattox K (eds.), *Sabiston's Textbook of Surgery: The Biological Basis of Modern Surgical Practice*, 16th ed. Philadelphia: W.B. Saunders; 2001, 929–973.

Scott-Conner CEH. In: Scott-Conner CEH (ed.), *Chassin's Operative Strategy in General Surgery*, 3rd ed. New York: Springer; 2002, 506–509.

CHAPTER 25

Anorectal Disease

Bridget M. Sanders, R. Barry Melbert, and Olaf B. Johansen

Questions

1. A 54-year-old male presents with complaints of a severe pain and tearing in his rectal area when he defecates. History elicits an occurrence of these same symptoms with partial resolution two times in the last year. His fiber intake is less than 10 g a day and he drinks only coffee and cola beverages. Your examination reveals the following (see Fig. 25-1) *initial* management should include

   (A) open or closed lateral internal sphincterotomy
   (B) anoscopy with dilatation under general anesthesia
   (C) dietary counseling to include 25–30 g of fiber per day, increasing intake of water, and application of topical nitrates
   (D) incision and drainage with seton placement
   (E) fistulotomy and debridement

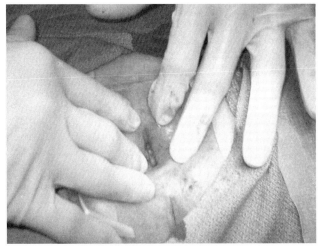

FIG. 25-1 Deep posterior anal fissure.

2. The same patient in Question 1 presents 2 months later with worsening pain and constipation. His physical examination had not significantly changed. The preferred treatment at this time is

   (A) open or closed lateral internal sphincterotomy
   (B) anoscopy with dilation under general anesthesia
   (C) dietary counseling to include 25–30 g of fiber per day, increasing intake of water, and application of topical nitrates
   (D) incision and drainage with seton placement
   (E) fistulotomy and debridement

3. A 22-year-old male construction worker is referred to your office complaining of an itching and burning rash around his anus that has worsened since he has started putting an over-the-counter hemorrhoid cream on it. The patient is asked to lie on his left side and examination reveals a diffuse erythematous rash surrounding the anus. There are no masses, fistula, hemorrhoids, or fissures evident. The patient states that it is getting worse since he has been sweating a lot at work. Appropriate recommendations should include

   (A) continue treating with over-the-counter hemorrhoidal cream for 6 weeks
   (B) washing the affected area with warm water, patting dry, and application of a steroid-based cream daily until symptoms are resolved
   (C) biopsy and preparation for wide local excision
   (D) incision and drainage with wet to dry dressing changes
   (E) colonic diversion

4. A 72-year-old female was found on routine hemorrhoidectomy to have a 3 cm lesion in the anal canal (see Fig. 25-2). Biopsy of the lesion is positive for moderately differentiated squamous cell carcinoma. All of the following are appropriate steps in treatment *except:*

(A) initial biopsy followed by chemoradiation therapy

(B) vigilant followup with repeat biopsy in 6–8 weeks after completion of therapy

(C) primary abdominal perineal resection for a 3 cm lesion at diagnosis

(D) second-line chemoradiation therapy for recurrent disease at first biopsy

(E) quoting a 5-year survival rate of 85% with a complete response of patients with appropriate therapy

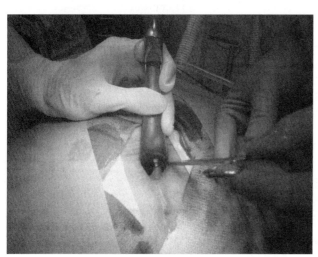

FIG. 25-2   A 3 cm anal canal lesion.

5. The role of endoscopic ultrasound (EUS) has an accuracy of 90% for preoperative staging of rectal cancer. All of the following are correct about endorectal ultrasound *except:*

(A) EUS delineates five separate layers of the rectum including mucosal surface, mucosal/muscularis mucosal, submucosa, mucosal propria, serosa and/or perirectal fat.

(B) EUS can predict lymph node involvement with an accuracy of 62–85%.

(C) Most incorrect staging is secondary to understaging of lesions.

(D) Only experienced physicians should interpret the results of EUS.

(E) Pelvic computed tomography (CT) is a poor predictor of tumor depth in rectal cancer.

6. Choice of hemorrhoid treatment depends not only on the grade of the hemorrhoid but also the location. Which of the following statements about external versus internal hemorrhoids is *correct?*

(A) External hemorrhoids are located in the anal canal and are of endodermal origin.

(B) Banding of grade 2 internal hemorrhoids in an office setting is feasible because they are located below the dentate line.

(C) Thrombosed hemorrhoids are typically located below the denate line and can cause exquisite pain.

(D) Grade 4 hemorrhoids can be easily controlled by simple ligation.

(E) Initial treatment for grade 1 hemorrhoids should include primary operative intervention.

7. Treatment of anal canal lesions less than 2 cm includes all *except:*

(A) initial wide local excision for melanoma

(B) initial wide local excision for carcinoid

(C) initial wide local excision for mucinous adenocarcinoma

(D) initial wide local excision for squamous cell carcinoma

(E) local fulguration for anal canal condyloma

8. Many anal margin lesions can be treated with wide local excision. For which of the following is wide local excision *not appropriate?*

(A) melanoma of the anal margin

(B) Bowen's disease of the anal margin

(C) noninvasive Paget's disease of the anal margin

(D) basal cell carcinoma of the anal margin

(E) all of the above can be treated surgically with wide local excision

9. Concerning embryologic origin, innervation, lymphatic, and venous drainage of the anal canal versus the rectum, which of the following is *correct?*

(A) The rectum is of ectoderm origin.

(B) The anal canal below the dentate line is insensitive to pain.

(C) The venous drainage for the rectum is the portal system.

(D) The lymphatic drainage for the rectum is the inguinal lymphatic system.

(E) The anal canal is lined with glandular mucosa.

10. A 33-year-old female presents with a perirectal abscess. She is exquisitely tender and you are unable to examine her adequately in the office. On evaluation under anesthesia, you find a fluctuant area surrounding an area of granulation tissue with associated purulence (see Fig. 25-3). Which of the following is *correct*?

(A) Perirectal abscess is the most common type of anorectal abscess accounting for approximately 40% of anorectal abscess.

(B) All perirectal abscesses must be drained under general anesthesia.

(C) Abscess and fistula do not occur with human immunodeficiency virus (HIV) as these patients are unable to mount a cellular response.

(D) If perirectal erythematic is present without apparent fluctuant mass, no incision and drainage is needed.

(E) Perirectal abscess is rare in hematologic abnormalities such as leukemia and lymphoma.

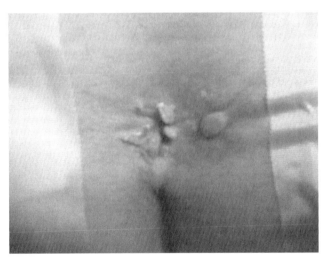

FIG. 25-3 Chronic external fistula with surrounding erythema.

11. The same patient in Question 10 undergoes incision and drainage. After draining the abscess, anoscopy is performed and a fistula is identified (see Fig. 25-4). Which of the following is *incorrect* regarding anal fistula?

(A) When the external opening lies anterior to the transverse plane, the internal opening usually is located radially.

(B) When the external opening lies posterior to the transverse plane, the internal opening tends to be located in the posterior midline.

(C) A transphincteric fistula is likely to occur in the posterior position secondary to a defect in the fusion of the longitudinal muscle and external sphincter in the posterior position.

(D) The internal opening should be easily identified by visualization alone.

(E) Intersphincteric fistulas tend to be superficial and transphincteric fistulas characteristically tend to be deep.

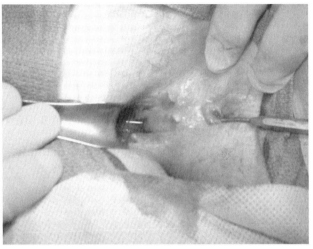

FIG. 25-4 Chronic anal fistula with probe demonstrating the internal and external anal openings.

12. Principles of surgical treatment of anal fistula should include all of the following *except*:

(A) After identification of external and internal fistula openings, the tract should be incised unless excessive overlying muscle is present.

(B) The granulation tissue exposed in the fistula tract should be treated with gentle curettage.

(C) If a large portion of external sphincter is involved, sphincter reconstruction, seton division, or endorectal flap advancement should be considered.

(D) Treatment of horseshoe fistula-in-ano should include complete resection of the entire fistula tract regardless of the extent of soft tissue involvement.

(E) The deep postanal space must be entered, curetted, and irrigated if the fistula is transphincteric.

13. A 52-year-old female is referred to your office for evaluation of foul smelling drainage from her vagina for 2 months. Pelvic examination revealed a small 2 mm opening in her vaginal vault with active drainage of stool consistency. Past surgical history was significant for an abdominal hysterectomy and bilateral oophorectomy for cervical cancer 3 years ago followed by radiation therapy. You are concerned about a rectovaginal fistula. Which of following is *incorrect* about rectovaginal fistulas?

   (A) A low rectovaginal fistula can be treated with a rectal advancement flap.
   (B) A high rectovaginal fistula may require a segmental resection such as a low anterior resection (LAR).
   (C) A vaginal fistulogram or barium enema can reveal anatomic data valuable to planning your operation.
   (D) Fibrin glue can be locally applied with good long-term results.
   (E) Etiology of rectovaginal fistulas can be congenital or acquired.

14. Which of the following is *incorrect* regarding staging of anal canal cancer?

   (A) Stage I includes any size less than 2 cm and no nodal involvement.
   (B) Stage II includes any T2 or T3 tumor with no nodal involvement.
   (C) Stage III includes any T with no nodal involvement.
   (D) Stage IV includes any T, any N, and any M1.

15. Anorectal manometry can be used in the evaluation of fecal incontinence. Which of the following statement regarding anal manometry is *incorrect*?

   (A) It is an objective method used to assess anal muscular tone, rectal compliance, and anorectal sensation.
   (B) Anorectal manometry can be used to verify the integrity of the rectoanal inhibitory reflex.
   (C) There is only one universally accepted method for obtaining and analyzing data for quality assurance.
   (D) Manometry can identify and document sphincter function before operative intervention that might require optimal continence.
   (E) Slow waves, ultraslow waves, and intermediate waves are examples of waveforms that might be encountered.

16. Regarding staging in rectal cancer, which of the following is *incorrect*?

   (A) Stage I rectal cancer has 80–90% 5-year survival rate.
   (B) In stage II rectal cancer, the primary tumor has extended either through the muscularis propria or into the pericolic fat with possible local extension into other organs.
   (C) Metastatic nodal involvement in stage III rectal cancer is classified as either N1 or N2, describing the number of nodes positive for metastatic cancer in the pericolic or perirectal position.
   (D) Stage IV rectal cancer is limited to a T4 lesion with any local lymph node involvement and distant metastasis.
   (E) Stage II rectal carcinoma has a 62–76% 5-year survival rate.

17. A 60-year-old female presents on referral from her primary care physician with a history of rectal prolapse and occasional bloody stools. Colonoscopy reveals no masses but a solitary ulcer of the rectum was noted. Biopsy was negative for malignancy. Which of the treatments listed below is *incorrect*?

   (A) Solitary rectal ulcer syndrome is usually seen in women.
   (B) Etiology of solitary rectal ulcer is unknown but chronic constipation and fecal impaction may play a role.
   (C) Treatment of solitary rectal ulcer syndrome is straightforward.
   (D) Solitary rectal ulcer is often confused with inflammatory bowel disease, neoplastic disease, and villous adenoma.
   (E) Initial therapy with high-fiber diet and bowel management is helpful in many individuals.

18. All of the following have been used to evaluate disorders of defecation *except*:

   (A) anorectal manometry and EUS
   (B) radiologic studies such as plain films and fluoroscopy
   (C) defecography or evacuation proctography
   (D) bowel transit studies and biofeedback
   (E) all of the above can be used for evaluation

19. Comparing the anorectal manifestation of Crohn's disease and ulcerative colitis, which of the following is *incorrect*?

(A) Perianal disease is common in Crohn's disease.

(B) Perirectal fistulas occur frequently in ulcerative colitis.

(C) Ulcerative colitis attacks always involve the rectum.

(D) Bloody stools are less common in Crohn's disease than in ulcerative colitis.

(E) Granulomas are a common finding on rectal biopsy in Crohn's disease.

20. A 60-year-old male with hypertension is referred to you for evaluation of rectal bleeding. He has had bloody diarrhea on and off for 6 weeks. He has lost 20 lb in the past 6 months but has been dieting. Antidiarrhea drugs have caused him to have crampy abdominal pain. Colonoscopy reveals a 4 cm lesion at 10 cm from the anal verge. Which of the following is *appropriate* for initial evaluation?

(A) endoscopic biopsy for pathology from the edge of the mass

(B) resection the lesion with endoscopic snare

(C) injection with hypertonic saline or alcohol for ablation

(D) termination of colonoscopy as diagnosis has been made

(E) application of methylene blue on the surface of the mass for easy intraoperative identification

21. Biopsy results of the above lesion reveal a poorly differentiated adenocarcinoma. Which of the following is the most useful in preoperative workup and staging of the cancer?

(A) magnetic resonance imaging (MRI) of the abdomen and pelvis

(B) EUS examination

(C) grade of the cancer

(D) CT of the abdomen and pelvis

(E) all of the above are useful in workup and staging of rectal cancer

22. The preoperative staging of the above patient is completed with perirectal lymphadenopathy but no distal metastatic lesions. All of the following is appropriate to consider in operative planning *except*:

(A) body habitus, gender, and age

(B) comorbidities including cardiomyopathy, coronary artery disease, and obstructive pulmonary disease

(C) distance of the tumor from the anal verge

(D) metastatic disease

(E) all of the above are important in operative planning

23. A 64-year-old female presents at your office with complaints of bleeding hemorrhoids. She describes them as always falling out no matter how many times she replaces them manually. A full colonoscopy reveals no other source of bleeding. Physical examination reveals grade 3 hemorrhoids with redundant mucosal prolapse circumferentially. Which of the following options would be best for this patient?

(A) dietary modification with increasing fiber and water intake

(B) rubber band ligation to all the hemorrhoidal bundles

(C) infrared coagulation (IRC) to all the hemorrhoidal bundles

(D) circumferential hemorrhoidectomy with removal of all hemorrhoidal tissue

(E) a stapled procedure for both the prolapsed mucosa and hemorrhoidal bundles

24. Melanoma of the anal canal can be discovered incidentally in hemorrhoid specimens. Which of the following is *incorrect* regarding melanoma?

(A) The anal canal is the most common site of the development malignant melanoma of the alimentary tract.

(B) 0.2% of all melanomas occur in the anal canal.

(C) All melanoma-in-ani are characteristically pigmented.

(D) Although abdominoperineal resection has traditionally been the surgical procedure of choice for melanoma of the anal canal, wide local excision is gaining acceptance.

(E) Supplemental therapy with chemotherapy, radiotherapy, and immunotherapy has been of no consistent benefit for survival.

25. A 52-year-old male presents at your office with complaint of a lump in his anus. He has little physical mobility and is wheel chair bound from advanced arthritis. You attempt to examine him in the office but he is unable to tolerate the examination without physical discomfort. He denies any other symptoms of rectal bleeding or constipation. He has no other medical problems. Colonoscopy under conscious sedation was undertaken in the last year but the examination was incomplete. Completion barium enema was performed and read as normal. You schedule him for examination under anesthesia and excision of the lesion. Your initial physical examination reveals the following: (see Fig. 25-5). Anoscopy reveals a large skin tag with a grade 3 left lateral hemorrhoid (see Fig. 25-6). What is the next appropriate step?

(A) Biopsy the skin tag and perform IRC of the hemorrhoid.

(B) Band the hemorrhoid and leave the skin tag intact.

(C) Perform open or closed hemorrhoidectomy and resect the skin tag.

(D) Perform a stapled procedure for hemorrhoid and prolapse.

(E) Biopsy the skin tag and perform a lateral sphincterotomy.

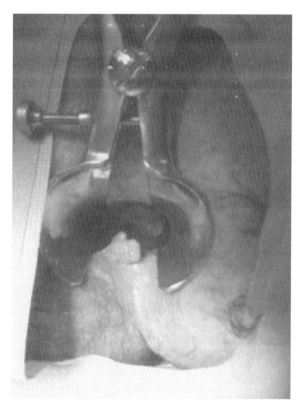

FIG. 25-6 Anoscopy discovers a large left lateral grade three hemorrhoid with the preexisting skin tag.

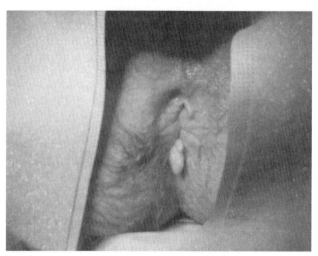

FIG. 25-5 Initial physical inspection of the perineum with a large sentinel skin tag.

26. Concerning local anesthesia and positioning for common anorectal procedures, which of the following is *false*?

(A) All procedure done in the prone jack-knife position must be done under general anesthesia.

(B) A perianal field block with bupivicaine and epinephrine is very effective at pain control and allows simple anorectal procedures to be done without general anesthesia.

(C) Prone jack-knife position is advantageous for anterior rectal lesions as well as for many anorectal procedures such as hemorrhoidectomy; high lithotomy is advantageous for posterior rectal lesions.

(D) Open or closed hemorrhoidectomy can be performed under spinal anesthesia as well as general anesthesia.

(E) Lateral sphincterotomy can be easily preformed with a perianal field block and conscious sedation.

Answers and Explanations

1. (C)

2. (A)

Explanations 1 and 2

Figure 25-1 reveals an anal fissure. The history of an acute anal fissure is usually sudden anal pain after defecation that might be described as a tearing sensation and minimal bright red bleeding. Chronic anal fissures present with a variable degree of pain, frequently along with symptoms of pruritis, a lump in the anal area, and drainage. The pain may cease shortly after the bowel movement but may persist for hours. If biopsied, the fissure will only show evidence of nonspecific inflammatory change and fibrosis through the internal sphincter; however, if a fissure appears atypical, is recurrent, or persistent, then biopsy of the edge of the fissure is appropriate. Examination in the office should be visual observation with the buttocks gently spread, as anoscopy may cause severe pain. The fissure consists as a crack, or split, in the lining of the anal canal that extends to various degrees up to the dentate line. The fissure may be heralded by a classic finding of a sentinel pile or skin tag (see Fig. 25-7) at the anal verge. Eighty to ninety percent of fissures are located in the posterior midline, 10–15% are located in the anterior midline, and 1–2% are located elsewhere. Women might present with anterior fissures because of laxity of the anterior external sphincter secondary to child bearing. Acute anal fissure can be successfully treated with conservative measures such as a high-fiber diet with 20–25 g of fiber intake a day, increasing nonalcoholic, noncaffeinated fluids to 64 oz a day, and application of topical nitrites. Topical trinitrate in glycerin can provide pain relief and relaxation of the internal sphincter. The patient should be instructed to wear gloves or finger cots as the topical nitrites can cause headache if systemically absorbed. Stool softeners and sitz baths

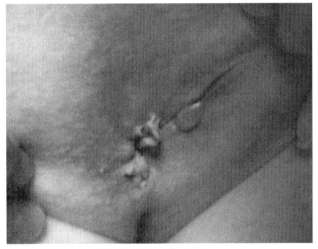

FIG. 25-7 Posterior skin tag.

can also provide some relief. A newer mode of anal fissure treatment is injection of botulinum toxin type A into the anal sphincter. The cost is high; however, the injection acts by blocking the release of acetylecholine at the presynaptic synapse and allowing the sphincter to relax out of spasm. The duration is usually 2 weeks, which may be enough time for the fissure to heal. Some transient incontinence has been reported.

If conservative measures fail, as with the patient in Question 1, the surgical procedure of choice is an open or closed lateral internal anal sphincterotomy. The internal sphincter has the involuntary action of maintaining the anal canal resting pressure. The internal sphincter may be partially divided without fear of significant incontinence if the external sphincter is spared. The open and closed methods are comparable and may be done under local in an outpatient setting. The distal one-third to one-half of the internal sphincter is divided.

Complications are minimal with anal fistula occurring in 1–2% and abscess in 2–3%. In the setting of refractory fissure or failure to heal, inflammatory bowel disease must be considered as well as adenocarcinoma causing atypical anal canal fissure and other malignancy such as basaloid or cloacogenic cancer. Biopsy would be appropriate with refractory of atypical fissures.

Anoscopy with dilation has no role in therapy because of the high rate of postoperative incontinence from 2 to 24% as the external fibers are also stretched. Incision and drainage with seton placement is indicated with a perirectal abscess with a transphincteric fistula. Fistulotomy with debridement should be considered in a superficial anal fistula.

Bibliography

Beck DE, Wexner SD. *Fundamentals of Anorectal Surgery*. London, UK: W.B. Saunders, 1998, 209–217.

Cohen AM, Sidney JW. *Cancer of the Colon, Rectum, and Anus*. New York, NY: McGraw-Hill, 1995, 1065.

Corman MI, Allison SI, Kuehne JP. *Handbook of Colon & Rectal Surgery*. Philadelphia, PA: Lippincott, Williams & Wilkins, 2002, 137–149.

3. **(B)** The patient in Question 2 has pruritis ani. Pruritis ani is a very common malady. Itching and burning is often the presenting complaint with reddened, irritated anoderm and surrounding skin on examination. Most patients are not found to have an associated anorectal pathology but contact dermatitis, yeast, diabetes, and pinworms (*Enterobius vermicularis*) have been associated with pruritis ani. Psoriasis of the anal verge must also be considered in the differential diagnosis. Certain foods such as cola, coffee, and tea have been suggested to promote pruritis. Reassurance of the patient that this is a manageable entity is paramount. Diphenhydramine may help with initial severe itching. No special studies have been helpful in the diagnosis although a lower threshold for internal sphincter relaxation has been observed in continence testing. Evaluation should consist of anoscopy and proctosigmoidoscopy to evaluate for local cause such as a draining fistula if suspicion is high. Most diagnosis is based on visual inspection. Conservative therapy with daily gentle cleansing, drying lightly with encouragement not to rub aggressively, and topical application of a mild-to-moderate potency corticosteroid alleviates symptoms in most cases. Hemorrhoidectomy can help with hygiene if prolapsed hemorrhoids are present on examination. Over-the-counter hemorrhoidal preparations are unlikely to help and may indeed worsen the condition if allergic dermatitis develops.

Biopsy will only reveal localized inflammation although skin scrapings can be used with a potassium hydroxide prep to evaluate for yeast. Wide local excision and colonic diversion have no place in the therapy for pruritis ani.

Bibliography

Cameron JL. *Current Surgical Therapy*, 7th ed. St. Louis, MO: Mosby, 2001, 295–297.

Corman MI, Allison SI, Kuehne JP. *Handbook of Colon & Rectal Surgery*. Philadelphia, PA: Lippincott, Williams & Wilkins, 2002, 302–307.

Gordon PH, Nivatvongs S. *Principles and Practice of Surgery for the Colon, Rectum and Anus*, 2nd ed. Quality Medical Publishing, 1999, 304–307.

4. **(C)** Anal canal carcinoma is by definition located in the area bounded inferiorly by the anal verge and proximal by the puborectalis muscle that is located approximately 2 cm above the dentate line. The anal canal is lined distally by nonhair bearing nonkeratanized, stratified squamous epithelium up to the dentate line. The 1.5–2 cm for proximal anal canal above the dentate line is first lined with cloacal (transitional) and then glandular mucosal. Cephalad to the proximal margin of the anal canal is the rectum proper. The rectum is lined with columnar mucosal. Lateral and caudad to the anal verge is the anal margin that is covered by keratinized, hair bearing, stratified squamous epithelium. Anal margin lesions are managed differently than anal canal lesions (see Question 8).

Anal canal cancer may present with nonspecific symptoms of difficulty with defecation, hematochezia, and different degrees of pain ranging from severe to minor discomfort. There frequently is a delay in diagnosis because of misdiagnosis with benign anal canal conditions such as hemorrhoids or fissures. Patients with persistent or unexplained complaints of pain, bleeding, tenesmus, or frequency should undergo a full perianal skin examination as well as anal canal, rectum, and perineum examination. The inguinal and femoral lymph nodes should be palpated for fullness or matting. A mass or fissure should be fully evaluated. A deep wedge biopsy or punch biopsy for more superficial lesion will be sufficient to make the diagnosis of cancer. Endoscopic ultrasound (EUS) is accurate for staging of anal canal carcinoma. Squamous cell carcinoma is the most common cancer of the anal canal.

Surgical therapy for anal canal carcinoma had historically been abdominal perineal resection with local recurrence rate of 50% and 5-year survival rates of approximately 40%. Dr. Norman Nigro from Wayne State University proposed a multimodality therapy for anal canal cancer, which is now considered standard of care with minimal modifications. Once the diagnosis of squamous cell carcinoma of the anal canal is made, the patient is treated with chemoradiation therapy using 5-fluorouracil (5-FU), mitomycin C, and pelvic irradiation of 5000 cGy. Followup anal biopsy 6–8 weeks after completion of therapy is frequently performed. If there is residual cancer, then second-line chemotherapy with completion radiation is initiated. Cisplatin is being evaluated as a second-line chemotherapeutic agent. A 90% complete response can be quoted with an 85% 5-year survival rate. Salvage abdominal perineal resection is offered only after second-line chemoradiation is failed with a long-term survival of 50%. Initial surgical resection might be adequate with very superficial well-differentiated squamous cell carcinoma that is confined above the submucosa.

Bibliography

Cameron JL. *Current Surgical Therapy*, 7th ed. St. Louis, MO: Mosby, 2001, 251–254.

Cohen AM, Sidney JW. *Cancer of the Colon, Rectum, and Anus.* New York, NY: McGraw-Hill, 1995, 1063–1071.

Corman MI, Allison SI, Kuehne JP. *Handbook of Colon & Rectal Surgery.* Philadelphia, PA: Lippincott, Williams & Wilkins, 2002, 574–591.

Feig BW, Berger DH, Fuhrman GM. *The M.D. Anderson Surgical Oncology Handbook*, 2nd ed. Philadelphia, PA: Lippincott, Williams & Wilkins, 1999, 212–217.

Gordon PH, Nivatvongs S. *Principles and Practice of Surgery for the Colon, Rectum and Anus*, 2nd ed. Quality Medical Publishing, 1999, 460–466.

5. **(C)** EUS provides an image of the sphincter mechanisms of the anus and the muscle and soft tissue of the rectum. The image is two dimensional and accurate. It can also be used in fecal continence evaluation and provides information with regard to complex fistulas, surveillance for anal cancers, and other congenital or acquired malformation of the rectum and anus. In a normal EUS there are five distinct layers of the anal canal or rectum. The inner most hyperechoic region is the mucosal surface, followed by the hypoechoic mucosal/muscularis mucosa. The next hyperechoic region is the submucosa, followed by the hypoechoic muscularis propria. The most distant hyperechoic region is the serosa or perirectal fat. EUS is widely used for staging of rectal cancers. EUS can predict lymph node involvement with an accuracy of 62–85%. Most incorrect staging is because of overstaging of a cancer. Experience in interpretation can increase accuracy. Pelvic CT is a poor predictor of depth in rectal cancer. Endoluminal magnetic resonance imaging and EUS have similar accuracy but EUS is far more cost-effective and accessible.

Bibliography

Beck DE, Wexner SD. *Fundamentals of Anorectal Surgery.* London, UK: W.B. Saunders; 1998, 286–290.

Cameron JL. *Current Surgical Therapy*, 7th ed. St. Louis, MO: Mosby, 2001, 236–237, 253–254, 299.

Corman MI, Allison SI, Kuehne JP. *Handbook of Colon & Rectal Surgery.* Philadelphia, PA: Lippincott, Williams & Wilkins, 2002, 478–479.

6. **(C)** Hemorrhoids are formed at an embryonic level as highly vascular cushions in the anal canal. They have been postulated to assist with anal continence. Hemorrhoids are usually referred to as pathologic once they prolapse or bleed. Squamous epithelial change and darkened mucosal may form with chronic symptoms. Hemorrhoids are designated external or internal depending on whether they originate above or below the dentate line.

External hemorrhoids are located distal to the dentate line. They are sensitive to pain and heat sensation and are of endodermal origin. Thrombosed external hemorrhoids may present with exquisite pain. Although conservative therapy is described, excision under local anesthesia may be indicated for acute thrombosed external hemorrhoids (see Table 25-1).

Internal hemorrhoids are further broken down into stage, grade, or degree—all describing degree of prolapse from 1 to 4, depending on the amount of prolapse. Table 25-1 describes the four stages of hemorrhoids with options for management.

All anal or rectal bleeding must be investigated to rule out cancer and other rectal and colonic lesions. Flexible sigmoidoscopy, colonoscopy, and barium enema are all methods of investigation on unanswered questions of etiology of lower gastrointestinal bleeding.

Bibliography

Gordon PH, Nivatvongs S. *Principles and Practice of Surgery for the Colon, Rectum and Anus*, 2nd ed. Quality Medical Publishing, 1999, 194–199.

Nyhus LM, Baker RJ, Fischer JE. *Mastery of Surgery*, 3rd ed. New York, NY: Little, Brown and Company, 1997, 1567–1573.

Sabiston DC Jr. *Textbook of Surgery*, 15th ed. Philadelphia, PA: W.B. Saunders, 1997, 1036–1038.

Schwartz SI. *Principles of Surgery*, 7th ed. New York, NY: McGraw-Hill, 1999, 1295–1298.

7. **(D)** Wide local excision is appropriate for most anal canal lesions. Aggressive initial surgical resection, such as abdominal perineal resection, has been found to have no survival benefit. Figure 25-8 demonstrates less than 3 cm anal canal mass biopsied as glandular carcinoma. Figure 25-9 is the wide-local excision specimen. Melanoma, carcinoid, and mucinous adenocarcinoma are often found incidentally with hemorrhoids on pathologic examination. The prognosis is often

TABLE 25-1 Four Stages of Internal Hemorrhoids and Thrombosed External with Options for Management

Stage, grade, degree	Signs and symptoms	Management
One	Small amounts of painless bleeding. No prolapse	Fully investigate other causes of bleeding. Increase dietary fiber to 20–25 g. Infrared coagulation. Rubber band ligation. Electrocautery
Two	Protrusion noticed with defecation-spontaneous reduction. Mild-to-moderate bleeding-blood streaked on stool.	Rubber band ligation. Infrared coagulation. Electrocautery
Three	Protrusion requiring manual reduction with defecation or straining. Mild-to-moderate bleeding-blood streaked on stool.	Rubber band ligation. Open or closed hemorrhoidectomy. Stapled procedure for hemorrhoids and prolapse.
Four	Irreducible and permanently prolapsed hemorrhoid. Mild-to-moderate bleeding-blood streaked on stool.	Open or closed hemorrhoidectomy.
Thrombosed external hemorrhoids	Exquisite tenderness. Edematous, grape-like, irreducible hemorrhoid.	Local anesthesia with lidocaine. Excision or conservative therapy

poor for melanoma and mucinous adenocarcinoma no matter what the surgical approach so wide local excision is the surgical treatment of choice, after biopsy, for local control. Carcinoid of the anal canal is rare and can be adequately treated with wide local excision for lesions less than 2 cm. Squamous cell carcinoma is the most common cancer of the anal canal. They are usually associated with chronic human papilloma virus. Squamous cell carcinoma of the anal canal should be treated in accordance to the Nigro protocol

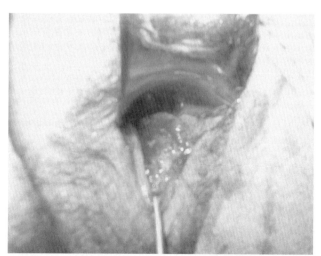

FIG. 25-8 A 2.5 cm anal canal lesion.

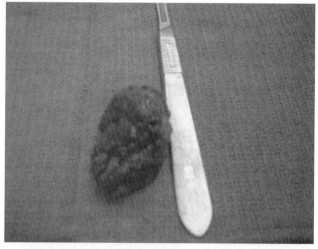

FIG. 25-9 The excised 2.5 cm anal canal lesion from Fig. 25-8.

TABLE 25-2 Physiologic and Embryonic Differences between the Anal Canal and the Rectum

	Anal canal	Rectum
Embryonic origin	Ectoderm	Endoderm
Pain/sensation	Sensitive to pain	Insensitive to pain
Cell type	Squamous epithelium	Glandular mucosa
Venous drainage	Systemic	Portal
Lymphatic drainage	Inguinal lymph nodes	Superior hemorrhoidal followed by paraaortic lymph nodes
Most common neoplasm	Squamous cell carcinoma	Adenocarcinoma

(see Question 4). Squamous cell carcinoma of the anal canal has over a 90% cure rate with initial chemoradiation treatment; abdominal perineal resection is only indicated for failure of second-line salvage chemotherapy. Condyloma of the anal canal should be fulgurated with electrocautery or bipolar cautery leaving the anoderm intact. Wide local excision of condyloma in the anal canal is unnecessary and carries a risk of anal stricture.

Bibliography

Cameron JL. *Current Surgical Therapy*, 7th ed. St. Louis, MO: Mosby, 2001, 251–255.

Cohen AM, Sidney JW. *Cancer of the Colon, Rectum, and Anus*. New York, NY: McGraw-Hill, 1995, 1023–1024.

Corman MI, Allison SI, Kuehne JP. *Handbook of Colon & Rectal Surgery*. Philadelphia, PA: Lippincott, Williams & Wilkins, 2002, 349–353.

8. **(E)** The anal margin lesions listed above have distinctly different pathologic findings but wide local excision can be used for adequate surgical resection.

    Melanoma of the anal margin is found on incidental hemorrhoidectomy at times. Bleeding is the overwhelming presenting complaint in 66% of patients with perianal melanoma. The anal margin melanoma may present as a small benign-looking grapelike growth. As anal margin melanoma has a very poor prognosis with only a 10–20% survival at 5 years, abdominal perineal resection has not been found to improve survival, thus, wide local excision of perianal melanoma is the standard of care. Perianal Bowen's disease is uncommon with very few cases reported to date. Bowen's disease is an intraepithelial squamous cell carcinoma *in situ*. Bowen's perianal disease can present with symptoms such as burning, itching, and bleeding. The lesions appear eczematous with scaly and crusted plaques. Wide local excision is the surgical treatment of choice. Perianal Paget's disease is a rare adenocarcinoma believed to come from apocrine cells. Noninvasive Paget's can adequately be treated with wide local excision. Basal cell carcinoma of the anal margin is a very rare entity consisting of less than 0.2% of anal margin cancers and can be adequately treated with wide local excision.

Bibliography

Beck DE, Wexner SD. *Fundamentals of Anorectal Surgery*. London, UK: W.B. Saunders, 1998, 270–274.

Cohen AM, Sidney JW. *Cancer of the Colon, Rectum, and Anus*. New York, NY: McGraw-Hill, 1995, 1007–1011.

Corman MI, Allison SI, Kuehne JP. *Handbook of Colon & Rectal Surgery*. Philadelphia, PA: Lippincott, Williams & Wilkins, 2002, 588–591, 362–368.

9. **(C)** The anal canal and the rectum have very different embryologic origin, innervation, lymphatic, and venous drainage. Table 25-2 reviews the difference in the anal canal and the rectum. The anal canal is located below the dentate line and is ectodermal in origin. The anal canal is very sensitive to pain and accounts for complaints of pain with thrombosed external hemorrhoids. The lining of the anus is squamous epithelium. The venous drainage of the anal canal is systemic and the primary lymphatic basin is inguinal. The most common neoplasm is squamous cell carcinoma. The distal rectum is located above the dentate line. There are no sharp pain receptors in the rectum although stretch is felt. The rectum is lined with glandular mucosa. The venous drainage of the rectum is via the portal system. The rectal lymphatics drain into the superior hemorrhoidal lymph node basin and then to the paraaortic lymph nodes. Adenocarcinoma is the most common neoplasia of the rectum.

Bibliography

Corman MI, Allison SI, Kuehne JP. *Handbook of Colon & Rectal Surgery*. Philadelphia, PA: Lippincott, Williams & Wilkins, 2002, 1–13.

Feig BW, Berger DH, Fuhrman GM. *The M.D. Anderson Surgical Oncology Handbook*, 2nd ed. Philadelphia, PA: Lippincott, Williams & Wilkins, 1999, 212–217, 185–191.

Gordon PH, Nivatvongs S. *Principles and Practice of Surgery for the Colon, Rectum and Anus*, 2nd ed. Quality Medical Publishing, 1999, 29–33.

10. **(A)** Perirectal (or perianal) abscess is the most common type of anorectal abscess accounting for 40–45% of cases reported. The black arrow in Fig. 25-3 reveals chronic external fistula with surrounding erythema. Physical examination reveals fluctuance around the fistula in this case. The patient usually complains of pain and fevers, and examination can reveal fluctuance, erythema, and cellulitis. Erythema may also be present without fluctuance; however, more often than not, an abscess is still present and incision and drainage is still required for treatment. If there is question of abscess, the erythematous or indurated may be needle aspirated under local anesthesia. Etiology of perirectal abscess and fistula has been theorized to be related to infected anal crypts. Perirectal abscess is also seen with some frequency in patients with HIV and Crohn's disease. Anorectal abscesses can be perirectal (perianal), ischiorectal, postanal, intersphincteric, and supralevator. Superficial perianal abscesses can usually be incised and drained under local anesthesia as an office procedure. A small gauze wick should be inserted initially. Postprocedure care should include frequent sitz baths and good hygiene. Antibiotics are usually unnecessary unless there is excessive cellulitis with fevers and leukocytosis in an immunocompromised patient. More complex anorectal abscesses may require general or spinal anesthesia for patient comfort and adequate exposure. Perianal abscess is often seen in patients with leukemia, lymphoma, and granulocytopenia representing up to 8% of hematology admissions. The usual presenting complaint is that of pain but fever, septicemia, and shock might also be present in a leucopenic patient. Fluctuance and pus may not be present. These patients are managed medically initially with antibiotic therapy and sitz baths until the hematologic disease can be better controlled. Fulminant sepsis, poor wound healing, and higher mortality rate can occur if operative intervention is undertaken without first initializing supportive therapy. However, operative intervention might be required for persistent abscess without resolution of symptoms with medical management.

Bibliography

Beck DE, Wexner SD. *Fundamentals of Anorectal Surgery.* London, UK: W.B. Saunders, 1998, 153–161.

Cameron JL. *Current Surgical Therapy*, 7th ed. St. Louis, MO: Mosby, 2001, 284–286.

Corman MI, Allison SI, Kuehne JP. *Handbook of Colon & Rectal Surgery.* Philadelphia, PA: Lippincott, Williams & Wilkins, 2002, 150–160.

11. **(D)**

12. **(D)**

Explanations 11 and 12

Perianal abscess and fistula-in-ano can occur synchronously in many cases. Patients who return with recurrent abscess after frequent incision and drainage require an examination under anesthesia for possible fistula.

Figure 25-4 reveals a transphincteric fistula that extends radially from an opening just anterior to the transverse line. Goodsall's rule describes the common characteristics of the fistula-in-ano tract: when the external opening of the fistula tract lies anterior to the transverse plane, the opening tends to be located radially. When the external opening lies posterior to the transverse plane, the internal opening is usually located in the posterior midline. Exceptions to the rule can occur, so rigorous evaluation of the anal canal for the internal opening is paramount. Vigorous probing can create fistula and should be discouraged.

The internal opening of the fistula tract can be difficult to identify and might require injection of hydrogen peroxide into the external tract to visualize the internal opening. A hypodermic syringe is filled with 3% hydrogen peroxide and a 20 gauge soft angiocatheter without the needle trocar is attached to the syringe. The external opening of the fistula is cannulized with the angiocatheter and the hypodermic is gently compressed while the retracted anal canal is being closely scrutinized for evidence of bubbling out of the internal opening. Other methods such as milk and dye have been used with less than optimal results. Fistula can be classified as intersphincteric, transphincteric, suprasphincteric, extraspincteric (trauma), and horseshoe.

Intersphincteric fistula can usually be treated with fistulotomy if superficial. More complex fistula including transphincteric might require seton placement for preservation of the external and internal sphincter complex. Figure 25-10 reveals a deep transphincteric fistula involving a significant amount of internal and external sphincter muscle. A black arrow is pointing to a vessel loop that has been passed through the fistula tract after exposing the internal and external opening. The skin was opened and the superficial portion of the tract debrided. The seton will be tightened at weekly intervals until the fistula tract has healed with preservation of the muscle complex.

Other options for treatment of deep fistulas include usage of an anorectal advancement flap to close the internal opening. Fig. 25-11 shows a completed anorectal advancement flap fully covering the internal opening of a chronic fistula. A lone-star

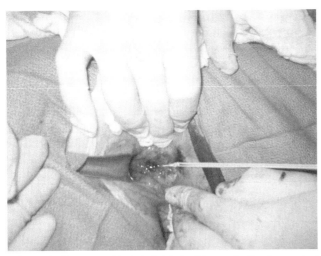

FIG. 25-10 Deep transphincteric fistula involving a significant amount of internal and external sphincter muscle.

retractor is ideal for exposure in reconstructive anal surgery.

Horseshoe fistula tunnel through extensive soft tissue and require multiple small incisions and packing to preserve soft tissue. This approach will decrease the morbidity associated with a large perianal wound that would result if the entire fistula were opened in entirety. A deep posterior anal abscess in association with the fistula must be opened, the granulation tissue must be debrided, and the area must be drained.

Bibliography

Beck DE, Wexner SD. *Fundamentals of Anorectal Surgery.* London, UK: W.B. Saunders, 1998, 161–170.

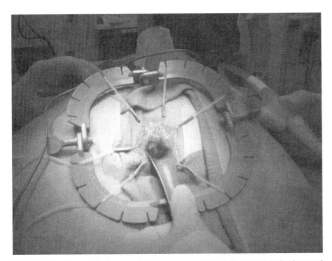

FIG. 25-11 Completed anorectal advancement flap fully covering the internal opening of a chronic fistula.

Cameron JL. *Current Surgical Therapy,* 7th ed. St. Louis, MO: Mosby, 2001, 284–289.
Corman MI, Allison SI, Kuehne JP. *Handbook of Colon & Rectal Surgery.* Philadelphia, PA: Lippincott, Williams & Wilkins, 2002, 161–183.

13. **(D)** Rectovaginal fistula most often occurs following trauma, including obstetric injury with up to 5% third and fourth degree laceration. Inflammatory bowel disease is the second most common cause. Other well-known causes include foreign body, radiation, infectious processes, diverticulitis, carcinoma, congenital, or any type of pelvic, perineal, and rectal surgery. The fistula can be described as low or high rectal depending on the location of the rectal opening. Anovaginal fistulas can also be observed. Low rectovaginal fistulas usually are identified on physical examination. A midlevel or high rectovaginal fistulas might be hard to identify. A barium enema could possibly assist with identification of the fistula if unable to readily see the internal vaginal opening. Other options include a methylene blue retention enema with endovaginal tampon in place. After an hour the tampon is removed and inspected for blue coloring. A fistulogram might assist in identifying the segment of bowel involved. Inspection of the proximal colon should be strongly considered before deciding on therapy.

Repair of high rectovaginal fistulas is approached transabdominally. The bowel involved is resected or repaired (for obstetrical injury) and a piece of omentum or fascia is interposed between the repair and the vaginal wall. Low rectovaginal fistulas can be approached either transvaginally in layers with a vaginal flap, transanally with an endorectal advancement flap, or perineal. Fistulotomy alone should be avoided, as there is usually a degree of full-thickness muscle involved which could cause some incontinence Fibrin glue alone has not been effective in long-term treatment of rectovaginal fistula.

Bibliography

Cameron JL. *Current Surgical Therapy,* 7th ed. St. Louis, MO: Mosby, 2001, 301–306.
Corman MI, Allison SI, Kuehne JP. *Handbook of Colon & Rectal Surgery.* Philadelphia, PA: Lippincott, Williams & Wilkins, 2002, 184–189.
Gordon PH, Nivatvongs S. *Principles and Practice of Surgery for the Colon, Rectum and Anus,* 2nd ed. Quality Medical Publishing, 1999, 401–420.

14. **(C)** Anal canal cancer is staged differently than rectal cancer. The TNM classification is outlined in Table 25-3 and the stage groups in Table 25-4. Stage I anal canal cancer is a small lesion less than 2 cm without regional nodal involvement or distant metastatic disease. Stage

TABLE 25-3   TMN Staging System for Anal Canal Cancers

T1	Tumor less then 2 cm
T2	Tumor 2–5 cm
T3	Tumor greater the 5 cm
N0	Tumor not involved with regional lymph nodes
N1	Tumor involvement of regional lymph nodes
M0	No distant metastasis
M1	Distant metastasis

II anal canal cancer is any lesion between 2 and 5 cm without nodal involvement or distant metastatic disease. Stage III anal canal is any size lesion with regional lymph node involvement and no distant metastasis. Stage IV disease is any size lesion with or without regional lymph node involvement in the presence of distant metastasis. The liver is the most common site of distant metastasis. The average survival for a patient who presents with liver metastasis is 9 months. Squamous cell (or epidermoid) carcinoma makes up the majority of the anal canal cancers followed by transitional (cloacogenic) cell and adenocarcinoma. Melanoma occurs in 0.5% of all tumors of the anorectum. Stage I–III squamous cell carcinoma has reported 5-year survival rates approaching 85% if treated with combination chemoradiation, even with locally advanced disease.

Bibliography

Cohen AM, Sidney JW. *Cancer of the Colon, Rectum, and Anus.* New York, NY: McGraw-Hill, 1995, 1069–1071.

Feig BW, Berger DH, Fuhrman GM. *The M.D. Anderson Surgical Oncology Handbook*, 2nd ed. Philadelphia, PA: Lippincott, Williams & Wilkins, 1999, 212–217.

Schwartz SI. *Principles of Surgery*, 7th ed. New York, NY: McGraw-Hill, 1999, 1375–1376.

15. **(C)** Anorectal manometry is a valuable tool in the complicated diagnosis and treatment of fecal incontinence. It is difficult to get an actual number measuring the extent of anal incontinence but is appears to have an incidence of 2.2%. Most are women over the age of 65; however, etiology can include surgical, obstetrical, congenital anomalies, colorectal disease, and neurologic conditions. Fistula surgery and internal anal sphincterotomy can cause partial fecal incontinence as

Table 25-4   Staging Groups Anal Canal Cancer

	TMN
Stage 1	T1N0M0
Stage 2	T2N0M0, T3N0M0
Stage 3	Any T, N1, M0
Stage 4	Any T, any N, M1

well as hemorrhoidal surgery. Understanding the mechanisms of the internal sphincter and the external sphincter is paramount to being able to diagnose and treat anal incontinence. The internal sphincter is composed of smooth muscle and is a continuation of the circular muscle of the rectum. The internal sphincter stays at near-maximal contraction at all times and relaxes in response to rectal distention. The external anal sphincter is composed of striated muscle and enables voluntary contraction. The response of the external sphincter to stimuli is contraction. The external sphincter must have voluntary inhibition of contraction. Anorectal manometry can be accomplished by any of the following methods including, macro and micro balloons, open or closed catheters. There is no universally accepted method for collecting and analyzing data. Only a physician that had been trained to perform and interpret the results should evaluate the data obtained. Anorectal manometry, when used in conjunction with the balloon expulsion test or photodefecography, is useful in evaluation of anorectal dysfunction including anorectal sensation, rectal compliance, and assessment of anal muscle tone. Slow waves, ultraslow waves, and intermediate waveforms might be obtained during testing.

Bibliography

Beck DE, Wexner SD. *Fundamentals of Anorectal Surgery.* London, UK: W.B. Saunders, 1998, 37–40.

Cameron JL. *Current Surgical Therapy*, 7th ed. St. Louis, MO: Mosby, 2001, 209, 261.

Corman MI, Allison SI, Kuehne JP. *Handbook of Colon & Rectal Surgery.* Philadelphia, PA: Lippincott, Williams & Wilkins, 2002, 65–68, 193–208.

16. **(D)** Colon and rectal cancer comprise 13% of all cancers in the United States. Rectal cancer is staged in accordance to guidelines for colon cancer with the TNM staging. Table 25-5 is a review of the TMN staging system. Rectal cancer presents most commonly with bleeding (35–40%). Diarrhea, change in bowel habits, rectal mass, and abdominal pain has also been reported at presentation. Biopsy is mandatory and is usually done at diagnosis of the lesion. The histology of the cancer is primarily adenocarcinoma. Surgical treatment of carcinoma of the rectum could include abdominal perineal resection, LAR, transanal excision, colostomy or ileostomy, and many other procedures depending on the stage of the lesion at diagnosis including presence of metastatic disease. Preoperative staging includes physical examination of the rectum and perineum, EUS to evaluate for regional lymphadenopathy and depth of tumor invasion, and computed tomography of the abdomen and pelvis to evaluate for metastatic disease. Table 25-6 outlines the

TABLE 25-5 TMN Classification for Rectal Cancer

Primary tumor (T)	T1	Tumor invades the submucosa
	T2	Tumor invades the muscularis propria
	T3	Tumor invades through the muscularis propria into the subserosa or nonperitonealized or perirectal tissues
	T4	Tumor perforates through the rectal wall and directly invades other structure
Lymph nodes (N)	N1	Metastasis in 1–3 perirectal lymph nodes
	N2	Metastasis in 4 or more perirectal lymph nodes
	N3	Metastasis in any lymph node along a named vascular trunk
Distant metastasis	MX	Presence of metastasis cannot be assessed
	M0	No distant metastasis
	M1	Distant metastasis present

current guidelines for staging. Dukes classification is still used by some physicians and correlates closely to the TNM staging. Stage I rectal cancer has an 80–90% 5-year survival rate. Stage II rectal cancer has a 62–76% 5-year survival rate. Stage III rectal cancer has a 30–40% 5-year survival rate followed by stage IV at 4–7% 5-year survival rate. Stage IV rectal cancer can involve any T lesion with local lymph node involvement and distant metastasis.

Bibliography

Cameron JL. *Current Surgical Therapy*, 7th ed. St. Louis, MO: Mosby, 2001, 235–239.

Cohen AM, Sidney JW. *Cancer of the Colon, Rectum, and Anus.* New York, NY: McGraw-Hill, 1995, 521–529.

Feig BW, Berger DH, Fuhrman GM. *The M.D. Anderson Surgical Oncology Handbook*, 2nd ed. Philadelphia, PA: Lippincott, Williams & Wilkins, 1999, 185–188.

Sabiston DC Jr. *Textbook of Surgery*, 15th ed. Philadelphia, PA: W.B. Saunders, 1997, 1028–1029.

TABLE 25-6 Current for Rectal Cancer Staging Guidelines

Staging rectal cancer	TNM	Dukes
Stage 1	T1-2, N0, M0	A
Stage 2	T3-4, N0, M0	B
Stage 3	Any T, N1-3, M0	C
Stage 4	Any T, 16 any N, M1	

17. (C) Solitary rectal ulcer syndrome is often confused with inflammatory bowel disease, neoplastic lesions, or polypoid disease. Symptoms can include constipation or diarrhea, rectal bleeding, or prolapse. The ulcer itself can be solitary or multiple. The ulcer is usually found on the anterior wall of the rectum at 6–8 cm. The ulcer can have induration with reddened, injected edges. The cause is unknown but is thought to be associated with chronic constipation and fecal impaction. On biopsy, there is microscopic replacement of normal lamina propria with fibroblast, but this also can be variable. Microscopic changes can be consistent with some inflammatory bowel findings such as mucosal thickening and inflammatory reaction of the submucosa. Management is not straightforward. Conservative therapy such as a high-fiber diet and increase in water intake should be initiated. Hydrocortisone enemas may be tried. Treatment of rectal prolapse may have some benefit. Excision with colostomy should be reserved for refractory massive bleeding. Close surveillance is a must for pathologic change.

Bibliography

Corman MI, Allison SI, Kuehne JP. *Handbook of Colon & Rectal Surgery.* Philadelphia, PA: Lippincott, Williams & Wilkins, 2002, 253–255.

Gordon PH, Nivatvongs S. *Principles and Practice of Surgery for the Colon, Rectum and Anus*, 2nd ed. Quality Medical Publishing, 1999, 1403–1408.

18. (E) Disorders of defecation present a source of social embarrassment and create hygiene issues for many patients. A fully functional colorectal physiology lab can perform anorectal manometry and EAUS to document the presence of muscular and sensory deficits, document sphincter function, and assist with the evaluation of constipation and diarrhea. Defecography or voiding proctography is performed to evaluate pelvic floor dysfunction. Defecography is performed in the sitting position with a double contrast barium and barium paste to outline the anus under fluoroscopy. Bowel transit studies are used to evaluate for severe constipation. The patient is given a single capsule containing 24 radiopaque rings and abdominal x-rays are taken on day 3 and 5 to evaluate transit time. If 80% of the markers are eliminated by the fifth day, the test is normal. EUS can identify sphincter anomalies that could be contributing to the incontinence. Biofeedback is also a very effective tool for those patients with adequate but weak voluntary external sphincter squeeze.

Bibliography

Corman MI, Allison SI, Kuehne JP. *Handbook of Colon & Rectal Surgery.* Philadelphia, PA: Lippincott, Williams & Wilkins, 2002, 63–76.

Gordon PH, Nivatvongs S. *Principles and Practice of Surgery for the Colon, Rectum and Anus*, 2nd ed. Quality Medical Publishing, 1999, 79–80, 371–376.

19. **(B)** The anorectal manifestations of Crohn's disease and ulcerative colitis are used for definitive diagnosis in some cases. Seventy-five percent of patients with Crohn's disease have associated anal disease including fissures and fistulas with sparing of the rectum. Bleeding is rare with Crohn's disease. Biopsy of a recurrent fissure or fistula will show granulomas in up to 20% of patients with Crohn's disease. Patients with ulcerative colitis always have rectal involvement from the anal verge cephalad to the proximal margin. Bleeding is very common with ulcerative colitis and may be refractory to steroid enemas and 5-ASA product. Fistula formation does not occur in association with ulcerative colitis.

Bibliography

Corman MI, Allison SI, Kuehne JP. *Handbook of Colon & Rectal Surgery*. Philadelphia, PA: Lippincott, Williams & Wilkins, 2002, 706–709.

Gordon PH, Nivatvongs S. *Principles and Practice of Surgery for the Colon, Rectum and Anus*, 2nd ed. Quality Medical Publishing, 1999, 950–956.

Sabiston DC Jr. *Textbook of Surgery*, 15th ed. Philadelphia, PA: W.B. Saunders, 1997, 926, 928, 1006–1007.

20. **(A)**

21. **(E)**

22. **(E)**

Explanations 20 through 22

The patient in Question 20 is presenting with common symptoms found in rectal cancer. Bleeding is the most common complaint followed by diarrhea or constipation, and abdominal pain. Any patient who presents with unknown etiology of rectal bleeding should undergo a colonoscopy or flexible sigmoidoscopy with completion barium enema. If a lesion is too large, usually greater than 2 cm, to be completely removed by snaring, a biopsy should be obtained. Tattooing the lesion with methylene blue should not be necessary in low-lying rectal carcinoma. A complete colonoscopy should always be performed, if possible, to evaluate for other polyps or masses.

Once the diagnosis of poorly differentiated adenocarcinoma has been made, staging of the cancer should take place. Local recurrence of aggressive poorly differentiated tumors is much greater than with well differentiated. Thorough physical examination with digital examination of the rectum, careful palpation of the perineum for nodal involvement, as well as complete cardiac and respiratory examinations should be performed. EUS is very sensitive and specific (>90%) for bowel wall involvement. Lymph node involvement is detected with EUS with a specificity of approximately 85%. CT of the abdomen and pelvis is useful in identifying metastatic disease, however, is not especially useful in gauging depth of disease. Abdominal and pelvic MRI have not been shown to be superior to CT scan at this time in staging of rectal cancer but are starting to gain popularity when EUS is not readily available.

Low-lying carcinoma of the rectum has always been a point of discussion among surgeons. LAR can often be safely performed with lesions near 8 cm and above. Newer data supports the use of LAR for most rectal lesions except the ones invading or located at the internal and external sphincter where a 2 cm distal margin is unobtainable. Total mesorectal excision is paramount when performing a LAR as failure to excise the mesorectum can lead to local failure by leaving gross or microscopic residual disease.

Abdominal perineal resection is reserved for those cancers that are near the anal verge, or used at the surgeons discretion. Superficial T1 lesions may be adequately excised with transanal excision.

The presence of metastatic disease at diagnosis can lead to excision with colostomy or a Hartmans resection, or simple transanal excision for low-lying rectal cancers for local control of bleeding.

Operative planning should include evaluation of body habitus, gender, and age. The narrow male pelvis may be difficult to maneuver with bulky tumors to perform a complete mesorectal excision.

Comorbidities such as severe coronary or lung disease might affect decision making regarding the extent of resection needed versus the operative time and blood loss encountered. Optimization of heart and lung function preoperatively should be accomplished.

Adjuvant therapy with 5-FU-based chemotherapy and radiotherapy to the pelvis is given with the goal of decreasing the chance of distant failure (metastatic disease) and improving local control. Neoadjuvant radiation therapy is being studied for treatment in reduction of tumor size preoperatively or in decreasing risk of local recurrence.

Bibliography

Cameron JL. *Current Surgical Therapy*, 7th ed. St. Louis, MO: Mosby, 2001, 246–250, 236–243.

Cohen AM, Sidney JW. *Cancer of the Colon, Rectum, and Anus*. New York, NY: McGraw-Hill, 1995, 561–569.

Corman MI, Allison SI, Kuehne JP. *Handbook of Colon & Rectal Surgery*. Philadelphia, PA: Lippincott, Williams & Wilkins, 2002, 518–521, 568–573.

Feig BW, Berger DH, Fuhrman GM. *The M.D. Anderson Surgical Oncology Handbook*, 2nd ed. Philadelphia, PA: Lippincott, Williams & Wilkins, 1999, 202–209.

Wexner SD, Rotholtz, NA. Surgeon influenced variables in resectional cancer surgery. *Dis Colon Rectum* 2000; 43(11): 1606–1627.

23. (E) Dietary modification with increasing dietary fiber intake and water intake is useful in controlling symptoms of stage 1 and 2 hemorrhoids.

Rubber band ligation has been described with great success in stage 1 and 2 hemorrhoids and some select grade 3 hemorrhoids that have no external component. It is a relatively painless procedure that can be accomplished in an outpatient setting. Patients need to be cautioned about signs of impending pelvic sepsis such as urinary retention, fever, and worsening pain. If any of these symptoms occur, immediate follow-up in the emergency room needs to be undertaken. Figure 25-12 demonstrates two rubber banding devices with a long handled fine-toothed grasper. The hemorrhoid is grasped with the long handled grasper and the rubber banding device is passed over the hemorrhoid and two or three rubber bands are placed at the neck of the hemorrhoid. The patient should not experience any pain, but may complain of some transient "pressure" or rectal fullness. If the band causes significant pain, the hemorrhoid is probably below the denate line and should not be banded.

IRC with repeated applications up to three to four times per hemorrhoidal bundle has been reported successfully with stage 1 and 2 hemorrhoids. IRC has not been shown to be effective for large prolasping circumferential hemorrhoids. The anoscope is inserted gently to better visualize the hemorrhoid. The

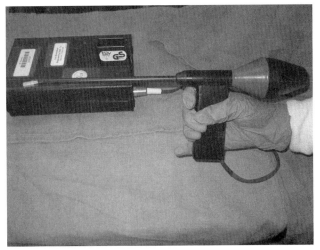

FIG. 25-13   Infrared coagulation device (IRC).

IRC is grasped and the tip is gently touched to the base of the hemorrhoid while depressing the trigger (see Fig. 25-13). The contact should be for 1–2 s.

Open or closed hemorrhoidectomy is indicated for grade 3 and 4 hemorrhoids. Grade 3 hemorrhoids with advanced mucosal prolapse might be better served with a stapled procedure to treat the prolase and the hemorrhoids. There are commercially available stapling systems for the treatment of prolapse and hemorrhoids. Figure 25-14 demonstrates a patient in prone jack-knife position with the surgeon and assistant holding out grade 3 hemorrhoids in the classical three quadrants of left lateral, right anterior, and right posterior. Figure 25-15 reveals the anal dilator that is sutured into place to attain stability.

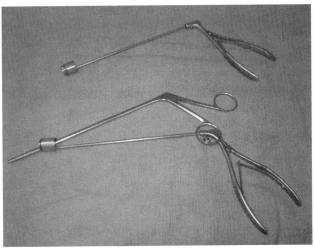

FIG. 25-12   Rubber banding devices.

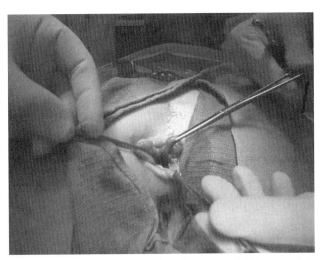

FIG. 25-14   Patient in prone jack-knife position with grade 3 hemorrhoids in the classical 3 quadrants: left lateral; right anterior; right posterior.

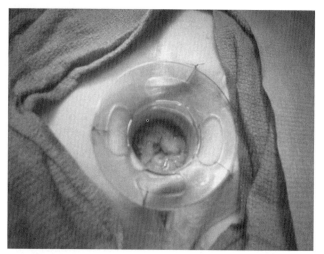

FIG. 25-15   Anal dilator being sutured into place to attain stability.

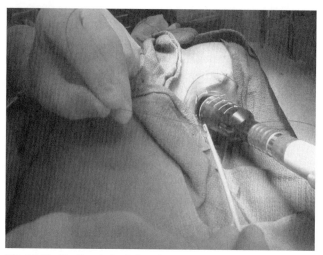

FIG. 25-17   Stapling device being placed with the pursestring pulled taut through the sides of the stapler.

The redundant prolapsed anal tissue is evident. Figure 25-16 demonstrates a nonabsorbable suture pursestring being placed 4 cm from the dentate line. Figure 25-17 demonstrates the stapling device being placed with the pursestring pulled taunt through the sides of the stapler. The tissue donuts are inspected for completion in Fig. 25-18. These patients do well and most go home after surgery as an outpatient.

Bibliography

Cameron JL. *Current Surgical Therapy*, 7th ed. St. Louis, MO: Mosby, 2001, 272–280.

Chung CC, Ha JP, Li MK, et al. Double-blind, randomized trial comparing harmonic scalpel ™ hemorrhoidectomy, bipolar scissors hemorrhoidectomy, and scissors excision:ligation technique. *Dis Colon Rectum* 2002; 45(6): 789–794.

Fleshman J. Advanced technology in the management of hemorrhoids: stapling, laser, harmonic scalpel, and ligasure. 2001 Consensus conference on benign anorectal disease. *J Gastrointest Surg* 2002;6(3):299–301.

Nyhus LM, Baker RJ, Fischer JE. *Mastery of Surgery*, 3rd ed. New York, NY: Little, Brown and Company, 1997, 1567–1573.

Sabiston DC Jr. *Textbook of Surgery*, 15th ed. Philadelphia, PA: W.B. Saunders, 1997, 1036–1038.

Schwartz SI. *Principles of Surgery*, 7th ed. New York, NY: McGraw-Hill, 1999, 1295–1298.

24. **(C)** Anal canal melanoma is the most common alimentary tract melanoma but is extremely rare accounting for 0.2% of all melanoma and 0.5% of all anorectal

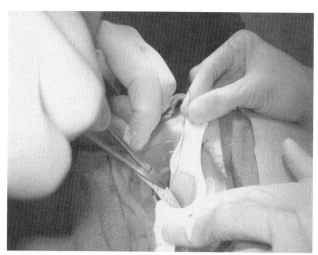

FIG. 25-16   A non-absorbable purse string suture pursestring being placed 4 cm from the dentate line.

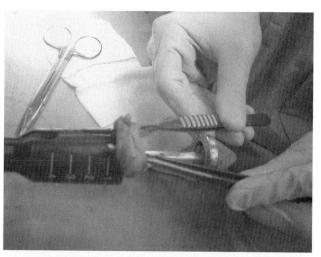

FIG. 25-18   Tissue donuts being inspected for completion.

tumors. Rectal bleeding is the most common complaint. One-tenth of patients with anorectal melenoma will have diagnosis on pathologic review of a hemorrhoid specimen. The melenoma may appear hemorrhoid-like or range from a deeply pigmented lesion to an amelanotic lesion. About 29% of anorectal melenoma are a melanotic.

Anorectal melanoma is rare but has a grim 5-year survival rate of less than 10% with most patients presenting with systemic metastatic disease and/or deeply invasive tumors. Abdominal perineal resection has been the classic treatment for anorectal melanoma; however, no real survival benefit has been proven versus wide local excision. Chemotherapy, radiotherapy, and immunotherapy are still being evaluated but also offer no consistent benefit for survival.

Bibliography

Bullard KM, Tuttle TM, Spenser MP. Surgical therapy for anorectal melanoma. *J Am Coll Surg* 2003;96(2):206–208.

Corman MI, Allison SI, Kuehne JP. *Handbook of Colon & Rectal Surgery*. Philadelphia, PA: Lippincott, Williams & Wilkins, 2002, 588–591.

25. **(C)** This patient is suffering from a grade 3 left lateral prolapsed hemorrhoid and has an incidental skin tag found on examination. A single quadrant symptomatic prolapsed hemorrhoid is amendable to either open or closed hemorrhoidectomy. Open hemorrhoidectomy with the harmonic scalpel or traditional closed hemorrhoidectomy should effectively treat the grade 3 hemorrhoid. The skin tag should be resected as it may cause symptoms postoperative that could be confusing to the patient and sent to pathology. A stapled procedure for prolapse and hemorrhoids would also be effective but is usually reserved for three quadrant prolapsed grade 3 or advancing grade 2 hemorrhoids and would not address the large redundant skin tag. Banding might also be an option but this hemorrhoid appears to have an external component also, and banding would not address the skin tag. IRC is not appropriate for grade 3 prolapsed hemorrhoids. Lateral sphincterotomy would not be appropriate as there is no evidence of an anal fissure.

Bibliography

Corman MI, Allison SI, Kuehne JP. *Handbook of Colon & Rectal Surgery*. Philadelphia, PA: Lippincott, Williams & Wilkins, 2002, 106–107.

Gordon PH, Nivatvongs S. *Principles and Practice of Surgery for the Colon, Rectum and Anus*, 2nd ed. Quality Medical Publishing, 1999, 193–206.

Khan S, Pawlak SE, Margolin DA, et al. Surgical treatment of hemorrhoids: prospective, randomized trial comparing closed excisional hemorrhoidectomy and the harmonic scalpel technique of excisional hemorrhoidectomy. *Dis Colon Rectum* 2001;44 (6):845–849.

26. **(A)** The inverted prone jack-knife position is extensively used in the United States for anorectal procedures. The exposure is unparalleled for many procedures such as hemorrhoidectomy, lateral internal sphincterotomy, and wide local excision of anal lesions. Both anterior and posterior anal and low rectal lesions can be exposed in the prone jack-knife position; however, high lithotomy might be advantageous for posterior lesions, whereas prone jack-knife position is excellent for anterior lesions. Of note, inverted jack-knife position should not be used for patients in late pregnancy, who have had recent abdominal surgery, severe cardiac arrhythmias, or retinal detachment/severe glaucoma. General anesthesia is not mandatory as conscious sedation and local/regional anesthesia can be used in a prone knife position. Local anesthesia is an important part of anorectal surgery. A combination of 0.5% lidocaine and 0.25% bupivocaine is ideal and a 1:200,000 epinephrine dilution can be added to prolong the anesthesia and minimize absorption. Signs and symptoms of local anesthetic can range from mild such as lightheadedness and dizziness to severe such as arrythmia and cardiac arrest. The anesthesiologist should be alerted to the surgeon injecting the local and every possible reaction, either allergic or toxic should be investigated. Figure 25-19 demonstrates a perianal field block being administered. A subcutaneous perianal wheal is raised and then deep injections are made into the intersphincteric groove in each of the four quadrants to paralyze the sphincter mechanism and create total perianal anesthesia. Slow steady injection can minimize the pain of administration. Warming and buffering the local anesthesia have also been advocated to decrease pain of injection.

Bibliography

Corman MI, Allison SI, Kuehne JP. *Handbook of Colon & Rectal Surgery*. Philadelphia, PA: Lippincott, Williams & Wilkins, 2002, 106.

Gordon PH, Nivatvongs S. *Principles and Practice of Surgery for the Colon, Rectum and Anus*, 2nd ed. Quality Medical Publishing, 1999, 98, 155–160.

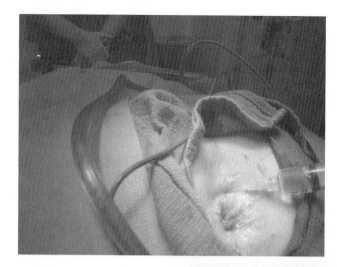
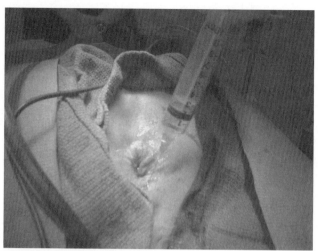
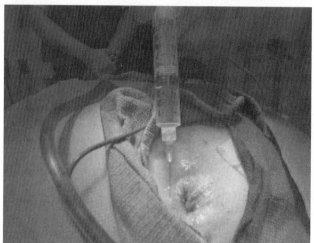

FIG. 25-19   Perianal field block being placed with local anesthesia.

CHAPTER 26

Acute Abdomen and the Appendix

Joao A. Lopes, Lucio Giovanni M. Palanca, and Clark J. Simons

Questions

1. A 23-year-old white male presents to the emergency room (ER) at night with abdominal pain beginning the prior afternoon. The pain is described as crampy with intermittent episodes of sharp pain, and non radiating. It is located in the right lower quadrant (RLQ) with an intensity of 8/10 which has progressively worsened since it started. He also has nausea and vomiting that began soon after the onset of pain. He denies fever, chills, or dysuria. Physical examination revealed RLQ tenderness, no palpable masses, a soft abdomen, with normal bowel sounds. He states no change in bowel habits. Lab studies reveal negative urine analysis (UA), WBC of 13,500, and Hgb of 16.0 gms/dl. The patient is taken to the operating room (OR) without obtaining a computed tomography (CT) scan of the abdomen and pelvis. Intra-operatively, the appendix appears normal. On further evaluation, the distal ileum appears inflamed with fat wrapping. You notice the cecum is not involved. What is your management at this time?

   (A) perform appendectomy

   (B) leave appendix and ileum as-is and close. Consult GI

   (C) perform appendectomy and distal ileum resection

   (D) perform appendectomy and stricturoplasty of the terminal ileum

   (E) run the small bowel to rule out Meckel's diverticulum

2. A 42-year-old white male presents to the ER at 10:00 p.m. with complaints of abdominal pain, nausea, and vomiting. He states the pain is 8/10 in intensity and began early in the morning. The pain is located in the left upper quadrant (LUQ) without radiation and is described as being achy and dull. There are no exacerbating or alleviating factors. He also complains of a low-grade fever and having no bowel movements in the last two days. There is no other significant medical history. Lab work reveals WBC 16,000 with left shift, UA is negative. Physical examination reveals tenderness in the lower border of the LUQ, with some guarding, but no rebound or rigidity. There are no palpable masses, no hepatosplenomegaly. A CT of the abdomen revealed malrotation with appendicitis. What is the most appropriate surgical option?

   (A) a Rocky-Davis incision with appendectomy

   (B) a midline mini-laparotomy incision with appendectomy

   (C) laparoscopic appendectomy

   (D) mini-laparotomy incision with appendectomy and excision of Ladd's bands

3. A 65-year-old African American female comes to the emergency room with a complaint of mild abdominal pain in the right, lower abdomen. She describes the pain as dull and persistent. It began two days ago and has not changed in intensity. She describes the pain now as 7/10 in intensity, with no exacerbating or alleviating factors. She admits to a 4-day history of constipation, as well as nausea and vomiting. Lab reveals WBC 10,000; UA shows *Escherichia coli* 50,000. The patient had a Foley catheter placed, yielding dark concentrated urine. Physical examination reveals the patient to be slightly tachycardic at 110 per minute, the remainder of the vital signs are stable. A mass was palpated in the RLQ. CT of the abdomen and pelvis showed an enlarge appendix. The patient was taken to the operating room where a Rocky-Davis incision was used and the tip of the appendix appeared to be neoplastic. Frozen section comes back as adenocarcinoma. What operative procedure is warranted?

   (A) appendectomy with culture and stain of peritoneal fluid

   (B) appendectomy with frozen section

   (C) create a midline incision to check for intraabdominal metastasis and perform appendectomy

   (D) perform a Fowler-Weir incision and perform right hemicolectomy and ileocolic anastomosis

4. An 18-year-old White female is referred to your surgery clinic from her family physician with a 5-day history of RLQ pain. She also complains of high-grade fevers of 39°C, which led her to see her primary care doctor earlier that morning. Lab reveals WBC of 18,000, urine pregnancy test is negative, and gynecology examination is negative. Her primary physician ordered a CT of the abdomen, which demonstrates a large phlegmon in the RLQ. What is the appropriate treatment for this patient?

   (A) exploratory laparotomy with drainage of abscess and appendectomy

   (B) RLQ incision, drainage, and appendectomy for small phlegmon

   (C) percutaneous placement of drain with ABX and elective appendectomy 6–8 weeks after resolution

   (D) conservative treatment with IV antibiotics for large abscesses

   (E) laparoscopy with drainage of abscess, appendectomy and placement of drain

5. A 30-year-old African American male presents with an acute onset of abdominal pain that he characterizes as sharp, in the RLQ for 4 days, which has become progressively worse. He states that it is currently 8/10 in intensity. He has associated anorexia, chills, fever, and yellowing of his skin. He has also noticed a darker color to his urine. Laboratory examinations reveal leukocytes of 18,000 with a left shift. His urinalysis is negative for infection, and blood, but positive for bilirubin. CT scan shows thrombosis and gas in the superior mesenteric and portal vein as well as appendicitis. What is the most likely diagnosis?

   (A) appendicitis

   (B) hepatic pyogenic abscess

   (C) parasitic infiltration secondary to ascaris causing appendicitis

   (D) pylephlebitis

6. A 42-year-old Hispanic female presents to her primary physician with 5-h history of nausea and vomiting accompanied by RLQ pain. She has just completed her menstrual cycle. She denies any changes on bowel habits or dysuria. She has a normal gynecological examination. Lab studies come back normal. She is sent to the ER where a CT of the abdomen and pelvis reveal enlargement of the distal appendix. After reviewing the studies you take the patient to the OR. On opening the peritoneum via RLQ incision, no purulent fluid is observed and there is a 2 cm mass visualized at the distal one-third of the appendix. You run the small bowel and find no areas to signify Meckel's, Crohn's, or mesenteric lymphadenitis. There is no purulent material surrounding the ovary and it is not cystic. What operation should you perform?

   (A) appendectomy

   (B) right hemicolectomy

   (C) close RLQ incision and create midline incision as to perform a search for metastasis

   (D) close incision and consult oncology for chemoradiation

7. A 50-year-old White male comes into the ER with upper gastrointestinal bleeding and hypotension. He has a 25-yr history of alcohol abuse, which has led to cirrhosis and subsequent development of ascites. The patient is adequately resuscitated with lactated Ringer's and packed red blood cells (PRBCs). Endoscopic therapy fails to halt the bleeding. What would be the next mode of therapy for controlling the esophageal variceal bleeding?

   (A) Sengstaken-Blakemore tube

   (B) Sugiura procedure

   (C) transjugular intrahepatic portosystemic shunt (TIPS)

   (D) Warren shunt

   (E) octreotide

8. An 80-year-old female presents to the emergency room with abdominal pain. She complains that the pain seems to be radiating to the right thigh, knee, and hip. She also has nausea and vomiting that is bilious in nature. Although this pain has been intermittent for the past year, she believes that this episode is more severe, which prompted her to seek assistance at the emergency room. She denies any history of prior surgery. However, she suffers from diabetes mellitus and had a myocardial infarction in the past. On physical examination, the patient is tachycardic, normotensive, and afebrile. Abdominal examination reveals a distended abdomen, with guarding, rebound, diffuse tenderness and high pitched bowel sounds. No obvious umbilical, nor inguinal hernias were detected. A palpable mass was discovered high in the medial aspect of the right thigh. What is your diagnosis?

   (A) femoral hernia

   (B) mesenteric ischemia

   (C) obturator hernia

   (D) ruptured appendicitis

   (E) lymphoma

9. A 65-year-old female complains of recurrent bouts of gnawing epigastric pain. She has occasional nausea and blood-streaked emesis. The pain has progressively worsened over the past 24 h and is aggravated by food intake. Moreover, medical management for peptic ulcer disease (PUD) has been unsuccessful. An esophagogastroduodenoscopy (EGD) shows an ulcer near the gastroesophageal junction. Choose the correct characteristics of the ulcer and operative management.

   (A) hyperacidity, truncal vagotomy and pyloroplasty

   (B) hyperacidity, vagotomy and antrectomy

   (C) hypoacidity, vagotomy and antrectomy

   (D) hypoacidity, Csendes procedure (Roux-en-Y esophagogastrojejunostomy)

   (E) hyperacidity, highly selective vagotomy

10. A 72-year-old female presents to the emergency room with abdominal distention, retching and complains of some chest pain. She complains of an acute onset of abdominal pain which she characterizes as sharp, epigastric in location, with 8/10 intensity. There are no exacerbating or alleviating factors. She has a history of gastroesophageal reflux (GERD) and atrial fibrillation. She continues to have normal bowel habits. Attempts at passing a nasogastric tube (NGT) were unsuccessful. She is febrile, tachycardic, and tachypneic. What is the diagnosis?

   (A) Boerhaave's syndrome

   (B) paraesophageal hernia

   (C) pancreatitis

   (D) perforated peptic ulcer disease

11. A 65-year-old male with a history of peptic ulcer disease presents with an acute onset of epigastric pain and hematemesis. He reports relief with antacids and proton pump inhibitors for 1 year. His past medical history is significant for hypertension and coronary artery disease. On physical examination, the patient is hypotensive, and tachycardic. His abdomen is soft and tender at the epigastric region, but otherwise

benign. Endoscopy reveals a large amount of clot in the stomach with an active arterial bleeder in the area of the duodenal bulb. Multiple attempts of endoscopic therapy failed. The patient continued to require additional IV fluids and blood products. He was taken to the operating room, where a laparotomy was performed. A longitudinal incision along the pylorus spanning 3 cm on each side of the great vein of Mayo was created. Traction sutures were placed superiorly and inferiorly prior to the enterotomy. The ulcer was readily identified at the posterior duodenal bulb and a clot was removed. What is the next step in the procedure?

   (A) sclerotherapy

   (B) perform a figure of eight stitch

   (C) vasopressin infusion

   (D) three suture ligation encompassing the proximal and distal branches of the gastroduodenal arteries and a U-type stitch to transfix the transverse branch of the pancreatic artery.

   (E) Kocherize the duodenum and perform a graham patch

12. A 50-year-old male presents to the emergency room with a history of melena, and most recently 3 episodes of hematemesis. The patient denies attacks of reflux or history of peptic ulcer disease. He has no other significant medical problems. He had a right inguinal hernia repair 10 years ago. The patient's vital signs are stable. Physical exam of the abdomen was unremarkable. Rectal examination reveals a positive fecal occult blood test. At this point in the exam, the patient retches and vomits approximately 250 cc of maroon emesis with specks of blood. Endoscopy reveals a large submucosal vessel along the lesser curvature that is not actively bleeding. What is the management for this condition?

   (A) endoscopic cauterization

   (B) vagotomy and antrectomy

   (C) wedge resection of gastric wall

   (D) distal gastrectomy without vagotomy

13. A 72-year old male presents with complaints of mild abdominal pain. On further questioning, the patient states that on the same day as the pain began, he had 2 bowel movements with blood-streaked stool and clots. He characterizes the abdominal pain as diffuse, colicky, with some mild tenesmus. Past history is significant for peripheral vascular disease, coronary artery bypass graft, congestive heart failure, diabetes mellitus, chronic obstructive pulmonary disease (COPD), and abdominal aortic aneurysm repair and left femoropopliteal bypass graft. On physical examination, he is normotensive and slightly tachycardic. Abdominal examination reveals no organomegaly, guarding, rebound, rigidity, nor any pulsatile mass. Rectal examination is heme positive without identification of any hemorrhoids. A nasogastric tube was passed, with only 50 cc of coffee-ground material aspirated. Endoscopy showed a defect in the duodenal mucosa with visualized synthetic graft. While waiting for a CT scan, the patient has massive amounts of hematochezia, and becomes hypotensive. What is the most likely diagnosis?

(A) bleeding duodenal ulcer

(B) perforated duodenal ulcer

(C) colon cancer

(D) AV malformation

(E) aortoenteric fistula

14. A 30-year-old male complains of abdominal pain, characterized as gnawing, epigastric in location, of 1 week duration. He also complains of diarrhea and a 20 lb weight loss in the last 6 months. Past medical history is significant for PUD which has been previously treated with antacids and triple therapy for *Helicobacter pylori*. He has no history of any prior surgery, alcohol intake, smoking, or any recent travel. On physical examination, mild epigastric tenderness with no rebound is noted. There is slight guarding at the hypogastric area. EGD showed esophagitis as well as ulcers in the second and third portion of the duodenum and gastric fundus. What is the imaging test of choice for localizing the above condition?

(A) endoscopic ultrasound

(B) somatostatin receptor scintigraphy

(C) CT scan

(D) magnetic resonance imaging (MRI)

(E) selective angiography

15. A 44-year-old male has sharp abdominal pain described as being located in the epigastrium, 10/10 intensity, radiating to the midthoracic region, with no exacerbating or alleviating factors. He has had several bouts of protracted vomiting. He denies any significant alcohol intake. Past surgical history consists of a cholecystectomy 10 years ago and nephrolithiasis. He denies any medication use or recent travel. He complains of chronic constipation and describes as arthritic pains in both his lower and upper extremities. Physical examination reveals the patient to be tachycardic, with dry mucous membranes. His abdomen is distended with some epigastric tenderness, no guarding, no palpable masses, and hypoactive bowel sounds. Laboratory analysis shows that he has leukocytosis of 16,500 cells/mm^3, a serum glucose of 250 mg/100 mL, serum lipase of 3000, and serum amylase of 800, aspartate aminotransferase (AST) of 40 U/100 mL, serum creatinine of 1.6 mg/dL, and lactic dehydrogenase (LDH) of 400 IU/L. A plain film of the abdomen shows the proximal colon cutoff sign at the midtransverse area. What diagnostic or laboratory modality would you choose to determine the cause of acute pancreatitis in this patient?

(A) CT scan of the abdomen

(B) endoscopic retrograde cholangiopancreatography (ERCP)

(C) basic metabolic profile, calcium, chloride, and phosphate values

(D) serum triglycerides

(E) ultrasound of the abdomen

16. The above patient was resuscitated with 5.5 L of LR and brought to the intensive care unit (ICU) where he later was intubated, because of a drop of PaO$_2$ to 50 mmHg. Laboratory studies showed a base deficit of 3 meq/L, with a blood urea nitrogen (BUN) increased from 10 mg/100 mL to 20 mg/100 mL, and a drop in hematocrit from 45 to 30. His serum calcium also dropped to 9 mg/100 mL. Based on the following lab values, what would be his mortality rate?

(A) 10%

(B) 25%

(C) 40%

(D) 80%

(E) 100%

17. A 48-year-old White male comes to the ER complaining of nausea, vomiting, and abdominal pain. He characterizes the pain as sharp, previously epigastric in location, now diffuse, and radiating to the back. He recalls a night of binge drinking prior to the occurrence of the pain. It is 9/10 in intensity, and leaning forward affords temporary relief. He also complains of being lethargic and denies any fevers or chills. He admits to a 20-year history of drinking alcoholic beverages, but denies the use of any drugs. He has no known comorbidities. He had cholecystectomy 10 years ago for cholelithiasis. Physical examination reveals tachycardia in the 120s, BP is 90/58 mmHg, RR is 26 breaths/min, and he is afebrile. Abdominal examination shows a distended abdomen, diffusely tender, guarding and rebound tenderness, with periumbilical, and bilateral flank and inguinal ecchymosis. Laboratory studies revealed a lipase of 3500, amylase of 1200, AST of 200, and ALT of 100, Hgb of 6 g/dL, and a normal coagulation profile. The patient is resuscitated with 2 L of crystalloid solution and 4 units of PRBC, but the patient continues to be hypotensive despite resuscitative efforts. What would be the next step in managing this patient?

(A) exploratory laparotomy with lavage and pancreatic resection

(B) angiogram with embolization

(C) admit to ICU and continue with supportive care

(D) EGD

18. A 21-year-old female comes in complaining of vague midepigastric pain that started 2 days prior. She describes this to be continuous, 5/10 in severity, with no exacerbating or alleviating factors. She has associated nausea and vomiting for approximately 1 day, but denies any fever, dysuria, or any change in bowel movements. She denies any significant past medical or surgical history. On physical examination she is a well-nourished female. Abdominal examination reveals moderate distention with slight guarding in the epigastric area, but no rebound, or rigidity. Laboratory studies reveal normal LFTs, with a lipase of 1200 and amylase of 350. Ultrasound of the RUQ showed no cholelithiasis, with no biliary dilatation. The patient is admitted and placed on NPO with IVF support. Attempts at feeding were unsuccessful because of exacerbation of the pancreatitis. ERCP showed that the major duct was draining into the minor papilla. What is the etiology for this acute episode of pancreatitis?

(A) gallstone pancreatitis

(B) annular pancreas

(C) sphincter of Oddi dysfunction

(D) pancreatic divisum

19. A 19-year-old female with history of anorexia nervosa has been complaining of abdominal pain for over a year. She has been seen by numerous physicians and attributes her pain to her psychologic condition. However, this recent bout of pain is unlike the pain in the past. In addition, she has experienced significant weight loss in the last 6 months. She has no other medical illness and denies any prior surgery. On physical examination, she is thin with normal vital signs. Her abdomen is distended, with no masses, with moderate tenderness over the upper abdomen and normoactive bowel sounds. Laboratory examinations show a hypokalemic, hypochloremic metabolic alkalosis. Upper GI series showed obstruction of the third portion of the duodenum. What is the most likely diagnosis?

(A) malrotation

(B) median arcuate syndrome

(C) annular pancreas

(D) superior mesenteric artery (SMA) syndrome

20. A 65-year-old male with a history of hypertension and diabetes presents to the ER with hematemesis. He claims to have no history of PUD, or significant weight loss. Two weeks ago he underwent debridement and drainage for an infected pancreatic pseudocyst, for which external drains were placed. He also underwent a recent colonoscopy with findings of benign polyps. On physical examination, he is afebrile, with vital signs showing a BP of 90/60 mmHg, HR 120 bpm, RR of 21 breaths/min. Abdominal examination revealed a soft abdomen, two Jackson-Pratt (JP) drains over the left hemiabdomen draining brownish material, slightly tender over the drain site, with a palpable spleen near the umbilicus with normoactive bowel sounds. An NGT was inserted and revealed fresh nonclotting blood. Laboratory examinations showed a hemoglobin of 6.1 g/dL. IVF and blood products given and a CT scan was performed which showed nonenhancing pancreas, no free air, no intraabdominal fluid or abscess but did show splenomegaly and splenic vein thrombosis. An EGD was performed which showed no ulcers, no erosions, but gastric varices were noted with no stigmata of recent bleed. Over the next 2 days, the patient stabilized, but then had another episode of GI bleed. Urgent endoscopy was performed which showed bleeding gastric varices. No attempts at endoscopic therapy were performed. Later that evening, the patient becomes hypotensive with a Hgb of 7 g/dL, BP of 80/60 mmHg, and HR of 120 bpm. What is the therapeutic modality of choice?

(A) splenectomy and wedge resection of the gastric varices
(B) subtotal gastrectomy
(C) splenectomy
(D) repeat EGD
(E) angiogram with arterial embolization

21. A 17-year-old male arrives by ground to the observation section of the ER with signs and symptoms of an acute abdomen. He states that this occurred approximately 1 h after leaving school after his wrestling practice. He gives no history of trauma. He states that he just had a mild upper respiratory tract infection 2 weeks earlier. He has been in good health with no other medical or surgical history. On physical examination his blood pressure is 90/67 mmHg with a HR of 120 bpm, and a RR of 22 breaths/min, shallow, and afebrile. Abdominal examination reveals a mildly distended abdomen, with guarding and rebound tenderness, with no palpable masses, and hypoactive bowel sounds. Laboratory studies show a Hgb of 9 g/dL, with a normal WBC of 8000. The patient receives 2 L of normal saline and his blood pressure responds transiently. A CT scan of the abdomen and

pelvis is performed (Fig. 26-1). What would be the treatment modality of choice?

(A) splenectomy
(B) IVF with continued observation
(C) angiogram with embolization
(D) laparoscopy
(E) transfusion of two units of packed red blood cells

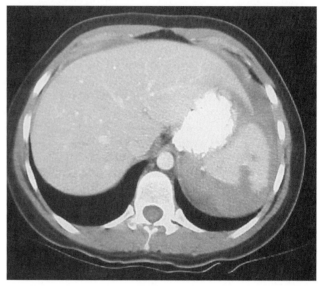

FIG. 26-1

22. A 68-year-old female with abdominal pain for about a week presents to the ER with fever and chills, increased abdominal pain and lethargy. On further questioning, she claims to have no change in bowel habits, no upper respiratory problems, but anorexia. She adds that she had surgery for injury to her bile ducts after a complicated cholecystectomy 3 years earlier. On physical examination, BP is 100/40 mmHg, HR is 110 bpm, RR is 21 breaths/min, and febrile at 38°C. She has icteric sclerae with no stigmata of portal hypertension. Her lungs are clear. The abdomen has a well-healed midline abdominal scar, it is soft with rebound tenderness over the RUQ with no masses, and hypoactive bowel sounds. Rectal examination is negative for blood. Laboratory examination shows Hgb 10 g/dL, WBC of 18,000 with a left shift, total bilirubin 2, with an increased direct fraction, and an alkaline phosphatase of 320. A CT of the abdomen and pelvis showed intrahepatic biliary dilatation with air fluid levels in a 3-cm diameter pocket in the right lobe of the liver. Based on the clinical scenario presented, what are the most common organisms causing this infection?

(A) *Staphylococcus*
(B) *Candida*
(C) *E. coli*

(D) *Klebsiella*

(E) cytomegalovirus (CMV)

23. A 65-year-old female, known hypertensive and diabetic, presents with abdominal pain of a few hours duration, with accompanying hematemesis. On further questioning, she claims that the pain has no exacerbating or alleviating factors and is more severe over the right upper quadrant. She claims to have associated nausea and vomiting, but no fever, and no change in bowel habits. Her past medical history is significant for peripheral vascular disease. Her past surgical history is significant for a carotid endarterectomy 2 years ago and a bypass graft of her right leg. On physical examination, her BP is 160/90 mmHg, HR is 100 bpm, RR is 20 breaths/min, and she is afebrile. She has icteric sclera. Her abdomen is soft, not distended, with a negative Murphy's sign, no palpable masses, and normoactive bowel sounds. She does have RUQ tenderness. Rectal examination is guiac positive. She was admitted and made NPO. An elective EGD was performed the following day which showed grade II esophagitis, normal stomach with some blood in the proximal duodenum and no evidence of mucosal ulceration, but blood tinged bile was noted from the sphincter of Oddi. Abdominal x-ray showed calcifications at the inferior edge of the liver. CT scan of the abdomen showed a 3 cm calcified common hepatic artery with no evidence of acute cholecystitis, no liver abscesses, and no other intraabdominal pathology. What is the treatment of choice for this patient?

(A) aneurysectomy

(B) hepatic lobectomy

(C) observation with followup

(D) heparin

(E) angiography and embolization

24. A 50-year-old male with a history of factor V Leiden deficiency presents with abdominal pain. He claims that this pain has been occurring for over a year. He has seen his primary physician, who has performed numerous tests with no specific diagnosis or intervention. Over the last few hours, he has become more lethargic and has noted an increase in his abdominal distention. The pain is diffuse with accompanying nausea. He denies any change in bowel habits, but admits to an increase in body weight in the last 3 months. His past medical history is significant for hypertension, and CAD. His denies any surgery in the past. On physical examination, his blood pressure is 160/90 mmHg, HR is 100 bpm, RR 20 breaths/min, and he is afebrile. He has pink conjunctivae, with anicteric sclerae. His abdomen is markedly distended

with RUQ tenderness without rebound, with spider angiomas, and a palpable nontender liver which spans 5 cm below the right subcostal margin. The patient also has a positive fluid wave. Initial laboratory examinations show elevated serum transaminases, Hgb 17 g/dL, and prolonged coagulation studies. CT scan of the abdomen and pelvis shows massive ascites with hepatomegaly, especially in the caudate lobe, and pooling of IV contrast in the periphery of the liver. The hepatic vasculature was not well visualized. He then underwent hepatic venography which showed a "spider web" picture. After correcting the coagulopathy, and decompressing the abdomen by performing a paracentesis, a percutaneous liver biopsy was performed which showed sinusoidal congestion, centrilobular necrosis, and lobular collapse. What would be the initial surgical management of this condition?

(A) TIPS

(B) mesovacal shunt

(C) mesoatrial shunt

(D) hepatic resection

(E) denver shunt

25. A 65-year-old female nursing home resident presents with crampy abdominal pain. She also has accompanying nausea and vomiting. She claims to have had difficulty in evacuating her stool since her stroke and has relied on laxatives. Her medical history is significant for a CPA 1 year ago with residual weakness of her left side which has kept her bed-ridden. Her past surgical history is significant for a previous cholecystectomy and total abdominal hysterectomy and bilateral salpingo-oophorectomy (TAH-BSO). On physical examination, BP is 160/80 mmHg, HR is 110 bpm, RR is 20 breaths/min, and she is afebrile. Her abdomen is distended, diffusely tender with high-pitched bowel sounds. No rebound, masses, or hernia is appreciated. An abdominal x-ray reveals a "bent inner tube sign" directed to the RUQ. A barium enema showed a "bird's beak deformity" at the proximal recto-sigmoid junction. A rigid sigmoidoscopy was performed with successful reduction of bowel and it showed no ischemic changes. What is the standard of care for this patient?

(A) observation and diet as tolerated

(B) repeated sigmoidoscopic decompression when it reoccurs

(C) placement of rectal tube with subsequent sigmoidectomy on same hospitalization after a bowel prep

(D) Hartmann's procedure on same day of hospitalization

(E) sigmoidectomy on same day of hospitalization

26. A 33-year-old White male comes into the ER complaining of abdominal pain for the past 4 days. He characterizes the pain as being initially crampy, but has now progressed to being sharp and diffuse with no radiation, severe in intensity, and exacerbated with movement. His last bowel movement was 3 days ago, which was of normal consistency. He denies any fever or chills, nausea or vomiting. He has a medical history which is significant for a factor V Leiden deficiency, and a cerebrovascular accident a year ago secondary to occlusion of the vertebral artery. He denies any surgical history. He also denies any use of illicit drugs, smoking, or alcohol use. On physical examination, his BP is 110/70 mmHg, HR is 120 bpm, RR is 21 breaths/min, and he is afebrile. Abdominal examination reveals a distended abdomen, diffusely tender with rebound tenderness. CT scan showed dilated loops of bowel with thickened wall and an enlarged portal and superior mesenteric vein with a central area of low attenuation. During the contrast phase there was a "bulls-eye" appearance of the vein wall. On laboratory examination he has leukocytosis and acidosis. The patient was taken emergently for exploratory laparotomy. Intraoperatively, a 2-ft segment of small bowel was found to be necrotic and was resected. The patient was then transferred to the ICU. What is the next step in the treatment for this patient with mesenteric venous thrombosis (MVT)?

(A) begin anticoagulation 2 days postoperatively

(B) no anticoagulation required since the involved bowel segment has been already resected

(C) begin anticoagulation immediately postoperatively

(D) give aspirin per rectum until patient resumes oral intake

Answers and Explanations

1. **(A)** The patient presented with a classic history for appendicitis. Twenty percent of all explorations for appendicitis turn out to be negative; therefore, other sources of pain must be sought. On exploration, the patient had classical signs of Crohn's disease, including fat wrapping, which is pathognomonic for Crohn's disease. Differentiating Crohn's from appendicitis is extremely difficult, especially without preoperative CT of abdomen/pelvis. The history of previous episodes of colicky abdominal pain with bouts of diarrhea may lead to a suspected diagnosis of Crohn's. Management of disease intraoperatively is to perform appendectomy if no cecal involvement in order to eliminate possibility of appendicitis versus Crohn's in the future. If the cecum is involved you do not perform appendectomy because of risk of fistula formation. Stricturoplasty is not indicated secondary to the lack of obstructive symptoms.

Bibliography

Silen W. *Appendicitis.Cope's Early Diagnosis of Acute Abdomen*, 19th ed. New York: Oxford; 1996, vol. 6, 70–87.

Townsend CM, Harris JW. *Sabiston's Textbook of Surgery*, 16th ed. Philadelphia, PA: W.B. Saunders Co, 2001, vol. 44, 893.

2. **(D)** This is a rare presentation of appendicitis within this age group. Malrotation is most commonly found within the pediatric population secondary to obstruction. The small bowel lacks appropriate fixation to the posterior wall and therefore the cecum fails to migrate to the RLQ as well as the colon not attaching to the lateral abdominal wall. The may lead to right upper quadrant (RUQ) position of the cecum which may extend bands (Ladd's bands) across the duodenum which may lead to obstruction. The surgical correction is to perform an appendectomy as well as a Ladd's procedure. This is extremely difficult through a Rocky-Davis incision and therefore best performed through a midline incision.

Bibliography

Fukuya T, Brown BP, Lu CC. Midgut volvulus as a complication of intestinal malrotation in adults. *Dig Dis Sci* 1993;38:438–434.

Townsend CM, Harris JW. *Sabiston's Textbook of Surgery*, 16th ed. Philadelphia, PA: W.B. Saunders Co, 2001, vol. 72, 1643.

3. **(D)** Primary adenocarcinoma of the appendix is rare and encompasses three types: mucinous adenocarcinoma, colonic adenocarcinoma, and adenocarcinoid. Typical presentation is that of appendicitis which may also present with ascites or palpable mass. Recommended treatment is right hemicolectomy, which can be performed with medial extension of a Rocky-Davis incision through the anterior and posterior rectus sheaths. These tumors have a tendency for early perforation although this does not necessarily worsen the prognosis. Patients have 55% 5-year survival. These patients are also at risk for synchronous and metachromnous neoplasms within the GI tract. Ten percent of patients have metastasis at diagnosis, which is not commonly diagnosed preoperatively. About half of the cases present with acute appendicitis and 15% have appendiceal abscess. Five-year survival is 60% after a right hemicolectomy and 20% for appendectomy alone. The later group includes patients with distant metastasis at the time of operative intervention.

Bibliography

Conte CC, et al. Adenocarcinoma of the appendix. *Surg Gynecol Obstet* 1988:166:451.

Harris GJ, et al. Adenocarcinoma of the vermiform appendix. *J Surg Oncol* 1990:44:218.

Lenriot JP, Hughuier M. Adenocarcinoma of the appendix. *Am J Surg* 1988:155:470.

Schwartz SI, Schires GT, Spencer FC, Daly JM, Fischer JE, Galloway AC. *Principles of Surgery*, 7th ed. New York: McGraw-Hill, 1999, vol. 27, 1392.

4. **(C)** Small abscesses can be treated by conservative therapy consisting of antibiotics, IV fluids, and keeping the patient NPO. Larger phlegmons should be managed via percutaneous drainage with interval appendectomy and antibiotic treatment, while complex or noncontained abscess cavities should be treated by surgical therapy with or without appendectomy. Because of the risk of cecal carcinoma perforation, people over 50 should undergo barium enema or colonoscopy prior to interval appendectomy.

For percutaneous drainage, drains are removed when output is no longer purulent and less than 50 mL per day to ensure resolution. Antibiotics are continued orally for a total of 14 days. Ten percent of patients, particularly in the younger age group, develop recurrent appendicitis; hence it is recommended that interval appendectomy be performed for this subset of patients.

Bibliography

Arnbjornsson E. Management of appendiceal abscess. *Curr Surg* 1984;41:4.

Baker RJ, Fischer JE. *Masters of Surgery*, 4th ed. Philadelphia, PA: Lippincott, Williams & Wilkins, 2001, vol. 125, 1469.

Schwartz SI, Schires GT, Spencer FC, Daly JM, Fischer JE, Galloway AC. *Principles of Surgery*, 7th ed. New York: McGraw-Hill, 1999, vol. 27, 1386.

Townsend CM. *Sabiston's Textbook of Surgery*, 16th ed. Philadelphia, PA: W.B. Saunders, 2001, 926.

5. **(D)** This patient presents with hallmarks of appendicitis complicated with pylephlebitis. Pylephlebitis is an infective suppurative thrombosis of the portal vein. It occurs as a complication of an intraabdominal infection, which is drained by the portal vein, which is most commonly from diverticulitis but can also occur from appendicitis. Thirty-one percent are associated with a hypercoagulable state and may lead to bowel ischemia or portal hypertension. Eighty-eight percent of cases have bacteremia, most commonly polymicrobial, of which the most common organism is *Bacteroides fragilis*. Symptoms include abdominal pain, fever, chills, and abnormal liver function tests (LFTs). Diagnosis is via ultrasound or CT scan. CT scan is the best means of detecting thrombosis and gas in the portal vein, but in equivocal cases, intraoperative ultrasound may also be beneficial. Treatment entails broad-spectrum antibiotics and correction of the primary disorder (i.e., appendectomy). Some authors advocate anticoagulation, but the time to start it is still controversial. Complications are hepatic abscess, bowel infarction, with a mortality rate of 11–32%.

Bibliography

Baril N, Wren S, et al. The role of anticoagulation in pylephlebitis. *Am J Surg* 1996;172(5):449–453.

Farin P, Paajanen H, Miettinen P. Intraoperative US diagnosis of pylephlebitis (portal vein thrombosis) as a complication of appendicitis: a case report. *Abdom Imaging* 1997;22: 401–403.

Way L. *Current Surgical Diagnosis and Treatment*, 7th ed. St. Louis, MO: Mosby, 1994, Chapter 29, 610–620.

6. **(B)** This is an example of carcinoid tumor of the appendix. Carcinoid tumors that arise at the stump of the appendix should receive right hemicolectomy; likewise, tumors that are greater than 2 cm regardless of location receive right hemicolectomy. Carinoids that are located in the distal appendix and are less than 2 cm may be treated with appendectomy. If it invades the mesentery, perform a right hemicolectomy. Distant metastasis are rare for tumors less than 2 cm (2% incidence) with a 5-year survival of 94% for localized lesions and 34% for distant mets. Fifteen percent have synchronous noncarcinoid tumors are other sites. This tumor is very common in children and presents as acute appendicitis. Carcinoid syndrome is rare in carcinoid of the appendix. The appendix is the most common site for carcinoid tumor and only 3% metastasize from this location. Grossly these tumors are small, firm, submucosal nodules that are yellow on cut surface. Carcinoids are also associated with MEN I in 10% of cases.

Bibliography

Bowman GA, Rosenthal D. Carcinoid tumors of the appendix. *Am J Surg* 1983;146:700.

Deans GT, et al. Neoplastic lesions of the appendix. *Br J Surg* 1995;82(3):299–306.

Moertel CG, Weiland LH, Nagorney DM, Dockerty MB. Carcinoid tumor of the appendix: treatment and prognosis. *N Engl J Med* 1987;317:1699–1701.

7. **(E)** Once the patient is resuscitated and the diagnosis of esophageal varices is confirmed, the next therapeutic modality would be drug therapy. Vasopressin was the first medication used with successful results. It would cease active bleeding in about 50–70% of patients. Once the drug is halted, recurrent bleeding is common. Side effects of vasopressin are hypertension, bradycardia, arrhythmias, myocardial ischemia, acute pulmonary edema, and water retention. This was the reason why nitroglycerin was added to vasopressin infusion. The current drug of choice is somatostatin and its analogue octreotide. These have been shown to reduce blood flow and to decrease both portal venous pressure and glucagon levels in patients with cirrhosis. Side effects of these medications are minimal, which may be mild abdominal pain, hot flashes, and diarrhea. Both vasopressin and octreotide have equal efficacy.

Bibliography

Mallory A, Schaefer JW, Cohen JR, et al. Selective intra-arterial vasopressin infusion for upper GI tract hemorrhage: a control trial. *Arch Surg* 1980;115:30.

Rodriguez-Perez E, Groszmann RJ. Pharmacologic treatment of portal hypertension. *Gastroenterol Clin North Am* 1992;21:15.

Zuidema GD. *Shackelford's Surgery of the Alimentary Tract*, 5th ed. Philadelphia, PA: W.B. Saunders, 2002, vol. 3, 348–349.

8. **(C)** Obturator hernias accounts for less than 5% of all mechanical bowel obstructions. It is most commonly found in females, on the right side, in the seventh and eighth decade of life. The hernia passes through the obturator canal, bounded by the superior pubic ramus and the obturator membrane. The obturator vessels and nerve passes through the canal and they lie posterolateral to the hernia sac. There are four cardinal features of this hernia, the most common being intestinal obstruction; another is the Howship-Romberg sign (pain down the inner surface of thigh, knee joint, and hip). This is referred pain from the cutaneous branch of the anterior division of the obturator nerve, which is compressed by the hernia in the canal. The next feature is a palpable mass high in the medial aspect of the thigh at the origin of the adductor muscles. The mass is best felt with the thigh flexed, adducted, and rotated outward. The last feature is repeated attacks of intestinal obstruction that pass spontaneously. Treatment entails operative intervention as soon as possible, secondary to the high rate of strangulation. The three preferred operative approaches are a midline transperitoneal approach, midline extraperitoneal approach, and exposure in the thigh. The former two are better since these hernias can be bilateral and therefore one can explore the other side if needed. Figures 26-2 and 26-3 show the classical

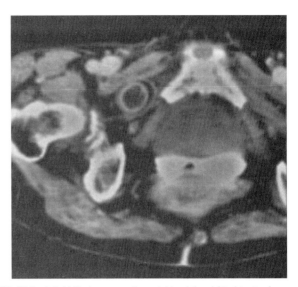

FIG. 26-3 A fluid-filled mass on the outside of the right obturator foramen. Radiologic findings demonstrate an *incarcerated obturator hernia* causing small bowel obstruction.

radiologic findings of an *incarcerated obturator hernia* causing small bowel obstruction.

Bibliography

Gray SW, Skandalakis JE. Strangulated obturator hernia. In: Nyhus LM, Codon RE (eds.), *Hernia*, 2nd ed. Philadelphia, PA: JB Lippincott, 1978, 427.

Hennington-Kiff JG. Obturator hernia and elusive diagnosis. *Jr Soc Med* 1992;85:508.

Martin MC, Welch TP. Obturator hernia. *Br J Surg* 1974;61: 547.

Yip AWC, Ahcheong AK, Lam KH. Obturator hernia: a continuing diagnostic challenge. *Surgery* 1993;113:266.

9. **(D)** Peptic ulcer disease is broken down into five types: type 1 is found in the lesser curvature and it is associated with hyperacidity and type A blood. Therapy is distal gastrectomy. Type 2 is found in the lesser curvature in combination with a duodenal ulcer and it is associated with hyperacidity and blood type O. Treatment is vagotomy and antrectomy. Type 3 is found in the prepyloric or pyloric area, and is seen with hyperacidity, type O blood, and treatment is also a vagotomy and antrectomy. Type 4 gastric ulcer is found by the G-E junction and is seen with hypoacidity and type O blood, and it is also known as a Csendes ulcer. Treatment is a Csendes procedure. Histologic studies have shown proximal migration of gastric nonparietal mucosa along the lesser curvature up to the G-E junction. Therefore, type 4 ulcers likely represent very high type 1 ulcers. The preferred operation for most type 4 ulcers is the Pauchet procedure which consists of a distal gastrectomy combined with a resection of a tongue of tissue extending up the lesser curvature and incorporating the ulcer itself. Another

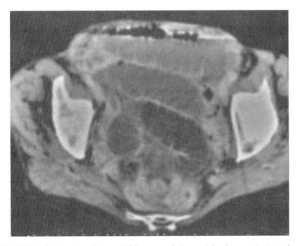

FIG. 26-2 Contrast-enhanced CT scan of the pelvis demonstrates signs of small bowel obstruction with dilated and collapsed loops.

alternative is the Kelling-Madlener procedure, which is used when the ulcer is in a location or of size not amenable to removal. It consists of distal gastrectomy, multiple biopsies of the ulcer, and leaving the ulcer in place. One last option for type 4 ulcers is vagotomy with pyloroplasty and biopsy of the ulcer. Type 5 ulcers can be found anywhere in the stomach and is associated with nonsteroidal anti-inflammatory drug (NSAID) use.

Bibliography

Csendes A, Braghetto I, Smok G. Type 4 gastric ulcer: a new hypothesis. *Surgery* 1987;101:361.

Eisenberg JI, McQuaid K, Laine L, et al. Acid peptic disorders. In: Yamada T, et al. (eds.), *Textbook of Gastroenterology*, 2nd ed. Philadelphia, PA: JB Lippincott, 1995, 1347.

Zuidema GD, Yeo CJ. Shackelford's: Surgery of the Alimentary Tract, 5th ed. Philadelphia, PA: W.B. Saunders, 2002, vol. II, 78.

10. **(B)** This is an example of a complication of paraesophageal hernia. There are four types of hiatal hernias. Type 1 "sliding hiatal hernia," which is an upward dislocation of the cardia in the posterior mediastinum with the G-E junction in the chest. This is the most common type, accounting for more than 90% of these hernias. It is associated with GERD. Type 2 or pure paraesophageal hernia "rolling type." This is most commonly seen in females, and is characterized by an upward dislocation of the gastric fundus along the normally positioned cardia. It is life threatening in 20% of individuals owing to the stretch of the stomach causing a decrease in blood supply which results to ischemia and possibly gastric volvulus, which is also known as an "upside-down stomach." The G-E junction is within the abdomen, while the fundus moves upward. Type 3 paraesophageal hernia, "mixed hernia," has the upward dislocation of both the cardia and fundus as well as the G-E junction. Type 4 paraesophageal hernia is a sliding hernia of any of the intraabdominal organs such as the colon, spleen, or small bowel. The patient described has a diagnosis of gastric volvulus, which is recognized by Borchardt's triad (acute epigastric pain, violent retching, and inability to pass an NG tube). The diagnosis is confirmed by the presence of a large, unusual gas-filled viscus in the chest or abdomen on plain abdominal film. Confirmation is by barium swallow. Surgical treatment involves untwisting the stomach, checking for viability of the stomach, reducing the hernia, cruroplasty (primarily or with mesh), and fundoplication or tube gastrostomy. There are reports of endoscopic reduction followed by percutaneous endoscopic gastrostomy tube (PEG) placement.

Bibliography

Carlson MA, Condon RE, Ludwig KA. Management of intrathoracic stomach with polypropylene mesh prosthesis reinforced transabdominal hiatus hernia repair. *J Am Coll Surg* 1998;187:227.

Dalgaard JB. Vovulus of the stomach. *Acta Chir Scand* 1952;103:131–153.

Perdikis G, Hinder RA, Philipi CJ, et al. Laparoscopic paraesophageal hernia repair. *Arch Surg* 1997;132:586.

11. **(D)** This is an example of a bleeding duodenal ulcer in the posterior wall. There are some studies that state that the incidence of emergent or urgent operations for bleeding duodenal ulcers has remained unchanged over the past years. Most patients with this disorder are successfully treated with medical or endoscopic management. Endoscopy remains the initial standard of care for the diagnosis and treatment of bleeding duodenal ulcers. Surgery is indicated when there is active hemorrhage which is refractory to endoscopic techniques. Initial management should include replacement of blood volume by large bore IVs as well as continuous monitoring of vital signs and urinary output. Emergent surgery is also indicated when transfusion is in excess of 6 units in a 24-h period. Antrectomy and vagotomy was historically considered the gold standard for this condition secondary to low recurrence rate, but has been replaced by the three suture technique, which has a significantly lower morbidity and mortality in the elderly, and unstable patient. With this technique, we add pyloroplasty and truncal vagotomy. A highly selective vagotomy can be done for the young, hemodynamically stable patient with minimal comorbidities.

Bibliography

Baker RJ, Fischer JE. *Mastery of Surgery*, 4th ed. Philadelphia, PA: JB Lippincott, 2001, 958.

Johnston D, Lyndon PJ, Smith RB, et al. Highly selective vagotomy without drainage procedure in the treatment of hemorrhage, perforation, and pyloric stenosis due to peptic ulcer. *Br J Surg* 1973;60:790.

Kochran TA. Bleeding peptic ulcer: surgical therapy. *Gastroenterol Clin North Am* 1993;22:751.

Ohmann C, Imhof M, Roher HD. Trends in peptic ulcer bleeding and surgical treatment. *World J Surg* 2000;24:284.

12. **(C)** This is an example of Dielafoy's lesion, which is a vascular malformation and a rare cause of upper GI hemorrhage. It is also called "caliber-persistent artery." The malformation is a large submucosal or mucosal vessel that may bleed when there is erosion into it. It is usually found along the lesser curvature, middle aged individuals, and no association with any vascular, or peptic ulcer disease. The hemorrhage produced from the lesion can be massive and can cease spontaneously at times. It is difficult to diagnose endoscopically because there is no ulcer surrounding the lesion. Diagnosis is best

achieved by performing endoscopy at the time of bleeding and visualizing a pinpoint mucosal defect with blood. Once the lesion is identified, the area is marked with India ink to delineate the area during surgical resection. Definitive management calls for wedge resection of the gastric wall, rather than an extended blind gastric resection. Vagotomy is not required since it is not associated with peptic ulcer disease. Endoscopic ablation with sclerotherapy or electrocoagulation has proved unsuccessful for this lesion. Surgery is required because of recurrent bouts of hemorrhage. Angiography and embolectomy are now also being used as first line therapy.

Bibliography

Townsend CM. *Sabiston Textbook of Surgery*, 16th ed. Philadelphia, PA: W.B. Saunders, 2001, 828.

13. **(E)** Aortoenteric fistula is a rare condition; it develops from an inflammatory tract between the aorta and GI tract caused by infectious aortitis, inflammatory aortic aneurysm, or aortic repair with a synthetic graft. The most common of these, is because of a AAA repair with a synthetic graft. Aortoenteric fistula complicates these repairs in up to 1% of patients. It most commonly involves the proximal of the anastomosis to duodenum or jejunum. Diagnosis is considered in any patient with acute GI bleed and history of aortic surgery. The herald bleed or "sentinel bleed" is an episode of acute bleed that ceases spontaneously, that occurs hours to days prior to massive exsanguination that ensues if not diagnosed and treated urgently. Treatment depends on the degree of retroperitoneal contamination. If there is minor contamination, and it is because of either infectious aortitis, or an inflammatory aortic aneurysm, treatment entails resection of the involved intestine and aneurysm with *in situ* graft replacement and omental interposition. When secondary to a AAA repair, it usually involves the suture line of an aortic graft with false aneurysm formation. Therapy in this case encompasses proximal vascular control, with graft excision and extraanatomic bypass (axillo-femoral) with resection of the involved bowel as the modality of choice. The aortic stump is debrided, closed in two layers, and buttressed with omentum.

Bibliography

Daugherty M, Shearer GR, Ernst CB. Primary aortoduodenal fistula: extranatomic vascular reconstruction not required for successful management. *Surgery* 1979;86:399–401.
Ricotta JJ, Faggioli GL, Stella AM, et al. Total excision and extra anatomic bypass for aortic graft infection. *Am J Surg* 1991;162:145–149.
Sweeney MS, Gadcz TR. Primary aortoduodenal fistula: manifestations, diagnosis and treatment. *Surgery* 1984;91:492–497.

14. **(B)** Zollinger-Ellison's (ZE) syndrome "gastrinoma" was first reported in 1955 by Zollinger and Ellison. It is caused by a pancreatic or duodenal neuroendocrine tumor which elaborates excessive amounts of gastrin. It occurs in sporadic (80% of cases) and familial (20% of cases) forms. The latter is associated with MEN I syndrome. It accounts for 0.1–1 % of cases with PUD. More than 60% of gastrinomas are malignant. Symptoms and signs are dyspepsia, GERD, dysphagia and diarrhea. Eighty percent are found in the gastrinoma triangle, as well as stomach, spleen, ovary, and heart. The diagnosis is by EGD, gastrin levels (fasting serum gastrin levels >100 pg/mL), increased basal acid output (>15 mm meq/h or >5 meq/h with history of antiulcer surgery for PUD), and secretin stimulation test (increase in gastrin levels >20 pg/mL). Localization procedures include ultrasound (sensitivity of 30%, specificity of 92%), CT scan (dependent on size, less than 1 cm is seldom visualized, while 1–3 cm are seen 30% of the time), endoscopic ultrasound (operator dependent, and invasive with a sensitivity of 53–75%), angiography (successful in diagnosing 60% of tumors and previously the imaging study of choice), and somatostatin receptor scintigraphy (with octrotide, first used in 1993). The radiolabeled somatostatin analogue has a high affinity for type 2 somatostatin receptor, which is expressed in most gastrinomas. Ninety percent of tumors are imaged with this modality with a specificity of 100% and a sensitivity exceeding all other imaging studies combined. Medical therapy includes omeprazole, lanzoprazole, with intermittent measurements of basal acid output. Surgical management entails enucleation of the lesion or resection of the involved organ.

Bibliography

Gibril F, et al. Somatostatin receptor scintigraphy: its sensitivity compared with that of other imaging methods in detecting primary and metastatic gastrinomas: a prospective study. *Ann Intern Med* 1996;125:26.
Krenning EP, et al. Somatostatin receptor scintigraphy with octreotide: the Rotterdam experience with more than 1000 patients. *Eur J Nucl Med* 1993;20:716.
Zollinger RN, Ellison EH. Primary peptic ulceration of the jejunum associated with islet cell tumors of the pancreas. *Ann Surg* 1955;142:709.

15. **(C)** The different etiologies for acute pancreatitis include alcohol and gallstones as the most common causes. Other causes include medications such as lithium, antacids, vitamin A, vitamin D, thiazides, and azathioprine among others. Hyperlipidemia is another risk factor. Trauma, ERCP, neoplasms, pancreatic divisum, and scorpion venum encompass most but not all of the other etiologies. Given the patient's denial of

any history of significant alcohol intake, no history of any trauma, recent travel, any intake of any medication, and a prior cholecystectomy, we can rule out most of these risk factors. With his associated symptoms, such as constipation, abdominal pain, nausea, and vomiting with some hint of bone disease, and a history of nephrolithiasis, the most likely explanation is hypercalcemia secondary to primary hyperparathyroidism (HPTH). The most common cause of HPTH is adenoma (most commonly single gland), others include hyperplasia (MEN syndrome and chronic renal failure). Symptoms and signs of this condition include St. Goar's triad which is bones (osteitis fibrosa cystica or Von Recklinghausen disease of bone), stones (nephrolithiasis or nephrocalcinosis), and abdominal groans (pancreatitis). Diagnosis includes an elevated serum calcium, elevated PTH, and a positive "poor man's test," which is a chloride to phosphate ratio of >0.33. Hypercalcemia may also cause constipation. Definitive treatment includes parathyroidectomy.

Bibliography

Baker RJ, Fischer JE. *Mastery of Surgery*, 4th ed. Philadelphia, PA: JB Lippincott, 2001, 521.

Townsend CM. *Sabiston Textbook of Surgery*, 16th ed. Philadelphia, PA: W.B. Saunders, 2001, 1116.

Zuidema GD, Yeo CJ. *Shackelford's: Surgery of the Alimentary Tract*, 5th ed. Philadelphia, PA: W.B. Saunders, 2002, vol. III, 9–24.

16. **(C)** Prognosis in acute pancreatitis is determined by the Ranson's criteria. This was first described by Dr. Ranson in 1974. It is a set of criteria based on prognostic signs determined by laboratory studies and severity of the condition (Tables 26-1 and 26-2).

     Mortality rates can be calculated based on the number of points in the Ranson's criteria. With scores of 0–2, mortality rates are at 1%, 3–4, 16%, 5–6, 40%, and >7 approximates 100% mortality. This patient had a score of 6, which would give him a mortality rate of 40%.

TABLE 26-1   Criteria for Pancreatitis Not Because of Gallstones

At admission	During the initial 48 h
Age >55 years	Base deficit >4 meq/L
WBC >16,000 cells/mm^3	BUN elevation >5 mg/100 mL
Serum glucose >200 mg/100 mL	Fluid sequestration >6 L
AST >250 U/100 mL	Serum calcium fall <8 mg/100 mL
Serum LDH >350 IU/L	Hematocrit fall >10% points
	Arterial PO$_2$ <60 mmHg

TABLE 26-2   Criteria for Gallstone Pancreatitis

At admission	During the initial 48 h
Age >70 years	Base deficit >5 meq/L
WBC >18,000 cells/mm^3	BUN elevation >2 mg/100 mL
Serum glucose >220 mg/100 mL	Fluid sequestration >4 L
AST >250 U/100 mL	Serum calcium fall <8 mg/100 mL
Serum LDH >400 IU/L	Hematocrit fall >10% points

Bibliography

Blamey SL, Imrie CW, O'Neil J, et al. Prognostic factor in acute pancreatitis. *Gut* 1984;25:1340.

Ranson JHC. Etiological and prognostic factors in human acute pancreatitis: a review. *Am J Gastroenterol* 1982; 77:633.

Ranson JHC. Diagnostic standards for acute pancreatitis. *World J Surg* 1997;21:136.

Ranson JHC, Rifkind KM, Roses DF, et al. Prognostic signs and the role of operative management in acute pancreatitis. *Surg Gynecol Obstet* 1974;139:69.

17. **(A)** Hemorrhagic pancreatitis is a severe form of acute pancreatitis wherein there is an elaboration of pancreatic enzymes and modulators of inflammation. Because of the location of the pancreas, inflammation spreads easily. In severe cases, fluid containing toxins and enzymes leaks from the pancreas through the lining of the abdomen. This can damage blood vessels and lead to internal bleeding, which may be life threatening. Some signs of hemorrhagic pancreatitis include Cullen's sign which is periumbilical ecchymosis, Gray turner's sign which is flank eccymosis, or Fox's sign which is inguinal ecchymosis. All these represent a spread of retroperitoneal blood. Diagnosis is ascertained by a thorough history and physical and laboratory studies which suggest intraabdominal hemorrhage. Several prognostic scores like the Ranson's criteria and APACHE-II score have been developed to achieve a higher sensitivity detecting transition to severe pancreatitis. A prophylactic antibiotic therapy is recommended in patients with sterile necrosis whereas an infected necrosis requires organ preserving necrosectomy and retroperitoneal lavage.

Bibliography

American Gastroenterological Association. Medical position statement: treatment of pain in chronic pancreatitis. *Gastroenterology* 1998;115(3):763–764.

Haas S, Singer MV. Differential diagnosis and therapy of acute pancreatitis. *Schweizerische Rundschau fur Medizin/ Praxis* 2002;91(39):1595–1602.

Kivilaakso E, Lempinen M, Makelainen A, Nikki P, Schroder T. Pancreatic resection versus peritoneal lavation for acute fulminant pancreatitis. A randomized prospective study. *Ann Surg* 1984;199(4):426–431.

18. **(D)** Pancreatic divisum is the most common congenital anomaly of the pancreas. It results when the dorsal and ventral pancreatic ducts do not fuse. It occurs in about 4–14% of autopsy results and 2–7% of patients undergoing ERCP. About 5–23% with this congenital anomaly have a dorsal duct with no evidence of ventral duct of Wirsung, a type 2 divisum. The presence of two separate pancreatic ducts is type 1 divisum. A finding of a dominant dorsal duct with a small narrow connection between the dorsal and ventral ducts is type 3. The common denominator between all types of divisum is that most of the pancreatic secretion flows through the minor papillae "accessory papillae." The theory behind the development of pancreatitis is the finding of the bulk of pancreatic flow through the minor papillae is stenotic or too small to handle the amount of flow causing obstructive pancreatitis. It is not a total obstruction, therefore it accounts for the intermittent nature of attacks of pancreatitis. ERCP is the "gold standard" for the diagnosis of this condition, but magnetic resonance cholangiopancreatography (MRCP) can also be a diagnostic tool. IV secretin stimulation of pancreatic secretions during real time imaging of the pancreatic ducts can determine the physiologic relevance of the divisum. Functional stenosis of the minor papillae with secretion-induced proximal duct dilatation is characteristic of clinical significant divisum. This test is controversial with a 78% sensitivity. Other causes of pancreatitis should be excluded prior to invasive diagnostic intervention. Therapy may include endoscopic dorsal duct stenting with or without sphincterotomy in treating acute recurrent pancreatitis, chronic pancreatitis, and chronic abdominal pain syndrome when associated with divisum. There is a 15% complication rate with poor satisfactory long-term success. Operative dorsal duct sphincterotomy with or without spincteroplasty is the preferred surgical therapy. It is performed via a transverse duodenotomy then identifying the minor papillae, dilating it and performing sphincterotomy to the level of the circular fibers of the duodenal muscularis. Some surgeons also advocate performing spincteroplasty, though this may not be necessary. Concomitant cholecystectomy with sphincteroplasty of the ampulla of vater and ventral pancreatic duct orifice are also advocated by some surgeons. In the rare patient with chronic pancreatitis with divisum, a puestow procedure should be performed.

Bibliography

Adzick NS, Shamberger RC, Winters HS, et al. Surgical treatment of pancreas divisum causing pancreatitis in children. *J Pediatr Surg* 1989;24:54.

Bernard JP, Sahel J, Giovannini M, et al. Pancreas divisum as a probable cause of acute pancreatitis: a report of 137 cases. *Pancreas* 1990;5:248.

Lans JI, Geenen JE, Johanson JF, et al. Endoscopic therapy in patients with pancreas divisum and acute pancreeatitis: a prospective, randomized, controlled clinical trial. *Gastrointest Endosc* 1992;38:430.

Lehman GA, Sherman S, Nisi R, et al. Pancreas divisum: results of minor papillae sphincterotomy. *Gastrointest Endosc* 1993;39:1.

Warshaw AL, Simeone JF, Scharpiro RH, et al. Evaluation and treatment of the dominant dorsal duct syndrome. *Am J Surg* 1990;159:59.

19. **(D)** SMA syndrome "Wilkie's syndrome" is a rare condition characterized by compression of the third portion of the duodenum by the superior mesenteric artery as it passes over it. It is most commonly seen in the young and females. Risk factors are weight loss, spine immobilization, scoliosis, placement in a body cast (sometimes called the cast syndrome). This has been reported in association with anorexia nervosa, AAA repair, and spinal surgery. Diagnosis starts with a high index of suspicion with a history of recent acute weight loss. Many patients have been followed for a long time with an inaccurate diagnosis of functional or psychiatric problems. Upper GI or CT scan reveals a persistent dilation of the proximal duodenum with a delay in passage of contrast into the jejunum. Often there is a vertical linear extrinsic defect indenting the third portion of the duodenum. At times, assuming the prone or knee chest position relieves the defect in obstruction. CT angiography with three-dimensional reconstruction may have a complimentary diagnostic role similar to angiography. Therapy varies with conservative measures attempted initially, with increasing success with this modality over the past decade. When medical therapy fails or in severe acute cases, the operation of choice is side-to-side duodenojejunostomy with or without lysis of the ligament of treitz and dextropositioning of the duodeno-jejunal junction.

Bibliography

Ahmed AR, Taylor I. Superior mesenteric artery syndrome. *Postgrad Med J* 1997;73:776–778.

Gersin KS, Henniford BT. Laparoscopic duodeno-jejunostomy for the treatment of superior mesenteric artery syndrome. *J Soc Laparoendosc Surg* 1998;2:281–284.

Gustafsson L, Falk A, LukesPJ, Gamklou R. Diagnosis and treatment of superior mesenteric artery syndrome. *Br J Surg* 1984;71:499–501.

Lee CS, Mangla JC. Superior mesenteric artery compression syndrome. *Am J Gastroenterol* 1978;79:141–145.

20. **(C)** The splenic vein lies posterior to the body of the pancreas and runs to the neck where it joins the superior mesenteric vein to form the portal vein. This location increases the susceptibility to its involvement with pancreatic inflammatory disease. This may lead to damage to the venous intima or extrinsic compression from edema, fibrosis, mass, or lymphadenopathy. Anyone of these can lead to splenic vein thrombosis. CT scan has led to increased diagnosis of this entity in patients with chronic pancreatitis. Approximately 7–15% of patients with chronic pancreatitis develop thrombosis of the splenic vein, with 2–5% of having extension into the portal vein. Splenic vein thrombosis causes extrahepatic or left-sided portal hypertension. Obstruction by the thrombus causes obstruction of splenic vein outflow causing enlargement of collateral vessels along the short gastrics and gastroepiploic veins. This leads to formation of gastric varices along the fundus and greater curvature of the stomach. This occurs in less than 50% of patients with splenic vein thrombosis. Splenomegaly is a common finding in these patients. The most common complication of splenic vein thrombosis is upper GI bleed secondary to the varices, which occurs in less than 10% of patients with thrombosis. Another important manifestation of splenic vein thrombosis is excessive intraoperative blood loss secondary to enlarged venous collaterals. The treatment is splenectomy, which eliminates splenic artery inflow and venous outflow with immediate reduction of variceal blood flow. Some researchers claim a cure rate of >90% in an 11-month followup after splenectomy. Arterial embolization is reserved for patients with extensive comorbidities, and these patients have a higher risk of splenic abscess. No specific intervention is required for asymptomatic splenic vein thrombosis.

Bibliography

Bernades P, Baetz A, Levy P, et al. Splenic and portal vein obstruction in chronic pancreatitis. *Dig Dis Sci* 1992;37:340.

Evans GR, Yellin AE, Weaver FA, Stain SC. Sinistral (left-sided) portal hypertension. *Am Surg* 1990;56:758.

Moosa AR, Gadd MA. Isolated splenic vein thrombosis. *World J Surg* 1985;9:384.

Warshaw AL, Jin G, Ottinger LW. Recognition and clinical implications of mesenteric and portal vein obstruction in chronic pancreatitis. *Arch Surg* 1987;122:410.

21. **(C)** This patient has a splenic laceration from his wrestling match. This occurred because of his contracting infectious mononucleosis 2 weeks before and subsequent development of splenomegaly. Patients who contract this disease are usually advised to avoid contact sports for at least 2–3 months. Criteria for selection of nonoperative management in splenic injury include (1) absence of significant injury to another intraabdominal organ, (2) absence of shock, (3) stabilization with 1–2 L of IVF resuscitation, and (4) no coagulopathy. Patients should be placed on bed rest, NGT decompression for patients who are vomiting, wretching, or with gastric distention. Every 6–12 h abdominal and Hgb examinations should be done. CT scans are repeated in patients with persistent abdominal pain, tachycardia, or slowly declining Hgb. Patients who have a vascular blush on CT scan, high injury severity score, longitudinal splenic lacerations, and large perisplenic or intraabdominal bleeding, are more likely to fail nonoperative management. With proper selection criteria, nonoperative management is successful in 70–80% of patients. Splenic artery embolization has been an effective way to stop bleeding in selected patients, particularly those who have a vascular blush on CT scan.

Bibliography

Malangoni NA, Cue JI, Fallat NE, et al. Evaluation of splenic injury by CT scan and its impact on treatment. *Ann Surg* 1990;211:592.

Thaemert BC, Cogill TH, LambertPJ. Non operative management of splenic injury: are follow up CT scans of any value? *J Trauma* 1997;43:748.

Powell M, Courcoulas A, Gardner M, et al. Management of blunt splenic trauma: significant differences, between adults and children. *Surgery* 1996;122:654.

Davis KA, Fabian TC, Croce MA, et al. Improved success in non operative management of blunt splenic injuries: embolization of splenic artery pseudoaneurysms. *J Trauma* 1998;44:1008.

22. **(C)** This is an example of a hepatic pyogenic abscess. Its common causes are biliary tree infection, sepsis, diverticulitis, perforated appendicitis, regional enteritis, pelvic inflammatory disease, and immunodeficient states. Patients undergoing biliary enteric bypass (choledochojejunostomy) are at increased risk of abscess formation even when there is no stricture at the anastomosis. This patient developed stricture at the anastomotic site, which resulted in the intrahepatic biliary dilatation on CT scan as well as increased LFTs. Diagnosis is difficult and requires a high index of suspicion. Symptoms and signs are fever, abdominal pain, nausea, weight loss, jaundice, hepatomegaly, leukocytosis, and LFT abnormalities. Plain films of the chest and abdomen, may show right-sided atelectasis, pleural effusion with an elevated hemidiaphragm or a subdiaphragmatic air fluid collection. Ultrasound is the modality of choice when IV contrast is contraindicated or with suspected biliary tract disease with a

sensitivity range of 85–95%. CT scan of the abdomen is the most sensitive with a range of 95–100%. Liver scan with technetium-99m sulfur colloid scanning, which is engulfed by Kupffer cells, has been useful in the diagnosis of liver abscesses. It is limited by lesions smaller than 2 cm. and is unable to differentiate between solid and cystic lesions. Definitive treatment is antibiotics, and abscess drainage (percutaneous vs. open drainage). The most common offending microorganisms are *E. coli* (33%), *Klebsiella* (18%), *Bacteroides* (24%), and *Streptococcus* (37%). The presence of isolated colonies of *E. coli* or *Klebsiella* should raise suspicion of a biliary source, whereas anaerobes would suggest a colonic source.

Bibliography

Chen C, Chen PJ, Yang PM, et al. Clinical and microbiological features of liver abscess after transarterial embolization for HCC. *Am J Gastroenterol* 1997;92:2257.

Chu KM, Fan ST, Lai EC, et al. Pyogenic liver abscess: an audit of experience over the past decade. *Arch Surg* 1996;131:148.

Hwang C, Pitt HA, Lipsitt PA, et al. Pyogenic hepatic abscess. *Ann Surg* 1996;223:600.

23. **(A)** Hepatic artery aneurysms makes up 20% of all splanchnic aneurysms. Most common causes, in order of frequency, are arterial sclerosis, medial degeneration, trauma, and infection. Other rare causes are poliarteritis nodosa, cystic medial necrosis, and illicit drug use. It is most commonly seen in females and older patients. Eighty percent are extrahepatic, and lesions more than 2 cm are most commonly saccular and those less than 2 cm are fusiform. Sixty-three percent arise from the common hepatic artery, 28% in the right hepatic artery, and 5% in the left hepatic artery. Quincke's triad encompasses RUQ pain, jaundice, and hematobilia. The biliary tree may be compressed resulting in duct obstruction. Rupture can occur into the peritoneal cavity or hepatobiliary tree. Rupture into the bile ducts can cause hematobilia, hematemesis, and jaundice. Rarely is there a palpable mass or abdominal bruit. Abdominal x-rays may show calcifications. CT scan, arteriography, and MRI have increased the recognition of this disease entity. Mortality from rupture is around 35%. Treatment is surgery unless the patient is too ill to undergo operative management.

Bibliography

Baker RJ, Fischer JE. *Mastery of Surgery*, 4th ed. Philadelphia, PA: JB Lippincott, 2001, 2086–2089.

Carr SC, Pearce WH, Vogelzang RL, et al. Current management of visceral artery aneurysm. *Surgery* 1996;120:627.

Lunsden AB, Mattar SG, Allen RC, et al. Hepatic artery aneurysms: the management of 22 patients. *J Surg Res* 1996;60:345.

Zelenock JD, Stanley JC. Splanchnic artery aneurysms. In: Rutherford RB (ed.), *Vascular Surgery*, 5th ed. Philadelphia, PA: W.B. Saunders, 2000, 1369.

24. **(A)** Budd-Chiari syndrome (BCS) is a rare condition and its diagnosis is often missed but should always be considered in a patient with unexplained ascites. It results from hepatic vein occlusion secondary to thrombosis of the major hepatic veins. The most common causes are chronic myeloproliferative disorders (polycythemia rubra vera), paroxysmal nocturnal hemoglobinuria, and other hypercoagulable states (factor V Leiden deficiency, protein C and S deficiency), oral contraceptives and pregnancy. The mechanical etiologies include vena caval membranous webs (commonly seen with patients with positive hepatitis B surface antigen positivity) and extrinsic hepatic vein occlusion by liver tumors. Clinically, the patients present with an insidious course with ascites, hepatomegaly, and some RUQ abdominal pain. Unexplained ascites should raise suspicion for BCS and lead to ultrasound of the hepatic veins and liver biopsy. Sudden occlusion presents with a more dramatic picture with massive ascites, severe RUQ tenderness, and increased serum transaminases. Diagnostic evaluation is based on hepatic vein imaging, liver biopsy, and hematology evaluation. Ultrasound of the hepatic veins is a screening test, which would show a decrease flow in the hepatic veins. Liver biopsy must also be performed to determine the progression and severity of the disease. Hematologic evaluation is also essential to define the cause. Hepatic venography is used if the ultrasound fails to confirm the patency of the hepatic veins. Surgical management is often indicated for BCS. If the patient has compensated liver dysfunction with cirrhosis without a web, the treatment of choice is orthotopic liver transplant. If he does not have cirrhosis then a TIPS or shunt should be performed. In fulminant hepatic failure, as seen in the patient described above, a TIPS is done as a bridge to orthotopic liver transplant (definitive therapy).

Bibliography

Blum U, Rossle M, Haag K, et al. Budd Chiari syndrome: technical hemodynamics and clinical results of treatment with TIPS. *Interv Radiol* 1995;197:805.

Bourliere M, LeTreut YP, Arnoux D. Acute Budd Chiari syndrome with hepatic failure and obstruction of the inferior vena cava as presenting manifestations of hereditary protein c deficiency. *Gut* 1990;31:949.

Ganger DR, Klapman JB, Mcdonald V, et al. Transjugular, intrahepatic portosystemic shunt for Budd Chiari syndrome or portal vein thrombosis: a review of indications and problems. *Am J Gastroenterol* 1999;94:603.

Ringe B, Lang H, Oldhafer KJ, et al. Which is the best surgery for Budd Chiari Syndrome: venous decompression or liver transplantation? A single center experience with 50 patients. *Hepatology* 1995;21:1337.

25. (C) Volvulus is derived from the Latin word *volvere* which means "to twist upon." The colon must be mobile with sufficient length to rotate around the mesenteric base. Most common sites involved are the sigmoid (90%) and cecum (10%). Volvulus accounts for 10–15% of colonic obstruction in the United States. Sigmoid volvulus is an acquired entity while cecal volvulus is congenital (incomplete peritoneal fixation of the right colon). Clinically, it presents with crampy abdominal pain, distention, and obstipation, while peritoneal signs and elevated white count suggest a gangrenous colon. The volvulus may act as a closed loop obstruction with increasing intraluminal pressure causing ischemia. Torsion may compromise the mesenteric vasculature. Predispositions are prior abdominal surgery, chronic constipation, demented individuals, and institutionalized patients. Abdominal x-rays may show the "bent inner tube sign" or "coffee bean sign." Barium enema shows "bird's beak" at the site of twisting. Treatment for sigmoid volvulus is reduction with endoscopy and placement of a rectal tube for decompression. Resuscitation and bowel prep is given for elective sigmoid resection on the same hospitalization, because of a 40% recurrence rate. If peritoneal signs and gangrenous colon is encountered, a Hartmann's procedure is performed. Mortality rate for emergent surgery for sigmoid volvulus is 40% versus 10% in elective cases. Cecal volvulus is usually treated by operation. The choices are detorsion alone, detorsion with fixation, or resection. Resection is required for ischemic or perforated colon consisting of a right hemicolectomy. Recurrence with resection is 0% compared to 15% for cecopexy or detorsion alone.

Bibliography

Gibney EJ. Volvulus of sigmoid colon. *Surg Gynecol Obstet* 1991;173:243.

Halverson AL, Orkin EA. Operative thearpy for colonic volvulus. *Semin Rectal Surg* 1999;10:149.

Stamos MJ, Hicks T. non operative management of colonic volvulus. *Semin Rectal Surg* 1999;10:145.

Tejler G, Giborn H. Volvulus of ceacum: a report of 26 case and a review of literature. *Dis Colon Rectum* 1998;31:445.

26. (C) MVT was initially described in 1895 and accounts for 6% of cases of acute mesenteric ischemia. It is classified based on symptom duration: acute MVT when symptoms are present for less than 4 weeks, and chronic MVT for patients with prolonged symptoms or in patients who have symptom-free intervals. MVT causes a rise in portal and skeletal muscle ventricle (SMV) pressures which causes increased hydrostatic pressure in the small intestine leading to bowel wall edema. This results in hypovolemia and hemoconcentration which can contribute to vasoconstriction. Some progress to bowel infarction. MVT is related to numerous etiologies, some of which include hypercoagulable states, traumatic injuries, venous outflow obstruction, and intraabdominal infections. Most commonly, the patient is between 30 and 60 years old with a female predominance. CT has a sensitivity of more than 90%. Bowel wall thickening and ascites are also suggestive of MVT. Therapy includes immediate anticoagulation to minimize thrombus progression. In patients with a hypercoagulable state, long-term anticoagulation is suggested for this condition. Mortality is around 20–25% and recurrent MVT presents in 50% of patients.

Bibliography

Boley SJ, Kaleya RN, Brandt LJ. Mesenteric venous thrombosis. *Surg Clin North Am* 1992;72:183–201.

Harward TRS, Green D, Bergan JJ, et al. Mesenteric venous thrombosis. *J Vasc Surg* 1989;9:328–333.

Rhee RY, Gloviczki P, Medonca CT, et al. Mesenteric venous throbosis: still a lethal disease in the 1990's. *J Vasc Surg* 1994;20:688–697.

Rijs J, Depreitere B, Beckers A, et Al. Mesenteric venous thrombosis: diagnostic and therapeutic results. *Acta Chir Belg* 1997;97(5):247–249.

CHAPTER 27

Abdominal Wall and Retroperitoneum

Derek C. Lou

Questions

1. Which of the following is *not* an absolute contraindication to laparoscopic inguinal hernia repair?

   (A) presence of infection
   (B) previous radical prostatectomy
   (C) strangulated hernia
   (D) cirrhosis with portal hypertension
   (E) history of pelvic irradiation

2. Which of the following is characteristic of epigastric hernias?

   (A) They rarely contain preperitoneal fat.
   (B) The defect is usually large and solitary.
   (C) They occur as a defect in the aponeurotic fibers in between the rectus sheaths.
   (D) A true peritoneal sac is frequently found on exploration.
   (E) Ultrasound has no role in the diagnosis of epigastric hernias.

3. Umbilical hernias

   (A) are present in one-third of all newborns
   (B) will most likely spontaneously close by the age of 4 years if the defect is 3 cm or smaller
   (C) are three times more likely to occur in males than females
   (D) can be safely managed nonoperatively with abdominal binders if the patient is not a surgical candidate
   (E) if larger than 2 cm, warrant consideration for mesh repair

4. Which of the following is most often associated with the development of lumbar hernias?

   (A) partial nephrectomy via a flank incision
   (B) latissimus dorsi flap
   (C) drainage of tuberculous lumbar abscess
   (D) stab injury to the flank
   (E) iliac bone graft harvesting

5. The shelving portion of the inguinal ligament used for open inguinal hernia repair

   (A) is formed from the external oblique aponeurosis
   (B) arises from the transversalis fascia
   (C) inserts directly onto the cremasteric fascia
   (D) represents the superior border of the iliopubic tract
   (E) is usually sutured to the transversus aponeurotic arch (falx inguinalis), which lies inferiorly to it, to complete a primary open repair

6. The median umbilical ligament is the remnant of which of the following fetal structures?

   (A) vitelline duct
   (B) urachus
   (C) umbilical vein
   (D) umbilical artery
   (E) ductus venosus

7. Which of the following is *true* concerning the anatomy of the abdominal wall?

   (A) The origin of the external oblique muscle is from the lowest five ribs.
   (B) The embryologic origin of the rectus abdominis muscle is ectoderm.
   (C) The majority of the neurovascular structures that supply the abdominal wall lie in between the external and internal oblique muscles.
   (D) An abdominal wall hernia requires a defect in the transversus abdominis fascia.
   (E) Lymphatic drainage of the abdominal wall above the umbilicus passes through the ipsilateral axillary lymph nodes.

8. Which of the following is *not* true concerning congenital abnormalities of the abdominal wall?

    (A) Diastasis recti is a weakness of the linea alba in the upper midline.

    (B) Gastroschisis occurs lateral to the umbilicus and does not involve an amniotic sac.

    (C) A persistent omphalomesenteric duct has a low risk of intussusception or volvulus and should be managed conservatively.

    (D) Meckel's diverticulum is a true diverticulum and represents persistent intestinal portion of the omphalomesenteric duct.

    (E) Chronic umbilical drainage may indicate the presence of a urachal sinus.

9. Retroperitoneal fibrosis

    (A) is considered idiopathic in about one-third of all cases

    (B) has been associated with hydralazine, ergotamine, methyldopa, and alpha-blocking agents

    (C) is excluded if only one ureter appears to be involved

    (D) can be treated surgically with ureteral transposition, renal autotransplantation, or omental encasement

    (E) cannot be accurately diagnosed with intravenous pyelography

10. Primary retroperitoneal tumors

    (A) are malignant in 60–85% of all cases

    (B) are classified as either mesodermal or neurologic in origin, the latter of which comprises the majority of these tumors

    (C) can be clearly defined with a combination of magnetic resonance imaging (MRI) and computed tomography (CT); angiography, however, shows limited utility in their evaluation

    (D) can be effectively treated with partial resection and chemotherapy, with a significant improvement in median survival at 5 years

    (E) are mostly found to have low histologic grade and be of small (<5 cm) size at the time of diagnosis

11. According to current guidelines for the management of retroperitoneal hematomas

    (A) zone 3 hematomas due to penetrating injury in a stable patient should be managed nonoperatively, with pelvic angiography to determine potential sites for embolization

    (B) exploration of nonexpanding stable zone 2 hematomas due to blunt trauma increases the likelihood of renal injury and/or loss of the kidney

    (C) supramesocolic zone 1 hematomas should first be approached by gaining control of the abdominal aorta via the midline posterior peritoneum at the supraceliac aorta

    (D) the most common site of blunt trauma to the abdominal aorta is at the origin of the superior mesenteric artery (SMA)

    (E) infrarenal lacerations of the abdominal aorta are associated with the highest mortality rate

12. Rectus sheath hematomas

    (A) can be caused by coughing

    (B) are rarely associated with anticoagulative therapy

    (C) usually occur at the semicircular line of Douglas at the entry site of the superior epigastric artery into the rectus sheath

    (D) are infrequently palpable on physical examination

    (E) usually require operative drainage

13. The peritoneum

    (A) can absorb isotonic fluids such as saline at a rate of approximately 90–100 cc/h

    (B) contains a mesothelial lining that secretes fluid to lubricate the peritoneal surfaces, and normally 200–300 cc of free intraperitoneal fluid is present in an adult

    (C) can reabsorb approximately 90% of the red blood cells in the peritoneal cavity intact via fenestrated lymphatic channels in the undersurface of the diaphragm

    (D) air can normally be present in the peritoneum after laparotomy for 7–8 days

    (E) chylous ascites predisposes to intraperitoneal infection

14. Which of the following is true concerning primary peritonitis?

  (A) It occurs more frequently in adults than in children.

  (B) Pediatric patients with nephrotic syndrome and systemic lupus erythematosus (SLE) are at increased risk for this condition.

  (C) Risk in the pediatric population occurs at age 2–3 years.

  (D) It occurs when inflammation of the peritoneal cavity occurs with a documented source of contamination.

  (E) The bacteriostatic nature of ascites related to liver disease explains the decreased incidence of primary peritonitis in that patient population.

15. Which of the following is *true* concerning peritoneal fluid?

  (A) Chylous ascites increases the likelihood of infection due to its high fat content.

  (B) Vancomycin doses should be adjusted in patients with peritoneal dialysis.

  (C) Choleperitoneum can only occur as a result of injury to the biliary tract.

  (D) Intraperitoneal hemoglobin interferes with intraperitoneal bacterial clearance and thus interferes with the immune response.

  (E) Ruptured aortic aneurysm and traumatic vascular injuries are the most common cause of hemoperitoneum.

16. Mesenteric cysts

  (A) are usually filled with lymph

  (B) are only embryonic or traumatic in origin

  (C) are rarely palpable on physical examination

  (D) usually present as nontender, asymptomatic abdominal mass

  (E) have a characteristic lateral mobility on physical examination

17. Which of the following is *not* true concerning congenital intraperitoneal hernias?

  (A) Transmesenteric hernias can occur through the epiploic foramen, congenital defects of the mesentery, or the broad ligament of the uterus.

  (B) Mesocolic hernias occur more often in adults than children.

  (C) Right mesocolic hernias should be operatively corrected by restoring normal rotational anatomic positioning of the small bowel and colon.

  (D) Left mesocolic hernias do not occur from herniation through the paraduodenal fossa near the fourth portion of the duodenum.

  (E) Reduction of left mesocolic hernias should involve releasing of the entrapped bowel near the border of the inferior mesenteric vein.

18. Which of the following is *true* about the omentum?

  (A) Omental torsion is usually primary, is frequently seen in athletes and patients with recent dramatic weight loss and is thought to be related to low omental fat content.

  (B) Omental infarction can occur secondary to torsion, but is usually unrelated.

  (C) Collagen vascular disease is not related to omental torsion and/or infarction.

  (D) Omental torsion shows no preference of location, occurring equally on the left and right side of the omentum.

  (E) Patients with omental torsion usually have symptoms mimicking pleurisy.

Questions 19 through 22

A 43-year-old male with a history of chronic pancreatitis, status postmultiple pancreatic duct stent placements presents to the emergency room with severe left lower quadrant abdominal pain. He notes increasingly frequent attacks of sharp pain in the past several days, with the pain on presentation being constant and having been present for 12 h. He notes no emesis but has nausea, and notes no hematemesis or hematochezia. His last bowel movement was earlier in the day. Examination reveals severe left lower quadrant pain on palpation with evidence of guarding and equivocal signs of rebound. WBC count is 13,000 with a left shift and his temperature is 37.0°C. A CT scan is obtained which shows the following (Fig. 27-1):

19. Given the CT scan, what is the most likely diagnosis?

  (A) recurrent pancreatitis

  (B) biliary colic

  (C) strangulated epigastric hernia

  (D) incarcerated spigelian hernia

  (E) peptic ulcer disease

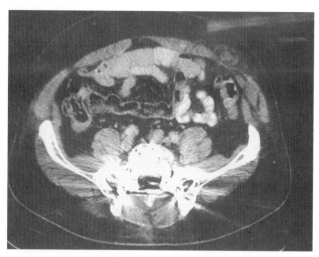

FIG. 27-1   CT abdomen.

20. Which of the following is *true* concerning spigelian hernias?

   (A) Preoperative diagnosis of spigelian hernias is made in over 75% of cases.
   (B) Regardless of the technique of repair, the recurrence rate for spigelian hernias is less than 10%.
   (C) Similar symptoms of pain can be produced by entrapment of the anterior cutaneous nerves of T10–T12.
   (D) Although ultrasound has no role in diagnosis, CT scan can be helpful in detecting small spigelian hernias.
   (E) None of the above.

21. Which of the following is *true* concerning the location of spigelian hernias?

   (A) It is more likely to occur below the semicircular line of Douglas because the aponeurotic fibers of the internal and external oblique muscles are parallel below the umbilicus.
   (B) They occur just medial to the semilunar line.
   (C) Spigelian hernias may occur inferior to the epigastric vessels.
   (D) A and B
   (E) B and C

22. Which of the following is *true* concerning repair of spigelian hernias?

   (A) Small spigelian hernias can most often be closed primarily.
   (B) Large hernias may require repair with prosthetic mesh.

   (C) Laparoscopic repair of nonincarcerated spigelian hernias is feasible, with a reduction in postoperative morbidity and length of hospital stay.
   (D) Some repairs may require reduction of herniated sigmoid colon.
   (E) All of the above is true.

Questions 23 through 26
A 37-year-old White male is 24-h postexploratory laparotomy for multiple gunshot wounds. Injuries required multiple bowel resections, repair of a liver laceration, and splenectomy; the patient has required over 10 L of fluid and blood product resuscitation. The patient is now oliguric with a tense, distended abdomen, and there is a high suspicion for abdominal compartment syndrome.

23. Which of the following would be the most likely set of findings for this patient?

   (A) CVP 6, peak airway pressure of 24, SVRI 500
   (B) CVP 20, peak airway pressure of 24, SVRI 1400
   (C) CVP 20, peak airway pressure of 44, SVRI 1400
   (D) CVP 20, peak airway pressure of 44, SVRI 500
   (E) CVP 6, peak airway pressure of 44, SVRI 500

24. Which of the following is *not* true concerning the etiology of this condition?

   (A) Elevated intrathoracic pressure is the result of elevation of the diaphragms.
   (B) Decrease in venous return to the heart results from compression of the intraabdominal IVC and is magnified by elevated intrathoracic pressure.
   (C) Oliguria results from decreased renal blood flow as well as from compression of the ureters.
   (D) Elevated intracranial pressures are associated with this condition.
   (E) Patients with this condition have an increased likelihood of thrombophlebitis and pulmonary embolism.

25. In which situation should immediate decompression be most likely warranted?

   (A) intravesicular pressure readings of 30 mmHg or 40 mmH$_2$O, urine output of 10 cc/h
   (B) intravesicular pressure readings of 25 mmHg or 20 mmH$_2$O, urine output of 40 cc/h
   (C) intravesicular pressure readings of 15 mmHg or 20 mmH$_2$O, urine output of 10 cc/h

(D) A and B

(E) A and C

26. Which of the following is *not* true about therapy for abdominal compartment syndrome?

 (A) Resolution of elevated peak airway pressures, decreased cardiac output, and oliguria always occurs immediately during operative intervention.

 (B) Frequently, fascial closure is not possible secondary to visceral and retroperitoneal edema.

 (C) If abdominal wall closure is not possible immediately, further attempts can reasonably be made within the following 3–4 days.

 (D) Abdominal closure techniques can include usage of sterile irrigation bags, polytetrafluoroethylene (PTFE) sheets, Vicryl mesh, and towel clip closure of the skin.

 (E) Abdominal wall component separation is a technique which can close a fascial defect of up to 15 cm.

Questions 27 through 30
A 54-year-old male is admitted to the hospital for suspected gallstone pancreatitis. CT scan on presentation reveals significant peripancreatic fluid, inflammation, and evidence of devitalized pancreatic tissue. He otherwise remains stable and afebrile, and is maintained on parenteral nutrition (TPN), IV broad-spectrum antibiotics, and bowel rest. After several weeks of stabilization, he is released to home with this continued therapy. Two weeks later, he presents with altered mental status, seizure activity, shortness of breath, substernal chest pain, and fever (39.0°C).

27. Which of the following is *not* part of the immediate workup?

 (A) CT scan of the head

 (B) CT scan of the chest, pulmonary embolus protocol

 (C) CT scan of the abdomen and pelvis

 (D) 12-lead electrocardiogram (ECG) and chest radiograph

 (E) electroencephalogram (EEG)

28. With other workup being negative, clinical attention focuses on continued pancreatic *complications* with this patient. Which of the following is *true* concerning the treatment of severe pancreatitis?

 (A) Nasoduodenal feeding with nonelemental formulas is recommended, as gastric feedings can stimulate pancreatic secretion.

 (B) Total parenteral nutrition is not associated with increased likelihood of infectious complications.

 (C) Piperacillin-tazobactam has the best tissue penetration of the pancreatic parenchyma.

 (D) Fungal organisms are the most common organisms found on aspiration of pancreatic fluid collections.

 (E) None of the above.

29. CT scan of the abdomen and pelvis reveal a large retroperitoneal fluid collection with evidence of air. Given the suspicion that this collection is infected, which of the following is *true*?

 (A) Pancreatic abscess, infected pseudocyst, and infected necrosis occur in up to 15% of patients with acute pancreatitis.

 (B) More than 50% of patients with six or more of Ranson's criteria will develop a pancreatic septic complication.

 (C) The double bubble sign signifies the presence of retroperitoneal, extraluminal air on plain abdominal radiograph.

 (D) CT scan is the gold standard for detecting pancreatic necrosis, with an accuracy of 95% when there is parenchymal necrosis of less than 10%.

 (E) None of the above.

30. The patient undergoes laparotomy with debridement of the necrotic pancreas and infected retroperitoneal collection. Concerning this therapy, which of the following is *true*?

 (A) There should be a low threshold for formal anatomic resection of the pancreas if open debridement of the pancreas is necessary.

 (B) Following operative debridement with sump drainage, mortality occurs in 5–50% of patients, averaging 30%.

 (C) The majority of patients with this condition can be managed conservatively with percutaneous drainage and antibiotics.

 (D) Minimally invasive techniques for pancreatic drainage have been proven to provide effective debridement of infected peripancreatic infected necrosis.

 (E) A cholecystostomy tube should be placed if operative intervention is necessary for biliary associated pancreatitis.

Answers and Explanations

1. **(D)** Laparoscopic hernia repair is a procedure which has been in common practice for over 10 years. There are currently two major techniques involved in a laparoscopic repair, known as the transabdominal preperitoneal (TAPP) and totally extraperitoneal (TEP) approaches. The TAPP involves laparoscopic dissection of the peritoneum off of the pelvic floor and hernia sac, placement of mesh around the defect, and closure of the peritoneum over the mesh. The TEP involves dissection between the peritoneum and transversalis fascia with a dissecting balloon, with subsequent creation of a pneumoextraperitoneum to allow visualization and reduction of the hernia. Mesh is placed over the defect once the hernia sac has been reduced or divided appropriately. Recurrence rate for both techniques range from 0 to 5%.

   Regardless of the technique used, appropriate selection of patients should be performed to determine the method of surgical correction. First, the ability to perform laparoscopy should gauge whether or not the laparoscopic approach even be offered. Evaluation of the patient should provide the initial determination whether a laparoscopic repair would even be feasible, as contraindications to general anesthesia may require open repair under local anesthetic. Laparoscopic repair would be favored with bilateral hernias, and has been shown to be advantageous for unilateral hernias in providing a quicker return to work. However, contraindications for laparoscopic inguinal hernia repair include previous preperitoneal surgery, history of radical prostatectomy, strangulation of the hernia, infection, and history of pelvic radiation. Cirrhosis with portal hypertension is considered only a relative contraindication to laparoscopic repair.

2. **(C)** Epigastric hernias can occur between the xiphoid process and the umbilicus. They occur through defects of the linea alba, the aponeurotic fibers between the rectus sheaths, and most often contain preperitoneal fat. They usually present with discomfort in the upper abdomen in the midline, and can often be palpated on physical examination. Ultrasound may also be needed to solve the diagnostic challenge provided by the anatomy of some patients. Often, upright positioning and synchronized valsalva maneuvers may assist in discovering the presence of epigastric hernias. Classic epigastric hernias rarely have a peritoneal sac, and are usually solitary and small in size, with the herniated tissues being much larger than the actual defect.

   The increased usage of the laparoscopy has provided a special type of epigastric hernia which is increasing in frequency. Incisional herniations just above the umbilicus may develop after trocar placement. These hernias usually will have a peritoneal sac and may involve other abdominal contents other than fat.

   Regardless of etiology, treatment of symptomatic hernias requires surgical intervention, and concomitant presence of an umbilical hernia should warrant conversion to a single large defect if one is palpated through the initial defect. The hernias can be closed primarily or with mesh depending on surgeon preference.

3. **(E)** Umbilical hernias overall are three times more common in females than males. Umbilical hernias are congenital in nature in children and most often acquired in the adult. In children, failure of the umbilical ring to close produces the hernia, which may occur in as many as 20% of newborns. If the umbilical hernia in the pediatric patient is less than 1.5 cm, it will more than likely close by the age of 4 years. Surgical candidates from this population are thus patients with large, complicated, or incarcerated/strangulated hernias, as well as children over the age of 4 with a persistent umbilical hernia.

   Adults usually acquire umbilical hernias from conditions that increase intraabdominal pressure. Persistent coughing (smokers) or abdominal straining (chronic constipation) can provide enough force over time to produce the hernia. Patients with ascites also frequently develop umbilical hernias. Small hernias are usually more symptomatic than larger ones. Over time, the herniated contents, usually bowel or omentum, adhere to the peritoneal sac, leading to incarceration. The classic adult patient is the multiparous obese, middle-aged female.

Management of umbilical hernias should favor surgical repair in patients who can tolerate it. An incarcerated or strangulated hernia could easily overwhelm the elderly patient with multiple comorbidities. Usage of abdominal binders has not been shown to adequately manage these hernias nonoperatively and should be avoided. Surgical management classically involved the Mayo repair ("vest over pants"), but recent years have heralded tension-free repairs using mesh. This is especially true for large umbilical hernias over 2 cm in size. Abdominal binders may be used postoperatively and may aid in reducing seroma formation.

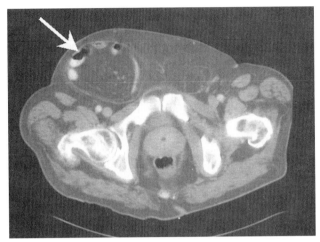

FIG. 27-2 Pelvic CT scan showing large right inguinal hernia containing small bowel.

4. **(A)** The lumbar hernia is classically defined as a hernia through one of two areas, the superior lumbar (Grynfelt-Lesshaft) and inferior lumbar (Petit) triangles. The superior triangle is formed superiorly from the 12th rib, medially from the paraspinous muscles, and laterally by the internal oblique muscle. The floor of the space is comprised of the lumbodorsal fascia, and covered by the latissimus dorsi muscle. The inferior lumbar triangle is formed by the latissimus dorsi medially, the external oblique muscle laterally, and the iliac crest inferiorly. Its floor is again the lumbodorsal fascia, but only subcutaneous tissue provides the cover in this location. Lumbar hernias are thought to occur more frequently through the superior lumbar triangle.

Lumbar hernias are classified either as congenital or acquired, the latter being the result of trauma, surgery, or spontaneous development. In spontaneous cases, it is thought that weaknesses of the lumbodorsal fascia possibly related to the perforations of the intercostal nerves are the etiology of lumbar hernias. Postoperative or iatrogenic causes of these hernias are most commonly the result of renal or adrenal surgeries via a flank incision. Latissimus dorsi flaps, drainage of lumbar abscesses, iliac bone graft harvesting, and blunt/penetrating trauma are less common causes.

5. **(A)** The anatomy of the inguinal canal is best visualized by considering its borders: the aponeurotic arch of the transversus abdominis (falx inguinalis) superiorly, the inguinal ligament inferiorly, the transversalis fascia posteriorly, and the external oblique aponeurosis anteriorly. The inguinal ligament runs from the

anterior superior iliac spine laterally to the pubic tubercle medially. The shelving portion of the inguinal ligament is formed when the external oblique aponeurosis travels inferiorly and posteriorly, cradling the spermatic cord. It thus inserts into the inguinal ligament, and runs along inferiorly to the iliopubic tract. Other named structures include the lacunar ligament, which is the medial extent of the inguinal ligament as it travels posteriorly to attach to the pectineal (Cooper's) ligament. The conjoined tendon is classically defined as the superiorly located fusion of the aponeurosis of the transversus abdominis to the internal oblique aponeurosis as they approach the midline. Although often discussed, Nyhus estimates its true presence in only 5% of patients. Regardless, it is the aponeurotic structures in this location which are usually sutured to either the shelving portion of the inguinal ligament or Cooper's ligament, both of which lie inferiorly to the falx inguinalis. If the distance between the superior conjoined tendon and the inferior shelving edge is too great to create a tension-free repair, relaxing incisions in the lateral rectus fascia may be necessary in order to complete the procedure. Normally, usage of these relaxing incisions results in increased postoperative pain and longer hospital stay (Fig. 27-2).

6. **(B)** The remnants of fetal structures and epigastric vessels are located in the extraperitoneal adipose layer of the abdominal wall between the endoabdominal fascia and the peritoneum. They become important during transabdominal laparoscopic hernia repairs in identifying structures of the lower abdominal wall. Along the abdominal wall the inferior epigastric vessels can be identified, traveling from the external iliac vessels to

the rectus sheath. The paired medial umbilical ligaments are remnants of the left and right umbilical arteries and lie between the epigastric vessels and the midline. The midline ligament, known as the median umbilical ligament, represents the obliteration of the urachus. The obliterated umbilical vein is located in the margin of the falciform ligament, and is known as the ligamentum teres. The vitelline duct is usually absent in the fully developed abdomen, although its presence can range from a fibrous band from the ileum to the umbilicus, a patent vitelline sinus of the umbilicus with obliteration before connecting to the bowel, a persistent vitelline duct with connection to the bowel (and subsequent umbilical drainage), or most commonly as a Meckel's diverticulum. The ductus venosus is a fetal vascular structure which connects the left umbilical vein to the upper inferior vena cava (IVC), allowing richly oxygenated placental blood to bypass the sinusoids of the liver. After birth, this structure, along with the umbilical vein, clots, and its obliteration eventually forms the ligamentum venosum within the falciform ligament.

7. **(E)** The abdominal wall components are derived from the mesoderm, and are recognizable by the seventh week of development. The abdominal wall is comprised of many layers: (from inside out) the parietal peritoneum, preperitoneal fat, transversalis fascia, transversus abdominis muscle, internal oblique, external oblique, Scarpa's fascia, subcutaneous tissue, and ending in skin.

The skin and subcutaneous tissue are fairly unremarkable, and it should be remembered that the subcutaneous tissue offers little to no strength to abdominal wall closure. Scarpa's fascia is more prominent in the lower abdominal wall, and although it provides little strength in closure, accurate reapproximation of this layer will produce a more aesthetically pleasing incisional scar.

The external oblique is the thickest and largest of the three abdominal wall muscles, and finds its origin from the lowest seven ribs, the thoracolumbar fascia, the iliac crest, and the inguinal ligament. Its fibers travel in a superolateral to inferomedial "hands in pockets" direction, producing a superolateral force of contraction. Its aponeurosis begins about the midclavicular line and travels anteriorly to the rectus sheath medially.

It is the internal oblique which originates from the lowest five ribs, as well as the iliac crest, thoracolumbar fascia, and lateral half of the inguinal ligament. Its fibers travel opposite to the external oblique. Of note, a small group of fibers travel with the testis as it descends into the scrotum; these

become the cremasteric muscle and serve to retract the testis from the scrotum when it contracts.

The transversus abdominis originates identically to the internal oblique, and its fibers travel in a transverse direction. Some of its aponeurosis fuses medially with the internal oblique aponeurosis to insert onto the os pubis; these two groups form the conjoined tendon, which most texts now agree is an infrequently formed structure. It should also be noted that the linea alba, formed from the aponeuroses of the muscular layer, provides the strongest layer for closure of the abdomen.

It is between the internal oblique and the transversus abdominis that the majority of the neurovascular structures lie, most notably anterior rami of T7–T11 and L1, which provide cutaneous sensation of the abdominal wall.

The transversalis fascia (or psoas fascia, named where it covers the psoas muscle) travels underneath the transversus abdominis. It is this layer which defines the integrity of the abdominal wall, and hernias are defined by whether or not there is a defect in the transversalis fascia. The iliopubic tract is also a part of this layer, running deep to and parallel with the inguinal ligament.

The preperitoneal fat contains the remnants of fetal structures (such as the medial and median umbilical ligaments) and the epigastric vessels. This layer also projects into the falciform ligament, forming its contents. The parietal peritoneum provides protection from infection for the peritoneum when it remains intact; however, it too provides little strength in closure of the abdomen.

The rectus abdominis muscles are a paired group traveling from the fifth rib to the pubic symphysis. They are enveloped in the rectus sheath and function to support the abdominal wall and flex the vertebral column. The sheath is formed anteriorly by the external oblique and internal oblique aponeuroses above the semicircular line of Douglas. Posteriorly and above the line, the sheath is strong and is comprised of internal oblique, transversus, and transversalis fibers. Below the semicircular line, the aponeuroses of the muscle layers pass anteriorly to the rectus abdominis, leaving only the transversalis fascia posteriorly.

Lastly, the lymphatic drainage of the abdominal wall follows two patterns: above the umbilicus, drainage is through the ipsilateral axillary lymph nodes. Below the umbilicus, drainage is through the ipsilateral superficial inguinal lymph nodes. This is roughly the pattern for venous drainage as well.

8. **(C)** Diastasis recti is defined as the protrusion of the abdominal wall in the midline above the umbilicus

between the rectus abdominis muscles. This is caused by a weakness of the linea alba, and does not represent a true hernia. Repair is not indicated unless a true epigastric hernia exists.

Omphalocoele is a congenital defect of the closure of the umbilical ring, and is classically represented by a midline herniation of abdominal contents within an amniotic sac. Gastroschisis, however, is a congenital defect in the closure of the abdominal wall during development, leading to a lateral defect leading to herniation of abdominal contents without an amniotic sac.

The omphalomesenteric (vitelline) duct is an embryologic structure connecting the fetal midgut to the yolk sac, and usually obliterates prior to birth. Remnants of the vitelline duct can present with a spectrum of conditions, from an umbilical polyp to a Meckel's diverticulum. Polyps are usually persistent umbilical growths resembling granulomas, except they remain after treatment with silver nitrate. When found, they should be excised. Umbilical sinuses result from the continued presence of the umbilical end of the vitelline duct, and should also be excised. Persistent vitelline ducts can be diagnosed by the passage of enteric contents via the umbilicus. Immediate laparotomy should be performed for excision in order to eliminate the high risk of intussusception or volvulus. Cystic remnants of the vitelline duct should be treated in the same fashion, although they are usually asymptomatic and are found at laparotomy for unexplained volvulus or obstruction. Meckel's diverticulum is a true diverticulum, and is formed when the intestinal end of the vitelline duct persists. If discovered, treatment is excision.

The urachus is a fetal structure which connects the bladder to the umbilicus, and it too usually obliterates prior to birth. A urachal sinus present with chronic umbilical drainage, as the umbilical end has not closed. Excision is warranted on diagnosis, as infection may ensue. Bladder diverticula may represent failure of closure of the bladder end of the urachus; these should also be excised once distal obstruction is ruled out. A persistent urachus is heralded by the leakage of urine from the umbilicus, and should also warrant excision.

9. **(D)** Retroperitoneal fibrosis is a rare condition, and is idiopathic in etiology in about two-thirds of all cases (usually called Ormond's disease). An association with various medications has been shown, which include methysergide, ergotamine, hydralazine, methyldopa, and beta-blocking agents. The key characteristic of retroperitoneal fibrosis is its effect on the ureters which pass through it. Constriction leading to obstruction is

the result of entrapment of the ureters, which will vary the presentation based on severity of the obstructive uropathy. Intravenous pyelogram (IVP) usually provides an accurate diagnosis, with characteristic signs of medial displacement, hydronephrosis/ hydroureter proximal to the lesion, and a long segment of affected ureter. The strictures are usually bilateral and symmetrical; however, only one ureter may be involved.

Mild cases with low-grade obstruction can be treated initially with medical management. This involves steroids and cessation of any associated medications. Failure of this regimen is seen by the lack of improvement over several weeks, and surgical management should be considered at this time. High grade or severe cases of obstruction will require surgical management and perhaps immediate nephrostomy if indicated. The cornerstone of surgical management is liberation of the ureters from the retroperitoneum. Concomitant intraperitoneal transposition of the ureters may be required, and encasement with omentum may also be necessary. Renal autotransplantation should also be considered, given its low complication risk.

10. **(A)** Retroperitoneal tumors are challenging both in diagnosis and in treatment. The majority of retroperitoneal tumors are discovered well after they have involved contiguous structures and organs. They are a rare phenomenon with an incidence of 0.3–3%, and are classified as either mesodermal or neural in origin. Overall, retroperitoneal tumors are malignant 60–85% of the time, with the majority of malignant tumors being mesodermal in origin. Diagnosis and determination of resectability is based on a combination of CT, MRI, and angiography. Evaluation of retroperitoneal soft tissue sarcomas has shown that the majority are greater than 10 cm in size (60%) and have a high-grade histology (64%) at presentation. Most common presenting symptoms include a palpable abdominal mass, lower extremity neurologic symptoms, and pain.

In terms of treatment, the primary treatment should be aimed at complete resection of tumor. Complete resection of primary disease provides a median survival time of 103 months, while incomplete and no resection provides a median survival of 18 months. Analysis of median survival times has shown that incomplete resection does not provide significant increase in survival than chemotherapy (doxorubicin based) and/or radiation therapy for unresectable tumors. However, partial resection has been shown to provide some symptomatic relief, and thus should be reserved for cases in which partial resection may provide palliation. Overall, high-grade histology, unresectability, and positive gross margin are the strongest factors negatively influencing survival for these tumors.

11. **(B)** The retroperitoneum is roughly divided into three major anatomic zones. Zone 1 is the midline retroperitoneum and contains the suprarenal abdominal aorta, IVC, superior mesenteric and proximal renal arteries. A hematoma in this area should warrant exploration for both blunt and penetrating trauma, as the likelihood of major vessel injury is high. The transverse mesocolon provides the boundary between the two types of zone 1 hematomas: supramesocolic and inframesocolic. This distinction is important as the approach will determine the fashion of vascular control and exposure for these hematomas. Supramesocolic hematomas usually arise from aortic, celiac, proximal SMA, or renal arterial injuries. Vascular control should begin with clamping of the abdominal aorta at the diaphragmatic hiatus and left-sided medial visceral rotation (Maddox maneuver). Inframesocolic hematomas generally arise from aortic or inferior vena caval injuries. Proximal control should be at the supraceliac aorta, with exposure via the posterior peritoneum in the midline similar to approaching an infrarenal aortic aneurysm.

Zone 2 of the retroperitoneum are the paired perinephric spaces, which contain the kidneys and renal vessels. Hematomas resulting from blunt trauma in zone 2 warrant exploration only if there is expansion or instability, as studies have shown an increase in subsequent loss of the kidney otherwise. Given the need for exploration, some centers advocate obtaining proximal control of the renal vessels at the aorta prior to incising Gerota's fascia. Other centers incise the fascia and clamp the hilum after medially rotating the kidney. Regardless, evaluation of injury along with watertight closure of the collecting system should remain the primary goals.

Zone 3 is the pelvic retroperitoneum, and contains the iliac vessels and the ureters. Blunt trauma resulting in nonexpanding stable hematomas are often secondary to pelvic fracture or bleeding which is most likely best controlled by angiographic embolization, and thus should not be explored. Blunt expanding hematomas and all penetrating trauma-related hematomas in this area should be explored given the likelihood of iliac vessel injury.

12. **(A)** Rectus sheath hematomas may mimic intraabdominal disease, and so care should be taken with diagnosis to avoid an unnecessary laparotomy. Trauma is the primary cause of rectus sheath hematomas, and may be caused by various blunt traumas or even vigorous paroxysms of coughing. Other causes include collagen vascular diseases, and infectious diseases like typhoid fever. Also, many patients with this condition are frequently on anticoagulative therapy or have some type of blood dyscrasia. Most often, the source of bleeding is usually from the inferior epigastric vessels and not the muscle proper. Logically, it occurs most often at the junction of the semicircular line of Douglas and the rectus sheath, where the inferior epigastric vessels enter the rectus sheath. Diagnosis can be made by palpation on physical examination, which can frequently be successful in revealing a tender mass over the rectus abdominis muscle. Likewise, abdominal CT scanning or ultrasonography should adequately reveal a rectus sheath hematoma. Management is most often nonoperative, although continued expansion of the hematoma may warrant operative therapy. This should usually involve simple evacuation, control of hemorrhage, and closure without drainage. Operative therapy is also indicated if more serious, intraabdominal conditions cannot be excluded in the process of diagnosis.

13. **(A)** The peritoneum is a mesodermally-derived structure, and serves many important functions. It provides a frictionless surface inside which intraabdominal organs can be contained. It also can secrete lubricating fluid from its mesothelial lining to assist in free movement of viscera. Given its structure, it also has bidirectional transport capabilities for water and solutes. This is driven largely in part by osmolar gradients; however, experimentally isotonic saline has been shown to be absorbed at a rate of 25–30 cc/h. Overall, there is approximately 100 cc of fluid that is normally present in the peritoneal cavity. This transport property of the peritoneum is the basis for peritoneal dialysis.

Air and gases can also be absorbed by the peritoneum. Normally, intraperitoneal air left after laparotomy is almost completely absorbed by 4–5 days. Of note, intraperitoneal blood can also be reabsorbed. Fenestrated lymphatic channels underlying the diaphragms serve to reabsorb red blood cells, to an extent that 70% of intraperitoneal red blood cells are resorbed intact and with a normal circulatory survival time. Chyle has bacteriostatic properties given its high lymphocytic content, and thus chylous ascites alone is not in fact a predisposing factor for the development of intraperitoneal infection.

14. **(B)** Primary peritonitis is defined as the inflammation of the parietal peritoneum without an evident source of infection. It is a condition which occurs more frequently in children and females. Incidence in the pediatric population shows a bimodal distribution in the neonatal period and again at 4–5 years of age.

Increased female incidence is thought to be the result of entry of organisms into the peritoneal cavity via the fallopian tubes. This condition is also associated with nephrotic syndrome and SLE in children; in adults, patients with liver disease have been shown to have an increased incidence of primary peritonitis. Also, previous upper respiratory tract infection or ear infection are not uncommonly found on taking the patient's history. Patients with this condition often present with fever, leukocytosis, and abdominal pain, which may be severe. Diagnosis can be made by paracentesis, culture, and exclusion of other sources of infection such as pneumonia or urinary tract infection. Organisms usually found with nephrotic syndrome or SLE are hemolytic streptococci or pneumococci. Liver disease more often associated with gram-negative rather than gram-positive organisms. Distinction between primary and secondary peritonitis may be difficult to establish, and sometimes may only be made after laparotomy or extensive investigation.

15. **(D)** The common causes of chylous ascites are from trauma, tumor involving lymphatic structures, spontaneous bacterial peritonitis, cirrhosis, abdominal surgery, tuberculosis, congenital defects, and peritoneal dialysis. Chyle appears to have bacteriostatic properties, and thus peritoneal infection is thus less likely.

Choleperitoneum is often the result of trauma or iatrogenic biliary tract injury or postoperative leak; however, spontaneous rupture of the bile duct can be seen in both adults and infants, and is the second most common cause of surgical jaundice in infancy. Bile produces an inflammatory response from the peritoneum due to its irritating properties. The increase of peritoneal fluid in response to bile is seen as biliary ascites. Infection of intraperitoneal bile requires urgent surgical intervention.

Hemoperitoneum is most often caused by hepatic or splenic trauma, although ruptured aortic aneursym and ectopic pregnancy are also common causes. Via the peritoneum, more than two-thirds of intraperitoneal red blood cells can be reabsorbed intact into the blood stream. However, efforts to evacuate as much blood as possible from the abdomen should be made during surgery, as hemoglobin has been shown to interfere with clearance of intraperitoneal bacteria and thus impair the immune response to peritonitis.

The peritoneum has the capability of bidirectional transport, thus making it a medium via which dialysis can be performed. Water, electrolytes, and various drugs can thus be removed with peritoneal dialysis. Most antibiotics do not require adjustment of dosing with peritoneal dialysis; this includes vancomycin. Antibiotics such as aztreonam, amikacin, cefaclor, ceftazidime, fluconazole, gentamicin, isoniazid, and kanamycin do require dosage adjustments.

16. **(E)** The mesentery develops with the embryonic gut. After the fifth week of development, the gut extends into the umbilical cord. The SMA provides the axis around which the duodenum rotates 270 degrees counterclockwise on its reentry into the abdominal cavity. The right colon also does the same, giving the normal anatomic positioning of the intestines. After the 12th week, the mesentery of the rotated gut begins to adhere to the posterior abdominal wall, although this may not be completed until birth. The root of the mesentery is formed with this fixation, spanning the transverse mesocolon in the left upper abdomen to the ileocecal junction in the right lower quadrant, thereby eliminating the risk of volvulus.

Mesenteric cysts are congenital lymphatic spaces, are most often filled with lymphatic fluid, and enlarge in size over time. They have been classified by their etiologies, which include embryonic/congenital, traumatic/acquired, neoplastic, and infective/degenerative cysts. They are often present as symptomatic abdominal masses, with pain, nausea, and/or vomiting, and can be often palpated on physical examination. Lateral mobility is a characteristic finding on palpation. Treatment consists of surgical resection, although they may often require partial bowel resection due to their proximity to the vascular supply of the bowel.

17. **(C)** There are two main classifications of congenital intraperitoneal hernias: transmesenteric and mesocolic. Transmesenteric hernias do not have a hernia sac, as they occur through potential defects of the mesentery, and present most often during childhood. The most common site of transmesenteric hernias occurs at the epiploic foramen, followed by congenital mesenteric defects and the broad ligament of the uterus. They can also occur secondary to trauma or iatrogenic mesenteric defects as well. Obstructive symptoms prevail in their presentation, and may range from chronic low-grade obstruction to high-grade or closed-loop symptoms. Operative reduction and correction of the defect is required for treatment, and care should be taken with the major blood vessels that are usually present at the perimeter of the constriction.

Mesocolic hernias have hernia sacs and are the result of abnormal rotation of the developing intestine. Their name derives from the fact that the hernia sac is mesentery, as due to malrotation, the small bowel becomes trapped behind either the right or the left side of the mesentery as it fixates to the posterior abdominal wall. They usually present in adults rather than children, and symptoms vary from vague abdominal pain to severe obstruction. In right mesocolic hernias, the duodenum rotates only 90 degrees while the colon rotates normally, trapping the small bowel behind the right mesocolon. Operative reduction involves releasing the right colon from the peritoneum, with placement of the colon on the left side of the abdomen and the small bowel on the right. Left mesocolic hernias were once thought to occur through the paraduodenal fossa near the fourth portion of the duodenum; however, they are most likely the result of malrotation placing the small bowel behind the left mesocolon. Operative reduction involves releasing the left mesocolon from its peritoneal attachments, which can be done by incising along the inferior mesenteric vein which usually marks the neck of the hernia sac.

18. **(B)** The greater and lesser omentum arise from different embryologic structures. The lesser omentum arises from remnants of the ventral mesogastrium, while the greater omentum is a two-layer structure formed by the merging of the transverse mesocolon and the dorsal mesogastrium. The omentum is rich in blood vessels and lymphatics, and serves a strong antibacterial function. This is achieved by release of macrophages and the compartmentalization of intraperitoneal sites of infection. Although once considered to be capable of motility to sites of infection, it has been shown that its movement is dependent on intestinal peristalsis and gravity. Omental dysfunction is seen in its torsion and infarction.

Omental torsion occurs as either primarily or secondary to adhesions, omental cysts, or omental tumors. The cause of primary torsion is unknown, and occurs much less frequently than conditions providing an omental leadpoint. Omental torsion does occur more often on the right than the left side of the omentum. Presentation of omental torsion mimics appendicitis, acute cholecystits, or ovarian torsion. Omental infarction is a rare condition, and although it can occur secondarily to torsion, it is usually unrelated. It is more often caused by abdominal trauma and is associated with collagen vascular disease. Resection of the portions of the omentum involved are usually adequate treatment for both conditions.

19. **(D)**

20. **(C)**

21. **(E)**

22. **(E)**

Explanations 19 through 22

The abdominal CT scan reveals evidence of a spigelian hernia on the left. These are a variation of ventral hernias that occur along the lateral edge of the rectus abdominis, medial to the semilunar line. Most often they occur inferior to the junction of the semilunar line of the rectus abdominis and the semicircular line of Douglas (arcuate line). This is consistent with the lack of posterior fascia below the arcuate line. They may occur at any level of the abdominal wall, and may also dissect between the internal and external oblique muscle layers.

Presenting symptoms are similar to those of standard ventral hernias, and include most often pain, palpable abdominal wall mass, and bowel obstruction. Entrapment of the anterior cutaneous nerves of T10–T12 can provide a similar distribution of pain. Preoperative diagnosis is usually possible in 50–75% of cases. Diagnosis is most often obtained by abdominopelvic CT scan; however, abdominal ultrasound can also provide the diagnosis. Sensitivity is increased with simultaneous valsalva maneuver during diagnostic testing.

Open surgical repair has been the traditional method of treatment for spigelian hernias. Hernia contents have been found most often to be nothing, small bowel, omentum, cecum, and sigmoid colon, in order of decreasing frequency. The vast majority is amenable to primary repair, but large hernias may require mesh placement. An extraperitoneal laparoscopic repair has been shown to provide improved results for length of stay and morbidity, and remains a viable option for elective repairs in the hands of the

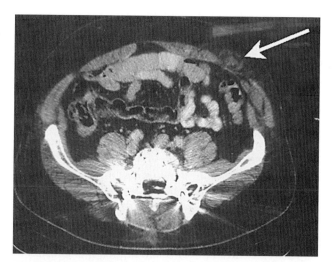

FIG. 27-3 Abdominopelvic CT scan showing a left-sided spigelian hernia. Note its position just lateral to the rectus abdominis. The hernia was found to contain fat and was closed primarily.

experienced surgeon. In a study of 76 patients, only 3 patients had recurrent hernias in an 8-year follow-up period (Fig. 27-3).

23. (C)

24. (C)

25. (E)

26. (A)

Explanations 23 through 26

Abdominal compartment syndrome (ACS) is used to describe the constellation of pulmonary, renal, and cardiac sequelae that results from increased abdominal pressure. Its etiology is multifactorial, and has been shown to be associated with many clinical syndromes, including hemorrhage, dilatation of bowel, acute ascites, mesenteric venous thrombosis, pelvic/retroperitoneal hematoma, necrotizing pancreatitis, and massive fluid resuscitation. It is important to note that although ACS is related to mostly intraabdominal processes, massive resuscitation alone from extremity or thoracic trauma, hypothermia, and sepsis may also be etiologic factors.

ACS most commonly occurs within 24–48-h post-injury, during the resuscitation period. The increased pressure is thought to produce several main effects: compression of both the kidneys and retroperitoneum, and elevation of the diaphragms. Direct compression of the retroperitoneum causes decreased venous return via the IVC, which in turn will result in decreased preload, leading to decreased cardiac output and stroke volume, with a resultant increase in systemic vascular resistance. The increased intrathoracic pressure also contributes to this. Elevation of the diaphragms results in increased intrathoracic pressure, which in turn causes increased peak airway pressures and decreased lung compliance, leading eventually to hypoxemia. Compression of the kidneys results in increased renovascular resistance, leading to decreased renal blood flow. This, in combination with a mild relative venous outflow obstruction, leads to oliguria. There is no significant compressive effect on the ureters. Interestingly enough, there also appears to be an association between ACS and increased intracranial pressure.

Diagnosis of ACS is made by a combination of clinical suspicion, measurement of cardiac/ventilatory parameters, and measurement of intraabdominal pressure. Clinical situations at risk of ACS should be evaluated, especially if abdominal distention, decreased cardiac output, oliguria, and elevated peak airway pressures occur. Intraabdominal pressure is directly measured by bladder pressures; this is performed via a Foley catheter. The bladder should be filled with approximately 50 cc of sterile saline with the drainage port clamped. As the bladder acts as a passive reservoir due to its low muscular tone, intraabdominal pressure can be measured with a manometer or by connecting a pressure transducer to the infusion port of the Foley catheter. The severity of ACS is based on a grading system: grade 1 (10–15 mmHg), grade 2 (16–25 mmHg), grade 3 (26–35 mmHg), and grade 4 (>35 mmHg). Regardless of the measurements, it is most important to consider the patient's clinical condition, and not basing all evaluation on the bladder pressure. ACS in some patients is manifested at levels as low as 10 mmHg, while others may tolerate pressures as high as 30 mmHg before symptoms occur.

The goal of therapeutic intervention for ACS lies in the reduction of abdominal pressure, which is achieved by surgical decompression via a midline incision. Resolution of hypoxemia, decreased cardiac output, and urinary output should occur quickly, however, not always immediately. Fascial closure is not an option given the retroperitoneal and visceral edema that these patients frequently have. There are many different options for closure, including simple skin closure of the abdomen, sterile irrigation or "Bogota" bags, PTFE sheets, Vicryl mesh, and towel clip closure of the skin. Regardless, the abdomen should be closed in 3–4 days to avoid development of intestinal fistulae. Should fascial closure still be difficult after several attempts at primary closure, mesh placement or abdominal wall component separation (which can close a fascial defect of up to 15 cm) can both be used to close the abdomen (Fig. 27-4).

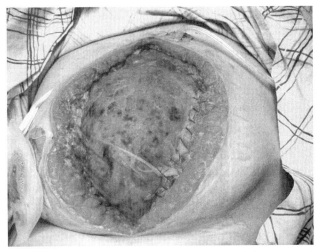

FIG. 27-4 Closure of abdomen in a patient with abdominal compartment syndrome due to severe pancreatitis.

27. **(E)**

28. **(E)**

29. **(B)**

30. **(B)**

Explanations 27 through 30

The standard treatment of acute pancreatitis is non-operative; however, operative intervention may be warranted for several reasons: (1) uncertainty of diagnosis, (2) correction of associated biliary tract disease, (3) progressive clinical deterioration given maximum supportive care, and (4) treatment of secondary pancreatic infections.

The advent of abdominopelvic CT scanning has facilitated the nonoperative diagnosis of acute pancreatitis; however, given the situation other surgical conditions cannot be excluded (perforated viscus or mesenteric ischemia, for instance), laparotomy may be warranted to elucidate the patient's condition. In exploration of the lesser sac, the pancreas can be evaluated for evidence of pancreatitis or necrosis. Should noncomplicated acute pancreatitis exist, no further surgical intervention is warranted. If concomitant biliary disease is suspected, cholecystectomy and/or intraoperative cholangiography may be needed. Also, if noninfected necrotizing pancreatitis is found, then gentle debridement of the necrotic tissue with wide sump drainage should be performed. Note that formal pancreatic resection is rarely warranted. Regardless, thoughts to placement of gastrostomy and/or jejunostomy tubes should be considered at the time of laparotomy, as studies have proven that postpyloric (jejunal or nasoduodenal) enteral feeding is superior to total parenteral nutrition, given the higher incidence of pneumonia and infectious complications with TPN.

Secondary pancreatic infections are classified as pancreatic abscess, infected pancreatic pseudocyst, and infected pancreatic necrosis; overall, only 5% of patients with acute pancreatits will develop an infectious pancreatic complication. Severity of pancreatitis is directly related to the incidence of infection. Patients with six or more Ranson's criteria have greater than 50% chance of developing pancreatic sepsis. The etiology is thought to derive from either hematogenous seeding or translocation of bacteria via adjacent bowel. Gram-negative organisms are most common, with fungal infections becoming more frequently identified. Imipenem has been shown to have the best parenchymal penetration of the pancreas, and is commonly thought to be the first line antibiotic of choice for prophylaxis.

Pancreatic sepsis should be considered in patients with known bacteremia, clinical deterioration after 7 days, or in those with pancreatitis which does not resolve after 7–10 days. Patients frequently present with symptoms of fever, tachycardia, abdominal pain, and distention. Radiographic findings usually begin with peripancreatic and/or retroperitoneal fluid collections, which often on CT scan are shown to dissect behind the right and left colon. The finding of gas (the so-called "soap bubble sign") within these collections is pathognomonic. Overall, CT scan is considered the gold standard of radiographic analysis, as the sensitivity is greater than 90% when more than 30% of the pancreatic parenchyma is involved. Laboratory abnormalities almost always show leukocytosis with concomitant elevations of liver function tests and serum amylase. Guided percutaneous needle aspiration may be warranted. Although it can demonstrate the presence of bacteria from within a peripancreatic fluid collection, some clinicians are concerned with the likelihood of seeding a previously sterile peripancreatic fluid collection with a percutaneous procedure, and often refrain from these invasive techniques to diagnose pancreatic infection.

Once the diagnosis is made, the treatment is primarily operative. Sometimes with well-defined pancreatic abscesses or infected pseudocysts, percutaneous drainage may be sufficient to adequately drain the lesion. There have also been efforts to endoscopically drain infected pancreatic necrosis. Often, however, there is a complex and loculated collection which is not amenable to these techniques

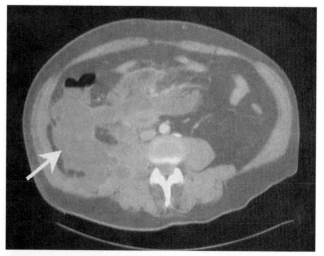

FIG. 27-5 Abdominopelvic CT scan showing a large peripancreatic fluid collection dissecting into the retroperitoneum behind the right colon. Note the absence of gas within this fluid collection.

alone. Open pancreatic debridement should be performed with several goals in mind. (1) Debridement should be *gentle*, avoiding vigorous debridement of the retroperitoneum, which could result in injury of retroperitoneal vascular structures resulting in life-threatening hemorrhage; (2) formal resection of the pancreas should be avoided; (3) wide sump drainage of the retroperitoneum via large-bore drains placed in dependent positions or open packing of the peri-pancreatic space should be performed; (4) given the presence of associated biliary tract disease, cholecystectomy with or without intraoperative cholangiogram should be performed.

Overall, 16–40% of patients requiring operative intervention will require reoperation for continued sepsis, and the mortality rate has been reported to be between 5 and 50%, averaging 30% (Fig. 27-5).

Bibliography

Artioukh DY, Walker SJ. Spigelian herniae: presentation, diagnosis, and treatment. *J R Coll Surg Edinb* 1996;41 (4):241–243.

Blackbourne LH (ed.). *Surgical Recall*, 3rd ed. Philadelphia, PA: Lippincott, Williams & Wilkins, 2002.

Cameron JL (ed.). *Current Surgical Therapy*, 7th ed. St. Louis, MO: Mosby, 2001.

Lewis JJ. Retroperitoneal soft-tissue sarcoma: analysis of 500 patients treated and followed at a single institution. *Ann Surg* 228(3):355–365.

Moreno-Egea A, Flores B, Girela E, Martin JG, Aguayo JL, Canteras M. Spigelian hernia: bibliographical study and presentation of a series of 28 patients. *Hernia* 2002;6 (4):167–170.

Sabiston DC Jr. (ed.). *Sabiston Textbook of Surgery*, 16th ed. Philadelphia, PA: W.B. Saunders, 2001.

Schwartz SI (ed.). *Principles of Surgery*, 7th ed. New York, NY: McGraw-Hill, 1999.

CHAPTER 28

Liver

Rabih A. Chaer and N. Joseph Espat

Questions

1. During fetal development

    (A) the liver primordium appears at the third month

    (B) the liver is derived from ventral thickening of the endoderm at the distal end of the foregut

    (C) a secondary caudal proliferation becomes the gallbladder and the cystic duct

    (D) the left umbilical vein drains into the left portal vein and passes through the ductus venosus into the inferior vena cava (IVC)

    (E) bile formation is evident as early as the third week

2. Regarding hepatic arterial supply

    (A) parallels the portal venous system intrahepatically

    (B) provides 70% of blood flow to the liver

    (C) normal anatomy is present in only 50% of individuals

    (D) the most important variations are a right hepatic artery and a common hepatic artery arising from a superior mesenteric trunk (replaced hepatic arteries)

    (E) the most common variant is origin of the right hepatic artery from the gastroduodenal artery

3. Which of the following statements about the anatomy of the liver is/are *true*?

    (A) The liver is divided into right and left lobes by the portal fissure (Cantlie's line).

    (B) The lobar anatomy of the liver is determined by the distribution of the hepatic veins and portal structures.

    (C) The caudate lobe is a portion of the right lobe.

    (D) The quadrate lobe is a portion of the medial segment of the left lobe.

    (E) The French segmental segment for hepatic anatomy is based mainly on hepatic venous drainage.

4. Which of the following is *true* regarding hepatic resections?

    (A) They usually involve dissection in the plane of the umbilical fissure.

    (B) Partial hepatectomy involves removal of the left or right lobe.

    (C) The anatomic division between right and left liver is the falciform ligament.

    (D) The nomenclature of liver resection is described by more than one classification system.

    (E) There are essentially five types of major resections.

5. Prior to hepatic resection, preoperative investigation and preparation should include

    (A) exact definition of the nature of the lesion

    (B) assessment of resectability

    (C) preoperative antibiotics for 24 h prior to the procedure

    (D) hepatic angiography

    (E) detailed cardiopulmonary workup

6. Liver resection is safely done

    (A) when only 50% of the liver volume is removed

    (B) in noncirrhotic livers only

    (C) if the reduction of the functional liver parenchyma is less than 50%

    (D) if the serum bilirubin is less than 2 mg/mL

    (E) in the context of clinically detectable ascites

7. Patients undergoing liver resection

   (A) should be well hydrated and have a central venous pressure (CVP) of 12 mmHg at all times
   (B) blood and infusion fluids should be warmed intraoperatively to avoid hypothermia
   (C) halothane is volatile anesthetic of choice
   (D) fentanyl is the ideal narcotic used to provide analgesia with minimal hypotension
   (E) hepatic isolation often requires the insertion of a pulmonary artery catheter and the administration of vasopressors

8. Which of the following strategies are useful to limit blood loss during major hepatic resection?

   (A) low CVP anesthesia
   (B) precise extrahepatic dissection of the major hepatic veins
   (C) portal triad clamping
   (D) induced hypothermia to minimize metabolic demand
   (E) occasional venovenous bypass

9. Which of the following statements is/are *true* regarding the anatomy and function of the portal vein?

   (A) It provides a minor part of hepatic blood flow.
   (B) It is the most posterior structure in the hepatoduodenal ligament.
   (C) It is formed by the junction of the inferior mesenteric vein and the splenic vein.
   (D) Its wall is hyperechoic on ultrasound.
   (E) The right portal vein branches sooner than the left portal vein.

10. Which of the following statements is/are *true* about portal vein tributaries?

   (A) They are usually physiologically significant.
   (B) They include connections to the renal and adrenal veins.
   (C) In certain diseased states, they develop into large channels with increased collateral flow.
   (D) They consist of pathologic portosystemic anastomoses.
   (E) They provide an anatomic explanation to distant hemorrhagic complications of advanced liver disease.

11. Which of the following statements is/are *true* about hepatic venous drainage and the anatomy of the hepatic veins?

   (A) The hepatic vein parallels the hepatic arterial system intrahepatically.
   (B) Hepatic venous drainage is through the right and left branch of the hepatic vein, each draining the right and left lobe of the liver, respectively.
   (C) The left hepatic vein drains the entire left lobe.
   (D) The right hepatic vein drains the entire right lobe.
   (E) None of the above.

12. Hypoxic injury primarily affects hepatocytes located in the following areas:

   (A) acinar zone I
   (B) acinar zone II
   (C) acinar zone III
   (D) the central acinar region
   (E) the central lobular region

13. Which of the following is *true* regarding liver regeneration?

   (A) it is essentially hypertrophy of the remaining hepatocytes
   (B) it is a continuous process throughout life
   (C) the liver can regain its normal size after a 75–90% hepatectomy
   (D) hepatocyte cell division after a hepatectomy is complete within 1 week
   (E) the mechanism of liver regeneration has been clearly identified

14. During fasting, the liver provides energy and substrates for metabolism by the following mechanisms:

   (A) glycogenolysis
   (B) gluconeogenesis
   (C) lipolysis
   (D) formation of ketone bodies from fatty acids
   (E) proteolysis

15. The basic histology and cellular physiology associated with liver function includes

   (A) a unique architecture with different hepatocyte function depending on the acinar zone
   (B) a heterogeneous hepatocyte plasma membrane with different regions and associated ultrastructures
   (C) a rich microcirculation with limited contact with the hepatocyte

(D) an intrinsic dependence on glucose metabolism

(E) cell-cell interaction at the level of the sinusoidal membrane

16. The cells involved in the reticuloendothelial function of the liver include

(A) ito cells

(B) Kupffer cells

(C) pit cells

(D) endothelial cells

(E) hepatocytes

17. Biotransformation reactions include

(A) oxidative reactions

(B) phase I and II reactions

(C) conjugation

(D) bile salt production

(E) reduction

18. Hepatic protein synthesis affects

(A) albumin regulation

(B) the coagulation cascade

(C) fibrinogen

(D) urea synthesis

(E) factor V

19. A 65-year-old man presents to the emergency room with 3 days history of fever, chills, and right upper quadrant pain. He is otherwise healthy and gives a history of prior cholecystectomy in the distant past. On physical examination, he is not jaundiced. He is febrile and tachycardic and has significant tenderness over the right upper quadrant. He denies any history of alcohol use or recent travel. An ultrasound is obtained and shows a hypoechoic intrahepatic lesion. The most likely diagnosis is

(A) hepatocellular carcinoma (HCC)

(B) a liver hemangioma

(C) acute hepatitis

(D) pyogenic liver abscess

(E) cholangitis

20. With the presumptive diagnosis of a pyogenic liver abscess, the initial management should include

(A) open incision and drainage

(B) laparoscopic exploration

(C) urgent endoscopic retrograde cholagiopancreatography

(D) intravenous antibiotics

(E) radiographically guided percutaneous drainage

21. Which of the following statements characterize an amebic abscess?

(A) Patients tend to be older than those affected with a pyogenic abscess.

(B) Primary treatment is pharmacologic.

(C) The diagnosis may be based on serologic tests and resolution of symptoms.

(D) Organisms most commonly reach the liver via the portal vein.

(E) Cultures of a percutaneous aspirate are usually sterile.

22. A 45-year-old man is found to have a 6 cm calcified cystic liver lesion containing daughter cysts in the right lobe of the liver. The initial preferred treatment includes

(A) right hepatic lobectomy

(B) pericystectomy

(C) a 2-week course of metronidazole

(D) percutaneous catheter drainage

(E) laparoscopic drainage

23. Schistosomiasis

(A) is a parasitic disease caused by tapeworms

(B) is a human disease because of poor sanitation

(C) is the most cause of portal hypertension worldwide

(D) is treated with mebendazole

(E) often requires surgical intervention

24. Characteristics of fulminant hepatic failure are as follows:

(A) It is rarely a medical emergency.

(B) It is a clinical syndrome representing a final common pathway for a wide variety of diseases.

(C) It is most commonly because of alcohol abuse.

(D) It has pathognomonic features making the diagnosis evident.

(E) Sometimes may not have an identifiable cause.

25. A 25-year-old female is brought to the local emergency room with signs and symptoms compatible with encephalopathy. Her family members report that she had been jaundiced over the past few days and had recently separated with her boyfriend. She had been otherwise healthy and on no medications. The most likely etiology and best treatment course include the following.

    (A) Hepatic failure in this setting is usually secondary to viral hepatitis.
    (B) The patient should receive broad-spectrum prophylactic antibiotics
    (C) Steroid therapy should be started immediately.
    (D) An evaluation for liver transplantation should be done as soon as possible.
    (E) Acetylcysteine should be administered.

26. A 33-year-old man tested positive for antibody to HCV when donating blood. His liver enzymes are within normal range. The patient is otherwise healthy, feels well, and denies any risk factors for HCV. His physical examination is unremarkable and shows no stigmata of chronic liver disease. Qualitative polymerase chain reaction (PCR) testing is positive for HCV RNA. Which of the following actions is most appropriate for this patient?

    (A) reassure the patient that he does not have chronic HCV infection and requires no further evaluation or treatment
    (B) recommend treatment with antiviral therapy for chronic HCV infection
    (C) recommend liver biopsy and initiate therapy accordingly
    (D) recommend yearly follow-up with liver enzymes monitoring and do not initiate any treatment at this time
    (E) recommend liver imaging consisting of an ultrasound or CT

27. A 26-year-old surgery resident is evaluated for malaise, fatigue, myalgia, and low-grade fever. He was previously well and denies illicit drug use, transfusions, or recent travel. He admits though to multiple needle stick accidents. Physical examination reveals jaundice and hepatomegaly. Laboratory studies are as follows: AST 1000 U/L, ALT 2000 U/L, INR 1.0, total bilirubin 4 mg/dL, IgG anti-HAV positive, IgM anti-HAV negative, HBsAg positive, IgG anti-HBc positive, IgM anti-HBc positive, anti-HCV negative.

The most likely diagnosis is

    (A) acute hepatitis C
    (B) acute hepatitis B
    (C) chronic hepatitis A
    (D) chronic hepatitis B
    (E) chronic hepatitis C

28. Eight weeks following a abdominal aortic aneurysm repair requiring several blood transfusions, a 55-year-old man notes tea colored urine, jaundice, fatigue, and anorexia. Examination shows icteric sclera and a mild hepatomegaly. Laboratory investigation reveals a bilirubin of 3 mg/dL, AST 550 U/L, ALT 650 U/L, negative HBsAg, anti-HBc, anti-HAV and anti-HCV assays. The most likely diagnosis is

    (A) ischemic hepatitis
    (B) acute viral hepatitis A
    (C) acute viral hepatitis B
    (D) acute viral hepatitis C
    (E) acute viral hepatitis D

29. Worldwide, the most important predisposing factor for HCC is

    (A) alcoholic cirrhosis
    (B) hepatitis B infection
    (C) chronic liver disease of any etiology
    (D) hepatitis C infection
    (E) repeated ingestion of aflatoxin

30. A 65-year-old man is diagnosed with HCC. The most likely presentation is

    (A) obstructive jaundice is the initial sign in 20–30% of patients
    (B) hepatomegaly is the most common sign at presentation
    (C) that of an occult process
    (D) most patients present with signs and symptoms of metastasis, most commonly to the lungs
    (E) the majority of patients are asymptomatic and the diagnosis is made incidentally

31. The most accurate procedure to diagnose HCC or other suspected liver tumors is

    (A) angiography
    (B) cholangiography
    (C) ultrasonography

(D) CT scan

(E) laparoscopy

32. A 66-year-old male patient is evaluated for jaundice and is found to have a hepatic mass. He has a history of long-term exposure to vinyl chloride. The most likely diagnosis is

(A) angiosarcoma

(B) fibrosarcoma

(C) leiomyosarcoma

(D) mesenchymal sarcoma

(E) rhabdomyosarcoma

33. Most primary and metastatic tumors to the liver derive nearly all their vascular inflow from branches of the

(A) portal vein

(B) collateral circulation

(C) hepatic artery

(D) celiac axis

(E) unnamed branches from the aorta

34. Regarding hepatic hemangioma

(A) it is the most common benign solid liver tumor in adults

(B) it carries a slight risk of malignant degeneration

(C) most patient are asymptomatic

(D) the most common symptom is jaundice

(E) it is best diagnosed by biopsy and histologic evaluation

35. During a laparoscopic cholecystectomy performed on a healthy young man, a 1-cm cavernous hemangioma is noticed on the surface of the left lobe of the liver. The most appropriate treatment for this lesion at this time is

(A) biopsy and frozen section analysis

(B) observation

(C) resection

(D) laparoscopic fulguration

(E) postoperative embolization

36. A 44-year-old man is found to have a small cystic liver lesion on ultrasound of the abdomen obtained for vague occasional epigastric pain. The patient is otherwise healthy and has no prior medical history. The next step should be

(A) elective open wedge resection

(B) diagnostic laparoscopy with possible resection

(C) CT guided needle biopsy

(D) observation

(E) percutaneous aspiration

37. Which of the following treatment options for HCC substantially prolongs survival?

(A) cryoablation

(B) ethanol injection

(C) liver transplantation

(D) resection

(E) radiofrequency ablation

38. In an otherwise healthy man with colorectal cancer and a 2-cm lesion metastatic to the liver, the treatment of choice is

(A) arterial chemoembolization

(B) cryoablation

(C) resection

(D) ethanol injection

(E) radiofrequency ablation

39. A 35-year-old woman with a history of a liver mass recently stopped oral contraceptives and became pregnant. She is evaluated for severe abdominal pain, tachycardia, and hypotension. She has a viable intrauterine pregnancy. She is found to have a liver lesion on ultrasonography. The most likely diagnosis is

(A) ruptured choledochal cyst

(B) rupture and hemorrhage of a FNH

(C) rupture and hemorrhage a hepatic adenoma

(D) rupture of HCC

(E) rupture of a hepatic hemangioma

40. Which of the following patients is more likely to have an elevated alpha fetoprotein (AFP) level?

(A) a patient with fulminant hepatitis B infection

(B) a patient with HCC

(C) a patient with a yolk sac tumor

(D) a patient with a teratocarcinoma

(E) a patient with cholangiocarcinoma

41. Which of the following is/are associated with the development of cholangiocarcinoma?

(A) chronic pancreatitis

(B) primary sclerosing cholangitis

(C) hepatolithiasis

(D) *Clonorchis sinensis* infestation

(E) inflammatory bowel disease

42. Which of the following is/are true regarding intra-hepatic cholangiocarcinoma?

    (A) Survival after resection is less than for distal cholangiocarcinoma.

    (B) Adjuvant chemotherapy is associated with improved survival.

    (C) Preoperative radiation therapy is associated with decreased local recurrence.

    (D) Resection is contraindicated unless histologically negative margins can be obtained.

    (E) Staging is by the TNM system.

43. A 66-year-old man is found to have an elevated carcinoembryonic antigen (CEA) 2 years after uneventful resection of a colon carcinoma. A metastatic liver lesion is identified. The workup and treatment options include the following:

    (A) CT scan

    (B) intraoperative ultrasound

    (C) liver resection

    (D) adjuvant hepatic arterial chemotherapy

    (E) adjuvant radiation therapy

44. Which of the following is true regarding the histology of HCC?

    (A) The fibrolamellar variant has a better prognosis than standard HCC.

    (B) The fibrolamellar variant occurs most commonly in the right lobe and accounts for 10–20% of case of HCC.

    (C) Carcinosarcoma is more commonly metastatic than standard HCC and has a worst prognosis.

    (D) The clear cell variant is often confused with metastatic clear cell lung cancer.

    (E) Childhood HCC is most commonly unilateral and unifocal.

45. Which of the following is true regarding FNH?

    (A) It is usually asymptomatic.

    (B) It has a central stellate scar.

    (C) It is easy to differentiate from a hepatic adenoma in most of the cases.

    (D) It may undergo malignant transformation.

    (E) Is clearly associated with the use of oral contraceptives.

46. A 53-year-old man has long-standing liver cirrhosis secondary to hepatitis C infection. The most appropriate screening regimen should include

    (A) yearly CT scan of the abdomen

    (B) a liver biopsy

    (C) liver ultrasound

    (D) AFP level

    (E) diagnostic laparoscopy

Answers and Explanations

1. **(B), (C), (D)** The liver primordium appears at around the third week of fetal development as a ventral thickening of the endoderm at the distal end of the foregut. This will mainly give rise to the hepatic parenchyma as well as the main bile duct. The gallbladder and the cystic duct on the other hand will develop from a secondary caudal proliferation. The left umbilical vein drains into the left portal vein and passes through the ductus venosus into the IVC. The ductus venosus as well as the left umbilical vein are obliterated after birth and form the ligamentum venosus and the ligamentum teres. As hepatocytes proliferate, the liver protrudes into the abdomen, with the bare area being a reminiscent of its origin. Bile production will happen as early as the third month, after bile ducts differentiate and join the extrahepatic biliary system.

Bibliography

Meyers WC, Jones RS. *Textbook of Liver and Biliary Surgery*. Philadelphia, PA: Lippincott, Williams & Wilkins, 1990.
Townsend CM, et al. *Sabiston Textbook of Surgery: The Biological Basis of Modern Surgical Practice*, 16th ed. Philadelphia, PA: W.B. Saunders, 2001.

2. **(A), (C)** The hepatic arterial supply is usually derived from the celiac axis by way of the proper hepatic artery, which becomes the common hepatic artery after giving off the gastroduodenal branch posterior and superior to the duodenum. It accounts for 25% of hepatic blood flow, the remainder being supplied by the portal vein. It subsequently bifurcates into the right and left hepatic branches within the hepatoduodenal ligament (Fig. 28-1).

    The extrahepatic arterial system does not parallel the portal channels, although the intrahepatic system does. Over 50% of the population has the same anatomic pattern. There are, however, significant variations in hepatic arterial anatomy. In 15–20% of individuals, the right hepatic artery arises from the superior mesenteric artery and is found in the posterolateral aspect of the hepatoduodenal ligament. In 15% of individuals, the left hepatic artery originates

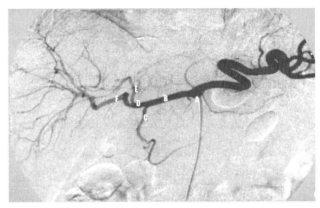

FIG. 28-1 Visceral angiogram illustrating "standard" hepatic artery anatomy. The celiac artery (A) gives rise to the proper hepatic artery (B); the gastroduodenal artery (C) arises perpendicular to the proper hepatic where it becomes the common hepatic artery (D); subsequently becoming the right (E) and left (F) hepatic arteries.

from the left gastric artery and is located in the gastrohepatic ligament. The most common situations in which aberrant hepatic arterial anatomy may be problematic are: during cholecystectomy when an aberrant right hepatic artery is mistaken for the cystic artery, during liver transplantation when aberrant branches are not recognized when coming off the aorta, superior mesenteric or gastric arteries, and during hepatobiliary resections or repairs when a replaced hepatic artery is erroneously ligated.

Bibliography

Blumgart LH, Fong Y. *Surgery of the Liver and Biliary Tract*, 3rd ed. Edinburgh: Churchill Livingstone, 2000.
Meyers WC, Jones RS. *Textbook of Liver and Biliary Surgery*. Philadelphia, PA: Lippincott, Williams & Wilkins, 1990.
Townsend CM, et al. *Sabiston Textbook of Surgery: The Biological Basis of Modern Surgical Practice*, 16th ed. Philadelphia, PA: W.B. Saunders, 2001.

3. **(A), (B), (D), (E)** The surgical anatomy of the liver is based on the distribution of the hepatic veins and portal structures. A plane called the portal fissure

(line of Cantlie) passes from the left side of the gall-bladder fossa to the left side of the IVC to divide the liver into right and left lobes. The left lobe consists of a medial segment, which lies to the right of the falciform ligament and umbilical fissure, and a lateral segment, which lies to the left of the falciform ligament. The right lobe consists of an anteromedial (segments V and VIII) and a posterolateral (segments VI and VII) sector, divided by a vertical plane containing the right hepatic vein.

According to the segmental nomenclature introduced by the French anatomists Soupault, Couinaud, and Bismuth, the liver is divided into eight segments: four on the right, three on the left, and one corresponding to the topographic caudate lobe. Segment I corresponds to the caudate lobe, and is considered anatomically independent of the right and left lobes, as it receives separate portal and arterial branches from both sides, and as hepatic venous drainage is by way of separate veins directly into the IVC. The left lobe is divided in posterosuperior (segment II), and inferoanterior sectors (segments III and IV) by the plane of the left hepatic vein (Fig. 28-2).

The quadrate lobe is a topographic description of the area between the gallbladder fossa, umbilical fissure, and portal triad. It is within the medial aspect of the left lobe (segment IV).

Bibliography

Blumgart LH, Fong Y. *Surgery of the Liver and Biliary Tract*, 3rd ed. Edinburgh: Churchill Livingstone, 2000.

Meyers WC, Jones RS. *Textbook of Liver and Biliary Surgery*. Philadelphia, PA: Lippincott, Williams & Wilkins, 1990.

Townsend CM, et al. *Sabiston Textbook of Surgery: The Biological Basis of Modern Surgical Practice*, 16th ed. Philadelphia, PA: W.B. Saunders, 2001.

4. **(D), (E)** The liver is divided into sectors that are formed from liver segments supplied by branches of the portal triads and drained by hepatic veins. Partial hepatectomy involves removal of one or more segments by isolation of the relevant portal pedicle and hepatic veins. The liver is divided into right and left lobes by the line of Cantlie, a line projected through a plane running from the medial margin of the gallbladder bed to the left of the IVC posteriorly (Fig. 28-3).

Each of these major right and left portions of the liver is divided into sectors and segments. That portion of the liver to the left of the ligamentum teres forms the left lobe and that to the right of the ligamentum teres the right lobe. The portal venous and hepatic arterial branches run within the segments, and between the sectors, the draining hepatic veins converge posteriorly toward the vena cava. Dissection is therefore not performed in the plane of the umbilical fissure to avoid injury to the portal vein.

There are five main types of major hepatic resections. There are two classification systems available, one based on the anatomic descriptions of Couinaud and Bismuth, and the more commonly used terminology of Goldsmith and Woodburne. A right hepatectomy in the Goldsmith terminology corresponds to segment V, VI, VII, VIII resection (right hepatectomy) in the Couinaud terminology, a left hepatic lobectomy in the Goldsmith nomenclature corresponds to segment II, III, IV resection (left hepatectomy) in the Couinaud system, an extended right

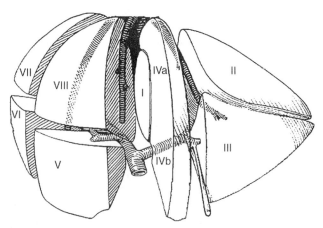

FIG. 28-2 The Couinaud segmental anatomy of the liver is based on the vascular supply to each anatomic segment. Under the most widely accepted system of anatomic classification the right lobe is composed of segments V–VIII and the left lobe of segments I–IV.

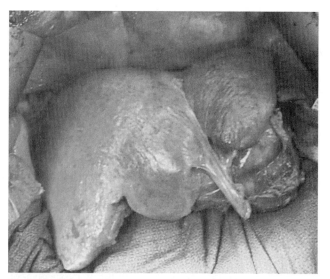

FIG. 28-3 Cantlie's line is the vascular demarcation of the midliver separating it into formal right and left lobes. This is defined as the imaginary plane between the middle of the gallbladder fossa (segment IVb/V) and the inferior vena cava. This photo illustrates the demarcation achieved in preparation for a left lobectomy.

hepatic lobectomy in the Goldsmith system corresponds to a segment IV, V, VI, VII, VIII, and sometimes I resection (right lobectomy) in the Couinaud system. A right lobectomy (extended right hepatic lobectomy) represents a right hepatectomy extended to segment IV and has been referred to by Starzl as right trisegmentectomy.

A left lateral segmentectomy in the Goldsmith system is a left lobectomy in the Couinaud system (segment II and III) resection, and an extended left lobectomy in the Goldsmith system is an extended left hepatectomy in the Couinaud system (segments II, III, IV, V, VIII, and sometimes I) resection. This was also referred to as a left trisegmentectomy by Starzl.

Bibliography

Blumgart LH, Fong Y. *Surgery of the Liver and Biliary Tract*, 3rd ed. Edinburgh: Churchill Livingstone, 2000.

Starzl TE, Bell RH, Beart RW, et al. Hepatic trisegmentectomy and other liver resections. *Surg Gynecol Obstet* 1975;141:429–437.

Strazl TE, Iwatsuki S, Shaw BW, et al. Left hepatic trisegmentectomy. *Surg Gynecol Obstet* 1982;155:21–27.

Townsend CM, et al. *Sabiston Textbook of Surgery: The Biological Basis of Modern Surgical Practice*, 16th ed. Philadelphia, PA: W.B. Saunders, 2001.

5. **(A), (B), (E)** Preoperative investigation should determine the nature of the lesion in preparation to surgical resection. This does not require a tissue diagnosis in all cases and this may actually not be advisable because of the associated risk of hemorrhage and tumor dissemination with to needle biopsy. A tissue diagnosis could be safely achieved with laparotomy or laparoscopy, with or without laparoscopic ultrasound. Respectability should be assessed on preoperative imaging first. Parenchymal liver lesions distant from major vascular structures and without evidence of metastatic disease are usually respectable, although some will have nodal disease or additional liver lesions on laparotomy or laparoscopy. On the other hand, evidence of multiple extensive bilateral disease implies irresectability. Cases where the tumor adheres to major hilar structures or compresses the vena cava are difficult to assess preoperatively and should not be declared unresectable based on preoperative imaging only, and this decision is often made intraoperatively after careful dissection.

Preoperative computed tomography (CT) scan is the test of choice and will usually provide accurate information regarding tumor location and involvement of hilar structures and the IVC. It should be obtained without contrast, then with an arterial and portal phase.

Magnetic resonance imaging (MRI) may show additional lesions not seen on initial CT scan and accurately shows vascular structures. The relationship of the tumor to the hepatic veins and vena cava could be therefore defined preoperatively by MRI angiography.

Ultrasonography is helpful in defining tumor size and extent of liver involvement and will differentiate solid from cystic lesions. Duplex ultrasonography is able to identify vascular structures including the hepatic veins and vena cava and is usually the next test obtained following the initial CT scan.

Hepatic angiography is no longer routinely performed with modern advances in MRI and duplex ultrasonography. It is usually obtained to define the extrahepatic arterial anatomy in patients expected to have a hepatic arterial infusion pump inserted.

Metastatic workup consisting of chest radiography or chest CT scan is also required.

Correction of anemia and coagulopathy is indicated, and a cardiopulmonary investigation is sought in patients over age 65 or as clinically indicated. Antibiotic prophylaxis consists of a single preoperative dose, repeated intraoperatively depending on the duration of the procedure (Fig. 28-4).

Bibliography

Townsend CM, et al. *Sabiston Textbook of Surgery: The Biological Basis of Modern Surgical Practice*, 16th ed. Philadelphia, PA: W.B. Saunders, 2001.

Blumgart LH, Fong Y. *Surgery of the Liver and Biliary Tract*, 3rd ed. Edinburgh: Churchill Livingstone, 2000.

6. **(C), (D), (E)** A noncirrhotic healthy liver may tolerate a resection of up to 75–85% of its volume. It is expected to regenerate within few weeks after major resection. This is feasible only if the reduction in the functional liver parenchyma is less than 50%. Besides the general condition of the patient and tumor resectability, preoperative hepatic reserve and function is the main prognostic factor. The best predictor of hepatic reserve is the indocyanine green (ICG-R15) clearance: normal retention at 15 min is <10%. Clinically, hepatic reserve is usually assessed by the Child-Pugh score or by the Child's classification. Mortality and morbidity are more significant in patients with Child's B or C than those with Child's A liver function. Moreover, liver resection should not be undertaken in patients with a serum bilirubin above 2 mg/mL or in the presence of clinically evident ascites. Cirrhosis is not an absolute contraindication to liver resection but entails much less effective liver regeneration and greater impairment of liver function.

Occasionally, preoperative portal vein embolization of the affected lobe allows hypertrophy of the

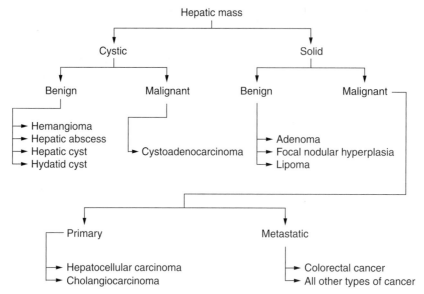

Hepatic mass

Cystic — Solid

Benign — Malignant   Benign — Malignant

Benign (Cystic):
→ Hemangioma
→ Hepatic abscess
→ Hepatic cyst
→ Hydatid cyst

Malignant (Cystic):
→ Cystoadenocarcinoma

Benign (Solid):
→ Adenoma
→ Focal nodular hyperplasia
→ Lipoma

Primary — Metastatic

Primary:
→ Hepatocellular carcinoma
→ Cholangiocarcinoma

Metastatic:
→ Colorectal cancer
→ All other types of cancer

FIG. 28-4 The preoperative patient evaluation should be guided by the presumptive diagnosis in addition to determining the physiologic capacity for the patient to tolerate a major operation. The algorithm proposed broadly divides the potential diagnoses to be considered in the patient with a hepatic mass.

contralateral side. It is indicated in the following circumstances:

1. resection of a large portion of nontumorous normal hepatic parenchyma (>60% of the functional liver)
2. resection of 40–60% of the functional liver in patients with abnormal ICG-R15 clearance ranging from 10 to 20% indicating mild impairment of liver function. It is contraindicated in patients whose clearance is over 20% since this indicates moderate to severe cirrhosis.
3. history of jaundice because of bile duct obstruction
4. concomitant resection of the head of the pancreas

Bibliography

Blumgart LH, Fong Y. *Surgery of the Liver and Biliary Tract*, 3rd ed. Edinburgh: Churchill Livingstone, 2000.

Kubota K, Makuuchi M, Kusaka K, Kobayashi T, Miki K, Hasegawa K, Harihara Y, Takayama T. Measurement of liver volume and hepatic functional reserve as a guide to decision making in resectional surgery for hepatic tumors. *Hepatology* 1997;26:1176–1181.

Miyagawa S, Makuuchi M, Kawasaki S, Kakazu T. Criteria for safe hepatic resection. *Am J Surg* 1995;169:589–594.

Townsend CM, et al. *Sabiston Textbook of Surgery: The Biological Basis of Modern Surgical Practice*, 16th ed. Philadelphia, PA: W.B. Saunders, 2001.

7. **(B), (D), (E)** Anesthetic planning prior to liver resection should include the possibility of major intraoperative bleeding. Hemorrhage during hepatic resection usually arises from the major hepatic veins or vena cava, hence the concept of low CVP anesthesia.

Indeed, preoperative fluid loading is practiced quite often in preparation for liver resection, resulting in a distended hepatic venous system, and a tense vena cava. Low CVP anesthesia aims at preventing caval distention and facilitating mobilization of the liver and dissection of the retrohepatic vena cava and major hepatic branches. Low CVP anesthesia therefore minimizes hepatic venous bleeding during liver resection and facilitates control of inadvertent venous injury. This reduced intraoperative blood loss translates into lower morbidity and mortality. The CVP is usually not allowed to rise above 5 mmHg. This is achieved by fluid restriction intraoperatively and by withholding preoperative overnight fluid replacement. Hemodynamic stability is maintained by occasional small fluid boluses. Moreover, this strategy has not led to an increase in postoperative renal failure. A minimum accepted intraoperative urine output is regarded as 25 mL/h. Dissection is also carried with the patient 15 degrees in the trendelenburg position. Not only does this obviate air embolism, it also improves venous return and helps maintain hemodynamic stability and renal function.

Anesthesia is maintained using a combination of isoflurane and narcotics. Isoflurane causes minimal myocardial depression, and the narcotic of choice is usually fentanyl because it provides analgesia with minimal hypotension. Halothane is usually avoided as a volatile anesthetic during liver resection because of the associated myocardial depression and the potential hepatotoxic effect.

In case prolonged inflow occlusion is anticipated, with or without hepatic vascular isolation, pulmonary artery catheters are usually inserted in anticipation of significant hemodynamic changes. Vascular isolation will decrease venous return with a resulting decrease in cardiac index. The CVP is kept elevated in this setting and vasopressor therapy may be required during the cross clamp period.

As in any major abdominal exposure and prolonged operation, blood and other infusion fluids are usually warmed to avoid hypothermia.

Bibliography

Blumgart LH, Fong Y. *Surgery of the Liver and Biliary Tract*, 3rd ed. Edinburgh: Churchill Livingstone, 2000.

Melendez JA, Arslan V, Fisher ME, et al. Perioperative outcomes of major hepatic resections under low central venous pressure anesthesia: blood loss, blood transfusion and the risk of postoperative renal dysfunction. *J Am Coll Surg* 1998;187:620–625.

Townsend CM, et al. *Sabiston Textbook of Surgery: The Biological Basis of Modern Surgical Practice*, 16th ed. Philadelphia, PA: W.B. Saunders, 2001.

Yanaga K, Kanematsu T, Takenaka K, Matsumata T, Yoshida Y, Sugimachi K. Hepatic resection for hepatocellular carcinoma in elderly patients. *Am J Surg* 1988; 155:238–241.

8. **(A), (B), (C), (E)** Bleeding from the hepatic veins and the vena cava during hepatic resection is a major concern. This is more likely to occur during parenchymal transection for high and posteriorly located tumors that are closely adherent or adjacent to the vena cava. A variety of intraoperative techniques have been developed in an attempt to avoid such complications. Clamping of the portal triad or the hepatic pedicle, the so-called Pringle maneuver, interrupts the arterial and venous inflow to the liver but has no effect on back bleeding from branches of the hepatic veins. It is indicated for both minor and major hepatic resections. This technique can be applied in either a continuous fashion until the hepatic parenchymal transection is finished, or in an intermittent fashion with 15–20 min of clamping followed by 5 min of unclamping. Although the liver tolerates better the intermittent strategy, blood loss is usually more significant because of parenchymal bleeding when the clamp is released. Yet the more important issue is tolerance of the liver to clamping, especially in patients with abnormal liver parenchyma (e.g., fatty liver and cirrhosis). Intermittent clamping is better tolerated and is usually recommended to avoid deterioration of postoperative liver function.

Persistent bleeding during a Pringle maneuver is usually secondary to incomplete inflow occlusion and/or back bleeding from the hepatic veins.

Backflow bleeding can be minimized in the majority of cases by maintaining the CVP below 5 mmHg.

Occlusion of the portal triad can be safely performed for up to 60 min under normothermic conditions and results in minimal hemodynamic changes and does not require any specific anesthetic management. However, in patients with right heart failure, pulmonary hypertension or significant tricuspid insufficiency who are preload dependent, a low CVP strategy may not be tolerated and total vascular exclusion should be considered.

Outflow control could be achieved by precise extrahepatic dissection of the major hepatic veins or by total vascular isolation techniques that obviate the risk of hemorrhage associated with hepatic venous control. Total hepatic vascular isolation requires occlusion of the IVC above and below the liver in addition to the Pringle maneuver, and may not be hemodynamically tolerated by some patients. Venovenous bypass has been applied by some to major hepatic resections and has been commonly used during hepatic transplantation.

Bibliography

Blumgart LH, Fong Y. *Surgery of the Liver and Biliary Tract*, 3rd ed. Edinburgh: Churchill Livingstone, 2000.

Cunningham JD, Fong Y, Shriver C, Melendez J, Marx WL, Blumgart LH. One hundred consecutive hepatic resections. Blood loss, transfusion, and operative technique. *Arch Surg* 1994;129:1050–1056.

Huguet C, Gavelli A, Chieco PA, Bona S, Harb J, Joseph JM, Jobard J, Gramaglia M, Lasserre M. Liver ischemia for hepatic resection: where is the limit? *Surgery* 1992;111: 251–259.

Man K, Fan ST, Path, et al. Prospective evaluation of the Pringle maneuver in hepatectomy for liver tumors by a randomized study. *Ann Surg* 1997; 226:704–713.

Townsend CM, et al. *Sabiston Textbook of Surgery: The Biological Basis of Modern Surgical Practice*, 16th ed. Philadelphia, PA: W.B. Saunders, 2001.

9. **(B), (D), (E)** The portal vein provides about 75% of the liver's blood supply. It is formed by the junction of the superior mesenteric and splenic veins, dorsal to the neck of the pancreas. It ascends dorsal to the common bile duct and hepatic artery in the hepatoduodenal ligament. It has no valves, which has several important clinical implications: portal vein pressure is similar to the pressure in portal vein tributaries, and the intrahepatic portal vein's low resistance sustains a large amount of flow.

The portal trunk divides into left and right hepatic branches in the portal fissure. The right branch divides into anterior and posterior segments approximately at the point of entry into the liver parenchyma. The left branch is longer and has two portions: a longer transverse portion (pars transversus) which

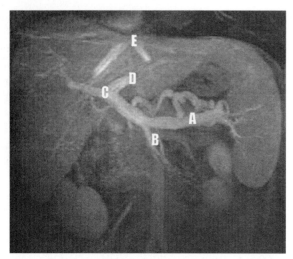

FIG. 28-5   This figure depicts the portal vein, which is the confluence of the splenic (A), inferior mesenteric and superior mesenteric (B) veins as it enters into the hepatic hilum past the pancreas. Intrahepatically the portal vein divides into the right (C) and left (D) portal veins. Also apparent (E) are middle and left hepatic veins.

traverses the base of segment IV, and the pars umbilicus which angulates anteriroly into the umbilical fissure, where it gives off branches to segment IV, and lateral branches to segments II and III (Fig. 28-5).

The portal vein and its branches have prominent hyperechoic walls on ultrasound. This has been attributed to the accompanying intrahepatic branches of the hepatic artery and bile duct, which are not usually individually seen on external ultrasound. In contradistinction, the hepatic veins appear "wall-less" hypoechoic structures that increase in caliber as they course toward the IVC.

Doppler ultrasonography further aids in the identification of flow patterns in the hepatic vessels. Portal venous flow is normally toward the liver (hepatopedal), is a continuous forward flow during diastole and is of low velocity. On the other hand, flow in the hepatic veins is hepatofugal and varies with the cardiorespiratory cycle.

Bibliography

Blumgart LH, Fong Y. *Surgery of the Liver and Biliary Tract,* 3rd ed. Edinburgh: Churchill Livingstone, 2000.

Meyers WC, Jones RS. *Textbook of Liver and Biliary Surgery.* Philadelphia, PA: Lippincott, Williams & Wilkins, 1990.

Townsend CM, et al. *Sabiston Textbook of Surgery: The Biological Basis of Modern Surgical Practice,* 16th ed. Philadelphia, PA: W.B. Saunders, 2001.

10. **(B), (C), (E)** Numerous tributaries of the portal vein connect outside the liver with the systemic venous system. The have no physiologic importance under normal circumstances but will develop into large channels with increased collateral flow in the setting of portal hypertension. These portosystemic anastomoses include the following.

1. Submucosal veins of the esophagus and proximal stomach, which can receive blood from the coronary and short gastric veins to drain into the azygous veins. This pathway forms the basis of gastric or esophageal varices or both in portal hypertension.
2. Umbilical and periumbilical veins, which are recanalized from the obliterated umbilical vein in the ligamentum teres hepaticus. These account for the physical finding of caput medusase or the Cruveilhier-Baumgarten bruit in portal hypertension.
3. The superior hemorrhoidal vein, which communicates with the middle and inferior hemorrhoidal veins of the systemic circulation and may result in large hemorrhoids and significant hemorrhage.
4. Retroperitoneal communications including communication with the renal and adrenal veins.

Bibliography

Blumgart LH, Fong Y. *Surgery of the Liver and Biliary Tract,* 3rd ed. Edinburgh: Churchill Livingstone, 2000.

Meyers WC, Jones RS. *Textbook of Liver and Biliary Surgery.* Philadelphia, PA: Lippincott, Williams & Wilkins, 1990.

Townsend CM, et al. *Sabiston Textbook of Surgery: The Biological Basis of Modern Surgical Practice,* 16th ed. Philadelphia, PA: W.B. Saunders, 2001.

11. **(E)** The hepatic venous drainage is through the three major hepatic veins: right, middle, and left. These begin in the liver lobules as the central veins and coalesce to form the major venous outflow (Fig. 28-6).

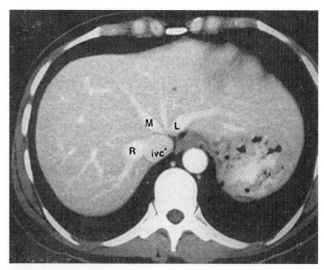

FIG. 28-6   Contrast enhanced CT image demonstrating the right (R), middle (M), and (L) hepatic veins arising from the inferior vena cava (IVC).

Each vein has a short extrahepatic course before draining in the IVC. They are of surgical importance because they define the three vertical scissura of the liver, and because the short extrahepatic segment makes surgical accessibility difficult, particularly for control of traumatic hemorrhage. The right vein is the largest and drains most of the right hepatic lobe. Its main trunk follows an intersegmental course between the French segments. Other several small veins also drain the right lobe directly into the IVC. The left vein drains the lateral segment of the left lobe and a portion of the medial segment as well. The left hepatic vein is joined by the middle hepatic vein in 80% of dissections. This vein lies in the portal fissure and drains the inferoanterior portion of the right lobe and the inferomedial segment of the left lobe. In the remainder of individuals, this vein drains directly into the vena cava.

Additional posterior inferior draining hepatic veins with a short course into the anterior surface of the IVC are sometimes encountered and may be large. These accessory veins should be recognized prior to liver resection and can be visualized on CT scan.

In addition, several small veins from the caudate lobe drain posteriorly directly into the IVC. These become especially important in Budd-Chiari's syndrome after thrombosis of the major hepatic veins.

Exact knowledge of the hepatic venous anatomy is key to a successful liver resection. A precise partial hepatectomy depends on control of the inflow vasculature, draining bile ducts and outflow hepatic veins. Liver regeneration will be prompt if the remaining liver segment has an excellent hepatic arterial and portal venous supply, as well as biliary drainage and unobstructed hepatic venous outflow.

Bibliography

Blumgart LH, Fong Y. *Surgery of the Liver and Biliary Tract*, 3rd ed. Edinburgh: Churchill Livingstone, 2000.

Meyers WC, Jones RS. *Textbook of Liver and Biliary Surgery*. Philadelphia, PA: Lippincott, Williams & Wilkins, 1990.

Townsend CM, et al. *Sabiston Textbook of Surgery: The Biological Basis of Modern Surgical Practice*, 16th ed. Philadelphia, PA: W.B. Saunders, 2001.

12. (C), (E) The liver consists of microscopic masses of cells functionally situated around terminal portal venules. The smallest functional unit of the liver is the acinus or hepatic lobule, first described by Rappaport. In the acinus, a hepatic arteriole, a bile ductule, a lymphatic, and nerves accompany a portal venule. Blood flows from the terminal portal venule into the hepatic sinusoids where it comes in contact with hepatocytes within the unit. It then drains into the terminal hepatic venule at the periphery of the acinar unit. The hepatic venules are at the center of the histologic lobule.

Solute concentration diminishes gradually toward the central veins as they are removed by hepatocytes along the way. The hepatocytes of the acinus are divided into three zones, with zone I being the area closest to the afferent portal venule where the sinusoids are smaller in diameter and have many collaterals. Zones II and III are farther away from the portal venule, with zone III being closest to the central acinar vein.

Within the acinus, there is a gradient of solute concentration and oxygen tension that is greatest near the portal venules at the center of the acinus The hepatocytes in zone I are therefore exposed to more oxygen, and the ones in zones II and III receive the least oxygen supply and are the first to be compromised in low flow states. This concept explains the centrilobular necrosis seen with hypotension. Zone III hepatocytes may also be less resistant to hepatotoxins since they receive nutritionally depleted blood. This heterogeneity in liver cells around the portal venule axis is reflected by the intracellular set up as well, with hepatocytes in zone I being richer in Golgi apparatus, much needed for bile salt transport.

Bibliography

Meyers WC, Jones RS. *Textbook of Liver and Biliary Surgery*. Philadelphia, PA: Lippincott, Williams & Wilkins, 1990.

Rappaport AM. The microcirculatory hepatic unit. *Microvasc Res* 1973;6:212.

Townsend CM, et al. *Sabiston Textbook of Surgery: The Biological Basis of Modern Surgical Practice*, 16th ed. Philadelphia, PA: W.B. Saunders, 2001.

13. (C) Compensatory enlargement of liver tissue as a response to partial resection has definite surgical implications. Liver regeneration is essential for recovery after liver surgery, and following hepatectomy, the liver can regain its normal size even if 75–90% has been resected, provided that the liver remnant is normal. Hepatocytes constitute the main cellular elements of the liver, and up to 95% of liver mass. They are highly differentiated cells, but not terminally differentiated and have the capacity to proliferate. Hepatocyte proliferation and turnover occurs in a complex special pattern and has not been fully elucidated yet. During the midlife of humans, the liver regenerates to a volume of 25 ± 1.2 mL/kg; however, the exact time course for this is not known, and regeneration to roughly 75% of the preoperative liver volume within 1 year is expected. It is also known that small livers will grow to the expected liver/body ratio after liver transplantation into a larger recipient.

It has been shown by serial CT scan imaging that there is an average increase of 70 mL per day of liver volume after transplantation until achievement of the volume consistent with the recipient's age, size, and gender. The opposite is not true though in the sense that reduction in liver size after transplantation is limited.

It is now believed that a synchronized series of events may restore the liver. Actual cell division occurs early on and this aspect of regeneration is actually complete within 72 h of hepatectomy. More than 70 diverse genes are implicated in liver regeneration. This is still an actively investigated field and more insight into the triggering events and the involved transcription factors and sequence of gene activation will allow for finite clinical applications as this work progresses.

Bibliography

Adson MA. The resection of hepatic metastases: another view. *Arch Surg* 1989;124:1023.

Blumgart LH, Fong Y. *Surgery of the Liver and Biliary Tract*, 3rd ed. Edinburgh: Churchill Livingstone, 2000.

Fausto N, Webber EM. 1994 liver regeneration. In: Arias IM, Boyer JL, Fausto N, Jakoby W, Schachter D, Hafritz D (eds.), *The Liver Biology and Pathobiology*. New York, NY: Raven Press, 1059–1084.

Townsend CM, et al. *Sabiston Textbook of Surgery: The Biological Basis of Modern Surgical Practice*, 16th ed. Philadelphia, PA: W.B. Saunders, 2001.

14. **(A), (D)** The liver plays a pivotal role in energy metabolism. It helps maintain homeostasis by detecting and altering components of both splanchnic and systemic blood. Indeed, most of the body's metabolic needs are regulated by the liver to some extent. The liver expends nearly 20% of the body's energy in order to accomplish this task, though it only constitutes 4–5% of the body weight. The main source of energy for the liver is ketoacids, yet it sometimes uses glycolysis during periods of glucose excess.

In the fasting state, the liver maintains homeostasis by glycogenolysis. The breakdown of stored glycogen will provide glucose, a critical energy source for red blood cells, the kidney, and the central nervous system; however, glycogen stores are depleted after 48 h and the liver relies on other sources to generate glucose. Amino acids mobilized mainly from muscle, primarily alanine, in addition to lactate and glycerol, serve as carbon sources for gluconeogenesis. Lactate produced by anaerobic metabolism is metabolized only in the liver. It will be converted to pyruvate and subsequently back to glucose. This shuttling of glucose and lactate between the liver and the peripheral tissues is part of the Cori's cycle.

Lipolysis occurs during prolonged fasting. The liver will oxidize fatty acids released from adipose stores into ketone bodies. These are important alternative sources of fuel for the brain and muscle.

Bibliography

Meyers WC, Jones RS. *Textbook of Liver and Biliary Surgery*. Philadelphia, PA: Lippincott, Williams & Wilkins, 1990.

Townsend CM, et al. *Sabiston Textbook of Surgery: The Biological Basis of Modern Surgical Practice*, 16th ed. Philadelphia, PA: W.B. Saunders, 2001.

15. **(A), (B)** The liver collects and transforms plasma substrates and proteins to meet the fuel requirement of other tissues in response to various metabolic signals. It is the only organ that produces acetoacetate for use by brain, kidney, and muscle but not itself. The liver also uses little glucose for its own requirement.

The functional histologic unit of the liver is the acinus at the center of which is a terminal branch of the hepatic arteriole, bile ductule, and portal vein. The acinar unit allows each cell to be in contact with sinusoidal blood and, at the same time, has an excretory pathway via a separate biliary component. The sinusoids are the major site for regulation of hepatic blood flow and solute exchange between the hepatocyte and blood. They are a low resistance system and lined by Kupffer cells along the luminal surface of the endothelium. Hepatocytes and membrane microvilli project through fenestrations in the endothelial cells, allowing significant access to blood and plasma. The fenestrae allow for free passage of plasma into the perisinusoidal space of Disse where it contacts the hepatocyte membrane; however, cells from different acinar zones behave differently because of different cell surface markers.

The sinusoidal membrane that borders the perisinusoidal space of Disse is covered with microvilli that project into the perisinusoidal space. Proteins, solutes, and other substances are actively transported across. On the other hand, the flat basolateral membrane connects the hepatocyte to adjacent cells and is essential for cell-to-cell interaction. Another specialized section of the hepatocyte membrane is the canalicular membrane that is involved in bile formation and excretion of various substances into bile. It comprises around 15% of the hepatocyte membrane and has a microvillous structure where enzymes such as alkaline phosphatase and 5'-nucleotidase are found.

Perisinusoidal cells consist of the Kupffer cells, important in phagocytosis and antigen presentation; ito cells or fat-storing cells important in collagen metabolism and vitamin A storage; and the rare pit cells that have neuroendocrine and natural killer activity.

Bibliography

Meyers WC, Jones RS. *Textbook of Liver and Biliary Surgery.* Philadelphia, PA: Lippincott, Williams & Wilkins, 1990.
Townsend CM, et al. *Sabiston Textbook of Surgery: The Biological Basis of Modern Surgical Practice*, 16th ed. Philadelphia, PA: W.B. Saunders, 2001.

16. **(A), (B), (D), (E)** The central location of the liver and the numerous immunologic cells confer to the liver a key role in host defense and immunology. The reticuloendothelial system functions to clear the circulation of particulate matter and bacteria. Splanchnic blood returns to the liver where initial host defenses become activated. The resultant defense mechanisms occur via Kupffer cells, neutrophils, ito cells, endothelial cells, or the hepatocytes themselves. Kupffer cells are primarily responsible for the reticuloendothelial function of the liver and, in addition to producing and controlling various cytokine and inflammatory regulators such as tumor necrosis factor and interleukin, they orchestrate the immunologic response by other cells. They also have a phagocytic function and engulf endotoxins or other microbials. Strategically located to perform this vital function, they line the hepatic sinusoids and process gut antigens through the splanchnic circulation.

Ito cells line the space of Disse and play an early role in cytokine and prostaglandin production. Endothelial cells promote migration and sequestration of other immune cells, and hepatocytes produce and degrade key cytokines and growth factors. These cells acting in concert constitute the hepatic defense against toxins and other pathogens.

Bibliography

Meyers WC, Jones RS. *Textbook of Liver and Biliary Surgery.* Philadelphia, PA: Lippincott, Williams & Wilkins, 1990.
Townsend CM, et al. *Sabiston Textbook of Surgery: The Biological Basis of Modern Surgical Practice*, 16th ed. Philadelphia, PA: W.B. Saunders, 2001.

17. **(A), (B), (C), (E)** Drug and toxin metabolism is primarily a hepatic function. Indeed, the liver is responsible for the biotransformation of endogenous and exogenous substances. For the most part, this is a protective function that detoxifies substances or biotransforms them to facilitate their elimination; however, in some instances, the byproducts of hepatic metabolism are more toxic metabolites.

Metabolic transformations performed by the liver are categorized into two broad headings:

1. Phase I reactions of oxidation, reduction, and hydrolysis. These are catalyzed by an enzyme system known as the cytochrome P-450 system.

2. Phase II reactions during which a compound is combined with an endogenous molecule to convert hydrophobic compounds into hydrophilic ones that are water-soluble. This conjugate is more easily excreted in bile or urine. These reactions involve an array of different enzymes.

The cytochrome P-450 system of enzymes could be up regulated or down regulated by different drugs and could significantly affect the elimination of other concomitantly administered medications.

Bibliography

Meyers WC, Jones RS. *Textbook of Liver and Biliary Surgery.* Philadelphia, PA: Lippincott, Williams & Wilkins, 1990.
Townsend CM, et al. *Sabiston Textbook of Surgery: The Biological Basis of Modern Surgical Practice*, 16th ed. Philadelphia, PA: W.B. Saunders, 2001.

18. **(A), (B), (C), (D)** Hepatic protein synthesis or catabolism is vitally important and involves at least 17 of the major human proteins. The liver is the only organ that produces albumin and alpha globulins and is responsible for most of the urea synthesis in the body. It is the principal site for conversion of ammonia to urea via the urea cycle.

Often used as an index of liver synthetic capacity, albumin is the most abundant serum protein and its level in the blood is determined by liver function, nutritional state, thyroid hormone, insulin, glucagon, and cortisol. Albumin loss is augmented in certain disease states such as sepsis, burn, nephrotic syndrome, and protein losing enteropathies.

Several proteins involved in the coagulation cascade are synthesized in the liver, including fibrinogen, the vitamin-K-dependent factors (II, VII, IX, X) and all the procoagulation factors except for Von Willebrand factor. Factor VII has the shortest half-life (5–7 h), and in patients with liver dysfunction, the synthetic ability of the liver can be assessed by monitoring the prothrombin time. Factor V, on the other hand, is synthesized by vascular endothelial cells.

Transferrin, which is also synthesized in the liver, has a shorter half-life than albumin. Changes in transferrin level therefore more accurately reflect acute changes in liver function than do changes in albumin level.

Bibliography

Meyers WC, Jones RS. *Textbook of Liver and Biliary Surgery.* Philadelphia, PA: Lippincott, Williams & Wilkins, 1990.
Townsend CM, et al. *Sabiston Textbook of Surgery: The Biological Basis of Modern Surgical Practice*, 16th ed. Philadelphia, PA: W.B. Saunders, 2001.

19. (D) The incidence of pyogenic liver abscess based on hospital admissions ranges from 0.029 to 1.47% and 0.3 to 1.4% in autopsy studies. There is a decline in the incidence of pyogenic liver abscess as well as a change in the relative frequency of pyogenic and amebic liver abscesses.

Pyogenic liver abscesses are almost always secondary to bacterial infection, although occasionally fungal infections may be the culprit. Positive cultures are documented in the majority of cases and mostly reveal intestinal organisms such as *Escherichia coli, Klebsiella, Proteus, Staphylococcus,* and *Streptococcus.* Polymicrobial cultures are uncommon.

Pyogenic liver abscesses result from

1. diseases of the biliary tract
2. infectious gastrointestinal disorders spreading via the portal vein. These are mostly accounted for by diverticulitis, perforated ulcers, and malignancies.
3. hematogenous spread via the hepatic artery. This occurs in the setting of systemic bacteremia, as in subacute bacterial endocarditis.
4. trauma
5. direct extension from intraabdominal infection

Diseases of the biliary tract are the most common cause of pyogenic liver abscesses. They account for about 40% of cases. Biliary obstruction from stones, strictures, or tumors leads to ascending cholangitis resulting in multiple liver abscesses.

Some cases remain of unknown etiology and are referred to as cryptogenic abscesses. These still account for up to 20% of cases.

A liver abscess forms once the offending organism overwhelms the hepatic defense systems. Bacteria entering the portal system are usually engulfed by Kupffer cells in the liver. Once the organisms exceed the capacity of Kupffer cells, or if the host is immunocompromised, a liver abscess may form.

Patients most commonly present with fever and chills. Other common manifestations include right upper quadrant pain, abdominal pain, jaundice, weight loss, nausea, and vomiting. Occasionally patients present with peritonitis after intraabdominal rupture.

Up to one quarter of patients will be septic. Leucocytosis, elevated serum bilirubin and alkaline phosphatase are common laboratory findings. Hepatic transaminases are mildly elevated.

Imaging techniques are essential for the diagnosis of hepatic abscesses. Indeed, prior to the introduction of high resolution imaging techniques, 30–50% of liver abscesses were diagnosed on postmortem examination.

Plain abdominal films may show gas in the abscess cavity in 10–20% of cases, and elevation of the right hemidiaphragm; however, ultrasonography should be the preferred initial diagnostic study when this entity is clinically suspected. It is 80–90% accurate in detecting abscesses larger than 2 cm in diameter, yet may be somewhat limited in delineating lesions located at the dome of the liver. Ultrasonographic findings include a hypoechoic lesion with irregular margins. The presence of microbubbles indicates gas within the abscess cavity.

CT has the advantage of detecting intrahepatic collections as small as 0.5 cm. This is essential in patients with multiple small pyogenic abscesses. The lesions on CT scan are seen as well-defined round or oval cavities, or poorly marginated lobulated lesions. Abscesses usually have a low internal density, yet contrast enhancement increase the ease of diagnosis (Fig. 28-7).

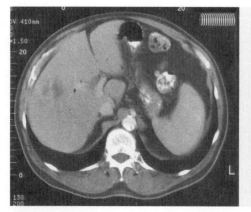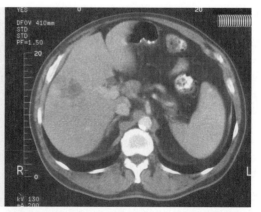

FIG. 28-7 Liver abscess is demonstrated; note the necrotic center of the lesion with apparent "air" within the central necrosis. The presence of "air" is useful in the differentiation between different pathologies; in this case, the patient had a fever and elevated WBC. Percutaneous placed drainage and intravenous antibiotics were successfully instituted in this case with complete resolution.

MRI is another well-established sensitive modality for the diagnosis of liver abscesses. It does not offer clear advantages over CT or ultrasound and is usually more expensive and not as readily available.

Bibliography

Meyers WC, Jones RS. *Textbook of Liver and Biliary Surgery.* Philadelphia, PA: Lippincott, Williams & Wilkins, 1990.

Pitt HA. Surgical management of hepatic abscesses. *World J Surg* 1990;14:498–504.

Townsend CM, et al. *Sabiston Textbook of Surgery: The Biological Basis of Modern Surgical Practice*, 16th ed. Philadelphia, PA: W.B. Saunders, 2001.

20. **(D), (E)** The mainstay of treatment of liver abscesses is drainage and systemic antibiotic therapy.

Drainage has been accomplished either surgically, by an open or laparoscopic technique, or percutaneously. Anesthetic risk of the patient, the presence or absence of a coexisting intraabdominal pathology, and the local expertise in the different available modalities are factors that determine the selection of drainage modality.

Ultrasonography or CT-directed percutaneous drainage is now considered the treatment of choice for patients without a surgically correctable disease. It has the advantage of avoiding a laparotomy and has a 70–90% success rate.

Surgical drainage of pyogenic liver abscesses should also eliminate the source of infection. Abscesses located in the dome of the liver can be drained via a transpleural approach. This approach provides limited exposure by avoiding peritoneal contamination. Intraoperative ultrasound may be helpful in localization during the procedure.

Laparoscopic drainage has also been advocated with a reported success rate of 85%. Laparoscopic ultrasound could also prove to be an invaluable tool for accurate localization.

No prospective randomized trials have compared the different modalities. The choice of drainage modality should therefore be individualized depending on the source and the patient's underlying clinical condition.

Targeted antibiotic therapy could be initially started if guided by pus aspiration. Broad-spectrum coverage should be otherwise used. It should include an aminoglycoside with either metronidazole or clindamycin, or a beta-lactam antibiotic with anaerobic coverage. Antibiotic therapy could be used as the only treatment modality in cases with solitary or microabscesses smaller than 2 cm in diameter, in patients in good clinical condition. The length of therapy should be individualized according to the clinical response and the number of abscesses.

Treatment for 4–6 weeks is usually recommended for patients with multiple abscesses.

Optimal management of pyogenic abscesses, however, involves not only treatment of the abscess, but correction of the underlying source as well.

Bibliography

Bertel CK, Van Herden JA, Sheedy PF. Treatment of pyogenic hepatic abscesses: surgical vs. percutaneous drainage. *Arch Surgery* 1986;121:554–558.

Chou FF, Sheen-Chen SM, Chen YS, et al. Prognostic factors for pyogenic abscess of the liver. *J Am Coll Surg* 1994;179:727–732.

Townsend CM, et al. *Sabiston Textbook of Surgery: The Biological Basis of Modern Surgical Practice*, 16th ed. Philadelphia, PA: W.B. Saunders, 2001.

21. **(B), (C), (D), (E)** Liver abscess complicates intestinal amebiasis in 3–10% of cases. Amebiasis is a disease with the highest incidence in subtropical and tropical climates and in areas with poor sanitation. It is more common in males and affects a younger population than pyogenic abscesses. It occurs as a result of infestation with *Entamoeba histolytica* via fecal-oral transmission. The cystic form of *E. histolytica* gains access to the host by oral ingestion of contaminated food or water. The trophozoites are then released into the gastrointestinal tract and can reach the liver via the portal system by entering the mesenteric venules. An amebic liver abscess results as the trophozoites cause cellular necrosis. It is usually solitary and surrounded by a thin walled granulation tissue. The right lobe is most commonly involved. These abscesses are usually sterile unless secondary bacterial contamination occurs.

Signs and symptoms are similar to those seen with pyogenic liver abscesses. The patients are usually younger though and have a history of travel to endemic areas. The most common symptoms are fever and abdominal pain. Diarrhea is present in 20–30% of cases. The most common signs include hepatomegaly and right upper quadrant tenderness.

Serology is the diagnostic test of choice. Indirect hemagglutination and gel diffusion precipitation are the most commonly used tests with a reported 85–95% sensitivity and specificity. Stool testing will show the cyst of the protozoon in only one-fourth of cases.

Imaging studies are essential to make the diagnosis. Ultrasonography reveals a round or oval hypoechoic lesion with well-defined margins in the setting of amebic liver abscess.

CT findings include a low-density lesion with smooth margins.

The most common complication of amebic liver abscesses is secondary infection. It occurs in 10–20%

of cases. Amebic abscesses can rupture into the pleura, lung, pericardium, or peritoneum. Those located in the dome of the liver may rupture through the diaphragm and result in empyema, pleural effusions or bronchopleural fistula in up to 7% of cases. Conversely, those located on the inferior surface tend to rupture into the peritoneal cavity in 7–11% of cases.

The first line of treatment of an amebic liver abscess is pharmacologic therapy. Metronidazole is the drug of choice and is effective against both the intestinal and hepatic phases. The dose is 750 mg three times a day and should be given for 7–10 days. The response to treatment is determined by the size of the abscess. Abscesses smaller than 5 cm in diameter respond better to metronidazole therapy. Pharmacologic therapy is still the treatment of choice in the setting of uncomplicated perforation, when the abscess perforates into the pleural or pericardial cavity, or even into the peritoneal cavity if there is no peritonitis.

Routine abscess aspiration is not recommended. It may be required for the treatment of larger abscesses and may be done under ultrasound or CT guidance.

Surgical open drainage is reserved for patients with complicated amebic liver abscesses with secondary infection or perforation with peritoneal irritation, or in patients who fail to respond to conservative methods.

Mortality for uncomplicated amebic abscesses should be less than 5%, in contrast to the 15–20% reported mortality rates for pyogenic abscesses.

Bibliography

Akgun Y, Tacyuluduz IH, Celik Y. Amebic liver abscess. Changing trends over 20 years. *World J Surg* 1999;23:102–106.

Donovon AJ, Yellin AE, Ralls PW. Hepatic abscess. *World J Surg* 1991;15:162–169.

Pitt HA. Surgical management of hepatic abscesses. *World J Surg* 1990;14:498–504.

Townsend CM, et al. *Sabiston Textbook of Surgery: The Biological Basis of Modern Surgical Practice*, 16th ed. Philadelphia, PA: W.B. Saunders, 2001.

22. **(B)** Hydatid disease is a zoonotic infection caused by the larval stage of the tapeworm *Echinococcus*. The disease has a worldwide distribution but is endemic in the Mediterranean and Baltic areas, Middle and Far East, South America, and South Africa. The only species of importance in human disease are *E. granulosus* and *E. multilocularis*. Infection occurs by fecal-oral transmission and is acquired by ingestion of the parasite eggs released in the feces of the definite host (carnivores and rodents) that harbors the adult worm in its gut. The eggs hatch after being ingested by the intermediate host (usually herbivores, accidentally humans). They migrate into different tissues and form multilayered cysts.

The liver is the most commonly involved organ in adults (50–70%). Lungs are the second most common site. In children, pulmonary involvement is the most common.

Clinical manifestations occur after an asymptomatic phase of variable duration. Symptoms are secondary to compression or complicated disease resulting in rupture or infection. Cyst rupture is a serious complication and can result in dissemination and hypersensitivity or anaphylactic reaction. Rupture most commonly occurs in the biliary tree and is the most common complication overall (25%). It can cause biliary obstruction by daughter cysts. There are no pathognomonic physical signs. Yet, the findings of fever, jaundice, right upper quadrant pain, and weight loss in endemic areas should raise the suspicion of hydatidosis.

Diagnosis is usually made by serologic testing. Indirect hemagglutination has a good sensitivity and has largely replaced the use of the complement fixation test.

The mainstay of radiologic diagnosis is by ultrasound because of its wide availability, low cost, and high diagnostic rate. CT scan of the chest and abdomen is not routinely done but is essential in planning for surgery as it gives a better definition of cyst size, number and relation to surrounding structures (Fig. 28-8).

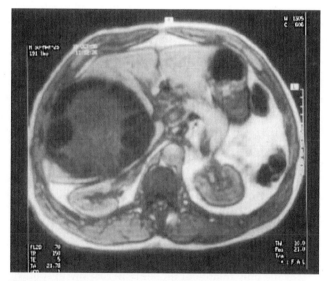

FIG. 28-8   This CT image demonstrates a heterogeneous mass in the liver of a patient from the Middle East. Hydatid (Echinococcus) cyst is the diagnosis by serological testing. The CT was obtained for surgical planning and the patient treated via pericystectomy with preservation of normal hepatic parenchyma.

Surgical therapy is the only curative approach, yet it is usually not necessary in very small cysts or calcified dead cysts.

Cysts could be radically excised by a partial hepatectomy or by a pericystectomy, which involves a nonanatomic liver resection.

Simple cystectomy is another option and consists of deroofing and evacuation of the cyst content. The cyst is usually aspirated before hand and injected with scolicidal agent in order to reduce spillage. These agents include 70–90% ethanol or 15–20% hypertonic saline or 0.5% silver nitrate and hydrogen peroxide. Their use is limited by the presence of a cysto-biliary fistula because of the possibility of chemical cholangitis and subsequent sclerosing cholangitis.

Albendazole is the drug of choice and is used in preparation for surgery, presumably to reduce the incidence of spillage and recurrence.

The best treatment of this disease is prevention. This is currently done by antihelmintic treatment of farm dogs.

Bibliography

Blumgart LH, Fong Y. *Surgery of the Liver and Biliary Tract*, 3rd ed. Edinburgh: Churchill Livingstone, 2000.

Townsend CM, et al. *Sabiston Textbook of Surgery: The Biological Basis of Modern Surgical Practice*, 16th ed. Philadelphia, PA: W.B. Saunders, 2001.

23. **(B), (C)** Schistosomiasis is a disease caused by trematodes belonging to the family Schistosomatidae. Three principal species are implicated in human disease and are: *Schistosoma mansoni*, prevalent in Africa, the Arabian Peninsula, Brazil, and Puerto Rico; *S. japonicum*, found mainly in the Far East: Japan, China, Taiwan, and the Philippines; and *S. haematobium*, centered in the Nile valley and Africa. It is estimated that more than 200 million of the world's population are affected with this disease.

Humans acquire the disease by exposure to water contaminated by the cercaria form of the organism, which emerges in large numbers from the snail host. Conditions that contribute to the prevalence of the disease include poor sanitation, contaminated water, and a snail host required to complete the life cycle. They penetrate the human skin and enter the peripheral venules. They are carried as metacercariae to the right side of the heart and lungs and subsequently enter the systemic circulation. They mature into the adult form after they reach the hepatic bed.

In endemic areas, the schistosome is the most frequent cause of hepatic fibrosis associated with portal hypertension and is the most common cause of portal

hypertension worldwide. It is mainly associated with *S. mansoni* and *S. japonicum*. Eggs that lodge in the portal areas form granuloma-like lesions, which, with the accompanying fibrosis, produce presinusoidal obstruction. Therefore, the wedged hepatic vein pressure will be normal. The disease course is slow and progressive and many patients are actually asymptomatic. Characteristic findings are hepatosplenomegaly and, in advanced stages, variceal bleeding associated with portal hypertension.

During the acute stage, the diagnosis may be made by finding the ova in freshly passed stools. A skin test and several serologic tests are available for diagnosis. The best is the complement fixation test; however, the reliance on serologic testing alone for diagnosis is hazardous because of the significant false positive and false negative reactions. In patients with liver involvement, needle biopsy will reveal portal and septal fibrosis and granulomatous lesions in association with the ova. The characteristic lesion is referred to as "pipe stem" fibrosis because of the extensive portal tract fibrosis.

Liver function, despite widespread involvement, appears to be much better than in other forms of cirrhosis. Treatment with praziquantel may reverse this fibrosis.

Surgical portal decompression may be considered for advanced stages with portal hypertension and recurrent bleeding varices.

Bibliography

Homeida MA, Tom IE, Nash T, et al. Association of the therapeutic activity of praziquantel with the reversal of Symmers' fibrosis induced by *Schistosoma mansoni*. Am J Trop Med Hyg 1991;45:360.

Mahmoud AAF, Wahab MFA. Schistosomiasis. In: Warren KS, Mahmoud AAF (eds.), *Tropical and Geographical Medicine*, 2nd ed. New York, NY: McGraw-Hill, 1990, 458.

24. **(B), (E)** Acute fulminant hepatic failure is an uncommon manifestation of liver disease that constitutes a medical emergency. It is because of loss of hepatic parenchyma secondary to a given insult and carries a grave prognosis (Fig. 28-9).

Fulminant hepatic failure has been defined by three criteria: (1) rapid development of hepatocellular dysfunction, (2) encephalopathy, and (3) no prior history of liver disease. It is therefore a clinical syndrome that could result from several different disease entities that cause liver injury. It is usually the end stage of hepatic cellular necrosis but could on occasions be the result of massive hepatocellular replacement as seen with malignant infiltration.

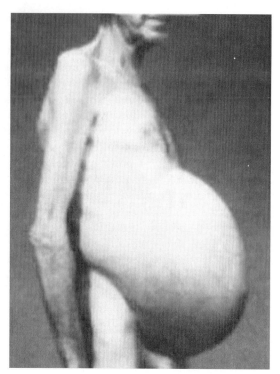

FIG. 28-9 Clinical hallmarks of hepatic cirrhosis associated with left-sided portal hypertension will include ascites, dilated periumbilical veins, thrombocytopenia, and significantly altered liver function. The presence of ascites is almost always a contraindication to liver resection, as it is a manifestation of the underlying poor hepatic function.

The time course of illness depends on the etiology and has prognostic significance. This relationship has lead to a stricter definition, reserving the term fulminant hepatic failure for cases in which encephalopathy develops within 2 weeks of the onset of jaundice, and using the term subfulminant hepatic failure to cases in which encephalopathy develops between 2 weeks and 3 months after the onset of jaundice.

The most common cause of fulminant hepatic failure is drug related it results from acetaminophen overdose. It is directly hepatotoxic and predictably produces hepatocellular necrosis with overdose (>12 g). Hepatic failure can even occur at recommended therapeutic doses (as low as 4 g) in patients with chronic alcohol abuse or those who chronically use drugs that induce cytochrome oxidases. Other implicated drugs include halothane, isoniazid, valproic acid, sulfonamides, phenytoin, and propylthiouracil. Fulminant hepatic failure in this setting is rare and usually idiosyncratic.

Viral hepatitis is another major cause of fulminant hepatic failure. Infection with hepatitis A virus rarely leads to fulminant liver failure and when it does, the prognosis is usually good. Hepatitis B virus (HBV) is the most common viral cause of fulminant hepatic failure, yet this is an uncommon manifestation. Hepatitis D virus infection has also been implicated and requires coinfection with hepatitis B virus. It can account for more than one-third of cases in patient seropositive for hepatitis B.

In some countries like Japan, infection with hepatitis C virus (HCV) has been implicated in fulminant hepatic failure. This association is quite rare in Western countries.

Fulminant hepatic failure of unknown etiology constitutes 20–40% of the total cases. This diagnosis is made in patients with negative viral hepatitis serology and no known cause.

Bibliography

O'Grady JG, Scalm SW, Williams R. Acute liver failure: redefining the syndromes. *Lancet* 1993;342:273.

Townsend CM, et al. *Sabiston Textbook of Surgery: The Biological Basis of Modern Surgical Practice*, 16th ed. Philadelphia, PA: W.B. Saunders, 2001.

Villamil FG, Hu KQ, Yu CH, et al. Detection of hepatitis C virus with RNA polymerase chain reaction in fulminant hepatic failure. *Hepatology* 1995;22:1379.

Wright TL, Mamish D, Combs C, et al. Hepatitis B and apparent fulminant non-A, non-B hepatitis. *Lancet* 1992;339:952.

25. **(D), (E)** The time course of fulminant hepatic failure has an etiologic and prognostic significance. An illness of 1 week or less before the development of failure is usually suggestive of hepatic ischemia or acetaminophen toxicity. On the other hand, illness longer than 4 weeks is more likely the result of viral hepatitis or hepatic failure of unknown etiology.

Patients who are ill for more than 8 weeks before they develop encephalopathy have a higher chance of developing portal hypertension, whereas patients with illness of shorter duration (<4 weeks) are more likely to develop cerebral edema. Encephalopathy preceded by 1 week of jaundice is a poor prognostic indicator.

Because of its easy availability, acetaminophen is a commonly used drug for suicide. This is also a problem with other over-the-counter remedies that contain acetaminophen as an active ingredient.

Although infectious complication may develop in up to 80% of patients with fulminant hepatic failure, prophylactic antibiotic therapy is still controversial. A wide variety of therapies have been proposed and used for the treatment of this disease, including corticosteroids, prostaglandins, and exchange transfusion, yet none have proved efficacious. Only the development of liver transplantation has allowed the salvage of patients with irreversible liver failure.

Patients should therefore be evaluated for liver transplantation as soon as possible and placed on the transplant waiting list. Treatment is otherwise supportive and includes prophylaxis for gastrointestinal bleeding in the setting of coagulopathy, correction of hypoglycemia, intracranial pressure (ICP) monitoring of intracranial hypertension, along with osmotherapy and barbiturates, hemodynamic monitoring and organ-directed support if multiorgan failure develops. Surveillance cultures should be routinely obtained and if infection is suspected, empirical therapy should be tailored to local hospital antimicrobial sensitivities and should cover *Staphylococcus* and gram-negative aerobes.

Bibliography

Gimson AES, O'Grady J, Ede RJ, et al. Late onset hepatic failure: clinical, serological and historical features. *Hepatology* 1986;6:288.

O'Grady JG, Alexander GJM, Thick M, et al. Outcome of orthotopic liver transplantation in the etiological and clinical variants of acute liver failure. *Q J Med* 1988; 69:817.

Rolando N, Harvey F, Brahm J, et al. Prospective study of bacterial infection in acute liver failure: an analysis of fifty patients. *Hepatology* 1990;11:49.

Townsend CM, et al. *Sabiston Textbook of Surgery: The Biological Basis of Modern Surgical Practice*, 16th ed. Philadelphia, PA: W.B. Saunders, 2001.

26. **(D)** Screening recommendations for HCV are currently practiced according to the Centers for Disease Control recommendations. The main transmission mode is following initiation of injection drug use, whereas the risk of sexual transmission is low. The accuracy of anti-HCV testing (enzyme immunoassay) depends on the pretest probability of disease. The predictive value in a patient with known parenteral exposure exceeds 90%, whereas the predictive value of a positive anti-HCV test in blood donors with a normal alanine aminotransferase (ALT) level and no risk factor for HCV infection is less than 50%. In this situation, direct measurement of HCV RNA by PCR assay is required.

Seventy to 85% of patients initially infected with HCV develop persistent infection. In approximately 15% of patients, HCV infection resolves within 1–6 months, possibly because of HCV-specific T-cell function. Of those patients with persistent infection, 20% have chronic viremia with normal liver enzymes. In this group of patients, risk of progression to cirrhosis is low. On the other hand, patients with a consistently or intermittently elevated ALT level have a 20% risk of developing cirrhosis over 20 years. The risk of hepatic decompensation manifesting as ascites, variceal bleed, encephalopathy, or loss of hepatic synthetic ability averages about 3–5% per year. Moreover, in the cirrhotic patient, the risk of hepatoma is in the range of 1–4% per year.

The decision to perform a liver biopsy should be individualized. It may provide useful information in a middle aged individual with long standing HCV infection and clinical features of advanced liver disease. Treatment is indicated for patients with significant inflammation or fibrotic disease. There are two Food and Drug Administration (FDA) approved therapies for chronic hepatitis C: interferon monotherapy and the combination of interferon with ribavirin. Sustained response after discontinuation of therapy is 5–15% with monotherapy and 35–40% with combination treatment.

Bibliography

Centers for Disease Control and Prevention. Recommendations for prevention and control of hepatitis C virus (HCV) infection and HCV-related chronic disease. *MMWR Morb Mortal Wkly Rep* 1998;47:1–39.

Dickson RC. Clinical manifestations of hepatitis C. *Clin Liver Dis* 1997;1:569–585.

McHutchison JG, Gordon SC, Schiff ER, Shiffman ML, Lee WM, Rustgi V, et al. Iterferon alfa-2b alone or in combination with ribavirin as initial treatment for chronic hepatitis C. *N Engl J Med* 1998;339:1485–1492.

Seeff LB. The natural history of chronic hepatitis C virus infection. *Clin Liver Dis* 1997;1:587–602.

27. **(B)** HBV is primarily transmitted by parenteral and mucous membrane exposure to infectious body fluids such as blood, serum, semen, and saliva. Risk factors include close personal or intimate exposure to an infected household contact or sexual partner, intravenous drug use, tattooing and body piercing, unapparent blood inoculations as with shared razor blades, blood transfusion or exposure to blood products, hemophilia and hemodialysis, and work in the health care profession. Because of improved screening of blood donors, and educational efforts to combat human immunodeficiency virus (HIV), the incidence of HBV infection has declined in the United States since 1991.

Diagnosis of acute hepatitis depends on the results of specific antiviral serology. Hospitalization is warranted for intractable symptoms of anorexia, vomiting, or severe impairment of liver function. Other symptoms include jaundice, weight loss, and malaise. Severe hepatic dysfunction manifests as renal failure, metabolic acidosis, encephalopathy, variceal bleeding or ascites.

In adults, more than 90% of HBV infection results in self-limited acute hepatitis with subsequent resolution of the disease in 3–6 months. Approximately 5% of patients will develop chronic hepatitis, and 1–2% will progress to fulminant hepatitis.

IgM antibody to hepatitis B core antigen is the most specific marker for diagnosis of acute hepatitis B. Development of antibody to hepatitis B surface antigen signifies resolution of the acute infection and is the marker for cure and immunity to HBV infection. The pattern of negative HBsAg, positive anti-HBsAg, and positive anti-HBc assays is seen during the recovery phase following acute hepatitis B. This antibody pattern may persist for years and is not associated with liver disease or infectivity. Coinfection with delta agent, an incomplete virus requiring HBsAg for replication, is associated with severe hepatitis and higher likelihood of fulminant hepatic failure.

Treatment is primarily supportive and consists of rest, fluids, and maintenance of adequate nutrition. Antiviral therapy is currently not recommended for acute hepatitis B in patients with preexisting HBsAg or anti-HBs. In patients with parenteral and sexual exposure, blood should therefore be tested for hepatitis B surface antigen and antibody to hepatitis B surface antigen prior to hepatitis B immune globulin (HBIG) administration.

Coadministration of hepatitis B vaccine with HBIG is recommended for susceptible individuals sustaining parenteral or sexual exposure and for all neonates born to HBV positive mothers.

Vaccination with the hepatitis B vaccine (genetically manufactured HBsAg particles with HBV DNA or core antigen) is universally indicated, with the initial dose given at birth and repeated at 1 and 6 months of age. It is associated with the development of anti-HBs antibody alone.

Bibliography

Lee W. Hepatitis B virus infection. *N Engl J Med* 1997;337:1733–1745.

Yuen MF, Lim WL, Cheng CC, Lam SK, Lai CL. Twelve-year follow up of a prospective randomized trial of hepatitis B recombinant DNA yeast vaccine versus plasma-derived vaccine without booster doses in children. *Hepatology* 1999;29:924–927.

28. **(D)** Postransfusion non-A, non-B hepatitis is usually because of hepatitis C infection. The incubation period is 5–10 weeks and the mean peak aminotransferase levels are 500–1000 U/L. Anti-HCV antibody is commonly not detectable until 18 weeks after the onset of symptoms; however, most cases of acute hepatitis C are asymptomatic and anicteric.

The risk factors for acute hepatitis C have changed over the last 10–20 years. Transfusion of blood products was previously a major risk factor. With the introduction of specific testing, this mode of transmission has virtually disappeared as a cause of hepatitis C. Intravenous drug use accounts for the majority of new cases of acute HCV infections nowadays.

At the onset of illness, antibody to HCV is usually negative, but HCV RNA is positive from the onset. Subsequent seroconversion to positive anti-HCV confirms the diagnosis.

The majority of patients with acute hepatitis C will progress to chronic hepatitis and potentially develop liver cirrhosis.

Immune globulin preparations are ineffective against HCV, and there is no HCV vaccine.

Prevention and universal precautions remain the most effective means of combating the disease.

Bibliography

Davis G. Treatment of acute and chronic hepatitis C. *Clin Liver Dis* 1997;1:61530.

Dickson RC. Clinical manifestations of hepatitis C. *Clin Liver Dis* 1997;1:569–585.

29. **(C)** Primary HCC, although less common in North America, is the most prevalent malignant disease in the world and accounts for the death of 1.25 million persons annually. HCC is the most common primary malignant liver tumor in adults, hepatoblastoma being the most common in young children. HCC is more common in males than in females, except in the group without preexisting liver disease where the ratio is 1:1. Endemic areas include sub-Saharan Africa, Southeast Asia, and Japan. It is also much more common is the Pacific islands, Greece, and Italy than it is in North America. Chronic liver disease of any cause probably plays a key role in the development of HCC in any part of the world.

Documented risk factors for HCC include alcoholic cirrhosis, as 8–10% of patients dying of alcoholic cirrhosis in the United States have HCC. Other risk factors are blood group B, hepatic adenoma, repeated ingestion of aflatoxin, Wilson's disease, hemochromatosis, and glycogen storage disease. Viral hepatitis is also associated with the development of HCC. Chronic infection with HBV confers a relative risk of developing HCC of 9.7. Whether HCC occurs as a consequence of chronic HBV infection or as a result of chronic liver disease is not certain. HBV does not contain an oncogene, but insertional mutagenesis is a potential mechanism. Indeed it is established that HBV DNA resides in the HCC cell genome, and progression form chronic active HBV to cirrhosis and subsequently HCC is well documented.

On the other hand, the case for HCV is less well established, and most of the evidence has been from Western civilizations. HCV infection is present in 51% of patients with HCC in Japan, as opposed to 26% with HBV infection. HCV is an RNA virus that does not become incorporated in host DNA, yet it results in chronic necroinflammatory liver disease, which may account for its carcinogenic effect.

Aflatoxins are the products of the fungus *Aspergillus flavus*, which can be found in dairy products, peanuts, wheat, soybeans, corn, rice, and oats. The FDA does limit the amount of aflatoxins allowed in peanut butter to 20 parts per billion because of this well-documented association.

Bibliography

Aoki K. Cancer of the liver: international mortality trends. *World Health Stat Rep* 1978;31:28.

Robinson WS. The role of hepatitis B virus in the development of primary hepatocellular carcinoma. *Int J Gastroenterol Hepatol* 1992;7:622.

Tanaka K, Sakai H, Hashizume M, Hirohata T. A long term follow-up study on risk factors for hepatocellular carcinoma among Japanese patients with liver cirrhosis. *Jpn J Cancer Res* 1998;89:1241–1250.

30. **(B), (C)** The symptom complex of HCC relates to advanced disease and late presentation. Indeed, constitutional symptoms such as weight loss, anorexia, and weakness are quite prevalent. The majority of patients are symptomatic mostly because of local mass effect. Biliary obstruction by either necrotic tumor emboli or extrinsic biliary tract compression accounts for the obstructive jaundice initially seen in 1–10% of patients. The majority of patients will develop right upper quadrant pain, tenderness, ascites, and peripheral edema; however, only 5% will present with symptoms pertaining to metastatic disease, most commonly pulmonary metastasis.

HCC is usually an occult process, yet a minority of patients will present with an acute event such as rupture of the tumor, hemorrhage, or fever of unknown origin. In endemic areas, HCC is a common cause of nontraumatic hemoperitoneum, and the incidence of spontaneous rupture has been reported to approach 8%.

The most common sign found in patients with HCC is hepatomegaly, and an arterial bruit can be heard in 10–20% of patients. Other physical findings depend on the stage of the disease, with up to two-thirds of patients showing signs of chronic liver disease such as spider angiomas and evidence of portal hypertension.

Some patients will present with a paraneoplastic manifestation, the most common of which is hypoglycemia. Others include hypertrophic pulmonary osteoarthropathy in the setting of hepatopulmonary syndrome, carcinoid syndrome, hypertension secondary to overproduction of angiotensin, and sensorimotor neuropathy affection in all extremities.

Bibliography

Stuart K, Anand A, Jenkins R. Hepatocellular carcinoma in the United States: prognostic features, treatment outcome and survival. *Cancer* 1996;77:2217–2222.

Tanaka K, Sakai H, Hashizume M, Hirohata T. A long term follow-up study on risk factors for hepatocellular carcinoma among Japanese patients with liver cirrhosis. *Jpn J Cancer Res* 1998;89:1241–1250.

31. **(E)** The goals of preoperative evaluation are intended to identify patients who can tolerate surgery and select those for whom liver-directed therapy would be useful. Preoperative evaluation usually begins with a comprehensive radiology evaluation in an effort to exclude the presence of extrahepatic cancer and to define the location and number of liver tumors. However, the diagnosis of the hepatic mass is distinct from the radiographic assessment of resectability in the planning of a potential surgical procedure for a specific diagnosis. Ultrasound should be the initial radiologic procedure. It is universally available, can be quickly obtained, and provides a substantial amount of information for a relatively moderate cost. It is accurate, noninvasive, and can detect lesions as small as 1 cm in diameter within the liver, evaluate the wall and contents of the gallbladder, and measure the ducts of the biliary system. Ultrasound readily distinguishes between solid and cystic lesions. The addition of Doppler ultrasound will assess the presence of vascular flow, thereby differentiating between simple cysts, hemangiomas, and other lesions.

Dynamic CT scan with an arterial and venous phase contrast imaging provides information regarding the anatomic location of the mass and is the most accurate and sensitive radiographic study for the detection of liver lesions. CT scan has emerged as the procedure of choice in most cases to define HCC. MRI will determine the tissue composition and architecture of the lesion, and will define its relationship to surrounding vascular and biliary structures.

Either CT scan or MRI could demonstrate extrahepatic disease.

On the other hand, neither angiography nor cholangiography are routinely obtained and are not usually required for the diagnosis of a liver tumor. Hepatic arteriography is occasionally helpful in determining the extent of the disease and, in particular, portal or arterial involvement. It may also be helpful in determining anatomic variations, especially

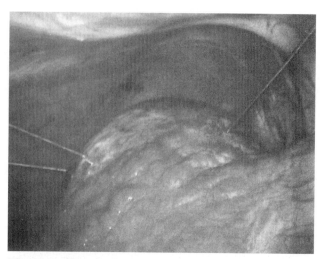

FIG. 28-10 Diagnostic laparoscopy enables the rapid and accurate diagnosis of hepatocellular cancer. In combination with laparoscopic ultrasound, biopsy can be safely performed, and as is demonstrated in this photograph, guided laparoscopic percutaneous ethanol ablation of an HCC lesion can be performed.

when the insertion of a hepatic arterial infusion pump is anticipated.

Percutaneous or retrograde cholangiography may be helpful in selected patients.

Diagnostic laparoscopy is an invaluable tool for the diagnosis of liver tumors as well as for the detection of patients with advanced disease. It is emerging as a procedure of choice in the diagnosis of HCC or other suspected liver tumors, and is particularly useful in the detection of occult metastases not demonstrated by other modalities. Indeed, diagnostic laparoscopy detects surface metastases as small as 1 mm on the peritoneal and liver surfaces that are undetectable by any imaging modality (Fig. 28-10).

The addition of laparoscopic ultrasonography further increases the ability to detect previously undetected small lesions in the liver and to identify and biopsy metastatic lymph nodes. It also offers an opportunity for limited treatment consisting of cryoablation, ethanol injection, resection, or a combination of therapies.

Bibliography

Bismuth H, Castaing D, Garden OJ. The use of operative ultrasound in surgery of primary liver tumors. *World J Surg* 1987;11:610.

Ferrucci JT. Liver tumor imaging: current concepts. *AJR Am J Roentgenol* 1990;155:473.

Helton WS. Diagnostic and therapeutic approaches to the patient with liver malignancy. In: Clavien PA (ed.), *Malignant Liver Tumors: Current and Emergent Therapies*, 1st ed. Oxford, UK: Blackwell Science, 1999, 62–84.

32. **(A)** Primary angiosarcoma of the liver accounts for up to 2% of all primary liver tumors and is the second most common primary malignant neoplasm of the liver. Approximately 10–20 new cases are diagnosed every year in the United States, and the prevalence varies from 0.14 to 0.25 per million. Hepatic angiosarcoma is three to four times more prevalent in men than in women, but in childhood, hepatic angiosarcoma occurs more often in girls; however, most hepatic angiosarcomas occur in adults.

One-fourth of all cases of hepatic angiosarcomas are associated with a previous exposure to chemical carcinogens. Environmental exposure to thorotrast was the first of these to be recognized, as early as in 1947. Subsequently, arsenic and vinyl chloride were also identified as causative factors in the development of hepatic angiosarcoma. Thorotrast is a 25% colloidal solution of thorium dioxide and was widely used in the past as a radiologic contrast medium. Its use was later discarded, because alpha emission of thorium occurs over a long period of time. The latency period of thorotrast-related tumors is about 20–42 years. These tumors occur principally in men. Thorotrast-induced hepatic angiosarcoma accounts for 25% of thorotrast-related tumors. Seven percent to 10% of hepatic angiosarcomas are thorotrast-related.

The environmental toxin next most commonly associated with hepatic angiosarcoma is vinyl chloride. This association was first described in employees of vinyl chloride polymerization facilities. The risk of hepatic angiosarcoma as a result of occupational vinyl chloride exposure is 10–15 times that of the general population.

Treatment protocols are debated. Various investigators have attempted different modalities, including surgery, radiotherapy, or chemotherapy, with limited results. Because most tumors are bilobar and multifocal, surgical resection is often not possible. Surgery may be an option when the angiogram has shown that the tumor is localized to one lobe and the remainder of the liver is not compromised.

The overall prognosis is dismal, with a median survival of only 6 months. The tumor is often unresectable at diagnosis. Only 3% of patients have been reported to survive for more than 2 years. The longest reported survival is 7 years in a patient who received radiotherapy.

Bibliography

Adson AM, Beart WR Jr. Elective hepatic resections. *Surg Clin North Am* 1977;57:339–358.

Alrenga DP. Primary angiosarcoma of the liver [review article]. *Int Surg* 1975;60:198–203.

Davenport M, Hansen L, Heaton ND, et al. Hemangioendothelioma of the liver in infants. *J Pediatr Surg* 1995;30:44–48.

Gargot D, Maitre F, Causse X, et al. Primary liver non-Hodgkin's lymphoma presenting as fulminant hepatic disease. *Eur J Gastroenterol Hepatol* 1994;6:843–846.

Levy DW, Rindsberg S, Friedman AC, et al. Thorotrast-induced hepatosplenic neoplasia: CT identification. *AJR Am J Roentgenol* 1986;146:997–1004.

MacMohan HE, Murphy AS, Bates MI. Endothelial cell sarcoma of liver following thorotrast injections. *Am J Pathol* 1947;23:585–611.

Tamburro CH. Relationship of vinyl monomer and liver cancers: angiosarcoma and hepatocellular carcinoma. *Semin Liver Dis* 1984;4:158–169.

Vianna NJ. Tumors in patients with angiosarcoma of the liver. *Ann Intern Med* 1981;95:185–186.

33. (C) The portal vein provides three-fourths of the liver's blood supply, whereas the rest is supplied by the hepatic artery. Metastatic tumors make up the largest group of malignant tumors in the liver, and reach the liver mostly as the result of shedding into the vascular system. This is most commonly caused by bronchogenic carcinoma, followed by prostate, colon, breast, pancreas, stomach, kidney, and cervix. This is explained by the fact that primary tumors that drain into the portal system contribute more hepatic metastases than tumors arising outside the portal drainage system. However, in contradistinction to liver parenchyma, liver metastases derive nearly all their vascular inflow from branches of the hepatic artery. The same concept applies to primary liver malignancies. This difference in blood supply between normal liver and malignant liver lesion is the basis for the use of dynamic CT scans for the detection of hepatic tumors. On the other hand, the fact that hepatic metastases greater than 3 mm in size derive their blood supply from the hepatic artery and not the portal vein provides the anatomic rationale for the use of liver-directed chemotherapy via a hepatic artery infusion (HAI) pump. In this setting, a fourfold increase in concentration of chemotherapeutic agent can be achieved in the liver when the drug is being delivered through the hepatic artery instead of being systemically infused (Fig. 28-11).

Bibliography

Ackerman NB. The blood supply of experimental liver metastases. Changes in vascularity with increasing tumor growth. *Surgery* 1974;75:589–596.

Townsend CM, et al. *Sabiston Textbook of Surgery: The Biological Basis of Modern Surgical Practice*, 16th ed. Philadelphia, PA: W.B. Saunders, 2001.

34. (A), (C) Hemangiomas are the most common benign solid tumors of the liver. They occur in two variants:

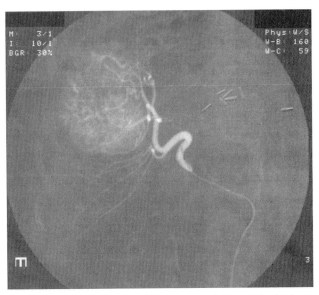

FIG. 28-11 The angiogram depicted is of a hepatic neuroendocrine tumor prior to selective embolization. Tumors in the liver bigger than 3 mm in size derive their blood supply for the hepatic artery and not the portal vein. This is an important factor in planning the treatment strategies for several types of hepatic tumors.

capillary and cavernous. Unlike other benign liver tumors, there has never been any documentation of malignant degeneration.

Capillary hemangiomas are the most common. They are usually small and have little clinical significance.

Cavernous hemangiomas are more clinically relevant because of the associated symptoms and potential complications. They occur in all age groups but are mostly seen in the third to fifth decades of life and have a predilection for women. They are found in 2–7% of livers at autopsy, making this the most common liver tumor encountered coincidentally at laparotomy. The origin is unclear though, and it is thought to represent progressive growth of congenital lesions.

This lesion can range in size from less than 1 mm to 30–40 cm, forming a so-called giant hemangioma. It is usually well demarcated from the surrounding liver tissue and may be partly necrotic or fibrotic. They have a sponge-like appearance and do not usually present a diagnostic dilemma. They are typically expansive rather than infiltrating, leading to compression of surrounding structures along the edge of the tumor, and forming a fibrous tissue plane for dissection.

Most patients with liver hemangiomas are asymptomatic and are diagnosed only at autopsy. Pain is usually the most common symptom, although other presentations have been reported such as nausea, vomiting, early satiety, increased abdominal girth, and fever. Some of these symptoms can be secondary to distension of Glisson's capsule or infarction within the tumor. Biliary-related symptoms seldom occur secondary to extrinsic compression by the tumor and include obstructive jaundice and biliary colic. The great concern about spontaneous rupture with life-threatening hemorrhage is unfounded since very few such cases have been reported in the world literature. Moreover, acute symptoms from a hepatic hemangioma are rare and are usually because of rapid expansion with stretching of the liver capsule or to thrombosis within the tumor.

Hemangiomas are occasionally present as non-tender palpable masses when they reach a large size, but the physical examination is usually unremarkable. A bruit can be sometimes heard over the liver on auscultation.

Diagnosis is usually made by noninvasive radiographic imaging and has largely replaced the need for biopsy and the associated risk of life-threatening hemorrhage.

Ultrasonography is usually the first study performed and shows a hyperechoic lesion clearly demarcated from the surrounding liver. CT scan is typically the next study obtained and shows a characteristic pattern of peripheral enhancement after contrast injection. Delayed image after several minutes show central filling of the lesion. The most sensitive test though is MRI and has largely replaced hepatic angiography and ^{99}Tc RBC scans. A hemangioma will yield a hyperintense pattern on T2-weighted images. The classic appearance of rim enhancement with centripetal filling on delayed images during the arterial phase is also demonstrated (Fig. 28-12).

In the patient for whom a definitive noninvasive diagnosis cannot be established, a diagnostic laparoscopy will establish the identity of a surface liver mass because of the characteristic appearance and the spongy texture.

Bibliography

Farges O, Daradkeh S, Bismuth H. Cavernous hemangiomas of the liver: are there any indications for resection? *World J Surg* 1995;19:19.

Ros P. Benign lesions of the liver. *Radiol Clin North Am* 1998;36:319.

Townsend CM, et al. *Sabiston Textbook of Surgery: The Biological Basis of Modern Surgical Practice*, 16th ed. Philadelphia, PA: W.B. Saunders, 2001.

35. (B) In nearly all cases of asymptomatic hemangiomas, observation is the most appropriate treatment since the risk of rupture is negligible and prophylactic resection

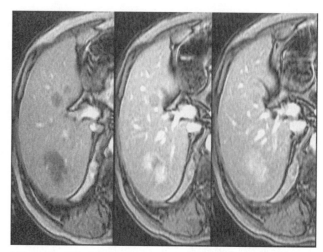

FIG. 28-12 Gallodinium enhanced MRI of liver with a posterior located abnormality demonstrating delayed uptake (left), peripheral enhancement after 3 min (middle image), and retained contrast after 5 min; consistent with a hemangioma (right). Hemangioma is also well characterized by ultrasound.

is not warranted. Indeed, the natural history of a liver hemangioma shows that 10% enlarge, 10% decrease in size, and the remainder remains stable. Follow-up should include ultrasound or CT scan at 6 months intervals to exclude an undetected malignancy manifesting as rapid enlargement of the lesion.

In general, the indications for resection of hepatic hemangiomas are as follows:

1. symptoms that are unequivocally attributed to the hemangioma
2. inability to obtain a noninvasive diagnosis and to exclude a malignant lesion
3. rupture with intraperitoneal hemorrhage

Size is not in itself an indication for elective resection, neither is the location of the lesion.

When surgery is indicated, the preferred procedure is enucleation of the lesion since the risk of recurrence is negligible and functional liver parenchyma is spared. This technique is also associated with less blood loss and postoperative complications and is applicable to most lesions since an avascular plane of dissection can often be developed between the hemangioma and the liver parenchyma. This is usually done through a right subcostal incision whereas the laparoscopic approach is applicable for surface lesions either for resection or diagnosis.

Formal anatomic resection may be safer in some cases, however, and is required if malignancy has not been excluded.

Resection is the most effective approach since more than 90% of patients report symptom relief after the operation. Reported mortality rates range from 0 to 4% and the procedure is well tolerated by the majority of patients.

In patients who are medically unfit, alternative nonoperative therapy is available with limited success though. External beam radiation therapy has been used and will result in involution of the hemangioma in some situations. Results are not always reproducible and recurrences have been reported.

Embolization or hepatic artery ligation has been described yet provide only transient symptom relief and should be mainly used to temporize uncontrollable hemorrhage following spontaneous rupture.

Corticosteroid therapy has been reported. The rationale for this approach is not fully understood and has met some success in the pediatric age group. Its use in the adult population has not been proven to be of any benefit.

Bibliography

Gedaly R, et al. Cavernous hemangiomas of the liver: anatomic resection vs. enucleation. *Arch Surg* 1999; 134:407.

Katkhouda N, et al. Laparoscopic management of benign solid and cystic lesions of the liver. *Ann Surg* 1999; 229:460.

Kuo P, Lewis W, Jenkins R. Treatment of giant hemangiomas of the liver by enucleation. *J Am Coll Surg* 1994; 178:49.

Weimann A, et al. Benign liver tumors: differential diagnosis and indications for surgery. *World J Surg* 1997;21:1983.

36. **(D)** The vast majority of benign liver masses are discovered incidentally during the course of a patient's evaluation for unrelated symptoms. The majority of benign hepatic lesions will be one of the following: a cyst, a hemangioma, focal nodular hyperplasia (FNH), or a liver cell adenoma. Based on characteristic radiologic appearance, it is almost always possible to make an accurate diagnosis without the need for a liver biopsy. A biopsy, whether percutaneous or radiographically guided, is often dangerous and contraindicated in these patients.

Liver lesions more likely to cause symptoms that are usually large, extend to the liver surface, occupy a large volume of the left lateral segment, or press on other viscera. In the absence of such features, the patient's symptoms are unlikely to be attributed to the liver mass and the search for other pathology should continue.

In general, benign liver tumors should undergo operative resection when they are symptomatic, they are actively bleeding or present a substantial risk for bleeding, they are at risk for malignant transformation, or when a malignancy cannot be confidently excluded radiologically or by biopsy when indicated.

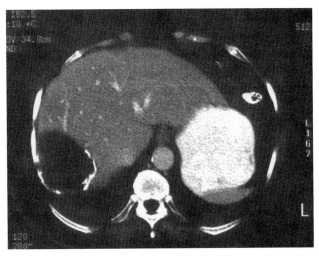

FIG. 28-13 Simple cysts are common findings during hepatic imaging. Simple cysts tend to "push" normal hepatic architecture out of the way (note the displaced liver parenchyma). A hallmark feature of these lesions is homogeneity on CT scan. Surgical treatment is only necessary if symptomatic and is accomplished by "un-roofing" and marsupialization of the cyst cavity. It is important to differentiate simple cysts from cystadenoma and cystadenocarcinoma.

Liver cysts are generally benign. They may be solitary or multiple and may or may not communicate with the hepatic ductal system. They are most commonly found in the right lobe of the liver, and are more frequent in males. They are usually small and asymptomatic, yet some can be quite large and can cause symptoms such as increased abdominal girth, vague pain, and rarely obstructive jaundice (Fig. 28-13).

Incidentally discovered small cysts require no treatment. Simple large cysts that cause symptoms usually never require resection since most can be adequately treated by laparoscopic marsupilization or ethanol injection. If pathology of a simple cyst wall reveals evidence of ovarian stroma, it is diagnostic of cystadenoma and resection is indicated because of the risk of malignant degeneration. Complex cysts with internal septae or fonds are indicative of cystadenoma or cystadenocarcinoma and resection is advised.

Bibliography

Blumgart LH, Fong Y. *Surgery of the Liver and Biliary Tract*, 3rd ed. Edinburgh: Churchill Livingstone, 2000.

Townsend CM, et al. *Sabiston Textbook of Surgery: The Biological Basis of Modern Surgical Practice*, 16th ed. Philadelphia, PA: W.B. Saunders, 2001.

37. **(D)** A variety of treatments exist for primary and secondary malignancies of the liver, including surgical resection; ablative therapies such as cryotherapy,

radiofrequency ablation, hepatic arterial embolization, ethanol injection and radiation, transplantation, and chemotherapy.

Local response to treatment is usually defined following the World Health Organization (WHO) criteria as follows:

Complete response (CR): complete disappearance of all known disease and no new lesions determined by two observations not less than 4 weeks apart.
Partial response (PR): >50% reduction in total tumor load of all measurable lesions determined by two observations not less than 4 weeks apart.
Stable disease (ST): does not qualify for CR/PR or progressive disease.
Progressive disease (PD): >25% increase in size of one or more measurable lesions or the appearance of new lesions.

There are no present data to propose a universal treatment algorithm to be implemented worldwide for the treatment of HCC. It is agreed on though that if the diagnosis is established early on, patients should be considered for any of the available options that provide a high rate of CR. These include surgical resection, liver transplantation, and percutaneous techniques. In general, radical surgical extirpation is the most effective therapy and should be the gold standard by which all other forms of therapy must be compared. Surgical resection provides excellent results for solitary HCC in patients with preserved liver function, with a 5-year survival reaching up to 70% in patients with normal bilirubin concentration and no evidence of portal hypertension. The main problem of surgical resection as compared to orthotopic liver transplantation is the high recurrence rate that may be as high as 70% at 5 years; however, the theoretical superiority of transplantation in terms of decrease recurrence is offset by the shortage of donors and cannot be currently recommended as a first line therapy. Whether living donor liver transplantation will meet this standard and overcome the lack of donors remains to be seen.

On the other hand, patients with decompensated cirrhosis or those with early multinodular disease (3 nodules ≤3 cm) should not undergo resection but should be offered liver transplantation as the first approach.

At present, ethanol injection should be considered the standard percutaneous technique. It is well tolerated with a high anti-tumoral efficacy. Percutaneous ethanol injection (PEI) is highly effective for tumors ≤3 cm in which an 80% CR rate can be expected. Recurrence after effective percutaneous treatment is as frequent as after surgical resection

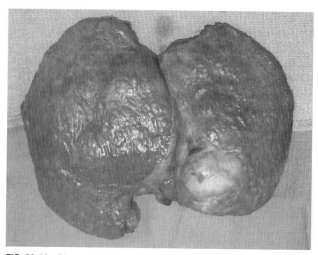

FIG. 28-14 Photograph of explanted cirrhotic liver with a large HCC lesion. While several treatment options are available for HCC, resection remains the only modality to significantly affect survival. It is important to recognize that it is only selected patients who are candidates for resection. The multifocal nature of disease and the underlying cirrhotic liver preclude resection in many patients.

(50% at 3 years and >70% at 5 years), and other more invasive percutaneous techniques such as cryoablation or radiofrequency ablation should at this time be compared with PEI through randomized controlled trials (RCT).

However, RCTs comparing the above three mentioned options associated with a high rate of CR are lacking, and similarly, there are no RCTs comparing surgical resection and ethanol injection. Therefore, PEI can be recommended for the time being only when surgery is precluded (Fig. 28-14).

Bibliography

Bismuth H, Majno PE. Hepatobiliary surgery. *J Hepatol* 2000;32:208–224.
Castells A, Bruix J, Bru C, Fuster J, Vilana R, Navasa M, et al. Treatment of small hepatocellular carcinoma in cirrhotic patients: a cohort study comparing surgical resection and percutaneous ethanol injection. *Hepatology* 1993;18:1121–1126.
Dibisceglie AM, Rustgi VK, Hoofnagle JH, et al. NIH conference: hepatocellular carcinoma. *Ann Intern Med* 1988;108:390–401.
Miller AB, Hoogstraten B, Staquet M, Winkler A. Reporting results of cancer treatment. *Cancer* 1981;47:207–214.

38. **(C)** Colorectal cancer metastases develop in up to two-thirds of the 140,000 patients newly diagnosed with colorectal cancer each year in the United States. Approximately 60% of these patients develop metastatic disease confined to the liver. Moreover, at the time of presentation with a colonic primary, 15–20% of

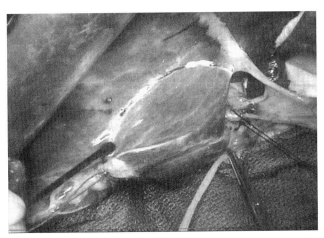

FIG. 28-15 Small peripherally located metastatic colorectal tumors can be safely resected during another procedure. The photograph depicts a metastasectomy employing a radiofrequency device to resect a lesion on the edge of segment IVb.

patients have a synchronous metastatic liver lesion. On the other hand, in patients without evidence of metastatic disease who undergo potentially curative colon resection, of those that recur, almost 80% recur within the liver.

Resection, if possible, remains the treatment of choice for metastatic colorectal cancer to the liver and is associated with low operative morbidity and mortality and a concomitant long-term survival benefit. Indeed, without treatment, 60–70% of patients die within 1 year and close to 100% die within 3 years. On the other hand, resection of a solitary metastatic lesion from a colorectal primary tumor can have as much as a 60% 5-year survival rate (Fig. 28-15).

When a synchronous hepatic metastasis if found during operation with a primary colorectal malignancy, the hepatic lesion may be removed simultaneously or at a second procedure. This decision depends on the magnitude of the planned procedure as well as the extent of hepatic metastases, the general health status of the patient and the experience of the surgeon with liver resections. In general, contraindications to major hepatic resection for metastatic disease include total hepatic replacement, advanced cirrhosis, invasion of the portal vein or vena cava, and extrahepatic metastasis.

However, complete resection of hepatic metastases can be achieved in only 10–20% of patients, and palliative resection has shown no survival benefit. Nonresective destructive techniques such as cryoablation, ethanol injection, or radiofrequency ablation are currently being used to focally ablate hepatic metastases via a percutaneous or laparo-

scopic approach. The benefits include improved operative morbidity and mortality and less destruction of normal hepatic parenchyma. They may also allow curative resections to be performed in patients with multiple tumors or tumors involving both hepatic lobes.

Bibliography

Scheele J, Stagl R, Attendorf A. Hepatic metastases from colorectal cancer carcinoma: impact of surgical resection on the natural history. *Br J Surg* 1990;77:1241.

Scudamore CH, et al. Radiofrequency ablation followed by resection of malignant liver tumors. *Am J Surg* 1999; 177:411.

Wagner JS, Adson MA, Van Heerden JA, et al. The natural history of hepatic metastases from colorectal cancer. A comparison with resective treatment. *Ann Surg* 1984;199:502–508.

Wingo PA, Ries LA, Rosenberg HM, et al. Cancer incidence and mortality, 1973–1995: a report card for the U.S. *Cancer* 1998;82:1197–1207.

39. (C) Hepatic adenomas are generally soft solitary lesions. They are typically small (less than 5 cm) but may vary in size up to 38 cm in diameter. Multiple lesions have been reported though and may cluster in families. Microscopically, a hepatic adenoma is made of closely approximated monotonous cords of hepatocytes with vacuolated sinusoidal borders, and is separate from adjacent normal hepatic parenchyma. Its center may undergo degenerative changes, yet it has an abundant blood supply. Unlike FNH, portal triads and bile ducts are absent, as well as Kupffer cells. The association between the use of oral contraceptive pills (OCP) and the development of hepatic adenomas is now well established, and the risk correlates with the duration of use and age above 30. Other risks factors are the use of anabolic steroids and certain glycogen storage disease (Fig. 28-16).

In patients who have used OCPs for more than 2 years, the incidence is 3–4 per 100,000. On the other hand, 90% of patients diagnosed with a hepatic adenoma have used OCPs in the past. The risk may indeed vary among different OCPs and depend on the amount of estrogen in the preparation. Hepatic adenomas usually persist, even after stopping OCP use. Although regression of the liver lesion has been documented, this is not universal.

The patient with an unresected adenoma who discontinues using oral contraceptives and becomes pregnant is at considerable risk for tumor rupture and hemorrhage. For this reason, women with an untreated hepatic adenoma should be advised to avoid pregnancy or to undergo resection before hand. All women with a hepatic adenoma should be

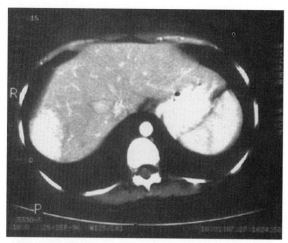

FIG. 28-16 Hepatic adenomas are vascular lesions of hypertrophic hepatic parenchyma. Generally devoid of normal hepatic architectural features, they can be confused with HCC or focal nodular hyperplasia.

advised to stop OCP use for life. On the other hand, any lesion suspected of being a hepatic adenoma should be resected if the patient can tolerate general anesthesia because of the risk for spontaneous rupture and bleeding as well as the real, but low risk, for malignant degeneration. Recurrence after resection is uncommon, provided that OCP are discontinued, and yearly follow-up imaging is recommended.

Enucleation may be an option in some patients, but the preferred approach is formal resection with adequate margins. While ablation therapy may be effective for such lesions, there is currently no long-term follow up with this approach and it should not be recommended for healthy patients. This may, however, be a reasonable option for elderly patient with significant medical comorbidities and with lesions less than 4 cm in size.

Bleeding from a ruptured hepatic adenoma may be controlled with hepatic artery embolization or hepatic artery ligation. Formal hepatic resection should be deferred in an unstable patient with ongoing hemorrhage.

Bibliography

De Carlis L, et al. Hepatic adenoma and focal nodular hyperplasia: diagnosis and criteria for treatment. *Liver Transpl Surg* 1997;3:160.

Foster JH, Berman MM. The malignant transformation of liver cell adenomas. *Arch Surg* 1994;129:712.

Jenkins RL, Johnson LB, Lewis WD. Surgical approach to benign liver tumors. *Semin Liver Dis* 1994;14:178.

Townsend CM, et al. *Sabiston Textbook of Surgery: The Biological Basis of Modern Surgical Practice*, 16th ed. Philadelphia, PA: W.B. Saunders, 2001.

40. (A), (B), (C), (D) AFP was the first described oncofetal antigen, identified initially as a useful marker in HCC and subsequently in nonseminomatous testicular cancer. AFP is a single chain polypeptide (molecular weight 64,000–74,000 Da) that is normally elevated in the fetus, rapidly falls to low levels after birth, and is elevated again during pregnancy. The half-life of circulating serum AFP is 4–6 days. Besides the yolk sac, AFP is synthesized by hepatic parenchymal cells as well as endodermally derived gastrointestinal tissue. The development of radioimmuno assays has significantly improved the sensitivity of detection of AFP, and routine commercially available tests are able to detect levels of 5 ng/mL.

Although abnormal serum levels usually occur in malignant neoplasms, benign disease of endodermally derived organs can cause increased levels including hepatitis, inflammatory bowel disease, and cirrhosis.

Approximately 75% of patients with HCC and cirrhosis have levels above 400 µg/L, whereas AFP is elevated in only about one-third of patients with HCC and a noncirrhotic liver. Sixty-five percent of patients with HCC secondary to alcoholic cirrhosis have an elevated AFP.

In the United States, three-fourth of patients with HCCs greater than 5 cm in diameter have an AFP level greater than 100 µg/L (normal level is 0–20 µg/L). A level greater than 400 µg/L is generally diagnostic of HCC.

Pronounced elevation of AFP can also be seen with teratocarcinoma, yolk sac tumors, fulminant hepatitis B infection, and occasionally metastatic pancreatic or gastric carcinoma. Mild elevation may be found in patients with chronic liver disease, acute viral hepatitis, and metastatic cancer.

AFP, along with ultrasound, is the recommended screening for patients at high risk for developing HCC. Serum levels may return to normal after liver resection and is a useful marker to follow.

Bibliography

Alpert ME, Uriel J, De Nechaud B. Alpha fetoglobulin in the diagnosis of human hepatoma. *N Engl J Med* 1968;27:984.

Taketa K. Alphafetoprotein: reevaluation in hepatology. *Hepatology* 1990;12:1420.

Tomasi TB. Structure and function of alpha-fetoprotein. *Annu Rev Med* 1977;28:453.

Townsend CM, et al. *Sabiston Textbook of Surgery: The Biological Basis of Modern Surgical Practice*, 16th ed. Philadelphia, PA: W.B. Saunders, 2001.

Wu AH, Sell S. Markers for hepatocellular carcinoma. *Immunol Ser* 1990;53:403.

41. (B), (C), (D), (E) It has been suggested that the term bile duct cancer be used for central lesions and cholangiocarcinoma for peripheral tumors, nonetheless the terms are interchanged in the literature.

Cholangiocarcinoma arises from the bile duct epithelium and can occur anywhere along the biliary tract. It is a rare tumor, with 2000–3000 cases diagnosed annually in the United States, and represents 5–20% of primary carcinomas of the liver. Most cases occur in patients in their fifth to seventh decade of life, and there is a 3:2 female predominance. Identified risk factors for the development of bile duct cancer include primary sclerosing cholangitis, ulcerative colitis, bile duct adenomas, choledochal cysts, Caroli's disease, hepatolithiasis, and exposure to the radio-opaque medium thorium dioxide (thorotrast). In Asia, infestation with the parasites *Opisthorchis viverrini* or *C. sinensis* is associated with increased risk. Indeed, *C. sinensis* infestation is associated with more than 90% of cholangiocarcinomas in Hong Kong.

Tumors arising from the extrahepatic bile ducts differ from those located intrahepatically in terms of their presentation, therapy, and prognosis. The intrahepatic type of cholangiocarcinoma is associated with chronic cholestasis, cirrhosis, hemochromatosis, and congenital cystic disease of the liver (Fig. 28-17).

Adenocarcinoma accounts for 95% of bile duct tumors. Other types include squamous cell carcinoma, small cell carcinoma, and mesenchymal tumors.

Cholangiocarcinomas are classified into three groups according to their anatomic location: (1) intrahepatic or peripheral (10% of cases), (2) perihilar (65% of cases), and (3) distal (25% of cases). Perihilar cholangiocarcinoma involving the confluence of the hepatic ducts is also known as Klatskin's tumor.

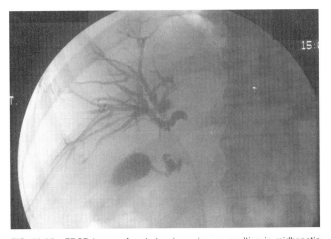

FIG. 28-17 ERCP image of a cholangiocarcinoma resulting in midhepatic duct obstruction.

The most common symptom is painless jaundice resulting from biliary obstruction. Other symptoms include pruritus, vague abdominal pain, and mild cholangitis. Physical examination is often unremarkable but may reveal slight hepatomegaly, jaundice, right upper quadrant tenderness, and a palpable gallbladder when the lesion is distal. Constitutional symptoms are usually present in advanced disease and include anorexia, weight loss, and fatigue.

Bibliography

Belmaric J. Malignant tumors in Chinese. *Int J Cancer* 1979;4:560.

De Groen PC, et al. Medical progress: biliary tract cancers. *N Engl J Med* 1999;341:1368.

Nakeeb A, et al. Cholangiocarcinoma: a spectrum of intrahepatic, perihilar, and distal tumors. *Ann Surg* 1996; 224:463.

Todani T, Tabuchi K, Watanabe Y, Kobayashi T. Carcinoma arising in the wall of congenital bile duct cysts. *Cancer* 1979;44:1134.

Townsend CM, et al. *Sabiston Textbook of Surgery: The Biological Basis of Modern Surgical Practice*, 16th ed. Philadelphia, PA: W.B. Saunders, 2001.

42. (A), (E) Bile duct cancers are staged using the TNM system. Stage I tumors (T1, N0, M0) are confined to the bile duct mucosa or muscularis, stage II tumors (T2, N0, M0) have invaded periductal tissue, stage III tumors (T1-2, N1, M0) have spread to regional lymphnodes, stage IV tumors have invaded adjacent organs (IVA, T3, N0-1, M0) or are associated with distant metastases (IVB, T1-3, N0-1, M1).

A useful classification system has been proposed by Bismuth et al. (Table 28-1).

Patients suspected of having cholangiocarcinoma should have a contrast spiral CT scan of the abdomen. The primary tumor is often not seen, but dilated hepatic ducts are appreciated. Cholangiography is the next test to obtain to define the proximal and distal extent of the tumor. This can be done as a percutaneous transhepatic cholangiography for intrahepatic and complex perihilar tumors, or endoscopically (ERCP) for distal tumors.

TABLE 28-1   Classification of Perihilar Bile Duct Cancers*

Type I: tumors below the confluence of the left and right hepatic ducts

Type II: tumors reaching the confluence

Type IIIA/IIIB: tumors involving the common hepatic duct and either the right or left hepatic duct, respectively

Type IV: tumors that are multicentric or involve the confluence and both the right and left hepatic ducts

*Adapted from Bismuth et al.

The treatment of choice is surgical resection, which provides the longest survival. Contraindications include bilateral or multifocal intrahepatic disease, invasion of the portal vein trunk or hepatic artery, bilateral involvement of hepatic arterial or portal venous branches, unilateral hepatic vascular invasion with contralateral spread and distant metastases. Severe cardiopulmonary disease and preexisting cirrhosis are patient-related contraindications to resection.

The prognosis is best for tumors of the distal bile ducts that can be resected by pancreaticoduodenectomy, with a 5-year survival of 30–40%. Indeed, most cures occur after resection of distal third tumors, and are unusual for proximal bile duct cancers. Klatskin's tumors are less often resectable, although a 20–25% 5-years survival can still be achieved. On the other hand, resection of intraheptic lesions is associated with a 20–40% 5-year survival.

Results of hepatic transplantation have been generally disappointing, primarily because of tumor recurrence.

Neither adjuvant or neoadjuvant chemotherapy has been shown to prolong survival or improve quality of life. Chemotherapy is currently considered an ineffective primary treatment modality although partial responses have been reported using various combinations of agents such as 5-fluorouracil, mitomycin, methotrexate, etoposide, doxorubicin, nitrosourea, and cisplatin.

On the other hand, external beam radiation and transcatheter brachytherapy may relieve pain and contribute to biliary decompression, yet no conclusive data is available on the effect on survival.

For unresectable disease, the median survival ranges from 6 to 7 months for intrahepatic lesions, and 5 to 8 months for hilar lesions. The primary management goal in this setting is palliation of symptoms of biliary obstruction and prevention of secondary hepatic failure.

Bibliography

Bismuth H, Nakache R, Diamond T. Management strategies in resection for hilar cholangiocarcinoma. *Ann Surg* 1992;215:31.

Gerhards MF, et al. Long term survival after resection of proximal bile duct carcinoma (Klatskin tumors). *World J Surg* 1999;23:91.

Launois B, et al. Proximal bile duct cancer: high respectability rate and 5-year survival. *Ann Surg* 1999;230:266.

Roayaie S, Guarrera JV, Ye MQ, et al. Aggressive surgical treatment of intrahepatic cholangiocarcinoma: predictors of outcome. *J Am Coll Surg* 1998;187:365–372.

43. **(A), (B), (C), (D)** A rise in CEA level in a patient after resection of colorectal carcinoma usually prompts a

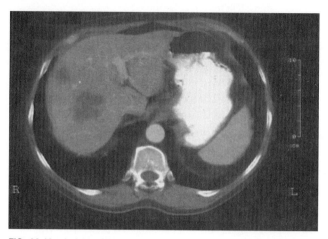

FIG. 28-18 A rising CEA in a patient with a history of colorectal cancer should prompt investigation for metastases. CT image demonstrates right lobe metastasis in a patient with history of node positive colon cancer previously resected.

search for metastatic disease. In addition to the routine history and physical examination, colonoscopy should be preformed if not done within the last 6 months, as well as a contrast CT scan of the chest, abdomen, and pelvis. Since ultrasonography does not provide good information regarding potential resectability, it should not be the first test to obtain in this setting. If anatomically feasible, a segmental hepatic resection should be performed to decrease the frequency of local recurrence and improve survival (Fig. 28-18).

Laparoscopic evaluation is used to assess the liver surface and intraabdominal tumor spread, and can detect lesion as small as 1 mm. Since approximately 90% of liver metastases are present on the surface, diagnostic laparoscopy is an essential tool for evaluation prior to hepatic resection. The addition of laparoscopic ultrasound will contribute further to the prevention of unnecessary laparotomies for unresectable lesions.

However, recurrence elsewhere within the liver remains a common cause of treatment failure. HAI chemotherapy has been used at the time of initial liver resection as well as for recurrences and as an adjuvant therapy in patients with unresectable disease. The rationale for this therapy is based on the hepatic arterial supply of hepatic metastases, the high concentration of chemotherapeutic agents that can be used, and the high clearance of some agents by the liver during the first pass, thus minimizing systemic toxicity. Several randomized trials have demonstrated higher partial and CR rates of intrahepatic versus systemic infusion in the treatment of hepatic metastases from colorectal cancer.

Indeed, it now appears that HAI chemotherapy after liver resection for more than a solitary metastasis is the standard of care in some centers. Not only has this been associated with improved quality of life, but also a survival advantage has been achieved in some institutions when HAI chemotherapy was combined with systemic therapy after liver resection.

Bibliography

Callery MP, et al. Staging laparoscopy with laparoscopic ultrasonography: optimizing respectability in hepatobiliary and pancreatic malignancy. *J Am Coll Surg* 1997; 185:33.

Fong Y, Cohen AM, Fortner JG, et al. Liver resection for colorectal metastases. *J Clin Oncol* 1997;15:938–946.

Allen-Mersh TG, Earlam S, Fordy C, et al. Quality of life and survival with continuous hepatic-artery floxuridine infusion for colorectal liver metastases. *Lancet* 1994; 344:1255–1260.

Kemeny N, Huang Y, Cohen AM, et al. Hepatic arterial infusion of chemotherapy after resection of hepatic metastases from colorectal cancer. *N Engl J Med* 1999; 341:2039–2048.

44. (A) The fibrolamellar variant of hepatocellular carcinoma (FLC) is relatively uncommon and accounts for less than 5% of noncirrhotic HCCs. It primarily occurs in younger patients with noncirrhotic livers as a very bulky lesion. Indeed, as many as 40% occur in patients younger than 35 years old.

Abdominal pain of variable duration is the most common presenting symptom. Other signs and symptoms include palpable abdominal mass, malaise, anorexia, and gynecomastia in male patients. Gynecomastia results from the production of the enzyme aromatase by the tumor. Aromatase converts circulating androgens to estrogens. Unlike conventional HCC, the serum AFP level is rarely elevated in patients with FLC. Indeed, serum AFP values are significantly elevated in only 10–15% of cases. No specific risk factors for FLC have been identified.

Whereas standard HCC has a male predominance, the fibrolamellar variant is believed by some to be more common in females; others believe it affects both sexes equally.

Histologically, it consists of sheets of well-differentiated hepatocytes separated by fibrous tissue. Gross features include a solitary mass sharply demarcated with scalloped borders. The lesion occurs in the left lobe in two-thirds of cases and has a central scar reminiscent of that seen in the benign process of FNH.

FLC is a slow-growing and often well-circumscribed tumor that develops in a noncirrhotic liver, allowing a successful hepatic resection to be performed in 50–75% of cases.

FLC carries a better prognosis when completely resected. Five-year survival rates of 35–56% can be achieved with resection; however, some authors believe that FLC carries the same prognosis as HCC stage per stage, and that the better prognosis associated with FLC is because of the fact that it is slow growing and detected at an earlier stage.

Childhood HCC is usually multifocal and bilateral, appears after the age of 10 in most cases, and can only be cured by surgical resection.

Carcinosarcoma may be associated with a higher rate of metastasis than standard HCC, yet it still carries a better prognosis.

The clear cell variant could be hard to differentiate from metastatic renal cell carcinoma, especially when the two coexist in the same patient. Patients with this variant may have a better prognosis than those with standard HCC.

Bibliography

Agarwal VR, Takayama K, Van Wyk JJ, et al. Molecular basis of severe gynecomastia associated with aromatase expression in a fibrolamellar hepatocellular carcinoma. *J Clin Endocrinol Metab* 1998;83:1797–1800.

Craig JR, Peters RL, Edmondson HA, et al. Fibrolamellar carcinoma of the liver: A tumor of adolescents and young adults with distinctive clinico-pathologic features. *Cancer* 1980;46:372–379.

Soreide O, Czerniak A, Bradpiece H, et al. Characteristics of fibrolamellar hepatocellular carcinoma. A study of nine cases and a review of the literature. *Am J Surg* 1986;151:518–523.

Townsend CM, et al. *Sabiston Textbook of Surgery: The Biological Basis of Modern Surgical Practice*, 16th ed. Philadelphia, PA: W.B. Saunders, 2001.

45. (A), (B) FNH is a benign, tumor-like condition that is predominantly (80–95%) diagnosed in women during their third to fifth decade of life, although it has been described in women in other age groups and in men as well.

FNH is the second most common benign tumor of the liver and, like hepatic adenoma, is most often found in women of reproductive age. It is usually asymptomatic and usually discovered incidentally. The association with OCP is not well established, and other than anecdotal reports, no firm data link pregnancy and changes in the size or symptoms of FNH.

Although FNH and hepatic adenoma are not always easily differentiated, important differentiating clinical and histologic features exist. Unlike hepatic adenoma, FNH carries little, if any, risk of spontaneous rupture and no risk of malignant transformation.

Macroscopically, FNH is a pale red to brown, firm lesion distinct from the surrounding liver.

Histologically, it is sharply demarcated from the normal liver but lacks a true capsule. Unlike hepatic adenoma, bile duct hyperplasia and Kupffer cells are prominent in FNH.

Radiographically, FNH is described as having a central stellate scar; however, the core of the lesion is neither necrotic nor fibrotic but is made up of a round cell infiltrate and thick-walled blood vessels divided by fibrous septae, giving the appearance of scar on imaging.

The blood supply to areas of FNH is quite different from that of hepatic adenomas, with most of the blood supply arising centrally rather than peripherally.

FNH is usually solitary, although 20% of patients have multiple lesions. CT scan may demonstrate a well-demarcated enhancing lesion with enhancement of the central scar during the portal venous phase (Fig. 29-19).

MRI is probably the most sensitive test. FNH is hypointense or even isointense on precontrast T1-weighted images and isointense to mildly hyperintense on T2-weighted images.

Symptoms and inability to exclude malignancy are the most common indications for resection.

If the diagnosis is known, enucleation is sufficient. Otherwise, a formal resection is required.

If asymptomatic and the diagnosis can be confidently made on imaging criteria, a trial of close observation with repeat imaging every 3–4 months is warranted. Resection should be considered if symptoms develop or the lesion enlarges.

Bibliography

De Carlis L, et al. Hepatic adenoma and focal nodular hyperplasia: diagnosis and criteria for treatment. *Liver Transpl Surg* 1997;3:160.

Kondo F. Focal nodular hyperplasia of the liver: controversy over etiology. *J Gastroenterol Hepatol* 2000;15:1229–1231.

Nguyen BN, Flejou JF, Terris B, et al. Focal nodular hyperplasia of the liver: a comprehensive pathologic study of 305 lesions and recognition of new histologic forms. *Am J Surg Pathol* 1999;23:1441–1454.

Townsend CM, et al. *Sabiston Textbook of Surgery: The Biological Basis of Modern Surgical Practice*, 16th ed. Philadelphia, PA: W.B. Saunders, 2001.

46. (C), (D) The risk factors for developing HCC are well documented and include the presence of cirrhosis, chronic active viral hepatitis associated with elevated AFP, age >50, male gender, family history of HCC, and previously resected or ablated HCC. Once cirrhosis has developed, HCC is estimated to occur at the rate of 1–4% per year. This well-documented risk for developing HCC has led to the practice of screening and surveillance of high-risk patients for HCC. Although there are no randomized trials comparing surveillance with no surveillance, a National Institute of Health Consensus Panel currently recommends the use of ultrasonography and AFP levels for early detection of HCC in high-risk populations (Fig. 28-20).

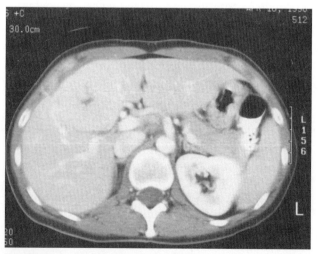

FIG. 28-19 Focal nodular hyperplasia (FNH) commonly is discernable on imaging by the centrally located stellate scar. Although considered a benign lesion, there is a potential for malignant degeneration; symptomatic or lesion >5 cm in size should be resected.

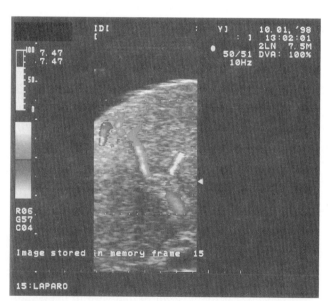

FIG. 28-20 Routine screening for HCC has been demonstrated not to be cost-effective; however, the wide availability of color-flow or power Doppler imaging provides a rapid noninvasive modality to serially examine the liver in patients at risk for the development of HCC. The image depicted illustrates an HCC lesion with a hallmark arterial feeding vessel visualized by color-flow Doppler imaging.

Serum markers other than AFP have no proven efficacy for early detection of HCC, and ultrasound has a reasonable sensitivity (60–78%) but is operator dependent. This combination should be done at 6 months intervals.

The identification of HCC by screening has marginal cost effectiveness. Despite this, screening for HCC in high-risk patients has become the standard of care and should be recommended when applicable.

When viewed from an individual patient's perspective, screening seems to be worthwhile for good surgical candidates who can undergo resection or transplantation.

The use of CT scan for this purpose is not cost-effective, and it is not currently recommended as a screening tool although some physicians use it in addition to AFP levels and ultrasound.

Liver biopsy and laparoscopy may establish the diagnosis of HCC in high-risk patients but should not be routinely obtained and have no role as screening tools.

Bibliography

Bruix J, Llovet J. Prognostic prediction and treatment strategy in hepatocellular carcinoma. *Hepatology* 2002;35 (3):519–524.

Di Bisceglie AM, et al. NIH conference: hepatocellular carcinoma. *Ann Intern Med* 1988;108:390–401.

Townsend CM, et al. *Sabiston Textbook of Surgery: The Biological Basis of Modern Surgical Practice*, 16th ed. Philadelphia, PA: W.B. Saunders, 2001.

Biliary Tract

Nicolas Villanustre and Thomas J. Howard

Questions

1. Regarding the extrahepatic biliary and vascular anatomy, which of the following is *true*?

   (A) The boundaries of the triangle of Calot include the common hepatic duct, cystic duct, and cystic artery.
   (B) The common duct courses downward posterior to the portal vein in the free edge of the lesser omentum.
   (C) The right branch of the hepatic artery crosses the main bile duct posteriorly.
   (D) The cystic artery usually crosses the common hepatic duct posteriorly.

2. All of the following provide blood supply to the extrahepatic biliary ducts *except*:

   (A) gastrodudenal artery
   (B) posterior superior pancreatoduodenal arteries
   (C) right hepatic artery
   (D) cystic artery
   (E) posterior inferior pancreatoduodenal arteries

3. Which of the following is a function of the gallbladder?

   (A) absorption
   (B) motor activity
   (C) secretion
   (D) storage of bile
   (E) all of the above

4. Which of the following is/are involved in the motor activity of the gallbladder? (More than one answer may be correct.)

   (A) vagal stimulation
   (B) splanchnic sympathetic activity
   (C) somatostatin
   (D) motilin
   (E) cholecystokinin

5. Which of the following is/are not functions of bile? (More than one answer may be correct.)

   (A) excretion of bile salt
   (B) excretion of cholesterol
   (C) facilitates lipid absorption
   (D) facilitates absorption of proteins
   (E) promotes absorption of vitamin B_{12}
   (F) facilitates absorption of vitamin K

6. What is the normal amount of bile produced by the liver daily?

   (A) 500–1000 cc
   (B) 1000–2000 cc
   (C) 1000–1500 cc
   (D) 200–400 cc

7. Regarding the enterohepatic circulation, mark the correct statement.

   (A) Terminal ileum resection will result in a decrease bile salt pool.
   (B) A patient with an external biliary fistula will have increased synthesis of bile by the liver.
   (C) During long fasting periods the total bile salt pool decreases.
   (D) Bacterial action in the colon over the primary bile salts (cholate and lithocolate), results in the formation of secondary bile salt (chenodeoxycholate and deoxycholate).

8. Concerning the function of the sphincter of Oddi, mark the correct answer.

(A) Antral distention in respond to food causes both gallbladder contraction and sphincter relaxation.

(B) The phase 3 of the MMC causes an increase in the sphincter pressure during fasting.

(C) Cholecystokinin action increases the activity of the sphincter of Oddi.

(D) Sphincter pressure elevates in response to a meal, preventing regurgitation of duodenal contents.

9. What is the most common type of gallstones in the United States?

(A) pigmented stones

(B) mixed cholesterol/Ca^+

(C) cholesterol stones

(D) Ca^+ stones

10. Mark the *incorrect* answer regarding cholesterol gallstones pathogenesis.

(A) Changes in the equilibrium between the amount of cholesterol and bile saturation capacity play a major role in stone formation.

(B) Decrease gallbladder motility results in less amount of bile available for cholesterol solubilization, predisposing to crystal formation.

(C) The formation of cholesterol stones is the result of specific alterations, congenital or acquired, in the hepatic metabolism.

(D) Mucin production in the gallbladder is known to be a pronucleating factor that predispose to stone formation.

11. A 30-year-old White male with a known hemolytic disorder comes to the surgery clinic with an ultrasound (US) that shows gallstones. What type of gallstones would you expect to find in this patient?

(A) cholesterol stones

(B) mixed cholesterol/Ca^+ stones

(C) brown pigmented stones

(D) black pigmented stones

(E) Ca^+ stones

12. A 42-year-old White female presents to the emergency room (ER) with 24-h history of right upper quadrant (RUQ) pain, fever, and a WBC count of 16,000. What is the most sensitive test in the diagnosis of acute cholecystitis?

(A) ultrasonography

(B) computed tomography (CT) scan of abdomen

(C) Kidney, ureter, and bladder (KUB) radiograph

(D) ^{99m}-Tc hepatobiliary scintigraphy (HIDA) scan

(E) oral cholecystography

13. Regarding the management of acute calculus cholecystitis. Mark the correct answer(s).

(A) Open cholecystectomy is the standard of care.

(B) The conversion rate in the acute setting (10–20%) is higher than in chronic cholecystitis.

(C) Laparoscopic cholecystectomy should be attempted soon after the diagnosis is made.

(D) The cholecystectomy should be delayed until the patient is afebrile and with normal WBC.

14. Which of the following is a contraindication for a laparoscopic cholecystectomy?

(A) previous upper abdominal surgery

(B) cholangitis

(C) cholecystoenteric fistula

(D) chronic obstructive pulmonary disease (COPD)

(E) pregnancy

(F) suspicious of gallbladder carcinoma

(G) morbid obesity

15. In which of the following patients would you consider open cholecystectomy?

(A) 60-year-old male with recent gallstones pancreatitis

(B) 25-year-old female, 10 weeks pregnant

(C) 65-year-old male with Child-Pugh class C disease

(D) 55-year-old female with gallbladder cancer

Questions 16 and 17

A 43-year-old White female comes to the ER complaining of abdominal pain, fever up to 102°F, yellow coloration of the skin, and dark urine for 36 h.

16. The patient undergoes an endoscopic retrograde cholangiopancreatography (ERCP) study (Fig. 29-1). What is the most likely diagnosis?

   (A) acute cholangitis secondary to periampullary tumor

   (B) acute cholangitis secondary to a biliary duct tumor

   (C) acute cholangitis secondary to a biliary-enteric fistula

   (D) acute cholangitis and cholecystitis secondary to hepatic duct obstruction

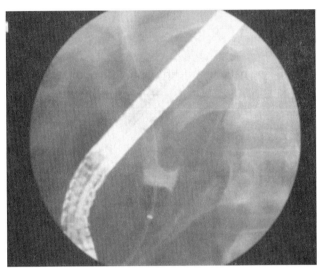

FIG. 29-1

17. What is the most appropriate treatment?

   (A) endoscopic sphincterotomy

   (B) percutaneous transhepatic placement of biliary drainage

   (C) open cholecystectomy and CBD exploration

   (D) laparoscopic cholecystectomy and CBD exploration

18. A 42-year-old White female comes to the ER complaining of RUQ abdominal pain for the last 36 h, associated with fever up to 39°C, bilious emesis, and jaundice. Direct bilirubin 2.2, alkaline phosphatase 450, WBC 19,000, AST 24, ALT 19.

What is the most probable diagnosis?

   (A) acute cholecystitis

   (B) acute cholangitis

   (C) pancreatic cancer

   (D) choledochal cyst

   (E) acute hepatitis

19. What would be the most common etiology for the diagnosis made in previous question?

   (A) primary pigment stones

   (B) secondary CBD stones

   (C) congenital abnormal development of the CBD

   (D) hepatitis virus

   (E) adenocarcinoma

20. Which of the following radiologic studies is not indicated for the diagnosis of this disorder?

   (A) abdominal CT scan

   (B) ERCP

   (C) percutaneous transhepatic cholangiography (PTC)

   (D) HIDA scan

   (E) abdominal ultrasound

21. What is the most common organism isolated from bile and blood cultures in patients with acute cholangitis?

   (A) *Enterobacter* spp.

   (B) *Bacteroides* spp.

   (C) *Escherichia coli*

   (D) *Enterococcus* spp.

   (E) *Candida albicans*

22. What would be the most appropriate antibiotic therapy for this patient?

   (A) cloxcicillin + tobramycin

   (B) piperacillin/tazobactam

   (C) cefazolin

   (D) ampicillin + clindamicin

   (E) metronidazol + ciprofloxacin

23. What is the most appropriate treatment for this patient?

   (A) antibiotics and urgent surgical biliary decompression

   (B) antibiotics and endoscopic biliary decompression

   (C) antibiotics and percutaneous transhepatic biliary decompression

   (D) antibiotics, surgical decompression, and cholecystectomy

24. Which of the following is/are considered a complication of cholangitis?

   (A) liver abscess
   (B) secondary sclerosing cholangitis
   (C) portal vein thrombosis
   (D) pancreatitis
   (E) sepsis
   (F) all of the above

25. What is the most sensitive test for the diagnosis of biliary dyskinesia?

   (A) abdominal CT scan
   (B) ERCP
   (C) cholecystokinin-Tc-HIDA scan
   (D) abdominal US
   (E) magnetic resonance cholangiopancreatography (MRCP)

26. Which of the following patients most likely has biliary dyskinesia?

   (A) 43-year-old Black female with 24 h of abdominal pain, fever, and gallstones by US
   (B) 60-year-old White male with RUQ pain, WBC 16, and diarrhea
   (C) 45-year-old White female with recurrent abdominal pain, gallbladder ejection fraction of 50% at 20 m
   (D) 30-year-old White female with chronic RUQ pain, normal US, and 30% ejection fraction at 10 m.

27. What is the appropriate treatment for biliary dyskinesia?

   (A) fat-free diet and decrease weight
   (B) ERCP with sphincteroplasty
   (C) cholecystectomy
   (D) prokinetic agents
   (E) NPO, antibiotics, and cholecystectomy

28. Regarding choledochal cysts, mark the *incorrect* answer.

   (A) The most common presentation in children is a RUQ abdominal mass, jaundice, and abdominal pain.
   (B) The most common type of choledochal cyst is confined to the extrahepatic biliary tree.
   (C) Caroli's disease is defined as dilatation of the intra- and extrahepatic biliary tree.

   (D) There are two histologic types of choledochal cyst: glandular and fibrotic.
   (E) If not treated they can progress to cholangiocarcinoma.

29. What is the most common type of choledochal cyst?

   (A) type I
   (B) type II
   (C) type III
   (D) type IV
   (E) type V

30. Which of the following is the most sensitive test for the diagnosis of choledochal cyst?

   (A) radionuclide HB scan
   (B) CT scan
   (C) percutaneous transhepatic cholangiogram
   (D) plain abdominal x-ray
   (E) upper gastrointestinal series

31. What type of choledochal cyst is seen in this ERCP study (Fig. 29-2)?

   (A) type I
   (B) type II
   (C) type II
   (D) type IV
   (E) type V

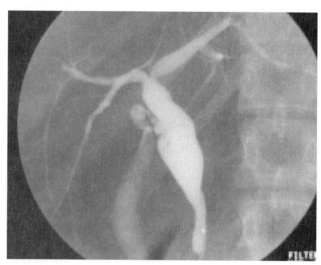

FIG. 29-2

32. What would be the surgical management of the cyst seen in the previous picture?

   (A) duodenopancreatectomy
   (B) hemihepatectomy
   (C) liver transplant
   (D) cystectomy and biliary-enteric Roux-en-Y anastamosis
   (E) transduodenal sphincteroplasty

33. About Caroli's disease, mark the correct answer(s).

   (A) It is characterized by intrahepatic bile duct atresia.
   (B) Abdominal mass and weight loss are the most common initial symptoms.
   (C) It is a developmental anomaly of the ductal plate characterized by saccular dilatations of the large bile ducts.
   (D) It is more commonly seen in adult females.
   (E) It is a risk factor for the development of cystadenocarcinoma of the bile duct.

34. Which of the following radiologic studies is *not* recommended for the diagnosis of Caroli's disease?

   (A) magnetic resonance imaging (MRI) abdomen
   (B) CT scan abdomen
   (C) abdominal US
   (D) HIDA scan
   (E) ERCP

35. Which of the following is *not* a complication of Caroli's disease?

   (A) stone formation
   (B) recurrent cholangitis
   (C) septicemia
   (D) cholangiocarcinoma
   (E) amyloidosis
   (F) renal disorders

36. A 30-year-old White male was recently diagnosed with Caroli's disease. The most appropriate management of this disease is

   (A) hepatic lobectomy
   (B) resection of the CBD and Roux-en-Y hepaticojejunostomy
   (C) internal drainage of the cyst into a Roux-en-Y jejunal limb

   (D) resection of the extrahepatic biliary duct and hepaticodoudenostomy
   (E) choledocal cyst resection

37. Which of the following (Fig. 29-3) is *not* considered a risk factor for cholangiocarcinoma development?

   (A) primary sclerosing cholangitis
   (B) Caroli's disease
   (C) choledocal cyst
   (D) biliary atresia
   (E) hepatolithiasis

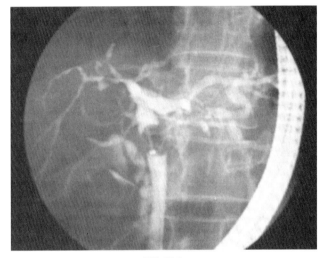

FIG. 29-3

38. What is the most common location of a cholangiocarcinoma?

   (A) right hepatic duct
   (B) left hepatic duct
   (C) hepatic ducts confluence
   (D) CBD

39. What is the appropriate treatment for a cholangiocarcinoma of the hepatic bifurcation?

   (A) right hepatic lobectomy
   (B) left hepatic lobectomy
   (C) pancreaticoduodenectomy (Whipple)
   (D) bile duct resection and hepaticojejunostomy + partial hepatectomy
   (E) radiation therapy + bile duct stenting.

40. Which of the following is *not* considered a risk factor for gallbladder cancer?

    (A) gallstones >3 cm
    (B) multiple small gallstones
    (C) porcelain gallbladder
    (D) biliary *Salmonella typhi* infection
    (E) gallbladder adenoma

41. What is the most common gallbladder tumor?

    (A) adenocarcinoma
    (B) papillary carcinoma
    (C) mucinous carcinoma
    (D) squamous cell carcinoma
    (E) oat cell carcinoma

42. After an uneventful laparoscopic cholecystectomy in a 55-year-old White male, the pathology review demonstrates a gallbladder carcinoma invading, but not penetrating the muscularis layer. What is the most appropriate next step in the management of this patient?

    (A) no more treatment needed
    (B) *en bloc* resection of gallbladder bed including segments four to five of the liver and regional lymph nodes
    (C) postoperative chemotheraphy
    (D) biliary stent placement to prevent future biliary obstruction
    (E) biliary-enteric bypass

43. A 50-year-old White male underwent a laparoscopic cholecystectomy for symptomatic gallstones. On postoperative day 4 he complains of abdominal pain and nausea. Laboratory studies showed WBC 10.000, direct bilirubin 2.5. What is the most appropriate first study?

    (A) magnetic resonance cholangiography
    (B) abdominal US
    (C) ERCP
    (D) HIDA scan
    (E) percutaneous transhepatic cholangiogram

44. The patient described above undergoes an ERCP study (Fig. 29-4). What is the most appropriate initial management?

    (A) total parenteral nutrition and antibiotics
    (B) urgent laparotomy and bile duct reanastomosis
    (C) percutaneous transhepatic cholangiogram and percutaneous biliary stents
    (D) sphincterotomy

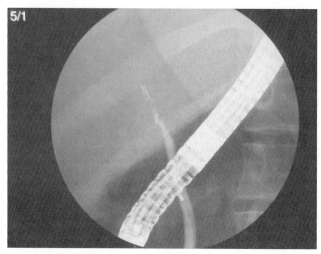

FIG. 29-4

45. What is the most appropriate treatment for the biliary injury seen in Fig. 29-4?

    (A) end-to-end anastamosis of the bile duct
    (B) Roux-en-Y hepaticojejunostomy
    (C) choledochoduodenostomy
    (D) choledocojejunostomy
    (E) ERCP and stent placement

46. A 40-year-old White female status post-laparoscopic cholecystectomy presents to the ER with abdominal pain and fever. After initial studies, an ERCP is obtained (Fig. 29-5). The treatment of choice is

(A) laparotomy and hepaticojejunostomy

(B) papillotomy and stent placement

(C) laparotomy with bile duct repair

(D) laparoscopic approach of the cystic duct and clip

(E) laparotomy and hepaticoduodenostomy

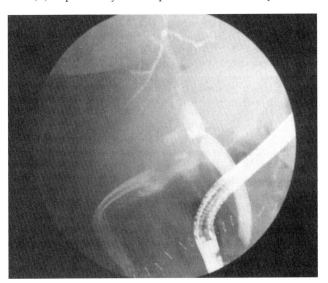

FIG. 29-5

47. A 60-year-old White female presents to the ER complaining of abdominal distention and intermittent abdominal pain for 4 days. A CT scan of the abdomen was obtained as shown in Fig. 29-6.

The treatment options include the following *except*:

(A) milking of the stone until passing the ileocecal valve

(B) push the stone proximally to a less edematous portion of intestine, then enterotomy and extraction

(C) extraction of the stone through an enterotomy and primary repair

(D) biliary-enteric fistula repair during initial surgery

(E) nasogastric tube decompression

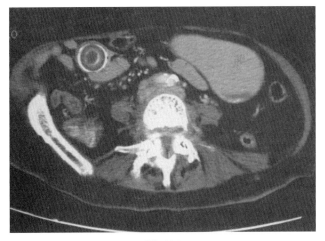

FIG. 29-6

Answers and Explanations

1. **(C)** The extrahepatic bile ducts are represented by the extrahepatic segments of the right and left hepatic ducts joining to form the biliary confluence and the main biliary channel training to the duodenum. The accessory biliary apparatus is comprised of the gallbladder and the cystic duct. The confluence of the right and left hepatic ducts takes place at the right of the hilar fissure of the liver anterior to the portal venous bifurcation and overlying the origin of the right branch of the portal vein.

The main bile duct, the mean diameter of which is about 6 mm is divided in two segments: the upper segment (common hepatic duct) is situated above the cystic duct, which joins it to form the common bile duct (CBD). The latter courses downward anterior to the portal vein in the free edge of the lesser omentum and is closely applied to the hepatic artery which runs upward on its left, giving rise to the right branch of the hepatic artery which crosses the main bile duct posteriorly, though in about 20% of the cases anteriorly.

The cystic artery arises from the right hepatic artery in 95% of the population and may cross the common hepatic duct posteriorly or anteriorly. The most commonly accepted definition of the triangle of Calot recognizes the inferior surface of the right lobe of the liver as the upper border and the cystic duct as the lower. Dissection of Calot's triangle is of key significance during cholecystectomy since in this triangle runs the cystic artery, often the right branch of the hepatic artery and occasionally a bile duct. There are a large number of anatomical variances. The most common occurs in 20% and involves one of the main tributaries of the right duct, usually the right anterior duct entering the common hepatic duct directly. In 12% of individuals there is a triple confluence formed by the right posterior, right anterior, and left hepatic ducts. One important variation is the presence of an anomalous subvesical duct, the duct of Luschka, which runs in the gallbladder fossa. It is found in 12–50% of individuals, drains a variable portion of the right liver and is potentially vulnerable to injury during a cholecystectomy.

Bibliography

Blumgart LH. Surgical and biologic anatomy of the liver and biliary tracts. In: Blumgart LH, Fong Y (eds.), *Surgery of the Liver and Biliary Tract*, 3rd ed. London, UK: WB Sanders, 2000, 3–33.

Britton J, Bickerstaff KI, Savage A. Benign diseases of the biliary tract. In: Morrys PJ, Malt RA (eds.), *Oxford Text Book of Surgery*. Oxford, UK: Oxford Medical Publications, 1994, 1209–1239.

Klein AS, Lillemoe KD. Liver, biliary tract, and pancreas. In: O'Leary JP (ed.), *The Physiologic Basis of Surgery*, 2nd ed. Baltimore, MD: Williams & Wilkins, 1996, 441–478.

2. **(E)** The joining of the right and left hepatic ducts forms the common hepatic duct. The accessory biliary apparatus, composed of the gallbladder and cystic duct, joins the common hepatic duct to form the CBD that drains bile into the duodenum. This constitutes the extrahepatic biliary system. The confluence takes place at the right of the hilus of the liver, anterior to the portal venous bifurcation and overlying the origin of the right branch of the portal vein. The arterial supply to the gallbladder is from the cystic artery. It can originate from the right hepatic, left hepatic, or the common hepatic artery, and can be posterior or anterior to the common hepatic duct. The blood supply to the CBD is divided in three segments. The supraduodenal has an axial blood supply, that originates from the retroduodenal artery, right hepatic artery, cystic artery, gastroduodenal artery, and the retroportal artery. Sixty percent of the blood supply occurs from the duodenal end of the duct, and 38% is from the hepatic end. Only 2% is nonaxial, arising from the main hepatic trunk. The second segment (retropancreatic) is supplied by the retroduodenal artery through a mural plexus around the duct. The third segment is the hilar duct, which receives its blood

supply from the surrounding blood vessels, forming a rich network.

Bibliography

Ahrendt S, Pitt HA. Biliary tract. In: Townsend, et al. (eds.), *Sabiston Textbook of Surgery.* London, UK: W.B. Saunders, 2001, 1076–1079.

Toouli J, Al-Jiffry B. Anatomy and physiology of the biliary tree and gallbladder. In: Clavien P-A, Baillie J (eds.), *On Diseases of the Gallbladder and Bile Ducts.* Oxford, UK: Blackwell Science, 2001, 3–11.

3. (E)

4. (A), (D), (E)

Explanations 3 and 4

The main function of the gallbladder is to concentrate and store hepatic bile during fasting state, allowing for its coordinated release in response to a meal. It also has absorptive, secretary, and motor capabilities. The usual gallbladder capacity is only 40–50 cc. Its absorptive capacity allows the gallbladder to manage the 600 cc of bile produced by the liver daily. The gallbladder mucosa has the greatest absorptive capacity per unit area of any structure in the body. Bile can be concentrated up to 10 folds by the absorption of water and electrolytes. The gallbladder epithelial cells secrete two important products: glycoproteins and hydrogen ions. They protect the mucosa against the effect of the highly concentrated bile. The acidification of the bile caused by the H^+ ions promotes Ca solubility, thereby preventing its precipitation as calcium salts. The release (motor activity) of stored bile from the gallbladder requires a coordinated motor response of gallbladder contraction and Oddi sphincter relaxation. This is mediated by humoral and neural factors. The main stimulus for emptying is the cholecystokinin, which is released by the duodenal mucosa in response to a meal. Vagal stimulation results in gallbladder contraction, and splanchnic sympathetic activity is inhibitory. Between meals the gallbladder empties as a result of phase 3 MMC secondary to the action of motilin. Defects in gallbladder motility, increasing residence time of bile in the gallbladder, play a central role in the pathogenesis of gallstones.

5. (D), (E)

6. (A)

7. (B)

8. (A)

Explanations 5 through 8

The formation of bile by the hepatocyte serves two functions. A route of excretion for certain solids, such as bilirubin and cholesterol and intestinal absorption of lipids and fat soluble vitamins (A, D, E, K). Bile excretion results from the active transport of solutes into the canaliculus followed by the passive flow of water (85% of bile volume).

The major organic solutes in bile are bilirubin, bile salt, phospholipids, and cholesterol.

The primary bile salts in humans, cholic, and chenodeoxycholic acid undergo bacterial conjugation in the intestine to form the secondary bile salts, deoxycholate, and lithocholate. The function of the bile salts is to solubilize lipids and facilitate their absorption.

The normal volume of bile secreted daily by the liver is 500–1000 cc. Bile flow depends on neurogenic, humoral, and chemical control. Vagal stimulation promotes bile secretion, while splanchnic stimulation causes vasoconstriction, decrease blood flow to the liver and, thus diminished bile secretion. Secretin, cholecystokinin, gastrin, and glucagon all increase bile flow, primarily by increasing water and electrolytes secretion.

The most important factor that regulates bile volume is the rate of bile synthesis by the liver, which is regulated by the return of bile salt to the liver by the enterohepatic circulation.

The enterohepatic circulation provides an important negative feedback system on bile synthesis. If the recirculation is interrupted by resection of the terminal ileum, or by primary ileal disease, large losses of bile salts can occur. The same happens if a large external biliary fistula is present. The hepatocyte regulates itself to maintain a constant bile salt pool size where synthesis matches losses.

During fasting periods 90% of the bile acid pool is sequestered in the gallbladder.

The sphincter of Oddi is a complex structure that is separated from the duodenal musculature. It creates a high pressure zone between the bile duct and the duodenum.

It regulates the flow of bile and pancreatic juice and prevents the regurgitation of duodenal contents. Neural and humoral factors influence its function. Under the effect of cholecystokinin after a meal we see a relaxation of the sphincter allowing the passage of bile and pancreatic secretions to the duodenum. During fasting (phase 3 MMC) the sphincter relaxes as the gallbladder contracts to allow the passive flow of bile into the duodenum. Antral distention stimulates the secretion of cholecystokinin causing contraction of the gallbladder and relaxation of the sphincter.

Bibliography

Klein AS, Lillemoe KD. Yeo CJ. Pitt HA. Liver, biliary tract and pancreas. In: O'Leary JP (ed.), *On the Physiologic Basis of Surgery*. Baltimore, MD: Williams & Wilkins, 1996, 441–451.

9. **(B)**

10. **(C)**

11. **(D)**

Explanations 9 through 11

Gallstones represent a failure to maintain certain biliary solutes, primarily cholesterol and Ca^+, in a solubilized state. They are classified by their cholesterol content as either cholesterol or pigment stones (black or brown). Pure cholesterol are uncommon (<10%), mixed cholesterol/Ca^+ (70–80%), and pigment stones (20–30%). The pathogenesis of cholesterol gallstones is multifactorial involving three stages: cholesterol saturation, nucleation, and stone growth. The hepatic metabolism is not involved in the pathogenesis of gallstones.

The process begins with excess cholesterol secretion, which surpasses the ability of the mixed micelles and cholesterol—phospholipids vesicles (carriers) to maintain cholesterol in solution, resulting in cholesterol supersaturation and subsequent precipitation.

Additional factors must be present in order to allow the gallstone formation. First is nucleation which is the process in which cholesterol crystals form and conglomerate. This process occurs more frequently in the gallbladder where the bile is more concentrated. Secondly is the actual stone growth. Growth of stones may occur in two ways: progressive enlargement of stones by deposition of additional insoluble precipitate or fusion of individual crystals or stones to form a larger conglomerate.

Pigment stones are classified as brown and black. The brown stones are more common in Asia, and are similar in composition to primary CBD stones, and occur as a result of infection. Bacteria are found in the brown stone matrix, but are consistently absent from either black pigment or cholesterol stones. Black stones are typically found in patients with hemolytic disorders or cirrhosis. This results from excessive load of bilirubin presented to the liver for excretion.

Bibliography

Klein AS, Lillemoe KD. Yeo CJ. Pitt HA. Liver, biliary tract and pancreas. In: O'Leary JP (ed.), *On the Physiologic Basis of Surgery*. Baltimore, MD: Williams & Wilkins, 1996, 441–451.

12. **(D)**

13. **(B), (C)**

Explanations 12 and 13

The HIDA scan is the most sensitive test available in the diagnosis of acute cholecystitis (98% sensitivity). It is able to provide reliable and accurate information regarding the patency of the bile duct and cystic duct, recognizing that cystic duct obstruction is the hallmark of the diagnosis of acute cholecystitis. This is diagnosed when there is normal imaging of the liver and CBD with prompt visualization of the duodenum but absence of label within the gallbladder. On the other hand HIDA scan examination does not demonstrate the presence of gallstones.

Ultrasonography is a very useful examination during the initial evaluation of a patient with suspected cholecystitis; however, it should be recognized that is most beneficial in identifying the presence or absence of gallstones, and not whether a patient has acute cholecystitis.

CT scan is not a first line test for the diagnosis of cholelithiasis or cholecystitis. It is very useful when the concern is extrahepatic obstruction owing to causes other than choledocholithiasis. Limiting factors include patient exposure to ionizing radiation and cost.

Bibliography

Karam J. Roslyn JJ. Cholelithiasis and cholecystectomy. In: Zinner MJ, Schwart S, Ellis H (eds.), *On Maingot's Abdominal Operations*, 10th ed., 1997, 1717–1753.

14. **(F)** The number of absolute and relative contraindications to performing laparoscopic cholecystectomy have decreased over the past 10 years as minimal invasive surgical equipment and skills have improved. Absolute contraindications include inability to tolerate general anesthesia or laparotomy, refractory coagulopathy, diffuse peritonitis with hemodynamic compromise, and potentially curable gallbladder cancer. Suspicion of gallbladder malignancy (porcelain gallbladder) mandates that standard open resection be undertaken. This is because of persistent concerns with adequacy of resection and reports of port site metastasis associated with the use of minimally invasive surgical techniques for the treatment of intraabdominal malignancies.

Relative contraindications are dictated by the surgeon's philosophy and experience. These include previous upper abdominal surgery with extensive adhesions, cirrhosis, portal hypertension, severe cardio pulmonary disease, morbid obesity, and pregnancy. Preexisting cardiac conditions mandate close observation for significant arrhythmias such as bradycardia and ventricular ectopy secondary to the establishment of a CO_2 pneumoperitoneum.

Pregnancy is a controversial relative contraindication because of the unknown effects of prolonged CO_2 pneumoperitonium of the fetus. We limit this intervention to the second trimester of gestation after organogenesis is complete and prior to the uterine fundus reaching a size and height that encroaches on the operative field.

Bibliography

Gertsch P. The technique of cholecystectomy. In: Blumgart LH, Fong Y (eds.), *Surgery of the Liver and Biliary Tract*, 3rd ed. London, UK: WB Sanders, 2000, 711–712.

15. (C), (D) Open cholecystectomy is rarely indicated; however, some cases require careful consideration for an elective open procedure. Patients with advanced liver disease should be considered for open cholecystectomy when its removal is necessary. Patients with Child-Pugh class C disease are at very high risk for complications. Portal hypertension recannulize umbilical veins, damage of this structure during camera insertion can be life threatening. Open cholecystectomy is recommended on patients with coagulopathy, portal hypertension, ascites, or thrombocytopenia.

During third trimester of pregnancy, open cholecystectomy is the most prudent approach. Port placements and insufflation can be dangerous and difficult during the latter part of pregnancy. Delivery of the fetus should be done first if possible.

If the diagnosis of gallbladder cancer is suspected, open surgery should be considered. Patient with calcified gallbladder (porcelain gallbladder) have a 30% chance of harboring cancer and warrants open cholecystectomy.

Open surgery is also indicated on patients who will not tolerate pneumoperitoneum.

When carbon dioxide is used there are two main changes in patients: (1) increase in blood CO_2 levels and (2) decrease preload to the heart secondary to increased intraabdominal pressure. Patients with COPD or congestive heart failure may not tolerate laparoscopic procedures. In this case minimal insufflation or gasless pneumoperitoneun or open procedures are indicated.

Bibliography

Rege RV. Jeyarejah DR. Open cholecystectomy: when is it indicated? In: Cameron JL (ed.), *Current Surgical Therapy*, 7th ed., 2001, 441–445.

16. (D)

17. (C)

Explanations 16 and 17

Mirizzi's syndrome is described as a hepatic duct obstruction because of cholelithiasis and cholecystitis. It is caused by an impacted gallstone in the cystic duct or the neck of the gallbladder that compresses the adjacent bile duct and results in complete or partial obstruction of the common hepatic bile duct.

Cholecystobiliary fistulas are a rare entity, usually seen in a later stage of Mirizzi's syndrome.

Currently three types are described:

Type A: External compression of the hepatic duct without fistula

Type B: Cholecystobiliary fistula with partial obstruction of the bile duct

Type C: Cholecystobiliary fistula with complete obstruction

Mirizzi's syndrome can be caused by a single large stone or multiple small stones impacted in Hartmann's pouch of the gallbladder or in the cystic duct. A long cystic duct parallel to the bile duct predisposes to the development of this syndrome. Recurrent attacks of cholecystitis may cause inflammation and adhesions in the CBD and may contribute to develop cholangitis. ERCP is the procedure of choice to establish the diagnosis and to classify the lesion. It is also important to determine the presence of a fistula preoperatively.

Percutaneous transhepatic cholangiogram can provide the same information; however, in cases of complete obstruction it is unable to visualize the distal CBD.

CT scan can also be helpful but the presence of periductal inflammation can be misinterpreted as carcinoma of the gallbladder.

The differential diagnosis includes cholangiocarcinoma, gallbladder carcinoma, pancreatic cancer, and sclerosing cholangitis. Surgery remains the treatment of choice for Mirizzi's syndrome. The kind of surgery is determined by whether a fistula is present or not. The common approach is laparotomy, cholecystectomy if possible and CBD exploration. If the CBD viability is questionable, a T-tube, choledocoduodenostomy, or hepaticojejunostomy are the recommended procedures. In any case excellent drainage should be achieved.

Bibliography

Clavien PA. Rudiger HA. Mirizzi's syndrome. In: Clavien PA, Baillie J (eds.), *On Diseases of the Gallbladder and Bile Ducts*, Oxford, UK: Blackwell Science, 2001, 187–195.

18. **(B)**

19. **(B)**

20. **(D)**

21. **(C)**

22. **(B)**

23. **(B)**

24. **(F)**

Explanations 18 through 24

Acute cholangitis is an inflammation/infection process that develops as a result of bacterial colonization and overgrowth within an obstructed biliary system. The obstruction and cholangitis result from impacted stones in 80% of the cases in the Western world. Such stones most commonly originate from the gallbladder (secondary to CBD stones). Primary stones, most commonly pigmented are seen in the East Asian countries. Other causes are benign strictures, neoplasms, papillary stenosis, sclerosing cholangitis, foreign bodies and so on.

Fifty to seventy percent of the patients will present with the Charcot's triad (abdominal pain, fever, and jaundice). The combination of confusion, hypotension, and the Charcot's triad constitutes the Reynold's pentad, which is invariably fatal if urgent biliary decompression is not done.

Chronic biliary obstruction may lead to liver abscesses and secondary biliary cirrhosis. Organ failure and sepsis, sclerosing cholangitis and strictures may develop.

Spread of the infection into the portal vein can cause pyelophlebitis and portal vein thrombosis.

Analysis of the bile and blood in prospective studies showed that *E. coli* (27–70%), *Klebsiella* spp. (17–14%), *Enterobacter* spp. (5–8%), and *Enteroccocus* spp. (17%) were the most common isolated organisms. *C. albicans* is the most common fungal cause in immunocompromised patients.

A combination of abdominal US, CT scan, and cholangiography complements and confirm the clinical diagnosis of cholangitis. Direct cholangiography (ERCP, PTC) is the gold standard for diagnosing acute cholangitis. ERCP is less invasive and has the advantage that offers therapeutic measures, including stone extraction and biliary drainage. PTC is used when ERCP failed or in patients with previous bilioenteric anastamosis.

The management begins with early recognition and aggressive antibiotic coverage.

Approximately 80% of the patients will improve with conservative therapy. The 20% remaining will require biliary drainage. Therapeutic endoscopy is the method of choice for biliary decompression, when it is not available or unsuccessful. Percutaneous transhepatic biliary decompression or surgery should be contemplated. High morbidity and mortality of immediate surgical decompression leaves this option as a last resource.

Once the acute event has resolved, a detailed treatment plan can be carried out electively to remove the underlying obstruction.

Bibliography

Ahrendt S. Pitt HA. Biliary tract. In: Townsend, et al. (ed.), *Sabiston Textbook of Surgery*, 17th ed. London, UK: W.B. Saunders, 2001, 1077–1111.

Yu AS. Leung JW. Acute cholangitis. In: Clavien PA, Baillie J (eds.), *On Diseases of the Gallbladder and Bile Ducts.* Oxford, UK: Blackwell Science, 2001, 205–225.

25. **(C)**

26. **(D)**

27. **(C)**

Explanations 25 through 27

Biliary dyskinesia is characterized by the presence of the typical symptoms of biliary colic including postprandial RUQ pain, fatty food intolerance, and nausea. These patients do not have gallstones disease on US examination. The cholecystokinin-Tc-HIDA scan has been useful in identifying patients with this disorder. Cholecystokinin is administered intravenously after the gallbladder is filled with the radionuclide. Twenty minutes after the injection, a gallbladder ejection fraction is calculated. An ejection fraction of less than 35% at 20 min is considered abnormal.

Patients with symptomatic and abnormal gallbladder ejection fraction should be managed with laparoscopic cholecystectomy. Between 85 and 94% of patients with proved biliary dyskinesia become asymptomatic or improve after the cholecystectomy. About 70% of these patients have pathologic evidence of chronic cholecystitis.

Bibliography

Ahrendt S. Pitt HA. Biliary tract. In: Townsend et al. (ed.), *Sabiston Textbook of Surgery.* London, UK: W.B. Saunders, 2001, 1076–1087.

28. (C)

29. (A)

30. (B)

31. (D)

32. (D)

Explanations 28 through 32

A choledochal cyst is defined as an isolated or combined congenital dilatation of the extrahepatic or intrahepatic biliary tree. In children the classic findings include a RUQ abdominal mass, jaundice, and abdominal pain. In adults it is usually confused with benign biliary and pancreatic diseases.

The most common type is confined to the extrahepatic biliary tree, starting just below the hepatic ducts bifurcation and extending into or near the pancreas (type I) (Fig. 29-7).

Other types include the following:

Type II: Saccular diverticulum of the extrahepatic bile duct

Type III: Dilatation of the extrahepatic bile duct within the duodenum (choledochocele)

Type IVa: Combined intra- and extrahepatic bile duct dilatation

Type IVb: Multiple extrahepatic cysts

Type V: Isolated intrahepatic biliary tree dilatation (Caroli's disease)

Histologically two types of cysts are described: glandular, characterized by a chronic inflammatory cell infiltrate and fibrotic, where the bile duct is

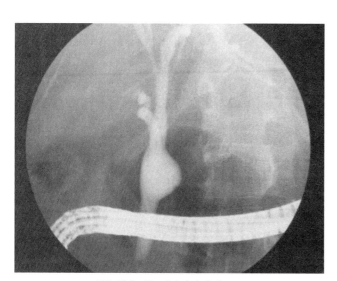

FIG. 29-7 Type I choledochal cyst.

thickened with well-developed collagen fibers and less inflammation. Although multiple studies are used for diagnosis—CT scan, cholangiography (ERCP, PTC), and ultrasonography are the most sensitive studies. ERCP is the most sensitive to diagnose the type of cyst and defining the lower ductal anatomy. US is very useful in determine size, contour, and location of the cyst especially in children. In the adult population, CT scan is the most accurate examination and is particularly useful in the diagnosis of other possible etiologies for biliary obstruction such as pancreatic or periampullary masses. It also delineates size, location, and extent of intra- and extrahepatic biliary tree involvement.

Choledochal cyst excision, with reconstruction via a Roux-en-Y hepaticojejunostomy is the procedure of choice for most type of choledochal cysts. One exception is the type III (choledochocele) cyst that can be treated with transduodenal sphincteroplasty or sphincterotomy. Also an exception is type V (Caroli's disease). If it is localized to one lobe, hepatectomy is the preferred treatment and if it is bilateral liver transplant is the procedure of choice.

Bibliography

Lipsett PA. Yeo CJ. Choledocal cysts. In: Zinner MJ, Schwartz S, Ellis, H (eds.), *On Maingot's Abdominal Operations*, 10th ed. Stamford, CT: Appleton & Lange, 1997, 1701–1713.

33. (C)

34. (D)

35. (F)

36. (A)

Explanations 33 through 36

Caroli's disease is an abnormal development of the intrahepatic bile ducts without an obstructive cause, characterized by saccular dilatations, resembling a picture of multiple cyst-like structures of varying size. Two types have been described: a type with bile duct abnormalities alone and a type with bile duct abnormality combined with periportal fibrosis, similar to congenital hepatic fibrosis. This combined type is also known as Caroli's syndrome and has been reported more frequently than the pure type, or Caroli's disease.

Caroli's disease is anatomically characterized for saccular dilatations of the bile ducts more frequently seen in the left side of the liver. In 30–40% of the cases this are confined to one segment of one side of the liver. Bilateral abnormalities are more common in the second type: Caroli's syndrome.

The most common complications are cholangitis, septicemia, amyloidosis, and cholangiocarcinoma (7–10% of patients). Caroli's syndrome is associated with renal disorders such as renal cysts and nephrospongiosis seen in 30–40% of patients. These disorders have not been seen in Caroli's disease.

The diagnosis is made by radiologic studies such as US, CT scan, ERCP, MRI where saccular or cystically dilated intrahepatic ducts are seen. Surgical treatment is indicated in order to reduce the risk of recurrent cholangitis, biliary cirrhosis, or cholangiocarcinoma. Hepatic lobectomy is indicated for localized bile duct abnormalities (Caroli's disease), while liver transplant should be considered in selected patients with generalized disease or concomitant liver fibrosis and portal hypertension (Caroli's syndrome).

Bibliography

Porte R, Clavien PA. Cystic diseases of the biliary system. In: *On Diseases of the Gallbladder and Bile Ducts.* Oxford, UK: Blackwell Science, 2001, 216–225.

37. (D)

38. (C)

39. (D)

Explanations 37 through 39

Cholangiocarcinoma is an uncommon cancer found in 0.01–0.2% of all autopsies. The majority of the patients are older than 65-year-old with a male predominance.

The etiology is unknown, but several predisposing conditions have been identified:

1. Primary sclerosing cholangitis have a 6–30% chance of developing it and 10–30% of patients who undergo liver transplant for PSC have an occult cholangiocarcinoma. (See Fig. 29-3.)
2. Congenital biliary cystic disease (Caroli's disease, choledochal cyst) have a 15–20% chance of cancer.
3. Hepatolithiasis (recurrent pyogenic cholangitiohepatitis or oriental cholangiohepatitis), prevalent in Japan, secondary to chronic portal bacteremia and portal phlebitis which may give rise to intrahepatic pigment stone formation.
4. Biliary parasites, especially *Clonorchis sinensis* and *Opisthorchis viverrini*, are associated with an increased risk.
5. Carcinogens such as thorium, radon, nitrosamines, dioxin, and asbestos.

Different classifications have been used to describe this tumor. Anatomically they can be divided in intra- and extrahepatics, where 94% of the cholangiocarcinomas are extrahepatics and perihiliar (67%).

The most commonly used classification is the Bismuth classification, which describes the tumor in perspective to the bile duct bifurcation and has direct implication on the surgical strategy.

> Bismuth 1: Tumor below hepatic bifurcation and can be treated with bile duct resection alone.
> Bismuth 2: Tumor that reaches the bifurcation. They usually require a caudate lobe resection, in addition to bile duct resection.
> Bismuth 3a: They may reach the second intrahepatic division of the right main duct.
> Bismuth 3b: They extend to the left main bile duct. Both require either a right or left hemihepatectomy with bile duct resection.
> Bismuth 4: Affects both main bile ducts. Surgery is not an option in this type of location.

Bibliography

Jarnagin WR. Blumgart LH. Cancer of the bile ducts: the hepatic ducts and common bile duct. *On Surgery of the Liver and Biliary Tract.* London, UK: W.B. Saunders, 2000, 1017–1058.

Selzner M, Clavien P-A. Cholangiocarcinoma. *On Diseases of the Gallbladder and Bile Ducts.* Oxford, UK: Blackwell Science, 2001, 277–282.

40. (B) Carcinoma of the gallbladder is a rare and fatal disease, with only 5% of patient surviving beyond 5 years. The association between cancer of the gallbladder and gallstones is well known. Ninety-five percent of the patients with cancer have gallstones. A single large stone >3 cm has a higher risk of cancer than multiple small stones. Calcified deposits in the gallbladder wall, known as porcelain gallbladder, also carries a high chance for cancer. Even asymptomatic patients should be offered cholecystectomy to prevent the development of cancer. Patients with chronic *S. typhi* infection in the biliary tree have increased incidence of gallbladder cancer. Gallbladder adenomas or polyps (>1 cm) have a higher chance to develop cancer than the rest of the population.

Bibliography

Cameron JL, Rosato FE. Gallbladder cancer. In: Cameron JL (ed.) *Current Surgical Therapy,* 7th ed., 2001, 489–493.

41. (A) The only histologic type with prognostic significance is the papillary adenocarcinoma which has a markedly improved survival compared to all other histologic types. There is some evidence to suggest that oat cell carcinomas and squamous carcinomas have the poorer survival rate. Gallbladder cancers have been separated into metaplastic and nonmetaplastic types based on the presence or absence of metaplastic changes in the tumor tissue. The metaplastic type showed a significantly improved survival rate.

Adenocarcinoma 89.4%
Papillary 5.7%
Mucinous 5.3%
Squamous cell 1.8%
Sarcoma 0.2%

Bibliography

Bartlett DL, Fong Y. Tumor of the gallbladder. In: Blumgart LH, Fong Y (eds.), *Surgery of the Liver and Biliary Tract*, 3rd ed. London, UK: WB Sanders, 2000, 997–998.

Bilimoria M. Benign and malignant gallbladder tumors. In: Pierre-Alain C, John B (eds.), *Diseases of the Gallbladder and Bile Duct*. Oxford, UK: Blackwell Science, 2001, 197–198.

42. **(A)** A cure for gallbladder cancer can only be achieved by a complete surgical resection. The extent of surgery for many stages of gallbladder cancer remains controversial.

The AJCC TMN and staging criteria are shown in Table 29-1.

The most accepted recommendations are as follows:

Stage 1 tumors (T1, N0, M0): simple cholecystectomy
Stage 2, 3, and 4a (T4, N0, M0): en bloc resection of the gallbladder, segments 4 and 5 of the liver and regional lymph node dissection
Stage 4b (distant mets): palliation

Patients with T1 tumor and cholecystectomy have a 5-year survival rate close to 100%. Cholecystectomy alone in T2 tumors offers a 40% survival rate and no survival for T3 lesions. Performance of a radical second operation improves the T2 5-year survival rate to 90%. Because of the small number of patients, there is no definitive conclusion regarding improvement survival after radical surgery for T3 and T4 patients.

There are no prospective, randomized studies examining the utility of adjuvant therapy. The tumor has been resistant to most forms of chemotherapy, and the mode of spread does not lend itself to radiation.

Bibliography

Bartlett DL, Fong Y. Tumor of the gallbladder. In: Blumgart LH, Fong Y (eds.), *Surgery of the Liver and Biliary Tract*, 3rd ed. London, UK: WB Sanders, 2000, 1002–1011.

Bilimoria M. Benign and malignant gallbladder tumors. In: Pierre-Alain C, John B (eds.), *Diseases of the Gallbladder and Bile Duct*. Oxford, UK: Blackwell Science, 2001, 198–199.

TABLE 29-1

Gallbladder Cancer Staging
TNM definitions
Primary tumor (T)
- TX: Primary tumor cannot be assessed
- T0: No evidence of primary tumor
- Tis: Carcinoma in situ
- T1: Tumor invades lamina propria or muscle layer
  - T1a: Tumor invades lamina propria
  - T1b: Tumor invades the muscle layer
- T2: Tumor invades the perimuscular connective tissue; no extension beyond the serosa or into the liver
- T3: Tumor perforates the serosa (visceral peritoneum) or directly invades one adjacent organ, or both (extension 2 cm or less into the liver)
- T4: Tumor extends more than 2 cm into the liver, and/or into two or more adjacent organs (stomach, duodenum, colon, pancreas, omentum, extrahepatic bile ducts, any involvement of the liver)
Regional lymph nodes (N)
- NX: Regional lymph nodes cannot be assessed
- N0: No regional lymph node metastasis
- N1: Metastasis in cystic duct, pericholedochal, and/or hilar lymph nodes (i.e., in the hepatoduodenal ligament)
- N2: Metastasis in peripancreatic (head only), periduodenal, periportal, celiac, and/or superior mesenteric lymph nodes
Distant metastasis (M)
- MX: Distant metastasis cannot be assessed
- M0: No distant metastasis
- M1: Distant metastasis
AJCC Stage Groupings
Stage 0
- Tis, N0, M0
Stage I
- T1, N0, M0
Stage II
- T2, N0, M0
Stage III
- T1, N1, M0
- T2, N1, M0
- T3, N0, M0
- T3, N1, M0
Stage IVA
- T4, N0, M0
- T4, N1, M0
Stage IVB
- Any T, N2, M0
- Any T, any N, M1

Used with the permission of the American Joint Committee on Cancer (AJCC), Chicago, Illinois. The original source for this material is the *AJCC Cancer Staging Manual, Sixth Edition* (2002) published by Springer-Verlag New York, www.springer-ny.com.

43. **(B)** Several modalities of radiologic and endoscopic investigation are available to evaluate symptoms suggestive of postcholecystectomy biliary injury. Ninety percent of cholecystectomies are done laparoscopically and most patients are discharge to home within 48 h of surgery. Immediate postoperative complications include hemorrhage, infection, bile leak or bile

duct injury. Initial investigation includes CBC, liver function tests, and serum amylase.

Abdominal US is the most useful imaging study in the early postoperative period, it will reveal fluid collections, abscess, bile leakage, and biliary dilatation.

Patients with large fluid collections and dilated bile ducts should undergo biliary imaging by PTC or ERCP.

ERCP has become the preferred technique for biliary duct visualization once the diagnosis of bile leak was made; allowing not only knowing what kind of injury is present, but also performing therapeutic interventions, such as stones extraction, stent placements, and sphincterotomies.

Magnetic resonance cholangiography is a noninvasive technique, with no need of intravenous contrast, allows detection of biliary and pancreatic pathology with a high degree of sensitivity (88%) and specificity (93%). Although its use during the evaluation of biliary injuries has not been fully investigated yet, it will probably become a strong tool for screening avoiding the ERCP complications.

Bibliography

Beckingham IJ, Rowlands BJ. Postcholecystectomy problems. In: Blumgart LH, Fong Y (eds.), *On Surgery of the Liver and Biliary Tract*, 3rd ed., 2000, 799–809.

44. (C)

45. (B)

Explanations 44 and 45

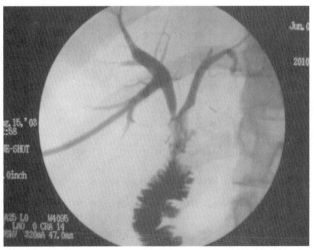

FIG. 29-8

Once a biliary injury is diagnosed and identified every attempt should be made to define the biliary anatomy by PTC and to control the bile leak with percutaneous biliary drainage. Immediate reexploration should be avoided. The inflammation associated with bile spillage and the retracted proximal bile duct make recognition and repair very difficult and unsafe. Delaying reconstruction by weeks helped by the percutaneous biliary decompression allows for optimal surgical results. The goal of operative management is the establishment of bile flow into the bowel in a way in which stone formation, cholangitis, development of a stricture, and biliary cirrhosis is prevented.

In order to obtain optimal results, healthy, nonischemic proximal bile duct and intestinal anatomy suitable for a Roux-en-Y anastomosis should be available to create a mucosal-mucosal biliary-enteric anastamosis (ERCP in Fig. 29-6).

Simple end-to-end anastomosis of the bile duct is very difficult to accomplish secondary to fibrosis associated with the injury. A hepaticojejunostomy constructed to a Roux-en-Y intestinal limb is the procedure of choice with a success rate greater than 90%.

Preoperative placement of percutaneous biliary catheters not only is essential in the early management of this patient but also in the intraoperative identification and manipulation of the proximal, injured bile duct. It is also important in the early postoperative period allowing decompression of the biliary tree, protection for possible bile leak, and ability to provide access for cholangiography.

Bibliography

Lillemoe KD. Benign biliary stricture. In: Cameron JL (ed.), *Current Surgical Therapy*, 7th ed., 2001, 454–461.

46. (B) Many complications related to laparoscopic cholecystectomy are similar to those occurring during traditional open cholecystectomy. These complications include hemorrhage, bile duct injuries, bile leaks, retained stones, pancreatitis, wound infections, and incisional hernias.

Complications secondary to pneumoperitoneum include gas embolism, vagal reaction, ventricular arrhythmias or hyper carbia with acidosis.

Most series demonstrates a bile duct injury rate of 0.3% or less during open cholecystectomy, compare with 0.4% during laparoscopic cholecystectomy.

Many surgeons attribute the cause of the injury to the direction of traction of the gallbladder, short cystic duct, or a large stone in Hartmann's pouch making the identification of the anatomy more difficult.

If a bile duct injury occurs during surgery an immediate repair should be performed. When a bile duct injury is discovered in the postoperative period, coordinated management between endocospists and surgeons offer the best outcome.

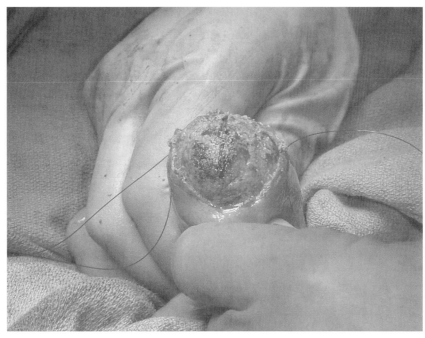

FIG. 29-9

Concerning this type of injury (type A, Bismuth classification), the intraperitoneal collection should be drained percutaneously. In order to control the leak, the intrabiliary pressure is reduced by endoscopic sphincterotomy with placement of a biliary stent. If ERCP fails, PTC may also be use to decompress the duct.

Bibliography

Steven S. Laparoscopic biliary injuries. In: Pierre-Alain C, John B (eds.), *Diseases of the Gallbladder and Bile Duct*. Oxford, UK: Blackwell Science, 2001, 226–242.

Underwood RA, Soper NJ. Laparoscopic cholecystectomy and choledocholythotomy. In: Blumgart LH, Fong Y (eds.), *Surgery of the Liver and Biliary Tract*, 3rd ed. London, UK: WB Sanders, 2000, 729–730.

47. **(D)** Gallstone ileus is a mechanical intestinal obstruction secondary to an impacted gallstone. The gallstone enters the bowel lumen through a biliary-enteric fistula. It accounts for 3% of all intestinal obstructions. A biliary-enteric fistula is a prerequisite for gallstone ileus. It results from a chronic inflammation of the gallbladder, causing necrosis of the gallbladder wall with perforation into the duodenum, colon or small bowel. Only large stones (>2.5 cm) can become impacted in the relatively narrow terminal ileum.

Abdominal pain, distention, cramping, nausea, and vomits that appear intermittently over several days may correlate with the "tumbling" of the stone as it moves distally. Bouveret's syndrome occurs when the stone impacts into the duodenum; nausea, nonbilious vomits, and no abdominal distention are the classical symptoms.

Multiple diagnostic tools are available, starting with an abdominal plain film where a classic obstructive pattern, pneumobilia (40%) and radiopaque stones (20%) are seen.

CT scan can be helpful when the KUB is not diagnostic; it is able to show air in the bile ducts and visualize the stone.

Exploratory laparotomy is the best approach. RUQ dissection should be avoided unless the obstruction is at the level of the duodenum (Bouveret's syndrome), in that case pushing the stone into the stomach, gastrotomy, and extraction is recommended.

If the stone is impacted distally it should be extracted either through an enterotomy, bowel resection (if not viable), or "milking" it until passing the ileocecal valve (Fig. 29-9).

Failure to remove all the stones increases recurrence rates. Management of the biliary-enteric fistula at the time of the initial surgery is not recommended. Most fistulas close spontaneously. Repairing of the fistula increases operative time and morbidity.

Bibliography

Levi DM, Levi JU. Gallstone ileus. In: Cameron JL (ed.), *Current Surgical Therapy*, 7th ed., 2001, 472–474.

CHAPTER 30

Pancreas

Cord Sturgeon and N. Joseph Espat

Questions

1. Which of the following statements regarding pancreatic anatomy is *true*?

   (A) The majority of the pancreas is drained through the major papilla by the duct of Santorini.

   (B) The minor papilla communicates with a small duct of Wirsung, draining the inferior head and uncinate process.

   (C) Nervous innervation of the pancreas arises in the superior mesenteric ganglion.

   (D) Venous drainage of the pancreas is into the inferior vena cava.

   (E) Heterotopic pancreas tissue has been identified in the stomach, duodenum, small bowel, and Meckel's diverticulum.

2. Which of the following is *not correct* regarding pancreatic exocrine secretions?

   (A) The total daily volume of pancreatic secretion can be as much as 3 L.

   (B) Somatostatin inhibits pancreatic enzyme secretion.

   (C) Cholecystokinin (CCK) stimulates gallbladder contraction and inhibits pancreatic enzyme secretion.

   (D) Secretin released in response to duodenal acidification stimulates pancreatic water and bicarbonate secretion.

   (E) The chloride and bicarbonate concentration in pancreatic fluid changes depending on the rate and volume of pancreatic secretion.

3. Which of the following is *false* regarding exocrine function of the pancreas?

   (A) Starches are broken down by amylase.

   (B) Fatty acids are hydrolyzed by lipase.

   (C) Proteins are broken down by trypsin and chymotrypsin.

   (D) Enzymes, in an inactive form, are made by the alpha, beta, and delta cells and are released into the pancreatic duct as zymogen granules.

   (E) Enterokinase activates trypsin (from trypsinogen), which in turn activates other digestive proenzymes.

4. Which of the following is *true* regarding the islets of Langerhans?

   (A) Alpha cells make glucagon and comprise the innermost aspect of the islet.

   (B) Beta cells produce insulin and are the smallest component of the islet volume.

   (C) Delta cells make somatostatin, and have a subtype that produces vasoactive intestinal peptide (VIP).

   (D) Islets comprise 25% of the pancreatic mass.

   (E) Islets in the head and uncinate process are replete with alpha cells, but poor in pancreatic polypeptide (PP) cells. The converse is true of islets in the body and tail.

5. Which is of the following statements about pancreatic adenocarcinoma is *false*?

   (A) The 5-year survival for pancreatic cancer is less than 5%.

   (B) The yearly U.S. incidence of pancreatic cancer is approximately 30,000 cases.

   (C) Familial predisposition and chronic pancreatitis are both risk factors for developing pancreatic cancer.

   (D) There is no association between cigarette smoking and pancreatic cancer.

   (E) Pain, jaundice, and weight loss are the most common presenting signs of pancreatic cancer.

6. A 67-year-old male presents to your office with pain-less jaundice. Courvoisier's sign is present. An abdominal ultrasound (US) is performed, followed by an abdominal computed tomography (CT) scan. You suspect that there is a neoplasm in the head of the pancreas. Which of the following CT scan findings does not rule out resectability?

   (A) encasement of the superior mesenteric artery (SMA) or celiac axis

   (B) dilated intra- and extrahepatic biliary ducts, with an engorged gallbladder

   (C) the confluence of the superior mesenteric vein (SMV) and portal vein is not patent

   (D) evidence of extrapancreatic disease

   (E) absence of a fat plane between the tumor and the SMA

7. Which of the following statements regarding the pathology of pancreatic cancer is *false*?

   (A) The vast majority of pancreatic exocrine tumors arise from ductal cells.

   (B) Ductal cells constitute approximately 80% of the mass of the pancreas.

   (C) More than three-fourths of pancreatic cancers are adenocarcinoma.

   (D) Approximately two-thirds of pancreatic adenocarcinomas arise in the head of the gland.

   (E) The incidence of diffuse involvement of the entire gland is approximately 20% in pancreatic adenocarcinoma.

8. A 64-year-old woman has an incidentally noted 3.0 cm pancreatic cyst in the uncinate process of the pancreas. She is asymptomatic. The cyst is homogenous, with no evidence of internal septations or adjacent organ invasion and the patient is entirely asymptomatic. Which of the following statements is *true* regarding this patient's disease?

   (A) This lesion is more common in men than women.

   (B) Benign cystic lesions of the pancreas are uncommon in women this age.

   (C) The patient should undergo a pancreatico-duodenectomy since this type of cyst has a significant malignant potential.

   (D) The CT should be repeated in 3 months and evaluated for change before surgically intervening.

   (E) The patient should undergo cholecystectomy since cholelithiasis is a risk factor.

9. A 50-year-old woman presents with a several week history of early satiety and left upper quadrant discomfort. On abdominal ultrasound (US) a complex heterogeneous mass is observed and CT imaging is recommended. Figure 30-1 is a representative section from the CT scan. Which of the following statements is *false* regarding to this patient and the CT image?

   (A) There is a heterogeneous abnormality between the posterior wall of the stomach and the spleen.

   (B) The abnormality most likely represents a pancreatic process located in the tail in gland, but will require a multiorgan resection.

   (C) There is no evidence of peritoneal or liver metastases.

   (D) The differential diagnosis would include mucinous tumor of the pancreas.

   (E) Use of endoscopic ultrasound (EUS) would be essential in establishing the diagnosis and in the decision-making process regarding an operation.

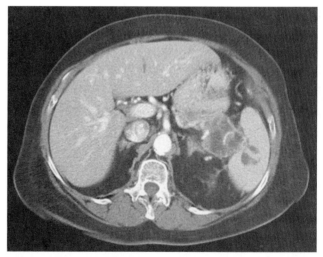

FIG. 30-1   CT abdomen.

10. Features of intraductal papillary mucinous neoplasms (IPMN) include all of the following *except*:

   (A) They may be benign, premalignant or malignant.

   (B) If IPMN is resected and found to contain adenocarcinoma, then the patient will have a more favorable outcome compared to non-IPMN pancreatic adenocarcinoma.

   (C) IPMN tumors can arise from either the main, primary, or secondary pancreatic ducts.

(D) Patients may experience of one ore more of the following; pancreatitis, abdominal pain, jaundice, or mucinous stools.

(E) A classic presentation for this disease is the findings by upper endoscopy or endoscopic retrograde cholangiography (ERCP) of "mucous" emanating from the ampulla.

11. Which of the following statements is *false* concerning modalities for staging pancreatic cancer?:

(A) CT scan is extremely sensitive and specific for demonstrating nonresectable disease.

(B) Laparoscopic staging is useful to differentiate between equivocal and resectable pancreatic cancer.

(C) Laparoscopic staging combined with laparoscopic US is superior at defining resectability compared to laparoscopy alone.

(D) CT guided fine needle biopsy should be performed prior to laparoscopic staging to confirm the diagnosis.

(E) CT scan is sensitive in the identification of vascular invasion in the selection of resectable pancreatic tumors.

12. Which is *true* about pancreatic microcystic adenoma?

(A) Macroscopically it is a single mass constituted of multiple cysts.

(B) Two-thirds of patients are asymptomatic.

(C) Angiography shows a hypovascular lesion.

(D) No relation exists with von Hippel-Lindau's syndrome.

(E) Enucleation rather than resection is the treatment of choice.

13. Intraductal papillary mucinous tumors (IPMT) are becoming more recognized in the Western world. What is the most common mode of presentation?

(A) recurrent episodes of pancreatitis

(B) incidental pancreatic nodule found on CT

(C) atypia of ERCP brushings

(D) asymptomatic

(E) no characteristic presentation

14. Which of the following is *true* of IPMT?

(A) Overall, patients have increasing risk of extrapancreatic cancer.

(B) Frozen section is not necessarily done at the time of resection.

(C) It is more common in men.

(D) No relationship exists with pancreatic carcinoma.

(E) K-ras oncogene mutation has no role.

15. In comparing nonpylorus preserving pancreaticoduo-denectomy (NPPPD) to pylorus preserving pancreate-ctomy (PPPD), which of the following statements is true?

(A) The gastric emptying time is faster in the early postoperative period for PPPD.

(B) PPPD has higher surgical morbidity.

(C) PPPD is more commonly associated with dumping syndrome at 6 months.

(D) When performed for pancreatic adenocarcinoma, there is no difference in survival between NPPPD and PPPD.

(E) In the 6-month perioperative period, NPPPD patients demonstrate improved nutritional parameters.

16. Current adjuvant chemoradiotherapy cooperative group study results for patients with resectable pancreatic cancer suggest a limited survival advantage to therapy. Which of the following statements is most accurate?

(A) Overall 5-year survival is 20%.

(B) The rate of loco-regional recurrence is reduced with chemoradiotherapy; however, patients succumb to metastatic disease.

(C) Most treatment failures occur within 6 months.

(D) 5-Fluorouracil (5-FU) alone is equivalent to 5-FU combined with radiation.

(E) Extended lymphadenectomy at the time of resection combined with chemoradiotherapy provides a survival advantage.

17. Which of the following is true with regard to palliative strategies for unresectable pancreatic cancer?

(A) Pancreatic adenocarcinoma is an asymptomatic disease.

(B) Celiac axis neurolysis is effective in 90% of patients over the short term.

(C) Gastric outlet obstruction (GOO) in the presence of unresectable disease is best treated by gastrojejunostomy.

(D) Presence of biliary obstruction is best treated with biliary-enteric anastomosis.

(E) Prophylactic gastrojejunal anastomosis is widely recommended.

18. A 54-year-old male presents to the emergency room with complaints of 3 days of severe, constant midepigastric pain, and vomiting. He attempted to treat the pain by drinking several pints of hard liquor, but it only made the pain worse. Which of the following findings are *not* consistent with acute pancreatitis?

    (A) sentinel loop sign on abdominal roentgenography
    (B) colon cutoff sign
    (C) pancreatic calcifications on plain abdominal roentgenography
    (D) hyperamylasemia
    (E) emesis that does not relieve abdominal pain

19. A 54-year-old male, well known to you from multiple admissions for exacerbations of chronic alcoholic pancreatitis, comes to clinic requesting your opinion regarding surgical treatment for his pancreatitis. Which of the following sequelae of chronic pancreatitis would prevent him from being a candidate for longitudinal pancreaticojejunostomy (modified Puestow procedure)?

    (A) disabling pain requiring the use of high doses of narcotics
    (B) obstruction of the intrapancreatic common bile duct
    (C) dilated pancreatic duct (6 mm) with no strictures
    (D) diabetes
    (E) multiple strictures along the entire length of a 9 mm duct

20. Which is *false* regarding the complication of pancreaticocutaneous fistulae following pancreatic surgery?

    (A) Low-output fistulae are defined as those draining less than 200 cc per day.
    (B) Fluid and electrolyte abnormalities are frequently encountered in these patients.
    (C) Most pancreaticocutaneous fistulae fail to close with conservative management.
    (D) Octreotide may be helpful in facilitating closure of fistulae.
    (E) Total parenteral nutrition is frequently required in the treatment of pancreatic fistulae.

21. A 45-year-old female with a history of gallstone pancreatitis presents to the emergency department with abdominal pain, early satiety, nausea, and vomiting. A CT scan of the abdomen is performed revealing a large fluid collection within the lesser sac. Which is *false* regarding this patient's condition?

    (A) The cyst wall lacks an epithelial lining.
    (B) These are the most common cystic lesions of the pancreas.
    (C) This fluid collection would be called a pseudocyst only if it is persistent 4 weeks after an attack of acute pancreatitis.
    (D) The preferred therapy is percutaneous drainage.
    (E) It is recommended that a 6-week period pass between the onset of pancreatitis and attempted surgical or endoscopic drainage.

22. Which of the following is *false*?

    (A) The insulin gene is located on chromosome 11.
    (B) Endogenous enzymatic cleavage of proinsulin yields equimolar amounts of insulin and C-peptide.
    (C) Commercially available pharmaceutical insulin contains 25–50% C-peptide.
    (D) The half-life of endogenous insulin is 3–6 min.
    (E) There is a greater rise in plasma insulin following oral glucose administration than there is following an equivalent intravenous glucose administration.

23. A 47-year-old female is referred to you by a psychiatrist. She has experienced early morning confusion and weakness, followed by paroxysms of extreme anxiety and palpitations. She has been treated for anxiety for approximately 2 years with no improvement. She notes that frequent meals obviate these symptoms. You believe that she may be manifesting Whipple's triad. Which of the following is *not* a component of Whipple's triad?

    (A) symptoms of hypoglycemia
    (B) plasma glucose levels less than 45 mg/dL
    (C) elevated plasma insulin levels ≥ 6 μU/mL.
    (D) relief of symptoms with administration of glucose

24. You believe that a patient is manifesting Whipple's triad. The patient undergoes a supervised 72-h fast, during which time serum glucose and insulin levels are measured every 6 h. The fast is terminated at 14 h because the patient develops symptoms of visual disturbances, confusion, and weakness. Blood and urine samples are obtained, and intravenous glucose is administered. Which of the following findings in this patient is *not* consistent with the diagnosis of insulinoma?

(A) blood glucose of 38 mg/dL

(B) elevated plasma insulin levels (≥6 μU/mL) during hypoglycemia

(C) elevated C-peptide levels (≥1.2 ng/mL)

(D) detectable urinary sulfonylurea

(E) symptoms of confusion, amnesia, and diplopia

25. Laboratory values from a patient with a positive 72-h fast reveal an elevated insulin to glucose ratio, and elevated proinsulin and C-peptide levels. No urinary sulfonylurea is detected. With the history and these findings, you make the diagnosis of insulinoma and schedule her for surgery. Which of the following is *false* regarding the localization of insulinomas?

(A) Approximately two-thirds are located to the left of the SMA in the body or tail of the pancreas.

(B) Intraoperative US can localize small tumors and their relationship to vascular and ductal structures.

(C) Transhepatic portal venous sampling can be used to differentiate between localized and diffuse hyperinsulinism.

(D) Because insulinomas have a poor blood supply, selective arteriography has never been useful.

(E) Selective arterial calcium injection with hepatic venous sampling can help locate the region of the insulinoma.

26. A 35-year-old man with a history of primary hyperparathyroidism treated by subtotal (three and one-half glands) parathyroidectomy presents with a recent onset of severe gastroesophageal reflux (GERD) and diarrhea. A secretin stimulation test is performed, yielding a serum gastrin elevation of 200 pg/mL over baseline. Somatostatin receptor scintigraphy suggests that there is a tumor in the region of the pancreas. Which of the following statements regarding this disease is *true*?

(A) Double-spiral CT scan is the imaging modality of choice for localizing these abdominal tumors, especially when they are smaller than 1 cm.

(B) These tumors arise in the head of the pancreas, and commonly metastasize to the duodenum.

(C) Ninety percent are benign.

(D) Diarrhea associated with this syndrome can be ameliorated by nasogastric suction.

(E) Three quarters of these tumors are found in association with MEN 1.

27. Which of the following statements about glucagon is *false*?

(A) Glucagon promotes the mobilization of glucose.

(B) Insulin, glucose, and free fatty acids decrease the synthesis of glucagon by the alpha cells of the pancreatic islet.

(C) Glucagon is secreted in response to hyperglycemia.

(D) Glucagon secretion is stimulated by the amino acids alanine and arginine.

(E) Infection, burns, and surgery increase glucagon secretion.

28. A 55-year-old woman presents to her family doctor with an extremely pruritic rash of the groin and lower extremities. Topical treatments were ineffective. Several weeks later she developed deep venous thrombosis and was admitted to a university hospital. During this admission she was also diagnosed with diabetes. A plasma glucagon level is obtained, and is found to be markedly elevated. Which of the following is *not* a common feature of this patient's syndrome?

(A) small, benign tumor of the head of the pancreas

(B) necrolytic migratory erythema

(C) diabetes mellitus

(D) deep venous thrombosis

(E) plasma glucagon levels above 1000 pg/mL

29. A 66-year-old male undergoes pancreaticoduodenectomy (Whipple procedure) for obstructive jaundice from a periampullary tumor. Immunohistochemical staining of the tumor is strongly positive for somatostatin. Which of the following is *not* a common feature of the somatostatinoma syndrome?

(A) tumor located in the pancreas or duodenum

(B) cholelithiasis

(C) diabetes mellitus

(D) deep venous thrombosis

(E) steatorrhea

30. A patient is admitted to the emergency room with severe, watery diarrhea and acute renal failure. The diarrhea is in excess of 3 L per day, and is found to be secretory in nature. The diarrhea is recalcitrant to standard medical therapy, and as part of the workup a plasma VIP level is obtained and found to be greater than 10-fold above normal. Which of the following is *not* a feature of this diarrhea-related syndrome?

(A) tumor located in the pancreas or duodenum

(B) flushing

(C) diabetes mellitus

(D) achlorhydria

(E) severe watery secretory diarrhea

31. All of the following are true about pancreas divisum *except*:

(A) Pancreas divisum is an anatomic variant occurring after the two primordial ductal systems fail to fuse.

(B) Definitive treatment for pancreas divisum is surgical resection.

(C) Pancreas divisum is found in 5–10% of patients undergoing ERCP for presumed benign pancreatic disease.

(D) The majority of patients are asymptomatic.

(E) Pancreas divisum is associated with abnormalities of the pancreaticobiliary junctions.

32. Pancreatic fistulae following pancreatic surgery remain problematic. Which of the following statements is most accurate?

(A) Randomized prospective studies using octreotide have conclusively shown to prevent pancreatic fistula.

(B) Postoperative pancreatic fistulae are reported to occur in as many as 30% of patients.

(C) Surgical sealants or glues to occlude pancreatic fistulae remain experimental.

(D) Reoperation is almost always contraindicated.

(E) CT scanning of the abdomen is not essential if a fistula develops.

33. Which is *true* about the surgical anatomy of the pancreas?

(A) The head lies over the first lumbar vertebra.

(B) The accessory duct enters the second part of the duodenum.

(C) The superior mesenteric vessels pass behind the uncinate process.

(D) The SMA lies to the right of the superior mesenteric vein.

(E) The superior mesenteric vein joins the portal vein behind the head of the pancreas.

34. During an exploratory laparotomy for the mechanism of injury by a low velocity gunshot wound to the abdomen, the surgeon finds duodenal disruption with necrosis of the middle segment and distal bile duct disruption within the head of the pancreas. The patient is hemodynamically stable. Which of the following procedures is most appropriate?

(A) Whipple

(B) duodenojejunostomy and placement of drains around the pancreas and bile duct

(C) pyloric exclusion, gastrojejunostomy, and wide pancreatic biliary drainage

(D) cholecystojejunostomy, tie off the distal bile duct and wide pancreatic biliary drainage.

(E) near-total pancreatectomy and biliary-enteric reconstruction

35. A 10-year-old child develops severe abdominal pain while in the hospital for a viral syndrome. The pain is better if she sits up and leans forward, laboratory studies demonstrate an amylase of 180 and WBC of 15,000. CT scan of the abdomen demonstrates an edematous pancreatic gland and retroperitoneal stranding. What is the most likely cause for her pancreatitis?

(A) gallstone pancreatitis

(B) coxsackie virus infection

(C) heterotopic pancreas

(D) drug-induced pancreatitis

(E) spherocytosis

Answers and Explanations

1. **(E)** The majority of the pancreas is drained through the minor papilla by the duct of Santorini. The major papilla communicates with a small duct of Wirsung, draining the inferior head and uncinate process. Nervous innervation of the pancreas is both sympathetic from the splanchnic nerves and parasympathetic from the vagus. Sympathetic nerves from the celiac ganglion are the main pathways for pain sensation, and are therefore targeted in splanchnicectomy for pain from chronic pancreatitis. Venous drainage of the pancreas is into the portal vein. Heterotopic pancreas tissue has been identified in the stomach, duodenum, small bowel, and Meckel's diverticulum.

Bibliography

Mulvihill S. Pancreas. In: Norton J, Bollinger R, Chang A, et al. (eds.), *Essential Practice of Surgery*. New York, NY: Springer-Verlag, 2003, 199–218.

Yeo C, Cameron J. Exocrine pancreas. In: Townsend C Jr, Beauchamp R, Evers B, Mattox K (eds.), *Sabiston Textbook of Surgery. The Biological Basis of Modern Surgical Practice*. Philadelphia, PA: W.B. Saunders, 2001, 1112–1143.

2. **(C)** The total volume of pancreatic secretion is variable and ranges from 1.5 to 3 L per day. Tonic inhibition by somatostatin minimizes pancreatic enzyme secretion between meals. Fat or amino acids in the duodenum after a meal leads to the release of CCK, which then stimulates gallbladder contraction and pancreatic enzyme secretion. Activated trypsin in the duodenum, conversely, inhibits CCK release. Secretin is found in the duodenal epithelium, is released in response to acid, and is the most potent stimulant of bicarbonate release. Although the concentration of the cations (sodium and potassium) is not related to the rate of pancreatic fluid secretion, the concentration of the anions (chloride and bicarbonate) changes with the secretory rate. Chloride concentration is inversely related to the bicarbonate concentration and volume of pancreatic secretion.

Bibliography

Mulvihill S. Pancreas. In: Norton J, Bollinger R, Chang A, et al. (eds.), *Essential Practice of Surgery*. New York, NY: Springer-Verlag, 2003, 199–218.

Yeo C, Cameron J. Exocrine pancreas. In: Townsend C Jr, Beauchamp R, Evers B, Mattox K (eds.), *Sabiston Textbook of Surgery. The Biological Basis of Modern Surgical Practice*. Philadelphia, PA: W.B. Saunders, 2001, 1112–1143.

3. **(D)** The digestive enzymes, amylase, lipase, trypsin, and chymotrypsin function, respectively to digest the starches, fatty acids, and proteins from a meal. Enzymes are made and stored in the pancreas in a form that requires activation. They are then packaged into zymogen granules and released into the central ductule of the acinus. Trypsinogen is cleaved by enterokinase from the duodenal brush border into its active form, trypsin. Trypsin can then activate other digestive proenzymes. The islets of Langerhans, composed of alpha, beta, and delta cells, secrete endocrine products related to glucose homeostasis, not digestive enzymes.

Bibliography

Mulvihill S. Pancreas. In: Norton J, Bollinger R, Chang A, et al. (eds.), *Essential Practice of Surgery*. New York, NY: Springer-Verlag, 2003, 199–218.

Thompson J, Townsend C Jr. Endocrine pancreas. In: Townsend C Jr, Beauchamp R, Evers B, Mattox K (eds.), *Sabiston Textbook of Surgery. The Biological Basis of Modern Surgical Practice*. Philadelphia, PA: W.B. Saunders, 2001, 646–661.

Yeo C, Cameron J. Exocrine pancreas. In: Townsend C Jr, Beauchamp R, Evers B, Mattox K (eds.), *Sabiston Textbook of Surgery. The Biological Basis of Modern Surgical Practice*. Philadelphia, PA: W.B. Saunders, 2001, 1112–1143.

4. **(C)** Alpha cells comprise 5–20% of the islet, make glucagon, and are found at the outermost aspect of the islet. Beta cells make up 50–80% of the islet volume, produce insulin, and are found at the core of the islet. Delta cells are less than 5% of the islet volume, make

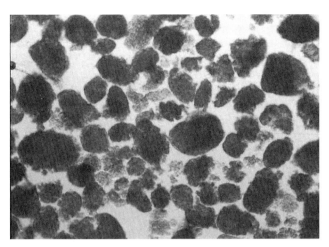

FIG. 30-2 Isolated pancreatic islet cell preparation; these cells have been harvested following "digestion" for islet cell autotransplantation.

somatostatin, and are found at the interface of the alpha and beta cells. A subtype of the delta cells, D_2 cells, make VIP. PP cells comprise 10–35% of the islet, make the inactive pancreatic polypeptide, and are found at the periphery of the islet. Islets occupy only approximately 2% of the pancreatic mass. Fortunately for patients who undergo a Whipple pancreaticoduodenectomy, islets in the head and uncinate process are rich in PP cells, but poor in alpha cells. Islets in the body and tail are rich in valuable glucagon producing alpha cells but poor in PP cells (Fig. 30-2).

Bibliography

Mulvihill S. Pancreas. In: Norton J, Bollinger R, Chang A, et al. (eds.), *Essential Practice of Surgery.* New York, NY: Springer-Verlag, 2003, 199–218.

Thompson J, Townsend C Jr. Endocrine pancreas. In: Townsend C Jr, Beauchamp R, Evers B, Mattox K (eds.), *Sabiston Textbook of Surgery. The Biological Basis of Modern Surgical Practice.* Philadelphia, PA: W.B. Saunders, 2001, 646–661.

5. **(D)** The 5-year relative survival for patients diagnosed with pancreatic adenocarcinoma (all races and all stages) from 1992 to 1998 was approximately 4%. Surveillance, epidemiology, and end results (SEER) data estimates the U.S. incidence of pancreatic adenocarcinoma to be 30,700 new cases in 2003. Even though it is relatively rare, it is the fourth leading cause of cancer deaths. Smoking cigarettes is believed to increase the risk of developing pancreatic cancer by three- to fourfold, and the risk appears to be correlated to the number of pack-years. Approximately 30% of cases of pancreatic cancer are believed to be related to cigarette smoking. Chronic pancreatitis also has been shown to be associated with the development of pancreatic cancer, and may be responsible for about 5% of cases. Between 5 and 8% of pancreatic cancers are familial. Pain, jaundice, and weight loss are the most common presenting signs of pancreatic cancer.

Bibliography

Bansal P, Sonnenberg A. Pancreatitis is a risk factor for pancreatic cancer. *Gastroenterology* 1995;109(1):247–251.

Jemal A, Murray T, Samuels A, et al. Cancer statistics, 2003. *CA Cancer J Clin* 2003;53(1):5–26.

Mulvihill S. Pancreas. In: Norton J, Bollinger R, Chang A, et al. (eds.), *Essential Practice of Surgery.* New York, NY: Springer-Verlag, 2003, 199–218.

Olsen GW, Mandel JS, Gibson RW, et al. A case-control study of pancreatic cancer and cigarettes, alcohol, coffee and diet. *Am J Public Health* 1989;79(8):1016–1019.

6. **(B)** Courvoisier's sign (palpable obstructed gallbladder) is only present in one-fourth to one-half of cases at presentation, and its presence does not implicate nonresectability. Approximately two-thirds of pancreatic adenocarcinomas arise in the head of the gland. About three-fourth of patients with adenocarcinoma of the pancreatic head present with weight loss, obstructive jaundice, and abdominal pain. Findings on CT that establish that the tumor is not resectable are the presence of extrapancreatic disease, tumor extension to the SMA or celiac axis, no fat plane between the tumor and these structures, and occlusion of the superior mesenteric vein (SMV)-portal vein junction. Endoscopic US is also valuable in the diagnosis and staging of pancreatic cancer, and in assessing the relationship between the neoplasm and SMA, SMV, and portal vein (Fig. 30-3).

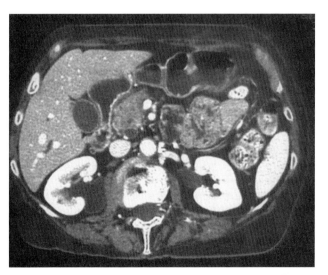

FIG. 30-3 Abdominal CT scan demonstrating distended palpable gallbladder (Courvoisier's sign) and pancreatic head mass with obvious dilated distal bile duct.

Bibliography

Bluemke DA, Fishman EK. CT and MR evaluation of pancreatic cancer. *Surg Oncol Clin North Am* 1998;7(1): 103–124.

Fuhrman GM, Charnsangavej C, Abbruzzese JL, et al. Thin-section contrast-enhanced computed tomography accurately predicts the resectability of malignant pancreatic neoplasms. *Am J Surg* 1994;167(1):104–111; discussion 111–113.

Rosch T, Braig C, Gain T, et al. Staging of pancreatic and ampullary carcinoma by endoscopic ultrasonography: comparison with conventional sonography, computed tomography, and angiography. *Gastroenterology* 1992;102(1):188–199.

Yeo C, Cameron J. Exocrine pancreas. In: Townsend C Jr, Beauchamp R, Evers B, Mattox K (eds.), *Sabiston Textbook of Surgery. The Biological Basis of Modern Surgical Practice.* Philadelphia, PA: W.B. Saunders, 2001, 1112–1143.

7. **(B)** Approximately 80–90% of pancreatic cancers arise from the ductules. The vast majority of these cancers are adenocarcinoma. Only 5% of the pancreatic mass is composed of ductal cells, even though the majority of pancreatic neoplasms arise from these cells. In contrast, approximately 80% of the gland is comprised of acinar cells, and acinar cell carcinoma is quite rare. Approximately two-thirds of pancreatic adenocarcinomas arise in the head of the gland, 15–20% arise in the body and tail, and 20% diffusely involve the entire pancreas.

Bibliography

Stojadinovic A, Brooks A, Hoos A, Jaques DP, Conlon KC, Brennan MF. An evidence-based approach to the surgical management of resectable pancreatic adenocarcinoma. *J Am Coll Surg* 2003;196(6): 954–964.

Yeo C, Cameron J. Exocrine pancreas. In: Townsend C Jr, Beauchamp R, Evers B, Mattox K (eds.), *Sabiston Textbook of Surgery. The Biological Basis of Modern Surgical Practice.* Philadelphia, PA: W.B. Saunders, 2001, 1112–1143.

8. **(D)** Pancreatic cysts are more common in women than men and generally occur in the fifth and sixth decades of life. Because these lesions are commonly asymptomatic they may be incidentally noted during abdominal imaging obtained for unrelated conditions. Pancreatic cysts can be divided into serous and mucin containing lesions. Serous cysts have a homogenous appearance and can be radiographically differentiated from their malignant counterparts, serous cystadenocarcinomas. Mucin containing cysts are more difficult to define, and the potential for some variant of an intraductal mucin producing neoplasm cannot be completely excluded. Endoscopic US may be useful at defining the contents of the cyst, and if indicated may be used to aspirate cyst contents for cytologic

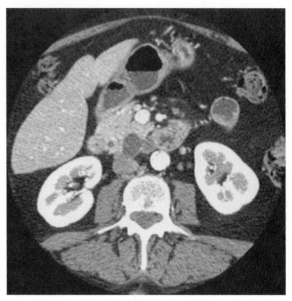

FIG. 30-4   A 3-cm cystic lesion is noted immediately anterior to the vena cava within the pancreatic uncinate. Note the homogeneity, a classic feature of a benign serous cyst.

examination. Asymptomatic cysts less than 5 cm in size do not carry an indication for pancreaticoduodectomy, particularly when radiographically they appear as benign serous fluid containing cysts. Given the patient's lack of symptoms and the favorable radiographic findings, homogeneity, size, and lack of adjacent organ invasion, a reasonable management plan would be to repeat the imaging in 3 months before proceeding with an invasive investigation. Should the cyst enlarge over that interval, then EUS or CT guided cyst aspiration may be indicated. While cholelithiasis is a risk factor for pancreatitis, which is associated with peripancreatic fluid, there is no role for cholecystecomy in this patient for this condition (Fig. 30-4).

Bibliography

Cohen-Scali F, Vilgrain V, Brancatelli G, Hammel P, Vullierme MP, Sauvanet A, Menu Y. Discrimination of unilocular macrocystic serous cystadenoma from pancreatic pseudocyst and mucinous cystadenoma with CT: initial observations. *Radiology* 2003;228(3):727–33.

Fernandez-del Castillo C, Targarona J, Thayer SP, Rattner DW, Brugge WR, Warshaw AL. Incidental pancreatic cysts: clinicopathologic characteristics and comparison with symptomatic patients. *Arch Surg* 2003;138(4): 427–423; discussion 433–434.

Song MH, Lee SK, Kim MH, Lee HJ, Kim KP, Kim HJ, Lee SS, Seo DW, Min YI. EUS in the evaluation of pancreatic cystic lesions. *Gastrointest Endosc* 2003;57(7):891–896.

9. **(E)** This patient has a mucinous cystadenocarcinoma. This CT image is the exact opposite of the finding in

the previous question, occurring in the same patient demographics. The CT demonstrates a >5 cm lesion with obvious multiorgan involvement. The posterior wall of the stomach is most likely invaded and the mass extends well into the splenic hilum. From the CT image we can deduce that the mass potentially arises from the tail of the pancreas, although this can't be appreciated fully. In order to confidently make this observation, the splenic vein must be visualized and the tumor must be above that point to confirm its origin in the pancreas; however, this resection will entail distal pancreatectomy, splenectomy, and gastric wedge resection. No evidence of peritoneal or hepatic metastasis is noted. EUS has only a descriptive role in this case. Regardless of the findings, the patient will need to undergo a procedure. EUS guided aspiration could only confirm the presence of malignancy, a negative aspirate would not preclude intervention given the hallmark findings of size, invasion, and septations.

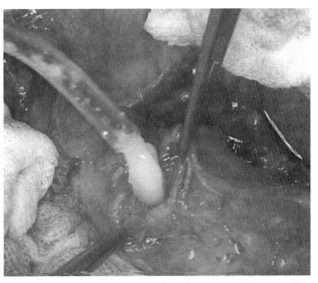

FIG. 30-5 Intraoperative evacuation of mucin-type material from a patient with IPMN tumor of the pancreas.

Bibliography

Fernandez-del Castillo C. Surgery of cystic neoplasms. *Gastrointest Endosc Clin North Am* 2002;12(4):803–812, ix.

Song MH, Lee SK, Kim MH, Lee HJ, Kim KP, Kim HJ, Lee SS, Seo DW, Min YI. EUS in the evaluation of pancreatic cystic lesions. *Gastrointest Endosc* 2003;57(7):891–896.

Frossard JL, Amouyal P, Amouyal G, Palazzo L, Amaris J, Soldan M, Giostra E, Spahr L, Hadengue A, Fabre M. Performance of endosonography-guided fine needle aspiration and biopsy in the diagnosis of pancreatic cystic lesions. *Am J Gastroenterol* 2003;98(7):1516–1524.

10. **(B)** Previously, this entity was an uncommon diagnosis. Increased awareness and likely the increase in endoscopic procedures that has occurred over the last decade has made this disease more common, although it still accounts for <2% of pancreatic neoplasms. A spectrum of disease presentation has been observed, ranging from the completely benign mucin producing tumor to those having *in situ* adenocarcinoma or invasive adenocarcinoma. While the natural history of the disease is still under investigation, most authors consider this to be a premalignant condition. Outcome for patients with pancreatic adenocarcinoma associated with IPMN is the same stage-for-stage as for pancreatic adenocarcinoma. Depending on the location of the mucin producing neoplasm, there can be a wide range of clinical symptoms. Pancreatic head tumors may lead to obstructive jaundice, pancreatitis, or abdominal pain. Heavy mucin secretion may present as diarrhea or "mucousy" stools. An endoscopy report describing the presence of mucous or that mucous emanates from the ampulla should prompt a further evaluation of the patient (Fig. 30-5).

Bibliography

Fukukura Y, Fujiyoshi F, Hamada H, Takao S, Aikou T, Hamada N, Yonezawa S, Nakajo M. Intraductal papillary mucinous tumors of the pancreas. *Acta Radiol* 2003;44(5):464–471.

Seki M, Yanagisawa A, Ohta H, Ninomiya Y, Sakamoto Y, Yamamoto J, Yamaguchi T, Ninomiya E, Takano K, Aruga A, Yamada K, Sasaki K, Kato Y. Surgical treatment of intraductal papillary-mucinous tumor (IPMT) of the pancreas: operative indications based on surgicopathologic study focusing on invasive carcinoma derived from IPMT. *J Hepatobiliary Pancreat Surg* 2003;10(2):147–155.

Sugiyama M, Izumisato Y, Abe N, Masaki T, Mori T, Atomi Y. Predictive factors for malignancy in intraductal papillary-mucinous tumours of the pancreas. *Br J Surg* 2003;90(10):1244–1249.

11. **(D)** CT scan has become a very adept modality for identifying patients with advanced or metastatic pancreatic adenocarcinoma that precludes staging laparotomy. CT demonstration of vascular invasion or peritoneal or hepatic metastases exclude patients from undergoing surgical exploration for staging. Laparoscopic staging techniques have been developed to mimic "open" staging laparotomy while obviating the need for a laparotomy. Advantages of laparoscopic staging that have been well described include direct vision biopsies, identification of subcentimeter disease, reduced hospital stay, and decreased interval until the commencement of chemotherapy. While CT guided biopsy may be a useful technique to establish a diagnosis, this should be reserved for patients in whom resectability has been excluded (Fig. 30-6).

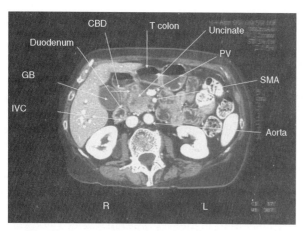

FIG. 30-6 CT demonstrated anatomy at the level of the pancreas in the evaluation of potential resectability.

Bibliography

Espat NJ, Brennan MF, Conlon KC. Patients with laparo-scopically staged unresectable pancreatic adenocarcino-ma do not require subsequent surgical biliary or gastric bypass. *J Am Coll Surg* 1999;188(6):649–655; discussion 655–657.

Minnard EA, Conlon KC, Hoos A, Dougherty EC, Hann LE, Brennan MF. Laparoscopic ultrasound enhances standard laparoscopy in the staging of pancreatic cancer. *Ann Surg* 1998;228(2):182–187.

Spanknebel K, Conlon KC. Advances in the surgical man-agement of pancreatic cancer. *Cancer J* 2001;7(4):312–323.

12. **(A)** Benign variants of pancreatic cysts include serous oligocystic or macrocystic and microcystic adenoma. Serous cystic adenoma accounts for 1–2% of all exocrine pancreatic tumors. There is a potential for malignant growth. It occurs more frequently in women than men. It involves the body and tail of the gland in up to two-thirds of cases. CT scan reveals an ovoid, multilocular mass with honeycomb-like cysts less than 2 cm in diameter. They often contain a central stellate scar or "sunburst calcification." Serous microcystic adenomas are associated with Evans' syndrome (autoimmune hemolytic anemia and idiopathic thrombocytopenic purpura) and von Hippel-Lindau's syndrome (hemangioblastomas, retinal angiomatosis, and renal cell cysts). The differentiation of serous cystic lesions from the mucinous neoplasms (cystade-noma or carcinoma and IPMT) is crucial because of the radically different biological characteristics of these two neoplasms.

Bibliography

Gazelle GS, Mueller PR, Raafat N, Halpern EF, Cardenosa G, Warshaw AL. Cystic neoplasms of the pancreas:

evaluation with endoscopic retrograde pancreatography. *Radiology* 1993;188(3):633–636.

Pyke CM, van Heerden JA, Colby TV, Sarr MG, Weaver AL. The spectrum of serous cystadenoma of the pancreas: clinical, pathologic, and surgical aspects. *Ann Surg* 1992; 215(2):132–139.

Sarr MG, Kendrick ML, Nagorney DM, Thompson GB, Farley DR, Farnell MB. Cystic neoplasms of the pancreas: benign to malignant epithelial neoplasms. *Surg Clin North Am* 2001;81(3):497–509.

13. **(A)**

14. **(A)**

Explanations 13 and 14

The first report of IPMT was in the 1980s. Females and males have equal risk. Clinical recognition of the disease is often delayed because it is confused with chronic pancreatitis or cystic neoplasms of the pan-creas. The classic appearance of the tumor is that of mucin emanating from the ampulla of Vater during ERCP. A spectrum of cellular atypia occurs with suspicious areas of invasive carcinoma. K-ras is a non-specific marker for the disease. Current recommen-dation is pancreatic resection although total pancreatectomy has been advocated by some. Frozen section taken at the time of resection should reveal negative margins. Up to 10% of patients with IPMT harbor another malignancy, particularly colorectal neoplasms (Fig. 30-7).

Bibliography

Paye F, et al. Intraductal papillary mucinous tumors of the pancreas: pancreatic resections guided by preoperative

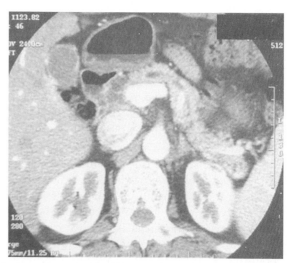

FIG. 30-7 CT demonstrated pancreatic uncinate neoplasm consistent with a mucinous tumor, pathologically determined to be IPMNT.

morphological assessment and intraoperative frozen section examination. *Surgery* 2000;127(5):536–544.

Sugiyama M, Atomi Y. Extrapancreatic neoplasms occur with unusual frequency in patients with intraductal papillary mucinous tumors of the pancreas. *Am J Gastroenterol* 1999;94:470–473.

15. **(D)** The pylorus-preserving pancreaticoduodenectomy (PPPD) was first described by Watson in 1944 and reintroduced by Traverso and Longmire in 1978 to improve the nutritional deficiencies associated with the classic Whipple (NPPPD). Delayed gastric emptying is found to be twice as common after PPPD (20–30%) compared to NPPPD. Multiple series have documented mortality rates well below 5% for both operations, although the morbidity rate for NPPPD is reported to be slightly higher. PPPD is associated with nutritional advantages, reduced likelihood of postgastrectomy dumping syndromes; including both dumping and bile reflux gastritis; however, the nutritional advantages are most evident in the early postsurgical period and become equivalent between operations over time. Unfortunately, there is no demonstrated improvement in survival between the procedures when performed for pancreatic adenocarcinoma.

Bibliography

Jimenez RE, Fernandez-del Castillo C, et al. Outcome of pancreaticoduodenectomy with pylorus preservation with anterectomy in the treatment of chronic pancreatitis. *Ann Surg* 2000;231:193–200.

Takada T, Yasuda H, Amano H, Yoshida M, Ando H. Results of a pylorus-preserving pancreatoduodenectomy for pancreatic cancer: a comparison with results of the Whipple procedure. *Hepatogastroenterology* 1997; 44(18):1536–1540.

Yeo CJ, Cameron JL, et al. Pancreaticoduodenectomy with or without extended retropertioneal lymphadenectomy for periampullary adenocarcinoma, comparison of morbidity, mortality and short term outcome. *Ann Surg* 1999;226:613–622.

16. **(B)** Pancreatic adenocarcinoma has an overall 5-year survival rate of 0.4% and has an annual mortality of approximately 28,000 in the United States. Potential predictors of survival include early stage disease, tumor grade and negative resection-margin; however, overall 5-year survival is approximately 5%. Several studies have demonstrated a beneficial role for neoadjuvant or adjuvant therapy to reduce the rate of local recurrence; however, the rate of distant metastases has been unaltered. Extended lymphadenectomy is suggested to provide a more complete and accurate staging of the disease for stratification of prognosis; however, no survival advantage has been demonstrated. The reader should be aware of the conclusions of three large cooperative group studies addressing the issue of pancreatic cancer and chemoradiotherapy, completed by the Gastrointestinal Study Group (GITSG), the European Organization for Research and Treatment of Cancer Study Group (EORTC) and the European Study Group for Pancreatic Cancer (ESPAC). The GITSG study concluded that the need for both chemoradiotherapy and chemotherapy is more effective than 5-FU alone. The EORTC study of adjuvant chemoradiotherapy with pancreatic cancer found no significant difference in median survival between adjuvant-treated patients and controls. The most recent ESPAC trial showed no survival benefit for adjuvant chemoradiotherapy but revealed a potential benefit for adjuvant chemotherapy, justifying the need for further controlled trials.

Bibliography

Evans DB, Hess KR, Pisters PW. ESPAC-1 trial of adjuvant therapy for resectable adenocarcinoma of the pancreas. *Ann Surg* 2002;236(5):694; author reply 694–696.

Neoptolemos JP, Dunn JA, et al. Adjuvant chemoradiotherapy and chemotherapy in resectable pancreatic cancer: a randomized controlled trial. *Lancet* 2001;358:1576–1585.

Pedrazzoli S, Dicarlo V, Dionigi R, et al. Standard versus extended lymphaedenectomy associated with pancreatoduodenectomy in the surgical treatment of adenocarcinoma of the head of the pancreas: a muticenter, prospective, randomized study. *Ann Surg* 1998;228:508–517.

17. **(C)** Approximately 80% of pancreatic cancer patients at first presentation have advanced unresectable disease; 40% will exhibit local spread, and 50% demonstrate distant disease. Pain is reported by 75% of patients. Transmission of painful sensation is via T5 to T11 through the sympathetic chain celiac ganglion. Neurolytic celiac plexus block is used to treat refractory cancer-associated pain of the upper abdomen as narcotic analgesics achieve satisfactory pain control for only 50% of patients. Pain relief is effective in the short term (3–6 months) for 90% of patients and in the long term for 23% of patients. In regards to obstructive jaundice, the data suggest an improved benefit from stent-biliary decompression rather than surgical bypass. This has been a paradigm shift as plastic stents have been replaced with metallic expandable wallstents. Metallic biliary stents have several advantages over plastic stents. They have a lower occlusion rate and a lower intervention rate. Wallstents allow for balloon tumorectomy or can be bypassed by placement of a second stent; however, metallic stents cannot be removed as easily as plastic stents (Fig. 30-8).

In contrast, gastric bypass remains controversial. The rate of GOO ranges from 3 to 19%. It is important

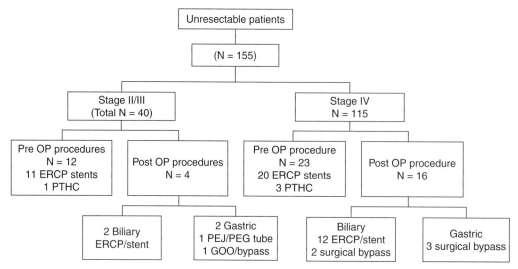

FIG. 30-8 Palliative nonsurgical procedures performed in a cohort of 155 patients with unresectable pancreatic adenocarcinoma. Note the low incidence of gastric bypass and the reliance on endoscopic biliary drainage.

to be aware that prophylactic gastric bypass for GOO remains recommended for laparotomy-based staging while not for laparoscopy-based staging. However, in the presence of unresectable pancreatic cancer with a demonstrated mechanical GOO, gastrojejunostomy is the procedure of choice.

Bibliography

Espat NJ, Brennan MF, Conlon KC. Patients with laparoscopically staged unresectable pancreatic adenocarcinoma do not require subsequent surgical biliary or gastric bypass. *J Am Coll Surg* 1999;188(6):649–655; discussion 655–657.

Molinari M, Espat NJ, Helton WS. Palliative strategies for locally advanced unresectable and metastatic pancreatic cancer. *Surg Clin North Am* 2001;81(3):651–666.

18. **(C)** Sentinel loop sign is the presence of a single dilated loop of small bowel in the midabdomen as visualized on a plain abdominal film (Fig. 30-9). Another sign of localized ileus, colon cutoff sign, is also seen on plain abdominal films and is the presence of a dilated proximal transverse colon with an abrupt change to normal caliber at the midline. Pancreatic calcifications are consistent with chronic pancreatitis from alcohol abuse, and are not seen in biliary or acute pancreatitis. These calcifications, although they are the hallmark of chronic pancreatitis, do not correlate with the degree of exocrine insufficiency. Despite these plain film findings, US of the right upper quadrant and CT scan provide more useful information in the radiographic evaluation of pancreatitis. Hyperamylasemia, although nonspecific, is expected early in the course of acute pancreatitis. The amylase level does not necessarily correlate with the severity of pancreatitis. In cases of chronic pancreatitis, amylase levels may be elevated, normal, or low. Elevated serum lipase levels are as sensitive, but are more specific for acute pancreatitis than serum amylase. Lipase also remains elevated longer than amylase. Vomiting that alleviates abdominal pain should suggest an alternative diagnosis.

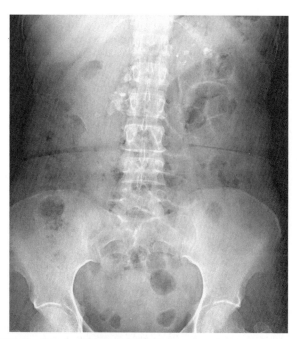

FIG. 30-9 KUB of patient admitted with acute pancreatitis. Note the pancreatic calcifications that suggest this is a recurrent problem. In the left upper quadrant a loop of small bowel is noted with air-fluid levels.

Bibliography

Mulvihill S. Pancreas. In: Norton J, Bollinger R, Chang A, et al. (eds.), *Essential Practice of Surgery*. New York, NY: Springer-Verlag, 2003, 199–218.

Yeo C, Cameron J. Exocrine pancreas. In: Townsend C Jr, Beauchamp R, Evers B, Mattox K (eds.), *Sabiston Textbook of Surgery. The Biological Basis of Modern Surgical Practice*. Philadelphia, PA: W.B. Saunders, 2001, 1112–1143.

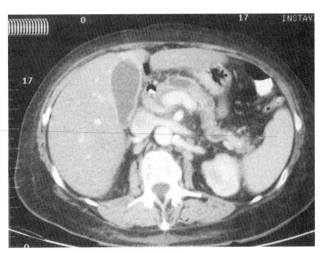

FIG. 30-10   CT scan demonstrating a distended gallbladder in a patient with a dilated, tortuous pancreas. The pancreatic duct has multiple strictures with an atrophic distal tail of the gland. Modified Puestow would not be indicated in this patient.

19. **(B)** Patients with chronic pancreatitis commonly seek medical attention for pain. Surgical treatment for pancreatitis is indicated in cases of severe disabling pain and obstruction of adjacent hollow viscera. Surgical options are myriad, and include the longitudinal pancreaticojejunostomy (modified Puestow procedure), caudal pancreaticojejunostomy (Duval procedure), pancreatic head resection (Beger and Frey procedures), pancreaticoduodenectomy (Whipple procedure), and various partial pancreatic resections. These operations can be broadly classified as either resections or ductal drainage procedures, and have different indications. The longitudinal pancreatectomy is indicated in patients with disabling pain, who have a dilated (>6 mm) pancreatic duct with or without strictures. In the longitudinal pancreaticojejunostomy, the surface of the pancreas is exposed, and the pancreatic duct is identified and opened along its length. An anastomosis is created between the opened duct and a Roux-en-Y limb. Relief of pain is anticipated in 80–90% of patients, especially if patients refrain from alcohol. Diabetes does not typically occur until 80% of the pancreas is destroyed; however, endocrine insufficiency is not a contraindication to surgery. Further loss of exocrine or endocrine function may, in fact, be delayed by performing a drainage procedure. Patients with obstruction of adjacent hollow viscera such as the common bile duct or duodenum are candidates for resectional surgery (Fig. 30-10).

Bibliography

Mulvihill S. Pancreas. In: Norton J, Bollinger R, Chang A, et al. (eds.), *Essential Practice of Surgery*. New York, NY: Springer-Verlag, 2003, 199–218.

Partington P, Rochelle R. Modified Puestow procedure for retrograde drainage of the pancreatic duct. *Ann Surg* 1960;152:1037–1043.

Puestow C, Gillesby W. Retrograde surgical drainage of pancreas for chronic relapsing pancreatitis. *Arch Surg* 1958;76:898–907.

20. **(C)** Although considered to be uncommon, fistulae may complicate as many as 25% of pancreatic operations. Fistulae are classified as low or high output based on whether the drainage exceeds 200 cc per day. Fluid and electrolyte abnormalities are common because of the loss of water, bicarbonate, and potassium. Severe skin breakdown and sepsis are also common sequelae of pancreaticocutaneous fistulae. Fistulae will usually close with broad-spectrum antibiotics, skin care, bowel rest, parenteral nutritional support, and drainage of abscess. Failure to close may be because of associated factors such as foreign body, radiation therapy, infection, epithelized tract, neoplasm, or distal obstruction (the FRIEND mnemonic). Somatostatin, in theory, should facilitate fistula closure because it inhibits motility of the stomach and small bowel and diminishes small bowel and pancreatic output, thereby decreasing the output form a fistula. The role of somatostatin has yet to be validated with level one data (Fig. 30-11).

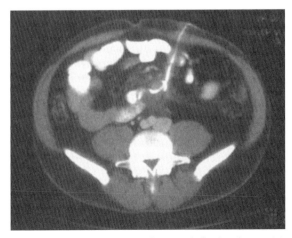

FIG. 30-11   Percutaneous drainage of pancreatic fistula subsequent to an exploratory laparotomy.

Bibliography

Yeo C, Cameron J. Exocrine pancreas. In: Townsend C Jr, Beauchamp R, Evers B, Mattox K (eds.), *Sabiston Textbook of Surgery. The Biological Basis of Modern Surgical Practice.* Philadelphia, PA: W.B. Saunders, 2001, 1112–1143.

21. **(D)** Pseudocysts are defined as persistent, contained collections of pancreatic fluid that remain for 4 weeks following an attack of acute pancreatitis. Pseudocysts are the result of a pancreatic duct disruption, and can occur in as many as 10% of patients following an episode of acute alcoholic pancreatitis. Pseudocysts may occur within the pancreatic parenchyma, or outside of the pancreas in an adjacent potential space. The cyst is formed by inflammation within the surrounding structures walling off the fluid. Pancreatic pseudocysts lack the epithelial lining that defines true cysts. Three-quarters of all cystic lesions of the pancreas encountered are pancreatic pseudocysts. Asymptomatic, uncomplicated acute pseudocysts should be expected to resolve with nonoperative treatment. Chronic pseudocysts with a mature cyst wall at presentation are less likely to resolve spontaneously. The preferred operative management of uncomplicated pancreatic pseudocysts is internal drainage. In the case of an acute pseudocyst, 6 weeks is allowed to pass from the time of the initial episode of pancreatitis to ensure adequate cyst wall maturation. External percutaneous drainage is indicated when the pseudocyst is infected, the patient is too ill to tolerate surgery, or if there is a rapidly enlarging fluid collection within an immature cyst wall. In these cases, a pancreaticocutaneous fistula inevitably follows which may persist and require continuous catheter drainage for days to months (Fig. 30-12).

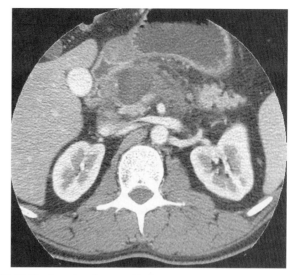

FIG. 30-12 Sequelae of pancreatitis demonstrated as a peripancreatic fluid collection extending into the lesser sac. Prior to a period of potential resolution and in the absence of clinical symptoms of infection, conservative nonoperative or radiologic management is recommended.

Bibliography

Mulvihill S. Pancreas. In: Norton J, Bollinger R, Chang A, et al. (eds.), *Essential Practice of Surgery.* New York, NY: Springer-Verlag, 2003, 199–218.
Yeo C, Cameron J. Exocrine pancreas. In: Townsend C Jr, Beauchamp R, Evers B, Mattox K (eds.), *Sabiston Textbook of Surgery. The Biological Basis of Modern Surgical Practice.* Philadelphia, PA: W.B. Saunders, 2001, 1112–1143.

22. **(C)** The gene that encodes insulin is located on chromosome 11 at 11p15. Preproinsulin is cleaved into proinsulin while still in the endoplasmic reticulum. In the rough endoplasmic reticulum and Golgi, proinsulin is cleaved into insulin and C-peptide. Mature insulin is then stored in secretory granules as inactive zinc-insulin crystals. Consumption of carbohydrates triggers a rapid insulin secretory response that is greater than an equivalent intravenous glucose administration. Hyperglycemia stimulates insulin secretion through a complex signaling pathway. GLUT2 transports glucose into the cell where it is phosphorylated by glucokinase. Adenosine triphosphate (ATP) is generated by the glycolytic pathway. As its intracellular concentration increases, the ATP sensitive potassium channel is inhibited, leading to depolarization of the cell membrane, an increase in cytoplasmic calcium, and exocytosis of the insulin secretory crystals. Equimolar amounts of insulin and C-peptide, along with a small amount of proinsulin, are released by exocytosis. Insulin is cleared from the circulation by the liver and kidney with a half-life of about 3–6 min. C-peptide has a longer half-life than insulin, resulting in a plasma C-peptide to insulin ratio of about 5:1. Commercially available insulin contains no C-peptide.

Bibliography

Kacsoh B. The endocrine pancreas. In: Dolan J (ed.), *Endocrine Physiology.* St. Louis, MO: McGraw-Hill, 2000, 189–250.

23. **(C)** Whipple proposed his triad prior to the development of laboratory testing more sophisticated than the measurement of serum glucose. The eponymous triad consists of documented glucose below 45 mg/dL, symptomatic hypoglycemia induced by fasting, and symptoms that are quickly ameliorated with the administration of glucose. Although elevated plasma insulin is a component of the diagnosis for insulinoma, it is not a component of Whipple's triad.

Bibliography

Dolan J, Norton J. Neuroendocrine tumors of the pancreas and gastrointestinal tract and carcinoid disease. In: Norton J, Bollinger R, Chang A, et al. (eds.), *Essential Practice of Surgery*. New York, NY: Springer-Verlag, 2003, 401–415.

Grant C. Insulinoma. In: Doherty G, Skogseid B (eds.), *Surgical Endocrinology*. Philadelphia, PA: Lippincott, Williams & Wilkins, 2001, 345–360.

Thompson J, Townsend C Jr. Endocrine pancreas. In: Townsend C Jr, Beauchamp R, Evers B, Mattox K (eds.), *Sabiston Textbook of Surgery. The Biological Basis of Modern Surgical Practice*. Philadelphia, PA: W.B. Saunders, 2001, 646–661.

Whipple A. The surgical therapy of hyperinsulinism. *J Int Chir* 1938;3:237.

Whipple A, Franz V. Adenoma of islet cells with hyperinsulinism. *Am Surg* 1935;101:1299–1335.

24. **(D)** Insulinoma is the most common islet cell tumor. The vast majority are solitary benign tumors. Five to 10% accompany the MEN 1 syndrome, and are multiple. The diagnosis of malignancy is clinical, based on local or distant metastases found during surgery. Detectable sulfonylurea in the urine suggests fictitious hypoglycemia, caused by the inappropriate ingestion of oral hypoglycemic medications. Exploration or even localization studies for insulinoma should not be considered before establishing the diagnosis clinically and biochemically. Since cleavage of endogenous proinsulin yields both active insulin and inactive C-peptide, elevated insulin levels without concomitant elevated C-peptide suggest fictitious hypoglycemia by an exogenous source of insulin. Hypoglycemia and neurologic signs which are ameliorated by the administration of glucose are the classic components of Whipple's triad.

Bibliography

Dolan J, Norton J. Neuroendocrine tumors of the pancreas and gastrointestinal tract and carcinoid disease. In: Norton J, Bollinger R, Chang A, et al. (eds.), *Essential Practice of Surgery*. New York, NY: Springer-Verlag, 2003, 401–415.

Grant C. Insulinoma. In: Doherty G, Skogseid B (eds.), *Surgical Endocrinology*. Philadelphia, PA: Lippincott, Williams & Wilkins, 2001, 345–360.

Thompson J, Townsend C Jr. Endocrine pancreas. In: Townsend C Jr, Beauchamp R, Evers B, Mattox K (eds.), *Sabiston Textbook of Surgery. The Biological Basis of Modern Surgical Practice*. Philadelphia, PA: W.B. Saunders, 2001, 646–661.

25. **(D)** Localization of insulinomas should not be attempted prior to establishing a biochemical diagnosis. Insulinomas are usually small (0.5–2 cm), solitary lesions, which have been found equally distributed across the head, body, and tail of the pancreas. Therefore, two-thirds are located to the left of the SMA. Most are benign. Malignancy is a clinical diagnosis, based on the finding of regional or hepatic metastases. Intraoperative US, when combined with palpation of the pancreas, is the most effective and cost-effective method to localize insulinomas; however, since there is an equal probability that these tumors will be found in any of the three regions of the pancreas, many surgeons desire preoperative regional localization. Multiple preoperative strategies have been employed in an attempt to localize these tumors, but most results have been unsatisfying. Unlike gastrinomas, insulinomas have few somatostatin receptors. CT, MR, transabdominal US, and octreotide scans are rarely useful. CT or MR are, however, good studies for evaluation of hepatic metastases. Endoscopic US has been shown to have a sensitivity of up to 85% and a specificity of up to 95% in the identification of pancreatic insulinomas in highly specialized centers. Insulinomas have a rich blood supply, and because of their rich vascularity, they can demonstrate a blush on selective arteriography. Since insulinomas (and other APUD tumors) are stimulated to release hormone by calcium injection, selective arterial calcium injection with hepatic venous sampling has been employed to localize these tumors. Success in localizing insulinomas using this modality has been nearly 90% in some series.

Bibliography

Dolan J, Norton J. Neuroendocrine tumors of the pancreas and gastrointestinal tract and carcinoid disease. In: Norton J, Bollinger R, Chang A, et al. (eds.), *Essential Practice of Surgery*. New York, NY: Springer-Verlag, 2003, 401–415.

Doppman JL, Chang R, Fraker DL, et al. Localization of insulinomas to regions of the pancreas by intra-arterial stimulation with calcium. *Ann Intern Med* 1995;123(4): 269–273.

Grant C. Insulinoma. In: Doherty G, Skogseid B (eds.), *Surgical Endocrinology*. Philadelphia, PA: Lippincott, Williams & Wilkins, 2001, 345–360.

Meko JB, Norton JA. Endocrine tumors of the pancreas. *Curr Opin Gen Surg* 1994:186–194.

Thompson J, Townsend C Jr. Endocrine pancreas. In: Townsend C Jr, Beauchamp R, Evers B, Mattox K (eds.), *Sabiston Textbook of Surgery. The Biological Basis of Modern Surgical Practice*. Philadelphia, PA: W.B. Saunders, 2001, 646–661.

26. **(D)** Zollinger and Ellison first reported the association of peptic ulcer disease with gastric acid hypersecretion and tumors of the islets of Langerhans in 1955. The gastrinoma which causes Zollinger-Ellison's syndrome (ZES) produces excessive amounts of gastrin,

thereby stimulating gastric acid secretion and causing the ulcer diathesis. ZES is rare, but should be suspected in patients with peptic ulcer disease or GERD in association with diarrhea. At least two-thirds of patients with MEN 1 have pancreatic neuroendocrine tumors (the majority of which are gastrinomas). Greater than 90% of gastrinomas express receptors for somatostatin. Consequently, somatostatin receptor scintigraphy is now the test of choice for localizing gastrinomas. Approximately 80% are found in the gastrinoma triangle. The duodenum is the primary site in 45–60% of patients. Approximately 70% of duodenal gastrinomas are located in the first portion, and 20% in the second portion. Although they are slow-growing, approximately 60% are malignant. Lymph node, liver, and distant metastases are not uncommon. Common presenting signs are abdominal pain, diarrhea, reflux, and dysphagia. The diarrhea associated with gastrinomas (40% of patients) is secretory and stops with nasogastric suctioning. Seventy-five to eighty percent of gastrinomas are sporadic. The remaining 20% are inherited and associated with MEN 1 syndrome.

Bibliography

Dolan J, Norton J. Neuroendocrine tumors of the pancreas and gastrointestinal tract and carcinoid disease. In: Norton J, Bollinger R, Chang A, et al. (eds.), *Essential Practice of Surgery*. New York, NY: Springer-Verlag, 2003, 401–415.

Jensen R. Zollinger-Ellison syndrome. In: Doherty G, Skogseid B (eds.), *Surgical Endocrinology*. Philadelphia, PA: Lippincott, Williams & Wilkins, 2001, 291–343.

Thompson J, Townsend C Jr. Endocrine pancreas. In: Townsend C Jr, Beauchamp R, Evers B, Mattox K (eds.), *Sabiston Textbook of Surgery. The Biological Basis of Modern Surgical Practice*. Philadelphia, PA: W.B. Saunders, 2001, 646–661.

Zollinger R, Ellison E. Primary peptic ulcerations of the jejunum associated with islet cell tumors of the pancreas. *Ann Surg* 1955;142:709–728.

27. **(C)** Glucagon is produced by the alpha cells of the pancreatic islets, and is secreted in response to fasting (hypoglycemia), stress, and protein-rich meals. The gene is located on chromosome 2q36, and has some expression in tissues other than the pancreatic islets. Glucagon acts primarily to counter regulate insulin in glucose homeostasis, and to mobilize energy sources. Glucagon has a plasma half-life of approximately 6 min and is cleared primarily by the liver. The target organs for the effects of glucagon are the liver and adipose tissue. Glucagon promotes the mobilization of glucose and achieves this primarily by stimulating lipolysis in adipose tissue, and glycogenolysis and gluconeogenesis in the liver.

Bibliography

Kacsoh B. The endocrine pancreas. In: Dolan J (ed.), *Endocrine Physiology*. St. Louis, MO: McGraw-Hill, 2000, 189–250.

28. **(A)** Glucagonomas are rare tumors of the alpha cells of the pancreatic islets that produce a distinct syndrome characterized by diabetes, migrating skin rash (necrolytic migratory erythema), hypoaminoacidemia, and malnutrition. Skin manifestations resolve with institution of total parenteral nutrition, and are believed to be linked to malnutrition. These patients are at high risk for the development of deep venous thrombosis, and should undergo prophylactic anticoagulation. Glucagon levels greater than 1000 pg/mL are diagnostic. Preoperative management includes the use of somatostatin analogues and nutritional supplementation. Glucagonomas are usually malignant, large at presentation, and have been found more frequently in the body and tail of the pancreas. In contrast to gastrinomas, they are always located in the pancreas. Imaging by CT scanning or somatostatin receptor scintigraphy is frequently successful in localizing primary and metastatic disease.

Bibliography

Doherty G. VIPoma, glucagonoma, and other rare islet cell tumors. In: Doherty G, Skogseid B (eds.), *Surgical Endocrinology*. Philadelphia, PA: Lippincott, Williams & Wilkins, 2001, 375–380.

29. **(D)** Somatostatinomas are rare tumors that produce somatostatin. They may be located in the pancreas or duodenum. The larger pancreatic tumors are usually in the head of the pancreas and are more frequently associated with the somatostatinoma syndrome. Diabetes, cholelithiasis, and steatorrhea comprise the classic triad. The diagnosis can be confirmed preoperatively by measuring elevated plasma levels of somatostatin, but it is often made postoperatively by pathologists, especially in the case of smaller duodenal tumors that present with local symptoms. These tumors frequently (>50%) have nodal and liver metastases at the time of diagnosis. Patients with localized disease should undergo pancreaticoduodenectomy.

Bibliography

Doherty G. VIPoma, glucagonoma, and other rare islet cell tumors. In: Doherty G, Skogseid B (eds.), *Surgical Endocrinology*. Philadelphia, PA: Lippincott, Williams & Wilkins, 2001, 375–380.

30. **(C)** Tumors that elaborate VIP are rare. The syndrome caused by excessive VIP secretion is known as Verner-Morrison's syndrome, or WDHA syndrome (acronym

for watery diarrhea, hypokalemia, and achlorhydria). The diagnosis is made by demonstrating an elevated fasting level of VIP concomitant with secretory diarrhea (>700 mL per day) and a pancreatic tumor. Although VIP is a neuropeptide that is normally distributed in the central and peripheral nervous systems, VIPomas are found in the pancreas, or rarely the duodenum. Flushing is sometimes seen because of the direct vasodilation effect of the hormone. Unlike other neuroendocrine tumors, diabetes is not a feature of this syndrome. Achlorhydria is because of the direct inhibitory effect that VIP has on gastric acid secretion. Treatment should be initiated with volume resuscitation, electrolyte (hypokalemia) normalization, and the administration of a somatostatin analog. Imaging by CT scanning or somatostatin receptor scintigraphy is frequently successful in localizing primary and metastatic disease. Complete resection is curative.

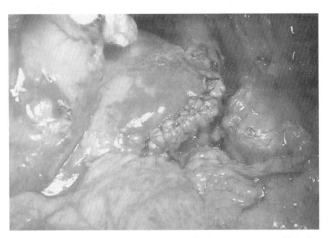

FIG. 30-13 Operative field subsequent to distal pancreatectomy. Note the oversewn pancreas; the placement of sutures themselves may result in pancreatic exocrine leakage; however, studies with sealants and fibrin-based tissue glues have not been positive.

Bibliography

Doherty G. VIPoma, glucagonoma, and other rare islet cell tumors. In: Doherty G, Skogseid B (eds.), *Surgical Endocrinology*. Philadelphia, PA: Lippincott, Williams & Wilkins, 2001, 375–380.

31. **(A)** Pancreas divisum is the most common congenital variant of pancreatic anatomy. Pancreas divisum occurs when the ventral and dorsal pancreatic ducts fail to fuse. As a result of this nonunion of the ducts, the major portion of the pancreatic exocrine secretions enters the duodenum via the dorsal duct and minor papilla. Affected patients also demonstrate a higher incidence of pancreaticobiliary anomalies. Most patients are asymptomatic and completely unaffected by the condition; however, a significant number present with recurrent attacks of acute pancreatitis. Pancreas divisum is identified in about 10% of patients. The initial treatment of choice in patients is ERCP including endoscopic sphincterotomy of the minor ampulla with or without sphincterotomy of the major ampulla, ductal balloon dilatation, and pancreatic duct stent placement. If sphincterotomy and stent placement fail, operative pancreatic resection or ductular drainage by longitudinal pancreaticojejunostomy may be required.

Bibliography

Coleman SD, Eisen GM, Troughton AB, Cotton PB. Endoscopic treatment in pancreas divisum. *Am J Gastroenterol* 1994;89(8):1152–1155.

Lehman GA, Sherman S, Nisi R, Hawes RH. Pancreas divisum: results of minor papilla sphincterotomy. *Gastrointest Endosc* 1993;39(1):1–8.

Yeo C, Cameron J. Exocrine pancreas. In: Townsend C Jr, Beauchamp R, Evers B, Mattox K (eds.), *Sabiston Textbook of Surgery. The Biological Basis of Modern Surgical Practice*. Philadelphia, PA: W.B. Saunders, 2001, 1112–1143.

32. **(B)** Pancreatic fistulae as a complication following pancreatic operation have been reported to be as high as 30%. Those that drain less than 200 cc/L over 24 h are defined as low output, while more than 200 cc/L are high output. Complications include sepsis, fluid and electrolyte abnormalities, and skin excoriation. CT can help identify the fistulous tract and demonstrate fluid collections for potential drainage. ERCP is most sensitive at demonstrating pancreatic duct connection or disruption. Endoscopic sphincterotomy or pancreatic duct stenting may be helpful by reducing the intrapancreatic duct pressure, allowing secretions to travel to the duodenum. Octreotide has been postulated to have benefit in closing external pancreatic fistulae; however, randomized studies have failed to support this suggestion. Similarly, fibrin sealant and glues have not been demonstrated to be of benefit. Surgical closure of fistulae is indicated when conservative means fail (Fig. 30-13).

In general terms, if surgery is contemplated, fistulae originating from the tail of the pancreas with relatively normal appearance of the proximal duct are best treated with distal pancreatectomy. If there are any abnormalities of the proximal duct in the head, neck, or body of the gland, fistulae are best managed with Roux-en-Y pancreaticojejunostomy to the fistula tract.

Bibliography

Buchler MW, Bassi C, Fingerhut A, Klempa I. Does prophylactic octreotide decrease the rates of pancreatic fistula and other complications after pancreaticoduodenectomy? *Ann Surg* 2001;234(2):262–263.

Suc B, Msika S, Fingerhut A, Fourtanier G, Hay JM, Holmieres F, Sastre B, Fagniez PL; and the French

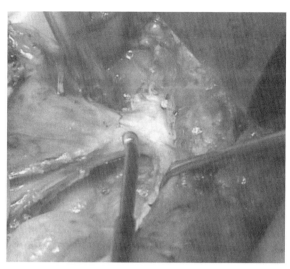

FIG. 30-14 Intraoperative view from right-to-left demonstrating uncinate process transection. The portal vein lies inferior to the pancreatic neck which has been divided during pancreaticoduodenectomy.

Association for Surgical Research. Temporary fibrin glue occlusion of the main pancreatic duct in the prevention of intra-abdominal complications after pancreatic resection: prospective randomized trial. *Ann Surg* 2003;237(1):57–65.

Voss M, Pappas T. Pancreatic Fistula. *Curr Treat Options Gastroenterol* 2002;5(5):345–353.

33. **(D)** The pancreas is a retroperitoneal organ at the level of L-2, posterior to the stomach and anterior to the vertebrae. The head of the pancreas is the portion between the duodenum and superior mesenteric vessels. The neck overlies the superior mesenteric vein. The exocrine drainage system is comprised of the main duct and accessory duct. The main pancreatic duct drains the tail, body, and most of the head of the pancreas. The lesser duct drains the superior of the pancreatic head into the second portion of the duodenum via the lesser papilla approximately 2 cm superior to the ampulla of Vater. The superior mesenteric vessels lie anterior to the uncinate process (Fig. 30-14).

Bibliography

Yeo C, Cameron J. Exocrine pancreas. In: Townsend C Jr, Beauchamp R, Evers B, Mattox K (eds.), *Sabiston Textbook of Surgery. The Biological Basis of Modern Surgical Practice.* Philadelphia, PA: W.B. Saunders, 2001, 1112–1143.

34. **(A)** Most pancreatic and duodenal injuries can be handled by simple repair and drainage. Injuries involving both organs that cannot be repaired require pancreaticoduodenectomy. Mortality is related to hemorrhage and associated injures, therefore hemostasis is of paramount importance. The surgeon should perform only the essential resections needed to obtain hemostasis and close the gastrointestinal (GI) tract. Postoperatively, hypovolemia, hypothermia, acidosis, and coagulopathy can be corrected. Definitive reconstruction when the patient has stabilized can be done in a delayed fashion. In other words, resect as necessary, stabilize then reconstruct. In this patient, a Whipple procedure is the most appropriate option when nonsalvageable duodenal injures and pancreatic duct injury occur, especially in a hemodynamically stable patient.

Bibliography

De Kerpel W, Hendrickx T, Vanrykel JP, Aelvoet C, De Weer F. Whipple procedure after blunt abdominal trauma. *J Trauma* 2002;53(4):780–783.

Koniaris LG, Mandal AK, Genuit T, Cameron JL. Two-stage trauma pancreaticoduodenectomy: delay facilitates anastomotic reconstruction. *J Gastrointest Surg* 2000; 4(4):366–369.

Tuech JJ, Pessaux P, Rege N, Bergamaschi R, Arnaud JP. Emergency pancreaticoduodenectomy with delayed reconstruction for bleeding: a life saving procedure. *Int J Gastrointest Cancer* 2001;29(1):59–62.

35. **(B)** Although biliary disease is a common cause of pancreatitis, cholelithiasis is an uncommon cause of pancreatitis in young children. Specific hematologic disorders such as hereditary spherocytosis or sickle cell anemia may predispose patients to early gallstone formation; however, pancreatitis is an uncommon presentation. Heterotopic pancreatic tissue or drug-induced pancreatitis are also reported but uncommon causes of pancreatitis in children. The most likely etiology in this young patient is coxsackie viral pancreatitis. There are two dozen viruses that may be associated with clinical pancreatitis and this uncommon syndrome may be associated with viral syndromes or vaccinations against specific viruses (i.e., mumps). Treatment is supportive and conservative.

Bibliography

Adler JB, Mazzotta SA, Barkin JS. Pancreatitis caused by measles, mumps, and rubella vaccine. *Pancreas* 1991;6(4):489–490.

Imrie CW, Ferguson JC, Sommerville RG. Coxsackie and mumps virus infection in a prospective study of acute pancreatitis. *Gut* 1977;18(1):53–56.

Ozsvar Z, Deak J, Pap A. Possible role of Coxsackie-B virus infection in pancreatitis. *Int J Pancreatol* 1992;11(2): 105–108.

CHAPTER 31

Spleen

Mimi Kim and Alan Ladd

Questions

1. Morphologic alterations in erythrocytes seen in individuals after splenectomy include all of the following *except* for:

   (A) Howell-Jolly's bodies
   (B) Heinz' bodies
   (C) Pappenheimer's bodies
   (D) stippling
   (E) Dohle's bodies

2. In agnogenic myeloid metaplasia, splenectomy

   (A) results in long-term improvement in thrombocytopenia and anemia in most cases
   (B) alleviates portal hypertension and lowers risk of variceal bleeding
   (C) has little proven benefit
   (D) results in resolution of the primary disease
   (E) is most commonly performed for life-threatening thrombocytopenia

3. In type I Gaucher's disease

   (A) most patients eventually require splenectomy
   (B) recent advances in medical therapies have largely obviated the need for surgical intervention
   (C) although partial splenectomy reduces the risk of overwhelming postsplenectomy sepsis (OPSI), it does not significantly affect glycolipid deposition in bone marrow
   (D) the most common clinical symptoms are related to hepatic cirrhosis and portal hypertension
   (E) genetic transmission is X-linked recessive

4. An otherwise healthy 18-year-old male underwent splenectomy for hereditary spherocytosis. He returned a month later with complaints of diffuse abdominal pain, diarrhea, vomiting, and fever. Examination revealed a lack of peritonitis or significant distention, and amylase and lipase were within normal limits. Blood cultures were negative. A computed tomography (CT) scan of the abdomen and pelvis shows evidence of portal vein thrombosis.

   The following therapy should be initiated:

   (A) complete bowel rest with total parenteral nutrition
   (B) exploratory laparotomy
   (C) observation
   (D) antiulcer therapy with a proton-pump inhibitor and empiric treatment for *Helicobacter pylori*
   (E) systemic heparinization followed by long-term oral anticoagulation

5. Splenic vein thrombosis

   (A) commonly presents with isolated esophageal varices
   (B) is usually accompanied by cirrhosis and portal venous hypertension
   (C) is usually a consequence of pancreatic pathology
   (D) should be managed initially with a course of thrombolytic therapy followed by systemic anticoagulation
   (E) is usually accompanied by hypersplenism and thrombocytopenia

6. The most common indication for splenectomy for a red cell enzymatic defect is

   (A) hereditary spherocytosis
   (B) glucose-6-phosphate dehydrogenase (G6PD) deficiency
   (C) pyruvate kinase deficiency
   (D) hereditary high red blood cell phosphatidylcholine anemia (HPCHA)
   (E) cold-agglutinin syndrome

7. Splenectomy is of proven benefit in the management of the following autoimmune conditions *except*:

   (A) Felty's syndrome
   (B) immune thrombocytopenic purpura (ITP)
   (C) cold-agglutinin syndrome (IgM autoimmune hemolytic anemia)
   (D) warm-agglutinin syndrome (IgG autoimmune hemolytic anemia)
   (E) systemic lupus erythematosus

8. A 25-year-old Black male presents to you with splenomegaly. He was previously healthy and has been otherwise asymptomatic except for mild fatigue. He denies any personal history of alcohol abuse, hematologic dysfunction, or travel. He was adopted as an infant, and family history is unknown. All laboratory studies, including peripheral smear, angiotensin converting enzyme levels, autoimmune antibody panel, hepatic panel, sickle cell and thalassemia assays, and HIV tests are normal. Platelet count is mildly depressed. A CT scan of the abdomen was performed and was completely unremarkable except for a large spleen. The next step in this patient's workup is

   (A) splenectomy
   (B) fine-needle aspiration
   (C) abdominal ultrasound
   (D) IV antibiotics
   (E) corticosteroid therapy

9. Each of the following is true regarding splenic circulation *except*:

   (A) The splenic vein and superior mesenteric vein join to form the portal vein.
   (B) The splenic vein typically runs superiorly to the artery.
   (C) The splenic artery gives rise to the left gastroepiploic artery.
   (D) The splenorenal ligament is the double-layered sheath containing the splenic vessels.
   (E) The inferior mesenteric vein usually empties into the splenic vein.

10. A 24-year-old woman presents with complaints of intermittent chronic abdominal pain for 3 months but no other significant problems. On abdominal examination you notice that she has a nontender mobile mass in the left lower quadrant. Her CT abdomen is shown in Fig. 31-1. The following statements regarding this disease are correct *except*:

    (A) The underlying defect involves absence or hyperlaxity of the ligamentous attachments of the spleen to the retroperitoneum, colon, and diaphragm.
    (B) An elongated vascular mesentery predisposes the organ to axial torsion and infarction.
    (C) It occurs most commonly among young women.
    (D) Treatment of choice is splenectomy.
    (E) Patients commonly present with an asymptomatic abdominal mass or varying degrees of pain.

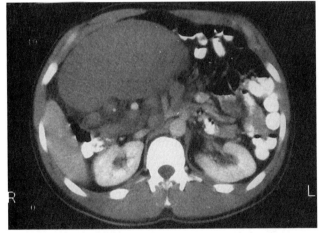

FIG. 31-1   CT of abdomen.

11. You are evaluating a 3-month-old patient with polysplenia for surgery. Each of the following anomalies is classically associated with this syndrome *except* for

    (A) interrupted IVC with azygous continuation
    (B) intestinal malrotation
    (C) common atrioventricular canal
    (D) bilateral trilobed lungs
    (E) bridging liver

Questions 12 and 13 refer to the following scenario:

A 19-year-old woman presents to clinic with complaints of intermittent episodes of acute knife-like midepigastric and left upper quadrant abdominal pain, nausea, and vomiting that have persisted over the last year. She also reports early satiety and progressive weight loss as well as the sensation of a heavy abdominal mass that is especially noticeable when she is supine. She denies any history of abdominal trauma, travel outside of North America, medication use, or any other significant medical history. Except for a palpable spleen, her physical examination is unremarkable. A CT abdomen is obtained (Fig. 31-2)

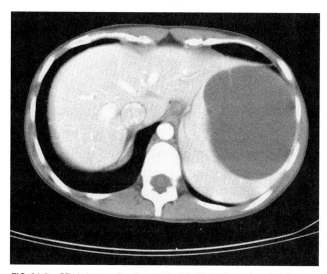

FIG. 31-2 CT abdomen. Courtesy of Dr. Erik Streib, Department of Surgery, Indiana University.

12. The following is most likely to be elevated:

    (A) CA 19-9
    (B) EBV IgM titer
    (C) p53
    (D) lipase
    (E) reticulocyte count

13. The following must be performed prior to operation:

    (A) *Echinococcus* serology
    (B) EBV IgM titer
    (C) evaluation for a primary source of infection
    (D) trial of medical therapy with bowel rest and total parenteral nutrition
    (E) bone marrow biopsy

14. A 65-year-old intoxicated male driver is brought to the trauma bay after a motor vehicle collision. On your assessment, he is confused and combative with obvious head trauma to the right occipital region. He has obvious instability of his left lower ribcage, but he is oxygenating well with breath sounds bilaterally. No other obvious deformities are present. On the initial evaluation, his blood pressure is 80/30 mmHg and heart rate is 140 bpm. On infusion of 2 L of crystalloid, blood pressure improves to 110/60 mmHg and heart rate drops to 100 bpm. The patient remains hemodynamically stable for the next 20 minutes and you decide to send the patient to the CT scanner to evaluate his head, chest, and abdomen. The most reliable predictor for the success of nonoperative treatment of splenic trauma in this patient is

    (A) hemodynamic status
    (B) grade of injury on CT abdomen
    (C) degree of hemoperitoneum on CT abdomen
    (D) coexistent head trauma
    (E) contrast blush on vascular phase of CT scan of spleen

15. Which of the following is true regarding partial splenectomy?

    (A) Selective ligation of vascular structures prior to parenchymal resection results in a consistently predictable amount of residual splenic mass.
    (B) Retained phagocytic function of splenic tissue is an indicator of intact immunologic function.
    (C) Splenic regrowth following partial splenic resection for hereditary spherocytosis results in recurrence of hemolysis.
    (D) For equivalent volumes of residual splenic tissue after partial splenectomy, among hemoglobinopathies, hereditary spherocytosis has the best preservation of splenic phagocytotic function.
    (E) Recent advances in immunologic testing demonstrate that immunization against encapsulated bacteria in patient who undergo partial splenectomy of 80% of original splenic mass is not warranted.

16. Splenectomy may increase long-term risk of each of the following *except*:

    (A) hypercoagulability
    (B) secondary atherosclerotic events
    (C) pneumococcal sepsis
    (D) pulmonary hypertension
    (E) pancreatitis

17. A 23-year-old woman in the first trimester of her pregnancy presents to the emergency department with complaints of acutely worsening left upper quadrant abdominal pain, nausea, and dizziness. She denied any fever, emesis, or any changes in bowel movements. She admits to a 5-month history of similar but milder pain in her midepigastrium and left upper abdomen which was treated with antacids. Your evaluation reveals a well-nourished, well-developed woman who appears uncomfortable but is normotensive and only mildly tachycardic. Her abdomen is moderately tender in the left upper quadrant and epigastrium. Laboratory studies, including complete blood count, platelets, chemistries, and lipase are appropriate. You obtain an acute abdominal series. The upright film is shown in Fig. 31-3. Which of the following is true?

(A) She should have splenectomy performed electively following delivery of her baby.

(B) Among patients with this problem, she is at relatively low risk for complications.

(C) The lesion poses a significant threat to the survival of the fetus.

(D) The most common time for complications to occur is at the time of labor and delivery.

(E) This lesion develops most commonly in patients with an alcohol abuse history or gallstones.

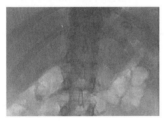

FIG. 31-3   Upright film. Courtesy of Dr. Michael Dalsing, Department of Surgery, Indiana University.

18. Risk and morbidity of bacteremia, meningitis, and pneumonia from encapsulated bacteria is significantly increased in asplenic individuals primarily because of

(A) decreased tuftsin levels resulting in deficient phagocytosis

(B) impaired binding of complement components to bacteria

(C) impaired immunologic memory

(D) impaired amplification of the immune response against known antigens

(E) impaired splenic neutralization of bacterial endotoxin

19. Immunologic function following splenectomy is most profoundly affected by defects in

(A) immunoglobulin-mediated opsonization of encapsulated bacteria

(B) properdin-mediated phagocytosis

(C) tuftsin-activated complement cascade

(D) lymphokine-mediated destruction of malignant cells

(E) CD4+ T-cell-mediated response to familiar antigens

20. A 45-year-old woman with Hodgkin's lymphoma is referred to you by her oncologist for staging laparotomy. You open the abdomen through a standard midline incision. Gross visual inspection of the abdominal cavity is unremarkable for any discrete lesions. You perform core needle biopsies of each lobe of the liver and then a wedge biopsy of the free edge of the left lateral segment. Frozen section is positive for lymphoma. What is the appropriate next step?

(A) close the abdomen and terminate the operation

(B) splenectomy

(C) lymph node sampling

(D) oophoropexy

(E) lymphangiography

21. A 25-year-old male being treated for advanced Hodgkin's disease presents to you for refractory pancytopenia. He is currently receiving a standard chemotherapy regimen and will require splenectomy to continue treatment. This patient most likely received all of the following agents *except* for:

(A) adriamycin

(B) bleomycin

(C) vinblastine

(D) dacarbazine

(E) taxol

22. The following statements regarding ITP are true *except*:

(A) Eighty-five percent of patients fail to respond to medical therapy.

(B) Eighty-five percent of patients undergoing splenectomy for ITP are successfully treated.

(C) Short-term thrombocytotic response to splenectomy is not a reliable predictor of long-term success or therapy.

(D) CNS bleeding is the primary indication for emergent splenectomy in ITP.

(E) Persistent postoperative thrombocytopenia mandates workup with nuclear medicine scanning prior to reinstituting aggressive medical therapy.

23. A 6-year-old male is found to have bilirubinate stones at the time of laparoscopic cholecystectomy. A CT abdomen obtained during a previous admission for abdominal pain shows a small shrunken spleen. This patient most likely has

   (A) thalassemia
   (B) sickle cell disease
   (C) thrombotic thrombocytopenic purpura with hemolytic-uremic syndrome
   (D) autoimmune hemolytic anemia
   (E) hereditary spherocytosis

24. Splenosis

   (A) usually results from failure of embryonic splenic lobules to fuse
   (B) results in splenetic tissue that in most cases derives its blood supply from a tributary of the splenic artery
   (C) results in tissue that differs histologically from the parent organ
   (D) often results in sufficient splenic tissue to clear intraerythrocytic inclusion bodies from the bloodstream
   (E) offers significant protection against OPSI

25. Which of the following factors does not correlate with increased morbidity in laparoscopic splenectomy?

   (A) splenic mass
   (B) blood transfusion
   (C) HIV status
   (D) hematologic malignancy
   (E) age

26. Which of the following splenectomized patients is at lowest risk for overwhelming postsplenectomy infection?

   (A) 25-year-old man who had splenectomy for traumatic rupture in a motor vehicle collision
   (B) 25-year-old man who had splenectomy for sequelae of thalassemia major
   (C) 5-year-old boy who had splenectomy for immune thrombocytic purpura
   (D) 25-year-old man who had splenectomy for staging of lymphoma
   (E) 25-year-old man who had splenectomy 8 years ago for hereditary spherocytosis

27. Asplenic individuals are at increased risk for severe fatal infections from all of the following *except*:

   (A) *S. pneumoniae*
   (B) *N. meningitidis*
   (C) *H. influenzae*
   (D) *E. coli*
   (E) *Candida albicans*

28. Immunizations for patients undergoing elective splenectomy

   (A) do not require boosters
   (B) are equally effective regardless of their timing in relation to the operation
   (C) are equally effective regardless of the age of the patient
   (D) provide complete protection against the major pathogens responsible for OPSI
   (E) can be improved by conjugation of polysaccharides to peptide adjuvants

29. Splenectomy is performed primarily for palliation in all of the following *except*:

   (A) non-Hodgkin's lymphoma
   (B) Hodgkin's lymphoma
   (C) chronic lymphocytic leukemia
   (D) chronic myeloid leukemia
   (E) hairy cell leukemia

30. You are asked to evaluate a 50-year-old kidney transplant patient hospitalized with recurrent sigmoid diverticulitis. After initial improvement, the patient deteriorated, requiring transfer to the intensive care unit, intubation, and pressors. White blood cell (WBC) count is 30,000. CT scan of the abdomen was obtained, demonstrating a unilocular heterogenous fluid collection in the splenic parenchyma. The following considerations are true regarding the appropriate management of this patient *except*:

   (A) This patient will likely require surgical intervention.
   (B) This patient will likely require colectomy in conjunction with management of splenic disease.
   (C) Broad-spectrum antibiotics including an antifungal agent is mandatory.
   (D) This process is likely a complication of diverticulitis.
   (E) Immunosuppression was a key predisposing factor in development of this problem.

Answers and Explanations

1. **(E)** The spleen plays an important role in processing erythrocytes as they pass through, attributable largely to its unique microstructure. In contrast to other organs in which the diameter of the smallest capillaries is slightly larger than that of red blood cells (RBCs), the splenic capillary bed terminates in the red pulp, a sieve-like network of sinuses and cords filled with macrophages through which only the most plastic of cells may pass. Here the circulation stagnates and permits prolonged contact of the bloodstream with cordal macrophages. Senescent cells are destroyed (culling), and weathered red cells that are salvageable are remodeled and repaired (pitting) as intracellular inclusion bodies are removed. Although other macrophage-rich organs such as the liver also take part in destruction of senescent cells, the spleen is more sensitive to damage in cells, so that even minimally damaged cells are removed, to the order of approximately 100 billion cells a day.

After splenectomy, the other macrophage-filled organs continue to remove damaged cells so that the overall survival of RBCs does not increase. At the same time, less damaged cells are not remodeled in the absence of the splenic filter, so that characteristic differences appear on peripheral blood smears of splenectomized individuals.

Heinz bodies, representing denatured hemoglobin; Howell-Jolly's bodies, the nuclear remnants of RBCs; Pappenheimer's bodies, from iron granules; target cells; spur cells and stippling are all characteristic findings in asplenic patients. Dohle's bodies are cytoplasmic inclusion bodies found in neutrophils in the setting of inflammatory diseases, infections, myelocytic leukemia, burns, cyclophosphamide therapy, and myeloproliferative syndromes.

Bibliography

Beauchamp RD, Holzman MD, Fabian TC. Spleen. In: Townsend CM, Beauchamp RD, Evers BM, et al. (eds.), *Textbook of Surgery: The Biological Basis of Modern Surgical Practice*, 16th ed. Philadelphia, PA: WB Saunders, 2001, pp. 1144–1164.

Blood studies. In: Fischbach FT (ed.), *Manual of Laboratory and Diagnostic Tests* [Book Online], 6th ed. Philadelphia, PA: Lippincott Williams & Wilkins, 2000. Available at: http://pco.ovid.com/lrppco/index.html. Accessed December 9, 2003.

Chapman WC, Newman M. Disorders of the spleen. In: Lee GR, Foerster J, Luken SJ, et al. (eds.), Wintrobe's *Clinical Hematology*, 10th ed. Baltimore, MD: Williams & Wilkins, 1999, pp. 1969–1989.

Weintraub LR. Splenectomy: who, when, and why? *Hosp Pract* 1994:27–34.

2. **(B)** Agnogenic myeloid metaplasia, a form of myelofibrosis with myeloid metaplasia, is characterized by reactive bone marrow fibrosis with associated ineffective erythropoiesis, extramedullary hematopoiesis, and hepatosplenomegaly. The exact mechanisms are unclear but the disease process appears to involve dysregulated secretion of growth factors with nonclonal proliferation of fibroblasts.

Patients are usually in the fifth decade of life, with complaints of fatigue, weight loss, and vague abdominal fullness or discomfort. Splenomegaly is virtually universal; 50–75% of patients develop hepatic fibrosis with consequent portal hypertension, hepatomegaly, varices, and ascites. Patients are anemic and may have either elevated or depressed leukocyte and platelet counts. Peripheral blood smear is diagnostic. In conjunction with medical therapy, patients with significant mechanical symptoms related to their splenomegaly and those with significant liver involvement may benefit from splenectomy by relief of portal hypertension and redistribution of portal flow into the liver with consequent decreased variceal bleeding and ascites. Severe thrombocytopenia is not a common indication for splenectomy in this population; in addition, the utility of splenectomy for management of transfusion-dependent anemia and severe thrombocytopenia is not clear. In a recent retrospective review of 223 patients, while durable remissions of portal hypertension (50%) and constitutional symptoms

(67%) were obtained, only 23% of patients had significant improvement in their anemia and none experienced improvement in their thrombocytopenia.

The leading causes of perioperative morbidity and mortality in the series above were bleeding, infection, thrombosis, and operative morbidity and mortality were 31 and 9%, respectively. External beam radiation to the spleen is an alternative to splenectomy; however, relief from splenomegaly is transient, myelosuppression may occur, and subsequent splenectomy is more difficult. Both treatments are palliative and do not ultimately improve survival, which is approximately 3–8 years. Stem cell transplant is potentially curative for a subset of patients.

Bibliography

Akpek G, McAneny D, Weintraub L. Risks and benefits of splenectomy in myelofibrosis with myeloid metaplasia: a retrospective analysis of 26 cases. *J Surg Oncol* 2001; 77:42–48.

Fraker DL. Spleen. In: Greenfield LJ, Mulholland MW, Oldham KT, et al. (eds.), *Scientific Principles and Practice of Surgery*, 3rd ed. Philadelphia, PA: Lippincott Williams & Wilkins, 2001, pp. 1236–1259.

Tefferi A, Mesa RA, Nagorney DM, et al. Splenectomy in myelofibrosis with myeloid metaplasia: a single institution experience with 223 patients. *Blood* 2000;95(7): 2226–2233.

3. **(B)** Gaucher's disease is the most common lysosomal storage disorder, resulting from an inherited deficiency in lysosomal glucocerebrosidase (hydrolase β-glucosidase) with accumulation of undegraded glycolipids. Uptake of glycolipids by the reticuloendothelial system results in infiltration of the bone marrow, spleen, and liver with associated bone dysplasia, pancytopenia, and organomegaly. Patients characteristically present with bleeding from hypersplenism-related thrombocytopenia, fatigue, anemia, and early satiety and weight loss because of mechanical compression of the stomach by the enlarged spleen. Although portal hypertension may occur with infiltration of the liver with Gaucher's cells and subsequent hepatic fibrosis, most patients experience no clinical manifestations.

The enzyme is encoded on chromosome 1 and transmission of the defect is autosomal recessive. Type I (nonneuronopathic) comprises 99% of all cases. Diagnosis can be made by assaying acid β-glucosidase activity in peripheral blood leukocytes or cultured fibroblasts. Mutation profiling with DNA analysis allows identification of the exact genotype. The exact clinical manifestations and individual response to therapy are highly variable and depend largely on the type of mutation combined with ethnic and environmental factors.

Formerly, surgical management was pivotal in management of severe cases and a large body of experience with partial splenectomy had been accumulated by the early 1990s. The spleen is the preferred reservoir for deposition of Gaucher's cells; therefore, in addition to risks related to postsplenectomy sepsis, total splenectomy may induce or aggravate bone marrow involvement.

Development of the human placenta-derived macrophage-targeted enzyme replacement therapy with alglucerase (Ceredase) in 1991, followed closely by the recombinant enzyme imglucerase (Cerezyme) has virtually obviated the need for operative intervention. Enzyme replacement therapy effectively normalizes hemoglobin levels in 90% of patients and substantially reverses organomegaly in most patients with 30–40% reduction in hepatomegaly after 5 years and 30–50% reduction in splenomegaly after 1–2 years of treatment. In addition, defective neutrophil chemotaxis is corrected with a decreased incidence of infections. Growth retardation is a marker in children for disease severity; one retrospective review of 56 patients demonstrated dramatic catch-up growth following initiation of enzyme therapy.

Therapy costs $100,000–300,000 annually per patient. Although cessation of enzyme replacement therapy does not typically result in clinical deterioration and relapse, severe rebound organomegaly has been reported. Current indications for splenectomy include inadequate response to high dose enzyme replacement therapy, inferior vena cava syndrome, splenic abscesses, severe abdominal pain crises, and life-threatening thrombocytopenia. In addition, because of the unique consistency of the spleen in this disorder, patients may be predisposed to life-threatening splenic injury after minor trauma, necessitating emergent splenectomy.

Bibliography

Dweck A, Abrahamov A, Hadas-Halpern I, et al. Type I Gaucher disease in children with and without enzyme therapy. *Pediatr Hematol Oncol* 2002;19:389–397.

Fraker DL. Spleen. In: Greenfield LJ, Mulholland MW, Oldham KT, et al. (eds.), *Scientific Principles and Practice of Surgery*, 3rd ed. Philadelphia, PA: Lippincott Williams & Wilkins, 2001, pp. 1236–1259.

Krasnewich D, Dietrich K, Bauer L, et al. Splenectomy in Gaucher disease: new management dilemmas. *Blood* 1998;91(8):3085–3087.

Stone DL, Ginns EI, Krasnewich D, et al. Life-threatening splenic hemorrhage in two patients with Gaucher disease. *Am J Hematol* 2000;64:140–142.

Tóth J, Erdos M, Maródi L. Rebound hepatosplenomegaly in type 1 Gaucher disease. *Eur J Haematol* 2003;70: 125–128.

Weinreb NJ, Charrow J, Andersson HC, et al. Effectiveness of enzyme replacement therapy in 1028 patients with type I Gaucher disease after 2 to 5 years of treatment: a report from the Gaucher registry. *Am J Med* 2002;113: 112–119.

4. **(E)** Previously believed to be a rare entity, in light of new evidence resulting from advances in diagnostic imaging and increased availability of CT, portal vein thrombosis following splenectomy may be more common than suggested by earlier studies. The risk of thrombosis is higher with splenectomy than with other upper abdominal operations. The syndrome is most commonly associated with splenectomy for myeloproliferative and hematologic indications but occurs also in the setting of splenectomy performed for trauma. In addition to the underlying indication for splenectomy, risk factors also include hypercoagulable state and splenomegaly, due to the proportionately larger diameter of the stump and consequent increased stasis. Other causes of stasis include increased viscosity associated with leukocytosis and thrombocytosis and decreased plasticity of erythrocytes from the high number of nuclear remnants in the absence of the filtering spleen. Although many patients remain asymptomatic and never come to clinical attention, others present with abdominal pain, diarrhea, nausea, vomiting or fever, or several years later with variceal bleeding because of portal hypertension. Occasionally the syndrome presents with extensive intestinal gangrene leading to death.

Patency of veins may be assessed by abdominal ultrasound with color flow Doppler imaging with a specificity of 99% and sensitivity of 93%. CT is less sensitive but is useful especially for imaging within the first postoperative week when ileus and bowel distention diminish the reliability of ultrasound. Each of these techniques is also helpful in concurrently evaluating other diagnoses with similar presentations such as acute pancreatitis, intraabdominal abscess, bilomas, and infected hematomas.

Failure to institute appropriate therapy expediently can result in complications such as bowel infarction or later portal hypertension with varices and bleeding. Treatment involves systemic heparinization followed by long-term oral anticoagulation. Some studies report use of thrombolytic therapy with success. Overall, successful recanalization appears to depend on prompt recognition and initiation of treatment. One study found complete recanalization in 40% of patients and partial recanalization in 60% after several months of anticoagulant therapy.

Measures to prevent thrombosis in predisposed individuals include subcutaneous prophylactic heparin perioperatively into the postoperative period and aspirin or dipyridamole started on the first postoperative day. Routine preoperative and interval postoperative Doppler ultrasound evaluation in high-risk individuals such as those with myeloproliferative or hematologic disorders has been suggested, but the efficacy of this has not been established.

Bibliography

Chaffanjon PCJ, Brichon PY, Ranchoup Y, et al. Portal vein thrombosis following splenectomy for hematologic disease: prospective study with Doppler color flow imaging. *World J Surg* 1998;22:1082–1086.

Hassn AMF, Al-Fallouji MA, Ouf TI, et al. Portal vein thrombosis following splenectomy. *Br J Surg* 2000;87: 367–368.

Petit P, Bret PM, Atri M, et al. Splenic vein thrombosis after splenectomy: frequency and role of imaging. *Radiology* 1994;190(1):65–68.

Rattner DW, Ellman L, Warshaw AL. Portal vein thrombosis after elective splenectomy: an underappreciated, potentially lethal syndrome. *Arch Surg* 1993;128:565–570.

Schwartz SI. Splenectomy and splenorrhaphy. In: Baker RJ, Fischer JE (eds.), *Mastery of Surgery*, 4th ed. Philadelphia, PA: Lippincott Williams &Wilkins, 2001, pp. 1691–1699.

Vant RM, Burger JWA, van Muiswinkel JM, et al. Diagnosis and treatment of portal vein thrombosis following splenectomy. *Br J Surg* 2000;87:1229–1233.

Winslow ER, Brunt LM, Drebin JA, et al. Portal vein thrombosis after splenectomy. *Am J Surg* 2002;184:631–636.

5. **(C)** Isolated thrombosis of the splenic vein occurs most commonly as a consequence of an underlying pancreatic inflammatory process or from infiltration by a neighboring pancreatic malignancy. Pancreatitis may externally compress the vein by glandular enlargement, by adjacent pseudocyst, or by fibrosis and encasement by surrounding tissues. The vessel may thus be patent but functionally occluded or actually thrombosed because of stasis, intimal injury from pancreatitis, or by systemic hypercoagulability.

Flow is consequently diverted to the short gastric veins with dilation of the cardiac and fundal submucosal venous plexus. While many patients remain asymptomatic, a significant proportion develop sinistral (left-sided) portal hypertension with isolated gastric varices, or less commonly, coexistent esophageal and gastric or isolated esophageal varices. Esophageal varices develop in this situation only if drainage of the coronary vein is distal to the point of obstruction in the splenic vein. The liver is characteristically normal without cirrhosis and the remainder of the portal system patent. When symptoms develop, the most common clinical presentation is with acute upper gastrointestinal (GI) bleeding, often with the patient in extremis.

In the case of acute bleeding, the diagnostic test of choice is upper endoscopy, especially in patients with known chronic pancreatitis because of alcohol abuse who need evaluation for more common etiologies as the cause of hemorrhage. Isolated gastric varices on endoscopy are pathognomonic. Splenic vein thrombosis is often an incidental finding on abdominal CT performed for other reasons. Although not essential for diagnosis, celiac angiography is considered the gold standard. Magnetic resonance imaging (MRI) and high-resolution ultrasonography may also be used to establish the diagnosis. Evaluation for coexistent pancreatic pathology should also be strongly considered if an underlying etiology is not evident because of the potential for a malignant cause of the occlusion.

Splenectomy is curative and results in reversal of the sequelae of sinistral hypertension including varices by elimination of blood flow into the spleen. Even if splenic thrombosis is discovered incidentally in the absence of symptoms, elective splenectomy is recommended, especially in alcoholic and questionably compliant patient populations. Other interventions such as splenic artery embolization and endoscopic gastric variceal sclerotherapy are under investigation; at the present time these should be considered temporizing measures for the poor operative candidate or unstable patient since the underlying process remains unaddressed and because of the theoretically increased risk of abscess formation.

Bibliography

Fraker DL. Spleen. In: Greenfield LJ, Mulholland MW, Oldham KT, et al. (eds.), *Scientific Principles and Practice of Surgery*, 3rd ed. Philadelphia, PA: Lippincott Williams & Wilkins, 2001, pp. 1236–1259.

Sakorafas GH, Sarr MG, Farley DR, et al. The significance of sinistral portal hypertension complicating chronic pancreatitis. *Am J Surg* 2000;179:129–133.

6. **(C)** Mature erythrocytes rely solely on the anaerobic metabolism of glucose through glycolysis (Embden-Meyerhof's pathway; Fig. 31-4) as their source of energy. Defects in the enzymes that catalyze these reactions may have profound effects on the energetics and behavior of erythrocytes. The most common hereditary enzymatic red cell defect is G6PD deficiency, with over 400 million cases, followed by pyruvate kinase deficiency. Both of these disorders manifest with nonspherocytic hemolytic anemia, although each with a wide range of clinical severity. In G6PD deficiency, defects in glucose metabolism produce less elastic erythrocytes that are trapped by the splenic sinusoids and destroyed. Although anemia may occur, splenomegaly is rare and splenectomy is not beneficial.

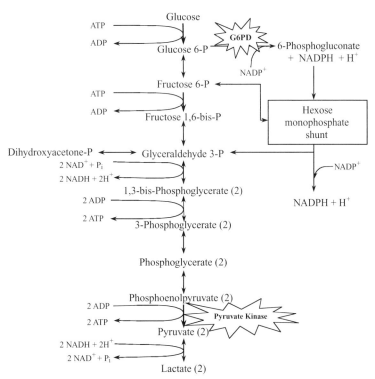

FIG. 31-4   Embden-Meyerhoff's pathway of glycolysis.

Pyruvate kinase converts phosphoenolpyruvate to pyruvate in glycolysis. Four isoenzymes exist, only one (R-PK) of which is normally present in mature erythrocytes. Inheritance is autosomal recessive; the mutated enzyme appears to be more susceptible to adenosine triphosphate (ATP) inhibition and less stable in the presence of heat. Patients often have mild-to-moderate splenomegaly because of sequestration of the less deformable cells. Splenectomy has been shown to decrease transfusion requirements presumably by preventing the trapping of reticulocytes and young red cells.

HPCHA is a rare hematologic disorder characterized by chronic hemolytic anemia of autosomal dominant inheritance. Levels of erythrocyte phosphatidylcholine are elevated while plasma levels are normal. In this situation, splenectomy is not indicated because while the hemolysis remains unaffected, the anemia worsens.

Although they are common indications for splenectomy, neither hereditary spherocytosis nor β-thalassemia are enzymatic disorders. Cold-agglutinin syndrome (IgM autoimmune hemolytic anemia) is an immunologic disorder, and splenectomy is of no benefit.

Bibliography

Gargiulo NJ III, Zenilman ME. Splenectomy for hematologic disorders. In: Cameron JL (ed.), *Current Surgical Therapy*, 7th ed. St. Louis, MO: Mosby, 2001, pp. 587–591.

McMullin MF. The molecular basis of disorders of red cell enzymes. *J Clin Pathol* 1999;52:241–244.

Otsuka A, Sugihara T, Yawata Y. No beneficial effect of splenectomy in hereditary high red cell membrane phosphatidylcholine hemolytic anemia: clinical and membrane studies of 20 patients. *Am J Hematol* 1990;34(1):8–14.

Schwartz SI. Role of splenectomy in hematologic disorders. *World J Surg* 1996;20(9):1156–1159.

7. **(C)** Felty's syndrome, ITP, IgG (warm) autoimmune hemolytic anemia, and systemic lupus erythematosus are acquired autoimmune disorders mediated by an IgG autoantibody against cellular membrane proteins. The spleen plays a dual role in these disorders: it produces IgG and because of its microstructure provides an environment conducive to cell destruction and removal. As cells pass through the spleen, they first encounter the white pulp where antibodies are produced and then the red pulp with its high macrophage content and low concentration of free IgG. Presumably free IgG binds to the macrophage Fc receptors, thus competing for binding sites with IgG opsonizing targeted cells; therapeutic high dose intravenous immunoglobulin may act by competitively inhibiting destruction of targeted cells.

Because of this unique feature of splenic anatomy, cells are thus first opsonized by IgG autoantibodies just prior to contact with macrophages that have receptors for the Fc (heavy chain) end of the IgG molecule. Sequestration and removal occurs preferentially in the spleen, although macrophages in the liver and bone marrow participate to a lesser degree. Splenectomy does not eliminate autoantibody production; it simply ameliorates cell destruction.

In ITP, the antibody targets platelet membrane glycoproteins, in most cases IIb/IIIa. Patients are typically in their 20s or 30s and clinically unremarkable except for nosebleeds, petechiae, or other bleeding with minor trauma. Splenomegaly is uncommon. When thrombocytopenia persists or recurs despite optimal medical management or if patients experience life-threatening complications of the thrombocytopenia such as intracerebral hemorrhage, splenectomy should be performed.

Systemic lupus erythematosus is characterized by production of a wide range of autoantibodies, and 15–20% of patients develop a form of secondary autoimmune thrombocytopenia that is similar to ITP. Similarly, many patients with thrombocytopenia refractory to steroids and immunosuppressive therapy as in ITP appear to have good success to splenectomy.

IgG is directed against the Rh antigen or against one of the minor Rh determinants (c or e) in IgG autoimmune hemolytic anemia. Splenectomy is indicated for patients who experience persistent or worsening anemia with medical therapy; a favorable response is achieved in 50–80% of patients.

Felty's syndrome refers to the syndrome of chronic severe rheumatoid arthritis with associated neutropenia and splenomegaly. The specific membrane protein in Felty's syndrome is not known, but accumulation of IgG on the surface of granulocytes has been observed, indicating the presence of a specific membrane antigen. Spleens in these patients have a relatively hypertrophic white pulp on gross examination with elevated concentrations of neutrophils in the white pulp, T-cell zone, and red pulp on microscopy.

Patients experience recurrent infectious complications because of neutropenia and chronic leg ulcers. Following splenectomy, neutropenia resolves in most patients within 2–3 days; at the very least, neutropenic response to infection improves so that 60% of patients experience decreased incidence of infections. The arthritis is unaffected by splenectomy.

IgM cannot directly opsonize its targets since macrophages lack receptors for the Fc fragment of IgM, instead binding complement to produce C3b, which indirectly opsonizes the targeted cell.

Hemolysis in IgM autoimmune hemolytic anemia is thus mediated by complement and takes place intravascularly rather than extravascularly with clinical manifestations resembling Raynaud's syndrome. For these reasons splenectomy plays no role in the management of IgM autoimmune hemolytic anemia.

Bibliography

Fraker DL. Spleen. In: Greenfield LJ, Mulholland MW, Oldham KT, et al. (eds.), *Scientific Principles and Practice of Surgery*, 3rd ed. Philadelphia, PA: Lippincott Williams & Wilkins, 2001, pp. 1236–1259.

Galindo M, Khamashta MA, Hughes GR. Splenectomy for refractory thrombocytopenia in the antiphospholipid syndrome. *Rheumatology* 1999;38(9):848–853.

Schwartz SI. Role of splenectomy in hematologic disorders. *World J Surg* 1996;20(9):1156–1159.

Weintraub LR. Splenectomy: who, when, and why? *Hosp Pract* 1994:27–34.

8. **(A)** Workup for splenomegaly should include a thorough history and examination including family history, past medical history, and history of substance abuse, travel or residence in a foreign country, medications as well as a history of any constitutional symptoms or history of bleeding. Early satiety or other mechanical symptoms may be reported if significant splenomegaly is present. Laboratory evaluation should include a complete blood count with platelet count, serum chemistries and liver function tests, autoimmune antibody panel, antibodies to Epstein-Barr virus (EBV), angiotensin converting enzyme levels (for sarcoidosis), peripheral smear, bone marrow biopsy. Flow cytometry and immunohistochemistry may also be helpful. CT or MRI should also be performed, especially if tumor is suspected.

Seven to fifteen percent of patients with splenomegaly have an undefined etiology despite exhaustive diagnostic evaluation. Dacie first described a syndrome of nontropical idiopathic splenomegaly in the absence of immune thrombocytopenia, B symptoms of lymphoma, or lymphadenopathy in 1969. Since then, multiple other retrospective studies have been performed, several in recent years, which confirm the high incidence of occult lymphoma in these patients discovered with diagnostic splenectomy ranging between 39 and 70%. Remarkably, most of these patients have no other manifestations of the underlying illness except for mild thrombocytopenia and anemia in some. Primary splenic lymphoma comprises less than 1% of all cases of lymphoma; these are predominantly B-cell non-Hodgkin's type of variable clinical behavior. Frequently analysis of bone marrow peripheral blood analysis and lymph nodes is negative. Caught early, these can often be treated successfully, frequently by splenectomy alone. In one recent series of 18 cases of splenomegaly with negative workup, splenectomy provided a diagnosis in 100% of patients, with a 22% minor morbidity rate and no major complications or mortalities. Thus, diagnostic splenectomy is a reasonable course of action in patients for whom an explanation cannot be found after a thorough evaluation. Although observation is an alternative, patients must be reliable and must be followed very closely. Aggressive pursuit of an etiology must follow in the absence of a definite diagnosis or clinical resolution within a short period of time.

Fine-needle aspiration is not routinely used for evaluation without a focal mass because of the potential for misdiagnosis among the diseases associated with isolated splenomegaly. Laparoscopic evaluation with biopsy and positron emission tomography (PET) scanning are options to consider but further study is needed to determine their effectiveness.

Other causes of idiopathic splenomegaly include sarcoidosis and a number of benign vascular tumors of the spleen. Diffuse splenic hemangiomatosis is angiomatous involvement of the entire spleen. Patients may present with minimal symptoms or with hypersplenism. Imaging may be nondiagnostic or may show a nonhomogenous texture on radionuclide studies, ultrasonography, or CT scan.

Bibliography

Carr JA, Shurafa M, Velanovich V. Surgical indications in idiopathic splenomegaly. *Arch Surg* 2002;137:64–68.

Kraus MD, Fleming MD, Vonderheide RH. The spleen as a diagnostic specimen: a review of 10 years' experience at two tertiary care institutions. *Cancer* 2001;91(11):2001–2009.

Shiran A, Naschitz JE, Yeshurun D, et al. Diffuse hemangiomatosis of the spleen: splenic hemangiomatosis presenting with giant splenomegaly, anemia, and thrombocytopenia. *Am J Gastroenterol* 1990;85(11):1515–1517.

9. **(B)** The splenic artery arises as one of the three branches from the celiac axis and courses laterally along the posterior wall of the omental bursa mostly external to the parenchyma of the pancreas, through the splenorenal (lienorenal) ligament and into the splenic hilum where it divides into six or more branches. The left gastroepiploic (gastroomental) artery originates from the splenic artery near the hilum. A massively enlarged spleen may parasitize vessels from the mesocolon of the splenic flexure, the diaphragm, or from the omentum.

The splenic vein emerges from the confluence of six or more veins from the splenic hilum. It then passes behind the pancreas below the artery and joins the superior mesenteric vein behind the pancreas to form the portal vein. The portal and systemic circulations intermingle through collateral vessels in this area, and this becomes clinically significant in portal hypertension. In the case of splenic vein occlusion or thrombosis with associated sinistral (left-sided) portal hypertension, drainage of the splenic outflow is diverted to the short gastric veins with subsequent dilation of the cardiac and fundal submucosal venous plexus resulting in isolated gastric varices. Esophageal varices are not typical since in the presence of normal portal pressures and patent coronary vein the esophageal bed is unaffected, but can occur if drainage of the coronary vein is distal to the point of obstruction in the splenic vein.

The spleen is affixed to the left upper quadrant by the splenorenal (lienorenal), gastrosplenic (gastrolienal), splenocolic suspensory ligaments, and more variably by the splenoomental and splenophrenic (phrenicolienal) attachments. The splenogastric ligament forms the mesentery between the spleen and stomach and contains the short gastric and left gastroepiploic vessels. The splenorenal ligament attaches the spleen to Gerota's fascia of the upper left kidney and contains the main splenic artery and vein. The splenophrenic, splenoomental, and splenocolic are considered relatively avascular but must be divided carefully because of small vessels that are often present, especially in disease states.

Bibliography

Fraker DL. Spleen. In: Greenfield LJ, Mulholland MW, Oldham KT, et al. (eds.), *Scientific Principles and Practice of Surgery*, 3rd ed. Philadelphia, PA: Lippincott Williams & Wilkins, 2001, pp. 1236–1259.

Pansky B (ed.). *Review of Gross Anatomy*, 6th ed. New York, NY: McGraw-Hill, 1996.

Sakorafas GH, Sarr MG, Farley DR, et al. The significance of sinistral portal hypertension complicating chronic pancreatitis. *Am J Surg* 2000;179:129–133.

10. **(D)** Wandering spleen, also called ectopic spleen, is a rare anomaly that results from absence or hyperlaxity of the normal ligamentous attachments to the retroperitoneum and neighboring structures that affix the organ in the left upper quadrant. The splenorenal and gastrosplenic ligaments are particularly critical in immobilizing the spleen. Its original cause is yet unknown. That 70–80% of patients are women of childbearing age supports the theory that hormonal changes lead to an acquired increased laxity of ligaments and excess mobility; however, a developmental etiology in which failure of dorsal mesogastrium fusion to the posterior abdominal wall during embryogenesis results in a wandering spleen is equally plausible, since its incidence is well documented among children. In addition, its association with gastric volvulus in

children has been well documented in the literature, suggesting a common etiology. The mechanical stress placed on attachments by enlarged spleens may also play a role; however, not all cases exhibit splenomegaly. Characteristically the vascular mesentery is elongated and serves as the sole attachment to the spleen, predisposing the organ to axial torsion and infarction. Symptoms of pain may develop chronically when capsular stretching leads to venous engorgement during intermittent episodes of mild torsion.

Clinical presentation varies considerably. Patients frequently present with an asymptomatic abdominal mass or abdominal pain that ranges from chronic intermittent and mild-to-acutely toxic with frank peritonitis because of torsion, infarction, and splenic necrosis. GI symptoms such as vomiting are also common. Acute pancreatitis from involvement of the tail of the pancreas in torsion has also been reported.

CT scan or ultrasonography can be used to establish a diagnosis. Decreased or absent flow may be present on Doppler examination and signifies torsion.

Treatment is operative. Conservative management carries a complication rate of 65%. Prior to discovery of the associated immunologic consequences, splenectomy was routinely performed; however, splenopexy is currently the procedure of choice in the absence of infarction or necrosis, and can be performed by formation of a retroperitoneal pouch, by suturing the spleen to the abdominal wall or diaphragm directly or by using synthetic or bioabsorbable mesh. Laparoscopic splenopexy has also been performed with success. Splenectomy is reserved for cases in which the spleen is nonviable.

Bibliography

Buehner M, Baker M. The wandering spleen. *Surg Gynecol Obstet* 1992;175:373–387.

Sayeed S, Koniaris LG, Kovach SJ, et al. Torsion of a wandering spleen. *Surgery* 2001;135:535–536.

Spector JM, Chappell J. Gastric volvulus associated with wandering spleen in a child. *J Pediatr Surg* 2000;35:641–642.

Steinberg R, Karmazyn B, Dlugy E, et al. Clinical presentation of wandering spleen. *J Pediatr Surg* 2002;37(10):1–4.

11. **(D)** Heterotaxia, or *situs ambiguus*, refers to the malposition and dysmorphism of viscera in the chest and abdomen. In contrast to *situs solitus*, or normal orientation of viscera and vasculature; and *situs inversus*, the complete mirror image of normal; visceral organization in heterotaxia is disorderly and variable among individuals along a wide spectrum. In asplenia (right isomerism, bilateral right-sidedness, double right-sidedness, Ivemark's syndrome) classically both lungs

are trilobar with bilateral minor fissures and eparterial bronchi. Polysplenia (left isomerism, bilateral left-sidedness) is associated with bilateral bilobar lungs.

The syndrome likely results from a disrupted lateralization leading to abnormal chiral development. Heritance appears to be multifactorial. Embryologically, the event occurs at 20–30 days gestation when the primitive heart and venous connections are forming, accounting for the high incidence of anomalies of the heart and great vessels. Incidence of congenital heart disease is estimated at 50–100%, in contrast to 0.6–0.8% in *solitus* and 3–5% in *inversus*. Asplenia has a stronger association with complex cyanotic cardiac malformations while anomalies in polysplenic patients are generally less severe, most commonly atrioventricular canal defects.

Intestinal nonrotation or malrotation is almost universal. The most consistent finding in polysplenic heterotaxia is interrupted inferior vena cava with azygous or hemiazygous continuation, often seen on chest x-ray. A bridging (midline) liver is common, more frequently found in patients with polysplenia than asplenia. Biliary atresia occurs in some patients with polysplenia. Central nervous system (CNS) malformations have also been reported.

Evaluation should include chest x-ray, echocardiography, abdominal ultrasound, and upper GI series. Certain structures must be evaluated to define situs: the atria; the aorta and great veins below the diaphragm with regard to their relationship to midline; the stomach and small bowel for the presence of malrotation; liver and gallbladder; location of the cardiac apex; the spleen or spleens, and lungs. Congenital asplenia should be suspected in any infant with abnormal abdominal viscera or complex congenital heart disease. Diagnosis may be established in a newborn by documentation of Howell-Jolly's bodies on peripheral smear in combination with scintigraphy.

Polysplenia is distinguished from splenosis by its congenital origin; splenosis is splenic autotransplantation and proliferation that most commonly follows trauma. While accessory spleen is a common condition affecting 10–20% of the population, polysplenia is rare and characteristically occurs in conjunction with other abnormalities; in addition the splenic elements each tend to be more substantial. Asplenic individuals have the same immune deficiency as with surgical splenectomy and thus should be given appropriate vaccinations and prophylaxis. Polysplenia is also associated with abnormal splenic function in certain children. Ladd's procedure should be performed in all stable patients with associated malrotation to prevent future midgut volvulus.

Bibliography

Applegate KE, Goske MJ, Pierce G, et al. Situs revisted: imaging of the heterotaxy syndrome. *Radiographics* 1999;19:837–852.

Noack F, Sayk F, Ressel A, et al. Ivemark syndrome with agenesis of the corpus callosum: a case report with review of the literature. *Prenat Diagn* 2002;22:1011–1015.

12. **(A)** This woman had an epidermoid cyst of the spleen. Cysts of the spleen may be classified into true cysts and pseudocysts and into parasitic or nonparasitic. True epidermoid cysts comprise 10–20% of all splenic cysts. They are usually congenital, and are typically solitary, unilocular, and have a squamous epithelial lining. Stratified squamous, transitional, cuboidal, or mesothelial cells may also line true cysts. The epithelial cells frequently produce the tumor markers CA 19-9 and carcinoembryonic antigen (CEA), elevating serum level; despite this, these cysts are benign and do not have an increased malignant potential.

Splenic pseudocysts account for 80% of all splenic cysts and occur most commonly following trauma. They lack an epithelial lining and are usually unilocular with thick, smooth walls composed of fibrous tissue. The incidence has risen in recent years because of the increased use of CT scanning and more widespread use of a nonoperative approach to blunt splenic injury.

Generally, symptoms are caused by the mass effect of the cyst so that cysts less than 8 cm are usually asymptomatic. Patients may present with abdominal fullness, left shoulder or back pain, early satiety, shortness of breath, pleuritic chest pain, or renal symptoms from mass effect. Complications include acute hemorrhage, rupture, or infection.

CT scan is the best modality for diagnosis of a splenic cyst. *Echinococcus* serology (ELISA or Western blot) must be performed prior to any invasive intervention to rule out a parasitic etiology because of the risk of anaphylactic shock with intraabdominal spillage of infective scolices.

Nonparasitic true cysts and pseudocysts should be treated if greater than 10 cm or symptomatic. Traditionally splenectomy has been the standard of care; however, spurred by the increased awareness of the immunologic consequences surrounding splenectomy and the rising popularity of minimally invasive surgery, techniques of splenic preservation are being used more frequently with encouraging results. Partial splenectomy, percutaneous aspiration, decapsulation, and partial cystectomy have all been used successfully to treat nonparasitic true cysts and pseudocysts; however, recurrence of epidermoid cysts following incomplete removal of the epithelial lining with partial cystectomy and marsupialization has been reported. Resected tissue should be evaluated by pathology since both benign and malignant primary cystic tumors of the spleen, although extremely rare, can mimic epidermoid cysts.

Under less favorable conditions, patients should receive immunizations against encapsulated bacteria prior to surgery in the event that splenectomy becomes necessary.

Reticulocytosis would be present in cases of hemolysis or blood loss not as a result of a splenic cyst. p53 and EBV IgM titer are not involved in the pathogenesis and are not routinely evaluated in such a patient.

13. **(A)** Most true splenic cysts are because of parasites and remain prevalent in areas of endemic hydatid infection. Worldwide, *Echinococcus* infection is the most frequent cause. Abdominal ultrasound and CT scan of the abdomen both typically demonstrates daughter cysts and cyst wall calcifications; associated hepatic cysts are also common. Although an uncommon cause of splenic cysts in North America, the diagnosis must be always be excluded by *Echinococcus* serology (ELISA or Western blot) prior to any invasive intervention to rule out the presence of parasites because of the risk of anaphylactic shock with intraabdominal spillage of infective scolices. Patients should undergo splenectomy with intraoperative injection of hypertonic saline, alcohol, or silver nitrate prior to removal.

Splenic abscess is a rare but potentially lethal condition. Immunocompromised patients and patients who abuse IV drugs are particularly susceptible. They develop by four basic mechanisms: metastatic hematogenous spread from a distant source such as osteomyelitis or infective endocarditis; following trauma or iatrogenic injury, especially with increasing use of nonoperative management; secondary infection following splenic infarction such as in sickle cell and splenic embolization; and by extension from a contiguous infective source such as a perinephric, pancreatic, or diverticular abscess. They are primarily unilocular in adults but multilocular in children. *Staphyloccoccus* and *Streptococcus* species account for 30% of cases; other common organisms include *Enterococcus*, *Salmonella*, and *Escherichia coli*. They tend to have a heterogeneous appearance on CT while cysts tend to be homogeneous. Patients should be treated promptly with broad-spectrum antibiotics. Unilocular abscesses may be percutaneously aspirated but multilocular abscesses usually require splenectomy. Partial splenectomy, splenotomy with drainage, and laparoscopic splenectomy have all been used with success. They may be complicated by

intraperitoneal rupture, rupture into adjacent organs, and with possible subsequent formation of a fistula. Given the patient's history and homogeneous appearance of the cyst on CT scan, a splenic abscess is highly unlikely.

Infectious mononucleosis may manifest with splenomegaly, fever, and adenopathy but rarely produces a cystic mass except possibly in the case of a traumatic pseudocyst resulting from subcapsular rupture. Symptomatic pseudocysts should be managed operatively or through percutaneous drainage. Again, the CT scan does not support this diagnosis nor does it suggest a hematologic malignancy.

Bibliography

Beauchamp RD, Holzman MD, Fabian TC. Spleen. In: Townsend CM, Beauchamp RD, Evers BM, et al. (eds.), *Textbook of Surgery: The Biological Basis of Modern Surgical Practice*, 16th ed. Philadelphia, PA: WB Saunders, 2001, pp. 1144–1164.

Ganti AL, Sardi A, Gordon J. Laparoscopic treatment of large true cysts of the liver and spleen is ineffective. *Am Surg* 2002;68(11):1012–1017.

Harris JA, Gadacz TR. Tumors, cysts, and abscesses of the spleen. In: Cameron JL (ed.), *Current Surgical Therapy*, 7th ed. St. Louis, MO: Mosby, 2001, pp. 591–595.

Sellers GJ, Starker PM. Laparscopic treatment of a benign splenic cyst. *Surg Endosc* 1997;11:766–768.

14. **(A)** Nonoperative management of blunt splenic injuries was stimulated by our growing understanding of the spleen's immunologic significance and the consequences surrounding its removal. Increasingly, prompted by the success with nonoperative management of splenic injuries in children, similar injuries in adults are now routinely treated nonoperatively. In the early trauma experience, only low-grade injuries were treated nonoperatively, but higher grade injuries are now increasingly managed conservatively with reasonable success. The current EAST guidelines for management of blunt injury to the liver and spleen conclude that in the hemodynamically stable patient, nonoperative management of splenic injuries in both children and adults is the treatment of choice regardless of the grade of injury. Nonoperative therapy avoids the risks and complications associated with abdominal surgery, transfusion, anesthesia as well as the additional financial burden involved with nontherapeutic operation. A number of studies indicate that the transfusion requirement is decreased with nonoperative therapy when compared to surgery.

Absolute contraindications to nonoperative management of splenic injuries include hemodynamic instability and concomitant serious intraabdominal injuries that require surgery. Major disruption of hilar vessels is another contraindication for splenic salvage. In addition, institutional resources such as available operating personnel and facilities and the ability for critical care monitoring should be available in case of acute bleeding requiring splenectomy.

While scintigraphy, diagnostic peritoneal lavage (DPL), laparoscopy, and ultrasound have all been used successfully in the assessment of splenic injury, the most specific, sensitive and accurate modality for determination of the severity and extent of injury is CT scan, which also provides the additional benefit of assessment of retroperitoneal injuries.

Hemodynamic status of a patient is the single most reliable criteria predicting the success of nonoperative therapy and in initial stages should be monitored continuously. Other indices such as age of the patient and the presence of a contrast blush on CT abdomen are also associated with an increased risk of failure but are less predictive and should not exclude a patient from a trial of conservative therapy. Grade of injury, hemoperitoneum on CT abdomen as well as concomitant head injury or extraabdominal injury are not accurate predictors of the outcome of nonoperative management.

Bibliography

Alonso M, Brathwaithe C, Garcia V, et al. Practice management guidelines on the nonoperative management of blunt injury to the liver and spleen. EAST Practice Management Guidelines Work Group. Accessed http://www.east.org/tpg/livspleen.pdf 9/12/03

Beauchamp RD, Holzman MD, Fabian TC. Spleen. In: Townsend CM, Beauchamp RD, Evers BM, et al. (eds.), *Textbook of Surgery: The Biological Basis of Modern Surgical Practice*, 16th ed. Philadelphia, PA: WB Saunders, 2001, pp. 1144–1164.

Coon WW. Surgical aspects of splenic disease and lymphoma. *Curr Probl Surg* 1998;35(7):543–546.

Omert LA, Salyer DS, Dunham M, et al. Implications of the "contrast blush" finding on computed tomographic scan of the spleen in trauma. *J Trauma* 2001;51:272–278.

15. **(D)** Severe hemolysis from splenic sequestration of abnormal red cells is a common problem among patients with congenital hemolytic anemia. Splenectomy abrogates the sequestration and destruction of erythrocytes, reducing hemolysis. In hereditary spherocytosis, though the underlying red cell structural abnormality persists, hemolysis resolves and anemia and the transfusion requirement improves.

Recent awareness of the immunologic consequences of splenectomy has fueled a growing interest in splenic conservation procedures such as partial splenectomy, particularly for children, who are at increased risk of overwhelming sepsis because of the lack of specific antibodies against bacteria that develop after exposure to antigens.

Phagocytosis accounts for the spleen's ability to remove intraerythrocytic inclusion bodies from red cells as they pass through its filter; splenectomy results characteristic changes in the peripheral smear because of the persistence of these in the absence of this function. The primary immunologic defect in the asplenic state is in antibody-mediated destruction of encapsulated bacteria. Antibody function and production and phagocytosis are independent functions of the spleen. Therefore, although animal studies suggest that partial splenectomy does confer some protection above the asplenic state, the level of immune competence cannot be inferred directly from the absence or presence of residual phagocytotic activity. In the case of splenosis, the posttraumatic autotransplantation of splenic fragments, even though phagocytosis remains intact judged by the absence of Howell-Jolly's bodies on peripheral smear, patients clearly remain susceptible to lethal postsplenectomy infections. No study thus far has been able to conclusively measure the level of immunologic protection remaining after selective arterial embolization or ligation or partial splenic resection.

For equivalent volumes of residual splenic tissue after partial splenectomy, among hemoglobinopathies, hereditary spherocytosis has the best preservation of splenic phagocytotic function.

Following splenectomy, hypertrophy of the remaining segment is the norm and occurs primarily during the first year after surgery. Even with regrowth to 75–100% of the original size of the spleen, hemolysis does not necessarily recur.

Selective ligation of vascular structures prior to parenchymal resection does not consistently result in a predictable amount of residual splenic mass because of the absence of discrete splenic lobules and the prevalence of aberrant arterial supply to the various segments. Because of the technically challenging nature of the operation, all patients should be also consented for total splenectomy and preoperatively receive immunizations against *Pneumococcus*, *Niseria meningitides*, and *Haemophilus influenzae*, optimally at least 2 weeks prior to surgery.

Bibliography

Bader-Meunier B, Gauthier F, Archambaud F, et al. Long-term evaluation of the beneficial effect of subtotal splenectomy for management of hereditary spherocytosis. *Blood* 2001;97:399–403.

Rice HE, Oldham KT, Hillery CA, et al. Clinical and hematologic benefits of partial splenectomy for congenital hemolytic anemia in children. *Ann Surg* 2003; 237(2):281–288.

Styrt B. Infection associated with asplenia: risks, mechanisms, and prevention. *Am J Med* 1990;88:5-33-40N.

16. (E) In addition to the risk of overwhelming septicemia from encapsulated bacteria, splenectomy may increase the long-term risk for a variety of other conditions.

Hypercoagulable states and thromboembolic disease appear to occur more frequently in a variety of inherited human hemolytic diseases and in a murine model of hereditary spherocytosis.

The increased risk of death from ischemic heart disease after splenectomy has been recognized since the 1970s. The exact pathophysiology is not known, but a number of factors are reasonable: the increased hematocrit, mild-to-moderate thrombocytosis, and elevated cholesterol levels in those with hereditary spherocytosis following splenectomy. In one review of 144 men with hereditary spherocytosis, a long-term increased incidence of arteriosclerotic events such as stroke, myocardial infarction, and coronary or carotid artery surgery was shown.

The incidence of pulmonary hypertension may be increased as a result of splenectomy. In one retrospective study, the prevalence of surgical asplenia among 61 patients with unexplained severe pulmonary hypertension was compared to that in a control group of 151 patients with pulmonary hypertension because of a variety of other diseases. In the study group, all other confounding factors were eliminated prior to comparison, including recurrent pulmonary embolism. Of the seven postsplenectomy patients, three with spherocytosis had persistent mild hemolysis and normal platelet counts at the time pulmonary hypertension developed. The prevalence of surgical asplenia was found to be 11.5% among the idiopathic group and 0% among controls. The expected prevalence of asplenia in the general population is estimated to be approximately 1%. On histologic analysis, lung tissue in the postsplenectomy patients demonstrated plexiform lesions, intimal fibrosis, and numerous thrombotic lesions. The underlying mechanism of disease remains unclear.

Although pancreatitis occurs in the immediate postoperative period in as many as 7% of cases, no association between splenectomy and the long-term risk of pancreatitis has been shown to exist.

Whether partial splenectomy offers protection against these potential risks is not yet clear.

Bibliography

Andrews DA, Philip SL. Role of red blood cell in thrombosis. *Curr Opin Hematol* 1999;6:76–82.

Bader-Meunier B, Gauthier F, Archambaud F, et al. Long-term evaluation of the beneficial effect of subtotal splenectomy for management of hereditary spherocytosis. *Blood* 2001;97:399–403.

Hoeper MM, Niedermeyer J, Hoffmeyer F, et al. Pulmonary hypertension after splenectomy? *Ann Intern Med* 1999; 130:506–509.

Schilling RF. Spherocytosis, splenectomy, strokes, and heart attacks. *Lancet* 1997;350:1677–1678.

17. (C) Aneurysms of the splenic artery are the most prevalent splanchnic artery macroaneurysm, accounting for 60% of cases. Although rare, improvements in radiologic imaging have resulted in an increased awareness of their significance. They are four times more common among women but occur in almost 10% of patients with portal hypertension with equal distribution among genders. Rarely, they may occur as a result of congenital anomalies of the foregut circulation. They occur most often external to the pancreatic parenchyma except when induced by periarterial chronic pancreatitis.

Three factors have been identified as fundamental to the development of these lesions: arterial fibrodysplasia, pregnancy with its hemodynamic changes and estrogen-related effects on elastic vascular tissue, and cirrhosis with portal hypertension. Pregnancy, especially with multiparity, is a major risk factor for both the development and rupture of aneurysms, with a rate of rupture approaching 95% in lesions identified during pregnancy. Aneurysms less commonly result from penetrating trauma, periarterial inflammation as in the case of chronic pancreatitis, or a systemic vasculitic process.

They are predominantly saccular, occur at vessel bifurcations, and occur multiply in 20% of cases. Pancreatic lesions tend to be solitary and occur proximally. Aneurysms are usually found incidentally during studies performed for other reasons and can be diagnosed with arteriography, MRI, color flow Doppler ultrasound, and CT scan. When seen on plain abdominal films they classically appear as signet ring calcifications in the left upper quadrant.

Patients may be asymptomatic or they may present with midepigastric or left upper quadrant pain. On rupture patients may remain hemodynamically stable if the bleeding remains confined to the lesser sac or they may present in extremis with free intraperitoneal rupture. Less commonly GI bleeding may be the presentation, resulting either from rupture of a pancreatitis-induced aneurysm into adjacent hollow viscera or from esophageal varices that form after rupture of the aneurysm into the neighboring splenic vein produces an arteriovenous fistula. Pregnancy-related lesions have a much higher rate of rupture compared to the 2% risk in other populations. Rupture typically occurs during the third trimester with a very high mortality rate for both the mother and fetus and thus mandates operative intervention.

Treatment of choice is simple aneurysm ligation or exclusion with vascular reconstruction. Distal pancreatectomy may be needed for the aneurysm imbedded within the pancreas. Splenectomy is another alternative; however, although formerly the standard of care, given the risks of OPSI, it should be avoided when possible.

Bibliography

Dave SP, Reis ED, Hossain A, et al. Splenic artery aneurysm in the 1990s. *Ann Vasc Surg* 2000;14:223–229.

Stanley JC, Henke PK. Splanchnic artery aneurysms. In: Greenfield LJ, Mulholland MW, Oldham KT, Zelenock GB, Lillemoe KD (eds.), *Scientific Principles and Practice of Surgery*, 3rd ed. Philadelphia, PA: Lippincott Williams & Wilkins, 2001, pp. 1834–1850.

Zarins CK, Hill BB, Wolf YG. Aneurysmal vascular disease. In: Townsend CM, Beauchamp RD, Evers BM, et al. (eds.), *Textbook of Surgery: The Biological Basis of Modern Surgical Practice*, 16th ed. Philadelphia, PA: WB Saunders, 2001, pp. 1357–1372.

18. (D)

19. (A)

Explanations 18 and 19

The spleen's cellular composition and microstructure account for its unique contribution to the body's immunologic defense that cannot be fully compensated for in its absence. The relatively stagnant flow of blood through the splenic microcirculation encourages prolonged contact and interaction between antigens and lymphocytes both for initiation and amplification of the immune response and for phagocytosis. It is a major site for formation of specific antibodies early in the course of infection. The spleen participates in both humoral- and cell-mediated immunity and helps to opsonize microorganisms through both the classic and alternate complement activation pathways. It is important in the primary response as well as in formation of immunologic memory for efficient subsequent responses to an antigen.

Lack of type-specific antibodies impairs the liver's ability to compensate for the absent spleen and is central to the immune deficiency experienced by asplenic patients against encapsulated bacteria. Serum complement activation is essential for bacterial uptake by the liver, the other major solid organ in the reticuloendothelial system. The complement components C3b and iC3b bind to foreign particles and to complement receptors on phagocytic cells. This is called immune adherence and leads to subsequent phagocytosis of the opsonized bacteria.

Antibodies facilitate hepatic clearance of organisms opsonized with complement primarily through their ability to mediate complement deposition on bacteria. Without a specific antibody, complement binds directly to the surface of bacterial cell wall through the alternate pathway. In this way, unencapsulated bacteria can be cleared almost totally by the liver; however, in the case of encapsulated bacteria, complement bound to the bacterial cell wall is inaccessible for immune adherence because of the thick polysaccharide capsule around the cell wall, preventing clearance. Opsonization of bacteria by anticapsular antibody allows C3b deposition by the classical pathway, that is, by interaction of complement with bound antibody.

Experimentally, while phagocytosis of encapsulated bacteria occurs in the liver in immunized animals, in the absence of anticapsular antibodies in nonimmune animals, clearance of these microorganisms takes place predominantly in the spleen through sequestration. In addition, clearance of organisms by the classical pathway is effectively triggered at levels of IgG far below the threshold for activation of complement. In this respect the spleen is more sensitive than the liver for clearance of bacteria in the nonimmune individual.

IgM is produced in the primary response to an antigen. IgG is the predominant antibody produced in the secondary response, that is, against subsequent exposures, and represents memory of the system to prior offenders to facilitate a bigger and faster response the second time. Gene rearrangement in B cells results in production of a clone of cells that produce antibodies of a different immunoglobulin class with identical antigenic specificity. This process is called type-switching and is central to the secondary response. Studies demonstrate that after splenectomy, although appropriate B cells exist, individuals have defective type-switching and insufficient maturation of the secondary response, producing IgM instead of IgG after secondary immunization by an antigen. Other investigators have shown quantitative deficiencies in IgM. Taken together, these data explain the particular susceptibility of these patients to infections with encapsulated bacteria characterized by their rapid proliferation and dissemination.

Tuftsin is a tetrapeptide derived from enzymatic cleavage of the heavy chain of IgG. It has been shown to enhance phagocytosis and plays an ancillary role in opsonization of bacteria; the deficiency seen in asplenic individuals (because of decreased IgG) may contribute to the impaired immune response seen in these patients. The spleen is a major source of properdin, another nonspecific opsonin;

following splenectomy, decreased levels are responsible for impaired alternative pathway activation.

T cells are not essential for initiating of the antibody response against capsular polysaccharides; however, they are important for regulating the magnitude of the response. Patients with Hodgkin's lymphoma may be at increased risk for secondary hematologic malignancies following splenectomy. Risk of cancer may be increased following splenectomy in patients with immunodeficiency states: kidney transplantation, primary immunodeficiency, AIDS, and autoimmune disease. In individuals with an otherwise intact immune system risk does not appear to be increased.

The spleen does not neutralize bacterial endotoxin.

Bibliography

Bohnsack JF, Brown EJ. The role of the spleen in resistance to infection. *Annu Rev Med* 1986;37:49–59.

Chapman WC, Newman M. Disorders of the spleen. In: Lee GR, Foerster J, Luken SJ, et al. (eds.), *Wintrobe's Clinical Hematology*, 10th ed. Baltimore, MD: Williams & Wilkins, 1999, pp. 1969–1989.

Styrt B. Infection associated with asplenia: risks, mechanisms, and prevention. *Am J Med* 1990;88:5-33-42N.

Sullivan JL, Ochs HD, Schiffman G, et al. Immune response after splenectomy. *Lancet* 1978:178–181.

20. **(A)** Hodgkin's disease has the distinct feature of a predictable stepwise progression from one lymphatic bed to the next, in a cephalad to caudal direction in 90% of cases. In other words, the cervical, chest, and mediastinal lymph nodes are characteristically involved before spreading to the abdominal nodes. Limitation of nodal involvement to the upper body means that often the disease can be treated exclusively by radiation therapy. Staging laparotomy is generally performed to determine whether a patient needs systemic chemotherapy and can be helpful if the status of abdominal involvement is not clear after CT scanning. With improvements in imaging, the need for traditional exploratory surgery for staging of Hodgkin's lymphoma has largely been obviated; however, in stage IA or IIA, a staging procedure can be used to make this determination. The development of minimally invasive techniques has significantly diminished the morbidity of the procedure and has revived interest in surgical staging of patients.

Staging laparotomy for Hodgkin's lymphoma is performed in a stepwise progression. Conventionally, an open technique had been used; however, with recent reports by multiple investigators of successful laparoscopic staging, a laparoscopic approach may become more common as the experience with this

grows. Preoperative lymphangiography should be performed to identify suspicious nodes. Intraoperatively, a core liver biopsy of each lobe is performed with a Tru-cut needle, followed by wedge biopsy of the free edge of the left lateral segment. If the frozen section shows hepatic involvement, the procedure is terminated, since this mandates chemotherapy. If the liver is clear, splenectomy is then performed and the spleen is evaluated histologically. In the presence of splenic involvement, because entire field lymph node irradiation can treat this, the procedure is aborted and the abdomen closed. In the absence of hepatic or splenic involvement, systematic sampling of the lymph nodes should next be performed: periaortic, internal iliac, portal, celiac, and mesenteric beds, as well as any suspicious nodes seen on preoperative lymphangiography. Clips placed at the time of removal of the last set of nodes allow intraoperative radiologic confirmation of their removal based on preoperative lymphangiography. Oophoropexy with placement of radioopaque clips to identify margins to mark fields helps to protect the ovaries from radiation and increases the likelihood that fertility will be preserved. Finally, iliac biopsy should be performed at the conclusion of the procedure to evaluate for marrow involvement.

Bibliography

Baccarani U, Carroll BJ, Hiatt JR, et al. Comparison of laparoscopic and open staging in Hodgkin disease. *Arch Surg* 1998;133:517–522.

Fraker DL. Spleen. In: Greenfield LJ, Mulholland MW, Oldham KT, et al. (eds.), *Scientific Principles and Practice of Surgery*, 3rd ed. Philadelphia, PA: Lippincott Williams & Wilkins, 2001, pp. 1236–1259.

Johna S, Lefor AT. Laparoscopic evaluation of lymphoma. *Semin Surg Oncol* 1998;15:176–182.

Walsh RM, Heniford BT. Role of laparoscopy for Hodgkin's and Non-Hodgkin's lymphoma. *Semin Surg Oncol* 1999;16:284–292.

21. **(E)** Prior to the development of combination chemotherapy in the 1960s, advanced stage Hodgkin's lymphoma was almost universally fatal. In large part because of the morbidity and mortality associated with staging laparotomy and potential delay in treatment, with few exceptions, in most centers both early- and late-stage disease is currently managed with chemotherapy, with or without radiation. Occasionally, patients may experience symptoms related to associated cytopenias; splenectomy may become necessary for completion of chemotherapy.

Outside of clinical trials, the agents used are adriamycin, bleomycin, vinblastine, and dacarbazine

(ABVD) and may be administered alone or in combination with radiation or as a hybrid regimen together with MOPP (mechlorethamine (nitrogen mustard), vincristine, procarbazine, and prednisone). Taxol (Paclitaxel) is not used in the management of Hodgkin's disease.

The major risk with ABVD therapy is pulmonary fibrosis and affects approximately 3% of individuals. Bleomycin has substantial pulmonary toxicity even years after treatment, and any history of therapy with the drug should prompt careful evaluation and perioperative fluid and ventilatory management. Its effects may be further potentiated if combined with thoracic radiation. Less commonly, it is associated with development of hemolytic-uremic syndrome. Adriamycin (doxorubicin) therapy is most notably associated with dose-dependent, irreversible cardiotoxicity that is also exacerbated by radiation therapy and is another long-term effect of chemotherapy, with a relative risk of death from cardiac disease after treatment of 3.1 times normal. Other sequelae include osteonecrosis and hypothyroidism.

MOPP is associated with significant toxicity, most notably myelosuppression, and carries an increased risk of myelodysplasia, leukemia, and infertility when used alone. It can be used for primary therapy; however, a significant number develop resistance. More commonly, it is used as hybrid therapy together with ABVD, and this regimen appears to have therapeutic equivalence with ABVD and does not appear to carry the same risks of acute leukemia or pulmonary fibrosis, although many still develop infertility.

Bibliography

Armitage A, Longo DL. Malignancies of lymphoid cells. In: Braunwald E, Fauci AS, Kasper DL, et al. (eds.), *Harrison's Principles of Internal Medicine*, 15th ed. New York: McGraw-Hill; 2001, pp. 715–727.

Fung HC, Nademanee AP. Approach to Hodgkin's lymphoma in the new millennium. *Hematol Oncol* 2002;20:1–15.

Schwartz SI. Role of splenectomy in hematologic disorders. *World J Surg* 1996;20(9):1156–1159.

22. **(C)** ITP is an autoimmune disorder in which the antibody targets platelet membrane glycoprotein IIb/IIIa. Patients are typically in their 20s or 30s and clinically unremarkable except for nosebleeds, petechiae, or other mucocutaneous bleeding with minor trauma. Approximately 50% of patients are children, characteristically presenting after a viral illness. Among adults, women are affected twice as frequently as men. Splenomegaly is uncommon except in children. The diagnosis is difficult to establish and remains one of exclusion. In adults, an underlying cause should be sought, including evaluation for other autoimmune diseases, lymphoproliferative disease, and viral infection. Certain medications such as quinidine and heparin are other etiologies of secondary ITP.

Medical therapy consists of high dose corticosteroids and intravenous immune globulin. In selected patients anti-D immune globulin may be helpful. Only 15% of patients respond to medical interventions and thus most adult patients require splenectomy.

Splenectomy is currently indicated (1) for persistent symptomatic thrombocytopenia after 4–6 weeks of medical therapy, (2) when toxic doses of steroids are necessary to induce remission, and (3) with recurrent thrombocytopenia following initial improvement with steroids. Intracerebral hemorrhage is a life-threatening complication and mandates emergent splenectomy. A favorable response to splenectomy is obtained in 85% of patients undergoing surgery. Predictors of success include initial response to medical therapy, younger age, short duration of disease, and prompt thrombocytosis after surgery.

ITP is typically self-limited in children and in most cases resolves within 12 months with medical management and activity restriction; 10–30% of cases become chronic but respond well to splenectomy.

Laparoscopic management has proven to be safe and cost-effective, with less postoperative pain, earlier return to regular diet and shorter hospitalization compared to the open procedure; results in ITP also compare favorably with laparoscopic splenectomy performed for other hematologic indications. The procedure has been reported to have a higher incidence of missed accessory spleens; thus a careful exploration should be performed at the start of the procedure. Any postoperative persistent thrombocytopenia should prompt careful workup with red cell scintigraphy to evaluate for residual splenic tissue before aggressive medical therapy is resumed. Reexploration for a missed accessory spleen appears to be effective with minimal associated morbidity. Preoperative scintigraphy and CT scanning for detection of accessory spleens has not proven sufficiently sensitive to be a cost-effective modality and is not recommended.

Bibliography

Cines DB, Blanchette VS. Immune thrombocytopenic purpura. *N Engl J Med* 2002;346(13):995–1008.

Cordera F, Long KH, Nagorney DM, et al. Open versus laparoscopic splenectomy for idiopathic thrombocytopenic purpura: clinical and economic analysis. *Surgery* 2003;134:45–52.

Gargiulo NJ III, Zenilman ME. Splenectomy for hematologic disorders. In: Cameron JL (ed.), *Current Surgical Therapy*, 7th ed. St. Louis, MO: Mosby, 2001, pp. 587–591.

Katkhouda N, Grant SW, Mavor E, et al. Predictors of response after laparoscopic splenectomy for immune thrombocytopenic purpura. *Surg Endosc* 2001;15(5): 484–488.

23. **(B)** Hemolytic anemia is an important cause of cholelithiasis and discovery of bilirubinate stones in a previously undiagnosed patient should prompt a search for an underlying etiology. Hemolysis can be diagnosed by the presence of reticulocytosis in the absence of bleeding. Other tests such as serum haptoglobin are less specific and are supplementary. Screening for sickle hemoglobinopathies is now routinely included in most neonatal screening programs.

The spleen often plays an important role in hemolytic disease, frequently sequestering abnormal or misshapen cells, leading to their early destruction. In sickle cell anemia, cells occlude the sinusoids and lead to splenomegaly, abscess formation, and infarction. After multiple episodes, the spleen may fibrose and cease to function. This is known as *autosplenectomy* and frequently occurs in children affected with sickle cell anemia by 1 year of age. Patients with sickle cell anemia are at extremely high risk for septicemia and must be treated as asplenic patients with careful attention to prophylactic oral penicillin and immunization against encapsulated bacteria. Prophylactic penicillin may reduce the risk of sepsis by as much as 84%.

β-Thalassemia is a heritable disorder which in its homozygous form is the most common cause of transfusion-dependent anemia in children worldwide. The primary defect is a quantitative deficiency in globin chain production that leads to microcytic and hypochromic anemia. Anemia develops after 3–4 months of life with the decline in production of fetal hemoglobin. Inadequate treatment results in massive hepatosplenomegaly, bony cortical thinning, and characteristic facial deformities. Diagnosis is by peripheral blood smear and hemoglobin electrophoresis. Treatment is primarily supportive with iron chelation and transfusion to maintain a hemoglobin of 9–10 g/dL. High transfusion requirements (greater than 200–250 mL/kg per year) often result in hypersplenism; requirements may be reduced significantly with splenectomy. Even with appropriate immunization and penicillin prophylaxis, among asplenic patients, these individuals have one of the highest rates of postsplenectomy sepsis.

In autoimmune hemolytic anemia, the body produces IgG or IgM directed against the Rh antigen or against one of the minor Rh determinants (c or e).

Splenectomy is indicated in IgG (warm) autoimmune hemolytic anemia if patients experience persistent or worsening anemia with medical therapy; a favorable response is achieved in 50–80% of patients. Surgery plays no role in the management of IgM (cold) autoimmune hemolytic anemia.

Thrombotic thrombocytopenic purpura is a disorder of unknown etiology that results in microvascular occlusion by subendothelial and luminal deposition of hyaline material. The classic clinical pentad consists of fever, hemolytic anemia, purpura, neurologic symptoms, and renal failure. Management is essentially medical, although splenectomy may be indicated in selected refractory cases.

Hereditary spherocytosis is an autosomal dominant disorder caused by a defect in spectrin, a membrane protein in red cells. It is the most common hemolytic anemia for which splenectomy is performed. Cells are less plastic and pass through the spleen with difficulty; trapping and sequestration result in mild-to-moderate hemolytic anemia, jaundice, and splenomegaly. Incidence of pigmented gallstones is estimated at 30–60% and in many patients cholecystectomy is performed at the time of splenectomy. Although splenectomy does not correct the membrane defect, anemia resolves because of hemolysis is stopped. Because of concerns of postsplenectomy sepsis, splenectomy should be postponed until children are 6 years old or above.

Of the above listed hemolytic disorders, sickle cell anemia alone characteristically results in a shrunken spleen. The others typically have a normal spleen or mild splenomegaly.

Bibliography

Lane PA, Nuss R, Ambruso DR. Hematologic disorders. In: Hay WH, Hayward AR, Levin MF, et al. (eds.), *Current Pediatric Diagnosis and Treatment*, 15th ed. New York: McGraw-Hill; 1999, pp. 741–792.

Schwartz SI. Role of splenectomy in hematologic disorders. *World J Surg* 1996;20(9):1156–1159.

Weintraub LR. Splenectomy: who, when, and why? *Hosp Pract* 1994:27–34.

Winslow GA, Nelson EW. Thrombotic thrombocytopenic purpura: indications for and results of splenectomy. *Am J Surg* 1995;170:182–187.

24. **(D)** Splenosis is the traumatic displacement, autotransplantation, and proliferation of fragmented splenic tissue. It may occur in as many as 75% of cases of splenectomy performed for trauma by some estimates. In elective splenectomy, splenosis correlates with splenic disruption and peritoneal contamination because of poor technique, especially during morcellation and extraction, and can be avoided by careful

dissection and handling of tissues. This condition is distinguished from accessory spleen and from polysplenia by its acquired nature. Histologically the splenetic tissue resembles the parent organ in that all components are present: white pulp, red pulp, and marginal zones. In addition, the fragments retain the ability to clear intraerythrocytic inclusion bodies. Although splenosis appears to correlate with elevated tuftsin levels, it does not appear to protect meaningfully against OPSI.

Polysplenia is a congenital abnormality found in some cases of heterotaxia, or *situs ambiguus*, the malposition and dysmorphism of viscera in the chest and abdomen. In contrast to *situs solitus*, or normal orientation of viscera and vasculature; and *situs inversus*, the complete mirror image of normal; visceral organization in heterotaxia is disorderly and variable among individuals along a wide spectrum. Patients with polysplenia have bilateral left-sidedness (left isomerism) and usually have other abnormalities such as bilateral bilobar lungs, congenital heart disease, and intestinal malrotation. Splenic elements each tend to be more substantial than in splenosis or accessory spleens; however, polysplenia may result in abnormal splenic function in certain children.

Accessory spleens result from incomplete embryologic fusion of splenic elements and have been reported to occur in as many as 15–40% of patients. Failure of splenectomy to treat hematologic disorders such as ITP is frequently because of a missed accessory spleen; thus a careful exploration should be performed at the start of the procedure. Any postoperative persistent thrombocytopenia should prompt careful workup with red cell scintigraphy to evaluate for residual splenic tissue before aggressive medical therapy is resumed. Preoperative scintigraphy and CT scanning for detection of accessory spleens has not proven sufficiently sensitive to be a cost-effective modality and is not recommended.

Bibliography

Applegate KE, Goske MJ, Pierce G, et al. Situs revisted: imaging of the heterotaxy syndrome. *Radiographics* 1999;19:837–852.

Chapman WC, Newman M. Disorders of the spleen. In: Lee GR, Foerster J, Luken SJ, et al. (eds.), *Wintrobe's Clinical Hematology*, 10th ed. Baltimore, MD: Williams & Wilkins, 1999, pp. 1969–1989.

Kaiser AM, Umbach TW, Katkhouda N. Predictors of outcome after laparoscopic splenectomy. *Probl Gen Surg* 2002;19(3):95–101.

Styrt B. Infection associated with asplenia: risks, mechanisms, and prevention. *Am J Med* 1990;88:5-33-42N.

25. **(C)** Laparoscopic splenectomy has rapidly become the standard of care for benign splenic disease in the last decade in both children and adults. Advantages include reduced postoperative pain, earlier mobilization, shorter hospitalization, reduced severity of wound-related complications, and improved postoperative pulmonary toilet. It has proved to be therapeutically equivalent to the open procedure and cost-effective. Lateral positioning, development of bipolar electrocautery and the harmonic scalpel, and standardization of techniques have all contributed to its success.

The application in treatment of malignant disease has been received less enthusiastically, particularly in cases of massive splenomegaly. Definitions of splenomegaly vary in the literature, but from a practical standpoint, a spleen larger than 1 kg results in increased technical difficulty of both open and laparoscopic procedures. Most patients with splenomegaly have a malignant diagnosis and tend to be older and more ill preoperatively so that these three factors tend to occur together. Increased splenic mass even in the absence of a malignant diagnosis substantially increases the technical difficulty of both the open and laparoscopic approaches. In a recent retrospective study, Patel and others found after multivariate analysis that splenic mass was the most powerful predictor of morbidity in 108 consecutive laparoscopic splenectomies, with a 14-fold increase in complications.

Blood transfusion also appears to correlate directly as an independent risk factor with the incidence of infectious complications in a linear, dose-dependent fashion. Other factors such as active perisplenitis, splenic infection, severe obesity, and abdominal adhesions also increase the difficulty of the procedure.

Splenectomy is often performed in HIV-positive patients for HIV-related ITP. HIV-positive status does not appear to adversely affect outcomes and splenectomy has proven effective therapy with a 93% remission rate in autoimmune thrombocytopenia. Of note, HIV-positive patients appear to improve following splenectomy, likely because of elimination of the large viral load carried by splenic lymphocytes, and have been observed to experience delay in onset of AIDS and elevation of CD4+ counts.

Bibliography

Goldstone J. Splenectomy for massive splenomegaly. *Am J Surg* 1978;135:385–388.

Hansen K, Singer DB. Asplenic-hyposplenic overwhelming sepsis: postsplenectomy sepsis revisited. *Pediatr Dev Pathol* 2001;4:105–121.

Kaiser AM, Umbach TW, Katkhouda N. Predictors of outcome after laparoscopic splenectomy. *Probl Gen Surg* 2002;19(3):95–101.

Patel AG, Parker JE, Wallwork B, et al. Massive splenectomy is associated with significant morbidity after laparoscopic splenectomy. *Ann Surg* 2003;238:235–240.

Sullivan JL, Ochs HD, Schiffman G, et al. Immune response after splenectomy. *Lancet* 1978;1(8057):178–181.

26. (A) OPSI is a syndrome of rapidly disseminating, fulminant bacterial sepsis that occurs in asplenic and hyposplenic patients. Encapsulated bacteria are most often responsible, with *Streptococcus pneumoniae* estimated to account for 50–90% of cases, but a wide range of other microorganisms such as *E. coli, Enterococcus, Salmonella, Staphylococcus,* and *Clostridium* species as well as nonbacterial organisms have been implicated. The risk does not appear to diminish with time, and cases several decades after splenectomy have been reported.

The spleen plays an important role in sequestration of microorganisms in the primary exposure to an antigen, and prolonged contact with immune cells in the splenic sinusoids facilitates the prompt manufacture of specific antibodies early in the course of infection and subsequent phagocytosis. Patients without a spleen have delayed amplification of the immune response in both primary and subsequent exposures, and are thus highly susceptible to infections by potent, rapidly disseminating organisms such as *S. pneumoniae.* In addition, while complement effectively opsonizes unencapsulated bacteria for uptake in the liver, complement bound to the cell wall in encapsulated bacteria is buried under the capsule and is thus inaccessible to hepatic phagocytes.

Children under 15 years of age are at highest risk (0.13–8.1%); the incidence in adults is estimated at 0.28–1.9%. The increased susceptibility stems partly from the relative naivety of their immune systems from lack of exposure to a sufficient range of antigens prior to the time of the hyposplenic or asplenic state. In addition, children do not appear to respond as efficiently to vaccination, indicating the involvement of factors innate to the developing immune system. For these reasons, splenectomy is delayed or avoided as much as possible and current recommendations advocate oral penicillin prophylaxis.

Incidence is also clearly related to the reason for the hyposplenic state, or in the case of postsurgical patients the diagnosis for which splenectomy was performed. Patients with thalassemia major, portal hypertension, and hematologic and lymphoproliferative malignancy are at greatest risk, and the lowest incidence is observed in patients who undergo splenectomy for trauma or incidentally as part of other procedures such as gastrectomy. Clinically, the disposition of patients with congenital absence of the spleen and sickle cell disease to developing OPSI is indistinguishable from that of postsurgical patients and these patients should be protected in a similar manner.

Bibliography

Davies JM, Barnes R, Milligan D. Update of the guidelines for the prevention and treatment of infection in patients with absent or dysfunctional spleen. *Clin Med JRCPL* 2002;2:440–443.

Hansen K, Singer DB. Asplenic-hyposplenic overwhelming sepsis: postsplenectomy sepsis revisited. *Pediatr Dev Pathol* 2001;4:105–121.

Styrt B. Infection associated with asplenia: risks, mechanisms, and prevention. *Am J Med* 1990;88:5-33-42N.

27. (E) The spleen plays an important role in defense against a wide range of microorganisms and its activities are mediated through multiple peculiarities unique to its anatomy. The immunologic functions of the spleen cannot be fully duplicated following its removal so that patients become vulnerable to severe, fulminant, life-threatening infection after splenectomy, most notoriously because of encapsulated bacteria. This may be manifested through pneumonia or meningitis; however, in many cases a focus of infection cannot be identified even in the presence of high-grade bacteremia.

The greatest risk is posed by encapsulated bacteria such as *S. pneumoniae (Pneumococcus), N. meningitides (Meningococcus),* and *H. influenzae,* although a multitude of other organisms have been implicated, including gram-negative rods such as *E. coli, Klebsiella, Enterobacter, Proteus, Pseudomonas, Serratia,* and *Salmonella* species; *Enterococcus;* and *Staphylococcus* and *Clostridium* species.

The basic mechanism behind the increased susceptibility to these bacteria is impaired synthesis of specific antibodies in the asplenic or hyposplenic state. Sequestration of microorganisms in the sinusoids results in prolonged contact of bacteria with immune cells as they pass first through the white pulp rich in lymphocytes and then through the red pulp where macrophages are in abundance. This arrangement facilitates the prompt manufacture of specific antibodies early in the course of infection and efficient phagocytosis. Inadequate type-switching from IgM to IgG and sluggish amplification of the specific immune response have also been noted. In addition, because hepatic phagocytosis is heavily dependent on complement-mediated opsonization, while unencapsulated bacteria can be easily opsonized, in the absence of type-specific anticapsular antibodies, complement bound to the cell wall in encapsulated bacteria is buried under the capule and is thus inaccessible to hepatic phagocytes. Hepatic uptake of these bacteria is thus suboptimal in the asplenic state.

The disproportionate risk posed by a select group of organisms in these high-risk patients is the driving rationale behind systematic immunization. All patients should receive immunization against the major organisms, optimally at least 2 weeks prior to splenectomy: *Pneumococcus*, *Meningococcus*, and *H. influenzae* type B vaccination. Prompt hospitalization and empiric intravenous antibiotic therapy is mandatory for any febrile illness and children should receive daily oral penicillin prophylaxis. Although the incidence of OPSI has diminished with rigorous vaccination programs and antibiotic chemoprophylaxis integrated with splenic conservation in surgical management and education, mortality with episodes of OPSI remains high.

Although defects in T-cell-mediated immunity have been reported, otherwise healthy individuals do not appear to be at substantially increased risk for mortality from candidal infection above the general population.

Bibliography

Davies JM, Barnes R, Milligan D. Update of the guidelines for the prevention and treatment of infection in patients with absent or dysfunctional spleen. *Clin Med JRCPL* 2002;2:440–443.

Lynch AM, Kapila R. Overwhelming postsplenectomy infection. *Infect Dis North Am* 1996;10(4):693–707.

Styrt B. Infection associated with asplenia: risks, mechanisms, and prevention. *Am J Med* 1990;88:5-33-42N.

28. **(E)** Immunity is serotype-specific, since specific antibodies are required to confer protection against each serotype. In addition, vaccines protect poorly against less immunogenic serotypes so that individuals remain susceptible despite careful adherence to protocols. Children under 2 years of age have suboptimal antibody responses to vaccination regardless of timing of vaccination because of the immaturity of their immune systems.

Conjugate vaccines are particularly effective in children and other patients with suboptimal immune competence. They are engineered using additional peptide adjuvants to a polysaccharide antigen to enhance immunogenicity. The current *Pneumococcus* vaccine incorporates 23 capsular polysaccharides responsible for 85% of infections and is estimated to have a 57% overall protective efficacy in patients over 5 years old. A conjugated form is not currently available. Asplenic patients who received the earlier

14-valent vaccine should be revaccinated. In addition, data show a decline over time in antibody titers, particularly in young children, and individuals should receive booster revaccination for *Pneumococcus* every 3–5 years, depending on the individual's degree of risk.

The conjugate *H. influenzae* type B vaccine has enhanced T-cell-dependent characteristics over the original unconjugated vaccine with excellent immunologic response even in infants. Integration of this vaccine in pediatric vaccination protocols has virtually eradicated invasive disease in young children and all previously unvaccinated adults should be immunized prior to splenectomy.

The vaccine against *Meningococcus* is a conjugate vaccine against four of the major capsular antigens: A, C, Y, and W135. Response to immunization against *Meningococcus* is more uniformly effective among all populations, even among children under 2 years of age. Serotype B is poorly immunogenic and although the incidence is approximately 60% of isolates, no vaccine exists at the present. Data currently does not support booster revaccination with *Meningococcus* or *H. influenzae* vaccines.

Although most patients have some degree of response to vaccines, data indicate that the response in asplenic individuals is subnormal, and thus current guidelines for vaccination recommend immunization of patients at the earliest possible time, at a minimum of 2 weeks prior to elective splenectomy. In patients immunized postoperatively following emergent splenectomy for trauma, delay of pneumococcal vaccination to 14 days postsplenectomy appeared to correlate with better functional antibody response against a number of serotypes. This benefit should be carefully weighed against the potential for loss to follow-up.

In addition to these measures, patients should receive annual influenza vaccination. Children should receive daily oral penicillin or erythromycin chemoprophylaxis. A high level of suspicion must be maintained for OPSI, and with any evidence of febrile illness, patients should be hospitalized and managed empirically with broad-spectrum systemic antibiotics while cultures are pending.

None of these measures protects completely against OPSI, and numerous cases of sepsis have been reported even with strict compliance with prescribed regimens. These interventions have, however, markedly reduced the incidence of OPSI.

Bibliography

Davies JM, Barnes R, Milligan D. Update of the guidelines for the prevention and treatment of infection in patients with absent or dysfunctional spleen. *Clin Med JRCPL* 2002;2:440–443.

DeBiasi RL, Simoes EAF. Immunization. In: Hay WH, Hayward AR, Levin MF, et al. (eds.), *Current Pediatric Diagnosis and Treatment*, 15th ed. New York: McGraw-Hill; 1999, pp. 215–248.

Keusch GT, Bart KJ. Immunization principles and vaccine use. In: Fauci AS, Braunwald E, Isselbacher KJ, et al. (eds.), *Harrison's Principles of Internal Medicine*, 14th ed., 1998, pp. 758–771.

Lynch AM, Kapila R. Overwhelming postsplenectomy infection. *Infect Dis North Am* 1996;10(4):693–707.

Shatz DV, Schinsky MF, Pais LB, et al. Immune responses of splenectomized trauma patients to the 23-valent pneumococcal polysaccharide vaccine at 1 versus 4 versus 14 days after splenectomy. *J Trauma* 1998;44(5):760–765.

29. (E) The primary indications for splenectomy in the management myeloproliferative and lymphoproliferative malignancies are symptomatic splenomegaly, cytopenias associated with hypersplenism, relief of pain from splenic infarction, and for staging to determine the need for chemotherapy. With the exception of diagnostic applications in Hodgkin's lymphoma, surgical intervention is therefore primarily palliative. Splenomegaly is common and frequently results in hypersplenism, the cellular trapping, and sequestration that lead to splenic enlargement, thrombocytopenia, and anemia. Patients tend to be older with greater morbidity and debilitation and are at higher risk for bleeding and complications than individuals undergoing splenectomy for benign causes. The increased risk of bleeding is related both to preexistent cytopenias as well as organomegaly. Some degree of immunosuppression is in most cases inherent in the primary disease process, and these patients are at particularly high risk for postsplenectomy sepsis. Nevertheless, splenectomy often provides significant relief as well as improvement in cytopenias and should be considered in symptomatic patients and those with refractory cytopenia.

Non-Hodgkin's lymphoma is distinguished from Hodgkin's lymphoma in that progression does not occur in a predictable stepwise fashion and frequently patients present with disseminated disease. Approximately 75% have hypersplenism and many experience correction of hematologic depression following splenectomy. Only in rare cases lymphoma may be limited to the splenic parenchyma and may require no further intervention beyond splenectomy. More commonly patients have splenic predominant features and low-grade disease; in these patients, splenectomy may improve short-term survival.

Although splenectomy is primarily of palliative value for relief of pain and cytopenia in all of the above indications, only in Hodgkin's lymphoma does it play a substantial role in diagnosis. The disease spreads in a predictable anatomic stepwise progression among nodal beds from cranial to caudal in 90% of patients. Staging laparotomy with splenectomy may be of benefit in selected early stage patients to help determine the need for systemic treatment for chemotherapy.

Bibliography

Beauchamp RD, Holzman MD, Fabian TC. Spleen. In: Townsend CM, Beauchamp RD, Evers BM, et al. (eds.), *Textbook of Surgery: The Biological Basis of Modern Surgical Practice*, 16th ed. Philadelphia, PA: WB Saunders, 2001, pp. 1144–1164.

Fraker DL. Spleen. In: Greenfield LJ, Mulholland MW, Oldham KT, et al. (eds.), *Scientific Principles and Practice of Surgery*, 3rd ed. Philadelphia, PA: Lippincott Williams & Wilkins, 2001, pp. 1236–1259.

Harris JA, Gadacz TR. Tumors, cysts, and abscesses of the spleen. In: Cameron JL (ed.), *Current Surgical Therapy*, 7th ed. St. Louis, MO: Mosby, 2001, pp. 591–595.

30. (E) Splenic abscess is a rare but potentially lethal condition. Immunocompromised patients and patients who abuse IV drugs are particularly susceptible. They develop by four basic mechanisms: metastatic hematogenous spread from a distant source such as osteomyelitis or infective endocarditis; following trauma or iatrogenic injury, especially with increasing use of nonoperative management; secondary infection following splenic infarction such as in sickle cell and splenic embolization; and by extension from a contiguous infective source such as a perinephric, pancreatic, or diverticular abscess. They may also develop in patients undergoing chemotherapy for diseases such as leukemia. They are primarily unilocular in adults but multilocular in children. *Staphyloccoccus* and *Streptococcus* species account for 30% of cases; other common organisms include *Enterococcus*, *Salmonella*, and *E. coli*. The growing population of immunosuppressed patients has increased the frequency of atypical pathogens such as *Mycobacterium* and *Actinomycoses* species as well as fungal infections with *Candida*, *Cryptococcus*, and *Aspergillus*.

The most common presenting symptoms are fever and abdominal pain in the left upper quadrant. Patients also frequently have splenomegaly, leukocytosis, and bacteremia. In the face of such a nonspecific presentation, imaging should be performed early for diagnosis, especially in the intensive care unit (ICU) setting and in immunosuppressed patients.

The imaging modality of choice is CT scan, on which lesions tend to have a heterogeneous appearance on CT while cysts tend to be homogeneous. Ultrasound may be helpful where CT is unavailable. Patients should be hospitalized and treated promptly with broad-spectrum systemic antibiotics including coverage for fungal agents if immunosuppressed.

Unilocular abscesses may be percutaneously aspirated; however, contents may be thick and tenacious, and with failure of percutaneous drainage, operative intervention should be performed early to avoid significant increases in morbidity and mortality. Percutaneous drainage has the advantage of splenic conservation with all of the associated immunologic implications, especially in young patients. Multilocular abscesses and those originating from a contiguous source usually require splenectomy. Relative contraindications to percutaneous management also include refractory coagulopathy, ascites, rupture with hemorrhage, and need for surgical intervention for another associated problem. Partial splenectomy, splenotomy with drainage, and laparoscopic splenectomy have all been used with success. Splenic abscesses may be complicated by intraperitoneal rupture, rupture into adjacent organs, and with possible subsequent formation of a fistula.

Although immunosuppressed patients are at higher risk for development of splenic abscesses, this patient is clearly able to mount an immune response judging from the marked leukocytosis and the recent history of clinical improvement of the diverticulitis. Depressed immune function would manifest first increased bacterial translocation across the gut mucosa into the portal system, and the presence of an isolated splenic abscess with no hepatic disease or other foci suggesting hematogenous dissemination further discounts this mechanism. More plausibly this process is a result of direct local extension of the sigmoid disease into the spleen or from rupture of a previously contained abscess.

Bibliography

Beauchamp RD, Holzman MD, Fabian TC. Spleen. In: Townsend CM, Beauchamp RD, Evers BM, et al. (eds.), *Textbook of Surgery: The Biological Basis of Modern Surgical Practice*, 16th ed. Philadelphia, PA: WB Saunders, 2001, pp. 1144–1164.

Harris JA, Gadacz TR. Tumors, cysts, and abscesses of the spleen. In: Cameron JL (ed.), *Current Surgical Therapy*, 7th ed. St. Louis, MO: Mosby, 2001, pp. 591–595.

Ooi LLPJ, Leong SS. Splenic abscesses from 1987 to 1995. *Am J Surg* 1997;174:87–93.

Phillips GS, Radosevich MD, Lipsett PA. Splenic abscesses: another look at an old disease. *Arch Surg* 1997;132:1331–1336.

CHAPTER 32

Vascular Surgery

Lori Rolando and Michael Dalsing

Questions

1. A 62-year-old man who underwent the procedure shown in Fig. 32-1 1 year ago presents with fever, abdominal pain, an ileus, and an elevated white blood cell (WBC) count. An Indium-labeled WBC scan confirms a graft infection. All of the following are true *except*:

   (A) The most common organism is *Staphylococcus epidermidis*.
   (B) The risk of graft infection in this location is relatively low—usually approximately 1–2%.
   (C) Treatment consists of 6 weeks of broad-spectrum antibiotic coverage only.
   (D) Excision of the graft with extra-anatomic bypass is indicated.
   (E) If surgery is performed, an extra-anatomic bypass should be constructed prior to graft excision if possible.

2. Figure 32-2 shows the aortogram of a 57-year-old male patient. Findings on history and physical examination could include all of the following *except*:

   (A) buttock and thigh claudication
   (B) impotence
   (C) absent femoral pulses
   (D) intestinal angina
   (E) decreased ankle-brachial index (ABIs)

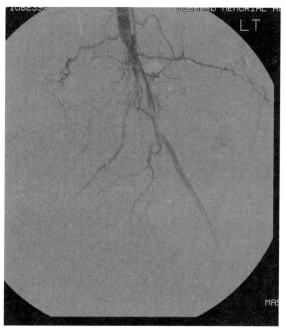

FIG. 32-2

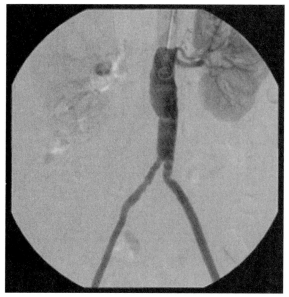

FIG. 32-1

3. Regarding reconstruction for this disease

   (A) aortobifemoral bypass patency rates approximate 60% at 5 years

   (B) patients with smaller vessels have higher patency rates

   (C) end-to-side proximal anastamosis may decrease risk of aortoenteric fistula

   (D) patients with a "hostile abdomen" may benefit from a thoraco-fem-fem bypass

   (E) axillary-bifemoral bypasses have lower patency rates than do axillary-unifemoral bypasses

4. A patient who required an aortobifemoral bypass graft for aortoiliac occlusive disease 3 years ago presents after an episode of severe hematemesis. His wife relates an episode of minor hematemesis 2 days prior. His hemoglobin is currently 7.2 and his systolic blood pressure (SBP) is 75. Nasogastric (NG) tube lavage illustrates profuse bright red blood. After appropriate resuscitation, the next step in management should be

   (A) GI consult for emergent esophagogastroduodenoscopy (EGD)

   (B) exploratory laparotomy

   (C) computed tomography (CT) scan

   (D) transfusion and admission to the intensive care unit (ICU)

   (E) angiography with embolization

5. A patient with a history of atrial fibrillation presents with a 6-h history of acute right lower extremity pain. On examination, the lower extremity is cool to the touch and the patient has pain on attempts to move his foot. The femoral pulse is palpable but pulses are absent, as are Doppler signals below this level. The next step in management should be

   (A) immediate embolectomy

   (B) arteriogram

   (C) anticoagulation and observation

   (D) amputation

   (E) femoral-femoral bypass

6. At the conclusion of the procedure mentioned above, fasciotomy is contemplated. Which of the following is true concerning a compartment syndrome and the use of a fasciotomy?

   (A) Compartment pressures below 30 mmHg essentially rule out the compartment syndrome.

   (B) In general, 2 or more hours of acute ischemic time is an indication for fasciotomy.

   (C) Fasciotomy skin incisions should always be closed after fascial release is completed.

   (D) Fluid resuscitation, diuretic use, and urine acidification are important measures to combat myoglobinuric renal failure.

   (E) Patients with myoglobinuric renal failure generally have favorable renal outcomes.

7. Which of the following is true regarding carotid artery stenosis?

   (A) The 5-year stroke rate for patients with equal or >60% asymptomatic lesion is 9% with surgery versus 26% with medical treatment.

   (B) The 2-year stroke rate for patients with an equal or >70% symptomatic lesion is 5% with surgery versus 11% with medical treatment.

   (C) The 5-year stroke rate for patients with an equal or >60% asymptomatic lesion is 5% with surgery versus 11% with medical treatment.

   (D) The 5-year stroke rate for patients with an equal or >70% symptomatic lesion is 11% with surgery versus 26% with medical treatment.

   (E) Stroke rates for medical versus surgical treatment in patients with an equal or >60% asymptomatic lesions is equivalent.

8. A patient presents to your office after an episode of L arm weakness. The arteriogram shown in Fig. 32-3 is obtained. Appropriate treatment would be

   (A) medical treatment with ASA 325 mg bid

   (B) right carcinoembryonic antigen (CEA) with shunt

   (C) left CEA followed by subsequent right CEA 2 weeks later

   (D) right CEA followed by subsequent left CEA 2 weeks later

   (E) right CEA without shunt

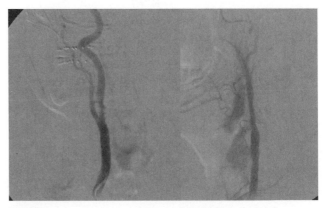

R carotid   L carotid (internal occluded)

FIG. 32-3

9. The most common cranial nerve injury after carotid endarterectomy is

   (A) vagus nerve
   (B) hypoglossal nerve
   (C) glossopharyngeal nerve
   (D) spinal accessory nerve
   (E) marginal mandibular nerve

10. A patient who underwent L CEA approximately one and half years ago presents for routine follow-up. Duplex of the carotids suggests recurrent stenosis of the L ICA, and arteriogram is performed. The images obtained are shown in Fig. 32-4. Which of the following is true?

   (A) This most likely represents myointimal hyperplasia.
   (B) The majority of these lesions are symptomatic.
   (C) Treatment of the lesion is best performed by repeat endarterectomy with primary closure.
   (D) Repeat operation carries a slightly lower risk of cranial nerve injury.
   (E) Recurrent stenosis occurs more often with the use of a patch than during primary repairs.

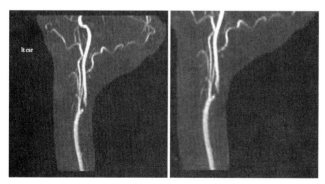

FIG. 32-4

11. Regarding findings in Fig. 32-5

   (A) kinks and coils can be found in children as well as adults
   (B) coils are more likely to be symptomatic than are kinks
   (C) coils are usually the result of atherosclerotic disease
   (D) definitive diagnosis can be made using duplex ultrasound
   (E) treatment involves pexy of the redundant vessel to eliminate the kink or coil

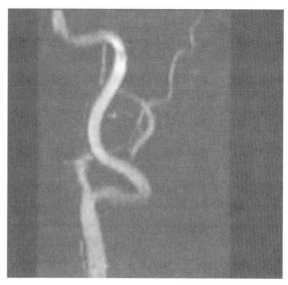

FIG. 32-5

12. A 45-year-old previously healthy female presents for a preoperative history and physical examination. She relates a history of heavy bleeding during her menstrual cycles as well as easy bruising and bleeding gums. Bleeding time is noted to be prolonged. All of the following are true regarding her condition *except*:

   (A) The disease is autosomal dominant.
   (B) Patients are high risk for spontaneous bleeding and hemarthrosis.
   (C) Ristocetin cofactor assay will be abnormal.
   (D) Treatment may be with cryoprecipitate or factor VIII concentrates.
   (E) Platelet counts are usually normal.

13. With regards to lower extremity arterial Doppler measurements

   (A) 0.9 is a normal ABI
   (B) diabetic patients often have artificially elevated ABIs
   (C) segmental pressure gradients >10 mmHg signify significant disease in the intervening segment
   (D) most accurate pressure measurements are obtained with cuffs that are 2× the diameter of the LE being measured
   (E) a change in ABI of >0.1 is clinically significant

14. With regard to the pathologic entity shown in Fig. 32-6

    (A) presence in one leg is associated with up to a 10% incidence of bilaterality
    (B) rupture is the most common complication
    (C) embolic phenomena are rare
    (D) asymptomatic lesions should be treated conservatively
    (E) patients presenting with ischemia have up to a 35% primary amputation rate

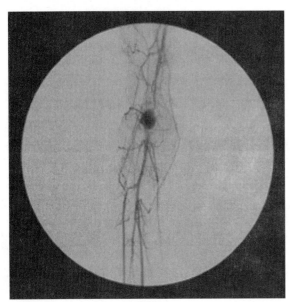

FIG. 32-6

15. Which of the following is false regarding subclavian steal?

    (A) The right subclavian artery is affected significantly more often than the left.
    (B) Clinical symptoms can be ischemic or vertebrobasilar in nature.
    (C) Prosthetic grafts (PTFE or Dacron) are more desirable than saphenous vein for use in bypass.
    (D) Symptomatic lesions can be treated with bypass, transposition, or—in some instances—stenting.
    (E) Transposition is contraindicated in patients with a prior left internal mammary artery (LIMA) coronary graft in place.

16. The treatment of choice for the lesion shown in Fig. 32-7 is:

    (A) embolectomy
    (B) replacement of the descending thoracic aorta
    (C) replacement of the aortic valve/aortic root
    (D) fenestration
    (E) aortoplasty

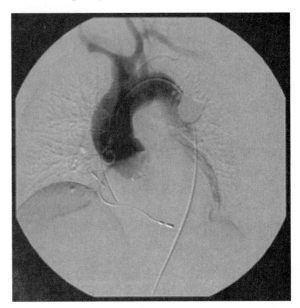

FIG. 32-7

17. Common causes of death from the lesion shown in Fig. 32-7 include all *except*

    (A) acute aortic valve regurgitation
    (B) coronary artery occlusion
    (C) aortic rupture
    (D) pericardial tamponade
    (E) stroke

18. Regarding thoracic outlet syndrome (TOS)

    (A) it maybe present with arterial, venous, or neurologic symptoms
    (B) arterial TOS is the most common form of the syndrome
    (C) thrombotic occlusion of the subclavian artery is the most common presentation of arterial TOS
    (D) resection of the middle scalene muscle is curative
    (E) thrombolysis is contraindicated in venous TOS

19. Embryologically, the pulmonary arteries develop from the

    (A) first arch arteries
    (B) second arch arteries
    (C) third arch arteries
    (D) fourth arch arteries
    (E) sixth arch arteries

20. Indications for the device shown in Fig. 32-8 include all of the following *except*:

   (A) pulmonary embolism in a patient with an INR 2.2

   (B) bleeding ulcer in a patient with an iliofemoral deep vein thrombosis (DVT) on heparin therapy

   (C) trauma patient with pelvic and femur fractures as well as a subdural hematoma

   (D) patient with a history of DVT with PE 1 year ago who develops left lower extremity (LLE) swelling. Duplex positive for DVT

   (E) free floating femoral DVT documented by duplex

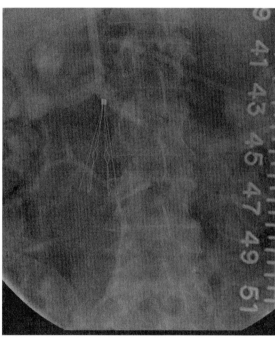

FIG. 32-8

21. Regarding the diagnosis and treatment of DVT, which of the following is true?

   (A) Venous ultrasound depends on augmentation of flow with proximal compression and obstruction of flow with distal compression during the examination.

   (B) Development of proximal lower extremity vein DVT should be treated with heparin and conversion to 6 weeks of coumadin therapy.

   (C) Patients treated for DVT whose platelet counts drop below 100,000 should have all heparin products immediately stopped.

   (D) Perioperative SCD use is the prophylactic measure of choice for patients at high risk of DVT.

   (E) Low-molecular weight heparins (LMWHs) exert their effect through inhibition of activated factor VIII.

22. Regarding the findings shown in Fig. 32-9, all of the following are true *except*:

   (A) The common or internal iliac artery is most commonly involved.

   (B) Bilaterality occurs in one-third of patients.

   (C) Should be repaired at >3 cm in size.

   (D) Most are symptomatic.

   (E) Treatment of disease isolated to the hypogastric artery is ligation of the proximal vessel neck.

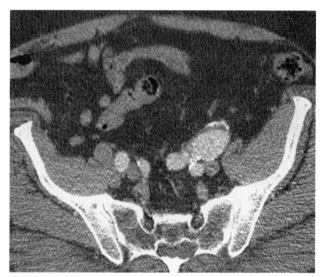

FIG. 32-9

23. A patient undergoes an uncomplicated aortic aneurysm repair. The next morning, the patient is noted to have a large maroon liquid bowel movement. The patient is otherwise stable. The next step in evaluation and management should be

   (A) immediate flexible sigmoidoscopy

   (B) stool sample for *Clostridium difficile*

   (C) intravenous fluids (IVF) hydration and observation

   (D) reexploration

   (E) obstruction series

24. Indications for arteriogram in a patient with the finding shown in Fig. 32-10 include all *except*:

(A) patient with a history of weight loss and postprandial epigastric pain

(B) patient with calf pain after walking half a block

(C) patient with BP 160/95 mmHg on three medications

(D) obese patient with inadequate imaging via abdominal ultrasound

(E) patient with a known horseshoe kidney

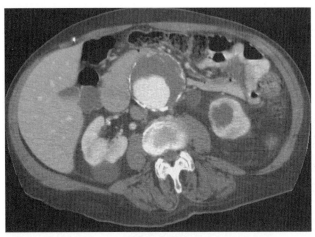

FIG. 32-10

25. Which of the following is true regarding aneurysmal disease of the aorta?

(A) The aorta is considered aneurysmal when its size is twice that of the normal proximal aorta.

(C) Women are generally affected more frequently than men.

(C) Aneurysm walls contain increased levels of collagen and elastin.

(D) The most common presentation of AAA is back pain.

(E) The risk of rupture increases with increasing size of the aneurysm.

26. Anatomic considerations in the placement of an endoluminal abdominal aortic aneurysm stent include all of the following *except*:

(A) proximal neck length

(B) proximal aortic diameter

(C) neck angulation

(D) aneurysm diameter

(E) iliac/femoral artery diameter

27. Regarding endoleaks

(A) they are defined as the inability to maintain blood flow around the endograft and into the lumbars or IMA

(B) they exist in three different types

(C) the main complication of an endoleak is graft thrombosis

(D) type II endoleaks involve back-bleeding from persistently patent lumbar vessels

(E) routing screening for endoleaks should be done with yearly angiography

28. All of the following are common causes of acute intestinal ischemia *except*:

(A) cardiac emboli

(B) thrombosis of a mesenteric artery

(C) hypotension

(D) celiac artery compression

(E) mesenteric venous thrombosis

29. With regard to the disease process pictured in Fig. 32-11

(A) symptoms arise only when three vessel disease is present

(B) acute abdominal pain is a common presenting symptom

(C) mesenteric angioplasty has replaced surgery as first-line treatment

(D) when surgery is performed, either greater saphenous vein or prosthetic graft may be used as a bypass conduit

(E) both the chronic and acute forms of this disease share atherosclerosis as the primary etiology

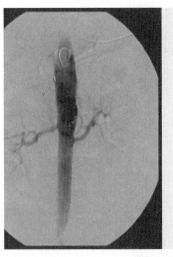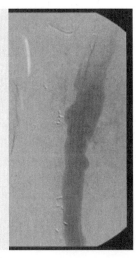

FIG. 32-11

30. Regarding cardiac risk assessment prior to peripheral vascular procedures, all of the following are independent predictors of postoperative MI *except*:

(A) angina

(B) age >70 years

(C) recent MI

(D) congestive heart failure (CHF)

(E) ectopy (>5 bpm)

31. Which of the following is true regarding the procedure shown here? (Fig. 32-12)

(A) should be considered an appropriate alternative to CEA for most patients with symptomatic lesions

(B) in early clinical trials, is noted to have a lower stroke rate than CEA

(C) is less costly than CEA

(D) is a viable alternative to CEA in high-risk patients

(E) should not be performed

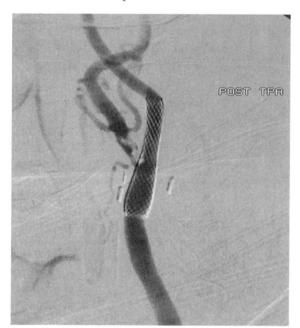

FIG. 32-12

32. Regarding lower extremity amputations, which of the following is true?

(A) Higher energy expenditure is required for ambulation after BKA than after AKA.

(B) Lower extremity digital amputations should be performed through the joint space to preserve smooth cartilaginous surfaces for granulation.

(C) Dependent rubor at a proposed level of amputation is a contraindication to amputation at that level.

(D) Guillotine amputation is inappropriate in the face of active infection.

(E) Diabetic patients who undergo amputation have up to a 10% risk of contralateral amputation within 5 years.

33. Regarding renal artery aneurysms, which of the following is true?

(A) The incidence is approximately 1%.

(B) Etiology is almost exclusively atherosclerosis.

(C) Risk of rupture is approximately 3%, with mortality of 10%.

(D) Repair should be undertaken when size approaches 1 cm or greater.

(E) Most are found intraparenchymally, making repair without nephrectomy difficult.

34. All are true of the entity illustrated in Fig. 32-13 *except*:

(A) Pancreatic lesions are likely secondary to prior episodes of pancreatitis.

(B) The most common visceral vessel involved with this particular pathology is the splenic.

(C) The majority of these lesions are the result of medial cystic degeneration.

(D) The hepatic artery is involved in approximately 40% of patients.

(E) Lesions of the gastric and gastroepiploic arteries have the highest risk of rupture.

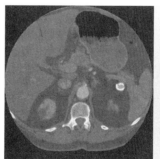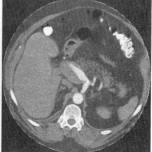

FIG. 32-13

35. All of the following are true regarding lymphedema *except*:

(A) Lymphedema praecox denotes primary lymphedema, while secondary lymphedema is also termed lymphedema tarda.

(B) Primary lymphedema has a marked female predominance.

(C) The most common world-wide cause of secondary lymphedema is filariasis.

(D) Lymphoscintigraphy is a reliable diagnostic tool for lymphedema.

(E) Methods of treatment include manual lymphatic drainage, compression devices, and surgery.

36. Regarding failing infrainguinal bypass grafts

(A) early failures are usually the result of progressive atherosclerotic changes

(B) critical stenoses are those which cause a 50% reduction in luminal area

(C) revision of grafts should be performed only after the graft has occluded

(D) grafts should be surveilled on a regular basis with duplex ultrasonography

(E) percutaneous angioplasty is contraindicated in the face of a failing graft

37. The patient with the arteriogram shown in Fig. 32-14 most likely suffers from

(A) diabetes

(B) hypertension

(C) tobacco abuse

(D) hypercholesterolemia

(E) hyperthyroidism

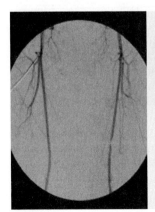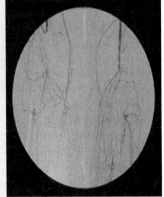

FIG. 32-14

38. A healthy 24-year-old male presented with the arteriogram after a posterior knee dislocation (Fig. 32-15). Which of the following is true?

(A) Presence of a pedal pulse reliably rules out significant arterial injury.

(B) All patients with known posterior knee dislocations should undergo diagnostic arteriogram to rule out arterial injury.

(C) Compartment syndrome is a rare complication of popliteal injury associated knee dislocation.

(D) In general, orthopedic repair should precede vascular repair in order to maintain lower extremity stability during arterial reconstruction.

(E) Primary repair or bypass—usually with contralateral saphenous vein—is indicated.

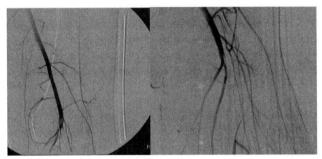

FIG. 32-15

39. Regarding superficial thrombophlebitis (ST), all of the following are true *except*:

(A) Deep venous involvement is rare.

(B) Treatment with warm compresses, anti-inflammatory agents, and elevation is often sufficient.

(C) Extended anticoagulation or ligation of the saphenous vein may be required for progressive ST or ST encroaching on the sapheno-femoral junction.

(D) Varicose veins are not risk factors for ST.

(E) Excision of the involved vein segment may be required in cases of suppurative ST.

Answers and Explanations

1. **(C)** Graft infections are a difficult problem for vascular surgeons. Fortunately, the incidence of aortobiiliac graft infection is fairly low—about 1.5%. Early graft infections (less than 4 months after bypass) are most often caused by *Staphylococcus aureus*, although later graft infections most often result from *S. epidermidis*. Antibiotics, usually 6 weeks in duration, are an important component of treatment, although antibiotics alone are insufficient treatment for an aortic graft infection. Aortic graft infections are best treated with graft excision and extraanatomic bypass. An extra-anatomic bypass, for example an axillobifemoral bypass, is often performed first with excision of the aortic graft subsequently performed in 1 or 2 days. This allows dissection in clean tissue planes without contamination by the infected graft and allows ultimate excision of the aortic graft without the necessity for heparinization with its inherent increased risk of bleeding. Of course, in the emergent situation of graft infection and rupture, aortic control is secured, with removal of the infected graft and the limb salvage procedure performed subsequently.

Bibliography

Ernst CB, Stanley JC. *Current Therapy in Vascular Surgery*, 4th ed. St. Louis, MO: Mosby, 2001.

Moore WS (ed.). *Vascular Surgery: A Comprehensive Review*, 6th ed. Philadelphia, PA: W.B. Saunders, 2002.

Rutherford RB (ed.). *Vascular Surgery*, 5th ed. St. Louis, MO: Mosby, 2000, vol. 1 and 2.

2. **(D)**

3. **(D)**

Explanations 2 and 3

LeRiche's syndrome is a specific triad of symptoms that can affect male patients with aortoiliac occlusive disease. This triad includes thigh and buttock claudication resulting from insufficient collateralization to compensate for the increased oxygen requirements needed during activity. Sexual dysfunction (impotence) can be a result of decreased arterial inflow. Femoral pulses will also be diminished as a result of the inflow disease. Pathology such as this can often be suggested by arterial Doppler studies. Abnormal arterial waveforms at the groin level, diminished thigh pulse volume recordings, and a decreased segmental pressure at the thigh level would signify disease at the aortoiliac level.

Intestinal angina would not be a symptom of distal aortoiliac disease, but rather would signify mesenteric arterial disease.

Revascularization of aortoiliac disease most often entails an aortobifemoral bypass. This repair is a very durable repair, with 5-year patency rates of up to 85%. Incorporating the profunda origin in the distal anastomosis has been noted to influence these increased patency rates by ensuring an adequate outflow, especially in patients who may have more distal (SFA) disease. Other factors influencing patency of an aortobifemoral bypass include size of the aorta and age. Patients with small aortas, especially those aortas smaller than 1.8 cm, and patients younger than 50 years have significantly decreased patency rates than do their older counterparts and those with aortas of larger diameter.

The proximal anastomosis of the bypass can be performed in an end-to-end or an end-to-side manner. Proponents of the end-to-end anastomosis cite easier ability to perform aortic endarterectomy, less chance of distal embolization from dislodgement of plaque from distal clamping, and less competitive flow down the native iliac vessels as benefits. Further, it is felt that end-to-end anastomosis may decrease the incidence of aortoenteric fistula, as the graft sits in a more anatomic position and there may be less protrusion of the graft anteriorly where the duodenum can lie against it.

However, certain situations may benefit from an end-to-side anastamosis. Patients with patent inferior mesenteric arteries may warrant this type of anasta-mosis to preserve flow to the IMA. In a similar man-ner, patients with distal iliac disease may preferen-tially undergo end-to-side anastamosis, as an end-to-end anastamosis may prevent any flow into the internal iliacs (prograde flow interrupted by the end-to-end nature of the anastamosis and retrograde flow prohibited by external iliac stenoses/occlusions).

If aortobifemoral bypass is not an ideal option, other alternatives exist. Axillofemoral bypasses are good options in high-risk patients. It should be noted, however, that axillobifemoral bypass has a higher patency rate than does axillounifemoral bypass. This is likely secondary to higher flow rates through the axillary limb in a bifemoral as opposed to a unifemoral graft. Patients with severely calcified aortas or multiple prior abdominal procedures may also benefit from a bypass using the descending tho-racic aorta as the inflow vessel. Long-term patency rates for this bypass approach 85%.

Bibliography

Ernst CB, Stanley JC. *Current Therapy in Vascular Surgery*, 4th ed. St. Louis, MO: Mosby, 2001.

Moore WS (ed.). *Vascular Surgery: A Comprehensive Review*, 6th ed. Philadelphia, PA: W.B. Saunders, 2002.

Rutherford RB (ed.). *Vascular Surgery*, 5th ed. St. Louis, MO: Mosby, 2000, vol. 1 and 2.

4. **(B)** This patient's presentation should raise concern for an aortoduodenal fistula. Patients with a known AAA or history of aortic graft placement who present with evidence of a GI bleed should be considered to have an aortoenteric fistula until proven otherwise. Aortoenteric fistulas are indeed a rather rare entity (approximately 2% of those with a GI bleed and aortic graft actually suffer from this entity); however, a mis-diagnosis is often fatal. Therefore, vigilant attempts to rule out this diagnosis should be undertaken. Patients with aortoenteric fistulas usually present with a "herald bleed"—mild GI bleeding (such as hemateme-sis, hematochezia, or melena) that does not cause insta-bility. If undiagnosed, however, further devastating, often fatal, hemorrhage can ensue. Thus, once presen-tation occurs, that window of opportunity should be taken to identify an aortoenteric fistula if present. In stable patients, prompt EGD with investigation of the third and fourth portions of the duodenum should be the first step. Findings such as extrinsic mass effect, duodenal wall bleeding, or a visible graft suture line are red flags for the diagnosis.

CT scan can compliment endoscopy, with such findings as perigraft fluid, gas bubbles, or pseudoa-neurysm helping to add weight to the diagnosis of aortoenteric fistula. Aortography can illustrate anastamotic aneurysms or kinks in grafts, which can heighten suspicion of the entity and can give further anatomic information; however, this diagnostic modality generally does not demonstrate the fistula itself.

Simple conservative management in the ICU with-out further investigation is a gross management error.

However, in the patient described, who has bled profusely and is hemodynamically unstable, emer-gent laparotomy for diagnostic and possibly thera-peutic intervention is most appropriate. In such patients, vascular control, repair of the GI fistula, removal of the graft, and revascularization if neces-sary (usually via extraanatomic bypass) is often war-ranted. Patients who are stable and are diagnosed with an aortoenteric fistula can often undergo extra-anatomic bypass first, with graft excision under more controlled circumstances a day or two later.

Bibliography

Ernst CB, Stanley JC. *Current Therapy in Vascular Surgery*, 4th ed. St. Louis, MO: Mosby, 2001.

Moore WS (ed.). *Vascular Surgery: A Comprehensive Review*, 6th ed. Philadelphia, PA: W.B. Saunders, 2002.

Rutherford RB (ed.). *Vascular Surgery*, 5th ed. St. Louis, MO: Mosby, 2000, vol. 1 and 2.

5. **(A)** In this instance, the patient has likely suffered an acute embolic occlusion of his right lower extremity. The most common source of such emboli is the heart. In this particular patient, atrial thrombus secondary to his atrial fibrillation is the likely culprit. Acute myocar-dial infarctions (MIs) or the presence of prosthetic heart valves with subsequent ventricular clot forma-tion is also a common cause. Aneurysmal disease of the aortoiliac system is a less common source of embolic occlusion. When emboli occur, they most often affect the lower extremities at bifurcations, such as the origin of the SFA or tibioperoneal trunk, which tends to block all collateral channels of distal flow.

Prevention of such potentially disastrous events with anticoagulation in at-risk patients is recommended.

Acute arterial occlusion of the lower extremity often presents with the six "p"'s: pulselessness, pallor, pain, paralysis, paresthesia, and poikilothermia. Motor changes are usually late manifestations of the disease, although worrisome earlier sensory deficits can be observed as loss of proprioception and light touch.

Patients who present with signs and symptoms of acute arterial occlusion should be treated as vas-cular emergencies, as timely diagnosis and treatment are important to potential limb salvage.

Following rapid resuscitation, revascularization should be the goal. Patients with advanced ischemia, immobile extremities, and lengthy periods of ischemia may best benefit from anticoagulation and primary amputation. All others, however, should have attempts at revascularization, as should this patient.

These patients should be heparinized while further intervention decisions are being made. Patients who present early in their course or who have known significant underlying disease may benefit from preoperative aortography to aid in planning operative procedures. Those in whom aortography would delay treatment unacceptably or in whom embolic disease is the likely etiology should undergo exploration without arteriography (with the understanding that intraoperative arteriography is always a viable option). This particular patient would best be served by immediate embolectomy, as he has had prolonged ischemic time and evidence of progressive sensorimotor deficits. In this case, the diagnosis is likely an acute embolus and aortogram would unacceptably prolong the treatment.

A fem-fem bypass likely would not help, as the occlusion is located below the iliac system.

Bibliography

Ernst CB, Stanley JC. *Current Therapy in Vascular Surgery*, 4th ed. St. Louis, MO: Mosby, 2001.

Moore WS (ed.). *Vascular Surgery: A Comprehensive Review*, 6th ed. Philadelphia, PA: W.B. Saunders, 2002.

Rutherford RB (ed.). *Vascular Surgery*, 5th ed. St. Louis, MO: Mosby, 2000, vol. 1 and 2.

6. **(E)** Compartment syndrome and its sequela are potentially life-threatening complications of acute limb ischemia. Acute ischemia causes depletion of cellular energy stores, which once repleted by reperfusion, can release toxic oxygen radicals. This can cause calcium influx and cellular disruption, releasing toxins such as potassium and myoglobin, as well as causing interstitial and cellular edema. Failure to recognize this syndrome of increased tissue pressure and release the affected compartments can cause further ischemia as the compartment pressure equalizes with the capillary pressure (as net blood flow approaches zero). The longer this condition goes untreated, the more tissue damage occurs.

Therefore, a high index of suspicion is necessary. Patients who have experienced approximately 6 h or more of acute ischemic time have a very high likelihood of suffering from compartment syndrome and potentially irreversible tissue damage.

Thus, fasciotomy to release compartments is an important step in treatment in high-risk patients. In those cases which are questionable, compartment pressures can be measured. It used to be felt that pressures above 30–40 mmHg indicated compartment syndrome, and pressures below this were safe; however, it is now understood that perfusion pressure—rather than only an absolute pressure—is important. Patients whose compartment pressures are within 20 mmHg of their diastolic blood pressure, or are within 30 mmHg of the mean arterial pressure, are at risk and should undergo fasciotomy.

Once fasciotomy is performed, skin incisions should be left open, as closure can compromise the pressures even if the fascia is released. Wounds should be carefully tended and allowed to gradually reapproximate. Skin grafts are sometimes required to close the wounds if significant swelling is seen.

Patients with reperfusion injury are at risk for acute renal failure (ARF) secondary to precipitation of myoglobin in the renal tubules. Careful attention to this is imperative, and creatine phosphokinase (CPK) levels, urine myoglobin levels, and urine pH should be monitored. Fluid resuscitation, as well as diuretic use, to keep urine output high (60–100 cc/h), in addition to bicarbonate for urine alkalinization, is often necessary to prevent renal damage. Mannitol is often recommended as a diuretic of choice secondary to its antioxidant effects. Those patients who ultimately do suffer ARF in this setting, however, generally do well long term.

Bibliography

Ernst CB, Stanley JC. *Current Therapy in Vascular Surgery*, 4th ed. St. Louis, MO: Mosby, 2001.

Moore WS (ed.). *Vascular Surgery: A Comprehensive Review*, 6th ed. Philadelphia, PA: W.B. Saunders, 2002.

Rutherford RB (ed.). *Vascular Surgery*, 5th ed. St. Louis, MO: Mosby, 2000, vol. 1 and 2.

7. **(C)** Treatment of patients with carotid stenosis has been the subject of multiple investigations over the years. The asymptomatic carotid atherosclerosis study (ACAS) investigated patients with asymptomatic lesions. This large study shows definitive benefit of surgical treatment over medical management of patients with asymptomatic lesions equal to or >60%. The 5-year stroke rate for those patients undergoing surgical treatment (endarterectomy) was 5%, while those in the medical arm had a stroke rate at 5 years of 11% (an absolute risk reduction of 6% and a relative risk reduction of 53%).

Patients with symptomatic lesions have also been the subject of numerous studies, the most significant of which may be the North American Symptomatic Carotid Endarterectomy Trial (NASCET). This randomized trial illustrated a significant benefit to surgical treatment of patients with an equal to or >70% symptomatic stenosis of the internal carotid artery. Patients undergoing medical treatment had a 2-year stroke rate of 26%, while those in the surgical arm had a 2-year stroke rate of 9%. This illustrates an absolute risk reduction of 17% and relative risk reduction of 65%. In point of fact, more recent information has been published as an extension of this initial NASCET trial, indicating a statistically significant benefit to repairing symptomatic lesions equal to or >50%, while lower-grade stenoses have no statistically significant benefit from surgical treatment versus medical treatment with aspirin.

Bibliography
Cameron JL (ed.). *Current Surgical Therapy*, 6th ed. St. Louis, MO: Mosby, 1998.

Moore WS (ed.). *Vascular Surgery: A Comprehensive Review*, 6th ed. Philadelphia, PA: W.B. Saunders, 2002.

Rutherford RB (ed.). *Vascular Surgery*, 5th ed. St. Louis, MO: Mosby, 2000, vol. 1 and 2.

8. **(B)** Determining surgical treatment of carotid disease involves many factors, including symptoms, clinical stability of the patient, and the degree of stenosis. This patient illustrates a symptomatic right-sided lesion with complete chronic occlusion of the contralateral carotid artery. As the left carotid is occluded and asymptomatic, surgical intervention is not warranted. The right side, however, is tightly stenotic and symptomatic. Therefore, surgical repair is advisable (2-year stroke rate for medical management of 26% vs. 9% with surgical treatment).

Intraoperatively, the decision to shunt a patient is very important, as up to 15% of patients without contralateral occlusion will have inadequate collateral circulation to supply the brain during carotid occlusion during surgery. Awake patients can be "tested" by occluding the common carotid artery, external and internal carotid arteries for 3 min. If no neurologic changes occur during this time, shunting can be safely forgone.

Patients who are under general anesthetic, however, should be investigated to determine if a shunt is indeed required. The most common method is measurement of "stump" or "back" pressures from the internal carotid artery after ipsilateral common carotid artery occlusion. A 22-gauge needle can be introduced into the common carotid artery distal to its clamp, and back pressures can be measured. Alternatively, some shunts are made to allow measurement of back pressures once the shunt is in place. Pressures of >30–50 mmHg have been used as a cutoff for performance of the endarterectomy without shunting. Pressures lower than this indicate the need for shunt placement.

There are exceptions, however. Patients with contralateral occlusion should be shunted, as should patients who have had a stroke in the past. Thus, the patient in this question should be shunted during CEA.

Bibliography
Ernst CB, Stanley JC. *Current Therapy in Vascular Surgery*, 4th ed. St. Louis, MO: Mosby, 2001.

Moore WS (ed.). *Vascular Surgery: A Comprehensive Review*, 6th ed. Philadelphia, PA: W.B. Saunders, 2002.

Rutherford RB (ed.). *Vascular Surgery*, 5th ed. St. Louis, MO: Mosby, 2000, vol. 1 and 2.

9. **(A)** Nerve injuries are a significant risk during CEA, as several important nerves run in very close proximity to the carotid artery.

The overall incidence of cranial nerve injuries can be up to 16% based on close clinical examination, and has been found to be up to 35–40% if more detained investigation by ear, nose, and throat (ENT)/speech pathology is undertaken. The vast majority are asymptomatic and/or temporary, resolving over the next 6 weeks. The most commonly injured nerve based on these studies is the vagus nerve or its recurrent branch (7–8% based on VA studies). Other studies set the incidence even higher, at up to 15%. The second most common injury is to the hypoglossal nerve, with other nerve injuries being much less common.

The majority of nerve injuries are noted to be traction injuries.

Clinically, vagus/recurrent laryngeal nerve injuries manifest themselves as hoarseness, usually secondary to paralysis of the vocal cord on the side of the injury. Once again, these injuries generally resolve, although determination of the extent of the injury becomes extremely important when planning a contralateral operation, as injury to both recurrent laryngeal nerves can have devastating effects.

Hypoglossal nerve injuries usually result in deviation of the patient's tongue to the side *ipsilateral* to the injury.

Bibliography
Moore WS (ed.). *Vascular Surgery: A Comprehensive Review*, 6th ed. Philadelphia, PA: W.B. Saunders, 2002.

Rutherford RB (ed.). *Vascular Surgery*, 5th ed. St. Louis, MO: Mosby, 2000, vol. 1 and 2.

10. **(A)** Recurrent carotid stenosis is believed to occur in anywhere from 1 to 21% of endarterectomized carotid arteries. The etiology of the disease differs depending on the time interval between operation and restenosis. In those patients with restenosis within the first 2 years after operation, the etiology is most often myointimal hyperplasia (collagen proliferation in the arterial wall). This is more common in women.

Those developing recurrent stenosis after 2 years are more likely to suffer from recurrent atherosclerotic disease.

Those patients who present with myointimal hyperplasia are most often asymptomatic, as there usually is a smooth surface which tends to preclude plaque formation, ulceration, and embolization. This is usually discovered on routine surveillance, and treatment of the asymptomatic lesion is usually preempted until the stenosis is equal to or >80%.

Those who suffer from recurrent atherosclerotic disease should be treated under the same guidelines as are those with primary carotid stenosis. Regardless of the etiology, recurrent stenosis should be treated with the use of patch angioplasty. The risk of restenosis after initial carotid endarterectomy has been shown to be significantly greater after primary arterial closure—especially of small vessels—than with patch (up to 21% vs. 7% in ACAS trials). Thus, on reoperation, the use of a patch is extremely important. One difference in the operative treatment of myointimal hyperplasia as opposed to recurrent atherosclerotic disease is the fact that myointimal hyperplasia rarely is amenable to repeat endarterectomy. The smooth surface usually makes it very difficult to find a dissection plane. Patching the artery is usually sufficient. Atherosclerotic lesions, on the other hand, require repeat endarterectomy to remove the plaque from the diseased vessel.

Bibliography

Ernst CB, Stanley JC. *Current Therapy in Vascular Surgery*, 4th ed. St. Louis, MO: Mosby, 2001.

Moore WS (ed.). *Vascular Surgery: A Comprehensive Review*, 6th ed. Philadelphia, PA: W.B. Saunders, 2002.

Rutherford RB (ed.). *Vascular Surgery*, 5th ed. St. Louis, MO: Mosby, 2000, vol. 1 and 2.

11. **(A)** Kinks and coils can be found in both children and adults, as they can be primary or acquired. Those found in children are often coils, and are the result of incomplete straightening of the carotid artery (from the third aortic arch/dorsal aorta) as the heart descends into the mediastinum during development. In adults, coils often result from progressive elongation of the vessel as a person ages. Kinks are usually secondary to atherosclerosis and therefore are more commonly symptomatic.

Kinks and coils are often initially found after examination notes a pulsatile mass in the neck suspicious for aneurysm. Noninvasive studies can be suggestive, but primary diagnosis requires angiogram.

Once symptomatic lesions are diagnosed, surgical treatment should be undertaken. Unfortunately, simply pexying the elongated artery is insufficient.

Treatment entails removal of the redundant segment of the vessel, which can be done via resection of the segment with reanastamosis, interposition, or reimplantation of the ICA to the CCA.

Bibliography

Ernst CB, Stanley JC. *Current Therapy in Vascular Surgery*, 4th ed. St. Louis, MO: Mosby, 2001.

Moore WS (ed.). *Vascular Surgery: A Comprehensive Review*, 6th ed. Philadelphia, PA: W.B. Saunders, 2002.

Rutherford RB (ed.). *Vascular Surgery*, 5th ed. St. Louis, MO: Mosby, 2000, vol. 1 and 2.

12. **(B)** This patient has von Willibrand's disease (vWD), an autosomal dominant disorder of coagulation. von Willibrand's factor (vWF) is produced by endothelial cells and megakaryocytes and is a necessary cofactor for platelet binding to vessel walls. Deficiency or defect in vWF causes minor bleeding symptoms such as menorrhagia, easy bruising, and bleeding gums. Severe bleeding such as spontaneous hemarthrosis is not usually seen with vWD, but rather with disorders such as hemophilia A and B. Platelet counts are usually normal, as this is a qualitative rather than a quantitative platelet disorder. Bleeding times will be prolonged secondary to a defect in platelet function. Because vWF with factor VIII binds together to form a complex, deficiency/defect in vWF can also decrease activity of factor VIII, thus altering the activated partial thromboplastin time (aPTT) as well.

Platelets will not aggregate in response to ristocetin, but addition of vWF to the assay will correct the problem and thus aid in diagnosis.

Treatment with vWF-rich cryoprecipitate can correct bleeding dysfunction, as can administration of factor VIII concentrates.

Bibliography

Moore WS (ed.). *Vascular Surgery: A Comprehensive Review*, 6th ed. Philadelphia, PA: W.B. Saunders, 2002.

Sabiston DC (ed.). *Textbook of Surgery: The Biological Basis of Modern Surgical Practice*, 15th ed. Philadelphia, PA: W.B. Saunders, 1997.

13. **(B)** ABI is often used as a noninvasive screening tool for lower extremity arterial disease. Upper extremity systolic BP measurements are obtained and compared with SBP measurements obtained at the posterior tibial and dorsalis pedis arteries. Normal ABIs are approximately 1 and anything below 0.92 is considered abnormal, indicating lower extremity arterial disease; however, medial wall calcification seen with diabetic patients can cause an inability to compress the vessels of the calf, leading to an artificially elevated ABI.

Inappropriate cuff size can also be the cause of erroneous measurements. Cuffs that are too small can lead to erroneously elevated pressures. Therefore, cuff size should be at least 1.5 times the diameter of the vessel to ensure more accurate measurements.

Serial ABIs can be used to follow progression of disease. There is inherent variability, however, from one measurement to the next, even with a single person doing the measurements. Variability of up to 0.15 has been reported; therefore anything greater than that should be considered clinically significant for disease progression.

In addition to ABIs, segmental pressures at different levels in the lower extremities can be measured to better delineate the level of disease. Measurements are sequentially taken at the thigh, upper calf, and ankle levels. Pressure differences of 30 mmHg or more (in lower extremities; 20 mmHg in upper extremities) indicated significant disease in the intervening segment. The larger the gradient, the more significant the disease.

Bibliography

Moore WS (ed.). *Vascular Surgery: A Comprehensive Review*, 6th ed. Philadelphia, PA: W.B. Saunders, 2002.
Rutherford RB (ed.). *Vascular Surgery*, 5th ed. St. Louis, MO: Mosby, 2000, vol. 1 and 2.

14. **(E)** Popliteal artery aneurysms are primarily associated with atherosclerosis. The presence of an aneurysm in one leg should precipitate an investigation for the presence of an aneurysm in the other popliteal, as bilaterality is common. Up to 60% of patients have bilateral popliteal aneurysms. Patients with popliteal aneurysms can present in several ways. The usual presentation is secondary to ischemic complications from thrombosis of the aneurysm or embolism of clot distally. Compression of venous or nervous structures adjacent to a large aneurysm can also lead to pain or swelling of the lower extremity. Rarely, aneurysms present as rupture.

Because patients who present with ischemic complications tend to ultimately do much worse (up to 35% primary amputation rate) than do those patients who undergo elective repair (up to a 95% limb salvage rate), early repair of popliteal aneurysms is important.

Symptomatic aneurysms should be repaired regardless of size. Treatment of asymptomatic aneurysms is a bit more controversial. Aneurysms 2 cm or greater in size, even if asymptomatic, are recommended for surgical repair, while some advocate repair of smaller asymptomatic aneurysms with thrombus precisely because the complications can be so devastating. Repair usually entails bypass of the aneurysmal segment with ligation above and below the aneurysm to prevent collateral flow and subsequent continued flow into the aneurysmal segment.

Bibliography

Ernst CB, Stanley JC. *Current Therapy in Vascular Surgery*, 4th ed. St. Louis, MO: Mosby, 2001.
Moore WS (ed.). *Vascular Surgery: A Comprehensive Review*, 6th ed. Philadelphia, PA: W.B. Saunders, 2002.
Rutherford RB (ed.). *Vascular Surgery*, 5th ed. St. Louis, MO: Mosby, 2000, vol. 1 and 2.

15. **(A)** Subclavian artery disease, while not common, can present with symptom constellations that require surgical correction. The left subclavian artery is more often affected than the right. Symptoms can develop in the form of upper extremity ischemia. Upper extremity "claudication" or rest pain can be the result of significant proximal stenosis. In addition, proximal subclavian stenotic lesions can embolize, leading initially to significant ischemia at the digital level and progressing proximally if diagnosis is delayed. This can lead to potential limb-threatening ischemia.

In addition to upper extremity ischemia, the clinical subclavian "steal" syndrome can be the first manifestation of proximal subclavian stenosis. In this situation, the patient, while asymptomatic at rest, cannot compensate for the increased blood flow requirements with use of the arm. Flow is then "stolen" from the ipsilateral vertebral artery. Vertebral artery flow reverses to supply the arm. As a result of the decreased vertebrobasilar perfusion, clinical symptoms of dizziness, drop attacks, vertigo, syncope, or ataxia may arise.

When clinical symptoms arise, surgical treatment is indicated. Aortography with views of the arch and extremity run-off is necessary to identify the location of the lesion and any affected distal vessels. Once decision to treat surgically is made, options include carotid-subclavian bypass, subclavian artery transposition, or stenting. Both bypass and transposition have excellent patency rates of >95%. Bypass with prosthetic materials—PTFE or Dacron—have a higher patency rate than vein (85–95% with prosthetic vs. approximately 65% with vein). Transposition (division of the subclavian artery proximally with anastamosis to the common carotid artery) is also a viable option, but is contraindicated in patients with LIMA coronary bypass grafts secondary to the coronary ischemia that would result from occlusion of the subclavian proximal to the take-off of the IMA vessel.

In selected patients with focal narrowings, angioplasty and stenting can also be a successful means of treatment. In experienced hands, initial success rates can approach 100%, with up to a 70% 2-year continued patency.

Bibliography

Ernst CB, Stanley JC. *Current Therapy in Vascular Surgery*, 4th ed. St. Louis, MO: Mosby, 2001.

Moore WS (ed.). *Vascular Surgery: A Comprehensive Review*, 6th ed. Philadelphia, PA: W.B. Saunders, 2002.

Moore WS, Ahn SS (eds.). *Endovascular Surgery*, 3rd ed. Philadelphia, PA: W.B. Saunders, 2001.

Rutherford RB (ed.). *Vascular Surgery*, 5th ed. St. Louis, MO: Mosby, 2000, vol. 1 and 2.

16. **(C)**

17. **(E)**

Explanations 16 and 17

The images in Fig. 32-7 illustrate an ascending aortic dissection—a type A dissection. Aortic dissections are classified based on the location of the origin of the intimal tear. The two main classifications are the DeBakey classification and the Stanford classification. The DeBakey classification includes types I, II, and III. Types I and II involve the ascending aorta, with type I also involving the descending aorta at least to some degree. Type II, however, is isolated to the ascending aorta. Type III is exclusively a descending aortic dissection. The Stanford classification consists of type A and B. Type A involves the ascending aorta (with or without the descending aorta), while type B involves only the descending aorta. This is a very important distinction, in that the location of the origin of the dissection determines the treatment strategy. Dissections of the descending aorta in the absence of acute ischemic complications can often be managed with close observation and control of hypertension. Evaluation with modalities such as transesophageal echocardiography (TEE), CT, magnetic resonance (MR), or angiogram can often reveal the diagnosis. In fact, TEE often is a quick, convenient modality and can readily assess cardiac status and valve integrity in type A aneurysms. Ultimately, those patients with type B dissections who are being managed conservatively should undergo arteriography to assess branch vessel patency and/or involvement with the dissection.

Those patients with a type A dissection, however, are almost uniformly considered in need of emergent surgical intervention. As the dissection starts at the aortic valve, operative repair usually consists of replacing the aortic valve and the proximal aorta. This usually will address the lead point of the dissection and the remaining false lumen will then be obliterated by flow through the true lumen. Close observation and studies should be undertaken to be sure any evidence of visceral or extremity ischemia resolves. Other methods of repair (e.g., replacement of the descending aorta or fenestration) are undertaken for type B dissections.

The most common life-threatening events that occur with type A dissections include free rupture of the aorta, acute occlusion of the coronary arteries, as the dissection extends to involve these vessels, causing massive MI, and rupture into the pericardial sac, contributing to pericardial tamponade. Finally, severe acute aortic regurgitation can result in cardiovascular decompensation and death. While cerebrovascular accident (CVA) can occur if a proximal dissection extends to involve the carotid arteries, death does not usually result from this alone.

Bibliography

Moore WS (ed.). *Vascular Surgery: A Comprehensive Review*, 6th ed. Philadelphia, PA: W.B. Saunders, 2002.

Rutherford RB (ed.). *Vascular Surgery*, 5th ed. St. Louis, MO: Mosby, 2000, vol. 1 and 2.

18. **(A)** TOS or symptomatic compression of upper extremity neurovascular structures, can manifest with neurologic, arterial, or venous symptoms, although the vast majority of patients present with neurologic symptoms (95%). Venous TOS accounts for only 2–3%, while arterial TOS is a rare occurrence, accounting for only about 1% of all cases.

Neurologic TOS presents with weakness, paresthesia, and/or pain in the affected upper extremity. Often it is seen after trauma and is associated with occipital headaches or paraspinous muscle pain. Arterial symptoms include a pulsatile mass in the supraclavicular area (indicative of a potential aneurysm) and clinically distal emboli. Thrombosis of the subclavian artery is rare. Venous TOS often presents as significant swelling and pain of the affected extremity, often in young males after strenuous activity (effort thrombosis). Venography is required to diagnose venous TOS and catheter-directed thrombolysis can be first-line treatment; however, this must be followed by a more definitive procedure to prevent recurrent/residual lesions and symptoms. Definitive treatment for TOS, whether it be neurogenic, arterial, or venous, is decompression of the thoracic outlet. This can be accomplished by first rib resection (with cervical rib resection if present). Often anterior scalenectomy can be performed to decompress the triangle, alone or in combination with first rib resection. Symptomatic improvement seems to be similar, regardless of whether scalenectomy, rib resection, or both are performed.

Bibliography

Ernst CB, Stanley JC. *Current Therapy in Vascular Surgery*, 4th ed. St. Louis, MO: Mosby, 2001.

Moore WS (ed.). *Vascular Surgery: A Comprehensive Review*, 6th ed. Philadelphia, PA: W.B. Saunders, 2002.

Rutherford RB (ed.). *Vascular Surgery*, 5th ed. St. Louis, MO: Mosby, 2000, vol. 1 and 2.

19. **(E)** The embryology of the vascular system is complex and is especially so for the aortic arch and its branches. There are embryologically six paired aortic arch arteries, which undergo development, regression, or alteration to become ultimately the aortic arch and its branches.

Early in gestation, the embryo develops paired dorsal aortaes which continue to about the C7–T1 level, where the heart is beginning to form. Below this, the aorta fuses. The paired arch arteries form from the paired dorsal aortae and ultimately fuse into the arch and its branch arteries.

The first arches develop into a part of the internal carotid arteries, while the second and fifth arches are essentially obliterated.

The third aortic arches form the common carotid arteries, while the fourth arched ultimately form the roots of the right and left subclavian arteries. The left fourth arch artery also forms the aortic arch. The sixth arch arteries form the pulmonary arteries after the left sixth artery helps form the ductus arteriosus.

Bibliography

Moore WS (ed.). *Vascular Surgery: A Comprehensive Review*, 6th ed. Philadelphia, PA: W.B. Saunders, 2002.

Rutherford RB (ed.). *Vascular Surgery*, 5th ed. St. Louis, MO: Mosby, 2000, vol. 1 and 2.

20. **(D)** Usually, patients with a DVT can be treated with anticoagulation to prevent propagation of clot or embolic complications. Heparinization and ultimate conversion to coumadin therapy with a target INR of 2–3 is desired.

There are, however, several instances when Vena Caval Filter placement as protection against PE is warranted. Patients who develop PE while adequately anticoagulated is one such indication.

Patients who develop bleeding complications that require discontinuation of anticoagulation also may necessitate inferior vena cava (IVC) filter placement.

Patients with contraindications to anticoagulation (such as neurologic or ocular injuries) or those patients with large free-floating clots are at increased risk of embolization and may represent reasons to place a vena caval filter. Patients with DVT who are not currently anticoagulated do not require IVC filter if no contraindications to anticoagulation exist. They

may, however, require longer—even indefinite—anticoagulation secondary to the recurrent nature of the disease.

Other indications for IVC filter include patients who have undergone pulmonary embolectomy or those whose illness severity would likely make them intolerant to the effects of a PE. Patients with septic emboli or propagating iliofemoral clots are also relative indications. A new use—as a purely prophylactic device against PE in patients with massive trauma and a high risk of DVT/PE is also being considered as an indication, even in the absence of documented DVT.

Bibliography

Ernst CB, Stanley JC. *Current Therapy in Vascular Surgery*, 4th ed. St. Louis, MO: Mosby, 2001.

Moore WS (ed.). *Vascular Surgery: A Comprehensive Review*, 6th ed. Philadelphia, PA: W.B. Saunders, 2002.

Rutherford RB (ed.). *Vascular Surgery*, 5th ed. St. Louis, MO: Mosby, 2000, vol. 1 and 2.

21. **(C)** DVT is a significant health concern with potentially fatal complications. Therefore, knowledge of diagnosis and treatment is very important. One of the mainstays of diagnosis is the duplex ultrasound. The Doppler probe is placed on the lower extremity to evaluate the venous signals. Flow with distal compression is augmented, while a proximal obstruction should cause dampened flow. Further information can be gained by duplex of the DVT, which uses the picture to evaluate presence of clot or compressibility of the vein.

Methods of prophylaxis are dependent on risk stratification of the patient. Low-risk patients require only early ambulation. Moderate risk patients require either SCDs or anticoagulation, often with LMWHs, which exert their effect via inhibition of factor X. High-risk patients, such as those patients over 40, obese, with a history of cancer or major trauma, or those undergoing major joint replacement, often require anticoagulation—with unfractionated heparin or LMWH.

Patients who develop DVT should be treated with anticoagulation if there are no contraindications. Either heparin—or in some cases, LMWH—should be initiated with conversion to coumadin therapy to a target INR of 2–3. Duration of coumadin treatment is subject of some debate; however, at least 3 months, and often 6 months is recommended to minimize the risk of recurrence and to prevent PE. Recurrent DVT after completion of therapy often leads to indefinite anticoagulation secondary to an up to 20% risk of further recurrences if the patient is not anticoagulated.

Heparin therapy is not without its risks, however. Heparin-induced thrombocytopenia (HIT), secondary to heparin associated antiplatelet antibodies, occurs in approximately 2–3% (and in some studies up to 10%) of those patients who receive heparin and is independent of the method of exposure (e.g., IV, subcutaneous, and so on). Because of the significant risk of thrombotic complications in patients who develop HIT, patients whose platelet count drops below 100,000 during heparin therapy should be suspected of suffering from this phenomenon. Usually this occurs 4–5 days after initial exposure and the platelet count usually responds rapidly to the cessation of ALL heparin products. Alternatives for anticoagulation, such as lepirudin or argatroban, can be used for IV anticoagulation, and coumadin can be used as an oral option in those patients suffering from HIT.

Bibliography

Ernst CB, Stanley JC. *Current Therapy in Vascular Surgery*, 4th ed. St. Louis, MO: Mosby, 2001.

Moore WS (ed.). *Vascular Surgery: A Comprehensive Review*, 6th ed. Philadelphia, PA: W.B. Saunders, 2002.

Rutherford RB (ed.). *Vascular Surgery*, 5th ed. St. Louis, MO: Mosby, 2000, vol. 1 and 2.

22. **(E)** Iliac artery aneurysms are, as isolated entities, rare, accounting for less than 2% of all aneurysms. Most often they are seen in combination with aortic aneurysmal disease and they most often involve either the common iliac artery, the internal iliac artery, or both. Approximately one-third of patients with iliac aneurysmal disease will have bilateral lesions. Although difficult to diagnose with certainty from history and physical examination, most iliac aneurysms are symptomatic, even when unruptured. Most commonly, abdominal, flank, or groin pain is the presenting complaint—and is often attributed to some other etiology. The aneurysm itself is often diagnosed during imaging studies for that other presumed pathology.

The larger the aneurysm, the higher the risk of rupture, and ruptured iliac artery aneurysms carry an extremely high mortality rate (approximately 40%). Thus, early detection and appropriate intervention is key. Isolated iliac artery aneurysms should be fixed if symptomatic or if asymptomatic at a diameter of 3 cm or greater. Lesser aneurysms should be addressed if in conjunction with repair of an AAA.

Treatment of iliac artery aneurysms is dependent on location. If isolated to the common iliac artery, it can often be treated with transabdominally by graft replacement. Internal iliac disease can be addressed via catheter-based coil embolization or endoaneurysmorrhaphy; however, simple ligation of the neck of the aneurysm is not adequate treatment, as collateral flow will still allow expansion of an internal iliac artery aneurysm.

Bibliography

Moore WS (ed.). *Vascular Surgery: A Comprehensive Review*, 6th ed. Philadelphia, PA: W.B. Saunders, 2002.

Rutherford RB (ed.). *Vascular Surgery*, 5th ed. St. Louis, MO: Mosby, 2000, vol. 1 and 2.

23. **(A)** One of the most devastating complications that can arise from AAA repair is colonic ischemia. Several factors can influence the development of ischemia. Ligation of the IMA or interruption of both hypogastric arteries in a patient with inadequate collateralization of the colon from the SMA, embolization during aneurysm manipulation, intraoperative hypotension, or direct compression from retractors can all have an effect.

Certain measures can be taken intraoperatively to help prevent ischemia. Minimal manipulation of the aortic neck, and prevention of hypotension or compression can help. Measurement of the back pressures within the IMA can usually be done from inside the opened aneurysm sac. Mean pressure >40 mmHg can be an indication for safe ligation of the IMA. Pressures lower than this would require reimplantation of the IMA.

Postoperatively, early diagnosis of colonic ischemia requires a high index of suspicion. Acidemia, elevated WBC, or increased fluid requirements can be early warning signs. Diarrhea, especially bloody or watery and especially in the first day or two after surgery, should also be aggressively investigated.

Patients with obvious peritoneal signs or evidence of hemodynamic instability should be taken emergently to the operating room; however, stable patients suspected of having colonic ischemia should undergo immediate flexible sigmoidoscopy, as the left colon and rectum are most often involved. Patients with full-thickness necrosis should be taken to the operating room for resection, while patients with ischemia limited to the mucosa should be treated supportively with NPO status, NG tube decompression, broad-spectrum antibiotics, and fluid resuscitation. Repeat endoscopy should be performed to document resolution or progression of the ischemia and appropriate subsequent action should be taken.

Bibliography

Ernst CB, Stanley JC. *Current Therapy in Vascular Surgery*, 4th ed. St. Louis, MO: Mosby, 2001.

Moore WS (ed.). *Vascular Surgery: A Comprehensive Review*, 6th ed. Philadelphia, PA: W.B. Saunders, 2002.

Rutherford RB (ed.). *Vascular Surgery*, 5th ed. St. Louis, MO: Mosby, 2000, vol. 1 and 2.

24. **(D)** Current technology has increased the available imaging modalities for evaluation of AAAs. The easiest and least invasive screening tool is abdominal ultrasonography. Ultrasound is considered the study of choice for evaluation of a suspected aneurysmal disease and for routine follow-up of asymptomatic, known aneurysms. There are drawbacks to ultrasound, however. Skill of the operator, as well as overlying bowel gas or significant obesity, can limit accuracy of ultrasound. Therefore, alternate imaging techniques are required; however, failure of ultrasound does not mandate aortography. Modalities such as CT scanning with three-dimensional reconstructions can demonstrate not only the size of an aneurysm, but also the extent of involvement of the aorta itself (e.g., thoracic or iliac involvement) as well as the aneurysm's relationship to other structures such as the renal or mesenteric arteries. Magnetic resonance imaging (MRI) has also emerged as a valuable tool in aneurysm evaluation. With these other, less invasive methods, arteriography is not a mandatory test for aneurysm repair. Indeed, arteriography—because it shows flow channels only—may in fact underestimate the size of an aneurysm that contains significant mural thrombus; however, there are indications for aortography prior to AAA repair.

For example, patients who present with symptoms of intestinal ischemia, such as weight loss, postprandial pain, or food fear, should be investigated with aortogram to rule out mesenteric occlusive disease. Patients with evidence of iliac or infrainguinal occlusive disease likewise may benefit from optimal evaluation of their arterial tree. Patients with evidence of renovascular hypertension or renal anomalies such as horseshoe kidney also should undergo arteriogram. In this way surgical correction of symptomatic renal artery stenosis may be planned or identification of important renal artery anomalies can be made and surgery planned accordingly.

Bibliography

Ernst CB, Stanley JC. *Current Therapy in Vascular Surgery*, 4th ed. St. Louis, MO: Mosby, 2001.

Moore WS (ed.). *Vascular Surgery: A Comprehensive Review*, 6th ed. Philadelphia, PA: W.B. Saunders, 2002.

Rutherford RB (ed.). *Vascular Surgery*, 5th ed. St. Louis, MO: Mosby, 2000, vol. 1 and 2.

25. **(E)** Aneurysmal disease is a fairly common disease. The aorta is considered aneurysmal when the diameter of the diseased aorta is dilated to a diameter 50% greater than that of the proximal, normal aorta. In a male, the average normal diameter of the abdominal aorta is approximately 2 cm, while in a female, it measures about 1.8 cm. Therefore, an aorta that measures approximately 3 cm in a male and 2.7 cm in a female would be considered aneurysmal. Once again, however, these "averages" are subject to some variability based on the normal aorta above the aneurysmal dilation.

AAAs affect both men and women, although males are affected much more frequently, with a male:female ratio of about 4–5:1. White ethnicity, increased age, positive family history, smoking, and hypertension are also associated with aneurysmal disease—with smoking being one of the most strongly associated factors.

Collagen and elastin are substances found in the aortic wall. These substances are noted to be significantly decreased in AAA formation. Aneurysmal aortas are noted to have increased levels of metalloproteases such as collagenase and elastase in relation to their inhibitors, such as alpha-1-antitrypsin. This imbalance leads to weakening of the aortic wall and aneurysmal changes.

While back or abdominal pain is the most common *symptom* of aortic aneurysmal disease, most AAAs are asymptomatic at presentation. In fact, 70% of patients with aneurysms are diagnosed as an incidental finding on physical examination or imaging studies performed for unrelated issues. Other symptoms include embolic phenomena, dissection, and rupture.

Indeed, rupture of an AAA is the most significant and indeed life-threatening sequela of aneurysmal disease. The risk of rupture of an AAA increases with increasing size of the aneurysm, with about a 5-year rupture rate of 25% for aneurysms 5–6 cm. This risk increases to approximately 50% for those aneurysms 6–7 cm and 80–100% at 7 cm or greater. Sudden, acute back, flank, or abdominal pain—especially when coupled with shock and/or pulsatile abdominal mass—should alert one to the presence of ruptured AAA.

Chronic obstructive pulmonary disease (COPD) and hypertension also have been found to be independent risk factors for aneurysm expansion and risk of rupture.

Bibliography

Ernst CB, Stanley JC. *Current Therapy in Vascular Surgery*, 4th ed. St. Louis, MO: Mosby, 2001.

Moore WS (ed.). *Vascular Surgery: A Comprehensive Review*, 6th ed. Philadelphia, PA: W.B. Saunders, 2002.

Rutherford RB (ed.). *Vascular Surgery*, 5th ed. St. Louis, MO: Mosby, 2000, vol. 1 and 2.

26. **(D)**

27. **(D)**

Explanations 26 and 27

When considering placing an endoluminal stent graft for aortic aneurysm repair, several anatomic considerations must be addressed. The neck of the aneurysm (the area between the renal arteries and the start of the aneurysmal dilatation) should ideally be at least 15 mm in length to prevent the graft from crossing the renal artery orifices and yet have a solid docking purchase. Endograft diameter is a maximum of 30 mm, therefore a neck diameter in excess of 28 mm precludes this type of repair. Aortic angulation in excess of 60 degrees also prevents proper deployment of the graft. And as the femoral route is used to deploy the devices, femoral and iliac artery diameter and tortuosity are important in that arteries that are too tortuous or too small to accommodate the 18–23 French diameter devices are contraindications to graft placement.

Once grafts are in place, close follow-up is required to identify endoleaks should they occur. The purpose of the stent graft is to exclude the aneurysm from the arterial system, thus preventing further enlargement. If for some reason, the aneurysm sees arterial flow and, therefore, pressure (an endoleak), enlargement and eventual rupture could occur. There are several types of endoleaks described.

A type I leak is an inability of the proximal or distal end of the device to completely seal, thus allowing blood flow into the aneurysm sac.

A type II leak occurs when lumbar vessels or the IMA remains patent, allowing continued pressure to be exposed to the aneurysm sac.

A type III leak occurs when component pieces of the endograft (such as an iliac extension) break apart, while type IV leaks occur secondary to graft porosity.

Endoleaks can occur at any time throughout the life of the graft; therefore yearly contrast-enhanced CT scans are required to evaluate for any such leak or expansion of the aneurysm with subsequent intervention if necessary.

Bibliography

Moore WS, Ahn SS (eds.). *Endovascular Surgery*, 3rd ed. Philadelphia, PA: W.B. Saunders, 2001.

28. **(D)** Acute intestinal ischemia is a surgical emergency, and as such, requires a high index of suspicion when circumstances are consistent with its possibility. Of the options listed above, all except celiac artery compression are common etiologies of acute ischemic changes.

Embolic phenomena (as shown in Fig. 32-16) are usually cardiac in origin and tend to occlude the SMA secondary to its relatively parallel course with the aorta. Preexisting atherosclerotic disease can also serve as a nidus for thrombus formation, causing acute occlusion of the vessel. Low flow states, often termed NOMI (nonocclusive mesenteric ischemia), are seen most commonly in situations that present

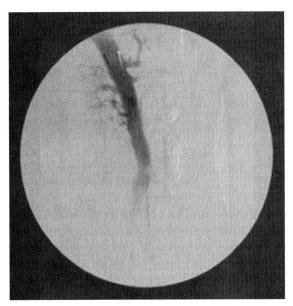

FIG. 32-16

with hypotension—such as sepsis or heart failure. Use of high doses of alpha agonists can compound this phenomena, as vasoconstriction in the face of already compromised blood supply can further risk ischemic damage to the bowel.

Mesenteric venous thrombosis causes ischemia secondary to the high back pressures caused by obstruction of venous outflow. The bowel subsequently becomes edematous and distended, and hemorrhagic infarction can occur.

Celiac artery compression (median arcuate ligament syndrome) does not usually cause acute ischemic events, but can be an uncommon contributing factor in chronic mesenteric ischemia.

Bibliography

Ernst CB, Stanley JC. *Current Therapy in Vascular Surgery*, 4th ed. St. Louis, MO: Mosby, 2001.
Moore WS (ed.). *Vascular Surgery: A Comprehensive Review*, 6th ed. Philadelphia, PA: W.B. Saunders, 2002.
Rutherford RB (ed.). *Vascular Surgery*, 5th ed. St. Louis, MO: Mosby, 2000, vol. 1 and 2.

29. **(D)** Unlike acute mesenteric ischemia, chronic mesenteric ischemia is caused by atherosclerotic progression in the vast majority of cases. As a result, the process is often insidious, usually not becoming symptomatic until two of the three mesenteric vessels become significantly stenotic. Often, large fully developed collateral vessels to the bowel can be seen as a result. The most common complaint of patients with chronic mesenteric ischemia is crampy, postprandial

pain—often called "intestinal angina." In fact, the pain associated with food intake often leads to "food fear" and weight loss develops, with significant malnutrition as the patient avoids food.

Duplex ultrasound can sometimes be used to aid in diagnosis, using elevated visceral artery peak systolic flow velocities as an indication of disease; however, this is operator-dependent, and therefore mesenteric angiography is still the study of choice for diagnosis.

Once diagnosed, treatment is planned. Angioplasty with/without stenting has been proposed as an alternative to surgical revascularization; however, the osteal location of many of the lesions and a relatively high restenosis rate have prevented endoluminal treatment from becoming more widespread. Further studies and longer follow-up are required to determine its place in the treatment of this condition.

Surgery in the form of aortomesenteric bypass is still the treatment of choice. Greater saphenous vein or prosthetic grafts may be used, although kinking of the GSV from the weight of the intestine can be an issue if improperly positioned during surgery.

Bibliography

Ernst CB, Stanley JC. *Current Therapy in Vascular Surgery*, 4th ed. St. Louis, MO: Mosby, 2001.
Moore WS (ed.). *Vascular Surgery: A Comprehensive Review*, 6th ed. Philadelphia, PA: W.B. Saunders, 2002.
Rutherford RB (ed.). *Vascular Surgery*, 5th ed. St. Louis, MO: Mosby, 2000, vol. 1 and 2.

30. **(A)** Patients with peripheral vascular disease have a high likelihood of having concomitant coronary disease (up to 50%). In fact, MI is the most common cause of perioperative morbidity and mortality in the vascular patient. Therefore, identifying those patients at risk is of extreme importance.

Elderly patients (>70 years), patients who have suffered an MI within the previous 6 months, those who have mitral regurgitation, ventricular ectopy, or severe CHF are at statistically significantly increased risk of perioperative MI than are their counterparts who do not suffer these symptoms. Patients with stable angina pectoris without evidence of the other risk factors mentioned above, however, are not at significantly higher risk for perioperative MI.

Of the factors listed, recent MI is the most important risk factor for perioperative cardiac events. Risk is up to 30% within 3 months of an MI, and finally levels off at 5% after 6 months' time.

Selective coronary angiography may be beneficial in identifying those patients at higher risk who would require further cardiac treatment prior to vascular interventions.

Bibliography

Moore WS (ed.). *Vascular Surgery: A Comprehensive Review*, 6th ed. Philadelphia, PA: W.B. Saunders, 2002.
Rutherford RB (ed.). *Vascular Surgery*, 5th ed. St. Louis, MO: Mosby, 2000, vol. 1 and 2.

31. **(D)** Endovascular approaches to lesions elsewhere in the vascular tree has spurred interest in potential endovascular approaches to carotid artery occlusive disease as well.

Carotid angioplasty and stenting is a very new treatment modality. Early studies have illustrated cumulative stroke rates of 7.7% for stenting versus 1.5% following an operative CEA. In addition, the cost of stenting is slightly higher—secondary to the cost of imaging required and devices used. Although there are not a large number of trials available, high success rates have been noted. It appears too early to give stenting recommendation *over* traditional CEA, although certain patients, such as those presenting after multiple neck operations or neck radiation, in whom the risk of an open surgical approach would be prohibitive, may benefit from stenting. Long-term outcomes are not yet available.

Bibliography

Moore WS, Ahn SS (eds.). *Endovascular Surgery*, 3rd ed. Philadelphia, PA: W.B. Saunders, 2001.

32. **(C)** Decisions regarding site of amputation can be difficult for the vascular surgeon, especially when differentiating between a BKA and an AKA. When amputation is required, it is important to remove all necrotic or infected tissue while providing enough blood flow to heal. If ambulation is a goal, BKA is preferable to AKA, as energy expenditure required to ambulate on a below-knee prosthesis is lower than that of an AKA (approximately a 40% increase for BKA vs. 70% increase for AKA).

It can be difficult to determine by clinical examination alone which level is appropriate for amputation. Often, further testing such as Doppler studies or $TCPO_2$ levels are obtained. One physical finding that can be useful, however, is presence of dependent rubor. This redness that occurs with the leg in the dependent position is an indication of tissue ischemia and any amputation through this level should be avoided.

Patients with active infection or gangrene can also pose special problems. Often formal amputation with skin closure is not optimal in patients with active infection or hemodynamic instability. In instances such as this, guillotine amputation can remove offending tissue, allowing stability of the patient and control of infection with definitive amputation several days later.

Technique and clinical judgment regarding amputations are not important only for major amputations, however. Toe amputations also require forethought. Amputation should be performed just distal or proximal to a joint space, as cartilage is avascular and does not allow for adequate granulation or healing.

Unfortunately for diabetics, the need for amputation of one lower extremity is a fairly significant risk factor for the loss of the other lower extremity, with a 5-year cumulative incidence of second amputation of up to 33%.

Bibliography

Ernst CB, Stanley JC. *Current Therapy in Vascular Surgery*, 4th ed. St. Louis, MO: Mosby, 2001.

Moore WS (ed.). *Vascular Surgery: A Comprehensive Review*, 6th ed. Philadelphia, PA: W.B. Saunders, 2002.

Rutherford RB (ed.). *Vascular Surgery*, 5th ed. St. Louis, MO: Mosby, 2000, vol. 1 and 2.

33. (C) Renal artery aneurysms are rare entities. The incidence in the general population is approximately 0.1%. Several etiologic factors play a role in the development of these aneurysms, including medial degeneration (as with other visceral artery aneurysms), hypertension, and even trauma. Atherosclerosis can be an etiologic factor, but is often a secondary result. The vast majority of these aneurysms are saccular aneurysms that are found extraparenchymally at first or second order branch points.

Despite the aneurysmal dilation, rupture is not common. Only approximately 3% of renal artery aneurysms rupture, and rupture carries a mortality rate of approximately 10%. One exception to this general rule is the pregnant patient. Pregnant women have a much higher mortality rate than do other patients with renal artery aneurysms. Mortality in these patients approached 40–50% for the mother and 80% for the fetus. It is, therefore, imperative that women of child-bearing age who plan on conceiving or are pregnant undergo repair of these aneurysms when diagnosed.

Other indications for repair include symptomatic aneurysms. Symptoms include rupture, embolization to the renal parenchyma (with worsening renal failure), renovascular hypertension, pain, or dissection. Increasing size of the aneurysm is also an indication for surgery. In the absence of these symptoms, however, size at which a renal artery aneurysm should be fixed has been somewhat controversial, but most now recommend repair at a size of 2 cm or greater.

Repair of these aneurysms often can be accomplished with simple resection of the aneurysm and primary patch angioplasty of the renal vessel (if the vessel is large enough, e.g., main renal artery) or renal artery bypass, usually with saphenous vein. Internal iliac artery can also be used. Nephrectomy is not usually necessary in these cases, but may be the only recourse for ruptured aneurysms. Rare intraparenchymal aneurysms may also require resection, but partial nephrectomy will usually suffice.

Bibliography

Ernst CB, Stanley JC. *Current Therapy in Vascular Surgery*, 4th ed. St. Louis, MO: Mosby, 2001.

Moore WS (ed.). *Vascular Surgery: A Comprehensive Review*, 6th ed. Philadelphia, PA: W.B. Saunders, 2002.

Rutherford RB (ed.). *Vascular Surgery*, 5th ed. St. Louis, MO: Mosby, 2000, vol. 1 and 2.

34. (D) Visceral artery aneurysms can affect just about any intraabdominal vessel, from the splenic artery, as shown here (the most commonly involved, at 60%) to the pancreaticoduodenal and pancreatic (at 1.5%). Other visceral vessels are variably involved with aneurysmal disease: hepatic (20%), SMA (5.5%), celiac (4%), gastric/gastroepiploic (4%), and intestinal (jejunal/ileal/colic 3%). The vast majority are the result of medial degeneration; atherosclerosis is usually a secondary event. Pancreaticoduodenal artery aneurysms are often the result of pancreatitis and its associated arterial necrosis.

Just as the incidence of these aneurysms is variable, so too is their rate of rupture. While splenic artery aneurysms are the most common visceral artery aneurysm, their rate of rupture is one of the lowest (at approximately 2%), while gastric and gastroepiploic artery aneurysms, although much more rare, have a rupture rate of up to 90%. Mortality from rupture of visceral artery aneurysms is about 50% for most aneurysms. A definite exception is the splenic artery aneurysm in the pregnant female, which carries a 70% maternal mortality and 75% fetal mortality.

Most aneurysms should be fixed when they are found. Surgical treatment usually involves resection of the aneurysm with arterial reconstruction. Gastric and intestinal aneurysms often require resection of a portion of the stomach or intestine along with the aneurysm if the aneurysm is intramural. Pancreatitis-related false aneurysms can often be ligated, as dissection in inflamed areas previously affected by pancreatitis may be difficult. Distal pancreatectomy may sometimes be required.

Bibliography

Ernst CB, Stanley JC. *Current Therapy in Vascular Surgery*, 4th ed. St. Louis, MO: Mosby, 2001.

Moore WS (ed.). *Vascular Surgery: A Comprehensive Review*, 6th ed. Philadelphia, PA: W.B. Saunders, 2002.

Rutherford RB (ed.). *Vascular Surgery*, 5th ed. St. Louis, MO: Mosby, 2000, vol. 1 and 2.

35. (A) Lymphedema constitutes a condition in which an abnormality in the lymphatic channels causes a build-up of protein-rich fluid in the interstitial space. Lymphedema can be classified as primary or secondary. Further primary lymphedema has several classifications. Congenital lymphedema is clinically present at birth or by age 2. Lymphedema praecox is primary lymphedema that presents itself before age 35, while lymphedema tarda presents after age 35. (The familial forms of lymphedema praecox and tarda are Milroy's and Meige's disease, respectively.) Lymphedema praecox is the most common form of primary lymphedema, and has up to a 10:1 female predominance.

Primary lymphedema is usually secondary to either a developmental abnormality in the lymphatics or a fibrotic obliteration of the lymph channels.

In contrast, secondary lymphedema denotes an acquired cause. Worldwide, the most common of these is infection with filariae. Bacterial infections causing lymphatic scarring and fibrosis, as will as tumor infiltration of lymphatics, are other secondary causes.

Several diagnostic methods can be used to evaluate lower extremity swelling, including CT scan and or MRI. CT findings can illustrate honeycomb appearance of the subcutaneous tissue, suspicious for lymphatic etiology, although it is not sensitive. Importantly, however, CT can help rule out tumor invasion as a cause for leg swelling. MRI is also useful and can be a good adjunct to lymphoscintigraphy.

Lymphoscintigraphy is an important diagnostic tool. Lymphoscintigraphy involves injection of radioactive tracer between the toes of the affected extremity. Uptake by the lymphatics occurs and images track the tracer up the extremity. In this way, findings such as absence of lymph channels, delayed uptake, or absence of nodes can be seen.

Treatment therapies include medical methods such as manual lymphatic therapy (a massage technique that can stimulate lymphatic flow), compression wraps or devices, and—in those cases refractory to medical management—surgical techniques such as lymphatic to lymphatic or lymphatic to venous anastamoses, or resection of affected tissue to reduce the size and volume of the extremity.

Bibliography

Ernst CB, Stanley JC. *Current Therapy in Vascular Surgery,* 4th ed. St. Louis, MO: Mosby, 2001.

Moore WS (ed.). *Vascular Surgery: A Comprehensive Review,* 6th ed. Philadelphia, PA: W.B. Saunders, 2002.

Rutherford RB (ed.). *Vascular Surgery,* 5th ed. St. Louis, MO: Mosby, 2000, vol. 1 and 2.

36. (D) Infrainguinal vein grafts should be carefully and closely monitored to ensure continued patency. Grafts that are "failing" are those that are affected by a defect that causes hemodynamically significant changes in the graft and ultimately put the graft at risk of occlusion if not corrected. Grafts can fail in the early or late postoperative period. Perioperatively (within 30 days), graft failure is usually secondary to a technical error or poor outflow vessels. Early failures (within 2 years) are usually secondary to intimal hyperplasia, whereas late failures (after 2 years) are usually secondary to progressive atherosclerotic changes. Narrowing of the graft to a point where it becomes hemodynamically significant is termed a "critical stenosis." This usually occurs at a diameter reduction of 50%, which corresponds to a crosssectional area reduction of approximately 75%. At this level, grafts are in danger of occluding if intervention is not undertaken. To ensure identification of these lesions, grafts should be surveilled on a regular basis with duplex studies to identify these lesions. Duplex can visually identify these areas, and velocity changes can also be used to localize areas of stenosis. Finding these lesions prior to graft occlusion is especially important, because grafts that are revised prior to progressing to total occlusion have a much better assisted patency rates than do those grafts that occlude.

Once the stenosis is identified, revision should be undertaken. Depending on the lesion, this can be accomplished by vein patch angioplasty, segmental bypass, or in some cases, angioplasty of the lesion. Lesions at the proximal or distal segment of the bypass are more amenable to angioplasty than are those in the midgraft, and shortsegment stenoses are better candidates for angioplasty than are longer lesions.

Bibliography

Moore WS (ed.). *Vascular Surgery: A Comprehensive Review,* 6th ed. Philadelphia, PA: W.B. Saunders, 2002.

Rutherford RB (ed.). *Vascular Surgery,* 5th ed. St. Louis, MO: Mosby, 2000, vol. 1 and 2.

37. (A) Many risk factors exist for peripheral arterial occlusive disease. The most significant risk factors include advanced age, hypertension, cigarette smoking, diabetes, hyperlipidemia, and homocysteinemia. Other factors that can be involved in the development of peripheral occlusive disease include male patients, high-fat diet, alcoholism, and hypercoagulability. Patients with diabetes often see a different pattern of peripheral arterial disease than do patients with other risk factors such as hypertension or tobacco use. Patients with these risk factors tend to develop aortoiliac and femoral occlusive disease; however, patients with diabetes tend to develop disease in the tibial vessels while the aortoiliac and femoral-popliteal segments remain relatively free of disease. If the femoral and popliteal arteries are involved, the lesions tend not to advance to occlusion; however, the tibial vessels become severely diseased, often throughout their course. This is likely secondary to increased calcification of the intima and thickening of capillary basement membranes. Hyperthyroidism is not a risk factor for peripheral occlusive disease.

Bibliography

Ernst CB, Stanley JC. *Current Therapy in Vascular Surgery*, 4th ed. St. Louis, MO: Mosby, 2001.

Moore WS (ed.). *Vascular Surgery: A Comprehensive Review*, 6th ed. Philadelphia, PA: W.B. Saunders, 2002.

Rutherford RB (ed.). *Vascular Surgery*, 5th ed. St. Louis, MO: Mosby, 2000, vol. 1 and 2.

38. **(E)** Popliteal artery injury is a very serious complication of knee dislocation. Injury can occur with both anterior and posterior dislocations (approximately 35% incidence), but is more common after posterior dislocation. Therefore, diagnosis and appropriate management are of the utmost importance, as undetected injury can lead to significant lower extremity ischemia and even amputation. A high index of suspicion is necessary. "Hard signs," such as lack of pulse, bruit, distal ischemia, or expanding hematomas, are clearly indicative of arterial injury; however, subtler examination findings cannot be overlooked. Pulse examination, both before and after reduction, is important and the presence of a *normal* pedal pulse can be a reliable indication of arterial integrity. Often, however, a palpable, but diminished, pulse may be present in the face of significant injury and should lead to suspicion of possible arterial injury. Contrary to previous beliefs, not every patient with a knee dislocation requires an arteriogram. Patients with a normal ABI and a normal examination can safely be observed with serial examinations. Likewise, patients with clear evidence of acute ischemia should not have repair delayed by arteriogram, but rather taken directly to the operating room. Those patients with suspected—but not proven—ischemia may benefit most from preoperative arteriography.

If arterial injury is identified, repair should be undertaken expeditiously. Primary repair may be selectively applied, but in the setting of more extensive arterial injury, vein bypass may be more appropriate. Most often, the contralateral saphenous vein is used secondary to the high incidence of concomitant deep venous injury associated with the knee dislocation.

In most instances, arterial repair should be undertaken first, to minimize ischemia time. Orthopedic repair—often in the form of external fixation—can then be undertaken with close attention to pulse examination during reduction and fixation. If orthopedic injury must be done first, often arterial shunting may be employed to prevent or minimize further ischemia time.

Compartment syndrome is common, secondary to acute edema/ischemia and associated reperfusion and increased index of suspicion is required. If any doubt, four-compartment fasciotomy should be performed.

Bibliography

Ernst CB, Stanley JC. *Current Therapy in Vascular Surgery*, 4th ed. St. Louis, MO: Mosby, 2001.

Moore WS (ed.). *Vascular Surgery: A Comprehensive Review*, 6th ed. Philadelphia, PA: W.B. Saunders, 2002.

Rutherford RB (ed.). *Vascular Surgery*, 5th ed. St. Louis, MO: Mosby, 2000, vol. 1 and 2.

39. **(D)** ST is a condition involving thrombosis of the superficial veins, usually of the lower extremity. Many risk factors exist, including trauma, varicose veins, pregnancy, hypercoagulable disorders, and malignancy. The most common symptoms include painful, hardened areas overlying the affected veins. Often, this is a self-limiting process that can be effectively treated with elevation, warm compresses, and anti-inflammatory agents. It is important, however, to ensure that the deep system is not involved. Duplex scanning to rule out associated DVT is prudent, as incidences of DVT from 12 to 44% have been noted (often these are asymptomatic).

Close follow-up is recommended, and progression of the thrombophlebitis toward the saphenofemoral junction (as noted by physical examination or serial duplex examinations) may warrant anticoagulation or ligation ± stripping of the vein to ensure that progression into the deep system does not occur. (It is important to remember, if stripping the saphenous vein in a patient with ST, to ligate the vein proximally prior to passing a stripper up the vein, as failure to do so has resulted in pulmonary embolus.)

Suppurative thrombophlebitis is often related to IV cannulation, and prompt treatment is important. Removal of the IV, systemic antibiotics, and—if gross purulence is noted from the vein—excision of the offending vein segment may be required.

Bibliography

Moore WS (ed.). *Vascular Surgery: A Comprehensive Review*, 6th ed. Philadelphia, PA: W.B. Saunders, 2002.

Rutherford RB (ed.). *Vascular Surgery*, 5th ed. St. Louis, MO: Mosby, 2000, vol. 1 and 2.

CHAPTER 33

Soft Tissue Sarcoma and Skin

Christian S. Hinrichs and Nathalie C. Zeitouni

Questions

1. Which of the following is *not* an appropriate surgical margin for melanoma excision?

   (A) melanoma *in situ* on the trunk—0.5 cm margin

   (B) 0.8 mm thick melanoma on the extremity—1.0 cm margin

   (C) 2 mm thick melanoma on the trunk—2.0 cm margin

   (D) 2 mm thick melanoma inferior to the lateral canthus—1.0 cm

   (E) all of the above are appropriate

2. Which of the following is *true* of biopsy for suspected melanoma?

   (A) Incisional biopsy is not acceptable.

   (B) Incisions on the extremities should be longitudinally oriented.

   (C) Shave biopsy should be performed for lesions in cosmetically sensitive locations.

   (D) A biopsy punch should never be used.

3. A 60-year-old, otherwise healthy, male presents 6 months after WLE of a melanoma from his ankle with 30 in-transit and cutaneous metastases scattered on his lower leg (Fig. 33-1).
   Which of the following is the *best* treatment?

   (A) amputation

   (B) WLE

   (C) isolated limb perfusion with melphalan

   (D) systemic therapy

   (E) none of the above

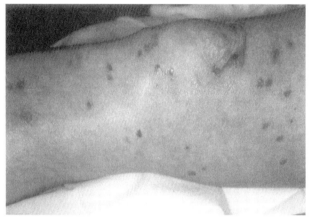

FIG. 33-1   In-transit metastasis from melanoma on leg of elderly male.

4. Which of the following is *true* about groin dissection for melanoma?

   (A) The greater saphenous vein is preserved in a superficial groin dissection.

   (B) The highest node removed in a radical (superficial and deep) groin dissection is Cloquet's node.

   (C) Sacrifice of the obturator nerve results in severe functional impairment in most patients.

   (D) In experienced hands wound complication rates are low.

   (E) None of the above.

5. Which of the following is *true* about sentinel lymph node (SLN) biopsy for melanoma?

   (A) Nonsentinel node metastases occur in the presence of a negative sentinel node in 15% of cases.

   (B) Sentinel node biopsy should be considered for melanomas greater than 1.0 mm thick.

   (C) Lymphatic mapping fails to identify the sentinel node in 10% of cases.

   (D) Patients with clinically involved lymph nodes should undergo SLN biopsy.

6. Which of the following is *true* of the American Joint Committee on Cancer (AJCC) staging system for cutaneous melanoma (sixth edition)?

   (A) Presence of ulceration raises T1 thickness tumors to T2.

   (B) In-transit metastasis are classified M1 disease.

   (C) Visceral metastases are substaged by site and presence or absence of elevated bilirubin.

   (D) All stage I and stage II disease is N0.

7. Which of the following is *true* of melanoma prognosis?

   (A) The most powerful prognostic feature of localized melanoma is tumor diameter.

   (B) Younger age, female gender, and site of disease on the trunk are all favorable prognostic indicators.

   (C) The number of metastatic nodes, tumor burden (microscopic vs. macroscopically positive nodes), and primary tumor ulceration are the most powerful predictors of survival in node positive disease.

   (D) Patients with lung metastases have a worse prognosis than those with metastases to other visceral sites.

8. Which of the following is *true* of retroperitoneal soft tissue sarcomas?

   (A) The most common histologic cellular type is malignant fibrous histiosarcoma.

   (B) Because of the risk of tumor seeding, preoperative biopsy is contraindicated.

   (C) Resection of contiguous organs that are not involved with tumor is indicated to obtain adequate margins.

   (D) Death usually results from distant metastases.

   (E) Lung is the most common site of distant metastases.

9. Which of the following is *true* of soft tissue sarcoma staging?

   (A) Malignant fibrous histiocytoma, rhabdomyosarcoma, synovial sarcoma, and angiosarcoma are grouped together for staging purposes.

   (B) The components of soft tissue sarcoma stage grouping are primary tumor, regional lymph nodes, distant metastasis, and histologic grade.

   (C) Retroperitonal, mediastinal, and pelvic sarcomas are staged by a different scheme than extremity sarcomas.

   (D) A malignant fibrous histiocytoma of the calf, 2 cm in diameter, superficial to the fascia, without regional node or distant metastasis, histologic grade 2 out of 3 is stage I disease.

   (E) Only 10% soft tissue sarcomas are node positive.

10. Which of the following is *true* of extremity soft tissue sarcoma?

    (A) Amputation provides better local control than WLE plus radiation.

    (B) At least 95% of patients presenting with soft tissue sarcomas of the extremities are effectively treated with limb preserving surgery.

    (C) The most common site of metastases is the liver.

    (D) There is no role for surgery in the treatment of distant recurrences.

    (E) Repeat excision of an incompletely excised sarcoma is futile and should rarely be attempted.

11. Which of the following is *true* of gastrointestinal stromal tumor (GIST)?

    (A) They arise from smooth muscle cells of the gastrointestinal tract.

    (B) They are immunohistochemically positive for CD117 and often CD34.

    (C) The small intestine is the most common primary site.

    (E) Primary therapy for unresectable tumors is doxyrubicin-based cytotoxic chemotherapy.

12. A 45-year-old lady has a biopsy proven, ill-defined morpheaform basal cell carcinoma (BCC) on the tip of the nose (Fig. 33-2). The best therapeutic option for this patient is

    (A) radiation therapy

    (B) surgical excision

    (C) electrodesiccation and curettage

    (D) cryosurgery

    (E) Mohs micrographic surgery

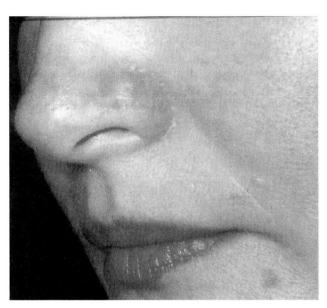

FIG. 33-2 Morpheaform basal cell carcinoma on nasal tip.

13. Which of the following is *not* true of immunotherapy for melanoma?

    (A) Vaccine therapies have not been demonstrated to induce regression of established metastatic melanoma.

    (B) Treatment with high-dose interleukin-2 results in less durable responses than treatment with combination chemotherapy.

    (C) Experimental treatment with adoptive cell transfer of tumor specific lymphocytes (TIL) in combination with high-dose interleukin-2 has shown objective response rates of greater than 40%.

    (D) High-dose interferon is approved by the FDA for adjuvant treatment of high-risk melanoma.

14. Which of the following is *not* considered to be a poor prognostic variable of subcutaneous squamous cell carcinoma (SCC)?

    (A) underlying immunosuppression

    (B) perineural invasion

    (C) associated with UV exposure

    (D) radiation-induced

    (E) arising from glabrous skin

15. Which of the following statements is *true* regarding treatment of cutaneous SCC?

    (A) achieving histological negative margins always eliminates the risk of local recurrence

    (B) local "in-transit" metastases are usually removed during surgical resection

    (C) clinically well-defined low-risk tumors less than 2 cm require approximately 2 cm surgical margins

    (D) adjuvant radiotherapy may be beneficial for high-risk SCC

16. Which of the following tumors is a type of verrucous carcinoma?

    (A) Buschke–Lowenstein's tumor

    (B) Ackerman's tumor

    (C) epithelioma curriculatum

    (D) cutaneous verrucous carcinoma

    (E) all of the above

17. A 69-year-old male with a previous history of skin cancer presented to his dermatologist with a new enlarging erythematous nodule on his nose (Fig. 33-3). A biopsy was performed and revealed Merkel cell carcinoma. What percent of patients will have regional lymph node disease?

    (A) 0%

    (B) 15%

    (C) 30%

    (D) 50%

    (E) 75%

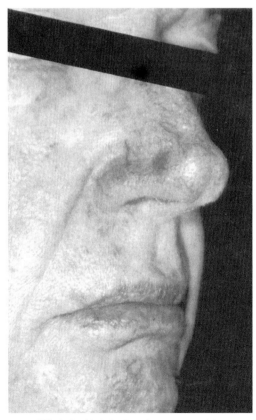

FIG. 33-3 Merkel cell carcinoma on nasal tip.

18. A 35-year-old male presented with a 5-year history of a scar-like lesion on his anterior shoulder (Fig. 33-4). Histopathology revealed a dermatofibrosarcoma protuberans (DFSP). What would be your initial management?

(A) local resection followed by XRT

(B) WLE and lymph node dissection

(C) radiation therapy then surgical resection

(D) local resection and SLN biopsy

(E) WLE with 2–3 cm margins alone

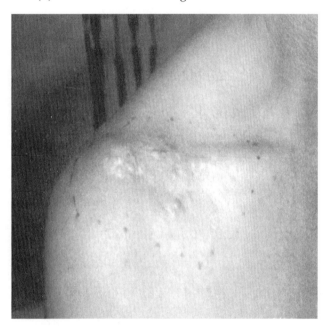

FIG. 33-4   Dermatofibrosarcoma protuberans of anterior shoulder.

19. Which of the following histologic or IHC findings is *not* characteristic of DFSP?

(A) invasion into fat with irregular tentacle-like projections

(B) significant cellular pleomorphism and mitotic figure

(C) storiform pattern of spindle cells

(D) CD34 positive, factor XIIIa negative

(E) variants include mxyoid, pigmented, and atrophic type

20. What is the most common site of origin of ocular sebaceous carcinoma?

(A) Meibomian gland

(B) gland of Zeis

(C) lacrimal gland

(D) caruncle

(E) multicentric origin

21. A 74-year-old female with a history of early stage breast cancer was treated with lumpectomy and radiotherapy 5 years ago. She now presents with ill-defined bruise-like patches, ulcerated nodules, and edema over her treated breast. What is the most likely diagnosis?

(A) Kaposi's sarcoma

(B) Steward-Treves' syndrome

(C) metastatic melanoma

(D) recurrent breast cancer

(E) radiation-induced angiosarcoma

22. Histologically, what does microcystic adnexal carcinoma (MAC) have a propensity for?

(A) invasion into bone

(B) high mitotic rate

(C) perineural invasion

(D) noncontiguous growth

(E) superficial growth

Answers and Explanations

1. **(E)** Guidelines for excision margins for cutaneous melanomas are suggested by the National Comprehensive Cancer Network (NCCN) Guidelines in Oncology. Table 33-1 shows recommended margins based on these guidelines. These margins may need to be adjusted to accommodate cosmetically or functionally sensitive areas, such as the face or hands. Melanoma involving a digit, as with subungual melanoma, generally requires amputation.

   These recommendations are supported by several randomized trials. 2 cm and 4 cm margins were demonstrated to provide equivalent local recurrence and survival for tumors 1–4 mm thick in the Intergroup Melanoma Surgical Trial. 2 cm margins were compared to 5 cm margins for tumors 0.8–2 mm thick in the Swedish Melanoma Study Group trial. No significant difference in local recurrence or survival was detected. The World Health Organization Melanoma Programme evaluated 1 cm versus 2 cm margins for melanomas less than 2 mm thick and found only 4 patients with local recurrence as a first relapse, all of whom had excision margins of 1 cm and tumors thicker than 1 mm. It is therefore generally accepted that margins of 1 cm are safe for tumors less than 1 mm thick. There is no randomized data that addresses margins for tumors greater than 4 mm thick, however, 2 cm margins are widely accepted as adequate.

   The technique for wide local excision (WLE) involves measuring and marking appropriate margin distance from the tumor or biopsy scar. The incision should be oriented longitudinally. Excision should be carried down to the underlying fascia. WLE excision wounds can almost always be closed primarily using a layered closure. It is rarely necessary undermine the skin significantly. Skin grafting or flap coverage may occasionally be required. Temporary immobilization of the affected limb may be required to allow adequate healing.

   ### Bibliography

   Balch CM, Soong SJ, Smith T, Ross MI, Urist MM, Karakousis CP, et al. Long-term results of a prospective surgical trial comparing 2 cm vs. 4 cm excision margins for 740 patients with 1-4 mm melanomas. *Ann Surg Oncol* 2001;8(2):101–108.

   Cohn-Cedermark G, Rutqvist LE, Andersson R, Breivald M, Ingvar C, Johansson H, et al. Long term results of a randomized study by the Swedish Melanoma Study Group on 2-cm versus 5-cm resection margins for patients with cutaneous melanoma with a tumor thickness of 0.8-2.0 mm. *Cancer* 2000;89(7):1495–1501.

   Houghton AN, Coit DG. Melanoma. 8-29-2001. National Comprehensive Cancer Network. *The Complete Library of Practice Guidelines in Oncology*, vol. 1, 2002.

   Veronesi U, Cascinelli N. Narrow excision (1-cm margin). A safe procedure for thin cutaneous melanoma. *Arch Surg* 1991;126(4):438–441.

2. **(B)** The approach to skin lesions suspected to be melanoma should address diagnosis and treatment in two separate processes. The diagnosis should be established first, and the histopathologic features and tumor thickness determined. After this information has been obtained, staging and definitive treatment may be accomplished. The biopsy technique must provide tissue that includes the full thickness of the tumor and skin at the thickest part of the tumor. Shave biopsies are not acceptable. Smaller lesions may be excised with 1–2 mm margins. Wider margins result in unnecessarily large incisions and may interfere with subsequent lymphatic mapping. Biopsy incisions should be planned to allow for subsequent WLE.

TABLE 33-1 Appropriate Margins for Excision of Melanoma Based on The National Comprehensive Cancer Network (NCCN) Practice Guidelines in Oncology

Tumor thickness	Recommended margins
In situ	0.5 cm
<1.0 mm	1.0 cm
1–2 mm	1.0–2.0 cm
>2 mm	≥2.0 cm

On the extremities they should be oriented longitudinally. Large lesions and those in cosmetically sensitive areas, such as the palm of the hand, sole of the foot, digits, and face or ears, should be approached with incisional biopsy. A punch or a knife may be used, but the biopsy must be full thickness. Multiple biopsies of a single lesion may be required to ensure adequate sampling.

Specimens should be examined by an experienced dermatopathologist. Depth of invasion (Breslow staging), Clarks's level, ulceration, regression, mitotic rate, tumor infiltrating lymphocytes, vertical growth pase, angiolymphatic invasion, satellitosis, neurotropism, and histologic subtype should be reported. These characteristics have prognostic significance and influence decisions about excision margins, staging with sentinel lymph node biopsy, and surveillance.

Bibliography

Houghton AN, Coit DG. Melanoma. 8-29-0001. National Comprehensive Cancer Network. *The Complete Library of Practice Guidelines in Oncology*, vol. 1, 2002. Ref Type: Report.

Kanzler MH, Mraz-Gernhard S. Treatment of primary cutaneous melanoma. *JAMA* 2001;285(14):1819–1821.

3. **(C)** Isolated limb perfusion (ILP) with melphalan-based chemotherapy is the treatment of choice for patients with limb recurrences that cannot reasonably be treated with excision. Melphalan is a cytostatic, alkylating agent that induces cross-linking of DNA strands in a cell-cycle indepedent manner, inhibiting transcription and DNA synthesis. ILP with this agent can result in complete response (CR) rates of greater than 50%. Of the patients who experience a CR, 24-25% will develop another limb recurrence. The median interval to recurrence after CR is, unfortunately, only 5–10 months. When recurrence after limb perfusion is limited in extent, it can be treated with local therapies, such as, excision, laser ablation, radiation, or topical immunotherapy. More extensive recurrences may be treated with repeat ILP with the expectation of CR rates of 44–74%. The rate of limb recurrence after repeat ILP is 71%, and the recurrence-free interval only 11 months.

Various strategies to increase the effectiveness of ILP have been explored. Use of hyperthemia with tissue temperatures increased to 41 to 42°C results in increased CR rates. Combination of melphalan with tumor necrosis factor-α (TNF-α) may result in increased CR rates; however, the combination regimen has not been compared to melphalan alone in random assignment trials. In one study a double-perfusions at 3–4-week intervals provided increased CR rates, but no significant differences in locoregional recurrence or recurrence-free intervals.

ILP has also been explored in the adjuvant setting. A randomized trial by the Swedish Melanoma Group looked at ILP in the setting of limb recurrence. It compared excision alone to excision plus ILP, and found improved disease-free-survival and decreased locoregional recurrences, but no overall survival benefit. ILP as an adjuvant to excision of primary tumors has also been evaluated. A trend toward a longer disease-free interval was noted, but with increased morbidity and treatment costs. At this time, ILP as adjuvant therapy has no role outside the setting of a clinical trial.

Bibliography

Hafstrom L, Rudenstam CM, Blomquist E, Ingvar C, Jonsson PE, Lagerlof B, et al. Regional hyperthermic perfusion with melphalan after surgery for recurrent malignant melanoma of the extremities. Swedish Melanoma Study Group. *J Clin Oncol* 1991;9(12):2091–2094.

Koops HS, Vaglini M, Suciu S, Kroon BB, Thompson JF, Gohl J, et al. Prophylactic isolated limb perfusion for localized, high-risk limb melanoma: results of a multicenter randomized phase III trial. European Organization for Research and Treatment of Cancer Malignant Melanoma Cooperative Group Protocol 18832, the World Health Organization Melanoma Program Trial 15, and the North American Perfusion Group Southwest Oncology Group-8593. *J Clin Oncol* 1998;16(9):2906–2912.

Kroon BB, Noorda EM, Vrouenraets BC, Nieweg OE. Isolated limb perfusion for melanoma. *J Surg Oncol* 2002;79(4):252–255.

Lienard D, Eggermont AM, Koops HS, Kroon B, Towse G, Hiemstra S, et al. Isolated limb perfusion with tumour necrosis factor-alpha and melphalan with or without interferon-gamma for the treatment of in-transit melanoma metastases: a multicentre randomized phase II study. *Melanoma Res* 1999;9(5):491–502.

Vrouenraets BC, Nieweg OE, Kroon BB. Thirty-five years of isolated limb perfusion for melanoma: indications and results. *Br J Surg* 1996;83(10):1319–1328.

4. **(E)** Groin dissection is commonly performed for treatment of regional nodal spread of melanoma of the lower extremities, perineum, genitalia, or lower abdominal wall. In a superficial groin dissection the inguinal nodes are removed. In a radical (superficial and deep) dissection the inguinal nodes plus the iliac and obturator nodes are resected *en bloc*.

The operation may begin with a transverse, oblique, "lazy-S," or vertical incision. The medial flap is raised to the pubic tubercle and the medial border of the adductor longus. The greater saphenous vein is divided. The spermatic cord is preserved. The femoral vein is exposed and the greater saphenous vein divided at the saphenofemoral junction. The lateral flap is elevated to expose the anterior superior iliac spine and the sartorius muscle. The lateral femoral cutaneous nerve is preserved if not grossly involved with tumor. Dissection is carried along the anterior surface of the superficial femoral artery and kept anterior to the femoral nerve.

To perform the deep dissection, the inguinal ligament is divided. The retroperitoneal space is entered and the peritoneum is lifted cephalad, exposing the external iliac vessels and lymphatics. The inferior epigastric artery and vein are divided. The dissection is carried up to the level of the bifurcation of the common iliac artery into the superficial and deep iliac arteries, the superior limit of the operation.

To dissect the obturator nodes, the ureter is bluntly swept medially while the internal iliac artery is exposed and the plane between the bladder wall and the obturator nodes is developed. The inferior epigastric vessels are again divided as they enter the space behind the rectus abdominis muscle. The obturator nerve, the innervation to the adductors, is preserved if possible, but may be sacrificed if involved with tumor. Its sacrifice is generally well tolerated, since in the standing position, gravity naturally draws the lower extremity into the adducted position. The resection is completed with dissection of the nodes from the internal iliac artery, the obturator nerve, and Cooper's ligament.

Drains are placed, the inguinal ligament reconstructed, and femoral canal closed with care taken not to impinge on the femoral vein. Different techniques of wound closure are described, but it is generally advisable to cover the femoral vessels with well-vascularized tissue, such as transposed sartorius muscle. Wound complication rates are high, ranging from 6 to 63%, even in experienced hands. Wound infection, flap necrosis, lymphocele, lymphorrea, or hematoma is common. Long-term morbidity consists primarily of lymphedema, which occurs in 7 to 46% of patients.

Bibliography

Baas PC, Schraffordt KH, Hoekstra HJ, van Bruggen JJ, van der Weele LT, Oldhoff J. Groin dissection in the treatment of lower-extremity melanoma. Short-term and long-term morbidity. *Arch Surg* 1992;127(3):281–286.

Bland KI, Copeland EM, Karakousis CP. Surgery for cutaneous melanoma. In: Bland KI, Karakousis CP, Copeland EM (eds.), *Atlas of Surgical Oncology*. Philadelphia, PA: W.B. Saunders, 1995, 71–128.

Spratt J. Groin dissection. *J Surg Oncol* 2000;73(4):243–262.

5. **(B)** Sentinel lymph node dissection (SLND) has been developed to stage regional lymphatic basins without the morbidity of a complete lymph node dissection. The sentinel node is the first node in a regional basin to which the lymphatics of the primary tumor

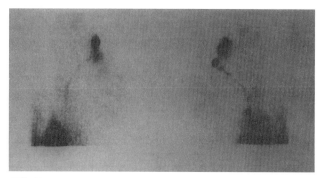

FIG. 33-5 Lymphoscintigraphy using technetium-99-labeled sulfur colloid.

drain. SLND consists of lymphatic mapping with resection of the sentinel node. Staging of regional lymphatics in this manner provides important prognostic information that influences decisions about adjuvant therapy and performance of a completion node dissection. Although randomized studies are lacking, it is generally accepted that the finding of a positive sentinel node should be followed by complete nodal dissection, for regional control. About 30% of patients will have an additional positive node in the completion lymphadenectomy specimen.

The technique of SLND begins with lymphatic mapping by injecting lymphazurin blue dye and/or technetium-99 labeled sulfur colloid intradermally around the tumor and tracing the drainage to the sentinel node or node (Figs. 33-5 and 33-6). Using the combination of blue dye and radioactive colloid, the sentinel node can be identified in 97% of cases. In most studies, the combination of the two types of injections is superior to blue dye alone. Nonsentinel node metastases in the presence of a negative sentinel node occur in less than 5% of SLNDs.

SLND is indicated for melanomas 1 to 4 mm thick. It should also be considered for tumors 0.76 to 0.99 mm thick, especially those with aggressive features such as Clark's level IV or V invasion, ulceration, high mitotic rate, angiolymphatic invasion, regression,

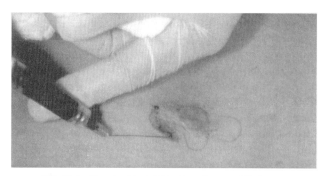

FIG. 33-6 Blue dye injected intradermally around the tumor.

vertical growth phase component, or axial location. While there is some controversy about tumors greater than 4 mm thick, SLND should be considered if there is no evidence of other disease.

Careful pathologic examination of the sentinel node to detect micrometastatic disease should be conducted. Serial sectioning and immunohistochemistry (IHC) for S-100 and HMB-45 should be performed routinely. Reverse transcriptase polymerase chain reaction (RT-PCR) is a highly sensitive method of detecting occult metastatic disease which is currently under investigation. Its clinical relevance remains to be determined at this time.

Bibliography

Cascinelli N, Belli F, Santinami M, Fait V, Testori A, Ruka W, et al. Sentinel lymph node biopsy in cutaneous melanoma: the WHO Melanoma Program experience. *Ann Surg Oncol* 2000;7(6):469–474.

Cochran AJ, Balda BR, Starz H, Bachter D, Krag DN, Cruse CW, et al. The Augsburg Consensus. Techniques of lymphatic mapping, sentinel lymphadenectomy, and completion lymphadenectomy in cutaneous malignancies. *Cancer* 2000;89(2):236–241.

Houghton AN, Coit DG. Melanoma. 8-29-0001. National Comprehensive Cancer Network. *The Complete Library of Practice Guidelines in Oncology*, vol. 1, 2001. Ref Type: Report.

Messina JL, Glass LF, Cruse CW, Berman C, Ku NK, Reintgen DS. Pathologic examination of the sentinel lymph node in malignant melanoma. *Am J Surg Pathol* 1999;23(6):686–690.

Morton DL, Thompson JF, Essner R, Elashoff R, Stern SL, Nieweg OE, et al. Validation of the accuracy of intraoperative lymphatic mapping and sentinel lymphadenectomy for early-stage melanoma: a multicenter trial. Multicenter Selective Lymphadenectomy Trial Group. *Ann Surg* 1999; 230(4):453–463.

Thompson JF, McCarthy WH, Bosch CM, O'Brien CJ, Quinn MJ, Paramaesvaran S, et al. Sentinel lymph node status as an indicator of the presence of metastatic melanoma in regional lymph nodes. *Melanoma Res* 1995;5(4):255–260.

6. **(D)** Accurate staging of melanoma provides important prognostic information and promotes consistency between clinical studies. Tables 33-2 and 33-3 show the AJCC staging system for cutaneous melanoma from the sixth edition *Staging Manual*. Tumor (T) classification is based on thickness using 1 or 2 mm increments to distinguish categories. The additional designation

TABLE 33-2   AJCC TNM Classification for Cutaneous Melanoma

T classification	Thickness	Ulceration/Clark's level
T1	<1.0 mm	a: without ulceration and level II/III b: with ulceration or level IV/V
T2	1.01–2.0 mm	a: without ulceration b: with ulceration
T3	2.01–4.0 mm	a: without ulceration b: with ulceration
T4	>4.0 mm	a: without ulceration b: with ulceration

N classification	No. of metastatic nodes	Nodal metastatic mass
N1	1 node	a: micrometastasis b: macrometastasis
N2	2–3 nodes	a: micrometastasis b: macrometastasis c: in-transit/satellite mets without metastatic nodes
N3	4, or matted nodes, or in-transit/satellite mets with metastatic nodes	

M classification	Site	Serum lactate dehydrogenase
M1a	Distant skin, subcutaneous, or nodal mets	Normal
M1b	Lung mets	Normal
M1c	All other visceral mets	Normal
	Any distant mets	Elevated

Used with the permission of the American Joint Committee on Cancer (AJCC), Chicago, Illinois. The original source for this material is the *AJCC Cancer Staging Manual, Sixth Edition* (2002) published by Springer-Verlag New York, www.springer-ny.com.

TABLE 33-3   AJCC Clinical and Pathologic Stage Grouping

Stage	Clinical TNM staging			Pathologic TNM staging		
	T	N	M	T	N	M
0	Tis	N0	M0	Tis	N0	M0
IA	T1a	N0	M0	T1a	N0	M0
IB	T1b	N0	M0	T1b	N0	M0
	T2a	N0	M0	T2a	N0	M0
IIA	T2b	N0	M0	T2b	N0	M0
	T3a	N0	M0	T3a	N0	M0
IIB	T3b	N0	M0	T3b	N0	M0
	T4a	N0	M0	T4a	N0	M0
IIC	T4b	N0	M0	T4b	N0	M0
III	Any T	N1	M0			
		N2	M0			
		N3	M0			
IIIA				T1-4 only a	N1a	M0
				T1-4 only a	N2a	M0
IIIB				T1-4 only b	N1a	M0
				T1-4	only b N2a	M0
				T1-4	only a N1b	M0
				T1-4	only a N2b	M0
				Any T	N2c	M0
IIIC				T1-4 only b	N1b	M0
				T1-4 only b	N2b	M0
				Any T	N3	M0
IV	Any T			Any T	Any N	M1

Used with the permission of the American Joint Committee on Cancer (AJCC), Chicago, Illinois. The original source for this material is the *AJCC Cancer Staging Manual, Sixth Edition* (2002) published by Springer-Verlag New York, www.springer-ny.com.

of "a" or "b" indicates the absence or presence of ulceration. The presence of ulceration is determined on pathologic examination by the absence of an intact epidermis overlying the primary melanoma. For T1 tumors, Clark's level II/III is designated T1a, and Clark's level IV/V is designated T1b. Tumors in the "b" classification group have a prognosis similar to those one T-stage higher (i.e., the prognosis is similar for T1b and T2a tumors).

Any positive lymph node without distant metastases is stage III disease. Pathologic staging allows further subdivision based on the number of positive lymph nodes. The additional "a" or "b" designation is given for micrometastasis or macrometastasis. Micrometastases are subclinical nodal metastasis detected by SLN biopsy or ELND. Macrometastases are clinically detectable nodal metastases confirmed by therapeutic lymphadenectomy or nodes demonstrating gross extracapsular extension on pathologic examination. In-transit metastases or satellite metastasis without metastatic nodes are designated N2c. In-transit metastases or satellite metastasis with metastatic nodes are designated N3.

Distant metastases are divided into subgroups based on the site of metastases (skin, subcutaneous, or nodal versus lung versus other visceral) and the presence of an elevated serum lactate dehydrogenase (LDH), which is an independent negative prognostic indicator.

The stage groupings for cutaneous melanoma group local disease into stage I and II, regional nodal disease into stage III, and distant disease into stage IV. Stage I and II subcategories are determined by tumor thickness and ulceration. Presence of ulceration upstages localized disease (i.e., T1 tumors with ulceration are grouped with T2 tumors without ulceration in stage IB). Regional nodal, or stage III, disease is subgrouped based on the number of involved nodes, macroscopic versus microscopic nodal disease, primary tumor ulceration, and satellite or in-transit metastases. The prognosis for stage III disease is variable, and inclusion of these criteria produce three distinct prognostic categories. Any metastatic disease is Stage IV.

Bibliography

Balch CM, Buzaid AC, Soong SJ, Atkins MB, Cascinelli N, Coit DG, et al. Final version of the American Joint Committee on Cancer staging system for cutaneous melanoma. *J Clin Oncol* 2001;19(16):3635–3648.

Balch CM, Soong SJ, Gershenwald JE, Thompson JF, Reintgen DS, Cascinelli N, et al. Prognostic factors analysis of 17,600 melanoma patients: validation of the American Joint Committee on Cancer melanoma staging system. *J Clin Oncol* 2001;19(16):3622–3634.

Melanoma of the skin. In: Frederick LG, David LP, Irvin DF, April GF, Charles MB, Daniel GH, et al. (eds.), *AJCC Cancer Staging Handbook*. New York, NY: Springer-Verlag, 2002, 239–254.

7. **(C)** Although numerous factors influence melanoma prognosis, the best validated and most widely accepted are the AJCC staging groups based on the Tumor Nodes Metastasis (TNM) criteria. For localized tumors, thickness is the single most predictive prognostic feature. Level of invasion (Clark's level) may add to the prognostic value of tumor thickness. For thin melanomas (less than 1 mm thick), Clark's level IV and V clearly predicts decreased survival. The prognosis for node positive disease depends on the number of positive nodes and the tumor burden (micrometastatic vs. macrometastatic), with greater number of nodes and macroscopic disease predicting worse survival. Other negative prognostic indicators include site of disease on the trunk (versus extremities), older age, and male gender, although these are not part of the AJCC staging criteria.

For both localized and regional disease, ulceration (Fig. 33-7) is an important prognostic indicator. Ulceration is a highly reproducible histopathologic feature defined by absence of epidermis overlying

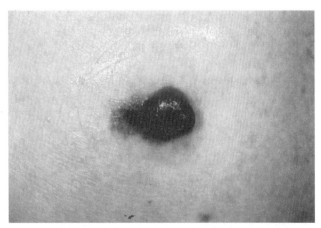

FIG. 33-7   Clinically ulcerated melanoma.

the tumor. It is a strong negative prognostic indicator, as evinced by the fact that thick, ulcerated, node negative melanomas carry a worse prognosis than some node positive disease.

Distant metastases indicate a grave prognosis, with 1-year survival of 41–59%. Metastases to skin, subcutaneous tissue, and lymph nodes have the best prognosis. Lung metastases are more favorable than those to other visceral sites. An elevated serum lactate dehydrogenase (LDH) is independently associated with worse prognosis for stage IV melanoma, and included in the AJCC staging scheme. Overall 10-year survival by stage is approximately: stage I-80%, stage II-50%, stage III-30%, stage IV 5%.

Bibliography

Balch CM, Buzaid AC, Soong SJ, Atkins MB, Cascinelli N, Coit DG, et al. Final version of the American Joint Committee on Cancer staging system for cutaneous melanoma. *J Clin Oncol* 2001;19(16):3635–3648.

Balch CM, Soong SJ, Gershenwald JE, Thompson JF, Reintgen DS, Cascinelli N, et al. Prognostic factors analysis of 17,600 melanoma patients: validation of the American Joint Committee on Cancer melanoma staging system. *J Clin Oncol* 2001;19(16):3622–3634.

Melanoma of the skin. In: Frederick LG, David LP, Irvin DF, April GF, Charles MB, Daniel GH, et al. (eds.), *AJCC Cancer Staging Handbook.* New York, NY: Springer-Verlag, 2002, 239–254.

8. **(C)** Sarcomas are a relatively uncommon and diverse family of tumors. The annual incidence in the United States is about 8300 cases, accounting for about 1% of adult malignancies and 15% of pediatric malignancies. Retroperitoneal sarcomas make up about 15–20% of soft tissue sarcomas. Most tumors in the retroperitoneum are malignant, and about one-third of them are soft tissue sarcomas. Because of their rarity, ideally, sarcomas should be treated in specialized centers, using a multidisciplinary approach and, whenever possible, enrolling patients in clinical trials.

Workup of retroperitoneal and visceral soft tissue sarcomas should include a history and physical, imaging of the tumor and abdomen with CT or MRI, chest imaging with x-ray or CT, and evaluation at a multidisciplinary review board. The need for biopsy is controversial, and depends on clinical suspicion of other malignancy, such as, germ cell tumor or lymphoma. The most common histologic cellular type for retroperitoneal sarcomas is liposarcoma. Biopsy should be planned so as to allow excision of the biopsy site with subsequent resection of the tumor. Biopsy must be with core needle or incisional biopsy. Fine-needle aspiration is inadequate for the diagnosis and histologic grading of sarcomas.

Standard primary therapy for resectable tumors is surgical resection. A liberal *en bloc* resection with the goal of obtaining negative margins should be performed. Contiguous organs that are not invaded but preclude adequate resection margin may need to be sacrificed as well. Because of their anatomic location it may be difficult to resect completely and with adequate margins. Therefore, unlike with extremity sarcomas, death from these tumors usually results from local recurrence. In one study median survival of patients undergoing complete resection was 103 versus 18 months for those with incomplete resection.

Adjuvant and neoadjuvant chemotherapy or radiation may be considered, but is best undertaken in the setting of a clinical trial. Tumors that are unresectable because of disseminated disease or technical considerations may be treated with chemotherapy with or without radiation. If the tumor becomes resectable following chemotherapy or radiation, resection should be performed. Recurrent disease should be resected whenever possible. Unresectable recurrent disease may be treated with chemotherapy with or without radiation as for primary unresectable disease. When distant metastases occur, the liver is the most common site.

Bibliography

Adult Soft Tissue Sarcoma. *Cancer.gov—Adult Soft Tissue Sarcoma (PDQ): Treatment* [Web Page]. March 14, 2003. Accessed June 7, 2003.

Demetri GD. Sarcoma. *Practice Guidelines in Oncology.* National Comprehensive Cancer Network, vol. 1, 2002. SARC-1-REF-3.

Heslin MJ, Lewis JJ, Nadler E, et al. Prognostic factors associated with long-term survival for retroperitoneal sarcoma: implications for management. *J Clin Oncol* 1997;15(8):2832–2839.

Jaques DP, Coit DG, Hajdu SI, Brennan MF. Management of primary and recurrent soft-tissue sarcoma of the retroperitoneum. *Ann Surg* 1990;212(1):51–59.

9. **(B)** Staging of soft tissue sarcomas has important prognostic and treatment implications. Staging workup should include history and physical examination, imaging of the primary tumor with magnetic resonance imaging (MRI) and/or computed tomography (CT), and chest x-ray or, for intermediate or high-grade tumors or tumors greater than 5 cm, chest CT. Biopsy specimens must be reviewed to determine histologic grade. The components of the AJCC staging system are primary tumor (T) size and depth, regional nodal involvement (N), distant metastasis (M), and histologic grade (G). Stage I consists entirely of low histologic grade sarcomas. Stage II includes high-grade tumors that are not greater than 5 cm and deep to the fascia. Stage III describes high-grade tumors greater than 5 cm and deep to the fascia. Stage IV sarcomas have regional lymph node or distant metastases. Overall survival for stage I, II, and III disease is approximately 90, 80, and 55%, respectively.

While tumor location (retroperitoneal, mediastinal, pelvic, or extremity) has important implications in prognosis and treatment, tumors of all locations are staged by the same system. Retroperitoneal, mediastinal, and pelvic tumors are classified as deep in location. Nodal metastases are rare with sarcomas, occurring in less than 3% of patients. The prognosis for node positive disease is poor, similar to that for distant metastases.

For soft tissue sarcomas included in the AJCC staging system, the histologic grade of the tumor has greater prognostic significance than the cellular classification. Tumor grade is determined by the number of mitoses per high-powered field, presence of necrosis, cellular and nuclear morphology, and the degree of cellularity. The most common histologic cellular type overall is malignant fibrous histiocytoma followed by liposarcoma. Clear cell sarcoma is included in the AJCC staging system; however, it has an increased propensity for nodal spread. Angiosarcoma is not included in this staging system, and has a generally poor prognosis.

Bibliography

Brennan MF. Staging of soft tissue sarcomas. *Ann Surg Oncol* 1999;6:8–9.

Coindre JM, Terrier P, Bui NB, Bonichon F, Collin F, Le D, V, Mandard AM, Vilain MO, Jacquemier J, Duplay H, Sastre X, Barlier C, Henry-Amar M, Mace-Lesech J, Contesso G. Prognostic factors in adult patients with locally controlled soft tissue sarcoma. A study of 546 patients from the French Federation of Cancer Centers Sarcoma Group. *J Clin Oncol* 1996;14:869–877.

Fong Y, Coit DG, Woodruff JM, Brennan MF. Lymph node metastasis from soft tissue sarcoma in adults. Analysis of data from a prospective database of 1772 sarcoma patients. *Ann Surg* 1993;217:72–77.

Pisters PW, Leung DH, Woodruff J, Shi W, Brennan MF. Analysis of prognostic factors in 1,041 patients with localized soft tissue sarcomas of the extremities. *J Clin Oncol* 1996;14:1679–1689.

Soft tissue sarcoma. In: Frederick LG, David LP, April GF, Charles MB, Baniel GH, Monica M (eds.), *AJCC Cancer Staging Handbook*. New York, NY: Springer-Verlag, 2002, 221–228.

10. **(B)** The extremities are the most common location for soft tissue sarcomas, accounting for about 50% of sarcomas. Treatment of these tumors presents a challenge in balancing preservation of limb function with adequate oncologic control. While extremity sarcomas were historically treated with amputation, limb-sparing resection with adjuvant radiation has since been proven safe and equally effective. Over 95% of extremity sarcomas may be adequately treated without amputation. Limb preservation is now a central concept in sarcoma surgery.

Adequate staging of extremity sarcomas includes a history and physical examination, imaging of the primary tumor with MRI and/or CT, incisional or core needle biopsy to establish histology and grade, and chest imaging with chest x-ray or CT. Primary therapy for all resectable tumors should be resection with margins of at least 1 cm. Unless necessary to obtain adequate margins, anatomic compartment excisions are not indicated. Low-grade, small, superficial (stage IA) sarcomas may be treated with surgical excision alone. All other resectable lesions generally should be treated with a combination of resection and radiation. Radiation timing (preoperative vs. intraoperative vs. postoperative) and method of delivery (external beam vs. brachytherapy) are the subjects of ongoing studies and debate. Sarcomas that cannot be resected without unacceptable loss of limb function can be treated with neoadjuvant radiation and/or chemotherapy in an effort to reduce the tumor to resectable status. The role of adjuvant chemotherapy also continues to be defined. Recent evidence suggests that it may prolong disease-free survival without affecting overall survival significantly. Doxyrubicin and ifosfamide are the most active agents presently available for systemic treatment of sarcomas.

Patients frequently present to referral centers following inadequate or incomplete excisions. Repeat resection is usually indicated. If repeat resection will be prohibitively morbid treatment with adjuvant radiation may be considered. Local recurrences should be treated as a primary tumor would, with repeat resection and radiation with or without chemotherapy as indicated. For recurrence at distant sites consideration may be given to metastasectomy depending on the patient's fitness for surgery, location of disease, extent of disease, biology of the tumor, symptoms, and wishes of the patient. The most common site of distant recurrence is the lungs. Chemotherapy may be indicated as well. Disseminated disease should be treated with chemotherapy, surgery, and radiation as needed to provide palliation.

Bibliography

Demitri GD. Sarcoma. *NCCN Practice Giudelines in Oncology*. National Comprehensive Cancer Network, vol. 1, 2002, SARC-1-REF-3.

Pollack A, Zagars GK, Goswitz MS, Pollock RA, Feig BW, Pisters PW. Preoperative vs. postoperative radiotherapy in the treatment of soft tissue sarcomas: a matter of presentation. *Int J Radiat Oncol Biol Phys* 1998;42(3):563–572.

Rosenberg SA. *Principles and Practice of the Biologic Therapy of Cancer*, 3rd ed. Philadelphia, PA: Lippincott, Williams & Wilkins, 2000.

Rosenberg SA, Tepper J, Glatstein E, et al. The treatment of soft-tissue sarcomas of the extremities: prospective randomized evaluations of (1) limb-sparing surgery plus radiation therapy compared with amputation and (2) the role of adjuvant chemotherapy. *Ann Surg* 1982;196(3): 305–315.

Yang JC, Chang AE, Baker AR, et al. Randomized prospective study of the benefit of adjuvant radiation therapy in the treatment of soft tissue sarcomas of the extremity. *J Clin Oncol* 1998;16(1):197–203.

11. **(B)** Gastrointestinal stromal tumors (GIST) are neoplasms of mesenchymal origin. They were previously considered to be leiomyosarcomas due to their histologic appearance similar to smooth muscle, but have since been identified as a distinct histologic type characterized by immunohistochemical positive staining for CD117 and frequently CD34 (Figs. 33-8 and 33-9). Although the cell of origin has not been identified

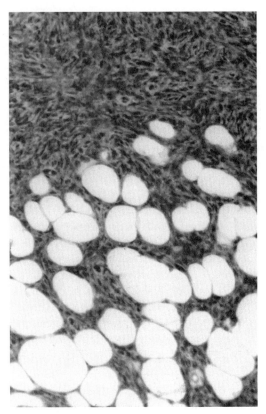

FIG. 33-9 Biopsy permanent section CD34 positive showing tumor excision into fat.

with absolute certainty, GISTs are thought to originate from the interstitial cells of Cajal which are also positive for CD117 and CD34. GISTs express the cell-surface transmembrane receptor KIT, detected by CD117 staining, which has tyrosine kinase activity and is the protein product of the proto-oncogene, *KIT*.

GISTs occur most commonly in the stomach (70%), followed by small intestine (20%), and esophagus, colon, and rectum (less than 10%). Median age at onset is about 55 years. Survival is best for esophageal and stomach tumors, and worst for small bowel primaries. Gastric GISTs are considered malignant when they exceed 5–10 cm, have a high mitotic index, or metastasize. Small bowel tumors are considered malignant if they have any mitoses or are greater than 2 cm.

Initial therapy for resectable GISTs should be surgical resection. For tumors that are unresectable or metastatic systemic therapy with imatinib mesylate (STI-571, Gleevec in the United States and Glivec in Europe [Novartis]) should be considered. Imatinib mesylate is a selective protein tyrosine kinase inhibitor initially targeted to the platelet-derived growth factor (PDGF) receptor, and found to inhibit the BCR-ABL tyrosine kinase of CML as well. It was subsequently discovered to inhibit the c-kit receptor tyrosine kinase of GISTs. In a recent study of the efficacy of imatinib

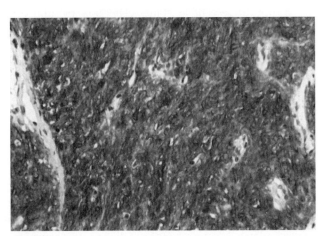

FIG. 33-8 Biopsy permanent section c-kit (CD117) positive. Courtesy of Richard Cheney.

mesylate in advanced GISTs, 54% of patients had a partial response and 30% of patients had stable disease. Traditionally, cytotoxic chemotherapy with agents such as doxyrubicin has yielded response rates less than 5%.

Bibliography

Demetri GD. Sarcoma. *National Comprehensive Cancer Network Clinical Practice Guidelines in Oncology.* National Comprehensive Cancer Network, 2002. SARC-1-REF-3.

Demetri GD, von Mehren M, Blanke CD, Van den Abbeele AD, Eisenberg B, Roberts PJ, Heinrich MC, Tuveson DA, Singer S, Janicek M, Fletcher JA, Silverman SG, Silberman SL, Capdeville R, Kiese B, Peng B, Dimitrijevic S, Druker BJ, Corless C, Fletcher CD, Joensuu H. Efficacy and safety of imatinib mesylate in advanced gastrointestinal stromal tumors. *N Engl J Med* 2002;347:472–480.

Pidhorecky I, Cheney RT, Kraybill WG, Gibbs JF. Gastrointestinal stromal tumors: current diagnosis, biologic behavior, and management. *Ann Surg Oncol* 2000;7:705–712.

Savage DG, Antman KH. Imatinib mesylate—a new oral targeted therapy. *N Engl J Med* 2002;346:683–693.

12. **(E)** Mohs micrographic surgery is a specialized technique, which offers high cure rates for skin cancers combined with preservation of normal tissue. Dr. Frederic E. Mohs developed the technique in the 1950s, while a general surgeon in Madison, Wisconsin. Initially, he would fix tissue *in situ* and then excise it with microscopic control. Later, he perfected the technique, which is called today the fresh-tissue technique. Mohs surgery is a precise process of serial excisions of malignant tumors, mapping of the operation field, and frozen section histologic control (Fig. 33-10).

Immediate reconstruction of the defect is generally performed by either primary closure, or any given flap or skin graft (Fig. 33-11).

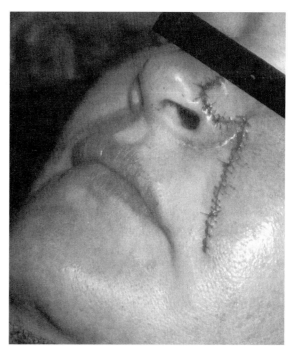

FIG. 33-11 Nasal labial flap reconstruction.

Mohs surgery is considered the first-line treatment for high-risk tumors, especially those located on the head and neck (Table 33-4).

BCC is the most common nonmelanoma skin cancer, with an estimated 30,000 new cases diagnosed each year in the United States. The tumor prevalence increases with age, UV light exposure, immunodeficiency, ionizing radiation, nonhealing wounds, and certain genetic syndromes. Morpheaform BCCs clinically appear as shiny scar-like papules or plaques. Often the tumors extend well beyond the clinical visible margin. Simple excisions may, therefore, be associated with high recurrence rates. Cure rates for patients who have undergone Mohs surgery are about 99% for primary BCC and between 93 and 98% for recurrent BCC. At 5 years, the recurrence rate of primary BCC are 1–7 and 4.8% for previously treated tumors. Mohs surgery has been shown to be as cost-effective as traditional surgical excision. Simple excision is suitable for small BCCs in non-high-risk

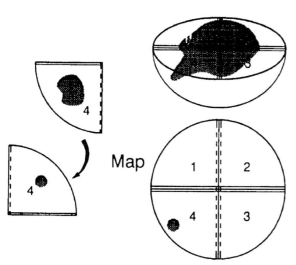

FIG. 33-10 Diagram of Mohs map.

TABLE 33-4   Indications for Mohs Surgery

Infiltrative pathology: micronodular, morpheaform
Incompletely excised tumor
Recurrent tumor
Indistinct clinical borders
Perineural invasion
Located in H-zone of face
>2 cm in size

areas, while radiation therapy is generally reserved for nonsurgical patients. Both cryosurgery and electrodesiccation with curettage are relatively inexpensive and time saving procedures for small BCC or non-high-risk sites, but both techniques fail to control for histologic margins, and may have unacceptable cosmetic outcome.

Bibliography

Kuijpers D, Thissen MRTM, Neumann MHA. Basal cell carcinoma: treatment options and prognosis, a scientific approach to a common malignancy. *Am J Clin Dermatol* 2002;3:(4)247–259.

Menaker GM, Chiu DS. Basal cell carcinoma. In: Steele GD, Phillips TL, Chabner BA, et al. (eds.), *American Cancer Society Atlas of Clinical Oncology Skin Cancer.* Hamilton, ON: BC Decker, 2001, 60–71.

Rowe DE, Carrol RJ, Day CL. Long-term recurrence rates in previously untreated (primary) basal cell carcinoma: implications for patient follow-up. *J Dermatol Surg Oncol* 1999;15:315–328.

Torres A, Pena JR, Saavedra A. Treatment of nonmelanoma skin cancer. In: Steele GD, Phillips TL, Chabner BA, et al. (eds.), *American Cancer Society Atlas of Clinical Oncology Skin Cancer.* Hamilton, ON: BC Decker, 2001, 271–299.

13. **(C)** The first clear evidence that immunotherapy can cause regression of established metastatic tumors came from the administration of high-dose interleukin-2 (IL-2) for the treatment of melanoma and kidney cancer. IL-2 is a cytokine secreted by T-helper lymphocytes that has profound effects on lymphocytes, including induction of expansion and activation. High-dose IL-2 for the treatment of metastatic melanoma has an objective response rate of about 15%, with a complete, and usually durable, response seen in about 50% of responders.

By comparison, chemotherapy with single agent dacarbazine (DTIC) or temozolomide (TMZ), both prodrugs of the active alkylating agent imidazole-4-carboximide (MTIC), is associated with response rates of around 20%. Unfortunately, durable complete responses with these drugs are rare. Treatment with combination chemotherapy also remains disappointing. Despite initial reports of increased efficacy with the Dartmouth regimen (combination [DTIC], carmustine [BCNU], cisplatin [DDP], and tamoxifen [TAM]), randomized trials have not consistently shown improved responses compared to single agent chemotherapy.

The ineffectiveness of chemotherapy has led to several experimental immunotherapies. These treatments can be classified as either active vaccine immunization or passive transfer of immune cells.

Active immunotherapy by vaccination with peptides derived from tumor antigens sometimes results in high numbers of circulating T cells directed against cancer antigens, but does not induce tumor regression. Passive immunotherapy by adoptive transfer of tumor infiltrating lymphocytes (TIL) recovered from resected tumors, expanded in vitro, and transferred with IL-2 back into the patient results in response rates of 35%. Lymphodepletion of the patient with nonmyeloablative chemotherapy prior to cell transfer results in improved response rates (>40%).

Immunotherapy has also been employed in the adjuvant setting. High-dose interferon alfa-2b is FDA approved for the adjuvant treatment of resected high-risk melanoma. Studies examining the ability of interferon to prolong survival have yielded conflicting results, and the therapy is associated with significant morbidity that may limit its use.

Bibliography

Bajetta E, Del Vecchio M, Bernard-Marty C, et al. Metastatic melanoma: chemotherapy. *Semin Oncol* 2002;29(5): 427–445. Review.

Dudley ME, Rosenberg SA. Adoptive-cell-transfer therapy for the treatment of patients with cancer. *Nat Rev Cancer* 2003;3(9):666–675. Review.

Rosenberg SA. Progress in human tumour immunology and immunotherapy. *Nature* 2001;411(6835):380–384. Review.

Sabel MS, Sondak VK. Pros and cons of adjuvant interferon in the treatment of melanoma. *Oncologist* 2003;8(5):451–458. Review.

Yang JC, Sherry RM, Steinberg SM, et al. Randomized study of high-dose and low-dose interleukin-2 in patients with metastatic renal cancer. *J Clin Oncol* 2003;21(16):3127-3132.

14. **(C)** The majority of SCCs develop on the head and neck region and are associated with prolonged, cumulative UV light exposure. SCC arising in sun-exposed sites carries overall a good prognosis. Several factors, however, have been documented to influence local recurrence rate and metastatic potential of these tumors.

1. *Anatomical site*: SCC of the lower lip has a metastatic rate of about 16 and 50% mortality rate as a result of metastases (Fig. 33-12). Tumors arising in non-sun-exposed sites, especially glabrous skin such as the glans penis as well as SCC of the ear have a high risk of metastases. Radiation-induced tumors and SCC developing in areas of chronic inflammation and ulceration or burn have an 18–20% rate of metastases.

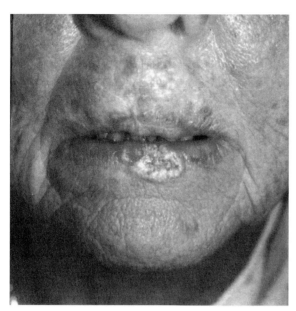

FIG. 33-12   SCC of lower lip in 70-year-old female.

2. *Size*: Tumors greater than 2 cm in diameter are 2x as likely to recur locally and nearly 3x as likely to metastasize as those tumors of smaller diameter. SCC greater than 4 mm in depth are at higher risk for local recurrence and metastasis (Fig. 33-13).

3. *Histology*: Poorly differentiated SCCs have double the local recurrence rate and triple the metastatic rate of well-differentiated tumors. Perineural involvement also raises both the recurrence and metastatic rate of tumors.

4. *Host immunosuppression*: Immunosuppressed patients tend to have a poor prognosis because of the tumor's invasiveness and the host's response to metastases.

5. *Previous treatment*: Locally recurrent SCCs have a higher risk for metastatic disease.

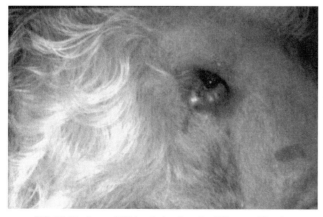

FIG. 33-13   Large SCC located on temple of 60-year-old male.

Bibliography

Motley R, Kersey P, Lawrence C. Multiprofessional guidelines for the management of the patient with primary cutaneous squamous cell carcinoma. *Br J Dermatol* 2002; 146:18–25.

Robinson JK. Squamous cell carcinoma. In: Steele GD, Phillips TL, Chabner BA, et al. (eds.), *American Cancer Society Atlas of Clinical Oncology Skin Cancer*. Hamilton, ON: BC Decker, 2001, 72–84.

Rowe DE, Carroll RJ, Day CI. Prognostic factors for local recurrence, metastasis and survival rates in squamous cell carcinoma of the skin, ear, and lip. *Am Acad Dermatol* 1992;25:1–25.

15. **(D)** Several treatment guidelines have been proposed in the management of cutaneous SCC. Surgery, either by local excision or, remains the treatment of choice for both primary and recurrent tumors.

For small, less than 2 cm, well-defined low-risk tumors, surgical resection with 4–5 mm margins is proposed. Confirmation of histologic negative surgical margins is always necessary. Despite negative assessment of the margins, however, conventional histopathology sectioning or "bread loafing" may miss certain tumor areas and increase the risk of local tumor recurrence. For high-risk tumors and for those tumor located in cosmetically challenging areas, Mohs surgery is recommended. With Mohs surgery, 100% of the histologic margins are examined, which reduces the rate of local recurrence.

In-transit metastases may develop from high-risk SCC lesions. Only wide surgical margins extending well beyond the primary tumor may include such metastases. Narrow margins may not remove in-transit metastases, which lead to tumor recurrence.

Radiotherapy may be used both as a primary treatment for selected cases of SCC or as adjuvant treatment after surgery. Tumors that are at high risk for recurrences such as those with perineural invasion or those with incomplete surgical margins would be considered for postoperative radiation.

Bibliography

Motley R, Kersey P, Lawrence C. Multiprofessional guidelines for the management of the patient with primary cutaneous squamous cell carcinoma. *Br J Dermatol* 2002;146:18–25.

Rowe DE, Carroll RJ, Day CI. Prognostic factors for local recurrence, metastasis and survival rates in squamous cell carcinoma of the skin, ear, and lip. *Am Acad Dermatol* 1992;25:1–25.

16. **(E)** Verrucous carcinoma is a rare, low-grade, SCC of the skin and mucous mucosa, which generally carries a favorable prognosis. Clinically, the tumor appears as

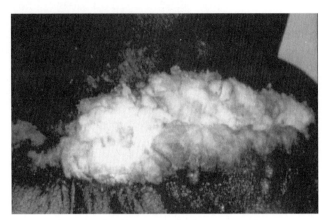

FIG. 33-14   Cauliflower-like mass of verrucous carcinoma.

Bibliography

Bezerra AL, Lopes A, Landman G, et al. Clinicopathologic features and human papillomavirus DNA prevalence of warty and squamous cell carcinoma of the penis. *Am J Surg Pathol* 2001;25(5):673–678.

Koch BB, Trask DK, Hoffman HT, Karnell LH, et al. National survey of head and neck verrucous carcinoma: patterns of presentation, care, and outcome. *Cancer* 2001;92(1):110–120.

Spiro RH. Verrucous carcinoma, then and now. *Am J Surg* 1998;176(5):393–397.

Zeitouni NC, Cheney R, Oseroff AR. In: Raghavan D, Brecher M, Johnson DH, Meropol NJ, Thigpen JT (eds.), *Textbook of Uncommon Cancer.* New York, NY: John Wiley & Sons, 1999, 199–219.

a cauliflower-like mass, which locally invades and which very rarely metastasize unless, longstanding and neglected (Fig. 33-14).

Based on anatomical site, four types of verrucous carcinoma have been described.

1. The Buschke-Lowenstein's tumor, or giant condyloma acuminatum, is found in the urogenital region. The tumor accounts for 5–24% of all penile cancers and is generally seen in uncircumcised men between 18 and 86 years old. Other anogenital sites include the perianal region, the vagina and cervix, and rarely the bladder. The main risk factor for the development of the Buschke-Lowenstein's tumor appears to be infection with HPV. Both nononcogenic HPV 6 and 11 and oncogenic HPV 16 and 18 have been found in these tumors.

2. The Ackerman's tumor, also called oral florid papillomatosis represents a verrucous carcinoma found in the aerodigestive region. The tumor represents 2–12% of all oral carcinomas. Most patients are men in their 50s and 60s. Etiological factors include tobacco chewing, alcohol or lye consumption as well as acid ingestion. HPV infection may also be a risk factor.

3. Epithelioma curriculatum, or carcinoma curriculatum, is a warty tumor located primarily on the palms and soles in middle-aged individuals. It can be initially mistaken for a verruca vulgaris, until the tumor invades the underlying soft tissue. Nononcogenic HPV is usually associated with this tumor.

4. Cutaneous verrucous carcinoma refers to all verrucous carcinomas in other anatomical sites.

Initial treatment of verrucous carcinoma is by surgery. Selected therapy with bleomycin, interferon, or etritinate may be helpful in selected cases. Adjuvant cases may respond to systemic chemotherapy.

17. **(C)** Merkel cell carcinoma is an aggressive cutaneous malignancy of neural origin. The tumor tends to develop both regional and distant metastasis. At presentation, 25–30% of patients will have regional nodal disease and within 2 years, and 50–70% of patients will develop lymph node metastasis. Disseminated disease will occur in 30% of patients, frequently to lung, liver, bone, and brain. The overall 5-year survival rate is between 50 and 68%. The incidence of Merkel cell carcinoma is unknown although over 1100 cases have been reported in the literature. The tumor typically presents in middle-aged to elderly patients with men and women being equally affected. Risk factors for Merkel cell carcinoma include ultraviolet radiation (UVR), immunosuppression, arsenicism, and possibly PUVA. The most common location includes the HEENT region (50%) followed by the extremities (40%) and the trunk (10%). Clinically, the tumor appears as a firm nodule with a violaceous hue and is generally asymptomatic. Histologically, Merkel cell carcinoma is a dermal tumor, invading underlying structures. The cells are arranged in a ball-in-mitt configuration with numerous mitosis, necrosis, and apoptosis. Histologic variants include the trabecular, intermediate, and small cell variant. IHC is positive in cytokeratins 18, 19, 20 neuron-specific enolase chromogranulin and synaptophysin.

Patients who present with palpable lymphadenopathy in the draining lymph node basin should undergo a CT scan and a fine needle aspirate of the node to confirm the diagnosis. A full lymph node dissection followed by adjuvant radiation therapy is indicated.

Patients who have clinical negative nodes should be considered candidates for lymphoscintigraphy and SLN biopsy (Figs. 33-15 and 33-16).

If the biopsy is positive, then regional lymph node dissection and radiotherapy is warranted. If the biopsy is negative then only radiotherapy is recommended. If the SLN biopsy is not available, then

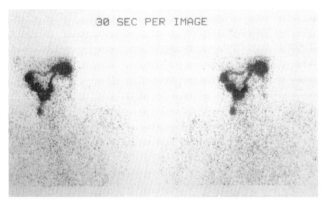

FIG. 33-15 Lymphoscintigraphy showing draining lymph node basin.

ELND and radiotherapy may be justified. According to several publications, SLN biopsy may be a strong predictor of disease recurrence.

Bibliography

Gruber SB, Wilson L. Merkel cell carcinoma. In: Miller SJ, Maloney ME (eds.), *Cutaneous Oncology*. Malden, MA: Blackwell Science, 1998, 710–722.

Mehrany K, Otley CC, Weenig RH, et al. A meta-analysis of the prognostic significance of sentinel lymph node status in Merkel cell carcinoma. *Dermatol Surg* 2002;28(2): 113–117.

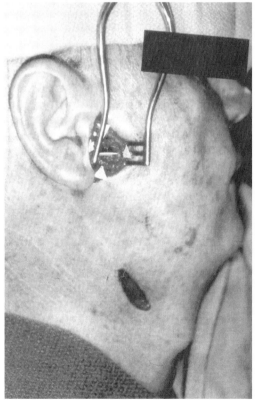

FIG. 33-16   SLN biopsies of right parotid and right neck.

Ratner D, Nelson BR, Brown MD, et al. Merkel cell carcinoma. *J Am Acad Dermatol* 1993;29:143–156.

Zeitouni NC, Cheney R, DeLacure MD. Lymphoscintigraphy, sentinel lymph node biopsy and Mohs micrographic surgery in the treatment of Merkel cell carcinoma. *Dermatol Surg* 2002;26:1–6.

18. **(E)** DFSP is a slow growing, low-grade spindle cell tumor. It is characterized by local invasion and a propensity to recur after surgical resection. It is typically seen in young to middle-aged adults with an equal male to female ratio. The trunk is the most common location followed by the proximal extremities and the head and neck region. The rate of metastasis is between 1 and 5%, seen especially with recurrent tumors, and tumors with fibrosarcomatous change.

Treatment of DFSP is by surgery. Local excision is associated with a high rate of local recurrence. Therefore, WLE with margins of 2–3 cm down to and including fascia is recommended. Confirmation of histologic-free margins is necessary for local control of this tumor. For tumors located on the head and neck region, where tissue sparing is important, many authors recommend the use of Mohs micrographic surgery. Mohs surgery has also been advocated for tumors elsewhere on the body, given the very local recurrence rate (1.6%) seen with this procedure.

The use of radiation therapy for DFSP is controversial because of reports of high-grade malignant transformation after radiation treatment. Chemotherapy does not appear to alter the prognosis of DFSP and is, therefore, not a management option.

Bibliography

Ah-Weng A, Marsden JR, Sanders DS, Waters R. Dermatofibrosarcoma protuberans treated by micrographic surgery. *Br J Cancer* 2002;87(12):1386–1389.

Minter RM, Reith JD, Hochwald SN. Metastatic potential of dermatofibrosarcoma protuberans with fibrosarcomatous change. *J Surg Oncol* 2003;82(3):201–208.

Nouri K, Lodha R, Jimenez G, Robins P. Mohs micrographic surgery for dermatofibrosarcoma protuberans: university of Miami and NYU experience. *Dermatol Surg* 2002; 28(11):1060–1064.

Oliveira-Soares R, Viana I, Vale E, Soares-Almeida LM, et al. Dermatofibrosarcoma protuberans: a clincopathological study of 20 cases. *J Eur Acad Dermatol Venereol* 2002;16(5): 441–446.

Vandeweyer E, De Saint Aubain Somerhausen N, Gebhart M. Dermatofibrosarcoma protuberans: how wide is wide in surgical excision? *Acta Chir Belg* 2002;102(6):455–458.

19. **(B)** Histopathology of DFSP reveals a dermal tumor composed of dense fascicles of spindle-shaped cells arranged in the characteristic fashion of cartwheel or storiform pattern. Extension into the subcutaneous fat

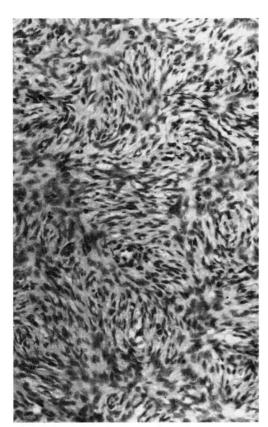

FIG. 33-17 Biopsy permanent section GIST (200x). Courtesy of Richard Cheney.

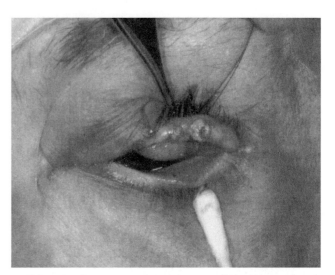

FIG. 33-18 Sebaceous carcinoma of upper eyelid in elderly female.

is also present in irregular tentacle-like projections (Fig. 33-17).

These projections that may extend well beyond the clinical visible margin and may explain the high rate of local recurrence of DFSP after standard surgical excision. Typically, cellular pleomorphism is rare. Mitotic figures and pleomorphism are uncommon. Very infrequently, small foci of fibrosarcomatous change can be noted, especially in recurrent DSFP.

Contrary to benign dermatofibromas that exhibit CD34 negatively and factor XIIIa positively, DFSP are CD34 positive and factor XIIIa negative on IHC. Histologic variants of DFSP include mxyoid, pigmented, and atrophic types. Not uncommonly DFSP may contain small areas of myxoid change but only rarely will the histologic pattern be almost entirely myxomatous. The pigmented variant, or Bednar tumor is also uncommon, and features pigmented dendric cells. The atrophic or sclerotic variant of DFSP exhibits large areas of dermal atrophy and may present clinically as a depressed plaque.

Bibliography

Gloster MW Jr. Dermatofibrosarcoma protuberans. *J Am Acad Dermatol* 1996;33:355–374.

Hattori H. Nodular sclerotic change in dermatofibrosarcoma protuberans: a potential diagnostic problem. *Br J Dermatol* 2003;148(2):357–360.

20. **(A)** Sebaceous carcinoma, also called Meibomian gland carcinoma, represents an aggressive primary malignancy of the adnexal epithelium of sebaceous glands. About 75% of sebaceous carcinomas are ocular in origin, while the remaining 25% of tumors are considered extraocular. Ocular sebaceous carcinomas account for 1.5–5% of all malignant eyelid neoplasms. The tumor most frequently develops on the upper eyelid of elderly patients (Fig. 33-18).

Clinically, the lesion may present as a firm yellowish nodule, resembling a chalazion, or may mimic an inflammatory condition such as blepharoconjunctivitis or keratoconjunctivitis. Often, the diagnosis is delayed from 1 to 3 years.

Between 51 and 70% of ocular sebaceous carcinomas originate from Meibomian glands of the tarsus. Less commonly, the tumor is either multicentric in origin or develops from the glands of Zeis, the lacrimal gland, or the caruncle.

Histologically, the tumor appears as an infiltrative, nonencapsulated dermal tumor composed of epithelioid cells with cytoplasmic vacuoles and nuclear scalloping. Occasionally, pagetoid spread is seen in the epidermis. Sebaceous carcinoma stains positive for lipids on Oil Red O and Sudan IV stains (Fig. 33-19).

Sebaceous carcinoma carries a poor prognosis because of its high recurrence rate and tendency to metastasize. At presentation, 25% of patients will already have regional lymph node involvement.

Early diagnosis and subsequent surgical therapy may lead to higher survival rates. Standard surgical

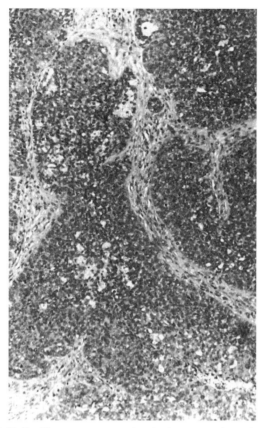

FIG. 33-19   Biopsy permanent section of sebaceous carcinoma (200x).

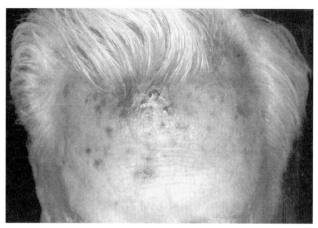

FIG. 33-20   Angiosarcoma of scalp in elderly male.

excision or Mohs surgery may be used as primary therapy. Radiation therapy is reserved for nonsurgical patients.

Bibliography

Misago N, Mihara I, Ansai S, et al. Sebaceous and related neoplasms with sebaceous differentiation: a clinicopathologic study of 30 cases. *Am J Dermatol* 2002;24(4): 294–304.

Nelson BR, Hamlet KR, Gillard M, et al. Sebaceous carcinoma. *J Am Acad Dermatol* 1995;33:1–15.

Zurcher M, Hintschich CR, Garner A, et al. Sebaceous carcinoma of the eyelid: a clinicopathological study. *Br J Dermatol* 1998;82(9):1049–1055.

Spencer JM, Nossa R, Tse DT, et al. Sebaceous carcinoma of the eyelid treated with Mohs micrographic surgery. *J Am Acad Dermatol* 2001;44:1004–1009.

21. **(E)** Angiosarcomas are a heterogeneous group of cutaneous and superficial soft tissue malignancies derived from vascular endothelial cells. They account for 1% of all sarcomas and generally carry a poor prognosis.

1. Angiosarcoma associated with prior radiation therapy is a rare occurrence. The tumor develops after high doses of radiation therapy for benign conditions or after therapeutic radiation of another malignancy.

The average time from irradiation to the development of angiosarcoma is 23 years for benign conditions and 12 years for malignant tumors.

2. Angiosarcoma of the scalp and forehead occurs predominantly in elderly individuals with men being affected twice as frequently as women (Fig. 33-20).

The tumor is often multifocal in nature and will locally invade and metastaize to regional lymph nodes and distant sites. Surgical intervention and postoperative radiotherapy are currently the best treatments available. Preoperative tumor mapping by taking multiple biopsies around the tumor before surgery may help in achieving complete excision.

3. Stewart-Treves' syndrome, or angiosarcoma associated with chronic lymphedema is seen in over 90% of cases in postmastectomy patients. Angiosarcoma secondary to other causes of chronic lymphedema such as lymph node dissection, congenital or idiopathic lymphedema or lymph secondary to infectious causes have also been reported. The prognosis is usually dismal although aggressive radical surgery may prolong survival in certain patients.

Bibliography

Aust MR, Olsen KD, Lewis JE, et al. Angiosarcomas of the head and neck: clinical and pathologic characteristics. *Ann Otol Rhinol Laryngol* 1997;106(11):943–951.

Parham DM, Fisher C. Angiosarcomas of the breast developing post radiation. *Histopathology* 1997;31(2):189–195.

Zeitouni NC, Cheney R, Oseroff AR. In: Raghavan D, Brecher M, Johnson DH, Meropol NJ, Thigpen JT (eds.), *Textbook of Uncommon Cancer*. New York, NY: John Wiley & Sons, 1999, 199–219.

22. **(C)** MAC, also known as sclerosing sweat duct carcinoma, is a locally aggressive neoplasm of both eccrine and follicular differentiation. Apocrine and sebaceous differentiation has also been described. The facial midline, or "T" zone, is most commonly affected with tumors developing in the perioral, periorbital, and nasal area. Ultraviolet light appears to be a risk factor for MAC development, given the high tumor incidence in sun exposed areas. Prior therapeutic facial irradiation also appears to predispose individuals to MAC, with an average latency period of 35–40 years following radiotherapy. Clinically, the tumor presents as an indurated, flesh-colored nodule or plaque of long-term duration. It can be asymptomatic or can be accompanied by symptoms of pain, numbness, tingling, or burning. These sensory changes are often because of the tumor's propensity for perineural invasion.

Histologically, the tumor is composed of poorly demarcated epithelial nests, strands and cords invading the deep dermis, subcutaneous fat and muscle.

Bony invasion is seen in only 13% of cases. Small keratinizing cysts and well-differentiated ductules may also be seen. Mitotic figures and pleomorphic cells are rare. Perineural invasion is, however, common. MAC may be very difficult to diagnose histologically especially if only a superficial biopsy is obtained. In about 27% of cases, the tumor is misdiagnosed as another neoplasm because of the superficial nature of biopsy. Excisional, incisional, or punch biopsies are required for adequate tissue examination.

Neurotropic invasion is believed to occur as the tumor spreads along the nerve, beyond the clinical visible margin. Local control of MAC by standard resection is challenging with no adequate guidelines regarding surgical margins. With Mohs micrographic surgery, however, tumor recurrence rate is low and this method should be considered first-line therapy. Radiation and chemotherapy have been used as primary and as adjuvant therapy but the data supporting these forms of treatment is generally lacking.

Bibliography

Friedman PM, Friedman RH, Jiang B, et al. Microcystic adnexal carcinoma: collaborative series review and update. *J Am Acad Dermatol* 1999;41:225–231.

Chiller K, Passaro D, Scheuller M, et al. Microcystic adnexal carcinoma: forty eight cases, their treatment, and their outcome. *Arch Dermatol* 2000;136:1355–1359.

Snow S, Madjar DD, Hardy S, Reizner G, et al. Microcystic adnexal carcinoma: report of 13 cases and a review of the literature. *Dermatol Surg* 2003;27(4):401–408.

Burns MK, Chen SP, Goldberg LH. Microcystic adnexal carcinoma: ten cases treated by Mohs micrographic surgery. *J Dermatol Surg Oncol* 1994;20:429–434.

Abbate M, Zeitouni NC, Seyler M, et al. Clinical course, risk factors, and treatment of microcystic adnexal carcinoma: a short series report. *Dermatol Surg* 2003;29:1–4.

CHAPTER 34

Pediatric Surgery

John A. Sandoval, Alan P. Ladd, and Fredrick J. Rescorla

Questions

1. Which of the following statements regarding neonatal physiology is *correct*?

   (A) The circulatory pattern of the fetus is two ventricles working in series, rather than in parallel as in an adult.

   (B) Rectal perforation due to rectal thermometry is common in infants.

   (C) Because of shivering thermogenesis, the infant is typically not vulnerable to hypothermia.

   (D) Infants are preferential nasal and diaphragmatic breathers.

   (E) A urinary output of 0.5 mL/kg/h is considered normal in infants.

2. Regarding immunologic function in the infant, which of the statements is most *accurate*?

   (A) By 1 month of age, most term infants can produce normal levels of specific antibodies to glycoprotein antigens.

   (B) Neonatal neutrophils ingest and kill bacteria as efficiently as their adult counterparts but adherence and migration to sites of infection is impaired.

   (C) The placental transfer of Ig is limited to the IgA isotype.

   (D) Risk factors associated with perinatal acquired neonatal bacterial infection are mainly related to neonatal factors (prematurity, low birth weight, and so on).

   (E) The susceptibility of neonates to infection results mainly from a deficiency in regulatory cytokines.

3. Select the *incorrect* statement.

   (A) Hypomagnesemia and pyridoxine deficiencies are a common cause of seizures in newborns.

   (B) Liver function in the newborn is immature.

   (C) Endocrine function in the full-term infant is near normal.

   (D) A neonate has increased insensible water losses compared to an adult.

   (E) A 12 kg infant requires approximately 44 mL of maintenance fluid per hour.

4. Which of the statements regarding nutrition best applies to an infant/child?

   (A) A neonate requires approximately 90 cal/kg per day and 1 g of protein/kg per day for growth.

   (B) Newborns lose weight during the first 1–2 weeks of life.

   (C) The preferred enteral diet for the full-term infant is formula milk, which provides more calories and minerals than human milk.

   (D) Enteral feeds are appropriate in patients with sepsis, hypotension, and episodes of apnea and bradycardia because rates of intestinal bacterial translocation increase in these situations.

   (E) With the advent of "more lipid soluble" total parenteral nutrition (TPN) solutions, the risk of cholestasis is rarely encountered as complication of TPN.

5. Match the numbered letters with the following statements.

    I. esophageal atresia (EA)/tracheo-esophageal (TE) fistula

    II. pyloric atresia

    III. duodenal obstruction (DO)

    IV. jejunal atresia

    V. ileal atresia

    VI. meconium ileus

    VII. aganglionic megacolon (Hirschsprung's disease, HD)

    (A) Usually infants are full term and have few associated anomalies. The cause is attributed to late intrauterine mesenteric vascular accident.

    (B) In 80% of cases, the rectosigmoid area is involved. Familial cases have been linked to ret-oncogene and others with endothelin B gene abnormalities.

    (C) Presents with emesis characterized by clear gastric juice at attempted feedings; the causative lesion is most likely a mucosal web.

    (D) Frequently presents with abdominal distension, bilious emesis, and failure to pass meconium. Common cause of distal small bowel obstruction in newborns.

    (E) Maternal polyhydramnios is observed in 30–50% of cases and the diagnosis can be detected by prenatal ultrasound (US).

    (F) Choking, coughing, cyanosis with first attempted feeding, the infant may also develop acute gastric dilation.

    (G) Afflicted bowel loop often has a soap bubble appearance on abdominal radiographs due to mixture of meconium and air.

6. A 5-day-old, 26-week premature baby develops sudden onset feeding intolerance and bloody stools. Over the proceding 12 h, abdominal distension ensues; abdominal radiograph is shown in Fig. 34-1. Regarding the pathologic process described, which of the following is *incorrect*?

    (A) The inflammatory mediators, platelet activating factor (PAF) and nitric oxide (NO), have been demonstrated to play a dominant role in the pathophysiology of this disease in animal models.

    (B) The ominous findings of pneumatosis intestinalis leads to surgery in virtually all cases.

    (C) Treatment for uncomplicated disease is medical, which includes bowel rest, electrolyte repletion, and serial radiographs to monitor for perforation.

    (D) Strong consideration should be given to bedside operation in the neonatal intensive care unit (NICU) in infants whose condition mandates surgery.

    (E) Postoperative complications are common; these may include sepsis, disseminated intravascular coagulation (DIC), wound infection, stomal complications, stricture, short bowel syndrome, and malnutrition.

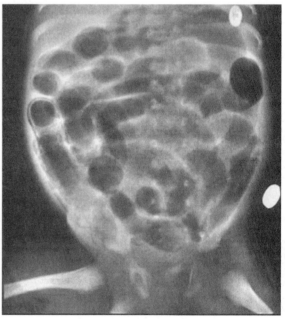

FIG. 34-1 Abdominal radiograph.

7. A 6-week-old child develops bilious emesis. Concerning this abnormality, which needs to be done emergently?

    (A) operative management

    (B) pH studies

    (C) radiologic evaluation

    (D) nutrition/dietician consultation

    (E) inform Child Protective Services of possible abuse

8. In counseling parents concerning abdominal wall defects, which of the following characteristics distinguishes an omphalocele from gastroschisis?

    (A) The abdominal wall defect is to the right of an intact umbilical cord.

    (B) There is no sac.

    (C) The liver and spleen rarely herniated through the defect.

(D) The mesentery of the herniated bowel may be compromised as it passes through the umbilical ring.

(E) Major associations with congenital malformations.

9. The chest radiograph (Fig. 34-2) demonstrates a surgically correctable cause of respiratory distress. Which is *true* regarding the possible differential diagnosis?

(A) A diaphragmatic eventration generally refers to the attenuation of the lateral portion of the diaphragm.

(B) Congenial diaphragmatic hernia can be diagnosed prenatally by US as early as 16 weeks gestation.

(C) Surgical intervention in an infant with asymptomatic pulmonary cystic adenomatoid malformation is usually associated with more postoperative complications.

(D) Congenital lobar sequestrations that demonstrate an extralobar lesion drain via the pulmonary veins.

(E) Cough, infection, and hemoptysis are the most important complications in infants and children with bronchogenic cysts, while compression symptoms occur later in life.

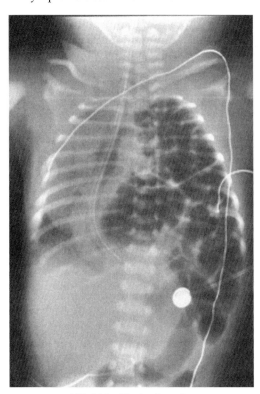

FIG. 34-2 Chest radiograph.

10. A 3-week-old, first-born male develops forceful, non-bilious emesis. Which of these findings establishes the diagnosis?

(A) ultrasonographic pyloric muscle thickness of 2.5 mm

(B) ultrasonographic pyloric:antrum ratio greater than 1.5 cm

(C) ultrasonographic pyloric diameter of 1.0 cm or less

(D) an UGI series showing a classic "double bubble" sign

(E) palpable pyloric mass (olive) midline of the abdomen

11. A 30-week-old infant presents with persistent symptoms consistent with irritability, frequent vomiting, apnea, history of aspiration pneumonia, and failure to thrive. Despite medical therapy, these symptoms continue. Regarding the disease process and treatment, which statement is most acceptable?

(A) Transient lower esophageal sphincter (LES) relaxation is the predominate mechanism and surgical therapy is indicated once intestinal malrotation has been ruled out.

(B) The majority of infants and children with this problem do not respond to medical management due to the hypertonicity of the esophageal sphincter mechanism.

(C) The etiology of this disease is related to pharyngogastric incompetence and treatment is related to bypassing this mechanism with insertion of a feeding gastrostomy tube.

(D) Most infants and children are not neurologically impaired and treatment is based on changing feeding volume and using feed thickeners to reduce liquid reflux.

(E) Promoting factors include a bout of viral gastroenteritis or upper respiratory infection and treatment is based on eradicating these infectious agents.

12. A mother brings her 9-month-old infant to a small town emergency department describing a 4-h period where the infant has been developing cycles of abdominal discomfort occurring every 5–10 min. Curiously, she notes that during the episodes of pain, the infant screams and draws up her legs. What is the next step in management for the patient described?

   (A) immediate operation
   (B) radiographic evaluation
   (C) hydrostatic barium enema
   (D) transfer to major pediatric hospital
   (E) treatment and release for presumptive viral gastroenteritis

13. Figures 34-3 and 34-4 demonstrate pathology consistent with what diagnosis?

   (A) nonsuppurative appendicitis
   (B) Meckel's diverticulum (MD)
   (C) urachal remnant
   (D) intussusception
   (E) enteric duplication

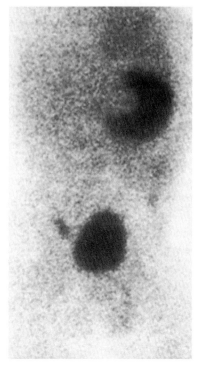

FIG. 34-4

14. An otherwise healthy 2-year-old female presents with a 3-week history of asymptomatic abdominal distension now complicated by pain, emesis, and anorexia. The patient underwent operative therapy after imaging studies revealed a causative abnormality. The OR findings shown in Fig. 34-5 indicate

   (A) ovarian cyst
   (B) choledochal cyst
   (C) mesenteric/omental cyst
   (D) cystic teratoma
   (E) intestinal duplication cyst

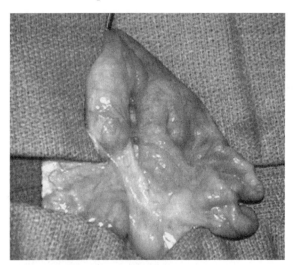

FIG. 34-3

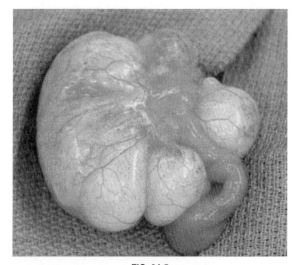

FIG. 34-5

15. When dealing with alimentary tract duplications (enteric duplications), the following apply (choose 2):

(A) Malignant transformation is not an issue.

(B) Complete resection is treatment of choice.

(C) The usual location is on the antimesenteric border of the viscera.

(D) The most common types are ileal, then esophageal and colonic duplications.

(E) The most common type of ectopic mucosa is respiratory epithelium.

(F) Associated anomalies can be found more commonly with esophageal duplications.

16. Gastrointestinal polyps in children. Match the numbered letters with the following statements?

I. Peutz-Jeghers syndrome (PJS)

II. Cronkite-Canada syndrome (CCS)

III. familial adenomatous polyposis (FAP)

IV. juvenile polyposis (JP)

V. Cowden's syndrome

VI. isolated juvenile polyps

VII. hereditary nonpolyposis colorectal cancer (HNPCC)

(A) Rare autosomal dominant disorder characterized by multiple hamartomatous polyps throughout the GI tract. Includes germline mutations in Smad4 and bone morphogenetic protein receptor (BMPR) 1A genes.

(B) Account for nearly 90% of colorectal polyps in children.

(C) Contains four major features: GI hamartomas, melanin pigmentation of the skin and mucous membranes, autosomal dominant, and significant risk for malignancy in multiple organs.

(D) The most common genetic polyposis syndrome. Mutational inactivation of the responsible gene results in accumulation of β-catenin, a protein involved in stimulation of cell growth.

(E) The most common genetic disorder leading to colorectal cancer risk in adults. Children have been reported to develop polyps with defects of mismatch repair genes.

(F) GI polyposis, alopecia, nail plate dystrophy (onychodystrophy), and diffuse pigmentation of palms, volar aspects of fingers, and dorsal hands characterize the syndrome.

(G) Syndrome associated with multiple phenotypic abnormalities and hamartomas in the intestines and other tissues. Germline mutations in the protein tyrosine phosphatase and tensin homologue (PTEN) gene are responsible for 80% of cases.

17. The appearance of cholestatic jaundice in the newborn period can be related to which of the following disorders *except*:

(A) cystic fibrosis (CF)

(B) ornithine transferase deficiency

(C) sphingomyelinase deficiency

(D) α1-antitrypsin (α1AT) deficiency

(E) congenital hypothroidism

18. A 3-week-old infant has had persistent jaundice since birth. The physical examination reveals an active infant with obvious jaundice, mild hepatomegaly, and the presence of acholic stools. Abdominal US results were equivocal. The HIDA scan shown in Fig. 34-6 suggests what abnormality?

(A) choledochal cyst (CC)

(B) biliary dyskinesis

(C) choledocholithiasis

(D) biliary fistula

(E) biliary atresia (BA)

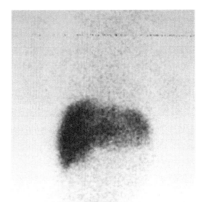

19 HR HIDA

FIG. 34-6

19. Regarding surgical treatment for the infant in Question 18, what is the appropriate operative management?

 (A) Since treatment for this ailment is hepatic transplantation, the timing depends on the availability of a donor liver.

 (B) The infant should undergo a hepaticoportoenterostomy (Roux-en-Y portoenterostomy) at approximately 4 months of age.

 (C) The infant should undergo a Roux-en-Y portoenterostomy prior to 2 months of age.

 (D) A Roux-en-Y hepaticojejunostomy should be performed within 2 months of life.

 (E) A cholecystectomy should be done emergently.

20. On ultrasonographic imaging, a pregnant woman learns that her 26-week fetus has prenatally diagnosed biliary disease. In cases of suspected CC, what should be done?

 (A) nothing, US is not sensitive enough to detect biliary abnormalities *in utero*

 (B) elective termination of the pregnancy

 (C) *In utero* fetal surgery to correct the abnormality

 (D) no significant difference exists in treatment for early versus delayed diagnosis of CC

 (E) once born, infants should undergo early surgical intervention to prevent the propagation of liver fibrosis

21. An 8-year old child is referred to a pediatric surgeon because of localized right lower quadrant pain. The pain has been ongoing for approximately 10 h and the child appears toxic. Which of the following is *incorrect* regarding appendicitis in children?

 (A) The classic presentation of appendicitis in children includes the onset of anorexia, nausea, and vomiting followed by the localization of right lower quadrant abdominal pain.

 (B) A recognized seasonal variation in appendicitis occurs during May to August due to parallel outbreaks in enteric infections caused by viral, bacterial, and parasitic infections.

 (C) The sensitivity and specificity of Rovsing's sign, psoas sign, and obturator sign have not been addressed in children.

 (D) The diagnostic accuracy of US and CT is greater than 90%; however, the history and physical are the most important features of a workup for appendicitis in a child.

 (E) Laparoscopic appendectomy in a child does not increase the complication rate in perforated/gangrenous appendicitis.

22. A child diagnosed with IBD can sometimes present with signs and symptoms of both Crohn's disease (CD) and ulcerative colitis (UC). Therefore, it is critical that the two diseases are differentiated properly for appropriate treatment. Which of the following is *true* regarding IBD in children?

 (A) Growth delay and malnutrition are particular important aspects of UC.

 (B) CD is heralded by the presence of blood and mucous mixed with stool.

 (C) The single most valuable imaging study for UC is an UGI series with small bowel follow through.

 (D) Excessive Th1 cell activity has been implicated in UC.

 (E) Serum levels of antineutrophil cytoplasmic antibody (ANCA) and anti-*Saccharomyces cerevisae* antibody (ASCA) can aid in differentiating UC from CD.

23. A 6-year-old child was struck by a car while attempting to cross the street in a residential neighborhood. The child presented to the hospital where he was immediately intubated for a Glasgow Coma Scale (GCS) of 4. Concerning the airway management of a child during trauma, which of the following statements is *correct*?

 (A) The pediatric airway does not differ from the adult airway.

 (B) Hypoxia is the most common cause of cardiopulmonary arrest in a child.

 (C) The narrowest portion of the pediatric airway is the vocal cords.

 (D) The pediatric larngeal/vocal cord complex is lower and more posterior as compared to an adult.

 (E) A protuberant pediatric tongue causes excessive neck flexion which can impact the structure of the airway.

24. EMS brings in a 3-year-old female infant who was ejected from the back of a vehicle after a 50-mile-an-hour head-on impact. The child is breathing spontaneously and the nurse reports that the child has a respiratory rate of 45. Oxygen saturations are 85% and blood pressure is 115/75 mmHg. Among the injuries, noted is a contused ecchymotic pattern over the left lower chest. Which of these statements reflects an important feature of breathing management in a child involved in trauma?

   (A) An infant requires approximately 12–18 breaths/min.

   (B) If this child is intubated for respiratory difficulty, tidal volume is 35 cc/kg.

   (C) Because of poorly developed intercostal muscles, infants rely on the diaphragm for breathing.

   (D) Because of an infant's adequate compensatory reserve, respiratory distress and failure are an infrequent issue during initial injury resuscitation.

   (E) The horizontal orientation of an infant's ribs allow the infant to increase chest expansion during respiration.

25. During the primary survey of a 5-year-old who was involved in a high impact fall off a second story apartment building, the trauma team is experiencing difficulty obtaining peripheral venous cannulation. What should be done next?

   (A) place a femoral central venous catheter

   (B) continue attempts at peripheral access

   (C) venous surgical cutdown of the saphenous vein

   (D) umbilical vascular access

   (E) proximal tibia intraosseous (IO) catheter placement

26. An 8-year-old female is thrown off her horse onto the ground striking her face and upper torso. Examination reveals an arousable child complaining of diffuse chest pain and shortness of breath. The chest radiograph in Fig. 34-7 shows the pathology responsible for the patient's symptoms. Regarding thoracic trauma in children, which of the statements is *correct*?

   (A) Rib fractures rarely serve as an injury severity marker.

   (B) Mediastinal injuries, while rare in children, may be complicated to diagnose on chest radiograph because of thymic prominence.

   (C) Pulmonary contusion is infrequently seen in children because of the pliability of children's ribs.

   (D) Hemorrhage, cardiac tamponade, pneumothorax, and pulmonary embolism can be differentiated on the basis of clinical grounds alone in children.

   (E) Blunt diaphragmatic rupture in children usually involves the left hemidiaphragm in the posteriomedial location

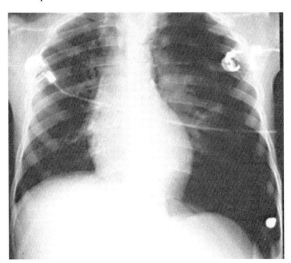

FIG. 34-7

27. Parents present to a children's hospital emergency department with their 11-year-old son who has been complaining of abdominal pain over the past 6 h. He apparently was a restrained backseat passenger involved in a motor vehicle accident earlier that day. No one was injured in the accident and he did not voice any complaints at the time of the accident. He was hemodynamically stable on arrival to the ER. Noted during the physical examination are a "seat-belt" sign over his lower abdomen and a mildly distended abdomen with diffuse pain with no guarding or rebound (Fig. 34-8). Abdominal x-rays show a nonspecific bowel gas pattern, with no associated free air. An abdominal CT demonstrated a grade II spleen injury with moderate free fluid (Fig. 34-9). Concerning diagnostic modalities in pediatric blunt abdominal trauma, what statement is *true*?

(A) The focused abdominal sonogram for trauma (FAST) examination in children is poor at identifying organ-specfic injury.

(B) There has not been any correlation to the abdominal CT pattern of free fluid following isolated blunt spleen or liver injury in the pediatric patient.

(C) Laparoscopy has not been shown to be a viable treatment option in selected pediatric blunt abdominal trauma.

(D) CT scan of the abdomen is reliable for the diagnosis of lumbar spine and intestinal injuries.

(E) Diagnostic peritoneal lavage (DPL) should not be used in children.

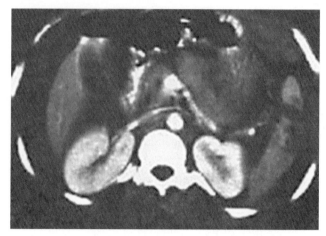
FIG. 34-9

28. A 15-year-old unrestrained passenger is "along for the ride" with friends in a recreational vehicle. Due to excessive speed, the driver loses control of the vehicle and strikes an embankment, causing the vehicle to roll many times. The patient is brought directly from the scene, intubated secondary to unresponsiveness and a GCS of 5. The evaluation of this pediatric head trauma patient includes all of the following *except*:

(A) Children often have more diffuse brain injury due to higher water content of the immature brain and incomplete axonal myelination.

(B) Hypoxia, hypotension, and intracranial hypertension are important factors that worsen prognosis in pediatric head trama.

(C) Children with traumatic head injury and a cerebral perfusion pressure (CPP) of greater than 40 mmHg have better outcomes.

(D) Continuous intracranial pressure (ICP) monitoring is recommended for pediatric patients with a GCS of less than or equal to 10.

(E) Hypertonic saline is a treatment modality used to reduce ICP in pediatric head trauma patients.

29. A 7-year-old child says he can swing from a tree like an acrobat. The child suffers a fall and states after the event that his legs feel "funny." Radiographs evaluating the spine and lower extremities find no local abnormality. Concerning traumatic spinal cord injuries in children, which one of the following applies?

(A) Anatomic differences are responsible for shifting resistence from the ligamentous attachments to the bony skeleton in a child.

(B) Injury prevention programs have not aided in decreasing risk-taking behavior associated with spinal cord injury.

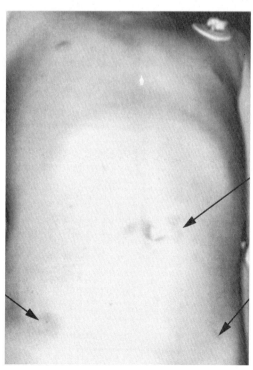
FIG. 34-8   Seat-belt sign.

(C) Spinal cord injury without radiographic abnormality (SCIWORA) is an entity most likely encountered in the pediatric population and its mechanism is due to lack of mineralization in bone.

(D) Misinterpretation of plain radiographs is uncommon in young children.

(E) Neck pain is often a hallmark of injury in young children.

30. An 18-month-old girl falls while her right hand is being held by her mother. She immediately screams and then refuses to use the right upper extremity. Musculoskeletal trauma in children is unique in that the growing bone has remarkable healing potential. Choose the *correct* statement.

(A) Only the endosteum (inner lining of the bone) is responsible for new bone formation during fracture healing.

(B) Plastic deformation of bone must be surgically corrected in children.

(C) Nursemaid's elbow (radial head subluxation) requires surgical intervention.

(D) The most common site of fracture in children is the humerus.

(E) Shoulder dislocations in children commonly are associated with neurologic and vascular injury.

31. A 3¹/₂-year-old child presents after his mother reports that the child fell off the couch and has been experiencing abdominal pain with nausea and vomiting. The child undergoes an abdominal CT scan which demonstrates the pathology (see Figs. 34-10 and 34-11). Of significance is the fact that the same child had presented to the ER five different times over the past year with bizarre injuries (bites, cigarette burns, rope marks). Concerning suspected child abuse, which is *incorrect*?

(A) Shaken baby syndrome consists of subdural hematoma, subarachnoid hemorrhage, retinal hemorrhage, and metaphyseal long bone fractures.

(B) Retinal hemorrhage is exclusive to child abuse.

(C) Other medical conditions that may be confused with abusive skeletal fractures include osteogenesis imperfecta, congenital syphilis, osteomyelitis, and infantile rickets.

(D) Brain injury is the most common etiology for fatal or near-fatal child abuse.

(E) Rib fractures in an infant most likely indicates physical abuse.

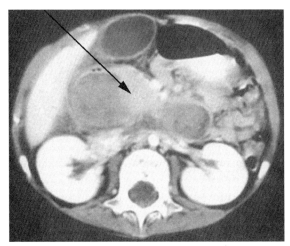

FIG. 34-10

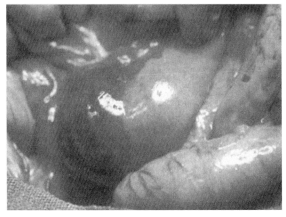

FIG. 34-11

32. A 12-year-old female presents for evaluation of a neck mass. Which of the following pairs are *correct*?

(A) branchial cleft cyst/sinus: most commonly involves the third branchial cleft remnant

(B) thyroglossal duct cyst (TGDCs): mesodermal remnants that produce lateral swelling over neck

(C) cystic hygroma: a salivary gland disorder related to a hypersecretory cyst

(D) torticollis: unilateral shortening of trapezius muscle

(E) medullary thyroid cancer: most common cause of death in multiple endocrine neoplasia (MEN) 2B

33. A 12-month-old full-term male is diagnosed with an inguinal and an umbilical hernia (ring diameter >2 cm). During the discussion of pediatric hernias with parents, select the *correct* statement.

   (A) The most common cause of indirect hernia in this age group is due to a connective tissue disorder.

   (B) Laparoscopy has aided in evaluation of the contralateral inguinal area for hernias; routine laparoscopic evaluation for a patent contralateral processus vaginalis should be advocated for all patients.

   (C) The inguinal hernia should be repaired and the umbilical defect left alone.

   (D) Repair of both inguinal and umbilical hernias (UH).

   (E) Femoral hernias (FH) in children are easier to detect as compared to an adult.

34. Worried parents bring in their full-term 18-month-old infant for evaluation of a unilateral UDT. On examination, normal male genitalia with scrotal asymmetry are noted. Despite maneuvers to detect a retractile testicle, a right testis is not palpable. What should be the next step in this patient's management?

   (A) the patient should be reexamined prior to 2 years of age because most patients undergo spontaneous descent of the testicle by 2 years of age

   (B) laparoscopy for presence and localization of the testicle

   (C) hormonal therapy with human chorionic gonadotropin (HCG)

   (D) imaging studies

   (E) scrotal exploration

35. A 5-year-old female presents with bilateral ecchymotic periorbital areas (see Fig. 34-12). Child abuse has been suspected and the primary team consults a pediatric surgeon as part of the workup. On physical examination an abdominal mass is appreciated. The abdominal CT shown in Fig. 34-13 demonstrates the diagnosis. Concerning the diagnosis, which statement is *incorrect*?

   (A) The tumor originates from neural crest cells and most likely arises from the adrenal medulla.

   (B) Cause of this malignancy has been directly linked to the tumor suppressor p53 gene product.

   (C) Younger patients (<1 year of age) usually experience more favorable outcomes as compared to older children (>1 year of age).

   (D) Amplification of N-myc oncogene, chromosome 1p deletion, and CD44 are biologic markers that aid with prognosis.

   (E) Mass screening using urinary catecholamines has not aided in decreasing mortality.

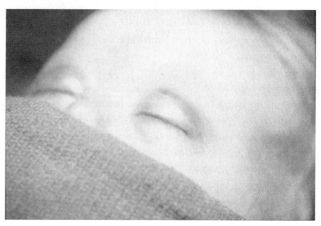

FIG. 34-12

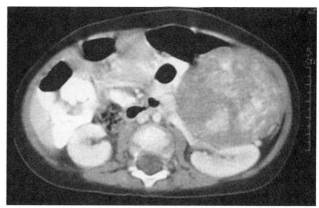

FIG. 34-13

36. A 3-year-old child presents for evaluation of an abdominal mass that was detected when the child was being bathed. An abdominal CT scan in Fig. 34-14 shows a solid lesion originating from the kidney. After determining that the primary tumor is resectable, the following applies during operative management:

   (A) The renal arteries lie anterior to the renal vein and the left renal vein is posterior to the origin of the inferior mesenteric artery.

   (B) Preresection percutaneous biopsy is superior to open operative exploration and biopsy.

   (C) Preoperative chemotherapy can obscure the postchemotherapy staging and inadequately define the risk of relapse or recurrence.

39. A 16-year-old female presents with increased abdominal girth and now pain. In the past, she has been treated with enemas and laxatives for constipation. Unfortunately her symptoms have progressed over the last 7 days. AFP, β-HCG, and CA-125 levels are normal. Plain abdominal radiographs reveal laterally displaced small and large bowel and areas of calcification within the central area of the abdomen and lower pelvis. A CT scan of the abdomen and pelvis confirms the diagnosis (Fig. 34-17). What surgical principle concerning this lesion should be *avoided*?

(A) laparotomy via midline or Pfannensteil incision

(B) laproscopic excision of lesion

(C) pelvic/retroperitoneal lymph node dissection with lymph node sampling

(D) inspect contralateral ovary

(E) US guided drainage of the lesion

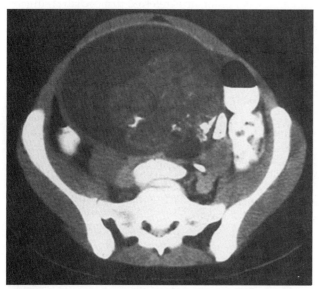

FIG. 34-17

40. A couple learns that on prenatal US imaging their 22-week-old fetus is highly suggestive of conjoined twins. On discussion of the embryology of conjoined twinning, which of the following is *correct*?

(A) because experimental human embryology is not feasible, there is no currently accepted theory

(B) the delayed fertilization theory

(C) fission development of the embryo

(D) spheroid/fusion theory

(E) environmental trigger theory

Answers and Explanations

1. (D) Neonatal and infant physiology is considerably different from an adult. The circulatory pattern of the fetus is unique in that the lungs are bypassed and intracardiac/extracardiac shunts enable blood to be oxygenated. Shunts (foramen ovale, ductus arteriosus, and ductus venosus) allow the fetus to receive blood from both ventricles, commonly referred to as parallel circulation. Adults experience a circulatory pattern in series that allows for an equal but separate output for each ventricle.

Thermoregulation in the infant is important to consider due to the fact that the infant can lose heat due to a relatively large body surface area, lack of hair and subcutaneous tissue, and increased insensible losses. Studies of neonatal rectal perforation due to rectal thermometry in the late '70s prompted the recommendation that rectal temperature measurement be discouraged. However, recent reports indicate that perforation has occurred in less than 1 in 2 million measurements. The validity of axillary temperature has been questioned with its lack of reliability and most authors use rectal thermometry for temperature measurement. Additionally in response to cold stress, an infant cannot shiver but relies on mobilization of brownian fat deposits in the neck, axilla, mediastinum, and perirenal area (*nonshivering thermogenesis*).

Pulmonary function is not fully mature until approximately 8 years of age. Because the intercostals muscles are underdeveloped in the infant age group, the diaphragm is the major muscle of breathing. Structure-function studies indicate that in contrast to adults, where the diaphragm acts as a piston within the rib cage, the diaphragm of the newborn infant acts as a bellow moving in the posterior segment. Of note, literature shows that infants are preferential nose breathers from birth to between 6 weeks and 6 months of age. This route of breathing in infants is preferred to the oral airway because of its ability to humidify, warm, and regulate the air coming into the lungs. Moreover, it stressed that if an infant requires a tube for gastric drainage, it should be inserted via the oral route rather than the nasal pathway.

The developing pediatric kidneys are provided with 2–4% (compared with 20–25% of an adult's cardiac output) of the fetus's combined ventricular output in the third trimester of pregnancy. This is due to the relatively high vascular resistance of the fetal kidney, which decreases within the first 48 h after birth. The decrease in vascular resistance is also responsible for increasing renal blood flow and glomerular filtration rate (full-term infant at birth GFR is 2–4 mL/min this increases to 8–20 mL/min within a few days postnatally). Because infants have a limited ability to concentrate urine due mostly to the limited concentration of urea, which is responsible for creating a hyperosmolar medulla and thus water reabsorption, measuring urine flow and concentration best assesses renal handling of water in an infant surgical patient. A urine output from 1 to 2 mL/kg/h, an osmolarity of 250–290 mOsm/kg, and a specific gravity of 1.010–1.013 is expected urine flow and concentration in term and premature infants.

Bibliography

Bergeson PS, Shaw JC. Are infants really obligatory nasal breathers? *Clin Pediatr* 2001;40:567–567.

Brown PJ, Christmas BF, Ford RP. Taking an infants's temperature:axillary vs. resctal thermometry? *N Z Med J* 1992;105(939):309–311.

Devlieger H, Daniels H, Marchal G, Moerman P, Casaer P, Eggermont E. The diaphragm of the newborn infant: anatomical and ultrasonic studies. *J Dev Physiol* 1991;16(6):321–329.

Frank JD, Brown S. Thermometers and rectal perforations in the neonate. *Arch Dis Child* 1978;53(10):824–825.

Heisler D. Pediatric renal function. *Int Anesthesiol Clin* 1993;31(1):103–107.

Morley CJ, Hewson PH, Thorton AJ, Cole TJ. Axillary and rectal measurements in infants. *Arch Dis Child* 1992;67(1): 122–125.

Rowe MI. The newborn as a surgical patient. In: O'Neil JA Jr, Rowe MI, Grosfeld JL, Fonkalsrud EW, Coran AG (eds.), *Pediatric Surgery*, 5th ed. St. Louis, MO: Mosby-Year Book, 1998, 43–70.

Stafford M. Cardiovascular physiology and care. In: O'Neil JA Jr, Rowe MI, Grosfeld JL, Fonkalsrud EW, Coran AG (eds.), *Pediatric Surgery*, 5th ed. St. Louis, MO: Mosby-Year Book, 1998, 103–133.

2. **(B)** The concept of "immunodeficiency of immaturity" has been proposed to encompass the decreased immune response in newborns as compared to adults. This increase in infection rate can be attributed to not only innate and specific immune defenses, but also neonatal and maternal factors.

For the most part, neonates have a reduced capacity to produce specific antibodies in the newborn period. By 1 year of age, most term infants can produce normal levels of specific antibodies to glycoprotein antigens. Antibody responses to polysaccharide antigens are delayed until after 2 years of age.

Innate immunity has certain quantitative deficiencies that can affect the newborn immune response. For example, neutrophils can function similar to adults with respect to engulfing and killing bacteria, but adhesion and migration are deficient secondary to functional deficiencies of the neutrophils themselves (decreased filamentous actin and increased neutrophil membrane fluidity) and decreased levels of complement-mediated chemoattractants, C3b and C5a.

Most of the newborn's serum immunoglobulin repertoir are derived from maternal transfer of IgG across the placenta during the third trimester of pregnancy. IgA, the principle antibody found in body secretions and mucosal surfaces, does not cross the placenta and is derived from the neonate; however, when the infant consumes breast milk, maternally-derived IgA contributes to gut immunity.

Obstetric and neonatal factors have been identified which are associated with increased risk of neonatal infection. Maternal risk factors include prolonged rupture of membranes >18–24 h, premature rupture of membranes (<37 weeks), maternal fevers ≥100.4°F, intraamniotic infection, maternal colonization with group B streptococcus (GBS), GBS bacteremia, previous infant with invasive GBS disease, and maternal urinary tract infection (UTI) at delivery. Neonatal risk factors include prematurity, low birth weight (<2500 g), male gender, 5 min Apgar <6, and multiple gestation.

Bibliography

Arkachaisri T, Ballow M. Developmental immunology of the newborn. *Immunol Allergy Clin North Am* 1999;19(2): 253–273.

Eichenwald EC. Perinatally transmitted neonatal bacterial infections. *Infect Dis Clin North Am* 1997;11(1):223–239.

Schelonka RL, Infante A. Neonatal immunology. *Semin Perinatol* 1998;22(1):2–14.

3. **(A)** The survival and growth of the newborn infant depends on successful adaptive changes that occur postnatally. From a metabolic/endocrine standpoint, the hypothalamic-pituitary-adrenal (HPA) axis is responsible for establishing metabolic/endocrine homeostasis. The neonate has been shown to mount a substantial endocrine/metabolic response in response to surgical stress. The HPA axis is functional in term infants and an immature HPA axis in premature infants may contribute to neonatal morbidity.

Additionally, the infant must maintain normoglycemia in an actively growing metabolic state. By activating hepatic glycogen stores, gluconeogenesis, and receiving exogenous glucose supply, the infant produces and receives the needed carbohydrate source that supply a number of organs and cells. Failure to accomplish this task may result in hypoglycemia and clinical manifestations. Hypoglycemia is the major cause of seizures in newborns and in infants who are small for their gestational age (GA) (secondary to inadequate glycogen stores). Hypocalcemia may also present with seizures in premature infants, while hypomagnesium and pyridoxine deficiencies are rare causes of seizures in newborns.

The liver is responsible for the enzymes that carry out glycogenolysis and gluconeogenesis. As a result, several of the hepatic metabolic enzymes are immature in the neonate. Some of these proteins include glucuronyl transferase (conjugates indirect to direct bilirubin), certain cytochromes, and glucuronidation enzymes involved in the detoxification of drugs and anesthetic agents.

Management of fluid/electrolyte status in the newborn can be challenging due to the large fluid fluctuations that occur postnatally. In an infant who requires surgery, these fluid shifts may be more dramatic perioperatively and postoperatively. Nevertheless monitoring the dynamic fluid balance in infants is based on administering a calculated maintenance rate. Maintenance fluids are calculated based on body weight using the 4-2-1 rule. The formula states that for the first 10 kg of body weight, 4 mLs of fluid are administered per hour. For the second 10 kg, 2 mLs/kg/h are given and for each additional kg over 20 kg, 1 mL/kg/h is administered. The formula originated from work done by

Holliday and Segar in the 1950s that correlated caloric expenditure with fluid loss. In general, a neonate has increased insensible water losses (30–35 mL/kg per day) as compared to an adult (15 mL/kg per day). Insensible water loss represents free water losses that occur through the skin and respiratory tract. Transepithelial water loss represents the majority of insensible loss. In reference to specific electrolyte requirements, sodium and potassium should be administered at 2–3 meq/kg per day.

Bibliography

Bolt RJ, van Weissenbruch, Lafeber HN, Delemarre-van de Waal HA. Development of the hypothalamic-pituitary-adrenal axis in the fetus and preterm infant. *J Pediatr Endocrinol Metab* 2002;15(6):759–769.

Brosnam PG. The hypothalamic pituitary axis in the fetus and newborn. *Semin Perinatol* 2001;25(6):371–384.

Engum SA, Grosfeld JL. Pediatric surgery. In: Townsend CM Jr, Beauchamp RD, Evers BM, Mattox KL (eds.), *Sabiston Textbook of Surgery*. Philadelphia, PA: W.B. Saunders, 2001, 1463–1517.

Gow PJ, Ghabrial H, Smallwood RA, Morgan DJ, Ching MS. Neonatal hepatic drug elimination. *Pharmacol Toxicol* 2001;88:3–15.

Holliday MA, Segar WE. The maintenance need for water in parenteral fluid therapy. *Pediatrics* 1957;19:823–832.

Okur H, Kucukaydin M, Ustdel KM. The endocrine and metabolic response to surgical stress in the neonate. *J Pediatr Surg* 1995;30(4):626–650.

Philipps AF. General metabolism and glucose. In: Polin R, Fox W (eds.), *Fetal and Neonatal Physiology*. Philadelphia, PA: W.B. Saunders, 1992, 373–384.

4. **(B)** A neonate has higher growth and energy requirements as compared to an adult. After approximately 3 months of age, growth rates gradually decline. Nevertheless, all newborns lose weight during the first 1–2 weeks of life as a result of postnatal diuresis. A similar trend occurs with caloric requirements in infants and children; the recommended dietary allowance (RDA) in the pediatric population decreases with age. Preterm infants require 120–130 kcal/kg per day and 3.0–4.0 g protein/kg per day; full-term infants require 110–120 kcal/kg per day and 2.0–2.5 g protein/kg per day; from 6 months to 3 years, 100 kcal/kg per day and 1.2–1.6 g protein/kg per day; by 7–10 years of age, 70 kcal and 1.0 g protein/kg per day. The final diet composition should provide 35–65% calories as carbohydrates, 7–16% as protein, and 30–50% as fat.

Enteral formula selection depends on many patient-specific factors such as age, intestinal function, and underlying disease. The preferred enteral diet for the full-term newborn is human milk (20 kcal/oz), which provides sufficient macronutrients, minerals, and water for normal growth. The preterm infant may

not grow as fast as human milk alone because of higher nutritional requirements. Using human milk fortifiers, 4 kcal/oz are added to provide 24 kcal/oz of fortified breast milk.

The enteral route of nutrition delivery has certain advantages over parenteral nutrition. Some of these include better maintenance/structural integrity of the gastrointestinal (GI) tract, decrease risk of bacterial translocation, and more efficient use of nutrient substrates. However, timing of initial enteral feeds should be optimized to improve chances for feeding tolerance. Clinical signs of acute sepsis, hypotension, significant apnea and bradycardia should be absent. Additionally, enteral nutrition should be avoided in necrotizing enterocolitis, bowel obstruction, intestinal atresia, severe inflammatory bowel disease (IBD), intestinal side effects of cancer therapy, and acute pancreatitis.

Pediatric patients who will withstand a period greater than 5–7 days without nutrition due to dysfunctional GI tract will necessitate parenteral nutrition. When highly concentrated carbohydrate solutions (>12.5 g/dL) are required, TPN must be administered to avoid thrombophlebitis in peripheral veins. Complications related to TPN can be categorized as mechanical, metabolic, nutritional, or infectious. While the field of parenteral nutrition continues to evolve in prevention of complications and refining nutrional needs, TPN associated intrahepatic cholestasis (TPNAC) remains a problem. The etiology of TPNAC is considered to be multifactorial and may be related to prematurity of bile flow/production, infection, lack of enteral feeding, total caloric overloading, and perhaps a free radical-mediated process. TPNAC eventually leads to irreversible cirrhosis and liver failure. The incidence of TPNAC in surgical neonates has decreased, yet the mortality remains at 3%. Data suggests that lipid supply may be a risk factor for TPNAC, however more lipid soluble solutions have not been investigated and studies with fish oil emulsions have been shown to attenuate TPN induced cholestasis in newborn piglets. Overall, the composition of parenteral nutrition solution may contribute to the development of this intrahepatic pathology.

Bibliography

Colomb V, Jobert-Giraud A, Lacaille F, Goulet O, Fournet JC, Ricour C. Role of lipid emulsions in cholestasis associated with long-term parenteral nutrition in children. *J Parenter Enteral Nutr* 2000;24(6):345–350.

Frantz FW. Enteral nutrition. In: Mattei P (ed.), *Surgical Directives Pediatric Surgery*. Philadelphia, PA: Lippincott, Williams & Wilkins, 2003, 25–33.

Kuboth A, Yonekura T, Hoki M, Oyanagi H, Kawahara H, YagI M, Imura K, Iiboshi Y, Wasa K, Kamata S, Okada A. TPN-associated cholestasis in infants: 25 years experience. *J Pediatr Surg* 2000;35(7):1049–1051.

Shulman RJ. New developments in TPN for children. *Curr Gastroenterol Rep* 2000;2(3):253–258.

Van Aerde JE, Duerksen DR, Gramlich L, Meddings JB, Chan G, Thomson A, Chandinin MT. Intravenous fish oil emulsion attenuates TPN-associated cholestasis in newborn piglets. *Pediatr Res* 1999;45(2):202–208.

5. **I (F), II (C), III (E), IV (A), V (D), VI (G), VII (B)** The clinical signs of different pathologic conditions causing intestinal obstruction in the newborn often aid in determining the site of obstruction. In general, maternal polyhydramnios, bilious emesis, abdominal distension, and failure to pass meconium in the first 24 h of life denote signs that are suspicious for an intestinal obstructive process that warrants further work-up in the newborn.

EA/TE fistula When clinically suspected, the diagnosis in confirmed with intranasal passage of a 10 French Replogle tube that stops at approximately 10 cm. Five variants (A–E, with C type being the most common) are recognized and 10% of patients have VACTERAL syndrome (abnormalities of vertebrae, anus, cardiovascular, trachea, esophagus, renal system, and limb buds). In Fig. 34-18, the radiographic observations in children with EA and/or TEF vary depending on the type of anomaly present. In this case, findings on posteroanterior chest radiograph suggest a diagnosis of EA by displaying a coiled nasogastric tube (placed for determination of EA) in the proximal esophageal pouch. Additionally, in EA a gasless abdomen may be depicted because air is normally present in the stomach 15 min after birth.

Pyloric atresia It is a rare cause of intestinal obstruction accounting for 1% of all cases of GI tract obstruction. Maternal polyhydramnios is present in >60% of cases and newborns present with repeated bouts of nonbilious emesis. Any pregnant female with amnionic fluid abnormalities should undergo prenatal ultrasonography to detect instances of GI tract obstruction, including EA without TE fistula, pyloric atresia, duodenal atresia (obstruction), and high jejunal atresia.

Duodenal obstruction The diagnosis of DO may be detected as early as 18 weeks gestation on fetal US. The findings of a dilated stomach and duodenum ("double bubble") on antenatal US with polyhydramnios can identify the diagnosis in experienced hands. In infants not diagnosed prenatally, infants present in the first few hours of life with bilious vomiting due to the duodenal obstruction located distal to the ampulla of Vater in 85% of cases. The differential of bilious emesis includes intestinal malrotation with volvulus, which must be made immediately with radiologic plain films and contrast studies. One adjunctive feature of DO is that in contrast to volvulus, infants with DO do not appear ill. The abdominal radiograph in Fig. 34-19 shows a double bubble sign, which represents dilatation of the stomach and duodenum. This configuration most commonly occurs

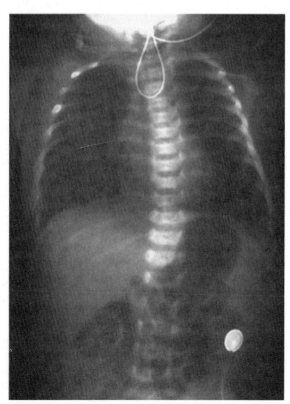

FIG. 34-18   Esophageal atresia (EA).

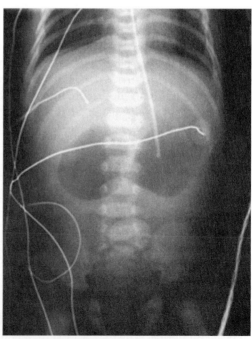

FIG. 34-19   Duodenal obstruction.

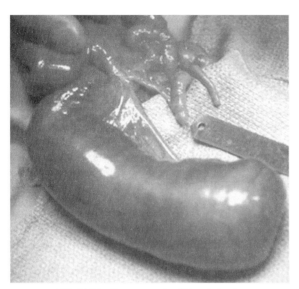

FIG. 34-20   Gross example of jejunal atresia.

with duodenal atresia or an annular pancreas with duodenal stenosis.

Jejunoileal atresia The prevalent theory of jejunoileal atresias is such that a late accident is responsible for the pathophysiology. Because of this notion, the presentation, treatment, and natural history of congenital atresia of the jejunum or ileum are similar. Differences include jejunal atresias are more likely to be multiple than ileal atresias and on presentation ileal atresias are more frequently seen with abdominal distension. Treatment and management is based on resection of the compromised small bowel segment while preserving bowel length. Four types of atresias exist. Figure 34-20 shows a type IIIa atresia. The atresia is characterized by both blind proximal and distal bowel segments with complete disconnection. The proximal blind end is markedly dilated and not peristaltic. The compromised bowel undergoes intrauterine absorption, and as a result, the bowel is variably shortened. Additionally, a V-shaped mesenteric defect is present.

Colonic obstruction The spectrum of colonic obstruction includes meconium plug syndrome, aganglionic megacolon (HD), colonic atresia, small left colon syndrome, neuronal colonic dysplasia, intestinal pseudoobstruction, and imperforate anus. Because of a similar clinical presentation, meconium ileus, which presents as a distal small bowel obstruction secondary to inspissated meconium, deserves mention in this category of colonic obstructive disorders. The clinical scenario for these ailments consists of failure to pass meconium within 24 h of life, abdominal distension, and bilious vomiting. While not all of these causes of distal neonatal bowel obstruction

mandate surgical attention, the role of diagnostic imaging helps determine the exact nature of the abnormality. Plain radiographs would typically show dilated air-filled loops of bowel consistent with a distal bowel obstruction. Abdominal films in meconium ileus would additionally demonstrate a ground-glass or soap bubble appearance (Neuhauser's sign) caused as the viscid meconium mixes with air. Moreover, neonates with complete low intestinal obstruction require a contrast enema examination. In cases of suspected HD, a rectal biopsy is required to confirm the diagnosis. A submucosal suction biopsy is adequate in identifying ganglion cells in Meissner's submucosal plexus in 90% of cases. Familial cases of HD have been associated with aberrant genes, such as chromosomes 10 (ret protooncogene) and 13 (endothelin B receptor). The treatment is decompression, resection of aganglionic bowel, and a pull through procedure of normally innervated bowel. While colonic atresia and meconium ileus are associated with microcolon, HD is characterized by normal or megacolon. Small left colon syndrome and meconium ileus are treated effectively with a gastrograffin enema. If this is unsuccessful, then surgical intervention will generally be required. Neuronal colonic dysplasia (hyperplasia of submucosal/myenteric plexus with increase in acetylcholinesterase activity) and pseudoobstruction (motor dysfunction of different sites and degrees in the GI tract) both can be challenging to diagnose/manage and involve a combination of bowel regimens and rectal irrigation to empty the colon. The initial diagnosis of imperforate anus can be made on physical examination; the absence of anal opening should raise the diagnosis.

Bibliography

Engum SA, Grosfeld JL. *Pediatric surgery.* In: Townsend CM Jr, Beauchamp RD, Evers BM, Mattox KL (eds.), *Sabiston Textbook of Surgery.* Philadelphia, PA: W.B. Saunders, 2001, 1463–1517.

Kiss P, Osztovics M. Association of 13q deletion and Hirschprung's disease. *J Med Genet* 1989;26:793–794.

Lyonnet S, Bolino A, Pelet A, Abel L, Nihoul-Fekete C, Briard ML, Mok-Siu V, Kaariainen H, Martucciello G, Lerone M, Puliti A, Luo Y, Weissenbach J, Devoto M, Munnich A, Romeo G. A gene for Hirschprung's disease maps to the proximal long arm of chromosome 10. *Nat Genet* 1993;4:346–350.

Nance ML. Neonatal intestinal obstruction. In: Mattei P (ed.), *Surgical Directives Pediatric Surgery.* Philadelphia, PA: Lippincott, Williams & Wilkins, 2003, 313–316.

Swischuk LE. Alimentary tract. In: Swischuk LE (ed.), *Imaging of the Newborn, Infant, and Young Child,* 4th ed. Baltimore, MD: Lippincott, Williams & Wilkins, 1997, 352–371.

6. **(B)** In this scenario, the appearance of pneumatosis in the abdominal radiograph (see Fig. 34-1) along with the clinical symptoms suggest the diagnosis of necrotizing enerocolitis (NEC). The single most common surgical emergency and major cause of death in the newborn period is NEC. NEC is a neonatal GI disease process that afflicts premature infants. Additional predisposing factors include enteral feeding and infections. While the exact pathogenesis remains elusive, animal models of NEC have shown that PAF and NO play a key role. PAF is an endogenous phospholipid mediator produced by inflammatory cells, endothelial cells, platelets, and bacteria of the intestinal flora. When PAF is injected into rats, the results show small intestinal necrosis of varying degree. Another mediator involved is NO. NO plays a function in gut mucosal protection and motility. In an adapted intraluminal piglet model of NEC, manipulation of the nitrergic system by providing the NOS substrate, L-arg, attenuated NEC induced intestinal damage without any systemic effects.

The most common clinical presentation of NEC includes GI symptoms such as feeding intolerance, abdominal distension, and bloody stools. Early radiographic evidence of NEC consists of generalized intestinal distension. The radiologic finding of pneumatosis intestinalis, or gas within the bowel wall, in a neonate is a prognostic sign for NEC. While the x-ray finding of pneumatosis by itself is not an indication for surgery, the presence of pneumoperitoneum should be acknowledged as an indication for operation. Additional indicators for operative management of NEC include portal venous gas and debris-filled ascites on peritoneal tap.

Uncomplicated NEC is a medically treated disease. Management includes bowel rest, orogastric decompression, IV hydration, and broad-spectrum antibiotics. Close observation is required along with serial abdominal x-rays to evaluate for resolution or progression of the disease.

Controversy exists in the surgical management of NEC including whether to resect intestine with or without primary anastomosis, intestinal diversion with limited resection or peritoneal drainage without resection. Nevertheless, if an infant shows indication for operative management, some have advocated bedside operation in the NICU. Serious physiologic deterioration, such as hypothermia, has been shown to occur during intrahospital transport of critically ill infants. In reference to NEC, Frawley and coworkers have evaluated neonates requiring laparotomy for NEC. His group has demonstrated temperature deterioration, decreasing arterial pO_2, and platelet count alterations on transfer to the operating room. Hospital survival for surgically treated patients with NEC averages 70%. The development of postoperative complications is common and includes recurrent NEC, sepsis, DIC, wound infection, stomal complications, enteric fistulae, and cholestasis. Long-term complications include intestinal strictures, malabsorption and short gut syndrome, and neurodevelopmental complications.

Bibliography

Chandler JC, Smith SD. Necrotizing enterocolitis. In: Mattei P (ed.), *Surgical Directives Pediatric Surgery*. Philadelphia, PA: Lippincott, Williams & Wilkins, 2002, 293–296.

Di Lorenzo M, Krantis A. Nitric oxide synthase isoenzyme activities in a premature piglet model of necrotizing enterocolitis: effects of nitrergic manipulation. *Pediatr Surg Int* 2002;18:624–629.

Frawley G, Bayley G, and Chondros P. Laparotomy for necrotizing enterocolitis: intensive care nursery compared with operating theatre. *J Paediatr Child Health* 1999;35(3):291–295.

Hsueh W, Caplan MS, Qu XU, Tan XD, De Plaen IG, Gonzalez-Crussi F. Neonatal necrotzing enterocolitis: clinical considerations and pathogenetic concepts. *Pediatr Develop Pathol* 2003;6(1):6–23.

Nadler EP, Upperman JS, Ford HR. Controversies in the management of necrotizing enterocolitis. *Surg Infect (Larchmt)* 2001;2(2):113–119.

Ricketts RR. Necrotizing enterocolitis. In: Ziegler MM, Azizkham RG, Weber TR (eds.), *Operative Pediatric Surgery*. New York, NY: McGraw-Hill, 2003, 661–670.

Wallen E, Venkataraman ST, Grosso MJ, Kiene K, Orr RA. Intrahospital transport of critically ill pediatric patients. *Crit Care Med* 1995;23(9):1588–1595.

7. **(C)** Malrotation with midgut volvulus most commonly occurs in the first month of life or before 1 year of age. It is further stressed that bilious vomiting in child under 1 year of age is assumed to be due to malrotation with volvulus until proven otherwise. Normal rotation of the midgut, which occurs during the 6th–12th week of embryonic development, is a process characterized by the herniation of the midgut into the body stalk, returning, and undergoing a counterclockwise rotation of the ligament of Trietz (duodenojejunal junction) 270 degress around the superior mesenteric artery such that the final position of the ligament of Trietz is to the left of the spine and at or above the pylorus. The ileocolic junction rotates 270 degrees counterclockwise around the superior mesenteric artery (SMA) to lie in the right lower quadrant. The major cause of midgut volvulus is due to nonrotation of the ligament of Trietz or cecocolic limb.

Radiologic evaluation is indicated when one suspects malrotation and several imaging studies are necessary in sequence in order to determine the position of the ligament of Trietz and its distance to the ileocecal junction. Plain abdominal radiographs are

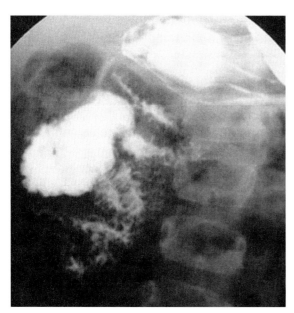

FIG. 34-21 Upper GI shows small bowel malrotation.

mostly nonspecific in patients with malrotation; therefore, further radiographic studies are needed. However, when obstruction is determined by x-rays or peritonitis is present, further studies are contraindicated and the patient should undergo emergent exploration. The upper gastrointestinal series (UGI) is the gold standard test to make the diagnosis of malrotation. Principle diagnostic findings on UGI include an abnormal right-sided position of the ligament of Trietz, obstruction of the duodenum, and right-sided filling of jejunal loops. The abnormal UGI on Fig. 34-21 demonstrates a spiral course ("corkscrew deformity") of the midgut loops in the right side of the abdomen, which is pathognomic for malrotation.

When an UGI is inconclusive for malrotation, barium enema should be performed to confirm the position of the cecum. This modality may also estimate the width of the mesenteric base from the ligament of Trietz to the cecum. However, caution must be taken when interpreting a normally located cecum because in 5–20% of cases, malrotation of the small bowel may be associated with a normal positioned cecum. Ultrasonography can be used to give anatomic details of the mesenteric vessels. The superior mesenteric vein (SMV) is normally to the right of the SMA. If malrotation is suspected, US can be helpful in that if the SMV lies anterior or to the left of the SMA, malrotation may be present. While these findings are inconsistent, US is mainly employed to rule out pyloric stenosis in a child with emesis. Additional imaging with computer tomography (CT), magnetic resonance imaging (MRI), or angiography

has been employed in some cases and relies on abnormal mesenteric vessel orientation.

The operative approach for the management of malrotation with midgut volvulus involves six steps: evisceration, counterclockwise detorsion of the volvulus, division of Ladd's bands, widening of the mesenteric base, relieving duodenal obstruction, and performing an incidental appendectomy.

Bibliography

Filston HC, Kirks DR. Malrotation-the ubiquitous anomaly. *J Pediatr Surg* 1981;16(Suppl 1):614–620.

Synder WH, Chaffin L. Embryology and pathology of the intestinal tract: presentation of 40 cases of malrotation. *Ann Surg* 1954;140:368–380.

Warner BW. Anomalies of intestinal rotation and fixation. In: Mattei P (ed.), *Surgical Directives*. Philadelphia, PA: Lippincott, Williams & Wilkins, 2002, 289–293.

8. **(E)** Congenital abdominal wall defects (omphalocele and gastroschisis) refer to an abnormal process where the abdominal wall fails to develop properly. While some may consider that omphalocele and gastroschisis have a common origin, they are referred to as separate entities. For instance, an omphalocele results from an incomplete fusion of the somatic folds that define the thoracic and abdominal walls at the umbilical ring, whereas gastroschisis is most likely related to improper formation of the umbilical coelom. Nevertheless, both conditions have distinct physical characteristics that enable proper diagnosis. Omphaloceles have a high incidence of associated conditions that can involve the cardiovascular, GI, musculoskeletal, or genitourinary systems as well as chromosomal anomalies (trisomies 13–15, 18, and 21). They are characterized by a central defect that can vary from 4 to 12 cm at the site of the umbilical ring. A translucent membrane sac with an attached umbilical cord covers eviscerated abdominal contents, which can include intestinal loops and the liver.

Gastroschisis is noted by a small defect, which is to the right of the midline with no sac. Additionally, the stomach and small/large intestines maybe eviscerated but not the liver. Management of both of these abdominal wall defects mandates operative intervention to close the abdomen. While the operative options for omphaloceles and gastroschisis differ, one of the most important issues in surgical management for the abdominal wall defect is related to whether to close the abdomen primarily or proceed with a staged silo closure. As a general rule, timing of closure depends on the patient's GA and birthweight, size of the defect, and associated congenital abnormalities (Figs. 34-22 and 34-23).

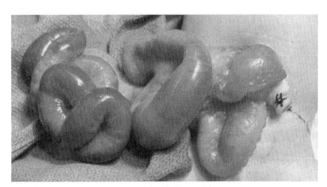

FIG. 34-22   Infant with gastroschisis.

Bibliography

Cooney DR. Defects of the abdominal wall. In: O'Neil JA Jr, Rowe MI, Grosfeld JL, Fonkalsrud EW, Coran AG (eds.), *Pediatric Surgery*, 5th ed. St. Louis, MO: Mosby-Year Book, 1998, 1045–1069.

Strovoff MA, Teague WG. Omphalocele and gastroschisis. In: Ziegler MM, Azizkhan RG, Weber TR (eds.), *Operative Pediatric Surgery*. New York, NY: McGraw-Hill, 2003, 525–536.

9. **(B)** The spectrum of congenital lung and diaphragm ailments amenable to surgical therapy are diverse. Congenital lung anomalies include lobar empysema, cystic adenomatoid malformation, bronchopulmonary sequestration, and bronchogenic cysts. Congenital diaphragm disorders consist of eventration and diaphragmatic hernia. While prenatal sonography has aided in diagnosing these disorders, there exists a high false negative rate of detection. For example, congenital diaphragmatic hernia (CDH), which results from the incomplete closure of the pleuroperitoneal reflection (forms the diaphragm by the 10th week of conception), can be detected between the 16th and 24th weeks of gestation. The most frequent *in utero* false negative factor in infants with CDH are US prior to 16 weeks GA, failure to document stomach position, failure to obtain a four-chamber view of the heart, and failure to appreciate mediastinal abnormalities. Moreover, it is important to pay careful attention to anatomic abnormalities of the GI tract and intrathoracic cavity in the appropriate GA infant in order to increase the sensitivity of US in these congenital disorders. The other pathology associated with the diaphragm is eventration. In eventration of the diaphragm, the diaphragm is an attenuated, thin amuscular sheet dividing the thoracic and abdominal cavities. The central portion of the diaphragm is most affected and allows the abdominal contents to push the diaphragm upward. Eventration is the result of either a congenital or acquired origin. While the congenital form is rare, the acquired form is due to injury to the phrenic nerve during intrathoracic surgery or trauma during birth. Treatment of choice is plication of the eventrated diaphragm. Obara and colleagues evaluated the histologic changes affecting the lung tissue in infants/children with diaphragmatic eventration. Biopsies showed atelectasis and pneumonia, which became increasingly diffuse and severe with age. They concluded that in order to reduce the pathologic changes of the lung, early surgical plication should be performed in patients if respiratory and digestive symptoms develop.

Congenital lobar emphysema (CLE) is abnormal inflammation of an anatomically normal lung. Babies are usually asymptomatic at birth but develop respiratory distress and tachypnea within the first few days of life. Treatment of choice for CLE is lobectomy of the afflicted lung. Brochopulmonary sequestration (BPS) refers to nonfunctioning lung tissue, which does not communicate with the normal tracheobronchial tree, and contains its own anomalous blood supply. Two types of sequestration exist: extralobar and intralobar. If the lung mass has its own pleural covering, then an extralobar pulmonary defect exists. A sequestrum that lies within the normal lung parenchyma is classified as an intralobar defect. Once the diagnosis has been established, surgical resection is mandated. It is important to establish blood supply, since vascular supply differs to these lesions. The most common origin of the arterial supply is the thoracic aorta. Venous drainage to these lesions is usually to the azygous veins for extralobar pathology and to the pulmonary veins for intralobar sequestrations. Congenital cystic adenomatoid malformation (CCAM) refers to intercommunicating

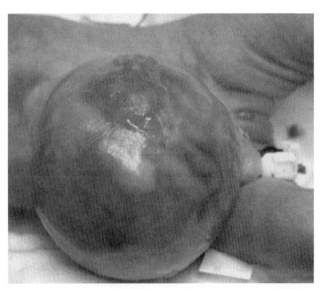

FIG. 34-23   Infant with a giant omphalocele (>10 cm).

cysts within the lung that develop as a consequence to increases/overgrowth of the terminal bronchioles in one lobe of the lung. Surgical excision is the management of CCAMs. There is some question as to whether to proceed with surgery in asymptomatic patient with a CCAM. Yet when definitive diagnosis is confirmed, studies suggest that surgical intervention in the asymptomatic infant is associated with shorter length of stay, fewer complications, and decreased medical cost as compared with intervening after symptoms have developed. Additionally is the rare risk of malignant degeneration with CCAM. Bronchogenic cysts (BC) originate form the foregut as do most congenital lung anomalies. BC are mucous-filled cysts which arise from the tracheobronchial tree. Clinical presentation of BC varies from respiratory distress at birth to infection (secondary to abnormal drainage of secretions) later in life. Main symptoms in infants and children are due to intrathoracic compression while cough, infection, and hemoptysis occur later in adulthood. Treatment involves excision of the cyst by segmentectomy or lobectomy. Asymptomatic cases warrant excision due to the high risk of complications including infection and malignant degeneration.

In the chest radiograph shown, typical findings in left-sided posterolateral CDH include air- or fluid-filled loops of the bowel in the left hemithorax and shift of the cardiac silhouette to the right.

Bibliography

Black TL. Pulmonary sequestration and congenital cystic adenomatoid malformations. In: Ziegler MM, Azizkhan RG, Weber TR (eds.), *Operative Pediatric Surgery*. New York, NY: McGraw-Hill, 2003, 445–454.

Lewis DA, Reikert C, Bowerman R, Hirschl RB. Prenatal ultrasonography frequently fails to diagnose congenital diaphragmatic hernia. *J Pediatr Surg* 1997;32(2):352–356.

MacKenzie TC, Flake AW. Congenital lung anomalies. In: Mattei P (ed.), *Surgical Directives Pediatric Surgery*. Philadelphia, PA: Lippincott, Williams & Wilkins, 2002, 481–484.

Marshall KW, Blane CE, Teitelbaum DH, van Leeuwen K. Congenital cystic adenomatoid malformation: impact of prenatal diagnosis and changing strategies in the treatment of the asymptomatic patient. *Am J Roentgenol* 2000;175(6):1551–1554.

Obara H, Hoshina H, Iwai S, Ito H, Hisano K. Eventration of the diaphragm in infants and children. *Acta Paediatr Scand* 1987;76(4):654–658.

Ribet ME, Copin MC, Gosselin BH. Bronchogenic cysts of the lung. *Ann Thorac Surg* 1996;61:1636–1640.

10. **(E)** Infantile hypertrophic pyloric stenosis (IHPS) is one of the most common surgical conditions of infancy. It occurs in 1–3 of every 1000 live births.

Boys are affected four times more often than girls. Pathogenesis involves pyloric muscle fiber hypertrophy causing a mechanical obstruction of the gastric outlet. The etiology of HPS remains elusive but family history, sex, birth order, and maternal feeding patterns all have been implicated. Various theories support the pathophysiology of HPS including compensatory work hypertrophy, neurodegeneration/immaturity, and abnormal endocrine signals. Some reports also link early erythromycin exposure and HPS. It is hypothesized that erythromycin interacts with motilin receptors inducing pyloric contractions that result in hypertrophy.

IHPS most commonly develops from 2 to 12 weeks (peak incidence of 3–6 weeks) of age in an otherwise healthy infant who feeds normally at birth. A pattern of vomiting ensues which varies but classically progresses to projectile nonbilious emesis. Diagnosis of HPS is primarily made by history and physical. Physical examination findings include peristaltic waves in the epigastric area and the presence of a palpable mass in the upper abdomen (Figs. 34-24 and 34-25). The absence of these findings with a strong history of HPS should prompt an US or an UGI contrast study. US criteria include a pyloric muscle thickness >4 mm, pyloric muscle diameter >14 mm, and a channel length >17 mm, but are adjusted by age. If US is nondiagnostic, an UGI contrast study can aid in ruling out reflux, malrotation, or obstruction. UGI finding consistent with HPS include a "string" sign, a "double track" sign, or "shoulders" at the proximal end of the pyloris. When

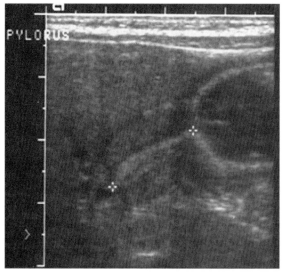

FIG. 34-24 Longitudinal sonogram of the pyloris in an infant with a surgically proven hypertrophic pyloric stenosis. Of importance are the thickened circular muscle, elongated pylorus, and narrowed pyloric channel.

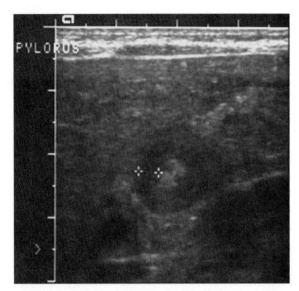

FIG. 34-25 Transverse sonogram demonstrating the target sign and heterogeneous echoic texture of the muscle layer in a patient with hypertrophic pyloric stenosis.

the diagnosis has been confirmed and the child's fluid and electrolyte status has been corrected, operative intervention is undertaken. The Ramstedt pyloromyotomy is the procedure of choice and can be performed via an open or laparoscopic approach.

Bibliography

Cooper WO, Griffen MR, Arbogast P, Hickson GB, Gautam S, Ray WA. Very early exposure to erythromycin and infantile hypertrophic pyloric stenosis. *Arch Pediatr Adolesc Med* 2002;156;647–650.

Harris SE, Cywes R. Laparscopic pyloromyotomy. *Pediatr Endo Innov Techn* 2001;15(5):405–410.

Murphy SG. Hypertrophic pyloric stenosis. In: Mattei P (ed.), *Surgical Directives Pediatric Surgery*. Philadelphia, PA: Lippincott, Williams & Wilkins, 2002, 269–272.

Ohshiro K, Puri P. Pathogenesis of infantile hypertrophic pyloric stenosis: recent progress. *Pediatr Surg Int* 1998;13:243–252.

11. **(A)** Antireflux procedures have become the third most commonly performed operation in pediatric surgery centers. Gastroesophageal reflux disease (GERD) occurs when a defective gastroesophageal junction causes significant symptoms or harm to the patient as a consequence of excessive gastric contents moving into the esophagus. Infant/childhood GERD causes irritability, frequent vomiting, apnea, aspiration, pneumonia, a failure to thrive, and even some cases of SIDS. The predominant mechanism of GERD is transient lower esophageal sphincter (LES) relaxation. The LES provides an antireflux barrier over an area of 3–7 cm. Transient relaxation of the LES leaves the distal esophagus open to episodic reflux of gastric contents. Additional factors that contribute to GERD include presence of hiatus hernia, esophageal dysmotility, delayed gastric emptying, elevated intraabdominal pressure, central nervous system (CNS) impairment, and the presence of a feeding gastrostomy tube. Management of GERD is initially approach nonoperatively. This usually includes upright positioning, small volume feeds or continuous tube feeds, thickened formula, prokinetic medication, and H2 antagonists/proton-pump inhibitors. The majority of neurologically intact children will respond to medical therapy.

When medical therapy fails to control GERD symptoms or complications arise (strictures, chronic pulmonary disease, worsening reactive airway disease, or failure to thrive), surgery is indicated. The diagnostic preoperative workup should include a contrast swallow to rule out anatomic abnormalities and obstruction of the esophagus, stomach, and duodenum and a 24-h pH monitoring to quantitate the frequency and duration of acid reflux over time. An esophagogastroduodenoscopy (EGD)/biopsy may be valuable in some cases for visualizing mucosal areas of injury [erosive esophagitis, peptic ulceration, stricture, active *Helicobacter pylori* infection, food intolerance (gluten enetropathy), and Barrett's disease] due to GERD. Other useful modalities are measuring gastric emptying rate, technetium labeled milk scan, and surface gastrography.

Surgery for GERD is aimed toward reestablishing the antireflux barrier while not obstructing food passage. The Nissen fundoplication (360° wrap) is most commonly used to increase pressure in the lower esophagus. Other procedures such as a Toupet (270° posterior wrap) and a Thal (180° anterior wrap) are also used to recreate the antireflux barrier. The approach to the fundoplication can be via the open or laparoscopic technique. Complications that develop after antireflux surgery include pneumonia, wound infection, small bowel obstruction, wrap disruption, dysphagia, hiatal hernia, gas bloat syndrome, vagus nerve injury, and chronic retching/vomiting.

Bibliography

Jolley SG. Gastroesophageal reflux disease. In: Ziegler MM, Azizkhan RG, Weber TR (eds.), *Operative Pediatric Surgery*. New York, NY: McGraw-Hill, 2003, 373–394.

Richards C, Spitz L. Gastroesophageal reflux disease. In: Mattei P (ed.), *Surgical Directives Pediatric Surgery*. Philadelphia, PA: Lippincott William & Wilkins, 2002, 245–249.

12. **(D)** Intussusception generally refers to a part of bowel invaginating into an adjacent section of bowel causing

intestinal obstruction and venous compression, which ultimately results in venous then arterial insufficiency and necrosis if left untreated. The condition is a common abdominal emergency between 3 months and 2 years of age with a peak incidence between 6 and 9 months. While most cases are idiopathic with a lead point due to an enlarged Peyer's patch (reported due to a viral infection), 5% are due to a polyp, Meckel's diverticulum (MD), duplication cyst, or tumor. The most common site of occurrence is the ileocecal junction.

Clinically a history of crampy, intermittent abdominal pain in an otherwise healthy infant should prompt the diagnosis of intussusception. A classical triad of acute abdominal pain, currant jelly stools, and a palpable abdominal mass is present in less than 50% of children with intussusception. Additionally intussusception may manifest solely with diarrhea or changes in mentation. Because of its many presentations, intussusception may avoid detection. Studies show that delay in diagnosis of greater than 12 h from initial medical contact is associated with increased mortality. Reports also suggest that management of intussusception outside tertiary centers is not uniform or standardized, further emphasizing the need to refer the patient to an appropriate pediatric hospital.

While intussusception may not be ruled out with clinical examination, radiography should be the next step in management if the patient is stable. Plain abdominal radiographs aid in excluding intussusception when clinical suspicion is low by visualizing the right colon filled with air or stool, confirming the diagnosis (right upper quadrant mass, target sign, or the meniscus sign), and excluding perforation or intestinal obstruction in cases of intussusception. In this particular case where clinical suspicion is high for intussusception, obtaining an abdominal radiograph may delay transfer/treatment and some investigators believe that it is not necessary to perform plain x-rays if symptoms are of short duration (<8 h).

When diagnostic confirmation is needed, barium enema (coiled spring sign) has been the standard of reference for intussusception. Another modality that has gained popularity is US, but critics note US is highly dependent on operator skill level. Nevertheless, once the diagnosis is made, IV fluids should be started and radiologic reduction with hydrostatic (fluid) or pneumatic (air) be performed. Nonoperative treatment of intussusception is possible in approximately 80% of cases. In patients who fail nonoperative reduction, surgery is mandated. Chung and colleagues found that risk factors leading

to surgical reduction were long standing duration of illness (>12 h); positive clinical triad of vomiting, colicky abdominal pain, and bloody stools; positive pathologic lead point; and radiologic finding of bowel obstruction. Generally, the surgical procedure is followed by making a transverse right lower quadrant incision and manually reducing the intussusception with retrograde milking of the intussuscepiens. Bowel resection is necessary when the intussusception cannot be reduced or bowel showing evidence of gangrene or perforation. Complications include the possibility of recurrence of intussusception (5%) and this is usually seen within 24 h of surgical intervention.

Bibliography

MacDonald IA, Beattie TF. Intussusception presenting to a paediatric accident and emergency department. *J Accid Emerg Med* 1995;12(3):182–186.

Calder FR, Tan S, Kitteringham L, Dykes EH. Patterns of management of intussusception outside tertiary centers. *J Pediatr Surg* 2001;36(2):212–315.

Daneman A, Alton DJ. Intussusception: issues and controversies related to diagnosis and reduction. *Radiol Clin North Am* 1996;34:743–756.

Chung JL, Kong MS, Lin JN, Wang KL, Lou CC, Wong HF. Intussusception in infants and children:risk factors leading to surgical resection. *J Formos Med Assoc* 1994;93(6): 481–485.

Whalen TV. Intussusception. In: Mattei P (ed.), *Surgical Directives Pediatric Surgery*. Philadelphia, PA: Lippincott, Williams & Wilkins, 2002, 331–334.

13. **(B)** Figure 34-3 shows a Meckel's diverticulum (MD). A positive ^{99m}Tc Meckel's scan (Fig. 34-4) completed prior to surgery confirms the presence of a MD as ectopic tissue present in the lower abdomen. MD is the most common congenital abnormality of the small intestine (2% of population) and is additionally the most common vitelline duct (VD) abnormality. The VD or omphalomesenteric duct is the *in utero* connection between the fetal gut and the yolk sac, which involutes during the seventh to eighth week of gestation. Most MDs are found along the antimesenteric border of the ileum within 100 cm of the ileocecal junction. The blood supply originates from the aorta from paired vitelline arteries, the right vitelline artery persists as the superior mesenteric artery and the left involutes.

The majority of MDs are asymptomatic and found incidentally, but may cause complications in children such as inflammation, bleeding, intestinal obstruction, perforation, volvulus, and intussusception. The diagnosis of a symptomatic MD may be difficult and more than 75% of symptomatic MDs occur in children younger than 10 years of age. Moreover children less than 2 years represent 50% of symptomatic MDs.

Ectopic mucosa (gastric mucosal tissue is the most prevalent) within the diverticulum is often the causative factor in 50% to 80% of symptomatic patients. Bleeding due to mucosal irritation in cases of MD represents the most common cause of significant lower GI hemorrhage in children. A ^{99m}Tc (technetium pertechnetate) Meckel's scan can be used to detect ectopic gastric mucosa and if negative, laparoscopy may be needed for diagnostic and therapeutic means of managing an MD. Intestinal obstruction due to MD may occur and is caused by the diverticulum itself or by fibrous bands that develop between the MD and the umbilicus that allow an extrinsic bowel obstruction to occur. Surgical intervention is needed to prevent late complications of strangulation and infarction of bowel. Inflammation of an MD is a condition that presents very similar to appendicitis. Yet inflammation of the diverticulum presents with a shifting tenderness as well as a shorter time course for development of diffuse peritonitis. Nevertheless, an operation for a suspected appendicitis would reveal a normal appendix and on further exploration an inflamed diverticulum in cases of Meckel's diverticulitis. The decision to perform a diverticulectomy versus a bowel resection for Meckel's diverticulitis is based on the following intraoperative factors: a wide-based diverticulum or a densely inflamed, adherent ileum. Completing an incidental appendectomy concludes the case.

The definitive treatment strategy of an asymptomatic MD is controversial. Some surgeons resect an asymptomatic diverticulum based on the presence of ectopic mucosa, male gender, preadolescent age, or a narrow base; since these factors have higher risks of complications. More importantly, however, are the indications for not removing an incidental MD. These would include patients undergoing surgery for life-threatening emergencies, elective procedures where the bowel is not opened, and in the presence of peritonitis.

Other VD remnants present as a myriad of umbilical abnormalities such as ectopic intestinal mucosa at the umbilicus, an umbilical sinus, subumbilical enteric cyst, an intrabdominal cyst in the midportion of the obliterated VD, and an umbilical-intestinal fistula. A challenge in diagnosing these entities is differentiating umbilical granuloma and urachal remnants from VD remnants. Umbilical granuloma is a local collection of granulation tissue at the umbilicus that persists after cord separation. Treatment is with topical application of silver nitrate. Failure to resolve should raise the diagnosis of VD remnant. Urachal remnants, such as a urachal fistula, can usually be suspected by urinary drainage at the umbilicus. A contrast study through sinus tract can aid in differentiating these abnormalities. The overall treatment of VD remnants is surgical excision.

Bibliography

Amoury RA, Synder CL. Meckel's diverticulum. In: O'Neil JA Jr, Rowe MI, Grosfeld JL, Fonkalsrud EW, Coran AG (eds.), *Pediatric Surgery*, 5th ed. St. Louis, MO: Mosby-Year Book, 1998, 1173–1184.

Emil SGS, Laberge JM. Meckel's diverticulum. In: Mattei P (ed.), *Surgical Directives Pediatric Surgery*. Philadelphia, PA: Lippincott, Williams & Wilkins, 2002, 327–330.

Onen A, Cigdem MK, Ozturk H, Otcu S, Dokucu AI. When to resect and when not to resect an asymptomatic Meckel's diverticulum: an ongoing challenge. *Pediatr Surg Int* 2003;19:57–61.

14. **(C)** Intraabdominal cysts are rare, usually benign entities, which can be detected prenatally, and be found in infants and children. A variety of different abdominal cystic masses occur in the fetus and the older child. Particular attention should be paid when the cyst size causes abnormal *in utero* organ development or when a large cystic mass interferes with respiratory or bowel function. Consequently, history, physical examination, or specific laboratory findings may not reveal the cystic abnormality and radiologic evaluation is usually mandated to reveal the abnormality. The modality used to demonstrate cystic elements of masses are abdominal US or CT scan.

Specifically, mesenteric/omental cysts are lymph-filled lesions that present in one-third cases in children under 10 years of age. While most are considered congenital in origin, these cysts may arise from trauma, infection, or neoplasm. Patterns of presentation relate to the size and location with most children presenting with abdominal distension and pain. Treatment of choice for these lesions consists of complete surgical excision.

Cystic teratomas of the abdomen are mainly retroperitoneal structures that most often contain large, chunky calcifications on imaging studies. Ovarian cysts (OC) may be difficult to differentiate from intestinal duplication cysts and mesenteric/omental cysts. Most OCs antenatally diagnosed resolve spontaneously. They most likely arise as a result of physiologic ovarian stimulation due to transplacental passage of maternal/placental hormones. Intervention is advocated for infants past 3–4 months with simple cysts larger than 5 cm due to concern for torsion. Because intestinal duplication cysts have characteristics similar to the intestine (thick, smooth, muscular wall), imaging studies would reveal a multilayered wall. A majority of choledochal cysts (CC) appear by the first decade of life and present with asymptomatic jaundice.

Bibliography

Appelbaum H. Abdominal cysts. In: Ziegler MM, Azizkhan RG, Weber TR (eds.), *Operative Pediatric Surgery*. New York, NY: McGraw-Hill, 2003, 713–718.

Beahrs OM, Judd ES Jr, Dockerty MD. Chylous cysts of the abdomen. *Surg Clin North Am* 1950;30:1081–1096.

Katz AL. Benign gynecologic disorders. In: Mattei P (ed.), *Surgical Directives Pediatric Surgery*. Philadelphia, PA: Lippincott, Williams & Wilkins, 2002, 765–770.

15. **(B)** and **(D)** Alimentary tract duplications are characterized as cystic/tubular structures within the GI tract that are lined by normal GI mucosa and contain intestinal smooth muscle walls. Duplications share a common blood supply, which is on the mesenteric side of the bowel [MD (VD remnant)-antimesenteric aspect]. The most common types of duplications, respectively, are ileal, esophageal, and colonic. The epithelium present may not be the same as the GI tract. The most common ectopic epithelium (20–25% of cases) lining the duplication are gastric and pancreatic. Since these anomalies can occur anywhere along the GI tract, chief complaints depend on age of the patient, type of mucosal lining, duration of disease, location and size of the duplication, and presence of complications such as obstruction, peptic ulcer, or perforation. A common feature, however, is the presence of an abdominal mass found on physical or radiologic evaluation. Ultrasonography is the diagnostic test of choice; a finding of an echogenic inner mucosal layer and a hypoechoic outer mucosal layer is suggestive of the pathology. Contrast studies, CT, and MRI may also be used in the workup in intestinal duplication. Surgical excision is the ideal treatment, but internal drainage, mucosal stripping, and staged excision are also options that may be used when complete excision is not possible. Malignant transformation has been reported in duplications typically after 30 years of age. Additionally, associated anomalies such as VACTERL, spina bifida, GU abnormalities, and imperforate anus can occur and are more commonly seen with colonic and rectal duplications.

Bibliography

Bond SJ, Groff DB. Gastrointestinal duplications. In: O'Neil JA Jr, Rowe MI, Grosfeld JL, Fonkalsrud EW, Coran AG (eds.), *Pediatric Surgery*, 5th ed. St. Louis, MO: Mosby-Year Book, 1998, 1257–1281.

Hebra A. Alimentary tract duplication. In: Mattei P (ed.), *Surgical Directives Pediatric Surgery*. Philadelphia, PA: Lippincott, Williams & Wilkins, 2002, 281–288.

16. **I (C), II (F), III (D), IV (A), V (G), VI (B), VII (E)** GI polyps in children are common and frequently present with painless rectal bleeding. Most GI polyps in children are juvenile polyps. These are isolated, benign lesions that do not predispose a child to malignant neoplasia; however, a child who presents with GI polyps and a strong family history of early colon cancer should be evaluated for a genetic polyposis disorder.

Juvenile polyps account for nearly 90% of colorectal polyps in children. Most appear during the first decade of life with asymptomatic hematochezia. Other less common presentations include abdominal pain, rectal polyp prolapse, diarrhea, and tenesmus. While the area of greatest predominance is the rectosigmoid area, the proximal colon is implicated in 25% of cases. Because of the wide possible distribution of juvenile polyps throughout the colon, the preferred method for diagnosis and treatment is complete colonoscopy with polypectomy. It is important to note that the discovery of five or more polyps may denote a polyposis syndrome; therefore the total number and pathology of each polyp must be evaluated. Neoplastic changes are rare and after removal of isolated polyps, no further treatment is usually necessary (unless rectal bleeding persists).

In contrast to juvenile polyps, children with juvenile polyposis (JP) show larger polyp loads varying in number from 10 to 200. JP is an autosomal dominant condition defined by hamartomatous polyps throughout the GI tract. These individuals tend to have a higher risk of carcinoma (17%) at an early age (mean age 35.5 years) and usually present with rectal bleeding, anemia, protein-losing enteropathy, malnutrition, and/or rectal prolapse. Because of anemia (chronic blood loss) and nutritional deficiencies (hypoproteinemia and electrolyte imbalances), multiple blood transfusions and parenteral nutrition are used to promote weight gain and growth. Surgical management is often individualized because of the number of polyps and location is variable. Nevertheless, treatment is based on removing the polyps via endoscopic techniques along with operative explorations with multiple enterotomies with polypectomy. Some also recommend resection of the terminal ileum and colon with ileal-rectal anastomosis to remove a large percentage of polyps and thus minimizing chronic blood loss and nutritional deficiencies. Recently, genetic analysis has revealed inactivating germline mutation in Smad4 and BMPR 1A genes to be responsible for JP. Defects in these genes promote unopposed growth stimulation and polyp formation by disturbing the transforming growth factor beta (TGF-β) pathway.

Multiple pedunculated GI hamartomatous polyps along with mucocutaneous pigmentation characterize PJS. PJS is an autosomal dominant inherited disease that carries a relatively slight increase in the neoplastic potential (adenomatous changes within the polyps) of GI lesions and approximately 48% of individuals develop extraintestinal cancers (breast, gonads, and pancreatobiliary). Specifically, PJS polyps are more common in the small intestine, usually as clusters within the jejunum/ileum. Melanotic spots occur on the lips, circumorally, or on the buccal mucosa. Symptoms in a child with PJS are related to episodes of small bowel obstruction secondary to intermittent SB/ileocolic intussusception and present with colicky abdominal pain and nausea/vomiting. Less common presentations include rectal bleeding, hematochezia, and polyp prolapse. Polyps larger than 0.5 mm should be removed and surgical treatment revolves around persistent GI obstruction and bleeding. Intestinal resection should be reserved for clusters of polyps within a short segment of bowel and irreducible intussusception. Cancer surveillance consists of upper/lower endoscopy and extraintestinal organ examination (abdominal US, breast examination, pelvic or testicular examination). Germline mutations in the STK11/LKB1 tumor suppressor gene account for 70% of individuals with PJS. The STK11/LBK1 protein is a serine-threonine kinase 11 that carries out apoptosis: inability to carry out this function results in unregulated cell growth.

FAP is the most common polyposis syndrome in childhood with approximately 50% of afflicted children presenting by the age of 16. Initial presentation of FAP is rectal bleeding or abdominal pain. Diagnosis is confirmed by the presence of hundreds to thousands of colonic adenomas. The 5q deletion in the adenomatous polyposis coli (APC) tumor suppressor gene is responsible for FAP. APC regulates β-catenin, a protein involved in the stimulation of cell growth. Mutational inactivation of APC leads to accumulation of β-catenin, cell proliferation, and tumor formation. Associated lifetime risk of colorectal malignancy in FAP is 100%, therefore, surgery is recommended prior to onset of malignant dysplasia. Options include total protocolectomy with permanent ileostomy, subtotal colectomy with ileorectal anastomosis, and protocolectomy with ileoanal pull-through. Moreover, it is important to note that following surgery, which eliminates the potential for colon cancer, the FAP child will continue to require surveillance for other malignancies (periampullary, thyroid, and adrenocortical carcinomas). Of note, variations of FAP exist that show specific extracolonic manifestations. Gardner's syndrome in addition to colonic adenomas shows epidermoid skin cysts, osteoid tumors, and desmoid tumors. Turcot's syndrome (brain tumor polyposis syndrome) is characterized by colonic adenomas and brain tumors (medulloblastomas, gliomas, and ependymomas).

HNPCC is the most common genetic disorder that leads to colorectal cancer in adults. Germline defects in DNA mismatch repair genes (repair errors in DNA sequences during replication) leads to this disorder. While this syndrome is exclusively a disease of adulthood, children as young as 6 years with colon cancer and HNPCC have been reported.

CCS is a nonfamilial syndrome resulting in GI polyposis and epidermal changes. GI polyps are hamartomas with intervening mucosal proliferation that results in malabsorption and protein-losing enteropathy. Epidermal characteristics include alopecia, nail plate dystrophy (onychodystrophy), and hyperpigmentation. The etiology of CCS is limited and patterns of inheritance have not been identified. An infant with JP who suffers from alopecia, clubbing, nail dystrophy, and hypoproteinemia has been termed as the infantile equivalent of CCS seen in adults.

Cowden's syndrome is characterized by GI polyps (which may be juvenile polyps, ganglioneuromas, or adenomas), mucocutaneous lesions, malignancy of the thyroid and breast, and genitourinary abnormalities with uterine leiomyomas. The clinical features of this rare autosomal syndrome present by 20 years of age. Germline mutations in PTEN gene make up for 80% of cases and the gene encodes for a lipid/protein phosphatase involved in apoptosis.

Bibliography

Daniel ES, Ludwig SL, Lewin KJ. The Cronkite-Canada Syndrome. An analysis of clinical and pathologic features and therapy in 55 patients. *Medicine* (Baltimore) 1982; 61(5):293–309.

Dillion PA. Gastrointestinal polyps. In: Ziegler MM, Azizkhan RG, Weber TR (eds.), *Operative Pediatric Surgery*. New York, NY: McGraw-Hill, 2003, 729–733.

Erdman SH, Barnard JA. Gastrointestinal polyps and polyposis syndromes in children. *Curr Opin Pediatr* 2002;14(5);576–582.

Lelli JL Jr, Coran AG. In: O'Neil JA Jr, Rowe MI, Grosfeld JL, Fonkalsrud EW, Coran AG (eds.), *Pediatric Surgery*, 5th ed. St. Louis, MO: Mosby-Year Book, 1998, 1283–1296.

Ruymann FB. Juvenile polyps with cachexia. Report of an infant and comparison with Cronkite-Canada syndrome in adults. *Gastroenterology* 1969;57(4):431–438.

17. **(B)** Jaundice in the newborn period is a relatively common occurrence in infants. For many newborn infants, jaundice may represent a manifestation of an ongoing adaptation to the extrauterine environment.

Nevertheless, it cannot be automatically assumed to be a mild or physiologic condition. Generally jaundice refers to an elevated blood concentration of bilirubin. Hyperbilirubinemia can be due to indirect or accumulation of unconjugated, lipid soluble bilirubin pigment in the serum or be due to direct bilirubin or conjugated, water soluble form. When the serum concentration of conjugated bilirubin and/or bile salts is elevated, it denotes a pathologic state (cholestasis) of reduced bile flow. While initial workup for the jaundiced infant is medically oriented, surgeons should be aware of the wide differential diagnosis of cholestatic jaundice and be cognizant of the surgically treated causes of cholestasis (biliary atresia, choledochocysts, congenital anomalies of the biliary tree, and perforation of the common bile duct). Cholestasis may develop due to a variety of insults. These include drugs (flecanide), parenteral nutrition (most common cause in the NICU), ECMO, infectious agents (e.g., bacterial sepsis, viral causes, and toxoplasmosis), inherited/metabolic causes, endocrine abnormalities, and chromosomal aberrations (trisomies 18 and 21).

For example, a lipid metabolic disorder such as Niemann-Pick's disease (NPD) (sphingomyelinase deficiency) can present with neonatal cholestasis. NPD is a heterogeneous group of lysosomal lipid storage diseases. Patients afflicted with NPD can present with neonatal cholestasis, hepatosplenomegaly, failure to thrive, and death between 3 and 9 months. Two metabolic classification groups exist: NP types A/B, which are primarily sphingomyelinase deficiencies, and type C, which refers to alterations of trafficking of endocytosed cholesterol. While liver pathology is unknown, histology resembles neonatal hepatitis. As the disease progresses, hepatic lobules become progressively distended with portal cholestasis.

CF may be confused with inspissated bile syndrome or ductal atresia and causes neonatal cholestasis. CF is most commonly caused by a mutation which results in deletion of phenylalanine at position 508 (delta F508 mutation). The gene product is cystic fibrosis transmembrane regulator (CFTR) and mutation in the protein results in the impaired ability of CFTR to increase chloride channel activity that leads to the paucity of water in mucous secretions.

α1AT deficiency results in neonatal cholestasis due to hepatocellular and bile duct injury. α1AT deficiency is the most common genetic cause of liver disease in children. α1AT, a member of the serine proteinase inhibitor superfamily, is the principle blood borne inhibitor of destructive neutrophil proteases which include elastase, cathepsin G, and proteinase 3. Most α1AT is synthesized in the liver where it translocates to the endoplasmic reticulum (ER).

When α1AT associates with a binding protein, it can fold into its native conformation and traverse the secretory pathway. Mutations in the gene responsible for α1AT result in misfolded molecules, which accumulate in the liver and cause hepatocyte injury due to resultant release of lysosomal enzymes and cause ductular proliferation and luminal bile plugging.

Endocrine diseases are frequently associated with liver abnormalities as a result of the important role of hormonal influence in normal hepatobiliary function in the infant. As a consequence, primary endocrinopathies such as hypothyroidism or panhypopituitarism can cause cholestasis.

On the other hand, ornithine transcarbamylase is a mitochondrial enzyme that is the most common urea cycle defect. The enzyme is responsible for converting ornithine and carbamoyl phosphate to citrulline and absence of the protein results in the clinical symptoms of feeding difficulties, lethargy, and respiratory distress. Biochemical analyses reveal hyperammonia, increased levels of glutamine and alanine, and decreased levels of citrulline. While hepatic disease is a rare manifestation in urea cycle enzyme defects, a hepatitic rather than a cholestatic pattern of liver dysfunction has been observed with this metabolic disorder.

Bibliography

Ellaway CJ, Silinik M, Cowell CT, Gaskin KJ, Kamath KR, Dorney S, Donaghue KC. Cholestatic jaundice and congenital hypopituitarism. *J Paediatr Child Health* 1995; 31(1):51–53.

Felber S, Sinatra F. Systemic disorders associated with neonatal cholestasis. *Semin Liver Dis* 1987;7(2):108–118.

Gordon N. Ornithine transcarbamylase deficiency: a urea cycle defect. *Eur J Paediatr Neurol* 2003;7:115–121.

Jevon GP, Dimmick JE. Histopathologic approach to metabolic liver disease: part 1. *Pediatr Dev Pathol* 1998;1(3): 179–199.

Pohl JF, Balistreri WF. Neonatal jaundice. In: Mattei P (ed.), *Surgical Directives Pediatric Surgery.* Philadelphia, PA: Lippincott Willliams & Wilkins, 2002, 536–541.

Ratjen F, Doring G. Cystic fibrosis. *Lancet* 2003;361:681–689.

Vanier MT. Prenatal diagnosis of Niemann-Pick diseases types A, B, and C. *Prenat Diagn* 2002;22:630–632.

18. **(E)** Persistence of neonatal jaundice beyond 2 weeks of age or once biochemical tests have confirmed pathologic jaundice (conjugated bilirubin greater than 2 mg/dL or over 15% of the total bilirubin concentration) warrants radiologic evaluation. US is usually the first modality used to evaluate pathologic jaundice. US can examine the liver, bile ducts, gall bladder, pancreas, spleen, and portal vein. In BA, US may show

hepatomegaly and increasing echogenicity, a small or absent gall bladder, and nonvisible biliary ducts. The presence of polyspenia also supports the diagnosis. CC at US appear as simple cysts (I, II, and III) in the region of the gall bladder. The presence of a dilated extrahepatic biliary tree in conjunction with a cyst highly suggests this pathology. Depending on the type of choledochal cyst, other intrahepatic cysts may be shown on US. Cholithiasis and choledocholithiasis in the newborn period is rare and if suspected on US, stones appear as freely movable, bright echoic shadowing foci within the gall bladder lumen while bright echoic structures within the biliary ducts is usually associated with ductal dilatation (the common bile duct should measure less than 1 mm in neonates, less than 2 mm in infants up to 1-year-old, less than 4 mm in older children, and less than 7 mm in adolescents). In most cases of biliary dyskinesia, the US is normal. Suspected biliary fistulas should be evaluated in patients who have sustained hepatic injury or undergone recent hepatobiliary surgery. An US may show free intraperitoneal fluid and subsequent paracentesis would reveal biliary fluid.

If US is unable to exclude hepatobiliary pathology, a nuclear hepatobiliary scan (HIDA scan) should be the next imaging test for studying the hepatic parenchyma and associated biliary tree. In BA, particularly early, the uptake of the nucleotide is rapid but excretion into the bowel is absent. Moreover, failure to show gut excretion is nondiagnostic and HIDA is unable to distinguish BA versus other causes of cholestasis. Cholangiography would be the next study to investigate exact areas in question; demonstration of duodenal contrast and intrahepatic ducts would exclude BA. In CC, HIDA and endoscopic retrograde cholangiography (ERCP) can be used after US in order to gain additional information concerning biliary anatomy. ERCP has the advantage of delineating biliary and pancreatic duct definition and may aid in preoperative decision making.

In cases of suspected choledocholithiasis, the most favorable treatment in children remains controversial. Options include an open cholecystectomy with simultaneous common bile duct (CBD) exploration, laparoscopic cholecystectomy with preoperative/postoperative ERCP with sphincterotomy and stone removal, or laparoscopic cholecystectomy and laparoscopic removal of CBD stones. Some consider the complication rate for pediatric ERCP higher and recommend strict selection criteria be done prior to subjecting a pediatric patient to ERCP, especially biliary lithiasis.

The advent of cholecystokinin (CCK)-HIDA has made the diagnosis of biliary dyskinesia more accurately. Using CCK (peptide hormone produced by the I cells of duodenum and upper jejunum that acts on the gall bladder wall musculature) to stimulate the gall bladder measures the degree of emptying (ejection fraction). An ejection fraction of <35% denotes biliary dyskinesia. Cholecystectomy should be considered in children with chronic upper abdominal pain and delayed ejection fraction on CCK-HIDA scintigraphy.

Hepatic biliary scanning (HIDA) is a sensitive test for documenting the presence or absence of biliary leaks (fistulas) because the tracer is concentrated and excreted into the biliary ductal system. Because it cannot pinpoint injuries to the extrahepatic ducts, cholangiography would be employed to detect exact injuries.

In this case, US fails to show a detectable sonographic abnormality yet the HIDA scan demonstrates inability to visualize radiolabelled iminodiacetic acid derivative into the small intestine after 19 h. The scan suggests a diagnosis of BA.

Bibliography

Al-Homaidhi HS, Sukerek H, Klein M, Tolia V. Biliary dyskinesia in children. *Pediatr Surg Int* 2002;18:357–360.

Gubernick JA, Rosenberg HK, Iiaslan H, Kessler A. US approach to jaundice in infants and children. *Radiograph* 2000;20:173–195.

Prasil P, Laberge JM, Barkun A, Flageole H. Endoscopic retrograde cholangiopancreatography in children: a surgeon's perpective. *J Pediatr Surg* 2001;36(5):733–735.

19. **(C)** BA is characterized by an extraobliteration or discontinuation of the biliary system that results in obstruction of bile flow. Infants appear well and active presenting with jaundice, clay colored stools, and hepatomegaly. Conjugated levels of bilirubin are elevated and greater than 15% of the total bilirubin. Early diagnosis is essential in BA because successful treatment depends on critical timing of surgical biliary reconstruction. Treatment options for BA are limited to surgery and include hepaticoportoenterostomy (Kasai procedure) or liver transplantation, both of which have been shown to provide long-term success for BA. The results for the Kasai procedure are best when the operation is performed before 2 months of age. Transplantation should be reserved for those infants greater than 4 months of age and those who fail to drain bile after portoenterostomy. The rationale for performing the Kasai procedure within 2 months of age is that in the first 2 months of life, histologic changes of the liver show preservation of the basic hepatic architecture with bile ductile proliferation, bile plugs, and mild periportal fibrosis in infants with BA.

As the infant ages, the fibrosis extends into the hepatic lobule resulting in cirrhosis.

Once the decision has been made to proceed with surgical intervention, diagnostic confirmation is the initial goal of surgery. In BA, gross involvement of the extrahepatic bile ducts is noted and cholangiography shows CBD occlusion. On inspection, the visualization of a fibrotic gall bladder with obliterated cystic duct mandates a Roux-en-Y hepaticoportoenterostomy (Kasai procedure). The general concept in the Kasai procedure is to remove the extrahepatic bile ducts *en bloc* and the exposed transected surface at the liver hilus is anastomosed to the intestine. Autoapproximation of the intestine and biliary ductal epithelial elements occurs and this attempts to provide biliary drainage for the liver. The major postoperative complication is cholangitis secondary to bile stasis and intestinal conduit bacterial contamination. Approximately one-third of patients with the Kasai procedure can be considered cured. Another one-third of patients will develop biliary cirrhosis due to minimal bile flow after reconstruction and the final third will develop bile cirrhosis with moderate drainage. Children who fail reconstruction will ultimately require liver transplantation.

In this scenario, the patient, who is less than 2 months old, should undergo a Kasai procedure for optimal treatment of suspected BA.

Bibliography

Karrer FM, Pence JC. Biliary atresia and choledochal cyst. In: Ziegler MM, Azizkhan RG, Weber TR (eds.), *Operative Pediatric Surgery*. New York, NY: McGraw-Hill, 2003, 775–787.

Neigut DA, Cigarroa FG. Biliary atresia. In: Mattei P (ed.), *Surgical Directives Pediatric Surgery*. Philadelphia, PA: Lippincott, Williams & Wilkins, 2002, 543–549.

Ohi R, Nio M. The jaundiced infant: biliary atresia and other obstructions. In: O'Neil JA Jr, Rowe MI, Grosfeld JL, Fonkalsrud EW, Coran AG (eds.), *Pediatric Surgery*, 5th ed. St. Louis, MO: Mosby-Year Book, 1998, 1465–1481.

20. (E) Overall CC can produce symptoms at any age, but usually present within the first decade of life. The classic triad of pain, jaundice, and a palpable mass is noted in less than one-third of afflicted individuals. Infants present with persistent asymptomatic jaundice, while children can present with advanced disease including cholangitis and pancreatitis. Diagnosis is usually achieved via US, yet HIDA and ERCP can be used to elucidate ductal anatomy in cases of uncertainty. Although treatment depends on the type of cystic malformation, surgical therapy is aimed at total cyst excision via a Roux-en-Y hepaticojejunostomy [types I, II,

IVb (multicystic disease that extends into the intrahepatic bilary ducts)]. Type III (choledochoceles) and type IVa (intraductal cysts) variants may require a lateral hilar dissection and fillet of the intrahepatic cyst. Type V is curable with only liver transplantation.

Advances in ultrasonographic imaging have allowed prenatal identification of biliary tree cystic malformations. Specifically, CC can be graded as "obstructed" or "unobstructed" based on US pattern. A large echoic or enlarging cyst is suggestive of an "obstructed" CC while an "unobstructed" CC appears as an echoic, small stable cyst. Moreover, prenatally diagnosed CC should undergo early exploration to rule out BA. Smith and colleagues have shown that the newborn cases of CC represent a special group of patients which demonstrate elevated values of serum bilirubin and grades of liver fibrosis; therefore, these children require early surgical intervention to prevent hepatic fibrosis.

Of note, CC cannot be treated by fetal surgery. Currently, cystic adenomatoid malformations and fetal sacrococcygeal teratomas in the fetus with hydrops have unequivocally benefited from fetal surgery. Other anomalies such as CDH, myelomeningocele, and obstructive uropathies have major questions as to whether fetal intervention can improve the natural history of the disease.

Bibliography

Flake AW. Surgery in the human fetus: the future. *J Physiol* 2003;547(1):45–51.

Karrer FM, Pence JC. Biliary atresia and choledochal cyst. In: Ziegler MM, Azizkhan RG, Weber TR (eds.), *Operative Pediatric Surgery*. New York, NY: McGraw-Hill, 2003, 775–787.

Suita S, Shono K, Kinugasa Y, Kubota M, Matsuo S. Influence of age on the presentation and outcome of choledochal cyst. *J Pediatr Surg* 1999;34(12):1765–1768.

21. (A) While appendicitis is a common surgical condition in childhood, pediatric appendicitis presents with a wide range of clinical manifestations and may make accurate diagnosis difficult. In 28–57% of children 12 years of age or younger, appendicitis was missed at initial clinical examination and in 100% of children younger than 2 years of age. Nevertheless, history and physical remain the hallmark of diagnosing this pathology. The classic constellation of symptoms of appendicitis includes initial periumbilical pain, which later localizes to the right lower quadrant, followed by anorexia, nausea/vomiting, and fever. Vomiting preceding abdominal pain is never secondary to appendicitis. While these classic symptoms are less often present in children, age-specific signs often correlate with symptoms. For example, in preschoolers (age

2–5 years), vomiting often precedes abdominal pain. Also of interest are the classic adult signs of appendicitis which include Rovsing's sign, psoas sign, and obturator sign. These physical findings have not been addressed within the pediatric literature as they relate to statistical significance, i.e., specificity and sensitivity.

The role of seasonal variation and appendicitis has revealed an epidemiologic recognition of increased number of cases of appendicitis from May to August. This has been shown to correlate to enteric infections caused by various infectious agents.

Radioimaging for appendicitis has assisted in decision making of patients who are difficult to evaluate. US is fast, inexpensive, and gives immediate results; sensitivity is from 80 to 92% and specificity reported from 86 to 98%. A diameter of greater than 6 mm, "target sign," appendicolith, appendiceal distension, and periappendiceal fluid are US findings suggestive of acute appendicitis. CT is more accurate than US and findings positive for appendicitis include appendiceal diameter greater than 6 mm, adjacent fluid collection, loculated gas, and pericecal inflammation or abcess. The sensitivity of CT is reported to be from 87 to 99% with a specificity ranging from 83 to 97%. However, it has continued to be stressed that while these radiograph adjuncts are not 100% accurate, the history and physical mandate the backbone for the workup of acute appendicits.

Operative approach for appendicitis can be performed by an open or laparoscopic means. However, some caution that laparoscopic appendicitis in children is not associated with the same advantages reported in adults; while others claim that laparoscopy in children does not increase the incidence of complications even with gangrenous or perforated cases. In any event, the decision for pursuing the laparoscopic route may depend on such variables as time of operation, access to proper equipment, and OR personnel familiarity with laparoscopic set up.

Bibliography

Arca MJ, Caniano DA. Acute appendicitis. In: Mattei P (ed.), *Surgical Directives Pediatric Surgery*. Philadelphia, PA: Lippincott, Williams & Wilkins, 2002, 395–398.

Callanhan MJ, Rodriguez DP, Taylor GA. CT of appendicitis in children. *Radiology* 2000;224(2):325–332.

Little DC, Custer MD, May BH, Blalock SE, Cooney DR. Laparoscopic appendectomy: an unnecessary and expensive procedure in children? *J Pediatr Surg* 2002; 37(3):310–317.

Meguerditchian AN, Prasil P, Cloutier R, Leclerc S, Peloquin J, Roy G. Laparoscopic appendectomy in children: a favorable alternative in simple and complicated appendicitis. *J Pediatr Surg* 2002;37(5):695–698.

Rothrock SG, Pagane J. Acute appendicitis in children: emergency department diagnosis and management. *Ann Emerg Med* 2000;36:39–51.

22. **(E)** IBD is an important cause of GI disease in children. Approximately 20% of adults with IBD develop symptoms during childhood with about 5% diagnosed prior to 10 years of age. Both CD and UC have defining histological and clinical features. Therefore, it is important to differentiate these diseases to adequately institute proper treatment.

CD may occur anywhere along the GI tract from oropharynx to perianal area. "Skip" areas of disease separate normal areas of bowel with accompanying transmural inflammation of the diseased segments. The most common location is the ileocecal area followed by the terminal ileum alone, diffuse small bowel disease, and isolated colon disease. The presentation of CD may be subtle. Symptoms include abdominal pain, diarrhea, weight loss, anorexia, or growth retardation. Malnutrition caused by patient limitation of caloric intake due to pain related to food consumption leads to growth delay and weight loss. Moreover, malnutrition and growth delay are particular important aspects of CD. Because of the subtleties associated with CD, delay in diagnosis is common. Diagnosis is often made with an UGI series with small bowel follow through (single most valuable study) which can show distinct radiographic stigmata of CD; rigid stenotic segments, skip areas, sinus tracts, or fistulae. Medical treatment and diet control many of the symptoms of CD, yet surgery has a role in CD in the face of specific complications (most common indication is general deterioration despite long-term medical management). It is also important to note that the disease is not cured by operative intervention. Strictureplasty has become a popular technique in a patient with multiple short obstructing segments. This intestinal sparing approach can be used to prevent the development of short gut syndrome in a child with CD.

In comparison to CD, the disease process in **UC** is confined to the colon and rectal mucosa. Characteristic histologic appearance of UC includes crypt abscesses, distortion of mucosal glands, and goblet cell depletion. Symptoms include intestinal and extraintestinal manifestations. The presence of blood and mucous mixed with stool with lower abdominal cramping (especially during passage of stool) mark key intestinal symptoms associated with UC. Growth delay (5–10% of patients), arthralgias, skin lesions, and primary sclerosing cholangitis are extraintestinal symptoms which can present with UC. Diagnosis is achieved via colonoscopy with biopsies (demonstrating nonspecific inflammation with hemorrhage without granulomas). Although medical treatment is used to provide relief of symptoms, UC can be cured by removal of diseased colon and rectum. Surgical options include pancolectomy with permanent ileostomy, abdominal colectomy with ileorectal anastomosis, or abdominal colectomy with rectal mucosectomy with/without ileal reservoir.

Nevertheless, while the defining morphologic changes that differentiate CD and UC are well described, it may be difficult to classify the type of inflammation present. For example, colonic CD may be difficult to distinguish from UC. The importance in making a diagnosis is such that UC is a potentially curable disease. One tool available to help in evaluating children for IBD is the evaluation of the types of inflammatory cells present. Reports have suggested that CD differs from UC in the inflammatory/immune response. CD4+ T cell populations can be classified as Th1 type cells or Th2 type cells on the basis of the cytokine secretion profile. Crohn's has been shown to be a Th1-mediated disease and excessive Th1 cell activity is a key component of CD. Less information is available describing the pathogenesis of UC but cytokine profile studies suggest that Th2 cells play a prominent role in UC.

An additional tool that has been demonstrated to aid in distinguishing these two diseases is serologic testing. Two markers have been employed to detect the presence of IBD: Antineutrophil cytoplasmic antibody (ASCA) for CD and perinuclear antinuclear cytoplasmic antibody (pANCA) for UC detection. When used separately, the value of these tests is limited, but when the tests are combined the statistical usefulness for these assays improves. For example, in cases of CD, a ASCA+ and pANCA– individual has a reported sensitivity of 64% and specificity of 94%. Whereas in UC cases, a pANCA+ and ASCA– result show a sensitivity and specificity of 51 and 94%. Overall the utility of these serologic assays can be used to support a diagnosis of IBD or as an aid to distinguish CD from UC, but it is cautioned that these markers should not be used solely to diagnose IBD.

Bibliography

Alexander F. Inflammatory bowel disease. In: Ziegler MM, Azizkhan RG, Weber TR (eds.), *Operative Pediatric Surgery*. New York, NY: McGraw-Hill, 2003, 691–698.

Dolgin SE. Crohn's disease. In: Mattei P (ed.), *Surgical Directives Pediatric Surgery*. Philadelphia, PA: Lippincott, Williams & Wilkins, 2002, 335–339.

Hendickson BA, Gokhale R, Cho JH. Clinical aspects and pathophysiology of inflammatory bowel disease. *Clin Micro Rev* 2002;15(1):79–94.

Linskens RK, Mallant-Hent RC, Groothuismink ZM, Bakker-Jonges LB, van der Merwe JP, Hooijkaas H, von Blomberg BM, Meuwissen SG. Evaluation of serologic markers to differentiate between ulcerative colitis and Crohn's disease: pANCA, ASCA, and agglutinating antibodies to anaerobic coccoid rods. *Eur J Gastroenterol Hepatol* 2002;14(9):1013–1018.

Warner BW. Ulcerative colitis. In: Mattei P (ed.), *Surgical Directives Pediatric Surgery*. Philadelphia, PA: Lippincott, Williams & Wilkins, 2002, 359–362.

23. **(B)** While the evaluation and resuscitation of an injured child is similar to ATLS protocols for an adult, anatomic and physiologic dissimilarities in children require special attention during the primary survey. With respect to the pediatric airway, several important differences exist between the normal pediatric airway and the adult airway. The inability to manage the pediatric airway leading to inadequate ventilation and hypoxia is the most common cause of cardiopulmonary arrest in a child. The laryngeal/vocal cord complex is quite different from an adult. The larynx is located higher in the neck (level C3-4), whereas the adult larynx is located at C4-5. The vocal cord attachments anteriorly are more inferior than the posterior attachments; this produces an anterocaudal angulation of the laryngeal/vocal cord complex in a child. The position of this complex can make visualizing the glottic opening more difficult during laryngoscopy. The narrowest portion of the pediatric airway is the subglottic or cricoid cartilage area while the vocal cords are the narrowest portion in an adult. An additional concern of the pediatric airway is the infant tongue. The relatively larger size tongue in combination with a more superior location makes airway obstruction a concern because the tongue apposes the palate more easily. The protuberant occiput of an infant is responsible for causing excessive neck flexion and promotes airway obstruction. A shoulder roll or neck roll aids in placing the infant's head in the proper position for mask ventilation and direct laryngoscopy. Additional differences include a larger and stiffer epiglottis and smaller nares (which can increase the resistance to air flow) in infants and children. These differences resolve as the child grows and by approximately 10 years of age, the upper child airway resembles an adult's airway.

Bibliography

Infosino A. Pediatric upper airway and congenital anomalies. *Anesthesiol Clin North Am* 2002;20:747–766.

Levy RJ, Helfaer MA. Pediatric airway issues. *Crit Care Clin North Am* 2000;16(3):489–504.

Stafford PW, Blinman TA, Nance ML. Practical points in evaluation and resuscitation of the injured child. *Surg Clin North Am* 2002;82:273–301.

TABLE 34-1   Vital Functions

Age group	Weight (kg)	Heart rate (bpm)	Blood pressure (mmHg)	Respiratory rate (breaths/min)	Urinary output (mL/kg/h)
Birth to 6 months	3–6	180–160	60–80	60	2
Infant	12	160	80	40	1.5
Preschool	16	120	90	30	1
Adolescent	35	100	100	20	0.5

Source.   Reproduced with permission from American College of Surgeons' Committee on Trauma, *Advanced Trauma Life Support for Doctors, Student Course Manual*, 6th ed. Chicago, IL: American College of Surgeons, 1997, 297.

24. **(C)** Once the airway has been assessed and secured, the respiratory status and work of breathing should be evaluated. Initially, supplemental oxygen should be delivered via face mask, nasal canula, or endotracheal tube. Important components of the evaluation include assessment of vital signs and mental status, auscultation of breath sounds (preferably in the axillary areas to reduce noise from the opposite chest), evaluation for use of accessory muscles and nasal flaring, and the presence of symmetric chest wall movement. Vital signs vary according to age and are used to gauge initial resuscitation efforts (see Table 34-1). With respect to respiration, the respiratory rate decreases with age (an infant requires 40–60 breaths/min whereas the older child breathes 20 times/min). Tidal volumes vary from 7 to 10 cc/kg for infants and children. The physical differences in the pediatric trauma patient regarding the pulmonary system include a decreased functional reserve capacity (increased tendency for atelectasis), limited respiratory reserve (more susceptible to respiratory distress and failure), greater chest wall compliance (low pressure for ventilation due to low chest wall resistance), and a more mobile mediastinum (infants/children less tolerant of a pneumothorax). These physiologic parameters, together with poorly developed intercostals muscles (infants rely on diaphragm for breathing) and horizontally oriented ribs (decreased chest expansion during breathing), can complicate initial resuscitation and lead to hypoxia. Additionally, one must be alert for life-threatening conditions that may compromise breathing such as tension pneumothorax, massive hemothorax, pericardial tamponade, flail chest, and massive pulmonary contusion.

Bibliography

American College of Surgeons: Pediatric Trauma. *Advanced Trauma Life Support Student Manual*, 1997, 289–312.

Kapklein MJ, Mahadeo R. Pediatric trauma. *Mt Sinai J Med* 1997;64(4–5):302–310.

Lynch JM. Pediatric trauma/child abuse. In: Peitzman AB, Rhoades M, Schwab CW, Yealy DM (eds.), *The Trauma Manual*. Philadelphia, PA: Lippincott-Raven, 1998, 431–442.

25. **(E)** Seriously injured children who are hypotensive and have decreased circulating volume may have obscured venous landmarks that make placement of peripheral intravenous catheters difficult. Some advocate a "60-second rule" when placing intravenous access; if intravenous access cannot be cannulated within 1 min, other routes are recommended. ATLS guidelines support IO catheter placement in children under 6 years of age when rapid venous access cannot be achieved after two attempts in a critically injured child. In children older than 6 years of age, either a venous cutdown may be performed at the ankle or a percutaneous femoral line should be placed. The intraosseus route for vascular access is based on the presence of noncollapsible veins that drain the medullary sinuses in the bone marrow. The vascular network empties into the central venous circulation via nutrient and emissary veins. As a result, drugs, crystalloid solutions, and blood products may be given by the IO route with almost immediate absorption. A 16- to 18-gauge bone aspiration needle is inserted through the skin 1–3 cm below and medial to the tibial tuberosity and advanced through the bone into the bone marrow. Contraindications to IO placement include lower extremity or pelvic fractures or if access to the tibia is not possible; other bones adequate for IO vascular access include the distal femur and the distal humerus. The IO line is considered a temporary maneuver; the child should have IO access discontinued once an appropriate IV line has been obtained. Complications related to IO access occur infrequently, yet rates increase with long-term use and include osteomyelitis, local cellulites, infiltration of fluid into the subperiosteal and subcutaneous tissues, and leakage at the insertion site. Of note, only newborns with an attached umbilicus are candidates for an umbilical venous catheter.

Bibliography

American College of Surgeons: Pediatric Trauma. *Advanced Trauma Life Support Student Manual*, 1997, 289–312.

Guy J, Haley K, Zuspan SJ. Use of intraosseus infusion in the pediatric trauma patient. *J Pediatr Surg* 1993;28(2):158–161.

Kapklein MJ, Mahadeo R. Pediatric trauma. *Mt Sinai J Med* 1997;64(4–5):302–310.

Strovroff M, Teague G. Intravenous access in infants and children. *Pediatr Clin North Am* 1998;45(6):1373–1393.

26. **(B)** Thoracic injury occurs in 4.5% of injured children. Because of a pliable skeleton that is surrounded by less fat and elastic connective tissues, rib fractures are uncommon in younger children and indicate a significant amount of energy transfer to the chest and thoracic contents. The presence of rib fractures should focus a clinician's attention to the risk of multiple serious injuries in a child with a history of trauma. Moreover, the identification of three or more fractured ribs is a sensitive marker of injury severity and multisystem injuries and fulfills criteria for transfer to a trauma center.

Pulmonary contusions are the most common thoracic injury in traumatized children. While initial chest radiographs may not reveal demonstrable pulmonary injury, a repeat chest film 48–72 h after the injury is diagnostic. The use of a chest CT frequently may show evidence of pulmonary contusion and hemopneumothorax that are sometimes not apparent on chest radiography. Chest CT is also useful for management of pulmonary contusion. A study by Wagner and colleagues showed that when greater than 28% of lung is involved, mechanical ventilation was required, but not needed when less than 18% was involved. Management of lung contusions is largely supportive (fluid administration, pain control, and pulmonary toilet) but may require more nontraditional modes of ventilation in more severe cases.

Mediastinal injuries, which involve the great vessels and the heart, are uncommon in children. The most common great vessel injury is aortic disruption and seen in older adolescents as a result of a high impact motor vehicle crash. Mechanisms of aortic disruption include sheer forces, compression of the aorta over the vertebral column, and intraluminal hyperextension. Diagnosis may be suggested by radiographic chest film demonstrating a "funny-looking mediastinum" and abnormal aortic knob contour (these two signs are the most reliable radiographic markers). Yet a prominent thymic shadow in young children can make mediastinal shape interpretation difficult.

In situations involving multiple trauma, it may difficult to differentiate causes of hypoxia and hypotension. Hemorrhage, cardiac tamponade, pulmonary embolism, and tension pneumothorax may all show similar clinical presentations and further diagnostic modalities (chest radiography and/or CT, echo, FAST) are needed if the child is stable. In a hemodynamically unstable child, a chest tube should be inserted to treat cases of tension pneumothorax and hemothorax. Beck's triad (hypotension, jugular venous distension, and muffled heart sounds) is infrequently present in children in cases of suspected cardiac tamponade. Pericardiocentesis should be performed in the trauma bay. If the patient is deteriorating rapidly, a left lateral thoracotomy must be performed. Echocardiogram is both sensitive and specific for tamponade. Additionally, pericardial fluid may also be detected in a focused abdominal sonogram for trauma (FAST) examination of an injured child. An OR thoracotomy should be the next step in cases of positive pericardiocentesis or FAST examination.

Diaphragm injuries from blunt trauma are often difficult to diagnose and as a consequence, management is delayed. Reports indicate that 40–50% are not diagnosed in the initial phase of trauma. The left hemidiaphragm is involved in two-thirds of cases (usually in the posterolateral location). When diaphragmatic rupture is suspected (visceral herniation, nasogastric tube within the hemithorax, or abnormal diaphram contour), operative exploration is indicated.

In the chest radiograph shown, a tension pneumothorax is responsible for the patient's clinical presentation.

Bibliography

Bliss D, Silen M. Pediatric thoracic trauma. *Crit Care Med* 2002;30(Suppl 11):S409–S415.

Garcia VF, Mooney D. Thoracic injuries. In: Ziegler MM, Azizkhan RG, Weber TR (eds.), *Operative Pediatric Surgery*. New York, NY: McGraw-Hill, 2003, 1115–1124.

Stafford PW, Blinman TA, Nance ML. Practical points in evaluation and resuscitation of the injured child. *Surg Clin North Am* 2002;82:273–301.

Wagner RB, Crawford WO, Schimpf PP. Quantitation and pattern of parenchymal lung injury in blunt chest trauma: Diagnostic and therapeutic implications. *J Comput Tomogr* 1988;12:270–281.

27. **(A)** Evaluation of a child with a history of intraabdominal trauma begins with a primary survey and a thorough secondary survey. Physical examination signs that are suspicious for intraabdominal injury

include adbominal wall abrasions and contusions, abdominal distension, and abdominal pain. In an unstable child, emergent surgical therapy is indicated. Several diagnostic approaches are available for the stable patient. Double contrast CT scanning of the abdomen/pelvis can reveal injury to the many solid organs (spleen, liver, kidneys, pancreas, adrenals, and the retroperitoneum). The spleen and liver are the most commonly injured intraabdominal organs in children. Nance et al. showed that following isolated blunt liver or spleen injury, there was a correlation between the severity of the injury and the association of free abdominal fluid. Abdominal CT scans were reviewed and injury grades to the spleen and liver were assessed. They found that as injury grades increased, so did the frequency of free fluid.

Identification of bowel injury can be difficult on CT scan. Extravasation of oral contrast, free intraperitoneal air, free fluid in the abdomen without solid organ injury, bowel wall thickening, and multiple loops of fluid-filled bowel are indicative of intestinal injury. CT is additionally poor at identifying Chance type (lumbar spine) fractures since the fracture plane is parallel to scanner plane.

FAST has emerged as an effective and inexpensive approach to identify intraabdominal fluid in adults. In children, its accuracy for detection of intraperitoneal fluid is less clear. Many children sustain intraabdominal injuries who do not demonstrate any free fluid. Additionally, FAST is poor at identifying organ specific injury. Nevertheless, FAST is advocated as a screening tool in the evaluation of abdominal injury in a child with multitrauma and no obvious sources of bleeding.

DPL is indicated in a child who is suspected of having an intraabdominal injury and will require operative intervention that will prevent subsequent examinations. Additional indications include children with seatbelt injuries with free intraperitoneal fluid with no evidence of organ specific injury on CT scan and selected children with abdominal stab wounds. Attention should be paid to bacteria and enteric contents since the presence of red blood cells (RBCs) (hemoperitoneum) does not mandate operative intervention in a hemodynamically stable child.

While all these imaging modalities have their strengths for detecting different types of intraabdominal injury, they have a low specificity for determining the need for laparotomy. Diagnostic laparoscopy may be used in selected cases to prevent delay in the detection of significant intraabdominal pathology. Advocates of diagnostic laparoscopy support the use of this tool not only for diagnostic purposes but for therapeutic means as well.

Bibliography

Gaines BA, Ford HR. Abdominal and pelvic trauma in children. *Crit Care Med* 2002;30(Suppl 11):S416–S423.

McKinely AJ, Mahomed AA. Laparoscopy in a case of pediatric blunt abdominal trauma. *Surg Endosc* 2002;16(2):358.

Nance ML, Mahboubi S, Wickstrom M, Prendergast F, Stafford PW. Pattern of abdominal free fluid following isolated blunt spleen or liver injury in the pediatric patient. *J Trauma* 2002;52(1):85–87.

28. **(D)** Children are more likely to suffer a head injury than an adult primarily due to the disproportionate size of a child's head as compared to an adult. Although children (>3 years) generally do better than an adult in terms of outcome, there are unique biomechanical and tissue properties of the pediatric brain that magnify resultant pathologic brain injury. Children often have more diffuse brain injury that is likely attributed to the higher water content of the immature brain and incomplete axonal myelination. This is supported by studies of postmortem pediatric brain injury patients that show venous congestion, edema, and diffuse axonal injury.

Second insults (hypoxia, hypotension, and intracranial hypertension) are events after the primary head injury that exacerbate and worsen the prognosis of pediatric brain injury. Avoiding hypoxia, ischemia, and cerebral edema prevents secondary brain injury. Maintaining CPP [CPP = MAP (mean arterial pressure) – ICP] lessens secondary injury and improves patient outcome. Reports evaluating optimal CPP in pediatric patients suggest that children with CPP of >40 mmHg had less mortality rates. In older children, CPP should be kept around 50–55 mmHg. Since low MAP or high ICP can affect CPP, efforts are undertaken to maintain mean arterial oxygen tension >80 mmHg and ICP below 15 in infants up to 6 years of age or below 20 for older children. ICP devices can be inserted to continuously monitor for elevated ICP. The guidelines for placing these devices are recommended for GCS ≤ 8.

Treatment of intracranial hypertension as evidence of elevated ICP consists of three major tier interventions (see Fig. 34-26). Of particular interest is the use of hypertonic, 3% NaCl after pediatric traumatic brain injury. The hypertonic saline may be given as a bolus or continuous infusion and results suggests that the osmolar effects may be greater and longer lasting than mannitol.

Bibliography

Mazzola CA, Adelson PD. Critical care management of head trauma in children. *Crit Care Med* 2002;30(Suppl 11):S393–S401.

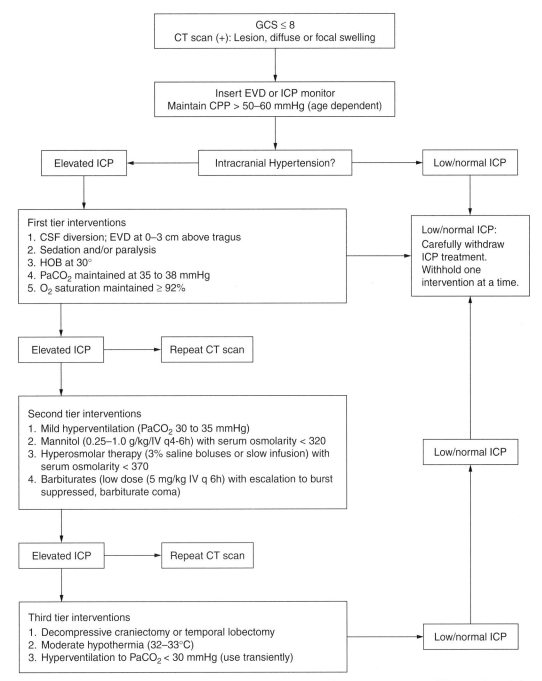

FIG. 34-26 Algorithm for the critical care setting. GCS, Glasgow Coma Score; CT, computer tomography; EVD, external ventricular drain; ICP, intracranial pressure; CPP, cerebral perfusion pressure; CSF, cerebrospinal fluid; HOB, head of bed; IV, intravenous; q, every.
Source. Reproduced with permission by Lippincott, Williams & Wilkins. Mazzola CA and Adelson PD. Critical care management of head trauma in children. Crit Care Med 2002;30(Suppl 11):S39–S40. Figure 1.

Queenan J, Mattei P. Head trauma. In: Mattei P (ed.), *Surgical Directives Pediatric Surgery*. Philadelphia, PA: Lippincott, Williams & Wilkins, 2002, 99–102.

Stafford PW, Blinman TA, Nance ML. Practical points in evaluation and resuscitation of the injured child. *Surg Clin North Am* 2002;82:273–301.

29. **(B)** Pediatric spinal cord injury accounts for approximately 5% of all spinal cord injuries. Because of age-related anatomic and physiologic differences, various types of spinal injuries are anticipated than those seen in adults because of the developmental phases of the pediatric spinal cord. For instance, children under 8 years of

age have a greater preponderance of cervical spine injuries while the injury patterns of children greater than 8 years old begin to reflect those seen in adults. Specifically, a larger head-to-body ratio and weak neck musculature are responsible for the higher fulcrum of motion (C2-3) in younger children (after the age of 8, the fulcrum changes to C5-6). Additional differences include incomplete ossification of the base of C2, anterior wedging of the vertebral bodies, horizontal orientation of the facets, and absence of the uncinate processes on the vertebral bodies. The overall result of these anatomic variations is that the ligaments have a greater degree of resistance to flexion and rotational forces than the bony skeleton; in other words, older children (>8 years old) have more fractures as compared to younger children. Younger children are predisposed to subluxation and spinal cord injury without radiologic abnormality (SCIWORA).

SCIWORA is predominately seen in children. Transient symptoms such as numbness, paraesthesia, or "shock like" sensations occur shortly after trauma. Delayed onset of neurologic injury is sometimes seen, usually within 48 h. The proposed mechanism is due to excessive elastic ligament dislocation and spontaneous reduction without radiographic abnormality seen on plain films. Other mechanisms recognized include ligamentous bulging, reversible subluxation, reversible disc protrusion, spinal cord concussion, and temporary occlusion of the vertebral or anterior spinal arteries. MRI should be performed to assess for spinal edema and ligament injury.

When evaluating a child for a possible spinal cord injury, radiographic assessment begins with a lateral cervical and anteroposterior plain radiographs. There are certain normal findings in the younger (<8 years) child that may be considered abnormal in the adult. These include apical ossification center of the dens, anteriorly wedged vertebral bodies, normal C2-3 pseudosubluxation, absent anterior ossification of the atlas, and a wider atlantodental interval of 3–5 mm. Because of these normal radiographic findings, misinterpretation is common with personnel unfamiliar with these common diagnostic variations.

The clearance of the pediatric cervical spine can be a challenge. While the hallmark of cervical column injuries in adults is neck pain, this is not true in children. Young children can be considered to be at risk for cervical spine injuries because of their inability to complain of pain. Additionally, a neurologic examination may be difficult to perform on children. Therefore, implementation of cervical spine management/clearance programs has been designed and studied to assess potential spine injuries in children

to decrease the morbidity associated with prolonged immobilization and missed injuries.

Because spinal cord injuries can be debilitating and devastating, injury prevention programs have been established to increase awareness and decrease risk-taking behavior associated with these types of injuries. While injury prevention programs have been shown to have an effect when aimed at elementary school children, a criticism with spinal cord injury prevention programs is that target audiences are too old (middle school). Awareness programs have not been effective for middle school aged students. A strategy that has been suggested is offering educational programs beginning in elementary school and demanding that government take a larger role in enforcing injury prevention laws.

Bibliography

Lee SL, Sena M, Greenholz SK, Fledderman M. A multidisciplinary approach to the development of a cervical spine clearance protocol: process, rationale, and initial results. *J Pediatr Surg* 2003;38(3):358–362.

Proctor MR. Spinal cord injury. *Crit Care Med* 2002;30(Suppl 11):S489–S499.

Rekate HL, Theodore N, Sonntag VKH, Dickman CA. Pediatric spine and spinal cord trauma. *Childs Nerv Syst* 1999;15:743–750.

Roche C, Carty H. Spinal trauma in children. *Pediatr Radiol* 2001;31:677–700.

30. **(B)** In a growing child, the bony skeleton is one organ system that is characterized with persistent growth, remodeling potential, elasticity, open physes, thick periosteum, and smaller anatomic structure. The basic anatomy of bone consists of several components that participate in fracture healing when bony disruption (fracture) occurs. The outer layer (periosteum) is thick and flexible and plays a major role in fracture healing due to the vascularity and bone forming capabilities associated with this layer. Under the periosteum, the hard cortex gives bone its shape and strength. A Haversian system (vascular passages running the length of the bone) and cellular elements such as osteocytes, osteoblasts and osteoclasts are present within this bony component. The inner lining of the bone (endosteum) additionally plays a role in new bone formation during fracture healing. The innermost structure, the medullary canal, contributes to the fracture healing cascade and progresses most rapidly. Finally, marrow elements within the cancellous bony canal are another factor in the healing potential of bone.

Different fracture patterns may result in children due to the varying amounts of cartilage residing in their immature bones. In pediatic skeletal trauma, plastic deformation of bone is a common finding. Persistent bony deformity results as the bone is bent beyond its elastic recoil potential, thus this type of bone deformity must be straightened or broken to effect reduction. Other types of fractures include torus or buckle fractures and greenstick fractures.

In terms of select injury fractures, the forearm is the most common site of fracture in children. The distal one-third of the radius and/or ulna is involved in 55% of all childhood fractures; 75% occur in the distal one-third of the radius, thereby making it the single most common fracture. Supracondylar humeral fractures make up approximately 60% of elbow fractures in children. The importance in identifying and immobilizing this type of injury in children is essential because of the high incidence of associated neurovascular injury. Additionally, particular attention should be directed toward the forearm compartments as forearm and elbow fractures can lead to compartment syndromes. Radial head subluxation (nursemaid's elbow) usually occurs in children less than 6 years old. Typically a history of a vigorous pull on the arm by a caretaker is elicited. The child usually holds the arm pronated and partially flexed, refusing to use the arm voluntarily. Treatment is geared toward reducing the trapped annular ligament, which is trapped between the radial head and the capitellum. This can usually be achieved by reducing the elbow through a series of nonsurgical maneuvers that allow that annular ligament to slide over the radial head to its normal position around the radial neck. While trauma is the cause of most anterior shoulder dislocations (posterior dislocations usually due to anatomic instability or epileptic seizure), brachial plexus and vascular injuries can occur but are rare.

Growth plate (physeal) injuries are a concern in the pediatric arena in that the injured area involves a functioning growth plate; if the open growth plate is sufficiently damaged, premature physeal arrest may occur leading to extremity deformity or shortening. For example, injury to the distal femoral physis can lead to partial or near-complete growth arrest and is more common than in any other similarly injured physis.

Overall management of pediatric orthopedic trauma includes considering future growth and bone remodeling potential, recognizing and minimizing physeal plate injury, and aggressive treatment of compartment syndromes.

Bibliography

Huurman WW, Ginsburg GM. Musculoskeletal injury in children. *Pediatr Rev* 1997;18(12):429–440.

Musgrave DS, Mendelson SA. Pediatric orthopedic trauma: principles in management. *Crit Care Med* 2002;30 (Suppl 11):S431–S443.

31. **(B)** The case reported describes a child with blunt abdominal trauma sustained secondarily to child abuse. Figure 34-10 is an axial CT abdominal image showing a soft tissue density and mild stranding surrounding the duodenum (arrow) consistent with a duodenal hematoma. While most patients with intramural hematomas of the duodenum respond well to conservative management, in this case the child remained obstructed over several days. The intraoperative photograph (Fig. 34-11) shows a large intramural hematoma over the duodenal wall. Operative intervention consisted of simple evacuation of the hematoma and closure of the serosal incision.

Because child abuse (nonaccidental trauma, NAT) remains prevalent in our society, it is imperative that, when injuries are inconsistent with a stated mechanism or time frame, physicians keep child abuse in their differential when examining a child. The manner in which child abuse patients present may be complex due to the various methods in which these children are injured, including shaking, slamming, throwing, and suffocating. While most abused children do not require surgery for their injuries, early abusive injuries may be seen as bruises, lacerations, bites, dental and ocular trauma, and fractures.

Serious brain injury is the leading cause of child abuse fatalities. Death is attributed to increased ICP and resultant cerebral edema. The term "shaken baby syndrome" is a serious form of abusive head trauma that occurs when a child is subjected to violent shaking with rapid acceleration, deceleration and rotational forces, with or without impact, resulting in a unique constellation of features which include subdural hematoma (with or without cerebral edema), subarachnoid hemorrhage, retinal hemorrhage(s), rib fracture(s), and metaphyseal fracture(s) of the long bones. Overall the victims of inflicted head trauma tend to have a higher morbidity when compared to accidental head trauma patients. The consequences of the inflicted trauma lead to a series of reactions that result in cerebral hypoxia, edema, increased ICP, and vasoocclusion.

While retinal hemorrhages are a strong indicator for suspected child abuse, other conditions have reported this finding. Examples include children with meningitis, bleeding disorders, after cardiopulmonary bypass, infants who have been recently delivered via vacuum assistance, vaginal or Cesarean-section, ECMO, in children with seizures, and in patients with the rare familial retinal arteriolar tortuosity disorder. Victims of accidental trauma rarely have retinal hemorrhages; if present they may be minor, unilateral, and ipsilateral to the side of injury.

Retinal hemorrhage in child abuse may be bilateral, unilateral, subretinal, intraretinal, or preretinal.

The radiologic manifestations of child abuse are found more commonly in infants and children than in older, physically abused children. Generally the finding of older, healing fractures on radiographs should be make any clinician suspicious of child abuse. Long bone injuries (metaphyseal fractures), skull fractures (linear, parietal region), and rib fractures (posterior in location) are highly characteristic for abuse. Of particular interest are rib fractures as an indicator of NAT in children. Studies show that the postive predictive value (PPV) of rib fractures as an indicator of NAT is 95%. The PPV increases to 100% once clinical history excludes other causes for rib fractures. Other suspicious fractures include scapular, spinous process, and sternal injuries. However, other medical conditions may show similar types of fractures and include osteogenesis imperfecta, congenital syphilis, osteomyelitis, and infantile rickets.

When suspected, child abuse cases require thorough documentation, including H&P (as well as photographs of the injuries) and radiologic survey for fractures so that appropriate legal and social service intervention will identify and prevent further abuse to other members of the family.

Bibliography

Barsness KA, Cha ES, Bensard DD, Calkins CM, Partrick DA, Karrer FM, Strain JD. The positive predictive value of rib fractures as an indicator of nonaccidental trauma in children. *J Trauma* 2003;54(6):1107–1110.

Care M. Imaging in suspected child abuse: what to expect and what to order. *Pediatr Ann* 2002;31(10):651–659.

Sutter FKP, Helbig H. Familial retinal arteriolar tortuosity: a review. *Surv Opthalmol* 2003;48(3):245–255.

Tayor L. Child abuse. In: Mattei P (ed.), *Surgical Directives Pediatric Surgery*. Philadelphia, PA: Lippincott, Williams & Wilkins, 2002, 129–132.

Zenel J, Goldstein B. Child abuse in the pediatric intensive care unit. *Crit Care Med* 2002;30(Suppl 11):S515–S523.

32. (E) Commonly encountered developmental neck abnormalities in children are of congenital origin yet may not cause problems or be detected until adulthood. While some of these neck lesions may appear asymptomatic at birth, they may precipitously become enlarged and disfiguring as a result of local or regional infection or hemorrhage. Developmental abnormalities of the branchial apparatus represent a common source of congenital lateral neck masses. Branchial anomalies may present as a cyst, sinus, or fistula. Branchial cleft anomalies arise most commonly (greater than 90%) from the second branchial cleft system. Eight percent arise from the first branchial anomaly whereas third and fourth branchial malfor-

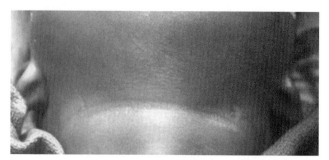

FIG. 34-27 A child with bilateral branchial cleft sinus.

mations are rare. Usually the second branchial cleft sinus or fistula presents with drainage from a small pit in the skin just anterior to the lower third of the sternocleidomastoid muscle. Treatment of choice is surgical excision due to the risk of infection (Fig. 34-27).

Thyroglossal duct cysts (TGDCs) represent the most common head and neck midline masses in children. It is reported that they account for about 70% of all congenital neck abnormalities. TGDCs are embryonic ectodermal rests that can present as midline structures as they follow the descent along the thyroid gland tract. Normally, the thyroglossal duct regresses once the thyroid gland reaches the anterior neck. Faulty thyroid migration or persistence of the thyroglossal duct can lead to the formation of lingual/ectopic thyroid tissue, pyramidal thyroid lobe, or a TGDCs. Since TGDCs are attached to the hyoid bone, clinical presentation typically shows a midline mass that moves with swallowing. Treatment is based on the Sistrunk procedure in which complete surgical excision of the cyst and tract up to the base of the tongue including the central portion of the hyoid bone is preformed (see Fig. 34-28).

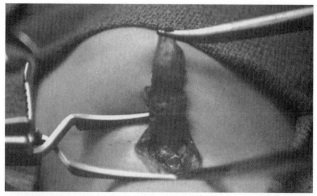

FIG. 34-28 Thyroglossal duct cyst excision including the central portion of the hyoid bone.

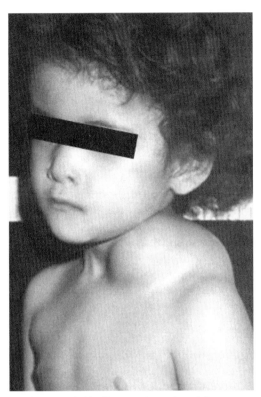

FIG. 34-29   Child with a posterior neck cystic hygroma.

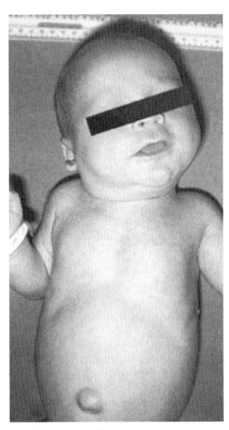

FIG. 34-30   An infant with torticollis.
Source. Reprinted from *Color Atlas of Pediatric Surgery*, 2/e, Leibert, PS, 59, (c)1996, with permission from Elsevier.

Lymphatic malformations commonly referred to as cystic hygromas are developmental abnormalities of the lymphoid system that occur at sites of lymphatic-venous connection, most commonly in the posterior neck (Fig. 34-29). The cysts may become enlarged and disfiguring not only as a result of infection or hemorrhage but also due to increases in fluid and endothelial cell growth. Imaging by US, CT, and MRI (for complex and extensive lesions) is mandated to determine whether involvement of deeper airway structures is present. This also gives pertinent clues as to the planning of the operative approach. When these lesions are diagnosed prenatally, the overall prognosis is poorer than those diagnosed after birth. Treatment of these lesions is primarily surgical but another therapy is injection sclerotherapy with such agents as bleomycin, OK-432, sodium morrhuate, 22.5% glucose, and triamcinolone. Sclerotherapy is usually reserved for extensive disease or recurrences.

Torticollis is a deformity characterized by the unnatural tilted or turned position of the head. The most common form is due to shortening of the sternocleidomastoid muscle, although a number of other conditions can potentially cause torticollis (cervical hemivertebrae, adenitis, fascitis, and oculomotor abnormalities). Birth trauma was once thought to

contribute to the cause of torticollis by injury to the sternocleidomastoid or the spinal accessory nerve, but this is rarely the case. The mother or primary physician usually notes the classic presentation of an otherwise healthy 2–8-week-old infant who preferentially turns their head to one side. Compete resolution of untreated torticollis occurs in 50–70% of cases by 6 months of age, but because it is difficult to predict which infants will develop an irreversible deformity, a passive range-of-motion exercise regimen is advocated. In cases that present with or develop facial hemihypoplasia, surgery to divide the sternocleidomastoid on the affected side is indicated (Fig. 34-30).

Medullary thryroid cancer can occur sporadically, in association with MEN types 2A or 2B, or with the familial medullary cancer syndrome. A mutation in the ret protooncogene in individuals with MEN and the familial variant predisposes family members (autosomal dominant inheritance) to the development of medullary thyroid cancer at an early age. This tumor is the first to develop in MEN children and is the most common cause of death. In these children, early thyroidectomy is advocated after the genetic mutation has been confirmed. MEN 2A children should undergo thyroidectomy prior to 5 years of age; whereas children of MEN 2B require thyroidectomy prior to 1 year of age due to the more virulent nature of the disease.

Bibliography

Azizkan RG, DeCou JM. Head and neck lesions. In: Ziegler MM, Azizkhan RG, Weber TR (eds.), *Operative Pediatric Surgery*. New York, NY: McGraw-Hill, 2003, 221–240.

Bruch SW. Thyroid disorders. In: Mattei P (ed.), *Surgical Directives Pediatric Surgery*. Philadelphia, PA: Lippincott, Williams & Wilkins, 2002, 171–174.

Cook SP. Thyroglossal duct cysts and related disorders. In: Mattei P (ed.), *Surgical Directives Pediatric Surgery*. Philadelphia, PA: Lippincott, Williams & Wilkins, 2002, 175–178.

Gallagher PG. Mahoney MJ, Gosche JR. Cystic hygroma in the fetus and newborn. *Semin Perinatol* 1999;23(4):341–356.

Mattei P. Torticollis. In: Mattei P (ed.), *Surgical Directives Pediatric Surgery*. Philadelphia, PA: Lippincott, Williams & Wilkins, 2002, 193–195.

Smith CD. Cysts and sinuses of the neck. In: O'Neil JA Jr, Rowe MI, Grosfeld JL, Fonkalsrud EW, Coran AG (eds.), *Pediatric Surgery*, 5th ed. St. Louis, MO: Mosby-Year Book, 1998, 757–771.

33. **(D)** The repair of pediatric hernias constitutes one of the most common congenital anomalies that pediatric surgeons are confronted with. The majority of inguinal hernias in infants and children are indirect and are a result of the failure of the processus vaginalis (a diverticulum of peritoneum) to involute as the process of gonad descent proceeds into the scrotum in males and the lower pelvis in females. The processus vaginalis is an anteromedial structure that appears to aid in testicular descent by providing the hydrolic force that positions the testis into the scrotum; it later regresses and thereby obliterates the entrance of the peritoneal cavity into the inguinal canal. Various other conditions are associated with inguinal hernias and include a positive family history, undescended testis (UDT), prematurity, ascites, hypospadias or epispadias, presence of a ventriculoperitoneal shunt, use of continuous peritoneal dialysis, ambiguous genitalia, and children with connective tissue disorders (Ehlers-Danlos and Hunter-Hurler syndrome). Because this type of hernia will not close spontaneously and of the high risk of incarceration (especially in infants under 1 year of age), inguinal hernias should be repaired within 4 weeks of diagnosis. While repair of inguinal hernias involves high suture ligation of the sac at the level of the internal ring, the issue of contralateral exploration continues to be a subject of debate. There seems to have evolved a selective approach to managing the opposite groin based on age, gender, and patent processes vaginalis. In children less than 2 years of age, the patency of the PV is high and some advocate contralateral exploration because of the frequent occurrence of unsuspected hernias. Recent studies have not shown significant differences in determining the presence of a contralateral PPV in cases of unilateral inguinal hernia. Laparoscopy has aided in detection of a contralateral PPV. Yet the issue of a PPV is that it is a potential factor for inguinal hernia development, it does not represent a true hernia. Spontaneous closure occurs in the majority of cases (60% by 2 years of age) and it appears that not all PPVs develop into inguinal hernias. Nevertheless, some justify a contralateral exploration in children who are at high anesthetic risk, when distance and transportation issues may impede the return of an infant to the hospital, and if the child is at risk for subsequent development for an inguinal hernia (children with VP shunts, connective tissue disorders, family history of bilateral inguinal hernias).

UH are a result of intestinal protrusion through an incompletely closed, contracting umbilical ring. Some conditions that predispose an infant to UH include low birth weight infants, Beckwith-Weidemann's syndrome (BWS), Down's syndrome, and ascites. Most UH close after birth and the risk of strangulation or incarceration is extremely low. Most pediatric surgeons defer treatment until 4 or 5 years of age before operating on asymptomatic patients. A relative surgical indication is related to size of the defect: a defect greater than 2 cm is not likely to close spontaneously. Additionally, elective repair is often sought when the patient will be undergoing general anesthetic for a concurrent minor procedure (i.e., inguinal hernia repair, ear tube, orthopedic case, etc.).

FH in infants and children are rare. Because of the similarity in clinical presentation to an indirect inguinal hernia, FH is easily misdiagnosed. Furthermore, the diagnosis may not be made until the patient returns to the clinic with a recurrent inguinal hernia. Thus, any child with recurrency after an adequate inguinal herniorrhaphy should be considered to have a femoral hernia. A high index of suspicion is needed especially when the absence of an expected indirect inguinal hernia is encountered in the operating room. Management consists of approaching the hernia that occupies the femoral canal just medial to the femoral vein; infrainguinal, transinguinal, suprainguinal open approaches are described and additionally laparoscopic diagnosis and repair have been noted.

In this case, the repair of the inguinal hernia should be undertaken in addition to the umbilical hernia due to the size of the umbilical hernia (UH) due to the size of the fascia defect (2 cm), and is therefore unlikely to spontaneously close.

Bibliography

Ikeda H, Suzuki N, Takahashi A, Kuroiwa M, Sakai M, Tsuchida Y. Risk of contralateral manifestation in children with unilateral inguinal hernia: should hernia in children be treated contralaterally? *J Pediatr Surg* 2000;35(12):1746–1748.

Kokoska ER, Weber TR. Umbilical and supraumbilical disease. In: Ziegler MM, Azizkhan RG, Weber TR (eds.), *Operative Pediatric Surgery.* New York, NY: McGraw-Hill, 2003, 537–542.

Lee SL, DuBois JJ. Laparoscopic diagnosis and repair of pediatric femoral hernia: initial experience of four cases. *Surg Endosc* 2000;14:1110–1113.

Lloyd DA. Inguinal and femoral hernias. In: Ziegler MM, Azizkhan RG, Weber TR (eds.), *Operative Pediatric Surgery.* New York, NY: McGraw-Hill, 2003, 543–554.

Nassiri SJ. Contralateral exploration is not mandatory in unilateral inguinal hernia in children: a prospective 6-year study. *Pediatr Surg Int* 2002;18:470–471.

Wolfson PJ. Inguinal hernia. In: Mattei P (ed.), *Surgical Directives Pediatric Surgery.* Philadelphia, PA: Lippincott, Williams & Wilkins, 2002, 521–525.

34. **(B)** UDT or cryptorchidism indicates a testis, which has failed to descend to the scrotum and is located at any point along the normal path of descent or at an ectopic site. The reported incidence is from 2 to 5% of all full-term newborn males, whereas the rate increases to 25% in premature and small-for-GA neonates. The mechanisms of normal testicular descent are multifactorial and include an intact hypothalamic-pituitary-testicular axis along with functional mechanical and neural components. The process of testicular descent has been proposed to occur in two steps; the first step is the movement of the testis from the retroperitoneum to the internal inguinal ring (controlled by Mullerian inhibiting substance from Sertoli cells). The secondary phase involves the migration of the testis from the internal inguinal ring to the scrotum (androgen dependent phase and mediated by genitofemoral nerve release of calcitonin gene-related peptide). Disorders that are associated with cryptorchidism include chromosomal syndromes, anterior abdominal wall abnormalities, cerebral and/or neuromuscular disorders, and endocrine dysfunction.

If unrecognized, the UDT will undergo degenerative changes and about one-third of UDT lack germ cells by the age of 2. Spermatic cord torsion and incarcerated inguinal hernias are also potential problems if the testicle is left untreated. The most important long-term complications of cryptorchidism are infertility and testicular germ cell cancer (the risk is highest in men who have had an intraabdominal testis). The malignancy risk does not lessen with orchidopexy in cases of delayed treatment.

The goal of diagnosis is to identify the presence or absence of a testis. The physical examination should evaluate the genitalia and the presence of scrotal asymmetry, which is suggestive of UDT. Because a retractile testis can be confused with cryptorchidism secondary to cremasteric muscle hyperactivity, the patient should be positioned to inhibit the reflex (upright, crossed-legged). Additional methods to reduce the cremasteric reflex include a warm environment, warm hands, and distracting the patient. An UDT is one that does not stay within the scrotal sac without overstretching the spermatic cord. UDT can be further classified in terms of whether they arrested in the normal line of descent (superficial inguinal pouch, canalicular, or intraabdominal), are ectopic, or are absent. Ectopic sites such as prepenile, femoral, and perineal locations should be examined in cases of a nonpalpable testicle. Infants, who are younger than 1 year of age, with suspected UDT should be reexamined at 3 and 6 months because spontaneous descent may occur in as many as one-third of patients due to the surge in testosterone, luteinizing hormone (LH), and follicle stimulating hormone (FSH) corresponding to the activation of the hypothalamic-pituitary-gonadal axis. Any testis that remains undescended past 1 year will necessitate treatment to attain scrotal position.

Some argue that preoperative localization of the nonpalpable testis is difficult and an unneeded tool. Specifically, scrotal US is appealing in that it is noninvasive and radiation exposure is negligible yet in the evaluation of an UDT, US has been demonstrated to lack benefit in most boys because it rarely localizes a true nonpalpable testis and when it is located, the testis is palpable in the clinician's office. Nevertheless, US is useful for documenting testicular size in secondary or recurrent cryptorchidism and in evaluating obese males with nonpalpable testes. An alternative that has received attention is gadolinium-infusion magnetic resonance angiogram (Gd-infusion MRA). Lam and colleagues have shown the usefulness of Gd-infusion MRA in the preoperative localization of nonpalpable undescended testes; when compared to conventional MRI, detection rates were 82% (MRI) versus 100% for MRA. Regardless of imaging, the most efficacious tool for locating a nonpalpable testis is laparoscopy.

Treatment options for UDT are either hormonal or surgical. Hormonal therapy with HCG has varied results. Some studies suggest that hormonal therapy is ineffective for UDT, yet HCG therapy is effective in aiding the final descent of retractile testes; thus hormonal therapy may be reserved in cases where retractile testes cannot be differentiated from truly undescended testes. Surgical therapy consists of inguinal orchidopexy for a palpable UDT while a laparoscopic approach may be used to confirm the presence or absence of a testis in nonpalpable cases, then an orchidopexy is performed if a testicle is visualized. The basic principles of an orchidopexy include identification of a testicle, mobilization of the spermatic vessels and vas deferens, isolation and high ligation of the processus vaginalis, and fixation of the testis in the subdartos pouch.

Bibliography

Barthold JS. Undescended testis. In: Mattei P (ed.), *Surgical Directives Pediatric Surgery*. Philadelphia, PA: Lippincott, Williams & Wilkins, 2002, 723–730.

Elder JS. Ultrasonography is unnecessary in evaluating boys with a nonpalpable testis. *Pediatrics* 2002;110(4): 748–751.

Husmann DA, Levy JB. Current concepts in the pathophysiology of testicular undescent. *Urology* 1995;46(2): 267–276.

Lam WW, Tam PK, Ai VH, Chan KL, Cheng W, Leong L. Gadolinium-infusion magnetic resonance angiogram: a new, noninvasive, and accurate method of preoperative localization of impalpable Undescended testes. *J Pediatr Surg* 1998;33(1):123–126.

Puri P. Cryptorchidism. In: Ziegler MM, Azizkhan RG, Weber TR (eds.), *Operative Pediatric Surgery*. New York, NY: McGraw-Hill, 2003, 555–562.

35. **(B)** Neuroblastoma (NB) is a childhood malignancy that has been described as "one of the most fascinating but frustrating of childhood neoplasms." With approximately 500 new cases diagnosed yearly, NB is known as the most common solid extracranial malignancy in children, accounting for 10–15% of pediatric neoplasms. The tumor originates from embryonal neural crest cells that can occur anywhere along the sympathetic nervous system from the neck to the pelvis. While the site of the tumor dictates clinical symptoms, in 50% of cases children present with an abdominal mass as the tumor arises from the adrenal gland. Diverse clinical variability is a hallmark of this malignancy; in children younger than 1 year of age, the tumor shows lower stage disease (1, 2, and 4s) and in a majority of cases spontaneously regresses whereas in children diagnosed older than 1 year of age NB presents as progressive, advanced stage disease (3 and 4) with poor prognosis. As a consequence, the progression of NB may follow one of three outcomes: (i) spontaneous regression, (ii) differentiation from malignant to benign, or (iii) progression to malignant disease. Specific biologic and genetic factors associated with NB have been identified and aid in determining not only clinical behavior but also directing therapy regimens, which may include surgery, chemotherapy, and/or radiotherapy depending on stage and age of presentation. Biologic factors associated with NB include serum ferritin, lactate dehydrogenase, nerve growth factor receptor TRK-A/B, and CD44. Other markers have been shown to be correlated with NB and include neuron-specific enolase, ganglioside GD2, neuronal peptide Y, chromogranin A, telomerase, and proliferating cell nuclear antigen (PCNA). Genetic analysis has provided important chromosomal aberrations correlating to NB the most common include DNA ploidy changes, deletions of chromosomal arms 1 p and 11q, amplification of MYCN oncogene, and gains of chromosome 17q.

Alteration in p53 is one of the most common biochemical findings in human malignancy. Mutant p53 fails to place restraints on cell growth and division allowing for unruly amplification and cellular inability to enter apoptosis, thus contributing to a neoplastic state. In NB, the role of p53 is less clear. p53 has not been shown to directly contribute to the pathogenesis of this disease. However, work on p73, a member of the p53 family of proteins, has recently shown that different isomers of this protein may be relevant to the role of NB formation and propagation. N-terminal truncated isoforms of p73 have shown to have oncogenic properties such that full-length variants induce apoptosis while shorter, truncated isoforms of p73 inhibit apoptosis and may induce neoplastic changes.

NB screening has been in place in Japan, Canada, and Europe to answer the question of whether prognostic improvement can be achieved in infants afflicted with NB. The screening tool, which is based on the observation that most NB produces catecholamines, consists of a urine sample from patients that is analyzed for catecholamine markers [vanillylmandelic acid (VMA) and homovanillic acid (HMA)]. Present results have determined that screening does not reduce mortality. These studies have shown that mass-screening negative, later presenting NB usually present with advanced disease. Future direction in the diagnosis of NB will be targeted toward identifying higher-risk patients early as survival remains dismal (barely above 30%) despite aggressive multimodal therapy.

While the clinical symptomology of NB varies on the primary location of the tumor, in the case presented the child has periorbital ecchymosis and proptosis (known as "panda eyes" or "raccoon eyes") which is consistent with intracranial tumor metastasis. The CT scan of the abdomen shows a retroperitoneal mass arising from the upper pole of the left kidney.

Bibliography

Brodeur GM, Maris JM, Yamashiro DJ, Hogarty MD, White PS. Biology and genetics of human neuroblastomas. *J Pediatr Hematol Oncol* 1997:19(2):93–101.

Hasse GM, La Quaglia MP. Neuroblastoma. In: Ziegler MM, Azizkhan RG, Weber TR (eds.), *Operative Pediatric Surgery.* New York, NY: McGraw-Hill, 2003, 1181–1191.

Romani M, Tonini GP, Banelli B, Allemanni G, Mazzocco K, Scaruffi P, Boni L, Ponzoni M, Pagnan G, Raffaghello L, Ferrini S, Croce M, Casciano I. Biological and clinical role of p73 in neuroblastoma. *Cancer Lett* 2003;197(1–2): 151–155.

Schilling FH, Spix C, Berthold F, Erttmann R, Fehse N, Hero B, Klein G, Sander J, Schwartz, Treuner J, Zorn U, Michaelis J. Neuroblastoma screening at one year of age. *N Engl J Med* 2002;346(14):1047–1053.

Suita S. Mass screening for neuroblastoma in Japan: lessons learned and future directions. *J Pediatr Surg* 2002;37(7): 949–954.

Woods WG, Gao RN, Shuster JJ, Robison LL, Bernstein M, Weitzman S, Bunin G, Levy I, Brossard, Dougherty G, Tuchman M, Lemieux B. Screening of infants and mortality due to neuroblastoma. *N Engl J Med* 2002;346(14): 1041–1046.

36. **(C)** The CT scan demonstrated shows a large, spherical intrarenal mass with a well-defined rim of compressed renal parenchyma consistent with WT. Nephroblastoma or WT is the most common malignant primary renal tumor of childhood and makes up approximately 6% of all pediatric cancers. The peak incidence of Wilms' is between 2 and 3 years of age with typical presentation of an abdominal mass appreciated by a parent while the child is being bathed or dressed. Other presenting signs and symptoms may include hypertension, hematuria, malaise, pain, weight loss, and left-sided varicocele (secondary to tumor extension into the left renal vein and subsequent obstruction of the spermatic vein). Several congenital disorders are often seen with WT. Conditions known to have an association with WT include WAGR (WT, aniridia, genitourinary malformations, and mental retardation) syndrome, BWS (omphalocele, visceromegaly, macroglossia, and gigantism), Denys-Drash's syndrome (WT, intersex disorders, and nephropathy), sporadic aniridia, isolated hemihypertrophy, and nephropathy with a female genotype/phenotype.

The genetic evaluation of Wilms' has revealed that there are two main loci that are responsible for both hereditary and sporadic forms of WT. Deletions in the band 13 on the short arm of chromosome 11 (WT1 gene) or the band 15 on chromosome 11 (WT2 gene) have been shown to not only be involved in the predisposition of WT but also some of the congenital syndromes associated with WT. Additional genes for WT include 16q, 1p, and 17p (p53).

Evaluation of a child with a suspected WT should begin with an US to determine if the mass is intrarenal or extrarenal and evaluation of the inferior vena cava (IVC) for flow and tumor thrombus. A CT should follow to evaluate the contralateral kidney, function of the kidneys, and for planning surgical and radiation therapy. Therapy is based on the stage of disease; factors guiding staging are disease extent, primary tumor respectability, lymph node status, adjacent organ involvement, presence of metastatic disease, and contralateral kidney involvement. Management of WT is based on protocols established by the National Wilms' Tumor Study Group (NWTSG) and the International Society of Pediatric Oncology (SIOP) cooperative groups.

Controversial areas in the management of WT are related to different therapeutic protocols; such issues include preresection biopsy, preoperative chemotherapy, preoperative imaging of the contralateral kidney, and partial nephrectomy. With regards to preresection biopsy, current protocols forego preoperative biopsy and proceed with either primary surgical therapy (NWTSG) or preresection chemotherapy (SIOP). However, in some cases (bilateral tumor, tumor expansion into the IVC above the hepatic veins, and tumor inoperability at exploration), biopsy is undertaken. Biopsy can be achieved open or percutaneously. Arguments against percutaneous biopsy are inability to collect adequate tissue specimen, needle tract reoccurrence, and lack of thorough exploration and inability to sample lymph nodes or inspect for tumor extension. Neoadjuvant chemotherapy is used in cases described above. Additionally, the benefits of preoperative chemotherapy include decreasing the incidence of tumor rupture, tumor debulking, and avoiding radiotherapy in the presence of metastatic disease. However, one of the major concerns with routine use of preoperative chemotherapy is the accuracy of posttherapy staging; unfavorable histology may result which could potentially lead to unnecessary intensification of therapy. Radiographic imaging to determine contralateral disease has been a subject of debate. The argument stems from whether the contralateral kidney can be reliably assessed with imaging or if surgical exploration is required. Seven percent of bilateral tumors have been reported to be missed by preoperative imaging and up to 50% of tumors measuring less than 1 cm cannot be detected by preoperative imaging techniques. Of importance is the surgical complication rate for this malignancy has been shown to increase when preoperative imaging fails to provide the correct diagnosis. Partial nephrectomy in WT is most commonly used for bilateral disease. Additionally, it is advocated for cases of WT complicated by a solitary kidney or renal insufficiency. The issue of parenchymal sparing procedures for unilateral WT is questionable. The incidence of renal dysfunction in patients with unilateral WT is low; however, one reason for pursuing renal preserving surgery is the concern for later developing renal dysfunction secondary to hyperfiltration damage to remaining nephrons. One dilemma for the subject of partial nephrectomy and unilateral disease is the potential for residual disease and higher rates of local reoccurrence compared with radical nephrectomy. Some advocate the role of preoperative chemotherapy as an integral component in achieving successful outcomes with unilateral WT and renal sparing surgery.

Nevertheless, while the issues of WT protocols continue to be further defined, the outcomes achieved from cooperative groups place WT among pediatric malignancies where survival rates are high.

Anatomically the kidneys are supplied by renal arteries, which branch directly from the abdominal aorta slightly inferior to the branching point of the SMA. The renal arteries travel to each kidney, each one *posterior* to its respective renal vein, which drain directly into the IVC. Of interest, the "nutcracker phenomenon" or left renal vein entrapment syndrome occurs when compression of the left renal vein between the abdominal aorta and the SMA as it passes medially to join the IVC (Fig. 34-31).

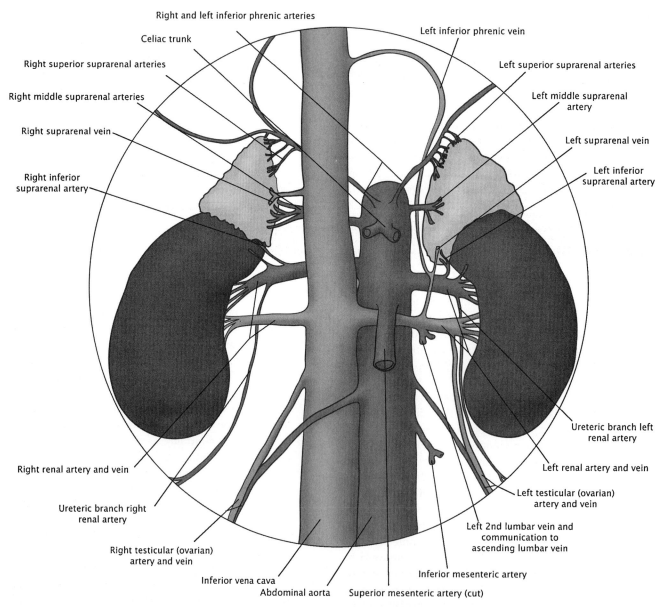

Right and left inferior phrenic arteries
Celiac trunk
Right superior suprarenal arteries
Right middle suprarenal arteries
Right suprarenal vein
Right inferior suprarenal artery
Right renal artery and vein
Ureteric branch right renal artery
Right testicular (ovarian) artery and vein
Inferior vena cava
Abdominal aorta

Left inferior phrenic vein
Left superior suprarenal arteries
Left middle suprarenal artery
Left suprarenal vein
Left inferior suprarenal artery
Ureteric branch left renal artery
Left renal artery and vein
Left testicular (ovarian) artery and vein
Left 2nd lumbar vein and communication to ascending lumbar vein
Inferior mesenteric artery
Superior mesenteric artery (cut)

FIG. 34-31   Renal and adrenal vasculature

Bibliography

Blakely ML, Ritchey ML. Controversies in the management of Wilms' Tumor. *Semin Pediatr Surg* 2001;10(3):127–131.

Davidoff AM, Shochat SJ. Nephroblastoma (Wilms' Tumor). In: Ziegler MM, Azizkhan RG, Weber TR (eds.), *Operative Pediatric Surgery*. New York, NY: Mcgraw-Hill, 2003, 1169–1180.

de Schepper A. "Nutcracker" phenomenon of the renal vein and venous pathology of the left kidney. *J Belge Radiol* 1972;55(5):507–511.

Farhat W, McLorie G, Capolicchio G. Wilms' Tumor. Surgical considerations and controversies. *Pediatr Urolog Clin North Am* 2000;27(3):455–462.

37. **(D)** RMS accounts for over 50% of all soft tissue sarcomas in children and are the third most common solid malignancy in children. While about 250 cases are diagnosed yearly, RMS constitutes one of the pediatric neoplasms that can present as a disseminated tumor in early childhood (other tumors that can present as disseminated masses are infantile myofibromatosis, NB, and lymphomas). In adults this malignancy (i.e., urinary bladder and CBD) generally arises in the extremities whereas in children RMS can occur anywhere in the body including in sites where there is no skeletal muscle (e.g., urinary bladder, CBD). The most common sites are the head and neck or the genitourinary system. Biologically, RMS is one of the small, round, blue-cell neoplasms that arises from the embryonal mesenchyme (NBs, Ewing's sarcoma, peripheral neural ectodermal tumors, non-Hodgkin's lymphoma, and soft tissue sarcomas are other small cell tumors). Five major subtypes of RMS exist (embryonal, alveolar, botryoid, spindle-cell, and pleomorphic) yet embryonal and alveolar are the two major subtypes.

As with most solid tumors, the site of RMS presentation usually reflects clinical symptoms. Nevertheless, diagnosis requires tissue examination, which may be attained by a variety of methods which include fine-needle, core biopsy, incisional biopsy, or endoscopic techniques. Specifically, extremity/truncal RMS lesions should be excised or biopsied through an incision in line with the anticipated incision for future resection. Therefore, a longitudinal biopsy incision should be made in a mass presenting on an extremity such that future resection is not hindered. Additionally, the regional lymph node status in patients with extremity RMS has important impact on survival, thus lymph nodes may be evaluated by lymphatic mapping with sentinel node biopsy; although limited information exists on sentinel node biopsy for children.

Cooperative groups [SIOP and Intergroup Rhabdomyosarcoma Study (IRS)] for RMS are used to classify and stage RMS and are employed to determine treatment protocols. While surgical intervention plays a key role in the management of this disease, surgery alone has been shown to have poor survival rates. The present management of RMS is multimodal which includes surgery, radiation, and chemotherapy. Survival rates are greater than 70% with multimodal therapy and operative procedures for RMS are less disfiguring and more conservative organ-sparing procedures.

Little is known regarding etiology of RMS, yet genetic evaluation has demonstrated that certain pathways are altered in this malignancy. For example, central regulatory components for RMS are c-Met (tyrosine kinase oncogene), pRB (retinoblastoma), and p53. Simultaneous disruption of these component pathways aggravates the regulation of myogenic growth and differentiation and promotes tumor formation. Additionally, RMS may be associated with Li-Fraumeni's syndrome, which is an autosomal dominant inherited condition due to a germline mutation of the p53 gene. The syndrome has a high incidence of soft-tissue or bony sarcomas, leukemia, brain or adrenal neoplasms, and maternal premenopausal breast cancer.

Bibliography

Cavenee WK. Muscling in on rhabdomyosarcoma. *Nat Med* 2002;8(11):1200–1201.

Neville HL, Andrassy RJ. Rhabdomyosarcoma. In: Mattei P (ed.), *Surgical Directives Pediatric Surgery*. Philadelphia, PA: Lippincott, Williams & Wilkins, 2002, 637–640.

Neville HL, Andrassy RJ, Lally KP, Corpron C, Ross MI. Lymphatic mapping with sentinel node biopsy in pediatric patients. *J Pediatr Surg* 2000;35:961–964.

Schalow EL, Broecker BH. Role of surgery in children with rhabdomyosarcoma. *Med Pediatr Oncol* 2003;41(1):1–6.

38. **(D)** In the case illustrated, the age of the patient and the findings on CT scan, which show a large intrahepatic mass with heterogenous attenuation and well-defined margins with multiple areas of reduced echogenicity, are suggestive of a HB. Primary pediatric hepatic tumors in the US are rare (approximately 120 cases per year), more than two-thirds of cases account for malignant disease. HB and HCC make up greater than 90% of hepatic neoplasms in children. Both of these malignancies have distinct features.

HB is an embryonal tumor that occurs in children less than 3 years of age (average 1 year). A male predominance is seen with HB, usually twice as many males as females. Presentation is typically with asymptomatic progressive abdominal growth within the right upper quadrant that is incidentally noted. Because these tumors present with few symptoms, greater than 60% of HB are diagnosed with advanced stage large, unresectable masses. A majority (90%) of these tumors produce AFP, which is sensitive although not specific marker for the presence of HB, that can be used clinically to monitor the effectiveness of treatment, disease progression, or detect tumor recurrence. Of significance, interpretation of AFP levels may be difficult in some cases due to fetal production of high levels of AFP yet these levels subsequently taper off within the first 8 months after birth. Associated anomalies are not uncommon with HB. The risk of HB is elevated with FAP and BWS suggesting that the genes responsible (chromosomes 5 and 11, respectively) may play a role in the pathogenesis for this malignancy. Initial radiographic evaluation for suspected hepatic malignancies may include US, CT, or MRI to discern whether the mass is benign versus malignant. Furthermore, imaging plays an important role as in other solid tumors not only in diagnosis but in staging and treatment protocols of patients with HB as well. Once malignancy has been suspected, accurate diagnosis is confirmed with an open, laparoscopic, or percutaneous needle biopsy. While several staging systems are used for HB, treatment is based on complete resection of the tumor with employment of neoadjuvant or adjuvant chemotherapy in selected patients with advanced disease. Approximately 75% of children with HB can be cured completely; nevertheless, large tumor burden, multifocal tumors, and metastic disease lead to poor prognosis.

In contrast to HB, HCC is more common in older children (between 12 and 15 years old) and often develops in the presence of underlying liver disease and cirrhosis; this includes viral diseases (especially hepatitis B), metabolic disorders (e.g., chronic cholestasis, tyrosinemia, hemochromatosis, and α-1 antitrypsin) and children with biliary obstructive processes (e.g., BA, primary biliary cirrhosis, and primary sclerosing cholangitis). Clinical signs include hepatomegaly that is occasionally associated with dull epigastric pain. Molecular evidence underlying HCC is limited and includes mutations in p53 and other cell cycle proteins such as pRB, p16, p21, and p27. As with HB, imaging and diagnostic approaches are similar yet treatment outcomes for these patients contrast sharply with HB patients. Treatment for HCC is complete tumor excision as standard chemotherapy is partially effective and response rates are complicated by the fact that HCC belongs to a family of chemoresistant tumors. Alternative therapies include transarterial chemoembolization, cryosurgery, thermotherapy, radiofrequency ablation, and liver transplantation.

Benign liver tumors represent a spectrum of pediatric liver disease for which liver resection may be indicated. Vascular malformations such as cavernous hemangiomas (most common vascular neoplasm of the liver) and hemangioendotheliomas may require resection secondary to development of mass effect with left-to-right cardiac shunting and platelet trapping (Kasabach-Merritt's syndrome). Other benign tumors which may undergo operative management due to symptoms or to establish diagnosis include mesenchymal hamartomas, adenomas, focal nodular hyperplasia, and cysts.

Hepatic metastasis in children is uncommon, yet liver resection is warranted for hepatic tumor extension or for isolated tumor deposits. Nephroblastomas, adrenal cortical carcinomas, pheochromocytomas, and germ cell tumors (GCT) are malignancies which have a tendency for rare hepatic involvement and may require operative resection.

Bibliography

Black CT. Hepatic tumors. In: Ziegler MM, Azizkhan RG, Weber TR (eds.), *Operative Pediatric Surgery*. New York, NY: McGraw-Hill, 2003, 1213–1225.

Czauderna P, Mackinlay G, Perilongo G, Brown J, Shafford E, Aronson D, Chapchap PP, Keeling J, Plaschkes J, Otte JB. Hepatocellular carcinoma in children: results of the first prospective study of the International Society of Pediatric Oncology Group. *J Clin Oncol* 2002;20(12): 2798–2804.

Schnater JM, Kohler SE, Lamers WH, von Schweinitz D, Aronson DC. Where do we stand with hepatoblastoma? A review. *Am Cancer Soc* 2003;98(4):668–678.

Shorter NA, La Quaglia MP. Hepatic malignancies. In: Mattei P (ed.), *Surgical Directives Pediatric Surgery*. Philadelphia, PA: Lippincott, Williams & Wilkins, 2002, 641–643.

39. **(E)** Ovarian tumors in children originate from one of three cell types; germinal epithelium of the urogenital ridge, stromal cell components of the urogenital ridge, or germ cells from the yolk sac. Of importance is age of presentation, since the frequency of tumor type is age-dependent. Age distribution of various ovarian tumors include the following: girls under 4 years typically have sex cord-stromal tumors (granulosa-theca cell and Sertoli-Leydig cell), older teenage females have epithelial tumors (serous or mucinous cystadenoma), and adenocarcinoma tends to occur more in adult females. Regardless, GCT make up from 60 to 74% of all ovarian tumors in females under 18 years of age. GCT represent the most common type of tumor in children. These usually present as an abdominal mass but pain is also a common symptom. Plain abdominal radiography may show coarse calcification, teeth, or bone consistent with a teratoma. US can also be used to visualize a mass or inspect for ovarian torsion. CT better characterizes a mass and aids in tumor extension.

Laboratory studies should include the tumor serum markers AFP, β-HCG, and CA-125. GCT subtypes exist which are based on degree of differentiation; dysgerminomas, endodermal sinus tumors, embryonal carcinomas, choriocarcinoma, and teratomas. Teratomas are the most common GCT and maybe immature, mature, or malignant. In children, the mature teratoma is the most predominant type. Usually, surgery alone is adequate therapy.

Surgical principles regarding ovarian lesions are based on adequately removing tumorous tissue and staging while preserving ovarian tissue if possible. Since it may not be possible to distinguish between benign versus malignant, it is important to recognize that a cancer operation may be necessary [salpingo-oophorectomy and contralateral ovary inspection/biopsy, lymph node sampling (both iliac and retroperitoneal), ascitic fluid cytology or peritoneal washings, peritoneal/diaphragm surface inspection, and infracolic omentectomy]. Entering the abdomen may be achieved by a midline approach or a Pfannensteil incision and some advocate the benefits of laparoscopy yet the verdict on the use of this modality for adenexal pathology is debatable. Aspiration of an ovarian mass with cystic features should never be done because of the uncertainty of malignancy. Parents should be carefully counseled about the risks of future fertility of their child, risks of laparotomy/laparoscopy (tumor spillage and adhesions), and recurrence/malignant tranformation.

In this patient, the large size of the ovarian mass displaced bowel and accounted for the complaints of abdominal pain and constipation. She underwent surgical removal of the lesion (unilateral salpingo-oophorectomy and contralateral biopsy via a Pfannensteil approach) and pathology demonstrated a benign cystic teratoma (see Fig. 34-32; Tables 34-2 and 34-3).

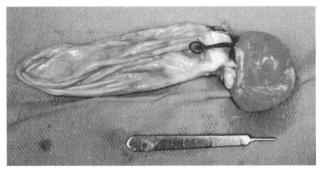

FIG. 34-32 A benign cystic teratoma of the ovary exhibiting multiple tissue types.

TABLE 34-2   Ovarian Tumor Markers and Incidence of Bilaterality*

Tumor	Markers	Bilaterality
Teratoma	+/– AFP	10%
Dysgerminoma	LDH-1	15%
Endodermal sinus tumor	AFP	LOW
Choriocarcinoma	β-HCG	LOW
Epithelial tumors	CA-125	15%

*Abbreviation: AFP, α-fetoprotein; LDH, lactate dehydrogenase; β-HCG, β-human chorionic gonadotropin.

Source.   Reproduced with permission from von Allmen D. Ovarian tumors. In: Mattei P (ed.), *Surgical Directives: Pediatric Surgery.* Philadelphia, PA: Lippincott, Williams & Wilkins, 2003.

Bibliography

Pokorny SF, Garza J. Pediatric and adolescent gynecology. In: Ziegler MM, Azizkhan RG, Weber TR (eds.), *Operative Pediatric Surgery.* New York, NY: McGraw-Hill, 2003, 945–964.

Templeman CL, Fallat ME, Lam AM, Perlman SE, Hertweck SP, O'Connor DM. Managing mature cystic teratomas of the ovary. *Obstet Gynecol Surv* 2000;55(12): 738–745.

von Allmen D. Ovarian tumors. In: Mattei P (ed.), *Surgical Directives Pediatric Surgery.* Philadelphia, PA: Lippincott, Williams & Wilkins, 2002, 653–656.

40. (D) Conjoined twins is one area in congenital malformations that brings much interest and attention to pediatric surgery. Conjoined twinning occurs in approximately 1 in 200,000 live births. The embryologic development of conjoined twins has been examined via experimental embryology of lower animals; the data from these studies have been used to shed light on human malformations. Nevertheless, stages in the early development of an embryo are important to the development of conjoined twinning. Specifically, only the postgestational third and fourth weeks are pertinent to the events of twinning. During this interval, the embryo, which appears as a disk, is growing most rapidly and changing in terms of size, shape, and relative position of one structure to another. By the end of the fourth week, except for the umbilical area, the entire embryo is covered by ectoderm. More importantly is the observation that intact ectoderm will not fuse to one another, thus the locations where there is ectodermal absence or where there are areas destined to break down are analogous to sites where conjoined twins will be united. These include the diaphragm, the heart, the oropharynx or cloacal membrane, neural tube, and the umbilicus. Ultimately these areas give rise to the eight types of twins, which can be organized into three groups based on orientation (ventral, lateral, and dorsal). The spherical theory has emerged to explain the theory of congenital twinning.

(D) The reliability of imaging contralateral tumors is firmly established in these tumors.

(E) Partial nephrectomy is never advocated in patients with unilateral Wilms' tumor (WT).

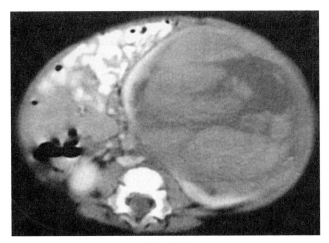

FIG. 34-14

37. A 4-year-old female presented to her primary care physician with fatigue and anorexia over a 2-week period. An abdominal mass was appreciated and a CT confirmed a solid, retroperitoneal lesion (Fig. 34-15). A presumptive diagnosis of NB was made. Intraoperatively, an ovarian mass was noted. Incisional biopsy confirmed the diagnosis of rhabdomyosarcoma (RMS). Which of the statements is *incorrect*?

(A) In adults this tumor occurs primarily in the extremities, while in children RMS can involve nonskeletal muscle sites.

(B) A longitudinal skin incision should be used to biopsy a mass on the upper leg of a 10-year-old boy.

(C) Intra-operatively, a pelvic retroperitoneal mass was noted.

(D) RMS is primarily a surgically treated disease.

(E) Sentinel lymph node biopsy has been used to assess lymph node status in children with RMS.

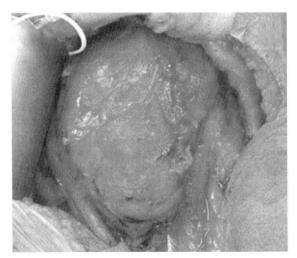

FIG. 34-15 Intraoperative retroperitoneal mass showing right ovarian tissue replaced with tumor.

38. A 2.5-year-old male is referred to a pediatric surgeon for progressive abdominal enlargement. Physical examination reveals a large intraabdominal mass within the right upper quadrant (Fig. 34-16). The lesion crosses the midline and extends toward the pelvis. AFP levels are markedly elevated. This lesion most likely represents

(A) a benign liver tumor

(B) metastatic disease

(C) teratoma

(D) hepatoblastoma (HB)

(E) hepatocellular carcinoma (HCC)

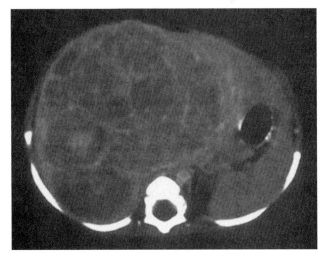

FIG. 34-16

TABLE 34-3   Description and Treatment of Ovarian Neoplams

Tumor	Pathology	Placement	Treatment
Epithelial			
Serous	Benign	20% Bilateral	Unilateral cystectomy, salpingo-oophorectomy, bx other ovary
Mucinous	10% Malignant	Unilateral	Unilateral cystectomy, salpingo-oophorectomy
SCST			
Pure granulosa	Malignant	Unilateral	Unilateral cystectomy, salpingo-oophorectomy
Granulosa/theca	Benign	Unilateral	Unilateral, cystectomy, salpingo-oophorectomy
Theca cell	Benign	Unilateral	Unilateral cystectomy, salpingo-oophorectomy
Sertoli-Leydig	Malignant	Unilateral	Unilateral cystectomy, salpingo-oophorectomy
Gonadoblastoma	Benign	33% Bilateral	Bilateral gonadectomy
Lipid cell	Benign	Unilateral	Unilateral salpingo-Oophorectomy
Germ cell			
Dysgerminoma	Malignant	10–20% Bilateral	Unilateral salpingo-oophorectomy, inspect other ovary, chemo
Endodermal sinus	Malignant	Unilateral	Stage I—Unilateral salpingo-oophorectomy Stage II and higher—Unilateral salpingo-oophorectomy and chemo
Choriocarcinoma	Malignant	Unilateral, with a tendency to be more diffuse	Stage I—Unilateral salpingo-oophorectomy Stage II and higher—TAH-BSO˙ and multi-agent chemo
Immature teratoma	Malignant	Unilateral	Stage I A/B—Unilateral salpingo-oophorectomy with nodal biopsy Stage II+ and grade III+ —Unilateral salpingo-oophorectomy with nodal biopsy
Mature teratoma	Benign	10% Bilateral	Removal of tumor/enucleation
Mixed cell	Mixed	Unilateral	Based on composition, but mostly surgical removal and chemo

˙Total abdominal hysterectomy-bilateral salpingo-oophorectomy.
Source. Used/Reproduced with permission from Pokorny SF, Garza J. Pediatric and adolescent gynecology. In: Ziegler MM, Azizkhan RG, Weber TR (eds.), *Operative Pediatric Surgery.* New York, NY: McGraw-Hill, 2003.

This theory proposes that two embryonic discs lying adjacent to one another at various angles and planes float on a the surface of one sphere (yolk sac) and become secondarily fused rostrally, caudally, laterally, or dorsally to result in all types of conjoined twins. Fission of the early fertilized ovum to produce two separate embryos results in monozygotic twins. There are some proponents that support an abnormal fission or division theory to account for conjoined twins but a major criticism of this theory is the mechanism to produce all types of twinning remains undefined.

Diagnosis of conjoined twins is usually made prenatally via US for maternal evaluation of large GA or polyhydramnios. At birth the infants are usually assessed for survivability and the presence of other anomalies. Postnatal evaluation may also include a wide array of radiographic studies to help delineate shared structures and organs. If stable, a well-orchestrated diagnostic and separation procedure may be planned. Surgical intervention is planned usually between 4 and 6 weeks of age in order for the twins to gain weight, pass the neonatal period, and allow for tissue expanders to be placed if required. Survival outcomes are encouraging for surgical separation of conjoined twins. Of vital success for these undertakings is the need to have an accurate preoperative evaluation, a multidisciplinary team of specialists, previous experience, and detailed operative and postoperative management.

Bibliography

Hilfiker ML. Conjoined twins. In: Ziegler MM, Azizkhan RG, Weber TR (eds.), *Operative Pediatric Surgery.* New York, NY: McGraw-Hill, 2003, 1063–1072.

Spencer R. Theoretical and analytical embryology of conjoined twins: part I: embryogenesis. *Clin Anat* 2000;13:36–53.

Spitz L, Kiely EM. Experience in the management of conjoined twins. *Br J Surg* 2002;89(9):1188–1192.

CHAPTER 35

Neurosurgery

Richard B. Rodgers and Julius M. Goodman

Questions

1. An 18-year-old male presents to the emergency room (ER) by ambulance after a motor vehicle accident. He was unconscious at the scene and given a Glasgow Coma Score (GCS) of 3. He was intubated and received 1 L of normal saline en route. On evaluation in the ER, he has obvious head trauma. With deep painful stimuli he will very briefly open his eyes, extend his right upper extremity, and reach for the painful stimulus with his left upper extremity. His lower extremities are flaccid and do not move with any stimulation. He does not follow commands. His GCS now is

   (A) 5
   (B) 6
   (C) 7
   (D) 8

2. A 21-year-old college student is admitted with a GCS of 5 after a motor vehicle accident. A computed tomography (CT) scan (Fig. 35-1) shows loss of cisterns. An intracranial pressure (ICP) monitor reveals a pressure of 35 torr. He is treated with ventricular drainage, mannitol, and high-dose barbiturate-induced coma. On day 3 his pupils are large and fixed and the ICP monitor reads 60 torr. Brain death is suspected and organ donation is being considered. The best method of declaring brain death would be

   (A) isotope flow study
   (B) isotope flow study after normalization of barbiturate level

   (C) normalization of barbiturate level and check for brain stem reflexes and absence of spontaneous respiration, then make clinical decision
   (D) normalization of barbiturate level and check for brain stem reflexes and absence of respiration, then perform electroencephalogram (EEG)

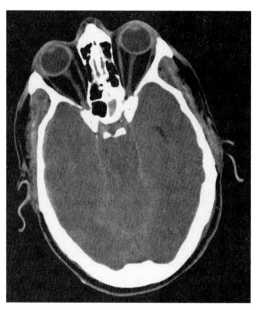

FIG. 35-1 Non-contrasted CT of the head, revealing absence of cerebrospinal fluid cisterns and loss of the normal gray matter-white matter interface.

Questions 3 and 4

A 35-year-old male is involved in a high-speed motor vehicle accident. There was a prolonged extrication, and he was intubated at the scene. On arrival to the emergency department, he is given a GCS of 4. Head CT scan is consistent with diffuse injury without operative hematoma, and basilar skull fracture. CT of the abdomen and pelvis reveals a liver laceration. He is hemodynamically stable after large volume resuscitation including two units of packed red blood cells. An ICP monitor is placed and he is admitted to the intensive care unit (ICU) with intravenous fluids 0.9NaCl with 20 meq KCl/L at 11/2 times maintenance. His ICP is 15–18 mmHg.

Eighteen hours after admission, the patient's urine output increases to 350 cc/h. Serum Na is 150 and urine specific gravity is 1.004. Central venous pressure by subclavian catheter is 7 mmHg.

3. The most likely explanation for the patient's current status is

    (A) syndrome of inappropriate antidiuretic hormone (SIADH)
    (B) neurogenic diabetes insipidus (DI)
    (C) normal diuresis after large volume resuscitation
    (D) cerebral salt wasting (CSW)

4. The most appropriate treatment for the above patient at this time is

    (A) continue 0.9NaCl with 20 meq KCl/L, decrease rate to maintenance
    (B) replace urinary water losses and treat polyuria as needed with aqueous vasopressin
    (C) change IVF to D5 0.45NaCl with 20 meq KCl/L at maintenance rate
    (D) continue current management, recheck electrolytes in 8 h

5. A 16-year-old boy is seen in the ER after falling out of a tree. He is awake and alert (GCS 15) but has blood draining from his right ear. There is swelling of the scalp in the right temporal area and a laceration over the occiput. He is neurologically intact. After several hours it is apparent that he is having spinal fluid otorrhea. It is elected not to start antibiotics. A CT scan of the head without contrast is normal. The following morning he is wide awake but he has had the acute onset of a left hemiplegia. There is a light ptosis of the right lid. The right pupil is slightly smaller than the left and the extraocular muscles are normal. The most likely diagnosis is

    (A) right epidural hematoma
    (B) right subdural hematoma
    (C) evolving right temporal lobe contusion
    (D) stroke of the right hemisphere

6. Appropriate treatment is begun in the above patient. Two days later his hemiplegia has not improved and he is now comatose. The right ptosis is worse and the right pupil is large, oval, and poorly reactive. A repeat CT scan (Fig. 35-2) shows massive swelling of the right hemisphere. The best chance for saving this patient would be

    (A) mannitol
    (B) ventriculostomy
    (C) high-dose dexamethasone
    (D) decompressive craniotomy

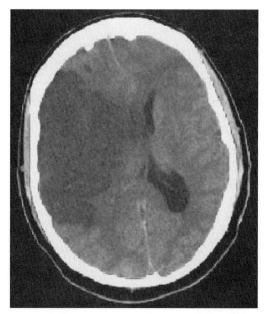

FIG. 35-2 Non-contrasted CT of the head.

Questions 7 through 9

An 18-year-old female is an unrestrained driver in a motor vehicle accident in which she struck her head and face on the windshield. She is neurologically intact after a brief loss of consciousness at the scene. A CT scan of the head reveals no evidence of brain injury, but there are nasal and facial fractures. She is admitted for observation. The following morning, she complains of bloody fluid leaking from her nose. You suspect the fluid is blood mixed with cerebrospinal fluid (CSF).

7. The *most specific* test to confirm CSF rhinorrhea in this situation is

    (A) clear halo around bloody drop on a gauze pad
    (B) fluid glucose level
    (C) fluid beta transferrin level
    (D) CT cisternogram

8. Your suspicions are confirmed in the above patient. The most appropriate treatment is

    (A) lumbar CSF drainage for 5 days
    (B) craniotomy for intradural repair of CSF fistula
    (C) transnasal repair of CSF fistula
    (D) observation with head of bed elevation

9. The plastic surgeon would like to repair her facial fractures. Which of the following is most appropriate?

    (A) proceed with facial fracture repair
    (B) wait for the CSF fistula to spontaneously resolve before operative repair of fractures
    (C) wait 2 weeks for repair of fractures due to increased risk of meningitis
    (D) combined procedure with facial fracture repair and repair of CSF fistula

10. A 32-year-old male presents to the emergency department complaining of redness and swelling of his right eye, right-sided headache, and double vision. In a motor vehicle accident 2 months ago he sustained a mild concussion and basilar skull fracture. On physical examination, he has right proptosis of 7 mm, the edema and hyperemia of the conjunctiva of his right eye, and complete external ophthalmoplegia. The most likely diagnosis is

    (A) carotid-cavernous sinus fistula
    (B) orbital pseudotumor
    (C) ethmoid sinusitis
    (D) traumatic aneurysm in the cavernous sinus

11. A 30-year-old woman presents with right-sided facial pain, transient loss of vision in the right eye, paralysis of the right side of the tongue, and a right Horner's syndrome. Results of CT of the head prompted cerebral angiography, which is shown in Fig. 35-3. The most important treatment for this patient is

    (A) heparin
    (B) endarterectomy
    (C) stent placement
    (D) aspirin

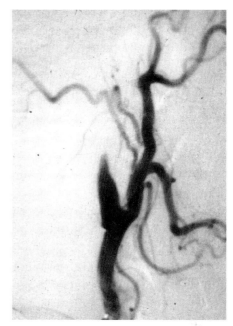

FIG. 35-3 Right common carotid arteriogram.

12. A very anxious 25-year-old male patient is 21 days s/p complete C6 spinal cord injury (SCI). He is on multiple medications. He develops sudden hypertension, sweating of the face, piloerection, and bradycardia. He is awake and alert, complaining of headache. The most appropriate intervention at this point would be

    (A) insert urinary catheter
    (B) stop haloperidol and treat neuroleptic malignant syndrome
    (C) order pulmonary ventilation/perfusion scan to check for pulmonary embolus
    (D) stop anticholinergic medications

13. A 65-year-old female is s/p right-sided carotid endarterectomy (CEA). The procedure was complicated by injury to the right hypoglossal nerve. Which of the following would be found on physical examination?

    (A) She would have no pin prick sensation on the right side of her tongue.
    (B) Her tongue would deviate to the left when sticking out.
    (C) Her tongue would deviate to the right when sticking out.
    (D) She would have no taste on the right side of her tongue.

Questions 14 and 15

A 17-year-old male undergoes a cervical lymph node biopsy. A diagnosis of Hodgkin's disease is made. When seen for suture removal, he complains of severe pain in his shoulder and he is unable to elevate the shoulder and abduct the right arm.

14. The most likely diagnosis is

    (A) injury to the upper trunk of the brachial plexus
    (B) injury to the axillary nerve
    (C) injury to the spinal accessory nerve
    (D) injury to the suprascapular nerve

15. After 3 months there is no clinical evidence of recovery. Which of the following statements is most appropriate?

    (A) Physical therapy with no attempt to repair the nerve because such a nerve injury causes minimal disability.
    (B) Electromyogram (EMG) shows electrical evidence of recovery. Observation should continue.
    (C) Explore the wound and do a primary repair if at all possible.
    (D) Explore the wound and be prepared to do a nerve graft if there is any tension on the anastomosis.

16. During exploration of a gunshot wound (GSW) to the elbow, there is noted to be complete transection of the ulnar nerve. Both severed ends are identifiable. The most appropriate treatment would be

    (A) primary nerve repair after extensive mobilization of proximal and distal ends to avoid any tension on suture line
    (B) primary nerve repair and immobilization of extremity in marked flexion to prevent tension on suture line

    (C) no repair, even though the proximal and distal stumps can be easily approximated in this fresh wound
    (D) nerve graft with sural nerve and transposition away from the damaged tissue

Questions 17 and 18

A 19-year-old college student serves as a pallbearer at the funeral of a friend who was killed in a motor vehicle accident. Shortly after the funeral he develops numbness in his fingers of the right hand. That night he has difficulty sleeping because of discomfort in the entire right upper extremity and worsening paresthesias of all of his fingers. He comes to the ER 6 days later because of weakness in his right hand and aching of the upper extremity. Paresthesias waken him at night and are accentuated by driving a car and holding up a book. He frequently shakes his hand for relief.

17. The most likely diagnosis is

    (A) median nerve neuropathy at the wrist
    (B) ulnar nerve neuropathy at the elbow
    (C) C7 radiculopathy
    (D) C8 radiculopathy

18. The best way to make this diagnosis would be

    (A) careful neurologic examination
    (B) EMG of the upper extremity
    (C) MRI of the cervical spine
    (D) x-rays of the right wrist

Questions 19 and 20

A 32-year-old woman slips on a wet floor in a supermarket and falls on her outstretched right arm. She has the immediate onset of pain in her wrist. When seen in the local ER examination reveals that all of her peripheral nerves are intact and the injury appears trivial. The patient's pain continues. Early and delayed x-rays of the wrist show no fracture. When seen in the pain clinic 8 weeks later, her symptoms seem out of proportion to the injury. She complains of burning pain in the right hand and discomfort of the entire upper extremity. Even a mild sensory stimulus to the hand produces severe pain (allodynia) and a mildly painful stimulus results in horrible discomfort (hyperpathia). She is anxious, depressed, and has difficulty sleeping. Repeat examination reveals all of the peripheral nerves remain intact. The forearm and hand are cool and dry, there is loss of hair, and the fingernails are long and uncut. Her joints are stiff and she refuses to use her hand. In fact, there appears to be spasms of the involved limb—the fourth and fifth fingers are flexed and the arm is held in adduction with the elbow flexed. She is considering litigation.

19. The most likely diagnosis is

(A) conversion reaction

(B) causalgia

(C) complex regional pain syndrome 1

(D) complex regional pain syndrome 2

20. Which of the following would probably have the *least* value to treating this patient?

(A) psychotherapy

(B) surgical sympathectomy

(C) dorsal column stimulation

(E) intrathecal baclofen

21. A 64-year-old diabetic male develops pain in the right back and hip followed several days later by severe sciatica. On examination he has weakness of the right quadriceps muscle and absence of the right knee and both ankle reflexes. The rest of his leg muscles have good strength. An MR scan is obtained (Fig. 35-4). The most likely diagnosis is

(A) a herniated disc at L5-S1 with S1 nerve root compression

(B) a herniated disc at L4-5 with L5 nerve root compression

(C) a herniated disc at L3-4 with L4 nerve root compression

(D) proximal diabetic neuropathy

22. A 72-year-old male has severe discomfort in both lower extremities when he attempts to walk more than half a city block. His symptoms are relieved by rest. He has no back pain. His neurologic examination is normal. His pedal pulses are very difficult to palpate, but Doppler vascular studies suggest only moderate vascular insufficiency. An MR of the lumbar spine (Fig. 35-5) reveals spinal stenosis at L3-4 and L4-5. The clinicians must decide whether the patient is suffering from vascular or neurogenic claudication. Which of the following would probably be most useful in this situation?

(A) myelogram followed by CT of lumbar spine

(B) aortogram with run off

(C) a more detailed history

(D) EMG and nerve conduction studies of the lower extremities

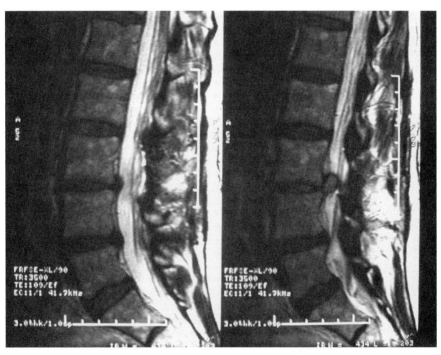

FIG. 35-4 Sagittal T2-weighted MRI of the lumbosacral spine.

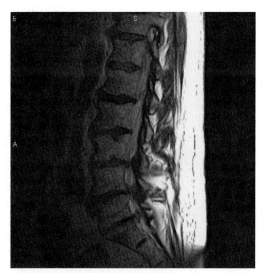

FIG. 35-5   Sagittal T2-weighted MRI of the lumbosacral spine.

23. A 26-year-old male undergoes a routine microlumbar discectomy at left L4-5. He is obese and there is considerable epidural bleeding. When he arrives in the recovery room the nurse notes that his blood pressure is 70/30 mm Hg and his pulse is 140. Emergency management should consist of

    (A) treatment for sepsis after drawing blood for cultures
    (B) immediate exploration of the wound
    (C) intense fluid resuscitation and observation
    (D) immediate laparotomy

24. A 37-year-old male with insulin-dependent diabetes mellitus has sudden onset of low back pain radiating down both legs and urinary incontinence. On physical examination, he has a left-sided foot drop and loss of bilateral Achilles reflexes. He has hypalgesia on the bottoms of his feet and in his perineum. Magnetic resonance imaging (MRI) of the lumbar spine is obtained (Fig. 35-6). The most likely diagnosis is

    (A) ependymoma of the filum terminale
    (B) epidural abscess
    (C) herniated L4-5 intervertebral disc
    (D) infarct of the conus medullaris

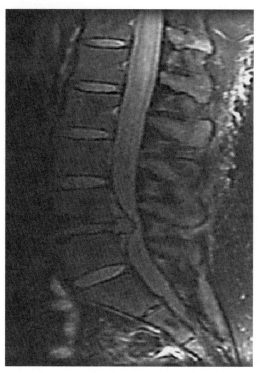

FIG. 35-6   Sagittal MRI of the lumbosacral spine.

25. A 47-year-old male with insulin-dependent diabetes mellitus and chronic renal failure on hemodialysis presents with fever, malaise, and localized signs of infection of his left forearm arteriovenous fistula. He is admitted and placed on intravenous antibiotics. On admission and throughout his hospitalization he has complained of neck pain requiring opioids. On the fourth hospital morning he is found to be quadriparetic. MRI is obtained (Fig. 35-7). The most appropriate next step in this patient's management is

    (A) steroids and high-dose antibiotics
    (B) anterior decompression of infected vertebral body
    (C) percutaneous aspiration
    (D) laminectomy

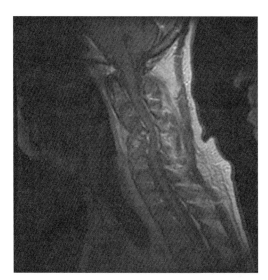

FIG. 35-7   Sagittal T1-weighted MRI with contrast of the cervical spine.

26. A 67-year-old male presents with occasional incontinence of urine. His urologist said his prostate and bladder are normal. He also states that he has been having trouble walking for a few weeks, like his feet are "glued to the ground." His family physician has found no evidence of paresis or spinal cord dysfunction on examination of his lower extremities. His wife tells you that during the past several months he has fallen once or twice a week, and he has trouble remembering recent events. He denies any headaches. This patient's history is most consistent with

  (A) brain tumor

  (B) chronic subdural hematoma

  (C) Alzheimer's disease

  (D) normal pressure hydrocephalus (NPH)

27. A 46-year-old female presents to the emergency department with the worst headache of her life. She has a 40 pack-year history of smoking, migraine headaches, mitral valve prolapse, and is 4 years s/p right-sided modified radical mastectomy followed by appropriate adjuncts for breast cancer. She has photophobia and also complains of neck pain and nausea. On physical examination she is drowsy but otherwise neurologically intact. There is a heart murmur, and electrocardiogram (ECG) is consistent with myocardial ischemia. CT scan of the head is obtained (Fig. 35-8). The most likely diagnosis for this patient is

  (A) ruptured intracranial aneurysm

  (B) carcinomatous meningitis from metastasic breast cancer

  (C) migraine headache

  (D) septic thromboemboli from valvular heart disease

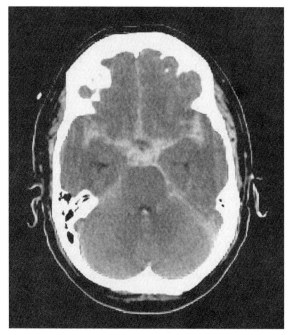

FIG. 35-8   Non-contrasted CT scan of the head.

28. A 29-year-old female who is 5 days postpartum presents with headache, confusion, and lethargy. She becomes unresponsive and has a generalized seizure. Noncontrasted head CT and MRI are shown in Figs. 35-9 and 35-10, respectively. The most appropriate management of this patient includes

  (A) anticoagulation

  (B) steroids

  (C) ventriculostomy

  (D) fresh frozen plasma

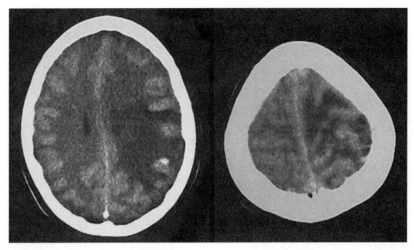

FIG. 35-9   Non-contrasted CT scan of the head, with hypodensity (left greater than right) with small focal hyperdensities in the left cortex.

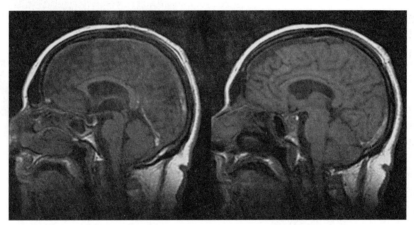

FIG. 35-10   Sagittal T1-weighted MRI without contrast of the brain (midline cuts).

Questions 29 and 30

A 52-year-old male who has always been in good health has the onset of severe paroxysms of facial pain when talking, chewing, brushing his right upper teeth, and eating. An imaging study is performed.

29. The most likely diagnosis is

    (A) a multiple sclerosis (MS) plaque in the pons

    (B) a arteriovenous malformation around the brain stem

    (C) a cerebellar-pontine angle tumor

    (D) compression of the trigeminal nerve by a normal blood vessel

30. The best treatment option for this patient would be

    (A) immunotherapy

    (B) carbamazepine

    (C) posterior fossa microvascular decompression

    (D) gamma knife radiosurgery

Questions 31 and 32

A 36-year-old female presents with pain and loss of vision in her right eye, worsening over 3 days. Her past medical history is significant for left TN treated with carbamazepime for 4 years and depression controlled with sertraline. On neurologic examination, her right eye vision in 20/400, left is 20/40. She has a Marcus-Gunn pupil (afferent pupillary defect) on the right. Her extraocular movements are intact although testing causes increased pain in the eye. Fundoscopic examination reveals no abnormality in either eye.

31. The most likely diagnosis for this patient is

(A) hysteria

(B) carbamazepime toxicity

(C) optic neuritis

(D) amaurosis fugax

32. The most appropriate next step in the above patient's management is

(A) psychologic evaluation

(B) serum carbamazepime level and liver function testing

(C) MRI of the brain and possible lumbar puncture

(D) carotid duplex imaging

33. A 19-year-old female presents to the emergency department via ambulance after having a 5-min long generalized tonic-clonic seizure. She has not yet recovered from the postictal state when she has another generalized seizure of 3 min duration. Her friend tells you that the patient recently immigrated to the United States from Iraq, has had epilepsy since childhood, and takes seizure medicine. You realize this is in status epilepticus (SE). All of the following should be instituted immediately *except*:

(A) lorazepam IV

(B) phenytoin IV

(C) intubation

(D) draw glucose and anticonvulsant levels

34. A 22-year-old female presents with complaints of intermittent bilateral hand tingling, "funny feeling" in her legs, and occasional loss of balance. Her mother says that she stumbles around and bumps into things. On physical examination, she has intact strength in upper and lower extremities. Sensation is intact to

light touch, pinprick, and proprioception on your testing. She has brisk reflexes at the knees and ankles, bilateral Hoffman's signs and equivocal Babinski signs. T2-weighted MRI is shown in Fig. 35-11. The most appropriate surgical intervention for this patient would be

(A) resection of spinal cord tumor

(B) syringosubarachnoid shunt

(C) syringopleural shunt

(D) posterior fossa and upper cervical decompression

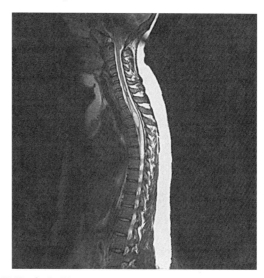

FIG. 35-11 Sagittal T2-weighted MRI from the craniocervical junction through the thoracic spine.

35. A 6-year-old male with hydrocephalus treated with VP shunt since birth presents to the emergency department with acute onset of right lower quadrant abdominal pain, anorexia, nausea, and vomiting. His temperature is 38°C, and peripheral WBC count is 13,000/mL. Abdominal ultrasound reveals an inflamed appendix with thickened mucosa and fecolith. There is no obvious peritoneal fluid collection. The most appropriate treatment would be

(A) appendectomy with externalization of the peritoneal portion of the shunt

(B) appendectomy without manipulation of the shunt

(C) appendectomy with conversion to ventriculo-gall bladder shunt

(D) appendectomy with conversion to ventriculoatrial shunt

36. A 10-month-old child is admitted to the hospital for lethargy, emesis, and failure to thrive. His height and weight are below the tenth percentile for his age. A thorough examination by the pediatrician reveals bilateral retinal hemorrhages, and these are documented by the ophthalmologist (Fig. 35-12). His fontanelle is slightly full. On laboratory evaluation he is anemic and baseline coagulation studies are normal. A CT scan of the head is performed (Fig. 35-13). The most appropriate consultation to assist in this patient's management is

(A) pediatric gastroenterology

(B) pediatric hematology/oncology

(C) medical genetics

(D) social worker and child protective services

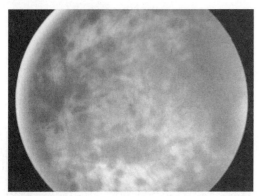

FIG. 35-12   Diffuse retinal hemorrhages, photograph taken with retinal camera.

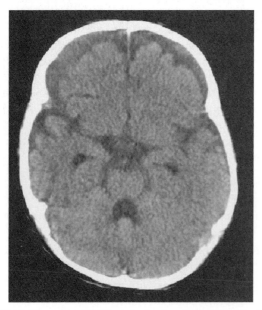

FIG. 35-13   Non-contrasted CT of the head, revealing bilateral subdural hypodense collections, right greater than left.

37. A 5-year-old boy is brought to the office by his parents, who tell you that he wakes with headache on most mornings, and sometimes in the middle of the night. After he is up for a while, he is able to pursue his normal playful activities. On examination, he is neurologically intact. MRI of his brain is shown in Fig. 35-14. All of the following dianoses are likely *except*:

(A) medulloblastoma

(B) ependymoma

(C) astrocytoma

(D) choroid plexus papilloma

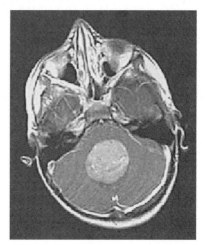

FIG. 35-14

Questions 38 and 39

A 34-year-old man presents with a 3-week history of headaches, lethargy, and vomiting. On examination his optic discs are flat. He has a mild left hemiparesis and a left extensor toe sign. An MR scan of the brain is performed with and without contrast enhancement (Fig. 35-15). The patient improves after starting high-dose dexamethasone.

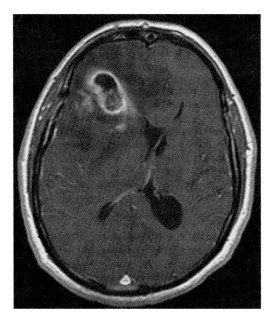

FIG. 35-15   Axial T1-weighted MRI with contrast of the brain, revealing a ring-enhancing lesion in the right frontal lobe, with considerable vasogenic edema and middle shift.

38. The next step in the patient's management should be

   (A) craniotomy with resection of the lesion

   (B) stereotactic needle biopsy and possible delayed craniotomy

   (C) open biopsy with neuronavigation

   (D) metastatic workup followed by an appropriate procedure

39. The patient's condition has stabilized after undergoing appropriate initial and definitive treatment, and he is ready to be released from the hospital. A repeat CT scan done 24 h after the procedure shows no contrast enhancement and complete excision of the lesion. All of the following statements are correct *except*:

   (A) Tumor cells have infiltrated beyond the area of previous enhancement and resection.

   (B) Radiation therapy is the most important next treatment that will prolong life.

   (C) Chemotherapy with carmustine (BCNU) should be administered.

   (D) The patient's young age makes the prognosis worse, even though the tumor appears to have been completely excised.

40. A 57-year-old male with a 60 pack-year smoking history presents with a seizure. His contrasted head CT is shown in Fig. 35-16. His past medical history is only significant for mild chronic obstructive pulmonary disease (COPD). Complete workup reveals a right middle lobe lung lesion. Bronchoscopic biopsy is consistent with adenocarcinoma. The lung lesion is felt to be completely respectable by the thoracic surgeon. There is no further evidence of metastases. The most appropriate management for this patient is

   (A) resection of brain lesion followed by resection of lung lesion, then appropriate adjuvant therapies

   (B) resection of lung lesion, radiation therapy for brain lesion

   (C) resection of lung lesion and radiosurgery for brain lesion

   (D) resection of brain lesion and radiation and chemotherapy for lung lesion

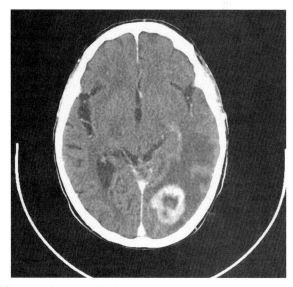

FIG. 35-16   Contrasted CT of the head, revealing enhancing lesion in the left occipital lobe, with surrounding vasogenic edema.

41. A 52-year-old woman with a long history of cigarette smoking presents with a cough and hilar mass. Workup reveals a nonresectable adenocarcinoma of the lung. She is treated with radiation therapy and chemotherapy. Eighteen months later she presents to the ER with a 4-week history of progressive painless paraparesis and dysesthesias in the lower extremities. On examination she is unable to lift her legs off the bed. The knee and ankle reflexes are hyperactive, clonus is present, and there is hypalgesia to pin prick in the lower extremities extending up to the level of the midabdomen. There is sphincter dysfunction. An MR scan shows swelling of the spinal cord in the midthoracic level with high signal intensity on T2-weighted images. There is ring enhancing intrathecal contrast enhancement. The most likely diagnosis is

(A) spinal cord tumor

(B) paraneoplastic necrotizing myelopathy

(C) radiation myelopathy

(D) metastasis to the spinal cord

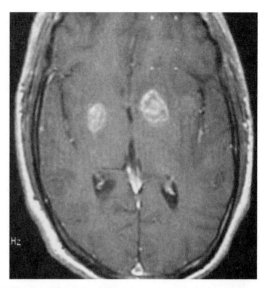

FIG. 35-17   Axial T1-weighted MRI with contrast of the brain, revealing multiple bilateral enhancing lesions of the deep white matter and basal ganglia.

42. A 34-year-old homosexual male presents to the ER with a 1-week history of headache, vomiting, and lethargy. A CT scan obtained in the emergency shows multiple low-density lesions in the basal ganglia and white matter (Fig. 35-17). All of the following should be considered in the differential diagnosis *except*:

(A) toxoplasmosis

(B) lymphoma

(C) diffuse glioma

(D) progressive multifocal leukoencephalopathy (PML)

43. A patient is brought to the ER 3 months following liver transplantation. The patient had been doing well until about 1 week prior to admission when he because confused, tremulous and complained of unsteadiness and difficulty with vision. An MR scan showed T2 hyperintense lesions in both occipital lobes (Fig. 35-18). The most likely diagnosis is

(A) Creutzfeldt-Jakob's disease (prion disease)

(B) cyclosporin toxicity

(C) PML

(D) posttransplantation lymphoma

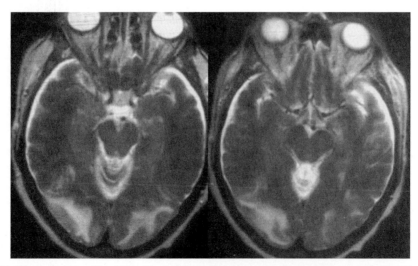

FIG. 35-18   Axial T2-weighted MRI of the brain, revealing white matter hyperintensity in both occipital lobes.

Answers and Explanations

1. (D) The GCS was developed as a means to quantify and communicate a patient's overall neurologic status. It is generally used in trauma situations, but also applies to medical illnesses affecting the nervous system. By no means does a documented GCS obviate the need for a thorough neurologic examination. Scoring is based on eye opening, verbal response, and motor response (Table 35-1).

Following the table, the minimum score is 3 and maximum is 15. Head injuries are often classified according to the GCS, with the postresuscitation GCS being more accurate than the GCS at the scene. GCS 13–15 is a mild head injury, 9–12 is moderate, and 3–8 is severe.

The score is designated by the best responses from the patient. This patient opens his eyes to pain, is intubated, and localizes to pain. Therefore, his GCS is 8.

Bibliography

Greenberg M, Greenberg MS. *Handbook of Neurosurgery*, 5th ed. New York, NY: Thieme, 2001, 118.

Teasdale G, Jennett B. Assessment of coma and impaired consciousness: a practical scale. *Lancet* 1974;2:81–84.

TABLE 35-1   Glasgow Coma Score

GCS	Eye opening	Verbal response	Motor response
1	None	None (or intubated)	None
2	To pain	Incomprehensible	Decerebrate posture
3	To voice	Inappropriate words	Decorticate posture
4	Spontaneous	Confused	Withdraws to pain
5		Normal, oriented	Localizes pain
6			Follows commands

2. (A) Brain death is suspected in this case because the patient has had a severe head injury, the CT scan is consistent with the ICP monitor showing high ICP that has not responded to aggressive treatment. The pupils then have become dilated and fixed. The diagnosis of brain death can be made clinically by history and certain well-established criteria—unresponsiveness, flaccidity, apnea with an appropriate level of CO_2 to drive respiration, loss of all brain stem reflexes, and mid or large fixed pupils to bright light in the absence of injury to the optic nerves. However, there must be no sedating drugs and absence of significant hypothermia. Withdrawing this patient from barbiturates would put him at risk if he were not brain dead. Also it would take at least several days for the barbiturate to reach nonsedating levels. In all cases of brain death, there is loss of significant cerebral blood flow. This was first shown by absence of intracranial blood flow during cerebral angiography. The contrast in the carotid and vertebral arteries would essentially stop at the base of the skull and remain in these vessels for over several minutes. The same phenomenon can be more safely and economically demonstrated by isotope scans, Doppler ultrasound, failure to visualize intracranial vessels on contrast enhanced CT and MR scans. The technique most widely used is a nuclear flow study. Most studies now are performed with Tc-99m HMPAO. This isotope is taken up normally by the cerebral hemispheres and cerebellum. In brain death, neither of these structures have uptake and the skull interior appears empty. In early brain death, occasionally there will be some uptake in the cerebellum. Invariably, a repeat scan will show no uptake. If Tc-99m HMPAO is not available, the flow study with Tc-99m-labeled human serum albumin may be used. In brain death using this isotope there is no intracranial arterial circulation. There may be some venous sinus visualization. Occasionally (2%) patients with clinical brain death will have arterial flow. If brain death is present, a repeat scan in 12–24 h will be confirmatory.

Bibliography

Goodman J, Heck L, Moore B. Confirmation of brain death with portable isotope angiography. A review of 204 consecutive cases. *Neurosurgery* 1985;16:492–497.

Greenberg MS. *Handbook of Neurosurgery*, 5th ed. New York, NY: Thieme, 2001, 128–131.

3. (B)

4. (B)

Explanations 3 and 4

This patient has developed DI, a well-known complication of severe traumatic brain injury. It is caused by injury to the hypothalamus and hypothalamic-pituitary axis secondary to diffuse axonal injury, and is heralded by polyuria (>30 cc/kg/h or >200 cc/h in adults), decreased urine-specific gravity/osmolarity, and increased serum Na/osmolarity.

Injury to the hypothalamus results in a *lack* of antidiuretic hormone (ADH), causing the patient to make large volumes of dilute urine independent of the current hemodynamic status. Onset after injury is usually delayed at least 6–8 h by circulating endogenous ADH. Due to large losses of free water, serum Na and osmolarity increase. Serum sodium and osmolarity, along with urine-specific gravity or osmolarity should be assessed with any large volume urine output in a head injured patient. Any administration of mannitol or diuretics should be taken into account, as they will alter these parameters. Treatment should be instituted quickly to avoid systemic complications from hypovolemia and hypernatremia, and includes replacement of calculated free water deficit and ongoing urinary losses with D5 0.225NaCl or D_5W. Urine output needs to be monitored hourly, and serum electrolytes checked every 4–6 h. Patients with complete DI will require administration of desmopressin (DDAVP, PO, or nasal spray) or vasopressin (SC, IV, or IM) to control urine output.

In the severely brain injured patient, early development of DI in indicative of profound diffuse injury and is highly predictive of mortality. It is also seen brain death.

SIADH and CSW are disorders that can occur in brain injury and result in increased urine output, but are associated with hyponatremia. The best way to clinically distinguish SIADH and CSW is to check central venous pressure, which is normal or elevated in SIADH and low in CSW. A test for serum ADH is available but rarely practical. The important parameters of each process are shown in Table 35-2.

TABLE 35-2   Disorders of Sodium Metabolism

	DI	SIADH	CSW
Volume status	Hypovolemia	Nl or hypervolemia	Hypovolemia
Serum Na	High	Low	Low
Urine volume	High	Low, Nl or high	High early, then low
Urine osmolarity	Low	High	High
Treatment	Water replacement, vasopressin	Fluid restriction	Sodium and fluids

Bibliography

Andrews BT. Fluid and electrolyte management in the head-injured patient. In: Narayan RK, Wilberger JR, Povlishock JT (eds.), *Neurotrauma.* New York, NY: McGraw-Hill, 1996, 335–339.

Nelson PB, Seif SM, Maroon JC, et al. Hyponatremia in intracranial disease. Perhaps not the syndrome of inappropriate secretion of antidiuretic hormone (SIADH). *J Neurosurg* 1981;55:938–941.

Wolf AL, Salcman M. Complications of head injuries in adults. In: Post KD, Friedman E, McCormack P (eds.), *Post-operative Complications in Intracranial Neurosurgery.* New York, NY: Thieme, 1993, 140.

5. (D)

6. (D)

Explanations 5 and 6

This patient became suddenly hemiplegic 1 day after a head injury secondary to an infarction of the left cerebral hemisphere. The factors in the history that lead to this diagnosis are the presence of a basilar skull fracture, the apoplectic onset of hemiplegia, and the fact that he remains awake and alert. Most patients who develop hemiplegia secondary to a mass lesion are obtunded or comatose. The mild ptosis is secondary to a partial Horner's syndrome. The other manifestations of a third nerve palsy are absent. The patient had dissection of the right carotid artery secondary to the basilar skull fracture in the area of the carotid canal (Fig. 35-19); however, most common location of carotid injury and dissection associated with trauma is in the neck, with the dissection beginning several centimeters above the bifurcation. The mechanism can be direct blunt trauma or stretching. In most patients symptoms develop within 1–24 h after trauma; however, in some patients may not have symptoms of cerebral ischemia for several or more days after injury. The sympathetic nerves, except those that cause sweating of the face,

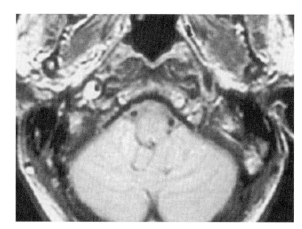

FIG. 35-19   Axial T1-weighted MRI without contrast, revealing bright crescent sign in the right internal carotid artery at the skull base.

travel around the carotid artery and are injured as the carotid is distended by the false lumen, resulting in the Horner's syndrome. Although cerebral angiography is the gold standard in diagnosing carotid dissection, the lesion can often be suspected on CT or MR scan, particularly the latter. On axial images the bright crescent signal in the wall of the carotid may be seen (Fig. 35-19). If this patient were obtunded or comatose when the hemiplegia developed, an acute epidural, subdural, or temporal lobe contusion could be present.

It was elected not to treat the otorrhea with antibiotics, because the incidence of meningitis is very low, and the organisms that cause meningitis on prophylactic antibiotics are often more difficult to deal with. Spinal fluid otorrhea usually stops spontaneously.

The patient's level of consciousness decreased several days after his stroke because of massive swelling of the infarcted brain, resulting in a marked right to left shift. Mannitol and ventriculostomy were probably used to treat hemisphere swelling in this young individual, but when all else fails, sometimes a life can be saved by massive decompressive craniotomy. The bone flap must be huge, the dura is left opened, and the scalp is closed. The bone flap can be frozen or buried in the anterior abdominal wall until the brain swelling resolves. Most neurosurgeons would not consider decompressive craniotomy with a massive infarct of the dominant hemisphere.

Bibliography

Ahmadi J, Levy M, Aarabi B. Vascular lesions resulting from head injury. In: Wilkins R, Rengachary S (eds.), *Neurosurgery*, 2nd ed. New York, NY: McGraw Hill, 1996, 2821–2840.

Morki B, Piepgras D, Houser O. Traumatic dissections of the extracranial internal carotid artery. *J Neurosurg* 1988;68:189–197.

7. (C)

8. (D)

9. (A)

Explanations 7 through 9

Confirmation that rhinorrhea is CSF can be difficult, especially when the amount is small and mixed with blood, and is usually presumptive based on the clinical features of the leak (increases with leaning forward and recumbency, salty taste) and the history (head injury, cranial surgery, tumor). However, there are tests available at the bedside and in the laboratory to assist with confirmation. Historically, CSF is described as having a clear halo around a bloody spot on a paper, gauze, or bed sheet. CSF contains glucose, but if there is contamination with blood (which there often is with trauma) the results of a glucose swab or lab test may be false positive. High resolution CT scan can reveal skull fractures that may be the site of a leak. This can be helpful in the late presentation of CSF leak when there is fluid density in a sinus adjacent to the fracture. The most specific and sensitive test is for beta transferrin, and the results are not altered by the presence of blood in the fluid. In some institutions, however, this test may require outside analysis.

Treatment of posttraumatic CSF fistula is conservative at first, since the majority will spontaneously resolve in 7 days or less. The head of the bed is elevated to approximately 45 degrees or higher, and the patient is instructed to avoid straining or coughing. If the leak continues after 4–7 days, lumbar spinal fluid drainage can be used to divert CSF until the fistula closes. Risks of lumbar drainage include pneumocephalus due to negative pressure, and meningitis, and it is contraindicated in patients with intracranial mass lesions due to risk of herniation. Occasionally surgery is required for persistent leaks, and the approach is based on the location and characteristics of the leak. Repair of facial fractures can take place at the convenience of the surgeons involved, and should not be altered by the presence of CSF rhinorrhea. Indeed, repair of the facial fractures may cause the fistula to close due to postoperative edema of the soft tissues. Patients with a CSF fistula are at increased risk for meningitis, but prophylactic antibiotics has not been shown to decrease this risk.

Bibliography

Geisler FH. Skull fractures. In: Wilkins RH, Rengachary SS (eds.), *Neurosurgery*, 2nd ed. New York, NY: McGraw-Hill, 1996, 2753–2754.

McCormack B, Cooper PR. Traumatic cerebrospinal fluid fistulas. In: Narayan RK, Wilberger JR, Povlishock JT (eds.), *Neurotrauma.* New York, NY: McGraw-Hill, 1996, 639–653.

10. **(A)** The carotid-cavernous fistula (CCF) is an abnormal connection from the internal carotid artery to the cavernous sinus. It is a rare but well-documented complication of head trauma and basilar skull fracture, but can also develop from spontaneous rupture of a cavernous carotid artery aneurysm. Symptoms of traumatic CCF can develop acutely or more often over weeks or months. Pulsatile proptosis, chemosis, ophthalmoplegia (partial or complete), and ocular bruit are the cardinal features. Often patients complain of retroorbital pain or ipsilateral headache. Ocular hypoxia from decreased ocular perfusion pressure and increased venous pressure may threaten vision. Diagnosis is confirmed with cerebral angiography, and endovascular treatment with detachable coils or balloons is the treatment of choice. An aneurysm of the cavernous carotid artery can result from trauma, and cranial neuropathies are more prominent signs than proptosis or chemosis. It is often associated with blindness at the time of injury secondary to ophthalmic artery injury or fracture in the area of the optic canal.

Orbital pseudotumor is a rare inflammatory process of unknown etiology. It is extremely painful. There is edema of the lids and conjunctiva. The inflammation is very steroid sensitive. Ethmoid sinusitis usually will cause lateral displacement of the globe, lid swelling, fever and other usual symptoms of sinusitis, and is less often associated with chemosis.

Bibliography

Gianotta SL, Gruen P. Vascular complications of head injury. In: Barrow DL (ed.), *Neurosurgical Topics: Complications and Sequelae of Head Injury.* Park Ridge, IL: American Association of Neurological Surgeons, 1992, 44.

Harris ME, Barrow DL. Traumatic carotid-cavernous fistulas. In: Barrow DL (ed.), *Neurosurgical Topics: Complications and Sequelae of Head Injury.* Park Ridge, IL: American Association of Neurological Surgeons, 1992, 13–29.

Lewis AI, Tomsick TA, Tew JM. Carotid-cavernous fistula and intracavernous aneurysms. In: Wilkins RH, Rengachary SS (eds.), *Neurosurgery,* 2nd ed. New York, NY: McGraw-Hill, 1996, 2529–2535.

Yee RD. Evaluation and treatment of vision loss, diplopia, and orbitopathies. In: Batjer HH, Loftus CM (eds.), *Textbook of Neurological Surgery.* New York, NY: Lippincott, Williams & Wilkins, 2003, 482–490.

11. **(A)** The clinical symptoms suggest a right carotid dissection, and the CT scan confirms the diagnosis by show clot in the wall of the carotid artery at the base of the skull. Most cases of carotid dissection are spontaneous, but they have been associated with fibromuscular dysplasia, Marfan's syndrome, and strenuous activity. Dissection is sometimes precipitated by minor trauma and occasionally occur following chiropractic manipulation. The dissection may occur intracranially or extracranially. The hallmark is extraluminal extravasation of blood. This patient's dissection took place in the neck, and the extravasation was between the media and adventitia. The amaurosis fugax was caused by emboli, the pain by distention of the carotid, and the tongue paralysis and partial Horner's syndrome by stretching of nerves adjacent to the suddenly enlarged carotid.

Most patients with carotid dissections are treated with heparin for several weeks and then oral anticoagulants. About 75% will do well with resolution of symptoms. An occasional patient will throw emboli from a pseudoaneurysm that form on the carotid when blood causes outpouching of the adventitia. If embolic symptoms continue with anticoagulation, options include ligation the cervical carotid with or without an extracranial-intracranial bypass, very occasionally a direct repair in the neck, and more recently by a stent placed by an endovascular technique.

Bibliography

Anson J, Crowell R. Cervicocranial arterial dissection. *Neurosurgery* 1991;29:89–96.

Morki B, Sundt T, Houser O. Spontaneous internal carotid artery dissection, hemicrania, and Horner's syndrome. *Arch Neurol* 1979;36:677–680.

12. **(A)** Autonomic dysreflexia (aka autonomic hyperreflexia, autonomic storm) is a syndrome of sympathetic overactivity which can occur in up to 85% of patients with SCI at T6 level or above, usually after the acute phase of injury (approximately 2 weeks). Symptoms occur when a noxious stimulus to an organ innervated by spinal nerves below the level of injury (e.g., distended urinary bladder) causes a spinal reflex to the adrenal glands. Due to interruption of descending inhibitory control from the injured spinal cord, there is massive sympathetic discharge resulting in hypertension, sweating, and piloerection. The hypertension can be extreme, and fatal intracranial hemorrhage has been reported. The bradycardia is a reflex response to severe hypertension mediated by carotid baroreceptors, and its presence is not necessary to make the diagnosis. Patients are often tachycardic in the early stages.

Autonomic dysreflexia is a *medical emergency.* Treatment involves immediate removal of the stimulus, which is by far most commonly a distended urinary bladder. Other common causes include fecal impaction, gastrointestinal (GI) or gastrourinary (GU) procedures, and urinary tract infection (UTI). It has also been reported with testicular torsion and birth labor. Care must be taken not to increase stimulation in attempt to remove the causative factor. For example, an anesthetic ointment or gel should be used when breaking up a fecal impaction.

Removal of the stimulus nearly always immediately resolves the hypertension; however, if it does not, pharmacologic therapy is indicated with such drugs as nitroprusside, nitroglycerine, or hydralazine. Patients with recurrent episodes may require prophylaxis with alpha-blockers such as phenoxybenzamine or clonidine.

Neuroleptic malignant syndrome, an idiosyncratic reaction to phenothiazine medications such as haloperidol, is characterized by autonomic dysfunction, hyperthermia, and extrapyramidal effects such as dystonia, muscle rigidity, and even catatonia. It can be treated with dopamine agonists (e.g., bromocriptine) and dantrolene sodium. An anticholinergic crisis presents as tachyarrhythmias, hypertension, mydriasis and altered level of consciousness, and is usually the result of overdose of medication (e.g., tricyclic antidepressants, antihistamines). Deep venous thrombosis and pulmonary embolism occur more frequently in the spinal cord injured patient, but do not present with a hypertensive crisis.

Bibliography

Cahill DW, Rechtire GR. The acute complications of spinal cord injury. In: Narayan RK, Wilberger JR, Povlishock JT (eds.), *Neurotrauma.* New York, NY: McGraw-Hill, 1996, 1210.

Lovejoy FH, Linden CH. Acute poisoning and drug overdosage. In: Isselbacher KJ, Braunwald E, Wilson JD, et al. (eds.), *Harrison's Principles of Internal Medicine,* 13th ed. New York, NY: McGraw-Hill, 1994, 2442.

Owens GF, Addonizio JC. Urologic evaluation and management of the spinal cord injured patient. In: Lee BY, Ostrander LE, Cochran GVB, et al. (eds.), *The Spinal Cord Injured Patient: Comprehensive Management.* Philadelphia, PA: W.B. Saunders, 1991, 130–131.

Petersdorf RG. Hypothermia and hyperthermia. In: Isselbacher KJ, Braunwald E, Wilson JD, et al. (eds.), *Harrison's Principles of Internal Medicine,* 13th ed. New York, NY: McGraw-Hill, 1994, 2476–2477.

13. (C) The hypoglossal nerve travels in a plane between the jugular vein and internal carotid artery (Fig. 35-20). It passes medially over the carotid usually distal to the bifurcation and proximal to the posterior belly of the digastric muscle. It is identified by following the superior root of the ansa cervicalis (often referred to as the descending hypoglossal nerve) superiorly to the point where it meets the hypoglossal nerve crossing the internal carotid. It can be mobilized superomedially to allow adequate exposure for CEA, and this may require transection of the superior root of the ansa cervicalis (this usually causes no noticeable loss of strap muscle function). Occasionally the hypoglossal nerve is not easily identified at surgery, as it can be hidden

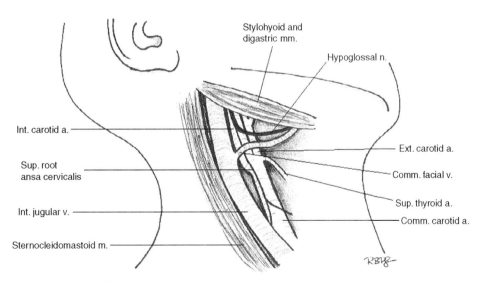

FIG. 35-20 The hypoglossal nerve in relation to carotid endarterectomy.

under the facial vein or digastric muscle. Accidental transection of the nerve is a rare complication. More often it is injured by prolonged retraction. Retraction injury will usually recover relatively quickly.

The hypoglossal is a pure motor nerve, responsible for the innervation of the intrinsic and extrinsic muscles of the tongue (except palatoglossus, innervated by the vagus nerve). When injured, there is weakness of ipsilateral tongue muscles, causing the tongue to protrude toward the side of injury.

Sensation of the anterior two-third of the tongue is mediated by the lingual nerve (a branch of the mandibular division of the trigeminal nerve). The posterior one-third is supplied by the glossopharyngeal nerve. Taste is a special sensation mediated by the facial, glossopharyngeal and vagus nerves.

The hypoglossal nerve descends in the neck in a plane between the internal jugular vein and internal carotid artery before swinging medially toward the tongue. It will cross the internal and external carotid between the bifurcation and the digastric muscle. The superior root of the ansa cervicalis can be mobilized off the common carotid and retracted medially or even sacrificed to allow superomedial retraction of the hypoglossal nerve. Occasionally the nerve is difficult to identify, as it may be fixed to the underside of the common facial vein or the digastric muscle.

Bibliography

Crowell RM, Ogilvy CS, Ojemann RG. Extracranial carotid artery atherosclerosis; carotid endarterectomy. In: Wilkins RH, Rengachary SS (eds.), *Neurosurgery*, 2nd ed. New York, NY: McGraw-Hill, 1996, 2107.

Pansky B. *Review of Gross Anatomy*, 5th ed. New York, NY: Macmillan, 1984, 62–63, 74–75.

14. (C)

15. (D)

Explanations 14 and 15

Injury to the spinal accessory nerve is one of the most common iatrogenic nerve injuries during a surgical procedure. Lymph node biopsy in the posterior triangle of the neck is the operation usually performed. The injury often goes unrecognized until the patient complains of pain, difficulty abducting the shoulder, and noticeable drooping of the shoulder. The injury is very serious and disabling. Prevention is critical when working in the posterior triangle of the neck for the well being of the patient as well as for the surgeon; injury to the spinal accessory nerve often has legal consequences. Although each patient must be individualized, some surgeons suggest doing lymph node biopsies in this area under general anesthesia without

muscle paralysis, use of a nerve stimulator, magnification, and minimal and/or bipolar coagulation.

This patient can be followed for several months to see if there is spontaneous recovery. EMG by a very experienced clinician can show signs of voluntary muscle contraction in all three portions of the trapezius, but if function is not evident clinically at 3 months, exploration of the wound should be undertaken because the EMG findings do not necessarily predict a good clinical outcome. The results of surgical repair may be excellent when performed at 3 months. At the time of reexploration, if the nerve appears to be in continuity, the nerve should be stimulated distal to the site of injury. If there is muscle contraction, then a neurolysis without repair should be considered. If the nerve had been divided, a primary anastomosis should be performed if there is no tension. Otherwise, a nerve graft is preferable. Finding the proximal and distal stumps can be difficult and confusion of the accessory nerve with sensory nerves in the area must be avoided. Knowledge of the anatomy is critical (Fig. 35-21).

The sternocleidomastoid and trapezius muscles and the clavicle define the posterior triangle of the neck. The spinal accessory nerve runs superficially through the triangle. Lymph nodes can be found along the border of the sternocleidomastoid and along the course of the nerve. The great auricular and lesser occipital nerves are sensory, and injury may not be as noticeable as injury to the spinal accessory nerve.

Bibliography

Nakamichi K, Shintaro T. Iatrogenic injury of the spinal accessory nerve. *J Bone Joint Surg* 1998;80-A:1616–1621.

Nason R, Abdurlrauf B, Stranc M. The anatomy of the accessory nerve and cervical lymph node biopsy. *Am J Surg* 2000;180:241–243.

Novak C, MacKinnon S. Patient outcome after surgical management of an accessory nerve injury. *Otolaryngol Head Neck Surg* 2002;127:221–224.

16. (C) With GSW to an extremity, tissue injury is determined by the projectiles direct course and by shock waves from its trajectory ("blast" injury). They frequently will require operative management. Immediate operative treatment consists of debridement of devitalized tissues, restoration of distal circulation, and stabilization of fractures.

Primary repair of transected nerves is not performed for GSW due to inability to determine the extent of the blast injury to the severed ends in the acute phase. The most appropriate treatment is to suture the proximal and distal stump to nearby clean tissue beds and marking them with suture that can be identified at delayed repair. Care should be taken to avoid extensive mobilization, especially of the

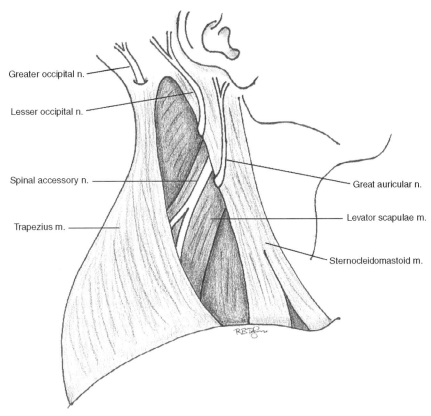

FIG. 35-21   The posterior triangle of the neck.

proximal stump (at debridement and at delayed surgery), as this may interrupt the vascular supply of the nerve and inhibit the axonal regeneration, which occurs from proximal to distal. Recovery of function with delayed surgical repair can be as high as 50%, but may take months or even years to return, and is dependent on many factors such as location and nature of nerve injury, need for nerve graft, and tension on the nerve. Nerves with primarily motor function (e.g., axillary and radial nerves) have better recovery rates than those with a large sensory component (e.g., median and ulnar nerves). In a GSW with neurologic deficit and no direct nerve injury at surgical exploration (or that which is treated nonoperatively), recovery is as high as 69%. This is likely due to axonotmesis, which is injury to the axon of the nerve without disruption of the nerve sheath, leaving a good path for axonal regeneration.

This management differs from laceration injury, in which primary repair is indicated.

Bibliography

Awasthi D, Hudson AR, Kline DG. Treatment strategies for the patient suffering from peripheral nerve injury. In: Benzel EC (ed.), *Neurosurgical Topics: Practical Approaches to Peripheral Nerve Surgery.* Park Ridge, IL: American Association of Neurological Surgeons, 1992, 35–36.

Friedman A. Restoration of extremity function. In: Benzel EC (ed.), *Neurosurgical Topics: Practical Approaches to Peripheral Nerve Surgery.* Park Ridge, IL: American Association of Neurological Surgeons, 1992, 214–220.

Omer GE. Peripheral nerve injuries and gunshot wounds. In: Omer GE, Spinner M, VanBeek AL (eds.), *Management of Peripheral Nerve Problems*, 2nd ed. Philadelphia, PA: W.B. Saunders, 1998, 398–404.

Omer GE. The prognosis for untreated traumatic injuries. In: Omer GE, Spinner M, VanBeek AL (eds.), *Management of Peripheral Nerve Problems*, 2nd ed. Philadelphia, PA: W.B. Saunders, 1998, 365–369.

17. (A)

18. (A)

Explanations 17 and 18

This patient's symptoms are classical for carpal tunnel syndrome except for the acute onset and rapid progression, which will be discussed below. Patients with carpal tunnel syndrome frequently complain of numbness in all of their fingers, even though the median nerve supplies sensation to the lateral four and a half fingers. Nocturnal paresthesias, paresthesias while driving or holding a book, and discomfort in the entire extremity are very common. Of the choices given, the best way to arrive at the diagnosis is by clinical examination. When examining for involvement of a peripheral nerve or nerve root, motor examination is usually more reliable then sensory examination. The median nerve supplies four intrinsic muscles of the hand—lateral two lumbricals, opponens pollicis, abductor pollicis brevis, and half the flexor pollicis brevis (LOAF muscles—a famous mnemonic). All the other intrinsic muscles of the hand are supplied by the ulnar nerve. The radial nerve does not supply any of the intrinsic muscles of the hand. The best muscle to test for carpal tunnel is the abductor pollicis brevis. The patient is asked to maintain abduction of the thumb at right angles to the palm against pressure by the examiner. Subtle weakness of the median nerve can be demonstrated in this way. When testing sensation, two-point discrimination is much better than pinprick.

Phalen's sign, also characteristic of carpal tunnel, is elicited by wrist flexion. Paresthesias are reproduced in less than a minute. Tinel's sign, paresthesias elicited by tapping over the median nerve at wrist, may also be present. EMG changes in the hand muscles would not appear for about 3 weeks after the onset of symptoms and therefore would not be helpful in this patient; however, the patient might have delayed sensory conduction (latency) across the wrist that could be demonstrated by electrophysiologic studies.

Ordinarily carpal tunnel surgery would not be undertaken with only a week of symptoms, but this young man's history suggests an acute process. He was explored and had a hematoma under the transverse carpal ligament secondary to an undiagnosed inherited coagulopathy. Aside from fractures, another cause of acute carpal tunnel syndrome is thrombosis of a persistent median artery.

Bibliography

Greenberg M. *Handbook of Neurosurgery*, 5th ed. New York, NY: Thieme, 2001, 535–539.

Rengachary S. Entrapment neuropathies. In: Wilkins R, Rengachary S (eds.), *Neurosurgery*, 2nd ed. New York, NY: McGraw-Hill, 1996, 3073–3098.

19. (C)

20. (A)

Explanations 19 and 20

Causalgia was a term introduced by Weir Mitchell during the Civil War to describe burning pain that occasionally appeared after partial nerve injuries. Autonomic symptoms and trophic changes were also part of the clinical picture. Causalgia major referred to high velocity missile injuries that involved a peripheral nerve and causalgia minor referred to less severe or nonpenetrating soft tissue injury. Early in the last century the pain was thought to be sympathetically mediated, and the term reflex sympathetic dystrophy (RSD) was introduced. Today most theories of this group of painful disorders do not involve the autonomic nervous system, and consequently the term complex regional pain syndrome (CRPS) is used to encompass a variety of clinical entities with somewhat similar symptoms with perhaps diverse etiologies. In CRPS 1 there is no nerve injury and in CRPS 2 there is a definable nerve injury.

CRPS 1 occurred in the above patient without a peripheral nerve injury after minor trauma. A similar symptom complex can be produced by mere immobilization of an extremity or by psychologic disuse and guarding.

It was initially thought symptoms were produced by ephaptic transmission between afferent pain fibers and efferent sympathetic fibers, but this theory is no longer accepted. Most contemporary theories do not involve the direct involvement of the sympathetic nervous system; the autonomic manifestation may merely be an epiphenomenon.

Symptoms of CRPS may begin within 24 h or days to weeks after injury. If there is a specific nerve injury, the median, ulnar, and sciatic nerves are most frequently implicated. The patient will have burning pain and allodynia and may resist having his/her hand or foot examined, particularly the palmar and plantar surfaces. The vasomotor tone can vary from a pink and warm to a cold and mottled extremity. The skin may be dry and scaly and the joints stiff. There may be hair loss or excess hair. There may be edema of the soft tissue and eventually atrophy. The attitude of this patient's extremity is probably secondary to a dystonic component of the syndrome.

There is no evidence that psychiatric support and physical therapy can cure CRPS, but most clinicians will use these modalities in managing such patients. There is controversy about the value of sympathetic blocks and peripheral sympathectomy in the treatment of CRPS. There is some literature claiming cure rates of 80–95%, but some authors claim that these results result from bias in defining the condition as RSD if they get benefit from sympathectomy. There is other data claiming that only 7% are cured with treatment directed toward the sympathetic nervous system. There is a very high response rate to placebo. Recently there has been evidence that dorsal column stimulation in carefully selected patients can reduce pain and improve quality of life when other treatments have failed. When there is a dystonic component, intrathecal baclofen may be useful in ameliorating some symptoms of CRPS.

Bibliography

Arguelles J, Burcdhiel K. Causalgia and reflex sympathetic dystrophy. In: Wilkins R, Rengachary S (eds.), *Neurosurgery*, 2nd ed. New York, NY: McGraw-Hill, 1996, 3209–3215.

Kelmer M, Barendse G, van Kleef M, et al. Spinal cord stimulation in patients with chronic reflex sympathetic dystrophy. *N Engl J Med* 2000;343:618–624.

Schwartzman R. New treatments for reflex sympathetic dystrophy. *N Engl J Med* 2000;343:654–656.

Van Hilten B, van d Beek W, Hoff J, et al. Intrathecal baclofen for the treatment of dystonia in patients with reflex sympathetic dystrophy. *N Engl J Med* 2000; 343: 625–630.

21. **(C)** The MR scan shows a herniated disk at L3-4 with compression of the L4 nerve root. The L4 nerve root supplies the quadriceps muscle, and along with L3 nerve root, is responsible for the knee reflex. Weakness of the quadriceps muscle is best demonstrated by having the patient step up on a platform about 15 in. high, first with the normal side and then with the involved side. Weakness not apparent on manual testing may be demonstrated by this maneuver. This patient's disk herniation is in a posterior lateral position. The L4 nerve root passes the L3-4 disk space and exits at the L4-5 neural foramen. A far lateral disk at L4-5 could also cause L4 nerve root compression. If the MR scan were normal, one would have to consider the diagnosis of diabetic proximal neuropathy, which might be the first manifestation of diabetes mellitus. In this disorder it is likely that, if an EMG were performed, the paraspinal muscles would not be involved, whereas the paraspinal muscles ordinarily would be involved in nerve root compression by a herniated disk. Proximal diabetic neuropathy causes hip and leg pain for 6–9 months and then usually subsides spontaneously, but the opposite side may become involved.

A herniated disk at L5-S1 usually compresses the S1 nerve root, which exists through the S1-S2 intervertebral foramen. With S1 nerve root compression, the ankle reflex is usually lost. In this case both ankle reflexes are absent because the patient is a diabetic. In the adult the two most common causes of absent ankle reflexes are diabetes and chronic alcoholism. A herniated disc at L4-5 usually compresses the L5 nerve root, which exists through the L5-S1 intervertebral foramen. There is no reflex to test for the L5 nerve root, but the extensor hallicus longus muscle is supplied almost exclusively by L5 and weakness of this muscle can usually be demonstrated.

Bibliography

Jorge A, Przybylski G. Herniated lumbar disc. In: Batjer H, Loftus C (eds.), *Textbook of Neurological Surgery*. Philadelphia, PA: Lippincott, Williams & Wilkins, 2003, 1657–1661.

Naftulin S, Fast A, Thomas M. Diabetic lumbar radiculopathy: sciatica without disc herniation. *Spine* 1993;18: 2419–2422.

22. **(C)** An elderly patient may have structural evidence of both lumbar spinal stenosis and vascular insufficiency of the lower extremities. In fact, 30% of elderly individuals have spinal stenosis on imaging studies but have no clinical symptoms. Both disorders can cause claudication type pain in one or both lower extremities with walking. Sorting out the etiology may be difficult and when these conditions coexist, but the subtle aspects of the clinical history can be helpful. The neurologic examination in symptomatic spinal stenosis is often normal and patients with symptomatic spinal stenosis may have poor pedal pulses. In vascular claudication, cramping symptoms can usually be reproduced by a specific amount of exercise, like walking 25 ft. The claudication-type symptoms in spinal stenosis vary from day to day as does the distance required to bring on the symptoms. Spinal stenosis symptoms are more apt to appear with just standing. Vascular claudication is not posture related. The pain in both disorders is relieved by rest. Vascular claudication is relieved almost immediately when ambulation is stopped. Relief is slower in neurogenic claudication, and the patient usually has to sit down. Patients with stenosis may also find relief with bending forward and they will occasionally walk this way. The anterior-posterior diameter of the spinal canal increases with flexion. Also in spinal stenosis back or leg discomfort can occur with bending or lifting. When spinal stenosis is severe, there may be some curling up of the nerve roots in the spinal canal, giving the appearance of spaghetti. When present, this imaging picture is very supportive of neurogenic claudication.

Treatment of spinal stenosis is by laminectomy, which involves removal of lamina and a portion of the facets. When there is evidence of spinal instability, such as degenerative spondylolisthesis due to disease of the facet joints, spinal stabilization at the time of laminectomy may be recommended.

Bibliography

Ciric I, Salehi S, Gravely L. Lumbar spinal stenosis and laminectomy. In: Batjer H, Loftus C (eds.), *Textbook of Neurological Surgery*. Philadelphia, PA: Lippincott, Williams & Wilkins, 2003, 1777–1684.

Epstein N. Symptomatic lumbar spinal stenosis. *Surg Neurol* 1998;50:3–10.

23. **(D)** This patient is in hypotensive shock. The wound is obviously too small for the profound blood loss required to produce shock after the incision is closed. Even if there is considerable epidural bleeding during

a single level disc operation under the microscope, the volume of blood lost is actually small and very rarely would transfusion be necessary. During lumbar diskectomy it is possible to injure the aorta or iliac artery with the bite of a rongeur that goes through the anterior annulus. In about 50% of cases there is no back bleeding from the disc space and the surgeon is unaware that a vascular injury has occurred. When examined in the recovery room, the hypotensive patient's flanks may become discolored and the abdomen distended. If there is some stability during fluid resuscitation, a CT scan of the abdomen could be obtained to confirm the diagnosis; however, more often the patient is *in extremis* and it is life saving to return the patient to the OR, open the abdomen, and secure the bleeding site. The vessel involved is usually the iliac artery, and the injury is usually more common with left-sided discectomy. It is good practice when doing disc surgery to palpate the anterior aspect of the disc space with an instrument to be sure there had been no perforation.

An occasional patient may present with anemia and tachycardia several days to weeks after lumbar disc surgery secondary to an accidental fistula created between an iliac artery and vein.

Bibliography

Anda S, Askhus S, Skaanes K, et al. Anterior perforation in lumbar diskectomies: a report of four cases of vascular complications and a CT study of the prevertebral lumbar anatomy. *Spine* 1991;16:54–60.

Lange M, Fink U, Philipp A, et al. Emergency diagnosis with spiral CT angiography in case of suspected ventral perforation following lumbar disc surgery. *Surg Neurol* 2002;57:15–19.

Pappas C, Harrington T, Sonntag V. Outcome analysis in 654 surgically treated lumbar disc herniations. *Neurosurgery* 1992;30:862–866.

24. **(C)** Cauda equina syndrome (CES) is an acute or chronic condition caused by compression of the nerve roots of the cauda equina (by ruptured intervertebral disc, tumor, trauma, postoperative hematoma, other mass lesion), and consists of a usually asymmetric distribution of pain and sensory and motor loss in the lower extremities. Saddle anesthesia and urinary sphincter problems are very common. The level of involvement can often be localized on physical examination. Rectal tone and sensation in the sacral dermatomes must be documented in any patient with suspected CES. There is urinary retention with resultant overflow incontinence in acute cases. Checking a postvoid residual is helpful in determining bladder function. The imaging modality of choice is the MRI, which can assist in surgical planning. Most agree that decompression for acute CES should take place as soon as possible, and usually within 24 h. Expeditious decompression gives the best chance for recovery of function, which is better for lower extremity function than for bladder function.

Acute epidural abscess in the lumbosacral area would typically present with excruciating low back pain, fever, and malaise and then progress to neurological deficit over the course of hours or days. Injury or infarct of the conus medullaris typically causes a symmetric syndrome of sensory and motor loss with sphincter dysfunction. Pain is less severe if present, and the motor finding less prominent than with cauda equina lesions.

Bibliography

Greenberg MS. *Handbook of Neurosurgery*, 5th ed. New York, NY: Thieme, 2001, 298–299, 491.

Rengachary SS. Examination of motor and sensory systems and reflexes. In: Wilkins RH, Rengachary SS (eds.), *Neurosurgery*, 2nd ed. New York, NY: McGraw-Hill, 1996, 155–156.

Shapiro S. Cauda equina syndrome secondary to lumbar disc herniation. *Neurosurgery* 1993;32:743–747.

25. **(B)** The most likely diagnosis based on this patient's current complaints, medical history, and imaging studies is spinal epidural abscess. Well-documented risk factors are diabetes mellitus, chronic renal failure, and intravenous drug abuse. Over half are from hematogenous spread. The clinical picture usually begins with localized pain (which may be excruciating) in the affected area of the spine, fever, malaise, and occasionally symptoms of meningeal irritation. Nerve root and then spinal cord symptoms (in lesions of the cervical and thoracic spine) ensue, and may progress to paralysis. Timing of progression varies according to organism from hours (acute bacterial infections) to months (mycobacterial and fungal infections). *Staphylococcus aureus* is the most commonly isolated organism in acute abscesses, with *Mycobacterium tuberculosis* in chronic cases. There is often associated discitis and osteomyelitis, and the presence of these may alter the surgical therapy. Sedimentation rate is usually elevated, but not specific. The MRI with gadolinium contrast is the imaging modality of choice, and usually will reveal a fluid-intensity enhancing mass in the epidural space. Straightforward spinal epidural abscesses are usually located dorsally, and removed via laminectomy. Those associated with discitis and/or osteomyelitis as in this case are usually anterior, and treatment likely will involve removal of infected disc and vertebral bodies with reconstruction and fusion. Percutaneous aspiration may reveal the causative organism, but will not

relieve or prevent further neurologic injury. The pathophysiology of SCI involves direct compression of the nervous structures, and more importantly thrombophlebitis of epidural and spinal veins causing venous infarction. Rates of recovery of deficits are very low, even with expeditious surgery, and mortality is as high as 23%. Early diagnosis is extremely important. Any patient with risk factors, fever, and local spine tenderness warrants investigation.

Bibliography

Allen MB, Flannery AM, Fisher J. Spinal epidural and subdural abscesses. In: Wilkins RH, Rengachary SS (eds.), *Neurosurgery*, 2nd ed. New York, NY: McGraw-Hill, 1996, 3327–3330.

Baker AS, Ojemann RG, Swartz MN, et al. Spinal epidural abscesses. *N Engl J Med* 1975;293:463–468.

Greenberg MS. *Handbook of Neurosurgery*, 5th ed. New York, NY: Thieme, 2001, 240–243.

Hlavin ML, Kaminski HJ, Ross JS, et al. Spinal epidural abscesses: a 10-year perspective. *Neurosurgery* 1990;27: 177–184.

26. (D) NPH is described as a classic triad of gait disturbance, urinary incontinence, and dementia. It is usually idiopathic, but may also be a long-term sequela of head injury or subarachnoid hemorrhage (SAH). The pathophysiology is not well understood, but is related to altered CSF dynamics. It is one of the few treatable causes of dementia. The onset usually begins with gait problems, progressing to a slow, unsteady wide-based shuffle, often describe as "magnetic." Urinary incontinence from lack of awareness and dementia of frontal-lobe type later ensue. There is no fecal incontinence. The diagnosis is made by history and physical examination, and other possible causes for the patient's condition are ruled out with CT and/or MRI. Further evidence of NPH can be obtained with a large-volume lumbar puncture followed by assessment for improvement in gait, but this is not a very sensitive test. Unfortunately there is no reliable confirmatory test to make the diagnosis. Therapy is with a ventriculoperitoneal (VP) shunt. Classically, the symptoms will improve in the same order in which they appear, i.e., improvement in gait followed by improved continence followed by improvement in mental status (which is rarely complete).

Alzheimer's disease is usually a progressive global dementia, with very late motor findings. A brain tumor can present with mental status changes, but the neurologic examination usually is more focal and the patient is likely to have headache. Chronic subdural hematoma is unlikely to present with incontinence unless the patient is obtunded.

Bibliography

Black PMcL. Hydrocephalus in adults. In: Youman JR (ed.), *Neurological Surgery*, 4th ed. Philadelphia, PA: Lippincott-Raven, 1996, 930–937.

Muhonen MG, Wellman BJ. Hydrocephalus and benign intracranial cysts. In: Grossman RG, Loftus CM (eds.), *Principles of Neurosurgery*, 2nd ed. Philadelphia, PA: Lippincott-Raven, 1999, 99–100.

27. (A) Although this patient has multiple medical problems, her presentation is classic for spontaneous SAH. The CT scan reveals blood in the basilar cisterns and subarachnoid spaces. The most common cause of nontraumatic SAH is by far a ruptured intracranial aneurysm, which will be found on four-vessel cerebral arteriography in 85% of cases. Definitive treatment of ruptured aneurysm is by craniotomy for clip ligation, endovascular coil embolization, or a combination of the two. Treatment is usually carried out very soon after the diagnosis is made to prevent a second hemorrhage. Risk factors for aneurysmal SAH include smoking, family history, and possibly hypertension. SAH carries significant morbidity and mortality. Approximately one-third of patients die in the first 24 h after hemorrhage, and only one-third of patients will have a good outcome. A lumbar puncture is the most sensitive test for SAH, but need only be performed in the rare patient with suspicious history and normal head CT.

There are ECG abnormalities and laboratory findings consistent with cardiac ischemia (elevated CK isoenzymes and troponin) in up to 70% of cases of patients with SAH. Many patients will even have cardiac wall motion abnormalities on echocardiography. Although it has been known for nearly 100 years that insults to the brain have cardiac effects, the phenomena are not well understood. Altered hypothalamic control of the autonomic nervous system may account for some of the pathophysiology.

Carcinomatous meningitis (breast, lung, melanoma are most common primaries) can present with headache and neck pain, but usually is associated with cranial neuropathies and will not have the appearance of SAH on CT. MRI with contrast and lumbar puncture assist with the diagnosis. Patients with migraine who present with SAH will almost always report that the headache is different from the usual migraine. Septic emboli from valvular heart disease will usually present with fever and stroke-like symptoms, but is a rare problem in the patient with other manifestations of endocarditis. Patients with bacterial endocarditis can develop bacterial (sometimes called mycotic) aneurysms of the cerebral arteries. These aneurysms are usually located in the distal branches, and present more often with intraparenchymal hemorrhage than SAH.

Bibliography

Elrifai AM, Dureza C, Bailes JE. Cardiac and systemic complications of subarachnoid hemorrhage. In: Bederson JB (ed.), *Neurosurgical Topics: Subarachnoid Hemorrhage: Pathophysiology and Management*. Park Ridge, IL: American Association of Neurological Surgeons, 1997, 87–105.

Greenberg MS. *Handbook of Neurosurgery*, 5th ed. New York, NY: Thieme, 2001, 469, 754–757.

Yao KC, Bederson JB. Subarachnoid hemorrhage. In: Andrews BT (ed.), *Intensive Care in Neurosurgery*. New York, NY: Thieme, 2003, 161–171.

28. (A) This patient is suffering from cerebral venous sinus thrombosis. It can present as in this case with elevated ICP without focal neurologic deficits, or as a focal deficit with or without increased ICP (implying occlusion of a cortical vein). Risk factors are extremes of age, especially men over 60, women between the ages of 20 and 35, and various states of abnormal blood flow (dehydration, CHF, polycythemia, or other hematologic disorder). It is also associated with trauma, infection of the paranasal and mastoid sinuses, and can be a result of obstruction of flow in the venous sinus from a meningioma. In young women, most cases are associated with pregnancy, the postpartum period, or oral contraceptives.

CT scan may reveal clot in the venous sinuses or cortical veins, venous infarcts, parenchymal hemorrhages, and small ventricles. Angiography will show prolonged circulation times and lack of filling of the affected venous sinuses. MRI is the imaging modality of choice for venous sinus thrombosis, as it is non-invasive, multiplanar, and can evaluate flow (or lack of) in the sinuses in addition to the effects on the brain parenchyma. This patient's images reveal thrombosis in the superior sagittal sinus, thrombosis of cortical veins and bilateral venous infarctions with hemorrhage on the left.

Goals of treatment are to prevent extension of the thrombosis, control symptoms from elevated ICP or seizures until recanalization, and remove any causative factor. Anticoagulation should be instituted immediately, even if there is evidence of hemorrhagic venous infarction, to prevent extension of thrombus until recanalization or formation of collaterals. Anticoagulation has been shown to improve the patient's condition without significant risk of increased hemorrhage. Endovascular treatment has been used to mechanically disrupt the thrombus and also to deliver thrombolytic medications. Adequate hydration is also important, and should be monitored with central venous pressure catheter. Antibiotics are given if there is an infectious cause, and surgical treatment of the infected site (e.g., mastoid sinus) is occasionally indicated. Surgery on the venous sinuses is reserved for thrombosis caused by

mass lesion such as a tumor. Ventriculostomy may be required to treat elevated ICP, but it is not first-line therapy. Steroids have no proven benefit.

Bibliography

Iskandar BJ, Kapp JP. Nonseptic venous occlusive disease. In: Wilkins RH, Rengachary SS (eds.), *Neurosurgery*, 2nd ed. New York, NY: McGraw-Hill, 1996, 2177–2190.

Soleau SW, Schmidt R, Stevens S, et al. Extensive experience with dural sinus thrombosis. *Neurosurgery* 2003;52:534–544.

Southwick FS, Swartz MN. Inflammatory thrombosis of major dural venous sinuses and cortical veins. In: Wilkins RH, Rengachary SS (eds.), *Neurosurgery*, 2nd ed. New York, NY: McGraw-Hill, 1996, 3307–3311.

29. (D)

30. (B)

Explanations 29 and 30

Trigeminal neuralgia (TN) is usually a disorder of older individuals, but it is not rare in middle age. A few percent of patients may have MS or a neoplasm as the cause of TN. Many neurosurgeons feel that the majority of cases of TN are probably due to compression of the trigeminal nerve by a normal blood vessel near the exit zone of the trigeminal nerve from the brain stem. MRI is obtained to rule out other causes of TN (tumor, MS, vascular malformation), but occasionally will reveal the offending vessel. One of the most successful procedures for treating TN is a posterior fossa craniectomy with examination of the trigeminal nerve under the microscope in search of vascular compression. The nerve is decompressed by placing a sponge between the vessel and nerve; however, drug therapy is the first-line treatment for TN and the most effective medication is carbamazepine. The initial response to carbamazepine is so good, that it can be considered as a diagnostic test for TN; however, there is eventually a 50% relapse rate. The patient should be instructed to take the lowest dose that relieves symptoms. The medication induces its own metabolism must be started gradually in order to avoid toxic symptoms. Rare idiosyncratic reactions can result in aplastic anemia or liver necrosis. Mild abnormal liver function tests and leukopenia can be observed and these abnormalities usually reverse when the medication is discontinued. An occasional patient will develop acute hyponatremia shortly after starting carbamazepine. Gabapentin and phenytoin also can be used in treating TN but are less effective. There is no perfect surgical treatment for TN. Posterior fossa microvascular decompression has the least recurrence and causes minimal sensory loss, but has the greatest surgical risk and is usually reserved for younger patients. Percutaneous procedures via a needle through the foramen ovale cause partial damage to the trigeminal nerve root and cause some facial sensory loss. The trigeminal root can also be partially injured by stereotactic radiation (gamma knife). Although this is the least invasive surgical technique, there is significant recurrence, some sensory loss, and least likely treatment to allow patients to be off all medication.

Bibliography

Greenberg, MS. *Handbook of Neurosurgery*, 5th ed. New York, NY: Thieme, 2001, 373–380.

Wilkins R. Trigeminal neuralgia. In: Wilkins R, Rengachary S (eds.), *Neurosurgery*, 2nd ed. New York, NY: McGraw-Hill, 1996, 3921–3929.

31. (C)

32. (C)

Explanations 31 and 32

This patient is suffering from optic neuritis. It has been described as a syndrome in which "the patient can't see anything and the doctor can't see anything," owing to a lack of findings on examination. This may lead the examiner to believe the patient is hysterical. The patient will have a relative afferent papillary defect (RAPD or Marcus-Gunn pupil), which is diagnosed with the swinging light test. The pupils are equal at baseline and constrict in the light; however, when swinging the light from the normal eye to the affected eye, the pupils will dilate. This is due to a relative decrease in afferent stimulation of the affected eye. Significant monocular vision loss does not occur without an RAPD.

Optic neuritis is the initial presentation of MS in 15% of cases, and 50% of patients with MS will develop optic neuritis at some point in their course. MS is a chronic demyelinating disease that is usually diagnosed in young adulthood, and affects women twice as often as men. Its cause is unknown. The diagnosis is made based on the history of neurologic symptoms combined with MRI evidence of lesions explaining the deficits. Lumbar puncture for elevated IgG index and oligoclonal bands. It can be a relapsing-remitting or chronic-progressive disease.

TN usually presents in the sixth decade. Its diagnosis in a young person should prompt a workup for MS.

Amaurosis fugax is usually very transient (minutes), painless, and the vision loss if often altitudinal, described by the patient as a shade being pulled over the eye.

Bibliography

Corbett JJ. Approach to the patient with visual loss. In: Biller J (ed.), *Practical Neurology.* Philadelphia, PA: Lippincott-Raven, 1997, 97–107.

DeMyer WE. *Technique of the Neurologic Examination*, 4th ed. New York, NY: McGraw-Hill, 1994, 143–144.

Greenberg MS. *Handbook of Neurosurgery*, 5th ed. New York, NY: Thieme, 2001, 69–71.

Miller JR. Multiple sclerosis. In: Rowland LP (ed.), *Merritt's Neurology*, 10th ed. Philadelphia, PA: Lippincott, Williams & Wilkins, 2000, 773–792.

33. (C) SE is usually defined as a seizure of more than 30 min duration, or two consecutive seizures without recovery from the postical state (some authors will define a seizure of 5 or 10 min as SE). The seizure activity is usually generalized tonic-clonic, but may be nonconvulsive in rare circumstances. Morbidity and mortality is due to continuous electrical discharges causing neuronal membrane damage and metabolic derangements from convulsive activity causing stress on cardiac, respiratory, renal, and nervous systems. Emergency treatment includes ABCs, thiamine and D50 (hypoglycemia is a life-threatening cause of seizures), and lorazepam (in adults, 4 mg over 2 min, may repeat in 5–10 min if necessary) or diazepam (10 mg over 2 min, may repeat in 3–5 min) early in the course. Regardless of response to benzodiazepine medications, the patient should be loaded with phenytoin. Treatment should be aggressive, as there is irreversible damage to the CNS in less than 20 min of SE. If uncontrolled within 30 min, the patient should be intubated and treated with barbiturates, midazolam, or even inhalation anesthetics.

The most common cause of SE in a patient with a seizure disorder is noncompliance or subtherapeutic anticonvulsant levels, but treatment should be instituted before serum glucose and anticonvulsant levels have returned from the laboratory. Other common causes include stroke and alcohol (intoxication or withdrawal) in adults and febrile illness in children.

Bibliography

Greenberg MS. *Handbook of Neurosurgery*, 5th ed. New York, NY: Thieme, 2001, 262–266.

Pedley TA, Bazil CW, Morrell MJ. Epilepsy. In: Rowland LP (ed.), *Merritt's Neurology*, 10th ed. Philadelphia, PA: Lippincott, Williams & Wilkins, 2000, 829–830.

Working Group on Status Epilepticus: treatment of convulsive status epilepticus. *JAMA* 1993;270:854–859.

34. (D) This patient has an Arnold-Chiari's malformation (also known as hindbrain herniation syndrome) with resultant syringomyelia, a cavitary CSF collection in the spinal cord. Most if not all of the patient's symptoms and physical examination finding are directly referable to the syrinx. In over 70% of cases, the cause of a cystic cavity in the spinal cord is a hindbrain abnormality. Multiple theories of the pathophysiology exist, and most deal with alterations in the CSF dynamics at the cervicomedullary junction. Therefore, definitive treatment is directed at the posterior fossa.

Surgical treatment of the Arnold Chiari's malformation with syringomyelia is with posterior fossa craniectomy and often requires upper cervical laminecmtomy. The dura is opened, arachnoid adhesions are taken down, and the dura is then patched with cervical fascia, fascia lata or artificial dural substitute. The syrinx is followed with serial images. If the symptoms or the syrinx do not improve after adequate posterior fossa decompression, fenestration or shunting of the syrinx into the subarachnoid or pleural space can be performed.

Syringomyelia can also be the result of any compressive lesion of the spinal cord (intramedullary or extramedullary tumor, prior trauma), or any tethering of the spinal cord (spina bifida, arachnoiditis). Appropriate imaging studies with contrast should be performed to rule out tumor. Even in these cases, initial treatment is still directed at the causative pathological process and not the syrinx.

Bibliography

Piper JG, Menezes AH. The relationship between syringomyelia and the Chiari malformations. In: Anson JA, Benzel EC, Awad IA (eds.), *Neurosurgical Topics: Syringomyelia and the Chiari Malformations.* Park Ridge, IL: American Association of Neurological Surgeons, 1997, 91–104.

Williams B. Management schemes for syringomyelia: surgical indications and nonsurgical management. In: Anson JA, Benzel EC, Awad IA (eds.), *Neurosurgical Topics: Syringomyelia and the Chiari Malformations.* Park Ridge, IL: American Association of Neurological Surgeons, 1997, 125–143.

35. **(B)** Patients with VP shunts can and often do have medical problems that are actually unrelated to the shunt. Even though the foreign body is an easy scapegoat, once a VP shunt has been in place for more than a few months, the chances of it being a source of fever or infection are extremely low. The exception is the shunted patient with the acute abdomen, because the shunt often is the culprit for the symptoms. Small bowel obstructions, enterocutaneous fistulae, and even bowel perforations have been reported. Ultrasound can be very important in assisting with the diagnosis.

The patient in this example has a classic case of appendicitis, and if there were no VP shunt, his management would be very straightforward. If the appendix were unruptured, surgical treatment is no different than in the patient without a shunt. The patient should undergo appendectomy and receive appropriate antibiotics. The shunt tubing should not be sought, and should be left undisturbed if in the surgical field. If there is gross peritonitis, the neurosurgeon should bring the abdominal catheter out through a separate incision and connect it to a drainage bag. The spinal fluid should be cultured. The risk of ascending infection of the shunt in this patient is extremely low. If the shunt tubing becomes infected, the entire shunt system will be removed and replaced after elimination of the infection and resolution of peritonitis. Postoperative complications include CSF pseudocyst due to decreased peritoneal absorption, and are rare. Conversion to a ventriculoatrial or ventriculopleural shunt may be performed in the uninfected shunt even before the peritonitis has resolved.

In patients without obvious cause for peritonitis, it is usually recommended that the distal portion of the shunt be externalized and antibiotics started. Abdominal symptoms related to shunt infection will usually resolve within 6 h.

Bibliography

Hadani M, Findler G, Muggia-Sullam M, et al. Acute appendicitis in children with a ventriculoperitoneal shunt. *Surg Neurol* 1982;18:69–71.

Pumberger W, Löbl M, Geissler W. Appendicitis in children with a ventriculoperitoneal shunt. *Pediatr Neurosurg* 1998;28:21–26.

Rekate HL, Yonas H, White RJ, et al. The acute abdomen in patients with ventriculoperitoneal shunt. *Surg Neurol* 1979;11:442–445.

36. **(D)** The fundoscopic pictures reveal retinal hemorrhages, which are seen in significant head trauma, traumatic birth, or acute altitude sickness. They have been rarely reported with other significant CNS insults such as aneurysmalSAH. They resolve quickly, so their presence is indicative of an acute injury. The head CT reveals bilateral subdural hematomas. They appear less dense (darker) than expected in this patient due to anemia. Nonaccidental trauma is the most common cause of subdural hematoma in infants and young children. MRI is better for differentiating acute from subacute or chronic blood because the intensity is based on the oxidative state of hemoglobin. This child has classic presentation for shaken baby syndrome (also referred to as shaken impact syndrome), and the CT and fundoscopy are nearly pathognomonic. Due to legal ramifications, a thorough evaluation is warranted, and should include a skeletal survey for fractures (acute or old), a workup for coagulopathy and

metabolic/genetic screen for glutaric aciduria (a rare metabolic disorder that causes neurologic decline and brain atrophy, and can be associated with subdural hematoma).

Any physician or caregiver that suspects child abuse is required by state and federal law to report these suspicions to the appropriate child protective services or to law enforcement personnel.

Bibliography

Duhaime A, Christian C. Child abuse. In: McLone DG (ed.), *Pediatric Neurosurgery: Surgery of the Developing Nervous System*, 4th ed. Philadelphia, PA: W.B. Saunders, 2001, 593–600.

Greenberg MS. *Handbook of Neurosurgery*, 5th ed. New York, NY: Thieme, 2001, 678–679.

37. (D) The axial T1 weighted MRI with contrast (Fig. 35-14) reveals a lesion in the posterior fossa, obliterating the fourth ventricle. Headache in a child is always a cause for concern, and this patient's history of postural headache is even more concerning. When lying down, the tumor obstructs flow of CSF through the cerebral aqueduct or through the foramina of Magendie and Luschka in the fourth ventricle, causing symptomatic hydrocephalus. Sitting or standing up relieves the obstruction and the hydrocephalus.

The differential diagnosis for a posterior fossa tumor in the pediatric population includes medulloblastoma, cerebellar astrocytoma, ependymoma, and brain stem glioma. These four account for about 90% of pediatric posterior fossa tumors. Presenting symptoms are usually related to hydrocephalus, as most of these are slow growing tumors. Focal deficits typically appear late, and are caused by infiltration of structures by the tumor or metastatic spread via the subarachnoid spaces. This tumor would be resected via posterior fossa craniotomy. If there is hydrocephalus, a ventriculostomy could be placed at the time of tumor resection or earlier if the patient is very symptomatic. This would be removed after resolution of hydrocephalus after tumor resection, or it can be converted to a VP shunt if the hydrocephalus does not resolve. MRI of the entire neuraxis and lumbar puncture is indicated for medulloblastomas and ependymomas due to their propensity for "drop mets," and the information obtained from these studies is used in staging and determination of adjunctive therapy.

Medulloblastomas comprise 29% of pediatric posterior fossa tumors, arise from the roof of the fourth ventricle, and are usually midline. They enhance with gadolinium-contrasted MRI. Postoperative treatment is with chemotherapy and radiation depending on age, stage, and extent of resection. The overall 5-year survival is approximately 60%. Cerebellar astrocytomas comprise over 25% of posterior fossa tumors in children, are often cystic, and enhance with contrast on MRI. They typically do not require postoperative adjunctive therapy, and may have over 95% 25-year survival rates with complete resection. Ependymomas arise from the floor or lateral recesses of the fourth ventricle, variably enhance on contrasted MRI, and account for 10% of posterior fossa tumors in children. Postoperatively they are treated with radiation. Unfortunately ependymomas are relatively chemoresistant. The 5-year survival rates are approximately 50%. Brain stem gliomas account for 27% of posterior fossa tumors. They are further subclassified by their appearance on imaging studies, and have different treatments and outcomes based on this subclassification.

Choroid plexus papilloma is a tumor of the choroid plexus, most commonly seen in the lateral ventricles of adults. A choroid plexus papilloma can occur in the fourth ventricle of a child, but it would be far less common than any of the above tumors.

Bibliography

Choux M, Lena G, Gentet JC, et al. Medulloblastoma. In: McLone DG (ed.), *Pediatric Neurosurgery: Surgery of the Developing Nervous System*, 4th ed. Philadelphia, PA: W.B. Saunders, 2001, 804–818.

Reddy AT, Mapstone TB. Cerebellar astrocytoma. In: McLone DG (ed.), *Pediatric Neurosurgery: Surgery of the Developing Nervous System*, 4th ed. Philadelphia, PA: W.B. Saunders, 2001, 835–842.

Tomita T. Ependymomas. In: McLone DG (ed.), *Pediatric Neurosurgery: Surgery of the Developing Nervous System*, 4th ed. Philadelphia, PA: W.B. Saunders, 2001, 822–832.

38. (A)

39. (D)

Explanations 38 and 39

The MR and clinical history are most compatible with glioblastoma multiforme (GBM). This tumor is the most malignant of all of the gliomas. Gliomas are tumors that arise from glial cells, which are the supporting cells of the brain. Some GBMs arise from lower grade gliomas, but most appear *de novo* associated with a short clinical history. MR scans show an irregularly ring enhancing lesion with a dark, necrotic center and surrounding edema. The histology consists of malignant appearing astrocytes, vascular hyperplasia, and areas of necrosis. The best place to biopsy is the enhancing rim biopsy, either closed or open without resection, will not relieve the mass effect and could precipitate hemorrhage or further swelling of the tumor, leading to transtentorial herniation. Also, because the nondominant hemisphere is involved, aggressive therapy should be undertaken to prolong life. The immediate threat to the patient is death from increased ICP secondary to the large mass effect. This patient needs a craniotomy with debulking of as much tumor as possible. Prior to the craniotomy, pretreatment with steroids to decrease cerebral edema is appropriate.

Since this patient is young, his prognosis is better than an elderly patient with a similar lesion. The extent of resection is best estimated by performing a CT scan in the very early postoperative period. Enhancing areas probably represent residual tumor. In later scans it may be difficult to distinguish scar from tumor. Even though the tumor may seem circumscribed, tumor cells always infiltrate beyond the enhancing margin.

The average life expectancy for this lesion with surgery, radiation, and chemotherapy is 12–18 months. Radiation therapy is the most important adjuvant therapy for GBM and should be given to the patient following resection. A dose of 6000 cGy is usually given in 33 fractions. Chemotherapy with alkylating agents such as BCNU and temozolomide are of some help and most neurooncologists would offer them to this patient, but there is no really good chemotherapy for malignant gliomas. The antineoplastic agents are weak. It is difficult for them to penetrate the blood-brain barrier to reach neoplastic cells. Also, tumor cells can develop drug resistance and there is risk to normal brain.

Bibliography

Binder D, Keles G, Aldape K, et al. Aggressive glial neoplasms. In: Batjer H, Loftus C (eds.), *Textbook of Neurological Surgery*. Philadelphia, PA: Lippincott, Williams & Wilkins, 2003, 1270–1280.

Shrieve D, Alexander E, Black P, et al. Treatment of primary glioblastoma multiforme with standard radiotherapy and radiosurgical boost: prognostic factors and long-term outlook. *J Neurosurg* 1999;90:72–77.

40. **(A)** This patient has lung cancer with a single metastasis to the brain, as is the case in approximately one-third of patients with brain metastases. The most common primaries of metastasis to the brain are lung, breast, colon, kidney, and melanoma. In general, the prognosis is poor, and an untreated patient will have a median life expectancy of approximately 1 month. Brain radiation therapy alone can be expected to add 3–6 months of life, and is used in all patients with metastases, single or multiple, operative or not.

Indications for surgery and outcomes depend on location of the metastases, extent of systemic disease, and type of primary. Randomized, prospective studies of surgery followed by whole brain radiation versus radiation alone reveal statistically significant increases in life expectancy and quality of life. Therefore, the patient with a surgically accessible single brain metastasis will usually undergo craniotomy for resection, followed by whole brain radiation therapy. The patient in this example may have an even better prognosis, as there is evidence that patients undergoing a curative procedure for a primary lung cancer have a statistically significant increased survival compared to those undergoing only palliative surgery or no resection of the primary. Radiosurgery (stereotactic-focused high-dose radiation) of a metastasis may be considered as an alternative to craniotomy in the patient with the surgically inaccessible lesion, the patient who is not medically able to undergo craniotomy, or in the patient who refuses to consider craniotomy. Radiosurgery does not impact on the patient's ability to receive adjuvant radiation therapy.

Bibliography

Galicich JH, Arbit E, Wronski M. Metastatic brain tumors. In: Wilkins RH, Rengachary SS (eds.), *Neurosurgery*, 2nd ed. New York, NY: McGraw-Hill, 1996, 807–821.

Patchell RA, Tibbs PA, Walsh JW. A randomized trial of surgery in the treatment of single metastases to the brain. *N Engl J Med* 1990;322:494–500.

Wróński M, Arbit E, Burt M, et al. Survival after surgical treatment of brain metastasis from lung cancer. A follow up study of 231 patients treated between 1976–1991. *J Neurosurg* 1995;83:605–616.

Young B, Patchell RA. Surgery for a single brain metastasis. In: Wilkins RH, Rengachary SS (eds.), *Neurosurgery*, 2nd ed. New York, NY: McGraw-Hill, 1996, 823–828.

41. **(C)** This patient most likely has radiation myelopathy. In a patient with lung carcinoma that presents with paraplegia, spinal cord compression from vertebral or epidural compression from metastasis is the most likely cause, but with extradural compression there is almost always severe pain. This patient has no pain. Radiation myelopathy results from inclusion of the spinal cord in the radiation field. It is usually painless and becomes symptomatic in about 18 months after the radiation therapy is completed. The upper level of spinal cord dysfunction is usually at the level of radiation. Although all the other diagnoses listed are possible, the time course from radiation and the rarity of other disorders makes radiation the likely culprit. In most cases of radiation myelopathy, the MRI is normal, but occasionally, as in this case, the cord can be swollen with signal change. The imaging studies can look similar in all of the above and may not absolutely establish the diagnosis. Eventually the spinal cord will atrophy. There is no proven effective treatment, but in some cases the neurologic deficits

will stabilize. There are anecdotal reports of response to steroids. The risk of developing radiation myelopathy increases with the total dose, the dose per fraction, and the length of the spinal cord radiated.

Bibliography

Black P, Nair S, Giannakopoulos G. Spinal epidural tumors. In: Wilkins R, Rengachary S (eds.), *Neurosurgery*, 2nd ed. New York, NY: McGraw-Hill, 1996, 1791–1804.

Cahill D. Malignant tumors of the boney spine. In: Batjer H, Loftus C (eds.), *Textbook of Neurological Surgery*. Philadelphia, PA: Lippincott, Williams & Wilkins, 2003, 1401–1421.

Dropcho E. Neurologic complications of radiation therapy. In: Biller J (ed.), *Iatrogenic Neurology*. Boston, MA: Butterworth-Heinemann, 1998, 469–470.

Eyster E, Wilson C. Radiation myelopathy. *J Neurosurg* 1970;32:414–420.

42. **(C)** Toxoplasmosis, lymphoma, and PML are the three most common cerebral lesions seen on imaging studies in a patient with AIDS. When an MR scan is obtained with contrast, toxoplasma abscesses and lymphoma may ring enhance and may be indistinguishable with any degree of certainty. Rather than perform a biopsy, some neurosurgeons prefer to treat the patient empirically with pyrimethamine and sulfadiazine for 2–3 weeks. If there is radiographic improvement, the patient should be maintained on these drugs for the remainder of life to control the infection. If there is no response to these drugs, biopsy is indicated. Other intracranial infections that can occur less frequently in AIDS are caused by *Cryptococcus neoformans, Candida, Coccidioidomycosis, Treponema pallidum* (syphilis), *M. tuberculosis*, and *Aspergillus*.

Primary CNS lymphoma associated with AIDS is treated with radiation therapy and the prognosis is worse than the lymphoma without AIDS.

PML is an infection of white matter in the immunocompromised patient caused by a papova virus. The lesions of PML characteristically do not enhance and often do not act like a mass. There is no satisfactory treatment. The AIDS virus can cause a subacute encephalitis manifested by dementia. Herpes simplex or herpes zoster encephalitis as well as a viral myelitis can also occur.

Bibliography

Greenberg M. *Handbook of Neurosurgery*, 5th ed. New York, NY: Thieme, 2001, 231–234.

Levy R, Russell E, Yungbluth M, et al. The efficacy of image-guided stereotactic brain biopsy in neurologically symptomatic acquired immuno-deficiency syndrome patients. *Neurosurgery* 1992;30:186–190.

43. **(B)** Cyclosporin toxicity can result in the posterior leukoencephalopathy syndrome. There are a variety of acute illnesses that can result in a reversible encephalopathy secondary to edema of the cerebral white matter, most prominently in the occipital and posterior parietal and temporal regions of the brain. Clinically the syndrome is manifested by the subacute onset of headache, lethargy, confusion, altered mental status, seizures, and difficultly with vision. The white matter edema is visible as decreased attenuation on CT scans and hypointensity on T1 and hyperintensity on T2 MR scans. Originally described in encephalopathy associated with malignant hypertension and eclampsia of pregnancy, the syndrome also occurs secondary to toxicity of cyclosporin and other immunosuppressants. White matter edema results from disruption of the blood-brain barrier. The mechanism for this disturbance is not entirely clear in cases of immunosuppression. The syndrome can occur with levels of drug in the therapeutic range and is probably the result of a vasculopathy caused by the medication. The syndrome is reversible by discontinuing or lowering the drug level. The radiologic abnormalities often resolve completely within several weeks.

Creutzfeldt-Jakob's disease is a prion (proteinaceous infectious particle) disease that results in an invariably fatal encephalopathy manifested by dementia, ataxia, myoclonic jerks, and visual symptoms. Creutzfeldt-Jakob's disease is not associated with immunosuppression. PML is a white matter infection of the brain caused by the polyomavirus in patients who are immunosuppressed and with certain malignancies. Mental symptoms as well as blindness can occur. The disease is rapidly progressive. Imaging studies show areas of white matter hypointensity on CT and low signal on T1 and high signal on T2 images. There is no enhancement and little if any mass effect. Primary central nervous system lymphoma occurs in patients with AIDS and in patients who have had organ transplantation and are immunosuppressed.

Bibliography

Hinchey J, Chaves C, Appignana B, et al. A reversible posterior leukoencephalopathy syndrome. *N Engl J Med* 1996;334:494–500.

Truwit C, Denaro C, Lake J, et al. MR imaging of reversible cyclosporin A-induced neurotoxicity. *Am J Neuroradiol* 1991;12:651–659.

CHAPTER 36

Anesthesia

*Michael D. Miller, David Camp, Anthony Keever,
Jason Lowrey, and Chansamone Saysana*

Questions

1. A 40-year-old male s/p renal transplant 2 years prior with juvenile onset diabetes mellitus presents to an ambulatory surgery center for debridement of an AV fistula used in the past for dialysis. In spite of tight glycemic control, the patient has diabetic retinopathy and neuropathy. His renal function is normal and is no longer on dialysis. The patient has no risk factors for aspiration.

    This patient's American Society of Anesthesiologists (ASA) physical status is

    (A) class I
    (B) class II
    (C) class IIE
    (D) class III
    (E) class IV

2. The above patient is brought to the operating suite, given an intravenous induction with fentanyl, propofol, and midazolam. The anesthesiologist makes an initial attempt at intubation but is unsuccessful. Mask ventilation is not adequate. The patient is repositioned and the laryngoscope blade is changed. The next attempt fails as well. The patient begins to wake up. The best approach at this juncture would be

    (A) allow the patient to wake up
    (B) paralyze the patient to facilitate mask ventilation
    (C) attempt a laryngeal mask airway (LMA)
    (D) attempt a light wand intubation
    (E) attempt intubation via fiberoptic bronchoscope

3. Which of the following factors is *not* unique to the pediatric airway?

    (A) large occiput
    (B) long, narrow epiglottis
    (C) short neck
    (D) short trachea
    (E) posterior larynx

4. Which of the following is *false* concerning neonatal physiology?

    (A) lower functional residual capacity (FRC) limits oxygen reserves
    (B) elevated respiratory rate
    (C) lower tidal volume per kg than adults
    (D) cardiac output dependent on heart rate (HR)
    (E) kidney function is normal by 12 months of age

Special thanks to Robert K. Stoelting, Professor and Chair, Department of Anesthesia, Indiana University School of Medicine.

5. A 74-year-old White male is being evaluated for carotid endarterectomy. Medical history includes transient ischemic attack (TIA) × 3, hypertension (HTN), adult onset diabetes requiring insulin for control, benign prostatic hyperplasia and mild osteoarthritis. He has a 50 pack-year history of tobacco use, but has not smoked for 12 years. His prescription medications include lisinopril, furosemide, K-dur, metoprolol, and insulin. He also takes over-the-counter medications including multivitamin, vitamin C, Saw Palmetto, baby aspirin, and PRN acetaminophen and naproxen. The patient relates he is quite active and has gradually increased the amount he exercises over the past 2 years at his doctor's suggestion. He swims 20 laps 3 times per week and plays doubles tennis 2 days per week. He denies shortness of breath, paroxysmal nocturnal dyspnea or history of myocardial infarction (MI), chest pain, or congestive heart failure (CHF). A 12-lead electrocardiogram (ECG) performed 15 months ago by his primary care physician is included with his records and shows sinus rhythm, 71 bpm, no block, no pathologic Q waves, but some nonspecific S-T changes in leads V1, V4 and V5. Which of the following cardiac tests or interventions should be performed prior to surgery?

   (A) repeat 12-lead ECG
   (B) treadmill stress testing
   (C) dobutamine stress echo
   (D) coronary angiography with subsequent percutaneous coronary intervention or coronary artery bypass graft (CABG) if stenotic lesions are detected
   (E) no further testing or intervention needed prior to surgery

6. Potential side effect(s) of succinylcholine include

   (A) hyperkalemia
   (B) rhabdomyolysis
   (C) malignant hyperthermia
   (D) myalgias
   (E) all of the above

7. Potential side effect(s) of nondepolarizing neuromuscular blockers include

   (A) histamine release
   (B) vagolysis
   (C) ganglionic blockade
   (D) allergic reaction
   (E) all of the above

8. All of these agents are nondepolarizing neuromuscular blocking agents *except*:

   (A) cisatracurium
   (B) succinylcholine
   (C) vecuronium
   (D) rocuronium
   (E) pancuronium

9. Patterns of nerve stimulation used to monitor neuromuscular function include

   (A) single twitch
   (B) train-of-four (TOF)
   (C) double-burst stimulation (DBS)
   (D) tetany
   (E) all of the above

10. A patient has undergone general anesthesia for an exploratory laparotomy. Pancuronium has been used for muscle relaxation. At the end of the procedure, there was evidence of residual neuromuscular blockade with use of a nerve stimulator. What combination of agents is best used to reverse this blockade?

   (A) edrophonium/atropine
   (B) neostigmine/atropine
   (C) neostigmine/glycopyrrolate
   (D) edrophonium/glycopyrrolate
   (E) none of the above

11. The mechanism of action of local anesthetics is best described as

   (A) binding of the cationic form of the local anesthetic molecule to extracellular local anesthetic receptors
   (B) binding of the neutral (basic) form of the local anesthetic molecule to cytoplasmic receptors
   (C) binding of the cationic form of the local anesthetic molecule to transmembrane sodium receptors in the inactivated-closed state
   (D) binding of the neutral (basic) form of the local anesthetic molecule to transmembrane sodium channels in the activated-open state
   (E) binding of the local anesthetic molecule to transmembrane potassium channels

12. In which of the following groups of conditions of local anesthetic, nerve fiber type and local pH at injection site would conduction blockade be expected to be established most rapidly (assume all other conditions equal)?

(A) lidocaine, highly stimulated preganglionic B fibers, pH 7.52

(B) lidocaine, infrequently stimulated C-fibers, pH 7.16

(C) lidocaine, moderately stimulated A-alpha fibers, pH 7.40

(D) mepivicaine, infrequently stimulated A-delta fibers, pH 7.23

(E) mepivicaine, highly stimulated A-alpha fibers, pH 7.38

13. An otherwise healthy, 80 kg 47-year-old male undergoes wide local excision of a suspected malignant melanoma along the right midaxillary line overlying the fifth rib. The incision is elliptically shaped, 8 cm long and 4 cm wide, and is able to be closed primarily. Which of the following represents the best choice for local infiltration to manage postoperative pain?

(A) 30 mL of 2% lidocaine with 1:200,000 epinephrine

(B) 40 mL of 1% lidocaine without epinephrine

(C) 5 mL of 0.25% mepivicaine without epinephrine

(D) 30 mL of 0.75% bupivicaine with 1:200,000 epinephrine

(E) 20 mL of 0.5% bupivicaine with 1:200,000 epinephrine

14. A 56-year-old female with a long history of rheumatoid arthritis and HTN is admitted through the emergency department. She presents with fever, malaise, and shortness of breath. She reports she began feeling ill 3 days prior to admission with sore throat, cough, and low grade fever. Her cough is productive of thick sputum. She reports allergies to penicillin, sulfa drugs and many cosmetics. Her vital signs are T 102.3°F, HR 105 bpm, RR 29 breaths/min, BP 130/75 mmHg. She appears uncomfortable but in no acute distress. Chest x-ray is strongly suggestive of left-sided pleural effusion. The decision is made to perform bedside thoracentesis with insertion of a chest tube if frank pus is returned. The patient complains of palpitations and increased malaise approximately 60 s after infiltration and intercostal block with a total of 5 mL of 1% lidocaine combined with 5 mL of 0.25% bupivicaine and 1:100,000 epinephrine. HR is found to be 145 bpm and BP is 175/110 mmHg. The most likely explanation is

(A) allergic reaction to lidocaine

(B) allergic reaction to bupivicaine

(C) accidental intravascular injection resulting in cardiac toxicity from lidocaine

(D) vascular absorption of the epinephrine-containing solution

(E) accidental intravascular injection resulting in cardiac toxicity form bupivicaine

Questions 15 and 16 refer to the following case scenario.

A 47-year-old Black male with insulin-dependent diabetes mellitus, HTN, and chronic renal failure presents for grafting of an AV fistula in the left upper extremity (LUE) in anticipation of a need for hemodialysis in the near future. On the morning of surgery the patient is feeling relatively well. He is appropriately NPO and did not take his morning insulin or ACE-inhibitor, but did take his normal dose of metoprolol (50 mg). Preoperative laboratory values (meq/L or mg/dL) include sodium 137, potassium 5.1, chloride 103, bicarbonate 25, blood urea nitrogen (BUN) 43, creatinine 3.1, and glucose 144. Preoperative ECG shows some nonspecific S-T changes but is otherwise unremarkable. Vital signs are T 97.4°F, HR 62 bpm, RR 12 breaths/min, BP 131/69 mmHg. The operative plan is to perform the procedure using an axillary block and IV sedation only if needed. The block is to be accomplished after connecting to the appropriate monitors and obtaining IV access using 50 mL of 0.5% mepivicaine with 1:200,000 epinephrine via a transarterial approach. Thirty milliliters of local anesthetic solution is injected posterior to the axillary artery in 3 mL doses with aspiration negative for heme between injections without difficulty. After moving the needle anterior to the axillary artery and again confirming negative heme on aspiration between 3 mL aliquots, the remainder of the local anesthetic injection is begun. During injection of the third aliquot (7–9 mL anterior to artery), the patient complains of a metallic taste in his mouth, a ringing in his ears, and a sense that "something is not right." The patient's periorbital muscles begin to twitch.

15. The sign or symptom of systemic toxicity that is most likely to occur next is

    (A) tonic-clonic seizures
    (B) CNS depression resulting in apnea and bradycardia
    (C) cardiovascular excitation resulting in tachycardia and HTN
    (D) blockade of the primary conducting system of the heart
    (E) CNS depression with decreased cerebral oxygen demand

16. Initial steps in management of the patient include all of the following *except*:

    (A) termination of injection of local anesthetic
    (B) instructing the patient to hypoventilate
    (C) administration of midazolam (2–5 mg) intravenously

    (D) consideration of rapid-sequence induction of general anesthesia with tracheal intubation and positive-pressure ventilation
    (E) preparation for cardiovascular support

17. A 23-year-old male victim of abdominal penetrating trauma is to be brought to the OR for exploratory laparotomy. On presentation to the emergency room (ER), the patient was in early stages of shock with HR 118 bpm, RR 26 breaths/min, BP 73/30 mmHg. External bleeding was controlled and the patient was aggressively resuscitated with 3 L normal saline and 2 units packed red blood cells (PRBCs). Post-resuscitation vitals have improved to HR 105 bpm, RR 22 breaths/min, BP 95/54 mmHg. Which of the following intravenous medications represents the best choice to induce general anesthesia and facilitate endotracheal intubation?

    (A) propofol 2 mg/kg
    (B) thiopental 5 mg/kg
    (C) etomidate 0.4 mg/kg
    (D) ketamine 1 mg/kg
    (E) midazolam 0.2 mg/kg

18. An 18-year-old White male presents with open fractures of the left femur and tibia as well as the right radius after a fall while rock-climbing. There is no head or neck injury. The patient is stable and awake, although clearly in discomfort despite intravenous morphine. The patient is able to relate that he is otherwise healthy and physically fit. This is to be the patient's first trip to the OR, but he had an uncle who died during a general anesthetic and his younger brother spent 6 days in the intensive care unit (ICU) following an elective knee arthroscopy. On further questioning, the patient states he believes he was told his brother had developed malignant hyperthermia during surgery. The decision is made to proceed to the OR, but to perform a "trigger-free" anesthetic with continuous infusions of cisatracurium, propofol, and a narcotic. Select the narcotic from which complete recovery from effects would be most rapid following a 5-h continuous infusion.

    (A) morphine
    (B) fentanyl
    (C) sufentanil
    (D) remifentanil
    (E) meperidine

19. Which of the following is *false* concerning the physiologic effects of volatile anesthetics?

    (A) decreased tidal volume
    (B) decreased blood pressure
    (C) decreased respiratory rate
    (D) bronchodilation
    (E) decreased sensitivity to the ventilatory stimulant effects of carbon dioxide

20. Appropriate anesthetic management of nonobstetric surgery during pregnancy includes all of the following *except*:

    (A) aspiration prophylaxis
    (B) use of nitrous oxide
    (C) postponement of elective surgery until after delivery
    (D) high inspired concentrations of oxygen
    (E) left uterine displacement position after 20 weeks gestation

21. Blood gas analysis of a patient with chronic obstructive pulmonary disease (COPD) reveals a pH 7.25, PCO_2 65, PO_2 65, on room air. What is the primary disorder?

    (A) metabolic acidosis
    (B) metabolic alkalosis
    (C) respiratory acidosis
    (D) respiratory alkalosis
    (E) none of the above

22. A 45-year-old female with epigastric pain is admitted to the ICU with recurrent pancreatitis. Examination of the arterial line waveform reveals variability in the amplitude of the waves. What is the most likely conclusion?

    (A) She also has peripheral vascular disease.
    (B) She has poor ventricular contractility.
    (C) There is a small clot in the catheter.
    (D) There is a kink in the catheter.
    (E) She is hypovolemic.

23. A 68-year-old male undergoes uneventful coronary artery bypass grafting with the use of cardiopulmonary bypass. On separation from bypass the following variables are noted by the use of a pulmonary artery catheter. CI = 2.1, PAOP = 21, SVO_2 = 0.50, CVP = 5, SVI = 20. Which of the following states best explains the above variables?

    (A) hypovolemia
    (B) hypervolemia

    (C) left ventricular failure
    (D) right ventricular failure
    (E) biventricular failure

24. Which of the following is *false* concerning basic monitoring?

    (A) Lead II contains the highest P waves on electrocardiography.
    (B) Criteria for ischemia includes 1 mm ST depression on electrocardiography.
    (C) The proper width of a blood pressure cuff is greater than the diameter of the extremity.
    (D) Automated blood pressure cuffs use Korotkoff sounds.
    (E) Systolic pressure readings increase with distance from the aorta.

25. Which of the following is *false* regarding pulse oximetry?

    (A) Presence of carboxyhemoglobin may lead to a falsely elevated pulse oximeter reading.
    (B) Pulse oximetry uses a single wavelength of light.
    (C) Presence of methemoglobin can result in a falsely low or high pulse ox reading.
    (D) Ear probes can detect changes in oxygen saturation faster than finger probes.
    (E) Pulse oximetry relies on the Lambert-Beer's law

26. A patient receives a spinal anesthetic at the T5 level. Which of the following physiologic effects is *not* likely to occur?

    (A) urinary retention
    (B) dilated and relaxed small bowel
    (C) decreased venous return
    (D) bradycardia
    (E) decreased ability to cough

27. A 27-year-old woman had a vaginal delivery under spinal anesthesia. On postoperative day 1, she complains of a severe frontal headache. Treatment of this condition may include which of the following?

    (A) intravenous caffeine
    (B) hydration
    (C) recumbent position
    (D) epidural autologous blood patch
    (E) all of the above

28. Which of the following statements regarding citrate intoxication following massive transfusion is *false*?

    (A) Patients undergoing liver transplantation are more likely to have it.
    (B) It may result in ECG changes.
    (C) It is associated with hypermagnesemia.
    (D) Treatment includes intravenous calcium chloride.
    (E) All of the above.

29. Which of the following statements regarding transfusion compatibility testing is *true*?

    (A) Patients with Rh-negative blood will have anti-D antibodies in serum.
    (B) Antibody screening is a check for anti-A and anti-B antibodies in donor serum.
    (C) Rh-negative patients given Rh-positive blood will always have hemolytic reactions.
    (D) Crossmatching of blood involves simulation of actual anticipated transfusion by mixing of recipient and donor blood.
    (E) All of the above.

30. A 37-year-old female undergoing total abdominal hysterectomy requires transfusion for unanticipated blood loss. After the third unit of PRBCs, she continues to have hypotension and tachycardia despite adequate blood replacement. The anesthesiologist later notes hemoglobinuria from the Foley catheter. Therapy of this reaction to transfusion may include all of the following *except*:

    (A) diphenhydramine
    (B) furosemide
    (C) dopamine
    (D) sodium bicarbonate
    (E) normal saline

31. The following statement regarding fluid management is *false*:

    (A) Glucose containing fluids are not recommended in non diabetic adult patients.
    (B) In patients with CHF, colloids have been shown to be superior to crystalloid during resuscitation.
    (C) Large doses of hydroxyethyl starch (>15 mL/kg) may cause a clinically significant coagulopathy.

    (D) Most patients mobilize the extracellular fluid compartment on postoperative day 3.
    (E) None of the above.

32. The following statement regarding the LMA is *true*:

    (A) The patient must be kept breathing spontaneously.
    (B) It is contraindicated in asthmatic patients.
    (C) It is not safe in patients with hiatal hernias.
    (D) It is associated with a significant increase in bronchospasm compared to a conventional endotracheal tube.
    (E) It should not be used if a traditional mask airway provides adequate ventilation.

Questions 33 and 34 refer to the following case scenario.

A 36-year-old female with a history of ulcerative colitis is admitted. Physical examination of the abdomen reveals right lower quadrant (RLQ) tenderness, high pitched bowel sounds, and rebound tenderness. A rapid-sequence induction of anesthesia is performed followed by a chest x-ray.

33. Rapid-sequence induction

    (A) is recommended in patients with bowel obstructions
    (B) avoids the use of neuromuscular blocking agents
    (C) uses direct laryngoscopy after positive pressure ventilation
    (D) does not involve the use of cricoid pressure
    (E) implies intubating the patient while awake

34. The chest x-ray reveals diffuse bilateral infiltrates consistent with ARDS. Which of the following statements regarding ARDS is *not* true?

    (A) The underlying pathology is an increase in capillary permeability.
    (B) Positive end expiratory pressure (PEEP) plays an important role in therapy.
    (C) Higher tidal volumes (10 mL/kg) have been shown to improve oxygenation.
    (D) Inhaled nitric oxide may be an effective modality in severe cases.
    (E) It is a severe version of acute lung injury with $PaO_2/FiO_2 < 200$

35. A 38-year-old female is to undergo a craniotomy for tumor resection. Which of the following agents would be least likely to be used in the delivery of anesthesia?

 (A) isoflurane
 (B) propofol
 (C) fentanyl
 (D) vecuronium
 (E) ketamine

36. A 7-year-old male with no prior surgeries is administered succinylcholine prior to intubation. Fifteen minutes into the surgery he develops elevation of end-tidal CO_2, tachycardia, and his body temperature increases 2°C over the next 5 min. Treatment of this disorder may include all of the following *except*:

 (A) dantrolene
 (B) gastric lavage with cold saline
 (C) calcium-channel blockers
 (D) mannitol
 (E) discontinuation of potential triggers

37. A 40-year-old female has undergone laproscopic cholecystectomy via general anesthesia. She had an uncomplicated surgical procedure. Propofol and succinylcholine were used for induction, and sevoflurane was used for maintenance. Rocuronium was used for muscle relaxation. Gentamicin was used for spontaneous bacterial endocarditis (SBE) prophylaxis. At the end of the procedure the patient was slow to awaken. Which of these agents would be least likely to be the cause for delayed awakening?

 (A) sevoflurane
 (B) rocuronium
 (C) succinylcholine
 (D) propofol
 (E) gentamicin

38. A 65-year-old patient is 4 days postliver transplantation. Her status is worsening and a recent arterial blood gas sample reveals a PaO_2 of 70 with an elevated CO_2 on supplemental oxygen by nasal cannula. The decision is made to intubate the trachea and place her on mechanical ventilation. Which mode of ventilation may lead to high airway pressures?

 (A) synchronized intermittent mandatory ventilation (SIMV)
 (B) pressure control (PC)
 (C) volume control (VC)
 (D) inverse ratio ventilation (IRV)
 (E) high frequency ventilation (HFV)

39. Which of the following does *not* increase the incidence of post operative nausea and vomiting?

 (A) propofol
 (B) morphine
 (C) pain
 (D) isoflurane
 (E) female gender

Answers and Explanations

1. **(D)** The American Society of Anesthesiologists (ASA) classification was developed in an effort to insure adequate comparisons between patient populations can be made between institutions for morbidity and mortality statistics. The ASA classes range from one; a normal healthy patient, to six; a brain dead organ donor. Those in between include: two, mild systemic illness with no physical limitations; three, systemic illness with physical limitations; four, systemic illness which is a constant threat to life; five, moribund patient expected to die within 24 hours without the operation. The designation "E" is added to procedures which are deemed emergent. The aforementioned patient is considered ASA class III because diabetes is limiting his physical status, i.e., vision and nervous system. Extremes in age carry a minimum of class II. Notice the ASA classification is independent of the surgical procedure. Accordingly, it does not imply preoperative risk.

Bibliography

Stoelting RK, Miller RD. *Basics of Anesthesia*, 4th ed. Philadelphia, PA: Churchill Livingstone, 2000, 113–114.

2. **(A)** The ASA established an algorithm which describes a systematic approach to the patient with known or unknown difficult airway. A difficult airway is defined as a "conventionally trained anesthesiologist experiences difficulty with mask ventilation (unable to keep oxygen saturation above 90% with FiO_2 100%), difficulty with tracheal intubation (requires more than three attempts or more than 10 min, or both). Since its initial publication in 1993, there have been advances in airway devices which can aid in the difficult airway. These include the LMA, intubating LMA, and light wand. Particularly important is the risk of aspiration. If the patient is judged to be at risk for aspiration, it is generally best to perform an awake procedure keeping the patients airway reflexes intact whenever possible. There are several advantages to the awake intubation: (1) maintenance of spontaneous ventilation, (2) increased size and patency of the pharynx, (3) forward placement of the tongue, (4) some maintenance of esophageal sphincter tone. Proper local anesthesia of the airway can make awake intubations surprisingly tolerable. There are no absolute contraindications to awake intubation. Many difficult airways can be managed with a traditional LMA thus eliminating the need for intubation all together. Obviously patient and procedure related factors may make an LMA not suitable for the case. The patient above should not be paralyzed until an airway can be reliably maintained. One option would be to give more propofol and attempt LMA placement, light wand intubation, or perhaps fiberoptic intubation. If these are unsuccessful, it would be prudent to allow the patient to wake up.

Bibliography

Barash, PG, Cullen BF, Stoelting RK. *Clinical Anesthesia*, 4th ed. Philadelphia, PA: Lippincott, Williams & Wilkins, 2001, 614–617.

3. **(E)** The pediatric airway differs from the adult airway in many aspects, requiring an understanding of these anatomical differences for proper mask ventilation and intubation. Infants and neonates have a proportionately larger head and tongue. The larynx is located more anterior and cephalad compared with adults. The epiglottis is long and narrow. The trachea and neck are short. Narrow nasal passages may preclude the use of nasal airways. Another important attribute is the cricoid cartilage, which is the narrowest part of the airway in children younger than 5 years of age. This is important for proper endotracheal tube selection, since a tube can be seen to pass through the vocal cords, but become stopped by the cricoid cartilage. Prominent adenoid and tonsillar tissue may also hinder visualization of the vocal cords.

Care must be taken to not collapse the submandibular tissue during mask ventilation. This will allow proper ventilation in infants and small children. Straight laryngoscope blades may aid in visualization of the vocal cords past the long epiglottis and anteriorly situated larynx. The large occiput tends to maintain the airway in a flexed position, which can be overcome with a towel placed under the shoulders.

Sizing of endotracheal tubes is much more important in the pediatric age group. The narrow trachea allows a higher incidence of edema from an oversized endotracheal tube. This can lead to postextubation stridor and airway obstruction. One formula used to choose proper endotracheal tube size involves taking the patients age divided by 4, and adding 4 to the result to obtain the internal tube diameter in millimeters. Correct size is confirmed by a positive leak at 10–25 cm H_2O. Proper length of insertion must also be determined. Too deep of an insertion can lead to an endobronchial intubation which may lead to atelectasis of the unventilated lung. One must always use auscultation as the final guide for depth of insertion.

Bibliography

Cravero JP, Rice LJ. *Pediatric anesthesia*. In: Barash PG, Cullen BF, Stoelting RK (eds.), *Clinical Anesthesia*, 4th ed. Philadelphia, PA: Lippincott, Williams & Wilkins, 2001, vol. 44, 1200.

Morgan GE Jr, Mikhail MS. *Clinical Anesthesiology*, 3rd ed. New York, NY: Lange Medical Books/McGraw-Hill, 1996, vol. 44, 729–730.

Stoelting RK, Miller RD. *Basics of Anesthesia*, 4th ed. Philadelphia, PA: Churchill Livingstone, 2000, 164.

4. **(C)** Successful care of neonates, infants, and children depends on knowledge of the physiologic characteristics which differentiate them from adults. Cardiac output in neonates and infants is dependent on HR, as stroke volume is relatively fixed by a noncompliant ventricle. This HR is higher than the average adult resting rate. Hypoxia can lead to a decline in HR and have profound effects on cardiac output. There is also a muted response to exogenous catecholamines, and a relative inability to use endogenous catecholamines during periods of hypotension. Therefore, fluid depletion is marked by a low blood pressure without concomitant tachycardia.

Respiratory rate is elevated in infants, while the per kilogram deadspace and tidal volume ratios are similar to adult values. Alveolar maturation is not complete until late childhood. These alveoli are less compliant than the cartilaginous chest wall of neonates and infants, leading to chest wall collapse during inspiration, and low residual lung volumes during expiration. This decrease in the FRC lowers oxygen reserves and increases the likelihood of atelectasis. Hypoxia and hypercarbia, while causing

increased respiratory drive in adults, lead to respiratory depression in neonates.

Pediatric patients have a larger surface area per kilogram than adults. This is responsible for rapid heat loss in this age group. Hypothermia has been linked with cardiac irritability, decreased respiratory drive, elevated pulmonary vascular resistance, and an altered response to medications. Excessive heat loss can be controlled with the use of warming blankets, warming IV fluids, and humidified gases.

Normal kidney function is usually in place by 12 months of age. Neonates may have a reduced creatinine clearance, with impaired sodium retention and bicarbonate reabsorption. Poor diluting and concentrating ability may also be present. Impaired glucose excretion in neonates is offset by a tendency toward hypoglycemia in premature neonates, infants small for gestational age, and those born to diabetic mothers. Strict glucose monitoring is required in this subset of patients.

Bibliography

Berry FA, Castro BA. Neonatal anesthesia. In: Barash PG, Cullen BF, Stoelting RK (eds.), *Clinical Anesthesia*, 4th ed. Philadelphia, PA: Lippincott, Williams & Wilkins, 2001, vol. 43, 1174, 1176–1177.

Morgan GE Jr, Mikhail MS. *Clinical Anesthesiology*, 3rd ed. New York, NY: Lange Medical Books/McGraw-Hill, 1996, vol. 44, 726–728.

Stoelting RK, Miller RD. *Basics of Anesthesia*, 4th ed. Philadelphia, PA: Churchill Livingstone, 2000, 364–365.

5. **(E)** Coronary artery disease (CAD) is prevalent throughout the United States. It is estimated that 40% of adult patients undergoing surgery annually in the United States will have or be at risk for CAD. Cardiovascular complications account for 25–50% of deaths following noncardiac surgery. All anesthetic techniques have the potential to cause changes in hemodynamics and coronary perfusion, and perioperative stress and pain can cause increased catecholamines and sympathetic tone resulting in increased myocardial oxygen demands. Several studies have shown that patients suffering a MI within 6 months prior to surgery are at increased risk for perioperative MI. Unfortunately there is a paucity of randomized, controlled trials to delineate optimal testing and management strategies for patients at risk for CAD undergoing noncardiac surgery. The American College of Cardiology (ACC) and American Heart Association (AHA) issued guidelines for perioperative cardiovascular examination for noncardiac surgery in 1996 and updated them in 2002. Recommendations are based largely on retrospective or observational

data and knowledge of management of cardiovascular disorders in nonoperative settings. The guidelines provide a framework in which to consider cardiac risk in noncardiac surgery in a variety of situations using a stepwise approach. The overriding theme of the guidelines is that preoperative intervention is rarely indicated simply to lower the risk of surgery unless the intervention is indicated irrespective of the preoperative context. The goal of preoperative evaluation is not to give "cardiac clearance," but to identify the most appropriate treatment and testing strategies to optimize short- and long-term care of the patient.

The stepwise approach to presurgical cardiac evaluation relies on assessment of clinical markers, prior cardiac evaluation and treatment, functional capacity, and surgery-specific risk. Emergent surgery needs to proceed to the operating room (OR) irrespective of prior cardiac evaluation, while patients undergoing urgent and elective surgery will generally benefit from more careful evaluation and testing. Noncardiac surgical procedures are stratified into three risk groups. High-risk surgeries (e.g., emergent major operations (especially in the elderly), aortic or other major vascular or peripheral vascular surgery, and long procedures with large blood loss or fluid shifts) often have reported perioperative cardiovascular risk of MI, heart failure or death of greater than 5%. Intermediate risk (CEA, head and neck, intrathoracic, intraperitoneal, prostate, and orthopedic) procedures generally have risks reported between 1 and 5%. Low-risk procedures (endoscopic, superficial, cataract, or breast surgery) generally have risks below 1%. The clinical predictors of increased perioperative cardiovascular risk are divided into major (unstable coronary syndromes such as MI within the past month or unstable angina, decompensated heart failure, significant arrhythmias or severe valvular disease), intermediate (mild angina pectoris, MI >1 month prior to surgery, compensated or prior heart failure, DM, and renal insufficiency) and minor (advanced age, abnormal ECG, rhythm other than sinus, low functional capacity, history of stroke or uncontrolled systemic HTN). Finally, functional capacity looks at activities a patient is able to do without angina or anginal equivalents such as shortness of breath, nausea, vomiting, diaphoresis, or fatigue. Functional capacity can be measured in metabolic equivalents (METs). Activities of daily living are considered to represent approximately 1 MET. Functional capacity is considered poor and perioperative cardiac risk is increased if a patient cannot meet a 4 MET demand in his/her daily activities. Activities requiring approximately 4 METs include walking up a flight of stairs while carrying a bag of groceries, walking >4 mph on level ground or heavy household chores (scrubbing, moving heavy furniture).

In this case, the patient is undergoing urgent or elective surgery. The surgical risk is intermediate and at least one intermediate clinical predictor of increased risk is present (DM). The patient clearly has good functional capacity. Following the algorithm in Fig. 36-1, this patient can proceed to the OR without further testing. If the patient were to undergo abdominal aortic aneurysm repair, further noninvasive testing would be indicated because of the high surgical risk. The most useful testing would be treadmill stress testing or stress echocardiography.

Bibliography

Eagle KA, Berger PB, Calkins H, et al. ACC/AHA guideline update for perioperative cardiovascular evaluation for noncardiac surgery : a report of the American College of Cardiology/American Heart Association task force on practice guidelines (committee to update the 1996 guidelines on perioperative cardiac evaluation for noncardiac surgery) *Circulation* 2002;105:1257–1267.

Morgan GE Jr, Mikhail MS, Murray MJ. Anesthesia for patients with cardiovascular disease. In: Morgan GE Jr, Mikhail MS, Murray MJ, et al. (eds.), *Clinical Anesthesiology*, 3rd ed. New York, NY: McGraw-Hill, 2002, 387–393.

Stoelting RK, Miller RD. Cardiovascular disease. In: Stoelting RK, Miller RD (eds.), *Basics of Anesthesia*, 4th ed. New York, NY: Churchill Livingstone; 2000, 248–253.

Wall RT. Anesthesia. In: Norton JA, Bollinger RR, Chang AE, et al. (eds.), *Surgery: Basic Science and Clinical Evidence.* New York, NY: Springer, 2001, 342–344.

6. **(E)** Succinylcholine is a depolarizing neuromuscular blocking agent that acts at postjunctional neuromuscular membrane to produce rapid skeletal muscle relaxation. Succinylcholine has a structure similar to acetylcholine and as such binds to nicotinic cholinergic receptors. Succinylcholine attaches to the two alpha subunits on the nicotinic cholinergic receptor and causes sustained opening of the nicotinic cholinergic receptor channel. This depolarization causes leakage of potassium ions from the intracellular stores to produce an average increase of 0.5 to 1 meq/L in serum potassium concentration in healthy patients. This increase may be exaggerated in patients who have proliferation of extrajunctional nicotinic receptors, which would include patients who have undergone denervation injury such as those with traumatic crush injury, unhealed third degree burns, and upper motor neuron disease. These patients are at risk of a hyperkalemic response to succinylcholine anywhere from a few days to 6 months after the injury. It is

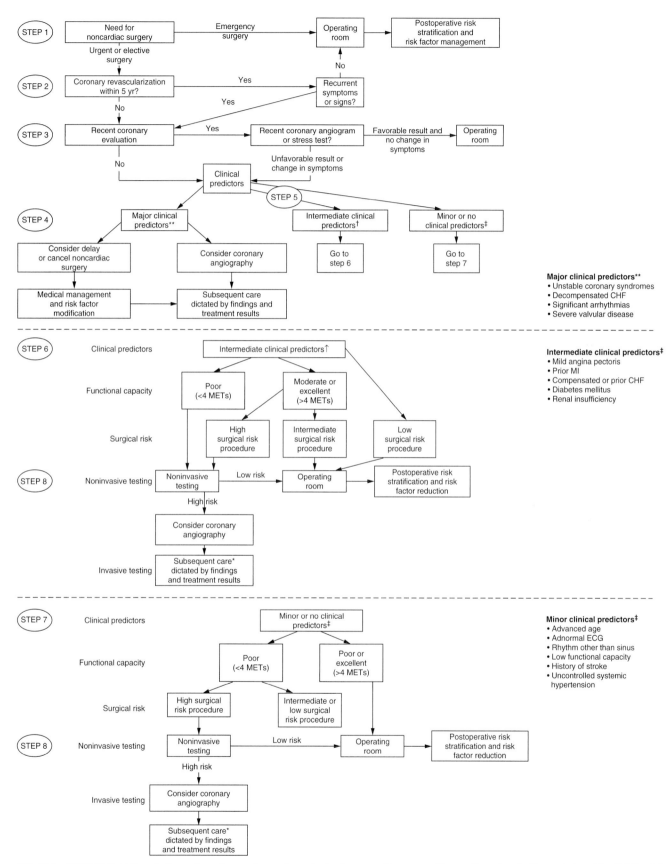

FIG. 36-1   ACC/AHA Guidelines for the perioperative cardiovascular evaluation for noncardiac surgery. (*Source:* Reproduced with permission. *J Am Coll Cardiol* 1996;27:910–948. Copyright 1996 by the American College of Cardiology and American Heart Association, Inc.)

advisable not to administer succinylcholine after 24 h to patients who have undergone denervation injury. Other patients who are predisposed to hyperkalemia include patients with severe intraabdominal infection or severe metabolic acidosis. Hyperkalemia in these patients may manifest as cardiac ventricular arrhythmia leading to arrest. Patients with undiagnosed myopathies such as Duchenne's muscular dystrophy may develop rhabdomyolysis, hyperkalemia, and cardiac arrest after succinylcholine administration. Because of this, succinylcholine is not routinely administered to children, especially males less than 5 years old or in nonemergent situations. Succinylcholine is also a known triggering agent for malignant hyperthermia and as such should be avoided in patients known to be susceptible to or have a strong family history of malignant hyperthermia.

Postoperative myalgias of the neck, back, and abdomen can occur after succinylcholine administration. These are thought to be secondary to fasciculation-induced muscle spindle stretch or prejunctional receptor motor firing. These fasciculations may result in muscle damage and myalgias postoperatively. Young muscular patients are more prone to develop these myalgias after succinylcholine. Small doses of a nondepolarizing agent as a pretreatment may attenuate this response secondary to suppression of the repetitive firing of muscle spindles.

Other potential side effects of succinylcholine include anaphylactic reaction, cardiac arrhythmia, transient increase in intraocular pressure, increase in intragastric pressure, and transient increase in intracranial pressure. Cardiac arrhythmias can range from bradycardia, junctional rhythm, and ventricular arrhythmia. This is most likely because of the similarity of structure between succinylcholine and acetylcholine. In addition to stimulation of the nicotinic receptors, succinylcholine may stimulate cardiac postganglionic muscarinic receptors in the sinus node. Increased intraocular pressure may be secondary to the contraction of the extraocular muscles. This may be relevant in open eye injuries where extrusion of ocular contents may lead to loss of vision. Increased intragastric pressure may be secondary to fasciculations of abdominal skeletal muscle. This may be reduced with pretreatment with nondepolarizing neuromuscular blocking drugs. Increased intracranial pressure may be of concern in patients with intracranial lesions after head injury. This effect may be attenuated with prior administration of thiopental or propofol or pretreatment with a nondepolarizing neuromuscular blocking drug.

Bibliography

Bevan DR, Donati F. Muscle relaxants. In: Barash PG, Cullen BF, Stoelting RK (eds.), *Clinical Anesthesia*, 4th ed. Philadelphia, PA: Lippincott, Williams & Wilkins, 2001, 419–447.

Morgan GE, Mikhail MS, Murray MJ. Neuromuscular blocking agents. In: Morgan GE, Mikhail MS, Murray MJ (eds.), *Clinical Anesthesiology*, 3rd ed. New York, NY: McGraw-Hill, 2002, 178–199.

Stoelting R. Neuromuscular-blocking drugs. In: Stoelting RK (ed.), *Pharmacology & Physiology in Anesthetic Practice*, 3rd ed. Philadelphia, PA: Lippincott-Raven, 1999, 182–223.

7. **(E)** Both depolarizing and nondepolarizing neuromuscular blockers have chemical structures similar to acetylcholine. This explains the pharmacologic activity at postsynaptic nicotinic membrane receptors. Nondepolarizers compete with acetylcholine receptors for binding sites on the alpha subunit of the nicotinic cholinergic receptors. As opposed to depolarizing neuromuscular blockers, the binding of nondepolarizers does not lead to depolarization of the postjunctional membrane. This leads to a competitive inhibition of acetylcholine at these receptors. Therefore, fasciculations do not occur with nondepolarizers. Additional cholinoceptive sites include nicotinic receptors of autonomic ganglia, muscarinic receptors in the sinus node of the heart, bowel, bladder, and other sites.

The benzylisoquinolinium compounds cause nonimmunologic release of histamine from mast cells. These agents include d-tubocurarine, metocurine, atracurium, and mivacurium. This histamine release is a function of both size of dose administered and rate of drug administration. The physiologic effects of histamine release include tachycardia and vasodilation. These effects generally last for a few minutes. Slow rate of infusion and administration of antihistamines may attenuate this response.

Vagolysis is secondary to muscarinic receptor blockade on the nodal cells of the heart. Pancuronium and gallamine particularly have significant vagolysis properties. This contributes to an increase in HR and predisposition to arrhythmias. This is secondary to vagal block and increased sympathetic tone. It may also be because of indirect sympathomimetic activation and atrioventricular nodal block greater than sinoatrial blockade. Autonomic ganglia are blocked by d-tubocurarine and metocurine, and as such these agents may impair autonomic reflexes and contribute to hypotension.

Allergic reactions to the nondepolarizers are rare. The antigenic group is believed to be the quaternary ammonia nitrogen molecule. The quaternary ammonia is present in both depolarizers and nondepolarizers, and as such there is theoretically a cross sensitivity in individuals truly allergic to those agents. In addition, the salt of the drug administered may contribute. For example, potential allergy may exist for patients with a history of seafood allergy or iodine allergy if they are given metocurine iodide or gallamine triethiodide.

Bibliography

Bevan DR, Donati F. Muscle relaxants. In: Barash PG, Cullen BF, Stoelting RK (eds.), *Clinical Anesthesia*, 4th ed. Philadelphia, PA: Lippincott, Williams & Wilkins, 2001, 419–447.

Morgan GE, Mikhail MS, Murray MJ. Neuromuscular blocking agents. In: Morgan GE, Mikhail MS, Murray MJ (eds.), *Clinical Anesthesiology*, 3rd ed. New York, NY: McGraw-Hill, 2002, 178–199.

Stoelting R. Neuromuscular-blocking drugs. In: Stoelting RK (ed.), *Pharmacology & Physiology in Anesthetic Practice*, 3rd ed. Philadelphia, PA: Lippincott-Raven, 1999, 182–223.

8. **(B)** Both depolarizing and nondepolarizing neuromuscular blockers have chemical structures similar to acetylcholine. The nondepolarizers compete with acetylcholine at nicotinic receptors at the postjunctional membrane. In contrast to the depolarizing neuromuscular blocker succinylcholine, nondepolarizers do not lead to depolarization of the postjunctional membrane, and these do not produce fasciculations. Succinylcholine is the only depolarizing muscle relaxant in general use today. Because of the competitive block of nondepolarizers, acetylcholine is prevented from binding to these receptors thus preventing the channels from opening. Nondepolarizing neuromuscular blockers can be categorized in terms of duration of action or chemical structure. Duration of action can be categorized as short, intermediate, or long acting. They are either benzylisoquinoliniums or aminosteroids. All nondepolarizers are hydrophilic. At physiologic pH, they are highly ionized. Because of this, they have a small volume of distribution and have limited ability to cross lipid membranes such as the blood-brain barrier, renal tubular epithelium, or placenta. Thus, nondepolarizing neuromuscular blocking drugs produce minimal central nervous system (CNS) effects, undergo minimal renal tubular reabsorption, and have little effect on a fetus when administered to parturients. Because of these features, nondepolarizing neuromuscular blocking drugs are eliminated by glomerular filtration via the kidney. It is when they are cleared by other mechanisms such

biliary excretion or liver metabolism that may shorten their duration of action.

The benzylisoquinoliniums include the short-acting mivacurium, the intermediate acting atracurium and cisatracurium, and the long-acting D-tubocurarine, metocurine, and doxacurium. The aminosteriods include the short-acting rapacuronium (currently unavailable because of market withdrawal), the intermediate acting vecuronium and rocuronium, and the long-acting pancuronium and pipecuronium. The choice of a particular nondepolarizing neuromuscular blocking agent used clinically depends on each drug's characteristics. These include onset, duration of action, metabolism, clearance mechanism, and side effects. These are related to the chemical structure of the drug. In general, steroidal compounds tend to be vagolytic, while the benzylisoquinoliniums tend to release histamine.

Cisatracurium is a single isomer of the 10 isomers that constitute atracurium. Both drugs are benzylisoquinoliniums and intermediate in duration. Both are metabolized independent of hepatic or renal function. Cisatracurium is metabolized by a spontaneous, nonenzymatic chemical degradation at physiologic pH and temperature known as Hofmann elimination. Atracurium relies on both Hofmann elimination and ester hydrolysis by nonspecific plasma esterases. Atracurium may cause significant histamine release, bronchospasm, transient hypotension, and tachycardia. It should be avoided in asthmatics. Cisatracurium does not produce clinically significant increases in histamine levels. Both drugs produce laudanosine as a metabolite from Hofmann elimination which has been associated with CNS excitation, including increasing microcystic adnexal carcinoma (MAC) and precipitation of seizures. This consideration appears to be clinically insignificant except in the presence of extremely high total doses and hepatic failure, as laudanosine is hepatically cleared.

Pancuronium, rocuronium and vecuronium are aminosteroid nondepolarizing muscle relaxants. Pancuronium is partially hepatically metabolized, and its metabolites possess some neuromuscular blocking activity. Excretion is primarily renal with a small amount of biliary excretion. Blockade is prolonged in renal failure. It may cause tachycardia and HTN because of vagal blockade and catecholamine release. These side effects also may cause increased ventricular dysrhythmias in predisposed individuals. Vecuronium resembles pancuronium minus a quaternary methyl group. This structural modification preserves potency while limiting side effects. Vecuronium is primarily excreted in the bile and secondarily by the kidneys. Liver failure does not typically prolong blockade except in high doses, however, while renal failure may produce some delay in recovery from effects. Even at two to three times the typical intubating dose vecuronium lacks significant cardiovascular effects. Rocuronium is an analogue of vecuronium and designed to provide rapid onset of action. It undergoes no metabolism and is excreted primarily by the liver. In doses of 0.9–1.2 mg/kg rocuronium has a rapid onset only slightly longer than succinylcholine, making it suitable for rapid-sequence induction.

Bibliography

Bevan DR, Donati F. Muscle relaxants. In: Barash PG, Cullen BF, Stoelting RK (eds.), *Clinical Anesthesia*, 4th ed. Philadelphia, PA: Lippincott, Williams & Wilkins, 2001, 419–447.

Morgan GE, Mikhail MS, Murray MJ. Neuromuscular blocking agents. In: Morgan GE, Mikhail MS, Murray MJ (eds.), *Clinical Anesthesiology*, 3rd ed. New York, NY: McGraw-Hill, 2002, 178–199.

Stoelting R. Neuromuscular-blocking drugs. In: Stoelting RK (ed.), *Pharmacology & Physiology in Anesthetic Practice*, 3rd ed. Philadelphia, PA: Lippincott-Raven, 1999, 182–223.

9. **(E)** Monitoring of neuromuscular function is important because of the high degree of variability in patients' sensitivity to neuromuscular blocking agents. This is especially important in patients who have received long or intermediate acting neuromuscular blocking agents. Neuromuscular monitoring is used routinely to determine the adequacy of neuromuscular blockade and the adequacy of relaxant reversal. This is done by applying various patterns of electrical stimulation via a peripheral nerve stimulator.

In the conscious patient, head lift is a sensitive test of neuromuscular function. A patient will not be able to lift the head if more than 33% of neuromuscular junction receptors are blocked; however, a patient can generate normal tidal volume when 80% of receptors are blocked. A reliable and accurate method to monitor neuromuscular function in patients undergoing anesthesia is with the use of a nerve stimulator.

A single twitch stimulation is a single pulse twitch delivered every second to every 10 s. The response depends on the frequency of the stimulus. As the rate increases, it may lead to a gradual decrease in the response. In general, increasing degree of blockade results in a decreased evoked response to stimulation. There is no difference in the characteristic of the twitch between a depolarizing and a nondepolarizing blocker except the depolarizing blocker has a faster onset.

TOF stimulation involves four successive 0.2 ms, 2 Hz stimuli in 2 s. The twitches in a TOF pattern progressively lessen as the degree of relaxation increases. A sensitive indication of a nondepolarizing blocker is to compare the ratio of the response of the first twitch to the fourth. Since it is difficult to determine this ratio, it is clinically more common to visually observe the sequential disappearance of the twitches. The disappearance of the fourth twitch correlates with a 75% blockade, the third with an 80% blockade, and the second with a 90% blockade. Clinical relaxation requires 75–90% blockade. When TOF ratio is greater than 0.7, a single-twitch height should be normal. In contrast to the nondepolarizing blockade, a depolarizing blockade does not lead to a decrease in the TOF ratio.

DBS involves two short bursts of 50-Hz stimulation separated by 750 ms. It is a variation of tetany. Nonparalyzed muscles will demonstrate equal responses to both bursts. During a nondepolarizing blockade, the second response is decreased. The ratio of the second to the first impulses in DBS correlates with the TOF ratio. The advantage of DBS is that the response may be easier to evaluate by tactile means.

Tetanic stimulation involves the rapid delivery of supramaximal stimuli at 50 or 100 Hz. In a nonparalyzed muscle, the response to stimulation is sustained contraction. If there is a nondepolarizing muscle relaxant in effect, there will be fade. There will be a decrease in twitch height and no fade with a depolarizing block unless there is a phase II block. A phase II block occurs when a large dose of succinylcholine is used or the duration of use is prolonged. This results in the postjunctional membranes to become repolarize but unable to respond to acetylcholine. This will have characteristics similar to a nondepolarizers blockade.

Bibliography

Bevan DR, Donati F. Muscle relaxants. In: Barash PG, Cullen BF, Stoelting RK (eds.), *Clinical Anesthesia*, 4th ed. Philadelphia, PA: Lippincott, Williams & Wilkins, 2001, 419–447.

Morgan GE, Mikhail MS, Murray MJ. Patient monitors. In: Morgan GE, Mikhail MS, Murray MJ (eds.), *Clinical Anesthesiology*, 3rd ed. New York, NY: McGraw-Hill, 2002, 86–126.

10. **(C)** Acetylcholinesterase breaks down acetylcholine into choline and acetic acid. Acetylcholinesterase inhibitors are commonly administered to accelerate the reversal of nondepolarizing neuromuscular muscle relaxant blockade. Because nondepolarizing neuromuscular blocking agents are competitive inhibitors at the postjunctional membrane receptor to

acetylcholine, administration of acetylcholinesterase inhibitors will increase the amount of acetylcholine available at the neuromuscular junction. With more acetylcholine available at the neuromuscular junction, acetylcholine will more likely bind to the receptor and thus antagonize the actions of the nondepolarizing neuromuscular blocker. At the same time acetylcholine is increased at the nicotinic cholinergic receptors at the postjunctional membrane. Acetylcholine is also increased at the muscarinic cholinergic receptors in the heart and other muscarinic receptors. This results in severe bradycardia, increased gastric secretions, and increased salivation. For this reason, an anticholinergic is given along with the cholinesterase inhibitor. Their chemical structures are such that their quaternary ammonia structures make them less lipid soluble so they do not cross the lipid membrane. This minimizes their CNS effects.

The factors that influence the choice of the anticholinesterase used to antagonize nondepolarizing neuromuscular blocking agents include the duration of action of the nondepolarizing agent used and the intensity of the blockade. Longer acting and more intense nondepolarizing neuromuscular blockade requires a longer acting acetylcholinesterase inhibitor.

The acetylcholinesterase inhibitors available in general use are neostigmine, pyridostigmine, and edrophonium. All of these agents have the quaternary ammonia structure. Because of the quaternary ammonia structure, these agents do not cross lipid membranes such as blood-brain barrier. In contrast, physostigmine is not used for nondepolarizing neuromuscular blockade reversal because it has a tertiary ammonia and it is able to cross the blood-brain barrier. Neostigmine and pyridostigmine bind to the acetylcholinesterase molecule via a carbonyl-ester linkage. As a result of the covalent bond, the degradation of bonding is slow and the duration of inhibition is thus longer. Edrophonium binds to the acetylcholinesterase molecule via an electrostatic bond, and thus the duration of action is brief. Neostigmine should be administered for the reversal of a nondepolarizing neuromuscular blocker that is intermediate or long acting. It is commonly coupled with glycopyrrolate because the delayed cardiac anticholinergic effects of glycopyrrolate closely parallel with the time of onset of the muscarinic effects of neostigmine. Since edrophonium has a shorter time of onset and shorter duration of action, it should be used when the nondepolarizing blocking agent has either short or intermediate activity and as such should be paired atropine because its shorter time of onset is similar to the short onset time for edrophonium.

The reversal of neuromuscular blockade should not be attempted until some recovery is demonstrated. If recovery is not demonstrated, the degree of neuromuscular blockade may be too intense that reversal by an anticholinesterase inhibitor may not be possible. In some cases, it may actually prolong the blockade.

Indicators of adequate muscle relaxant reversal can be shown by a 5-s continuous tetany and would correlate to a TOF ratio greater than 0.7. Other indicators are the ability to open eyes, grip strength, sustained head lift, and ventilatory parameters such as vital capacity.

Other considerations that may interfere with adequate reversal of neuromuscular blockade include patient temperature, acid-base status, or electrolyte abnormalities. Patients with renal or liver disease may have prolonged neuromuscular blockade as those agents are eliminated via those routes. Hypothermic patients tend to metabolize neuromuscular blockers slower. Hypermagnesemia, amnioglycoside antibiotics, and local anesthetic also potentiate neuromuscular blockers.

Bibliography

Bevan DR, Donati F. Muscle relaxants. In: Barash PG, Cullen BF, Stoelting RK (eds.), *Clinical Anesthesia*, 4th ed. Philadelphia, PA: Lippincott, Williams & Wilkins, 2001, 419–447.

Morgan GE, Mikhail MS, Murray MJ. Cholinesterase inhibitors. In: Morgan GE, Mikhail MS, Murray MJ (eds.), *Clinical Anesthesiology*, 3rd ed. New York, NY: McGraw-Hill, 2002, 199–206.

Stoelting R. Anticholinesterase drugs and cholinergic agonists. In: Stoelting RK (ed.), *Pharmacology & Physiology in Anesthetic Practice*, 3rd ed. Philadelphia, PA: Lippincott-Raven, 1999, 224–237.

11. **(C)** The clinically useful local anesthetics share the structure of a hydrophobic aromatic ring structure connected to a hydrophilic tertiary amine group via a short alkyl chain containing an amide or an ester bond. The aromatic side-chain provides the lipophilic properties of the molecule. Lipophilicity relates directly to potency, since the local anesthetic molecule must pass through the lipid-rich nerve cell membrane to gain access to the transmembrane sodium channel where it acts. The linking chain is the principal site of metabolism with esters undergoing rapid hydrolysis by plasma esterases, while amides are cleared more slowly by hepatic metabolism. The length of this chain is also important in properly aligning the aromatic and amine groups, as local anesthetic activity rapidly disappears if the chain is less than three or more than seven carbon-equivalents in length. Local anesthetics

are weak bases (pK_a's 7.6–9.1) and accept a proton at the tertiary amine at physiologic pH. It is the neutral (basic) form of the anesthetic which most easily crosses the cell membrane, but once intracellular it is the protonated (cationic) form of the molecule which is able to bind to the transmembrane sodium channel.

Local anesthetics block nerve conduction by interrupting sodium channel excitability and thereby sodium ion movement. Neuronal sodium channels cycle through activated-open, inactivated-closed, and rested-closed states at various points of an action potential. Opening of sodium channels (activated-open) allows sodium influx into the axolemma and depolarizes the transmembrane potential (–70 mV). If the threshold potential (–55 mV) is reached sodium conductance becomes even more rapid and an action potential is propagated. The protonated (cationic) form of the local anesthetic molecule gains access to the sodium ion channel when it is in the activated-open state, but selectively binds to the channel in the inactivated-closed state. This binding stabilizes the channel and prevents return to the rested-closed state, which must be cycled through before the channel can again become activated-open. Local anesthetics do not alter the resting transmembrane potential or the threshold potential. By stabilizing the inactivated-closed state, the rate of sodium influx and thus the rate of depolarization slows such that the threshold potential is not reached and nerve conduction is blocked.

Bibliography

Morgan GE Jr, Mikhail MS, Murray MJ. Local anesthetics. In: Morgan GE Jr, Mikhail MS, Murray MJ, . (eds.), *Clinical Anesthesiology*, 3rd ed. New York, NY: McGraw-Hill, 2002, 233–240.

Stoelting RK. Local anesthetics. In: Stoelting RK. (ed.), *Pharmacology and Physiology in Anesthetic Practice*, 3rd ed. Philadelphia, PA: Lippincott, Williams & Wilkins, 1999, 158–178.

Tetzlaff JE. The pharmacology of local anesthetics. *Anesthesiol Clin North Am.* 2000;18(2):217–233.

Wall RT. Anesthesia. In: Norton JA, Bollinger RR, Chang AE, et al. (eds.), *Surgery: Basic Science and Clinical Evidence*. New York, NY: Springer, 2001, 345–348.

12. **(A)** The pK_a is the pH at which 50% of a molecule exists in the basic form and 50% in the protonated form. The higher the pK_a of the local anesthetic, the greater the proportion of the drug existing in the protonated (charged) form at a given pH at any given moment (Table 36-1). Only the uncharged local anesthetic can cross the cell membrane and raise the intracellular concentration. Once intracellular, the equilibrium between charged and uncharged forms of the molecule continues, and, as above, it is the charged form which binds to sodium receptors causing conduction blockade. Local anesthetics with pK_a's closest to physiologic pH will have more optimal ratios between charged and uncharged forms and have more rapid onset of action. Local acidosis (as in tissue infection) will further increase the proportion of charged anesthetic, delaying onset of anesthesia. Solutions of local anesthetics are generally prepared as hydrochloride salts of the cation with a pH of 5.0–6.0 (2.0–5.0 if commercially prepared with epinephrine). Addition of sodium bicarbonate (e.g., 1 mL 8.4% sodium bicarbonate/10 mL 1% lidocaine) has been suggested to raise the local pH, increasing the proportion of nonionic local anesthetic (speeding onset) and reducing pain at the injection site during subcutaneous infiltration.

Nerve fiber type greatly affects onset of action and effectiveness of blockade. Fiber types are divided into myelinated A and B fibers and unmyelinated C fibers. A fibers are subdivided into alpha through delta types. The largest fibers (A-alpha) conduct motor impulses. A-beta fibers conduct light touch, pressure, and innervate some muscle. A-gamma fibers provide

TABLE 36-1   pK_a, Lipid Solubility, Potency and Ionized Fractions of Local Anesthetics at Various Local pH

	Lipid solubility	Potency	pK_a	% ionized at pH 7.2	% ionized at pH 7.4	% ionized at pH 7.6
Esters						
Procaine	Low	Low	8.9	98	97	95
Chloroprocaine	intermediate	Intermediate	8.7	97	95	93
Tetracaine	Very high	Very high	8.5	95	93	89
Amides						
Lidocaine	Low	Low	7.9	83	75	67
Etidocaine	Very high	High	7.7	76	67	56
Prilocaine	Low	Low	7.9	83	75	67
Mepivicaine	Low	Low	7.6	72	61	50
Bupivicaine	High	High	8.1	89	85	76
Ropivicaine	High	High	8.1	89	85	76

proprioception, while the smallest A fibers (A-delta) conduct pain and temperature sensation. All B fibers are smaller than A fibers and are preganglionic sympathetic fibers. C fibers are the smallest in the body, conducting temperature, pain and are postganglionic autonomic fibers. Larger fibers require higher concentration of local anesthetic and are slower to establish the same degree of conduction blockade. Myelination decreases the length of nerve necessary to be exposed to local anesthetic. If three successive nodes of Ranvier are blocked, conduction block will occur, whereas in unmyelinated nerves a full circumference as well as a greater length must be bathed by local anesthetic. These differences explain the observed differential conduction blockade, with B fibers the easiest fibers to block. In spinal anesthesia, sympathetic blockade is generally two levels higher than sensory blockade, which is two levels higher than motor blockade. This also explains why patients typically experience pressure and touch but not pain after local anesthetic infiltration.

The more frequently a nerve is stimulated, the more frequently the sodium channels cycle through the activated-open state. Since this is the state during which the local anesthetic gains access to the channel, the channel is susceptible to the local anesthetic more frequently. The higher potency of local anesthetics for nerves with a higher frequency of stimulation is termed "frequency-dependent" blockade.

Bibliography

Kleinman W. Spinal, epidural and caudal blocks. In: Morgan GE Jr, Mikhail MS, Murray MJ, et al. (eds.), *Clinical Anesthesiology*, 3rd ed. New York, NY: McGraw-Hill, 2002, 258–260.

Morgan GE Jr, Mikhail MS, Murray MJ. Local anesthetics. In: Morgan GE Jr, Mikhail MS, Murray MJ, et al. (eds.), *Clinical Anesthesiology*, 3rd ed. New York, NY: McGraw-Hill, 2002, 233–240.

Stoelting RK. Local anesthetics. In: Stoelting RK (ed.), *Pharmacology and Physiology in Anesthetic Practice*, 3rd ed. Philadelphia, PA: Lippincott, Williams & Wilkins, 1999, 158–178.

Tetzlaff JE. The pharmacology of local anesthetics. *Anesthesiol Clin North Am* 2000;18(2):217–233.

Wall RT. Anesthesia. In: Norton JA, Bollinger RR, Chang AE, et al. (eds.), *Surgery: Basic Science and Clinical Evidence.* New York, NY: Springer, 2001, 345–348.

13. (E) All local anesthetics have a maximum recommended dose for local infiltration, which can be found in package inserts, drug indices, and databases (Table 36-2). The purpose of these maximums is to limit or prevent systemic toxicity. A strong argument can be made that these limits are somewhat arbitrary and illogical, however, as toxicity is ultimately

TABLE 36-2 Maximum Recommended Doses, Protein Binding, and Approximate Duration of Action for Infiltration of Local Anesthetics

	Maximum recommended dose[a]	Relative protein binding	Approximate duration[b]
Esters			
Procaine	500	Very low	45–60
Chloroprocaine	600	Very low	30–45
Tetracaine	100	High	60–180
Amides			
Lidocaine	300	High	60–120
Etidocaine	300	Very high	240–480
Prilocaine	400	Moderate	60–120
Mepivicaine	300	High	90–180
Bupivicaine	175	Very high	240–480
Ropivicaine	200	Very high	240–480

[a](In mg) for infiltration in adults (without epinephrine).
[b](In min) (without epinephrine).

determined by plasma concentration and exposure of the CNS and cardiac tissue to local anesthetic. The site of injection plays a tremendous role in the rate of vascular absorption and therefore the plasma concentration of the local anesthetic. Intercostal blocks are associated with the highest blood levels of local anesthetic and subarachnoid injections with the lowest. The leading cause of systemic toxicity is accidental intravascular injection, in which case doses well below the recommended maximums are toxic. Addition of epinephrine maintains local anesthetic concentration in the vicinity of the nerve fibers and slows systemic absorption (prolonging duration of action) for all local anesthetics during local infiltration, but has variable effects depending on the local anesthetic when injected at other sites. The addition of epinephrine is also often used as a marker for accidental intravascular injection. Epinephrine should generally not be used in distal end-vascular sites (e.g., digits) where ischemia could result from vasoconstriction.

In calculating the dose to be injected one must consider both concentration and volume. For example, the maximum recommended dose of bupivicaine for infiltration in an adult is 175 mg. A 0.75% solution contains 7.5 mg/mL while a 0.25% solution contains 2.5 mg/mL, so the maximum dose is reached with 70 mL of the latter but only 23.3 mL of the former. The most prudent method to decide what strength solution to use would be to consider what volume of solution will be needed to adequately infiltrate the entire area needing to be anesthetized, and then determining what strength solution will approach but not exceed the maximum dose in that volume.

Individual patient factors should also be considered (physiology, size, weight, site of injection).

Finally, one must consider differences in duration of action of the different local anesthetics. Duration of action correlates directly to strength of protein binding. Highly protein bound anesthetics (bupivicaine) are tightly associated with proteins in the neuronal membrane (transmembrane sodium receptors). In contrast, poorly bound anesthetics (procaine) rapidly diffuse away from the neuronal proteins and have a much shorter duration of action.

Bibliography

Morgan GE Jr, Mikhail MS, Murray MJ. Local anesthetics. In: Morgan GE Jr, Mikhail MS, Murray MJ, et al. (eds.), *Clinical Anesthesiology*, 3rd ed. New York, NY: McGraw-Hill, 2002, 233–240.

Stoelting RK. Local anesthetics. In: Stoelting RK (ed.), *Pharmacology and Physiology in Anesthetic Practice*, 3rd ed. Philadelphia, PA: Lippincott, Williams & Wilkins, 1999, 158–178.

Scott DB. "Maximum recommended doses" of local anesthetic drugs. *Br J Anaesth* 1989;63(4):373–374.

Tetzlaff JE. The pharmacology of local anesthetics. *Anesthesiol Clin North Am.* 2000;18(2):217–233.

Wall RT. Anesthesia. In: Norton JA, Bollinger RR, Chang AE, et al. (eds.), *Surgery: Basic Science and Clinical Evidence.* New York, NY: Springer, 2001, 345–348.

14. **(D)** True allergy or anaphylactic reaction to local anesthetic solutions is very rare despite the common use of these drugs. An allergic mechanism is estimated to be the cause of less than 1% of all adverse reactions to local anesthetics. Rather, the most common cause of adverse responses is an excessive plasma concentration of local anesthetic. Of the local anesthetics, allergy is much more common in the ester class. This is because of one of the metabolites of ester local anesthetics, para-amino-benzoic acid (PABA), which is ubiquitous throughout the pharmaceutic and cosmetic industries. Amides do not produce this metabolite. Occasionally allergic reaction may occur after exposure to commercial solutions of either class because of the presence of methylparaben or similar substances as a preservative in multidose vials. These preservatives are structurally similar to PABA and can produce a cross-reaction. Because of the common metabolite (PABA), a patient with documented allergy to one ester local anesthetic should be assumed to be allergic to all ester local anesthetics. There would be no increased risk of allergy after administration of an amide local anesthetic, however, provided it is preservative free. Allergy to local anesthetics can be confirmed by intradermal testing with preservative-free solutions, but clinical history is usually sufficient. If a patient develops rash, urticaria, and laryngeal edema

with or without hypotension and bronchospasm, allergy is strongly suggested.

In the case above, the most likely explanation of both increased HR and blood pressure is the alpha-adrenergic effects of epinephrine. Histamine-mediated anaphylaxis would result in tachycardia with hypotension from vasodilation. Cardiac toxicity is unlikely to preceded CNS symptoms and would not be expected to produce HTN since toxicity results from cardiac depression. The patient should be closely monitored, but it should be safe to proceed with thoracentesis and possible chest tube as the adrenergic effects of epinephrine subside.

Bibliography

Liu SS, Hodgson PS. Local anesthetics. In: Barash PG, Cullen BF, Stoelting RK (eds.), *Clinical Anesthesia*, 4th ed. Philadelphia, PA: Lippincott, Williams & Wilkins, 2001.

Morgan GE Jr, Mikhail MS, Murray MJ. Local anesthetics. In: Morgan GE Jr, Mikhail MS, Murray MJ, et al. (eds.), *Clinical Anesthesiology*, 3rd ed. New York, NY: McGraw-Hill, 2002, pp 233–240.

Stoelting RK, Miller RD. Local anesthetics. In: Stoelting RK, Miller RD (eds.), *Basics of Anesthesia*, 4th ed. New York, NY: Churchill Livingstone, 2000, pp 80–88.

Stoelting RK. Local anesthetics. In: Stoelting RK (ed.), *Pharmacology and Physiology in Anesthetic Practice*, 3rd ed. Philadelphia, PA: Lippincott, Williams & Wilkins, 1999, pp 158–178.

Tetzlaff JE. The pharmacology of local anesthetics. *Anesthesiol Clin North Am* 2000;18(2):217–233.

15. **(A)** Systemic toxicity results from exposure of the CNS and cardiac tissue to increased plasma levels of local anesthetic. The toxic form of the local anesthetic is the nonionic, unbound portion in the blood which is able to cross the blood-brain barrier. Both the absolute concentration and the rate of change in concentration of local anesthetic affect the development of signs of toxicity. As plasma concentration increases, classically the first symptoms are numbness of the tongue and circumoral tissues, often described as a metallic taste. This is presumably because of increased delivery of anesthetic to these highly vascularized and innervated tissues. The first CNS symptoms to manifest are restlessness, vertigo, tinnitus, and blurred vision. As levels rise further, slurred speech and twitching of skeletal muscles (especially facial and extremity muscles) typically follows. Muscle-twitching usually signals the imminence of tonic-clonic seizures. Seizures may result from inhibition of the release of γ-aminobutyric acid (GABA) and other inhibitory neurotransmitters or selective depression of inhibitory cortical neurons, leaving excitatory pathways unopposed. Tonic-clonic seizures are classically followed by CNS depression which may cause hypotension and

apnea. Many practitioners will not perform nerve blocks associated with increased risk of systemic absorption in asleep patients, as the first warning signs of rising plasma levels will be muscle-twitching and seizures. The local anesthetics which are bound more tightly to proteins are slower to manifest symptoms of toxicity, but also have a narrower gap between the development of the first, milder symptoms and more dangerous massive reaction to CNS local anesthetic exposure. The more lipid soluble (potent) anesthetics also have a much narrower therapeutic index.

The cardiovascular system is more resistant to local anesthetic toxicity than is the CNS. The first effects may be profound hypotension because of direct myocardial depression (decreasing cardiac output) and relaxation of arteriolar smooth muscle (decreasing PVR). The direct cardiac toxicity is primarily because of binding and blockade of cardiac sodium channels. In lower concentrations this blockade explains the antidysrhythmic effects of these drugs, but in higher concentrations enough sodium channels are blocked that the normal conduction pathways and automaticity are disrupted. As this occurs, there is increased activity in reentrant pathways which may predispose the heart to ventricular arrhythmias. Local anesthetics also affect calcium-ion and potassium-ion channels and induce inhibition of cyclic adenosine monophosphate (cAMP) production which may contribute to cardiac toxicity. Of all local anesthetics, bupivicaine is most selective for cardiac toxicity, with the narrowest ratio between levels causing CNS and cardiac toxicity. It is the most likely to cause catastrophic cardiovascular collapse which may be refractory to resuscitation efforts. Pregnant patients are more susceptible to bupivicaine toxicity, presumably mediated by progesterone, decreased alpha$_1$-glycoprotein and albumin concentration (increased free drug), and impaired venous return during resuscitation efforts.

Bibliography

Liu SS, Hodgson PS. Local anesthetics. In: Barash PG, Cullen BF, Stoelting RK (eds.), *Clinical Anesthesia*, 4th ed. Philadelphia, PA: Lippincott, Williams & Wilkins, 2001.

Stoelting RK. Local anesthetics. In: Stoelting RK (ed.), *Pharmacology and Physiology in Anesthetic Practice*, 3rd ed. Philadelphia, PA: Lippincott, Williams & Wilkins, 1999, 158–178.

Tetzlaff JE. The pharmacology of local anesthetics. *Anesthesiol Clin North Am* 2000;18 (2):217–233.

Wall RT. Anesthesia. In: Norton JA, Bollinger RR, Chang AE, et al. (eds.), *Surgery: Basic Science and Clinical Evidence*. New York, NY: Springer, 2001, 345–348.

16. (B) The best means of avoiding systemic toxicity of local anesthetics is cautious use and prevention, bearing in mind that, despite their many benefits and wide spread use, local anesthetics are potentially lethal. In this example an adverse reaction occurred despite appropriate precaution. The most likely explanation for development of symptoms was the needle tip slipping back into the axillary artery after aspiration, with injection causing retrograde flow of local anesthetic and rapid rise in cerebral plasma concentration. In this scenario, progression to cardiac toxicity is unlikely, but preparations should still be made.

Systemic toxicity is primarily treated supportively. Obviously, injection should be terminated. In an awake patient it may be helpful to instruct the patient to hyperventilate to decrease cerebral blood flow and local anesthetic delivery, although this could theoretically slow clearance of already high plasma concentrations from cerebral tissue. Local anesthetic toxicity is potentiated by hypoxia, hypercarbia, and acidosis. Seizures will rapidly cause regional hypoxia and acidosis, thus rapidly worsening toxicity, so early administration of drugs to raise the seizure threshold (benzodiazepines, barbiturates) should definitely be considered. Supplemental oxygen should be administered to awake patients and consideration given to intubation and positive pressure ventilation, especially if seizures develop. Succinylcholine will stop muscular activity of tonic-clonic seizures (reducing development of acidosis, hypoxia, and hypercarbia), but will not terminate CNS seizure activity and increased cerebral oxygen demand.

Should they develop, cardiovascular symptoms from the less potent anesthetics such as mepivicaine are generally mild, resulting from myocardial depression and vasodilation. Symptoms of bradycardia and hypotension will usually respond to atropine and ephedrine or phenylephrine. The more potent anesthetics (bupivicaine) are more likely to cause malignant dysrhythmias which should be aggressively treated. They may be refractory to treatment with epinephrine and cardioversion. Bretylium (20 mg/kg) IV has been shown to reverse bupivicaine-induced myocardial depression in anesthetized dogs, but this drug may not be available.

Bibliography

Liu SS, Hodgson PS. Local anesthetics. In: Barash PG, Cullen BF, Stoelting RK (eds.), *Clinical Anesthesia*, 4th ed. Philadelphia, PA: Lippincott, Williams & Wilkins, 2001.

Morgan GE Jr, Mikhail MS, Murray MJ. Local anesthetics. In: Morgan GE Jr, Mikhail MS, Murray MJ, et al. (eds.), *Clinical Anesthesiology*, 3rd ed. New York, NY: McGraw-Hill, 2002, 233–240.

Stoelting RK, Miller RD. Local anesthetics. In: Stoelting RK, Miller RD (eds.), *Basics of Anesthesia*, 4th ed. New York, NY: Churchill Livingstone, 2000, 80–88.

Stoelting RK. Local anesthetics. In: Stoelting RK (ed.), *Pharmacology and Physiology in Anesthetic Practice*, 3rd ed. Philadelphia, PA: Lippincott, Williams & Wilkins, 1999, 158–178.

Tetzlaff JE. The pharmacology of local anesthetics. *Anesthesiol Clin North Am* 2000;18(2):217–233.

17. **(D)** All of the above intravenous anesthetics can be used in the above doses to induce anesthesia in healthy patients. Of these agents, however, ketamine has the most favorable pharmacologic profile in this scenario. Ketamine is a phencyclidine derivative with multiple effects throughout the CNS. It produces a "dissociative anesthesia" resembling a cataleptic state with unconsciousness, amnesia, and intense analgesia by "dissociating" the thalamus from the limbic system. The patient's eyes will typically remain open with nystagmic gaze. Ketamine is extremely lipid soluble with very rapid crossing of the blood-brain barrier and onset of anesthesia followed by redistribution. Hepatic microsomal enzymes metabolize ketamine to norketamine, which possess one-third to one-fifth the activity of ketamine and may contribute to prolonged effects following multiple doses or continuous infusion. Of all the above agents, ketamine is the only one not to interact with GABA receptors in the CNS, but rather interacts with *N*-methyl-D-aspartate, opioid, monoaminergic, and muscarinic receptors as well as voltage-sensitive calcium ion channels.

The major advantage of ketamine in this scenario is its effects on the cardiovascular system. These resemble sympathetic stimulation with increases in cardiac output, HR, systemic blood pressure, and pulmonary blood pressure. The most important mechanism seems to be direct stimulation of the CNS leading to increased sympathetic outflow. It is generally the induction agent of choice in acutely hypovolemic patients, but if endogenous catecholamine supplies have been depleted (e.g., decompensated shock) ketamine will cause myocardial depression. Although transient apnea may follow rapid IV administration or concomitant opioid administration, ketamine does not produce significant respiratory depression. Ketamine has bronchodilatory properties and may be useful in treating bronchospasm. The production of analgesia is unique to ketamine among the intravenous induction agents. In contrast to the other agents, however, ketamine increases cerebral blood flow, ($CMRO_2$), and (ICP). It should be used cautiously if at all in patients with increased ICP, pulmonary HTN, or CAD. Ketamine

can cause emergence delirium characterized by visual, auditory, proprioceptive, and confusional illusions, perhaps contributing to its less frequent use in outpatient procedures.

Propofol is a substituted isopropylphenol and is rapidly cleared from the circulation by redistribution and extensive, rapid hepatic metabolism. Thiopental is a barbiturate with increased lipid solubility (faster onset of action and redistribution) than its oxybarbiturate analog pentobarbital because of a sulfur atom on the number 2 carbon. Despite rapid redistribution, elimination from the body depends almost exclusively on metabolism. Etomidate is a carboxylated imidazole derivative which is nearly completely hydrolyzed to inactive metabolites. Midazolam is a benzodiazepine which has a short duration of action because of redistribution (lipid solubility) and is metabolized to an inactive metabolite by hepatic P450 3A4. In healthy patients, all of the above agents produce unconsciousness in less than 30 s except midazolam, which has a slower effect-site equilibration. Awakening is generally prompt after a single dose of all of the agents, although it may be delayed following midazolam. In contrast, the context sensitive half-lives of barbiturates, ketamine, and benzodiazepines may be prolonged, resulting in delayed awakening following multiple doses or continuous infusion. This is because of saturation of secondary sites with much more rapid redistribution than metabolism and/or active metabolites. Etomidate is considered "cardiovascular neutral" in that it does not greatly increase or decrease HR and blood pressure, so is useful for induction in patient's with compromised myocardial contractility. It is unique among the agents in producing dose-dependent suppression of the adrenal glands lasting 4–8 h after induction. This suppression may be desirable or undesirable depending on the stress to which the patient is exposed in the perioperative period. Other systemic effects of the above agents are compared in Table 36-3.

Bibliography

Morgan GE Jr, Mikhail MS, Murray MJ. Nonvolatile anesthetic agents. In: Morgan GE Jr, Mikhail MS, Murray MJ, et al. (eds.), *Clinical Anesthesiology*, 3rd ed. New York, NY: McGraw-Hill, 2002, 151–175.

Stoelting RK, Miller RD. Intravenous anesthetics. In: Stoelting RK, Miller RD (eds.), *Basics of Anesthesia*, 4th ed. New York, NY: Churchill Livingstone, 2000, 58–68.

Wall RT. Anesthesia. In: Norton JA, Bollinger RR, Chang AE, et al. (eds.), *Surgery: Basic Science and Clinical Evidence*. New York, NY: Springer, 2001, 348–350.

TABLE 36-3   **Comparative effects of selected intravenous anesthetics.**

	Propofol	Thiopental	Etomidate	Ketamine	Midazolam
Dose for IV induction	1.5–2.5mg/kg	3–5mg/kg	0.2–0.4 mg/kg	1–2 mg/kg	0.1–0.2 mg/kg
Onset	Fast	Fast	Fast	Fast	Intermediate
Induction	Smooth, possibly painful	Smooth	Painful, possible myoclonus	Smooth or excitatory	Smooth
Awakening following single dose	Rapid	Rapid	Rapid	Rapid	Intermediate
Recovery from effects	Rapid	Intermediate	Rapid	Intermediate	Intermediate
Heart rate	Unchanged to mild decrease	Moderate increase	Unchanged to mild increase	Moderate increase	Unchanged to mild increase
Mean arterial pressure	Marked decrease	Moderate decrease	Unchanged to mild decrease	Moderate increase	Unchanged to moderate decrease
Systemic vascular resistance	Marked decrease	Moderate decrease	Unchanged to mild decrease	Moderate increase	Unchanged to mild decrease
Ventilation	Marked decrease	Marked decrease	Mild decrease	Unchanged to mild decrease	Unchanged to mild decrease
Bronchodilation	No effect	Mild decrease	No effect	Marked increase	No effect
Cerebral blood flow	Marked decrease	Marked decrease	Marked decrease	Mild to marked increase	Unchanged to moderate decrease
$CMRO_2$	Marked decrease	Marked decrease	Marked decrease	Mild increase	Moderate decrease
Intracranial pressure	Marked decrease	Marked decrease	Marked decrease	Marked increase	Moderate decrease

18. **(D)** Opioids are exogenous substances (natural or synthetic) which bind specifically to opioid receptors and produce some type of agonist effect. Four main types of opioid receptors have been identified–mu (further subdivided into mu-1 and mu-2), kappa, delta, and sigma. The clinical effects of a given opioid depend on which receptor is bound, the binding affinity of the opioid for that receptor, and whether the drug functions as an agonist or antagonist at the given receptor type. Activation of mu receptors produces supraspinal analgesia (mu-1), respiratory depression (mu-2), physical dependence, and muscle rigidity. Kappa activation results in sedation and spinal analgesia. Delta receptor activation can cause analgesia, but may also result in behavioral changes and be epileptogenic, while sigma receptor activation is associated with dysphoria, hallucinations, and respiratory stimulation. Opioid receptors have been isolated from somatic and sympathetic peripheral nerves. Opioids exert their greatest effect within the CNS, however, where receptor activation inhibits presynaptic release and postsynaptic response to excitatory neurotransmitters from nociceptive neurons. Pain impulse transmission can also be interrupted at the level of the dorsal horn following intrathecal or epidural opioid administration.

All opioid agonists cause dose-dependent depression of ventilation, primarily through direct effects at brain stem respiratory centers. Nausea and vomiting can be caused by direct stimulation of dopamine receptors in the chemoreceptor trigger zone in the floor of the fourth ventricle. Opioids can cause biliary smooth muscle spasm, decrease bowel peristalsis, and increase pyloric sphincter and bladder sphincter tone, explaining the side effects of biliary colic, constipation, delayed gastric emptying, and urinary retention. Although rapid IV bolus with morphine can cause histamine release resulting in hypotension and both morphine and meperidine can produce orthostatic hypotension, opioid administration is unlikely to cause myocardial depression. Combination of opioids with benzodiazepines or nitrous oxide, however, may lower systemic blood pressure unlike when any of these drugs are used in isolation. Endogenous and exogenous opioid peptides cause modulations in immune function. Patients may develop tachyphylaxis, tolerance, and/or dependence in response to opioid agonists. Tolerance develops to essentially all effects and side effects except constipation and mydriasis. Rapid, high-dose opioid boluses may result in chest wall musculoskeletal stiffness which might be so severe as to impair ventilation. These side effects (as well as the beneficial effects) of opioids can be reversed with the opioid-receptor antagonist naloxone.

Morphine and meperidine are considered long acting, while fentanyl, sufentanil, alfentanil, and remifentanil are short-acting opioids. Clearance of opioids is principally by hepatic metabolism. Some metabolites have opioid agonist and/or partial agonist activity,

TABLE 36-4   Comparison of Opioid Agonists

	Equivalent potency	pK_a	Percent of drug nonionized at pH 7.4	Relative lipid solubility	Relative protein binding	Approximate elimination half time (hours)
Morphine	1	7.9	35	Very low	Very low	2.5
Meperidine	0.1	8.5	70	Low	High	4
Fentanyl	100	8.4	84	Very high	High	4
Sufentanil	750	8.0	93	Very high	Very high	3
Alfentanil	25	6.5	92	High	Very high	1.4
Remifentanil	100	7.3	58	Low	High to very high	0.2

so renal failure can result in impaired metabolite elimination and prolonged effects or side effects. Fentanyl, alfentanil, and sufentanil appear to be very fast acting and have short duration, but this fast on/fast off effect is primarily because of high lipid solubility and redistribution. As secondary tissue sites (fat, muscle) become saturated with repeat boluses or prolonged continuous infusion, return of drug from these sites to the plasma will keep plasma concentrations from falling rapidly after the drug is discontinued. In contrast, remifentanil contains an ester bond which is rapidly hydrolyzed by nonspecific plasma and tissue esterases (not pseudocholinesterase). Consequently, termination of action of remifenatnil remains constant (and rapid) regardless of length of infusion or the presence of hepatic or renal failure (Table 36-4).

Bibliography

Coda BA. Opioids. In: Barash PG, Cullen BF, Stoelting RK (eds.), *Clinical Anesthesia*, 4th ed. Philadelphia, PA: Lippincott, Williams & Wilkins, 2001.

Morgan GE Jr, Mikhail MS, Murray MJ. Nonvolatile anesthetic agents. In: Morgan GE Jr, Mikhail MS, Murray MJ, et al. (eds.), *Clinical Anesthesiology*, 3rd ed. New York, NY: McGraw-Hill, 2002, 164–169.

Stoelting RK. Opioid agonists and antagonists. In: Stoelting RK (ed.), *Pharmacology and Physiology in Anesthetic Practice*, 3rd ed. Philadelphia, PA: Lippincott, Williams & Wilkins, 1999, 77–112.

Stoelting RK, Miller RD. Opioids. In: Stoelting RK, Miller RD (eds.), *Basics of Anesthesia*, 4th ed. New York, NY: Churchill Livingstone, 2000, 70–79.

Wall RT. Anesthesia. In: Norton JA, Bollinger RR, Chang AE, et al. (eds.), *Surgery: Basic Science and Clinical Evidence*. New York, NY: Springer, 2001, 350–351.

19. **(C)** Inhaled anesthetics have very narrow margins of safety and require close monitoring of their physiologic effects. Concentrations that produce general anesthesia frequently cause significant CNS, cardiovascular, and respiratory depression.

The standard measure of potency for inhaled anesthetics is the minimum alveolar concentration (MAC). MAC is defined as the end-tidal anesthetic concentration (partial pressure at one atmosphere) that prevents movement in response to a noxious stimulus (such as surgical incision) in 50% of patients. At 1.3 MAC, 99% of patients do not move in response to surgical stimulation. MAC values are additive, such that a mixture of several anesthetics will have the same effect on the brain as a single agent at an equivalent MAC.

All volatile anesthetics depress the cardiovascular system. In general, blood pressure decreases as a result of a reduction in systemic vascular resistance and depressed myocardial contractility; however, the agents differ in the hemodynamic effects that lead to hypotension. Halothane decreases myocardial contractility and HR, whereas isoflurane, sevoflurane, and desflurane cause a drop in blood pressure primarily through decreased systemic vascular resistance. In contrast, nitrous oxide produces little effect on systemic blood pressure. Substituting it for a portion of volatile anesthetic will diminish the magnitude of cardiovascular depression caused by an equivalent MAC.

Use of inhaled anesthetics may also lead to significant changes in respiration. Spontaneous breathing is typically rapid and shallow. This increased respiratory rate is unable to compensate for the decreased tidal volume, leading to reduced overall minute volume and elevated $PaCO_2$ levels. Also, the ventilatory responsiveness to carbon dioxide and arterial hypoxia is blunted. These depressant effects can be treated by controlled ventilation during anesthesia.

In addition, volatile anesthetics cause a decrease in airway resistance by relaxing bronchial smooth muscle. This bronchodilation may have a beneficial effect in patients with reactive airway disease. During induction, however, isoflurane and desflurane can

TABLE 36-5 Factors that Modify MAC

Increase	Decrease
Infants	Neonates
Hyperthermia	Elderly
Alcohol habituation	Hypothermia
CNS stimulants	Acute alcohol use
MAO-I	Pregnancy
Cocaine	CNS depressants
Tricyclic antidepressants	Benzodiazepines
Amphetamines	Barbiturates
	Alpha$_2$-adrenergic agonists
	Narcotics
	Propofol
	Lithium

irritate the airway. Both will cause excessive secretions, coughing, and breath holding. Other agents such as halothane, sevoflurane, and nitrous oxide are better tolerated (Table 36-5).

Bibliography

Lockhart SH, Rampil IJ, Yasuda N, et al. Depression of ventilation by desflurane in humans. *Anesthesiology* 1991;74:484–488.

Merkel G, Eger EL. A comparative study of halothane and halopropane anesthesia. Including method for determining equipotency. *Anesthesiology* 1963;24:346–357.

Weiskopf RB, Cahalan MK, Eger EL, et al. Cardiovascular actions of desflurane in normocarbic volunteers. *Anesth Analg* 1991;73:143–156.

20. **(B)** The critical period of organogenesis occurs in the first 8 weeks of gestation. If at all possible, surgery should be postponed until the second trimester to reduce the risk of teratogenic drugs. Elective surgery should be postponed until after delivery; however, if surgery is necessary, it is preferable to choose drugs with a long history of safety in pregnancy. These include thiopental, morphine, meperidine, muscle relaxants, local anesthetics, and volatile anesthetics. The use of nitrous oxide and benzodiazepines is controversial. Anesthetic management must take into account potential effects on the growing fetus as well as pay close attention to physiologic changes that occur in every organ system during pregnancy.

An enlarging uterus forces the diaphragm upward. As a result, the FRC is decreased, leading to atelectasis and decreased oxygen reserve. In fact, marked decreases in PaO$_2$ can occur if intubation is prolonged. Also, minute ventilation is increased because of higher tidal volumes. This combination of increased minute ventilation and decreased FRC speeds both induction and emergence of parturients from anesthesia because of a faster rate of change in alveolar concentration of volatile anesthetics.

Pregnant patients have a higher incidence of difficult intubation because the upper airway is often edematous and friable. Weight gain in already obese patients can result in even more difficulty inserting the laryngoscope because of a short neck and large breasts. Gastrointestinal changes include delayed gastric emptying, increased intragastric pressure, relaxed lower esophageal sphincter, and decreased gastric pH. This causes pregnant patients to be at increased risk of reflux and aspiration pneumonia. Therefore, preoxygenation, cricoid pressure, and rapid-sequence induction is recommended prior to intubation.

Other changes that may impact perioperative management include decreased MAC for inhalational anesthetics and hypotension in the supine position from decreased venous return. The compression of the inferior vena cava can be lessened by positioning patients in left uterine displacement.

Bibliography

Ezri T, et al. Difficult airway in obstetric anesthesia: a review. *Obstet Gynecol Surv* 2001;56:631–641.

Hawkins JL. Anesthesia for the obstetric patient for nonobstetric surgery. *Anesth Analg* 1997;84:S60–S65.

21. **(C)** Measurement of arterial blood gas is used to assess ventilation, oxygenation, and acid-base status. Since systemic diseases frequently cause disturbances in the acid-base status, measurement of arterial blood gas allows for quantitative assessment of the cardiorespiratory system function. The major buffering system in the blood is the bicarbonate/carbonic acid buffer. With an acid-base disturbance, the initial correction is through the buffering system. Over the next several hours, compensation for the underlying acid-base disturbance is accomplished via the renal system for respiratory conditions and through the respiratory system for a metabolic acid-base abnormality.

Acid-base abnormalities involve a compensatory mechanism which minimizes the effect on pH. If there is an acute metabolic acidosis, bicarbonate decreases and respiratory compensation causes increased ventilation to decrease PaCO$_2$, and thus minimizes the change in pH. As a general rule, for every 10 mmHg change in PaCO$_2$, the pH will change 0.08 units in the opposite direction. If the pH change can be accounted for by this PaCO$_2$ change, then the acid-base disturbance is a respiratory disturbance. In this example, the pH change can be accounted for by the increase in PaCO$_2$. And as such, this represents an acute respiratory acidosis.

If the pH change cannot be accounted for by this, then it is a metabolic acid-base disturbance. More commonly there is a mixed metabolic-respiratory acid-base abnormality.

In evaluating oxygenation, the first thing to consider is whether hypoxemia is present. In most patients, hypoxemia exists if PaO_2 is less than 60 mmHg. This is the part on the oxyhemoglobin dissociation curve where the oxygen content of blood drops rapidly with a small decrease in the PaO_2. This is the area of the curve which is steep. The alveolar to arterial gradient is then determined. If the alveolar to arterial gradient is normal, then the hypoxemia is from hypoventilation or decreased inspired oxygen concentration. If the gradient is increased, then the hypoxemia is from a ventilation-perfusion mismatch, shunting, or diffusion impairment. Normal alveolar-arterial gradient is generally less than 10 mmHg. This is because of physiologic shunting through the bronchial and thebesian (coronary) veins that drain deoxygenated blood to the left side of the heart. The gradient is also dependent on the fraction of inspired oxygen. The gradient increases as the fraction of inspired oxygen increases.

Bibliography

Morgan GE, Mikhail MS, Murray MJ. Acid-base balance. In: Morgan GE, Mikhail MS, Murray MJ (eds.), *Clinical Anesthesiology*, 3rd ed. New York, NY: McGraw-Hill, 2002, 644–661.

Prough DS, Mathru M. Acid-base, fluids, and electrolytes. In: Barash PG, Cullen BF, Stoelting RK (eds.), *Clinical Anesthesia*, 4th ed. Philadelphia, PA: Lippincott, Williams & Wilkins, 2001, 165–170.

22. **(E)** Invasive blood pressure monitoring allows for precise beat-to-beat recording of a patient's blood pressure. This allows for more rapid diagnosis and treatment of hypotension and HTN. Invasive monitoring with an arterial catheter is indicated for patients with end-organ disease necessitating strict control of blood pressure. It is also useful for patients being mechanically ventilated and other situations which may require frequent blood draws. Contraindications to arterial catheter placement include vessels without adequate collateral flow or significant vascular insufficiency. If invasive monitoring is still required, then a more central location of catheter placement is warranted.

Several arteries are easily accessible for cannulation. These include the radial, brachial, femoral, dorsalis pedis, and posterior tibial arteries. The radial artery is most often chosen because of its superficial location and presence of adequate collateral flow. Allen's test may aid in assessing collateral flow, but is not completely reliable. Collateral flow can also be assessed by palpation, Doppler, or pulse oximetry.

Complications associated with the placement of an arterial catheter include arterial thrombosis, damage to the vessel, and nerve damage. Infection, or skin necrosis overlying the catheter is also possible. Prolonged cannulation, repeated insertion attempts, and use of vasopressors may increase these complications. These risks may be minimized with a minimal catheter to artery ratio, strict aseptic technique, and continuous heparinized saline flush at 2–3 mL/h. One may assess adequate perfusion with a pulse oximeter distal to catheter placement.

Accuracy of measurements depends on correct calibration of the transducer, which converts mechanical pressure to electrical energy for display. The transducer can be placed at the midaxillary line, or at the level of the ear to determine cerebral pressure. The shape of the arterial wave can be valuable. Contractility is indicated by the rate of upstroke, while peripheral vascular disease can be assessed by the rate of downstroke. Hypovolemia is suggested if the amplitude of the waves is variable.

Bibliography

Murphy GS, Vender JS. Monitoring the anesthetized patient. In: Barash PG, Cullen BF, Stoelting RK (eds.), *Clinical Anesthesia*, 4th ed. Philadelphia, PA: Lippincott, Williams & Wilkins, 2001, vol. 25, 673–674.

Morgan GE Jr, Mikhail MS. *Clinical Anesthesiology*, 3rd ed. New York, NY: Lange Medical Books/McGraw-Hill, 1996, vol. 6, 79–80.

Stoelting RK, Miller RD. *Basics of Anesthesia*, 4th ed. Philadelphia, PA: Churchill Livingstone, 1994, vol. 15, 214–215.

23. **(C)** The basic design of a pulmonary artery catheter consists of four lumens integrated into a 7F catheter which is 110 cm long. The lumens consist of an air channel for inflation of the balloon, wiring for the thermistor probe for evaluation of cardiac output, a proximal passage for infusions, and a distal passage for mixed venous sampling and measurements of pulmonary artery pressure.

Insertion is guided by a pressure waveform, as well as markings on the catheter. A central venous tracing is seen at approximately 15 cm as the catheter enters the right atrium. An increase in the systolic pressure indicates passage of the catheter into the right ventricle. Entry into the pulmonary artery occurs at 35–45 cm and is signified by an increase in the diastolic pressure. A wedge pressure is identified by small amplitude waves after minimal advancement into the pulmonary artery.

Hemodynamic variables derived from a pulmonary artery catheter include central venous pressure (CVP), total peripheral vascular resistance (TPVR), stroke volume (SV), cardiac output (CO), pulmonary artery pressure (PAP), as well as cardiac and ventricular indices. Pulmonary catheters allow more precise estimations of preload than central venous cannulation, by pulmonary capillary wedge pressure (PCWP) estimations of the left ventricular end diastolic pressure. Estimations of left ventricular end diastolic pressure (LV EDP) via PCWP may be inaccurate in the case of mitral valve disease, or changes in left atrial or ventricular compliance. Cardiac output measurements are by thermodilution technique, involving the injection of a known volume and temperature of fluid into the proximal infusion port, and measuring the temperature of this fluid at the distal end of the catheter. The degree of temperature change is inversely proportional to cardiac output.

Certain conditions can be diagnosed with interpretation of the data collected. Hypovolemia results in low CVP and pulmonary diastolic pressures. Hypervolemia results in the elevation of these variables. Left ventricular failure produces low cardiac output measurements and a decrease in stroke volume. Isolated left ventricular failure occurs in the absence of an elevated CVP.

Bibliography

Murphy GS, Vender JS. Monitoring the anesthetized patient. In: Barash PG, Cullen BF, Stoelting RK (eds.), *Clinical Anesthesia*, 4th ed. Philadelphia, PA: Lippincott, Williams & Wilkins, 2001, vol. 25, 675–678.

Morgan GE Jr, Mikhail MS. *Clinical Anesthesiology*, 3rd ed. New York, NY: Lange Medical Books/McGraw-Hill, 1996, vol. 6, 85–91.

Stoelting RK, Miller RD. *Basics of Anesthesia*, 4th ed. Philadelphia, PA: Churchill Livingstone, 2000, 217–218.

24. (D) See answer following Question number 25.

25. (B) Basic patient monitoring includes a noninvasive blood pressure cuff, ECG monitor, and pulse oximeter. These monitors are mandated by the ASA for intraoperative use, and are routinely used for monitoring ward patients. An understanding of the technology behind these monitors assures optimal care of patients.

Automated blood pressure monitors use oscillometry. Arterial pulsations create small oscillations in cuff pressure which are maximal at mean arterial pressure. A microprocessor uses algorithms to derive systolic and diastolic pressures. The sampling site can affect measurements, with greater systolic and diastolic differences the more distal the cuff is from the aorta. These differences are increased further by the use of vasodilating drugs such as nitroglycerine. Blood pressure measurements can also be altered by the presence of peripheral vascular disease. Care

should be taken to avoid placing blood pressure cuffs on the same extremity with any vascular abnormality, including dialysis access grafts.

Manual blood pressure readings are taken using Korotkoff sounds, which is the sound of turbulent flow in an artery. The cuff is inflated to a pressure which collapses the underlying artery. Systolic pressure is noted at the appearance of sound after deflation of the cuff. Diastolic pressure is heralded by the muffling or disappearance of sound. Proper cuff size is assured with the cuff bladder extending at least halfway around a patient's arm. The width of the cuff should be 20–50% greater than the diameter of the extremity.

Electrocardiography is a reading of the electrical potential of myocardial cells. Silver chloride electrodes contact the patient through a conductive gel which lowers the skin's electrical resistance. Two channels are routinely monitored intraoperatively. Lead II is used for detection of rhythm abnormalities, while V5 is used for the detection of anterolateral ischemia. The axis of lead II parallels the atria, resulting in the greatest P-wave amplitudes in this lead. Esophageal leads may provide better rhythm detection, but have not yet gained widespread acceptance.

Artifact can be caused by lead wire movement and electrocautery. Monitoring filters can be used to circumvent this artifact, but can lead to exaggerated changes in ST segments, limiting its usefulness in ischemia detection. Criteria for ischemia include flat or downsloping ST depression greater then 1 mm, occurring 60–80 ms after the J point. ST elevation or T-wave inversion can also signal ischemia. Continuous ST monitoring allows for early detection of ischemia. Certain conditions such as Wolff-Parkinson-White, bundle branch block, and pacemaker capture preclude the use of ST analysis for the detection of ischemia.

Pulse oximetry employs the Lambert-Beer's law to noninvasively measure arterial blood oxygen saturation. This law states that oxygenated and deoxygenated hemoglobin absorb red and infrared light differently. Two light emitting diodes produce different wavelengths of light which travel through tissue, and are detected at a sensor opposite the diodes. The wavelengths used are in the red and infrared parts of the spectrum. Oxyhemoglobin absorbs more infrared light, while deoxyhemoglobin absorbs red light more effectively. The difference in absorption is detected by the sensor and resultant oxygen saturation is displayed. Plethysmography is used to filter out light absorption from venous blood and other tissues, using only those of arterial pulsations. The amplitude of the waveform produced can be used as a measure of tissue perfusion. Ear probes can detect changes in oxygen saturation sooner than finger probes by virtue of a shorter circulation time. Carboxyhemoglobin absorbs infrared light as effectively as oxyhemoglobin which can lead to a falsely elevated reading. Methemoglobin absorbs the light of both wavelengths equally, causing a saturation reading of 85%. This reading is falsely low if saturation is greater than 85%, or falsely high if saturation is lower than 85%.

Mixed venous oxygen saturation is an application of pulse oximetry obtained from the placement of a specially designed fiberoptic sensor in the pulmonary artery. The resulting measurements can be used with other variables obtained from a pulmonary artery catheter to make an assessment of a patient's hemodynamic state.

Bibliography

Monitoring. In: Stoelting RK, Miller RD (eds.), *Basics of Anesthesia*, 4th ed. Philadelphia, PA: Churchill Livingstone, 2000.

Morgan GE Jr, Mikhail MS. *Clinical anesthesiology*, 3rd ed. New York, NY: Lange Medical Books/McGraw-Hill, 1996, vol. 6, 73–78, 83–84, 93–95.

26. **(B)** Spinal anesthesia is the placement of local anesthetic solution into the subarachnoid space. Many operations on the lower extremities, pelvis, and lower abdomen can be managed safely with spinal blocks alone, or they may be used simultaneously with general anesthesia for postoperative pain management. Adverse reactions do occur, however, and range from self-limited back pain to severe cardiovascular effects and even death. Table 36-6 lists contraindications to spinal anesthesia.

The physiologic effects of spinal anesthesia depend on the level of anesthesia. For example, a low spinal will produce little or no change in blood pressure, but a high spinal may result in profound hypotension. Blockade of preganglionic sympathetic nerves results in vasodilatation and pooling of blood in the large veins of the lower extremities and abdomen. This leads to a reduction in preload and decrease in stroke volume. Normally, patients can compensate by increasing HR and contractility; however, many patients (such as the elderly), cannot compensate because of reduced physiologic reserve. In addition, if the block is sufficiently high to block the cardioaccelerator nerves (T1-T4), bradycardia may also contribute to hypotension. Therapy for spinal-induced hypotension includes fluids, head down position, and pharmacologic therapy with atropine, ephedrine, and other pressors as the situation dictates.

High spinal can also cause significant alteration on respiratory physiology. The effects are greater on expiratory function than on inspiratory function. This is related to the different muscles involved with each action. The principle muscles of inhalation are the diaphragm, the external intercostals, and the accessory muscles (sternocleidomastoid and scalene). The diaphragm and accessory muscles are innervated by the upper cervical nerves. Thus, even high thoracic levels of spinal anesthetic are unlikely to cause a significant decrease in inspiratory capacity. On the other hand, the principle muscles of exhalation are the abdominal and internal intercostal muscles. These muscles are innervated by thoracic spinal nerve roots which easily can be blocked by high spinal. As a result, expiratory reserve volume and the ability to cough effectively are markedly reduced. This may lead to atelectasis and hypoxia in patients with pulmonary disease.

Spinal anesthesia may also affect several other organ systems. First, sympathetic outflow to the gastrointestinal tract originates at the T5-L1 level. It serves to decrease peristalsis and maintain sphincter tone. Therefore, neuraxial blockade at this level would allow unopposed parasympathetic tone and result in a contracted bowel with active peristalsis. Also, at the lumbar and sacral levels, both sympathetic and parasympathetic control of bladder function is affected. This results in contracted sphincters and urinary retention requiring use of a urinary catheter until the block wears off. And finally, a T11 sympathectomy can block the adrenal response to surgical stress. This may be helpful by diminishing hyperglycemia, HTN, and catecholamine release.

Bibliography

Critchley LA. Hypotension, subarachnoid block and the elderly patient. *Anaesthesia* 1996;51:1139–1143.

Liu SS, McDonald SB. Current issues in spinal anesthesia. *Anesthesiology* 2001;94:888–906.

Pollard JB. Cardiac arrest during spinal anesthesia: common mechanisms and strategies for prevention. *Anesth Analg* 2001;92:252–256.

TABLE 36-6   Contraindications to Spinal Anesthesia

Absolute
Patient refusal
Coagulopathy
Infection at site
Severe hypovolemia
Increased intracranial pressure

Relative
Sepsis
Preexisting neurologic deficits
Aortic stenosis

27. (E) Postdural puncture headache may occur after lumbar puncture, spinal anesthesia, or intraoperative spinal drainage. It is thought to result from leakage of cerebrospinal fluid and decreased intracranial pressure. With decreased support, gravitational traction of brain structures in the upright position causes tension on pain sensitive structures. The classic presentation involves onset 1–2 days after dural puncture, increased severity when sitting or upright, and an occipital or frontal location. Auditory and visual disturbances are very rare.

The incidence of postdural puncture headache increases when a larger diameter spinal needle is used, as well as insertion of the needle bevel oriented perpendicular to the dural fiber axis. In addition, a history of any of the following can indicate a higher risk: young age, female sex, pregnancy, previous spinal headache, or history of motion sickness.

The headache usually resolves spontaneously in a few days to a week in most patients. Recumbent position, bed rest, hydration, and analgesics are the mainstay of treatment. Intravenous caffeine has also been shown to produce symptomatic relief. In severe cases that do not respond to conservative treatment, an epidural blood patch can be done. Autologous blood is drawn from the patient and injected into the epidural space near the original puncture. It is believed that this works by sealing the dura and preventing further cerebrospinal fluid leakage. Symptom relief occurs within 24 h in greater than 90% of patients. If a headache persists even after two epidural blood patches, another etiology may be responsible. Rarer, more serious causes of headache that need to be considered are subdural hematoma, meningitis, tumor, or any cause of increased intracranial pressure.

Bibliography

Holst D, Mollmann M, Ebel C, et al. In vitro investigation of cerebrospinal fluid leakage after dural puncture with various spinal needles. *Anesth Analg* 1998;87:1331–1335.

Liu SS, McDonald SB. Current issues in spinal anesthesia. *Anesthesiology* 2001;94:888–906.

Morewood GH. A rational approach to the cause, prevention, and treatment of postdural puncture headache. *CMAJ* 1993;149:1087–1093.

Vakharia SB, Thomas PS, Rosenbaum AE, et al. Magnetic resonance imaging of cerebrospinal fluid leak and tamponade effect of blood patch in postdural puncture headache. *Anesth Analg* 1997;84:585–590.

28. (C) Storage of blood products is responsible for many of the complications associated with massive transfusion (10 units or more). During storage, red blood cells lyse, potassium increases, pH drops, 2,3-diphosphoglycerate (2,3-DPG) decreases, platelet count decreases, and factors V and VII degrade.

Coagulation disorders manifest as hematuria, microvascular bleeding, or bleeding from IV sites. The most common cause of abnormal bleeding is dilutional thrombocytopenia. After 24 h, blood stored at 4°C has virtually no viable platelets remaining. In acute thrombocytopenia, bleeding may occur with a platelet count less than 50,000 cells/mm³. Treatment with platelet concentrate will typically increase platelet count by 10,000 cells/mm³ per unit transfused.

Factor V, factor VIII, and fibrinogen also decrease following massive transfusion; however, because only 20% of factor V and 30% of factor VIII are needed for hemostasis during surgery, this is rarely a problem. Fresh frozen plasma is the treatment of choice when the prothrombin time or partial thromboplastin time is elevated. Other disorders that must be considered are disseminated intravascular coagulopathy, hemolytic transfusion reactions, and preoperative coagulation defects.

The citrate found in blood preservative binds both calcium and magnesium. Hypocalcemia from massive transfusion is rare in patients who are not hypothermic and have normal hepatic function. In fact, the administration of calcium is not indicated until evidence of hyocalcemia is present (prolonged QT, measurement of decreased ionized calcium). This may occur in very rapid transfusions, patients with liver disease, and neonates. Hypomagnesemia is often overlooked, and may manifest as tachyarrhythmias, torsade de pointes, or ventricular fibrillation.

Other metabolic abnormalities can occur and treatment should be based on frequent arterial blood gas and electrolyte results. Metabolic acidosis may be associated with large transfusions because of increased hydrogen ions in preservatives and continued metabolism of red blood cells. Metabolic alkalosis can result from the conversion of citrate to bicarbonate. Hyperkalemia can be seen because of elevated potassium in stored blood, but rarely occurs. And finally, decreased 2,3-DPG could cause a left shift of the oxygen-hemoglobin dissociation curve leading to tissue hypoxia.

Bibliography

Goodnough LT, Brecher ME, Kanter MH, et al. Transfusion medicine. *N Engl J Med* 1999;340:438–447.

Murray DJ, Olson J, Strauss R, et al. Coagulation changes during packed red cell replacement of major blood loss. *Anesthesiology* 1988;69:839.

29. (D) Type, screen, and crossmatch are compatibility tests used to detect harmful antigen-antibody interactions and prevent transfusion reactions. Determination of ABO-Rh types of both donor and recipient is the first and most important step, because the most serious reactions are caused by accidental transfusion of ABO-incompatible blood. Anti-A and anti-B antibodies are formed when an individual lacks either or both of the A and B antigens. Thus, a patient with type A blood will make anti-B, and a patient with type B blood will make anti-A. On the other hand, when a patient is Rh-positive (the D antigen is present), anti-D antibodies are not made. This is because the D antigen is not ubiquitous in our environment as the A and B antigens are; however, Rh-negative patients can still produce antibodies when exposed to donor (or fetal) red blood cells with the D antigen.

The next step is the antibody screen. This is a test to determine the presence of abnormal red cell antibodies in recipient serum to clinically significant antigens. Examples of antigens that have been implicated in transfusion reaction are D, C, E, c, e, Duffy, Kell, and Kidd.

The type and screen is used most often when the patient is unlikely to require transfusion during the planned surgical procedure, but blood should be readily available. The next step, crossmatch, is a simulation *in vitro* of the actual anticipated transfusion. In the first phase, donor red blood cells are mixed with the recipient's serum and examined for macroscopic agglutination. This tests for ABO, M, N, P, and Lewis incompatibilities. Next, the products of the first phase are incubated at 37°C in low ionic strength saline or albumin to enhance incomplete antibodies. In the final phase, the indirect antiglobulin test, antiglobulin serum is used to detect antibodies which may be attached to donor red blood cells.

Bibliography

Goodnough LT, Brecher ME, Kanter MH, et al. Transfusion medicine. *N Engl J Med* 1999;340:438–447.

Heiss MM. Risk of allogeneic transfusions. *Br J Anaesth* 1998;81:16–19.

Petz LD. The surgeon and the transfusion service: essentials of compatibility testing, surgical blood ordering, emergency blood needs, and adverse reactions. In: Speiss BD, Counts RB, Gould SA (eds.), *Perioperative Transfusion Medicine*. Baltimore, MD: Williams & Willkins, 1998, 45–49.

30. **(A)** Transfusion reactions can be divided into febrile, allergic, and hemolytic. Febrile reactions are more common and likely represent an alteration of the thermoregulatory set point by chemical mediators released by donor leukocytes in response to recipient antibodies. Patients often have fever only, but also may experience chills, myalgia, headache, nausea, or dyspnea.

If a febrile reaction occurs, the transfusion should be slowed and antipyretics administered.

Next, mild allergic reactions to blood products can occur by IgE-mediated histamine release. Patients typically present with fever, urticarial rash, and generalized pruritis. In severe cases transfusion may need to be stopped. In most cases, however, patients can be treated symptomatically with diphenhydramine and the transfusion continued.

Hemolytic transfusion reactions occur when incompatible blood is administered (often because of clerical errors) and are life threatening. Antibodies and complement in the recipient attack donor red blood cells leading to hemolysis. The antibodies that commonly produce immediate hemolysis are anti-A, -B, Kell, Kidd, Lewis, and Duffy. Release of hemoglobin and cytokines leads to shock, disseminated intravascular coagulation (DIC), and acute renal failure. Many of the signs and symptoms of a hemolytic transfusion reaction may be masked by anesthesia. In an awake patient, signs include fever (most common), chills, chest/back pain, nausea, flushing, dyspnea, and headache; however, under general anesthesia, the first signs may be tachycardia and hypotension despite adequate blood replacement. Unfortunately these are common in surgery, and the diagnosis is often not made until diffuse bleeding secondary to DIC or hemoglobinuria is noted later on.

When a reaction is suspected, the transfusion should be immediately discontinued. Hypotension can be treated with fluids, dopamine, and compatible blood if necessary. High urine output should be maintained with crystalloid solution and administration of furosemide or mannitol. Also, the use of sodium bicarbonate to alkalinize the urine has been suggested.

Bibliography

Capon SM, Goldfinger D. Acute hemolytic transfusion reaction, a paradigm of the systemic inflammatory response: new insights into pathophysiology and treatment. *Transfusion* 1995;35:513–520.

Goodnough LT, Brecher ME, Kanter MH, et al. Transfusion medicine. *N Engl J Med* 1999;340:438–447.

Santoso JT, Lin DW, Miller DS. Transfusion medicine in obstetrics and gynecology. *Obstet Gynecol Surv* 1995;50:470–481.

31. **(B)** Total body water (TBW) consists of intracellular volume (40% of body weight) and extracellular volume (20% of body weight). Of the extraceullar volume, 20% is plasma and 80% is interstitial fluid. Both crystalloid and colloid are distributed into the extracellular volume

when administered. TBW is regulated thirst, hormonally by antidiuretic hormone (ADH), aldosterone, and naturetic peptides, and also hemodynamically by atrial and carotid baroreceptors. These mechanisms are triggered by decreases in extracellular volume or increase in tonicity. A healthy adult will lose water from three sources: gastrointestinal 200 cc per day, urine 1 L per day, and insensible 1 L per day (half because of respiration and half because of skin). The replacement of the normal water loss or maintenance can be calculated using a weight-based formula. It provides 4 cc/kg/h for the first 10 kg, 2 cc/kg/h for the second 10 kg, and 1 cc/kg/h for each kg above 20 kg. For example, maintenance fluid requirement for a 50 kg person would be $(4 \times 10) + (2 \times 10) + (1 \times 30) = 90$ cc/h. Multiply the maintenance values by the number of hours NPO to calculate the NPO deficit. Surgical patients require replacement of maintenance, losses from NPO periods, wounds, burns, ascites, trauma, blood loss, and tissue manipulation. Surgical stress is associated with a hyperglycemic response; therefore, glucose containing solutions are used only in pediatric patients and patients taking glucose altering medicines. Dehydration from any source develops more rapidly and is more severe in the young because the ratio of extracellular fluid to intracellular fluid is greater than in the adult population. Postoperatively, the mobilization of fluid from the interstitial compartment to the intravascular compartment typically occurs on the third postoperative day. Pulmonary edema and cardiac events can occur with this mobilization if cardiovascular and/or renal function is impaired. Colloid solutions, such as albumin and hydroxyethyl starch, theoretically increase the plasma volume without the concomitant increase in the interstitial compartment and; thus, minimizing the volume given thereby reducing the fluid needing to be mobilized postoperatively. However, research has not been able to prove definitively any advantage between colloid versus crystalloid. Hydroxyethyl starch, however, has been shown to produce laboratory evidence of coagulopathy if given in large amounts (>15 cc/kg).

Bibliography

Barash PG, Cullen BF, Stoelting RK. *Clinical Anesthesia*, 4th ed. Philadelphia, PA: Lippincott, Williams & Wilkins, 2001, 170–172.

Stoelting RK. *Pharmacology and Physiology in Anesthetic Practice*, 3rd ed. Philadelphia, PA: Lippincott, Williams & Wilkins, 1999, 586–587.

32. **(C)** The LMA is a substitute for a mask airway used in cases in which endotracheal intubation is not warranted or when traditional mask ventilation is not adequate. At least 20% of all cases in the United States use an LMA. It comes in different sizes and is chosen according to patient size. When inserted properly, the distal tip of the device will be seated just above the upper esophageal sphincter and the inflated rim seated tightly in the hypopharynx. Although the LMA does not reliably seal the esophageal inlet and thus does not fully protect against aspiration, the actual number of reported aspiration events in low-risk patients approaches the incidence of non-LMA general anesthetics (2~10,000). Those considered high risk for aspiration include the obese, hiatal hernia, Trendelenberg position, intraabdominal surgery, patients with dementia, emergency surgery, and difficult airways. Other contraindications include poor lung compliance, high airway resistance, glottic airway obstruction, and poor mouth opening. Although traditional use of the LMA required a spontaneously breathing patient; positive pressure ventilation on a paralyzed patient can safely performed through a well-fitted LMA. Given its lack of tracheal stimulation, the LMA may actually be preferable to endotracheal tube placement in the asthmatic. This, together with the fact that inhaled anesthetics are bronchodilators, makes the LMA a valuable tool in the treatment of patients with asthma. It has also been valuable in the management of the difficult airway. After proper insertion, blind, fiberoptic, and direct intubation attempts can be made with the LMA still in place. The LMA Fasttrach is an apparatus in which a conventional endotracheal tube can be placed through this customized LMA and into the trachea blindly with good success. Complications of LMA are rare and include nerve injury, laryngospasm, bronchospasm, vocal cord dysfunction, and other problems associated with airway instrumentation. These complications are nearly always reversible and without permanent sequelae.

Bibliography

Barash PG, Cullen BF, Stoelting, RK. *Clinical Anesthesia*, 4th ed. Philadelphia, PA: Lippincott, Williams & Wilkins, 2001, 599–601.

33. **(A)** Induction of general anesthesia in patients with full stomachs or incompetent lower esophageal sphincters can result in aspiration of gastric contents. High-risk groups include the obese, pregnant, diabetics with gastroparesis, emergent procedures, and patients with gastroesophageal reflux. Clinically significant aspiration can occur when pH <2.5 or gastric volume >25 cc. Several pharmacologic agents are available which increase gastric pH or decrease gastric volume including histamine blockers, prostaglandin E analogs, proton-pump inhibitors, and metoclopramide. The goal of rapid-sequence induction is to

limit the time in which the airway is unprotected after induction. It is performed by administering an intravenous anesthetic followed immediately by a neuromuscular blocker with a rapid onset. Cricoid pressure is generally held and direct laryngoscopy is performed when neuromuscular blockade is confirmed. Cricoid pressure occludes the esophageal lumen preventing the passage of gastric contents into the pharynx. Cricoid pressure is contraindicated in actively vomiting patients (possibility of esophageal perforation), cervical spine fracture, and laryngeal fracture. Generally positive pressure mask ventilation is avoided during rapid-sequence induction; however, gentle positive pressure ventilation may be used if there are difficulties in securing the airway.

Bibliography

Barash PG, Cullen BF, Stoelting RK. *Clinical Anesthesia*, 4th ed. Philadelphia, PA: Lippincott, Williams & Wilkins, 2001, 609–610.

34. **(C)** The adult respiratory distress syndrome (ARDS) is term applied to a common endpoint for which there are a myriad of causes. It is characterized by decreased lung compliance, refractory hypoxia, diffuse bilateral pulmonary infiltrates. At the alveolar level, its hallmark is an increase in lung water secondary to an increase in capillary permeability. At the cellular level, there are accumulations of neutrophils and leukocytes releasing inflammatory mediators such as leukotrienes, thromboxanes, and prostaglandins. Compliment activation occurs causing local inflammation and destruction of alveolar architecture. Platelet and coagulation abnormalities also play a role in microembolic phenomena in the pulmonary vasculature which correlates with the severity of lung injury. Early recognition and treatment of primary insult is essential. Hypoxia is generally correctable early on. As alveoli are destroyed, a right-to-left shunt occurs limiting the effectiveness of supplemental oxygen. When adequate oxygenation cannot be achieved, mechanical ventilation should be used. PEEP therapy continues to be an important component in the treatment of ARDS. PEEP improves oxygenation by decreasing FRC and dead space ventilation and increasing lung compliance. Lower lung volumes (5–6 cc/kg) with titration of PEEP to optimize lung compliance avoid volutrauma and shear stress which has been shown to improve outcome. PEEP can also have detrimental hemodynamic effects. It impairs venous return, increases pulmonary vascular resistance, and alters ventricular compliance curves. Complications include pneumothorax, pneumomediastinum, and interstitial edema. Inhaled nitric oxide is a potential option in severe ARDS. It has been shown to decrease oxygen requirements thereby limiting toxicity and decrease both pulmonary edema and barotrauma.

Bibliography

Barash PG, Cullen BF, Stoelting RK. *Clinical Anesthesia*, 4th ed. Philadelphia, PA: Lippincott, Williams & Wilkins, 2001, 1468–1469.

35. **(E)** Signs and symptoms of a space occupying lesion are related to the mass effect on intracranial pressure. The anesthetic management for patients undergoing surgical resection of an intracranial tumor has the goal of minimizing changes in intracranial blood flow and thus minimizing changes in intracranial pressure. The normal cerebral blood flow is approximately 50 mL/100 g/min. The factors which can alter cerebral blood flow include $PaCO_2$, temperature, and anesthetic drugs. Cerebral blood flow is linearly related to $PaCO_2$. Cerebral blood flow will increase 1 mL/100 g/min for every 1 mmHg increase in $PaCO_2$. The cerebral blood flow remains relatively constant between mean arterial pressure of 60–150 mmHg. This is because of autoregulation where the cerebral vasculature is able to vasodilate or vasoconstrict in response to arterial blood pressure to maintain the cerebral blood flow. This autoregulation may be impaired in the presence of a tumor or anesthetic agents. Isoflurane, like all inhaled anesthetic agents, increases cerebral blood flow in a dose-dependant manner in a dose above 0.6 MAC. This is most likely because of cerebral vascular dilation.

Isoflurane has the least effect on cerebral blood flow as compared to other inhaled anesthetic agents. Another effect of volatile anesthetic agents is a decrease in cerebral metabolic oxygen requirement. Normally as cerebral blood flow increases, the cerebral metabolic oxygen requirement increase. Volatile anesthetics uncouple this by decreasing cerebral metabolic rate while increasing cerebral blood flow.

Propofol decreases cerebral blood flow via cerebral vasoconstriction. It also decreases the cerebral metabolic oxygen requirement. As such, propofol, thiopental, and etomidate all decrease intracranial pressure.

Fentanyl, like other opioids, may minimally decrease cerebral blood flow and thus decrease intracranial pressure. One must use this with caution because side effects such as hypoventilation and hypercapnia may worsen increased intracranial pressure. But when used with volatile anesthetics and controlled ventilation, opioids may enable administration of volatile anesthetics to less than 0.6 MAC; and thus may be helpful in decreasing intracranial pressure.

Succinylcholine and all nondepolarizing neuro-muscular blocking drugs can be administered to patients undergoing resection for cranial tumors. The problem with succinylcholine is the mild, transient increase in intracranial pressure associated with its administration. It is used when rapid control of the airway is desired. All nondepolarizers are considered safe to administer, except when histamine release may cause an increase in intracranial pressure. Neuromuscular blockade prior to laryngoscopy may prevent coughing which may increase intracranial pressure.

Ketamine is generally not used in patients with intracranial tumors where increased intracranial pressure is a concern. This is because of ketamine's ability to increase cerebral blood flow and thus increase intracranial pressure.

Other methods used to decrease intracranial pressure include changes in head position to facilitate venous drainage, hyperventilation, induced hypothermia, and surgical decompression or drainage of cerebral spinal fluid. Other drugs used to decrease intracranial pressure include osmotic diuretics such as mannitol, loop diuretics, and corticosteroids.

Bibliography

Bendo AA, Kass IS, Hartung J, et al. Anesthesia for neurosurgery. In: Barash PG, Cullen BF, Stoelting RK (eds.), *Clinical Anesthesia*, 4th ed. Philadelphia, PA: Lippincott, Williams & Wilkins, 2001, 743–789.

Morgan GE, Mikhail MS, Murray MJ. Anesthesia for neurosurgery. In: Morgan GE, Mikhail MS, Murray MJ (eds.), *Clinical Anesthesiology*, 3rd ed. New York, NY: McGraw-Hill, 2002, 567–582.

Morgan GE, Mikhail MS, Murray MJ. Neurophysiology and anesthesia. In: Morgan GE, Mikhail MS, Murray MJ (eds.), *Clinical Anesthesiology*, 3rd ed. New York, NY: McGraw-Hill, 2002, 552–566.

Stoelting RK, Dierdorf SF. Diseases of the nervous system. In: Stoelting RK, Dierdorf SF (eds.), *Anesthesia and Coexisting Disease*, 4th ed. New York, NY: Churchill Livingstone, 2002, 233–244.

36. (C) Malignant hyperthermia is an inherited disorder characterized by hyper metabolism of skeletal muscle. It is autosomal dominant with variable expression and is more common in males and the pediatric population. Untreated, this disorder has an 80% mortality; however, the use of dantrolene has lowered this rate to below 10%.

Triggers include all potent volatile anesthetics and succinylcholine. Barbiturates, opioids, benzodiazepines, propofol, local anesthetics, nitrous oxide, and nondepolarizing neuromuscular blocking drugs do not trigger malignant hyperthermia. Onset of clinical signs may be immediately following the introduction of a trigger, but also may be significantly delayed. Early signs include increased end-tidal CO_2 levels, tachycardia, and tachypnea (if patient is unparalyzed).

More than 20 mutations responsible for malignant hyperthermia have been identified. The unifying theme is a defect in calcium release/control leading to increased intracellular calcium. Calcium pumps then attempt to maintain homeostasis, which leads to an increased metabolic state. The rigidity occurs when myofibrillar calcium approaches the contractile threshold. Dantrolene likely decreases the amount of calcium released from the sarcoplasmic reticulum. After symptoms are under control, continue dantrolene 1 mg/kg IV every 6 h do not give calcium-channel blockers. The combination of these with dantrolene results in hyperkalemia and myocardial depression (Tables 36-7 and 36-8).

Bibliography

Denborough M. Malignant hyperthermia. *Lancet* 1998;352:1131–1136.

Loke J, MacLennan DH. Malignant hyperthermia and central core disease: disorders of Ca^{2+} release channels. *Am J Med* 1998;104:470–486.

Morgan KG, Bryant SH. The mechanism of action of dantrolene sodium. *J Pharmacol Exp Ther* 1977;201:138–147.

Saltzman LS, Kates RA, Corke BC, et al. Hyperkalemia and cardiovascular collapse after verapamil and dantrolene administration is swine. *Anesth Analg* 1984;63:473–478.

TABLE 36-7   Clinical Signs of Malignant Hyperthermia

Tachycardia
Tachypnea
Masseter muscle rigidity
Increased ET CO_2
Metabolic and respiratory acidosis
Rhabdomyolysis
Arrhythmias
Sweating
Hypertension
Increased temperature

TABLE 36-8   Treatment of Malignant Hyperthermia

1. Call for assistance
2. Immediate discontinuation of succinylcholine or volatile anesthetics
3. Hyperventilate patient with 100% oxygen
4. Administer dantrolene 2 mg/kg IV, with repeat doses every 5–10 min until symptoms are controlled or a cumulative dose of 10 mg/kg IV is reached
5. Attempt to decrease temperature with cold saline, gastric lavage, and surface cooling
6. Treat metabolic acidosis with sodium bicarbonate
7. Maintain urine output with hydration and diuretics if necessary

37. (D) Recovery from anesthesia and wakefulness requires diffuse cortical activation via the reticular activating system. After general anesthesia, there is a continuum of arousal with the ability to follow commands returning before the ability to converse. Delayed awakening from general anesthesia can be pharmacologic, metabolic, or neurologic. The rate of emergence correlates with timing, total doses of drugs given, and bioavailability. All agents when given together can potentiate each other and prolong awakening. Delivery of a high concentration of inhaled agent for long periods of time coupled with hypoventilation may prolong awakening. Propofol is unlikely in this case of a young healthy adult to prolong awakening. Like other induction agents propofol rapidly undergoes redistribution with a half-life of 2–8 min and total elimination with a half-life of about an hour. The concentration of propofol decreases rapidly following the intravenous bolus because of redistribution. Awakening from a single bolus dose of propofol can occur within minutes.

Sevoflurane can cause a delay in awakening especially when coupled with hypoventilation. In addition, when delivery is prolonged and at high concentration, there may be saturation of sevoflurane in fat and other tissues to delay its effects.

Rocuronium can be implicated if there is inadequate muscle relaxant reversal. The patient may be weak or have hypoventilation. Hypercarbia and incomplete washout of volatile agents would result.

Succinylcholine can be implicated if the patient has an atypical plasma cholinesterase. Since succinylcholine is metabolized by plasma cholinesterase, patients with atypical enzymes are less able to metabolize succinylcholine and thus have prolonged effects leading to muscle weakness and hypoventilation. These patients may have muscle weakness that lasts for hours after succinylcholine administration. A way to diagnose the presence of atypical plasma cholinesterase is with the use of the dibucaine number. Dibucaine is a local anesthetic which inhibits normal plasma cholinesterase. The dibucaine number is a reflection of the quality of a patient's available plasma cholinesterase enzyme. The normal dibucaine number is 80 because normal plasma cholinesterase enzyme is inhibited 80% by dibucaine. Heterozygous patients with atypical plasma cholinesterase have a dibucaine number between 40 and 60. In these patients, the duration of action of succinylcholine would be about 30 min. The incidence of this is 1:480. Patients who are homozygous for atypical plasma cholinesterase have a dibucaine number of about 20. In these patients, the duration of succinylcholine would be up to a couple of hours. The incidence of this is 1:3200.

Gentamicin could also be a cause of delayed awakening because of its potentiation of nondepolarizing muscle relaxants. Other causes could be metabolic, such as hypothermia or decreased liver or kidney function. These may lead to slower excretion of drugs. Hypoglycemia can also delayed awakening as do electrolyte abnormalities such as hypomagnesemia, hypovolemia, and hyponatremia. Neurologic causes such as hypoperfusion from low cardiac output states or thromboembolic phenomenon may play a role.

Bibliography

Bevan DR, Donati F. Muscle relaxants. In: Barash PG, Cullen BF, Stoelting RK (eds.), *Clinical Anesthesia*, 4th ed. Philadelphia, PA: Lippincott, Williams & Wilkins, 2001, 419–447.

Mecca RS. Postoperative recovery. In: Barash PG, Cullen BF, Stoelting RK (eds.), *Clinical Anesthesia*, 4th ed. Philadelphia, PA: Lippincott, Williams & Wilkins, 2001, 1377–1402.

Morgan GE, Mikhail MS, Murray MJ. Postanesthesia care. In: Morgan GE, Mikhail MS, Murray MJ (eds.), *Clinical Anesthesiology*, 3rd ed. New York, NY: McGraw-Hill, 2002, 936–950.

Stoelting R. Inhaled anesthetics. In: Stoelting RK (ed.), *Pharmacology & Physiology in Anesthetic Practice*, 3rd ed. Philadelphia, PA: Lippincott-Raven, 1999, 36–76.

Stoelting R. Neuromuscular-blocking drugs. In: Stoelting RK (ed.), *Pharmacology & Physiology in Anesthetic Practice*, 3rd ed. Philadelphia, PA: Lippincott-Raven, 1999, 182–223.

Stoelting R. Nonbarbituate induction drugs. In: Stoelting RK (ed.), *Pharmacology & Physiology in Anesthetic Practice*, 3rd ed. Philadelphia, PA: Lippincott-Raven, 1999, 182–223.

38. (C) Mechanical ventilation is selected for patients with poor ventilation or oxygenation after using supplemental oxygen. It is almost exclusively provided with positive pressure delivered through an endotracheal tube. This positive pressure can lead to elevated airway pressures resulting in barotrauma. Venous return may also be hampered by these elevated pressures. Lastly, positive pressure may create V/Q defects secondary to preferentially ventilating more compliant areas of the lung, while blood flow is greatest in the noncompliant, dependent areas of the lung.

Positive pressure ventilators create a pressure difference between the gas circuit and the alveoli, periodically allowing inspiratory gas flow. Exhalation is a passive process. Four phases are inherent in ventilators. These include inhalation, exhalation, and the changeover between these phases.

Ventilators are most often classified by inspiratory phase characteristics, and cycling characteristics. Ventilator cycling refers to the event which changes phases from inspiration to exhalation. Time cycled ventilators end inspiration after a set time. Volume cycled ventilators deliver a set volume before ending the inhalation phase. Pressure cycled ventilators end inspiration after a certain airway pressure is achieved. Pressure support refers to a supplemental gas flow which allows a patient to overcome the resistance of the breathing circuit. PEEP is the pressure applied to alveoli after exhalation in an attempt to stent open the alveoli and improve oxygenation.

The ventilation mode is the method a ventilator uses to cycle from exhalation to inhalation. During controlled ventilation the inspiratory phase begins after a selected amount of time which thus controls the respiratory rate. It is best used for patients with little effort. Assist control ventilation allows for the patient to trigger another ventilator breath if a certain negative pressure is achieved, while maintaining a constant minimum background rate. Synchronized intermittent mandatory ventilation allows for a patient to ventilate spontaneously between a set number of breaths. It is routinely used as a weaning technique. Inverse ratio ventilation involves reversing the normal ratio of inspiration to exhalation to greater than a 1:1 ratio. It is used to improve oxygenation. SIMV, HFV, IRV, and PC ventilation are all ways to alleviate high airway pressures. Volume controlled ventilation may lead to elevated airway pressures, if high resistance is present.

Bibliography

Brown M. ICU: critical care. In: Barash PG, Cullen BF, Stoelting RK (eds.), *Clinical Anesthesia*, 4th ed. Philadelphia, PA: Lippincott, Williams & Wilkins, 2001, vol. 56, 1469–1472.

Morgan GE Jr, Mikhail MS. *Clinical Anesthesiology*, 3rd ed. New York, NY: Lange Medical Books/McGraw-Hill, 1996, vol. 44, 807–812.

Stoelting RK, Miller RD. *Basics of Anesthesia*, 4th ed. Philadelphia, PA: Churchill Livingstone, 2000, 440–443.

39. (A) Nausea and vomiting is a very important contributor to delays in discharge and unanticipated admissions following outpatient surgery. Prophylactic treatment and choice of anesthetic technique can reduce the morbidity involved with this condition. Identification of those patients who are at increased risk is the first step. A good history includes any predisposition to motion sickness and history of postanesthetic nausea. Women, especially in pregnancy, and obese patients have an increased risk. Type of surgery is also important. Procedures that lead to a higher incidence of nausea include: laparoscopy; ear, nose, and throat surgery; lithotripsy; breast augmentation; ophthalmologic procedures; and any surgeries that lead to blood in the stomach or peritoneal irritation.

Certain anesthetic techniques and agents should be avoided if possible in those patients identified by history to be at higher risk. Opioids can stimulate the chemoreceptor trigger zone, thus activating the vomiting center of the brain (lateral reticular formation). Volatile anesthetic gases and nitrous oxide have been implicated in postoperative nausea, as well as regional blockade. In contrast to those anesthetics, propofol and benzodiazepines appear to have a relatively low incidence of nausea as a side effect.

In high-risk patients, many pharmacologic agents have been used preoperatively or intraoperatively to prevent this condition. Most of these act as antagonists of the major receptor types implicated in nausea and vomiting. These include dopamine, acetylcholine (muscarine), histamine, and serotonin receptors. Dopamine antagonists such as promethazine are effective and are associated with sedation, which also can be helpful. Another dopamine antagonist, droperidol, has limited use because of significant side effects such as extrapyramidal symptoms, anxiety, and potential serious proarrhythmogenic effects (torsade de pointes). Serotonin antagonists such as ondansetron have been shown to be effective with minimal adverse effects. Anticholinergic medications include scopolamine or atropine. In addition, dexamethasone has been shown to decrease postoperative nausea and vomiting, especially in the pediatric population after tonsillectomy. And finally, an H2 receptor antagonist or metoclopramide may be indicated in patients at risk for aspiration.

If prevention fails and nausea and vomiting occurs in the post anesthesia care unit (PACU), treatment should be directed at evaluating any underlying causes such as hypotension, hypoxia, anxiety, pain, or hypoglycemia. Supine positioning and avoidance of sudden movements or bright lights can help, as can administration of one of the numerous antiemetic agents on the market.

Bibliography

Aouad MT, et al. The effect of dexamethasone on postoperative vomiting after tonsillectomy. *Anesth Analg* 2001;92:636–640.

Gan TJ. Postoperative nausea and vomiting—can it be eliminated? *JAMA* 2002;287:1233–1236.

Sinclair DR, Chung F, Mezei G. Can postoperative nausea and vomiting be predicted? *Anesthesiology* 1999;91:109–118.

Visser K, et al. Randomized controlled trial of total intravenous anesthesia with propofol versus inhalation anesthesia with isoflurane—nitrous oxide: postoperative nausea and vomiting and economic analysis. *Anesthesiology* 2001;95:616–626.

CHAPTER 37

Orthopedics

Terrence J. Endres

Questions

1. A 31-year-old man is involved in a motor vehicle accident (MVA). He is transported to the emergency room (ER) in stable condition. The patient is unable to flex or extend his right hip, and there is concern expressed for a possible posterior hip dislocation. The anteroposterior (AP) pelvis radiograph and computed tomography (CT) scan shown in Fig. 37-1a and b, respectively, confirm the clinical suspicion. On clinical examination, the right lower extremity would most likely be in which of the following positions?

    (A) flexed, adducted, internal rotation
    (B) flexed, abducted, internal rotation
    (C) flexed, adducted, external rotation
    (D) flexed, adducted, external rotation
    (E) flexed, adducted, neutral rotation

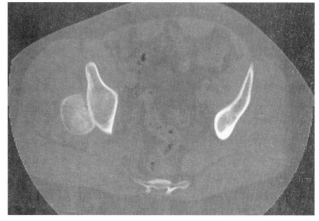

FIG. 37-1b Axial CT scan of pelvis

2. A 25-year-old male has severe pain and is unable to ambulate on his left knee following a car accident. A posterior knee dislocation was diagnosed at an outlying hospital and reduced. An initial AP radiograph is shown in Fig. 37-2a and a postreduction lateral radiograph in Fig. 37-2b. The patient is now evaluated 6 h postinjury following the transfer. The examination now reveals an extremely swollen and painful knee and evidence of ischemia. Posterior tibial and dorsalis pedis pulses are diminished. The next best course of action should be?

    (A) obtain an emergent arteriogram
    (B) obtain emergent magnetic resonance imaging (MRI) scan to assess the ligamentous injuries
    (C) perform a comprehensive examination to assess the ligamentous stability
    (D) perform surgical repair or bypass of the injured popliteal vessels
    (E) perform surgical repair or ligamentous reconstruction

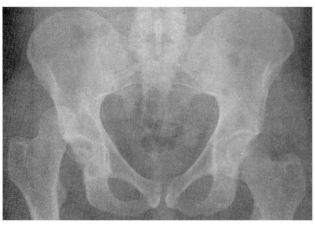

FIG. 37-1a AP pelvis

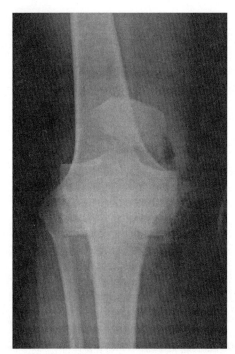

FIG. 37-2a   AP radiograph knee

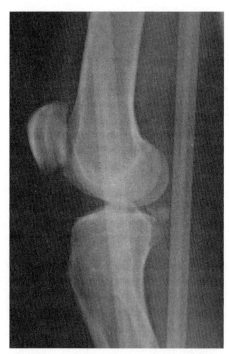

FIG. 37-2b   Post-reduction lateral radiograph of knee

3. A 19-year-old sustained a left arm injury in a motor-cycle accident. Initial examination in the ER reveals a Glasgow Coma Scale (GCS) of 15 and no hemodynamic instability. Radiographs of the closed, isolated injury to the left arm are shown in Fig. 37-3*a* and *b*. Which of the following deficits are most likely to be identified on a detailed physical assessment?

(A) extension of the wrist and radial deviation

(B) flexion of the thumb interphalangeal (IP) joint

(C) abduction and adduction of the fingers

(D) sensory loss over the dorsal web space of the thumb with no motor deficits

(E) sensory loss over the tip of the thumb and index finger with no motor deficits

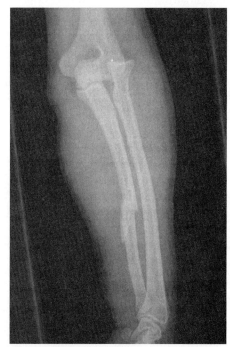

FIG 37-3a   AP forearm radiograph

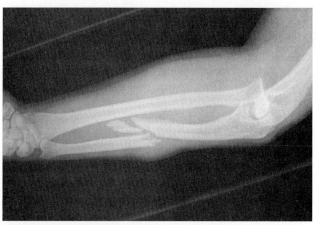

FIG. 37-3b   Lateral forearm radiograph

4. A 16-year-old student-athlete reported sudden onset of low back pain while weight training for football. The initial examination revealed no abnormalities in muscle strength, sensation, or reflexes; however, muscle spasms and a positive straight leg raise test were noted. The x-rays were unremarkable. Now, several weeks later the symptoms have persisted. The next course of action should include

(A) electromyogram (EMG) and nerve conduction studies

(B) an MRI scan

(C) repeat x-rays

(D) physical therapy

(E) bed rest followed by decreased activity

5. A 23-year-old man sustains an injury to his chest as a result of an auto accident. He complains of sternal pain after being struck on the driver's side. He noted difficulty with breathing and swallowing immediately following the accident. Now the symptoms have improved. The best test to further evaluate a potential sternoclavicular injury would be

(A) CT scan

(B) angiogram

(C) shoulder x-ray

(D) chest x-ray

(E) clavicle x-ray

6. A 35-year-old who sustained a blow to the anterior region of his left shoulder in a car accident is unable to abduct the arm above shoulder level. The examination also reveals pain and limitation in external rotation. Figure 37-4 reveals the initial radiograph. Which of the following would be the next appropriate course of action?

(A) physical therapy

(B) bone scan

(C) MRI

(D) EMG

(E) axillary radiograph

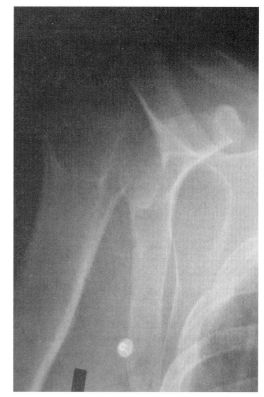

FIG. 37-4 AP shoulder radiograph

7. Figure 37-5*a* and *b* show the radiographs of a 40-year-old man who was riding a bicycle and was struck by a car. Treatment should consist of

(A) cemented total hip arthroplasty

(B) protected weight bearing until union

(C) bed rest until union

(D) ORIF

(E) cemented hemiarthroplasty

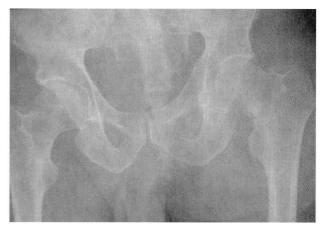

FIG. 37-5*a* AP pelvis radiograph

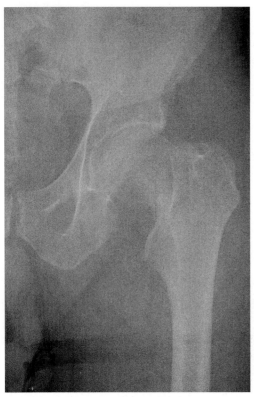

FIG. 37-5b   AP hip radiograph

8. Which of the following findings on physical examination is the least likely to be associated with the significant pelvic injury shown in Fig. 37-6?

(A) scrotal or labial swelling

(B) blood at the meatus

(C) inability to pass a Foley catheter

(D) excessive external rotation of the lower extremities

(E) no motion with anterior superior iliac compression

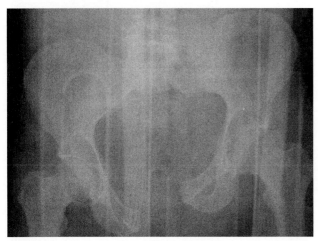

FIG. 37-6   AP pelvis radiograph

9. An 18-year-old injured his left shoulder playing rugby. He has his left arm supported by his right hand. Radiographs are shown in Fig. 37-7a and b. What would be the best course of treatment for this patient's injury?

(A) surgical stabilization with plate and screws

(B) surgical stabilization with an percutaneous intramedullary screw

(C) closed reduction and cast treatment

(D) sling for comfort and restricted activity with the extremity

(E) biopsy and culture, followed by appropriate antibiotics

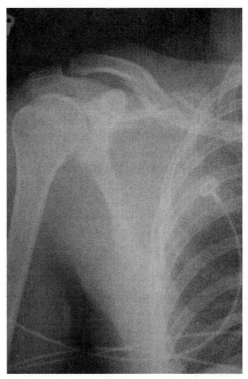

FIG. 37-7a   AP shoulder radiograph

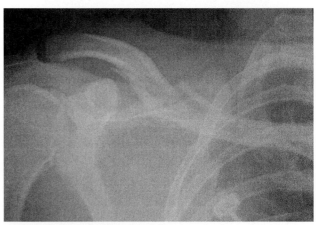

FIG. 37-7b   AP clavicle radiograph

10. A 20-year-old male injured his left shoulder in a football-related accident. Physical examination reveals decreased external rotation and inability to abduct his shoulder. A neurovascular examination determines the patient has numbness over the proximal-lateral aspect of his upper arm. What is the explanation for the numbness on the arm?

    (A) injury to the axillary nerve
    (B) injury to the musculocutaneous nerve
    (C) injury to the ulnar nerve
    (D) injury to the medial brachial cutaneous nerve
    (E) injury to the lateral antebrachial cutaneous nerve

11. A 28-year-old male is brought to the ER 2 h after a car accident. He is unable to move his lower extremities. Radiographs reveal a flexion-distraction injury. A subsequent MRI is shown in Fig. 37-8 and confirms cord injury at the level of the fracture. Which of the following is the most appropriate course of pharmacologic treatment for this patient's spinal cord injury?

    (A) methylprednisolone bolus 30 mg/kg, then infusion 5.4 mg/kg/h for 72 h
    (B) methylprednisolone bolus 30 mg/kg, then infusion 5.4 mg/kg/h for 24 h
    (C) methylprednisolone bolus 30 mg/kg, then infusion 5.4 mg/kg/h for 48 h
    (D) no benefit from treatment with methylprednisolone
    (E) naloxone infusion for 48 h

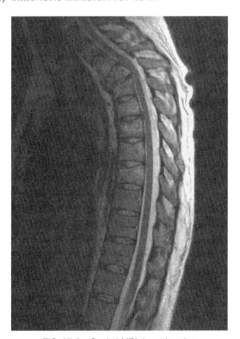

FIG. 37-8 Sagittal MRI thoracic spine

12. The radiograph and CT scan shown in Fig. 37-9a and b are from the right hip of a 20-year-old female who has been having pain in her groin. Although she has not had any fevers or night sweats, the pain seems to be worse at night. She has been taking aspirin with some relief of the pain. The most likely diagnosis is

    (A) osteosarcoma
    (B) osteoblastoma
    (C) multiple myeloma
    (D) myositis ossificans
    (E) osteoid osteoma

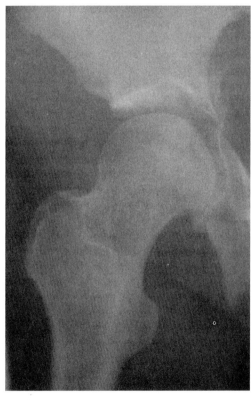

FIG. 37-9a AP hip radiograph

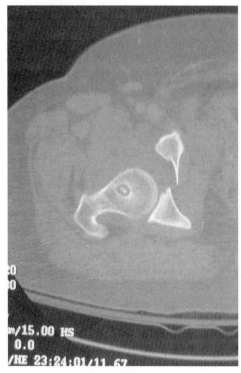

FIG. 37-9b   Axial CT scan of hip

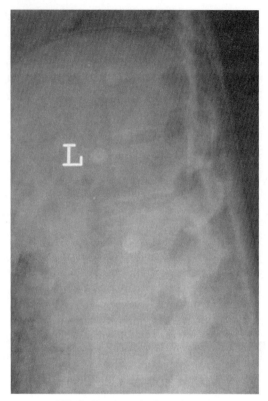

FIG. 37-10a   Lateral spine radiograph

13. Which nerve roots are responsible for innervation of the diaphragm?

(A) C1-C3

(B) C1-C8

(C) C1-T1

(D) C3-C5

(E) C4-C6

14. What type of spinal fracture is shown in these figures? Figure 37-10a is a lateral lumbar radiograph, and an axial CT scan of the thoracic spine in shown in Fig. 37-10b.

(A) compression fracture

(B) flexion-distraction

(C) fracture-dislocation

(D) extension injury

(E) burst fracture

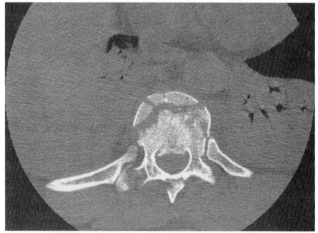

FIG. 37-10b   Axial CT scan thoracic spine

15. What type of pelvic ring injury, such as that displayed in Fig. 37-11, is associated with the greatest average transfusion requirements?

    (A) lateral compression
    (B) vertical shear
    (C) sacral fractures
    (D) superior and inferior rami fractures
    (E) AP compression

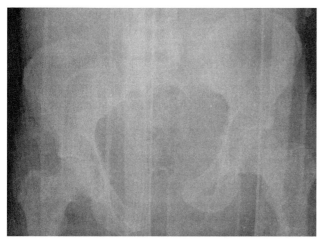

FIG. 37-11   AP pelvis radiograph

16. The injury severity score (ISS) is determined based on which of the following?

    (A) the sum of the squares from the three highest abbreviated injury scale (AIS) scores
    (B) the sum of the three highest AIS scores
    (C) the sum of all nine sections from the AIS
    (D) the sum of the scores from all six body regions used in the ISS
    (E) the sum of the squares from all nine sections of the AIS

17. Vertebral body fractures associated with osteoporosis (OP) are associated with which of the following?

    (A) related to the high bone turnover and trabecular bone loss
    (B) related to the high bone turnover and cortical bone loss
    (C) related to the high bone turnover and disc disease
    (D) related to facet arthritis
    (E) related to the poor circulation associated with OP

18. A 28-year-old man is seen following a gunshot wound to the back. Examination reveals 5/5 strength in both upper extremities. He has 5/5 strength in the left lower extremity; however, there is decreased sensation in the left lower extremity. The right lower has normal sensation, but significant motor weakness. Which of the following conditions best describes his neurologic injury?

    (A) central cord syndrome
    (B) anterior cord syndrome
    (C) brown-Sequard's syndrome
    (D) cauda equina syndrome
    (E) a complete spinal cord syndrome

19. A lesion on MRI reveals a very homogeneous characteristic. It reveals bright signal intensity (SI) on T1 and there is high signal with no increase on T2 images. Based on these characteristics the lesion most likely represents a

    (A) lipoma
    (B) normal muscle
    (C) synovial sarcoma
    (D) liposcarcoma
    (E) desmoid

20. Which Salter–Harris fracture type best describes a transverse fracture through the entire length of the growth plate without involving the metaphysis?

    (A) Type I
    (B) Type II
    (C) Type III
    (D) Type IV
    (E) Type V

21. An 11-year-old boy injured his left leg while tackling an opponent in a football game. He was treated to stabilize the fracture and postoperative radiographs are shown in Fig. 37-12. What is the most likely diagnosis?

    (A) unicameral bone cyst
    (B) metastatic tumor
    (C) Ewing's tumor
    (D) nonossifying fibroma
    (E) osteosarcoma

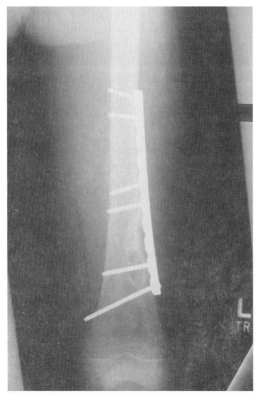

FIG. 37-12a   Post-operative AP radiograph of distal femur

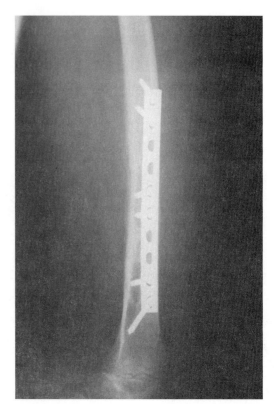

FIG. 37-12c   Post-operative lateral radiograph of distal femur

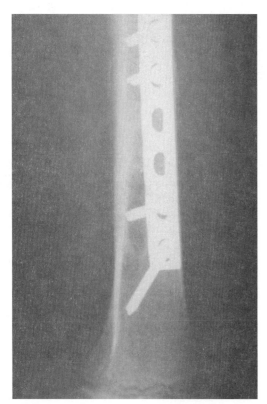

FIG. 37-12b   Post-operative close up lateral radiograph distal femur

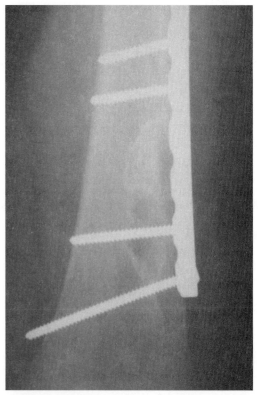

FIG. 37-12d   Post-operative close up AP radiograph of distal femur

22. A 28-year-old man sustains a laceration and degloving to the volar and ulnar surface of his dominant left forearm. Figure 37-13 shows the clinical photo prior to surgical debridement. Preoperatively, the median nerve is best evaluated initially by

  (A) checking reflexes in the right arm compared to the uninjured left arm
  (B) asking the patient to cross his fingers
  (C) order urgent nerve conduction studies and an EMG
  (D) asking the patient to extend his thumb at the IP joint
  (E) assessing the thumb for abduction and opposition

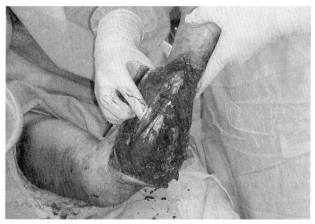

FIG. 37-13   Pre-operative forearm degloving injury

23. A 39-year-old female was involved in a MVA and sustained multiple injuries including a splenic laceration, left forearm fracture, and a closed right midshaft femur fracture. At initial evaluation she was hemodynamically stable, alert, and oriented. The patient was transferred from an outlying hospital for definitive care. Later that evening the patient has become confused and petechiae are noted in the conjunctiva and on the chest. An arterial blood gas (ABG) reveals a PaO_2 of 51 mmHg and vital signs include a heart rate of 125 bpm and a respiratory rate of 25 breaths/min. Management should include

  (A) emergent stabilization of the femur fracture with intramedullary nailing
  (B) ventilatory support
  (C) emergent Doppler ultrasound examination of both lower extremities
  (D) treatment with albuterol nebulizers as needed
  (E) urgent helical CT scan of the chest followed by low-molecular weight heparin

24. A 19-year-old is injured in an industrial accident. He sustains a closed femur fracture, and a distal radius fracture. Radiographs are shown in Fig. 37-14. The chest radiograph reveals a pneumothorax and multiple rib fractures. He has a GCS of 15 and a normal neurovascular examination in his extremities. Vital signs reveal a pulse rate of 100/min, respirations of 24 breaths/min, and a blood pressure of 144/92 mmHg. An ABG reveals a PaO_2 of 75 mmHg, a $PaCO_2$ of 33, and a normal pH. The femoral shaft fracture is best managed with

  (A) External fixation as definitive treatment
  (B) Skeletal traction only
  (C) Intramedullary nailing
  (D) Skeletal traction until stable and then external fixation
  (E) Skeletal traction until stable and then intramedullary nailing

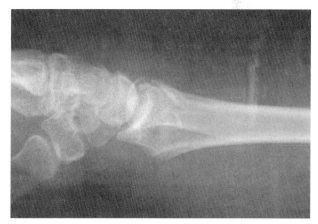

FIG. 37-14a   Lateral wrist radiograph

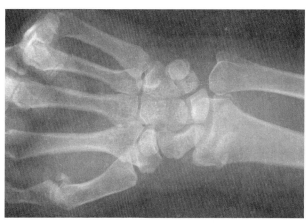

FIG. 37-14b   AP wrist radiograph

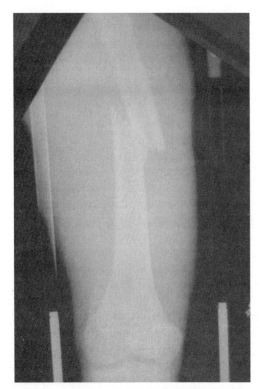

FIG. 37-14c AP femur radiograph

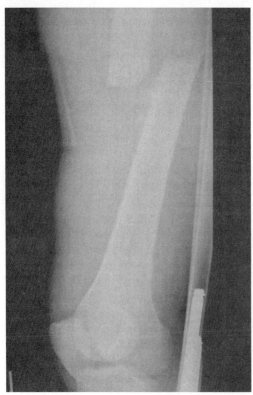

FIG. 37-14d Lateral femur radiograph

25. A 47-year-old man sustains an injury to his right arm in a work-related fall. You are asked to consult for a left humerus fracture, and there is concern for potential injury to his radial nerve at the fracture site. A radiograph of the right humerus is shown in Fig. 37-15. Clinical findings supporting an injury to the radial nerve would include

(A) inability to flex the thumb at the IP joint

(B) decreased sensation over the volar surface of the index finger and thumb

(C) loss of sensation over the ulnar border of the ring and small fingers

(D) loss of sensation over the lateral border of the arm extending from the fracture site to the wrist

(E) inability to extend the wrist and fingers

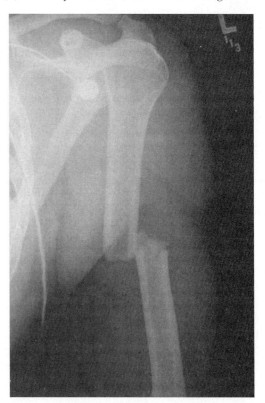

FIG. 37-15 AP humerus radiograph

26. A 26-year-old undergoes a closed reduction of a hip dislocation in the ER. A postreduction AP pelvic radiograph and CT scans are shown in Fig. 37-16. The next best step in the course of treatment would be

  (A) MRI scan

  (B) traction followed by restricted weight bearing for 6 weeks

  (C) arthrotomy for removal of loose body

  (D) immediate progressing weight bearing as tolerated

  (E) examination under anesthesia

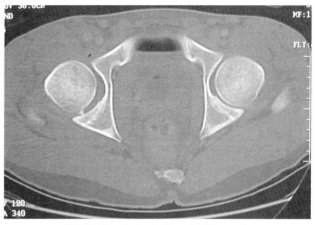

FIG. 37-16*c*   Post reduction axial CT scan hip

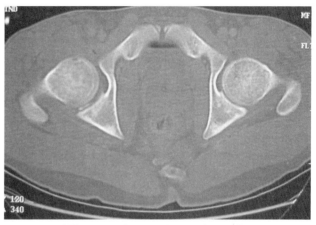

FIG. 37-16*d*   Post reduction axial CT scan hip

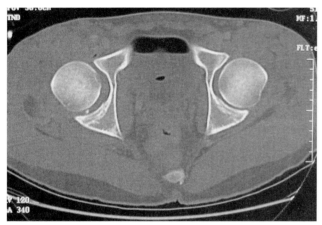

FIG. 37-16*a*   Post reduction axial CT scan hip

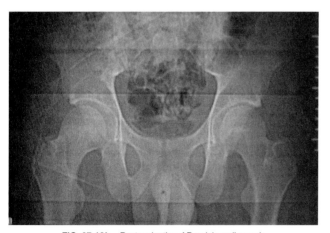

FIG. 37-16*b*   Post reduction AP pelvis radiograph

27. A 22-year-old male sustained pelvic injuries in an auto accident. An AP and an outlet pelvis radiograph are shown in Fig. 37-17. Examination reveals perineal swelling, a scrotal hematoma, and blood at the meatus. The patient complains of inability to void and pelvic pain. The next step in management would include

   (A) intravenous pyelogram (IVP)
   (B) external fixation to stabilize the pelvis
   (C) careful insertion of a Foley catheter
   (D) CT scans of the abdomen
   (E) retrograde urethrogram

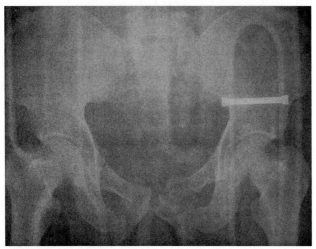

FIG. 37-17a   AP pelvis radiograph

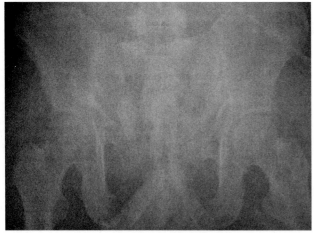

FIG. 37-17b   Outlet pelvis radiograph

28. A patient is transported to the ER following a fall from a ladder. The GCS can categorize the patient's neurologic status by assessing motor response, verbal response, and which of the following?

   (A) pupil response to light
   (B) orientation to person and place

   (C) withdrawal to pain
   (D) eye-opening response
   (E) CT scan assessment

29. The most common direct cause of mortality in patients with pelvic fractures is

   (A) head and thorax injuries
   (B) pelvic fracture directly
   (C) associated extremity injuries
   (D) genitourinary injury
   (E) bowel injury

30. A patient sustained an open tibial fracture in a work-related accident. The initial treatment involved intramedullary nailing with a free-flap for soft tissue coverage. The patient has gone on to develop a delayed union. The most important factor in fracture healing in this and all patients is

   (A) blood supply
   (B) rigid fixation
   (C) fracture pattern
   (D) age of the patient
   (E) mechanism of injury

31. Figure 37-18 shows a radiograph of a patient with a posterior hip dislocation and associated femoral head dislocation. Following closed reduction, there is 4 mm displacement on a postreduction CT scan. The next course in treatment should include

   (A) MRI
   (B) closed reduction under anesthesia
   (C) ORIF
   (D) excision of the fragment
   (E) protective progressive weight bearing

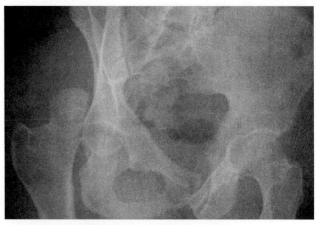

FIG. 37-18a   AP pelvis radiograph

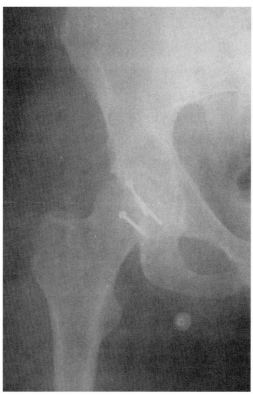

FIG. 37-18b   Post operative AP hip radiograph

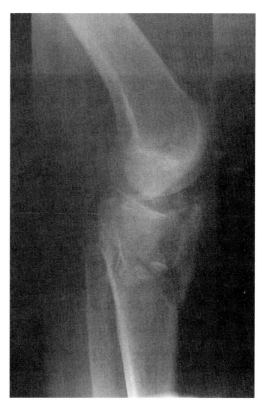

FIG. 37-19b   Lateral knee radiograph

32. A 40-year-old male is transported to the ER with bilateral tibia fractures. He is combative and requires sedation and subsequent intubation. You are called to evaluate the patient and notice the left lower leg is tense and swollen, but the posterior tibial and dorsalis pedis pulses are palpable. Radiographs of the left proximal tibia are shown in Fig. 37-19. Which of the following is the next best step in management of this patient?

   (A) measurement of compartment pressures
   (B) elevation above heart level to reduce swelling
   (C) serial observation for improvement of soft tissue and swelling
   (D) ORIF of tibia fracture with plates and screws
   (E) closed reduction and casting of tibia fracture

33. A 32-year-old male injures his left ankle while snowboarding. The initial AP and lateral radiographs are shown in Fig. 37-20a and b. A subsequent CT scan is shown in Fig. 37-20c. The next best course of treatment for this patient is

   (A) ORIF
   (B) closed reduction and casting
   (C) treatment with an external fixator spanning the ankle
   (D) delayed internal fixation to allow swelling to subside
   (E) air cast and gradual mobilization

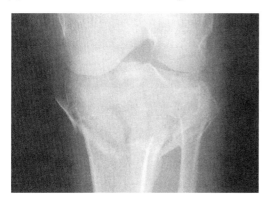

FIG. 37-19a   AP knee radiograph

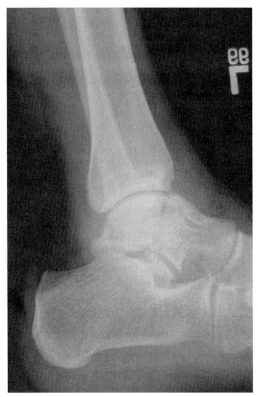

FIG. 37-20a   Lateral ankle radiograph

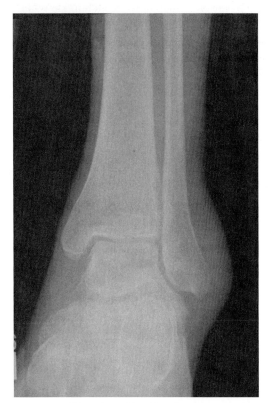

FIG. 37-20b   AP ankle radiograph

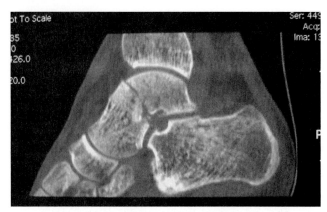

FIG. 37-20c   CT scan of ankle

34. A 26-year-old man undergoes a lymph node biopsy from the side of his neck. He is diagnosed with lymphoma. Following the biopsy, he is unable to elevate his shoulder and has pain in the shoulder region. Which of the following structures has likely been injured?

(A) supraspinatus
(B) suprascapular nerve
(C) axillary nerve
(D) trapezius muscle
(E) cranial nerve XI

35. A 41-year-old female presents with the injury shown in Fig. 37-21. Her neurovascular examination was normal. She then underwent irrigation and debridement followed by intramedullary nailing of the tibia fracture. She required a free-flap for wound coverage. Which of the following most appropriately describes this injury?

(A) type I open fracture
(B) type II open fracture
(C) type III A open fracture
(D) type III B open fracture
(E) type III C open fracture

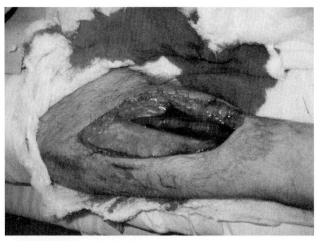

FIG. 37-21   Preoperative clinical picture open tibia fracture

36. A 30-year-old male sustains a closed fracture of his tibia. Radiographs are shown in Fig. 37-22*a* and *b*. The patient is treated with an intramedullary nail. Which of the following is considered the most common complication following this choice of treatment for this patient?

    (A) nonunion
    (B) infection
    (C) malunion
    (D) knee pain
    (E) CS

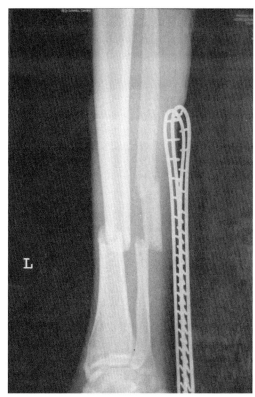

FIG. 37-22*b*   AP tibia radiograph

37. A pathologic fracture secondary to metastasis from which of the following common primary tumors requires a preoperative angiogram prior to surgical stabilization?

    (A) kidney
    (B) lung
    (C) breast
    (D) thyroid
    (E) prostate

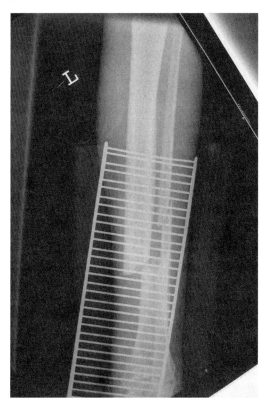

FIG. 37-22*a*   Lateral tibia radiograph

38. An axial MRI image of the L4-L5 level is shown in Fig. 37-23. The arrow identifies which structure?

(A) L5 vertebral body

(B) spinal cord

(C) L5 nerve root

(D) L4 nerve root

(E) L4 pedicle

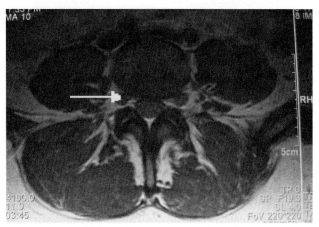

FIG. 37-23a Axial MRI of L4-L5 level

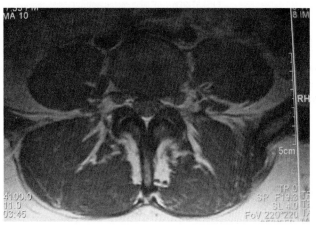

FIG. 37-23b

39. A 26-year-old male is transported to the ER after sustaining multiple injuries in a fight. The patient is awake and alert. Multiple facial contusions are identified, and a laceration over the fifth metacarpal phalangeal joint of the right hand is noted. The best course of treatment for the hand laceration wound be

(A) antibiotics in the ER followed by local debridement and wound closure

(B) antibiotics in the ER followed by discharge to home with wound care instructions

(C) local debridement and wound closure, followed by discharge to home

(D) local debridement followed by discharge to home with wound care instructions

(E) irrigation and debridement in the OR followed by IV antibiotics

40. A patient sustains a complete cervical cord injury secondary to a cervical burst fracture. The radiographs reveal injury at the C6-C7 level. Assuming a complete cord injury at this level, which of the following findings on physical examination would not correlate with this level of injury?

(A) absent patellar tendon reflexes

(B) weakness with ankle plantar flexion

(C) weakness with elbow flexion

(D) weakness with finger abduction/adduction

(E) weakness with shoulder abduction

Answers and Explanations

1. **(A)** Hip dislocations are generally the result of a high-energy injury, commonly a MVA in which the knee strikes the dashboard and forces the hip out of the acetabulum. This may often be associated with an acetabulum fracture as well, specifically a posterior wall fracture. The position of the hip and leg at the time of the accident will influence the direction of the dislocation. A hip that is flexed, adducted, and internally rotated at the time of impact will result in a posterior hip dislocation. A hip that is flexed and abducted at the time of injury will result in an anterior hip dislocation. Most dislocations are posterior dislocations, whereas anterior dislocations are relatively rare.

   The key structures at risk during dislocation of a hip are the circulation to the femoral head and the sciatic nerve. The posterior vascular supply to the femoral head provides the majority of the circulation. An extracapsular ring originates at the base of the neck and traverses the capsule to the head. Injury to this region can result in acute disruption of the vessels that are closely associated with the capsule, stretching or compression of the vessels, and venous occlusion of the vascular outflow. All of these may contribute to the risk of developing subsequent avascular necrosis (AVN). The sciatic nerve is in close proximity to the posterior capsule and can be injured directly as the femoral head displaces posteriorly out of the acetabulum. A complete sciatic nerve injury can result, or more commonly the peroneal distribution is affected. A varied clinical outcome can range from isolated dorsal foot numbness to complete motor and sensory loss for the entire foot.

   With a posterior dislocation, the hip lies in a flexed, internally rotated, and adducted position. The leg is shortened and the patient is unable to extend the hip. With an anterior dislocation, the hip lies in a flexed, abducted, and externally rotated position. These patients also are unable to extend the leg into a neutral position. Radiographs may reveal a head that appears larger in anterior dislocation or smaller in a posterior dislocation.

   This injury is an orthopedic emergency. The incidence of osteonecrosis has been reported in 1–20% of hip dislocations. Prompt reduction, within 6 h, can reduce the incidence of osteonecrosis. This should be performed under conscious sedation with adequate muscle relaxation. If reduction is not completed on the first attempt, repeated attempts are not indicated and reduction should be performed under general anesthesia to ensure adequate muscle relaxation. Following reduction, patients should be allowed to weight bear as tolerated to the limits of pain. There is currently no evidence to support the belief that delayed weight bearing has any impact on the outcome of isolated hip dislocations. Extremes of motion should be avoided to allow capsular healing.

   Acute sciatic nerve injuries occur in 8–20% of hip dislocations. Most of these are neuropraxias, and 60–80% of patients will recover to a level in which good function can be obtained; however, full recovery of strength is unusual, and use of an appropriate ankle-foot orthosis and a rehabilitation program are critical during the recovery phase. Development of posttraumatic arthritis is the most common long-term complication. This is more likely after posterior dislocations than anterior, and is related to age, severity of the injury, and activity of the patient.

   Bibliography

   Egol KA, Koval KJ. Hip: trauma. In: Koval KJ (ed.), *Orthopaedic Knowledge Update 7*. Rosemont, IL: American Academy of Orthopaedic Surgeons, 2002, 410–412.

   Goulet JA, Levin PE. Hip dislocations. In: Browner BD, Jupiter JB, Levine AM, Trafton PG, et al. (eds.), *Skeletal Trauma*, 3rd ed. Philadelphia, PA: W.B. Saunders, 2003, 1657–1690.

   Heckman JD (ed.). *Rockwood and Green's Fractures in Adults*, 5th ed. Philadelphia, PA: Lippincott, Williams & Wilkins, 2001, 1547–1576.

   Leighton RK, Lammens P. Hip dislocations and fractures of the femoral head. In: Kellam JF, Fischer TJ, Tornetta P III (eds.), *Orthopaedic Knowledge Update: Trauma 2*. Rosemont, IL: American Academy of Orthopaedic Surgeons, 2000, 311–314.

Motley GS, Eddings TH III, Moore RS. Adult trauma. In: Miller MD, Brinker MR (eds.), *Review of Orthopaedics*, 3rd ed. Philadelphia, PA: W.B. Saunders, 2000, 476–477.

2. **(D)** The traumatic dislocation of the knee is uncommon, but should be considered an orthopedic emergency. Capsular disruption often prevents a tense hemarthrosis from developing and spontaneous reductions are common. Both of these contribute to occasional missed diagnosis. It is critical to closely evaluate and document the neurovascular status of the limb during examination. Emergent reduction should be performed with appropriate sedation and analgesia. The limb should then be immobilized in the position of greatest stability, usually 15–20 degrees of flexion. The goals of treatment are a painless, stable knee, with normal strength and range of motion.

Associated injuries are common, and injury to the popliteal artery has been reported in up to 30% of dislocations. It is most common in anterior and posterior dislocations because of the course of the popliteal artery as it traverses the popliteal fossa of the knee. It is tethered at the adductor hiatus proximally and by the soleal arch distally. Clinical signs associated with vascular injury include diminished pulses or capillary refill, neurologic deficit, hypotension, or hematoma. More obvious signs include absent pulses, coolness or cyanosis, active bleeding, expanding hematoma, and bruits or thrill. The knee does not have the collateral circulation to remain viable in the presence of a popliteal artery injury. Therefore, vascular spasm is not a valid clinical assessment, and any vascular insufficiency, including diminished pulses, implies arterial injury until proven otherwise. In the presence of satisfactory perfusion following reduction, obtaining an arteriogram on an urgent basis may be an acceptable option. However, as in this patient, surgical repair or restoration of flow to the extremity should not be delayed to obtain an arteriogram. If necessary, an arteriogram can be obtained in the operating room (OR).

This particular patient has evidence of ischemia that is approaching 6 h. This should be considered a vascular emergency. The risk of muscle necrosis, contracture, and amputation rise significantly when ischemia exceeds 6 h. Amputation rates approach 30% if repair is not accomplished within the first 7–12 h and approach 0% when done within the first 6 h. No delays are acceptable in this patient. Ligamentous assessment can be assessed clinically, and confirmed by MRI, following the arterial repair. Ligamentous reconstruction should be delayed until vascular stability and soft tissue healing has been achieved.

Peroneal nerve injuries can be associated with knee dislocations as well and have been reported from 14 to 35%. This injury carries a poor prognosis and primary or secondary repairs and grafting have resulted in poor results. Bracing or tendon transfers are often required.

Bibliography

Bush-Joseph C, Cater TR, Miller MD, et al. Knee and leg: soft-tissue trauma. In: Koval KJ (ed.), *Orthopaedic Knowledge Update 7*. Rosemont, IL: American Academy of Orthopaedic Surgeons, 2002, 495–498.

Kremcheck TE, Welling RE, Kremcheck EJ. Traumatic dislocation of the knee. *Orthop Rev* 1989;18:1051–1057.

Motley GS, Eddings TH III, Moore RS. Adult trauma. In: Miller MD, Brinker MR (eds.), *Review of Orthopaedics*, 3rd ed. Philadelphia, PA: W.B. Saunders, 2000, 484–485.

Reckling FW, Peltier LF. Acute knee dislocations and their complications. *J Trauma* 1969;9:181–191.

Schenck RC. Injuries of the knee. In: Bucholz RW, Heckman JD (eds.), *Rockwood and Green's Fractures in Adults*, 5th ed. Philadelphia, PA: Lippincott, Williams & Wilkins, 2001, 1914–1928.

Siliski JM. Dislocations and soft tissue injuries of the knee. In: Browner BD, Jupiter JB, Levine AE, et al. (eds.), *Skeletal Trauma*, 3rd ed. Philadelphia, PA: W.B. Saunders, 2003, 2045–2073.

Wascher DC. High velocity knee dislocation with vascular injury: treatment principles. *Clin Sports Med* 2000;19: 457–477.

3. **(A)** This patient's x-rays reveal a fracture pattern commonly referred to as a Monteggia fracture. In 1814, Monteggia described a fracture of the proximal third of the ulna and dislocation of the radial head at the proximal radioulnar joint. Bado has classified these into four types:

Type 1: Anterior (65%) radial head dislocation—anterior ulna angulation

Type 2: Posterior (18%) radial head dislocation—posterior angulation

Type 3: Lateral (16%) radial head dislocation—ulna fracture just distal to coronoid

Type 4: Both bone fracture (1%) radial head dislocation—anterior dislocation with proximal fracture of both radius and ulna

Monteggia fractures require early open reduction and internal fixation (ORIF) of the ulna. Restoring length to the forearm generally leads to reduction of the radial head. The arm is immobilized in the proper position to allow healing of the radioulnar joint. This is based on the degree of stability during examination, and is usually a position of flexion and supination. If there is an associated fracture of the radial head or neck, all attempts to reconstruct or to replace the radial head should be made. There is often an injury to the interosseous membrane and simple excision can lead to proximal migration of the radius.

This question indirectly asks which nerve is the most commonly injured with this fracture pattern. It is logical that the radial nerve is the most commonly injured because of its proximity to the radial neck. Specifically this would involve the motor component or posterior interosseous nerve (PIN). On examination this would manifest as extensor weakness of the wrist and fingers. The only appropriate answer would be **A**. Flexion of the thumb is the result of the flexor pollicis brevis, which is innervated by the median nerve. Flexion at the interphalangeal joint of the thumb specifically, is from the flexor pollicis longus, which is innervated by the anterior interosseous nerve. Finger adduction and abduction is powered by the interosseoi and lumbricals. The ulnar nerve innervates all the interosseoi and the ulnar two lumbricals. The median nerve innervates the radial two lumbricals. The sensory branch of the radial nerve provides sensation to the dorsal web space of the thumb, however, this branches prior to the nerves passing around the radial neck. The PIN is closely associated with the radial neck and isolated injury to the sensory branch is much less common than motor involvement. The median nerve provides the sensory distribution over the tips of the thumb and index fingers.

Bruce et al. (1974) identified six nerve palsies in 35 patients (17%) with Monteggia injuries. Of these, three were isolated complete radial nerve palsies (motor and sensory) and one was a pure PIN (motor) palsy. The others had additional deficits. All had complete spontaneous recovery of nerve function. After treatment, five other patients (14%) were noted to have nerve palsies. Two lost radial nerve function (sensory and motor) after closed reduction. One adult and one child had PIN palsies after treatment. Another patient after intramedullary nail (IM) rodding had radial, median, and ulnar nerve palsies and required neurolysis at 8 months postoperation. All five of these patients with "iatrogenic" nerve injury had complete recovery except for paresthesias in two.

Bibliography

Bruce HE, Harvey JP, Wilson JC Jr. Monteggia fractures. *J Bone Joint Surg* 1974;56A;1563–1576.

Hotchkiss RN. Displaced fractures of the radial head: internal fixation or excision? *J Am Acad Orthop Surg* 1997;5:1–10.

Jupiter JB, Kellam JF. Diaphyseal fractures of the forearm. In: Browner BD, Jupiter JB, Levine AE, et al. (eds.), *Skeletal Trauma*, 3rd ed. Philadelphia, PA: W.B. Saunders, 2003, 1381–1387.

Marsh JL. Elbow and forearm: trauma. In: Kasser JR (ed.), *Orthopaedic Knowledge Update 5*. Rosemont, IL: American Academy of Orthopaedic Surgeons, 1996, 274–276.

Richards RR. Fractures of the shafts of the radius and ulna. In: Bucholz RW, Heckman JD (eds.), *Rockwood and Green's Fractures in Adults*, 5th ed. Philadelphia, PA: Lippincott, Williams & Wilkins, 2001, 900–916.

4. **(B)** The majority of low back pain and back-related leg pain are generally self-limited and respond favorably to a short period of 24–48 h of rest, decreased activity, and physical therapy. In any individual with back pain that fails to respond to rest and activity restriction, nonspinal etiologies for back or radiating pain must always be considered, especially in children. These include abdominal or pelvic pathology, sciatic joint pathology, and hip pathology.

Using these same initial recommendations, the natural history of lumbar disc herniation is progressive resolution of symptoms without the need for surgical intervention. Approximately 50% of patients recover in 1 week and up to 90% of patients within 1–3 months. A positive contralateral straight leg-raising test is the most specific test for a herniated disc, and although nerve root tension signs are generally very reliable in patients younger than age 30 years, they are not absolute. When an adolescent who is involved with weight lifting complains of persistent low back pain, a herniated disc must be considered. Activities which load the spine with significant shear stresses are associated with a higher rate of central disc herniation, and lumbar herniated discs in adolescents may not present with the more typical findings in adults such as radicular symptoms, sensory deficits, or even motor deficits. Therefore, when an adolescent who lifts weights has low back pain that has failed to respond to rest and activity restriction, an MRI scan is the next study of choice to evaluate for a herniated disc. Regular x-rays are generally not helpful in the initial evaluation of low back pain or in the diagnosis of a herniated disc and can be deferred for 6 weeks. However, x-rays are warranted in a patient with greater than 6 weeks of symptoms and in those with a history of cancer, constitutional symptoms, or significant trauma. Repeat x-rays in a short time span are certainly of no benefit. The use of physical therapy is part of the initial phase of treatment combined with rest and decreased activity. These would be continued as part of the treatment plan once other causes have been eliminated.

Herniated lumbar discs most commonly affect the L4-L5 disc space, followed by the L5-S1 disc. Most herniated discs are posterolateral. The nerve root affected is the lower nerve root, or traversing root. The root from the upper level is already exiting

TABLE 37-1   Lumbar Disc Herniations

Level	Nerve Root	Motor	Sensory	Reflex
L3-L4	L4	Quadriceps, Tibialis anterior	Medial calf	Knee Jerk
L4-5	L5	EHL, EDL	Dorsal foot, medial calf	None
L5-S1	S1	Gastroc/Soleus	Plantar foot, Posterior calf	Ankle Jerk

beneath the pedicle at the level of the disc herniation. Central herniations are often only accompanied by pain. Table 37-1 summarizes the more typical findings with lumbar disc herniations.

Bibliography

Epstein JA, Epstein NE, Marc J, et al. Lumbar intervertebral disk herniation in teenage children: recognition and management of associated anomalies. *Spine* 1984;9: 427–432.

Hashimoto K, Fujita K, Kojimoto H, et al. Lumbar disc herniation in children. *J Pediatr Orthop* 1990;10:394–396.

Lauerman WC, Goldsmith ME. Spine. In: Miller MD, Brinker MR (eds.), *Review of Orthopaedics*, 3rd ed. Philadelphia, PA: W.B. Saunders, 2000, 359–362.

Spivak JM, Bendo JA. Lumbar degenerative disorders. In: Koval KJ (ed.), *Orthopaedic Knowledge Update 7*. Rosemont, IL: American Academy of Orthopaedic Surgeons, 2002, 630–634.

5. **(A)** The sternoclavicular joint has little inherent stability and its stability relies on the ligamentous support of the capsule, costoclavicular ligaments, interclavicular ligaments, and intraarticular disc ligament. Sternoclavicular dislocations are classified as anterior and posterior. The anterior are more common, and the diagnosis is usually made clinically based on the prominent deformity at the medial end of the clavicle, and associated pain. The AP chest radiograph may be suggestive of an injury, as in this patient; however, it is not always obvious. Occasionally a "Serendipity" view radiograph (40 degree cephalic tilt) is obtained; however, only CT scan is accurate enough to fully characterize the injury.

Since the medial clavicle physis is the last to close, in patients younger than 25 years of age, these injuries may constitute a Salter-Harris type I or type II physeal injury. This distinction is difficult with any study other than a CT scan. Anterior dislocations are inherently unstable and tend to redislocate after closed reduction. Despite this, closed reduction should be attempted. Management consists of closed reduction under general anesthesia followed by symptomatic treatment, and little functional disability usually results.

Diagnosis of a posterior dislocation is similar; however, these require more rapid diagnosis and management because of the potential for injury to the vulnerable mediastinal structures. The trachea, esophagus, brachial plexus, and major vascular structures are all at risk. As a result, patients may complain of dysphagia or dyspnea, and a careful neurologic assessment is mandatory. As with anterior dislocations, plain radiographs are often inadequate. The injury can easily be missed because of the overlap of the ribs and difficulty in obtaining images in the correct plane to display the deformity. Therefore, CT scanning is the study of choice to confirm a potential posterior dislocation, and to evaluate the mediastinal structures. All posterior dislocations must be reduced under general anesthesia in the OR with a chest surgeon available. If this is unsuccessful, open reduction is indicated. These generally remain stable following closed reduction, and treatment following reduction usually involves a figure-of-8 strap for 4–6 weeks.

Complications are usually related to injuries of associated structures. Chronic dislocations respond well to surgical resection of the medial 1–1.5 cm of the clavicle. Any greater resection can lead to increased instability.

Bibliography

Blachut PA, Broekhuyse HM. Fractures of the scapula and clavicle and injuries of the acromioclavicular and sternoclavicular joints. In: Kellam JF, Fischer TJ, Tornetta P III (eds.), *Orthopaedic Knowledge Update: Trauma 2*. Rosemont, IL: American Academy of Orthopaedic Surgeons, 2000, 10.

Higgins LD, McCann PD, Warner JP. Shoulder instability. In: Beaty JH (ed.), *Orthopaedic Knowledge Update 6*. Rosemont, IL: American Academy of Orthopaedic Surgeons, 1999, 287–297.

Motley GS, Eddings TH III, Moore RS. Adult trauma. In: Miller MD, Brinker MR (eds.), *Review of Orthopaedics*, 3rd ed. Philadelphia, PA: W.B. Saunders, 2000, 494–495.

Ring DR, Jupiter JB. Injuries to the shoulder girdle. In: Browner BD, Jupiter JB, Levine AE, et al. (eds.), *Skeletal Trauma*, 3rd ed. Philadelphia, PA: W.B. Saunders, 2003, 1245–1289.

Wirth MA, Rockwood CA. Injuries to the sternoclavicular joint. In: Bucholz RW, Heckman JD (eds.), *Rockwood and Green's Fractures in Adults*, 5th ed. Philadelphia, PA: Lippincott, Williams & Wilkins, 2001, 1245–1289.

6. **(E)** The anterior shoulder dislocation is the most common shoulder dislocation. Most of these injuries are the result of athletic-related trauma or a fall. The arm is usually in an abducted and externally rotated position, resulting in disruption of the anterior capsule and labral complex. This is referred to as the Bankart lesion. The shoulder has little intrinsic stability. The

capsuloligamentous structures provide static stability and the muscles provide dynamic stability. Acute anterior dislocations are initially managed with gentle, closed reduction. The need and duration for postreduction immobilization remains controversial. Associated injuries may include fractures, rotator cuff tears, or neurovascular injury. The younger the patient, the higher the recurrence rate of repeat dislocation. Those who fail conservative treatment are candidates for surgical repair of the torn capsulabral complex. Although acute surgical stabilization can be considered for young high-demand patients, conservative treatment remains the standard for first time dislocations.

An AP radiograph, as shown in Fig. 37-24 may be adequate to initially diagnose a shoulder dislocation; however, an axillary view should be part of the standard radiographic assessment of any shoulder injury. The recommended series is three views in the plane of the scapula including an AP, an axillary, and a scapular lateral (Y view). This becomes extremely important in the patient, such as this one, with a posterior shoulder dislocation. The history of an anterior blow and the limitation in rotation and abduction on clinical examination are classic for a posterior shoulder dislocation. Clinically, there may also be posterior prominence and anterior flattening of the

shoulder, and the coracoid is also often prominent. The diagnosis of a posterior dislocation is often delayed and can be missed on an AP radiograph. An AP radiograph such as that in Fig. 37-24 does reveal some signs that suggest the injury, however. The normal elliptical shadow and overlap of the humeral head on the glenoid is distorted. Normally on an AP radiograph, the humeral head will fill an even portion of the glenoid fossa. In this case, the majority of the glenoid is vacant and there is an apparent increase in the space between the anterior rim of the glenoid and the medial aspect of the humeral head. This is referred to as the "vacant glenoid" or "positive rim sign." The AP radiograph may reveal significant internal rotation and the margins of the greater tuberosity are no longer visible; however, it fails to reveal the displacement, which is directly posterior. An axillary radiograph is the most effective means to assess the position of the humeral head relative to the glenoid.

Axial CT scans could also be useful, but are less cost-effective. They would be helpful in the case of suspected fractures to help quantify displacement. Similarly, an MRI may be helpful later in the course of treatment to assess for intraarticular pathology. It is of limited use acutely, however. The other options would not help to confirm the diagnosis. Although the majority of shoulder dislocations are anterior, a posterior dislocation should be suspected with a history of an anterior blow, electrocution, or seizure disorder.

Management consists of gentle reduction under appropriate sedation. These dislocations can often become locked on the posterior glenoid, and force or excessive internal rotation at the time of reduction can result in an iatrogenic humerus fracture. Immobilization in a position of stability, which may include slight extension, and limited, internal rotation is used in the initial healing phase followed by range of motion and strengthening.

Fractures of the glenoid rim or proximal humerus are relatively common with posterior dislocations. Compression of the anteromedial aspect of the humeral head is referred to as a "reverse Hill-Sachs lesion." Fractures of the lesser tuberosity may also occur. These should be identified at the time of injury and addressed if they are related to recurrent instability.

Bibliography

Green A, Norris TR. Glenohumeral dislocations. In: Browner BD, Jupiter JB, Levine AE, et al. (eds.), *Skeletal Trauma*, 3rd ed. Philadelphia, PA: W.B. Saunders, 2003, 1598–1614.

Matsen FA, Thomas SC, Rockwood CA, et al. Glenohumeral instability. In: Rockwood CA, Matsen FA (eds.), *The Shoulder*, 2nd ed. Philadelphia, PA: W.B. Saunders, 1998, 649–675.

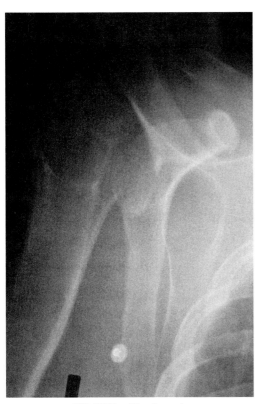

FIG. 37-24   AP radiograph

Schmidt AH. Fractures of the proximal humerus and dislocation of the glenohumeral joint. In: Kellam JF, Fischer TJ, Tornetta P III (eds.), *Orthopaedic Knowledge Update: Trauma 2*. Rosemont, IL: American Academy of Orthopaedic Surgeons, 2000, 19–20.

Wirth MA, Rockwood CA. Subluxations and dislocations about the glenohumeral joint. In: Bucholz RW, Heckman JD (eds.), *Rockwood and Green's Fractures in Adults*, 5th ed. Philadelphia, PA: Lippincott, Williams & Wilkins, 2001, 1109–1162.

7. **(D)** The radiographs reveal a displaced femoral neck fracture. Femoral neck fractures are found in two different clinical scenarios: the elderly patient who sustains a low energy fall, and the patient usually less than age 50 who sustains an injury from a high-energy traumatic event. The Garden classification system is the most widely used; however, there is significant interobserver variability. The most reliable classification categorizes fractures into displaced and nondisplaced, or impacted fractures. The management is different. Treatment of nondisplaced or impacted fractures is generally performed using multiple lag screws, or occasionally with a large compression screw and side plate. Nonunion and AVN are uncommon, following nondisplaced fractures occurring in less than 5 and 10% of cases, respectively.

These radiographs reveal a displaced fracture. This injury in a young patient should be considered an orthopedic emergency and ORIF is warranted. The concern involves the risk for developing AVN of the femoral head. A network of vascularity that includes the lateral and medial femoral circumflex arteries and the obturator artery supplies the femoral head. The treatment of displaced fractures remains somewhat controversial; however, achieving anatomic reduction is the most critical factor in maintaining reduction, and avoiding nonunion or AVN. Some individuals advocate performing a capsulotomy or aspiration at the time of ORIF to release the hemarthrosis that develops. They feel this elevated pressure may be the pathophysiologic mechanism, which may influence the circulation to the femoral head and contribute to the development of AVN. This has been shown to improve femoral head blood flow in laboratory animal models; however, this has not been conclusively proven in clinical trials. Nonunion and AVN are more common following displaced fractures. The incidence of nonunion ranges from 10 to 30% and the incidence of AVN ranges from 15 to 33%.

Prosthetic replacement with hemiarthroplasty is reserved for older and less active individuals. Total hip replacement would be indicated in patients with significant preexisting arthritis involving the acetabulum. Bed rest can be associated with significant complications including decubitus ulcers, pneumonia, and deep vein thrombosis. Bed rest, therefore, is only indicated if patients are not considered surgical candidates. Protected weight bearing is not a consideration in displaced fractures.

Bibliography

Asnis SE, Wanek-Sgaglione L. Intracapsular fractures of the femoral neck: results of cannulated screw fixation. *J Bone Joint Surg* 1994;76A:1793–1803.

Baumgaertner MR, Higgins TF. Femoral neck fractures. In: Bucholz RW, Heckman JD (eds.), *Rockwood and Green's Fractures in Adults*, 5th ed. Philadelphia, PA: Lippincott, Williams & Wilkins, 2001, 1583–1602, 1609–1610.

Frandsen PA, Andersen E, Madsen F, et al. Garden's classification system of femoral neck fractures: an assessment of interobserver variation. *J Bone Joint Surg* 1988;70B:588–590.

Koval KJ, Zuckerman JD. Trauma: hip. In: Callaghan JJ, Dennis DA, Paprosky WG, et al. (eds.), *Orthopaedic Knowledge Update: Hip and Knee Reconstruction*. Rosemont, IL: American Academy of Orthopaedic Surgeons, 1995, 97–108.

Swiontkowski MF. Intracapsular hip fractures. In: Browner BD, Jupiter JB, Levine AE, et al. (eds.), *Skeletal Trauma*, 3rd ed. Philadelphia, PA: W.B. Saunders, 2003.

8. **(E)** A conscious trauma patient will alert the examiner to a potential pelvic injury. In an unconscious trauma patient, however, associated injuries may not initially be obvious, and a detailed examination is indicated to successfully identify and manage these injuries. Urologic injuries occur in up to 15% of pelvic fractures. Blood at the meatus and a high-riding prostate are indicative of urethral disruption. Hematuria may also be found, and may be suggestive of a bladder injury. In males, a retrograde urethrogram should be obtained prior to passing a Foley if one of these findings is identified. In a female, a catheter may be passed because the urethra is very short.

Additional findings during physical examination that are associated with a pelvic ring injury include scrotal or labial swelling and ecchymosis, open lacerations, or other soft tissue injuries around the pelvis. These findings may indicate an open pelvic fracture. Therefore, all patients with significant pelvic injuries require a rectal and, in females, a vaginal examination. The lumbosacral plexus is very closely associated with the inner pelvis and injury has been reported to occur in 8–56% of patients. An abnormal position to the lower extremity with excessive shortening or rotation can indicate an "open book" type pelvic injury or possibly a sacroiliac injury.

The standard AP pelvis x-ray may reveal a skeletally unstable injury. Abnormal motion or pain on provocative testing may further confirm these suspicions. The anterior superior iliac spine compression test involves placing the hands on the patient's anterior superior iliac spines (ASIS) and gently rocking the pelvis from side to side. If free motion is detected the patient has a mechanically unstable pelvic injury. Subtle instability may require radiographic stress testing in the OR. No motion is considered a normal finding. If an injury is identified, repeated stressing of the pelvis is contraindicated to minimize possible disruption of an established clot.

If an unstable injury is identified, stabilization can be performed in the ER by wrapping a sheet around the iliac wings for AP compression injuries or by using an external fixator with or without traction. Providing pelvic fracture stability helps decrease blood loss by opposing fracture ends, closing the pelvic volume to allow tamponade, and by protecting initial clot formation.

Bibliography

Dickson KF. The acute management of pelvic ring injuries. In: Kellam JF, Fischer TJ, Tornetta P III (eds.), *Orthopaedic Knowledge Update: Trauma 2*. Rosemont, IL: American Academy of Orthopaedic Surgeons, 2000, 229–230.

Jones AL, Burgess AR. Fractures of the pelvic ring. In: Bucholz RW, Heckman JD (eds.), *Rockwood and Green's Fractures in Adults*, 5th ed. Philadelphia, PA: Lippincott, Williams & Wilkins, 2001, 1482–1498.

Kellam JF, Mayo K. Pelvic ring disruptions. In: Browner BD, Jupiter JB, Levine AE, et al. (eds.), *Skeletal Trauma*, 3rd ed. Philadelphia, PA: W.B. Saunders, 2003, 1102.

Tornetta P III, Templeman D. Pelvis and acetabulum: trauma. In: Koval K (ed.), *Orthopaedic Knowledge Update 7*. Rosemont, IL: American Academy of Orthopaedic Surgeons, 2002, 395–396.

9. (D) This man has an isolated clavicle fracture. Fractures of the clavicle are among the most common seen among adults. These fractures are classified based on the location of injury. Typically they occur in the middle one-third (85% of fractures) of the clavicle. This portion of the clavicle is vulnerable for a couple of reasons. First, it is in a subcutaneous position, and second, it has no muscular attachments. A cephalic and caudal tilt radiograph can be obtained to supplement the standard AP radiograph used to diagnose a clavicle fracture.

Most of these injuries are managed nonsurgically with a figure-of-8 bandage or sling for up to 6 weeks with gradual increases in range of motion. Healing is usually evident on radiographs by 6 weeks; however, up to 12 weeks may be needed for full return to function. There has been no difference shown between use of a sling or figure-of-8 bandage. Treatment with casting is of historical interest only. The long-term results of isolated clavicle fractures managed with sling or immobilizer is excellent. Full functional return is expected and the incidence of nonunion is between 0.1 and 5%. More recent studies have shown a link between displaced fracture and nonunion. Shortening can occur in displaced fractures; however, this has been shown to not affect functional outcome.

Indications for acute surgical management include open fractures, associated vascular injury, polytrauma, and ipsilateral scapula fracture. Fractures which are tenting the skin and it appears that skin compromise is imminent are also considered in this group. Some have advocated displacement of greater than 2 cm as an indication for surgery, to avoid the higher risk of nonunion is this select group.

If surgery is indicated, attempts are made to avoid the supraclavicular nerves, which cross the incision. Plate fixation is the most commonly used method, which requires precise contouring of the plate to match the shape of the clavicle. Intramedullary fixation with larger diameter threaded pins is another alternative. Small diameter, smooth K-wires, however, should never be used. Complications include infection, nonunion, and hardware migration. A higher complication rate has been reported following internal fixation of acute fractures (over 20% in one study), and routine ORIF of isolated middle one-third clavicle fractures is not supported by the literature.

Bibliography

Blachut PA, Broekhuyse HM. Fractures of the scapula and clavicle and Injuries of the acromioclavicular and sternoclavicular joints. In: Kellam JF, Fischer TJ, Tornetta P III (eds.), *Orthopaedic Knowledge Update: Trauma 2*. Rosemont, IL: American Academy of Orthopaedic Surgeons, 2000, 8–9.

Bostman O, Manninen M, Pihlajamak H. Complications of plate fixation in fresh displaced midclavicular fractures. *J Trauma* 1997;43:778–783.

Dirschl DR. Shoulder trauma: bone. In: Koval K (ed.), *Orthopaedic Knowledge Update 7*. Rosemont, IL: American Academy of Orthopaedic Surgeons, 2002, 264–265.

Hill JM, McGuire MH, Crosby LA. Closed treatment of displaced middle third fractures of the clavicle gives poor results. *J Bone Joint Surg* 1997;79B:537–539.

Lazarus M. Fractures of the clavicle. In: Bucholz RW, Heckman JD (eds.), *Rockwood and Green's Fractures in Adults*, 5th ed. Philadelphia, PA: Lippincott, Williams & Wilkins, 2001, 1044–1054.

Nordqvist A, Peterson CJ, Redlund-Johnell I. Mid-clavicle fractures in adults: end result study after conservative treatment. *J Orthop Trauma* 1998;12:572–576.

10. (A) This patient has an anterior shoulder dislocation. Most of these injuries are the result of athletic-related trauma or a fall. The injury usually occurs when the arm is in an abducted and externally rotated position, resulting in disruption of the anterior capsule and labral complex. The shoulder has little intrinsic stability. The capsuloligamentous structures provide static stability and the muscles provide dynamic stability. Acute anterior dislocations are managed with gentle, closed reduction.

Other shoulder girdle injuries can be associated with dislocations. Among these are fractures, rotator cuff tears, and nerve and vascular injuries. The position of the brachial plexus and peripheral nerves in the axilla, places them at risk at the time of injury. Brachial plexus and axillary nerve injuries are the most common. The axillary nerve arises from the posterior cord of the brachial plexus. It is tethered both anteriorly and posteriorly to the glenohumeral joint and is vulnerable to injury as it passes through the quadrangular space in conjunction with the posterior humeral circumflex artery. The nerve divides into a superior and inferior branch. The superior branch passes around the humeral neck to innervate the deltoid muscle. The inferior branch supplies the teres minor muscle and some posterior fibers of the deltoid. It then continues on to provide cutaneous innervation to the lateral arm as the superior lateral brachial cutaneous nerve.

The musculocutaneous nerve provides only motor innervation in the upper arm. It continues into the forearm as the lateral antebrachial cutaneous nerve providing sensory innervation to the anterior-lateral forearm. The ulnar nerve has no innervation in the upper arm. In the forearm, the ulnar sensory components involve the small finger and the ulnar border of the ring finger. The medial brachial cutaneous nerve is a branch off the medial cord of the brachial plexus. It travels beside the brachial artery to the middle arm where it pierces the fascia and provides sensation to the posterior surface of the lower third of the upper arm extending to the olecranon. These sensory innervations are easily summarized in Fig. 37-25.

Bibliography

Green A, Norris TR. Glenohumeral dislocations. In: Browner BD, Jupiter JB, Levine AE, et al. (eds.), *Skeletal Trauma*, 3rd ed. Philadelphia, PA: W.B. Saunders, 2003, 1598–1614.

Matsen FA, Thomas SC, Rockwood CA, et al. Glenohumeral instability. In: Rockwood CA, Matsen FA (eds.), *The Shoulder*, 2nd ed. Philadelphia, PA: W.B. Saunders, 1998, 649–675.

Netter FH. *The Ciba Collection of Medical Illustrations. Volume 8—Musculoskeletal System, Part I: Anatomy Physiology and Metabolic Disorders.* Summit, NJ: Ciba-Geigy, 2001, 20–26.

Schmidt AH. Fractures of the proximal humerus and dislocation of the glenohumeral joint. In: Kellam JF, Fischer TJ, Tornetta P III (eds.), *Orthopaedic Knowledge Update: Trauma 2.* Rosemont, IL: American Academy of Orthopaedic Surgeons, 2000, 19–20.

Wirth MA, Rockwood CA. Subluxations and dislocations about the glenohumeral joint. In: Bucholz RW, Heckman JD (eds.), *Rockwood and Green's Fractures in Adults*, 5th ed. Philadelphia, PA: Lippincott, Williams & Wilkins, 2001, 1109–1162.

11. (B) Spinal cord injury occurs up to 65% of the time in the cervical region. Common mechanisms include MVAs, falls, and gunshot wounds. Spinal cord injury occurs from two distinct processes. The primary injury is the result of the mechanical injury at the time of the initial insult. This primary injury is followed by a cascade of events, which leads to secondary injury and increased cell death as a result of the pathophysiologic response.

Surgical stabilization of the spine can prevent further mechanical injury to the cord. Additionally, removing compression such as a herniated disc or encroaching fragments of bone might further assist in the functional recovery. Over the past several years, the pharmacologic treatment of spinal cord injury has been used in an attempt to reduce or minimize the secondary injury. It is felt that interrupting the cascade of events that leads to the secondary injury has the potential to limit cell damage and improve functional outcome. Methylprednisolone is the only agent in randomized clinical trials, which has been shown to have favorable effects on the neurologic recovery following injury. It has, therefore, become the standard for acute care of the patient with a spinal cord injury.

The National Acute Spinal Cord Injury Study (NASCIS) trials were large scale, randomized clinical trials that evaluated the use of methylprednisolone in spinal cord injury patients. The most recent NASCIS III trial recommendations are:

Methylprednisolone bolus of 30 mg/kg followed by infusion 5.4 mg/kg
Infusion for 24 h when bolus given within 3 h of injury
Infusion for 48 h when bolus given between 3 and 8 h from time of injury
No benefit when methylprednisolone started more than 8 h after injury
No benefit from naloxone
No benefit from tirilazad

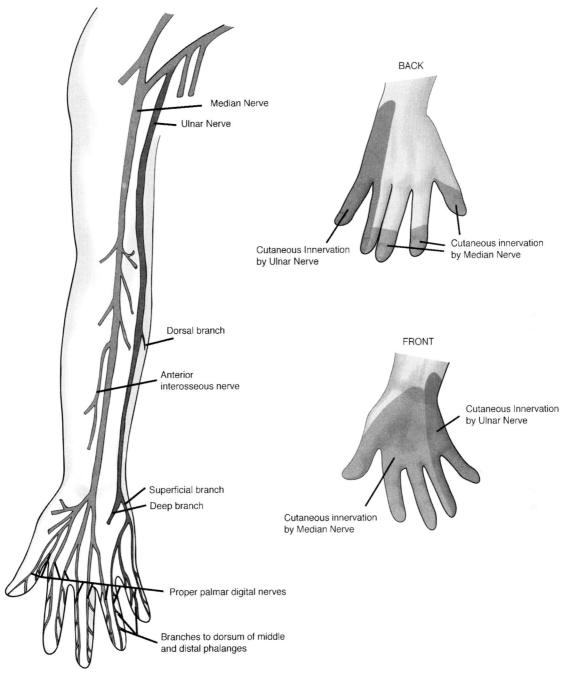

FIG. 37-25 Sensory innervation of median and ulnar nerves

Bibliography

Bracken MB, Shepard MJ, Holford TR, et al. Administration of methylprednisolone for 24 or 48 hours or tirilazad mesulate for 48 hours in the treatment of acute spinal cord injury. Results of the Third National Acute Spinal Cord Injury Randomized Controlled Trial National Acute Spinal Cord Injury Study. *JAMA* 1997;277: 1597–1604.

K-B Tay B, Eismont F. Cervical spine fractures and dislocations. In: Fardin DF, Garfin SR, Abitbol J, et al. (eds.), *Orthopaedic Knowledge Update: Spine 2*. Rosemont, IL: American Academy of Orthopaedic Surgeons, 2002, 251–253.

Mirza SK, Chapman JR, Grady MS. Spinal cord injury: pathophysiology and current treatment strategies. In: Kellam JF, Fischer TJ, Tornetta P III (eds.), *Orthopaedic Knowledge Update: Trauma 2*. Rosemont, IL: American Academy of Orthopaedic Surgeons, 2000, 359–368.

12. (E) Osteoid osteoma is one of three lesions in which the tumor cells produce osteoid. It is a self-limiting, benign, painful vascular lesion of uncertain etiology. It occurs most commonly in younger patients, ages 5–30. The pain usually increases with time and most patients will have night pain. The pain is often significantly improved with aspirin or salicylates. Common sites include the proximal femur, tibial diaphysis, and the spine. The lesion may be difficult to identify on plain radiographs; however, findings include reactive bone and a radiolucent nidus. For this reason, special studies may be warranted. Bone scans are always positive and MRI or CT scan can help to further define the location. By definition the nidus is always less than 1.5 cm. The reactive area of bone, however, may be larger.

Microscopically, there is a distinct differentiation between the nidus and the reactive bone. The nidus consists of osteoid trabeculae with varied mineralization. The organization is haphazard and the greatest mineralization is in the center of the lesion.

Treatment consists of surgical removal of the complete lesion through excision of the entire lesion or curettage of the nidus. Nonoperative treatment with the use of aspirin or nonsteroidal anti-inflammatory drugs (NSAIDs) may alleviate the pain in some patients. Up to 50% of these patients treated medically with have the pain resolve secondary to burn out of the lesion. A newer technique of percutaneous radiofrequency ablation under CT guidance is gaining popularity. This has resulted in about 90% success rates of treatment.

Osteoblastoma is very similar to osteoid osteoma; however, it is not self-limited like osteoid osteoma, and can attain a large size. As noted earlier, osteoid osteoma is by definition less than 1.5 cm. Osteosarcoma is a malignant bone-forming tumor. Multiple myeloma is a plasma cell disorder and not a bone-forming tumor. Although they do present with pain, it occurs more commonly in an older patients between 50 and 80 years of age. In addition, the classic radiographic appearance is that of a punched-out lytic lesion. Myositis ossificans occurs following a traumatic event. It is most common over long bones in the midportion of muscles. This should not be confused with osteoid osteoma. Radiographically there is no similarity, and the microscopic pattern, which reveals mature, trabecular bone at the periphery and immature tissue at the center, is the opposite of that found in osteoid osteoma.

Bibliography

Frassica FJ, Frassica DA, McCarthy EF. Orthopaedic pathology. In: Miller MD, Brinker MR (eds.), *Review of Orthopaedics*, 3rd ed. Philadelphia, PA: W.B. Saunders, 2000, 379–440.

Springfield DS, Bolander ME, Friedlaender GE, et al. Molecular and cellular biology of inflammation and neoplasia. In: Simon SR (ed.), *Orthopaedic Basic Science*. Rosemont, IL: American Academy of Orthopaedic Surgeons, 1994, 262–275.

Temple HT, Clohisy DR. Musculoskeletal oncology. In: Koval K (ed.), *Orthopaedic Knowledge Update 7*. Rosemont, IL: American Academy of Orthopaedic Surgeons, 2002, 159–171.

13. (D) The diaphragm is innervated by the phrenic nerve, which is formed from branches off of nerve roots C3-C5. This is critical in patients with cervical spine fractures and associated spinal cord injuries. Those with high cervical injuries are often ventilator dependant, where as those with lower injuries rarely need respiratory support.

The functional level of a patient with a spinal cord injury is determined from the most distal, intact sensory and motor (grade 4/5) levels. Many factors surrounding a patient's independence with mobility and activities of daily living can be predicted based on the level of injury (Table 37-2).

Sacral sparing is an indication of an incomplete spinal cord injury. The neurologic level established by the American Spine Association standards is defined as the most caudal level with normal motor and sensory function bilateral. Spinal shock refers to the first 24–72 h period of paralysis, hypotonia, and areflexia. This concludes with the progressive onset of spasticity, hyperreflexia, and clonus, which develop over days to weeks. The return of the bulbocavernosus reflex signifies the end of spinal shock and the likelihood of improvement in neurologic function of a patient with a complete injury is minimal. The prognosis in an incomplete injury is unaffected by the bulbocavernosus reflex.

TABLE 37-2   Functional Level after Spinal Cord Injury

Functioning Level	Working	Not Working	Mobility/ADLs
Above C4		Diaphragm, Upper extremity muscles	Respirator dependent
C4	Diaphragm, Trapezius	Upper extremity muscles	Wheelchair, chin/puff
C5	Elbow flexors	Below elbow	Electric wheelchair
C6	Wrist extensors	Elbow extensors	Manual wheelchair, flexor hinge
C7	Elbow extensors	Grasp	Manual wheelchair–independent, Cut meat
L2	Iliopsoas	Knee/ankle	KAFO, Household ambulation
L3	Quadriceps	Ankle	AFO, Community ambulation

Neurogenic shock is the result of loss of sympathetic tone. This is commonly confused with spinal shock.

Bibliography

Gottschalk F. Rehabilitation: gait, amputations, prosthetics, orthotics. In: Miller MD, Brinker MR (eds.), *Review of Orthopaedics*, 3rd ed. Philadelphia, PA: W.B. Saunders, 2000, 458–459.

Lauerman WC, Goldsmith ME. Spine. In: Miller MD, Brinker MR (eds.), *Review of Orthopaedics*, 3rd ed. Philadelphia, PA: W.B. Saunders, 2000, 357–359.

14. **(E)** The Denis classification divides the vertebra into three columns: anterior—anterior longitudinal ligament, anterior annulus and disc, and anterior half of vertebral body; middle—posterior disc and annulus, posterior longitudinal ligament and posterior half of vertebral body; posterior column—posterior bony arch including lamina, pedicles, facets, and spinous process. Lumbar spine fractures generally occur from four mechanisms or a combination of them. These forces include compression, flexion, distraction, and shear. The resulting injuries include compression, burst, flexion-distraction, and fracture-dislocation. Compression fractures are the result of flexion forces on the anterior column. When the anterior compression is <50%, the middle and posterior columns are usually intact. An intact middle column defines a compression fracture and distinguishes a compression fracture from a burst fracture, which involves axial compression failure of the anterior and middle columns with either an intact or disrupted posterior column. Important factors to consider in the treatment of burst fractures are spinal canal compromise, the degree of angulation, and presence or absence of neurologic deficit; however, controversy still exists regarding the most beneficial means of management of these fractures. Surgical treatment is generally preferred if there is greater than 50% canal compromise or more than 30 degrees of kyphosis at the level of injury, even if there are no neurologic deficits. If a neurologic deficit is present, surgical management is again usually preferred, nonoperative management can be considered, even if a neurologic deficit is present, only if the fracture pattern is stable and there is no spinal cord compression. Neurologic deficit must consider not only lower extremity motor and sensory function. Perineal sensation, and bladder and bowel function must be evaluated and a rectal examination is mandatory.

Compression fractures are generally stable injuries because of the intact posterior structures, and most are managed nonoperatively with a brace for up to 3 months or longer. Fractures dislocations are high-energy injuries involving failure of all three columns from a combination of forces. They are unstable injuries and are associated with the highest incidence of neurologic injury. These injuries require surgical stabilization. The seat belt injury is the classic flexion-distraction injury, which involves tension failure of the middle and posterior columns, and either tension or compressive failure of the anterior column depending on the site of the axis of rotation. These injuries can occur through either the bony or soft tissue elements. The fractures through bone have a better prognosis for healing, whereas the injuries through the ligamentous or soft tissue structures are less predictable and should be considered unstable.

The radiographs of the lumbar spine show obvious involvement of the anterior and middle columns and therefore this injury is consistent with a lumbar burst fracture.

Bibliography

Bolesta MJ, Rechtine GR III. Fractures and dislocations of the thoracolumbar spine. In: Bucholz RW, Heckman JD (eds.), *Rockwood and Green's Fractures in Adults*, 5th ed. Philadelphia, PA: Lippincott, Williams & Wilkins, 2001, 1405–1415.

Kwok DC. Thoracolumbar injuries: The posterior approach. In: Kellam JF, Fischer TJ, Tornetta P III (eds.), *Orthopaedic Knowledge Update: Trauma 2*. Rosemont, IL: American Academy of Orthopaedic Surgeons, 2000, 393–400.

Motley GS, Eddings TH III, Moore RS. Adult trauma. In: Miller MD, Brinker MR (eds.), *Review of Orthopaedics*, 3rd ed. Philadelphia, PA: W.B. Saunders, 2000, 469–470.

Vaccaro AR, Singh K. Thoracolumbar injuries: nonsurgical treatment. In: Kellam JF, Fischer TJ, Tornetta P III (eds.), *Orthopaedic Knowledge Update: Trauma 2*. Rosemont, IL: American Academy of Orthopaedic Surgeons, 2000, 383–387.

Vaccaro AR, Jacoby SM. Thoracolumbar fractures and dislocations. In: Fardin DF, Garfin SR, Abitbol J, et al. (eds.), *Orthopaedic Knowledge Update: Spine 2*. Rosemont, IL: American Academy of Orthopaedic Surgeons, 2002, 273–276.

15. **(E)** Pelvic ring injuries can be classified according to location, stability, or mechanism of injury. Each classification system has advantages and disadvantages, but the mechanism of injury system is the most helpful in the acute setting with injury recognition and prediction of blood loss. The Young and Burgess classification system is mechanism based and classifies injuries into AP compression, lateral compression, or vertical shear injuries. The APC-I is a stable injury with disruption of the symphysis only, with less than 2.5 cm of diastases. There is no significant posterior injury identified. The APC-II occurs as forces increase and the sacrospinous and sacrotuberous ligaments are

disrupted, creating greater rotational instability. The pelvis is being opened like a book and the adjacent vascular structures are at risk. Finally, when the posterior ligamentous structures are disrupted, significant posterior diastases results in a completely unstable APC-III injury.

The LC-I injury results from a lateral blow often seen in drivers of MVAs. The impact occurs at the lateral aspect of the iliac wing or pelvis. This results in superior and inferior rami fractures often oriented in the horizontal plane, and a compression injury on the sacrum. This injury pattern is often stable. Increasing displacement results in greater instability usually from a fracture or dislocation involving the iliac wing and sacroiliac joint (LC-II). The greater force creates a point of rotation around the anterior sacrum. There may be a compression failure along the anterior sacrum, and there is an associated bone or soft tissue injury involving the posterior aspect of the sacroiliac joint. As forces continue, the hemipelvis is pushed across to the opposite side and there is disruption of the contralateral pelvis. This creates a windswept appearance of the pelvis (LC-III). Vertical shear injuries result in disruption of the pelvis anteriorly and posteriorly.

AP injuries are associated with a higher incidence of pelvic vascular injury and subsequently a greater incidence of shock, sepsis, ARDS, and death. Lateral compression injuries are associated with a higher incidence of brain and visceral injury, but a lower incidence of pelvic vascular injury. LC-I and LC-II injuries have a 50% incidence of brain injury. LC-III injuries, however, have a lower association with brain injury because the mechanism is usually a rollover versus a lateral crush. Death from an AP injury is usually from a combination of pelvic blood loss and visceral injuries, whereas death associated with a lateral compression injury is usually from severe brain injury or intraabdominal injury, or both. The average blood loss from an APC-III injury is 14.8 units, and the average loss from a LC-III injury is only 3.6 units. As stated earlier, APC injuries have a higher association with pelvic vascular injury.

The radiograph in this case depicts an APC-III type injury. These are associated with the greatest average transfusion requirements.

Bibliography

Burgess AR, Eastridge BJ, Young JW, et al. Pelvic ring disruptions: effective classification system and treatment protocols. *J Trauma* 1990;30:848–856.

Dalal SA, Burgess AR, Siegel JH, et al. Pelvic fracture in multiple trauma: classification by mechanism is key to pattern of organ injury, resuscitative requirements, and outcome. *J Trauma* 1989;29:981–1002.

Dickson KF. The acute management of pelvic ring injuries. In: Kellam JF, Fischer TJ, Tornetta P III (eds.), *Orthopaedic Knowledge Update: Trauma 2*. Rosemont, IL: American Academy of Orthopaedic Surgeons, 2000, 229–234.

Kellam JF, Mayo K. Pelvic ring disruptions. In: Browner BD, Jupiter JB, Levine AE, et al. (eds.), *Skeletal Trauma*, 3rd ed. Philadelphia, PA: W.B. Saunders, 2003, 1059–1060.

Whitbeck MG Jr, Zwally HJ II, Burgess AR. Innominosacral dissociation: mechanism of injury as a predictor of resuscitation requirements, morbidity, and mortality. *J Orthop Trauma* 1997;11:82–88.

16. **(E)** The ISS provides a numerical description of the overall severity of injury and chance of mortality in multiple injured patients. The ISS was derived from the AIS. Injuries to six body regions are graded as (1) mild, (2) moderate, (3) severe, (4) critical—outcome usually favorable, and (5) critical—outcome usually fatal. This scale is based on threat to life, expected impairment, treatment period, and energy dissipation. The ISS is defined as the sum of the squares of the highest AIS grade in each of the three most severely injured areas. The ISS uses the six body regions of injury head/neck, face, chest, abdominal or pelvic contents, extremities and bony pelvis. Scores range from 1 to 75 as any patient with a score of six is assigned an ISS of 75.

Becker et al. (1974) studied over 2000 victims of MVA, pedestrians, or other road users. Multiple trauma patients are defined by an ISS >18. When the ISS is 25 or greater, a patient who is considered polytraumatized and is at risk for multiorgan failure will benefit from specialized trauma care. An ISS <30 is usually indicative of a good prognosis unless associated with a severe head injury. An ISS >60 is usually fatal. In the initial report there were no deaths in an ISS <10. The highest surviving score was 50. Age significantly affected death rate; with an ISS 10–19 death rates were eight times greater in patients over 70 compared to those under 50. With an ISS <20 one-half of the deaths occurred in the first week. With an ISS >50 all deaths occurred in the first week and 75% within 1 h.

ISS has limitations since it can underestimate the injury severity of a patient with multiple injuries in the same body region. It also tends to overweigh combined nonlethal injuries.

Example

Isolated severe head AIS-5 = ISS 25

Liver laceration AIS-4,
   femur fracture AIS-3 = ISS 25

Mortality, complication rate, and resource uses are probably very different in these two patients.

Bibliography

Baker SP, O'Neil B, Haddon W Jr, et al. The injury severity score: a method for describing patients with multiple injuries and evaluating emergency care. *J Trauma* 1974; 14:187–196.

Roberts CS, Gleis GE, Seligson D. Diagnosis and treatment of complications. In: Browner BD, Jupiter JB, Levine AE, et al. (eds.), *Skeletal Trauma*, 3rd ed. Philadelphia, PA: W.B. Saunders, 2003, 452–453.

17. **(A)** OP is a condition of reduced bone mass in the absence of a mineralization defect. This leads to bone fragility and an increased risk of fracture. OP is a quantitative defect, not a qualitative defect. The precise mechanism is unclear but involves the hormonal mediators such as estrogen and osteoblasts and osteoclasts.

Riggs and Melton have subclassified primary OP based on the pattern of bone loss and fracture. Type I or postmenopausal OP occurs in women of ages 51–65 and involves predominantly trabecular bone. It is characterized by vertebral and Colles' fractures. Estrogen deficiency plays a primary role. Type II, known as senile OP, involves predominantly cortical bone and occurs in both men and women age >75. Clinically, fractures of the hip, pelvis, proximal humerus, and proximal tibia are seen. Causes are the aging process itself and chronic calcium or vitamin deficiency. Sedentary, thin White women of northern European descent are at increased risk for developing OP. Other risk factors include smoking, heavy alcohol use, low body weight, and steroid use.

Diagnosis is made through the measurement of bone density. Secondary bone loss must be ruled out and the use of routine or even specialized laboratory studies may be useful in some osteopenic conditions. However, these studies are usually normal in OP. Plain radiographs are not helpful unless the bone loss is in excess of 30%. Dual-energy x-ray absorptiometry (DEXA) is considered the gold standard the most accurate method with less radiation to evaluate the extent of OP. Patients with bone densities of 1–2.5 standard deviations below the mean peak bone mass measurements (T-score) are considered to be osteopenic. Bone densities greater than 2.5 standard deviations below the mean are used to define OP.

The spine is composed of primarily trabecular bone. Compared with cortical bone it has a high surface to volume ratio. Because remodeling occurs on bone surfaces, trabecular bone in general and vertebral bodies in particular are resolved preferentially in times of loss. The histology reveals thinning of trabeculae, decreased osteon size, and enlargement of the haversian and marrow spaces. The differential resorptions result in the timing and patterns of fractures associated with OP. Therefore, answer **A** is correct as the vertebral body fractures in OP are related to the high bone turnover and trabecular loss, not the cortical bone loss as in answer E.

Answers B, C, and D are all incorrect as disc disease, facet arthritis, and circulation are all independent of OP.

Bibliography

Bernstein J, Lane JM. Metabolic bone disorders of the spine. In: Rothman RH, Simeone FA (eds.), *The Spine*, 3rd ed. Philadelphia, PA: W.B. Saunders, 1992, 1381–1427.

Brinker MR. Basic sciences: section 1—bone. In: Miller MD, Brinker MR (eds.), *Review of Orthopaedics*, 3rd ed. Philadelphia, PA: W.B. Saunders, 2000, 32–35.

Lucas TS, Einhorn TA. Osteoporosis: the role of the orthopaedist. *J Am Acad Orthop Surg* 1993;1:48–56.

Riggs BL, Melton LJ III. The prevention and treatment of osteoporosis. *N Engl J Med* 1992;327:620–627.

18. **(C)** It is the responsibility of the physician to perform a thorough neurologic evaluation in every patient, and especially in a patient with a suspected spinal cord injury. The extent of injury must be determined, as a patient with an incomplete injury has a reasonable prognosis for some gains in functional recovery; however, a functional recovery is only seen in 3% of patients with complete injuries in the first 24 h, and never after 24–48 h. According to the American Spinal Injury Association (ASIA), a complete injury is one in which no motor and/or sensory function exists more than three segments below the neurologic level of injury. An incomplete injury is one in which some neurologic function is spared more than three levels below the level of injury. The level of injury is defined as the most caudal segment that tests at least grade 3 (antigravity) out of 5 for motor and the next level above is graded 4 out of 5.

Sacral sparing is defined as perianal sensation, great toe flexor activity, and rectal tone. Sacral sparing is important because it indicates that there is at least partial continuity of the spinal tracts within the cord. This presence indicates an incomplete cord injury. This may be the only finding on initial examination so documentation of this finding is important. It is vital, however, to rule out spinal shock. Spinal shock is that initial period of complete spinal areflexia that develops after severe spinal cord injuries. This is evaluated by testing the bulbocavernosus reflex. The completeness of a spinal cord injury cannot be determined until the bulbocavernosus reflex returns, usually within the first 24 h.

This patient's clinical examination is consistent with an incomplete spinal cord injury. Incomplete spinal cord syndromes have a variable prognosis for recovery. Greater recovery can be expected in patients in whom there is greater initial sparing of function below the level of injury. Brown-Sequard's syndrome is a lesion caused by hemitransection of the cord usually from penetrating trauma. It results in ipsilateral motor and proprioception loss below the level of injury, and contralateral loss of pain and temperature sensation beginning one to two levels below the injury level. This carries the best prognosis for recovery of all the incomplete syndromes. Central cord syndrome occurs essentially in the cervical region and involves injury to the central portion of the cord. This results in sacral sparing (preservation of perianal sensation and rectal tone) and greater weakness in the upper extremities with sparing of the motor function in the lower extremities. This injury pattern reflects the topographic organization of the motor tracts within the spinal cord in which the upper extremity tracts are located in a more central position within the cord. Overall this carries the second best prognosis for recovery with the lower extremities often recovering better function than the upper. Anterior cord syndrome results from damage to the anterior spinal artery and involves damage to the anterior two-third of the cord and sparing of the posterior columns. Patients will have minimal if any motor function distally, and pain and temperature sensation is lost as well; however, proprioception, deep pressure, and vibratory sensation are preserved. The prognosis for motor recovery is poor. Cauda equina syndrome involves injury to the lumbosacral nerve roots within the spinal canal resulting in an areflexic bladder, bowel, and lower limbs.

Bibliography

Bohlman HH. Acute fractures and dislocations of the cervical spine. *J Bone Joint Surg* 1979;AM61:1119–1142.

Stauffer ES. Neurological recovery following injuries to the cervical spinal cord and nerve roots. *Spine* 1984;9: 532–534.

Vaccaro AR, Jacoby SM. Thoracolumbar fractures and dislocations. In: Fardin DF, Garfin SR, Abitbol J, et al. (eds.), *Orthopaedic Knowledge Update: Spine 2*. Rosemont, IL: American Academy of Orthopaedic Surgeons, 2002, 239–253.

19. **(A)** MRI has become the most useful modality for the definition of soft tissue masses. Tissues display different SI on T1 and T2 images. The MRI provides excellent definition of normal muscle, fascial boundaries, and the tumor mass. Both T1 and T2 weighted sequences are essential to detect and characterize soft tissue lesions. MRI cannot accurately predict the histology or whether a lesion is benign or malignant. Two exceptions to this rule are lipomas and hemangiomas. Lipomas are often very homogeneous and have signal characteristics that exactly match the surrounding fat thus establishing the diagnosis. They show bright SI on T1 and do not increase in SI on T2 or fat suppression images. Hemangiomas contain numerous blood vessels and present with a recognizable pattern.

Synovial sarcoma is low to intermediate on T1 and homogeneously bright on T2. Desmoid tumors are characterized by low SI fibrous bands, which demonstrate low to intermediate SI on T1 and high SI on T2 images. MFH features on MRI are nonspecific. Inhomogeneity with low to intermediate SI on T1 and high SI on T2 is found. Liposarcomas are more inhomogeneous than lipomas. The focal areas of malignant change demonstrate low to intermediate SI on T1 and high SI on T2.

Bibliography

Imaging beyond conventional radiology. In: Beaty JH (ed.), *Orthopaedic Knowledge Update—6*. Rosemont, IL: American Academy of Orthopaedic Surgeons, 1999, 81–87.

Brinker MR. Basic sciences: section 7—imaging and special studies. In: Miller MD, Brinker MR (eds.), *Review of Orthopaedics*, 3rd ed. Philadelphia, PA: W.B. Saunders, 2000, 115–116.

Moser RP, Madewell JE. Radiologic evaluation of soft tissue tumors. In: Enzinger FM, Weiss SW (eds.), *Soft Tissue Tumors*, 3rd ed., St. Louis, MO: Mosby, 1995, 39–88.

20. **(A)** Physeal fractures make up 15–30% of all childhood fractures. Injury to the physis is rare younger than age 5, and peaks in early adolescence, age 11–12. Boys are affected twice as often as girls. Salter and Harris developed a classification system of fractures, which involve the physeal plate. The five types in this system can be very useful in predicting the effects of the fracture on the physis and the effect on future growth.

Type I fractures involve a transverse fracture through the entire length of the growth plate without involvement of the metaphysis. Prognosis is generally excellent with the exception of the distal femur, or after severely displaced fractures, which were subsequently difficult to reduce. Type II injuries account for 75% of all physeal fractures. This fracture passes through the growth plate, but then exits through the metaphysis prior to passing the full length as in a type I fracture. This results in a metaphyseal bone fragment attached to the epiphyseal segment.

The prognosis for these is again good with growth disturbances occurring in 10–30% of cases. Type III injuries involve a fracture line transverse through part of the growth plate and then crossing the epiphysis to exit the articular surface. Anatomic reduction is indicated and prognosis is dependent on the vascularity of the physis and damage to the germinal zone. Type IV fractures are vertical fractures which cross all regions of the physis. These traverse the metaphysis, physis, epiphysis, and exit the articular surface. Despite an anatomic reduction, the prognosis for normal growth is poor. Type V involves a compressive mechanism with a crushing force. Growth arrest is common. This injury can occur in combination with any of the other patterns. Type VI has been added by Rang. This is a peripheral injury to the perichondrial ring. Localized growth disturbances can occur.

Fractures through the physis tend to pass through the hypertrophic zone. This region consists of cartilage, which is weaker than bone. Although this region is responsible for conversion of cartilage to bone, it is not the site of growth and cell multiplication. This occurs in the regions more nearer the epiphysis; however, any trauma to the region surrounding or involving the physis can result alteration in growth. This may be from damage to the vascularity, damage to the germinal cells, or from formation of a physeal bar or bony bridge that tethers the epiphysis to the metaphysis.

In summary, type I and II fractures are the least likely to interfere with growth because they do not pass through the growth zone; however, all bones respond differently, and the mechanism of injury may involve a compression component to the injury not initially appreciated. This may account for some of the higher-than-expected growth disturbances seen with some type II injuries. Type III and IV fractures cross the growth zone, are intraarticular, and are more likely to develop growth disturbances. Type IV fractures are more likely to develop a bony bridge, therefore these fractures must be anatomically reduced. Type V fractures can occur in association with any other pattern as implied above, or they may occur independently. These type V fractures may not always be easily recognized on initial radiographs. This classification provides assistance in predicting the potential of growth disturbance, but definitive prediction is not possible. For this reason, close clinical follow-up with radiographs is mandatory for these patients.

Bibliography

Paterson H, Madhok R, Benson J, et al. Physeal fractures. Part 1. Epidemiology in Olmsted County, Minnesota, 1979–1988. *J Pediatr Orthop* 1994;14:423.

Price CT, Phillis JH, Devito DP. Management of fractures. In: Morrissy RT, Weinstein SL (eds.), *Lovell and Winter's Pediatric Orthopaedics*, 5th ed. Philadelphia, PA: Lippincott, Williams & Wilkins, 2001, 1323–1326.

Rang M. *The Growth Plate and its Disorders*. Baltimore, MD: Williams & Wilkins, 1969.

Salter R, Harris W. Injuries involving the epiphyseal plate. *J Bone Joint Surg Am* 1963;45:587.

21. **(D)** Nonossifying fibroma or metaphyseal fibrous defect is a very common benign lesion in young patients. Most patients are asymptomatic and lesions are found incidentally. It has a characteristic appearance on x-ray. Most (90%) are located in the distal femur and proximal and distal tibia. The lesion is metaphyseal, lytic, and eccentric. It is scalloped and surrounded with a sclerotic rim and the cortex may be slightly thinned or expanded. Treatment of this lesion is observation as most of them will resolve. The diagnosis can be made by the characteristic appearance. Surgery, curettage, and bone grafting, is indicated if there is risk for pathologic fracture, if the patient is symptomatic, or if more than 75% of the cortex is involved.

Ewing's tumor is a small round cell sarcoma. It is a malignant tumor found in children and young adults who usually present with pain and may have fevers. The most common locations include the pelvis, distal femur, proximal tibia, femoral diaphysis, and proximal humerus. The radiographs reveal a destructive lesion that may be purely lytic or have some reactive new bone. There is often a large soft tissue component and the periosteum may be lifted off in layers, creating the classic radiographic onion-skin appearance. Treatment involves multiagent chemotherapy, irradiation, and surgical resection. Ewing's is associated with a translocation of chromosomes 11 and 22 resulting in a fusion protein, EWS-FLI 1, which is a transcription factor.

Giant cell tumor is a benign tumor; however, it can be locally aggressive, and can rarely metastasize to the lungs. It is most common in the third and fourth decade of life. It is most commonly found in the epiphysis of long bones. Patients may present with pain, and radiographs reveal a purely lytic, well-circumscribed lesion within the metaphysis. Treatment involves careful removal of the lesion, with preservation of the surrounding joint. Giant cell tumor has a high incidence of local recurrence.

Osteosarcoma is a malignant primary bone tumor, second only to multiple myeloma. It most commonly occurs about the knee (distal femur and proximal tibia) in children and young adults. Most patients will present with pain. Most tumors are high-grade, destructive bone-forming lesions. They often penetrate the cortex early and form a large soft tissue component. Radiographs reveal a poorly defined lesion with bone destruction and bone formation. Lesions involve the medullary canal and have periosteal reaction, such as Codman's triangle or sunburst pattern, which is indicative of rapid growth. On microscopic examination, there is osteoid production, and the cells are obviously malignant. Following appropriate staging, treatment involves multiagent chemotherapy and surgical resection. Osteosarcoma can also occur in older patients who have received radiotherapy in the past or in patients with Paget's disease.

Fibrosarcoma is a malignant soft tissue sarcoma or fibrous tumor. Patients usually present with a mass that is enlarging and relatively painless. Plain radiographs are often normal except in advanced cases where there is involvement of the bone resulting in destructive changes. Treatment involves wide local excision and radiation therapy for larger tumors greater than 5 cm.

These particular radiographs reveal a lesion that has a typical appearance for a nonossifying fibroma/metaphyseal fibrous defect. It has sclerotic, scalloped margins, and has a benign appearance. It is not aggressive in appearance as would be expected with osteosarcoma or Ewing's. The fact that the patient presented with a pathologic fracture and no prior symptoms supports the slow growing, less aggressive nature of this lesion. Giant cell tumors are epiphyseal in location and uncommon in children with open physes. Fibrosarcoma is similar in appearance to osteosarcoma and is found in patients of ages 30–80 years.

Bibliography

Frassica FJ, Frassica DA, McCarthy EF. Orthopaedic pathology. In: Miller MD, Brinker MR (eds.), *Review of Orthopaedics*, 3rd ed. Philadelphia, PA: W.B. Saunders, 2000, 379–440.

Springfield DS, Bolander ME, Friedlaender GE, et al. Molecular and cellular biology of inflammation and neoplasia. In: Simon SR (ed.), *Orthopaedic Basic Science*. Rosemont, IL: American Academy of Orthopaedic Surgeons, 1994, 262–275.

Temple HT, Clohisy DR. Musculoskeletal oncology. In: Koval K (ed.), *Orthopaedic Knowledge Update 7*. Rosemont, IL: American Academy of Orthopaedic Surgeons, 2002, 159–171.

22. **(E)** Any time there is soft tissue injury or fracture of an extremity, a thorough neurologic assessment of the peripheral nerves is critical once the appropriate advanced trauma life support (ATLS) protocols have been followed. This should include a detailed assess-

ment of motor, sensory, and vascular status. This particular patient has a significant soft tissue injury involving the volar and ulnar aspects of the forearm. This creates suspicion for injury to the median nerve as well as the ulnar nerve based on their locations within the forearm. The median nerve enters the forearm by splitting the heads of the pronator teres muscle. It then runs down the forearm deep to the flexor digitorum superficialis and on the surface of the flexor digitorum profundus muscle. It provides sensory distribution to the hand as outlined in Fig. 37-14b. Motor innervation is provided proximally to the flexor carpi radialis (FCR), flexor digitorum superficialis (FDS), flexor digitorum profundus ([FDP] index and long). Distally, the motor innervation continues to the thenar eminence including the abductor pollicis brevis, flexor pollicis brevis, and opponens pollicis. The anterior interosseous is an important branch from the median nerve in the proximal aspect of the forearm. This courses distally to innervate the flexor pollicis longus, pronator quadratus, and the flexor digitorum profundus to the index and long fingers. The median nerve function cannot be evaluated by specific reflex testing.

The ulnar nerve travels along the medial aspect of the forearm on the flexor digitorum profundus muscle and deep to the flexor carpi ulnaris muscle. It lies in close proximity to the ulnar artery, which is just lateral. A dorsal cutaneous branch emerges from the ulnar nerve approximately 5–10 cm above the wrist. The intrinsic muscles of the hand allow the patient to cross his fingers and are innervated by the ulnar nerve. Urgent nerve conduction studies and an EMG are not practical in the ER and are unnecessary. Asking the patient to extend his thumb at the IP joint specifically involves the extensor pollicis longus, which is innervated by the radial nerve.

Only by assessing the most distal innervation of the median nerve, the abductor pollicis brevis, and by assessing sensation in the appropriate distribution can the integrity of the median nerve be evaluated. The motor and sensory innervations described above are summarized in Fig. 37-25.

Bibliography

Netter FH. *The Ciba Collection of Medical Illustrations. Volume 8—Musculoskeletal System, Part I: Anatomy Physiology and Metabolic Disorders*. Summit, NJ: Ciba-Geigy, 2001, 45–58.

23. **(B)** Fat embolism is the unexpected development of hypoxia, confusion, and petechiae within a few days after long bone fractures. It is usually seen 24–72 h following trauma. It occurs in 3–4% of patients with long

TABLE 37-3   Gurd and Wilson Criteria

Major Criteria	Minor Criteria
Hypoxemia (PaO2 < 60mm Hg)	Tachycardia > 110
CNS depression	Decreased hematocrit
Petechiae	Fever > 38.3 C
Pulmonary edema	Retinal emboli on fundoscopy
	Fat in urine
	Fat in sputum
	Thrombocytopenia

bone fractures and can be fatal in 10–15% of patients. FES seems to affect young adult patients with lower extremity fractures. Often the fractures are closed. FES consists of the triad of symptoms described above. Additional symptoms include tachypnea and tachycardia. Sixty percent of cases are seen in the first 24 h, and 90% appear within 72 h. Gurd and Wilson's criteria for FES are commonly referenced (Table 37-3). The diagnosis is made when one major and four minor signs are present in addition to macroglobulinemia. Use of these criteria is often criticized for not considering blood gas in the criteria. Lindeque et al. subsequently added this to their criteria. Clinically when PO_2 is less than 60 mmHg, the patient is in the early stages of FES.

Embolization of fat and marrow contents is part of the inciting events in FES; however, other events occur to cause the injury to the lungs, brain, and other tissues. Although these exact pathomechanics of FES have not been completely defined, two prevailing theories exist. The mechanical theory suggests that fat droplets enter the circulation and create a mechanical obstruction of the pulmonary vasculature because the droplets are larger than the small vessels in the lungs. The biomechanical theory postulates that mediators from the fracture site create a cascade of events that leads to activation of the clotting cascade and chemical injury to the vascular endothelial cells and subsequent increased pulmonary permeability.

Prevention is the key, and the development of FES can be prevented. Proper fracture splinting, use of oxygen in the postinjury period, and early surgical stabilization of long bone fractures are three measures that can reduce the incidence of FES. Large doses of steroids immediately after injury may have a beneficial effect on FES, most likely by reducing damage from free fatty acids; however, routine use of steroids is not without significant risks, which may outweigh the benefits. Therefore, currently treatment methods are mainly with oxygen and ventilatory support. High levels of positive end expiratory pressure (PEEP) are frequently required, and

early recognition is the key to preventing a potential devastating course of events.

Bibliography

Brinker MR. Basic sciences: section 6—perioperative problems. In: Miller MD, Brinker MR (eds.), *Review of Orthopaedics*, 3rd ed. Philadelphia, PA: W.B. Saunders, · 2000, 109.

Gurd AR, Wilson RI. The fat embolism syndrome. *J Bone Joint Surg* 1974;56:408–416.

Roberts CS, Gleis GE, Seligson D. Diagnosis and treatment of complications. In: Browner BD, Jupiter JB, Levine AE, et al. (eds.), *Skeletal Trauma*, 3rd ed. Philadelphia, PA: W.B. Saunders, 2003, 437–441.

Schemitsch EL, Bhandari M. Complications. In: Bucholz RW, Heckman JD (eds.), *Rockwood and Green's Fractures in Adults*, 5th ed. Philadelphia, PA: Lippincott, Williams & Wilkins, 2001, 479–489.

24. **(C)** Displaced femoral shaft fractures are best treated with intramedullary nailing. Closed intramedullary nailing involves minimal soft tissue dissection and provides stable fixation. An intramedullary nail is a load-sharing device and union rates of 99% with few complications. The nails should be locked statically. This does not impact fracture healing, and Brumback and associates have shown 10% of cases thought to be stable and locked dynamically resulted in rotation or shortening. A statically locked, antegrade intramedullary nail is the current standard of care for femoral shaft fractures.

Reaming of the femoral canal results in pulmonary embolization of fat and bone marrow contents. This leads to concern regarding exacerbation of an underlying pulmonary injury; however, technique, reamer design, and reamer sharpness all affect this degree of embolization, and the clinical significance is debated. This patient definitely has pulmonary injury. He has a pneumothorax, multiple rib injuries, and findings consistent with a pulmonary contusion. However, these findings should not prohibit the treatment of this patients femoral shaft fracture with an intramedullary nail. Although some concern has continued to focus on the possible negative effects of intramedullary nailing in trauma patients with an associated pulmonary injury, studies indicate that there is no effect on pulmonary injury with regard to the implant used. A delay in stabilization of the femur, however, limits mobilization of the patient, prolongs the hospital stay, and may subsequently worsen the pulmonary injury. Charash and associates have supported these findings. Bosse and associates looked at polytrauma patients with femoral shaft fractures with and without pulmonary injuries. Patients were managed at two institutions. One treated the femurs with plates and the other with reamed intramedullary nails. No difference was identified in the incidence of pulmonary complication. Additionally, an animal model has shown no significant difference in peak pressures generated within the canal comparing reamed to nonreamed nails.

Skeletal traction is rarely indicated as the only form of treatment. It is a rapid means to provide length and stability as a temporizing measure in unstable trauma patients. Definitive treatment with traction predisposes a patient to the added risks of remaining in bed. These risks are even magnified in the trauma patient. External fixation, likewise, is rarely indicated as definitive treatment. It is generally used acutely only as a temporary method of stabilization in a patient who has a vascular injury or may be hypothermic or coagulopathic, and requires further resuscitation. Once the patient is stabilized the external fixator is removed and converted to intramedullary fixation. External fixation may be used definitively in children, where open physes, preclude the use of intramedullary nails.

Bibliography

Bosse MJ, Mackenzie EJ, Riemer BL, et al. Adult respiratory distress syndrome, pneumonia, and mortality following thoracic injury and a femoral fracture treated either with intramedullary nailing with reaming or with a plate: a comparative study. *J Bone Joint Surg* 1997;79A:799–809.

Boulanger BR, Stephen D, Brenneman FD. Thoracic trauma and early intramedullary nailing of femur fractures: Are we doing harm? *J Trauma* 1997;43:24–28.

Brumback RJ, Reilly JP, Poka A, et al. Intramedullary nailing of femoral shaft fractures. Part 1. Decision making errors with interlocking fixation. *J Bone Joint Surg* 1988;70A:1441–1452.

Brumback RJ, Uwagie-Ero S, Lakatos RP, et al. Intramedullary nailing of femoral shaft fractures. Part II. Fracture healing with static interlocking fixation. *J Bone Joint Surg* 1988;70A:1453–1462.

Charash WE, Fabia TC, Croce MA. Delayed surgical fixation of femur fractures is a risk factor for pulmonary failure independent of thoracic trauma. *J Trauma* 1994;37:667–672.

Neudeck F, Wozasek GE, Obertacke U, et al. Nailing versus plating in thoracic trauma: an experimental study in sheep. *J Trauma* 1996;40:980–984.

25. **(E)** Humeral shaft fractures are a relatively common orthopedic occurrence. A variety of methods are available for the treatment of these fractures with good results. Increased concern develops when there is an associated neurovascular injury. The proximity of the brachial plexus and vascular structures of the shoulder make them vulnerable in an injury to the shoulder girdle. The radial nerve is the most vulnerable nerve in a shaft fracture because of its location as it spirals around the humerus as it descends through the upper arm. Radial nerve injury with a shaft fracture occurs in up to 18% of patients. The distal third, oblique shaft fracture (Holstein-Lewis) is the most widely associated with radial nerve injury; however, it is the middle third fracture that actually has the highest incidence of radial nerve palsy. Most nerve injuries are true "palsies" or neuropraxias. Electromyography studies can help evaluate the degree of nerve injury and follow the recovery; however, most recover in 3–4 months. For this reason the treatment of a closed fracture with a nerve palsy is not an indication for surgery and most fractures will heal with nonoperative treatment and most of the nerve deficits will resolve. Historically, a nerve palsy that develops following manipulation has been considered an indication for open treatment; however, observation is currently recommended. The only absolute indication for surgical treatment is an open fracture with a nerve injury. Surgical exploration of a nerve injury is generally recommended after 3–4 months if there has been no recovery.

The radial nerve begins as the terminating branch of the posterior cord of the brachial plexus. It contains nerve bundles from nerve roots C5 to T1, the entire brachial plexus. It passes with the deep brachial artery through the triangular interval formed by the long and lateral heads of the triceps and the lower border of the teres major muscles. It then comes in close proximity to the bone as it lies in the groove for the radial nerve on the posterior aspect of the humerus. It is here where it can become lacerated by fracture fragments or become entrapped between fracture fragments.

An accurate understanding of radial innervation allows a thorough examination and subsequent management if a deficit is identified. The radial nerve provides no innervation in the proximal arm. The sensory distribution is most reliably tested in the dorsal web space between the thumb and index finger. The motor innervation generally involves all extensors of the wrist and hand, and any deficit in extension of the wrist or fingers is indicative of injury to the radial nerve. Inability to flex the thumb at the IP joint indicates anterior interosseous nerve injury and loss of the flexor pollicis longus. This is seen in supracondylar humerus fractures in children. Decreased sensation over the volar aspect of the thumb and index finger represents the median nerve distribution. The ulnar nerve innervates the small finger and ulnar border of the ring finger. Injury to this nerve may occasionally be seen in injuries about the elbow. The lateral antebrachial cutaneous nerve, the terminal branch of the musculocutaneous nerve, innervates the lateral border of the forearm.

Bibliography

Dirschl DR. Shoulder trauma: bone. In: Koval KJ (ed.), *Orthopaedic Knowledge Update 7*. Rosemont, IL: American Academy of Orthopaedic Surgeons, 2002, 267–269.

Gregory PR Jr. Fractures of the shaft of the humerus. In: Bucholz RW, Heckman JD (eds.), *Rockwood and Green's Fractures in Adults*, 5th ed. Philadelphia, PA: Lippincott, Williams & Wilkins, 2001, 991–992.

Netter FH. *The Ciba Collection of Medical Illustrations. Volume 8—Musculoskeletal System, Part I: Anatomy Physiology and Metabolic Disorders*. Summit, NJ: Ciba-Geigy, 2001, 28–31, 38–39, 53.

Schemitsch EL, Bhandari M. Complications. In: Browner BD, Jupiter JB, Levine AE, et al. (eds.), *Skeletal Trauma*, 3rd ed. Philadelphia, PA: W.B. Saunders, 2003, 1504–1505.

26. **(C)** This patient sustained a posterior hip dislocation. The postreduction pelvic radiograph shows asymmetry in the medial hip joint space. The CT scan confirms that there is an interposed fragment between the femoral head and posterior wall of the acetabulum. In this situation the appropriate management would include an arthrotomy to retrieve to loose body or possibly hip arthroscopy to remove the fragment.

    Traction followed by restricted weight bearing would place the patient at risk for the multiple complications associated with prolonged bed rest, and still do nothing to alleviate the incarcerated fragment. An MRI scan may be helpful in the future if a patient with otherwise normal radiographs continues to have problems following a hip dislocation. It may identify a labral tear or other soft tissue irregularity. Acutely, however, this would only confirm what is already visible on the CT scan. Immediate progressive weight bearing is the treatment for a patient with an uncomplicated hip dislocation. Examination under anesthesia would likewise not alleviate the entrapped loose body.

Bibliography

Ebraheim NA, Savolaine ER, Skie MC, et al. Soft-tissue window to enhance visualization of entrapped osteocartilaginous fragments in the hip joint. *Orthop Rev* 1993; 22:1017–1021.

Egol KA, Koval KJ. Hip: trauma. In: Koval KJ (ed.), *Orthopaedic Knowledge Update 7*. Rosemont, IL: American Academy of Orthopaedic Surgeons, 2002, 410–412.

Epstein HC, Wiss DA, Cozen L. Posterior fracture dislocation of the hip with fractures of the femoral head. *Clin Orthop* 1985;201:9–17.

Goulet JA, Levin PE. Hip dislocations. In: Browner BD, Jupiter JB, Levine AE, et al. (eds.), *Skeletal Trauma*, 3rd ed. Philadelphia, PA: W.B. Saunders, 2003, 1657–1690.

Leighton RK, Lammens P. Hip dislocations and fractures of the femoral head. In: Kellam JF, Fischer TJ, Tornetta P III (eds.), *Orthopaedic Knowledge Update: Trauma 2*. Rosemont, IL: American Academy of Orthopaedic Surgeons, 2000, 311–314.

Motley GS, Eddings TH III, Moore RS. Adult trauma. In: Miller MD, Brinker MR (eds.), *Review of Orthopaedics*, 3rd ed. Philadelphia, PA: W.B. Saunders, 2000, 476–477.

Tornetta P III. Hip dislocations and fractures of the femoral head. In: Bucholz RW, Heckman JD (eds.), *Rockwood and Green's Fractures in Adults*, 5th ed. Philadelphia, PA: Lippincott, Williams & Wilkins, 2001, 1547–1576.

27. **(E)** High-energy pelvic injuries are associated with significant injury to the surrounding soft tissues, and can lead to disruption of the pelvic floor. This should lead to suspicion for a possible urethral injury. Associated urologic injury occurs in up to 15% of pelvic fractures, and is more common in males. The most common physical findings of urethral disruption are high riding prostate and blood at the meatus. Hematuria may also be found and is more indicative of bladder injury. Occasionally inability to freely pass a Foley may be the first sign of injury. In a hemodynamically stable male patient, a retrograde urethrogram should be obtained prior to placing a Foley catheter. In a hemodynamically unstable male patient, one attempt at placement of a Foley catheter is considered. Placement of a Foley catheter can be attempted in females without obtaining an urethrogram because the urethra is short.

    This patient has a pelvic fracture with associated perineal swelling, a scrotal hematoma, and blood at the meatus; therefore, a retrograde urethrogram should be obtained prior to inserting a Foley catheter. Inserting a Foley catheter should only be performed after a urethral injury has been ruled out, and this is most accurately done through a retrograde urethrogram. This patient's retrograde urethrogram (Fig. 37-18c) confirms the suspected genitourinary injury.

    An IVP would not provide sufficient information about the lower genitourinary tract. A pelvic external fixator is a key component of management of a hemodynamically unstable patient, but would not assist in evaluating the lower genitourinary tract. It would provide stability to the pelvis; however, this could be temporarily performed with use of a sheet or pelvic binder. The placement of an external fixator or definitive open reduction and fixation of the pelvic fracture should be coordinated with the urologist. Proper communication will allow simultaneous management and hopefully definitive care of the urologic injury and the fracture. CT scans of the abdomen without contrast do not adequately image general urinary tract trauma.

Bibliography

Jones AL, Burgess AR. Fractures of the pelvic ring. In: Bucholz RW, Heckman JD (eds.), *Rockwood and Green's Fractures in Adults*, 5th ed. Philadelphia, PA: Lippincott, Williams & Wilkins, 2001, 1495–1496.

Kellam JF, Mayo K. Pelvic ring disruptions. In: Browner BD, Jupiter JB, Levine AE, et al. (eds.), *Skeletal Trauma*, 3rd ed. Philadelphia, PA: W.B. Saunders, 2003, 1102.

Moorhouse DD. Injuries to the urethra and urinary bladder associated with fractures of the pelvis. *Can J Surg* 1988;31:85–88.

Tornetta P III, Templeman D. Pelvis and acetabulum: trauma. In: Koval KJ (ed.), *Orthopaedic Knowledge Update 7*. Rosemont, IL: American Academy of Orthopaedic Surgeons, 2002, 395–396.

Watnik NF, Coburn M, Goldberger M. Urologic injuries in pelvic ring disruptions. *Clin Orthop* 1996;329:37–45.

28. **(D)** The most widely used system or scale to assess traumatic brain injury is the GCS. The scores range from 3 to 15 with 15 being normal. The scale is summarized in Table 37-4. The GCS is also used in the revised trauma score, which can help project patient outcome.

Bibliography

Brautigam RT, Ciraulo DL, Jacobs LM. Evaluation and treatment of the multiple-trauma patient. In: Browner BD, Jupiter JB, Levine AE, et al. (eds.), *Skeletal Trauma*, 3rd ed. Philadelphia, PA: W.B. Saunders, 2003, 122.

Teasdale G, Jennett B. Assessment of coma and impaired consciousness: a practical scale. *Lancet* 1974;2:81–84.

29. **(A)** The orthopedic surgeon should become involved in the care of a patient with a pelvic fracture as soon as possible, and preferably in the ER. In a review of 210

TABLE 37-4   Glasgow Coma Scale

Level of Consciousness		Score
Eye Opening	Opens spontaneously	4
	Opens to voice	3
	Opens to painful stimuli	2
	No eye response	1
Best Verbal Response	Oriented conversation	5
	Confused conversation	4
	Inappropriate words	3
	Incomprehensible sounds	2
	No verbal response	1
Best Motor Response	Obeys simple commands	6
	Localizes painful stimuli	5
	Withdraws painful stimuli	4
	Decorticate	3
	Decerebrate	2
	No motor response	1

pelvic fracture patients, only two patients died directly from the pelvic injury. Although the most common direct cause of mortality in patients with pelvic fractures is head and thorax injuries, pelvic bleeding can be a significant contributing factor and did contribute to the death in 10 additional patients. Normotensive pelvic injury patients have a 3% mortality rate; patients with a systolic pressure <90 mmHg have a 38% mortality rate.

The management of an unstable pelvic injury begins in the field with appropriate resuscitation and some form of external support. Although military anitshock trousers can be used, a towel or sheet with a clamp can be just as effective. The pneumatic devices can be associated with impaired ventilation and compartment syndrome (CS) of the lower extremity. Careful deflation is also required to avoid a rapid increase in intravascular space and the subsequent development of shock. Most pelvic bleeding is venous in nature and use of sheet and towel clamp, traction, an external fixator, or a combination can help to stabilize a mechanically and hemodynamically unstable pelvic injury. The external fixator is an effective means of temporary stabilization, and Riemer has shown patients with similar ISSs showed a decrease in mortality with the use of an external fixator in patients with pelvic fractures.

Surgeons must be familiar with the pelvic anatomy prior to attempting external fixation. Fluoroscopic assistance can also be used as a guide for placement. Studies have shown a reduced rate of mortality and transfusion requirements with the use of an emergency external fixator in unstable patients. When possible, the fixator should ideally be placed before any surgical procedures begin, including patients about to undergo laparotomy; however, it should never delay emergency laparotomy.

Continued unexplained hemodynamic instability despite fracture stabilization and adequate resuscitation requires angiography. A heightened sense of awareness and suspicion for arterial injury can facilitate preparation and allow for timely embolization of arterial bleeders. The definitive treatment of a mechanically unstable pelvic fractures requires ORIF.

Bibliography

Burgess AR, Eastridge BJ, Young JW, et al. Pelvic ring disruptions: effective classification system and treatment protocols. *J Trauma* 1990;30:848–856.

Flint L, Babikian G, Anders M, et al. Definitive control of mortality from severe pelvic fracture. *Ann Surg* 1990;211:703–707.

Pohlemann T, Gansslen A, Bosch U, et al. The technique of packing for control of hemorrhage in complex pelvic fractures. *Tech Orthop* 1994;9:267–270.

Poole GV, Ward EF, Muakkassa FF, et al. Pelvic fracture from major blunt trauma: outcome is determined by associated injuries. *Ann Surg* 1991;213:532–539.

Riemer BL, Butterfield SL, Diamond DL, et al. Acute mortality associated with injuries to the pelvic ring: the role of early patient mobilization and external fixation. *J Trauma* 1993;35:671–677.

Templeman D, Lang R, Harms B. Lower-extremity compartment syndromes associated with the use of pneumatic antishock garments. *J Trauma* 1987;27:79–81.

30. **(A)** At the time of fracture, there is mechanical failure of the bone. In addition, the blood supply to the bone at the fracture site is disrupted. The surrounding soft tissues become a critical component in the healing process. The biology of fracture repair is actually a regenerative process in which the injured bone is replaced by bone rather than scar tissue as in most other organs of the body. This regeneration of bone goes through four stages: inflammation, soft callous, hard callous, and remodeling.

Inflammation begins at the time of injury with the development of clot, hematoma, and the appearance of osteoprogenitor cells at the fracture site. Blood vessels of the surrounding periosteal callus develop in the beginning stages of angiogenesis. The soft callus phase of healing begins when pain and swelling subside and lasts until the bony fragments are united by fibrous or cartilaginous tissue, and there is no longer free motion between the segments. This period involves are large increase in vascularity at the fracture site. Stage 3, hard callus, is a continuum from stage 2 as the callus is converted from cartilaginous tissue to woven bone. The final stage, bone remodeling, involves the conversion of woven bone to lamellar bone and reconstitution of the medullary canal. This final stage may take years as the bone remodels according to Wolf's law.

The mechanism of injury often relates to the fracture pattern and can indirectly affect the healing process; however, this is through its impact on the blood supply. This becomes evident when there is significant soft tissue injury, such as an open fracture. In this situation, meticulous soft tissue handling and limited exposure at the time of ORIF can protect the remaining soft tissues and associated blood supply. Oxygen is needed for cell viability, and this is directly related to blood supply. No matter how rigid the fixation, bone cannot heal without an adequate blood supply. While the other options may influence healing, the most important factor is clearly blood supply.

Bibliography

Buckwalter JA, Einhorn TA, Simon SR (eds.), *Orthopaedic Basic Science: Biology and Biomechanics of the Musculoskeletal System*, 2nd ed. Rosemont, IL: American Academy of Orthopaedic Surgeons, 2000, 372–399.

31. **(E)** Hip dislocations must be assessed with a high index of suspicion for a femoral head fracture. Posterior femoral head dislocations are associated with a 7% incidence of femoral head fracture. Although much rarer, anterior dislocations are associated with a higher rate of fracture. Radiographs should include an AP pelvis and AP and lateral views of the injured hip. By uncovering some overlap of the hip and pelvis, Judet-views may uncover a fracture not easily visible on the initial films.

The most important task is prompt reduction of the femoral head. Like hip dislocations, femoral head reduction should be considered an orthopedic emergency and reduction should be accomplished as quickly and atraumatically as possible. This may be performed with adequate conscious sedation in the emergency department; however, generally anesthesia is warranted if any difficulty is encountered. Care must also be taken to avoid possible displacement of an associated nondisplaced femoral neck fracture. If a hip dislocation is irreversible and associated with a femoral head fracture, treatment requires open reduction, usually from the direction of the dislocation. Following reduction, an AP radiograph can evaluate concentricity of the hip joint. A CT scan is necessary to assess the quality of reduction in addition to evaluate any potential loosed body within the joint.

The most commonly used classification system is that of Pipkin (Table 37-5). This system divides the femoral head fractures at the fovea, and identifies the location of the fracture, which correlates with initial treatment. The preferred treatment is anatomic reduction. When this is achieved following closed reduction, nonoperative treatment can be successful. ORIF is otherwise the standard (Fig. 37-18*b*), as opposed to excision of the fragment. Any step off or deformity at the fracture is not well tolerated and can lead to increased risk of posttraumatic arthritis. Type III fractures require fixation of the femoral neck fracture, followed by ORIF of the femoral head. In type IV fractures, the treatment depends on the type of acetabulum fracture. The risk of posttraumatic

TABLE 37-5 Pipkin Classification of Femoral Head Fractures

Class	Description	Initial Treatment
Type I	Fracture of the femoral head below the fovea	Closed reduction
Type II	Fracture of the femoral head above the fovea	Closed reduction
Type III	Type I or II associated with a femoral neck fracture	Open reduction
Type IV	Type I, II, or III associated with an acetabulum fracture	Closed reduction

arthritis and osteonecrosis are high. Type I fractures and type II fractures have rates similar to simple dislocations. Type III fractures have a poor prognosis with 50% rate of posttraumatic osteonecrosis. Type IV fractures have about the same prognosis as the acetabular fracture.

Bibliography

Egol KA, Koval KJ. Hip: trauma. In: Koval KJ (ed.), *Orthopaedic Knowledge Update 7*. Rosemont, IL: American Academy of Orthopaedic Surgeons, 2002, 407–408.

Leighton RK, Lammens P. Hip dislocations and fractures of the femoral head. In: Kellam JF, Fischer TJ, Tornetta P III (eds.), *Orthopaedic Knowledge Update: Trauma 2*. Rosemont, IL: American Academy of Orthopaedic Surgeons, 2000, 314–316.

Motley GS, Eddings TH III, Moore RS. Adult trauma. In: Miller MD, Brinker MR (eds.), *Review of Orthopaedics*, 3rd ed. Philadelphia, PA: W.B. Saunders, 2000, 477.

Swiontkowski MF. Intracapsular hip fractures. In: Browner BD, Jupiter JB, Levine AE, et al. (eds.), *Skeletal Trauma*, 3rd ed. Philadelphia, PA: W.B. Saunders, 2003, 1700–1714.

Tornetta P III. Hip dislocations and fractures of the femoral head. In: Bucholz RW, Heckman JD (eds.), *Rockwood and Green's Fractures in Adults*, 5th ed. Philadelphia, PA: Lippincott, Williams & Wilkins, 2001, 1547–1576.

32. **(A)** Acute CS is defined as elevated tissue pressures within a closed, nondistensible space or compartment. This can reduce muscle and nerve tissue perfusion below levels necessary for tissue viability. The most common causes are fractures, soft tissue trauma, arterial injury, limb compression, burns, and bleeding disorders. Chronic exertional compartment syndrome (CECS) is a reversible elevation of tissue pressure brought on by exercise and returning to normal between periods of activity. It is most common in long distance runners and military recruits. Iatrogenic CS can result from tight closure of fascial defects, excessive traction of fractured limbs, IV infiltration, and circumferential casts/splints.

Although the mechanism of ACS and CECS may differ, the pathogenesis is similar. Swelling and edema within the compartment cause increased tissue pressure. Increased tissue pressure leads to increased local venous pressure. As venous pressure increases the A-V pressure gradient is decreased and can result in decreased local blood flow. Capillary basement membranes may become leaky compounding the problem. If blood flow drops below metabolic demands, the tissues become ischemic and viability is compromised. Clinically, this results in pain, dysfunction, dysaesthesia, and potentially muscle necrosis.

The clinical diagnosis of CS may be obvious; however, the variability in signs and symptoms may make the diagnosis difficult. It remains, however, primarily a clinical diagnosis. Severe pain out of proportion to injury is the hallmark of acute CS. A swollen and tense compartment that is painful to palpation is also a finding. Pain with passive stretch is a reliable sign in an alert patient. Parasthesias or weakness because of nerve or muscle ischemia is a late finding. Intracompartmental pressures rarely exceed systolic blood pressure, so peripheral pulses are present and an absent pulse is never a finding unless there is an associated arterial injury. In addition, digital capillaries may drain into extracompartmental veins, so capillary refill is not a good indicator of tissue perfusion within a compartment. Capillary refill may be slow but is often normal.

Diagnosis becomes more difficult in an unconscious or obtunded patient. Without the benefit of appropriate history and assessment from examination, measurement of compartment pressures becomes the only means to diagnose the condition. There are several methods of measurement available; however, uniform consensus as to when fasciotomy is warranted is lacking. Normal pressures range from 0 to 10 mmHg, and pressures from 30 to 45 mmHg have been recommended as threshold for decompression. Others have recommended decompression when pressures are within 10 to 30 mmHg of the patient's diastolic pressure. The use of 30 to 35 mmHg as an absolute pressure may be adequate; however, the patient's clinical status and diastolic blood pressure must be considered. McQueen and Court-Brown have shown the difference between diastolic pressure and the measured pressure is the most reliable.

It is critical to remove any tight or constricting dressings on a patient with symptoms of CS. Limb position should be at the level of the heart to promote arterial inflow. It has been shown that elevation reduces mean arterial pressure and as a result reduces blood flow to the compartment.

CS is the most common in the leg, but may occur in the forearm, hand, foot, thigh, arm, shoulder, and buttocks. Management is by surgical decompression of the involved compartments. Skin, fat, and fascial layers must all be decompressed. Fasciotomy wounds should be left open, and repeat inspection and debridement is performed after 48 h. There are various mechanical methods available to assist with closure, but this is ultimately by delayed skin closure or split thickness skin grafts.

Pain associated with a tense and swollen compartment and worsening pain with passive stretch are the earliest findings in an acute CS. Surgical decompression is the standard treatment for CS, and if delayed, irreversible damage to muscle or nerves may occur.

Bibliography

Amendola A, Twaddle BC. Compartment syndromes. In: Browner BD, Jupiter JB, Levine AE, et al. (eds.), *Skeletal Trauma*, 3rd ed. Philadelphia, PA: W.B. Saunders, 2003, 268–290.

Heppenstall RB, McCombs PR, DeLaurentis DA. Vascular injuries and compartment syndromes. In: Bucholz RW, Heckman JD (eds.), *Rockwood and Green's Fractures in Adults*, 5th ed. Philadelphia, PA: Lippincott, Williams & Wilkins, 2001, 331–350.

Lang GJ. Fractures of the tibial diaphysis. In: Kellam JF, Fischer TJ, Tornetta P III (eds.), *Orthopaedic Knowledge Update: Trauma 2*. Rosemont, IL: American Academy of Orthopaedic Surgeons, 2000, 185–186.

Lang GJ. Knee and leg: bone trauma. In: Koval KJ (ed.), *Orthopaedic Knowledge Update 7*. Rosemont, IL: American Academy of Orthopaedic Surgeons, 2002, 487.

Miller MD. Sports medicine. In: Miller MD, Brinker MR (eds.), *Review of Orthopaedics*, 3rd ed. Philadelphia, PA: W.B. Saunders, 2000, 213.

Motley GS, Eddings TH III, Moore RS. Adult trauma. In: Miller MD, Brinker MR (eds.), *Review of Orthopaedics*, 3rd ed. Philadelphia, PA: W.B. Saunders, 2000, 463.

Netter FH. *The Ciba Collection of Medical Illustrations. Volume 8—Musculoskeletal System, Part I: Anatomy Physiology and Metabolic Disorders*. Summit, NJ: Ciba-Geigy, 2001, 98–103.

33. **(A)** More than 60% of the surface of the talus is covered with articular cartilage, and there are no muscles that attach to the talus. It is supported by its bony architecture and ligamentous restraints between the tibia and the calcaneus. Three major arteries supply the talar body by forming a vascular ring at the neck of the talus. The artery of the tarsal canal arises from the posterior tibial artery. The deltoid artery may be the only remaining circulation in many fractures of the talus. The third, the sinus tarsi artery arises from the anterior and peroneal arteries. The circulation to the talar body is vulnerable in fractures and dislocations. This is in part because of the retrograde flow that must occur to supply the body from the circulation at the neck.

Fractures may occur in any part of the talus, but more than 50% involve the neck. The Hawkins classification system is the most commonly used. Displaced talar neck fractures are an orthopedic emergency, and urgent reduction is required to restore circulation. Anatomic alignment of the fracture is one of the most important factors affecting outcome, and there is debate as to whether a nondisplaced talar neck fracture truly exists.

The preferred approach uses medial and lateral incisions to restore anatomic alignment, assess the degree of comminution, explore, and debride the subtalar joint of any debris, and finally insert hardware. Early range of motion is encouraged, and patients are kept nonweightbearing until union at the fracture site.

Among the complications encountered include delayed union and nonunion, arthritis, malunion, and osteonecrosis. Delayed union occurs when there is no healing evident at 6 months and nonunion with no healing at 12 months. Arthritis has been reported to occur 50% in the subtalar joint, 33% tibiotalar joint, and 25% both. Malunion involves varus malposition, which results in hindfoot varus and forefoot adduction. Patients are forced to walk on the lateral border of their foot. A custom orthosis may relieve the subsequent pain, but often osteotomy or fusions are required and can be unpredictable. Finally, osteonecrosis is related to the severity of the injury and subsequent disruption of circulation. During follow-up, an AP radiograph of the ankle at 6–8 weeks may reveal subchondral lucency (Hawkins sign) within the talus. This is a positive finding indicating there is restoration of circulation to the talar body. Absence of the sign, however, does not absolutely indicate osteonecrosis. If osteonecrosis is diagnosed after 3 months, patients are not kept nonweightbearing. There is no evidence indicating that outcome is improved with prolonged nonweightbearing. If patients go on to develop collapse, salvage is usually with a tibiotalar or tibiocalcaneal fusion.

Bibliography

Baumhauer JF, Geppert MJ, Michelson JD, et al. Ankle and foot: trauma. In: Koval KJ (ed.), *Orthopaedic Knowledge Update 7*. Rosemont, IL: American Academy of Orthopaedic Surgeons, 2002, 553.

DiGiovanni CW, Benirschke SK, Hansen ST. Foot injuries. In: Browner BD, Jupiter JB, Levine AE, et al. (eds.), *Skeletal Trauma*, 3rd ed. Philadelphia, PA: W.B. Saunders, 2003, 2379–2397.

Heckman JD. Fractures of the talus. In: Bucholz RW, Heckman JD (eds.), *Rockwood and Green's Fractures in Adults*, 5th ed. Philadelphia, PA: Lippincott, Williams & Wilkins, 2001, 2091–2128.

Motley GS, Eddings TH III, Moore RS. Adult trauma. In: Miller MD, Brinker MR (eds.), *Review of Orthopaedics*, 3rd ed. Philadelphia, PA: W.B. Saunders, 2000, 491–493.

Stephen DJG. Ankle and foot injuries. In: Kellam JF, Fischer TJ, Tornetta P III (eds.), *Orthopaedic Knowledge Update: Trauma 2*. Rosemont, IL: American Academy of Orthopaedic Surgeons, 2000, 210–213.

34. **(E)** The most likely structure injured during this dissection for the lymph node biopsy is the cranial nerve XI, which is the spinal accessory nerve. It exits the cranium through the foramen magnum and supplies the motor innervation to the sternocleidomastoid and trapezius muscles. A significant function of the trapezius is shoulder elevation, and injury would lead to

loss of this function. The supraspinatus muscle is an important component of the rotator cuff that functions to initiate shoulder abduction and stabilize the shoulder during continued abduction. It is unlikely dissection would continue to the level of the supraspinatus and shoulder abduction would be impacted greater than elevation. The suprascapular nerve passes over the scapula deep to the transverse ligament at the suprascapular notch and then through the spinoglenoid notch innervating the supraspinatus and infraspinatus muscles. Compression results in posterior shoulder pain and weakness in external rotation. Injury to this nerve would lead to loss of function in these respective muscles and subsequent weakness with abduction and external rotation. The axillary nerve remains deep in the axilla beneath the humeral head anteriorly. It then courses laterally around the proximal humerus to innervate the deltoid and teres minor muscles. Injury would be extremely unlikely and would lead primarily to loss of abduction from deltoid weakness. It is unlikely that injury to the trapezius muscle directly would be significant enough to result in damage to the entire muscle and complete loss of function. Electromyographic studies could be used in this case to help confirm the clinical diagnosis.

Bibliography

Chandawarkar RY, Cervino AL, Pennington GA. Management of iatrogenic injury to the spinal accessory nerve. *Plast Reconstr Surg* 2003;111(2):611–617.

Novak CB, Mackinnon SE. Patient outcome after surgical management of an accessory nerve injury. *Otolaryngol Head Neck Surg* 2002;127(3):221–224.

Yavuzer G, Tuncer S. Accessory nerve injury as a complication of cervical lymph node biopsy. *Am J Phys Med Rehabil* 2001;80(8):622–623.

35. **(D)** An open fracture involves one in which a break in the skin and underlying soft tissues leads to direct communication with the bone. An open fracture found on the same extremity with a confirmed fracture should be considered open until proven otherwise. As with any extremity, the neurovascular status should be thoroughly documented. Following this, any deformity or dislocation should be immediately reduced. If there are obvious foreign bodies or debris in the wound they should be removed with a sterile instrument. The wound should then be dressed with a sterile dressing and an appropriate splint applied. If there will be significant delay before entering the OR a brief irrigation may be performed prior to dressing the wound. The sterile dressing should then be left in place until the patient enters the OR. No further wound inspection is necessary. Digital or polaroid photos can be used to communicate findings on inspection. Studies have found a 4.3% infection rate in open wounds covered immediately and an 18% infection rate in wounds that were left exposed until the time of surgery. The only exception is when a patient is transferred with an inappropriate dressing or splint and this must be changed. The use of betadine or providine dressings may interfere with osteoblasts function so it should be used only in cases of extreme contamination. Cultures of the wound are no longer indicated.

Open fractures are classified based on the Gustilo classification system. Type I result from low energy and the wound is 1 cm or less. Type II involves higher energy and the wound is less than 10 cm. Type III open fractures are subclassified. Type IIIA injuries result from high energy, and the wounds are greater than 10 cm. Type IIIB is a wound that requires a soft tissue procedure for coverage, and type IIIC injuries have an associated vascular injury. Any significant contamination, comminution, or known high-energy injury is automatically classified as type III because treatment and outcome parallel a type III injury versus a type I or type II. Although this system uses wound size, the degree of energy with which the injury occurred and the amount of injury to the surrounding soft tissue is probably more critical.

Treatment ultimately is with surgical irrigation and debridement is a systematic fashion involving the skin, subcutaneous tissues, fascia, muscle, and ultimately bone. Care to preserve the remaining soft tissues is vital fracture healing as well as potential wound closure. The initial treatment begins with the dressing and antibiotics, which should be considered therapeutic not prophylactic. The goal is to kill bacteria that have contaminated the wound, and to prevent growth to a point where the number of organisms is below the threshold level of developing an infection. The antibiotics do not take the place of an adequate debridement.

In the ER, a first generation cephalosporin antibiotic is recommended for all type I and type II fractures. The use of an aminoglycoside is recommended for all type III fractures. If suspicion is high for possible anaerobic contamination, penicillin or Flagyl is added. The duration of use is debated, but often antibiotics are continued anywhere from 24 to 72 h after wound closure.

Bibliography

Gustilo RB, Anderson JT. Prevention of infection in the treatment of one thousand and twenty five open fractures of long bones: retrospective and prospective analyses. *J Bone Joint Surg* 1976;58:453–458.

Gustilo RB, Mendoza RM, Williams DN. Problems in the management of type III (severe) open fractures: a new classification of type III open fractures. *J Trauma* 1984;24:742–746.

Kaysinger KK, Nicholson NC, Ramp WK, et al. Toxic effects of wound irrigation and solutions on cultured tibiae and osteoblasts. *J Orthop Trauma* 1995;10:298–303.

Lee J. Efficacy of cultures in the management of open fractures. *Clin Orthop* 1997;339:71–75.

Olson SA, Finkemeier CG, Moehring HD. Open fractures. In: Bucholz RW, Heckman JD (eds.), *Rockwood and Green's Fractures in Adults*, 5th ed. Philadelphia, PA: Lippincott, Williams & Wilkins, 2001, 285–314.

Tscherne H, Gotzen L. The management of open fractures. *Fractures with Soft Tissue Injuries*. New York, NY: Springer-Verlag, 1984.

36. **(D)** Tibial shaft fractures can result from low-energy mechanisms such as a twist and fall or from the more common high-energy mechanisms such as a fall from a height, or motor vehicle or motorcycle accident. This is the most common long bone fracture. The treatment of tibial shaft fractures tends to parallel the injury. The higher the energy, the more likely surgical intervention is indicated. Low energy, minimally or nondisplaced fractures are amenable to cast treatment. Soft tissue management is very important in the treatment of this fracture.

Closed treatment guidelines commonly referred to include angular alignment of 5 degrees or less, rotational alignment of 10 degrees or less, and 10 mm or less of shortening. Among the indications for surgery include failure of closed treatment or unacceptable alignment, polytrauma patients, ipsilateral femoral shaft fracture, open injuries, and fractures with vascular injury or CS. Plate fixation has been less commonly used for shaft fractures because of slowed healing rates and increased time to weight bearing. External fixation can be used in open fractures with severe soft tissue injuries including burns and CS or in patients with multiple injuries to provide rapid stabilization. The most common complication is pin tract infection, reported in up to 50% of patients. Obtaining bone-to-bone contact at the factor is the most critical factor that impacts stability of the construct. Intramedullary nailing is considered the gold standard of operative treatment. Reaming is generally standard for closed fractures; however, it is debatable for open fractures.

Nonunion and delayed union rates increase with the bone loss, associated fibula fractures, comminution, and open fractures. Reports range from 2 to 5%. Infection rates are often related to the degree of soft tissue injury and range from 1 to 3%. CS is occasionally associated with tibial shaft fractures. The incidence ranges from 1 to 9%. This can occur in both open and closed fractures, and is more common in the high-energy group. Malunion can lead to degenerative changes within the knee and ankle as a result of the malalignment. With proper surgical technique the rates are from 2 to 5%.

Knee pain is now recognized as the most common complication following intramedullary nailing of tibial fractures, and was first described by Keating, and by Court-Brown and associates. Some studies report rates from 40 to 56%. It can often lead to removal of hardware in these patients following fracture union. In one study, this lead to resolution of pain in 45%, partial relief in 35%, and no relief in 20% of patients. The other complications described above occur much less commonly.

Bibliography

Court-Brown CM, Gustilo T, Shaw AD. Knee pain after intramedullary tibial nailing: its incidence, etiology, and outcome. *J Orthop Trauma* 1997;11:103–105.

Keating JF, Orfaly R, O'Brien PJ. Knee pain after tibial nailing. *J Orthop Trauma* 1997;11:10–13.

Lang GJ. Fractures of the tibial diaphysis. In: Kellam JF, Fischer TJ, Tornetta P III (eds.), *Orthopaedic Knowledge Update: Trauma 2*. Rosemont, IL: American Academy of Orthopaedic Surgeons, 2000, 177–186.

Motley GS, Eddings TH III, Moore RS. Adult trauma. In: Miller MD, Brinker MR (eds.), *Review of Orthopaedics*, 3rd ed. Philadelphia, PA: W.B. Saunders, 2000, 489–491.

Sarmiento A, Sharpe FE, Ebramzadeh E, et al. Factors influencing the outcome of closed tibial fractures treated with functional bracing. *Clin Orthop* 1995;315:8–24.

Van der Schoot DKE, Den Outer AJ, et al. Degenerative changes at the knee and ankle related to malunion of tibial fractures. *J Bone Joint Surg.* 1996;78B:722–725.

Watson JT. Treatment of unstable tibial fractures of the shaft of the tibia. *J Bone Joint Surg* 1994;76A:1575–1584.

37. **(A)** A pathologic fracture is one that occurs in abnormal bone. These fractures often result from minimal to no trauma, and may even occur during events of everyday normal activity. This history should raise suspicion for an underlying pathologic condition. OP is the most common condition associated with pathologic fractures. Other conditions include Paget's disease, osteomalacia, osteogenesis imperfecta, osteopetrosis, a primary bone lesion, and metastatic bone lesions.

Plain radiographs should be closely evaluated. The lesion may have an obvious diagnosis; however, the entire extent of the bone should be examined, and often the remainder of the skeleton when the lesion appears metastatic. Impending fractures at other sites can easily be missed. The spine, ribs, pelvis, femur, and humerus are the most common sites of metastasis to bone. Plain radiographs of these sites will help to further evaluate the skeleton.

Further identification of the primary lesion is important. A bone scan can be obtained as a screen for the entire skeleton. It is the most efficient means to identify occult metastatic sites. Additional hot spots should be more closely evaluated. A chest radiograph, breast examination, and mammogram can assess for metastatic breast and lung carcinoma, the two most common metastases to bone. Renal, thyroid, and prostate are the other three tumors also found as metastatic lesions to bone. A careful physical examination, baseline laboratory studies, PSA, and abdominal ultrasound or chest CT scan will further identify most of these primary sites. Biopsy will ultimately confirm these findings.

In pathologic fractures the goal is to provide surgical stabilization. This is more difficult in the diseased bone. In addition, pathologic bone heals more slowly than normal bone. Often there may be hardware failure prior to healing. All patients should also receive adjuvant irradiation beginning about 3 weeks after surgery. This does not seem to increase the incidence of nonunions. Long bone fractures are generally stabilized with an intramedullary implant when available, as this provides a load sharing construct as well as prophylactic fixation for the entire length of the bone. Another component of preoperative assessment includes the need for embolization. Renal cell carcinoma is extremely vascular and can result in significant intraoperative blood loss. In this situation a known primary or suspicion of renal cell carcinoma requires an angiogram and embolization.

Bibliography

Springfield DS. Pathologic fractures. In: Bucholz RW, Heckman JD (eds.), *Rockwood and Green's Fractures in Adults*, 5th ed. Philadelphia, PA: Lippincott, Williams & Wilkins, 2001, 557–580.

38. **(C)** MRI is excellent and has become the standard to evaluate soft tissues and bone marrow. It is especially useful in imaging the spine to evaluate for nerve root impingement from disc herniation, from stenosis of the central canal, and from the intervertebral foramina as well. It is commonly used to evaluate osteonecrosis, tumors, and infections as well. MRI can display images in any plane without the use of radiation. Some tissues appear differently on T1- and T2-weighted MRI scans. Generally T1 images are ideal for evaluating anatomic structure, whereas the T2 images are more useful in contrasting normal and abnormal tissue.

The arrow is pointing at the right L5 nerve root. It is important to remember that the nerve roots in the lumbar spine exit beneath the pedicle of the same vertebra. At the level of the L4-L5 intervertebral disc, the nerve root from the above level (L4) has already exited just beneath the pedicle (L4) above. The lower nerve root (L5) is seen traversing the intervertebral

disc (L4-L5) at this level. It then proceeds to exit just beneath the pedicle of the L5 vertebral body.

A patient with a disc herniation at this level would complain of pain and have sensory and motor findings associated with the L5 level.

Bibliography

Brinker MR. Basic sciences: section 7—imaging and special studies. In: Miller MD, Brinker MR (eds.), *Review of Orthopaedics*, 3rd ed. Philadelphia, PA: W.B. Saunders, 2000, 115–116.

39. **(E)** Any injury to the hand sustained in a fight should raise suspicion for a bite injury, regardless of the history. These injuries commonly result from striking teeth with a clenched fist. With a clenched fist injury, the tendon is injured exposing the joint to inoculation. The tendon of the flexed hand then slides proximally as the fingers are extended and the joint becomes sealed. This provides a favorable environment for the introduced bacteria. For this reason, all patients with injuries over the metacarpal phalangeal (MCP) joint should be considered to have a tooth injury regardless of the history. The involved pathogens are the flora of the human mouth. The most commonly isolated organisms are alpha- and beta-hemolytic *Streptococci*, *Staphylococcus aureus, Staphylococcus epidermidis, Eikenella corrodens*, and *Neisseria*. Although *Eikenella* is becoming more prevalent in reports, *S. aureus* is still the most common pathogen.

Bite wounds account for up to 40% of hand infections. The potential complications are significant and serious. Infection can lead to destruction of the joint and surrounding soft tissues and extensor mechanism as well as osteomyelitis. Therefore, these wounds should be treated aggressively with exploration, irrigation, and debridement. Patients should receive tetanus prophylaxis in addition to antibiotics. Aerobic and anaerobic cultures should be obtained at the time of debridement with special attention to *E. corrodens*. The antibiotic of choice includes ampicillin-sulbactam or augmentin. Other recommendations include penicillin G, ampicillin, carbenicillin, or tetracycline for *E. corrodens* and a cephalosporin for *Staphylococcus* organisms. The antibiotics should be adjusted appropriately based on culture and sensitivity results. Bite wounds should never be closed primarily. Delay more than 24 h before debridement and inadequate initial debridement are two factors that increase the risk of developing osteomyelitis.

Bibliography

Brinker MR. Basic sciences: section 5—orthopaedic infections and microbiology. In: Miller MD, Brinker MR (eds.), *Review of Orthopaedics*, 3rd ed. Philadelphia, PA: W.B. Saunders, 2000, 100.

Neviaser R. Acute infections. In: Green DP, Hotchkiss RN, Pederson WC (eds.), *Green's Operative Hand Surgery*, 4th ed. Philadelphia, PA: Churchill Livingstone, 1999, 1045.

40. **(E)** This patient has a burst fracture at the C6-C7 level with complete cord injury. A complete cord injury indicates loss of motor and sensory function at all levels below the level of injury (Table 37-6). Therefore, patellar tendon reflexes and ankle plantar flexion would be lost. Finger abduction and adduction are primarily functions of T1 so this would also be lost. Elbow flexion is primarily derived from C5 and C6 so some weakness could be detected with resisted testing. Shoulder abduction, however, is primarily from C5 so this likely would be spared.

TABLE 37-6

Level	Sensory	Major Motor	Reflex
C5	Lateral Arm	Deltoid, Biceps	Biceps
C6	Lateral Forearm	Biceps, Wrist Extensor	Brachioradialis
C7	Middle Finger	Triceps, Wrist Flexors, Finger Extensors	Triceps
C8	Medial Forearm	Finger Flexors, Interossei	None
T1	Medial Arm	Interossei	None

Bibliography

Netter FH. *The Ciba Collection of Medical Illustrations. Volume 8—Musculoskeletal System, Part I: Anatomy Physiology and Metabolic Disorders.* Summit, NJ: Ciba-Geigy, 2001, 29.

CHAPTER 38

Plastic and Reconstructive Surgery

Jeffrey E. Schreiber and Navin K. Singh

Questions

1. A 62-year-old female shows up in clinic for her post-operative check following a lumpectomy for ductal carcinoma *in situ* (DCIS). Her daughter is with her and is concerned about her own risk for breast cancer because 2 years ago she underwent augmentation mammoplasty with silicone implants. She also asks you if the implants will make mammograms harder to read. Do silicone breast implants cause breast cancer?

   (A) no
   (B) yes
   (C) only if placed before 1990
   (D) only if placed after 1990
   (E) only if placed after 1995

2. What is the blood supply for a pedicled transverse rectus abdominus muscle (TRAM) flap?

   (A) superior epigastric artery
   (B) inferior epigastric artery
   (C) rectus abdominis perforators
   (D) internal iliac artery
   (E) intercostal artery

3. After performing a bilateral reduction mammoplasty, the recovery room nurse calls to tell you that the right nipple is turning blue. What is the most appropriate next step?

   (A) remove more breast tissue
   (B) convert to a free nipple graft
   (C) release the sutures
   (D) start IV heparin
   (E) apply leeches

4. What is the central zone of a burn called?

   (A) zone of stasis
   (B) zone of hyperemia
   (C) zone of necrosis
   (D) zone of coagulation
   (E) zone of dermolysis

5. Which of the following is not part of the rule of tens regarding cleft lip repair?

   (A) age greater than 10 weeks
   (B) weight about 10 lbs
   (C) hemoglobin of at least 10 g/dL
   (D) cleft lip defect greater than 10 mm
   (E) none of the above

6. What is the incidence of cleft palate with or without cleft lip?

   (A) 1 in 500 live births
   (B) 2 in 1000 live births
   (C) 1 in 10,000 live births
   (D) 1 in 1000 live births
   (E) 1 in 750 live births

7. A wrestler from a local high school visits you in clinic complaining of swelling in his right ear after practice that afternoon. You notice that he has a large, doughy mass with overlying ecchymosis on his ear. What is the current treatment?

   (A) observe only
   (B) drainage with a 16 gauge needle
   (C) compression bandage only
   (D) drainage with a 16 gauge needle, followed by a compression bandage
   (E) drainage through a small incision followed by a compression bandage

8. How many bones make up the orbit?

(A) 7
(B) 8
(C) 9
(D) 6
(E) 4

9. While you're obtaining consent from a patient to excise and graft a third degree burn injury to his leg you explain to him that he will eventually need a skin graft to cover the defect. He asks you how a piece of skin could possibly survive once it has been totally detached from the body. Which of the following is not one of the mechanisms for graft survival?

(A) imbibition
(B) inosculation
(C) revascularization
(D) reepithelialization
(E) none of the above

10. When a hair follicle is in the telogen stage of the growth cycle, what is it doing?

(A) growing
(B) turning gray
(C) resting
(D) dividing
(E) becoming infected

11. A concerned mother brings in her 7-month-old infant and states that she has noticed the rapid growth of a red "tumor" on the infant's cheek and she wants it removed immediately. What is the lesion?

(A) café-au-lait spot
(B) Spitz nevus
(C) hemangioma
(D) juvenile melanoma
(E) basal cell carcinoma

12. A patient comes to you for keloid resection and wants it permanently removed. Can you guarantee permanent removal?

(A) yes
(B) no
(C) only with steroids
(D) only with radiation
(E) only with silicone gel sheeting

13. On walking into a patient's clinic room, you notice that he has tattoos all over his body. After introducing yourself, he asks you if you are able to remove his purple and yellow tattoos. Which laser would you use?

(A) Q-switched ruby
(B) carbon dioxide
(C) argon
(D) frequency doubled Q-switched Nd:YAG
(E) copper vapor

14. In an obese patient setting, what has happened to the adipocytes?

(A) hypertrophied
(B) replicated
(C) became squamous cells
(D) lysed
(E) A and B

15. Lidocaine is used very commonly as a local anesthetic. Which cell membrane channel does it block?

(A) bicarbonate (HCO^-_3)
(B) chloride (Cl^-)
(C) calcium (Ca^{2+})
(D) magnesium (Mg^{2+})
(E) sodium/potassium (Na^{2+}/K)

16. In open tibial fractures, which Gustilo classifications require plastic surgery consultation?

(A) II
(B) II and III
(C) IV
(D) IIIA
(E) IIIB and IIIC

17. What is the most common cause of lymphedema?

(A) *Wuchereria bancrofti*
(B) *Entamoeba histolytica*
(C) *Clonorchis sinensis*
(D) *Cyclospora cayetanensis*
(E) *Ixodes scapularis*

18. A patient presents to you with a brownish-black lesion on his arm that is 7 mm in diameter and has been bleeding occasionally. What is the appropriate therapy for this patient?

(A) fine-needle aspiration

(B) incisional biopsy

(C) excisional biopsy

(D) laser

(E) cryotherapy

19. The dominant pedicle of the latissimus dorsi flap consists of which artery and vein?

(A) thoracodorsal

(B) internal mammary

(C) subscapular

(D) suprascapular

(E) axillary

20. In the operating room, your assistant accidentally cuts the main pedicle of your forehead flap. What vessels did he cut?

(A) supratrochlear and superficial temporal

(B) occipital and supraorbital

(C) posterior auricular and superficial temporal

(D) supratrochlear and supraorbital

(E) angular and infratrochlear

21. One hour after rhinoplasty the patient is complaining of shortness of breath and the pulse oximeter reads 87%. What is the leading diagnosis?

(A) sinusitis

(B) pain

(C) faulty pulse oximeter

(D) anxiety

(E) pneumothorax

22. Which structure is not affected by Fournier gangrene?

(A) genital

(B) perineal

(C) perianal

(D) periumbilical

(E) none of the above

23. During tissue expansion, what happens to the skin over the expander?

(A) It only stretches.

(B) It undergoes partial necrosis and then regenerates.

(C) It generates new skin.

(D) It undergoes de-epithelialization.

(E) It undergoes columnar metaplasia.

24. What is the most common type of collagen in the body?

(A) I

(B) II

(C) III

(D) IV

(E) V

25. When prosthetic mesh is contraindicated for large hernia reconstruction (for example, presence of fistula, ostomy, and intraoperative enterotomy), which of the following is *not* a method for abdominal wall reconstruction?

(A) separation of components

(B) tensor fascia lata graft

(C) Gortex

(D) alloderm

26. Gynecomastia presenting in the teenage years needs the following workup:

(A) liposuction

(B) needle biopsy

(C) observation

(D) amputation with free nipple graft

27. A panniculectomy can be performed safely on an

(A) outpatient basis

(B) inpatient basis

(C) inpatient with ICU observation

(D) cannot be safely performed

28. Which of the following is a contraindication to autologous breast reconstruction?

(A) abdominal liposuction

(B) abdominoplasty

(C) inadequate tissues in abdomen

(D) none of the above

29. From mild-to-moderate size breast reduction, which of the following are appropriate surgical techniques?

(A) liposuction

(B) anchor-shaped breast reduction

(C) vertical pattern breast reduction with short scar technique

(D) all of the above

30. After healing of acute burns, resurfacing for improved functional and cosmetic outcomes can be accomplished by

    (A) split-thickness skin graft
    (B) full-thickness skin graft
    (C) debridement and granulation
    (D) cultured epithelial autographs

31. Which of the following is required for addressing any pressure sore?

    (A) antibiotics
    (B) pressure reduction
    (C) hyperbaric oxygen
    (D) flap coverage

32. A 32-year-old man comes into the emergency department after a motor vehicle accident. He has a cervical spine injury, scalp laceration (Fig. 38-1), and is hypotensive with a blood pressure of 80/40 mmHg and a pulse of 145. The most likely cause of his hypotension is

    (A) hypovolemic shock
    (B) neurogenic shock
    (C) hypothermic shock
    (D) cardiogenic shock

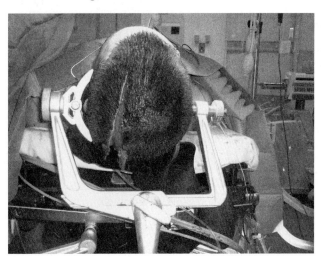

FIG. 38-1

33. After a routine three vessel coronary artery bypass grafting (CABG) including the left internal mammary artery, a 72-year-old type II diabetic female develops a sternal click and a fever. On examination, she is found to have a small area of wound dehiscence with thick drainage. On computed tomography (CT) scan she has a substernal fluid collection. Previously, this woman has undergone a gastrectomy for gastric cancer. The

diagnosis of sternal osteomyelitis is undertaken and jointly with the cardiac surgery service and plastic surgery service she undergoes chest wall reconstruction. Which of the following flaps is most appropriate?

    (A) omental flap
    (B) right pectoralis major turnover
    (C) left pectoralis major turnover
    (D) left rectus abdominis flap

34. A 52-year-old hypertensive vasculopathic patient undergoes left leg revascularization with a aorto-bifemoral bypass graft. On postoperative day 2 he is noted to have wound dehiscence of his left groin with clear fluid drainage. The most appropriate management is

    (A) wet to dry dressings
    (B) rectus femoris flap
    (C) sartorius muscle flap
    (D) application of a V.A.C. sponge

35. Depicted in Fig. 38-2 is an 18-year-old male whose left eye was struck with a baseball. He complains of double vision, a headache, and tenderness in his left cheek. The most likely injury is

    (A) orbital floor fracture
    (B) intracranial hemorrhage
    (C) retinal detachment
    (D) LeFort III fracture

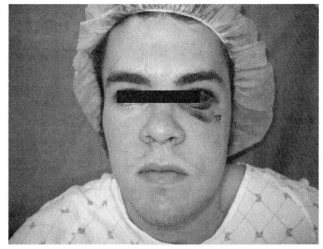

FIG. 38-2

36. After suffering a dog bite to the tip of her nose, a 15-year-old woman is brought to the emergency room in stable condition with a 3.5 cm × 3.5 cm piece of amputated skin from her nasal tip. The part has been retrieved from the dog and placed on iced saline slurry and brought into the emergency room. After antibiotics

and tetanus prophylaxis have been administered, what is the most appropriate next step? (Fig. 38-3)

(A) microsurgical reimplantation

(B) discarding the piece and performing a forehead flap

(C) composite graft

(D) full-thickness skin graft from supraclavicular skin

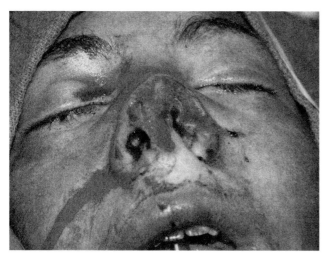

FIG. 38-3

37. Which one of the following structures is *not* part of the contents of the carpal tunnel?

(A) median nerve

(B) flexor digitorum superficialis tendons

(C) flexor digitorum profundus tendons

(D) flexor pollicis longus tendon

(E) flexor pollicis brevis tendon

38. Which bacterium is most commonly encountered with a hand bite from a human?

(A) *Pasteurella multocida*

(B) *Neisseria gonorrhoeae*

(C) *Streptococcus*

(D) *Eikenella corrodens*

(E) *Staphylococcus aureus*

39. To what artery(ies) can the Allen test be applied?

(A) radial

(B) ulnar

(C) common digital

(D) all of the above

(E) none of the above

40. What are the two most commonly injured nerves during a rhytidectomy?

(A) facial and ophthalmic

(B) facial and great auricular

(C) mental and supraorbital

(D) supratrochlear and supraorbital

(E) facial and auriculotemporal

41. A patient presents to the emergency department with an amputation through the tip of his left index finger. What is the treatment of choice?

(A) replantation

(B) revision amputation

(C) toe to finger transfer

(D) pollicization

Answers and Explanations

1. **(C)** Silicone breast implants do *not* cause breast cancer or autoimmune disease. Despite the previous media frenzy and lawsuit regarding silicone breast implants and breast cancer, the definitive report from the Institute of Medicine shows no causal link. In fact, two large studies have shown that a lower incidence of breast cancer occurs in augmented women compared to nonaugmented women. One study included 11,676 women from Alberta, Canada followed for 13 years and another based in Los Angeles followed women with silicone breast implants for 15.5 years. The lower incidence may be because of the possibility that smaller breasted women are less likely to develop breast cancer, and the silicone may actually be protective against cancer based on animal studies.

As far as mammograms are concerned, implants do interfere with the amount of breast tissue that can be seen (56% for subglandular placement and 75% for submuscular). However, the implants may be displaced via the Eklund technique allowing greater visualization (64% for subglandular and 85% for submuscular).

Several different incisions may be used to insert the implant. The inframammary approach is simple and provides good access, but may be noticeable. The periareolar approach is less noticeable, but may alter areolar sensation, form cysts from injured ducts, and create microcalcifications on mammogram. The transaxillary incision leaves no scar on the breast mound, but provides poor exposure, places the intercostobrachial nerve at risk for injury, and the subclavian vein at risk for thrombosis. The transumbilical breast augmentation (TUBA) technique is quite new. It leaves no incision on the breast mound, but the difficulty level is high, and if the surgeon cannot do it via this approach another one must be used.

Contraction of the implant may occur, and the Baker classification addresses the amount. Class I: no contraction, the implant cannot be felt. Class II: the implant can be felt, but no contraction. Class III: a palpable implant with noticeable contraction. Class IV: the breast is hard, tender, painful, cold, and distorted.

Bibliography

Berkel H, Birdsell D, Jenkins H. Breast augmentation: a risk factor for breast cancer? *N Engl J Med* 1992;326(25): 1649–1653.

Deapen D, Bernstein L, Brody G. Are breast implants anticarcinogenic? A 14-year follow-up of the Los Angeles Study. *Plast Reconstr Surg* 1997;99(5):1346–1353.

Eklund G, Busby R, Miller S, Job J. Improved imaging of the augmented breast. *Am J Roentgenol* 1998;151(3): 469–473.

Nelson N. Institute of medicine finds no link between breast implants and disease. *J Natl Cancer Inst* 1999; 91(14):1191.

Silverstein M, Handel N, Gamagami P. The effect of silicone-gel-filled implants on mammography. *Cancer* 1991; 68(Suppl 5):1159–1163.

Slavin S. Augmentation mammoplasty and its complications. In: Aston SJ, Beasley RW, Thorne CHM (eds.), *Grabb and Smith Plastic Surgery*, 5th ed. New York, NY: Lippincott-Raven, 1997.

Spear S, Baker J Jr. Classification of capsular contracture after prosthetic breast reconstruction. *Plast Reconstr Surg* 1995l;96(5):1119–1123.

Su C, Dreyfuss D, Krizek T, Leoni K. Silicone implants and the inhibition of cancer. *Plast Reconstr Surg* 1995; 96(3):513–518.

2. **(A)** A pedicled TRAM flap is based off the blood supply from the superior epigastric artery while the deep inferior epigastric artery supplies the free TRAM flap once it is anastamosed to the donor artery. Donor arteries can be either the thoracodorsal or internal mammary. Free TRAMs have demonstrated less partial flap loss and fat necrosis compared to pedicled TRAMs, but the learning curve is steep. Figures 38-4 through 38-6 represent a patient with a free TRAM (with skin sparing mastectomy), Figs. 38-7 and 38-8

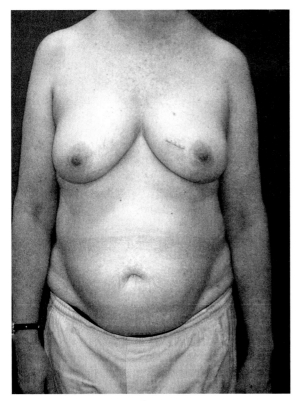

FIG. 38-4

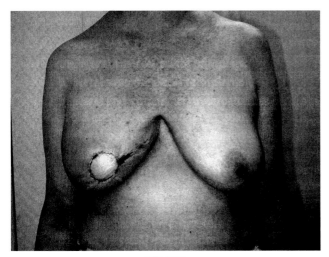

FIG. 38-5

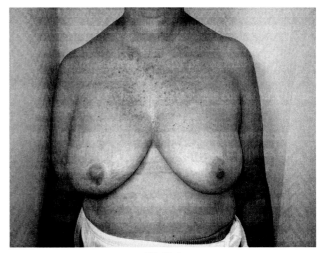

FIG. 38-6

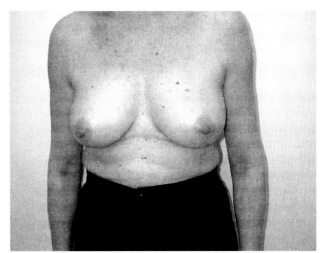

FIG. 38-7

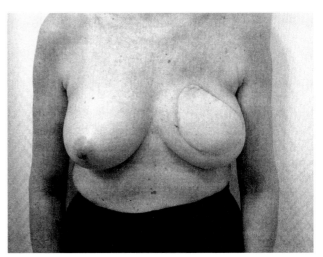

FIG. 38-8

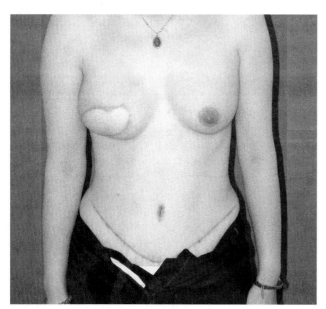

FIG. 38-9

represent another free TRAM (without skin sparing mastectomy), and Fig. 38-9 is an example of the abdominal donor site scar. Patients may inquire about abdominal function after a TRAM flap. Previous flaps included much of the rectus abdominis muscle, but with the new muscle-sparing techniques almost no deficit is seen.

Other flaps used include the latissimus, superior gluteal, and inferior gluteal flaps. Implants may also be used for breast reconstruction following mastectomy for breast cancer, but they carry the normal implant risks (infection, rupture, contraction, and so on) and don't fare well with radiation. Nipple-areolar complex reconstruction is performed as a separate procedure and one of several different flaps can be used for the nipple (star, skate, mushroom, and so on) and the areola is almost always tattooed.

Most breast cancers are either noninvasive or invasive. Noninvasive includes DCIS and lobular carcinoma *in situ* (LCIS). DCIS develops from the terminal mammary ducts, is usually palpable, and may be treated with lumpectomy, lumpectomy with radiation or total mastectomy depending on severity of disease. LCIS arises from lobules and occasionally fills distal ducts. It's a sinister disease for the following reasons: it's never palpable, usually found in both breasts, and one in four will develop into invasive disease. Bilateral mastectomy with immediate reconstruction should be considered with LCIS.

Invasive breast carcinoma is usually infiltrating ductal carcinoma or invasive lobular carcinoma. Infiltrating ductal carcinoma is the most common

(70%) and is detectable via mammogram. Invasive lobular carcinoma (10%) usually occurs in the upper outer quadrant of the breast. Of the other variants of invasive carcinoma, angiosarcoma is the most malignant.

Bibliography

Baldwin B, Schusterman M, Miller M, Kroll S, Wang B. Bilateral breast reconstruction: conventional versus free TRAM. *Plast Reconstr Surg* 1994;93(7):1410–1416.

Drever J. The lower abdominal transverse rectus abdominis myocutaneous flap for breast reconstruction. *Ann Plast Surg* 1983;10(3):179–185.

Nahabedian M, Dooley W, Singh N, Manson P. Contour abnormalities of the abdomen after breast reconstruction with abdominal flaps: the role of muscle preservation. *Plast Reconstr Surg* 2002;109(1):91–101.

Schwartz SI, et al. Breast: carcinoma of the breast. *Schwartz's Principles of Surgery*, 7th ed. New York, NY: McGraw-Hill, 1999. Retrieved January 28, 2003, from STAT!Ref Online Electronic Medical Library.

Schwartz SI, et al. Plastic and reconstructive surgery. *Schwartz's Principles of Surgery*, 7th ed. New York, NY: McGraw-Hill. Retrieved January 28, 2003, from STAT!Ref Online Electronic Medical Library.

3. **(C)** The most likely cause is kinking of the pedicle, and the first thing you should do is release the sutures. If the pedicle is not kinked, then more breast tissue might need to be removed; however, if removing more breast tissue does not help, free nipple grafts should be your next consideration. Other complications include tissue necrosis, hematoma, asymmetry, hypertrophic scarring, decreased nipple-areola complex sensation, and altered mammography. The blood supply to the breast is derived from the following arteries: internal mammary, lateral thoracic, thoracodorsal, thoracoacromial, and intercostal artery perforators. The nipple receives its blood supply from the subdermal plexus and is innervated by the lateral cutaneous branch of T4. The rest of the breast is innervated by the anteromedial and anterolateral branches of the thoracic intercostal nerves T3-T5. Also, the supraclavicular nerves from the cervical plexus innervate the superior and lateral breast.

Concerning mammography, patients older than 35 should get pre- and postoperative studies for baseline comparison. Patients can breast feed after reduction but may need to supplement. Nipple-areolar complex sensation may be altered depending on the type of reduction and amount of breast tissue removed. Many different types of reduction have been described. Basically, the goal is to significantly reduce the amount of breast tissue while preserving enough tissue for blood supply and innervation. Examples of reduction include the vertical bipedicle (McKissock, 1976), the horizontal bipedicle (Strombeck, 1960), and the lateral pedicle (Skoog, 1963).

Women get breast reduction for symptoms of gigantomastia that include back, neck, and shoulder pain, intertrigo, inability to play sports, and shoulder notching. Breast reduction surgery relieves these symptoms in all patients and eliminates them in 25%. Congenitally asymmetric breasts may also be treated by reduction mammoplasty in the larger one with the optional use of an implant in the smaller one.

Bibliography

Danikas D, Theodorou S, Kokkalis G, Vasiou K, Kyriakopoulou K. Mammographic findings following reduction mammoplasty. *Aesth Plast Surg* 2001;25(4): 283–285.

Gonzalez F, Brown F, Gold M, Walton R, Shafer B. Preoperative and postoperative nipple-areola sensibility in patients undergoing reduction mammoplasty. *Plast Reconstr Surg* 1993;92(5):809–814.

Gonzalez F, Walton R, Shafer B, Matory W Jr, Borah G. Reduction mammoplasty improves symptoms of macromastia. *Plast Reconstr Surg* 1993;91(7):1270–1276.

Harris L, Morris S, Freiberg A. Is breast feeding possible after reduction mammoplasty? *Plast Reconstr Surg* 2001;89(5):836–839.

Kerrigan C, Collins E, Kneeland T, et al. Measuring health state preferences in women with breast hypertrophy. *Plast Reconstr Surg* 2000;106(2):280–288.

Schwartz SI, et al. Breast: anatomy and development. *Schwartz's Principles of Surgery,* 7th ed. New York, NY: McGraw-Hill, 1999. Retrieved January 30, 2003, from STAT!Ref Online Electronic Medical Library.

4. **(D)** After sustaining a burn, three zones develop: zone of coagulation (center), zone of stasis (middle), and zone of hyperemia (outer). The zone of coagulation is nonviable tissue and the zone of stasis will die unless adequate resuscitation begins and perfusion is maintained. For fluid resuscitation, the Parkland's formula is commonly used as Ringer's lactate 4 cc/kg/%TBSA burned. Half is given within the first 8 h, and the other half is given over the following 16 h. It is paramount to maintain a urinary output of at least 30 cc/h.

When the patient presents to the emergency department with blisters, unroofing them is a common practice in many hospitals; however, this is controversial owing to the fact that the fluid underneath the blister is rich in electrolytes. Keeping them intact also helps with pain control. Therefore, infection is usually the only indication for debridement. Topical antimicrobials are a mainstay of burn care today since sepsis is the leading cause of death in burn patients. Three formulas are typically used: silver sulfadiazine, silver nitrate, and mafenide acetate (sulfamylon).

Silver sulfadiazine (Silvadene) is the most commonly used and inhibits growth of gram-positive and gram-negative organisms, *Candida albicans*, and possibly herpes viruses. Application is minimally painful, penetrates intermediately (toxicity is rare), but may cause leukopenia which reverses with discontinuation. Silver nitrate is widely antimicrobial, but only penetrates minimally making its use prophylactic only instead of in the face of established infection. Its concentration (0.5%) is in distilled water making it hypotonic. This may sequester serum electrolytes and mandates careful monitoring of them. Silver nitrate stains everything it touches black, is painless on application, but must be kept wet at all times to prevent cytotoxic concentrations from occurring (>2%). Mafenide acetate is also broadly antimicrobial and penetrates deeply making it ideal for eschars and cartilage (burned noses and ears). Caution must be exercised with judicious use because of the fact that mafenide acetate is a carbonic anhydrase inhibitor and may cause an alkaline diuresis. If polyuria develops, a hyperchloremic metabolic acidosis may ensue leading to hyperventilation and pulmonary compromise in an already critically ill patient.

Most chemical burns must be washed thoroughly regardless of acid/base status. Lime is one exception to this since it reacts with water to produce a burn. Therefore, lime powder should be brushed off and solid pieces of lime should be removed before flushing with water. Oral and intravenous antibiotics in the burn setting should only be used for documented infection, not prophylactically.

Bibliography

Baker J, Tarantino D Jr, Miller M. Lime disease? *Arch Dermatol* 2000;136(10):1277–1278.

Burn wound. *Histological Assessment (Zones of Injury)*, 2000. [Data file] Available from Burnsurgery.org site, http://www.burnsurgery.org

Durtschi M, Orgain C, Counts G, Heimbach D. A prospective study of prophylactic penicillin in acutely burned hospitalized patients. *J Trauma* 1982;22(1):11–14.

Heggers J, Ko F, Robson M, Heggers R, Craft K. Evaluation of burn blister fluid. *Plast Reconstr Surg* 1980;65(6): 798–804.

Nissen D. Section II: drug information. *Mosby's Drug Consult*™, 13th ed. St. Louis, MO: Mosby, 2003. Retrieved January 30, 2003, from STAT!Ref Online Electronic Medical Library.

Schwartz SI, et al. Burns: fluid management. *Schwartz's Principles of Surgery,* 7th ed. New York, NY: McGraw-Hill, 1999. Retrieved January 30, 2003, from STAT!Ref Online Electronic Medical Library.

5. **(D)** The rule of tens means that a cleft lip is repaired when the infant's age is greater than tens weeks, his weight is about 10 lbs, and he has a hemoglobin of at least 10 g/dL. The following are several characteristics of a cleft lip: a shortened columella on the cleft side, the medial crus of the cleft side alar cartilage is moved

posteriorly, the lateral crus is widened spans the width of the cleft, the cleft side nostril has a horizontal axis compared to the vertical axis of the noncleft nostril, the cleft side philtrum is shortened, the Cupid's bow peak is too high, and the dome of the nose is pulled down on the cleft side.

Cleft lip occurs at a rate of 1 in 1000 live births in Whites, with the highest rate being 1 in 500 births in Asians, and the lowest at 1 in 2000 births in Blacks. The only known cause of cleft lip is the use of phenytoin during pregnancy (10-fold increase). Although, smoking is associated with double the incidence of cleft lip compared to nonsmoking mothers.

Historically, Chinese physicians first reported surgical correction of a cleft lip, but it wasn't until 1955 that Ralph Millard described the most frequently used technique today. He described the rotation-advancement technique where the Cupid's bow rotates downward into a normal position via release of the medial lip while the lateral lip is advanced into the space left by the previous rotation. Repair of the orbicularis oris muscle is also performed to allow for normal lip function and eversion of the lip border.

Intrauterine repair of a cleft lip has been done in animals, but the risk of fetal loss is still too high to attempt this in humans. Along the same lines, neonatal cleft lip repair poses too many perioperative risks for a purely psychologic benefit to the parents.

Bibliography

Chung K, Kowalski C, Kim H, Buchman S. Maternal cigarette smoking during pregnancy and the risk of having a child with cleft lip/palate. *Plast Reconstr Surg* 2000; 105(2):485–491.

Das S, Runnels R Jr, Smith J, Cohly H. Epidemiology of cleft lip and cleft palate in Mississippi. *South Med J* 1995;88(4): 437–442.

Kim S, Kim W, Oh C, Kim J. Cleft lip and palate incidence among the live births in the Republic of Korea. *J Korean Med Sci* 2002;17(1):49–52.

Massey K. Teratogenic effects of diphenylhydantoin sodium. *J Oral Ther Pharmacol* 1996;2(5):380–385.

Millard D Jr. A primary camouflage of the unilateral Harlook. In: Skoog T (ed.), *Transactions of the First International Congress of Plastic Surgery, Stockholm, 1955*. Baltimore, MD: Williams & Wilkins, 1957, 160.

Vrebos J. Harelip surgery in ancient China: further investigations. *Plast Reconstr Surg* 1992;89(1):147–150.

Schwartz SI, et al. Plastic and reconstructive surgery: head and neck. *Schwartz's Principles of Surgery*, 7th ed. New York, NY: McGraw-Hill, 1999. Retrieved January 30, 2003, from STAT!Ref Online Electronic Medical Library.

Stelnicki E, Lee S, Hoffman W, et al. A long-term, controlled-outcome analysis of in utero versus neonatal cleft lip repair using an ovine model. *Plast Reconstr Surg* 1999;104(3):607–615.

6. (D) The answer is 1 case in 1000 live births. Most (50%) are cleft lip and palate with 38% being unilateral. This is a fairly common problem and much work has been done regarding its treatment. Ultrasonography can detect a cleft palate as early as the 17th week of gestation. The etiology of cleft palate, environmental or genetic, is still a mystery; however, the highest frequency of cleft palates are seen in American Indians, 3 cases per 1000 live births, compared to the lowest occurrence rate in Blacks, with 0.72 cases per 1000 live births.

The anatomy of a cleft palate varies with severity of the cleft. Yet, the basic concept is that the barrier between the nasal and oral cavities is incomplete. The palate is divided into the hard palate anteriorly and the soft palate posteriorly with its blood supply coming from the internal maxillary artery. The internal maxillary artery divides into the greater palatine artery to supply the hard palate via the greater palatine foramen, and the lesser palatine artery to supply the soft palate via the lesser palatine foramen. The nerve supply to the palatal muscles is from the maxillary branches of the trigeminal nerve. Cranial nerves VII and IX are also present. The soft palate (velum) is muscular while the hard palate is not. It is these muscles which play vital roles in speech, facial growth, and dentition. The muscles are the tensor veli palatini, palatoglossal, palatophyarngeal, uvular, superior constrictors, palatothyroideus, and salpingopharyngeus. The soft palate provides an anchoring point for these muscles, and when a cleft is present their positions are incorrect which lead to problems.

For example, feeding becomes problematic with a cleft palate; however, simple maneuvers such as making the bottle nipple opening bigger, squeezing the bottle, and placing the baby in a semiupright position can alleviate many problems. Breast feeding is also a valid option. Airway obstruction can occur from the tongue blocking the pharynx or nasal cavity. Prone positioning, lip-tongue adhesion, and tracheotomy can be done according to severity of obstruction. Further, otitis media can become chronic and lead to hearing loss. Therefore, grommet tubes (ear tubes) can be placed to facilitate drainage and prevent otitis media.

Surgical correction is based on creating an airtight and watertight seal between the oral and nasal cavities. The following are some of the techniques that have been developed: von Langenbeck, bipedicle mucoperiosteal flaps; Schweckendiek, 2 stages, soft palate first with a three-layer closure of the nasal mucosa, levator muscles, and oral mucosa followed by hard palate closure with a vomer flap; two-flap technique, based on two posterior flaps, three-flap/V-Y (Wardill-Kilner-Veau) technique using a V-Y advancement flap; and the Furlow technique using a double reverse Z-plasty. A common potential complication is fistula formation, quoted as high as 34%. Closure of asymptomatic fistulas may be amenable to a palatal obturation prosthesis, but symptomatic fistulas should be surgically corrected no sooner than 6–12 months after the initial procedure to allow for complete tissue healing and reestablishment of an adequate blood supply.

About 400 syndromes include a cleft palate as one feature, and cleft palates are usually part of a syndrome (30%). When a baby is born and a cleft palate is present but not obvious, its presence can be manifested by feeding difficulties. Parents become concerned with this and usually want something done as soon as possible. The easy answer to this problem is surgery, but the difficult answer is when. Today, most major clefts palates are repaired before 1 year of age to avoid any problems with speech development.

Bibliography

Sipek A, Gregor V, Horacek J, Masatova D. Facial clefts from 1961 to 2000—incidence, prenatal diagnosis and prevalence by maternal age. *Ceska Gynekol* 2002;67(5): 260–267.

Coddington D, Hisnanick J. Midline congenital anomalies: the estimated occurrence among American Indian and Alaska Native infants. *Clin Genet* 1996;50(2):74–77.

Croen L, Shaw G, Wasserman C, Tolarova M. Racial and ethnic variations in the prevalence of orofacial clefts in California, 1983–1992. *Am J Med Genet* 1998;79(1):42–47.

Schweckendiek W. Early veloplasty and its results. *Acta Otorhinolaryngol Belg* 1968;22(6):697–703.

Furlow L. Cleft palate repair by double opposing Z-plasty. *Plast Reconstr Surg* 1986;78:724.

Honnebier M, Johnson D, Parsa A, Dorian A, Parsa F. Closure of palatal fistula with a local mucoperiosteal flap lined with buccal mucosal graft. *Cleft Palate Craniofac J* 2000;37(2):127–129.

Bauer B, Patel P. Cleft palate. In: Georgiade G, Riefkohl R, Levin L (eds.), *Georgiade Plastic, Maxillofacial and Reconstructive Surgery*, 3rd ed. Baltimore, MD: Williams & Wilkins, 1997.

7. **(E)** Blunt trauma to the ear, especially around the helix, results in a hematoma that requires drainage. If the hematoma is subperichondrial and is not adequately drained, it may calcify or fibrose causing a permanent mass to form which is known as "cauliflower ear." Drainage is performed through a small incision followed by a compression dressing against the ear which is secured with a bandage placed around the head. Ear reconstruction following trauma is greatly facilitated by the excellent blood supply to the ear. The posterior auricular artery off the external carotid is the main source with the superficial temporal, deep auricular, and occipital arteries as additional sources.

Furthermore, ear reconstruction involves unique methods of tissue advancement and flaps. Examples include helical advancement, contralateral and ipsilateral chonchal cartilage grafts, preauricular, banner, and chondrocutaneous composite flaps. Split earlobes are also a common concern, and available techniques for repair include Z-plasties and the Pardue repair where one edge is transposed to the other while creating a hole for immediate earring use. When reviewing ear anatomy, a commonly asked question involves the auricular tubercle of Darwin. This structure is often observed and is a small "bump" seen on the helix as it turns downward.

Many times congenital ear anomalies will be encountered. The Tanzer classification groups these as follows:

I. Anotia
II. Complete hypoplasia (microtia)

   a. With atresia of the external auditory canal
   b. Without atresia of the external auditory canal

III. Hypoplasia of the middle third of the auricle
IV. Hypoplasia of the superior third of the auricle

   a. Constricted (cup or lop) ear
   b. Cryptotia
   c. Hypoplasia of the entire superior third

V. Prominent ear

Bibliography

Brent B. Auricular repair with autogenous rib cartilage grafts: two decades of experience with 600 cases 1992;90(3):355–374.

Gajiwala K. Repair of the split earlobe using a half Z-plasty. *Plast Reconstr Surg* 1998;101(3):855–856.

Giffin C. Wrestler's ear: pathophysiology and treatment. *Ann Plast Surg* 1992;28(2):131–139.

Pardue A. Repair of torn earlobe with preservation of the perforation for an earring. *Plast Reconstr Surg* 1973;51(4):472–473.

Park C, Lineaweaver W, Rumly T, Buncke H. Arterial supply of the anterior ear. *Plast Reconstr Surg* 1992;90(1): 38–44.

Tanzer RC. *Reconstructive Plastic Surgery*, 2nd ed. Philadelphia, PA: W.B. Saunders, 1977.

Tolleth H. Artistic anatomy, dimensions, and proportions of the external ear. *Clin Plast Surg* 1978;5(3):337–345.

8. **(A)** The following seven bones make up the orbit: frontal, zygoma, maxilla, palatine, greater and lesser wings of the sphenoid, lacrimal, and ethmoid bones. Of note, the nasal and temporal bones do not contribute. Orbital anatomy is very intricate, and surgery on or around the eye requires thorough knowledge of it. The optic nerve passes through the optic foramen.

The superior orbital fissure, located between the greater and lesser wings of the sphenoid, permits passage of cranial nerves III, IV, V_1, and VI. The greater wing of the sphenoid is separated from the orbital floor by the inferior orbital fissure that provides passage of the infraorbital artery, V_2, branches of the inferior ophthalmic vein to the pterygoid plexus, and branches of the sphenopalatine ganglion. The supraorbital vessels and nerve are transmitted through the supraorbital notch/foramen, while the infraorbital vessels and nerve travel via the infraorbital notch.

Five orbital fat compartments exist in the eyelids: two in the upper lid and three in the lower lid. These are manipulated and/or removed during blepharoplasty, but excessive removal may cause a hollowed-out appearance. Hemostasis is key during a blepharoplasty as blindness is likely to ensue following an untreated hematoma. You may be called into the recovery room after a blepharoplasty because the patient is complaining of excessive pain around the eye, lack of the ability to see light, or the nurse notices excessive edema. It is imperative to release the sutures and take the patient back to the operating room and remove any hematoma. Further, if no hematoma is found and all possible bleeding points are stable, then a lateral canthotomy is indicated to relieve any retrobulbar pressure. The incidence of blindness following blepharoplasty is very small (<0.1%), but its prevention is still paramount.

Another complication following blepharoplasty, although not as severe as blindness, is ectropion. This is defined by an outward turning or eversion of the eyelid and in the case of blepharoplasty is usually caused by excessive removal of skin, fat, or muscle, damage to the orbicularis oculi muscle, lid edema, hematoma, proptosis, or scar contracture. Treatment includes massage of the lower eyelid, application of cool compresses, and if persistent may require full-thickness skin grafting or tightening and/or shortening of the lateral canthus.

Lacerations of the eyelid require meticulous repair to prevent any cosmetic or functional problems. Three layers of the eyelid exist: the skin, tarsus, and conjunctiva. Repair of a laceration should start with a suture at the end through the skin and tarsus that, with gentle traction, aligns the wound edges. Next, the pretarsal muscle is repaired with an absorbable suture followed by a nylon for skin approximation. To prevent scarring, suture removal should occur after 3–4 days.

Bibliography

Carraway J, Mellow C. The prevention and treatment of lower lid ectropion following blepharoplasty. *Plast Reconstr Surg* 1990;85(6):971–981.

Gray H. *Anatomy of the Human Body*, 20th ed. Philadelphia, PA: Lea & Febiger, 2000. Retrieved January 31, 2003 from Bartleby.com.

Shamoun J, Ellenbogen R. Blepharoplasty, forehead, and eyebrow lift. In: Georgiade G, Riefkohl R, Levin L (eds.), *Georgiade Plastic, Maxillofacial and Reconstructive Surgery*, 3rd ed. Baltimore, MD: Williams & Wilkins, 1997.

9. **(D)** Split-thickness skin grafts, such as the one that will likely be applied to his burn site, survive via three mechanisms: imbibition, inosculation, and revascularization. During the first 2–3 days, the graft undergoes imbibition. Basically, the skin "imbibes" or "drinks" from the nutrient-rich wound exudate via capillary action of the absorbent dermis and blood vessels in the graft. Following this, a period of inosculation occurs where the blood vessels in the wound bed and the graft make contact to establish blood flow. Lastly, new blood vessels actually grow into the skin graft by day 6 or 7 during a process of revascularization.

Harvest of a split-thickness skin graft results in shrinkage of the graft. This is because of the elastin present in the dermis and is called primary contracture. Several weeks after application, secondary contracture may occur from the action of myofibroblasts. Because they have more dermis and therefore more elastin, full-thickness skin grafts have greater primary contraction, but less secondary contraction compared to split-thickness skin grafts. After application of a split-thickness skin graft, a xeroform or op-site dressing is usually applied as these dressings are the least expensive and cause the least amount of pain. Another technique, called pinch grafting, is the process of placing small pieces of split-thickness skin graft into a large wound bed with granulation tissue to promote epithelialization.

A full-thickness skin graft requires a bolster dressing (xeroform and mineral oil soaked cotton) to maximize graft adherence and prevent hematoma and/or seroma formation. The mineral oil prevents blood clotting which allows any remaining blood to drain. Unfortunately, several things may cause failure of skin grafts. These include hematoma, seroma, inadequate vascularity of the recipient bed (bone, cartilage, foreign material, or tendon), infection, and most commonly, shear (mechanical disruption).

Bibliography

Schwartz SI, et al. Plastic and reconstructive surgery: skin grafts. *Schwartz's Principles of Surgery*, 7th ed. New York, NY: McGraw-Hill, 1999. Retrieved January 31, 2003, from STAT!Ref Online Electronic Medical Library.

10. (C) Each hair follicle goes through three phases of growth during its cycle: anagen, catagen, and telogen. Anagen is the phase when the follicle is actively growing. About 85% of all hair follicles are in this stage which lasts approximately 3–4 years. Catagen is the next stage and represents regression. Affecting about 1–2% of the follicles, it lasts 3–4 weeks during which the base of the follicle becomes keratinized, the melanocytes stop producing melanin, and the follicular bulb is eventually destroyed. Finally, telogen, lasting 3–4 months and representing approximately 10–15% of the follicles, is the resting phase of the growth cycle. During this stage, the dermal papilla is released from its epidermal attachment and a new hair begins formation in the anagen phase. Every hair follicle is divided into three parts: the infundibulum (upper), isthmus (middle), and bulb (lower).

Hair loss is very common among men and women and affects more than half of them in the United States. The percentage of women who lose hair is the same as men, but hormones allow them the benefit of not losing as much volume. Forms of hair loss include traumatic alopecia, alopecia areata (patchy reversible hair loss), drug-induced alopecia (warfarin, allopurinol), and the most common form, androgenic alopecia or male-pattern baldness. Androgenic alopecia can affect females as well and is defined by increased sensitivity to dihydrotestosterone (DHT) which shortens anagen causing the hair follicles to become progressively thinner. Other causes of alopecia include lupus, syphilis, cancers, liver and kidney failure, poor nutrition, and stress. 5-Alpha reductase converts testosterone to DHT and male-pattern baldness may be treated with synthetic 5-alpha reductase inhibitors (finasteride).

Male-pattern baldness is categorized by the Hamilton-Norwood classification with type I being minimal hairline recession progressing to type VII, the most severe form with only a small horseshoe-shaped band of hair posterior to the ears and around the occiput. Before the late 1980s and early 1990s, physicians were rotating flaps of hair around the scalp, using tissue expanders, excising pieces of scalp, or transplanting strips or plugs of hair to treat hair loss. These techniques frequently resulted in donor site defects, flap necrosis, and were aesthetically unattractive. Recently, however, the technique of hair grafting involves placing small grafts with 1–2 hair follicles per graft in a pattern on the scalp that appears natural. This procedure does not involve flaps, has very little donor site defect, and is the way most hair transplantation is performed today.

Bibliography

Aldhizer G. *The Doctor's Book on Hair Loss.* Englewood Cliffs, NJ: Prentice-Hall, 1983.

Griffin E. Hair transplantation. The fourth decade. *Dermatol Clin* 1995;13(2):363–387.

Hamilton J. Patterned loss of hair in man: types and incidence. *Ann N Y Acad Sci* 1951;53:708–728.

Kligman A. The human hair cycle. *J Invest Dermatol* 1959; 33:307–316.

Rittmaster R. Finasteride. *N Engl J Med* 1994;330(2): 120–125.

11. (C) The lesion is most likely a hemangioma and treatment is observation only. Hemangiomas have three stages of growth: rapid, then at the same rate as the child's growth, then involution. By age 5, 50% of hemangiomas involute completely followed by 70% at age 7. Further involution occurs until the ages of 10–12; however, around 20% of hemangiomas require treatment other than observation because they are somehow dangerous to the child (e.g., airway obstruction, visual disturbance, or diversion of blood flow). Treatment for these hemangiomas ranges includes intralesional or systemic steroids, interferon, laser, or surgery.

Hemangiomas are commonly confused with vascular malformations. In 1982, Mulliken classified these two entities on a cellular level. Hemangiomas have endothelial hyperplasia, multilaminated basement membranes, and a history of rapid growth followed by regression. Vascular malformations, on the other hand, have normal structural integrity, grow proportionately with the child, and consist of a mixture of capillary, lymphatic, and venous elements. An example of a vascular malformation is a port-wine stain. This lesion is usually treated with an argon or flash-lamp pumped pulsed dye laser, tuned to the absorption frequency of oxyhemoglobin.

Along the same lines, arteriovenous malformation (AVMs) range from simple lesions to life-threatening ones. These should be treated initially by correcting any coagulopathies with possible embolization followed by complete excision as any remaining tissue may lead to recurrence. These lesions may even require hypotensive anesthesia or cardiopulmonary bypass with deep hypothermic circulatory arrest to prevent fatal hemorrhage from occurring during excision. An AVM may become even more threatening with ligation of the feeding vessel as this may not be the only source. Hence, this should never be done.

Certain syndromes include hemangiomas as one of their main characteristics. For example, Sturge-Weber's syndrome involves vascular lesions of the upper facial dermis, choroids plexus, and ipsilateral leptomeninges. Kasabach-Merritt describes thrombocytopenia in the face of a large hemangioma (GI, pleural, CNS, or peritoneal). Anderson-Fabry's disease is associated with telangiectasias around the waist and thighs often with fatal renal failure.

Bibliography

Mulliken J. Vascular anomalies. In: Aston SJ, Beasley RW, Thorne CHM (eds.), *Grabb and Smith Plastic Surgery*, 5th ed. New York, NY: Lippincott-Raven, 1997.

Mulliken J, Glowacki J. Hemangiomas and vascular malformations in infants and children: a classification based on endothelial characteristics. *Plast Reconstr Surg* 1982; 69(3):412–422.

12. **(B)** A keloid can be resected, but one cannot guarantee that it will be permanently removed. In fact, it may recur and be worse, which is why conservative therapy is usually initiated before surgery. Therefore, indications for surgery include failure of conservative therapy, cosmetic deformity, and functional impairment. Examples of conservative therapy include topical silicone sheeting, intralesional steroids, and pressure garments.

Keloids (Figs. 38-10 through 38-13) are an excessive form of healing as are hypertrophic scars. They occur in about 10% of wounds and are 10 times more common in nonWhites. No definite genetic mode of transmission has been assigned to keloid formation as it has been reported as autosomal dominant and autosomal recessive; however, a genetic association exists between certain HLA types, blood type A, and abnormal scar formation. The difference between keloids and hypertrophic scars is that keloids grow beyond the original scar margin, and hypertrophic scars do not. The time interval for appearance is

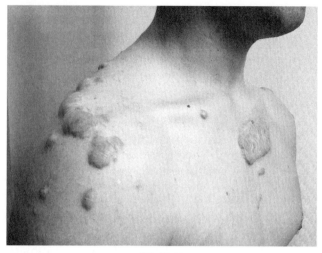

FIG. 38-11

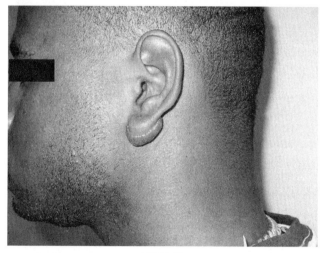

FIG. 38-12

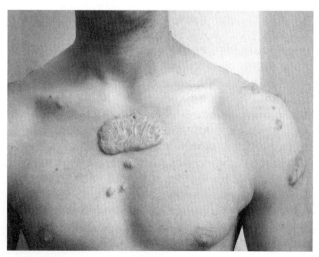

FIG. 38-10

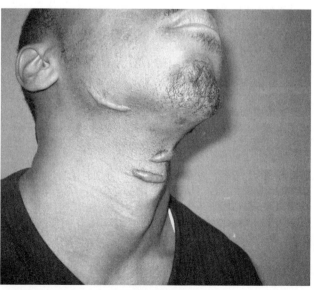

FIG. 38-13

usually 1 week for hypertrophic scars, while keloids can develop up to 1 year later. Both keloids and hypertrophic scars have thickened epidermal layers and rich vasculature. The composition of keloids includes excessive mucinous ground substance, irregular and malaligned collagen fibers with 20 times the amount of collagen synthesis compared to normal skin. Hypertrophic scars also have abnormal collagen fibers with three times the amount of collagen synthesis compared to normal skin. If one is unsure about the diagnosis of a keloid or hypertrophic scar, an excisional biopsy is indicated to rule out malignancy.

The mechanism of action of silicone sheeting involves the occlusive hydration effect while pressure devices act by producing local tissue hypoxia. Scar volume as well as intralesional steroids decrease the amount of connective tissue. Lasers, radiation, colchicine, and interferon are still under study for therapeutic benefit.

Bibliography

Alhady S, Sivanantharajah K. Keloids in various races: a review of 175 cases. *Plast Reconstr Surg* 1969;44(6):564–566.

Berman B, Flores F. The treatment of hypertrophic scars and keloids. *Eur J Dermatol* 1998;8(8):591–595.

Glat P, Longaker M. Wound healing. In: Aston SJ, Beasley RW, Thorne CHM (eds.), *Grabb and Smith Plastic Surgery*, 5th ed. New York, NY: Lippincott-Raven, 1997.

Gold M. Topical silicone gel sheeting in the treatment of hypertrophic scars and keloids: a dermatologic experience. *J Dermatol Surg Oncol* 1993;19(10):912–916.

Santucci M, Borgognoni L, Reali U, Gabbiani G. Keloids and hypertrophic scars of Caucasians show distinctive morphologic and immunophenotypic profiles. *Virchows Archives* 2001;438(5):457–463.

13. (D) Many different lasers are available for use in plastic surgery. For tattoos, lasers are chosen based on the pigments used. Blue, green, and black amateur tattoos are removed with the Q-switched ruby laser because all of the energy is absorbed by the pigments and spares the epidermis. The frequency doubled Q-switched Nd:YAG laser can remove red, orange, purple, yellow, and brown tattoo inks. Tattoo removal usually requires multiple visits for completion.

The word *laser* stands for "light amplification by stimulated emission of radiation" and was developed based on Einstein's quantum theory of radiation. Their use in plastic surgery is relatively recent, but many different conditions are amenable to laser therapy. For instance, wrinkles may be treated with the CO_2 laser. Alster et al. reviewed their experience of treating facial wrinkles in 259 patients and found that periorbital wrinkles were the easiest to treat with deeper wrinkles such as those found in the forehead were the hardest. Lasers can also be used to treat infantile hemangiomas. Compared to observation alone, lasers produced better volume and texture while at the same time alleviating the psychologic stress found at school age. Port-wine stains are capillary malformations and are also amenable to laser therapy, specifically the flash-lamp pulsed dye laser and results are excellent with virtually no scarring. Interestingly enough, better results may be achieved in infancy and childhood and even though pain is minimal, intralesional lidocaine or topical eutectic mixture of local anesthesia (EMLA) cream may be used. Many other lesions may be treated with lasers, such as hemangiomas, blue nevi, café-au-lait macules, surgical and acne scars, striae distensae, and warts.

Safety in laser use is very important since the vapor produced with laser use may carry viable bacteria and viruses. Vacuum suction should be placed 1–2 in. away from the vapor source, masks should be worn that can filter particles as small as 0.3 mm, protective eyewear is essential, reflective surfaces should be removed from the operating field, special anodized instruments should be used to minimize laser reflection, and fire safety is mandatory as lasers pose a very high flammable potential. Patients with infectious diseases (HIV, HPV, hepatitis B, and the like) can potentially infect those in the operating room who do not follow all safety precautions.

Bibliography

Achauer B, Chang C, Vander Kam V. Management of hemangioma of infancy: review of 245 patients. *Plast Reconstr Surg* 1997;99(5):1301–1308.

Alster T, Garg S. Treatment of facial rhytides with a high-energy pulsed carbon dioxide laser. *Plast Reconstr Surg* 1996;98(5):791–794.

Garden J, Polla L, Tan O. The treatment of port-wine stains by the pulsed dye laser: analysis of pulse duration and long-term therapy. *Arch Dermatol* 1988;124(6):889–896.

Grossman M, Kauvar A, Geronemus R. Cutaneous laser surgery. In: Aston SJ, Beasley RW, Thorne CHM (eds.), *Grabb and Smith Plastic Surgery*, 5th ed. New York, NY: Lippincott-Raven, 1997.

Kuperman-Beade M, Levine V, Ashinoff R. Laser removal of tattoos. *Am J Clin Dermatol* 2001;2(1):21–25.

14. (E) In the initial setting of obesity, the adipocytes hypertrophy, but when the total body fat exceeds 40 kg, new adipocytes are produced. During gestation, mesenchymal cells differentiate into preadipocytes and become mature fat cells or remain in the precursor cell stage. If they mature, replication is not possible unless they become ischemic or malnourished allowing them to dedifferentiate into preadipocytes and replicate if needed.

Liposuction is the second most common aesthetic surgery procedure performed in the United States today with Botox injections being first. The amount suctioned varies widely, and large-volume liposuction has received media attention because of complications including death. How much is "large"-volume liposuction? In 1998, the American Society of Plastic Surgery Task Force on Lipoplasty and the Plastic/Cosmetic Surgery Committee of the Medical Board of California both defined large-volume liposuction as greater than 5000 cc. In a review of 76,000 surgeries involving liposuction, the complication rate was 0.1% with two deaths, one from a pulmonary embolus and the other from a fat embolus. Large-volume liposuction should be performed by a plastic surgeon in a hospital setting with an anesthesiologist along with an overnight hospital stay for cardiac and volume status monitoring.

When liposuction is performed, fluid is injected subcutaneously to assist with hemostasis and ease of suctioning the fat. Solutions vary in composition, but usually include epinephrine, lidocaine, and lactated ringers. The tumescent technique involves injecting enough fluid (with epinephrine and lidocaine) to cause skin turgor. General anesthesia is not required. Concerning fluid resuscitation, nothing is better than sound clinical judgement and constant communication between the surgeon and anesthesiologist; however, one current guideline involves maintenance fluid only for less than 4 L removed, but maintenance plus 0.25 cc crystalloid/cc aspirate for greater than 4 L removed.

Bibliography

Albin R, de Campo T. Large-volume liposuction in 181 patients. *Aesth Plast Surg* 1999;23(1):5–15.

Klein J. The tumescent technique. Anesthesia and modified liposuction technique. *Dermatol Clin* 1990;8(3):425–437.

Teimourian B, Rogers W 3rd. A national survey of complications associated with suction lipectomy: a comparative study. *Plast Reconstr Surg* 1989;84(4):628–631.

The American Society for Aesthetic Plastic Surgery survey. (n.d.) Retrieved February 4, 2003, from http://surgery.org/news_releases/feb2002stats.html

Trott S, Beran S, Rohrich R, Kenkel J, Adams W Jr, Klein K. Safety considerations and fluid resuscitation in liposuction: an analysis of 53 consecutive patients. *Plast Reconstr Surg* 1998;102(6):2220–2229.

15. **(E)** Lidocaine, and other local anesthetics, block the sodium channels in the cell membrane thus inhibiting nerve conduction. The total amount of lidocaine one can give is 4–6 or 8 mg/kg if epinephrine is added. Lidocaine should not be taken lightly and toxicity can lead to death. Symptoms of lidocaine toxicity are initially central nervous system (CNS) related (headache, numbness of the lips and tongue, tinnitus, lightheadedness, and facial twitching). As severity progress, one may see loss of consciousness, seizures, apnea, cardiovascular collapse, or even v-fib arrest. If your patients begins to seize, secure an airway, hyperventilate with 100% oxygen, and administer diazepam. Other signs or symptoms require supportive care as needed. A tourniquet may be used to delay further lidocaine absorption.

Today, many patients inquire about EMLA cream for superficial skin procedures. EMLA cream is most commonly a mixture of lidocaine and prilocaine and it works very well, but takes 1–2 h to work. After application for 2 h, anesthesia can reach to a depth of 5 mm and last up to 4 h. Caution must be exercised with EMLA cream use as lidocaine toxicity can occur. Usual adult dose is 1.5 g/10 cm^2.

In the emergency department, suturing an extensive laceration in a child can best be done under conscious sedation. Fentanyl with midazolam or ketamine are the anesthetics best suited for this. After many operations, the anesthesiologist will ask you to inject marcaine. It provides great local anesthesia (4–6 h) and may be dosed as 3 mg/kg, 200 mg maximum.

The major risk with its use is reentrant tachycardia or v-fib. Epinephrine is helpful to prevent bleeding during laceration repair. A concentration of 1:100,000 provides excellent vasoconstriction (greater concentrations do not improve duration or amount of bleeding), a minimum of 7 min is required for its onset of action, and it should be avoided in the fingers, toes, ears, penis, and nose.

Bibliography

Siegel R, Vistnes L, Iverson R. Effective hemostasis with less epinephrine. An experimental and clinical study. *Plast Reconstr Surg* 1973;51(2):129–133.

Thorne A. Local anesthetics. In: Aston SJ, Beasley RW, Thorne CHM (eds.), *Grabb and Smith Plastic Surgery*, 5th ed. New York, NY: Lippincott-Raven, 1997.

16. **(E)** The incidence of lower extremity trauma is very prevalent during wars and in countries with ongoing military exchanges; however, in countries not at war the incidence appears to be increasing. Open tibial fractures have a wide range of severity, and lower limb injuries commonly require plastic surgical intervention because of the limited skin and muscle availability in that area. The Gustilo classification is as follows:

 I: Open fracture with a wound <1 cm
 II: Open fracture with a wound >1 cm without extensive soft tissue damage
 III: Open fracture with extensive soft tissue damage

IIIA: III with adequate soft tissue coverage

IIIB: III with soft tissue loss with periosteal stripping and bone exposure

IIIC: III with arterial injury requiring repair

Consultation with a plastic surgeon concerning coverage of the fracture should occur with classifications IIIB and IIIC. Options for coverage vary widely, but mainly depend on what skin, muscle, arteries, and veins are available, the location of the defect, and whether or not the nerves have been damaged. Nerve damage to the foot can be a relative contraindication to reconstruction. For instance, if the posterior tibial nerve is destroyed, the patient will lose plantar flexion of the foot as well as sensation on the planar aspect of the foot leading to a step-off in ambulation, a loss of position sense, and an increased risk of chronic wounds on the bottom of the foot. Fasciocutaneous flaps are useful for covering large superficial defects involving tendon and bone. Examples in the lower leg include the peroneal, anterior tibial, posterior tibial, and sural artery flaps. Fasciocutaneous flaps in the foot include the dorsalis pedis, flexor digitorum brevis, abductor digiti minimi, and abductor hallucis flaps, as well as the lateral and medial plantar artery flaps.

Muscle flaps may be used for more extensive local wounds and include the lateral and medial gastrocnemius flaps and the soleus flap. Free flaps are another option when local tissue is inadequate, deep defects are present after excessive bony debridement, and when local flaps have failed. Chronic venous and diabetic ulcers of the lower extremity should not deter one from salvaging the lower extremity if bacterial contamination is controlled and vascular inflow has been maximized.

Bibliography

Gustilo R, Anderson J. Prevention of infection in the treatment of one thousand and twenty-five open fractures of long bones: retrospective and prospective analysis. *J Bone Joint Surg* 1976;58:453.

Gustilo R, Chapman M. *Management of Type III Open Fractures*. Orthopedic Surgery Viewpoints' 83 (Monograph). Indianapolis, IN: Eli Lily.

Kasabian A, Karp N. Lower extremity reconstruction. In: Aston SJ, Beasley RW, Thorne CHM (eds.), *Grabb and Smith Plastic Surgery*, 5th ed. Philadelphia, PA: Lippincott-Raven, 1997.

17. **(A)** Worldwide, the most common cause is infection with the parasite *W. bancrofti* causing filariasis. In the United States, tumor invasion, radiation, and surgery are the leading causes. Lymphedema is either primary or secondary, with the primary form divided into three subtypes: congenita, praecox, and tarda. Lymphedema congenita is present at birth, lymphedema praecox is the most common of the primary types (80%) and occurs during adolescence, and the onset of lymphedema tarda is after the age of 35. A familial form of lymphedema praecox is known as Milroy's disease and is X-linked dominant. Secondary lymphedema includes filariasis, tumors, surgery, and radiation.

The treatment of lymphedema has perplexed surgeons throughout history and many different ideas and techniques have been developed. Basically, treatment can be divided into medical and surgical, with surgical involving drainage or excisional procedures. Currently, medical therapy is implemented first and consists of wearing compressive garments, massage, pneumatic compression devices, antibiotics, good hygiene, and limb elevation. Strict compliance is mandatory for efficacious medical therapy. Diuretics are not therapeutic. When medical treatment fails, surgery is indicated and usually only for severe cases. Surgical techniques aimed at lymphatic drainage include lymphatic to venous anastamoses, deepithelialized dermal flaps, and the creation of fascial windows. Excisional procedures are more commonly performed and include removal of the affected tissue with skin grafts using the skin of the removed tissue. Unfortunately, surgery is mostly palliative instead of curative. A commonly performed procedure with a high rate of resultant lymphedema is mastectomy with axillary dissection. The rate of occurrence is anywhere from 6 to 30% and again, treatment is conservative with surgery only for severe cases with failed medical therapy. Scrotal lymphedema is initially treated with elevation, but this only works for mild cases. Instead, this is one of the few instances where surgical therapy is initiated early and has reproducible results.

Bibliography

Larson D, Weinstein M, Goldberg I, et al. Edema of the arm as a function of the extent of axillary surgery in patients with stage I-II carcinoma of the breast treated with primary radiotherapy. *Int J Radiat Oncol Biol Phys* 1986; 12(9):1575–1582.

Miller T, Wyatt L. Lymphedema. In: Aston SJ, Beasley RW, Thorne CHM (eds.), *Grabb and Smith Plastic Surgery*, 5th ed. New York, NY: Lippincott-Raven, 1997.

18. **(C)** A punch or excisional biopsy will provide the necessary information for diagnosis and further therapy. If the lesion is melanoma, further workup is indicated and is described in the following text.

Melanoma is a disease with a rapidly rising incidence. Over the past 40 years, the incidence has more than tripled in the White population and by the year 2010, the lifetime risk for developing melanoma is estimated to be 1 in 50. And with its dismal prognosis of advanced disease, melanoma should not be taken lightly.

Four types of melanoma exist: superficial spreading, nodular, acral lentiginous, and lentigo maligna. Each type has certain unique characteristics. For example, superficial spreading is the most common type (70%), nodular rapidly grows (weeks to months), acral lentiginous can occur on the palms and soles, and lentigo maligna grows slowly (5–20 years) and usually occurs on the head and neck. The diagnosis of melanoma follows the well-known ABCD criteria: A—asymmetry; B—border irregularity; C—color variation; and D—diameter >6 mm. In 2002, staging of melanoma underwent major changes by the American Joint Committee on Cancer (AJCC) after review of over 17,000 patients. The new criteria include several salient points. First, Breslow thickness is the number one prognostic indicator. Second, ulceration is now the number two prognostic indicator. Third, Clark's level of invasion only applies to thin (≤1 mm depth) primary tumors and only regarding prognosis. Finally, the number of lymph nodes involved instead of their size is included as a prognostic factor. Overall, stage I melanoma has a high 5-year survival rate (89–100%) depending on the subtype, but stage IV melanoma usually indicates fatal disease (7–9% 5-year survival rate).

If the patient in the question above does have melanoma, what should be the margin of resection? It depends on the Breslow thickness. The following are the current recommendations for resection: melanoma *in situ* = 0.5cm; <1 mm thick = 1 cm; 1–4 mm thick = 2 cm; and >4 mm = 2 cm, but may be more to achieve local control. Further, the recent AJCC modifications also addressed the question of sentinel lymph node dissection (SLND) versus elective lymph node dissection (ELND). Generally, SLND should be performed for all lesions ≥1 mm thick without palpable nodes followed by completion lymph node dissection for positive results. ELND should only be performed at the same time as wide local resection if occult metastases are discovered.

Finally, some benefit has been demonstrated with interferon-alpha therapy for high-risk melanoma patients and certain vaccines are undergoing trials. Hence, medical oncology consultation should be obtained for patients with advanced disease.

Bibliography

Balch C, Buzaid A, Atkins M, et al. A new American Joint Committee on Cancer staging system for cutaneous melanoma. *Cancer* 2000;88(6):1484–1491.

Roses D. Surgical management of malignant melanoma. In: Aston SJ, Beasley RW, Thorne CHM (eds.), *Grabb and Smith Plastic Surgery*, 5th ed. New York, NY: Lippincott-Raven, 1997.

19. **(A)** Microsurgery is one of the great recent developments in surgical technique pioneered by the father of microsurgery, Dr. Harry Buncke, and has revolutionized hand, plastic, and ENT surgery. The actual technique involves meticulous planning pre-, intra-, and postoperatively. For instance, preoperatively the patient should be able to tolerate at least 8 h of surgery, an alternative flap should be available as a back-up, and the planned recipient vessel should be located out of the zone of injury. Intraoperatively, one should avoid vasoconstrictors and maintain a normal body temperature in the patient to avoid vasospasm. Postoperatively, flap monitoring is so vital to the success of the procedure that it almost always warrants admission to an intensive care setting so as to allow close observation by the nurses and supporting staff. Flap failure is most commonly because of venous thrombosis and/or hematoma. Therefore, the success of saving a flap if it fails depends on effective monitoring. Many different modalities of monitoring flaps have been developed and include laser Dopplers, temperature probes, and ultrasound Dopplers; however, the most effective way to monitor a flap is with hourly clinical assessment of skin color, turgor, capillary refill, and temperature.

If a flap does, in fact, appear to be failing there are several ways of saving it. First, several immediate steps include releasing any constricting sutures, removal of compressive dressings, and patient repositioning to alleviate any compression. If these maneuvers don't work, then immediate reexploration is required. Salvage of free flaps intraoperatively includes evacuating any hematoma, release of several anastamotic sutures for clot removal, and there have been several reports of successful flap salvage with streptokinase and tissue plasminogen activator (TPA).

An array of free flaps have been described, but a certain group of them is worth mentioning because of their versatility, durability, ease of harvest, and common use. First, the rectus abdominis flap, supplied by the deep inferior and superior epigastric arteries and veins, provides a large muscle mass with the option of a skin paddle. Second, the radial forearm flap, supplied by the radial artery, venae comitantes and cephalic vein, has a long, useful vascular pedicle with thin, pliable skin. Third, the gracilis flap, supplied by the ascending branch of the medial circumflex femoral artery and vein, may assist with facial paralysis or extremity muscle function as it has both motor (obturator) and sensory (femoral cutaneous) innervation. Fourth, the great toe flap, supplied by the first dorsal metatarsal artery and vein, can be used for thumb replacement. Lastly, the latissimus dorsi flap, supplied by the thoracodorsal artery and vein, is a very reliable flap with a large muscle mass and a long vascular pedicle. In fact, it can be made even larger if the serratus anterior and/or scapular muscles are included as a "chimeric" flap.

Finally, free flaps may be designated as muscular, musculocutaneous, fasciocutaneous, or osteofasciocutaneous flaps depending on their composition. For example, the fibula flap is an osteofasciocutaneous flap with its blood supply from the peroneal artery.

Bibliography

Buncke H. Forty years of microsurgery: what's next? *J Hand Surg* 1995;20(3 Pt 2):S34–S45.

Serafin D. *Atlas of Microsurgical Composite Tissue Transplantation*. Philadelphia, PA: W.B. Saunders, 1996.

Shenaq SM, Sharma SK. Principles of microvascular surgery. In: Aston SJ, et al. (eds.), *Grabb and Smith's Plastic Surgery*, 5th ed. New York, NY: Lippincott-Raven, 1997, 73–77.

20. **(D)** The dominant pedicle is the supratrochlear artery, with the minor pedicle being the supraorbital artery. The flap may survive via connections from the angular, infratrochlear, and dorsal nasal arteries as flap survival has been reported after division of the supratrochlear and supraorbital arteries.

The history of nasal reconstruction dates back to 600–700 BC, with Sushruta in India having performed the first recorded plastic surgery procedure. Tagliacozzi also made contributions to nasal reconstruction in 1597 with his description of staged transfer of skin from the arm to the nose. Historically, efforts were encouraged by the results of hand-to-hand combat and by the cutting off of one's nose as criminal punishment. Today, however, nasal reconstruction is most commonly undertaken after removal of nasal skin cancer, particularly basal cell carcinoma.

The anatomy of the nose is very intricate, involving an internal layer of mucosa and an external layer of skin supported by bone and cartilage, resulting in a structure with a truly unique shape. The nose can be divided into nine subunits based on shadows produced by normal lighting. The subunit borders allow for excellent concealment of scars, and the subunits are as follows: the dorsum, 2 nasal side walls, the tip, 2 ala, 2 soft tissue triangles, and the columella. For defects greater than 50% of the corresponding nasal subunit,

a general rule dictates that the defect should be enlarged to include the entire subunit for the best cosmetic result. Anything less than 50% should be treated without making it larger.

Nasal reconstruction can be done with a variety of flaps and grafts or just allowing the deficit to heal by secondary intention. The forehead flap is the ultimate flap for nasal reconstruction as it can be used to replace any or all of the nasal subunits. However, the patient must be stable enough to tolerate the two-stage procedure. The nasolabial flap is useful for defects between the nasal tip and alar lobule. Reconstructing the nasal lining is performed with the septal mucosal flap with vascular inflow coming from the superior labial artery. Defects located near the medial canthus are best treated with healing by secondary intention. Also, healing by secondary intention is recommended for defects 10 mm or less located on the nasal dorsum or lateral nasal walls. Larger deficiencies are amenable to a bilobed, paramedian, or cheek advancement flap. Total nasal reconstruction is possible with forehead flaps, rib grafts for the dorsum and lateral nasal walls, and conchal cartilage grafts to recreate the alar lobules. Patients who snort cocaine may present with ischemic necrosis of the septal cartilage and/or septal perforation. Antibiotics and debridement may be required initially followed by reconstruction with a mucosal flap and possible bone or cartilage grafts.

Bibliography

Burget G, Menick F. The subunit principle in nasal reconstruction. *Plast Reconstr Surg* 1985;76(2):239–247.

Rohrich R, Barton F, Hollier L. Nasal reconstruction. In: Aston SJ, et al. (eds.), *Grabb and Smith's Plastic Surgery*, 5th ed. New York, NY: Lippincott-Raven, 1997, 73–77.

21. **(E)** Rib cartilage is sometimes used as a graft in rhinoplasty and a pneumothorax may result during harvest. Therefore, it should be determined if rib cartilage was used in the patient above and if so, a chest x-ray should be ordered, a chest tube thoracostomy set obtained, and if the patient's status continues to decline, needle decompression should be performed for possible tension pneumothorax.

In addition to aesthetic reasons, rhinoplasty or septoplasty is also performed for functional problems, such as dyspnea from nasal obstruction and recurrent sinusitis. Several causes of cosmetic deformities include traumatic, iatrogenic from previous rhinoplasty, intranasal cocaine use, and certain medical illnesses leading to cartilagenous destruction in the nose (Wegener granulomatosis, polychondritis, leprosy, syphilis, and ectodermal dysplasia).

Prior to incision, local anesthesia with 1% lidocaine with 1;100,000 epinephrine is injected for regional pain and hemostasis. The trigeminal nerve provides sensation to the nose via the ophthalmic and maxillary divisions. Vascular inflow comes from the infraorbital, angular, superior labial, supratrochlear, and anterior ethmoidal arteries. Septal procedures usually require nasal packing soaked in 2% lidocaine with epinephrine or neosynephrine or 5% cocaine.

Rhinoplasty can be approached with an open or closed approach. The open approach involves a skin incision with nasal flap elevation, while the closed approach uses a transcartilaginous incision without flap elevation. The advantages of the open rhinoplasty include better visualization, more accurate repair of defects, and improved hemostasis; however, it may lead to displacement of the lateral crura, excess edema of the nasal tip, and unwarranted manipulation of a normal dome. As in the question above, implants may be used to repair nasal defects. Choices range from autogenous materials like bone and cartilage or alloplastic implants such as polyamide mesh, expanded polytetrafluoroethylene (ePTFE), and porous high-density polyethlylene. Cartilage is usually used first, bone second (greater morbidity and resorption than cartilage), and alloplasts last as their infection and extrusion rates are higher.

Bibliography

Adams J. Grafts and implants in nasal and chin augmentation. A rational approach to material selection. *Otolaryngol Clin North Am* 1987;20(4):913–930.

Daniel R. Rhinoplasty. In: Aston S, Beasley R, Thorne C (eds.), *Grabb and Smith's Plastic Surgery*, 5th ed. New York, NY: Lippincott-Raven, 1997, 651–668.

22. **(D)** Fournier gangrene is polymicrobial necrotizing fasciitis of the genital, perianal, or perineal areas. The skin may be erythematous, gangrenous, or malodorous, and air may be present on imaging studies. *Escherichia coli* (most common aerobe) and *Bacteroides* (most common anaerobe) usually cause it. Fournier gangrene is a urologic surgical emergency requiring aggressive debridement, hyperbaric oxygen, and intravenous antibiotics. Gas gangrene is caused by *Clostridium perferingens* and causes infection that spreads along muscle planes.

Tetanus is a disease involving generalized muscle spasms, usually involving the jaw and neck. Patients present with trismus most commonly, but may also manifest dysphagia, muscle rigidity, laryngeal spasms, and risus sardonicus (extreme contracture of the facial musculature causing a distorted grin). Tetanus is caused by the anaerobe *Clostridium tetani*, a spore-forming gram-positive bacillus that

releases tetanospasmin, a substance that prevents neurons from inhibiting motor reflex responses. Treatment involves elective intubation for airway protection, intensive care unit (ICU) admission, antibiotics, and possible surgical debridement.

Rabies is a viral disease that affects the CNS. Signs and symptoms vary, but initial presentation may involve high fevers, mental status changes, paralysis, or incoordination with late presentation manifesting as cardiac arrhythmias or arrest, hypotension, or coma. The bullet-shaped RNA virus may cause infection through a bite or aerosol exposure from an infected animal. Human rabies immunoglobulin and vaccine are the mainstay of therapy, and the method of exposure, patient vaccination status, and successful capture of the animal dictates their use.

A brown recluse spider bite manifests itself 6–12 h after a painless and unrecognized bite as an erythematous halo around the bite that develops into a clear or hemorrhagic vesicle progressing to a dark eschar as the final lesion. The venom is cytotoxic and hemolytic and may lead to systemic symptoms such as renal failure, coagulopathy, hemolysis, and, rarely, death. Treatment includes local wound care with the possible use of dapsone when G-6-PD deficiency has been excluded.

A black widow spider bite also presents as an erythematous halo around a pale area, but does not form vesicles. The venom affects the nervous system and may cause chest pain and abdominal cramps mimicking pancreatitis, appendicitis, ulcer, or gallbladder pain. Treatment is generally aimed to treat the symptoms, but antivenin may be required for severe cases only as its anaphylactic potential is high.

Bibliography

Schwartz SI, et al. Infectious disease & environmental and toxicology emergencies. *Schwartz's Principles and Practice of Emergency Medicine*, 4th ed. New York, NY: McGraw-Hill, 1999. Retrieved February 6, 2003, from STAT!Ref Online Electronic Medical Library.

23. **(C)** Skin undergoing active expansion generates epidermal mitotic division and new skin formation. The process of tissue expansion has provided plastic surgeons with an extremely useful option for a wide range of cases requiring reconstruction. The first recorded use of a tissue expander occurred in 1957 when Neumann placed a rubber balloon in a subcutaneous pocket, gradually expanded it with air, and used the newly generated skin to cover an ear defect. Now, expanders are available in different shapes (round, rectangular, crescentic, and so on) and sizes to provide the required amount of skin for adequate coverage while at the same time being in a position that

allows the skin to be easily oriented into the defect. Expanders can be placed either subcutaneously (wound coverage) or submuscularly (breast reconstruction). For wound coverage, the diameter of the expander base should equal the diameter of the wound.

Tissue expanders are made of a silicone shell and are intermittently filled with saline via an internal or external port with patient discomfort being the usual indicator to stop filling. The expander should be filled until enough skin is generated to cover two times the area of the wound as this will compensate for the skin contracture that occurs after expander removal. Two terms associated with tissue expansion are "creep" and "stress relaxation." When the force of the growing expander causes the skin to stretch via its viscoelastic properties, this is called "creep." As the skin is stretched with a constant force, the amount of force necessary to stretch the skin decreases over time and this is termed "stress relaxation." Concerning the vascular supply of the expanded skin, it's actually increased because the process of expansion acts as a delay. The capsule that forms on top of the expander adds to the vascular integrity of the skin flap and therefore should be included during flap inset. The expanded skin has thickened epidermis, thin dermis, atrophic, but functional muscle, and permanently atrophied fat. Complications of tissue expanders include extrusion, infection, and flap necrosis. The expander should be removed in these cases unless expansion is almost complete and the majority of the flap is not in jeopardy.

Bibliography

Bengtson B, Ringler S, George E, DeHaan M, Mills K. Capsular tissue: a new local flap. *Plast Reconstr Surg* 1993;91(6):1073–1079.

Berrino P, Galli A, Santi P. New options in breast reconstructive surgery: alternatives to the latissimus dorsi musculocutaneous flap. *Aesth Plast Surg* 1986;10(4):237–241.

Cherry G, Austad E, Pasyk K, et al. Increased survival and vascularity of random pattern skin flaps elevated in controlled, expanded skin. *Plast Reconstr Surg* 1983;72:680.

Jackson I, Sharpe D, Polley J, et al. Use of external reservoirs in tissue expansion. *Plast Reconstr Surg* 1987;80:226.

Johnson T, Lowe L, Brown M, Sullivan M, Nelson B. Histology and physiology of tissue expansion. *J Dermatol Surg Oncol* 1993;19(12):1074–1078.

Manders E, Schenden M, Furrey J, Hetzler P, Davis T, Graham W III. Soft-tissue expansion: concepts and complications. *Plast Reconstr Surg* 1984;74(4):493–507.

Mustoe T, Bartell T, Garner W. Physical, biomechanical, histologic, and biochemical effects of rapid versus conventional tissue expansion. *Plast Reconstr Surg* 1989;83(4):687–691.

Neumann C. The expansion of an area of skin by progressive distention of a subcutaneous balloon. *Plast Reconstr Surg* 1957;19:124.

Pasyk K, Argenta L, Austad E. Histopathology of human expanded skin. *Clin Plast Surg* 1987;14(3):435–445.

Pasyk K, Argenta L, Hassett C. Quantitative analysis of the thickness of human skin and subcutaneous tissue following controlled expansion with a silicone implant. *Plast Reconstr Surg* 1988;81:516.

Santoro J, Radovic P, Grumbine N. Use of the subcutaneous tissue expander for delayed primary closure of flaps. *J Foot Surg* 1989;28(3):225–232.

24. **(A)** Type I collagen is the most common type and it is present in skin, bones, tendons, and ligaments. In wound healing type III is the most common, but the ratio of type III to type I is low. As the wound completes maturation, type I collagen predominates.

Wound healing is a complex series of events that is adversely affected by many different disease processes and has been the focus of intense research for many years. The four stages of wound healing include hemostasis, inflammation, granulation, and remodeling. Hemostasis begins with vasoconstriction and involves the release of adenosine diphosphate (ADP) and several different cytokines from platelets, such as transforming growth factor-beta (TGF-β), platelet factor IV, and platelet-derived growth factor. Beginning immediately and lasting up to a few days, hemostasis ends with a fibrin mesh essential to coagulation. Next, inflammation ensues lasting 6–8 h and is based on the action of polymorphonuclear leukocytes (PMNs) and macrophages. Generally, PMNs clear the wound of debris while macrophages also clean the wound, but are vital to successful healing as they produce various growth factors (tumor necrosis factor, TNF; interleukin-1, IL-1; TGF; and cytokines). Following this stage, granulation begins and may last up to 4 weeks. This is when collagen formation and deposition begins in addition to neovascularization. The wound will gain maximum tensile strength at 12 weeks, but its final strength will only be about 80% of the original skin. Remodeling is the final stage of wound healing and is based on more orderly collagen deposition and collagen cross-linking with the actual amount of collagen remaining the same.

Wound healing is inhibited by infection (most commonly when the bacterial count is 10^5 organisms/gram tissue), corticosteriods, diabetes, smoking, and chemotherapy. To reverse these effects and reestablish adequate wound healing, many different remedies have been developed. Yet, few of these have proven significant benefit in all aspects of impaired wound healing. Wound care or plastic surgical consultation is therefore recommended in these settings as different therapies are applied to the impaired wound setting depending on the adverse factors involved and the present state of the wound. One therapeutic modality that has proven benefit for many nonhealing wounds and is becoming more popular is the vacuum-assisted closure (V.A.C.) dressing. It's basically a sponge placed on the wound, sealed to prevent leaks, and connected to a continuous vacuum. Its mechanism of improved wound healing involves removing chronic edema from the wound thus allowing increased blood flow and improved deposition of granulation tissue. Topical growth factors and hyperbaric oxygen also play roles in improving wound healing.

Bibliography

Glat P, Longaker M. Wound healing. In: Aston S, Beasley R, Thorne C (eds.), *Grabb and Smith's Plastic Surgery*. Philadelphia, PA: Lippincott-Raven, 1997, 3–12.

Morykwas M, Argenta L, Shelton-Brown E, McGuirt W. Vacuum-assisted closure: a new method for wound control and treatment: animal studies and basic foundation. *Ann Plast Surg* 1997;38(6):553–562.

25. **(C)** In any algorithmic approach to abdominal wall reconstruction, one must consider the initial problem. If the problem is a loss of domain, then tissue must be added. One of the primary choices in abdominal wall reconstruction includes autologous tensor fascia lata harvested from the thigh. This includes the disadvantage of a separate donor incision, the potential for knee instability, and a contour deformity of the thigh. Studies have shown that tensor fascia lata (TFL) is just as durable as native fascia and because it is autologous tissue, becomes revascularized (Figs. 38-14 through 38-18). The advantage to TFL is that it can be reoperated through. Another option is the addition of alloderm which is a processed cadaveric source of dermis. Because it is biological tissue, it becomes revascularized and has a potential for long-term healing (Figs. 38-19 through 38-21).

The separation of components method as described by Ramirez and Dellon should be the first choice in reconstruction where there is loss of domain. By undermining the skin and soft tissues to expose the fascia, mobility of the fascia is gained. Further, by release of the external oblique aponeurosis from the level of the costal margin to the arcuate line allows an additional 3–5 cm of advancement on each side. Occasionally, there is significant loss of domain and free flaps might be used for this type of reconstruction. Such a durable free flap is a TFL musculocutaneous free flap with microvascular anastomosis to the gastroepiploic vessels along the greater curvature of the stomach.

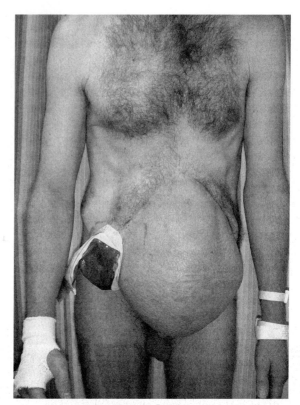

FIG. 38-14

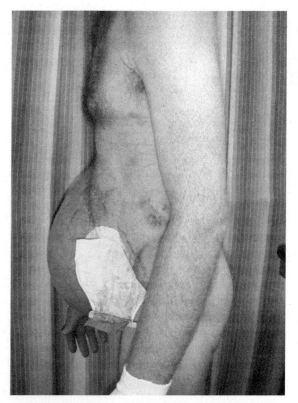

FIG. 38-15

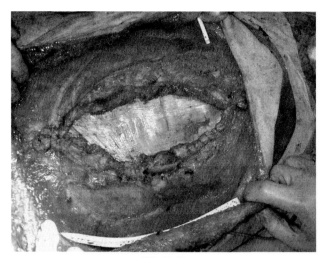

FIG. 38-16

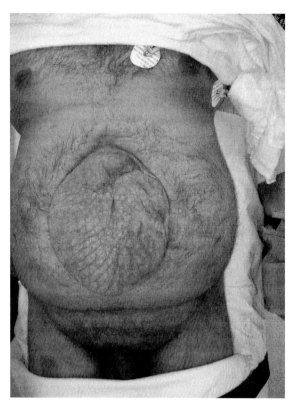

FIG. 38-19

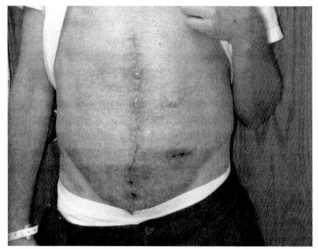

FIG. 38-17

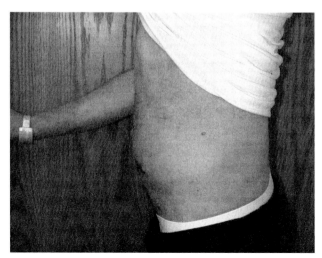

FIG. 38-18

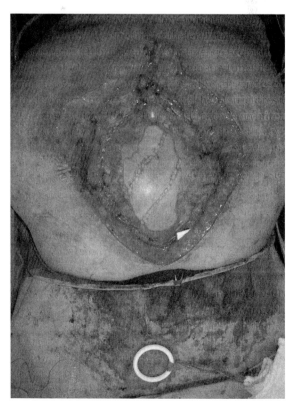

FIG. 38-20

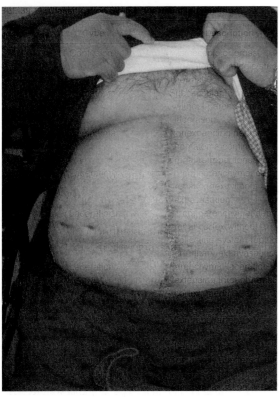

FIG. 38-21

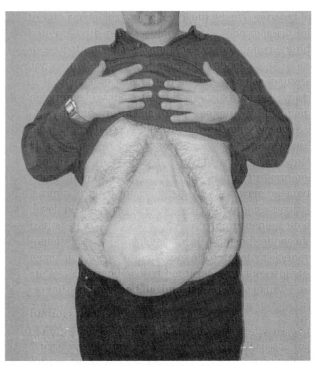

FIG. 38-22

If there are no contraindications to prosthetic devices, dual Gortex mesh is usually the material of choice. It has great structural integrity, minimizes risks for adhesions on the peritoneal surface, and if it is appropriately "corduroyed" on the superficial surface then it can adhere into the skin (Figs. 38-22 through 38-26). Risk of infection remains if there is contamination such as an intraoperative enterotomy, presence of a fistula, or presence of infection preoperatively. Seromas because of the nonadherent properties of Gortex can also develop and are short-term complications.

Bibliography

Girotto J, Ko M, Redett R, Muehlberger T, Talamini M, Chang B. Closure of chronic abdominal wall defects: a long-term evaluation of the components separation method. *Ann Plast Surg* 1999;42(4):385–394.

Nagy K, Perez F, Fildes J, Barrett J. Optimal prosthetic for acute replacement of the abdominal wall. *J Trauma* 1999;47(3):529–532.

Ramirez O, Ruas E, Dellon A. "Components separation" method for closure of abdominal-wall defects: an anatomic and clinical study. *Plast Reconstr Surg* 1990; 86(3):519–526.

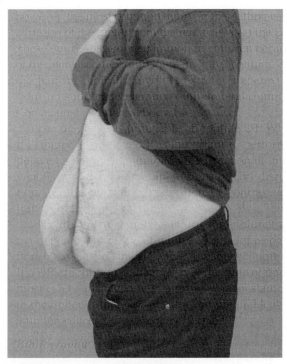

FIG. 38-23

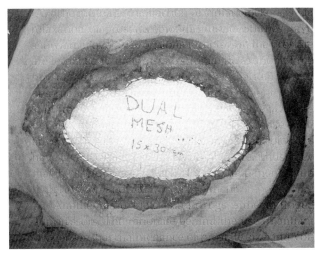

FIG. 38-24

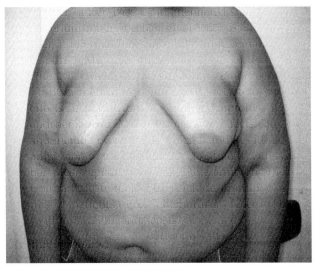

FIG. 38-27

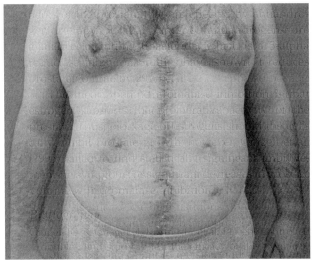

FIG. 38-25

Weinstein L, Kovachev D, Chaglassian T. Abdominal wall reconstruction. *Scand J Plast Reconstr Surg* 1986;20(1): 109–113.

White D, Pearl R, Laub D, DeFiebre B. Tensor fascia lata myocutaneous flap in lower abdominal wall reconstruction. *Ann Plast Surg* 1981;7(2):155–162.

Williams J, Carlson G, Howell R, Wagner J, Nahai F, Coleman J. The tensor fascia lata free flap in abdominal-wall reconstruction. *J Reconstr Microsurg* 1997;13(2):83–90.

26. **(C)** Gynecomastia (Figs. 38-27 through 38-31) is seen physiologically at the following two periods: (1) perinatal because of the high levels of circulating maternal

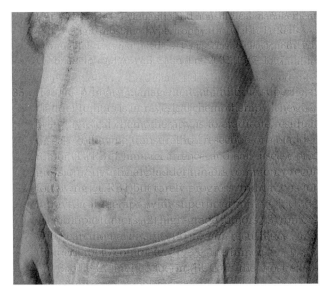

FIG. 38-26

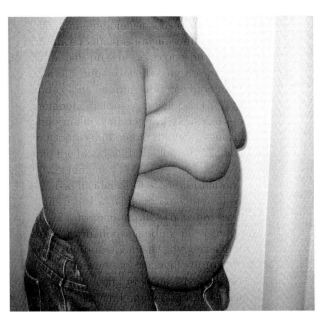

FIG. 38-28

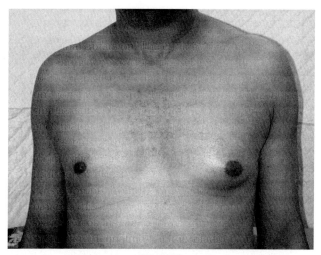

FIG. 38-29

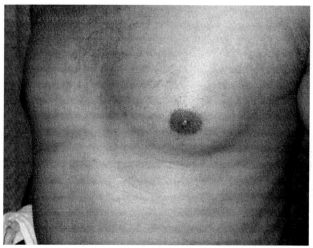

FIG. 38-30

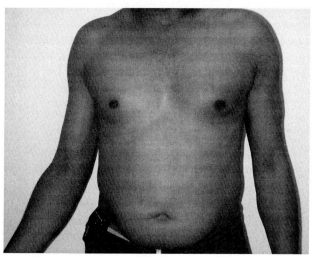

FIG. 38-31

hormones and (2) peripubertal because of hormonal fluxes. During these two times it is considered to be physiologic and needs no further workup. Most of this is expected to abate with tincture of time. During other times a thorough general physical examination must first be undertaken with specific attention paid to the abdomen looking for hepatomegaly and signs of liver disease and if needed a hormone level assay should be obtained. A medical history must also be conducted to rule out endocrinologic causes or hormones such as anabolic steroids, medications such as spironolactone, or drug use such as marijuana. Once these have been appropriately addressed or corrected including correctable conditions such as obesity, treatment can be undertaken based on the degree of deformity. Breast cancer is unlikely and has no correlation with gynecomastia. In fact, less than 1% of all cancers in men originate from the breast. Corrective surgeries may include liposuction, which has been shown to decrease the redundant skin as well as the granular and fatty components, and reduce the nipple-areola complex diameter. Other surgeries such as debulking, minimal incision, or radical excision with free nipple graft may be indicated.

Bibliography

Courtiss E. Gynecomastia: analysis of 159 patients and current recommendations for treatment. *Plast Reconstr Surg* 1987;79(5):740–753.

Volpe C, Raffetto J, Collure D, Hoover E, Doerr R. Unilateral male breast masses: cancer risk and their evaluation and management. *Am J Surg* 1999;65(3): 250–253.

27. **(C)** A panniculectomy is often performed on morbidly obese patients who have a significant overhang of skin and subcutaneous tissue (Figs. 38-32 through 38-35). Because of hydrostatic pressures, the abdominal wall pannus often will develop lymphedema, recurrent bouts of lymphangitis which worsen the lymphedema, dilated and tortuous varicosities, and skin excoriations. Aside from problems of personal hygiene, these patients often develop intertrigo or *C. albicans* rashes in the grooves associated with the pannus. Ambulation becomes difficult because of this increase in mass which is held far away from the center of axis and load bearing of the body, namely the spinal axis. Often times this is accompanied with either occult or evident ventral herniations.

Panniculectomy can be safely performed under a general anesthetic. But, because of the frequent accompaniment of sleep apnea in the morbidly obese, the potential for a difficult airway with a retruded chin and "bull" neck, associated morbidities such as diabetes and hypertension, this is most often performed

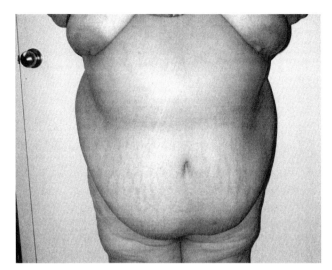

FIG. 38-32

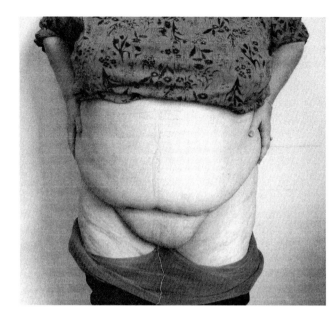

FIG. 38-34

with a postoperative ICU bed reserved for the patient. Although transfusions are not frequently necessary, the estimated blood loss from a panniculectomy can vary from 150 to 3500 cc.

Specifically, surgical technique encompasses a wedge-shaped resection with minimal undermining and closure over multiple drains. Meticulous attention is devoted to hemostasis. Patients can expect a nearly 100% risk of some delayed healing, poor healing, fat necrosis, or other complications. They should be maintained on deep vein thrombosis (DVT) prophylaxis via subcutaneous heparin, sequential compression stockings, or an inferior vena cava filter. Typically "a big boy" bed is needed both for the operation and for postoperative convalescence, with the use of physical therapy for assistance with early ambulation. Patients can be advised that they will most likely loose the umbilicus during the procedure.

Bibliography

Pearl M, Valea F, Chalas E. Panniculectomy and supraumbilical vertical midline incisions in morbidly obese gynecologic oncology patients. *J Am Coll Surg* 1998;186(6): 649–653.

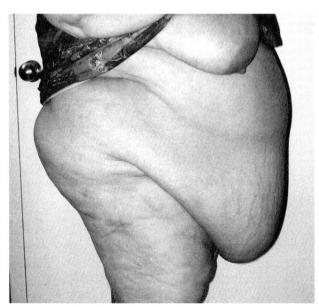

FIG. 38-33

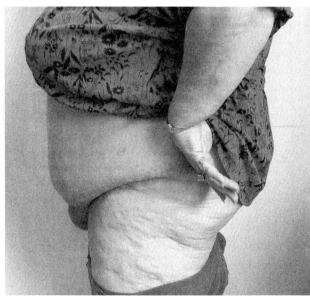

FIG. 38-35

28. **(D)** Autologous reconstruction typically takes tissue from the lower abdominal wall for reconstruction of the breast mound. Because of its fatty nature and the average age of the woman undergoing such an operation, adequate soft tissues are usually found here to reconstruct like tissue with like. That is, the soft and fatty nature of the breast is reconstructed with abdominal fat that creates lifelike feel and motion of the breast; however, this is not the only donor site available. Previous liposuction, although not a strict contraindication to a TRAM operation, can diminish the reservoir effect needed. Similarly, abdominoplasty not only diminishes abdominal wall fatty tissues, but is also a contraindication to a free TRAM operation, as all the perforators have been divided previously by the operation. A paucity of local tissue in a very thin woman is similarly a contraindication to recruitment of tissues from the abdomen.

However, autologous tissue does not rely solely on the abdominal site for a donor reservoir. Other modalities in reconstructing the breast include the latissimus dorsi muscle flap which recruits muscle and subcutaneous soft tissue padding from the back, the S-GAP flap which uses tissues from the buttock region based on the perforator of the superior gluteal artery. Other less used areas of donor areas include the tensor fascia lata from the trochanteric region or a pedicled omentum.

Bibliography

Blondeel P. The sensate free superior gluteal artery perforator (S-GAP) flap: a valuable alternative in autologous breast reconstruction. *Br J Plast Surg* 1999;52(3):185–193.

Emeri J, Krupp S, Doerfl J. Is a free or pedicled TRAM flap safe after liposuction? *Plast Reconstr Surg* 1993;92(6):1198.

Hartrampf C, Scheflan M, Black P. Breast reconstruction with a the transverse abdominal island flap. *Plast Reconstr Surg* 1982;69: 216.

Heitmann C, Pelzer M, Menke H, Germann G. The free musculocutaneous tensor fascia lata flap as a backup procedure in tumor surgery. *Ann Plast Surg* 2000;45(4): 399–404.

Phillips C. Breast reconstruction after classic radical mastectomy: use of omental pedicled grafts and fascia lata. *South Med J* 1982;75(3):270–273.

Ribuffo D, Marcellino M, Barnett G, Houseman N, Scuderi N. Breast reconstruction with abdominal flaps after abdominoplasties. *Plast Reconstr Surg* 2001;108(6): 1604–1608.

Schneider W, Hill H Jr, Brown R. Latissimus dorsi myocutaneous flap for breast reconstruction. *Br J Plast Surg* 1977;30(4):277–281.

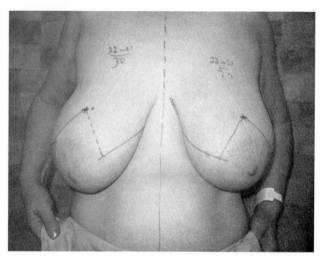

FIG. 38-36

29. **(D)** For mild-to-moderate breast reductions without significant nipple-areola complex ptosis, any of the above techniques are well suited. Whereas liposuction to reduce breasts in this range is acceptable, long-term follow-up is needed. Similarly, the short scar technique or the vertical breast reduction involves limitation of the scar to just around the nipple-areola complex and a vertical component. Drs. Lejour and Lassus champion this technique. The traditional anchor-shaped or Wise pattern (Fig. 38-36) breast reduction is the long held technique. It provides adequate shaping as well as reduction of the breast. The skin pattern is very versatile and useful in all sizes of breast reduction (Figs. 38-37 through 38-40). However, this technique of breast reduction does leave very significant

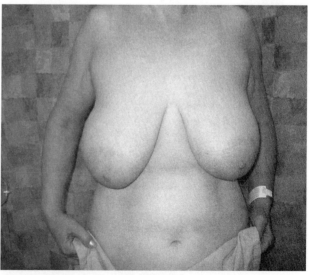

FIG. 38-37

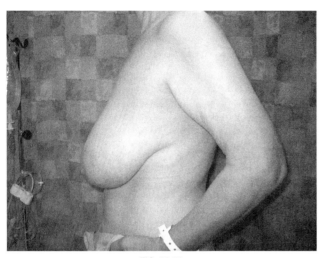

FIG. 38-38

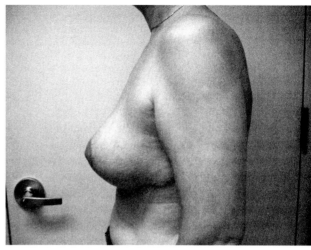

FIG. 38-40

scars, and it is especially unattractive to the young patient. The scars include one around the nipple-areola complex, a vertical scar, and an inframammary scar which is often approximately 30 cm in length.

Bibliography

Gray L. Liposuction breast reduction. *Aesth Plast Surg* 1998;22(3):159–162.

Lejour M, Abboud M, Declety A, Kertesz P. Reduction of mammaplasty scars: from a short inframammary scar to a vertical scar. *Ann Chir Plast Esthet* 1990;35(5): 369–379.

Matarasso A, Courtiss E. Suction mammaplasty: the use of suction lipectomy to reduce large breasts. *Plast Reconstr Surg* 1991;87(4):709–717.

Wise R. A preliminary report on a method of planning the mammaplasty. *Plast Reconstr Surg* 1956;17:367.

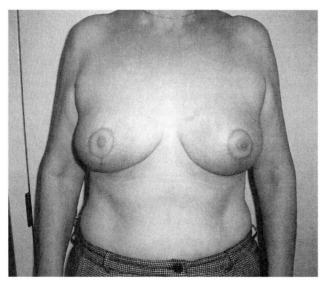

FIG. 38-39

30. **(B)** After the acute recovery phase is completed and the patient's burn wound is healed, a period of time is permitted to allow softening and maturation of the scars. Typically, secondary burn reconstruction can begin 3–12 months after the injury. Best results are obtained using full-thickness skin grafts. Because the donor sites for full-thickness skin grafts are limited, tissue expansion may be undertaken. Tissue expanded areas can be used as full-thickness skin grafts or expanded transposition flaps to achieve resurfacing. The best color match for the face typically comes from skin available from behind the ear, the upper eyelids, the front of the ear as in a facelift, or the supraclavicular area. Thus, donor sites are limited to the head/neck region and the groin crease. Full-thickness skin grafts offer the least secondary contracture and when they are used to cover areas across joints, limitation of function is not typically encountered.

Split-thickness skin grafts typically show the greatest degree of secondary contracture and deformation. These are not suitable for reconstruction across functional regions or in areas of aesthetic concerns, such as the head and neck region or genitalia. Debridement and granulation is not a suitable alternative since it will cause far poorer results than split-thickness skin grafting. Cultured epithelial autograft is reserved for patients with large burn surface areas and limited donor sites. It is used for immediate coverage and not suitable for secondary reconstruction. It is also prohibitively expensive.

Bibliography

Iwuagwu F, Wilson D, Bailie F. The use of skin grafts in postburn contracture release: a 10-year review. *Plast Reconstr Surg* 1999;103(4):1198–1204.

O'Connor NE, Mulliken JB, Banks-Schlegel S, Kehinde O, Green H. Grafting of burns with cultured epithelium prepared from autologous epidermal cells. *Lancet* 1981; 10;1(8211):75–78.

Spence R. Experience with novel uses of tissue expanders in burn reconstruction of the face and neck. *Ann Plast Surg* 1992;28(5):453–464.

31. **(B)** Pressure reduction is absolutely required in any attempts to treat a pressure sore. A pressure sore develops because of undue pressure either because of an acutely compromised or chronically compromised state. Acutely, one might see an otherwise healthy person who has been medically debilitated either because of a stroke, severe trauma, or acute exacerbation of a preexisting condition. Once they recover from their acute illness and neurologic function has been restored, these areas will start to heal as pressure is reduced. For severe pressure sores during this time, musculofascial flap coverage may be developed to shorten the time period for convalescence and to restore function early.

Patients in a chronically compromised state, such as that sustained from a neurologic injury that leaves them debilitated and insensate, are a profound risk factor for pressure sores. There is no expectation of reversal, so diligent pressure reduction is the key to prevention. For the wheelchair-bound it not only requires improved cushions, but also requires shifting the weight of and changing positions of the patient every 20 min. If this is not religiously adhered to, pressure sores will develop. For those that are bed confined, similar methods of pressure reduction of varying degrees are available. Nonetheless, pressure reduction via position changes is paramount.

Pressure sores do not often get infected, therefore antibiotics are not critical; however, mechanical debridement with wet to dry dressings, chemical debridements with enzymatic debriders (Accuzyme), surgical debridement, or biological debridement (maggots) can help to improve the wound. Flap coverage using musculofasciocutaneous flaps is important in closing wounds. Nonetheless, the wound will break down again if pressure reduction is not maintained throughout. Flaps must be used parsimoniously in the chronically impaired individual, understanding that they have a 70% chance of developing repeat pressure ulcerations because of their insensate nature. Hyperbaric oxygen is a useful adjunct, as are antibiotics, but they are not critical for closure of such wounds.

Bibliography

Disa J, Carlton J, Goldberg N. Efficacy of operative cure in pressure sore patients. *Plast Reconstr Surg* 1992;89(2): 272–278.

Fischer B. Low pressure hyperbaric oxygen treatment of decubiti and skin ulcers. *Proc Annu Clin Spinal Cord Inj Conf* 1966;15:97–107.

Griffith B. Myocutaneous flaps for repair of pressure sores. *Plast Reconstr Surg* 1977;60(3):441.

Rodeheaver G. Pressure ulcer debridement and cleansing: a review of current literature. *Ostomy Wound Manage* 1999;45(1A Suppl):80S–85S.

Stotts N, Hunt T. Pressure ulcers. Managing bacterial colonization and infection. *Clin Geriatr Med* 1997;13(3): 565–573.

32. **(A)** Patients will typically lose one to two units of blood from a large scalp laceration at the scene. Even deaths have been reported in the medical literature from isolated scalp laceration exsanguination. Although scalp laceration bleeding frequently stops spontaneously or with the application of pressure, if bleeding does not stop immediately, surgical attention must be directed to the wound promptly. Typically, this involves something as simple as suture ligation of bleeding vessels from the occipital artery or the temporal artery. Then, the wound is closed, as this will further achieve hemostasis. In a patient with any traumatic injury, hypovolemic shock must be anticipated and treated immediately if it occurs. Scalp lacerations can become life threatening if they continue to bleed; they must be paid attention to and not relegated to a junior member of the surgical team.

Bibliography

Limongelli W, Ogle O, Clark M, Williams A. Fatal massive edema of the head and neck secondary to scalp laceration: report of case. *J Oral Surg* 1977;35(3):215–218.

Turnage B, Maull K. Scalp laceration: an obvious 'occult' cause of shock. *South Med J* 2000;93(3):265–266.

33. **(B)** One flap available after debridement of the nonviable sternum includes the omentum. This is based on the right or left gastroepiploic arteries; however, since this woman has previously had a gastrectomy, those vessels are likely to be absent and the omentum may have been resected. The workhorses for obliteration of the defect are the pectoralis major muscle flaps. The axial blood flow is based on the thoracoacromial vessels and they can be advanced from either the left or right side to obliterate the defect. Secondary sources of blood supply for these flaps are perforators from the internal mammary artery. Based on these, the thoracoacromial pedicle can be divided and the muscle turned over into the defect based on the internal mammary perforators. Since the left internal mammary artery has been redirected to revascularize the coronaries in the above patient, a left

pectoralis major turnover flap is not an option. On the right side the pectoralis major may be turned over to obliterate the defect. Similarly, the left rectus abdominis cannot be turned into the defect since its superior blood supply is the superior epigastric which is a continuation of the internal mammary. In this patient, the right rectus can be turned up to obliterate the defect.

Overall, risk factors for sternal dehiscence include diabetes, prolonged surgery time, extended ICU stay, and harvest of the internal mammary artery, especially if both the left and right internal mammary arteries are harvested. Females with large pendulous breasts have an additional risk factor as the breasts place immense lateral traction on the sternum.

Bibliography

Copeland M, Senkowski C, Ulcickas M, Mendelson M, Griepp R. Breast size as a risk factor for sternal wound complications following cardiac surgery. *Arch Surg* 1994;129(7):757–759.

Gummert J, Barten M, Hans C, et al. Mediastinitis and cardiac surgery—an updated risk factor analysis in 10,373 consecutive adult patients. *Thorac Cardiovasc Surg* 2002;50(2):87–91.

Jurkiewicz M, Bostwick J III, Hester T, et al. Infected median sternotomy wounds: Successful treatment by muscle flaps. *Ann Surg* 1980;191:738.

Neale H, Kreilein J, Schreiber J, Gregory R. Complete sternectomy for chronic osteomyelitis with reconstruction using a rectus abdominis myocutaneous island flap. *Ann Plast Surg* 1981;6(4):305–314.

Texier M, Preaux J, Baruch J, Banzet P, Dufourmentel C. Treatment of thoracic radiodermatitis by pediculated autoplasty of the omentum following by cutaneous graft (Kiricuta's technic). *Chirurgie* 1973;99(4):262–267.

34. (C) The sartorius muscle can be easily mobilized with minimal donor site morbidity to cover overexposed prostheses in the groin. The rectus femoris is also a potential flap as are rectus abdominus and gracilis flaps. The donor site related to the rectus femoris in an elderly person can lead to impaired ability to stand upright from a recumbent position. The rectus abdominis donor site can lead to truncal instability, abdominal wall laxity, and even hernia formation.

The rectus abdominis is not a good choice if the patient has had extensive external iliac artery dissection, such as in the case of an aorto-bifemoral graft. Since the blood supply to the rectus abdominis comes off as the deep inferior epigastric artery from the external iliac, this will likely have been ligated in an extensive mobilization of the iliac and after division of the inguinal ligament. If a lymph leak is discovered intraoperatively, the source and location for this can be identified by injecting lymphazurin into

one of the foot followed by looking for extravasation of the blue dye. The source of the lymph leak can then be oversewn.

Bibliography

Babayan R. Soft tissue defects of the groin and their treatment with myocutaneous flaps of m. rectus femoris. *Zentralbl Chir* 1986;111(1):53–56.

Parkash S. The use of myocutaneous flaps in block dissections of the groin in cases with gross skin involvement. *Br J Plast Surg* 1982;35(4):413–419.

35. (A) This most likely represents an orbital floor fracture. A black eye finding on physical examination is not an innocuous finding. It must be followed through with a thoroughly directed head/neck examination including cranial nerves II through XII, palpation for tenderness, and an ophthalmologic consultation. A CT scan with coronal and axial scanning cuts is recommended (Figs. 38-41 and 38-42). Typically after localized trauma to the periorbital region, bony sheer forces create an orbital floor blowout fracture. Periorbital muscles and fat can become herniated and trapped in the fracture line along the orbital floor causing restriction of eye movement resulting in diplopia. Intraocular hemorrhage, such as hyphema, may accompany the bony injury. An orbital floor fracture can also be part of a series of fractures such as in the case of a zygomatical maxillary complex fracture.

In this case, the physical findings do not represent a LeFort III fracture since there is no contralateral spectacle hematoma. Since his only complaints are that of double vision and a headache, these do

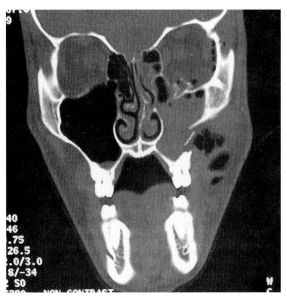

FIG. 38-41

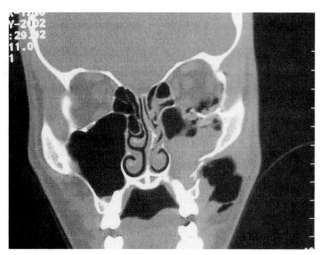

FIG. 38-42

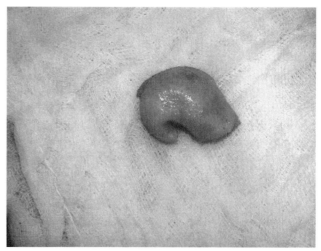

FIG. 38-43

not increase the suspicion for an intracranial hemorrhage. There is also no evidence of retinal detachment at this point.

Bibliography

DeHaven C, Harle T. Orbital blowout fracture; a "black eye". *Texas Med* 1966;62(9):71–74.

Manson P. Facial fractures. In: Aston S, Beasley R, Thorne C (eds.), *Grabb and Smith's Plastic Surgery*, 5th ed. Philadelphia, PA: Lippincott-Raven, 1997, 383–412.

36. **(C)** Principles of management concerning amputated body parts are as follows: prehospital treatment including retrieval of the part, preservation of tissue with cooling, and early replantation within 6 h. Furthermore, the principle of spare parts states that even if the bulk of the tissue cannot be adequately salvaged, portions such as tendons, nerves, or skin may be used. While this is generally more applicable in hand surgery, it nonetheless applies everywhere with amputated parts. Microsurgical techniques can also be undertaken if a suitable artery and vein are found to replant the part. This is possible for large blocks of tissue such as an ear, a finger, a hand, or an entire limb. Microsurgical replantation is not suitable for a small portion of the nose.

In this case, placement of the tissue back on the nose after debridement as a composite graft is most appropriate (Figs. 38-43 through 38-45). The tissue, if it is less than 2 cm × 2 cm, might be expected to survive almost entirely including all of its constituent parts (cartilage, fat, and skin). The success of this depends on the youth of the patient and the size of the amputated part (smaller is preferable). In this case, no bridges are burnt if the entire piece is thinned and replaced as a composite graft. Depending on how much might survive, further reconstruction might

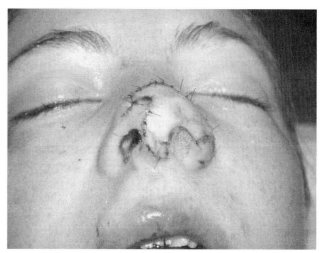

FIG. 38-44

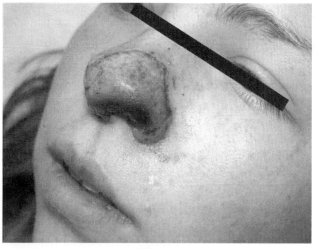

FIG. 38-45

vary from very little to full reconstruction. If the piece was too large or too mangled to be considered for replacement as a composite graft, constituent tissues such as a full-thickness skin graft can be harvested and placed on the wound for at least temporary coverage.

Bibliography

Rohrich R, Barton F, Hollier L. Nasal reconstruction. In: Aston S, Beasley R, Thorne C (eds.), *Grabb and Smith's Plastic Surgery*, 5th ed. New York, NY: Lippincott-Raven, 1997, 513–528.

37. (E) Inside the carpal tunnel, one will find 10 structures: the median nerve, the 4 flexor digitorum superficialis tendons, the 4 flexor digitorum profundus tendons, and the flexor pollicis longus tendon. The flexor carpi radialis and flexor carpi ulnaris tendons do not cross the carpus.

Several key structures associated with hand anatomy are described in the following text. When dividing the hand into regions, one will find the wrist, palm, digits, and thumb. Starting with the wrist, it is made up of eight carpal bones: (proximal row, lateral to medial) scaphoid, lunate, triquetrum, and pisiform; (distal row, lateral to medial) trapezium, trapezoid, capitate, hamate. The extensor retinaculum, located on the dorsum of the wrist, transmits the extensor tendons through six extensor compartments: first—abductor pollicis longus and extensor pollicis brevis; second—extensor carpi radialis longus and brevis; third—extensor pollicis longus; fourth—extensor digitorum communis and extensor indicis proprius; fifth—extensor digiti minimi; and sixth—extensor carpi ulnaris. The radial artery passes through the anatomical snuff box located between the first and third compartments.

Key structures in the palm include the five metacarpal bones and four groups of intrinsic muscles (the lumbricals, interossei, thenar, and hypothenar). The lumbricals flex the metacarpophalangeal (MP) joints and extend the interphalangeal (IP) joints, while the interossei abduct and adduct the digits. Two deep spaces in the palm include the thenar and midpalmar.

The thumb is unique in that it has dorsal and volar arterial inflow. It consists of only two phalangeal bones but has an incredible range of motion because of its saddle joint between the thumb metacarpal and trapezium.

The digits can flex because of two tendons: the flexor digitorum profundus (inserts into the epiphysis of the distal phalanx) and the flexor digitorum superficialis (inserts into the epiphysis of the middle phalanx). Once the extensor tendons reach the digits, they divide into three slips: one intermediate (inserts into the middle phalanx) and two collaterals (insert into the distal phalanx).

The hand is innervated by the median, radial, and ulnar nerves, each providing movement and sensation to various parts of the hand with some redundancy. Vascular inflow comes from the radial and ulnar arteries. They provide enough inflow individually that the hand can usually survive with only one of them if the palmar arch is complete. Surface anatomy is also important to hand anatomy in that it helps to locate certain structures. For example, the metacarpophalangeal crease is located about halfway between the first digital phalanx. For a complete review of hand anatomy, please access one of the sources referenced.

Bibliography

Moore K. *Clinically Oriented Anatomy*, 2nd ed. Baltimore, MD: Lippincott, Williams & Wilkins, 1985.
Williams P, Warwick R. *Gray's Anatomy*, 37th ed. Edinburgh: Churchill Livingstone, 1989.

38. (D) Human bites frequently transmit the bacterium *E. corrodens* while cat bites are associated with *P. multocida*. All bites should be irrigated copiously and any human bite that invades a joint space should be washed out and debrided in the operating room. Antibiotic coverage for a human bite should include a first-generation cephalosporin or penicillin while cat bites require ampicillin/sulbactam.

Hand infections are a common occurrence in the emergency room, and special attention should be given to those patients with diabetes or some other immunocompromised state. Tetanus prophylaxis is mandatory. Several specific types of infections are described in the following text. Paronychia involves infection around the fingernail. *Staphylococcus aureus* is the most common organism, and treatment involves incision and drainage with a low threshold to remove the fingernail in order to achieve adequate debridement. Chronic paronychia is associated with *C. albicans* infection and is seen in patients who frequently immerse their hands in water (dishwashers). Therefore, behavior modification and a topical antifungal comprise the treatment of choice.

A *felon* is infection in the distal pulp of a digit or thumb. Again, incision, drainage, and antibiotics are used for treatment. The incision should be longitudinal and on the side of the digit or thumb instead of directly in the middle as this results in the fewest complications.

Flexor tenosynovitis is also commonly encountered and carries high morbidity if not adequately treated in a timely manner. The presence of Kanavel's signs are highly indicative of flexor tenosynovitis and include (1) extreme tenderness over the flexor tendon sheath, (2) erythema and edema of the involved digit with a "sausage" digit, (3) a flexed position of the digit, and (4) pain with passive extension of the digit. Treatment is operative and includes an incision in the distal palm to access the proximal portion of the tendon sheath. After the distal portion has been exposed with a midaxial incision over the distal digit, an irrigation catheter is inserted into the sheath followed by copious irrigation intraoperatively and for 48 h on the floor.

Bibliography

Antosia R, Lyn E. The hand. In: Marx J, Hochberger R, Walls R (eds.), *Rosen's Emergency Medicine: Concepts and Clinical Practice*, 4th ed. St. Louis, MO: Mosby, 1998, 662–665.

Hausman M, Lisser S. Hand infections. *Orthop Clin North Am* 1992;23(1):171–185.

Kanavel A. Tuberculous tenosynovitis of the hand: a report of fourteen cases of tuberculous tenosynovitis. *Surg Gynecol Obstet* 1923;37:635.

39. **(D)** The Allen test can be used to assess the radial, ulnar, and common digital arteries along with the superficial palmar arch. To evaluate the radial and ulnar arteries with the Allen test, ask the patient to clench his hand, occlude the radial and ulnar arteries, have the patient open his hand, release one of the arteries, and observe for capillary refill.

Neurologic examination of the hand involves the ulnar, median, and radial nerves. To evaluate ulnar sensory function, test two-point discrimination over the small finger and ulnar half of the ring finger. Ulnar motor function is tested by having the patient open his extended fingers against resistance. Median sensory function involves the thumb and medial 2 $1/2$ digits. Thumb flexion assesses median motor function. The radial nerve provides sensation to the dorsal surface of the radial 3 $1/2$ digits. Extension of the digits tests radial nerve motor function. Dermatomes attributed to the hand include C6 (thumb and index finger), C7 (middle finger), and C8 (ring and little fingers). To test sensory function in children, immerse the hand in water. Wrinkling of the skin indicates intact sensory function.

The joints should be evaluated for any range of motion deficits. To assess the flexor digitorum superficialis tendon, have the patient flex each finger while the others are held in extension. Flexor digitorum profundus function is evaluated by holding the PIP in place while the patient tries to flex the DIP. Extensor pollicis longus function is evaluated by telling the patient to place his hand on a table and then attempt to lift the thumb. In the uncooperative

or comatose patient, the cascade of the digits and the tenodesis effect may be used to confirm that the tendons are intact.

Three view radiographs of the hand should be obtained in all hand injuries to assess bony defects and to detect any foreign bodies. Keep the patient NPO in case the injury requires a trip to the operating room. During the history and physical, it is important to ask which hand is dominant and what the position the hand was in during the injury.

Bibliography

Orthoteers. *Hand Examination*, 2000. [Data file] Available at: http://www.orthoteers.co.uk

Wheeless' Textbook of Orthopaedics. *Hand and Wrist: Physical Exam*, 2002. [Data file] Available at: http://wheeless.orthoweb.be

40. **(B)** A rhytidectomy, or facelift, can be done using several different techniques, such as the subcutaneous plane, superficial musculoaponeurotic system (SMAS), deep plane, composite, or subperiosteal. The subcutaneous facelift is the easiest to perform, poses little risk to the facial nerve, provides the ability to tighten the skin, but does not provide access to any of the deep tissues for more definitive maneuvers. In the face exists a unique fascial layer that divides the subcutaneous fat into two layers. It joins the temporoparietal fascia superiorly, the orbicularis oris anteriorly, and the platysma muscle inferiorly. Pulling on the SMAS give more definition to the jawline, but deepens the nasolabial fold. The deep plane technique allows relaxation of the nasolabial fold, provides more vascularity than the subcutaneous technique, but poses a higher risk to the facial nerve. The composite facelift uses the deep plane, but also tightens the platysma and orbicularis oculi muscles. Finally, the subperiosteal facelift uses the temporal fascia as an anchor for tightening the facial tissue, but this technique can cause excessive facial swelling, produce a "mask effect" for a few months, and also places the facial nerve at high risk for damage. The most common complication following a facelift is a hematoma, followed by injury to the great auricular and facial nerves.

Recent FDA approval has allowed the use of Botox (botulinum toxin type A) injections to treat facial wrinkles. Actually, eight types of toxins exist and the mechanism of action involves inhibiting acetylcholine release at the neuromuscular junction. Onset of action is 5–7 days and the antiwrinkle effect usually lasts 4–6 months. Care must be taken during injection as complications include diplopia, ecchymoses, eyebrow ptosis, retrobulbar hemorrhage, and globe perforation.

Facial contour may be augmented with alloplastic implants and their use in the operating room is simple and fast with very good results. The cheek, malar, and submalar areas are commonly augmented to correct deficiencies resulting from trauma, congenital asymmetry, or aging. Placement may be performed intraorally or through a facelift or subciliary incision. The intraoral approach is scarless, but exposure to oral flora raises the risk for infection. Also, subciliary placement may result in ectropion.

Bibliography

Eppley B. Alloplastic implantation. *Plast Reconstr Surg* 1999;104(6):1761–1783.

Ivy E, Lorenc Z. Aston SJ. Is there a difference? A prospective study comparing lateral and standard SMAS face lifts with extended SMAS and composite rhytidectomies. *Plast Reconstr Surg* 1996;98(7):1135–1143.

Kamer F, Frankel A. SMAS rhytidectomy versus deep plane rhytidectomy: an objective comparison. *Plast Reconstr Surg* 1998;102(3):878–881.

Matsudo P. Botulinum toxin for correction of fronto-glabellar wrinkles: preliminary evaluation. *Aesth Plast Surg* 1996; 20(5):439–441.

41. (B) Digital tip amputations without exposed bone should undergo revision amputation or be left to heal by secondary intention. If bone is exposed, skeletal shortening with a rongeur should be done to provide enough skin for primary or secondary closure. If a large portion of the finger pad has been amputated, several flaps may be performed for sensate wound coverage (V-Y advancement, lateral V-Y, cross-finger pedicle, or thenar flaps). The thumb is of special consideration in all amputations in that every effort should be made to preserve length and sensation. Therefore, tip amputations of the thumb may warrant a local flap (volar Moberg flap) to provide sensate coverage.

Amputations through the DIP and PIP joints should be closed after roungeuring the volar and lateral condylar prominences for aesthetic appearance. If the digit is amputated distal to the insertion of the flexor digitorum superficialis into the epiphysis of the middle phalanx, length should be preserved with minimal skeletal shortening for adequate primary closure or replantation should be attempted if possible. However, if the amputation is proximal to the FDS insertion, skeletal shortening to the PIP should be performed. Any amputation at or near the metacarpophalangeal joint warrants a ray amputation to prevent the problem of dropping objects through the defect.

Incredible technological advances in microsurgery have allowed us the possibility of replantation. Instances where replantation should be attempted include amputations in children, amputations of multiple digits or the thumb, and amputations at the palm, wrist, or forearm. Attempts at replantation should be avoided with crush injuries, gross contamination, amputation through or distal to the DIP, and multilevel injuries. When replantation is attempted, efforts should be aimed at restoring function instead of solely cosmetic appearance. All amputated pieces should be transported with the patient as they may be useful for bone or tendon pieces. The parts should be wrapped in a saline-soaked gauze, placed in a dry plastic bag, and this bag should be placed on ice. A 90% success rate has been reported with replantation efforts.

Bibliography

Kutler W. A new method for finger tip amputation. *JAMA* 1947;144:29.

Soucacos P, Beris A, Touliatos A, et al. Current indications for single digit replantation. *Acta Orthop Scand Suppl* 1995;264:12–15.

Gurdin M, Pangman W. The repair of surface deficits of fingers by transdigital flaps. *Plast Reconstr Surg* 1950;5: 368–371.

Gatewood A. A plastic repair of finger defects without hospitalization. *JAMA* 1926;87:1479.

Moberg E. Aspects of sensation in reconstructive surgery of the upper limb. *J Bone Joint Surg* 1964;46A:817–825.

Louis D. Amputations. In: Green D (ed.), *Green's Operative Hand Surgery*, 1st ed. New York, NY: Churchill Livingstone, 1982, 55–112.

CHAPTER 39

Urologic Surgery

Peter Lawrence, Tyler Emley, and Mike Koch

Questions

1. A 19-year-old male undergoes a left radical orchiectomy for a painless left testicular mass. Pathology reveals embryonal carcinoma (40%), yolk sac (20%), and teratoma (40%). Serum alpha-fetoprotein (AFP) and beta-HCG were both elevated preoperatively. A computed tomography (CT) scan revealed moderate paraaortic lymphadenopathy and he received three courses of platinum-based chemotherapy. Following chemotherapy his tumor markers normalized and a follow-up CT is shown in Fig. 39-1. What is the most appropriate next step?

   (A) observation
   (B) repeat tumor markers and CT in 3 months
   (C) administer one additional cycle of platinum-based chemotherapy
   (D) administer two additional cycles of platinum-based chemotherapy
   (E) retroperitoneal lymph node dissection (RPLND)

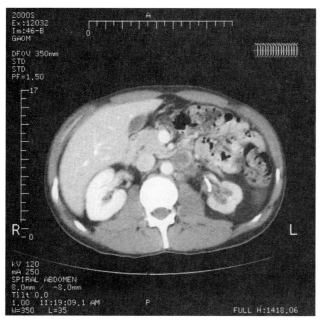

FIG. 39-1

2. Which of the following is the most important prognostic factor for patients with renal cell carcinoma?

   (A) tumor size
   (B) nuclear grade
   (C) histologic subtype
   (D) performance status
   (E) pathologic stage

3. A 32-year-old male presents for evaluation prior to a vasectomy. Physical examination reveals a normal phallus and the testicles are descended bilaterally without any palpable masses. The right vas deferens is normal but the left is absent. What is the most appropriate next step?

   (A) scrotal ultrasound
   (B) renal ultrasound
   (C) pelvic CT
   (D) transrectal ultrasound
   (E) right vasogram

4. A 20-year-old male sustains a gunshot wound to the abdomen with a low caliber handgun. He undergoes an emergent laparotomy and is found to have a complete transection of the left ureter at the pelvic brim. Which technique of repair is most appropriate?

   (A) ureteral reimplantation
   (B) primary reanastomosis
   (C) transureteroureterostomy
   (D) end cutaneous ureterostomy
   (E) ureteronoecystotomy with Boari flap

5. A 12-year-old male presents to the emergency room with acute scrotal pain and swelling for 4 h. On examination his left hemiscrotum is edematous, erythematous, and exquisitely tender to touch (T 99.9°F, HR 125 bpm, BP 126/60 mmHg). An ultrasound with Doppler is obtained and is shown in Fig. 39-2. What is the most likely diagnosis?

    (A) epididymitis
    (B) testicular cancer
    (C) acute testicular torsion
    (D) torsion of appendix testis
    (E) orchitis

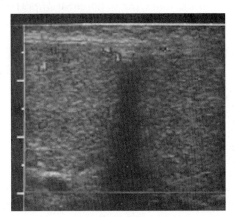

FIG. 39-2

6. Which of the following statements concerning urinary tract infections (UTIs) during pregnancy is *true*?

    (A) The prevalence of bacteruria is increased in pregnant females when compared to nonpregnant females.
    (B) The prevalence of bacteruria is decreased in pregnant females when compared to nonpregnant females.
    (C) Sulfa preparations can be safely used during the third trimester of pregnancy.
    (D) The incidence of acute clinical pyelonephritis is increased in pregnant women with bacteruria.
    (E) The risk of bacteruria decreases with the duration of pregnancy.

7. Which of the following bacteria is most commonly associated with infected renal calculi?

    (A) *Escherichia coli*
    (B) *Ureaplasma urealyticum*
    (C) *Staphylococcus epidermidis*
    (D) *Klebsiella pneumonia*
    (E) *Proteus mirabilis*

8. A 50-year-old female undergoes a radical hysterectomy for invasive endometrial carcinoma. The operation was complicated by excessive bleeding during division and ligation of the right uterine artery. On postoperative day 3 she develops persistent right flank pain, nausea, and vomiting. Physical examination reveals significant discomfort in the right upper quadrant and severe CVA tenderness (T 102.1°F, BP 91/46 mmHg, HR 119 bpm). An intravenous pyelogram is obtained and is shown in Fig. 39-3. What is the most appropriate next step?

    (A) percutaneous nephrostomy tube
    (B) observation
    (C) reexploration and open repair
    (D) ureteroscopy
    (E) pain medication and antiemetics

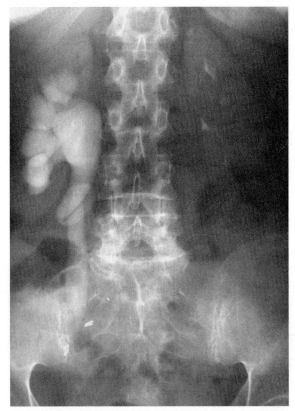

FIG. 39-3

9. A 42-year-old female has an arteriogram for uncontrollable hypertension (Fig. 39-4). What is the most likely diagnosis?

    (A) medial fibroplasia
    (B) intimal fibroplasia
    (C) perimedial fibroplasia
    (D) fibromuscular hyperplasia
    (E) none of the above

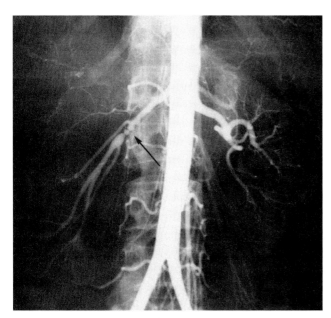

FIG. 39-4

10. A 7-year-old female is diagnosed with bilateral moderate (grade III) vesicoureteral reflux after developing a febrile UTI. A renal ultrasound reveals normal kidneys bilaterally and she is started on prophylactic antibiotics. Three months later she develops a temperature of 39°C. A urine culture done at that time grows >100k colomy forming units (CFU) *E. coli*. The most appropriate management is to treat the active infection and

   (A) observation
   (B) unilateral vesicoureteral reimplant
   (C) bilateral vesicoureteral reimplants
   (D) bilateral end cutaneous ureterostomies until she is old enough to undergo reimplants
   (E) bilateral percutaneous nephrostomy tubes to decompress the kidneys

11. Which of the following statements concerning enteroceles is *false*?

   (A) The diagnosis of an enterocele is made on the basis of physical examination.
   (B) Enteroceles may occur in association with rectoceles.
   (C) Dyspareunia and vaginal discomfort are commonly associated symptoms.

   (D) During the rectovaginal examination, the mass is classically found anterior to the cervix.
   (E) Surgical repair of an enterocele can be performed abdominally or vaginally.

12. Which of the following statements concerning undescended testicles is *true*?

   (A) In diagnostic laparoscopy, the observation of blind ending spermatic vessels indicates a vanishing testis and requires no further exploration.
   (B) Orchiopexy reduces but does not eliminate the risk of cancer in an undescended testicle.
   (C) The incidence of cryptorchidism in premature males is 3–5%.
   (D) The most common location of an undescended testicle is in the superficial inguinal pouch between the internal oblique and external oblique aponeurosis.
   (E) Fertility rates are not reduced in patients with cryptorchidism if orchiopexy is performed before puberty.

13. A 71-year-old man with a known solitary right kidney presents with a 3-week history of intermittent gross hematuria. His medical history is significant for hypertension and non-insulin-dependent diabetes mellitus. His serum creatinine is 1.4 mg/dL and an IVP (Fig. 39-5) revealed a filling defect in the right midureter. Biopsy of the lesion showed a grade 1/3 Ta transitional cell carcinoma (TCC). Which of the following is the most appropriate management?

   (A) open radical nephroureterectomy with bladder cuff excision
   (B) laparoscopic radical nephroureterectomy with bladder cuff excision
   (C) segmental ureterectomy with ureteroureterostomy
   (D) subtotal ureterectomy with psoas hitch ureteroneocystotomy
   (E) ureteroscopy with endoscopic resection and laser ablation of the tumor

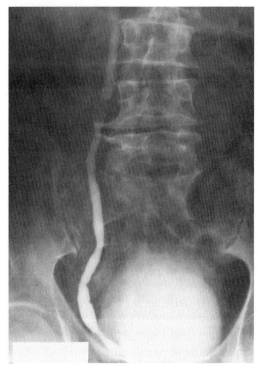

FIG. 39-5

14. A newborn is delivered by spontaneous vaginal delivery at 39 weeks gestation. The mother is a healthy 26-year-old female who reports normal prenatal care. The child is discharged home on the second day of life; however, returns 4 days later with lethargy, vomiting, and poor oral intake. Physical examination reveals a normal sized phallus with chordee and proximal hypospadias. Neither testicle is palpable.

Laboratory evaluation reveals:

Na: 119 meq/L
K: 6.5 meq/L
CO_2: 16 meq/L

What is the most likely diagnosis?

(A) 21-hydroxylase deficiency
(B) 11-beta-hydroxylase deficiency
(C) 3-beta-hydroxylase deficiency
(D) 20,22-desmolase deficiency
(E) 17-alpha-hydroxylase deficiency

15. Which of the following best describes the mechanism of action of sildenafil citrate (Viagra)?

(A) selective inhibitor of phosphodiesterase-5 (PDE-5)
(B) alpha$_1$-adrenergic antagonist
(C) alpha$_2$-adrenergic antagonist

(D) dopaminergic agonist
(E) beta-adrenergic agonist

16. A 36-year-old female with Crohn's disease requires a partial small bowel resection. Six months later she develops left flank pain and a CT scan reveals a 3 mm calculus in the left midureter. What is the most likely composition of the ureteral stone?

(A) calcium oxalate
(B) uric acid
(C) struvite
(D) cystine
(E) ammonium acid urate

17. An ultrasound of a newborn with an abdominal mass is shown in Fig. 39-6. What is the most likely diagnosis?

(A) Wilm's tumor
(B) neuroblastoma
(C) hepatoblastoma
(D) multicystic-dysplastic kidney (MCDPK)
(E) ureteropelvic junction (UPJ) obstruction

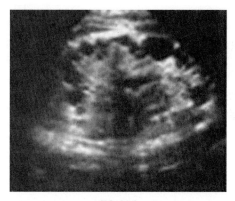

FIG. 39-6

18. A 50-year-old woman presents with right flank pain following blunt abdominal trauma. She is hemodynamically stable with a SBP of 120/70 mmHg, HR of 82 bpm, and RR of 13 breaths/min. Physical examination reveals mild right flank tenderness but is otherwise unremarkable. Her urine is grossly clear but urinalysis reveals 15 RBC/hpf. What is the most appropriate next step?

(A) abdominal/pelvic CT scan
(B) renal ultrasound
(C) intravenous pyelogram
(D) observation
(E) magnetic resonance imaging (MRI)

19. A 53-year-old male with a history of tobacco abuse is found to have 10 RBC/hpf on routine urinalysis. The remaining portion of the urinalysis is normal and culture revealed no growth of bacteria. Which of the following is the most appropriate next step?

(A) observation

(B) repeat urinalysis in 6 months

(C) IVP and cystoscopy

(D) voided cytology

(E) cystogram

20. A 56-year-old male presents with long-standing complaints of a decreased urinary stream. He reports a remote history of urethritis for which he did not seek medical attention. A urethrogram is obtained and is shown in Fig. 39-7. Which of the following organisms is most likely responsible for this process?

(A) *Neisseria gonorrhoeae*

(B) *Ureaplasma urealyticum*

(C) *Chlamydia trachomatis*

(D) *Trichomonas vaginalis*

(E) *Calymmatobacterium granulomatis*

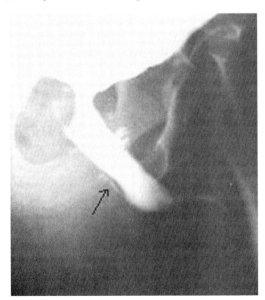

FIG. 39-7

21. A 58-year-old male presents for evaluation of an elevated prostate-specific antigen (PSA) at 5.8. Digital rectal examination reveals a firm, palpable nodule on the right lobe of the prostate. Transrectal ultrasound guided biopsy reveals high-grade prostatic intraepithelial neoplasia (PIN). What is the next most appropriate step?

(A) observation

(B) repeat prostate biopsy

(C) repeat PSA in 6 months

(D) radical prostatectomy

(E) external beam radiation

22. A 52-year-old Black male presents to the emergency department with a painful erection which has been present for approximately 8 h. Aspiration of the corpora reveals dark blood with a pH of 7.23, PO_2 of 26 mmHg, and a PCO_2 of 65 mmHg. Which of the following is least likely to represent the etiology of this patient's priaprism?

(A) sickle cell disease

(B) intracavernosal injection therapy

(C) total parenteral nutrition

(D) perineal trauma

(E) trazodone therapy

23. A healthy 60-year-old male was evaluated for microhematuria. An IVP was obtained and revealed an abnormality in the upper pole of the left kidney. The follow-up CT scan is illustrated in Fig. 39-8. What is the most appropriate management of this lesion?

(A) observation

(B) percutaneous biopsy

(C) left partial nephrectomy

(D) left radical nephrectomy

(E) left radical nephrectomy with excision of bladder cuff

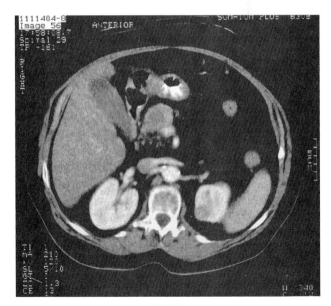

FIG. 39-8

24. A 51-year-old female is evaluated for severe hypertension and headaches. As part of the workup a 24-h urine was collected and revealed a significant elevation in the levels of epinephrine, norepinepherine, and vanillylmandelic acid (VMA). A T2-weighted MRI was obtained and is illustrated in Fig. 39-9. Which of the following is *not* a familial syndrome associated with this neoplasm?

(A) multiple endocrine neoplasia 2 (MEN-2)

(B) Von Recklinghausen's disease (neurofibromatosis)

(C) Von Hippel-Lindau (VHL)

(D) autosomal dominant polycystic kidney disease

(E) tuberous sclerosis

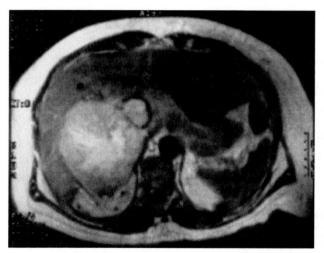

FIG. 39-9

25. A 30-year-old male presents with a 2-week history of right renal colic. He reports a history of passing several small calculi but has never required surgical intervention. An IVP is obtained and is shown in Fig. 39-10. Which of the following represents the most likely diagnosis?

(A) medullary sponge kidney

(B) megacalycosis

(C) hydrocalycosis

(D) renal tubular acidosis

(E) hyperparathyroidism

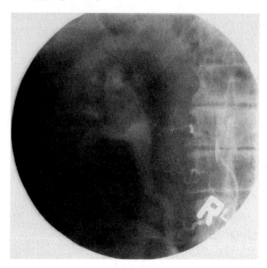

FIG. 39-10

26. A 46-year-old male presents with complaints of right flank pain. Urinalysis reveals 100 RBCs/hpf and 75 WBC/hpf. A kidney, ureter, and bladder (KUB) is obtained and is shown in Fig. 39-11. Which of the following is the most appropriate management?

(A) extracorporal shock wave lithotripsy (ESWL)

(B) ureteroscopy and laser lithotripsy

(C) chemolysis with sodium bicarbonate

(D) percutaneous nephrostolithotomy (PCNL)

(E) anatrophic nephrolithotomy

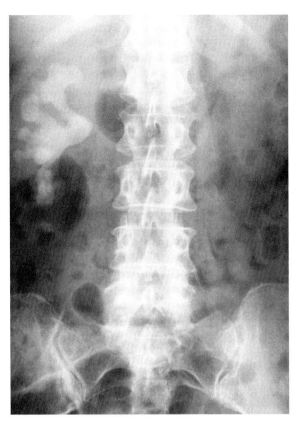

FIG. 39-11

27. A 35-year-old female with hypertension is found to have a bruit on abdominal auscultation. An arteriogram was obtained and is shown in Fig. 39-12. Which of the following predisposes this lesion to rupture?

(A) size greater than 1 cm
(B) pregnancy
(C) coexisting hypotension
(D) complete calcification
(E) none of the above

28. An 18-year-old male presents after a high-speed motor vehicle accident. On physical examination he has severe pelvic pain but the abdomen is benign. A plain radiograph reveals a fracture of the lateral portion of the right ileum. A Foley catheter is inserted with return of 75 cc of bloody urine and a retrograde cystogram is obtained (Fig. 39-13). Which of the following is the most appropriate management of this patient?

(A) continued catheter drainage
(B) CT cystogram
(C) suprapubic cystostomy tube
(D) flexible cystoscopy
(E) open operative repair

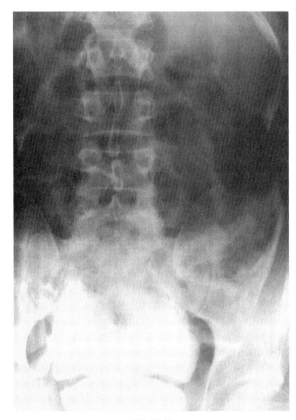

FIG. 39-13

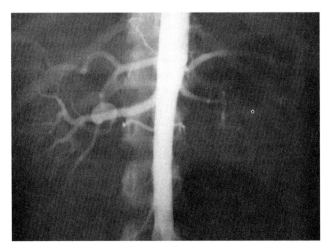

FIG. 39-12

29. An 18-year-old male with a history of seizures and mental retardation presents with vague abdominal pain. Physical examination reveals a palpable left flank mass. He is also noted to have multiple angiofibromas concentrated in the malar region of his face. A CT scan is obtained and is illustrated in Fig. 39-14. What is the most likely diagnosis?

   (A) VHL disease
   (B) Sturge-Weber's disease
   (C) Beckwith-Wiedemann's syndrome
   (D) prune belly syndrome
   (E) tuberous sclerosis

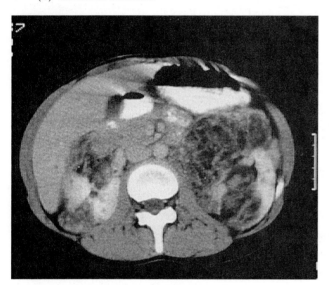

FIG. 39-14

30. A 38-year-old male is involved in a head-on motor vehicle accident. Initial radiographs reveal bilateral inferior pubic rami fractures. On physical examination, he is noted to have blood at the urethral meatus and a retrograde urethrogram is obtained (Fig. 39-15). Which of the following statements concerning this injury is *true*?

   (A) This represents a urethral stretch injury (type I urethral disruption).
   (B) This represents a supramembraneous urethral disruption (type II urethral disruption).
   (C) This represents a transmembraneous urethral disruption (type III urethral disruption).

   (D) Immediate open repair with primary alignment minimizes the risk of impotence.
   (E) Immediate open repair with primary alignment minimizes the risk of incontinence.

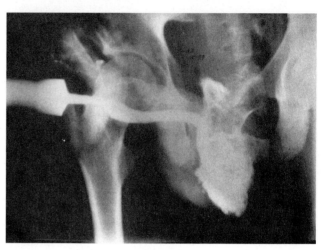

FIG. 39-15

31. A 46-year-old male presents after a high-speed motor vehicle accident. He has remained hemodynamically stable (BP 110/70 mmHg, PR 102, RR 13 breaths/min). Physical examination reveals diffuse abdominal tenderness and right flank eccymosis. A CT scan of the abdomen and pelvis is obtained and is shown in Fig. 39-16.

   Lab data shows the following:

   Hct: 30 mg/dL
   Na: 136 mmL/dL
   K: 4.1 mmL/dL
   Cl: 110 mmL/dL
   CO_2: 22 mg/dL
   BUN: 11 mg/dL
   Cr: 1.3 mg/dL

   Which of the following represents the most appropriate management of this injury?

   (A) hospital admission, bedrest, and serial CBCs
   (B) selective right renal arteriogram
   (C) selective segmental artery embolization
   (D) cystoscopy and right ureteral stent placement
   (E) transabdominal renal exploration

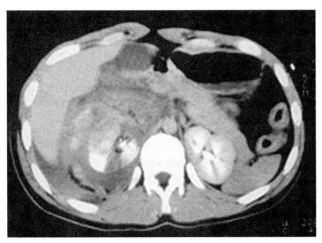

FIG. 39-16

32. A 42-year-old construction worker presents to the emergency department after falling from the roof of a two-story house. Physical examination reveals right upper quadrant and right flank tenderness. A CT scan is obtained and is illustrated in Fig. 39-17. What is the most likely diagnosis?

   (A) segmental renal artery injury
   (B) segmental renal vein injury
   (C) main renal artery injury
   (D) main renal vein injury
   (E) UPJ disruption

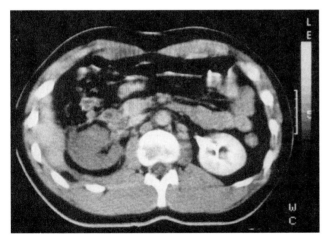

FIG. 39-17

33. A 7-year-old girl presents after being struck by a motor vehicle. She is hemodynamically stable and physical examination reveals point tenderness over the L1 and L2 vertebrae. A CT scan with delayed images is shown in Fig. 39-18. What is the most likely diagnosis?

   (A) renal artery injury
   (B) renal vein injury

   (C) disruption at the UPJ
   (D) renal contusion
   (E) renal cortical laceration

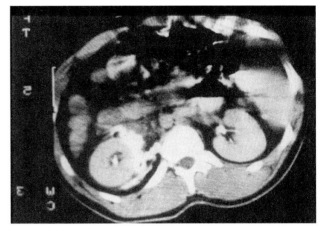

FIG. 39-18

34. What is the mechanism of action of alpha blockers in the treatment of benign prostatic hypertrophy (BPH)?

   (A) relaxation of prostate smooth muscle
   (B) inhibition of 5-alpha reductase
   (C) inhibition of androgen binding
   (D) aromatase inhibition
   (E) beta-adrenergic blockade

35. A 65-year-old male is evaluated for hematuria and is found to have three small bladder tumors on cystoscopy. Transurethral resection demonstrates grade 1/3 superficial (Ta) TCC. What is the next most appropriate step in this patient's management?

   (A) bone scan
   (B) abdominal/pelvic CT scan
   (C) external beam radiation
   (D) radical cystectomy with urinary diversion
   (E) intravesical chemotherapy

36. Which of the following is a potential complication of using intestinal segments in urinary diversion procedures?

   (A) electrolyte abnormalities
   (B) conduit stone formation
   (C) osteomalacia
   (D) sepsis
   (E) all of the above

37. Which of the following contributes to postoperative urinary retention?

    (A) bladder overdistention
    (B) traumatic instrumentation
    (C) decreased bladder contractility
    (D) preexistent pathology
    (E) all of the above

38. A male is born by spontaneous vaginal delivery at 38 weeks EGA. Prenatal ultrasound had revealed bilateral hydronephrosis and oligohydramnios. A repeat renal ultrasound on day 3 of life confirmed severe bilateral hydronephrosis. A voiding cystourethrogram (VCUG) is obtained and is shown in Fig. 39-19. What is the most likely diagnosis?

    (A) retroperitoneal fibrosis
    (B) posterior urethral valves (PUV)
    (C) urethral stricture
    (D) neurogenic bladder
    (E) prune belly syndrome

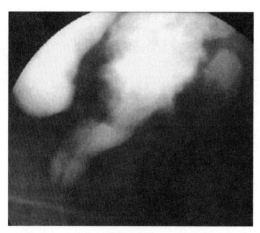

FIG. 39-19

39. Which of the following statements regarding risk factors for the development of bladder cancer is *false*?

    (A) Patients with history of smoking have a higher risk for developing TCC.
    (B) It is more common amongst Black males when compared to White males.
    (C) Industrial exposure increases the risk of developing TCC.
    (D) Long-term indwelling bladder catheters increase the risk of developing squamous cell carcinoma.
    (E) Patients treated with certain chemotherapeutic agents have an increased incidence of TCC.

40. Which of the following values on semen analysis is indicative of male infertility?

    (A) ejaculate volume of 3 mL
    (B) 80% of sperm viable
    (C) pH of 7.2
    (D) 60% motility
    (E) 5×10^6 sperm per ejaculate

Answers and Explanations

1. **(E)** The CT scan reveals persistent paraaortic lymphadenopathy following chemotherapy. Approximately 30% of patients with metastatic testis cancer who receive cisplatin-based chemotherapy will experience a partial remission. This is defined as normalization of tumor markers but persistent radiographic disease in the retroperitoneum, chest, mediastinum, neck, or elsewhere. Histologically, this persistent disease is either necrosis, teratoma, or carcinoma.

   Postchemotherapy RPLND provides both staging and therapeutic benefits. If persistent carcinoma is discovered, then additional chemotherapy is indicated. Removal of teratoma is therapeutic because it is not chemosensitive and can degenerate into nongerm cell cancer. Furthermore, it can also grow and cause morbidity merely by its size.

   The technique of RPLND has also evolved to decrease morbidity. Mapping studies of the retroperitoneum have revealed that not all patients with low volume metastatic disease require a full bilateral RPLND. Modified nerve sparing RPLND allows for the preservation of retroperitoneal sympathetic fibers and virtually eliminates the risk of anejaculation.

Bibliography

Foster RS, Donohue JP. Retroperitoneal lymph node dissection. In: Vogelzang NJ, Scardino PT, Shipley WU, et al. (eds.), *Comprehensive Textbook of Genitourinary Oncology*. Philadelphia, PA: Lippincott, Williams & Wilkins, 2000, 955–959.

2. **(E)** Various tumor-related factors such as size, nuclear grade, and histologic subtype have proved to be useful prognostic factors for patients with renal cell carcinoma. However, multiple studies have shown that pathologic stage is the single most important prognostic factor. These studies demonstrate a 70–90% 5-year survival for organ confined disease. Survival drops by 15–20% with tumor invasion of the perirenal fat. Therefore, the extent of regional or systemic disease at the time of diagnosis is the primary determinant of outcome.

Bibliography

Novick A, Campbell S. Renal tumors. In: Walsh P, Retik A, Vaughan E, et al. (eds.), *Campbell's Urology*, 8th ed. Philadelphia, PA: W.B. Saunders, 2002, 2701–2704.

3. **(B)** The vas deferens and the ureter share an embryologic origin through the mesonephric duct. During the fifth week of gestation, the ureteric bud appears on the posteromedial aspect of the mesonephric duct. The ureteric bud grows toward the sacral portion of the intermediate mesoderm known as the metanephric blastema. The ureteric bud interacts with the metanephric blastema to induce nephrogenesis. During the eighth week of gestation, testosterone acts on the distal mesonephric duct to develop into the male genital ducts (epididymis, vas deferens, and seminal vesicles). Therefore, patients with a congenital absence of the vas deferens are also at risk for renal agenesis. Ipsilateral renal anomalies are present in up to 80% of men with unilateral absence of the vas deferens. Therefore, renal ultrasonography should be considered in all patients with an absent vas deferens.

Bibliography

Cuckow P, Nyirady P. Embryology and pathophysiology of the kidneys and urinary tracts. In: Gearhart J, Rink R, Mouriquand P (eds.), *Pediatric Urology*. Philadelphia, PA: W.B. Saunders, 2001, 5–10.

Sigman M, Jarow J. Male infertility. In: Walsh P, Retik A, Vaughan E, et al. (eds.), *Campbell's Urology*, 8th ed. Philadelphia, PA: W.B. Saunders, 2002, 1495.

4. **(B)** Most partial and complete transactions of the ureter resulting from gunshot wounds can be repaired by primary ureteroureterostomy. Nonviable tissue should be debrided from both the proximal and distal ureteral segments. These segments should be mobilized with care to avoid devascularization. Once the length of the defect is established, a ureteroureterostomy should only be attempted if a tension-free anastomosis can be performed. The anastomosis is usually

performed over a double J stent and retroperitoneal drainage should be provided.

Bibliography

Presti J, Carroll P. Ureteral and pelvic trauma: diagnosis and management. In: McAninch J (ed.), *Traumatic and Reconstructive Urology*. Philadelphia, PA: W.B. Saunders, 1996, 173–175.

5. **(C)** Testicular torsion is a urologic emergency and requires prompt diagnosis and treatment to salvage the testis. It is most common in adolescence and has an estimated incidence of 1 in 4000 males under the age of 25; however, it can be seen at any age and a high level of clinical suspicion must be maintained. The pathogenesis of testicular torsion is thought to be due to a narrowed mesenteric attachment between the cord and the testis. This allows the testis to rotate on its axis leading to torsion. A pubertal testis is at a higher risk for torsion because the testis increases in volume at this time which further exacerbates the narrowness of the mesenetery.

Also in the differential diagnosis of the acute scrotum is torsion of the appendix testis and epididymitis. A torsed appendix testes is the most common cause of an acute scrotum in this age group and usually presents with a firm, tender mass at the upper pole of the testis. Occasionally, the classic "blue dot sign" is visualized because of venous congestion and necrosis. In patients with epididymitis, the pain may be localized directly to the epididydmis. Dysuria and urethral discharge may also be present; however, scrotal edema and patient discomfort may make distinguishing the epidydimis and the testis difficult. Radiologic evaluation is often quite helpful in establishing the correct diagnosis in an acute scrotum.

Ultrasonography is a noninvasive, rapid study which will help differentiate between epidydimitis and testicular torsion. In patients with torsion, ultrasound with Doppler will show an absence of blood flow to the affected testis (as illustrated in Fig. 39-2). However, patients with epidydimitis will have increased blood flow to the epidydimis and normal blood flow to the testicle. Nuclear medicine perfusion studies can also be used to evaluate testicular blood flow.

The treatment for testicular torsion must be prompt. Testis survival is best if the patient is operated on within 6 h of the onset of symptoms. If torsion of the testis cannot be ruled out, surgical exploration must be performed. Manual detorsion has been described by rotating the testis laterally, like "opening a book," as most torsions occur with an inward rotation. However, this should be seen as a maneuver to gain time as

exploration and orchiopexy will still be required. At surgery the torsed testicle should be evaluated for viability and resected if not viable. At the same time a contralateral orchiopexy should be performed as prophylaxis against torsion on that side. If the diagnosis of torsed appendix testis can be firmly established, no operative intervention is needed.

Bibliography

Sigman M, Jarow J. Male infertility. In: Walsh P, Retik A, Vaughan E, et al. (eds.), *Campbell's Urology*, 8th ed. Philadelphia, PA: W.B. Saunders, 2002, 1506–1507.

6. **(D)** The prevalence of bacteruria found in screening pregnant females is the same as that in nonpregnant females; however, because of certain anatomic and physiologic alterations, the incidence of acute clinical pyelonephritis is significantly increased in pregnant women with bacteruria. Of pregnant women who develop pyelonephritis, approximately two-thirds will develop it during the third trimester of pregnancy. This is the phase in which hydronephrosis and urinary stasis are most pronounced. Therefore, it is important to adequately treat bacteruria during pregnancy, even if the patient is asymptomatic. Furthermore, pregnant women with acute pyelonephritis should be admitted to the hospital for treatment with parenteral agents.

Bibliography

Schaeffer A. Infections of the urinary tract. In: Walsh P, Retik A, Vaughan E, et al. (eds.), *Campbell's Urology*, 8th ed. Philadelphia, PA: W.B. Saunders, 2002, 580–583.

7. **(E)** Infected renal calculi are typically composed of magnesium ammonium phosphate. They also contain varying amounts of carbonate appatite, which crystallizes in the presence of urease producing organisms. The enzyme urease catalyzes the formation of ammonia and carbon dioxide from urea through the following reaction:

$$NH_2 - C - NH_2 \xrightarrow{\text{urease}} CO_2 + 2NH_3$$

$$NH_3 + H_2O \longrightarrow NH_4 + OH^-$$

These products alkalinize the urine (pH >7.2) which in turn results in struvite crystal formation. Some species of *Klebsiella*, *Pseudomonas*, and *Staphylococcus* produce urease but *Proteus* species are by far more commonly associated with infected stones.

Bibliography

Menon M, Resnick M. Urinary lithiasis: etiology, diagnosis and medical management. In: Walsh P, Retik A, Vaughan E, et al. (eds.), *Campbell's Urology*, 8th ed. Philadelphia, PA: W.B. Saunders, 2002, 3260–3264.

8. **(A)** The IVP shows complete obstruction of the right ureter down to the level of the pelvic brim. Surgical clips are present in this region, likely indicating a ligation injury. If the injury is recognized within 3–5 days of the procedure, immediate repair can be performed if the patient is afebrile and without signs of sepsis. An injury of this nature may simply require deligation but can require debridement and ureteral reimplantation if the segment is ischemic. If the diagnosis is delayed beyond 5–7 days, ureteral stent placement should be attempted; however, patients who are febrile or have other signs of sepsis should be temporarily diverted with a percutaneous nephrostomy tube. This will provide adequate drainage of the obstructed kidney while allowing time for the patient to convalesce prior to definitive repair.

Approximately 70% of intraoperative ureteral injuries occur during gynecologic procedures. Abdominal hysterectomy is the most common with a ureteral injury rate of 2–3%. Presenting signs and symptoms include flank pain, nausea, vomiting, prolonged ileus, and leukocytosis. Anuria may occur if a patient has a solitary kidney or if both ureters are injured. Drainage from the vagina or wound may be indicative of a ureterovaginal or ureterocutaneous fistula.

The leading cause of nongynecologic ureteral injury is abdominoperineal resection. The majority of injuries occur when dividing the lateral ligaments of the rectum. For this reason, many advocate prophylactic ureteral catheters.

Bibliography

Gulmi F, Felsen D, Vaughan E. Pathophysiology of urinary tract obstruction. In: Walsh P, Retik A, Vaughan E, et al. (eds.), *Campbell's Urology*, 8th ed. Philadelphia, PA: W.B. Saunders, 2002, 426–428.

Payne C, Raz S. Ureterovaginal and related fistulas. In: McAninch JW (ed.), *Traumatic and Reconstructive Urology*. Philadelphia, PA: W.B. Saunders, 1996, 218–221.

9. **(A)** The arteriogram reveals medial fibroplasia involving the main renal artery with the characteristic "string of beads" appearance. Medial fibroplasia is the most common fibrous lesion accounting for 75–80% of the fibromuscular dysplasias. The string of beads appearance results from the presence of collangenous rings alternating with aneurysmal dilations. These involve the media of the main renal artery and often extend into smaller branches.

These lesions tend to occur in women between the ages of 25 and 50. The lesion does not dissect and complete occlusion has not been reported. Schreiber and colleagues studied the natural history of this lesion and followed a group of patients for a mean of 65 months. Progressive renal artery stenosis developed in 33% of patients regardless of age; however, serial decreases in renal function or size of the kidney rarely occurs in patients with progressive medial fibroplasia. This suggests that patients who are managed medically have a small risk of losing renal function. If surgical treatment is required, correction of the lesion by angioplasty is recommended.

Bibliography

Novick A, Fergany A. Renovascular hypertension and ischemic nephropathy. In: Walsh P, Retik A, Vaughan E, et al. (eds.), *Campbell's Urology*, 8th ed. Philadelphia, PA: W.B. Saunders, 2002, 233.

Schreiber M, Pohl M, Novick A. The natural history of atherosclerotic and fibrous renal artery disease. *Urol Clin North Am* 1984;11:383.

Vaughan E, Sosa R. Renovascular hypertension and ischemic nephropathy. In: Gillenwater J, Grayhack J, Howards S, et al. (eds.), *Adult and Pediatric Urology*, 4th ed. Philadelphia, PA: Lippincott, Williams & Wilkins, 2002, 974–975.

10. **(C)** Because of a flap valve mechanism in the anatomically normal ureterovesical junction (UVJ), urine in the bladder should not reflux back into the ureter; however, in patients with reflux the ureter typically enters the bladder at more of a right angle, decreasing its intramural course. Structural anomalies and lower tract abnormalities which increase bladder pressure can also cause reflux. The majority of mild-to-moderate vesicoureteral reflux will spontaneously resolve with time; however, absolute indications for surgical correction include breakthrough UTI and patient noncompliance with antibiotic therapy. Relative indications for correction include the presence of high-grade reflux (grade IV or V), impaired renal growth or function, and reflux associated with structural abnormalities such as a paraureteral diverticulum.

Bibliography

Park J, Retik A. Surgery for vesicoureteral reflux. In: Gearhart J, Rink R, Mouriquand P (eds.), *Pediatric Urology*. Philadelphia, PA: W.B. Saunders, 2001, 421–429.

11. **(D)** An enterocele occurs as a result of the herniation of peritoneum and its contents at the level of the vaginal apex. Symptoms may include a feeling of fullness in the perineum, dyspareunia, vaginal discomfort, as well as low back pain. Enteroceles often coexist with rectoceles and cystoceles which may result in constipation and urinary complaints. The diagnosis is typically made on the basis of physical examination. With the patient in lithotomy position, straining often allows palpation of the hernia sac against the fingertip. The

mass is located posterior to the cervix in women who have not undergone a hysterectomy. Surgical repair can be performed abdominally or vaginally and should be dictated by surgeon's preference and whether there is concomitant vaginal or abdominal pathology.

Bibliography

Chopra A. Enterocele and vault proplapse. In: Raz S (ed.), *Female Urology*, 2nd ed. Philadelphia, PA: W.B. Saunders, 1996, 465–473.

Shull B. Enterocele and rectocele. In: Walters MD, Karran MM (eds.), *Urogynecology and Reconstructive Pelvic Surgery*, 2nd ed. St. Louis, MO: Mosby, 1999, 221–233.

12. **(A)** The incidence of cryptorchidism in premature boys is 9.2–30%. The incidence drops to 3–5% in term males. Abnormal descent can cause a testicle to occupy an aberrant position outside the scrotum. The most common site of ectopia is in the superficial inguinal pouch between the external oblique aponeurosis and Scarpa's fascia. Patients with an undescended testicle have a 40-fold increased risk of developing a testicular cancer. Orchiopexy does not reduce the risk of malignancy but allows for better examination of the scrotal testis and earlier detection. The most significant pathologic feature of the cryptorchid testis is a reduced number of germ cells. Even after orchiopexy, fertility is impaired in 50–70% of males.

Bibliography

Baker L, Silver R, Docimo S. Cryptorchidism. In: Gearhart JP, Rink RC, Mouriquand PD (eds.), *Pediatric Urology*. Philadelphia, PA: W.B. Saunders, 2001, 738–753.

Kogan S, Hudziselimovic F, Howards S, et al. Pediatric andrology. In: Gillenwater J, Grayhack J, Howards S, et al. (eds.), *Adult and Pediatric Urology*, 4th ed. Philadelphia, PA: Lippincott, Williams & Wilkins, 2002, 2591–2601.

13. **(E)** TCC of the ureter represents 2% of all urothelial malignancies in the urinary tract. Ureteral tumors are twice as common in men, but women have a 25% higher chance of dying from the disease. Risk factors include smoking, analgesic abuse, cyclophosphamide, and certain chemical exposures. Ureteral tumors are more commonly located in the lower ureter and least commonly in the upper ureter. More than 90% of upper tract tumors are TCC. Other less common tumors include squamous cell carcinoma (0.7–7%), adenocarcinoma (<1%), and inverted papillomas.

The treatment of upper tract malignancies is evolving. The gold standard has been radical nephroureterectomy (with bladder cuff excision) and is still recommended for large, high-grade, invasive tumors of the renal pelvis and proximal ureter. This is now routinely performed laparoscopically with favorable results; however, more conservative nephron sparing surgery is being advocated for distal ureteral tumors and less invasive papillary tumors of the renal pelvis and ureter. This is especially true in patients such as this, who will have compromised renal function with nephroureterectomy.

Multiple studies have shown the safety and efficacy of endoscopic treatment of upper tract TCC. The tumors can be approached in an antegrade or retrograde fashion. The holmium YAG laser is particularly useful in the ureter because tissue penetration is less than 0.5 mm. The primary concern with this method of treatment is recurrence. The overall recurrence rate for ureteral tumors is 30% and is primarily dependent on tumor grade. Therefore, treatment decisions must balance the risk of recurrence against the morbidity of radical surgery and the potential quality of life risks associated with dialysis.

Bibliography

McDougall E, Clayman R, Figenshau RS. Endourology of the upper urinary tract: noncalculous applications. In: Gillenwater J, Grayhack J, Howards S, et al. (eds.), *Adult and Pediatric Urology*, 4th ed. Philadelphia, PA: Lippincott, Williams & Wilkins, 2002, 783–787.

Messing E. Urothelial tumors of the urinary tract. In: Walsh P, Retik A, Vaughan E, et al. (eds.), *Campbell's Urology*, 8th ed. Philadelphia, PA: W.B. Saunders, 2002, 2765–2769.

Sagalowsky A, Jarrett T. Management of urothelial tumors of the renal pelvis and ureter. In: Walsh P, Retik A, Vaughan E, et al. (eds.), *Campbell's Urology*, 8th ed. Philadelphia, PA: W.B. Saunders, 2002, 2845–2866.

14. **(A)** Female pseudohermaphrodism is the most common cause of ambiguous genitalia. It is characterized by a 46,XX karotype, nonpalpable gonads, and a varying degree of virilization of the external genitialia. More than 95% of the cases of female pseudohermaphrodism are caused by congenital adrenal hyperplasia (CAH). A deficiency of the enzyme 21-hydroxylase is responsible for more than 90% of the cases of CAH. This enzyme is responsible for converting progesterone to deoxycorticosterone in the pathway for aldosterone synthesis. It also catalyzes the formation of deoxycortisol from 17-OH progesterone in cortisol synthesis. This blockade results in increased adrenocorticotrophic hormone (ACTH) production through the loss of cortisol-induced negative feedback inhibition of the pituitary. This drives the adrenal gland to produce more cortisol and ultimately increases the concentration of 17-hydroxyprogesterone and 17-hydroxypregnenolone. These precursors are then metabolized to androgens and result in virilization of the fetus.

Varying forms of 21-hydroxylase deficiency exist but the classic form combines virilization and salt wasting. The diagnosis is usually made on metabolic evaluation and confirmed by karotype and radiographic evaluation. Prompt diagnosis is essential as infants can develop vomiting, dehydration, hyperkalemia, and circulatory collapse because of decreased cortisol and aldosterone production.

Bibliography

Hasmann D. Intersex. In: Gillenwater J, Grayhack J, Howards S, et al. (eds.), *Adult and Pediatric Urology*, 4th ed. Philadelphia, PA: Lippincott, Williams & Wilkins, 2002, 2544–2546.

15. **(A)** Sildenafil citrate has been a significant advancement in the medical management of erectile dysfunction. The mechanism of action is through the selective inhibition of PDE-5. This enzyme breaks down cyclic guanosine monophosphate (cGMP) which is an intracellular messenger that is responsible for corporal smooth muscle relaxation. The inhibition of PDE-5 results in the accumulation of cGMP which promotes smooth muscle relaxation needed for erection.

Bibliography

Benson G, Boileau M. The penis: sexual function and dysfunction. In: Gillenwater J, Grayhack J, Howards S, et al. (eds.), *Adult and Pediatric Urology*, 4th ed. Philadelphia, PA: Lippincott, Williams & Wilkins, 2002, 1954–1955.

Broderick G, Lue T. Evaluation and nonsurgical management of erectile dysfunction and priaprism. In: Walsh P, Retik A, Vaughan E, et al. (eds.), *Campbell's Urology*, 8th ed. Philadelphia, PA: W.B. Saunders, 2002, 1653–1654.

16. **(A)** Patients with inflammatory bowel disease or a history of small bowel resection have varying degrees of fat malabsorption. This results in increased luminal fat which binds to calcium, forming soaps. Therefore, less calcium is available to bind oxalate resulting in increased oxalate absorption and hyperoxaluria. There is also evidence that malabsorbed fatty acids or bile acids increase the colonic permeability to oxalate. The incidence of nephrolithiasis in inflammatory bowel disease is 2–3%, but ileal resection increases the risk to 10%.

Bibliography

Jenkins A. Calculus formation. In: Gillenwater J, Grayhack J, Howards S, et al. (eds.), *Adult and Pediatric Urology*, 4th ed. Philadelphia, PA: Lippincott, Williams & Wilkins, 2002, 369–370.

17. **(D)** MCDPK is one of the most common causes of an abdominal mass in neonates. The etiology is unknown but is likely because of an antenatal obstructive uropathy which occurs early in fetal development. The kidney is severely dysplastic and classically has the appearance of a "bunch of grapes." Evaluation of the entire urinary tract should be performed because of the high incidence of associated anomalies. The more common anomalies include a contralateral UPJ obstruction and a contalateral UVJ obstruction. Treatment of MCDPK is generally conservative. Many multicystic kidneys will involute over time, which may occur either antenatally or postnatally. Should the MCDPK become large enough to cause symptoms by its sheer size, then surgical intervention should be considered. Two other concerns of MCDPK are hypertension and malignant degeneration. There is presently insufficient data to support prophylactic nephrectomy to prevent malignant degeneration. Also, the literature is equivocal about whether hypertension in a patient with MCDPK resolves with nephrectomy.

The ultrasound shown in figure typical features of a multicystic dysplastic kidney. There are multiple, noncommunicating cysts throughout the kidney. Note that there is no evidence of renal parenchyma and the smaller cysts are centrally located. Ultrasound is usually diagnostic, but confusion can occur with hydronephrotic kidneys because of a UPJ obstruction. In this case, the diagnosis of MCDPK is confirmed by the lack of function on renal scan.

Bibliography

Glassberg K. Renal dysgenesis and cystic disease of the kidney. In: Walsh P, Retik A, Vaughan E, et al. (eds.), *Campbell's Urology*, 8th ed. Philadelphia, PA: W.B. Saunders, 2002, 1960–1965.

18. **(D)** McAninch et al. reviewed 1588 adult patients with blunt abdominal trauma who presented with microhematuria and no evidence of shock. There were only three significant renal injuries detected and each were diagnosed in the process of evaluating other intraabdominal injuries. Therefore, radiographic evaluation is not necessary in this type of patient. If renal trauma is suspected, the criteria for which radiographic assessment is recommended includes (1) penetrating trauma to the flank or abdomen, regardless of the degree of hematuria, (2) blunt trauma in adults with either gross hematuria or microhematuria and shock (SBP <90 mmHg), (3) deceleration injuries, (4) major associated intraabdominal injuries and microhematuria, and (5) flank or abdominal trauma in all pediatric patients.

Bibliography

Miller K, McAninch J. Indications for radiographic assessment in suspected renal trauma. In: McAninch J (ed.), *Traumatic and Reconstructive Urology*. Philadelphia, PA: W.B. Saunders, 1996, 91–94.

19. (C) Asymptomatic microscopic hematuria is common and studies estimate the prevalence to be between 0.19 and 16.1%. Urothelial cancers are the most commonly detected malignancies in patients with microscopic hematuria. Imaging can be used to detect TCC in the collecting system or ureter, renal cell carcinoma, infection, and urolithiasis. IVP has been the traditional modalitiy of choice but CT scans have gained recent popularity; however, imaging is unable to adequately evaluate the bladder and cystoscopy is necessary to rule out bladder pathology. Cystoscopic evaluation is currently recommended for all adults with microscopic hematuria over the age of 40 and those under the age of 40 with risk factors for the development of bladder cancer. Those risk factors include smoking, occupational chemical exposure (aniline dyes), cyclophosphamide, radiation, and history of chronic cystitis.

Bibliography

Grossfeld G, Wolf J, Litwin M, et al. *American Urologic Association Best Practice Policy: The Evaluation of Asymptomatic Microscopic Hematuria in Adults.* AUA update series, vol. XXI, lesson 9, 2002.

20. (A) The image shows an anterior urethral stricture because of gonococcus. Gonorrhea is a sexually transmitted disease which can cause urethritis, epidydimitis, and rarely systemic complications from disseminated bacteremia. It typically causes a purulent urethral discharge with dysuria. Swabs for culture and Gram stain should be obtained from within the uretha. A positive Gram stain will reveal intracellular gram-negative diplococci. The treatment of choice is a single IM dose of ceftriaxone plus azithromycin or doxycycline.

The overall incidence of gonorrhea has been decreasing over the past 15 years; however, it remains the most commonly reported communicable disease in the United States. Postgonococcal urethral strictures are because of the intense inflammatory reaction set up by the bacteria and are generally located in the anterior urethra. The incidence of these strictures has been decreasing with the advent of effective antibiotics; however, strictures have been reported up to 30 years after the initial infection. The role of *Chlamydia* and *Ureaplasm* in the development of urethral strictures is unclear. There is presently no definite association between nongonococcal urethritis and the formation of anterior urethral strictures.

The radiograph demonstrates findings typical of an anterior urethral stricture. The posterior urethra is dilated because of the distal obstruction. The paraurethral glands (arrow) are dilated and filled with contrast. The bladder also appears trabeculated from longstanding obstruction.

Bibliography

Berger R, Lee J. Sexually transmitted diseases: the classic disease. In: Walsh P, Retik AB, Vaughan E. *Campbell's Urology,* 8th ed. Philadelphia, PA: W.B. Saunders, 2002, 673–674.

Davidson J, Hartman DS. *Radiology of the Kidney and Urinary Tract,* 2nd ed. Philadelphia, PA: W.B. Saunders, 1994, 649–657.

Jordan G, Schlossberg S. Surgery of the penis and urethra. In: Walsh P, Retig A, Vaughan E (eds.), *Campbell's Urology,* 8th ed. Philadelphia, PA: W.B. Saunders, 2002, 3916.

Kreiger J. Sexually transmitted disease. In: Tanagho EA, McAninch J (eds.), *Smith's General Urology,* 15th ed. New York, NY: McGraw-Hill, 282–285.

21. (B) PIN consists of benign prostatic acini which are lined with cytologically atypical cells. In patients who develop adenocarcinoma of the prostate, there is an increased incidence of high-grade PIN as compared to patients without carcinoma. Likewise, patients with increasing amounts of high-grade PIN also have a higher incidence of multifocal carcinomas. The largest studies report a 23–35% risk of cancer in patients with PIN who undergo a repeat biopsy. Furthermore, PIN alone does not give rise to elevated serum PSA values. Therefore, the most appropriate management of this patient would be to repeat the biopsy.

Bibliography

Epstein J. Pathology of prostatic neoplasia. In: Walsh P, Retik A, Vaughan E, et al. (eds.), *Campbell's Urology,* 8th ed. Philadelphia, PA: W.B. Saunders, 2002, 3025–3026.

22. (D) Priaprism is a prolonged penile erection that persists beyond or is not related to sexual stimulation. The etiology is either because of compromised venous outflow (low-flow priaprism) or high sustained arterial inflow (high-flow priaprism). It is important to make the correct diagnosis as low-flow priaprism beyond 4 h requires emergent medical intervention.

Causes of low-flow priaprism include sickle cell disease, leukemia, TPN (20% fat emulsion), intracavernosal injection therapy, malignant penile infiltration, oral medications (especially antidepressants and antipsychotics), and neurogenic causes. The diagnosis of low-flow priaprism is made when aspiration of the corpora reveals dark blood which is typically acidotic with a low PO_2. Therapy is dependent on the etiology but most commonly consists of corporal irrigation with saline and an alpha-adrenergic agonist. If this does not result in detumescence, a surgical shunt procedure should be performed.

High-flow priaprism is almost always because of perineal or penile trauma. Injury to the cavernosal artery results in a cavernous artery to corporal body fistula. Because of unregulated arterial inflow, aspiration reveals bright red arterial blood without hypoxia or acidosis. Treatment is not urgent as the penis is well perfused. Most patients with high-flow priaprism are treated conservatively or with arterial embolization.

Bibliography

Benson G, Boileau M. The penis: sexual function and dysfunction. In: Gillenwater J, Grayhack J, Howards S, et al. (eds.), *Adult and Pediatric Urology*, 4th ed. Philadelphia, PA: Lippincott, Williams & Wilkins, 2002, 1962–1964.

Leu T. Physiology of penile erection and pathophysiology of erection dysfunction and priaprism. In: Walsh P, Retik A, Vaughan E, et al. (eds.), *Campbell's Urology*, 8th ed. Philadelphia, PA: W.B. Saunders, 2002, 1610–1613.

23. **(C)** The CT scan reveals a small enhancing mass in the upper pole of the left kidney. Any renal mass that enhances with contrast on CT should be considered a renal cell carcinoma until proven otherwise. Biopsy of renal masses is not recommended because of the high rate of false negatives.

Renal sparing surgery is indicated in situations in which radical nephrectomy would obligate the patient to dialysis. These situations include a solitary kidney, bilateral renal tumors, poor renal function, and diseases which threaten the function of the contralateral kidney. Multiple studies have also confirmed the role of partial nephrectomy for patients with localized renal cell carcinoma and a normal contralateral kidney. Patients who present with a solitary tumor less than 4 cm have a 5-year cancer-specific survival rate of 87–90%. These survival rates are similar to those obtained with radical nephrectomy.

Bibliography

Novick A. Surgery of the kidney. In: Walsh P, Retik A, Vaughan E, et al. (eds.), *Campbell's Urology*, 8th ed. Philadelphia, PA: W.B. Saunders, 2002, 3602–3603.

24. **(D)** The MRI illustrates a large right pheochromocytoma. Tank and coworkers estimated that 95% of pheochromocytomas are sporadic and the remaining 5% are familial (10% is often reported). Several different types of genetic abnormalities are responsible for familial pheochromocytomas.

MEN-2 is an autosomal dominant syndrome resulting from mutations in the RET protooncogene. The clinical triad consists of pheochromocytoma, medullary carcinoma of the thyroid, and parathyroid adenomas. Pheochromocytomas are also part of MEN-2B which also includes mucosal neuromas, alimentary tract ganglioneuromatosis, medullary carcinoma of the thyroid, and thickened corneal nerves.

Thirty distinct mutations in the VHL gene are associated with pheochromocytomas. Patients with VHL and pheochromocytomas are classified as VHL type 2. Partial adrenalectomy should be considered in the patients because of the high incidence of bilateral disease.

There is also a group of neuroectodermal dysplasias which are familial and associated with pheochromocytoma. These include Von Recklinghausen's disease, tuberous sclerosis, Sturge-Weber's syndrome, and VHL.

Bibliography

Bukowski R, Klein E. Adrenal neoplasms. In: Vogelzang N, Scardino P, Shipley W, et al. (eds.), *Comprehensive Textbook of Genitourinary Oncology*. Philadelphia, PA: Lippincott, Williams & Wilkins, 2000, 1091.

Tank E, Gelbard M, Bland B. Familial pheochromocytomas. *J Urol* 1982;128:1013.

Vaughan ED, Blumenfield JD, Pizzo JD. The adrenals. In: Walsh P, Retik A Vaughan E, et al. (eds.), *Campbell's Urology*, 8th ed. Philadelphia, PA: W.B. Saunders, 2002, 3542–3543.

25. **(A)** Medullary sponge kidney is a benign entity which is diagnosed radiographically. In general, the diagnosis is made on IVP and the characteristic features include (1) enlarged kidneys (often with calcifications), (2) elongated papillary tubules which fill with contrast medium, and (3) persistent medullary opacification. The dilated ducts often have the appearance of bristles on a brush.

Of patients undergoing IVP, the incidence of medullary sponge kidney is 0.5%. It is most commonly diagnosed from 20 to 50 years of age. The typical presentation is renal colic (50–60%), gross hematuria (10–18%), or UTI (20–33%).

Infection and calculus formation are the major complications which require treatment. Approximately 60% of patients with medullary sponge kidney will pass calculi at some time. One-third to one-half of these patients have hypercalcemia which can be caused by increase parathyroid hormone, renal calcium leak, or increased intestinal absorption of calcium. Stone prevention can be attempted with thiazide diuretics which decrease hypercalcuria.

Bibliography

Glassberg K. Renal dysgenesis and cystic diseases of the kidney. In: Walsh P, Retik A, Vaughan E, et al. (eds.), *Campbell's Urology*, 8th ed. Philadelphia, PA: W.B. Saunders, 2002, 1974–1976.

Lippert M. Renal cystic disease. In: Gillenwater J, Grayhack J, Howards S, et al. (eds.), *Adult and Pediatric Urology*, 4th ed. Philadelphia, PA: Lippincott, Williams & Wilkins, 2002, 863–864.

26. **(D)** The radiograph illustrates a large right staghorn calculus. The treatment of staghorn calculi remains a technical challenge for urologists. Staghorn calculi are usually composed of magnesium ammonium phosphate (struvite) and are typically infectious stones; however, stones consisting of cystine, uric acid, and calcium oxalate monohydrate can also form a staghorn configuration. Definitive treatment of these stones is essential as conservative management can lead to renal failure, sepsis, and death. Blandy and Singh reported a 28% mortality rate at 10 years with untreated staghorn calculi.

There is currently no universally accepted approach to the treatment of staghorn calculi; however, most experts agree that percutaneous stone removal provides a less invasive, less morbid procedure that results in a high success rate. Stone-free rates following PCNL vary widely but exceed 85% in experienced hands. The overall risk of acute complications following PCNL is 7.4%. Complications include bleeding, lung injury, renal pelvic injury, ureteral strictures, and sepsis.

Shock wave lithotripsy monotherapy can be considered in patients with nondilated collecting systems; however, the stone-free rate is only 50% when the stone surface area is greater than 500 m². Retrograde ureteroscopic laser lithotripsy is also an option but would be difficult in this patient because of the amount of stone burden. This approach can be particularly useful in anticoagulated patients. Anatrophic nephrolithotomy can be considered in patients with extremely large staghorn calculi and complex collecting system anatomy; however, this approach is associated with a longer hospital stay, longer convalescence, and is not necessary in this case.

Bibliography

Assimos D, Martin J. *Treatment Options for Staghorn Calculi*. AUA Update Series, vol. XXI, lesson 1.

Blandy J, Singh M. The case for a more aggressive approach to staghorn stones. *J Urol* 1976;115:505–506.

Lingeman J, Lifshitz D, Evan A. Surgical management of urinary lithiasis. In: Walsh P, Retik A, Vaughan E, et al. (eds.), *Campbell's Urology*, 8th ed. Philadelphia, PA: W.B. Saunders, 2002, 3364–3372.

Tillem S, Smith A. Treatment of staghorn calculi. In: Smith A, Badlani G, Bagley D, et al. (eds.), *Smith's Textbook of Endourology*. St. Louis, MO: Quality Medical Publishing, 1996, 1522–1526.

27. **(B)** The arteriogram reveals an aneurysm of the main renal artery at its bifurcation. The overall incidence of renal artery aneurysms is between 0.09 and 0.3%. They occur with equal frequency in both sexes and have been reported in all age groups (1 month to 82 years). Renal artery aneurysms can be categorized into four basic types: saccular, fusiform, dissecting, and intrarenal.

The image illustrates a saccular aneurysm which is a localized outpouching that communicates with the arterial lumen by either a narrow or wide opening. This is the most common type of aneurysm accounting for 93% of all aneurysms. They typically occur at the bifurcation possibly because of an inherent weakness in this region. These lesions often become involved with atherosclerotic degeneration or intramural calcification. Incompletely calcified aneurysms may become thin and ulcerated between areas of calcification, predisposing them to rupture.

Most renal artery aneurysms are small and asymptomatic. Well-calcified, small (<2 cm) aneurysms in an asymptomatic normotensive patient can be followed with serial radiographs. However, surgical intervention is indicated for aneurysms: (1) associated with local symptoms such as flank pain or hematuria, (2) dissecting aneurysms, (3) aneurysms occurring in a woman of child bearing age who is likely to conceive, (4) aneurysms causing renal ischemia, (5) aneurysms occurring with functionally significant renal artery stenosis, (6) aneurysms with radiographic evidence of expansion on serial radiographs, and (7) aneurysms containing a thrombus with evidence of distal embolization.

Bibliography

Koff S, Mutabagani K. Anomalies of the kidney. In: Gillenwater J, Grayhack J, Howards S, et al. (eds.), *Adult and Pediatric Urology*, 4th ed. Philadelphia, PA: Lippincott, Williams & Wilkins, 2002, 2149–2150.

Novick A, Fergary A. Renovascular hypertension and ischemic nephropathy. In: Walsh P, Retik A, Vaughan E, et al. (eds.), *Campbell's Urology*, 8th ed. Philadelphia, PA: W.B. Saunders, 2002, 261–262.

28. **(E)** The cystogram reveals an intraperitoneal bladder rupture. Extravasated contrast can be visualized lining multiple loops of small bowel and can also be seen in the left paracolic gutter. Bladder injuries typically occur in high energy accidents such as motor vehicle accidents. The vast majority of patients with bladder injuries also have an associated pelvic fracture (83–100%).

The diagnosis is usually made with either retrograde cystography or CT cystography. With either imaging modality, it is important to adequately fill the bladder with contrast. It is recommended that 350 cc of contrast be instilled to ensure adequate filling (unless the patient complains of pain at lower volumes). It is also important to obtain postdrainage films on cystograms as 13% of bladder ruptures are diagnosed on the drainage film.

In contrast to extraperitoneal bladder rupture, intraperitoneal rupture should be managed with open operative repair. These injuries are often much larger than they appear on cystography and conservative management can often lead to persistent urinary leakage. Furthermore, leaking of urine into the peritoneal cavity can result in peritonitis and even death.

Bibliography

McAninch J, Santucci R. Genitourinary trauma. In: Walsh P, Retik A, Vaughan E, et al. (eds.), *Campbell's Urology*, 8th ed. Philadelphia, PA: W.B. Saunders, 2002, 3721–3725.

29. **(E)** Tuberous sclerosis is an autosomal dominant disorder caused by defects in genes on chromosomes 9 and 16. The classic triad for patients with tuberous sclerosis consists of epilepsy (80%), mental retardation (60%), and adenoma sebaceum (75%). Adenoma sebaceum consists of multiple papules of angiofibroma which are typically prevalent in the malar region. Central nervous system (CNS) lesions usually consist of cortical hamartomas. These lesions also appear in the kidneys and retina of patients with tuberous sclerosis.

    The renal lesions seen on CT are characteristic of angiomyolipomas. These lesions are benign renal neoplasms that contain varying amounts of fat, smooth muscle, and blood vessels. The visualization of fat within the lesion confirms the diagnosis (fat density measurements range from −10 to −50 HU). Angiomyolipomas occur in 40–80% of patients with tuberous sclerosis. Lesions greater than 4 cm are especially prone to hemorrhage and many authors advocate prophylactic embolization or surgical excision.

    Renal cysts also develop in approximately 20% of patients with tuberous sclerosis. Renal failure can develop but usually not before the fourth decade. These patients are also at an increased risk of developing renal cell carcinoma (2%) which typically occurs at a younger age.

Bibliography

Glassberg K. Renal dysgenesis and cystic disease of the kidney. In: Walsh P, Retik A, Vaughan E, et al. (eds.), *Campbell's Urology*, 8th ed. Philadelphia, PA: W.B. Saunders, 2002, 1955–1958.

Ramchandani P, Rowling S. Computed tomography. In: Gillenwater J, Grayhack J, Howards S, et al. (eds.), *Adult and Pediatric Urology*, 4th ed. Philadelphia, PA: Lippincott, Williams & Wilkins, 2002, 107–108.

30. **(C)** The retrograde urethrogram demonstrates a type III prostatomembranous urethral disruption. The proposed mechanism is that shearing forces are generated in this region because of sudden cephalad migration of the bladder and prostate. More than 90% of these injuries are a result of blunt trauma. They are also a common sequelae of pelvic fractures, particularly bilateral rami fractures.

    The classic triad of physical findings with urethral disruption is (1) blood at the meatus, (2) inability to urinate, and (3) a palpable full bladder. A retrograde urethrogram should be obtained if any of these findings are present prior to attempting to place a urethral catheter. Colapinto and McCallum (1977) developed a classification scheme to describe the location of posterior urethral distraction injuries:

    Type I: Urethral stretch injury

    Type II: Urethral disruption proximal to the genitourinary diaphragm

    Type III: Urethral disruption both proximal and distal to the genitourinary diaphragm

    The treatment of urethral distraction injuries has been somewhat controversial; however, most experts favor early endoscopic realignment in which the gap is bridged with a urethral catheter. The rates of impotence, anejaculation, and incontinence are not worsened with this approach. Urethral strictures develop in 50–65% of patients managed with endoscopic realignment but the majority of these strictures can be managed with dilation or direct vision internal urethrotomy.

Bibliography

Dixon C. Diagnosis and acute management of posterior urethral disruptions. In: McAninch J (ed.), *Traumatic and Reconstructive Urology*. Philadelphia, PA: W.B. Saunders, 1996, 347–354.

McAninch J, Santucci R. Genitourinary trauma. In: Walsh P, Retik A, Vaughan E, et al. (eds.), *Campbell's Urology*, 8th ed. Philadelphia, PA: W.B. Saunders, 2002, 3725–3731.

31. **(A)** The CT scan reveals a grade IV renal injury. Of all injuries to the genitourinary tract following blunt trauma, renal injuries are by far the most common. The American Association for Trauma Surgery's Organ Injury Scaling Committee devised the most widely accepted classification system for renal injuries (see Table 39-1).

TABLE 39-1   Classification System for Renal Injuries

Grade	Type	Description
I	Contusion	Microscopic or gross hematuria, urologic studies normal
	Hematoma	Subcapsular, nonexpanding without parenchymal laceration
II	Hematoma	Nonexpanding perirenal hematoma confined to renal retroperitoneum
	Laceration	<1 cm parenchymal depth of renal cortex without urinary extravasation
III	Laceration	>1 cm parenchymal depth of renal cortex without collecting system rupture or urinary extravasation
IV	Laceration	Parenchymal laceration extending through renal cortex, medulla, and collecting system
	Vascular	Main renal artery or vein injury with contained hemorrhage
V	Laceration	Completely shattered kidney
	Vascular	Avulsion of renal hilum, devascularization of the kidney

Only a small percentage of renal trauma cases are significant injuries (grade II–V); however, these injuries can usually be managed conservatively in hemodynamically stable patients. Overall 98% of renal injuries can be managed nonoperatively. Absolute indications for renal exploration include (1) persistent renal bleeding, (2) an expanding perirenal hematoma, and (3) a pulsatile perirenal hematoma. Relative indications include (1) urinary extravasation, (2) nonviable tissue, (3) segmental arterial injury, (4) incomplete staging, and (5) delayed diagnosis of an arterial injury. Complications following these injuries include urinoma, delayed bleeding, perinephric abcess, and renin-induced hypertension.

Bibliography

McAninch J, Santucci R. Genitourinary trauma. In: Walsh P, Retik A, Vaughan E, et al. (eds.), *Campbell's Urology*, 8th ed. Philadelphia, PA: W.B. Saunders, 2002, 3707–3714.

32. (C) The CT scan demonstrates lack of renal enhancement in the presence of a normal renal contour. These findings are consistent with an injury to the main renal artery. Approximately 25% of all major renal injuries include injuries to the renal vasculature. These patients are more prone to complications and are more likely to suffer renal loss and even death when compared to patients with nonvascular injuries. The majority of these patients have other associated injuries and approximately 70% will present in shock.

Outcome in patients with renal vascular injury is determined by the extent of associated injuries which often dictates treatment. Repair of injuries to the main renal artery have yielded the lowest rates of success. Haas and associates reviewed their 15-year experience and found that surgical revascularization in renal artery thrombosis was seldom successful. Furthermore, a significant percentage of patients who were repaired developed hypertension; however, surgical revascularization should always be attempted in patients with a solitary kidney or bilateral injuries. The indications for repair in patients with a normal contralateral kidney are less clear and should be dictated by the patient's overall condition and the time lapsed since injury.

Bibliography

Carrol P. Injuries to major abdominal arteries, veins and renal vasculature. In: McAninch J (ed.), *Traumatic and Reconstructive Urology*. Philadelphia, PA: W.B. Saunders, 1996, 121–124.

Haas C, Dinchman K, Nasrallah P, et al. Traumatic renal artery occlusion: a 15-year review. *J Trauma* 1998; 45: 557–561.

McAninch J, Santucci R. Genitourinary trauma. In: Walsh P, Retik A, Vaughan E, et al. (eds.), *Campbell's Urology*, 8th ed. Philadelphia, PA: W.B. Saunders, 2002, 3713–3718.

33. (C) Ureteral injury following blunt trauma is rare; however, the most common injury in this setting is the avulsion of the ureter from the renal pelvis at the UPJ. These injuries are more common in children because of the increased flexibility of their spinal column. The mechanism typically involves extreme hyperextension and sudden deceleration with ureteral compression against a vertebral body.

The diagnosis is unreliable on routine CT. When this injury is suspected it is important to perform a delayed scan at 5–8 min following injection of intravenous contrast. Radiographic signs of UPJ disruption include medial extravasation of contrast and transverse process fractures.

The treatment of ureteral injuries after blunt trauma depends on (1) site of injury, (2) time of recognition, (3) associated injuries, and (4) patient condition. If a UPJ disruption is diagnosed at the time of injury most can be managed with a primary reanastamosis to the ureter. If there is not sufficient ureteral length, a ureterocalicostomy can be performed.

Bibliography

Casale A. Urinary tract trauma. In: Gearhart J, Rink R, Mouriquand P (eds.), *Pediatric Urology*. Philadelphia, PA: W.B. Saunders, 2001, 931–934.

34. (A) The mechanism of action of alpha blockers is via relaxation of prostate smooth muscle. Studies have shown that over 90% of alpha receptors in the prostate are localized to the prostate stroma. Relaxation of the prostate smooth muscle decreases bladder outlet obstruction with subsequent improvement in the symptoms of BPH. Alpha blockers have a dose-dependent effect on BPH symptoms. They have a relatively rapid clinical response and most alpha blockers have an effect of lowering blood pressure. Thus, they may be useful as single drug therapy in patients with hypertension and BPH.

Another available class of drugs is the androgen suppressors. The rationale behind the use of antiandrogens is that maintenance of prostate size and volume is an androgen-dependent process. By blocking androgens, prostate size the symptoms of BPH may be improved. It is primarily the epithelial components of the prostate that are effected by antiandrogen therapy. Several types of antiandrogens are available, including finasteride, which is a 5-alpha reductase inhibitor. Studies have shown it reduces prostate volume by 20%.

The theory behind aromatase inhibition is that estrogen supports the proliferative activity of the prostate. Thus, blockage of estrogens should theoretically inhibit prostate growth; however, Gingell et al. (1995) failed to find statistically significant improvements in symptoms or significant decreases in prostate volume with aromatase inhibition.

Bibliography

Gingell JC, Knonagel H, Kurth KH, et al. Placebo controlled double blind study to test the efficacy of the aromatase inhibitor atamestane in patients with benign prostatic hyperplasia not requiring operation. *J. Urol* 1995; 154: 399–401.

Lepor H, Lowe F. Evaluation and nonsurgical management of benign prostatic hypertrophy. In: Walsh P, Retik A, Vaughan E, et al. (eds.), *Campbell's Urology*, 8th ed. Philadelphia, PA: W.B. Saunders, 2002, 1347–1367.

35. (E) The primary management of multiple superficial bladder tumors is intravesical chemotherapy. The goal of intravesical chemotherapy is to eradicate residual disease following transurethral resection of a bladder tumor (TURBT), limit recurrence, and halt disease progression. Superficial bladder tumors commonly recur following TURBT but rarely progress. Indications for intravesical therapy with superficial tumors include (1) multiple tumors, (2) high-grade tumors, (3) tumors with carcinoma *in situ*, (4) recent recurrence, and (5) inability to completely resect the tumor.

Bacille-Calmette-Guerin (BCG) is the most effective intravesical agent for the treatment of superficial bladder cancer. BCG is an attenuated strain of mycobacterium and its mechanism of action is unclear; however, it likely induces a cellular tumorcidal immune response. Multiple studies have shown that BCG is effective in delaying or preventing tumor recurrence.

BCG therapy is commonly associated with side effects such as irritative voiding symptoms, malaise, and hematuria. More serious side effects can occur and include BCG sepsis, which mandates immediate admission to the hospital and treatment with antituberculosis agents and aggressive antibiotic therapy. Contraindications to BCG include immunocompromised patients, gross hematuria, recent TURBT (within 1 week), and sepsis.

Bibliography

Malkowicz S. Management of superficial bladder cancer. In: Walsh P, Retik A, Vaughan E, et al. (eds.), *Campbell's Urology*, 8th ed. Philadelphia, PA: W.B. Saunders, 2002, 2785–2792.

Messing E. Urothelial tumors of the urinary tract. In: Walsh P, Retik A, Vaughan E, et al. (eds.), *Campbell's Urology*, 8th ed. Philadelphia, PA: W.B. Saunders, 2002, 2759–2760.

36. (E) All of the above complications may be seen with the use of intestinal segments in urinary diversion. Different electrolyte abnormalities occur depending on what segment is used. For diversions using gastric segments, a hypochloremic metabolic alkalosis can develop. With jejunal segments, metabolic acidosis occurs in the presence of hyperkalemia and hyponatremia. This is because of an excessive secretion of sodium and chloride with increased absorption of hydrogen and potassium. This carries with it an obligate water loss and the patient becomes dehydrated. The renin-angiotensin axis is stimulated and urine is produced which is low in sodium and high in potassium. This presents as a concentration gradient to the jejunum, thus exacerbating the problem. With ileal and colon conduits, a hyperchloremic, hypokalemic metabolic acidosis develops. The etiology of this abnormality is thought to be because of ammonium transport. Ammonium chloride is effectively absorbed into the blood with the loss of carbonic acid into the bowel lumen.

The incidence of stone formation in colon conduits is 3–4%, while those with ileal conduits have a 10–12% formation rate. There are several factors for stone formation including persistent infection with urea splitting organisms, hypercalciuria, and foreign bodies (such as permanent sutures or staples). The majority of conduit stones are composed of calcium, magnesium, and ammonium phosphate.

Osteomalacia is most commonly seen with uretero-sigmoidostomies but may be seen with other types of intestinal diversion. The etiology is usually because of the underlying acidosis caused by the diversion. The body attempts to buffer the hydrogen ions with calcium ions which are obtained by resorbing bone. A smaller subset of patients develops a vitamin D resistance that is independent of the acidosis.

Patients with a urinary diversion are at higher risk for infection, ranging from bacteruria to pyelonephritis to sepsis. Most patients become colonized but have no symptoms from their infection; however, in some patients this will progress to bacteremia and even sepsis. The reasons are not clear but may be because of the different qualities of the bladder and intestinal epithelium.

Bibliography

Koch MO, McDougal WS. The pathophysiology of hyperchloremic metabolic acidosis after urinary diversion through intestinal segments. *Surgery* 1985;98:561–570.

Mcdougal WS. Use of intestinal segments and urinary diversion. In: Walsh P, Retik A, Vaughan E, et al. (eds.), *Campbell's Urology*, 8th ed. Philadelphia, PA: W.B. Saunders, 2002, 3777–3784.

37. **(E)** Postoperative urinary retention is a relatively common condition with multiple etiologic factors. The incidence is estimated at anywhere between 4 and 25% and it is more common following pelvic surgery. Anesthesia and analgesia are two main contributing factors, especially in decreasing bladder contractility. Two studies have shown that postoperative bladder decompression with an indwelling catheter significantly decreases the incidence of retention when compared to clean intermittent catheterization. This is likely because of the avoidance of acute bladder distention postoperatively. Prophylaxis with phenoxybenazamine, an alpha blocker, has been shown to decrease the incidence of postoperative urinary retention. The mechanism is uncertain but may be related to either a decrease in uretheral outlet resistance or a blockage of sympathetic pathways to the bladder.

Bibliography

Wein A. Neuromuscular dysfunction of the lower urinary tract and its management. In: Walsh P, Retik A, Vaughan E, et al. (eds.), *Campbell's Urology*, 8th ed. Philadelphia, PA: W.B. Saunders, 2002, 960–961.

38. **(B)** Posterior urethral valves present in numerous ways and at different times, depending on the degree of obstruction. Newborns with PUV often have a palpably distended bladder and severe hydronephrosis. Additionally, they may be noted to have oligohydramnios on prenatal ultrasound and may develop respiratory distress secondary to pulmonary hypoplasia. They generally have a thick walled bladder (as can be seen on the above VCUG), along with high-grade ureteral reflux. Patients who present later in life generally have preserved renal function at the time of birth. They typically present with UTIs and voiding dysfunction. If unrecognized, they may continue to slowly develop worsening bladder and renal function which can ultimately lead to renal failure.

PUV are broken down into three subtypes. The most common is type I, which accounts for 95% of the cases of PUV. In this case the valve radiates distally from the posterior edge of the verumontanum before inserting anteriorly at the proximal margin of the membranous urethra. Type II valves were initially described as radiating proximally from the verumontanum to the bladder neck. This is a historical designation, as they are no longer considered obstructive. Type III valves are felt to be persistent remnants of the urogenital sinus located distal to the verumontanum.

Timely diagnosis is crucial in order to preserve renal function. The obstructing valves generate very high bladder pressures which are in turn transmitted to the kidneys. This constant high pressure eventually leads to glomerular dysfunction and deterioration of renal function. Immediate treatment should include placement of a urethral catheter to decompress the bladder and upper tracts. The patient should then be fluid resuscitated and have electrolyte abnormalities corrected. Surgical therapy includes cystoscopy with valve ablation. Urinary diversion with a vesicostomy in infants or a suprapubic tube in older children is also an option.

Bibliography

Gonzales E. Posterior urethral valves and other urethral anomalies. In: Walsh P, Retik, AB, Vaughan E, et al. (eds.), *Campbell's Urology*, 8th ed. Philadelphia, PA: W.B. Saunders, 2002, 2210–2222.

39. **(B)** TCC is the most common histologic subtype of bladder cancers in the United States. It is two times more common in White than in Black males; however, when it occurs in Black males it generally presents at a later stage and has a lower 5-year survival rate than that seen in White males (71% vs. 84%). Some studies have shown that the increased risk for Whites is generally in developing superficial cancers.

Cigarette smoking has been shown to be a clear risk factor for developing TCC. The risk appears to be directly proportional to the amount and the length of tobacco abuse. The degree of the increased risk appears to be upward of fourfold. Also, the increased risk of developing TCC is sustained even in the face of smoking cessation. It takes nearly 20 years of a smoke-free lifestyle to reach a baseline age adjusted risk of TCC development.

There have been multiple chemical and industrial toxins implicated in the development of TCC. Aromatic amines are the most commonly implicated bladder carcinogen. They are found in many industries including dye plants, dry cleaners, and paper manufacturers. It is estimated that 20% of all cases of TCC have their origins in occupational exposure.

Cyclophosphamide, a chemotherapeutic agent, has been implicated in the development of high-grade, invasive TCC. It is believed that they have up to a ninefold increase in the risk of TCC. A metabolite of cyclophosphamide, acrolein, is excreted in the urine is believe to be the offending agent. Cyclo-phosphamide is also known to cause hemorrhagic cystitis, although development of this condition is not necessarily linked with the development of TCC.

Other risk factors for the development of TCC include pelvic irradiation, prolonged immunosuppression, and ingestion of large quantities of analgesics containing phenacetin. Infection with *Schistosoma haematobium* (common in the middle east) and chronic indwelling catheters are risk factors for the development of squamous cell carcinoma of the bladder. This is because of a metaplastic response from constant irritation.

Bibliography

Messing E. Urothelial tumors of the urinary tract. In: Retik AB, Vaughan E, Wein A (eds.), *Campbell's Urology*, 8th ed. Philadelphia, PA: W.B. Saunders, 2002, 2732–2741.

40. (E) The World Health Organization refers to the following values as standards on semen analysis:

1. Volume of 2.0 mL or greater
2. pH of 7.2 or more
3. Sperm concentration of 20×10^6 sperm per ejaculate
4. Total sperm number of 40×10^6 spermatozoa per ejaculate
5. Motility of 50% or greater with grade A + B motility or greater than 25% with grade A motility
6. Normal morphology of greater than 15%
7. Viability of more than 75%
8. WBC of less than 1 million/mL

Infertility is defined as failure to conceive after 1 year of unprotected intercourse. Ninety percent of all normal couples will be able to conceive at the end of 1 year. When looking at all cases of infertility, 20% of cases are caused solely by male factors and male factors will play a role in another 30–40% of cases. The initial workup should include a careful history, physical examination, and semen analysis. Factors that may be identified on history include a history of cryptorchidism, prior pelvic or retroperitoneal surgery, prior sexually transmitted diseases, steroid abuse, history of diabetes, chemotherapy, or radiation therapy. Physical examination should assess testicular size, volume, and presence of a spermatic cord. Patients with a known solitary kidney should be evaluated carefully as there is an association between renal agenesis and agenesis of the vas deferens. The presence of varicoceles should also be assessed as they are a leading cause of male factor infertility.

Semen analysis is an important part of the workup of male infertility. Several characteristics of semen are evaluated including volume, sperm count, sperm motility, sperm morphology, and pH. Low volume ejaculates can be because of multiple etiologies including androgen deficiency, vas deferens obstruction, or the absence or disruption of sympathetic pathways. Sperm agglutination may be indicative of the presence of antisperm antibodies, while a sample with all nonmotile sperm may have defects with the function or structure of their flagella. Sperm morphology points to the quality of spermatogenesis. The acid-base balance of semen is dependent on the relative inputs of the acidic prostatic secretion and the alkaline seminal vesicle input.

The initial workup will allow for classification of male infertility into several broad groups including azoospermic, oligospermic, asthenospermic (defect with sperm movement), low ejaculate volume, and those with a normal workup who are infertile. Once this classification has been made, further evaluation to identify the specific cause is much more cost effective and time efficient.

Bibliography

Sigman M, Jarow J. Male infertility. In: Walsh P, Retik AB, Vaughan E, et al. (ed.), *Campbell's Urology*, 8th ed. Philadelphia, PA: W.B. Saunders, 2002, 1475–1489.

Obstetrics and Gynecology

Marisa A. Mastropietro, Patrice M. Weiss, and Valerie Schissler

Questions

1. The vulva contains all the following components *except*:

   (A) labia majora
   (B) hymen
   (C) vestibule
   (D) Skene's glands
   (E) broad ligament

2. A 30-year-old, gravida 2 para 1, female is undergoing a Cesarean section at term secondary to known placenta previa. After delivery of the infant and placental extraction, uterine atony is noted with increased hemorrhage. Ligation of which of the following pelvic arteries would safely reduce hemorrhage?

   (A) ovarian artery
   (B) internal pudendal artery
   (C) hypogastric artery
   (D) inferior mesenteric artery
   (E) umbilical artery

3. A 50-year-old, gravida 2 para 2, female who is status postsurgical menopause by total abdominal hysterectomy (TAH), bilateral salpingo-oophorectomy (BSO) secondary to myomatous uterus presents with a 6-month history of pelvic pain and pressure. What is the most likely diagnosis?

   (A) Bartholin's gland duct cyst
   (B) vaginal vault prolapse
   (C) urethral diverticulum
   (D) vaginal neoplasm

4. The leading cause of trauma during pregnancy in industrialized nations is

   (A) falls
   (B) motor vehicle accidents (MVA)
   (C) domestic violence
   (D) homicide

5. The diagnosis of appendicitis in a pregnant female is associated with increased difficulty secondary to

   (A) the absence of fever
   (B) the colicky nature of pain
   (C) location of pain
   (D) lack of radiologic confirmation

6. A 3-year-old girl presents to the office with her mother who reports "her bottom is stuck together." You examine the girl and diagnose labial agglutination. The first line of treatment is

   (A) surgical repair
   (B) topical estrogen cream
   (C) physical separation in the office
   (D) expectant management

7. A mother presents to your office with her 14-year-old daughter who has been experiencing monthly cyclical abdominal pain. Menarche has not yet occurred. During physical examination, an introital opening could not be identified. Rectal examination revealed a palpable anterior vaginal fullness and a palpable uterus. The correct diagnosis is

   (A) vaginal agenesis
   (B) imperforate hymen
   (C) vaginal septum
   (D) leiomyoma

8. Physiologic changes of pregnancy are associated with all of the following anesthetic risks *except*:

   (A) maternal hypotension
   (B) increased risk of aspiration
   (C) increased difficulty with endotracheal intubation
   (D) increased risk of fetal and maternal hypoxia
   (E) slower emergence from general anesthesia

9. Of the following methods of analgesia/anesthesia for labor, which is considered the most effective and least depressing to the central nervous system?

(A) paracervical block

(B) general anesthesia

(C) parenteral opioids

(D) epidural

10. Regional anesthesia, specifically epidural anesthesia, has been associated with all of the following risks *except*:

(A) an increase in maternal temperature

(B) prolonged labor

(C) increased incidence of Cesarean section

(D) transient back ache

(E) postdural puncture headache

Questions 11 through 13 refer to the following scenario:

A 33-year-old, gravida 2 para 1, pregnant obese female at 26 weeks gestation presents complaining of increasing nausea for 3 days with decreased appetite and one episode of emesis this morning. She also admits to abdominal pain but denies similar symptoms with her first pregnancy. Past medical history is significant only for obesity. Past obstetric history includes one prior spontaneous vaginal delivery at full term without complications. Physical examination reveals a temperature of 100°F and normal fetal heart tones at 140 bpm without uterine contractions.

11. Abdominal examination reveals right upper quadrant tenderness without uterine tenderness. Fundal height is appropriate to gestational age and cervical examination reveals a normal nondilated, firm cervix. Your next step in evaluation is

(A) serial cervical examinations

(B) abdominal ultrasound

(C) urinalysis

(D) antiemetic therapy with observation

12. Abdominal ultrasound, and specifically right upper quadrant ultrasound, reveals multiple small gallstones with biliary sludge present. The best treatment for this patient should include

(A) hospitalization with parenteral nutrition

(B) oral bile acid therapy

(C) laparoscopic cholecystectomy

(D) extracorporeal shock wave lithotripsy

13. Cholelithiasis in pregnancy is associated with all of the following *except*:

(A) preterm labor

(B) urinary tract infection

(C) acute pancreatitis

(D) asymptomatic disease

14. All of the following laboratory tests should be performed routinely in pregnant women presenting for prenatal care *except*:

(A) thyroid-stimulating hormone (TSH)

(B) syphilis screen

(C) rubella titer

(D) blood group and Rh type

15. Laboratory diagnosis of thyroid disease in pregnancy is most affected by

(A) increasing human chorionic gonadotropin (hCG) levels

(B) decreased maternal iodide levels

(C) increased levels of thyroid binding globulin

(D) decreased concentration of thyroid binding globulin

16. When evaluating a pregnant woman for thyroid disease, either hypothyroidism or hyperthyroidism, which of the following lab tests is useful?

(A) TSH

(B) FT4

(C) TT4

(D) RT3U

(E) all of the above

Questions 17 and 18 refer to the following scenario:

You are the general surgeon on call at a community hospital and are paged to labor and delivery to assist the obstetrician with a Cesarean section. On arrival to the labor and delivery operating room, the obstetrician reports the patient's history. The patient is a 32-year-old, gravida 5 para 5, who was delivered by Cesarean section secondary to arrest of labor. A liveborn 4000 g male infant was delivered followed by extraction of the placenta. After delivery of the infant and placenta, increased hemorrhage is noted with greater than 1 L of blood loss. Vital signs are as follows: pulse rate, 100bpm; blood pressure, 140/96 mmHg; and temperature, 99°F.

17. The most likely etiology for postpartum hemorrhage in this case scenario is

 (A) uterine atony
 (B) vaginal laceration
 (C) chorioamnionitis
 (D) prolonged labor

18. The next step in management is

 (A) abdominal hysterectomy
 (B) methylergonovine maleate (Methergine 0.2 mg intramuscularly)
 (C) uterine massage
 (D) intramuscular prostaglandin 15-methyl $F_{2\alpha}$ ($PGF_{2\alpha}$) 0.25 mg
 (E) interventional radiology for arterial embolization

19. In the normal female menstrual cycle, which of the following statements are *true*?

 I. The follicle-stimulating hormone (FSH) acts primarily on granulosa cells to stimulate ovarian follicular growth.
 II. The onset of the luteinizing hormone (LH) surge is the most reliable indicator of impending ovulation, occurring 34–36 h prior to follicle rupture.
 III. The follicular phase is the major determinant of the menstrual cycle length.
 IV. The ovarian luteal phase occurs simultaneous with the uterine proliferative phase, which is progesterone dominant.

 (A) I, II, and III
 (B) I and III
 (C) IV only
 (D) II and IV

20. Postmenopausal hormone therapy (HT) is indicated for which of the following:

 I. prevention of heart disease
 II. treatment of vasomotor symptoms
 III. prevention of colon cancer
 IV. treatment of vulvovaginal atrophy

 (A) I, II, and III
 (B) I and III
 (C) IV only
 (D) II and IV

21. All of the following statements regarding the WHI are true *except*:

 (A) It was not designed to assess the treatment of menopausal vasomotor symptoms.
 (B) The primary outcomes studied were coronary heart disease and invasive breast cancer.
 (C) HT users had a statistically significantly increased cumulative risk for mortality.
 (D) There were less hip fractures in the HT group than the placebo.

22. Conservative treatment with intravenous antibiotics for a TOA is considered a "failure" if clinical response is not seen in what time frame:

 (A) twenty-four hours of IV antibiotics
 (B) thirty-six hours of IV antibiotics
 (C) forty-eight hours of IV antibiotics
 (D) seventy-two hours of IV antibiotics
 (E) ninety-six hours of IV antibiotics

23. All of the following are risk factors for TOA *except*:

 (A) multiple sexual partners
 (B) postmenopausal status
 (C) previous episodes of PID
 (D) low socioeconomic status

Questions 24 through 27 are based on the following clinical scenario:

A 26-year-old nulliparous female presents to the emergency room with sudden onset of right lower quadrant pain. She recently stopped her oral contraceptives as she desires pregnancy. She had been using oral contraceptives for several years to control her irregular periods. Her last menstrual period was 5 weeks ago. She denies any vaginal bleeding or fever, but does report nausea and vomiting. Her past medical history otherwise is unremarkable.

On physical examination, she is afebrile, normotensive, and nontachycardic. She is noticeably uncomfortable, but physical examination reveals no abdominal rebound tenderness. Bimanual examination reveals marked voluntary guarding and a fullness in the right lower quadrant as well as cervical motion tenderness.

24. Differential diagnosis in this patient includes all of the following *except*:

 (A) ectopic pregnancy
 (B) adnexal torsion
 (C) mittelschmerz
 (D) acute appendicitis
 (E) acute pancreatitis

25. Appropriate next steps include

 (A) complete blood count (CBC)

 (B) urine pregnancy test

 (C) pelvic ultrasound

 (D) all of the above

26. The results of the pelvic ultrasound demonstrate an 8-cm right adnexal mass with minimal fluid in the cul-de-sac. CBC is normal and urine pregnancy test is negative. Abnormal (markedly decreased) right ovarian arterial blood flow is noted on Doppler ultrasound. The most likely diagnosis now is

 (A) adnexal/ovarian torsion

 (B) ruptured hemorrhagic cyst

 (C) TOA

 (D) fallopian tube carcinoma

27. The most appropriate management of this patient at this time is

 (A) laparoscopic evaluation of the adnexa

 (B) inpatient intravenous antibiotics

 (C) exploratory laparotomy

 (D) obtaining a serum Ca-125 level

28. Regarding the management of asymptomatic leiomyomas, which statement is *correct*?

 (A) Hysterectomy should be performed when postmenopausal.

 (B) Rapid enlargement is cause for concern.

 (C) nonsteroidal anti-inflammatory drug (NSAIDs) may increase blood flow and blood loss with menses.

 (D) Myomectomy should be performed if uterine size is greater than 12 weeks.

29. Leiomyosarcomas

 (A) are malignant sarcomas that can mimic benign leiomyomas

 (B) are diagnosed by pathologic and histologic examination

 (C) are characterized by rapid uterine enlargement

 (D) have a worse prognosis if patient is postmenopausal

 (E) are all of the above

30. What are the two most common gynecologic findings diagnosed in women undergoing laparoscopy for evaluation of chronic pelvic pain?

 I. hydrosalpinx
 II. ovarian mass
 III. endometriosis
 IV. adhesions

 (A) I and II

 (B) II and III

 (C) III and IV

 (D) I and IV

31. All of the following are risk factors for endometrial adenocarcinoma *except*:

 (A) early menarche

 (B) diabetes

 (C) obesity

 (D) use of combination oral contraceptives, either presently or in the past

32. All of the following are physiologic changes which occur in pregnancy *except*:

 (A) respiratory alkalosis secondary to increased minute ventilation

 (B) hypervolemia resulting from increased blood volumes at or near term

 (C) decreased absorption of iron from the gastrointestinal tract resulting in iron deficiency anemia

 (D) an increase in the glomerular filtration rate

33. A 42-year-old para 3 presents for her routine yearly physical examination. She is having no problems. She recently had a normal mammogram and reports regular menses with slightly lessening flow. Her close friend was recently diagnosed with ovarian cancer. She expresses concern about her own chances of having ovarian cancer and wants to be thoroughly screened for it.

You share with her which of the following information:

 (A) Ovarian cancer is the most common gynecologic malignancy.

 (B) Ovarian cancer is the leading cause of death because of gynecologic malignancy.

 (C) Transvaginal ultrasound has a limited role in ovarian cancer screening because of its inability to accurately visualize the ovaries in pre- and postmenopausal women.

 (D) The prevalence of ovarian cancer decreases over 50 years of age.

34. Which statement is *false*?

(A) Abruptio placenta is the most common cause of fetal compromise following trauma during pregnancy.

(B) MVAs are the most common cause of trauma in pregnancy.

(C) Because of the enlarged gravid uterus, abdominal rebound tenderness and guarding may be more difficult to elicit following trauma during pregnancy.

(D) CT is contraindicated in pregnancy.

35. All of the following regarding amniotic fluid embolism are true *except*:

(A) A hypertonic uterus associated with oxytocin use in a pattern of vigorous labor has been established as the etiology of amniotic fluid embolism.

(B) It is characterized by an abrupt onset of hypotension, hypoxia, and consumptive coagulopathy.

(C) It classically occurs in the late stages of labor or immediately postpartum.

(D) There is no data that any type of intervention improves maternal prognosis in the presence of an amniotic fluid embolism.

Questions 36 through 39 refer to the following scenario:

A 28-year-old G1 presents to the emergency room with vaginal bleeding and right lower quadrant pain. Last menstrual period was 8 weeks ago and she had a positive home urine pregnancy test 2 weeks ago. Her past medical history is noncontributory except she and her husband have been trying to conceive for 6 months. Past surgical history is significant for a laparoscopic right ovarian cystectomy 2 years ago for a mature teratoma. Physical examination reveals stable vital signs, a palpable right adnexal fullness with voluntary guarding. Mild cervical motion tenderness is noted, especially when moving the cervix to the patient's left. The cervix is closed and thick. There is a small amount of dark blood in the vagina but no acute active bleeding.

36. Appropriate workup at this point includes

(A) type and screen

(B) quantitative serum beta hCG

(C) CBC

(D) pelvic ultrasound

(E) all of the above

37. The most likely diagnosis at this point is:

(A) Incomplete abortion.

(B) Threatened abortion.

(C) Hemorrhagic cyst.

(D) Ectopic pregnancy.

38. Management options of this patient include

I. intramuscular methotrexate
II. uterine dilation and curettage
III. laparoscopic salpingostomy
IV. expected management

(A) I, II, and III

(B) I and III

(C) II and IV

(D) IV only

(E) all of the above

39. All of the following are indications for methotrexate therapy for ectopic pregnancy *except*:

(A) absence of hemoperitoneum

(B) hemodynamically unstable

(C) absence of fetal cardiac activity

(D) desire for future fertility

Questions 40 through 42 refer to the following scenario:

A 40-year-old, gravida 2 para 1, at 8 weeks gestation is referred to you for evaluation of a left breast mass. The patient first noticed it just prior to learning she was pregnant. She has never had a mammogram. On physical examination, her breasts are with bilateral tenderness. The left breast contains a mass 1–2 cm in size, firm, nonmobile and, in your opinion, warrants further investigation.

40. Regarding mammography, you inform the patient:

(A) Mammography sensitivity in pregnancy for evaluation of breast masses is increased.

(B) Mammography should be delayed until the patient reaches her second trimester.

(C) Because histologic types of breast cancer are different in the pregnant versus nonpregnant patient, mammography should be replaced by excisional biopsy.

(D) Mammography with abdominal shielding results in less than 1 rad exposure per breast.

41. Mammography reveals a mass with several characteristics suspicious for malignancy. The appropriate next step(s) include which of the following:

   I. needle biopsy
   II. observation with repeat mammogram in the second trimester when sensitivity and specificity of mammography are improved
   III. excisional biopsy
   IV. CT of the chest with abdominal shielding

   (A) I, II, and III
   (B) I and III
   (C) II and IV
   (D) IV only
   (E) all of the above

42. Which of the following statements regarding breast cancer in pregnancy is/are *true*?

   I. Pregnancy itself does not increase the rate of growth or spread of breast cancer.
   II. Pregnant patients are more likely to present with positive lymph nodes.
   III. Prognosis and survival rates stage for stage are similar between pregnant and nonpregnant women.
   IV. If stage I malignancy is confirmed histologically, therapy should be delayed until delivery.

   (A) I, II, and III
   (B) I and III
   (C) II and IV
   (D) IV only
   (E) all of the above

Questions 43 through 45 refer to the following scenario:

You are paged to the emergency room to see a 34-year-old, gravida 1 para 1, patient with right breast pain and fever. The E.R. physician informs you she is 3 weeks postpartum and breastfeeding. Her temperature is 101.4°F, pulse 100, respirations 18. On physical examination, the right breast is tender and warm to the touch with a palpable 2 cm mobile mass.

43. The most likely diagnosis is

   (A) galactocele
   (B) abscess
   (C) fat necrosis
   (D) fibroadenoma

44. The appropriate next step in the management of this patient is

   (A) outpatient oral antibiotics
   (B) analgesics and warm compresses
   (C) excision and drainage of the mass
   (D) excisional biopsy of the mass

45. The patient emphasizes that she wishes to continue breastfeeding. The patient should be instructed to

   (A) discard all breast milk while on antibiotics because of potential effects on the infant
   (B) continue breastfeeding on the unaffected side
   (C) continue breastfeeding after the infant has been treated with therapy for thrush
   (D) pump and discard all breast milk until her fever resolves

Questions 46 through 49 refer to the following scenario:

A 23-year-old G0 female is referred to you for evaluation of a labial lump. Five years ago you had removed a lipoma from her back, and her primary care physician now seeks your opinion regarding this finding. She reports two prior similar episodes which spontaneously resolved within a few days. She states she noticed this present labial fullness after intercourse 1 day ago. She denies any pain, fever, chills, or sweats. Her last menstrual period was 2 weeks ago, and she uses condoms for contraception. Past medical and surgical history is significant only for the above lipoma excision. On physical examination, she is afebrile and you note a unilateral, tense, nonpainful 3 cm mass located at the region of the left labia minora.

46. The most likely diagnosis is

   (A) Bartholin's gland abscess
   (B) Gartner's duct cyst
   (C) Bartholin's gland cyst
   (D) vaginal mesonephric cyst

47. Treatment options for this patient include all of the following *except*:

   I. insertion of a Word catheter
   II. excision of underlying gland
   III. marsupialization of the mass
   IV. hot sitz baths accompanied by broad-spectrum antibiotics

   (A) I, II, and III
   (B) I and III

(C) II and IV

(D) IV only

(E) all of the above

48. If this patient's age were 50 and she presented with the identical history and physical examination, the recommended treatment would be

(A) obtain an IVP to assess the urinary collecting system

(B) incision and drainage of mass

(C) excision or biopsy of underlying gland

(D) expectant management because spontaneous resolution is more common in older patients

49. All of the following are true regarding vulvovaginitis *except*:

(A) A cottage cheese-like discharge is associated with candidiasis.

(B) A strong fishy or musty vaginal odor suggests bacterial vaginosis (BV) or trichomonas.

(C) The presence of hyphae on KOH prep in diagnosing candidiasis is less important than the presence of pruritus and a thick, white discharge.

(D) Trichomonas is considered a STD and treatment of the sexual partner is necessary.

(E) Candidiasis is usually associated with a vaginal pH of less than 4.5.

50. Regarding a hydatidiform mole, which of the following is/are *true*?

I. With complete moles, all cells are derived from the sperm (androgenesis).

II. Incomplete moles have a triploid karyotype.

III. Rh immunoglobulin is recommended for all Rh negative patients regardless if a complete or incomplete mole is present.

IV. An enlarged uterus is a more common finding than is vaginal bleeding.

(A) I, II, and III

(B) I and III

(C) II and IV

(D) IV only

(E) all of the above

Answers and Explanations

1. **(E)** The organs of the female reproductive tract are classically divided into external and internal genitalia. The vulva is a collective term for the external female genital organs that are visible on the perineal area. The vulva consists of the following: mons pubis, labia majora, labia minora, hymen, clitoris, vestibule, urethra, Skene's glands, Bartholin's glands, and vestibular bulbs. The internal genital reproductive organs are located in the true pelvis and include the following: vagina, uterus, cervix, oviducts, ovaries, and surrounding supporting structures including the broad ligament.

The mons pubis is a rounded eminence located anterior and superior to the pubic symphysis after pubertal development. This region becomes hair-bearing with the typical female hair pattern being triangular.

The vulva consists of two paired labia, labia majora and minora. Like the mons pubis, the labia majora are hair-bearing and extend from the mons pubis to the posterior fourchette. The labia majora are continuous folds largely made up of adipose and fibrous tissue containing both sebaceous and apocrine glands. The skin of the outer surface is typically pigmented on the sides of the labia majora, will vary with fat content, and typically atrophy in the postmenopausal female. The labia majora are embryologically homologous to the male scrotum.

Medial to the labia majora are two small continuous folds, namely the labia minora. Differentiating from the labia majora, the labia minora are thinner, shorter, nonpigmented, non-hair-bearing, and contain only sebaceous glands. They are composed of dense connective tissue with erectile and elastic fibers. Embryologically, the labia minora are homologous to the penile urethra and part of the skin of the male penis.

The hymen is a thin membrane at the vaginal orifice covered by stratified squamous epithelium and consists of fibrous tissue. This membrane is usually perforated and varies in both structure and shape. If completely or incompletely perforated, girls may experience difficulty with pain or primary amenorrhea with menarche because of outflow obstruction.

The clitoris is a short erectile organ embryologically homologous to the male penis. Anatomic dimensions may change with previous childbearing but is not influenced by age, weight, or contraceptive use. The clitoris consists of a base of two crura, the body and the glans.

The vestibule is the visualized cleft between the labia minora when the labia minora are held apart and extends from the clitoris to the posterior fourchette. Opening into the vestibule are the orifices of the urethra, vagina, and ducts of the Bartholin's glands.

The female urethra is a conduit for urine from the urinary bladder to the vestibule and typically measures 3.5–5.0 cm in length. The mucosa varies along the length of the urethra with the proximal two-thirds including stratified transitional epithelium in contrast to the distal one-third which consists of stratified squamous epithelium.

Skene's glands are branched, tubular, paraurethral glands. The ducts may open into the vestibule but more often empty into the urethra. Skene's glands are the largest of the paraurethral glands and are embryologically homologous to the male prostate. Infection with subsequent duct obstruction and coalescence may lead to formation of paraurethral cysts or diverticula. The presence of paraurethral cysts or diverticula may result in symptoms of dysuria, postvoid dribbling, dyspareunia, or discharge.

The Bartholin's glands are vulvovaginal glands with ducts opening into the vestibule at the four and eight o'clock position. Embryologically, the Bartholin's glands are homologous to the male Cowper's glands. The Bartholin's gland is typically nonpalpable, however, may become painfully symptomatic because of mechanical duct obstruction with subsequent cystic dilatation and infection of the gland. Bartholin's gland cysts may be asymptomatic or result in acute pain.

The vestibular bulbs are paired elongated erectile tissue on either side of the vaginal orifice immediately below the bulbocavernosus muscle. The distal ends are adjacent to the Bartholin's gland and are embryologically homologous to the bulb of the male penis.

The broad ligament is a double-layered reflection of peritoneum extending from the lateral pelvic side walls to the uterus and is intimately associated with the internal organs of the uterus, fallopian tubes, and ovaries. Despite its name, the broad ligament provides extremely minor support to the uterus.

Bibliography

Droegemueller W. Reproductive anatomy. In: Stenchever MA, Droegemueller W, Herbst AL, Mishell DR Jr (eds.), *Comprehensive Gynecology*, 4th ed. St. Louis, MO: Mosby, 2001, 40–43.

2. **(C)** The female reproductive organs are supplied by a network of arteries. The arteries are generally paired bilaterally and have multiple, collateral connections resulting in an extensive anastomotic network. The arteries generally enter their respective organs laterally and unite with the vessels from the contralateral side near the midline. Venous drainage is complex and accompanies the arterial system.

    The ovarian arteries originate from the aorta just below the renal vessels. During their course in the retroperitoneal space, the ovarian arteries will cross anterior to the ureter and enter the infundibulopelvic ligament to supply the ovary and oviduct. The ovarian artery will then unite with the ascending branch of the uterine artery just under the suspensory ligament of the ovary.

    After the bifurcation the common iliac artery divides into the external iliac and hypogastric (internal iliac) arteries. The hypogastric arteries are approximately 3–4 cm in length and throughout their course are in close association with the ureters. Each hypogastric artery branches into an anterior and posterior division. The posterior division divides into three parietal branches: iliolumbar, lateral sacral, and superior gluteal arteries. The anterior division has nine branches including three parietal and six visceral branches: the obturator, internal pudendal, and inferior gluteal comprise the parietal branches, whereas the umbilical, medial vesical, inferior vesical, middle hemorrhoidal, uterine, and vaginal arteries comprise the visceral branches. The superior vesical artery often arises from the umbilical artery. In situations of hemorrhage, surgical ligation of the anterior division of the hypogastric arteries distal to the posterior parietal branch either unilaterally or bilaterally is effective in controlling hemorrhage. Because of the extensive collateral circulation, this procedure results in reduction of pulse pressure which allows clot formation without producing hypoxia. An alternative approach to ligation is arterial embolization with assistance from interventional radiology.

Bibliography

Droegemueller W. Reproductive anatomy. In: Stenchever MA, Droegemueller W, Herbst AL, Mishell DR Jr (eds.), *Comprehensive Gynecology*, 4th ed. St. Louis, MO: Mosby, 2001, 51–54.

3. **(B)** Pelvic organ prolapse is a common diagnosis affecting millions of American women. Risk factors in the development of pelvic organ prolapse include the following: childbirth, smoking, menopause, chronic medical conditions such as collagen vascular diseases, chronic obstructive pulmonary disease, obesity, prior pelvic surgery, and other social or environmental factors associated with chronic increased abdominal pressure. The common exposure in these conditions is increased abdominal pressure which leads to nerve and muscle devascularization along with ligamentous stretching and tearing, resulting in pelvic floor laxity and dysfunction.

    The vagina is a fibromuscular tube extending from the vestibule to the uterus in the standing position. The upper vagina runs horizontally. It is commonly at a 90-degree angle with the uterus. The vagina is held in its position by the surrounding endopelvic fascia and ligaments. Endopelvic fascia is a fine meshwork of collagen, elastin, and neural fibers.

    The uterus is a thick-walled, hollow muscular organ located centrally in the female pelvis. Anterior to the uterus is the bladder with the rectum posteriorly and broad ligaments laterally. The dome-shaped upper portion of the uterus is termed the fundus. The short area of constriction in the lower uterus is termed the isthmus below which is the uterine cervix which extends into the upper portion of the vagina. The uterus has three layers including the external serosa, the middle muscular layer, and the inner mucous membrane of the endometrium. Extending outward from the uterine fundus are paired oviducts or fallopian tubes. The oviducts are approximately 10–14 cm in length and are divided into four anatomic sections. The uterine intramural, or interstitial, segment is 1–2 cm in length and is surrounded by myometrium. The isthmic segment begins as the tube exits the uterus and is approximately 4 cm in length. This segment is narrow and approximately 1–2 mm in inside diameter. The ampullary segment is 4–6 cm in length and approximately 6 mm in inside diameter. This segment is wider and more tortuous in its course and is normally where ovum fertilization occurs. The infundibulum is the distal trumpet-shaped portion of the oviduct terminating in multiple finger-like projections termed fimbriae.

Extending from the uterus are five pair of ligaments. The pelvic ligaments, however, are not classic ligaments but are thickenings of retroperitoneal fascia and consist primarily of blood and lymphatic vessels, nerves and fatty connective tissue. The retroperitoneal fascia is referred to by surgeons as endopelvic fascia. Extending from the superior portion of the uterus are the paired round ligaments and uteroovarian ligaments. The round ligament provides minimal support to the uterus but is an important surgical landmark in making the initial incision into the parietal peritoneum, allowing access to the retroperitoneal space. The round ligament is composed of fibrous tissue and muscle fibers and runs via the broad ligament to the lateral pelvic side wall, entering into the inguinal canal and terminally inserting into the labia majora. The uteroovarian ligament is one of three ligaments which provide anatomic mobility to the ovary. This is a narrow, short, fibrous band extending from the lower pole of the ovary to the uterus. The broad ligaments are a double reflection of peritoneum, stretching the lateral pelvic side wall to the uterus which become contiguous with the uterine serosa. These peritoneal folds enclose a loose connective tissue termed the parametrium. The broad ligaments provide minor support to the uterus but are conduits to many important anatomic structures of the pelvis. The uterosacral ligaments extend from the upper portion of the cervix posteriorly to the third sacral vertebra. They are thickened anteriorly near the cervix and run a curved course around the lateral aspect of the rectum. Along with the cardinal ligaments, the uterosacral ligaments provide the major support to the uterus and cervix. The cardinal ligaments extend from the lateral aspect of the upper portion of the cervix and vagina to the pelvic side wall.

Support to the uterus, cervix, and vagina is often described in three levels as described by DeLancey. Level I support includes the uterus and upper vagina as provided by the uterosacral cardinal ligament complex. Level II support includes the middle third of the vagina, including the lateral attachment of the vagina with the endopelvic fascia to the arcus tendinious fascia pelvis. Level III is the distal or lower third vaginal support associated with the urethral attachment in apposition with the pelvic and urogenital diaphragms.

In this case presentation, the patient's surgical history is the risk factor toward development of pelvic organ prolapse. Clinical presentations of pelvic organ prolapse include cystocele, rectocele,

TABLE 40-1   Clinical-Anatomic Correlation

Level	Structure	Function	Effect of damage
Level I: Suspension	Upper paracolpium	Suspends apex to pelvic walls	Prolapse of vaginal apex
Level II: Attachment	Lower paracolpium	Supports bladder and vesical neck	Cystocele-urethrocele
	Pubocervical fascia		Rectocele
	Rectovaginal fascia	Prevents anterior expansion of rectum	
Level III: Fusion	Fusion to perineal membrane, perineal body, musculi levator ani	Fixes vagina to adjacent structures	Urethrocele or deficient perineal body

enterocele, uterine prolapse, and vaginal vault prolapse. These terms describe the relaxation of the anterior, posterior, and middle or superior compartments, respectively. Numerous surgical procedures have been described in order to restore the pelvic support anatomy. As seen in this case presentation, symptoms of discomfort, pain, and pressure in the vaginal area are common and may also be associated with bowel and bladder dysfunction including urinary and fecal incontinence and urinary retention (Table 40-1).

Bibliography

DeLancey J. Anatomic aspects of vaginal eversion after hysterectomy. *Am J Obstet Gynecol* 1992;166:1717–1728.

Droegemueller W. Reproductive anatomy. In: Stenchever MA, Droegemueller W, Herbst AL, Mishell DR Jr (eds.), *Comprehensive Gynecology*, 4th ed. St. Louis, MO: Mosby, 2001, 51–54.

4. **(B)** Trauma, either accidental or intentional, is the leading cause of death in women of reproductive age. Trauma is also the leading cause of nonobstetric maternal death. Similarly it has become one of the leading causes during pregnancy. According to the American College of Obstetricians and Gynecologists, 1 in 12 pregnancies is associated with physical trauma. Of the many causes of physical trauma, approximately two-thirds of all trauma during pregnancy is because of MVAs. Other frequent causes include falls, homicides, and physical and sexual abuse often associated with domestic violence.

When considering MVAs, car accidents account for the majority of these deaths which might be prevented by the use of three-point restraints. Proper seat belt use in crash severity were the best predictors of maternal fetal outcomes. One-third of women do not use seat restraints or use them incorrectly during pregnancy. The effect of air bag deployment in pertinent drivers or passengers is unclear.

Physical abuse in the form of domestic violence is estimated to affect five million women each year. Factors for physical abuse in pregnancy include social instability, unhealthy lifestyle, and physical health conditions. Sixty percent of women report two or more episodes of physical abuse during pregnancy, often with a resultant increase in physical abuse postpartum.

Bibliography

Obstetric Aspects of Trauma Management. *American College of Obstetricians and Gynecologists Education Bulletin*, vol. 251, 1998.

Critical care and trauma. In: Cunningham FG, Gant NF, Leveno KJ, et al. (eds.), *Williams Obstetrics*, 21st ed. New York, NY: McGraw-Hill, 2001, 1171–1777.

5. (C) Suspected appendicitis is one of the most common indications for surgical abdominal exploration during pregnancy. A Swedish registry from 720,000 reported deliveries revealed appendectomy as the indication in about 1 in 1000 pregnancies. The diagnosis was confirmed in 65%.

Difficulty in diagnosis is most attributable to the similar symptom complex of pregnancy and appendicitis. Anorexia, nausea, and vomiting that often accompany normal pregnancy are common symptoms of appendicitis. In addition, mild leukocytosis is often present in normal pregnancy. This may, therefore, obscure acute changes. Other conditions often associated with pregnancy such as pyelonephritis, renal colic, and placental abruption must also be considered. Of most importance is the anatomic change of the appendix during pregnancy and its contribution to the symptom complex of appendicitis. As the uterus enlarges with advancing gestational age, the appendix commonly moves upward and outward toward the flank. The change of position may, therefore, alter the location of pain and tenderness from the right lower to right upper quadrants. As the enlarging uterus results in a cord displacement of the appendix, infection and subsequent rupture may lead to increased generalized peritonitis as containment by the omentum is decreased. In general, prognosis worsens with later gestations. Increased fetal or maternal morbidity and mortality is most often because of surgical delay.

When suspecting the diagnosis of appendicitis, persistent abdominal pain and tenderness are the most reproducible findings. Radiologic studies including both ultrasound and computed tomography (CT) may assist in diagnosis. Treatment, however, in suspected appendicitis, should always include immediate surgical exploration. Both surgical approaches of laparotomy and laparoscopy are acceptable in the pregnant patient. Laparotomy and laparoscopy have held comparable perinatal outcomes with gestations less than 20 weeks.

Even with appropriate diagnosis and management of appendicitis, obstetric complications may occur, such as spontaneous abortion or preterm labor. This is particularly increased in the presence of peritonitis and increased gestational age (beyond 20 weeks). No association with subsequent infertility has been demonstrated.

In the nonpregnant female, differential diagnosis of the acute abdomen when considering appendicitis should also include salpingitis, tubo-ovarian abscess (TOA), ectopic pregnancy, or ruptured ovarian cyst. In the older female, particularly torsion or rupture of the adnexa, acute cholecystitis, perforated ulcer, and acute diverticulitis should also be considered. These conditions may be distinguished according to location of pain.

Bibliography

Gastrointestinal disorders. In: Cunningham FG, Gant NF, Leveno KJ, et al. (eds.), *Williams Obstetrics*, 21st ed. New York, NY: McGraw-Hill, 2001, 1281–1283.

Mazze RI, Källén B. Appendectomy during pregnancy: a Swedish registry study of 778 cases. *Obstet Gynecol* 1991;77:835.

Reedy MB, Källen B, Kuehl TJ. Laparoscopy during pregnancy: a study of five fetal outcome parameters with the use of Swedish Health Registry. *Am J Obstet Gynecol* 1977;177:673.

6. (B) The above case scenario specifically describes a common case of adhesive vulvitis. This has often been described as a self-limiting consequence of chronic vulvitis in the pediatric gynecologic patient. It occurs secondary to denudation of the epithelium of the adjacent labia minora. These epithelial changes result in agglutination and fusion, creating a distorted flat appearance of the vulva. Although not a serious condition, this area may be mistaken for congenital absence of the vagina. Various stages of agglutination may occur. Mild cases demonstrate agglutination only in the posterior aspects of the labia. More advanced cases may demonstrate complete fusion with urethral and vaginal orifice obstruction. The majority of cases are asymptomatic; however, if urethral obstruction occurs, voiding dysfunction and urinary tract infections may result.

Although no treatment is necessary unless voiding difficulties occur, most mothers prefer active treatment of the condition. Spontaneous separation in approximately 2–3 weeks results from topical application of estrogen cream. Forceful physical separation during an office visit is unnecessarily traumatic and should not be performed. Similarly, surgical separation is not required. Most importantly, if agglutination does not resolve with time or estrogen cream application, referral to a gynecologic endocrinologist is recommended to rule out congenital anomaly.

Bibliography

Droegemueller W. Pediatric gynecology. In: Stenchever MA, Droegemueller W, Herbst AL, Mishell DR Jr (eds.), *Comprehensive Gynecology*, 4th ed. St. Louis, MO: Mosby, 2001, 278–279.

7. **(B)** Congenital anomalies of the female reproductive tract are often caused by genetic error or by teratologic event during embryonic development. Minor abnormalities are often of little consequence, but major abnormalities may lead to severe impairment of menstrual and reproductive functions.

One of the common abnormalities of the external genitalia includes imperforate hymen. The hymen is a thin membrane at the vaginal orifice covered by stratified squamous epithelium and consists of fibrous tissue. It represents the junction of the sinovaginal bulbs with the urogenital sinus. Perforation of the hymen ordinarily occurs during embryonic life to establish connection between the vaginal canal and vestibule. As this is an abnormality of the external genitalia, the internal genitalia are intact.

In the pediatric patient, the diagnosis of imperforate hymen is rarely made before puberty, as primary amenorrhea is the major symptom. At puberty, the patient may experience cyclic cramping; however, because of outflow obstruction, no menstrual flow is evident. This may result in hematocolpos and/or hematometrium as is seen in the above case scenario with a palpable vaginal fluid collection. Diagnosis is often made by history and clinical examination demonstrating a bulging membrane at the introitus. Therapy is surgical and consists of a cruciate incision into the hymen extending to the 10, 2, and 6 o'clock positions.

Vaginal agenesis occurs with both Rokitansky-Küster-Hauser's syndrome and testicular feminization syndrome. In both syndromes, there is complete absence of the uterus, therefore, ruling out these diagnoses in the above case scenario. Rokitansky-Küster-Hauser's syndrome is the congenital absence of both vagina and uterus and is associated with the genotype of 46,XX. The ovaries and fallopian tubes are usually present. Twenty-five percent of these patients may have a short vaginal pouch. This disorder does not appear to be an inherited condition.

Testicular feminization syndrome (also known as androgen insensitivity) demonstrates a 46,XY karyotype. This is usually associated with complete vaginal agenesis or the presence of a short vaginal pouch. These patients have undescended testicles and male sex ducts and, therefore, no internal female genitalia are present. The testes in these patients should be removed after puberty to prevent the risk of seminomas. These disorders are often associated with additional urologic and skeletal abnormalities and should, therefore, be screened.

Vaginal septum is incorrect as this is associated with incomplete canalization of the vaginal canal and would be associated with a shortened vaginal pouch.

Bibliography

Stenchever MA. Congenital anomalies of the female reproductive tract. In: Stenchever MA, Droegemueller W, Herbst AL, Mishell DR Jr (eds.), *Comprehensive Gynecology*, 4th ed. St. Louis, MO: Mosby, 2001, 254–260.

8. **(E)** The pregnancy state is associated with multiple physiologic changes in all systems which play a role in all aspects of care of the mother and fetus. Integral in this medical care is pain management during labor. Understanding physiologic changes and their effect on anesthetic management will aid in optimizing patient comfort while minimizing internal or neonatal morbidity and mortality (Table 40-2).

Bibliography

Analgesia and anesthesia. In: Cunningham FG, Gant NF, Leveno KJ, et al. (eds.), *Williams Obstetrics*, 21st ed. New York, NY: McGraw-Hill, 2001, 362–380.
Obstetric Analgesia and Anesthesia. *American College of Obstetricians and Gynecologists Practice Bulletin*, vol. 36, 2002.
Zuspan K. Obstetrical anesthesia (lecture). *Columbus Comprehensive Review*. Perinatal Resources, 2002.

9. **(D)** Labor results in severe pain for many women. Uterine contractions and cervical dilatation result in visceral pain T10-L1. As labor progresses, somatic pain transmitted by the pudendal nerve (S2-S4) results from fetal head descent and associated pressure on the pelvic floor, vagina, and perineum. Goals of obstetric analgesia and anesthesia are the relief of both sources of pain. Multiple methods are available including parenteral medications, local, regional, and general anesthesia.

The use of systemic opioids is one of the most common means of labor analgesia in the United States. These agents can be given in intermittent doses on patient request or via patient controlled administration. The analgesic effect of these agents is limited, as the primary mechanism of action is sedation. Randomized trials comparing intermittent opioid agents with regional anesthesia resulted in significantly higher visual analog

TABLE 40-2   Physiologic Changes of Pregnancy and Their Effect on Anesthetic Management

System and change	Anesthetic significance
Respiratory	
Respiratory mucosa more vascular and edematous	Creating an increased risk of *difficult intubation*, thus, use smaller endotracheal tube (e.g., 6.0 or 7.0); avoid nasal intubation.
Lowered functional residual capacity; increased oxygen consumption; hyperventilation present	Significantly increases the risk of *fetal and maternal hypoxia*. This increases the risk of respiratory arrest in cases of difficult intubation. Thus, preoxygenation is essential for general anesthesia. Give O$_2$ by face mask for 3 min or four deep breaths before induction. For regional anesthesia use supplemental O$_2$.
Cardiovascular	
40% increase in cardiac output	More rapid induction and emergence from general anesthesia.
Engorgement of venous plexus (e.g., veins in epidural space)	Causes an increased risk of intravascular placement of epidural catheter; also decreases the size of epidural space so less drug is needed to obtain epidural block.
Reproductive	
Increased size and weight of uterus	Patients in the supine position are at increased risk of *aortocaval compression* leading to maternal hypotension and decreased uteroplacental blood flow. Use a wedge typically under the patient's right hip to give left lateral uterine displacement to help alleviate. 10% of patients require a right lateral uterine wedge.
Gastrointestinal	
Increased intragastric pressure; delay in gastric emptying; relaxation of gastroesophageal sphincter tone; decreased gastric and intestinal mobility	One-third of all maternal deaths due to anesthesia are because of the complications of *aspiration*. Prevention and prophylaxis are essential.

pain scores. Administration of these parenteral agents are also associated with fetal and neonatal sedation, affecting fetal heart rate variability and increasing the need of neonatal Naloxone therapy. With increasing doses of parenteral agents, patients are exposed to increased risk of aspiration and respiratory arrest.

Paracervical block when used for pain relief during labor may result in fetal bradycardia with associated fetal metabolic acidosis and neonatal depression. The etiology is unclear and, therefore, this technique is relatively contraindicated in the obstetric patient.

Of the various methods used for pain relief during labor and delivery, regional analgesia techniques including epidural, spinal, and combined spinal epidural block are the most flexible, effective, and least depressing to the central nervous system. In the obstetric patient, regional analgesia refers to a partial or complete loss of pain sensation below the T8-T10 level. A varying degree of motor blockade may be present depending on the anesthetic agents used. Epidural analgesia offers the most effective form of pain relief and is used by most women in the United States. Medical indication for epidural analgesia include anticipated difficulty in intubation, a history of malignant hypothermia, selected forms of cardiovascular and respiratory disease, and prevention or treatment of autonomic hyper-reflexia in patients with a high spinal cord lesion. The advantage of this method is that medication can be titrated over the course of labor as needed and can be used for cesarean delivery or postpartum tubal ligation. Spinal analgesia alone or in combination with epidural analgesia may be used to provide pain relief during labor and delivery. Benefits of spinal analgesia include rapid onset, ease of technique, minimal drug exposure, and high effectiveness with the possibility of patient ambulation.

Because general anesthesia results in loss of maternal consciousness, it must be accompanied by airway management by trained anesthesia personnel. The use of intravenous agents followed by rapid sequence induction is used to minimize the risk of aspiration. All inhaled anesthetic agents cross the placenta readily and have been associated with neonatal depression. This places importance on minimizing induction to delivery time when general anesthesia is used.

Additional anesthetic options include various local anesthetic agents for infiltration of the perineum and vagina for analgesia during episiotomy and laceration repair. Rapid acting agents will provide local anesthesia for a duration of 20–40 min. Toxic effects are rare and is highest with inappropriate intravascular injection. Local anesthetic agents can also be used for a pudendal block to aid in operative vaginal deliveries.

Most importantly, all available methods of anesthesia and analgesia should be considered in light of the laboring patient's medical history. It is the responsibility of the physician providing labor and delivery care to provide pain relief in the most safe, effective manner, in consultation with anesthesia colleagues.

Bibliography

Intrapartum and postpartum care of the mother. In: Gilstrap LC, Oh W (eds.), *Guidelines for Perinatal Care*. Washington, DC: American Academy of Pediatrics, American College of Obstetricians and Gynecologists, 2002, 138–142.

Obstetric Analgesia and Anesthesia. *American College of Obstetricians and Gynecologists Practice Bulletin*, vol. 36, 2002.

Optimal Goals for Anesthesia Care in Obstetrics. *American College of Obstetricians and Gynecologists Committee Opinion*, vol. 256, 2001.

Pain Relief during Labor. *American College of Obstetricians and Gynecologists Committee Opinion*, vol. 231, 2000.

10. **(C)** Epidural analgesia is associated with a mild increase in maternal temperature of approximately 0.1°C/h starting about 45 h after the epidural is initiated. The mechanism of fever is not known. Theories include thermoregulation and chorioamnionitis. Although epidural related fever carries no increased risk of neonatal sepsis, studies have shown a statistically significant increase in neonatal sepsis evaluations.

While controlled prospective studies continue to demonstrate that epidurals managed appropriately may be associated with only slight prolongation of the first or second stages of labor, other studies have shown conflicting results. Level C evidence supports that the decision when to place epidural analgesia should be made individually with each patient, with additional factors such as parity being considered. Women in labor should not be required to reach a specific cervical dilatation of 4–5 cm before receiving epidural analgesia. Although total prolongation of labor is usually less than 1 h, increases as much as 40–90 min have been demonstrated.

Labor epidurals are associated with transient back aches in 30–50% of patients immediately postpartum; however, no association with long-term back ache has been demonstrated.

One possible complication of epidural catheter placement includes subarachnoid placement which may then lead to occurrence of postdural puncture headache.

Early studies which demonstrated prolonged labor also demonstrated an increased risk for Cesarean section with epidural analgesia. Recent several large prospective randomized studies now clearly demonstrate no increased risk for Cesarean section. Similarly, metaanalysis in 1998 confirmed that regional anesthesia for labor does not increase the incidence of operative vaginal delivery or Cesarean section.

Bibliography

Bofill JA, Vincent RD, Ross EL, et al. Nulliparous active labor, epidural analgesia, and cesarean section for dystocia. *Am J Obstet Gynecol* 1997;177(6):1465–1470.

Halpern SH, Leighton BL, Ohlsson A, et al. Effect of epidural vs. parenteral opioid analgesia on the progress of labor; a meta-analysis. *JAMA* 1998;280(4):2105–2110.

Obstetric Analgesia and Anesthesia. *American College of Obstetricians and Gynecologists Practice Bulletin*, vol. 36, 2002.

Sharma SK, Sidawi JE, Ramin SM, et al. Cesarean delivery: a randomized trial of epidural versus patient-controlled meperidine analgesia during labor. *Anesthesiology* 1997;87(3):487–494.

Zhang J, Klebanoff MA, DerSimonian R. Epidural analgesia in association with duration of labor and mode of delivery: a quantitative review. *Am J Obstet Gynecol* 1999;180(4):970–977.

11. **(B)**

12. **(C)**

13. **(B)**

Explanations 11 through 13

Gallbladder disease including cholelithiasis is common in the United States and affects upward of 20% of women over the age of 40. Gallstones are commonly cholesterol predominant. Oversecretion into the bile is a major factor in pathogenesis. Biliary sludge which has been shown to increase during pregnancy state is also an important precursor to gallstone formation. As the cumulative risk for surgery remains low at approximately 1–2% per year, prophylactic cholecystectomy is not recommended for asymptomatic gallstones. Similarly, in pregnancy and the puerperium, the incidence of asymptomatic gallstones on ultrasound approaches 10%; therefore, as in the nonpregnant patient, cholecystectomy is not recommended for silent stones.

Multiple nonsurgical approaches for gallstone disease are available. These options include oral bile acid therapy, extracorporeal shock wave lithotripsy, and contact dissolution; however, no experience with these methods during pregnancy is available. Therefore, they are not recommended in the obstetric patient.

Pregnancy is associated with an increased risk of gallstones. This is supported by findings including increased gallbladder volume during fasting and residual volumes postprandially.

Cholecystitis holds a high recurrence rate during the same pregnancy. With recurrence later in gestation, complications of this disease including preterm labor and biliary pancreatitis are more likely.

Similarly, surgical management including cholecystectomy becomes technically more difficult. Because of these factors, more aggressive surgical approach is recommended. Cholecystectomy, both open and laparoscopic, has been demonstrated to be equally safe throughout pregnancy. In the patient with concomitant pancreatitis, cholecystectomy should be considered after inflammation subsides.

Bibliography

Gastrointestinal disorders. In: Cunningham FG, Gant NF, Leveno KJ, et al. (eds.), *Williams Obstetrics*, 21st ed. New York, NY: McGraw-Hill, 2001, 1295–1297.

14. **(A)** Comprehensive prenatal care should include preconceptional care and antepartum care. The goal of preconceptional care is to identify those conditions that could affect a future pregnancy or fetal outcome. Antepartum care should be initiated as soon as there is a reasonable likelihood of pregnancy. The major goals of antepartum care are to define the health status of the mother and fetus, to determine the gestational age of the fetus, and to initiate the plan for continuing obstetrical care. The initial prenatal care visit should include a complete medical history, internal physical examination, risk assessment, determination of estimated due date, along with patient education and laboratory screening tests. Recommended routine laboratory tests should include hematocrit, urinalysis, urine culture, blood grouping, Rh type, antibody screen, Rubella status, syphilis screen, Pap smear, hepatitis B screening along with offering of HIV testing. Thyroid function tests in the asymptomatic pregnant patient without a predisposing medical history are not recommended.

Bibliography

Antepartum care. In: Gilstrap LC, Oh W (eds.), *Guidelines for Perinatal Care*. Washington, DC: American Academy of Pediatrics, American College of Obstetricians and Gynecologists, 2002, 73–121.

Prenatal care. In: Cunningham FG, Gant NF, Leveno KJ, et al. (eds.), *Williams Obstetrics*, 21st ed. New York, NY: McGraw-Hill, 2001, 222–244.

Thyroid Disease in Pregnancy. *American College of Obstetricians and Gynecologists Practice Bulletin*, vol. 37, 2002.

15. **(C)** Thyroid disease is a common endocrinologic disease affecting women of reproductive age. Hyperthyroidism and hypothyroidism may initially manifest during pregnancy. Similarly, obstetric conditions may affect function of the thyroid gland. It is, therefore, important for physicians caring for women, nonpregnant and pregnant, to clearly understand thyroid disease and to interpret laboratory evaluation correctly.

Thyrotoxicosis is a clinical and biochemical state resulting from an excess production and exposure to thyroid hormone. It is associated with symptoms of weight loss despite increased appetite, sweating with heat intolerance, tachycardia, emotional lability, and tremor. Hyperthyroidism is thyrotoxicosis caused by hyperfunctioning of the thyroid gland. This occurs in 0.2% of pregnancies, and Grave's disease accounts for 95%. Inadequately treated disease is associated with miscarriage, a greater risk of preterm delivery, severe preeclampsia and heart failure, along with low birthweight infants and possible fetal loss. Hypothyroidism, on the other hand, is caused by inadequate thyroid hormone production. Etiology may be congenital or acquired and include iodine deficiency, chronic thyroiditis, and autoimmune disease. Classic signs and symptoms are fatigue, constipation, hair loss, dry skin, cold intolerance, muscle cramps, and prolonged relaxation phase of deep tendon reflexes. Similar to hyperthyroidism, untreated hypothyroidism is associated with increased risk of preeclampsia, a higher incidence of low birthweight neonates. When present in the infant, congenital hypothyroidism results in cretinism (growth failure, mental retardation, and additional neuropsychologic deficits).

Thyroid function tests change with normal pregnancy and in both the hyperthyroid and hypothyroid states. Estrogen stimulation of thyroid binding globulin synthesis along with reduced hepatic clearance results in increased concentration of thyroid binding globulin in the pregnant patient. Therefore, those test results that change significantly in pregnancy are those that are most influenced by thyroid binding globulin concentration, namely total thyroxine (TT4), total triiodothyronine (TT3), and resin triiodothyronine uptake (RT3U). hCG stimulation may transiently increase free thyroxine (FT4) and free thyroxine index (FTI); however, these increases usually do not result in levels beyond the normal nonpregnant range. Although plasma iodide levels decrease during pregnancy because of fetal use of iodide and increased maternal renal clearance, this has only been associated with a physical increase in thyroid gland size and no change in thyroid function tests has been seen (Table 40-3).

Bibliography

Endocrine disorders. In: Cunningham FG, Gant NF, Leveno KJ, et al. (eds.), *Williams Obstetrics*, 21st ed. New York, NY: McGraw-Hill, 2001, 1340–1348.

Thyroid Disease in Pregnancy. *American College of Obstetricians and Gynecologists Practice Bulletin*, vol. 37, 2002.

TABLE 40-3   Changes in Thyroid Function Test Results in Normal Pregnancy and in Thyroid Disease

Maternal Status	TSH	FT4	FTI	TT4	TT3	RT3U
Pregnancy	No change	No change	No change	Increase	Increase	Decrease
Hyperthyroidism	Decrease	Increase	Increase	Increase	Increase or no change	Increase
Hypothyroidism	Increase	Decrease	Decrease	Decrease	Decrease or no change	Decrease

*Abbreviations: TSH, thyroid-stimulating hormone; FT4, free thyroxine; FTI, free thyroxine index; TT4, total thyroxine; TT3, total triiodothyronine; RT3U, resin T3 uptake.

16. **(E)** The American Association of Clinical Endocrinologists and the American Thyroid Association recommend TSH as the initial test for the screening and evaluation of symptomatic disease. The free component is biologically active and not affected by pregnancy changes. If FT4 is unavailable, the FTI can be calculated as the product of TT4 and RT3U.

Bibliography

Thyroid Disease in Pregnancy. *American College of Obstetricians and Gynecologists Practice Bulletin*, vol. 37, 2002.

17. **(A)**

18. **(C)**

Explanations 17 and 18

Postpartum hemorrhage is a serious complication of labor and delivery, and requires a coordinated and rapid response. Possible etiologies for postpartum hemorrhage are uterine atony, retained placenta, genital tract lacerations, maternal coagulopathy, uterine inversion or rupture, and low-lying placenta. General risk factors for the development of postpartum hemorrhage include both obstetric and medical disorders. Obstetric risk factors include multiparity, prolonged labor, preeclampsia, the use of antepartum oxytocin, chorioamnionitis, low-lying or retained placenta, uterine overdistention secondary to polyhydramnios or multifetal pregnancy, and operative vaginal delivery. Similarly, the use of uterine relaxants either for tocolysis in the setting of preterm labor or halogenated inhalational agents for anesthesia have also been associated with increased hemorrhage.

This patient has uterine atony for which she has three risk factors. She has had five obstetric deliveries (multiparity) and just delivered a large neonate after a probable prolonged labor which resulted in arrest. Vaginal laceration in this patient is unlikely, as she was delivered by Cesarean section. Similarly, chorioamnionitis in the afebrile patient is less likely.

Prolonged labor is a risk factor for uterine atony and not an etiology for postpartum hemorrhage. Inspection of the surgical field should be performed to verify hemostasis at all suture lines. In addition, lacerations or extension of the uterine incision should be identified and repaired.

Initial treatment for uterine atony should include vigorous uterine fundal massage along with intravenous oxytocin (20 units in 1000 mL of lactated Ringer or normal saline at 10 mL/min). If inadequate response is noted, ergot derivatives may be used to stimulate uterine contraction. The agent most commonly used is methyler-gonovine maleate (Methergine) 0.2 mg intramuscularly. Methylergonovine is contraindicated in the hypertensive patient. If no response persists, prostaglandin derivatives including $PGF_{2\alpha}$ can be given either intramuscularly or intramyometrially and is the best next step. The initial recommended dose is 250 µg and this may be repeated at 15–90 min intervals up to a maximum of eight doses. If bleeding continues to be unresponsive to uterotonic agents, reevaluation for lacerations or retained placenta is necessary. Additional resuscitative efforts including two large bore intravenous catheters should be used to administer intravenous crystalloid while the patient is type and cross-matched for possible blood transfusion. Coagulation profile should also be evaluated. Surgical management is then indicated for failed medical therapy. This may include initially uterine artery ligation or hypogastric artery ligation or hysterectomy. If available, consideration for interventional radiologic treatment with arterial embolization may be considered.

Bibliography

Obstetrical hemorrhage. In: Cunningham FG, Gant NF, Leveno KJ, et al. (eds.), *Williams Obstetrics*, 21st ed. New York, NY: McGraw-Hill, 2001, 635–652.

19. **(A)** The female menstrual cycle occurs as a result of coordinated hormone and steroid function resulting in simultaneous ovarian and uterine, specifically

endometrial, changes. In order to understand the physiologic mechanisms involved in regulation of the normal menstrual cycle, it is helpful to divide it into three phases: follicular, ovulation, and luteal phase. During the follicular phase, an orderly sequence of events takes place, then ensures the proper number of follicles is ready for ovulation. In the human ovary, follicular development usually results in one surviving mature follicle. Follicular development typically occurs over 10–14 days. Adequate function of the hypothalamic-pituitary-ovarian axis results in normal menstrual function with hypothalamic release of gonadotropin releasing hormone (GnRH) in the normal pulsatile fashion. The pituitary is stimulated to synthesize and release both LH and FSH from its anterior lobe. In the ovary, FSH stimulates granulosa cell growth and initiates steroidogenesis in the granulosa cell of the follicle. Steroidogenesis in the granulosa cell occurs by a luteinization of androgens to produce estrogen. LH, on the other hand, acts on the theca cells of the follicle producing androgens which can then be converted to estrogens in the granulosa cells. Increasing levels of estrogen result in negative feedback at the hypothalamic pituitary level to suppress other follicles from developing. FSH induces LH receptor development on the granulosa cells of the large follicles. Increasing levels of estrogen stimulate LH release during the midfollicular phase. Ovulation typically occurs 34–36 h after the LH surge. After ovulation, the granulosa and theca cells become luteinized. Under the influence of LH, the corpus luteum produces progesterone. In case of fertilization and conception, the production of progesterone in the corpus luteum continues under stimulation from hCG. Levels of progesterone will continually increase after ovulation, reaching a plateau approximately 1 week luteal phase. Increasing levels of progesterone and estrogen exert a negative feedback on FSH and LH secretion.

As a result of the hormonal milieu, the endometrial lining of the uterus will go through various phases; proliferative, secretory, and menstrual. The endometrium can be divided morphologically into the upper two-thirds functionalis layer and lower one-third basalis. It is the purpose of the functionalis layer to prepare for implantation and is, therefore, the site of proliferation, secretion, and subsequent degeneration of menstruation. The proliferative phase of the endometrium is associated with the ovarian follicular phase and increased estrogen secretion. During this growth phase of the endometrium, the glandular epithelium significantly expands. All tissue components including glands, stroma, and endothelium will proliferate, peaking on days 8 through 10 of the cycle, corresponding to peak estradiol levels systemically.

During proliferation, the endometrium may expand up to 3.5–5.0 mm in height. After ovulation, the endometrium responds to combined estrogen and progesterone activity. Proliferation typically ceases 3 days postovulatory inhibition, predominantly because of progesterone. The glandular elements become more tortuous as the stroma is increasingly edematous. In the absence of fertilization and implantation, the corpus luteum of the ovary will undergo degeneration with decreasing estrogen and progesterone levels. This withdrawal will similarly impact the endometrium as evidenced by decreasing tissue height. Endometrial tissue breakdown will involve various enzymatic actions including collagenases and proteinases with continued tissue disorganization. Ischemic breakdown ensues with cell necrosis, leading to menstrual flow.

Ninety percent of women have menstrual cycles with an interval of 24–35 days. The typical duration of menstrual flow is 4–6 days with normal volume of menstrual blood loss approximately 30 mL, greater than 80 mL being abnormal.

Bibliography

Mishell DR. Reproductive endocrinology. In: Stenchever MA, Droegemueller W, Herbst AL, Mishell DR Jr (eds.), *Comprehensive Gynecology*, 4th ed. St. Louis, MO: Mosby, 2001, 83–109.

Regulation of the menstrual cycle. In: Speroff L, Glass RH, Kase NG (eds.), *Clinical Gynecologic Endocrinology and Infertility*, 6th ed. Baltimore, MD: Lippincott, Williams & Wilkins, 1989, 201–238.

The uterus. In: Speroff L, Glass RH, Kase NG (eds.), *Clinical Gynecologic Endocrinology and Infertility*, 6th ed. Baltimore, MD: Lippincott, Williams & Wilkins, 1989, 123–144.

20. (D) Postmenopausal HT is currently approved for the treatment of vasomotor symptoms (hot flashes, night sweats) and vulvovaginal atrophy. Standard doses of HT [0.625 conjugated equine estrogen (CEE) combined with 2.5 mg medroxyprogesterone acetate (MPA)] effectively reduce the incidence of severity of hot flashes within 3 weeks of commencing therapy. Recently, lower doses of HT (0.45 mg CEE/1.5 mg MPA) have been demonstrated to be equally effective to standard doses in relieving vasomotor symptoms.

Vulvovaginal atrophy is a result of estrogen deficiency and can result in dyspareunia, urinary symptoms, and vaginal bleeding. Oral HT in both the standard and lower doses significantly increases the percentage of superficial cells from baseline by 6 months. Treatment solely for urogenital atrophy commonly consists of topical estrogen creams.

Several studies looking at HT have shown that HT is not effective in the primary or secondary prevention of cardiovascular disease. The women's health initiative (WHI), a primary prevention trial, demonstrated an increase in coronary heart disease events (relative risk 1.29) and stroke (relative risk 1.41) in HT users versus placebo over a 5-year time frame. The HERS trial, Heart and Estrogen/Progestin Replacement Study, was a randomized, postmenopausal, double-blind placebo-controlled secondary prevention trial. Two thousand seven hundred sixty-three postmenopausal women with a mean age of 66.7 years with known coronary artery disease were studied. The treatment group received CEE 0.625 mg + MPA 2.5 mg daily. The primary study end point was non-fatal myocardial infarction or coronary heart disease death. HERS I had a follow-up of 4.1 years. The HERS trial, published prior to the WHI, demonstrated an increased incidence in recurrent cardiovascular events in patients taking HT versus placebo in the first year, followed by a significant reduction in years 4 and 5. HERS II, was an open-label continuation of HERS I for an additional 2.7 years. HERS II, however, did not demonstrate a continued reduction in the incidence of cardiovascular events after years 4 and 5.

For these reasons, HT is not indicated for prevention, either primary or secondary, of cardiovascular disease. While the WHI showed a decrease in the incidence of colorectal cancer (0.63 RR), HT is currently not indicated by the FDA for prevention of colorectal cancer.

Bibliography

Grady D, et al. Heart and estrogen-progestin replacement study II. *JAMA* 2002;288:49–57.

Hulley S, et al. Heart and estrogen-progestin replacement study I. *JAMA* 1998;280:605–613.

Utian WH, et al. Relief of vasomotor symptoms and vaginal atrophy with lower doses of conjugated equine estrogens and medroxyprogesterone acetate. *Fertil Steril* 2001;75:1065–1079.

Writing group for Women's health initiative investigators. *JAMA* 2002;288:321.

21. **(C)** The WHI was a randomized, double-blind, placebo-controlled primary prevention trial. Sixteen thousand six hundred eight postmenopausal women, mean age 63.3, without vasomotor symptoms were enrolled. The treatment group received CEE 0.625 mg and MPA 2.5 mg. The primary study end points were nonfatal myocardial infarction or coronary heart disease death. The study duration was planned for 8.5 years but was terminated early at an average of 5.2 years because of a statistically significant increase in cardiovascular events (1.29 hazard ratio) (HR) and invasive breast cancer

(1.26 HR) in the treatment group. Additionally, the incidence of strokes (1.41 cumulative HR) and venous thromboembolic events (2.11 cumulative HR) were increased.

However, the all cause mortality was not significantly different between the study group and the placebo group (HR = 0.98; placebo = NS).

The incidence of colorectal cancer (HR = 0.63) and hip fracture (HR = 0.66) was decreased in the treatment group. HT is indicated for the prevention of osteoporosis but not the prevention of colorectal cancers.

The estrogen-progestin arm of the study was halted at an average of 5.2 years. The estrogen only arm is still ongoing.

Baseline characteristics of the study participants have contributed to criticisms of the WHI as a primary cardiovascular prevention trial. These characteristics include average participant age of 63.3 years, mean body mass index of participants 28.5 kg/m^2, approximately 36% of participants had hypertension, nearly 7% were taking statins and nearly 2% had a history of myocardial infarctions. It has been argued that based on the above baseline characteristics, the WHI more closely parallels the HERS trial than a primary prevention trial.

Nonetheless, conclusions from the WHI include the following:

- ET/HT should not be used for the prevention of cardiovascular disease.
- There is an increased risk of coronary heart disease, stroke, venous thromboembolic events and invasive breast cancer in HT users.
- There is a risk reduction for hip fracture and colon cancer in HT users.
- HT needs to be prescribed selectively, appropriately and individualized based on each patient's unique benefits and risk profile.

Bibliography

Hulley S, et al. Heart and estrogen-progestin replacement study I. *JAMA* 1998;280:605–613.

Writing Group for Women's health initiative investigators. *JAMA* 2002;288:321.

22. **(D)** TOA is the most serious consequence of salpingitis and pelvic inflammatory disease (PID). TOA is a collection of pus involving the fallopian tubes, ovaries, and adjacent organs (bowel, bladder, uterus, omentum). Long-term sequelae, present in up to 25% of patients with TOA, include adhesions, pelvic pain, infertility, and increased incidence of ectopic pregnancy.

Mortality rates approach 9% with intraabdominal rupture of a TOA. Traditional treatment was surgical and aggressive via a TAH/BSO. Availability of broad-spectrum antibiotics, improved diagnostic imaging modalities, and minimally invasive surgical procedures have permitted conservative management of TOA.

Antibiotic therapy for TOA must cover gram-negative aerobes, gram-positive aerobes and gram-negative anaerobes. *Neisseria gonorrhea* and *Chlamydia trachomatis* are the major pathogens in the etiology of PID and TOA, but are rarely isolated at the time of culture. The antibiotic treatment must also cover these two organisms.

The polymicrobial nature of TOA requires broad-spectrum coverage such as second generation cephalosporins. Clindamycin and metronidazole provide excellent anaerobic coverage and abscess cavity-penetrating ability.

Clinical response to IV antibiotic therapy may not be evident prior to 72 h of treatment. Patients not demonstrating clinical improvement (resolving abdominal pain, decreasing WBC count, and resolving fever) within 72 h are considered treatment failures. Ultrasound or CT-guided percutaneous drainage or surgical removal of a TOA should be considered once treatment failure has occurred. Similarly, patients who decline clinically or develop an acute abdomen need immediate surgical intervention. The surgical procedure of choice is based on the patient's clinical status, intraoperative findings, patient's age, and reproductive desires. Exploratory laparotomy with TAH/BSO is usually performed in the presence of an intraabdominal rupture of a TOA.

Bibliography

Krivak TC, Propst A. Tubo-ovarian abscess. *Female Patient* 2001;26:43–49.

23. **(B)** TOA is a serious complication of PID and has similar risk factors; low socioeconomic status, multiple sexual partners, lack of condom use, previous episodes of PID in adolescence. Often the initial offending organisms (*N. gonorrhea* and *C. trachomatis*) are asymptomatic or silent in females. Therefore, patients presenting with TOA may have no known history of previous PID episodes.

PID accounts for nearly 350,000 hospitalizations and 150,000 surgeries per year; however, TOA is uncommon in postmenopausal women. Approximately 1.7% of TOA occur in postmenopausal women. The differential diagnosis of a pelvic abscess in a postmenopausal woman must include malignancy (gastrointestinal or gynecologic) and a perforated viscus. The treatment of choice in a postmenopausal woman with TOA is an exploratory laparotomy with a TAH/BSO.

Bibliography

Krivak TC, Propst A. Tubo-ovarian abscess. *Female Patient* 2001;26:43–49.

24. **(E)**

25. **(D)**

26. **(A)**

27. **(A)**

Explanations 24 through 27

Acute abdominal pain in a reproductive age female can be gynecologic, gastrointestinal, genitourinary, or musculoskeletal in origin. The evaluation should address all of these systems. Ectopic pregnancy, adnexal torsion, Mittelschmerz, and acute appendicitis can present as acute onset lower abdominal pelvic pain, particularly in the location of the right lower quadrant. Acute pancreatitis, though, is commonly associated with right- and left-sided upper quadrant pain, not lower quadrant pain.

Ectopic pregnancy is a possibility, as the patient is late for her monthly menses and has an adnexal fullness/pain. Based on the patient's history of irregular menses, the pain could also represent mittelschmerz or a ruptured ovarian cyst. Equally likely is adnexal torsion and acute appendicitis. For this reason, high clinical suspicion and appropriate diagnostic tests will aid in obtaining the correct diagnosis in the most timely fashion.

Ectopic pregnancy has a classic symptom triad of pain, amenorrhea, and vaginal bleeding; however, only 50% of patients with an ectopic pregnancy will have this symptom group. There is no pathognomonic pain that is diagnostic for an ectopic pregnancy. While the severity and location can vary, abdominal pain is the most common complaint on presentation. On physical examination, the uterus may be slightly enlarged. The abdominal examination can vary from nontender to differing degrees of tenderness with or without rebound. Cervical motion tenderness may or may not be present. An adnexal mass may be palpated up to 50% of the time. Additionally, the examination will vary depending if rupture of the ectopic pregnancy with intraabdominal hemorrhage has occurred. Tachycardia and hypotension are associated with intraabdominal hemorrhage. A serum beta hCG and/or transvaginal ultrasound is frequently required to accurately diagnose an ectopic pregnancy. Mittelschmerz is midcycle pain believed to be because of ovarian follicular rupture during ovulation; however, the actual mechanism is not clearly understood. Both mittelschmerz and a ruptured ovarian cyst can present with acute onset of pelvic pain; however, following the results of the pelvic ultrasound, mittelschmerz or a ruptured hemorrhagic ovarian cyst is unlikely, as the patient is noted to have a right adnexal mass and minimal fluid in the cul-de-sac. Typically, there is marked fluid in the cul-de-sac following a ruptured ovarian cyst, and an adnexal mass or cyst is not present.

Acute appendicitis is a possible diagnosis in any age group. The pain usually begins in the periumbilical region and then localizes to the right lower quadrant. Anorexia or nausea and vomiting generally are present with an acute appendicitis. Voluntary guarding is frequently present, and rebound can be a sign of rupture. A CBC will usually show an elevated white blood cell count.

Based on the differential diagnosis, the workup needs to include a CBC, urine pregnancy test or a serum beta hCG, and a pelvic ultrasound.

Ovarian torsion is an uncommon cause of lower abdominal pain but diagnosis is imperative to prevent severe vascular compromise. Conservative operative management is possible in 75% of cases when early diagnosis occurs. The majority of torsion can occur in young women of reproductive age (average age midtwenties), further making conservative management by gently untwisting the adnexa ideal.

Patients with ovarian torsion or adnexal torsion, if the fallopian tube is involved, present with acute, severe, unilateral lower abdominal and pelvic pain. Two-thirds of patients have nausea and vomiting, making a distinction between torsion and acute appendicitis difficult. More than 90% of patients with torsion have a unilateral, extremely tender, adnexal mass on bimanual examination. While patients most often report acute onset of severe pain, many patients note intermittent episodes of similar pain for several days or weeks prior to the severe current episode.

Factors that increase the patient's likelihood of developing adnexal torsion include pregnancy, enlarged ovaries secondary to ovulation induction, and ovarian tumors. Approximately one-half of women with ovarian torsion are found to have an ovarian tumor. Dermoids, paraovarian cysts, solid benign ovarian tumors, and serous cysts are the most common ovarian findings in adnexal or ovarian torsion. Rarely, torsion of a malignant ovarian tumor occurs. Interestingly, torsion of the right ovary is more common than the left ovary.

Ultrasound is useful in confirming the presence of an ovarian mass as well as defining the characteristics of the mass (solid, cystic, complex). Doppler ultrasound assists in diagnosis of ovarian or adnexal torsion by evaluating ovarian arterial blood flow. While nearly 50% of women with surgically confirmed torsion have normal Doppler blood flow, abnormal color flow Doppler is strongly correlated with ovarian/adnexal torsion.

Because of the patient's age and her desire for fertility, conservative surgical management is appropriate. A laparoscopic approach with gentle untwisting of the pedicle with observation for restored vascular integrity to the ovary is acceptable and, in this patient, desirable. Concomitant ovarian cystectomy may help prevent recurrent torsion. If severe vascular compromise has occurred, unilateral salpingo-oophorectomy is necessary. The ureter may be incorporated into the torsed pedicle, making determination of ureteral location essential to avoid ureteral injury.

Bibliography

Stenchever MA. Differential diagnosis of major gynecologic problems by age groups. In: Stenchever MA, Droegemueller W, Herbst A, et al. (eds.), *Comprehensive Gynecology*, 4th ed. St. Louis, MO: Mosby, 2001, 160–163.

Stovall TG, McCord ML. Early pregnancy loss and ectopic pregnancy. In: Berek JS, Adashi EY, Hillard PA (eds.), *Novak's Gynecology*, 12th ed. Baltimore, MD: Williams & Wilkins, 1996, 496.

28. **(B)** Uterine leiomyomas, also known as fibroids, are the most common pelvic tumors in females. Approximately 20–25% of reproductive age women have fibroids. Interestingly, postmortem examinations of women revealed a 50% presence of fibroids. Because most leiomyomas are asymptomatic, the true prevalence is unknown. Two-thirds of women with a leiomyoma will be found to have multiple leiomyomas. Leiomyomas are more commonly found in Black women. Leiomyomas are the most common indication for hysterectomy.

A leiomyoma is a benign, smooth muscle tumor of the uterus. Leiomyomas are believed to be unicellular in origin. Histologically, they are characterized by bundles of smooth muscle cells arranged in a whirl-like pattern with fibroblasts and collagen. The nuclei have a uniform rod-shaped appearance. Mitotic figures are uncommon and nuclear atypia is never present. This is in contrast to leiomyosarcomas where mitotic figures and nuclear atypia are a characteristic feature.

The development and growth of leiomyomas is influenced by estrogen and progesterone. Exposure to estrogen will promote the growth, while progesterone or progesterone-like substances may decrease the size by exerting an antiestrogen effect. Leiomyomas may range in size from a few millimeters to very large tumors weighing more than 100 lbs.

While the majority of fibroids are asymptomatic, the most common symptom associated with fibroids is abnormal bleeding; usually menorrhagia. Pelvic pressure, increasing abdominal girth and less commonly pain are also reported by some patients. As leiomyomas grow, impingement on adjacent organs can result in increased urinary frequency (compression of bladder), urinary retention (impingement of urethra or bladder neck), hydronephrosis (ureteral compression), and constipation (bowel compression).

For the majority of asymptomatic patients, expectant or observational management is appropriate. Serial clinical examinations and ultrasound studies are required to reassure the physician enlargement is not occurring. Initially, follow-up should be at 1–3-month intervals. If the size appears stationary and the patient remains asymptomatic, evaluation can be at 6-month intervals and then yearly. If rapid growth is noted, then surgical intervention is warranted as this may be a leiomyosarcoma.

Bibliography

Burrows LJ, Elkins TE. Leiomyoma. In: Ransom SB, Dombrowski MP, McNeeley SG, et al. (eds.), *Practical Strategies in Obstetrics and Gynecology*. Philadelphia, PA: W.B. Saunders, 2000, 51–56.

Whelan JG, Vlatios NE, Wallach EE, Ransom RB, et al. Contemporary management of leiomyomas. In: Ransom SB, Dombrowski MP, Evans MI, et al. (eds.), *Contemporary Therapy in Obstetrics and Gynecology*. Philadelphia, PA: W.B. Saunders, 2002, 367.

29. **(E)** Leiomyosarcoma is a smooth muscle malignancy of the uterus. Of all the uterine sarcomas that can occur, leiomyosarcomas are the most common, but the overall incidence is very rare. Approximately 0.1% of uterine leiomyomas are noted to have a malignant change consistent with a leiomyosarcoma. The signs and symptoms of a leiomyosarcoma are similar to those of a leiomyoma; abnormal bleeding, pressure, and abdominal fullness. However, rapid enlargement of a presumed benign leiomyoma, particularly in a perimenopausal or postmenopausal patient, should heighten the clinician's suspicion for a leiomyosarcoma. Leiomyosarcomas often occur in patients in their fifties and in conjunction with leiomyomas. Once thought to be a result of malignant degeneration of benign leiomyomas, leiomyosarcomas are now thought to arise *de novo*.

One study by Leibsohn et al. evaluated hysterectomy specimens from 1423 patients with a uterine size 12 weeks or greater. The incidence of sarcoma was 0.4% for patients in their thirties. The incidence increased for patients in their fifties to 1.4%. In addition to the increased incidence of leiomyosarcomas in postmenopausal patients, the prognosis and survival is decreased in the postmenopausal population. Histologically, a triad of hypercellularity, nuclear atypia, and numerous mitotic figures is seen in leiomyosarcomas. Differentiation between a leiomyoma and leiomyosarcoma is based on the microscopic evaluation of the level of mitotic activity and the cellular atypia. Five mitotic figures/10 hpf with cytological atypia confirms the diagnosis of leiomyosarcoma. Vascular invasion, extrauterine spread, and greater than 10 mitotic figures/10 hpf all worsen the prognosis. The overall 5-year survival is 20% but increases to approximately 40% in patients with stage I or stage II disease.

TAH/BSO is the most important treatment for leiomyosarcomas and, in reality, diagnosis is made and confirmed at the time of hysterectomy. Distant metastases to the lung, liver, and bone do occur but lymph node metastases are uncommon. Radiotherapy and chemotherapy have been used each with fair results.

Bibliography

Burrows LJ, Elkins TE. Leiomyoma. In: Ransom SB, Dombrowski MP, McNeeley SG, et al. (eds.), *Practical Strategies in Obstetrics and Gynecology*. Philadelphia, PA: W.B. Saunders, 2000, 53.

Herbst AL. Neoplastic diseases of the uterus. In: Stenchever MA, Droegemueller W, Herbst A, et al. (eds.), *Comprehensive Gynecology*, 4th ed. St. Louis, MO: Mosby, 2001, 943–944.

Whelan JG, Vlatios NE, Wallach EE. Contemporary management of leiomyomas. In: Ransom SB, Dombrowski MP, Evans MI, et al. (eds.), *Contemporary Therapy in Obstetrics and Gynecology*. Philadelphia, PA: W.B. Saunders, 2000, 367.

30. **(C)** Chronic pelvic pain is defined as cyclic or non-cyclic pain for 6 months or more in duration that localizes to the pelvic region and impairs functional ability of the patient. It accounts for 10% of all outpatient visits to a gynecologist, 40% of laparoscopies, and 10–15% of hysterectomies. Approximately 15% of the adult female population in the United States reports chronic pelvic pain as a common complaint. Chronic pelvic pain can be a difficult and frustrating symptom for both the patient and health care provider.

The most important component of evaluating a woman with chronic pelvic pain is the history and physical examination. Often a pain questionnaire is mailed to the patient prior to her initial visit to elicit a focused and complete history. A thorough description of the pain including its character, palliative and provocative features is necessary. Equally challenging is that the etiology of chronic pelvic pain can have a single or multiple origin, and a differential diagnosis is vast. Several organ systems must be included in the differential diagnosis, including gynecologic, gastrointestinal, genitourinary, myofascial, skeletal, and psychologic disorders. Gynecologic disorders include endometriosis, adhesions, and chronic PID. Gastrointestinal diseases include irritable bowel syndrome, constipation, diverticulitis, and diverticulosis. Genitourinary diseases that can contribute to chronic pelvic pain include interstitial cystitis, bladder dyssynnergia, and chronic urethritis. Myofascial disorders including fasciitis, nerve entrapment syndrome, and hernias can contribute to chronic pelvic pain. Skeletal disorders such as scoliosis and lumbar disc disorders must also be considered in the differential diagnosis. Psychologic disorders including somatization, psychosocial dysfunction, and depression may be a cause of persistent pain. Similarly though, depression and psychologic distress may also be a consequence rather than a cause of persistent pain. The health care provider treating patients with chronic pelvic pain must consider all these possible etiologies when evaluating a patient.

For those patients who undergo laparoscopy as part of their evaluation of chronic pelvic pain, less than 50% of the women were found to be helped by diagnostic or operative laparoscopy as it relates to their symptoms of chronic pelvic pain. Forty percent of the women with chronic pelvic pain had no apparent pathology at the time of laparoscopy; however, endometriosis and more specifically, atypical endometriotic findings, are likely missed at the time of diagnostic laparoscopy because of its abnormal nontypical appearance. In those patients who do have abnormal surgical findings, the most common gynecologic problems noted in women undergoing laparoscopy for evaluation of chronic pelvic pain are endometriosis and pelvic adhesions. Laser and cautery methods may effectively treat superficial endometriotic lesions; however, they do not adequately treat deeply infiltrating endometriotic lesions. GnRH agonists used postoperatively significantly prolong the pain-free interval after laparoscopy in patients with endometriosis. GnRH agonists alone may effectively show complete responses in minimal or mild endometriosis; however, long-term use of this medication is associated with significant side effects including hot flashes and bone demineralization.

When abnormal findings are noted at the time of laparoscopy, pelvic adhesions in addition to endometriosis are commonly seen; however, the long-term benefit of adhesiolysis is questionable because adhesion reformation begins nearly immediately following surgery. Patients though who did benefit from adhesiolysis were those patients with severe adhesions involving the intestinal tract.

Bibliography

Gelbaya TA, El-Halwagy HE. Focus on primary care: chronic pelvic pain in women. *Obstet Gynecol Surv* 2001; 56:757–764.

Scialli AR. Evaluating chronic pelvic pain. A consensus recommendation. *J Rep Med* 1999;44:945–952.

31. **(D)** Endometrial carcinoma is the most common gynecologic malignancy in the United States. One out of 50 women in the United States will develop endometrial cancer in her life. This is 1.3 times the likelihood of developing ovarian cancer and twice that of developing cervical cancer.

Postmenopausal bleeding is the presenting symptom in approximately 90% of patients with endometrial adenocarcinoma. By definition, postmenopausal bleeding is vaginal bleeding which occurs 1 year after the last normal menstrual period. In the premenopausal patient, endometrial cancer can be associated with menorrhagia, metrorrhagia, or menometrorrhagia. Sampling of the endometrium (either via endometrial biopsy or dilatation and curettage) is indicated. Transvaginal ultrasound to evaluate the thickness of the endometrial lining in a postmenopausal patient is helpful in the diagnosis of endometrial hyperplasia or adenocarcinoma. A thickness greater than 5 mm on transvaginal ultrasound warrants histologic evaluation in a postmenopausal patient not taking HT.

The main risk factor for endometrial adenocarcinoma is endometrial stimulation by unopposed estrogen. The postmenopausal patient taking estrogen alone has a four- to eight-time increased risk of developing endometrial adenocarcinoma. Patients with breast cancer taking tamoxifen are also at an increased risk. Tamoxifen is a selective estrogen receptor modulator with both estrogen and antiestrogen properties. The use of a progestin in addition to estrogen therapy decreases the risk of endometrial cancer. Likewise, there is a decreased risk of endometrial adenocarcinoma in patients taking combination oral contraceptives. Other risk factors include obesity, nulliparity, late menopause (after age 52 years) and diabetes. Hypertension has often been reported as a risk factor but has not been established as an independent risk factor; obesity and hypertension are frequently seen in the same patient.

The staging of endometrial adenocarcinoma is based on surgical and pathologic findings. The primary therapy for endometrial adenocarcinoma is exploratory laparotomy, pelvic washings, and TAH/BSO. High grade lesions (grade II and III), depth of myometrial invasion, cervical involvement and histology consistent with papillary serous or clear cell carcinoma increase the risk of lymphatic spread. The benefit of complete surgical staging has been debated, and lymph node sampling may be reserved for the above high-risk findings.

Bibliography

Deppe G, Mankarah AR. In: Ransom SB, Dombrowski MP, McNeeley SG, et al. (eds.), *Practical Strategies in Obstetrics and Gynecology*. Philadelphia, PA: W.B. Saunders, 2000, 471–475.

Herbst AL. Neoplastic diseases of the uterus. In: Stenchever MA, Droegemueller W, Herbst A, et al. (eds.), *Comprehensive Gynecology*, 4th ed. St. Louis, MO: Mosby, 2001, 919–921.

32. **(C)** Numerous maternal adaptations occur during pregnancy. An understanding of these changes will prevent the medical care provider from misinterpreting normal pregnancy adaptations as a disease process. Similarly, laboratory values that would be considered abnormal in a nonpregnant state may actually represent normal physiologic changes in the pregnant state.

Pulmonary changes occur normally in pregnancy, including increase in tidal volume and minute ventilation. Functional residual capacity and residual volume are decreased because of the elevated diaphragm. Unchanged are the respiratory rate and lung compliance. Dyspnea and increased awareness of a desire to breathe suggest a pulmonary or cardiac abnormality in the nonpregnant state; however, in pregnancy, physiologic dyspnea may result from increased tidal volume which slightly lowers the PCO_2 causing dyspnea.

Maternal blood volume in pregnancy increases by 40–45% by term. An increase in both plasma and erythrocytes contribute to the increase in the blood volume. This pregnancy-induced hypervolemia assists in meeting the vascular demands of the hypertrophied uterus and protect against the adverse effects of blood loss at time of delivery. Cardiac output and ventricular performance increase as a result of decreased systemic vascular resistance. The resting heart rate increases by approximately 10 bpm. Blood volume and plasma volume increases exceed that of

the increase in RBC mass, and hemoglobin and hematocrit decrease slightly during pregnancy; the so-called dilutional anemia of pregnancy.

Although gastrointestinal tract absorption of iron moderately increases during pregnancy, iron deficiency anemia is common in pregnancy. The amount of iron absorbed from the diet as well as that mobilized from stores is commonly insufficient to meet the demands imposed by pregnancy. The iron requirements of normal pregnancy total around 1000 mg. Two hundred milligrams of this iron is lost through normal excretion. These losses are obligatory and occur even if the mother is iron deficient. Three hundred milligrams of iron is actively transferred to the fetus and placenta. Iron requirements average 6–7 mg per day during the second half of pregnancy. Most women's body stores cannot accommodate this iron requirement amount. Without supplemental iron, the hemoglobin concentration and hematocrit fall markedly as the maternal blood volume naturally increases. However, even when the mother has severe iron deficiency anemia, sufficient amounts of iron are obtained via the placenta for the fetus to establish and maintain normal fetal hemoglobin levels.

Bibliography

Maternal adaptations to pregnancy. In: Cunningham FG, Gant NF, Levino KJ, et al. (eds.), *Williams Obstetrics*, 21st ed. New York, NY: McGraw-Hill, 2001, 167–197.

33. **(B)** Ovarian cancer is the leading cause of death because of gynecologic malignancies. Endometrial cancer is the most common gynecologic malignancy. Ovarian cancer accounts for 4% of all new cancers diagnosed in women and 14,000 deaths occur each year from ovarian cancer.

Seventy-five percent of all ovarian cancers are diagnosed at an advanced stage and survival is based on histologic grade and extent of disease at time of diagnosis. Overall 5-year survival for all stages of ovarian cancer is 50%, but decreases to 28% with stage 3 or stage 4 at initial diagnosis. If detected and treated at stage 1, 5-year survival approaches 95%. Early diagnosis is the key to survival and successful treatment; however, early clinical symptoms rarely occur. For this reason, ovarian cancer screening using ultrasound and serum tumor markers has gained increased attention.

Ultrasonography can detect early morphologic changes in ovarian cancer and has been used as a screening tool. Transvaginal ultrasound has improved the resolution of ovarian imaging because the transvaginal transducer is in a closer proximity to the ovaries than a transabdominal transducer.

Transvaginal ultrasonography can accurately visualize the ovaries in approximately 95% of premenopausal women and 85% of postmenopausal women. However, high false positive rates of abnormal ovarian ultrasound findings and an inability to show a decrease in ovarian cancer deaths by screening for ovarian cancer with ultrasound has limited the usefulness of ovarian ultrasound as a universal screening tool.

A radioimmunoassay is used to detect serum tumor marker Ca-125. It is elevated in over 80% of stage 3 and stage 4 ovarian cancers, but an elevated Ca-125 is not specific for ovarian cancer. Other conditions such as endometriosis, leiomyomas, smoking, PID, inflammatory bowel disease, diverticulitis, and several nongynecologic malignancies are also associated with an elevated Ca-125. When combining elevated serum Ca-125 with abnormal pelvic ultrasound findings, surgical intervention yielded an ovarian cancer specificity of 99.9% and a positive predictive value of 26.8%.

The lifetime risk of a woman developing ovarian cancer is 1:70, and increases to 1:20 with one affected first-degree relative and 1:14 with two or more affected first-degree relatives. Focusing on high-risk populations may improve the yield of ovarian cancer screening. A family history consistent with hereditary ovarian cancer syndrome put a woman at the highest risk for developing ovarian cancer. Women with site-specific familial ovarian cancer, breast ovarian cancer syndrome, or a predisposition to developing ovarian, endometrial and/or colon cancer (Lynch's syndrome II) have been reported to develop ovarian cancer as early as age 30–40 years.

The prevalence of ovarian cancer is highest in women over age 50. There is a greater than threefold risk increase in ovarian cancer between the age of 40 years compared to 75 years. There is also an increase in ovarian cancer mortality in women over 65 years of age.

Bibliography

Platt LD, Karlan BY, Greene NH, et al. Screening for ovarian cancer. In: Ransom SB, Dombrowski MP, Evan EI, et al. (eds.), *Contemporary Therapy in Obstetrics and Gynecology.* Philadelphia, PA: W.B. Saunders, 2002, 399–403.

34. (D) MVA account for nearly 60% of all pregnancy trauma cases. Domestic violence and assaults range from 4 to 20% of all cases. MVAs are the leading cause of death in women age 15 through 24 and the second leading cause of death for women age 25–44 years. While pregnant women may be less likely to wear seat belts than their nonpregnant counterpart, the use of restraints dramatically reduces both maternal and

fetal complications from MVA. The use of seat belts should be discussed with pregnant patients throughout the entire pregnancy.

Placental separation, abruptio placenta, compromises 20–50% of severe trauma cases and is the most common cause of fetal compromise following trauma in pregnancy. Abruption can result from direct abdominal trauma or deceleration forces. These can result in placental shearing from the decidua. Uterine contractions and/or a nonreassuring fetal heart rate tracing following trauma may signal the presence of an abruption; however, frequent uterine contractions, uterine tenderness, and ultrasound are not specific predictors of placental separation. Therefore, trauma patients at risk for placental separation should be monitored for a minimum of 4 h for maternal and fetal wellbeing once fetal viability has been reached.

The abdominal examination of the pregnant patient becomes more difficult with advancing maternal age. At 12 weeks of gestation, the uterus rises out of the pelvis and above the pubic bone. In advancing gestations, the intraabdominal contents will be displaced into the upper abdomen. Not only may peritoneal signs be more difficult to elicit during pregnancy, but injuries to the upper abdomen may result in extensive bowel injuries, splenic rupture, or retroperitoneal hemorrhage.

Most trauma patients, pregnant or nonpregnant, require radiographic evaluation. With exposures of 5 rads or less, few fetal concerns exist regardless of gestational age. The threshold for developmental consequences from radiation in the first trimester is approximately 15–20 rads. The exposure doses of radiation producing adverse neurologic outcomes is much higher in the second and third trimester. While the radiation dose to the fetus with a CT scan exceeds 5 rads, by limiting the number of slices and the thickness of slices, the exposure can be reduced to less than 5–10 rads. Therefore, CT can be used as a radiologic diagnostic tool when indicated in the pregnant patient.

Bibliography

Gunter J. Trauma in pregnancy. In: Ransom SB, Dombrowski MP, Evan EI, et al. (eds.), *Contemporary Therapy in Obstetrics.* Philadelphia, PA: W.B. Saunders, 2002, 128–131.

35. (A) Amniotic fluid embolism is a disorder that classically occurs in women in the late stages of labor or immediately postpartum. A woman begins gasping for air, becomes hypotensive and often within minutes suffers a cardiorespiratory arrest and a seizure. Amniotic fluid embolism management is further complicated by the occurrence of disseminated intravascular coagulation, massive hemorrhage, and death. While classically this disorder is characterized by the abrupt onset of hypotension, hypoxia, and consumptive coagulopathy, there is great variation in the clinical presentation of this condition, making the immediate and accurate diagnosis challenging. The estimated frequency of amniotic fluid embolism is about one case per 20,000 deliveries. While the occurrence of an amniotic fluid embolism is uncommon, maternal death is likely to occur with an amniotic fluid embolism.

Because most cases of amniotic fluid embolism occur in association with labor, a pattern of a hypertonic uterus, vigorous labor, and the use of oxytocin have been implicated in the past in the pathogenesis of this condition. However, recently cardiovascular collapse seen in the presence of amniotic fluid embolism appears to be the effect of the amniotic fluid embolism rather than the cause. Also, uterine blood flow ceases completely when intrauterine pressures exceed 35–40 mmHg, making the presence of hypertonic contractions the least likely time for a fetal-maternal exchange to occur. It was also demonstrated that the use of oxytocin was not increased in women who experienced an amniotic fluid embolism.

Often death occurs rapidly in women who experience an amniotic fluid embolism, but for those women who survive beyond the initial cardiovascular collapse, a secondary noncardiogenic pulmonary edema (adult respiratory distress syndrome) (ARDS) or acute tubular necrosis may occur. Survival and maternal prognosis is based on early recognition; however, currently there is no data that any type of intervention including circulatory support, blood component replacement therapy improves maternal prognosis in the presence of an amniotic fluid embolism. Maternal mortality rate has been reported anywhere from 60 to 90%, with death occurring as rapidly as 30 min. For those women who do survive, profound neurologic impairment is common. While overall neonatal survival is approximately 70%, residual neurologic impairment is seen in over 50% of the neonates. Neonatal outcome is related to "arrest to delivery" interval.

As stated previously, no type of intervention has been shown to improve maternal prognosis with amniotic fluid embolism; however, treatment when an amniotic fluid embolism is recognized, is directed toward three goals: (1) oxygenation, (2) maintenance of cardiac output and blood pressure, and (3) treatment of the coagulopathy.

Bibliography

Amniotic fluid embolism. In: Clark SL, Cotton SB, Hankins GDV, et al. (eds.), *Handbook of Critical Care Obstetrics*. Boston, MA: Blackwell Scientific, 1994, 209–214.

Obstetrical hemorrhage. In: Cunningham FG, Gant NF, Leveno KJ, et al. (eds.), *Williams Obstetrics*, 21st ed. New York, NY: McGraw-Hill, 2001, 660–662.

36. (E) The beta hCG is 6000 mIU/mL, CBC is within normal limits, blood type is A negative, and pelvic ultrasound shows no intrauterine pregnancy, minimal amount of fluid in the cul-de-sac and a 3.0 cm mass in the right adnexa.

37. (D)

38. (B)

39. (B)

Explanations 37 through 39

The incidence of ectopic pregnancy has steadily increased in the United States. Currently, approximately 20 per 1000 pregnancies are an ectopic pregnancy. While the incidence of ectopic pregnancy has increased, maternal mortality has decreased. This is mainly because of increased diagnostic modalities and an earlier diagnosis prior to rupture. Standard treatment of ectopic pregnancy had been surgical; however, medical management of tubal pregnancy has become an option using intramuscular methotrexate for selected ectopic pregnancies. This option allows outpatient treatment of ectopic pregnancies and allows avoidance of surgery.

Risk factors for ectopic pregnancy include a history of PID, particularly PID caused by *C. trachomatis*, prior ectopic pregnancy, cigarette smoking, and prior tubal surgery. Increasing age is also associated with an increased incidence of ectopic pregnancy. The classic triad of ectopic pregnancy includes the following symptoms: abdominal pain, absence of menses, and irregular vaginal bleeding. Abdominal pain is present in approximately 90–100% of patients with an ectopic pregnancy. The location may be unilateral, bilateral, or generalized, and can be severe or colicky in nature. If rupture of the oviduct occurs, the pain usually becomes intense. Syncope occurs in approximately one-third of patients who experience tubal rupture with an ectopic. Regarding absence of menses, there is usually a 6-week or more interval of amenorrhea that is reported by patients with ectopic prior to them experiencing vaginal bleeding. The bleeding is classically spotting but may be similar to the patient's normal menstrual flow. Rarely though is it as heavy as that which occurs in a spontaneous abortion. Approximately half of the women with ectopic pregnancies will have a palpable adnexal mass on bimanual examination. Temperature elevation is rare and tachycardia and hypotension are usually seen only with oviduct rupture and profuse blood loss.

Laboratory evaluations that can aid in the diagnosis and management of ectopic pregnancies include a CBC, specifically evaluating the hematocrit and the leukocyte count. For patients with a ruptured ectopic pregnancy, hematocrit of less than 30% is found in one-quarter of these patients. The leukocyte count will be normal in approximately 50% of patients with an ectopic pregnancy. Quantitative beta hCG helps confirm the state of pregnancy, date the pregnancy, and help direct the use of ultrasonography. A discriminatory value of 6500 mIU/mL has become a useful figure when using abdominal ultrasonography. For patients with a quantitative beta hCG greater than 6500 mIU/mL and no gestational sac seen in the uterus on abdominal ultrasound, nearly all women had an ectopic pregnancy. With the development of transvaginal ultrasound and transvaginal transducer probes, more precise imaging of the pelvic organs in early pregnancy has become possible. Specifically, an intrauterine gestational sac is able to be identified when hCG levels reach 1500 mIU/mL. When no intrauterine sac is seen with hCG levels exceeding this value, a pathologic pregnancy—either an ectopic or a nonviable intrauterine pregnancy—is most likely present. Of note, nearly two-thirds of women presenting with symptoms consistent with an ectopic pregnancy will have beta hCG levels greater than 2500 mIU/mL. With this level of beta hCG, the diagnosis of ectopic pregnancy can usually be made using transvaginal ultrasonography when no intrauterine sac is identified. Type and screen is also imperative not only if oviduct rupture has occurred and blood loss is profuse, but also to determine based on the patient's Rh status if RhoGAM is required. Rh negative pregnant patients with abnormal bleeding or an ectopic pregnancy are required to receive RhoGAM.

With a beta hCG of 6000 mIU/mL in this patient, transvaginal ultrasound should demonstrate an intrauterine pregnancy if, in fact, it exists. Minimal fluid in the cul-de-sac suggests that oviduct rupture and profuse blood loss has not occurred. The 3 cm mass in the right adnexa most likely represents an ectopic pregnancy in the fallopian tube. Based on the patient's positive beta hCG and her ultrasound findings, the most likely diagnosis is ectopic pregnancy;

specifically, a right fallopian tube ectopic pregnancy. Incomplete and threatened abortion are very unlikely because no intrauterine pregnancy or sac is visualized.

Dilatation and curettage of the uterus is not a management option at this time, as no gestational sac is seen within the uterus. Expectant management is an option in some ectopic pregnancies; however, spontaneous resolution is greatest in patients whose initial beta hCG level is less than 200 mIU/mL. Patients opting for expectant management must be willing to accept the potential risks of hemorrhage and tubal rupture. This patient's beta hCG is well above 200 mIU/mL and spontaneous resolution of her ectopic pregnancy is low. Optimal management options for this patient include intramuscular methotrexate and laparoscopic salpingostomy. A definitive diagnosis of ectopic pregnancy by direct visualization of the pelvis with laparoscopy can nearly always be made. Difficulty in visualizing the pelvic organs may be because of hemoperitoneum, adhesions, or obesity. There is no evidence of hemoperitoneum in this patient based on transvaginal ultrasound, so diagnostic laparoscopy with laparoscopic salpingostomy is a treatment option for this patient. Exploratory laparotomy is generally reserved for patients who are hemodynamically unstable, oviduct rupture with profuse blood loss, inability to adequately visualize the pelvic organs with laparoscopy, or lack of expertise in laparoscopic surgery. Intramuscular methotrexate provides a nonsurgical medical management option for patients with ectopic pregnancy. Patients who are candidates for medical management with methotrexate must be hemodynamically stable, able to return for follow-up care, no history of hepatic, renal or hematologic dysfunction, no preexisting blood dyscrasias such as leukopenia, thrombocytopenia or significant anemia, and no known sensitivity to methotrexate. Intramuscular methotrexate also provides a treatment option to patients in whom general anesthesia poses a significant risk. Single-dose methotrexate for ectopic pregnancy has a reported success rate of approximately 84%. Factors decreasing the effectiveness of methotrexate include gestational sac size greater than 3.5 cm, the presence of fetal cardiac activity on ultrasound, and a beta hCG level exceeding 15,000 mIU/mL.

For patients who receive methotrexate, they should be counseled to expect to experience vaginal bleeding or spotting and mild abdominal pain, as well as medication related side effects including nausea, vomiting, stomatitis, diarrhea, gastric distress, and dizziness. Patients who experience sudden onset of severe abdominal pain or worsening of current abdominal pain should be evaluated immediately by the physician, as rupture of an ectopic pregnancy has been reported following methotrexate injection. Likewise, dizziness, syncope, or tachycardia also warrant evaluation of the patient. Additionally, patients should be instructed to avoid alcoholic beverages, nonsteroidal anti-inflammatory drugs, and sexual intercourse. Because methotrexate is a folinic acid antagonist that inhibits dihydrofolic acid reductase, thereby interfering with DNA synthesis repair and cellular replication, patients should also be instructed to avoid vitamins containing folic acid, particularly their prenatal vitamin.

Bibliography

Medical management of tubal pregnancy, ACOG Practice Bulletin, #3, December 1998. *Compendium of Selected Publications.* Washington, DC: ACOG Distribution Center, 2003, 463–469.

Mishell D. Ectopic pregnancy. In: Stenchever MA, Droegemueller W, Herbst AL, et al. (eds.), *Comprehensive Gynecology*, 4th ed. St. Louis, MO: Mosby, 2001, 443–475.

40. (D)

41. (B)

42. (A)

Explanations 40 through 42

Breast cancer is diagnosed in one of 3500–10,000 pregnancies. About 3% of all breast cancers occur during pregnancy. Detection of a mass is difficult as the breasts have increased nodularity and firmness because of the pregnancy. These may increase with increasing breast hypertrophy as the pregnancy progresses, emphasizing the importance of a baseline breast examination at the first prenatal visit.

Any persistent mass with suspicious characteristics on physical examination warrants a thorough evaluation. Mammography is a noninvasive test that can be performed safely at a low radiation dose with abdominal shielding (less than 1 rad per breast). However, because of the changes in breast tissue, including increased density, vascularity and water content, mammography is not a sensitive screening test during pregnancy. Suspicious masses warrant biopsy. If expertise and experienced personnel are available, needle biopsies performed under local anesthesia are indicated. If not, then an excisional biopsy is required.

Early diagnosis of breast cancer, whether pregnant or nonpregnant, greatly improves the response to treatment and survival. Pregnancy itself does not significantly influence the spread or course of breast cancer. The 5-year survival rate in breast cancer is primarily dependent on the stage of disease at diagnosis; however, serious delays in diagnosis and treatment of pregnant women with a breast cancer have been reported. As stated previously, the pregnant breast is subject to hormonally induced changes which may obscure a mass. Sadly, 75% of pregnant women diagnosed with breast cancer have positive lymph nodes versus 37% positive lymph nodes in nonpregnant patients. In addition to the delayed diagnosis of breast cancer in pregnant women, the increased vascularity and lymphatic drainage from the breast may contribute to the advanced stage of diagnosis. Also, breast cancer in young patients tends to be more aggressive and usually pregnant patients are young.

Optimal therapy for breast cancer in pregnancy is debated because of a lack of randomized control trials. Initial treatment is surgery ranging from a simple mastectomy, modified mastectomy or radical mastectomy. "Delay in surgical intervention until fetal viability has not been shown to be of benefit to the mother or the fetus." For early stage disease (I and II), therapy consists of a modified radical mastectomy or lumpectomy followed by radiation. These two approaches have been shown to be equal in efficacy. There is a 1% spontaneous abortion rate with a mastectomy. With chest radiation, there can be significant local scatter but this should not prohibit timely intervention. If nodal involvement is present, chemotherapy following surgery is indicated. There is potential teratogenicity with most chemotherapeutic agents. Particularly in early pregnancy and with organogenesis occurring, therapeutic abortion should be considered. By waiting even 6 months for delivery or fetal viability, therapeutic efficacy of adjuvant chemotherapy may be lost. For advanced local disease (stage III), chemotherapy is required. For metastatic patients (stage IV), therapy is palliative and may be delayed until documentation of fetal lung maturity is made and delivery is achieved.

Bibliography

Brewster WR, DiSaia PL. Cancer in pregnancy. In: Ransom RB, Dombrowski MP, McNeeley SG, et al. (eds.), *Practical Strategies in Obstetrics and Gynecology*. Philadelphia, PA: W.B. Saunders, 2000, 525–527.

Dance VD, Krueger MD, Ma W. Breast disease. In: Ransom SB, Dombrowski MP, Evans MI, et al. (eds.), *Contemporary Therapy in Obstetrics and Gynecology*. Philadelphia, PA: W.B. Saunders, 2002, 343–343, 372.

Neoplastic diseases. In: Cunningham FG, Gant NF, Leveno KJ, et al. (eds.), *Williams Obstetrics*, 21st ed. New York, NY: McGraw-Hill, 2001, 1442–1443.

Williams SF, Schilsky RL. Neoplastic disorders. In: Barrow WM, Lindheimer MD (eds.), *Medical Disorders during Pregnancy*, 3rd ed. St. Louis, MO: Mosby, 2000, 400–401.

43. (B)

44. (C)

45. (B)

Explanations 43 through 45

Breast abscesses are suspected when therapy for puerperal mastitis fails to result in clinical improvement after 48–72 h of antibiotic therapy or there is a development of a palpable mass in the affected breast. Mastitis is characterized by a high fever (>38.5°C), chills, erythema, pain, increased local skin temperature, and myalgias. It commonly occurs during the first 3 weeks of postpartum breastfeeding. *Staphylococcus aureus* is the most common etiologic organism. Treatment consists of frequent feeding from both breasts with the affected breast being offered first. Rest and oral antibiotics for 10–14 days are also indicated. Dicloxacillin and first-generation cephalosporins are optimal choices for treatment of mastitis. Erythromycin is prescribed to penicillin allergic patients. No clinical improvement in 48–72 h suggests a breast abscess.

This patient's diagnosis is most consistent with a breast abscess. Though a galactocele may be tender, it is usually not accompanied with fevers, chills, myalgias, or skin warmth. A galactocele is a cystic area filled with breast milk and results from ductal obstruction. A galactocele is usually seen following cessation of lactation. Warm showers, heat, and massage to the area will help relieve the ductal obstruction and resolve the galactocele.

Fat necrosis of the breast commonly follows breast trauma; usually in the form of breast surgery or radiation therapy. Its characteristics are similar to those of breast cancer; firm, palpable mass with skin or nipple retraction. Biopsy is required to rule out cancer, but if left untreated the mass will eventually resolve.

Fibroadenomas are one of the most common benign lesions found in the breast. On examination a round, firm, usually mobile, nontender mass is palpated. Size can range up to 5 cm. Excisional biopsy or fine-needle aspiration for cytology will confirm the diagnosis. Enlarging fibroadenomas must be removed to rule out malignancy. In younger women (under age 25), close observation of small fibroadenomas is acceptable.

Surgical drainage is essential and necessary for treatment of a breast abscess. To enhance cosmetic results, the incision should be made in the circumareolar location or in the direction of Langer's lines if further out in the breast. The incision and drainage is performed under general anesthesia as vigorous debridement and disruption of loculations is required. The surgical cavity is then packed with gauze and replaced with fresh gauze in 24 h. Multiple abscesses may require multiple incisions. The patient should also receive antibiotic treatment for up to 14 days.

There is no consensus regarding breastfeeding continuation on the affected side. Postoperative discomfort itself may eliminate this as an option early on. If the patient wishes to continue breastfeeding, it is advisable for her to continue from the unaffected breast. There is no reason why the breast milk needs to be discarded for any period of time while the patient is using dicloxacillin, a first-generation cephalosporin or erythromycin, or has a fever. Similarly, thrush is not a contraindication to breastfeeding nor is it the most likely etiologic agent in mastitis or breast abscess.

Bibliography

Dance VD, Krueger MV, Ma W. Breast disease. In: Ransom SB, Dombrowski MP, Evans MI, et al. (eds.), *Contemporary Therapy in Obstetrics and Gynecology*. Philadelphia, PA: W.B. Saunders, 2002, 339–341.

Johnston C. Diseases of the breast. In: Ransom SB, Dombrowski MP, McNeeley SG, et al. (eds.), *Practical Strategies in Obstetrics and Gynecology*. Philadelphia, PA: W.B. Saunders, 2000, 172–174.

The peurperium. In: Cunningham FG, Gant NF, Leveno KJ, et al. (eds.), *Williams Obstetrics*, 21st ed. New York, NY: McGraw-Hill, 2001, 414.

46. (C)

47. (C)

48. (D)

Explanations 46 through 48

A Bartholin's gland cyst is an obstruction of the duct usually secondary to trauma or nonspecific inflammation. Following obstruction of the duct, there is continued secretion of fluid by the gland and this results in cystic dilation. The incidence of adult women who develop Bartholin's gland cyst is approximately 2%. When present, it is commonly seen in women during their reproductive years. In fact, of women who develop a Bartholin's gland cyst, 85% of them are in their reproductive years.

Normally, the Bartholin's glands cannot be palpated. They are located deep in the perineum at the 5 and 7 o'clock position at the entrance of the vagina.

When ductal obstruction occurs, Bartholin's gland cysts are located in the labia majora near the hymen.

Most women who develop a Bartholin's cyst are asymptomatic with the exception of them noticing a fullness in the labia. On physical examination, a non-tender, unilateral, tense cyst is noted.

Obstruction of the duct and formation of the Bartholin's cyst usually occurs without an infection or abscess; however, an abscess of the cyst may develop rapidly over 2–4 days. Physical findings of a Bartholin's gland abscess differ from that of a simple Bartholin's gland cyst in that patients report acute pain and tenderness. On physical examination, there is marked erythema, pain on palpation of the mass, and occasionally cellulitis in the adjacent subcutaneous tissues. In this patient, the physical findings and the patient's history are most consistent with a Bartholin's gland cyst as findings of an abscess are not present.

Mesonephric cysts of the vagina are generally more anterior in the vagina whereas the Bartholin's gland cyst is more caudal. A Gartner's duct cyst does not involve the labia but occurs in a cephalad portion of the vagina approaching the apex and on the lateral vaginal wall. On physical examination, a nontender cystic-like protrusion of either side vaginal wall near the cervix is noted.

Treatment options for a Bartholin's gland duct cyst include warm soaks and expectant management, insertion of a Word catheter or a marsupialization of the duct to create a fistulous tract. However, in this patient, because the Bartholin's gland cyst is recurrent, expectant management with warm soaks is not appropriate. Simple incision and drainage of the cyst will immediately alleviate the fullness; however, the tendency for recurrence is high. Because this patient has had recurrent Bartholin's gland duct cysts, insertion of a Word catheter or marsupialization of the duct is the most appropriate treatment. A Word catheter is a short catheter with an inflatable Foley balloon at the distal end which is inserted into the cyst after a stab incision is made. This can be performed under local anesthesia. Ideally, the Word catheter is left in place for 4–6 weeks, during which time a tract will form which will help prevent further duct obstruction and recurrence of a Bartholin's gland duct cyst. Often though, the Word catheter will spontaneously fall out prior to the 4–6-week time period. Care must be taken when inserting a Word catheter to keep the stab incision of a size just big enough to insert the tip of the Word catheter. This will help with premature extraction of the catheter before the 4–6-week time frame. Marsupialization is performed in the operating room and is the classical

surgical treatment. Marsupialization of the duct will help develop a fistulous tract in an attempt to prevent recurrence. An elliptical incision is made overlying the protruding Bartholin's cyst, and the tissue is removed. Marsupialization is then performed by suturing the edges of the everted duct to the surrounding skin. This has a success rate of approximately 90% in preventing recurrent Bartholin's gland duct cysts.

Because this patient does not have an obvious Bartholin's gland abscess, broad-spectrum antibiotics are not indicated; however, in the case of Bartholin's gland abscess, broad-spectrum antibiotics with aerobic and anaerobic coverage are indicated. Cultures from Bartholin's gland abscess contain anaerobic, aerobic, and facultative anaerobic organisms and typically are classified as polymicrobial. It was once believed that Bartholin's gland cysts or abscesses were pathognomonic with a gonococcal infection. This is no longer believed to be true, as bacterial cultures of Bartholin's cysts and abscess have revealed polymicrobial infections. In fact, in the majority, therefore, Bartholin's gland cysts or infection is not felt to be caused by a sexually transmitted disease (STD) or a sexually transmitted infection.

While asymptomatic Bartholin's gland cysts in women under age 40 do not require treatment, excision of a Bartholin's gland duct cyst is indicated in women over the age of 40. If complete excision is not possible, biopsy of the gland is required to rule out adenocarcinoma of the Bartholin's gland. Excision of the Bartholin's gland is also indicated for persistent deep infection, multiple recurrences of Bartholin's gland cyst or abscess and despite marsupialization. However, particularly in those patients over age 40, histologic examination of the Bartholin's gland required as adenocarcinoma has been noted in this age group.

Bibliography

Droegemueller W. Infections of the lower genital tract. In: Stenchever MA, Droegemueller W, Herbst AL, et al. (eds.), *Comprehensive Gynecology*, 4th ed. St. Louis, MO: Mosby, 2001, 645–647.

49. (C) Vaginal infections, vaginitis, are the most common reason for gynecologic visits, accounting for more than 10 million office visits per year. The three most common vaginal infections are candidiasis (yeast), BV, and trichomonas vaginitis. Obtaining the accurate and complete diagnosis requires a complete history and a thorough examination involving a pelvic examination, vaginal pH testing, wet mount, and a KOH "whiff" test. Relying solely on the patient's symptoms or the clinician's visual examination is not sufficient to provide an accurate diagnosis because different vaginal infections can present in similar ways. Hence, the importance of performing the wet mount (saline and KOH) testing.

Patients with candidiasis will commonly complain of a white, cottage cheese-like discharge which has no odor. They also can have vulvovaginal pruritus; however, basing a diagnosis purely on the presence of the appearance of the discharge is not sufficient. The diagnosis of vulvovaginal candidiasis should be based on the observation and presence of budding hyphae on the KOH wet prep. While yeast infections are not associated with serious health risks, medical conditions such as diabetes and human immunodeficiency virus infection can increase a patient's likelihood to have a yeast infection. Similarly, the recent use of antibiotics, oral contraceptives, and pregnancy can also increase the likelihood of a patient having a yeast infection. Treatment of the patient's sexual partner has not been shown to decrease the frequency of recurrence of the infection nor improve the initial response to therapy.

BV is commonly associated with an unpleasant fishy or musty vaginal odor. This is present in approximately 50–75% of patients, and this odor may also be associated with trichomoniasis. The odor is because of the anaerobic metabolism of various amine byproducts. Patients may often notice this odor following sexual intercourse or during menstruation. Visually, the discharge is usually gray or white, homogeneous and thin. Vaginal pruritus and irritation may also be present. Diagnosis is based on the findings of a pH greater than 4.5, a positive KOH "whiff" test, the presence of clue cells on a saline slide as observed under microscopic observation and the presence of a homogeneous discharge as described previously. Numerous complications have been associated with BV, including PID, endometritis, postoperative infections, premature rupture of the membranes, and preterm delivery. Treatment of the sexual partner is not recommended nor required, as this has not influenced a woman's response to therapy nor recurrent infections.

Trichomonas vaginalis also can have a foul, fishy odorous discharge. This discharge though is usually yellow-green and frothy, and the cervix is described as having a classical strawberry-like appearance with numerous cervical petechia. The patient may also have dysuria, dyspareunia, and severe vulvovaginal pruritus. Diagnosis is made by observing motile trichomonads on the saline smear of the wet prep.

Risk factors for trichomonas include a history of previous STD, coinfection with other STDs or *N. gonorrhea* and multiple sexual partners. Trichomonas

is considered a STD and treatment of the sexual partner is necessary.

In summary, a thorough evaluation for vaginal infections includes a pelvic examination with visual evaluation of the whole genital area, pH testing as a pH greater than 4.5 can indicate BV or trichomonas, a pH less than 4.5 is usually associated with *Candida* infections. However, douching or recent intercourse may alter the pH. A wet mount consisting of a saline slide and a KOH slide is the most important test for an accurate diagnosis of vaginal infections. The KOH "whiff" test consists of adding vaginal fluid secretions to a mix of KOH and then detecting a foul, strong, fishy odor. This is usually indicative of BV or trichomonas.

Bibliography

Diagnosis of vaginitis. *APGO Educational Series in Women's Health Issues*, 1996.

50. **(A)** A hydatidiform mole is a cystic swelling of the chorionic villi which results from an abnormal pattern of fertilization which accounts for the chromosomal origin of complete and partial moles. A hydatidiform mole is classically described as a delicate friable mass of thin-walled, translucent, cystic, grape-like structures found within the uterus. In a complete mole, one or two sperm (dispermy) fertilize an egg that is devoid of chromosomal material. Because the egg is without any maternal DNA material, all cells are derived from the sperm; androgenesis. It is postulated that either two sperm fertilize an egg without any maternal DNA or that a single sperm fertilizes an egg without any maternal DNA and then duplicates the chromosomes found in the sperm. The most common karyotype of a complete mole is 46,XX. With an incomplete mole, the egg has its usual 23,X (haploid status) and is either fertilized by one diploid sperm or two haploid sperm. In either situation, the karyotype is triploid, either 69,XXY or 69,XXX. This is in contrast to the maternal egg that is devoid of genetic material in the formation of a complete mole.

Hydatidiform mole is more common in the extremes of age, with maternal age over 35 a significant risk factor for developing a complete mole. If the maternal age is over age 35, the relative risk of having a complete mole is 2, and if maternal age is over 40, the relative risk is 7.5. There also appears to be an association with a maternal blood type A, and a prior hydatidiform mole increases the risk for a subsequent molar pregnancy to 1%.

Vaginal bleeding in the first trimester is the most common presentation seen in patients with a hydatidiform mole. It occurs in approximately 97% of cases. This bleeding can be heavy and is associated with anemia in half of the cases. An enlarged uterus, with size greater than dates, is also considered a classic sign but is present in only half of patients. There can also be passage of clear, watery fluid, sometimes with grape-like tissue. Patients with a hydatidiform mole are also at an increased risk of developing preeclampsia, hyperemesis gravidarum, hyperthyroidism, and respiratory distress.

Pelvic ultrasound can aid in the diagnosis of a hydatidiform mole as a classic "snow storm pattern" representing swollen villi. Quantitative levels of beta hCG are also another useful tool. Levels of beta HCG will be elevated out of proportion to the gestational age and rise more rapidly than seen in a normal pregnancy. The combination of first trimester bleeding, excessive uterine size, markedly elevated quantitative beta hCG and findings on pelvic ultrasound are sensitive in detecting and diagnosing a molar pregnancy.

Treatment consists of uterine curettage to evacuate the uterus of the trophoblastic tissue. Excessive blood loss can occur at the time of curettage, and oxytocin given intraoperatively will decrease the blood loss. If the patient is Rh negative, it is recommended that she receives Rh immunoglobulin at the time of curettage, regardless if it is a partial or complete mole, as trophoblastic cells express Rh positive. Hysterectomy is an option for treatment if the woman does not desire future fertility; however, hysterectomy has not been shown to prevent recurrence of disease. Follow-up of these patients is essential, as beta hCG levels should be monitored weekly until they are normalized for 3 weeks. Serum beta hCG levels should be checked monthly until normal for 6 months to 1 year. Pregnancy is not recommended in the first year following treatment, as a rising beta hCG of pregnancy could obscure the diagnosis of invasive gestational trophoblastic disease. Therefore, contraception is recommended and essential for 1 year.

Malignant forms of a hydatidiform mole include an invasive mole and choriocarcinoma. An invasive mole penetrates the uterine wall and increases the risk of uterine rupture. Irregular uterine growth, irregular bleeding, and persistently elevated beta hCG levels aid in the diagnosis of an invasive mole. Fortunately, this tumor is responsive to chemotherapy.

Choriocarcinoma is an epithelial malignant neoplasm of trophoblastic cells. It is characterized by early vascular dissemination and metastatic spread. Thirty to fifty-five percent of choriocarcinomas arise from hydatidiform moles and is more common following a complete mole and very rarely associated with a partial mole. Approximately 2% of complete moles will progress to a choriocarcinoma. Interestingly, approximately 20% of all choriocarcinomas are diagnosed following a normal pregnancy. Beta hCG levels may be increased or, if the trophoblastic tissue is necrosed and nonhormone producing, the beta hCG level may not be increased. Vaginal bleeding and a foul odorous discharge are associated with a choriocarcinoma. Unfortunately, metastasis can be a common finding at the time of diagnosis. Usual sites of metastases are the lungs (50–80%), vagina (30%), and brain, liver, and kidney. Treatment varies with the metastatic staging at time of diagnosis, but chemotherapy regimens have curative rates in the 90th percentile.

Bibliography

Berkowitz RS, Goldstein DP. Gestational trophoblastic disease. In: Berek JS, Adashi EY, Hillard PA (eds.), *Novak's Gynecology*, 12th ed. Baltimore, MD: Williams & Wilkins, 1996, 1261–1279.

Herbst AL. Gestational trophoblastic disease. In: Stenchever MA, Droegemueller W, Herbst AL, et al. (eds.), *Comprehensive Gynecology*, 4th ed. St. Louis, MO: Mosby, 2001, 1039–1062.

Sulzman A. Choriocarcinoma after hydatidiform mole. *Am J Obstet Gynecol* 2000;183(1):257.

CHAPTER 41

Minimally Invasive Surgery and Bariatrics

Don Seltzer and Andrew C. Eppstein

Questions

1. According to the National Institutes of Health (NIH) Consensus Development Conference Statement, patients interested in weight loss surgery for treatment of clinically severe obesity must satisfy several qualifications prior to consideration. Which one of the following is *not* a qualification for bariatric surgery determined by the NIH?

   (A) body mass index (BMI) greater than 35 kg/m² with a medical comorbidity related to morbid obesity

   (B) BMI greater than 40 kg/m²

   (C) age <18

   (D) poor outcomes with nonsurgical methods including dieting, exercise, and behavioral modifications

   (E) understanding of the surgical risks and demonstrated follow-up with previous methods of weight loss

2. Which of the following patients does *not* qualify for weight loss surgery?

   (A) 40-year-old female with no medical comorbidities and a BMI of 42 kg/m²

   (B) 55-year-old male with diabetes mellitus, a BMI of 38 kg/m², and failed nonsurgical weight loss techniques for 12 months

   (C) 48-year-old male with BMI of 65 kg/m² who suffers from arthritis, sleep apnea, and gastroesophageal reflux

   (D) 25-year-old female with BMI of 40 kg/m² with depression and hyperparathyroidism

3. Several surgical weight loss procedures have been performed during the development of bariatric surgery. Roux-en-Y gastric bypass procedure (GBP) is the most commonly performed bariatric procedure in the United States. Outcomes following weight loss procedures are frequently reported in excess body weight (EBW) loss. EBW is equal to the difference of a patient's presurgical weight and his or her ideal body weight. How much EBW can a patient expect to lose at 2 years following a Roux-en-Y GBP?

   (A) 15%

   (B) 31%

   (C) 65%

   (D) 86%

   (E) 100%

4. Adjustable gastric banding (AGB) is performed around the world for treatment of clinically severe obesity. Benefits of the AGB include all of the following *except*:

   (A) easy reversibility

   (B) adjustable to desired weight loss

   (C) limited risk of malnutrition and vitamin deficiencies

   (D) low risk of gastrointestinal leak

   (E) equally successful in all patient populations

5. AGB has gained significant exposure in Europe and Australia since the development of a laparoscopic approach. It is becoming more popular in the United States, but results in the United States do not coincide with results seen abroad. Proponents emphasize the benefits of gastric banding compared to the time honored GBP. Which of the following comparisons is *not* accurate?

   (A) Gastric banding is more easily reversible compared to Roux-en-Y GBP.

   (B) Long-term weight loss (5 years) following successful gastric band is similar to the weight loss following Roux-en-Y GBP.

(C) Mortality and gastrointestinal leak are higher following Roux-en-Y GBP.

(D) AGB provides similar weight loss results as GBP in the super obese patient with BMI >55 kg/m².

(E) Medical comorbidities improve equally well following gastric banding and GBP.

6. Jejunoileal bypass (JIB), a malabsorptive weight loss procedure, involves a surgical bypass of the majority of the jejunum and ileum, including the terminal ileum. Which of the following long-term complications was *not* seen following the JIB?

(A) constipation

(B) liver disease with steatohepatitis

(C) oxalate kidney stones

(D) osteoporosis, osteomalacia, and even pathologic fractures

(E) peripheral neuropathy

7. A 35-year-old female with a BMI of 45 kg/m² and no significant medical comorbidities underwent Roux-en-Y GBP. On the morning of postoperative day number 1, she has a heart rate of 110 bpm and a temperature of 38.5°C. Oxygen saturation on 2 L per nasal cannula is 98% and her blood pressure is 140/80 mmHg. What is the most appropriate first step in management of this patient?

(A) administer an acetaminophen suppository per rectum, monitor the patient's vital signs, and encourage incentive spirometry

(B) start a clear liquid diet without concentrated sweets

(C) perform an exploratory laparotomy to identify and treat a gastrointestinal leak

(D) obtain a computerized tomographic (CT) scan to evaluate for intraabdominal abscess or fluid collection

(E) schedule an immediate water-soluble contrast study to evaluate postoperative anatomy

8. According to institutional protocol, the patient in Question 7 undergoes a gastrografin swallow approximately 3 h later as shown in Fig. 41-1. The patient's heart rate remains elevated at 125 bpm with a temperature of 38.2°C. Her oxygen saturation is 96% on 4 L per nasal cannula and her blood pressure is 100/60 mmHg. What is the next step in management of this patient?

(A) upper endoscopy is necessary to identify and treat the source of these findings

(B) surgical exploration to evaluate, drain, and possibly repair the swallow study findings

(C) CT guided placement of percutaneous drainage catheters

(D) administer broad-spectrum intravenous antibiotics and begin intravenous hyperalimentary fluid

(E) insert a nasogastric tube to decompress the gastric pouch and proximal small intestine

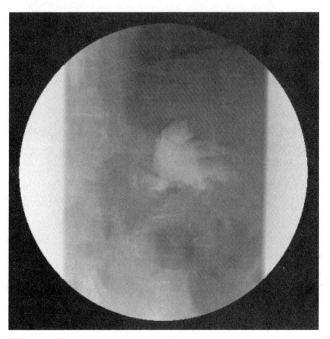

FIG. 41-1 Gastrografin swallow study from patient one day after Roux-en-Y gastric bypass with heart rate of 125 and temperature of 38.2°C.

9. Four weeks after undergoing a laparoscopic Roux-en-Y GBP, a 38-year-old man develops intolerance of solids and most liquids. Preoperatively, he weighed 127 kg (280 lbs) and he had a BMI of 42.5 kg/m². His current weight is 114 kg (251 lbs) and his BMI is 38 kg/m². Consumption of a 2 oz meal leads to dysphagia and subsequent emesis. Upper endoscopy is performed. The endoscopic image is shown in Fig. 41-2. Which of the following is the most appropriate therapy?

(A) nasogastric decompression of the gastric pouch and proximal small intestine

(B) take down of the GBP with reestablishment of normal anatomical intestinal continuity

(C) insertion of central venous access with administration of intravenous hyperalimentary fluid

(D) dilation of the gastrojejunostomy anastomosis followed by observation and supportive care

(E) administration of a proton-pump inhibitor and antibiotic therapy for *Helicobacter pylori*

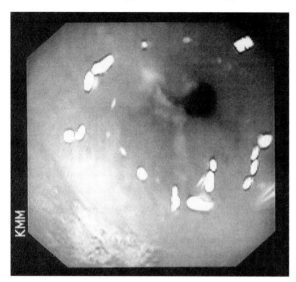

FIG. 41-2 Upper endoscopy image for patient intolerant of solids and most liquids following gastric bypass.

10. A 28-year-old man underwent laparoscopic Roux-en-Y GBP and cholecystectomy 18 months prior to his presentation to an emergency room for sudden onset of abdominal pain. His preoperative weight was 185 kg and his BMI was 58.5 kg/m². He now weighs 101 kg with a BMI of 32 kg/m². He is compliant and has kept appropriate postoperative follow-up appointments, takes his supplements, and maintained an active lifestyle with a controlled diet. He has no other health problems. The pain extends "like a band" across his midabdomen and causes him to double over. Abdominal examination demonstrates minimal tenderness in the left upper quadrant of the abdomen and no signs of peritonitis. A kidney, ureter, and bladder (KUB) is shown in Fig. 41-3. Lab tests including complete blood count and comprehensive chemistry panel are normal. What is the most likely cause for his pain?

(A) anastomotic stricture

(B) internal herniation

(C) marginal ulcer

(D) dumping syndrome

(E) gastrointestinal leak

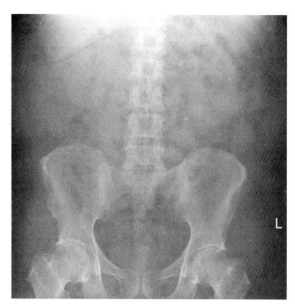

FIG. 41-3 Abdominal flat plate film for patient 18 months after Roux-en-Y gastric bypass with abdominal pain.

11. Following a divided Roux-en-Y GBP performed for treatment of morbid obesity, patients are prone to develop specific vitamin and mineral deficiencies. Which of the following micronutrients is *least* likely to be deficient in a patient who has undergone a Roux-en-Y GBP?

(A) calcium

(B) iron

(C) vitamin K

(D) folic acid

(E) vitamin B$_{12}$

12. Which of the following medications is used postoperatively to prevent gallstone formation after bariatric surgery?

(A) cholestyramine

(B) ursodiol

(C) octreatide

(D) simvastatin

(E) misoprostol

13. A 43-year-old woman undergoes an uneventful laparoscopic insertion of an AGB. Her band reservoir is left empty on insertion. She undergoes a postoperative swallow study as demonstrated in Fig. 41-4. Her preoperative weight was 286 lbs with a BMI of 46.3 kg/m². She now weighs 253 lbs with a BMI of 41 kg/m² 1 year after surgery. Her weight loss has reached a plateau. She presents for a band adjustment. Fluoroscopic evaluation is performed including a barium swallow. An image from the study is demonstrated (Fig. 41-4). The patient has no complaints, excluding her inability to continue to lose weight. Which of the following has most likely lead to this patient's weight plateau?

    (A) maladaptive eating behavior
    (B) band slippage
    (C) gastrogastric fistula
    (D) inadequate band reservoir inflation
    (E) esophageal dilatation

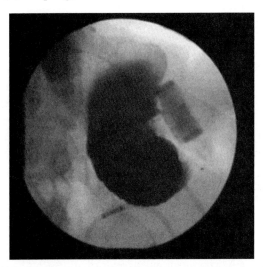

FIG. 41-4 Swallow study following adjustable gastric band placement with plateau of weight loss.

14. Which of the following is *not* a reason for the shift from vertical banded gastroplasty (VBG) to other weight loss operations?

    (A) mesh band erosion
    (B) maladaptive eating behavior
    (C) recurrent vomiting
    (D) vitamin and mineral malnutrition
    (E) gastrogastric fistula

15. Although multiple variations of bariatric procedures are performed around the world, three basic procedures are performed commonly: Roux-en-Y GBP, AGB, and biliopancreatic diversion (BPD). What is the appropriate order of average percent excess weight loss 1 year after laparoscopic surgery for a patient with a BMI >50?

    (A) GBP > AGB > BPD
    (B) GBP > BPD > AGB
    (C) AGB > GBP > BPD
    (D) BPD > GBP > AGB
    (E) none of the above

16. What is the appropriate order of average percent excess weight loss 5 years after laparoscopic surgery for a patient with a BMI > 50?

    (A) GBP > AGB > BPD
    (B) GBP > BPD > AGB
    (C) AGB > GBP > BPD
    (D) BPD > GBP > AGB
    (E) none of the above

17. During insufflation of the abdomen, your anesthesiologist notices that the patient has become more cyanotic, is having ventricular arrhythmias, and the end-tidal CO_2 on the monitor has decreased. Which of these treatments is *not* indicated?

    (A) cessation of insufflation
    (B) positioning the patient head-down and left lateral
    (C) hyperventilation
    (D) hypoventilation
    (E) aspiration of gas through central venous catheter

18. A pneumoperitoneum of less than 20 mm Hg is associated with which of the following observed changes in the following cardiac parameters: mean arterial pressure (MAP), systemic vascular resistance (SVR), and central venous pressure (CVP)?

    (A) increased MAP, increased SVR, increased CVP
    (B) decreased MAP, decreased SVR, increased CVP
    (C) increased MAP, decreased SVR, decreased CVP
    (D) decreased MAP, decreased SVR, decreased CVP
    (E) increased MAP, increased SVR, decreased CVP

19. You are insufflating the abdomen of an otherwise healthy 35-year-old female for laparoscopic cholecystectomy when the patient becomes severely bradycardic. What should be your next course of action?

    (A) continue with laparoscopic cholecystectomy
    (B) administer 1 mg epinephrine
    (C) deflate the abdomen
    (D) place the patient in Trendelenburg position
    (E) administer 10 mg rocuronium

20. Insufflation of the peritoneum with CO_2 has several effects on CO_2 excretion and arterial CO_2. Which of the following effects is *correct*?

    (A) linearly increasing CO_2 excretion; linearly increasing $PaCO_2$

    (B) increase, then plateau of CO_2 excretion; linearly increasing $PaCO_2$

    (C) increase, then plateau of CO_2 excretion; increase, then plateau of $PaCO_2$

    (D) unchanged CO_2 excretion, unchanged $PaCO_2$

    (E) decreased CO_2 excretion, increasing $PaCO_2$

21. Which of the following factors is *not* associated with postoperative nausea and vomiting?

    (A) postoperative opioids

    (B) female gender

    (C) previous history of postoperative nausea

    (D) history of migraine

    (E) smoking

22. All of the following are possible complications of incorrect veress needle placement *except*:

    (A) crepitus of neck, face, perineum, or extremities

    (B) medial displacement of the ureters

    (C) retroperitoneal gas accumulation

    (D) ventral hernia

    (E) cardiovascular collapse

23. While performing a laparoscopic Nissen fundoplication, the patient becomes markedly hypotensive, hypoxic, and difficult to ventilate. The anesthesiologist notes that the patient's breath sounds are now diminished on the left. What intervention should *not* be considered?

    (A) placing an angiocatheter in the left chest

    (B) placement of a left tube thoracostomy

    (C) desufflation of the abdomen

    (D) dissecting through the diaphragmatic crura into the parietal pleura

    (E) discontinuing nitrous oxide ventilation

24. Which one of the following sets of gases used for laparoscopy and their adverse effects is *correct*?

    (A) helium—respiratory acidosis

    (B) nitrous oxide—intraperitoneal combustion

    (C) carbon dioxide—respiratory alkalosis

    (D) air—hypercarbia

    (E) none of the above

25. While performing a laparoscopic cholecystectomy for acalculous cholecystitis, you see an adhesion between the gallbladder and the duodenum. You take down the adhesion with electrocautery. The remainder of the cholecystectomy is uneventful. Five days after discharge, the patient presents to the emergency room with severe epigastric pain, rigid abdomen, and fever. Which of the following is the most likely cause of this patient's illness?

    (A) duodenal necrosis

    (B) gallstone pancreatitis

    (C) localized ileus

    (D) Mallory-Weiss' tear

    (E) Barrett's esophagus

26. The following are advantages of bipolar cautery over monopolar cautery *except*:

    (A) decreased tissue damage

    (B) decreased smoke

    (C) improved hemostasis

    (D) elimination of grounding pad burns

    (E) reduced risk of insulation failure

27. You are consulted to see a patient with CT scan findings suspicious for malignancy. The patient refuses exploratory laparotomy, saying that he would rather have laparoscopy to avoid a large, painful incision. All of the following would preclude him from undergoing diagnostic laparoscopy *except*:

    (A) distended bowel

    (B) congestive heart failure

    (C) abdominal wall sepsis

    (D) coagulopathy

    (E) multiple prior abdominal surgeries

28. The preceding patient does not have any contraindications to laparoscopy. He is scheduled for diagnostic laparoscopy. Given his suspected malignancy, which of the following measures should be taken to minimize morbidity?

    (A) use of carbon dioxide insufflation

    (B) use of sequential compression devices

    (C) placement in Trendelenburg position

    (D) insufflation to 20 mmHg

    (E) all of the above

29. You are performing a laparoscopic cholecystectomy for a patient with suspected choledocholithiasis and, on performing an intraoperative cholangiogram, you notice a filling defect proximal to the duodenum. Which of the following options should be considered for relief of biliary obstruction intraoperatively?

    (A) lithotripsy
    (B) glucagon administration
    (C) holmium laser stone obliteration
    (D) ERCP
    (E) none of the above

30. A 24-year-old woman presents with right lower quadrant tenderness and guarding, fever, anorexia, and leukocytosis of 17,000. She is also in the second trimester of her pregnancy. Ultrasound is highly suspicious for appendicitis. You consider laparoscopic appendectomy. Which of the following statements is *true* regarding laparoscopic appendectomy during pregnancy?

    (A) Laparoscopic appendectomy is contraindicated in pregnancy.
    (B) The patient should be positioned with her left side down.
    (C) Pneumoperitoneum pressure should reach 15 mmHg.
    (D) Laparoscopic appendectomy cannot be performed in the second trimester.
    (E) Fetal loss is 10% in nonperforated appendicitis.

31. A 47-year-old man presents to your office with problems 3 months after laparoscopic Nissen fundoplication. You suspect the fundoplication has failed. Which of the following signs and symptoms is *not* associated with a slipped wrap?

    (A) hourglass-shaped stomach on upper GI study
    (B) shortened esophagus
    (C) breakdown of sutures between the fundoplication and distal esophagus
    (D) improvement in symptoms over time
    (E) regurgitation and dysphagia

32. A 53-year-old woman presents to clinic with continued reflux symptoms despite a Nissen fundoplication and two revisions. During the course of workup, it is evident that the fundoplication has failed again. What is the most reasonable option for this patient?

    (A) laparoscopic Nissen revision
    (B) open Nissen revision
    (C) convert the Nissen to a Toupet fundoplication
    (D) esophageal dilation
    (E) truncal vagotomy with gastric resection

33. Which of the following structures forms the medial border of the "triangle of doom" to be avoided in laparoscopic inguinal herniorrhaphy?

    (A) inferior epigastric vessels
    (B) vas deferens
    (C) spermatic vessels
    (D) iliac vessels
    (E) lateral femoral cutaneous nerve

Answers and Explanations

1. (C) The NIH Consensus Development Conference Statement summarizes the conclusions obtained following a 2-day conference in March 1991. Several basic patient selection criteria were recommended and included the following: BMI ≥40 kg/m2 or BMI ≥35 kg/m2 with a minimum of one medical comorbidity related to obesity (e.g., sleep apnea, Pickwickian's syndrome, diabetes mellitus, joint disease, gastroesophageal reflux disease, and so on), a demonstrated low probability to be successful with nonsurgical weight loss measures, and demonstrated ability to participate and maintain follow-up on a long-term basis.

The consensus panel was unable to agree on any conclusions regarding surgical weight loss treatment of children or adolescents, even subjects with BMI >40 kg/m². Although several centers perform weight loss surgery on adolescents, the appropriate treatment for these patients is not determined. Many feel the gastric bypass (GBP) is too radical an approach; however, obesity during the important development stage of adolescence may lead to significant psychologic sequela currently underestimated by the medical community. Continued study is necessary.

Bibliography

Garcia VF, Langford L, Inge TH. Application of laparoscopy for bariatric surgery in adolescents. *Curr Opin Pediatr* 2003;15:248–255.

Gastrointestinal surgery for severe obesity. *NIH Consens Dev Conf Statement* 1991;9(1).

Sugerman HJ, Sugerman EL, DeMaria EJ, et al. Bariatric surgery for severely obese adolescents. *J Gastrointest Surg* 2003;7:102–108.

2. (D) NIH guidelines have become the primary method of determining eligibility for surgical weight loss procedures. According to these guidelines, patients with a BMI ≥40 kg/m² or BMI ≥35 kg/m² with one obesity-associated medical comorbidity are surgical candidates. In addition, these patients must demonstrate consistent attempts at nonsurgical methods of weight loss with good follow-up and compliance and failure to maintain weight loss. Patients must understand the benefits and risks of the surgical procedure and be good operative candidates.

Other guidelines followed by the American Society of Bariatric Surgeons (ASBS) require preoperative psychologic evaluation to confirm that patients with obesity, who frequently suffer from psychopathology, are able to provide adequate informed consent. In addition, an endocrine etiology for weight gain must be addressed prior to surgical intervention. This may include patients with multiple endocrine neoplastic syndrome (MEN I) that have a pituitary adenoma, hyperparathyroidism, and a possible pancreatic islet cell insulinoma.

Bibliography

Brolin RE. Gastric bypass. *Surg Clin North Am* 2001;81(5):1077–1095.

Gastrointestinal surgery for severe obesity. *NIH Consens Dev Conf Statement* 1991;9(1).

3. (C) The common goal for all bariatric surgical procedures is achieving weight loss and obtaining its beneficial effects on the treatment or prevention of obesity related medical comorbidities including hypertension, coronary artery disease, and diabetes mellitus. Roux-en-Y GBP, initially described by Mason and Ito, is currently the most commonly performed bariatric procedure. It uses a restrictive gastric pouch with a small outlet. This pouch is drained by a Roux intestinal limb that causes malabsorption as food bypasses the distal stomach, entire duodenum, and the proximal jejunum. Although both a traditional open and a laparoscopic approach are both available, weight loss results appear to be similar.

On average, patients experience an initial loss of approximately 60–70% EBW at 2 years after the procedure. The most precipitous weight loss occurs during the first 6–12 months. This is followed by a slower period of weight loss or even a plateau. Long-term results suggest a slight weight gain several years following the procedure. Patients may experience a gain of 10–15% weight at 5 years following the procedure.

Bibliography

Brolin RE. Gastric bypass. *Surg Clin North Am* 2001; 81(5): 1077–1095.

Buchwald H. A bariatric surgery algorithm. *Obes Surg* 2002; 12:733–746.

Cottam DR, Mattar SG, Schauer PR. Laparoscopic era of operations for morbid obesity. *Arch Surg* 2003; 138: 367–375.

Mason EE, Ito C. Gastric bypass. *Ann Surg* 1969; 170(3): 329–336.

4. **(E)** AGB was first described by Kuzmak in the early 1980s, but it was not commonly performed until it was adapted to a laparoscopic approach in the early 1990s. An AGB is a synthetic plastic ring with an inflatable balloon that allows the internal diameter to be altered for differing degrees of gastric restriction. More inflation leads to more restriction and more weight loss.

Many controversies surround the use of AGB for clinically severe obesity. The excellent results of weight loss following insertion of AGB in patients at large European and Australian centers are not reproducible at centers in the United States. Failure of weight loss in specific patient groups including sweet eaters and frequent revision operations needed to reposition or remove the band have caused many surgeons to limit the use of AGB.

However, AGB has many benefits over GBP and other bariatric procedures. AGB does not involve division of the gastrointestinal tract. So, gastrointestinal leak occurs very infrequently. Removal of the band can be performed laparoscopically and essentially leads to reversibility of the restrictive procedure. Increased inflation of the band balloon leads to a small internal band diameter and greater restriction. This can effectively allow adjustability to a desired weight loss. No segments of the intestine are bypassed, so micronutrient malnutrition and dumping syndrome are not a significant concern after AGB.

Bibliography

O-Brien PE, Dixon JB, Brown W, et al. The laparoscopic adjustable gastric band (Lap-Band®): a prospective study of medium-term effects on weight, health and quality of life. *Obes Surg* 2002;12:652–660.

Schauer PR, Ikramuddin S. Laparoscopic surgery for morbid obesity. *Surg Clin North Am* 2001;81(5):1145–1179.

Zinzindohoue F, Chevallier JM, Douard R, et al. Laparoscopic gastric banding: a minimally invasive surgical treatment for morbid obesity. *Ann Surg* 2003;237(1): 1–9.

5. **(D)** Use of AGB remains controversial in the United States for treatment of clinically severe obesity. Results provided by large centers located in Europe and Australia demonstrate excellent long-term weight loss and resolution of medical comorbidities. However, frequent reoperation and lack of reproducibility in patient populations in the United States have lead to a slow acceptance for the AGB.

Removal of the AGB can be performed laparoscopically and essentially reverses many of the effects of the AGB. In addition, long-term weight loss results for AGB rival those provided by open GBP. The literature is wanting for good long-term results of the laparoscopic GBP, but weight gain 2–5 years following laparoscopic GBP is likely to mimic the open surgical procedure. In addition, insertion of the AGB does not require division of the stomach or intestine. So, risk of gastrointestinal leak is much less following AGB. Mortality is much less after AGB because of its limited nature; however, AGB appears to be most effective in patients with a lower BMI. Patients with BMI >55 kg/m² lose more weight following GBP than AGB. Other patient populations appear to respond differently to the band as well including males and Black patients.

Bibliography

Cottam DR, Mattar SG, Schauer PR. Laparoscopic era of operations for morbid obesity. *Arch Surg* 2003;138:367–375.

Favretti F, Cadiere GM, Segato G, et al. Laparoscopic banding: selection and technique in 830 patients. *Obes Surg* 2002;12:385–390.

Greenstein RJ, Martin L, MacDonal K, et al. The Lap-Band system as surgical therapy for morbid obesity: intermediate results of the USA, multicenter, prospective study. *Surg Endosc* 1999;13:S1–S18.

6. **(A)** JIB was once a commonly performed weight loss procedure. This procedure included a surgical bypass of the majority of the jejunum and ileum, including the terminal ileum. Patients lost weight through caloric malabsorption.

JIB has not been routinely performed for approximately 20 years; however, approximately 100,000 patients underwent this operation in the United States during the 1960s and 1970s, and they continue to require medical care today. Although many patients who underwent this operation benefited from this procedure with weight loss, others suffered complications and continue to require reversal of the intestinal bypass.

The most common indication for reversal of the JIB was severe medical and nutritional complications. Liver dysfunction, a common life-threatening complication after JIB, ranged from mild disease to end-stage disease with cirrhosis. Biopsies frequently revealed hepatic steatosis. In addition, patients experience hyperoxaluria with oxalate kidney stones, calcium, and vitamin D deficiency with osteomalacia and pathologic fractures, arthritis, and peripheral neuropathy related to vitamin B_{12} and folate deficiency. Malabsorption leads to frequent loose stools and commonly diarrhea with associated electrolyte abnormalities.

Bibliography

Buchwald H, Buchwald JN. Evolution of operative procedures for the management of morbid obesity 1950–2000. *Obes Surg* 2002;12:705–717.

Dean P, Joshi S, Kaminski DL. Long-term outcome of reversal of small intestinal bypass operations. *Am J Surg* 1990;159:118–124.

Economou TP, Cullen JJ, Mason EE, et al. Reversal of small intestinal bypass operations and concomitant vertical banded gastroplasty: long-term outcome. *J Am Coll Surg* 1995;181:160–164.

7. (E)

8. (B)

Explanations 7 and 8

This patient has undergone a Roux-en-Y GBP. An infrequent, but life-threatening complication is gastrointestinal leak. Obese patients make physical examination a difficult and inaccurate method of determining intraabdominal processes. Therefore, postoperative recovery with abnormal findings requires a high index of suspicion for complications, especially a gastrointestinal leak.

Initially, this patient demonstrated tachycardia, fever, and diminished respiratory capacity. These physical findings are common in obese patients with gastrointestinal leak following GBP; however, they are also associated with multiple benign postoperative sources including atelectasis and postoperative pain. It is imperative that an immediate fluoroscopic water-soluble contrast swallow study is performed to assist with the diagnosis of a leak. It's important to recognize that this study is not helpful in evaluating the enteroenterostomy or distal anastomosis in a Roux limb.

This patient's study demonstrates a leak of contrast from the region of the gastric pouch or gastrojejunostomy. Treatment in this patient, that is beginning to demonstrate signs of sepsis, includes resuscitation and reoperation. During the reoperation, attempts to define the leak are performed, but they are frequently unsuccessful. If a leak is identified, primary repair may be performed. Extensive internal drainage is necessary. During the same surgical reexploration, many surgeons will introduce an enteral feeding tube in the gastric remnant or jejunum. With restricted oral intake, proper internal drainage, and supplemental enteral tube feeding or parenteral alimentation, patients with a leak from the gastric pouch or gastrojejunostomy will frequently experience spontaneous resolution of the leak without further surgical intervention.

Bibliography

Byrne TK. Complications of surgery for obesity. *Surg Clin North Am* 2001;81(5):1181–1193.

Hamilton EC, Sims TL, Hamilton TT, et al. Clinical predictors of leak after laparoscopic Roux-en-Y gastric bypass for morbid obesity. *Surg Endosc* 2003;17(5):679–684.

Marshall JS, Srivastava A, Gupta SK, et al. Roux-en-Y gastric bypass leak complications. *Arch Surg* 2003;138:520–524.

9. **(D)** One of the most common complications following Roux-en-Y GBP is stricture of the gastrojejunostomy. It occurs from 5 to 12% following open and laparoscopic GBP. Patients frequently present with an increasing or even sudden inability to tolerate solids or even liquids. Patients experience earlier than normal satiety and vomiting. Mechanisms to obtain a diagnosis include upper gastrointestinal swallow study; however, upper endoscopy is helpful in making a diagnosis, ruling out marginal ulcer, and treating the stricture with balloon dilation.

The image provided of the strictured gastrojejunostomy is stereotypic. As shown in Fig. 41-5, balloon dilation of a stenotic anastomosis is efficient and very effective. Rigid dilators passed transorally may also be used to dilate the anastomosis, but these

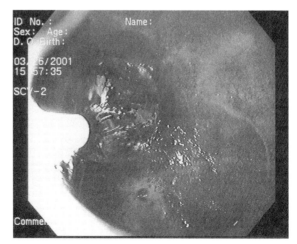

FIG. 41-5 Ballon dilation of gastrojejunostomy stricture following Roux-en-Y gastric bypass.

dilators are difficult to pass and must be inserted blindly. Balloon dilation is effective and can be performed quickly with limited sequela and immediate symptomatic relief.

Bibliography

Byrne TK. Complications of surgery for obesity. *Surg Clin North Am* 2001;81(5):1181–1193.

Cottam DR, Mattar SG, Schauer PR. Laparoscopic era of operations for morbid obesity. *Arch Surg* 2003; 138:367–375.

10. **(B)** All of the complications listed above occur following Roux-en-Y GBP and are associated with abdominal pain; however, gastrointestinal leak typically occurs within a 1–2-week period following surgery. Dumping syndrome is associated with flushing, abdominal cramping, nausea, headache, and diarrhea. This patient does not carry the stereotypical presentation for dumping syndrome.

Anastomotic stricture frequently occurs during the healing phase of the gastrojejunostomy. During the initial 6 weeks after GBP, the gastrojejunostomy stoma may diminish in diameter from larger than 1 cm to only millimeters; however, after the initial 6 weeks following surgery, anastomotic stricture is an uncommon occurrence. In addition, a stricture is typically not associated with abdominal pain. It causes vomiting and inability to tolerate oral intake.

Marginal ulcer may be associated with abdominal pain, but typically it is associated with gastrointestinal bleeding, melena, or gastric pouch outlet obstruction. Again, this patient does not appear to have these symptoms.

Internal herniation occurs in varying degrees following GBP and may occur in different locations based on the technique used. It occurs in approximately 2.5–5% of patients following GBP. The most common locations of internal hernia occur in the mesocolic window following a retrocolic Roux limb creation or through Petersen's defect following an antecolic Roux limb creation. Petersen's defect is defined by the Roux limb mesentery sweeping over the transverse colon and its mesentery (Fig. 41-6). Figures 41-6 and 41-7 demonstrate the mesenteric window created by the antecolic Roux limb. Weight loss during the 18 months after surgery allows the potential defect to enlarge and permit passage of intestine as shown in Fig. 41-6. Treatment requires surgical intervention to reduce the hernia and close the defect.

Bibliography

Byrne TK. Complications of surgery for obesity. *Surg Clin North Am* 2001;81(5):1181–1193.

Cottam DR, Mattar SG, Schauer PR. Laparoscopic era of operations for morbid obesity. *Arch Surg* 2003;138: 367–375.

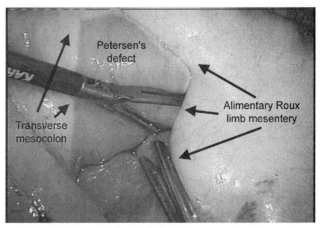

FIG. 41-6 Demonstration of Petersen's defect during Roux-en-Y gastric bypass.

Higa KD, Boone KB, Ho TC. Complications of the laparoscopic Roux-en-Y gastric bypass: 1,040 patients—what have we learned? *Obes Surg* 2000;10:509–513.

11. **(C)** Roux-en-Y GBP leads to weight loss with both a restrictive component and a malabsorptive component. The distal stomach, entire duodenum, and proximal jejunum are bypassed. Iron and calcium are absorbed most effectively in the duodenum and risk for deficiencies in these minerals is over 50% in patients following GBP. Even with supplementation, patients may experience a 20–25% chance of clinically significant calcium or iron deficiency.

The distal stomach allows vitamin B_{12} to bind intrinsic factor. Binding intrinsic factor is necessary for preparation of vitamin B_{12} absorption in the terminal ileum. GBP prevents the binding of the intrinsic factor to vitamin B_{12}. Therefore, a patient must

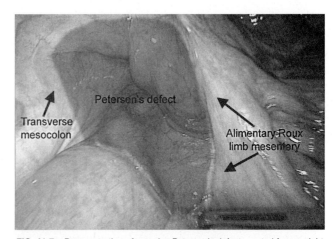

FIG. 41-7 Demonstration of massive Petersen's defect created from weight loss following Roux-en-Y gastric bypass.

receive supplementation of vitamin B$_{12}$ to prevent deficiency after GBP.

Folic acid is less commonly associated with deficiency after GBP, but it is a recommended supplement as well. Folate deficiency is seen in as many as 38% of patients following GBP.

Vitamin K, a fat-soluble vitamin, is absorbed in the terminal ileum. Like all the fat-soluble vitamins including vitamins A, D, and E, vitamin K is at minimal risk for deficiency following a GBP.

Bibliography

Elliot K. Nutritional considerations after bariatric surgery. *Crit Care Nurs Q* 2003;26(2):133–138.

Halverson JD. Micronutrient deficiencies after gastric bypass for morbid obesity. *Am Surg* 1986; 52:594–598.

MacLean LD, Rhode BM, Shizgal HM. Nutrition following gastric operations for morbid obesity. *Ann Surg* 1983; 198(3):347–354.

12. **(B)** Bypass of the gastric body and duodenum leads to biliary stasis. Biliary stasis, in conjunction with the rapid weight loss observed following Roux-en-Y GBP, leads to a high rate of acute cholecystitis in postoperative patients. Controversy remains over the most appropriate management of preoperative cholelithiasis; however, study results recommend the use of medical therapy postoperatively to prevent the development of gallstones.

A randomized controlled trial demonstrated that ursodeoxycholic acid, or ursodiol, at a dose of 300 mg administered orally twice daily was effective at limiting the development of gallstones during the rapid weight loss seen following GBP. Although currently produced in the laboratory, ursodeoxycholic acid was originally obtained from the gallbladder of the Chinese black bear. It has been used for centuries to treat liver disease. The structure of ursodiol is demonstrated in Fig. 41-8. Its mechanism of action is twofold. It inhibits synthesis of cholesterol in the liver and limits the intestinal absorption of cholesterol. These two actions lead to decreased release of cholesterol by the liver and prevent cholesterol stone formation in the gallbladder. Ursodiol is also used to treat primary biliary cirrhosis, congenital cholestasis, viral hepatitis, and many more hepatic pathologies.

Bibliography

Sugerman HJ, Brewer WH, Brolin RE, et al. A multicenter, placebo-controlled, randomized, double-blind, prospective trial of prophylactic ursodiol for the prevention of gallstone formation following gastric-bypass-induced rapid weight loss. *Am J Surg* 1995;169(1):91–97.

13. **(B)** Laparoscopic insertion of an AGB is a commonly performed procedure abroad and increasingly in the United States. Weight loss results demonstrated by centers in Europe and Australia show a significant change in rate of reoperation following a change in surgical technique.

One of the main reasons for reoperation is gastric band slippage. Band slippage occurs when the gastric wall herniates through the band and allows the proximal gastric pouch to enlarge as demonstrated in the swallow study. The enlarged pouch leads to less restriction of oral intake and diminished weight loss. An enlarged gastric pouch and AGB slippage are demonstrated in Fig. 41-4. Normal alignment of an AGB provides a small gastric pouch as demonstrated by the barium swallow seen in Fig. 41-9.

During the early and mid-1990s, AGBs were inserted following creation of a transmesenteric window adjacent to the lesser gastric curve. In addition, the lesser peritoneal sack was routinely entered and the band was secured only in an anterior location

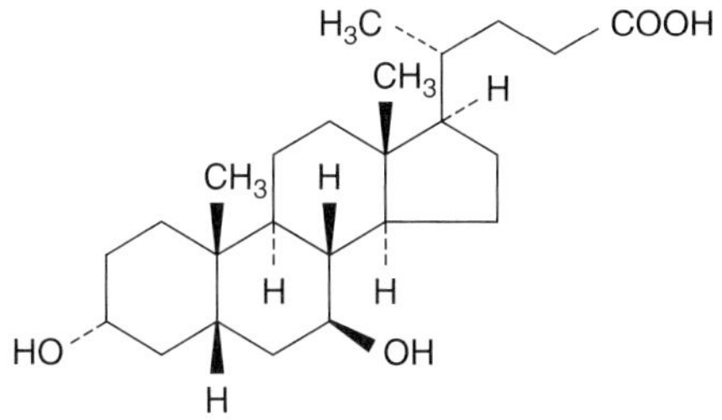

FIG. 41-8 Molecular diagram of ursodiol, commonly used to prevent development of gallstones following weight loss surgery.

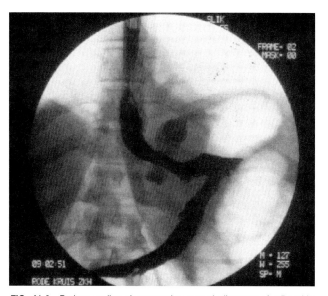

FIG. 41-9 Barium swallow demonstrating normal alignment of adjustable gastric band and size of small gastric pouch.

with a limited number of sutures. During the late 1990s, a significant shift in surgical technique lead to creation of the transmesenteric window through the pars flaccida and dissection was limited to the retroperitoneal space above the lesser sack. In addition, several sutures were used to secure the band anteriorly. All of these changes have significantly reduced rate of reoperation and improved results.

Bibliography

Angrisani L, Furbeta F, Doldi SB, et al. Lap Band® adjustable gastric banding system: the experience with 1863 patients operated on 6 years. *Surg Endosc* 2003; 17: 409–412.

Weiner R, Blanco-Engert R, Weiner S, et al. Outcome after laparoscopic adjustable gastric banding—8 years experience. *Obes Surg* 2003;13:427–434.

14. **(D)** VBG was first described by Mason in 1982. VBG is performed by creating a transgastric window with a circular stapler. A linear stapler, in addition to a transorally inserted bougie dilator, was used to create a vertical staple line. A band is created from synthetic material, typically polyester or polypropylene, and placed around the base of the proximal gastric pouch. This band is passed through a transmesenteric window and the transgastric window. The mesh is sutured to itself to allow for a 4.5–5.0 cm external diameter. The resulting gastric pouch measured only 20 mL in size. The band was used to maintain stoma size and prolong restriction of oral intake.

VBG was once the most commonly performed weight loss procedure; however, it is now performed at a limited number of centers both in the United States and abroad. Patient and surgeon dissatisfaction with the VBG has led to this change in bariatric surgical preference. Now, the most commonly performed procedure is the Roux-en-Y GBP.

Complications relating to the band lead to the dissatisfaction. The synthetic material of the mesh irritated the gastric serosa and lead to a 1–2% risk of band migration or erosion through the gastric wall. In addition, the staple line used to create the vertical border of the pouch frequently disrupted and allowed communication with the gastric remnant. These gastrogastric fistulae decreased the restriction provided by the band and decreased weight loss.

Quality of life following VBG was initially found to improve dramatically as patients were successful in losing weight; however, as time progressed, patients grew frustrated with the feeling of fullness and satiety created by the band. Certain food stuffs, including breads and meats, fill the proximal pouch

with limited quantities; however, persistent hunger caused the patients to continue to eat, distend the proximal pouch, and suffer the consequences of regurgitation or emesis. Patients developed maladaptive eating behaviors as high caloric liquids, like milk shakes, were easily consumed in high quantities without repercussion. This ultimately led to poor weight loss. Poor weight loss, in addition to the maladaptive eating behavior, caused quality of life to decrease several years following the procedure.

The benefit of the VBG, similar to other gastric restrictive procedures, is the lack of an intestinal bypass procedure. Therefore, concern for micronutrient malnutrition postoperatively is limited.

Bibliography

Balsiger BM, Poggio JL, Mai J, et al. Ten and more years after vertical banded gastroplasty as primary operation for morbid obesity. *J Gastrointest Surg* 2000;4:598–605.

Lee WJ, Yu PJ, Wang W, et al. Gastrointestinal quality of life following laparoscopic vertical banded gastroplasty. *Obes Surg* 2002;12:819–824.

Mason EE. Vertical banded gastroplasty. *Arch Surg* 1982; 117:701–706.

Mason EE, Doherty C, Cullen JJ, et al. Vertical gastroplasty: evolution of vertical baned gastroplasty. *World J Surg* 1998;22:919–924.

15. **(D)**

16. **(E)**

Explanations 15 and 16

By convention, obesity is measured by BMI and weight loss is reported as change in BMI and percentage of EBW loss. EBW is the difference of ideal body weight from the patient's preoperative weight.

Each of the listed procedures leads to weight loss in different ways. AGB is a gastric restrictive procedure. A synthetic band with an inflatable balloon allows adjustment of the internal diameter with injection of saline through a subcutaneous reservoir. The band is placed high on the stomach and creates a proximal gastric pouch approximately 20–30 cc in size. Injection of saline leads to a reduced internal diameter of the ring, more restriction on oral intake, and slower gastric pouch emptying. More restriction limits oral caloric intake and weight loss occurs.

GBP uses both a restrictive and a malabsorptive method of weight loss. A small gastric pouch approximately 20–30 cc in size is drained by a Roux-en-Y limb. The pouch restricts oral intake and the stoma between the gastric pouch and the small intestine slows pouch emptying. The Roux limb causes food to bypass the distal stomach, entire duodenum, and proximal jejunum. This leads to caloric malabsorption. The two methods of restriction and malabsorption cause weight loss.

Finally, the BPD, developed over 20 years ago, leads to weight loss by primarily malabsorptive methods. Two forms of the BPD are currently performed. The classic form of BPD includes a hemigastrectomy drained by a Roux limb that causes bypass of the entire duodenum, jejunum, and proximal ileum. Pancreatic juices and bile mix with food stuffs in a short segment of terminal ileum that measures 50–100 cm long. Duodenal switch is another popular form of the BPD that includes formation of a gastric tube and division of the duodenum 1–2 cm from the pylorus. The proximal duodenal stump is drained by the distal Roux limb that bypasses the remaining duodenum, jejunum, and proximal ileum. Both forms of BPD limit digestion of oral intake, cause malabsorption, and lead to weight loss.

Patients lose weight precipitously following GBP and BPD. During the first 6–12 months following these procedures, patients experience the majority of weight loss. At 1 year, AGB patients experience approximately 40% EBW loss. GBP patients experience a 60–70% EBW loss, while BPD patients experience 70–80% EBW loss. At 5 years, data is less prevalent and percentages appear to change. Over 20% of AGB patients undergo reoperation for band repair/reposition or removal secondary to dissatisfaction or lack of weight loss. The remaining patients continue to experience weight loss during the second and third years following surgery and may see a 50–60% EBW loss at 5 years. At 2 years after GBP, patients typically experience maximum weight loss. They then regain 10–15% EBW. This leads to a total EBW loss of approximately 50–60% on average. Laparoscopic BPD long-term outcomes are limited, but weight regain is also seen with a 65–70% EBW loss observed at 5 years.

Bibliography

Anthone GJ, Lord RVN, DeMeester TR, et al. The duodenal switch operation for the treatment of morbid obesity. *Ann Surg* 2003;238(4):618–628.

Kim WW, Gagner M, Kini S, et al. Laparoscopic vs. open biliopancreatic diversion with duodenal switch: a comparative study. *J Gastrointest Surg* 2003;7:552–557.

Schauer PR, Ikramuddin S, Gourash W, et al. Outcomes after laparoscopic Roux-en-Y gastric bypass for morbid obesity. *Ann Surg* 2000;232(4):515–529.

Weiner R, Blanco-Engert R, Weiner S, et al. Outcome after laparoscopic adjustable gastric banding—8 year experience. *Obes Surg* 2003;13:427–434.

Zinzindohoue F, Chevallier JM, Douard R, et al. Laparoscopic gastric banding: a minimally invasive surgical treatment for morbid obesity. *Ann Surg* 2003;237(1):1–9.

17. **(D)** The scenario illustrated is of CO_2 embolism caused by direct injection of CO_2 into the systemic circulation. The hallmarks are cardiovascular collapse, including cyanosis, increased venous pressures, pulmonary edema, ventricular arrhythmias, and decreased end-tidal CO_2. The gas insufflation should be stopped, the patient should be hyperventilated, placed in Trendelenburg position, and the gas aspirated via central catheter to remove it from the circulation. A high clinical suspicion should lead to immediate measures for diagnostic confirmation. Transesophageal echocardiography may be performed during the surgical procedure with limited morbidity and good sensitivity.

Bibliography

Fahy BG, Hasnain JU, Flowers JL, et al. Trans-esophageal echocardiographic detection of gas embolism and cardiac valvular dysfunction during laparoscopic nephrectomy. *Anesth Analg* 1999;99:500–504.

Schmandra TC, Mierdl S, Bauer H, et al. Trans-esophageal echocardiography shows high risk of gas embolism during laparoscopic hepatic resection under carbon dioxide pneumoperitoneum. *Br J Surg* 2002;89:870–876.

Zucker K. *Surgical Laparoscopy*, 2nd ed. Philadelphia, PA: Lippincott, Williams & Wilkins, 2001, Chapter 2, 18.

18. **(A)** Creation of pneumoperitoneum to an intraabdominal pressure of less than 20 cm H_2O is associated in the supine position with increased MAP, SVR, and cardiac filling pressures. These effects stem from direct mechanical effects of the pneumoperitoneum, myocardial and vasodilatory effects of carbon dioxide, and sympathetic stimulation.

The increased cardiac filling pressures are reflective of increased preload. CVP, pulmonary artery wedge pressure, and pulmonary vascular resistance, all increase secondary to increased intrathoracic pressure transmitted via the elevated diaphragm from the increased intraabdominal pressure created during pneumoperitoneum. Although the filling pressures appear to have increased, in fact, they are decreased. True filling pressures are determined by calculating the difference of the intrathoracic pressure from the observed CVP. The increase in intrathoracic pressure is greater than the increased in CVP will leads to decreased filling pressures.

SVR increases secondary to increased venous resistance, compression of the intraabdominal arterial tree by the pneumoperitoneum, and sympathetic or other chemical actions leading to increased afterload. Increased SVR helps create an increased MAP.

In addition to these changes, cardiac output is decreased. Stroke volume is limited secondary to chemical mediators, specifically hypercarbia, that restrict cardiac contractility. For all these reasons, laparoscopic surgery with pneumoperitoneum is still used cautiously in the frail and elderly patients with limited cardiac or respiratory reserve.

Bibliography

Chandrakanth A, Talamini MA. Current knowledge regarding the biology of pneumoperitoneum-based surgery. *Probl Gen Surg* 2001;18(1):52–63.

Zucker K. *Surgical Laparoscopy*, 2nd ed. Philadelphia, PA: Lippincott, Williams & Wilkins, 2001, Chapter 2, 16.

19. **(C)** The scenario referred depicts a vagal response to the stimulation created during peritoneal insufflation. This may result in bradycardia and even asystole or atrioventricular block. The first course of action is to stop the procedure and desufflate the abdomen to remove the source of vagal stimulation. An anticholinergic agent, such as glycopyrrolate, may be administered for vagolytic activity.

One study, performed on gynecologic patients, describes regular use of preemptive glycopyrrolate prior to insufflation of the abdomen. This is not regularly performed, because bradycardia is an uncommon occurrence. In addition, it frequently resolves after the initial attempt to insufflate the abdomen. Simply desufflating the abdomen, allowing the patient to recover, and performing another attempt to insufflate, perhaps with a lower pressure limit, is generally sufficient to prevent another vagal response.

Bibliography

Ambrose C, Buggy D, Farragher R, et al. Pre-emptive glycopyrrolate 0.2 mg and bradycardia during gynaecological laparoscopy with mivacurium. *Eur J Anaesthesiol* 1998;15(6):710–713.

Zucker K. *Surgical Laparoscopy*, 2nd ed. Philadelphia, PA: Lippincott, Williams & Wilkins, 2001, Chapter 2, 16.

20. **(B)** Excretion of CO_2 increases as insufflation pressure increases from 0 to 10 mmHg, but then plateaus with insufflation pressure greater than 10 mmHg. CO_2 excretion is proportionally related to absorption, and the increase and plateau in CO_2 excretion may be caused by the initial increase in peritoneal surface area exposed to the CO_2, which then stabilizes as the peritoneum becomes distended and has no more surface area to absorb additional CO_2. $PaCO_2$, however, increases continuously as insufflation increases from 0 to 25 mmHg as dead space increases.

Bibliography

Zucker K. *Surgical Laparoscopy*, 2nd ed. Philadelphia, PA: Lippincott, Williams & Wilkins, 2001, Chapter 2, 21–22.

21. **(E)** The most important predictor of postoperative nausea and vomiting is previous history of postoperative nausea. Other predictors include postoperative opioids, female gender, history of migraines, history of motion sickness, length of operation, and history of nonsmoking.

Bibliography

Zucker K. *Surgical Laparoscopy*, 2nd ed. Philadelphia, PA: Lippincott, Williams & Wilkins, 2001, Chapter 2, 23–24.

22. **(D)** Placement of the veress needle in the extraperitoneal space can lead to crepitus of the abdomen and chest, with large volumes of air extending the crepitus to the neck, face, perineum, or extremities. Posterolateral extension of extraperitoneal insufflation can displace the ureters medially, which may increase the risk of ureteral injury. Passage of the insufflation needle in the retroperitoneal space may result in gas in the retroperitoneum, mesentery, and bowel. Viscus perforation is also possible, as is cardiovascular collapse from CO_2 embolism. Ventral hernia is not a complication of veress needle placement.

Bibliography

Jager RM, Wexner SD (eds.). *Laparoscopic Colorectal Surgery. Anesthetic and Positional Complications*. New York, NY: Churchill Livingstone, 1996, 45–47.

23. **(D)** The scenario described is that of a tension pneumothorax, which may be secondary to intraabdominal gas passing through diaphragmatic defects into the pleural or mediastinal space. Deflation of the abdomen is indicated, as well as standard treatment of a pneumothorax, including placing a needle into the chest or placing a chest tube thoracostomy. Nitrous oxide should be discontinued, and the patient placed on 100% oxygen. Entering the parietal pleura may not relieve the pneumothorax, and may actually lead to parenchymal injury of the lung, worsening the situation.

Pneumothorax is a common complication following advanced laparoscopic foregut procedures. Hemodynamic compromise is a rare occurrence. Intraoperative care routinely includes increased percentage of inspired oxygen, as mentioned above, with completion of the procedure at a lower pressure pneumoperitoneum. Patients are monitored postoperatively with continuous oxygen saturation, and the pneumothorax resolves without further intervention.

Bibliography

Jager RM, Wexner SD (eds.). *Laparoscopic Colorectal Surgery. Anesthetic and Positional Complications*. New York, NY: Churchill Livingstone, 1996, 47.

Leong LM, Ali A. Carbon dioxide pneumothorax during laparoscopic fundoplication. *Anaesthesia* 2003;58(1):97.

Pohl D, Eubanks TR, Omelanczuk PE, Pellegrini CA. Management and outcome of complications after laparoscopic antireflux operations. *Arch Surg* 2001;136(4):399–404.

24. **(B)** At high concentrations, nitrous oxide supports combustion, which may occur with electrocautery or laser use. Nitrous oxide, once used regularly for creation of pneumoperitoneum during the 1970s was abandoned because of these concerns. However, new technology allows dissection without electrical current sources and has allowed many procedures to be performed with limited morbidity and no evidence of combustion.

    Helium is inert, which decreases risk of respiratory acidosis. Carbon dioxide causes hypercarbia and respiratory acidosis unless countered by the anesthesiologist with an increased set respiratory rate. Air was associated with combustibility, and is no longer used.

Bibliography

Jager RM, W SD (eds.). *Laparoscopic Colorectal Surgery. Physiology of Pneumoperitoneum.* New York, NY: Churchill Livingstone, 1996, 76–77.

Tsereteli Z, Terry ML, Bowers SP, et al. Prospective randomized clinical trial comparing nitrous oxide and carbon dioxide pneumoperitoneum for laparoscopic surgery. *J Am Coll Surg* 2002;195(2):173–179.

25. **(A)** Inadvertent injury from errant grounding of electrocautery may present as a delayed complication following laparoscopic procedures. Damaged insulation or movement outside of the videoscopic field with electrified instruments may lead to intestinal or other injuries. Full-thickness wounds may demonstrate immediate leak of intestinal contents; however, partial thickness burns of the intestinal wall may progress to full-thickness over the course of several days and provide a delayed presentation.

    Along these lines, duodenal necrosis can occur from electrocautery injury, especially if the adhesion is narrowly based at the duodenum and widely based at the gallbladder. In this case, current travels to both the gallbladder and duodenum, but is concentrated at the duodenum. The resulting burn injury takes a few days to cause necrosis of the duodenum, which may then perforate.

Bibliography

Wu MP, Ou CS, Chen SL, et al. Complications and recommended practices for electrosurgery in laparoscopy. *Am J Surg* 2000;179(1):67–73.

Zucker K. *Surgical Laparoscopy*, 2nd ed. Philadelphia, PA: Lippincott, Williams & Wilkins, 2001, Chapter 5, 56–57.

26. **(C)** Bipolar cautery is less effective at hemostasis than monopolar cautery because of smaller area of current dispersal and therefore less depth of tissue penetration. However, this lower tissue penetration can decrease tissue damage and necrosis and decrease smoke production. As the current only travels between the two leads of the bipolar, grounding pads are not needed and this eliminates the risk of grounding pad burns. And, as each lead is separately insulated, the risk of insulation failure is decreased.

Bibliography

Wu MP, Ou CS, Chen SL, et al. Complications and recommended practices for electrosurgery in laparoscopy. *Am J Surg* 2000;179(1):67–73.

Zucker K. *Surgical Laparoscopy*, 2nd ed. Philadelphia, PA: Lippincott, Williams & Wilkins, 2001, Chapter 5, 62–63.

27. **(E)** Multiple prior abdominal surgeries are not a true contraindication for diagnostic laparoscopy, though adhesive disease may limit its value. Two major concerns initially lead surgeons to limit offering laparoscopic surgery to patients with prior surgery: intestinal or mesenteric injury during initial access for laparoscopy and injury to intraabdominal contents during an extensive lysis of adhesions. With growing experience, the concerns have dramatically reduced.

    Initial abdominal access may be gained with veress needle or an open technique. Performing initial access at a site remote from the previous surgical field may help to decrease risk of intraabdominal injury. An open technique provides the added benefit of allowing examination of the peritoneal compartment prior to insertion of the laparoscopic port. Surgeon preference remains the determining factor for method of initial port introduction. Improved instrumentation and optics allow better visualization and manipulation of tissue to perform lysis of adhesions. Moreover, surgeon experience has grown providing more confidence of performing an extensive lysis of adhesions.

    As for medical comorbidities, laparoscopy should be avoided in patients with congestive heart failure, severe coronary artery disease, distended bowel, abdominal wall sepsis, and uncorrected coagulopathy. Patients with limited physiologic reserve frequently do not tolerate creation of the pneumoperitoneum and the longer operative times associated with laparoscopic procedures.

Bibliography

Curet MJ. Special problems in laparoscopic surgery: previous abdominal surgery, obesity, and pregnancy. *Surg Clin North Am* 2000;80(4):1093–1110.

Zucker K. *Surgical Laparoscopy*, 2nd ed. Philadelphia, PA: Lippincott, Williams & Wilkins, 2001, Chapter 8, 104.

28. (B) Controversy still surrounds the use of laparoscopy in treatment of malignant disease processes. However, it is gradually lessening as surgical experience with laparoscopic procedures improves and complications diminish. One of the most significant concerns stems from port site metastases. Early reports of laparoscopic treatment of colorectal cancer demonstrated a 21% development of cancer at the location of former laparoscopic port sites. Many theories developed regarding the reasons and multiple methods of prevention were developed. Large trials involving a comparison of laparoscopic versus open traditional colorectal resections have demonstrated port site recurrence percentages similar to historically accepted open surgery rates. Ongoing trials in the United States and Europe will help demonstrate outcomes of laparoscopic colorectal resection for malignancy.

Deep venous thrombosis prophylaxis with sequential compression devices and/or subcutaneous heparin may decrease the risk of malignancy-associated thrombotic disease. Carbon dioxide insufflation is controversial, as some have suggested that it may stimulate tumor growth. Placement in reverse Trendelenburg position allows ascites to flow to the pelvis and the bowel to float cephalad, minimizing the risk of bowel injury if using the veress needle and providing confirmation of intraperitoneal placement by ascetic fluid drainage. The abdominal insufflation should be limited to 15 mmHg or less. Hemodynamic and pulmonary sequela of pneumoperitoneum rise dramatically after pressure of the pneumoperitoneum rises about 10–12 mmHg.

Bibliography

Greene FL. Pneumoperitoneum in the cancer patient: advantages and pitfalls. *Semin Surg Oncol* 1998;15:151–154.

Schiedeck THK, Schwandner O, Baca I, et al. Laparoscopic surgery for the cure of colorectal cancer: results of a German five-center study. *Dis Colon Rectum* 2000;43(1):1–8.

Zucker K. *Surgical Laparoscopy*, 2nd ed. Philadelphia, PA: Lippincott, Williams & Wilkins, 2001, Chapter 8, 104–105.

29. (B) Glucagon administration is the easiest intraoperative measure to relieve biliary obstruction by relaxing the sphincter of Oddi. Following administration of 1 mg of glucagon, normal saline administered through the cholangiogram catheter may be used to flush the common bile duct. A repeat cholangiogram is then performed to reassess the duct. Simple flushing with saline is frequently unsuccessful in clearing the duct of stones. A common bile duct exploration is then necessary to clear the stones. This is a technically demanding procedure when performed both open and laparoscopically. Laparoscopic techniques include a transcystic duct approach. This frequently involves insertion of wire stone retrieval baskets through the cystic duct. The baskets are following with fluoroscopic guidance. The stones are either withdrawn through the cystic duct or pushed into the duodenum. Other methods include creation of a choledochotomy with insertion of a flexible choledochoscope allowing direct visualization of the stone for removal. In skilled hands, series have demonstrated a 75% or greater success rate at clearance of the common duct. Lithotripsy and holmium laser therapy are not typically used for gallstones, but are useful for nephrolithiasis. Endoscopic retrograde cholangiopancreatography (ERCP) may be performed postoperatively, but is not typically performed during laparoscopic cholecystectomy.

Bibliography

Ferguson CM. Laparoscopic common bile duct exploration: practical application. *Arch Surg* 1998;133(4):448–451.

Lauter DM, Froines EJ. Laparoscopic common duct exploration in the management of choledocholithiasis. *Am J Surg* 2000;179(5):372–374.

Zucker K. *Surgical Laparoscopy*, 2nd ed. Philadelphia, PA: Lippincott, Williams & Wilkins, 2001, Chapter 10, 127–128.

30. (B) The patient should be placed with left side down to avoid vena cava compression. Laparoscopic appendectomy is reasonable in the first two trimesters, and there is no increase in fetal or maternal morbidity; however, fetal loss is reported to be 1.5% in nonperforated appendicitis but as much as 35% in perforated appendicitis. When performing laparoscopic appendectomy, placement of the umbilical trocar should be performed using open technique and the pneumoperitoneum pressure should be 10 mmHg to avoid injury to the gravid uterus and prevent impediment to placental blood flow.

Bibliography

Curet MJ. Special problems in laparoscopic surgery: previous abdominal surgery, obesity, and pregnancy. *Surg Clin North Am* 2000;80(4):1093–1110.

Zucker K. *Surgical Laparoscopy*, 2nd ed. Philadelphia, PA: Lippincott, Williams & Wilkins, 2001, Chapter 19, 235.

31. (D) A slipped wrap occurs when proximal stomach slips proximal to the wrap, resulting in an hourglass-shaped stomach. It is commonly associated with shortened esophagus or failure or breakdown of sutures tying down the fundoplication to the distal esophagus. The most common complaints include heartburn and/or dysphagia, while bloating, nausea and vomiting, diarrhea, chest pain, abdominal pain, or shoulder

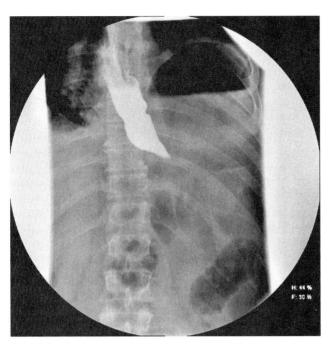

FIG. 41-10   Gastrografin swallow following laparoscopic Nissen fundoplication with dehiscence of cruroplasty and slippage of the stomach into the chest.

pain is also possible though less common. Symptoms of a slipped wrap progress rather than diminish over time, so early surgical intervention is warranted to prevent worsening of the disorder. The swallow study demonstrates a Nissen wrap that has slipped into the chest (Fig. 41-10).

Bibliography

Hunter JG, Smith D, Branum GD, et al. Laparoscopic fundoplication failures: patterns of failure and response to fundoplication revision. *Ann Surg* 1999;230(4):595–606.

Soper NJ, Dunnegan D. Anatomic fundoplication failure after laparoscopic antireflux surgery. *Ann Surg* 1999; 229(5):669–677.

Zucker K. *Surgical Laparoscopy*, 2nd ed. Philadelphia, PA: Lippincott, Williams & Wilkins, 2001, Chapter 36, 458–459.

32. (E) Patients with three or more failed fundoplications are unlikely to benefit from revision of their fundoplications, as resulting adhesions and scarring will make further revisions near impossible and greatly increase the likelihood of another failure. Symptom relief may be attempted with truncal vagotomy to decrease gastric acid production, with or without associated gastric resection and esophagojejunostomy.

Bibliography

Hunter JG, Smith D, Branum GD, et al. Laparoscopic fundoplication failures: patterns of failure and response to fundoplication revision. *Ann Surg* 1999;230(4):595–606.

Soper NJ, Dunnegan D. Anatomic fundoplication failure after laparoscopic antireflux surgery. *Ann Surg* 1999;229(5):669–677.

Zucker K. *Surgical Laparoscopy*, 2nd ed. Philadelphia, PA: Lippincott, Williams & Wilkins, 2001, Chapter 36, 436.

33. (B) When looking toward the pelvis during extraperitoneal inguinal herniorrhaphy, the triangle of doom is bordered medially by the vas deferens, laterally by the spermatic vessels, and inferiorly by the iliac vessels. The inferior epigastric vessels lie superior to the triangle of doom, while the lateral femoral cutaneous nerve is lateral to the epigastric vessels. While not part of the triangle of doom, they should be avoided as well. In addition, the space lateral to the triangle of doom along the anterior surface of the psoas muscle contains the genitofemoral and iliophypogastric nerves. Dissection in this region may lead to paresthesias or numbness.

Bibliography

Townsend CM (ed.). *Sabiston Textbook of Surgery*, 16th ed. Philadelphia, PA: W.B. Saunders, 2001, Chapter 40, 792.

CHAPTER 42

Medical Malpractice
Medical Liability

John P. Clark

Nearly all physicians will face the threat of a lawsuit at some point during a career. While relatively few medical malpractice lawsuits actually go to trial (estimates vary, but are probably on the order of around five percent or less), the stress of being involved in litigation can take its toll regardless of the point at which the complaint ends—with a verdict, settlement, or hopefully dismissal.

"Medical Liability" is a broad term covering the fields of medical malpractice, contract liability, responsibility for those under your supervision (called *respondeat superior*), and risk management. Though a complete treatment of all these is not possible or intended in this chapter, it is hoped the reader will develop a solid groundwork for understanding the way the law views and interprets various aspects of medical practice. Awareness of some legal issues facing our clinical practices every day will provide a basis for further learning and avoidance of legal pitfalls.

A *tort* is a legal wrong, usually interpreted as some sort of harm or injury caused by one party and suffered by another. *Negligent torts* are injuries wherein one party acts in a way that creates an unreasonable risk of danger to another party, or fails to act in a way that would avoid such danger. This is differentiated from *intentional torts*, which require intent to harm or knowledge that harm is likely to occur. Medical malpractice "actions" (or "cases" or "complaints") are negligent torts in which a medical provider through an act of commission or omission placed the patient at an unreasonable risk of harm, and the patient actually suffered some sort of injury.

In order to bring a successful malpractice action the patient-plaintiff must prove four elements. First, there must be a duty. A legal duty exists when there is any recognizable relationship between two parties. This is generally easily fulfilled in the context of the doctor-patient relationship

wherein one party, the patient, seeks the advice and care of the other, the physician. The law deems this a *fiduciary* relationship, or one characterized by a substantial difference in knowledge and/or a specialized skill. By the nature of this relationship the physician is charged with acting always in the best interests of the patient, and bringing to that relationship the requisite skill, knowledge, and expertise possessed by others similarly situated in his or her field.

Second, there must be a breach of the duty owed. It must be shown that the physician somehow failed to use a level of knowledge, skill, and expertise possessed by a reasonably diligent physician of similar training and experience. This breach of duty is commonly known as a violation of the *standard of care*. In the past, a local standard of care was determined for each malpractice action. This had the practical effect of holding a rural practitioner who may not have the benefit of a large hospital and cutting-edge technology to a different standard than, say, a physician at a large urban teaching institution. Recent trends in malpractice litigation have shown a shift toward a more national or less relative standard of care, for better or worse. Further, the advent and popularity of a dizzying array of guidelines and practice parameters have served to further dilute the idea of a local or regional standard in favor of a more homogenous, generic, nationwide standard of care.

Next, the breach of duty or violation of the standard of care must have been both the actual and proximate cause of the patient's injury. Actual cause is also known as "cause in fact," and embraces the traditional notion of causation, meaning that one event was the direct result of another, preceding event. Proximate cause is a legal invention requiring that the harm suffered by the patient be foreseeable in terms of the risk created by the physician's negligence. This concept is effectively a policy decision seeking to limit causation. By way of example, a retained laparotomy sponge is both the actual cause of the patient's chronic abdominal pain and the proximate cause of that pain, but the fact that the sponge caused pain sufficient to keep the patient in the hospital one day longer which led her to miss her daughter's piano recital is not the proximate cause of the daughter's emotional pain and suffering because of the mother's absence. The otherwise endless ripples of causation must stop somewhere; proximate cause is the method for stopping such ripple effect.

Lastly, there must be some harm suffered by the patient. A medical mistake or mishap that leads to no pain, injury, or suffering is not actionable, meaning a lawsuit may not be instituted on the basis of that mistake.

Negligence does not occur in a void; acts, omissions, and harms must occur for a patient-plaintiff to get paid.

A final comment on the concept of *reasonableness* is warranted. The whole of liability determination in tort or injury law is based on the elusive concept of the "reasonable person." In the context of medical malpractice the standard is that which a reasonably prudent physician of similar knowledge, training, and experience would do under the same or similar circumstances. If the conduct of a particular physician either by act or omission seems to be outside the bounds of a reasonable and prudent course of action, that physician is more likely exposed to allegations of malpractice should the patient come to any harm. That which is reasonable is defensible, grounded in substantial medical knowledge and experience, and should thereby be beyond reproach. If nothing else, be reasonable.

Questions

1. Mrs. Smith is well known to the staff of your hospital. She is a frequent visitor to the Emergency Room (ER) for abdominal pain with pseudo-obstructive symptoms and a heavy user of medical services, probably related to the dozen or so laparotomies she's had in the past twenty years. She frequently "fires" physicians, is irregular in following-up with after care, and has outstanding bill for unpaid office services with many of the groups in town. As the preeminent surgical scholar in your hospital, she has been sent to you for her chronic abdominal pain syndrome. After five office visits in a month, several late-night phone calls for opioid prescription refills, and a half a dozen missed appointments it becomes clear to you there is little hope for a therapeutic relationship with this patient and you wish to terminate your relationship with her. You should:

   (A) Instruct your receptionist not to schedule the patient for appointments hoping she'll stop seeing you

   (B) Tell the patient there is nothing more you can do for her and tell her to see another doctor

   (C) Send her a letter by Certified mail, return receipt requested, listing the names of other local physicians in your field and ask that she schedule an appointment with one of them in a month, after which time you'll no longer be able to see her

   (D) Deny her prescription refills, ignore her phone messages, and instruct your office staff to be evasive about your availability

2. Which of the following would probably NOT be considered patient abandonment?

   (A) Failing to see your hospitalized patients for one day because you've contracted a highly infectious *E. coli* diarrhea

   (B) Failing to see a patient whose leg you set for two days while you're on vacation then discharging that patient without a pre-discharge examination

   (C) Discharging a patient home after a laparotomy for a large bowel obstruction when the patient is still showing feculent emesis

   (D) Sending a patient home from the ER after casting his leg but not giving any discharge or aftercare instructions.

3. Mrs. Abrams has been sent to you for surgical management of her peptic ulcer disease, which has been quite refractory to aggressive and ongoing medical therapy. You propose a vagotomy and pyloroplasty procedure. During the course of answering the patient's questions which of the following statements, if made, could unintentionally constitute a contract with the patient?

   (A) "Patients in my practice experience a 95% reduction in symptoms after this procedure."

   (B) "You'll be able to eat three-alarm chili again."

   (C) "Almost everyone is able to go off their stomach medicines after the procedure."

   (D) "I've never had a patient develop an infection after this surgery, but there is a very small chance it could happen."

4. You have been treating Mr. Able for a chronic, non-healing ulcer on his left calf for more than six months. The lesion has no doubt been exacerbated by the patient's obesity, sedentary lifestyle, and diabetic vascular disease. After a period of intensive treatment the patient misses several follow-up appointments despite your staff's reminder messages left at his home. After a four-month absence, Mr. Able returns to the clinic with a remarkably swollen, erythematous left lower extremity, and the formerly well-controlled ulcer now probes to dull, soft, grey bone. You suspect advanced osteomyelitis and recommend amputation. The patient leaves in a fit of rage.

   A few weeks later you receive notice from Mr. Able's attorney accusing you of malpractice in "allowing" his chronic ulcer to become so serious. Which of the following types of information would be most likely to mitigate damages, or perhaps exonerate you completely?

   (A) Obese, sedentary patients often develop osteomyelitis in spite of good medical care

   (B) Osteomyelitis often requires amputation even with appropriate treatment

   (C) The patient failed follow-up appointments on several occasions

   (D) The patient was uninsured, and poor access to health care has been shown to increase complications of chronic diseases.

5. During the routine postoperative removal of a Jackson–Pratt drain you discover that the tip of the drain appears to be sheared off. Remembering back to the operation it seems you might have used the dull end of the scalpel to hold the tip in place while suturing the deep tissues back together, but you are not sure. Despite subsequent X-rays and CT scans, no foreign body is found.

   You should:

   (A) Realize the drain tip is exceedingly unlikely to cause this patient any harm and determine what she doesn't know won't hurt her

   (B) Convince yourself that the tip should have shown up on the radiographs and forget the whole incident

   (C) Admit your uncertainty and convince the patient a small piece of plastic in the abdomen is unlikely to cause any harm

   (D) Consult with the patient after she is sufficiently recovered and offer a candid and open discussion of the situation and her options for further evaluation

6. You are in the midst of a routine laparotomy when the anesthesiologist suddenly exclaims, "he's crashing!" and institutes a cardiac arrest protocol. The patient survives but has a long postoperative course complicated by an inability to walk correctly and memory loss. On later review of the chart the small T-waves are obvious, and frankly you feel someone would have detected his underlying hypokalemia sooner but for the patient's failure to mention he was on furosemide preoperatively.

   How would a jury *most likely* treat the patient's failure to notify you of his medications?

   (A) Consider this a substantial factor in his injury and reduce damages, if any

   (B) Consider this something the anesthesiologist should have discovered and let you off the hook

   (C) Consider the whole episode the patient's fault and deny him any remuneration for his injury

   (D) Ignore this fact and focus on his injury secondary to the cardiac arrest

7. You are seeing a mildly overweight but otherwise healthy 32-year old woman with cholecystitis. She is a low surgical risk and you feel laparoscopic cholecystectomy is the most appropriate procedure. Which of the following is *inappropriate*?

   (A) A discussion of risks associated with laparoscopic procedures in general

   (B) A discussion of risks and benefits associated with delaying the procedure

   (C) A discussion of the risks associated with general anesthesia

   (D) A discussion of laparoscopy only, without mention of the risks and benefits of open cholecystectomy

8. A multiply injured trauma patient presents to the emergency department during your call night. He consents to laparotomy to treat his abdominal injuries but refuses blood or blood products, citing religious grounds. Unfortunately, his hemorrhage is extensive and he dies on the table. How is a court most likely to treat his refusal of the lifesaving transfusion?

   (A) Uphold the patient's right of refusal and find the surgeon liable for wrongful death

   (B) Deny the patient had any right to refuse lifesaving treatment and find the surgeon liable for wrongful death

(C) Find the patient partly responsible for his death through the refusal of transfusion but blame the surgeon for the death itself

(D) Find the patient completely responsible for his death through the refusal of transfusion

9. As part of a routine preoperative workup on a sixty year-old gentleman you order a chest X-ray and electrocardiogram (ECG). You review the studies briefly, note nothing grossly abnormal, and send them through the system to be over-read by radiology and cardiology respectively. The day before surgery reports come across your desk indicating a 1.5 cm solitary pulmonary nodule and borderline QRS prolongation. Who holds ultimate responsibility to ensure these abnormalities are addressed appropriately?

(A) The primary care physician, to whom you sent copies of the results

(B) The patient's cardiologist, to whom you sent copies of the results

(C) The anesthesiologist, who routinely reviews the preoperative record for abnormalities

(D) You, the ordering physician

10. As director of your institution's Peer Review Committee you have received a letter from a patient's attorney demanding all information relevant to a recent peer review proceeding regarding a physician on your staff. The letter informs you of a pending malpractice complaint against that physician and threatens a court order if you do not produce the Peer Review Committee's minutes, notes, and final report.

Knowing that peer review proceedings are protected from such disclosures by state law, you may confidently withhold all but which of the following documents?

(A) Notice to Physician of Peer Review Proceeding

(B) Report of Peer Review Findings

(C) Recommendation of Peer Review Committee

(D) Notes of a discussion between the hospital administrator and a nurse complaining against that physician in this matter

11. A surgical colleague at your hospital has a reputation for using unconventional surgical methods and the newest treatment modalities, even if they aren't well supported in the literature. Remarkably, he has the lowest complication rate on the staff. To no one's great surprise he is eventually sued for malpractice after a rare postoperative complication.

To prove his technique fell below the standard of care, the patient-plaintiff must do which of the following at trial?

(A) Establish the relevant standard of care through expert testimony

(B) Show exactly how his technique exposed her to an unreasonable risk of harm

(C) Show how his departure from the standard of care caused her injuries

(D) All of the above

12. It's 2 a.m. You have just finished "putting out fires" for postoperative ICU patients during another busy call night when a "code" is called overhead. You arrive at the room to realize you are the first physician there. The patient, an ill-appearing man that must be at least ninety, is unconscious and the monitor is flat line. The chart is not immediately at the bedside.

What is the most reasonable course of action?

(A) Ask for the chart to verify the patient's code status.

(B) Spend a brief moment trying to determine the patient's code status then institute Advanced Cardiac Life Support (ACLS) protocols

(C) Immediately institute ACLS protocols regardless of the ready availability of the chart at the nurse's station

(D) Verify the diagnosis of asystole in at least one other lead and pronounce death.

13. During a routine laparotomy you are working with a surgical technician with whom you've not worked before. The case is fairly routine, and in preparation for closing you ask for 10 cc of saline to rinse the surgical field. After a short delay, a syringe appears in your hand, and you flush. A moment later the monitor shows an accelerated supraventricular rhythm. You then realize the tech must have misheard your order for "saline" and handed you atropine by mistake.

Who is most likely to be correctly blamed for this mishap?

(A) The hospital for negligently failing to train and supervise the surgical tech properly

(B) You, the surgeon, for negligently administering the wrong drug

(C) The shift charge nurse, for negligent supervision and failing to see that the instrument table was set up properly

(D) The surgical technician for negligently failing to ask about a mumbled or nonsensical order by you, the physician

14. When recommending a medication for a patient, you feel strongly about discussing pertinent risks, benefits, and side effects of the drug. You also feel strongly about not wasting your time or the patient's covering every idiosyncratic reaction ever observed with a medication. Given the relatively uncommon but potentially serious side effects of the medication you have in mind, what should you discuss with the patient?

(A) Common, mild, transient side effects

(B) Serious, potentially life-threatening or permanent side effects

(C) Common side effects and more uncommon though potentially very serious side effects

(D) Every side effect listed in your copy of the Physician's Desk Reference©

15. You are performing a routine laparotomy for removal of a small colonic lesion discovered during colonoscopy. You anticipated taking only a relatively small portion of the distal colon with appropriate margins, and appropriately discussed this with the patient preoperatively. During the procedure you run the colon and discover three other intraluminal masses that are very likely to be malignant. The patient consented to "sigmoid colectomy with other procedures as indicated." What should you do?

(A) Proceed with subtotal colectomy and appropriate lymph node biopsy

(B) Proceed with the operation to which the patient consented and discuss your findings with the patient when she is recovered

(C) Stop the operation, close the incision, and discuss total colectomy with the patient after she has recovered

(D) Perform a radical colectomy with lymph node and mesenteric biopsies

16. You begin a routine open herniorrhaphy on a young, otherwise healthy adult male patient. Quite unexpectedly, the patient's right lower quadrant abdominal mass does not resolve with reduction of the hernia. You then discover a low-lying abscessed appendix disguised by the hernia sac. What is the most prudent course of action at this point in the operation?

(A) Repair the hernia, remove the appendix, drain the abscess, and insert an external drain as necessary

(B) Repair the hernia, wait for the patient to recover, then discuss the need for appendectomy

(C) Repair the hernia, remove the appendix, drain the abscess, then proceed with laparotomy to explore the abdomen for other pathology

(D) Repair the hernia and ignore the diseased appendix; the patient had been asymptomatic and would probably do well even with the abscess

17. After an appropriate exam you diagnose an ER patient with acute appendicitis and recommend appendectomy. After a review of the chart you determine the ER physician has given the patient 4 mg of morphine. The patient is alert, awake, eloquent, and seemed to comprehend the informed consent discussion you just had with him. Still, you wonder about the effect of the morphine on his ability to consent.

Which of the following is true?

(A) The patient is legally incapable of consenting to surgery after receiving opioid medication

(B) The patient is not legally capable of consenting to surgery until eight hours after opioid administration

(C) This patient's consent is valid because there is no objective evidence his judgment has been impaired by the opioid medication

(D) This patient's consent is effective, but the ER doctor will be to blame if anything goes wrong because of his decision to administer opioid medication before your exam

18. During routine preoperative counseling, what sort of information should you provide to the patient to assist her decision-making process as to the advisability of the procedure you propose?

(A) Whatever information the patient feels is material to her decision to accept or reject the proposed treatment

(B) The most statistically common and likely complications of the proposed treatment

(C) Whatever information the physicians in your community would routinely give in this situation

(D) Whatever information you feel is material, according to your knowledge and expertise

19. As part of your practice in a teaching institution you routinely involve surgical residents in your cases. Also, good business sense has led your group to employ a Physician's Assistant for help with routine cases and postop rounds. For the actions of which of the following personnel might you be liable?

    (A) The resident, while acting under your direction and control

    (B) The operating room nurses for their actions during your case, even though they are hospital employees

    (C) The Physician's Assistant while acting under your direction, though technically an employee of the group and not you personally

    (D) All of the above are potential sources of liability

20. The case was a disaster from the start. The anesthesiologist chipped one of the patient's teeth during the initial intubation. The OR personnel didn't have the correct tray open and had to search for the right equipment, unnecessarily prolonging the procedure. The patient's multiple prior procedures had set up a web of adhesions throughout the abdomen and pelvis. The colleague you called in to assist with this technically nightmarish case inadvertently cut the ureter on the side on which he was working. To further add to this comedy of errors, an independent physician with whom you share call inexplicably put the patient back on her estrogen replacement one night in spite of her postoperative deep venous thrombosis (DVT).

    You sense the summons to a lawsuit is coming. For what other physician's actions are you likely liable?

    (A) The anesthesiologist; under the "captain of the ship" doctrine you "control" OR personnel

    (B) The partner you called in to the case; as the lead surgeon you are responsible for the surgery, even if your partner was operating independently

    (C) The independent physician in your call group, because you are responsible for the postoperative care of your patient

    (D) None of the above

21. What is the most radiation legally allowed during pregnancy?

    (A) The equivalent of ten x-rays or one abdomino-pelvic CT scan

    (B) 500 millirads

    (C) 1000 millirads

    (D) No legal standard for radiation during pregnancy exists

22. The Preopera-tive Informed Consent form at your hospital lists your name "and assistants" on the "Operation to be Performed by" line. To whom does this consent almost certainly apply?

    (A) Your equally qualified surgical partner

    (B) Your Physician Assistant, who assists in many of your cases (though the patient doesn't know this)

    (C) A qualified colleague in your call group

    (D) A resident at your institution

23. The disclosure of confidential patient information to third parties usually makes the disclosing physician liable for an invasion of privacy. In which of the following instances would the disclosure of confidential information likely *not* lead to liability for the physician?

    (A) To the patient's employer, when you are performing a work-related physical

    (B) To the patient's spouse, when he or she has a legitimate interest in the matter

    (C) To an identified third party, when you are aware of a specific threat to that person

    (D) All of the above are probably acceptable disclosures

Answers and Explanations

1. (C) Abandonment (sometimes referred to as "constructive abandonment") is the unilateral termination of the doctor-patient relationship by the physician without notice to the patient at a time when medical care is still needed by the patient.[1] This may occur intentionally, as when a physician declares outwardly that he or she will no longer be involved in the care of the patient, unintentionally, as when the physician goes on leave or otherwise fails to see the patient for ongoing care and does not provide a replacement physician for ongoing care, or due to some extenuating factor such as personal illness by the physician.

Two kinds of doctor-patient relationships exist. "General" relationships are formed when the physician is responsible for addressing any medical condition that might arise while he or she has a relationship with the patient; this is typically the case for relationships with primary care physicians. "Special" relationships are formed with consultants and in most cases surgeons, wherein the duration of the doctor-patient relationship is for the duration of an illness or condition seen through to its resolution. Accordingly, surgeons are of course responsible for continuing to care for the patient through the peri- and post-operative periods until the patient is "cured of the operation."[2]

The doctor-patient relationship may only be terminated in narrow circumstances, namely by mutual consent of the patient and the physician (a "parting of ways"), by discharge of the physician by the patient, or when the services of the physician are no longer needed.[3] Any other severance of the doctor-patient relationship can be deemed abandonment and liability in the form of a lawsuit and potential damages may result.

Generally, a patient may be discharged from a practice safely, ethically, and legally with adequate notice and provision for continuing care. First, the medical record should contain some notation as to the legitimate reason for the termination; failure to pay bills, failure to attend appointments, any mention of the patient's character, demeanor, or habits, and certainly failure to improve symptomatically are all inappropriate and potentially risky reasons for discharging a patient. Notation merely stating "end of therapeutic benefit," "resolution of surgical condition," or "no longer able to care for this patient's needs" are sufficient. Next, a list of providers in the area that are competent to care for the patient's medical needs and currently accepting patients must be provided to the patient. No exact number is required, merely a "reasonable" number; eight or ten names should be sufficient in most geographic areas. The letter of discharge must specifically inform the patient that you will no longer be able to provide medical or surgical service for the patient after a specified date, usually thirty days from *receipt* of the letter. This information must be clearly provided to the patient by means of certified mail, preferably with delivery confirmation and return receipt requested.

During the thirty-day period surrounding discharge the physician must continue to care for the patient on an emergency basis and address ongoing medical issues that have formed the basis of the doctor-patient relationship in the past. Care should be taken neither to refuse to see the patient in this interim nor fail to return phone messages as either could be construed as abandonment. Further, the physician should be meticulous in not scheduling the patient for an office visit to discuss a new problem; this could be interpreted as creating a new doctor-patient relationship for the care of that problem and tolling the thirty-day discharge period until the new problem is fully addressed.

Finally, it is possible that the discharged patient may again be encountered for an acute problem when the discharging physician is on call. In this case the usual responsibilities of on-call physicians supersede the patient's discharge from your practice and care should be provided. It is prudent to state in

---

[1]*See generally* 57 ALR 2d 432
[2]*Id.,* §4.
[3]*Id.,* §3.

the *first* progress note on the patient chart that the duration of this relationship arose from an on-call duty and will continue only until appropriate care by another qualified provider can be secured. Be sure also to give the patient notice of the conditional nature of this relationship and that another qualified physician will be assuming her care as soon as practical; failure to give the patient notice of a change in caregivers has been deemed abandonment.[4]

2. **(A)** Abandonment can occur when the physician fails to provide appropriate postoperative or continuing care for the patient's medical issues. As with any tort (injury) action, a duty must be present (here, the duty of a doctor to act in the best interest of the patient), that duty must be breached through an act of commission or omission (to do or not do that which is appropriate), and that breach must be the cause of some harm suffered by the patient.

Abandonment is often construed for inadequate or incompetent postoperative care, physician unavailability for no apparent reason, inappropriate discharge from inpatient care, and inadequate discharge instruction.

Answer "a" carves out an exception to the abandonment theory for the physician's own compelling illness.[5] It could be argued that an aggressive *E. coli* infection would be a greater risk to fragile postoperative patients than missing a visit for one day. Of course, a competent colleague must provide coverage.

Failure to provide ongoing postoperative care led to the permanent disability for the patient in answer "b." While the soon to be defendant surgeon was on vacation another surgeon saw the patient for complaints of pain and swelling in the extremity, bivalved the cast, and appeared to have at least temporarily ameliorated the developing compartment syndrome. On the first surgeon's return, the patient was discharged without further examination and developed necrosis at the ankle distal to the cast.[6]

Despite eighteen days of feculent emesis the attending physician did not see the patient in answer "c" postoperatively. He eventually suffered perforation of both stomach and proximal small intestine that formed a fistula communicating to skin. The fistula of course required further surgical care two years later, when the patient was able to secure the services of another surgeon.[7]

Lastly, the patient in answer "d" was provided no aftercare instructions for his lower extremity fracture and suffered non-union, an aggressive wound infection, and eventual amputation of the extremity that could have been avoided with proper medical care.[8]

3. **(B)** In the apocryphal case *Cirafici v. Goffen*,[9] a dentist's representations to a patient in reference to a proposed surgical procedure were so specific as to go beyond the usual therapeutic reassurances and act as a binding promise. This promise was found to create a contract between the dentist and the patient, so when those representations were found to be false, the patient sued and won on a breach of contract complaint.

Key to this concept is the idea of concrete promises for a specific outcome. Most of what is said between the doctor and patient is considered in the spirit of providing reassurance and support for a troubled patient. The line crossed is that which in effect guarantees a particular result to a particular patient. This goes beyond the tongue-in-cheek guarantee of being "one gallbladder lighter" after cholecystectomy. Patients take seriously statements by trusted medical professionals about definitely being able to stop certain medications, eat particular foods, or participate in important activities.

These pitfalls can easily be avoided with factual information and qualified statements. In the above example, use of the terms "ninety-five percent," "almost," and "but" remove the discussion from the realm of an oral contract[10] and back to therapeutic reassurances.

4. **(C)** Patients are obligated to exercise a reasonable degree of care for themselves in the interests of their better health. The law does not obligate physicians to force patients to take medication or care properly for their diabetes. Some onus of proper care is placed on the patient.[11]

Evidence of the patient's failure to return on an appropriate basis for ongoing medical care has been allowed as a defense in medical malpractice cases under the theory of *comparative negligence*. Comparative negligence seeks to apportion fault resulting

---

[4]*Id.*, §23.
[5]57 ALR 2d 432, §20.
[6]*Vann v. Harden*, 47 SE2d 314 (1948).
[7]*Gross v. Partlow*, 68 P2d 1034 (1937).

[8]*Beck v. German Klinik*, 43 NW 617 (1889).
[9]407 N.E.2d 633 (1980); he promised she'd be able to eat corn on the cob again
[10]A contract need not be written, signed, or witnessed to be enforceable. Basically a contract is a set of promises between two or more parties supported by consideration. Consideration is something of legal value to one party and/or legal detriment to another. We make oral contracts every day; care should be taken not to make them with patients for specific outcomes.
[11]*See generally* 84 A.L.R.5th 619

in harm to those who are responsible, including the injured party if it can be shown that he or she directly contributed to his or her injury or failed to take steps to prevent further injury. If the physician-defendant can prove by a "preponderance of the evidence" that the patient's behaviors were a substantial factor in causing his or her harm, the patient-plaintiff may be barred completely from recovery.

In a case similar to ours, a patient complained to his physician of a poorly healing lower extremity lesion with a probable underlying osteomyelitis but failed to return for regular visits as directed. He was lost to follow-up for a period of months, then returned and was diagnosed with advanced osteomyelitis requiring amputation of his foot. When the jury found for the plaintiff and awarded damages, the verdict was thrown out and a new trial granted because the jury verdict was against the "overwhelming weight of the evidence."[12]

Two other cases demonstrate similar principles of patient responsibility. A patient's widow was denied recovery for her husband's death when it was shown that he refused a lipid profile and failed to follow-up with his physician for chest pain. He died of an acute myocardial infarction a short time later.[13] Another patient was denied recovery for failing to follow-up when a breast lump she pointed out to her physician continued to grow. An extensive resection was eventually required. Because her physician was meticulous about documenting his discussion regarding the curability of such a lump had she returned as directed, the patient recovered nothing.[14]

Courts are not usually so unforgiving to injured patients, however. Typically, evidence of a patient-plaintiff's failure to exercise ordinary care in his or her own interest will reduce the amount of recovery but not exonerate the health care provider completely. For example, after suffering significant chest and abdominal trauma, including a ruptured diaphragm and a liver fracture, a mechanic returned to work before being released by his physician. He was found to be 60% at fault for subsequent injuries related to going back to work prematurely, and his jury award was reduced by 60%.[15]

Although answers "a" and "b" are accurate, it is still the responsibility of the physician to adequately educate and inform the patient of the seriousness of his condition and the importance of regular and proper follow-up. Information like that mentioned in answer "d" should never be raised by the defense in a malpractice action.

States vary in their interpretations of the comparative negligence doctrine. Most states follow the rule exactly, as in the last case: 60% fault means 60% reduction in award. Some states have adopted a modified comparative negligence statute, whereby a patient-plaintiff that is more than 50% responsible for his own injuries will not recover anything. Finally, a few jurisdictions still retain the venerable contributory negligence doctrine, where patients that are even 1% to blame for their injuries are barred from recovery.[16]

5. **(D)** The Statute of Limitations is just that, a statute or law that has been passed by a state legislature to limit the time in which a lawsuit can be instituted after an injury. Generally, the statute of limitations begins to run at the time of the injury, and once that time limit has been exceeded a lawsuit, no matter how strong, cannot be begun.

An important exception to this rule is for that of retained foreign bodies, specifically surgical ones. Although a few states still retain the old rule of starting the statute of limitations from the moment of injury (i.e. when the sponge was left in the abdomen, for example), most states are now tolling the statute until the *injury* caused by the foreign body is or by reasonable diligence could be discovered by the patient (as when the sponge first causes a bowel obstruction). Most states disregard the statute of limitations if it can be shown the surgeon knew of a retained foreign body and was silent or deceptive on the issue, which amounts to a fraudulent concealment of an injury. An alternative approach adopted my many states begins the statute of limitations at the moment the doctor-patient relationship ceases.[17]

A few representative cases:

- A surgical leg wound failed to heal for over ten years. A second operation revealed this was because of a surgical sponge left over from the first procedure.[18]
- A failed tubal ligation was not discovered until the patient became pregnant years later.[19]
- The cause of recurrent abdominal pain was found to be a wing nut from a retractor that had fallen apparently unnoticed into the surgical field.[20]

[12]*Durphy v. Kaiser Foundation Health Plan*, 698 A.2d 459, 468 (1997).
[13]*Fall v. White*, 449 N.E.2d 628 (1983).
[14]*Chudson v. Ratna*, 548 A.2d 172 (1988).
[15]*Wister v. Hart*, 766 P.2d 168 (1988).

[16]Virginia, Maryland, North Carolina, and the District of Columbia still follow contributory negligence.
[17]*See generally* 70 A.L.R.3d 7
[18]*Frazor v. Osborne*, 414 S.W.2d 118 (1966).
[19]*Tomlinson v. Siehl*, 459 S.W.2d 166 (1970).
[20]*Fernandi v. Strully*, 173 A.2d 277 (1961).

In every instance where a surgical foreign object may have been left in a patient's body every reasonable measure should be taken to identify and of course remove the object. A candid discussion with the patient and family, perhaps with the aid of the hospital's risk manager, will likely avoid future litigation. At that point the patient must act in her own best interests or risk losing all chance of recovery under comparative negligence, above.[21]

6. **(A)** Patients have a duty to exercise ordinary care for themselves and as part of this duty are obliged to volunteer any information that he knows or should reasonably know is important to his medical care and which the physician has failed to ascertain.[22] Particularly important are medication allergies and adverse reactions, current medications being taken, and any known medical conditions that could in any way impact care.

In a very few cases, patients have been found to be contributorily negligent for failing to mention pertinent medical facts to their physicians and being injured as a result of that failure to divulge. *Contributory negligence* is a concept that the defendant-physician must raise in his or her defense. This defense asserts that a patient has done something to worsen his injury or failed to do something to mitigate his injury. This defense will either reduce a patient-plaintiff's award for an injury or prevent recovery for the injury altogether.[23]

For example, an award for damages in a case of inappropriate treatment of a breast lump was reduced for the patient's failure to mention prior diagnoses and treatments for breast lumps.[24] The damage award was also reduced for a man admitted to the hospital claiming to be suffering from heroin withdrawal. In fact, he was withdrawing from alcohol and polydrug abuse and suffered a fatal reaction when given Methadone® twice for his withdrawal symptoms.[25] Finally, a hospital was relieved of a malpractice claim entirely when a patient suffered a cardiac arrest during surgery and sustained extensive brain damage as

a result. He failed to tell the anesthesiologist he was taking furosemide.[26]

The defense of contributory negligence is not absolute. A physician was held liable for a patient's death due to complications of barbiturate addiction. On admission, the patient admitted she was taking barbiturates but did not reveal she was addicted to them.[27]

Although patients can sometimes be found to have contributed to their own harms, there is no substitute for a good history and physical examination and no better defense than thoughtful, appropriate patient care.

7. **(D)** Though few physicians find enthusiasm for the topic of informed consent, the preoperative consultation is a critical juncture in the physician-patient relationship. It is at this point the patient should receive information from the physician on probable and alternative diagnoses, proposed and alternative treatments, and risks and benefits attendant to those alternatives. It is also at this point that a minor breakdown in communication between physician and patient can be later amplified by unfavorable outcomes in to a malpractice lawsuit.

Informed Consent is a process whereby a reasonable patient agrees to a procedure or intervention after having been supplied with appropriate information regarding the risks, benefits, alternatives, and expectations of a procedure. An obvious example would be a discussion of the relative risks and benefits of open versus laparoscopic cholecystectomy as alternatives to a course of watchful waiting. The expectation of either procedure would be improvement of the patient's abdominal pain, if not complete resolution.[28]

Informed Consent can fail if a patient is not given an option between alternatives, even more complicated or dangerous alternatives.[29] When a gallbladder was injured during a needle biopsy of the kidney, the referring urologist was held liable for failing to inform the patient that open kidney biopsy was an alternative even though it was a more complicated and potentially more hazardous procedure. The internist who referred the patient to that urologist was found to have no duty to explain the procedure or alternatives.[30]

---

[21]Foreign body cases illustrate a personal pet peeve against the old "if it wasn't documented, it wasn't done" maxim. Of course the lost sponge wasn't documented; if the count was wrong, we would have looked for it. Does that mean it never happened?—*JC*

[22]*See generally* 33 A.L.R.4th 790

[23]In four jurisdictions (MD, VA, NC, DC) a finding of contributory negligence is a complete bar to recovery, i.e. the patient will not receive any award for his injury. In the other forty-seven jurisdictions evidence that a patient contributed to his harm may reduce the award or, depending on the percentage of fault, prevent recovery altogether. See the discussion, above.

[24]*Jamas v. Krpan*, 568 P.2d 1114 (1977).

[25]*Rochester v. Katalan*, 320 A.2d 704 (1974).

---

[26]*Mackey v. Greenview Hosp.*, 587 S.W.2d 249 (1979).

[27]*O'Neil v. State*, 66 Misc.2d 936 (1971).

[28]Care must be taken of course not to promise a specific outcome that is only likely; see the note above regarding promises of specific outcomes and contract formation.

[29]*See generally* 38 A.L.R.4th 900

[30]*Logan v. Greenwich Hosp. Assn.*, 465 A.2d 294 (1983); curiously, the radiologist who performed the procedure was exonerated.

Liability was clearly established against the surgeon who did not warn the patient of the risks of infection or incisional hernia associated with an open cholecystectomy. The patient suffered multiple wound infections and required operative repair of a substantial incisional hernia.[31] Similarly, a patient who suffered a recurrent laryngeal nerve injury after thyroidectomy was successful in suing her surgeon for failing to discuss non-operative treatment of her thyroid tumor.[32]

An important exception for Informed Consent is made for emergency situations. All persons are legally held to consent to lifesaving emergency treatments absent an advanced directive to the contrary. Even though alternatives existed, a patient multiply injured after a motor vehicle accident was denied recovery his physicians' failure to discuss those alternatives.[33] The court felt it was not necessary for the surgeon during an emergency situation to discuss options that were unnecessarily risky or not feasible.

Lastly, it is important to realize that courts regard the discussion leading to Informed Consent to be a non-delegable duty, even if hospitals do not. That is, the final responsibility to ensure the patient is "informed" and has in fact "consented" lies with the physician performing the procedure, not a signature on a form, a nurse, the primary care physician[34], or the anesthesiologist (except for risks of anesthesia). Simply writing "obtain consent for [procedure]" in the chart's orders section does not relieve the operating surgeon of responsibility or liability should the patient not understand his procedure or the risks associated with it.[35]

8. **(D)** The doctrine of *comparative fault* seeks to allocate an injured person's losses proportionately among the parties that caused those losses. In the medical malpractice setting, comparative fault recognizes that sometimes patients are responsible for at least part of the harms they suffer. This fault may be for specific actions, inactions, or a failure to minimize the injury suffered.

Patients who object to specific interventions or treatments on moral, religious, or any reasonable grounds may be forced to bear part responsibility for their injuries.[36] Courts generally recognize a further doctrine of "avoidable consequences," which prevents injured patients from recovering for harms that would have been avoided but for their religious objections. For example, the estate of a Jehovah's Witness was prevented from recovering any damages in a suit against the patient's surgeons and the hospital for failing to prevent his death after a motor vehicle accident. The patient suffered rib and pelvic fractures, a large retroperitoneal hemorrhage, and a lacerated intrathoracic artery. He died after refusing blood transfusions.[37] Similarly, a Christian Science practitioner was denied any award from his medical doctor after receiving only Christian Science treatments for his prostatitis; he was ill for ten days.[38]

Religious objection is not always a bar to recovery for injuries. In one case, a Jehovah's Witness developed fevers after a segmental colectomy and was given aspirin. After seven days on aspirin the patient developed coffee-grounds emesis and subsequently died of hemorrhagic shock after refusing consent for a blood transfusion. The surgeon was held partly responsible for ordering the drug.[39] Similarly, a Jehovah's Witness who died of hemorrhagic shock after a dilation and curettage procedure was found to be 75% responsible for her death for refusing a transfusion, so her damage award was reduced by 75%.[40] In both of these cases the medical team was found to be responsible for the condition that led to the necessity to receive blood transfusion and so was held partly liable for the patient's death.

The law will support a competent individual's right to refuse lifesaving treatment so long as he or she is fully informed of the risks of refusing the treatment. The law will not, however, hold others responsible for the consequences of such refusals.

9. **(D)** The duty of physicians to inform patients of test results should be obvious. To what point that duty extends, however, is sometimes unclear. Physicians are responsible for informing patients of the results of all tests he or she orders; this is not a duty that should be assumed to be covered by the consultant or primary care physician. This duty is to disclose "all facts which materially affect the patient's rights and interests."[41]

---

[31]*Harwell v. Pittman,* 428 S.2d 1049 (1983).

[32]*Archer v. Galbraith,* 567 P.2d 1155 (1977).

[33]*Downer v. Veilleux,* 322 A.2d 82 (1974).

[34]*Panea v. Isdaner,* 773 A.2d 782 (2001); responsibility to obtain informed consent is non-delegable, even to another physician.

[35]No nurse, technician, or primary care physician understands the procedure and risks associated as well as the operating physician. You wouldn't let those people operate for you; don't risk your reputation on their ignorances. The patient with confidence in and involvement with the decision-making process is far less likely to sue.—JC

[36]*See generally,* 3 A.L.R.5th 721

[37]*Munn v. Algee,* 924 F.2d 568 (1991).

[38]*Baumgartner v. First Church of Christ, Scientist,* 490 N.E.2d 1319 (1986).

[39]*Corlett v. Caserta,* 562 N.E.2d 257 (1990).

[40]*Shorter v. Drury,* 698 P.2d 116 (1985).

[41]*Wohlgemuth v. Meyer,* 293 P.2d 816 (1956).

As with any malpractice claim the patient must have suffered some kind of harm as a direct consequence of the physician's failure to inform him of his test result in order to recover any damages. For example, a patient was given no recovery for his physician's failure to notify him of normal (or inconsequential) test results.[42] In stark contrast, another physician was found guilty of malpractice for failing to notify a patient of the suspicious lung nodule on an X-ray. It later turned out to be cancerous and could have been treated more successfully had it been addressed at the time of the initial X-ray.[43]

Exactly where this duty to notify ends is not clear. In one case an X-ray reading suggested acute appendicitis but the patient was not informed of this fact. The court found that suggested or improbable diagnoses did not have to be discussed with the patient after a test, absent a clinical indication for doing so.[44] In fact, discussion of all possible diagnoses may do more harm than good, constituting "bad medical practice."[45]

Lastly, a physician was found innocent of malpractice when a patient gave a wrong address and phone number to which her (abnormal) pap results was sent. The patient contributed to her injury by providing inaccurate information.[46]

As a general rule, a physician will be held responsible for the results of any test he or she orders. This responsibility may not be assumed to be that of the primary care or consulting physician; if you order it, you have to do something about the results. Courts are more sympathetic to injured patients than to careless physicians.

10. **(D)** Laws protecting peer review proceedings serve to protect the public interest by encouraging physicians to engage in candid review of their peers. In nearly all states these laws prohibit discovery of a peer review proceeding by a patient-plaintiff's lawyer, who is undoubtedly looking for evidence of past wrongdoing on the part of the physician-defendant.

To confidently participate in peer review activities it is important to have an accurate idea of what exactly constitutes a peer review proceeding.[47] Generally, the peer review process involves a standing committee of staff physicians, department heads, hospital administrators, hospital risk management personnel, and/or other hospital personnel. Review of an event can be triggered by a hospital incident report, patient complaint, insurance or guarantor inquiry, or even a casual discussion with a member of the peer review committee. An investigation is then made, evidence gathered, and information presented to the physician with opportunity to respond. Subject matter of peer review can range from an inconsequential missed radiographic finding to suggestion of intentional or grossly negligent injury to a patient. Peer review actions may range from filing a notice of a missed finding in a physician's credentialing file to expulsion from the medical staff and termination of privileges.

Documents outlining the peer review process as well as those pertaining to a particular peer review action are generally *privileged*, that is, not available to an attorney or party outside the peer review committee other than the physician being reviewed.[48] These may include minutes of the peer review hearing (if a hearing was had), incident reports relevant to the review, reports, findings, and recommendations for specific credentialing or privileging actions.[49] Any action taken on recommendation of the peer review committee, however, is not privileged information, as this is considered to have occurred after the peer review process has ended.[50] Also, nurse and patient complaints against a physician are often not privileged,[51] as these are generated before the peer review process begins, although they are later incorporated in to it.

Other information that is accessible to a plaintiff's attorney regarding a peer review proceeding includes investigation by an individual before the formal peer review proceeding begins (even if that individual is a member of the peer review committee)[52] and informal discussions with the hospital administrator regarding the subject of an upcoming peer review.[53] Such information gathering outside the auspices of peer review may subject both the investigator and interviewee to deposition (pre-trial interview) by both attorneys as to the content and outcome of the conversation, or even being called to testify at trial.[54]

---

[42]*Cady v. Fraser*, 222 P.2d 422 (1950).

[43]Ind. Sup. Ct. No. 49S05-0004-CV-231; 726 N.E.2d 272 (2000).

[44]*Sinkey v. Surgical Associates*, 186 N.W.2d 658 (1971).

[45]*Natanson v. Kline*, 350 P.2d 1093 (1960).

[46]*Ray v. Wagner*, 176 N.W.2d 101 (1970).

[47]This section, like the entire chapter, is intended to provide an overview of general principles, not to serve as an authoritative reference tool. State statutes can and do vary in these matters.

[48]*See generally* 69 A.L.R. 5th 559.

[49]*Id.*, 590-605.

[50]*Id.*, 621-24.

[51]*Leanhart v. Humana, Inc.*, 933 S.W.2d 820 (1996).

[52]*Roach v. Springfield Clinic*, 623 N.E.2d 246 (1993).

[53]*Grandi v. Shah*, 633 N.E.2d (1994).

[54]At least one state (New York) has a recent series of cases allowing peer review information to be discovered at trial, including statements made by the subject physician, notes taken at the peer review hearing by that physician, and his written responses to peer review inquiries. 69 A.L.R.5th 616-21. This is a disturbing trend away from the confidentiality and hence candor of peer review proceedings and is contrary to the policy and spirit of peer review proceedings.

Peer review is an important tool in the quality assurance process for physicians and hospitals alike. Medical staff members should be encouraged to participate in and cooperate with peer review proceedings within the boundaries of the peer review process. Individual efforts to circumvent the legally recognized boundaries of this process may subject the investigator to additional, unwanted liability.

11. **(D)** As discussed at the outset of this chapter, medical malpractice is a subset of personal injuries known as negligence. Negligence is a failure to exercise due care for the safety of self or others under the circumstances. This is differentiated from other harms such as assault and battery by lack of an element of *intent*. To be negligent one must not have intended to harm the plaintiff but acted in such a way as to allow harm to happen.

As with any negligence claim a patient-plaintiff must prove the physician-defendant owed him a duty of care, that the duty was breached by the physician-defendant either through action or inaction, that the breach caused the patient-plaintiff's harm, and that a harm did in fact result. Duty is shown by the existence of a doctor-patient relationship. From the time of the first consultation the physician owes that patient a duty of reasonable care, which is to use the judgment, skill, and knowledge of a reasonable physician in a similar situation. When the patient feels as though the requisite care, knowledge, and skill has not been used in his case, a complaint of malpractice may ensue.

The legal concept of *breach of duty* is the medical equivalent of care that falls below a recognized standard of care. In this sense our medical "standard of care" is the care a reasonable physician of similar knowledge, training, and experience would use in the same or similar circumstances. The common-law practice comparing physicians in similar practice situations (eg. solo vs. group, rural vs. urban, private vs. academic) has been abandoned in favor of a more regional or national "standard of care." This standard must be proven at trial for a plaintiff to succeed in his or her malpractice lawsuit. This is done through the introduction of expert testimony. In one apocryphal case, a physician was freed from liability for the death of a mother and her newborn after failing to timely diagnose and treat the patient's toxemia because the patient's attorney did not produce an expert to testify to the relevant standard of care, instead relying on a cross-examination of the physician-defendant and excerpts from "learned medical treatises."[55]

Further, to be sufficient to establish negligence expert testimony must establish the manner in which the physician-defendant breached the standard of care. Courts recognize that " ... medicine is not an exact science [but] ... the exercise of individual judgment within the framework of established procedures."[56] In that case, a surgeon was found not to be liable for a recurrent laryngeal nerve injury following thyroidectomy. Because the location of the recurrent laryngeal nerve was uncertain, his choice was to make a wide incision to avoid areas of scar tissue from a prior operation. Though the plaintiff's expert testified he would have used a different incision, the expert was unable to show that the strategy employed by the physician-defendant was manifestly unreasonable or contrary to an established standard of care.[57] Without a violation of a standard of care, no liability can be found.

A case failing any of these four elements of duty, breach, causation, and damages will not succeed, exonerating the physician.

12. **(B)** Do Not Resuscitate (DNR) orders are a daily part of the practice of medicine. In recent years it has become standard practice to inquire about advanced directives of all hospitalized patients on admission. This practice has had the effect of granting patients, families, and physicians permission to discuss end of life care and act in a manner consistent with the patient's wishes.

Courts have recognized the benefits to both the individual patient and society with the advent of the DNR order. The right of a competent adult to determine that which is to be done to his or her body is one of the cornerstone concepts in our legal system.[58] The individual benefits through his or her right of self-determination and a right to avoid prolonged suffering and maintain a sense of dignity. Society benefits from restraint in providing futile care to maintain the life of the organism, rather than the person. As such, the legal and medical standards of care are the same: full resuscitative efforts should be instituted absent evidence of a prior DNR order or evidence of medical futility.[59] Conversely, courts have

---

[55]*Smith v. Knowles*, 281 N.W.2d 653 (1979).

[56]*Walski v. Tiesenga*, 381 N.E.2d 279 (1978).

[57]*Id.*

[58]Paraphrased from Justice Cardozo, *Schloendorff v. Society of New York Hospital*, 105 N.E. 92 (1914), "every human being of adult years and sound mind has a right to determine what shall be done with his own body; and a surgeon who performs an operation without his patient's consent commits an assault, for which he is liable in damages."

[59]As an example from my years in the emergency department: resuscitative efforts were not instituted on an MVA victim whose skull and brain were substantially traumatically absent; to have done so would have been medically futile.—JC

been reticent to hold physicians liable for following a prior DNR order in good faith.[60]

"Good faith" determinations are generally straightforward. If a physician sees the DNR order on the chart (or similar notation) or if the resuscitation team is summoned and thereafter the chart reveals a DNR order the physicians in attendance will not be held responsible for the patient's death. An important exception was found in a case where the sister of a seriously (but not terminally) ill patient requested a DNR order be placed on the chart. The patient subsequently arrested and died. The physician who issued the DNR order was held responsible for medical negligence for failing to determine whether or not the family member requesting the DNR order had legal authority to do so (e.g. through a legal guardianship, healthcare power of attorney, or the like).[61] It is important to note that the physicians responding to the "code" would not be liable, just the physician responsible for issuing the DNR order.

Two cases producing interesting results deserve mention. In the first, a patient was admitted to a hospital with a DNR order that the family later requested removed. On review, the hospital's internal "Optimum Care Committee" reinstituted the DNR order and the patient subsequently expired. Predictably, the family sued. The court found that even though the committee reinstituted the DNR order improperly, resuscitation would have been futile and thus no damages were due.[62] The second case involved a patient who requested a DNR and subsequently went in to cardiac arrest. The duty nurse that day was apparently unaware of the DNR order and successfully resuscitated the patient. The patient then lived nearly two years more, but suffered a stroke with hemiplegia and incontinence after the resuscitation. Again, the patient sued for the nurse's failure to follow the DNR order. The patient was denied recovery for "wrongful resuscitation" because the state in which she sued (like most) does not recognize "wrongful life" as an injury. The court did say, however, that because the resuscitation was against the patient's wishes the nurse and hospital could be sued for injuries suffered during the resuscitation itself.[63]

Finally, two points should be made regarding minors. One case involved a seventeen-year old patient with muscular dystrophy and multiple complications. His parents requested a DNR order be issued; the patient later expired. The parents then sued alleging the patient, as a "mature minor," should have been consulted prior to issuing the order. The court agreed.[64] In the view of the civil common law (as opposed to criminal law), children fourteen years and older are presumed capable of making many of their own decisions. Final authority rests with the parent or guardian, but the child's wishes should be discussed and documented.

Finally, when parents disagree on the appropriateness of a DNR order, don't issue one. This should be readily apparent, but the wishes of a non-custodial parent in opposition to a DNR order can be a basis for a malpractice suit.[65]

13. **(D)** Medication administration errors have been identified as a major source of adverse events occurring in hospitals.[66] With few exceptions physicians are responsible for the medication administration errors of those under their supervision.[67] Again, this is considered under the legal doctrine of *respondeat superior*, or "captain of the ship." The supervising physician has been held responsible both for the actions of a nurse[68] and an office assistant[69] under his direction even when it is not clear that the physician gave an order for use of the harmful medications in question.

Physicians have been exonerated for the mistakes of ancillary personnel in some narrow circumstances. A physician barely escaped liability for a nurse's mistaken use of a harmful compound during bladder irrigation. The court found that the patient's symptoms could be explained by factors other than the mistaken medication and was denied restitution for the error.[70] A surgeon was released from liability when he injected a patient with ethyl alcohol he had been handed in a syringe; the nurse thought it was novocain. The court recognized a duty on the part of the physician to question the medication if he had reason to suspect it was not the one he'd ordered.[71] In circumstances similar to these, surgeons are generally exonerated from liability for administering the wrong medication when a nurse or assistant passes

[60]46 A.L.R. 5th 793, 800.
[61]*Payne v. Marion General Hosp.*, 549 N.E.2d 1043 (1990).
[62]*Gilgunn v. Massachusetts General Hosp.*, (April 21, 1995 Mass. Super.) No. 91-4820-H.
[63]*Anderson v. St. Francis-St. George Hosp.*, 671 N.E.2d 225 (1996).

[64]*Belcher v. Charleston Area Medical Center*, 422 S.E.2d 827 (1992). Apparently the parents felt no obligation to consult with their son prior to requesting the DNR order; one can only assume feelings of guilt and responsibility led to a desire for retribution.
[65]*In re Doe*, 418 S.E.2d 3 (1992).
[66]"To Err Is Human: Building a Safer Health System." The Institute of Medicine. The National Academies Press, 2001.
[67]*See generally* 23 A.L.R. 3d 1334 *and* 51 A.L.R. 2d 970
[68]*Schulz v. Feigal*, 142 N.W.2d 84 (1966).
[69]*Myrkie v. Hill*, 236 N.W. 287 (1931).
[70]*Simons v. Jennings*, 46 P.2d 704 (1935).
[71]*Abercrombie v. Roof*, 28 N.E.2d 772 (1940).

incorrect medications to them.[72,73] In our scenario, the surgical technician though technically the only party at fault is unlikely to have assets significant enough to enforce a judgment against him. The hospital, as the "deep pocket," is likely to bear the brunt of liability.

As with any malpractice allegation, reasonableness is key. If a surgeon reasonably should question a medication given to him or her by a nurse, that surgeon is under a duty to do so in the interest of patient safety. Further, reasonable steps should be taken by physicians to minimize the chance of error in medication administration and hence exposure to liability.[74]

14. **(C)** Medication side effects, adverse reactions, and allergies are an inevitable part of the practice of medicine. As such courts recognize that the occurrence of a side effect, even a serious or life-threatening one, is not in itself evidence of malpractice.[75]

Courts are divided in the matter of physician liability for failure to discuss common, serious, and/or potentially life-threatening side effects with patients prior to prescribing a particular drug.[76] Innumerable cases have found the physician liable for negligent failure to warn a patient of the risks associated with use of medications. Among these specifically are the risk of avascular necrosis from prednisone,[77] cerebrovascular accident from oral contraceptive medications,[78] Zyderm® and autoimmune syndromes,[79] and tardive dyskinesia from neuroleptic medications.[80] Alternatively, many cases have exonerated physicians from liability for failing to mention particular side effects of medication, including avascular necrosis from Decadron,[81] toxic hepatitis from isoniazid,[82] priapism from MINIPRESS,[83] and peripheral neuropathy from metronidazole.[84] In the first two cases, courts found the relatively unlikely side effects listed would not have prevented patients

from consenting to their use given the seriousness of the primary medical conditions being treated, pseudotumor cerebri and tuberculosis respectively. The latter two cases were thought to be representative of such rare side effects that discussion of them was not within the standard medical practice and therefore a physician should not be liable for the harms that resulted.

One court provided an excellent framework for determining the importance of discussing a particular side effect with a patient. First, the manifestation of the side effect should be considered, for example mortal pain over minor discomfort. Second, permanency of the side effect should be taken into account. Next, the availability of an effective cure is important. Fourth, seriousness of the condition must be considered. Lastly, the "overall effect" of a reaction should be taken into account.[85]

Medication allergies present a special case. When a patient is not known to be hypersensitive to a drug the physician is not responsible for harms resulting from an allergic reaction.[86] Courts recognize that not every hypersensitivity test can (or should) be done on every patient, and that hypersensitivity tests don't exist for most drugs.[87] When a physician or hospital is aware of a drug allergy, responsibility for harms resulting from administration of the drug will attach. A hospital was held responsible for an anaphylactic reaction to cephalexin when the patient told her nurse she was allergic to penicillin. Her chart listed both drugs as allergies.[88] A primary care physician notified the hospital his patient was allergic to penicillin; the surgeon ordered penicillin perioperatively and was thereby responsible for the severe reaction that resulted.[89]

Most physicians commonly use only a few dozen medications. To know their indications, potential side effects, and possible cross-reactivity will significantly reduce exposure to liability.[90]

15. **(A)** Informed consent is usually obtained for a specific procedure for treatment of a specific condition.

---

[72]*Hallinan v. Prindle*, 62 P.2d 1075 (1937).

[73]*Bugden v. Harbor View Hospital*, 2 D.L.R. 338 (1947).

[74]For example, the hospital with which I am affiliated specifically prohibits easily confused abbreviations such as "MSO4" (which could be mistaken for "MgSO4"), "U" for Units (interpreted as a trailing zero, "10U" or "100") and "QD" (mistaken for "QID").—JC

[75]*Campos v. Weeks*, 53 Cal. Rptr. 915 (1966).

[76]*See generally* 47 A.L.R. 5th 433.

[77]*Hutchinson v. United States*, 915 F.2d 560 (1990).

[78]*Hamilton v. Hardy*, 549 P.2d 1099 (1976).

[79]*Mears v. Marshall*, 905 P.2d 1154 (1995).

[80]*Barclay v. Campbell*, 704 S.W.2d 8 (1986).

[81]*Niblack v. United States*, 438 F. Supp. 383 (1977).

[82]*Jackson v. State*, 428 So.2d 1073 (1983).

[83]*Marchione v. State*, 598 N.Y.S. 2d 592 (1993).

[84]*Wu v. Spence*, 605 A.2d 395 (1992).

[85]*Barclay*, 704 S.W.2d.

[86]*Tangora v. Matansky*, 42 Cal. Rptr. 348 (1964); *Campos*, 53 Cal. Rptr.

[87]*Slack v. Fleet*, 242 So.2d 650 (1970).

[88]*Baylis v. Lourdes Hosp.*, 805 S.W.2d 122 (1991).

[89]*Yorston v. Pennell*, 153 A.2d 255 (1959).

[90]Incidentally, the Physicians Desk Reference can and will be used against you. Courts have allowed admission of PDR data as definitive evidence of the standard of care (*Garvey v. O'Donoghue*, 530 A.2d 1141 (1987); *Thompson v. Carter*, 518 So.2d 609 (1987)) or at least some evidence of the standard of care (*Ellington v. Bilsel*, 626 N.E.2d 386 (1993); *Morlino v. Medical Center of Ocean County*, 706 A.2d 721 (1998); *Ramon v. Farr*, 770 P.2d 131 (1989)).

Often, a catchall phrase such as "and other procedures as necessary" is appended to the patient consent form. This practice evolved largely from the rejection of the common-law doctrine of general consent, whereby the patient's consent is thought to entail a blanket assent to any and all interventions his physician deems necessary.[91]

The more modern view adopted by today's courts is that of specific and limited consent to the operation discussed.[92] Should the surgeon decide to perform procedures not discussed in advance with the patient, he or she could be accused of battery or criminal trespass, both of which involve an unconsented touch that is harmful or offensive. Procedures outside the scope of the operation to which the patient has consented or those that require an incision beyond that required for the consented operation are a potential source of liability for the surgeon.

This general rule was restated against a surgeon who performed procedures in excess of the patient's consent. There, a patient suffering from a recurrent laryngeal nerve palsy sued alleging the surgeon performed an anterior cervical diskectomy at a level other that the one to which she had consented.[93] In an even more ridiculous case, a surgeon was found liable for battery for performing a superficial mole removal during an oophorectomy,[94] again because this exceeded the consent given by the patient.

Courts are willing to recognize an exception for potentially life- or limb-threatening conditions that were otherwise concealed and later discovered at surgery. A surgeon was exonerated for removing an unexpected colonic mass, albeit with postoperative complications.[95] The scope of this discretion, however, is limited. Another surgeon was fined $1000 for removing a diseased Fallopian tube and inflamed diverticulum during a laparotomy performed for the sake of determining the source of the patient's abdominal pain.[96] In yet another case, a surgeon was found guilty of battery by reason of exceeding the patient's consent for performing a quadrantectomy of the breast. The patient had consented to a "lumpectomy, possible quadrantectomy" based on the results of intraoperative pathology. The pathology came back "inconclusive," so the surgeon took the whole breast quadrant.[97]

In short, the surgeon's professional judgment as to what procedures are truly "medically necessary" in any patient's case must be taken in light of the relatively higher standard of that which is imminently life- or limb-threatening. To allow a more liberal interpretation of medical necessity is to flirt with malpractice liability.

16. **(A)** The law of course recognizes the potential for emergency situations to arise and life threatening conditions to be found during the course of an otherwise routine operation. As discussed more generally in the section on informed consent, above, all persons are assumed to have consented for those interventions that are necessary to prevent loss of life or limb absent specific evidence to the contrary. Thus, the surgeon that discovers a gangrenous appendix during a routine herniorrhaphy is justified in removing the diseased organ even thought the patient has not consented specifically for an appendectomy, because it may be assumed the patient would consent to treatment of the life-threatening situation were he given the opportunity to do so.[98]

Exactly how far this implied consent for correction of emergency conditions goes is the subject of some debate. Most jurisdictions hold the surgeon to that of another surgeon of similar training, skill, and experience acting reasonably in a patient's best interests, or that which is usual and customary in the community.[99]

Finally, should the patient have a guardian or medical decision-maker easily accessible to the surgeon, it would be appropriate and prudent to obtain actual consent from that person to extend the operation.[100] If that person is not readily available, the surgeon's best judgment and the community standard should guide him or her.

17. **(C)** Like the medical profession, the law presumes all persons of adult years to be sane and mentally competent absent evidence to the contrary. The practical effect of this assumption is the ability of adults to decide that which is to be done to and with their bodies and to what treatments they will submit. A layer of complexity is added to the discussion of consent

---

[91]*See generally* 56 A.L.R.2d 695 (& Supp.)

[92]*Id.*, §2.

[93]*Washburn v. Klara*, 561 S.E.2d 682 (2002)

[94]*Lloyd v. Kull*, 329 F.2d 168 (1964)

[95]*Babin v. St. Paul Fire & Marine Insurance Co.*, 385 So.2d 849 (1980)

[96]*Guin v. Sison*, 552 So.2d 60 (1989). Of note, $1000 is a preposterously small amount for a malpractice award. The court seemed to recognize an obligation to admit the technical battery but was not willing to go so far as to award the plaintiff-patient any substantial amount. This sends a mixed message to physicians and their defense attorneys: should an operation be extended for the ultimate benefit of the patient, or should the incision be closed, the patient recovered, and consent for a second operation obtained with the attendant risks and discomfort taken as "legally" necessary?—JC

[97]*Hernandez v. Schittek*, 713 N.E.2d 203 (1999)

[98]*See generally* 56 A.L.R.2d 695 (& Supp.)

[99]*Id.*, §3

[100]41 Am. Jur.2d, Physicians and Surgeons, §110

when a patient has received sedative or narcotic medications.[101]

The standard of proof for an adult's incompetency after receiving sedatives and narcotics was determined to be "clear, cogent, and convincing evidence."[102] Accordingly, a surgeon was relieved of a malpractice claim for obtaining the patient's consent to septoplasty after sedative and narcotic medications had been administered because the surgeon had no clear evidence that the patient was in any way impaired.[103] Another surgeon was similarly exonerated from a patient's claim that her consent to hysterectomy was invalid because sedative medications had been administered prior to that consent.[104]

While it is always advisable to obtain the patient's consent to a procedure before the patient is sedated, there are grounds to uphold consent obtained after medications have been given should the surgeon reasonably believe the patient is not significantly impaired and does in fact understand the nature, risks, benefits, and alternatives to the proposed treatment.

18. **(A)** Answers "c" and "d" are expressions of the older, now superseded standards for obtaining informed consent. In the past, great deference was given to professional opinion, and a physician could posit just about any discussion as fulfilling the community standard of informed consent if he or she were able to find another physician in the area to testify to that fact. In recent years courts have shifted to what is described as a more patient-oriented and less physician-oriented standard for the informed consent discussion. This has been commonly articulated as the "patient's need for information material to his decision whether to accept or reject the proposed treatment."[105]

The practical effect of this shift in the legal standard for physicians conscientious about informed consent discussions is little. Patients who are given an opportunity to ask questions, especially those that are prompted for any further or specific concerns they might have about the proposed procedure have, by definition, received all information material to the making of a reasonable, informed decision. This standard was more precisely articulated in the apocryphal *Canterbury* case: 1.) Every human of adult years and sound mind has the right to determine that which will be done to his own body, 2.) True

consent is an opportunity to knowledgeably evaluate risks of a proposed procedure and options to it, and 3.) The average person is dependent on his physician to impart medical knowledge toward the patient's better understanding of the proposed procedure.[106]

This duty is measured by the patient's need for information material to the decision to accept or reject a proposed treatment. For example, a patient undergoes a routine excision of a symptomatic duodenal ulcer. Incident to that surgery, his spleen is injured, necessitating a later splenectomy. Later, complications from the splenectomy require the patient to undergo subtotal gastrectomy. The patient may reasonably assert that the possibility of significant injury to other abdominal organs was material to his decision to consent to the first operation and should have been discussed with him. The court agreed.[107] This duty was extended to require a higher level of discussion for complicated cases, especially elective ones.[108]

The current legal trend is toward a standard of "materiality" in determining what information should be shared with a patient to obtain truly "informed" consent. By covering usual, routine operative risks and prompting the patient for specific concerns about the procedure the physician's legal and moral duties to the patient will be fulfilled.

19. **(D)** As mentioned in the introduction most states[109] recognize the "captain of the ship" or *respondeat superior* doctrine in the context of medical negligence. This principle dictates the operating surgeon or physician in charge of a medical encounter will generally be held liable for the actions of any personnel under his or her direction and control. The law views actions of those personnel as direct extensions of your professional activities and therefore actions for which you should be held liable.[110]

Despite the varied and sometimes complex relationships between persons in various roles during any medical encounter, the general rule of responsibility (and hence liability) for others' actions is mercifully simple: you are responsible for those under your direction and control. If you are able by custom or rule to direct the actions and behaviors of other personnel, you are responsible for their actions.

---

[101]*See generally* 25 A.L.R.3d 1439.
[102]*Grannum v. Berard*, 422 P.2d 812 (1967).
[103]*Id.*
[104]*Wheeler v. Barker*, 208 P.2d 68 (1949).
[105]88 A.L.R.3d 1008, §2.

[106]*Canterbury v. Spence*, 464 F.2d 772 (1972)
[107]*Cobbs v. Grant*, 502 P.2d 1 (1972)
[108]*Riedinger v. Colburn*, 361 F.Supp. 1073 (1973), in this case an anterior C5-6 diskectomy.
[109]Wisconsin is a notable exception.
[110]*See generally* 85 A.L.R.2d 889 (& Supp.)

This principle is most often applied in cases of employees, agents, assistants, and house officers. Employees are generally held to be under the control of employers, which in fact forms the basis of *respondeat superior*, formerly known as "master and servant." So, persons such as Physicians' Assistants, Nurse Practitioners, private scrub nurses, and office personnel are under your control and hence a potential source of liability. Further, a patient or onlooker might reasonably presume that the operating room personnel are under your direction and control due to the nature of interactions between you and them. You may direct them to perform, refrain from performing, or perform their duties in a particular way. This makes the surgeon vicariously liable for OR personnel under the "borrowed servant" doctrine, even though they are employees of the hospital. Again, the issue is direction and control, or more accurately, who is directing and controlling other persons.

The apocryphal *Ybarra* case continues to be a cornerstone in demonstrating the principles of *respondeat superior*. There, a patient suffered what was likely a brachial plexus injury during a routine abdominal operation. In the months following the operation his right arm became paralytic, atrophied, contractured, and a source of ongoing pain and discomfort. Because the patient was anesthetized he was unable to identify which of the operating room personnel were responsible for the injury and because he was not a medical professional he was unable to determine who should be responsible for ensuring his safety while anesthetized. The court held as a matter of policy (and since then, precedent) that the nurses and OR personnel were temporarily under the control of the surgeon and therefore the surgeon was responsible for ensuring the patient's safety and liable for injuries that resulted from the operation, whether directly related to the procedure or not.[111] Similarly, surgeons have been found responsible when assistants leave sponges in patients[112] and even for the acts of other physicians who are assisting but still under the control of the chief operating surgeon.[113]

The same "borrowed servant" doctrine is applicable to floor nurses, other hospital personnel, and sometimes residents.[114] Again the issue is one of direction

and control: should you direct a nurse, other hospital employee, or house officer to act in a certain way you will likely be held responsible for those acts regardless of who technically employs that person.[115] Routine duties not specifically under your control will usually not create liability on your part for the actions of hospital employees, for example acts of residents involved in routine postoperative care[116,117] unless you actively supervised the resident or gave him or her negligent or improper instructions that led to the injury.[118]

In practical terms, the physician will be held responsible for the acts of any other person who could be construed to be under his or her supervision, direction, or control. It is therefore wise to maintain close, congenial relationships with those under your direction and encourage candor, honesty, and openness to prevent mistakes from being concealed and your liability expanded.

20. (D) With the complexity and multiplicity of relationships between physicians in the hospital setting it is appropriate to wonder for what physicians' actions besides your own might you be held liable. The answer again is mercifully straightforward: none.[119]

Physicians are recognized under the law as independently licensed professionals and therefore only responsible for the actions of those whom they control. Generally, physicians do not control the actions

---

[111]*Ybarra v. Spangard*, 154 P.2d 687 (1944)

[112]*Ales v. Ryan*, 64 P.2d 409 (1936)

[113]*Morey v. Thybo*, 199 F. 760 (1912); here, a second surgeon was hired independently by the patient to assist a complex operation, but was found to be under the control of the chief operating surgeon therefore creating liability to the chief surgeon for the acts of the assistant.

[114]85 A.L.R. 2d 889, §§ 3-5, 14, 15

[115]One practical matter deserves mention. When a patient is injured, his or her attorney is likely to name everyone in sight as a potential defendant and bring multiple allegations of wrongdoing. This is an outgrowth of a procedural rule requiring all claims related to an event (or chain of events) to be brought together for the sake of efficiency, fairness, and in the interest of a "just, speedy, and inexpensive determination of every [lawsuit]" (Fed. R. Civ. Proc. 1). For that reason a patient-plaintiff is likely to claim both the operating surgeon and the hospital-employer are responsible for the injurious actions of a nurse. Unfortunately, this 'pleading in the alternative' is allowed, if not encouraged (Fed. R. Civ. Proc. 8(a)). When the patient-plaintiff's attorney determines who is the "deep pocket" (i.e. which party has larger assets), the claim against the other party is likely to be dropped. This produces the anomalous result of actually arguing against *respondeat superior* on the part of the surgeon, because the hospital is likely to have greater assets than the surgeon. This does not however prevent a hospital found responsible for the actions of a nurse from counter-suing the surgeon who had actual control of the nurse's actions at the time of the injury. In the interests of medical staff harmony this is not likely to happen, but is something of which you should be aware.—JC

[116]*Parmelee v. Kline*, 579 So.2d 1008 (1991)

[117]85 A.L.R 2d, Id., §14.

[118]*Barrette v. Hight*, 230 N.E.2d 808 (1967)

[119]Narrow exceptions for negligent referral and concerted action are noted in the text.

of other physicians[120] and are therefore not liable for the actions of other physicians acting independently.[121] Exceptions are rare, as noted above.

This principle applies to the sending of a substitute physician to complete care of a patient (as in a change of inpatient service or going on leave), anesthesiologists and surgeons for the acts of each other, and acts of other physicians in your call group,[122] even when they injure your patients.[123] In at least one case the acts of a surgical resident were not attributable to the supervising surgeon (who was on vacation) because the problem was of a kind the resident would typically have acted independently to correct.[124] Also, a neurosurgeon and orthopedic surgeon were exonerated from responsibility for their patient's perioperative myocardial infarction because fault was more properly attributed to the internist performing the preoperative cardiac evaluation.[125]

The same principle applies to intra-operative consultation with another physician, whether a member of your specialty or not.[126] The consulting physician is generally not liable for acts performed by the consultant, nor is the consultant liable for acts performed prior to his or her arrival on the case.[127] An important exception exists in the realm of concerted action. If the operation is performed negligently by one or both surgeons (either consulting or consulted) *both* may be held liable for the negligence (injury) suffered by the patient. A physician's duty to act in the best interests of his or her patients extends to protecting them from harms about which he or she knew or should have known, regardless of who inflicted those harms. In other words, if either physician on a case knew or should have known of the other's negligence, both will share in the blame.

A further caveat: the consulting physician may be held liable for negligent consultation if the consultant he or she brings in on the case is known to be incompetent. For example, if a surgeon is aware that a particular colleague has a suspiciously high complication rate or is (or should be) aware of a substance abuse problem by that physician, then the first surgeon would be liable for injuries inflicted by the second if the first consults him. Again, this is an extension of every physician's responsibility to act in the best interests of his or her patients and a

willingness to penalize those physicians who do not do so.

Special note should be made of business organizations. Members of a true partnership share in assets, liabilities, and culpabilities equally. This means that each partner will be held personally liable for injuries inflicted by his or her partners, even to the extent that a judgment against one partner may be completely enforced against any other partner.[128] This is only applicable, however, to activities that form the basis of the partnership (e.g. providing medical services) and not to unrelated activities (for example, your partner's auto accident).[129] Members of a Limited Liability Partnership (L.L.P.) or shareholders in a Professional Corporation (P.C.), however, are not liable for the acts of other partners or shareholders.[130] These latter forms of business associations are for that reason greatly preferable.

In short, physicians will generally not be held liable for actions of other physicians not under their direct supervision or control. Each professional should and will be responsible first and foremost for his or her own acts.

21. (D) Physicians rightly feel some degree of trepidation when approaching the pregnant patient with a potentially surgical abdomen. Anecdotal evidence to support "safe" levels of radiation during pregnancy is hard to come by, and published guidelines on the topic are far from coming. Even case law dealing with radiation during pregnancy is thin, and no treatises or other analytical materials on the matter could be found.[131]

Case law may be divided into those in which the physician was found liable for harm to the fetus resulting from prenatal radiation and those in which the physician was exonerated. A few cases fall outside these categories, as when a malpractice suit was brought against a physician for failure to diagnose a Large for Gestational Age (LGA) infant because he *did not* perform x-ray pelvimetry on the patient.[132] Also, a physician was found liable for failure to diagnose the patient's breast malignancy by *not* ordering a mammogram during her pregnancy; by the time of biopsy, the malignancy was metastatic.[133]

---

[120]*But see Morey v. Thybo, supra*
[121]*See generally* 85 A.L.R.2d 889
[122]*Id.*, §§6-11.5 (& Supp.)
[123]*Reeck v. Huntington Hosp.*, 215 A.D.2d 464 (1995)
[124]*Parmelee, supra*
[125]*Brooker v. Hunter*, 528 P.2d 1269 (1974)
[126]85 A.L.R.2d 889, §§6, 8
[127]*Mayer v. Hipke*, 197 N.W. 333 (1924)

[128]For example, the responsible physician may be insolvent, absent, or otherwise judgment-proof.
[129]85 A.L.R.2d 889, §11(a)
[130]*Id.*, §§11, 11.5, & Supp.
[131]Searching was done on both Westlaw and Lexis, in the sections of Federal and State Cases (combined), Jurisprudence, Restatements, and Law Reviews (Combined).
[132]*Dinner v. Thorp*, 338 P.2d 137 (1959); the physician was exonerated.
[133]*Tiernan v. Heinzen*, 104 A.D.2d 645 (1984)

Prior to the 1970's x-ray pelvimetry on pregnant women was a relatively common practice. This practice was judicially all but terminated in the textbook *Salinetro* case.[134] There, a patient received x-rays of her back for complaints of pain after a motor vehicle accident. She was later found to be pregnant and advised by her Obstetrician to have a therapeutic abortion due to known adverse effects of radiation on the fetus.[135] The physician was exonerated because the patient-plaintiff admitted that she didn't know she was pregnant at the time of the x-rays and that even if the defendant-physician *had* asked if she were pregnant she would have answered "no."[136] This decision made it clear, however, that courts would thereafter recognize radiation during pregnancy was a source of harm to the fetus for which physicians would be held liable. A string of similar cases followed in which a patient was irradiated without prior ascertainment of pregnancy, underwent a therapeutic abortion, then sued the physician ordering the x-rays for negligence. Generally, the patients have won.[137]

Many cases, however, have exonerated defendant physicians for the patient-plaintiff's failure to establish a causal connection between the radiation exposure and the injury suffered[138,139,140] or in at least one case because no injury to the fetus could be shown at all.[141]

A disturbing trend has begun in at least a few malpractice cases relating to radiation during pregnancy. Mothers in at least two cases have been allowed to sue physicians for mental anguish after radiation during pregnancy. Both mothers claimed to be distraught over worry about what injury might befall their unborn children; in neither case was actual harm to the children proven.[142]

Little exists in the way of clinical guidelines for the clinician faced with a potentially surgical abdomen in the pregnant patient.[143] The law has similarly been reticent to establish a standard of radiation exposure during pregnancy below which physicians may be assured innocence.[144] For further discussion of specific surgical problems in pregnancy, see Dr. Gabbe's excellently written chapter on the matter.[145]

22. **(B)** A *battery* is described in the law as an unconsented bodily touch that is harmful or offensive. Patients who discover that the surgeon to whom they gave consent for an operation did not actually perform the operation, those patients may have a valid basis for injury in battery.[146]

The term "other personnel" on a consent form was found a valid expression of consent to have the surgeon's PA perform saphenous vein cutdown during a vascular operation.[147] Surgical assistants including physicians with whom the consented surgeon is operating are also usually covered.[148]

Rules for teaching institutions are mixed. Consent for involvement of residents and medical students generally has been determined to be valid when their involvement is part of the usual "practice and custom" of the institution.[149] A medical student was covered by the patient's consent for a bone marrow biopsy procedure.[150] Battery claims against residents have been upheld, however,[151] especially when the patient specifically asked that a resident not be involved.[152]

An important differentiation should be made. As discussed in the opening comments to this chapter medical malpractice is based on the theory of *negligence*, demonstrated by acting unreasonably under the circumstances or failing to act when action would have been reasonable under the circumstances. Contrast this with *battery*, which is the intentional unconsented touch that is harmful or offensive. Because an operation that is technically performed

[134]*Salinetro v. Nystrom,* 341 So.2d 1059 (1977)

[135]*Id.*

[136]*Id.*

[137]*Ex. Deutsch v. Shein,* 597 S.W.2d 141 (1980); *Gamble v. Mintz,* 1991 Tenn. App. LEXIS 47.

[138]*Poulin v. Fleming,* 782 So.2d 452 (2001); causal connection between CXR plus LGI series and resultant schizencephaly not shown.

[139]*Page v. Gilbert,* 598 So.2d 1110 (1992); causal connection between x-rays after MVA and son's subsequent learning disability not shown.

[140]*Cox v. Dela Cruz,* 406 A.2d 620 (1979); medical professionals differ on what dose of radiation is "safe," therefore neurosurgeon could not be held presumptively liable for x-rays taken during pregnancy.

[141]*Gilphilin v. Ware,* 205 A.D.2d 353 (1994)

[142]*Paintiff v. Parkersburg,* 345 S.E.2d 564 (1986); *Jones v. Howard University, Inc.,* 589 A.2d 419 (1988)

[143]The National Guideline Clearinghouse maintains recommendations promulgated by more than 150 organizations. Two hundred seventy-four guidelines referring to pregnancy were reviewed; none mentioned appropriate radiation doses in pregnancy. *Available at* www.guidelines.gov.

[144]*Cox, supra.*

[145]Stephen Gabbe, ed. *Obstetrics—Normal and Problem Pregnancies, 4th ed.,* Copyright 2002 Churchill Livingstone, Inc. Chapter 19: Specific Surgical Problems in Pregnancy.

[146]*See generally* 39 A.L.R.4th 1034 &Supp.

[147]*Cardio TVP Surgical Assoc. v. Gillis,* 528 S.E.2d 785 (2000)

[148]*Larche v. Rodriguez,* 765 So.2d 388 (2000)

[149]*Henry v. Bronx Lebanon Medical Center,* 384 N.Y.S.2d 772 (1976)

[150]*Bowlin v. Duke University,* 423 S.E.2d 320 (1992)

[151]*Guebard V. Jabaay,* 452 N.E.2d 751 (1983)

[152]*Gove v. St. Joseph's Hosp. Health Center,* 662 N.Y.S.2d 675 (1997)

competently cannot by definition be negligent, surgeons who allow others (including residents) operate for them cannot be liable for malpractice if all goes well. There is a basis for a battery claim against the operating physician, however, even if the operation is an uncomplicated success.[153] This is because the patient gave consent to a particular surgeon, but another surgeon actually performed the procedure. It is a technical point but an important one. Surgeons have been held liable for battery in these cases many times.[154] Further, patients have been allowed to claim mental anguish for the substitution of surgeons[155] and breach of contract against the surgeon to whom consent was validly given.[156] Fraud was even found against a surgeon who allowed a second surgeon to operate with him after the patient had expressly refused the second surgeon's participation in the procedure.[157]

The privilege to determine who touches one's own body extends in to the physician-patient relationship. Surgeons who allow others to operate for them to whom the patient has not given consent for operation risk both tort (injury) and contract (breach) liability.

23. **(D)** Confidentiality of patients' medical records has become a growing public concern with the widespread use of electronic information technologies. The implementation of the Health Insurance Portability and Accountability Act (HIPAA) seeks to safeguard confidential patient medical information by providing a uniform federal statute by which violations might be measured. Surprisingly, although nearly all courts recognize invasion of privacy by disclosure of confidential information as a legal injury for which a patient may sue, there is no common-law duty of legal confidentiality for a patient.[158]

Courts are quick to find liability on the part of physicians who breach confidentiality to inappropriately reveal patient information to third parties.[159] The usual test involves weighing any legitimate public concern against mental suffering, shame, or humiliation suffered by the patient.[160]

In a number of cases, however, physicians have been exonerated because of the particular facts involved. For example, disclosures of medical information by company physicians to the patient's employer or by an independent physician who has

been contracted by the employer to provide care for work-related injuries are allowed.[161] This has included results of a drug screen in the course of employment[162] and even full disclosure of relevant medical conditions when the patient authorized only part disclosures about his alcoholism.[163] Physicians have been found liable for damages for disclosing medical conditions to an employer that are irrelevant to a patient's employment.[164] Of course, medical records relevant to Worker's Compensation claims may be disclosed to the employer and relevant state agency without liability.[165]

Photographs or film of an operation may be an invasion of privacy even if the patient consents to the photographing or filming if intent exists to show the images publicly or for commercial gain.[166] A surgeon's use of pre- and post-operative films, even without identifying patient information, was found to have breached the patient's privacy. The surgeon displayed the images on a local television news program and in a department-store display,[167] though even a less egregious display of a patient's likeness is likely to be a source of liability, too.

Spouses may have a legitimate interest in confidential information.[168] While confidences made to a psychiatrist or counselor may not be appropriate to share with a spouse,[169] information regarding a substance abuse problem going to the patient's fitness as a parent may be disclosed.[170]

A key case in 1976 created a duty by physicians particularly to warn any identified third party toward whom a patient has expressed a present intent to harm. In the landmark *Tarasoff* case, a student expressed intent to kill his girlfriend; his psychiatrist took no action. After the patient murdered that girlfriend, her parents sued the physician (among others) alleging a failure to warn an identified party of imminent harm and taking reasonable steps to protect her. The California Supreme Court found that physicians and patients have a "special relationship" that creates a duty by physicians to warn identified third parties of imminent harm.[171] This essentially means that when a patient tells a physician that he or she presently intends to harm a

---

[153]39 A.L.R.4th 1034 &Supp.
[154]*Perna v. Pirozzi*, 457 A.2d 431 (1983); *Pugsley v. Privette*, 263 S.E.2d 69 (1980); et. al.
[155]*Perna, supra*
[156]*Id.*
[157]*Johnson v. McMurray*, 461 So.2d 775 (1984)
[158]*See generally* 48 A.L.R.4th 668
[159]*Id.*, §§3, 8
[160]*Horne v. Patton*, 287 So.2d 824 (1973)

[161]48 A.L.R.4th 668, §4
[162]*Neal v. Corning Glass Works Corp.*, 745 F.Supp. 96 (1989)
[163]*Clark v. Geraci*, 208 N.Y.S.2d 564 (1960)
[164]*Horne v. Patton*, 287 So.2d 824 (1973)
[165]*Acosta v. Cary*, 365 So.2d 4 (1978)
[166]48 A.L.R.4th 668, §4(g)
[167]*Vassiliades v. Garfinckel's, Brooks Bros.*, 492 A.2d 580 (1985)
[168]48 A.L.R.4th 668, §5(b)
[169]*Id.*
[170]*Mikel v. Abrams*, 541 F.Supp. 591 (1982)
[171]*Tarasoff v. Regents of University of Calif.*, 551 P.2d 334 (1976)

particular person, the physician has a duty to take reasonable steps to warn the potential victim and/or avert the harm. The public and the identified individual both have a compelling interest in being made aware of specific threats to individuals.

Absence of malice or intent to do harm has been allowed as a defense to unauthorized disclosure of confidential information.[172] This is perhaps the physician's best defense to a good-faith effort to act in the patient's best interests. For example, family relationships are often complicated and extensive. Obtaining the patient's consent to discuss the case with family members in advance of the procedure is preferable, but circumstances arise when it is necessary to discuss the patient's case with a next of kin. Generally, spouses are default next of kin as are custodial parents for minors. Information about the patient may of course be shared with a medical or legal power of attorney. Beyond that is a grey area of relation, including adult children, siblings, extended family, and close neighbors. Courts will sympathize with a good-faith interest to act in your patient's best interests, though discretion should be of paramount concern.

---

[172] *Eckhardt v. Charter Hosp. of Albuquerque, Inc.*, 953 P.2d 722 (1997)

Index

Page numbers followed by "f" or "t" denote figures or tables, respectively.

Jason Heckman, M.D.